Cohen's Comprehensive Thoracic Anesthesia

Cohen's Comprehensive Thoracic Anesthesia

Edmond Cohen, MD, FASA

Professor of Anesthesiology and Thoracic Surgery
Director of Thoracic Anesthesia
Department of Anesthesiology, Perioperative and Pain Medicine
Icahn School of Medicine at Mount Sinai
New York, New York

ELSEVIER

Elsevier

1600 John F. Kennedy Blvd.
Ste 1800
Philadelphia, PA 19103-2899

COHEN'S COMPREHENSIVE THORACIC ANESTHESIA ISBN: 978-0-323713016

Library of Congress Control Number: 2021944589

Content Strategist: Sarah E. Barth/Kayla Wolfe
Content Development Specialist: Deborah Poulson
Publishing Services Manager: Deepthi Unni
Project Manager: Beula Christopher
Design Direction: Ryan Cook

Printed in the United States of America.

Last digit is the print number: 9 8 7 6 5 4 3 2

Dedicated to my parents, Naomi and Eliyahu Cohen and my brother Avraham. May their memory be a blessing.

To my family, my wife Myra and children Jennifer and Adam, whose endless support and love made this book possible.

Preface

When I began my anesthesia practice, thoracic anesthesia was not considered an independent subspecialty. Today, 40 years later, it is one of the most challenging subspecialties, with innovations that include devices for lung isolation and monitoring capability, new understanding of the intraoperative managing of one lung ventilation, and a significant innovation in postoperative pain management. Over the years, thoracic workshops and thoracic symposiums have become integral during global anesthesia conferences. Thoracic anesthesia literature is now indispensable to many practicing clinician's libraries.

My intentions when editing this book were not to replace any thoracic anesthesia book, but rather to offer something slightly more comprehensive in the critical and rapidly expanding subspecialty of the anesthetic practice. I conceptualized this volume to serve as a true contribution to the field of thoracic anesthesia, appealing to clinicians who require the necessary skills and updated principles of thoracic anesthesia. The book is unique in that it redefines how we, as anesthesiologists, can achieve superior patient care. The perioperative care is discussed linearly, just as we encounter these situations in the hospital environment.

The book contains 55 chapters divided into six sections. The first section covers topics of pre-operative assessment including anatomic correlation of the respiratory system, radiology, and classifications of thoracic tumors from the surgeon's perspective, as well as pulmonary pathophysiology and the role of hypoxic pulmonary vasoconstriction. The second and the third sections cover preoperative evaluation and preparation, monitoring of oxyanion and hemodynamics, and the role of bronchoscopy and high frequency ventilation during thoracic procedures. The fourth section describes the intraoperative management of one-lung ventilation, methods of lung separation, ventilatory strategies, fluid management, and pediatric patient care. The fifth section reviews the multimodal approach to acute and chronic pain management and postoperative complications including the use of extracorporeal ventilatory therapy. The sixth section contains a large number of specifics in clinical scenarios and case management such as video-assisted thoracoscopy, robotic surgery, tubeless procedures, and management of both geriatric and cardiac patients for lung resection. Other procedures include surgical and endoscopic lung volume reduction, esophageal surgery, cystic fibrosis, lung transplantation, tracheal resection, mediastinoscopy, tracheal stents, and enhanced recovery after surgery during thoracic surgery. Finally, the use of transesophageal echocardiography and ultrasound for thoracic procedures is discussed.

I would like to thank the contributors for their fine and meticulous work, many of whom are directors of the thoracic division in their institutions. The team is truly international, with participants hailing from a vast array of countries, such as the United Kingdom, Canada, Germany, Spain, Italy, Turkey, Saudi Arabia, Belgium, Switzerland, The Netherlands, and China. This diverse team of contributors provides a wide range of perspective, with all contributors adhering to the goal of this book, namely, keeping the focus for practicing clinicians. They have managed to simplify difficult concepts within thoracic anesthesia. Each has succeeded admirably and helped produce what we hope will contribute positively to the field of anesthesiology.

This book would not have been possible without the support of the editorial staff from Elsevier. I would like to thank Sarah Barth, Publisher, who enthusiastically supported the project, navigating through the complexity to make this book a reality. I would also like to thank Deborah Poulson, Content Development Specialist, for her advice and leadership throughout the process. Additionally, I would like to thank Beula Christopher, Senior Project Manager, who oversaw production and printing.

Finally, thank you to my wife Myra and my children Jennifer and Adam, who welcomed this book into our family rather than viewing it as an intruder.

Foreword

THE GROWTH OF THORACIC ANESTHESIA

Cardiothoracic anesthesia is the largest and most complex subspecialty of anesthesiology. The patients often are very high risk, with pulmonary, cardiac, and systemic comorbidities, and the surgical procedures may produce significant physiologic challenges to the anesthesiologist. Within the broad field of cardiothoracic anesthesia, thoracic anesthesia has developed into a field of its own, separate from cardiac anesthesia. This direction became obvious to me in the 1980s, with the increasing number of more complex operations for lung and esophageal cancers, and new approaches to other intrathoracic diseases including mediastinal masses, tracheal lesions, and thoracic trauma. This led to the first edition of my textbook entitled *Thoracic Anesthesia* published in 1983, which was dedicated to improving the care of patients undergoing noncardiac thoracic surgery. It described the anesthetic agents used at the time such as thiopental and halothane, and anesthetic techniques using reusable red rubber double-lumen tubes. *Thoracic Anesthesia* served as a companion to my earlier *Cardiac Anesthesia* text, published in 1979. These books gave straightforward, distinct names to the new subspecialties in an era when subspecialization in anesthesiology was controversial and most practitioners were generalists. Over the ensuing four decades, other textbooks by Marshall, Benumof, and Slinger, dealing with anesthesia for thoracic surgery, have described further developments in the field, and now *Cohen's Comprehensive Thoracic Anesthesia* presents the modern state of the art in this well-recognized subspecialty.

From 1983 to 1998, I served as Professor and Chairman of the Department of Anesthesiology at the Mount Sinai School of Medicine and Mount Sinai Hospital in New York City. Dr. Cohen was one of our early residents, who then decided to take a cardiothoracic fellowship year with our very popular program in which most of the fellows were focused on anesthesia for cardiac surgical procedures. Recognizing the potential growth of thoracic surgery, I suggested that he focus on the noncardiac thoracic procedures as a thoracic anesthesia specialist. The rest is history, as Dr. Cohen has become a full professor and one of the educational leaders in the field who has lectured around the world, organized technical workshops at all the major anesthetic meetings, and published extensively in the field, culminating with this important and timely textbook.

The 55 chapters of *Cohen's Comprehensive Thoracic Anesthesia* cover the entire perioperative experience from the preoperative care through the intraoperative period and into the postoperative management of these patients. The preoperative preparation of patients with extensive pulmonary disease has always been a challenging area that has not had enough attention paid to it. Recently, thoracic prehabilitation, including chest physiotherapy and exercise training, has been introduced and appears to help reduce respiratory complications and hospital length of stay, as well as improve outcomes. During many thoracic surgeries, lung separation is critical. Dr. Cohen introduced one of the new bronchial blockers for this purpose. These types of bronchial blockers, or the new disposable double-lumen tubes, are placed with fiberoptic bronchoscopic guidance for newer procedures such as video-assisted or robotic thoracic surgery, as well as for standard open thoracic surgery. All of these techniques and their related physiologic changes are discussed in detail throughout this book.

Thoracic surgery can produce one of the most painful acute postoperative experiences for a patient and may be followed by a chronic pain syndrome. Thoracic epidural anesthesia, paravertebral blocks, and intercostal blocks have been used for years to try to alleviate the postoperative pain, with some degree of success. However, in recent years, new fascial plane blocks, such as the serratus anterior plane block and the erector spinae plane block, have been introduced and have replaced some of the older techniques in many practices. These new blocks appear to be easier to perform, are safer, and highly effective for many patients. They are now becoming part of the enhanced recovery after surgery protocols in many institutions.

Over the past few years, the world has experienced the COVID-19 pandemic, and this pandemic has had an enormous impact on anesthesia for thoracic surgery. Multiple international organizations have created guidelines for the management of these patients and their surgeries. Aerosol-generating procedures, such as intubation and extubation, have placed all of us at increased risk, and have led to the introduction of many new isolation devices for operating rooms and intensive care units. COVID-19 has further expanded the expertise and increased the respect of the skilled practitioners caring for these very sick patients in the operating rooms and critical care units of our hospitals.

The *Journal of Cardiothoracic and Vascular Anesthesia (JCVA)*, for which I serve as Editor-in-Chief, is now in its 35th year, and Dr. Cohen has served as a senior member of the editorial board for most of that time, while helping to expand the publications in thoracic anesthesia. He has been a very active participant as author and editor as the field has further expanded into new techniques for lung transplantation and extracorporeal membrane oxygenation for intraoperative and postoperative support. I fully appreciate all that he has done for the subspecialty of thoracic anesthesia including his leadership as an editor of the *JCVA*, and, now as the editor of the most comprehensive textbook on anesthesia for thoracic surgery and related procedures.

Joel A. Kaplan, MD
Professor of Anesthesiology
University of California San Diego
Dean Emeritus, School of Medicine
University of Louisville

Contributors

Anoushka M. Afonso, MD, FASA
Assistant Professor
Department of Anesthesiology and Critical Care
Memorial Sloan Kettering Cancer Center
New York, New York

Felice Eugenio Agrò
Professor of Anesthesia and Intensive Care
Chairman of Postgraduate School of Anesthesia and Intensive Care
Director of Department of Anesthesia, Intensive Care and Pain Management
Policlinico Universitario "Campus Bio-Medico" of Rome
Rome, Italy

David Amar, MD
Professor of Anesthesiology
Director of Thoracic Anesthesia
Program Director, Thoracic Anesthesia Fellowship
Memorial Sloan Kettering Cancer Center;
Weill Cornell Medical College
New York, New York

Omar Ben Amer, MS, MD
Clinical Assistant Professor of Anesthesiology
Department of Anesthesiology
Sidney Kimmel Medical College at Thomas Jefferson University
Philadelphia, Pennsylvania

Wolfgang Baar, MD
Department of Anesthesiology and Critical Care
Medical Center-University of Freiburg
Freiburg, Germany

Elizabeth Cordes Behringer, MD
Professor of Anesthesiology
Cardiac Surgical Intensivist-Anesthesiologist
Division of Cardiovascular Surgery and Critical Care
Kaiser Permanente Los Angeles Medical Center
Los Angeles, California

Astrid Bergmann, MD, PhD, DESA
Senior Consultant in Cardio-Thoracic Anesthesia
Department of Anesthesiology and Intensive Care Medicine
Otto-von-Guericke-University
Magdeburg, Germany;
Research Anesthesiologist
Department of Medical Sciences
Hedenstierna Laboratory
Uppsala University
Uppsala, Sweden

Daniel Blech, MD
Anesthesiology Fellow
Department of Anesthesiology
Icahn School of Medicine at Mount Sinai
New York, New York

Marcelle Blessing, MD
Assistant Professor of Anesthesiology
Department of Anesthesiology
Yale University School of Medicine
New Haven, Connecticut

Jay B. Brodsky, MD
Professor of Anesthesiology
Department of Anesthesiology, Perioperative and Pain Medicine
Stanford University School of Medicine
Stanford, California

David Bronheim, MD
Professor of Anesthesiology
Director of the Post Anesthesia Care Unit
Department of Anesthesiology, Perioperative, and Pain Medicine
Icahn School of Medicine at Mount Sinai
Mount Sinai Hospital
New York, New York

Javier H. Campos, MD
Professor and Executive Medical Director
Perioperative Services
Department of Anesthesia
University of Iowa Health Care
Iowa City, Iowa

Maria Castillo, MD
Assistant Professor
Department of Anesthesiology, Perioperative and Pain Medicine
Icahn School of Medicine at Mount Sinai
New York, New York

Michael Charlesworth, MBChB, FRCA, FFICM
Consultant
Department of Cardiothoracic Anaesthesia
Critical Care and ECMO
Wythenshawe Hospital, Manchester University
NHS Foundation Trust
Manchester, United Kingdom

Grant H. Chen, MD, MBA
Assistant Attending
Department of Anesthesiology and Critical Care Medicine
Memorial Sloan Kettering Cancer Center
New York, New York

Edmond Cohen, MD, FASA
Professor of Anesthesiology and Thoracic Surgery
Director of Thoracic Anesthesia
Department of Anesthesiology, Perioperative and Pain Medicine
Icahn School of Medicine at Mount Sinai
New York, New York

Anahita Dabo-Trubelja, MD, FASA
Associate Attending
Anesthesiology and Critical Care
Memorial Sloan Kettering Cancer Center
New York, New York

Marcelo Gama de Abreu, MD, MSc, PhD, DESA
Professor of Anesthesiology
Department of Anaesthesiology and Intensive Care Medicine
Pulmonary Engineering Group
University Hospital Carl Gustav Carus at Technische Universität Dresden
Dresden, Germany

Dawn P. Desiderio, MD
Professor of Anesthesiology
Anesthesiology and Critical Care Medicine
Memorial Sloan Kettering Cancer Center
New York, New York

Qinglong Dong, MD
Professor of Anesthesiology
Director of Anesthesia
Department of Anesthesiology
Guangzhou Medical University 1st Affiliated Hospital
Guangzhou, China

Lily Eaker, BA
Clinical Research Coordinator
Department of Orthopedic Surgery
Icahn School of Medicine at Mount Sinai
New York, New York

James B. Eisenkraft, MD
Professor of Anesthesiology
Department of Anesthesiology, Perioperative and Pain Medicine
Icahn School of Medicine at Mount Sinai;
New York, New York

Mohamed R. El Tahan, MD, Msec, MBBch
Professor of Anesthesiology
Department of Anaesthesia and Surgical Intensive Care
Mansoura University
Mansour, Egypt

Gregory W. Fischer, MD, FASA
Professor and Chairman
Department of Anesthesiology and Critical Care Medicine
Memorial Sloan Kettering Cancer Center
New York, New York

Raja Flores, MD
Ames Professor of Cardiothoracic Surgery
Chairman, Department of Thoracic Surgery
Department of Thoracic Surgery
Icahn School of Medicine at Mount Sinai
Mount Sinai Health System
New York, New York

Jonathan Gal, MD, MBA, MS, FASA
Associate Professor
Department of Anesthesiology, Perioperative, and Pain Medicine
Icahn School of Medicine at Mount Sinai;
System Director, Clinical Revenue Initiatives
Department of Clinical Business Intelligence and Implementation
Mount Sinai Health System
New York, New York

Funda Gök
Associate Professor of Anesthesiology
Anesthesiology and Reanimation
Necmettin Erbakan University
Meram School of Medicine
Konya, Turkey

Diego Gonzalez-Rivas, MD, FECTS
Consultant Thoracic Surgeon
Thoracic surgery and lung transplantation unit
Coruña University Hospital
Coruña, Spain;
Chief Thoracic surgery
Thoracic Surgery
Shanghai Pulmonary Hospital
Shanghai, China

Manuel Granell Gil, MD
Professor of Anesthesiology
University of Valencia;
Chief Section of Anesthesiology
Anesthesiology, Critical Care and Pain Relief
Consorcio Hospital General Universitario of Valencia
Valencia, Spain

Nicole Ginsberg, MD
Clinical Assistant Professor
Department of Anesthesiology, Perioperative Care and Pain Medicine
New York University Langone Medical Center
New York, New York

Amitabh Gulati, MD
Associate Attending
Memorial Sloan Kettering Cancer Center
Department of Anesthesiology and Critical Care Medicine
New York, New York

Thomas Hachenberg, MD, PhD
Professor of Anesthesia
Chair, Department of Anesthesiology and Intensive Care Medicine
Otto-von-Guericke-University
Magdeburg, Germany

Paul Ryan Haffey, DO
Anesthesia Pain Medicine
Department of Anesthesia
New York Presbyterian/Weill Cornell Medicine Tri-Institutional Pain Fellowship
New York, New York

Andres Hagerman, MD
Physician
Division of Anaesthesiology
Department of Anaesthesiology, Pharmacology, Intensive Care, and Emergency Medicine
Geneva University Hospitals
Geneva, Switzerland

Timothy J. Harkin, MD
Associate Professor of Medicine, Pulmonary, Critical Care and Sleep Medicine
Departments of Medicine and Thoracic Surgery
Icahn School of Medicine at Mount Sinai
New York, New York

Jianxing He, MD, PhD
Professor of Thoracic Surgery
Director of Thoracic Surgery
Department of Anesthesiology
Guangzhou Medical University 1st Affiliated Hospital
Guangzhou, China

Jiaxi He, MD, PhD
Attending Thoracic Surgeon
Thoracic Surgery
Guangzhou Medical University 1st Affiliated Hospital
Guangzhou, China

Patrick Hecht, MD, FRCPC
Clinical Assistant Professor
Department of Anesthesiology, Pharmacology and Therapeutics
University of British Columbia
Vancouver, Canada

Johannes Hell, MD
Department of Anesthesiology and Critical Care
Medical Centre University of Freiburg
Freiburg, Germany

Karl D. Hillenbrand, MD
Assistant Professor of Anesthesiology
Department of Anesthesiology
University of Virginia
Charlottesville, Virginia

Leila Hosseinian, MD
Associate Professor
Anesthesia and Critical Care
Loyola University
Chicago, Illinois

Benjamin M. Hyers, MD
Anesthesiology Fellow
Department of Anesthesiology, Perioperative and Pain Medicine
Icahn School of Medicine at Mount Sinai
New York, New York

Jacob C. Jackson, MD
Assistant Attending
Anesthesiology and Critical Care Medicine
Memorial Sloan Kettering Cancer Center
New York, New York

Daniel Kalowitz, MD, MBA
Attending Anesthesiologist
Anesthesia Associates of Morristown
Morristown Medical Center
Morristown, New Jersey

George W. Kanellakos, MD, FRCPC
Assistant Professor
Department of Anesthesia, Pain Management and Perioperative Medicine
Faculty of Medicine
Dalhousie University
Halifax, Canada

Waheedullah Karzai, MD
Professor of Anesthesiology
Head, Department of Anesthesia, Critical Care and Emergency Medicine
Zentralklinik Bad Berka
Bad Berk, Germany

Steven P. Keller, MD, PhD
Assistant Professor of Medicine
Division of Pulmonary and Critical Care Medicine
Johns Hopkins Hospital
Baltimore, Maryland

Mark S. Kim, MD
Clinical Assistant Professor of Anesthesiology
Co-Director of Liver Transplantation Anesthesiology
Department of Anesthesiology
Sidney Kimmel Medical College at Thomas Jefferson University
Philadelphia, Pennsylvania

Alf Kozian, MD, PhD
Professor of Anesthesiology
Department of Anesthesiology and Intensive Care Medicine
Otto-von-Guericke-University
Magdeburg, Germany

Moritz A. Kretzschmar, MD, PhD, DESA
Clinical Professor of Anesthesiology
Anesthesiology and Intensive Care Medicine
Otto-von-Guericke University
Magdeburg, Germany

Dong-Seok Lee, MD
Assistant Professor of Thoracic Surgery
Department of Thoracic Surgery
Icahn School of Medicine at Mount Sinai
Mount Sinai Health System
New York, New York

Jonathan Leff, MD, FASE
Professor of Anesthesiology
Montefiore Medical Center
Albert Einstein College of Medicine
Bronx, New York

Eric Leiendecker, MD
Assistant Professor of Anesthesiology
Department of Anesthesiology, and Critical Care Medicine
Emory University and the Emory Critical Care Center
Atlanta, Georgia

Shuben Li, MD, PhD
Professor of Thoracic Surgery
Guangzhou Medical University 1st Affiliated Hospital
Guangzhou, China

Lixia Liang, MD
Professor of Anesthesiology
Department of Anesthesiology
Guangzhou Medical University 1st Affiliated Hospital
Guangzhou, China

Marc Licker, MD
Professor of Anesthesiology
Division of Anaesthesiology
Department of Anaesthesiology, Pharmacology, Intensive Care, and Emergency Medicine
Geneva University Hospitals
Geneva, Switzerland

Hui Liu, MD
Attending Anesthesiologist
Department of Anesthesiology
Guangzhou Medical University 1st Affiliated Hospital
Guangzhou, China

Jens Lohser, MD, MSc, FRCPC
Clinical Professor of Anesthesiology
Department of Anesthesiology, Pharmacology and Therapeutics
University of British Columbia
Vancouver, Canada

Baron Lonner, MD
Professor of Orthopedic Surgery
Chief of Minimally Invasive Scoliosis Surgery
Icahn School of Medicine at Mount Sinai
Mount Sinai Hospital
New York, New York

Torsten Loop, MD
Professor of Anesthesia
Department of Anesthesiology and Critical Care
Medical Center-University of Freiburg;
Faculty of Medicine
University of Freiburg
Freiburg, Germany

Karen McRae, MDCM
Associate Professor of Anesthesiology
Department of Anesthesia and Pain Management
Toronto General Hospital;
University of Toronto
Ontario, Canada

Massimiliaino Meineri, MD, FASE
Professor of Anesthesiology
Director, Perioperative Echocardiography
Director, Arnold and Lynne Irwin Cardiovascular Anesthesia imaging Centre
University Health Network - Toronto General Hospital

Jacob Michael Lurie, MD, MPH
Physician
Department of Anesthesiology
NewYork Presbyterian/Weill Cornell Medical Center
New York, New York

Jeffrey J. Mojica, DO
Clinical Assistant Professor of Anesthesiology
Department of Anesthesiology
Sidney Kimmel Medical College at Thomas Jefferson University
Philadelphia, Pennsylvania

Nicole Morikawa, MD
Montefiore Medical Center
Albert Einstein College of Medicine
Bronx, New York

Jo Mourisse, MD, PhD
Professor of Anesthesiology
Cardio-thoracic Anesthesiologist
Radboud University Medical Centre
Anesthesiology, Pain and Palliative Medicine
Radboud University Medical Centre
Nijmegen, Netherlands

Allen Ninh, MD
Department of Anesthesiology, Perioperative, and Pain Medicine
Icahn School of Medicine at Mount Sinai
Mount Sinai Hospital
New York, New York

John Pawlowski, MD, PhD
Assistant Professor of Anesthesiology
Department of Anesthesia
Beth Israel Deaconess Medical Center
Harvard School of Medicine
Boston, Massachusetts

Alessia Pedoto, MD, FASA
Clinical Professor of Anesthesiology
Department of Anesthesia and Critical Care Medicine
Memorial Sloan Kettering Cancer Center
New York, New York

Elena Biosca Pérez, MD
Anesthesiology and Critical Care Specialist
Anesthesiology, Critical Care and Pail Relief
Consorcio Hospital General Univesitario of Valencia
Valencia, Spain

Chiara Piliego, MD
Department of Anesthesia, Intensive Care and Pain Management
Policlinico Universitario "Campus Bio-Medico" of Rome
Rome, Italy

Ruth Martínez Plumed
Anesthesiology and Critical Care Specialist
Anesthesiology, Critical Care and Pail Relief
Consorcio Hospital General Univesitario of Valencia
Valencia, Spain

Wanda M. Popescu, MD
Professor of Anesthesiology
Department of Anesthesiology
Yale School of Medicine
New Haven, Connecticut

Neal Rakesh, MD, MS
Anesthesia Pain Medicine
Department of Anesthesia
New York Presbyterian/Weill Cornell Medicine Tri-Institutional Pain Fellowship
New York, New York

Alessandra Della Rocca, MD
Anesthesiology
Department of Surgical, Medical and Molecular Pathology and Critical Care Medicine
University Pisa
Pisa, Italy

Giorgio Della Rocca, MD
Professor of Anesthesiology
Department of Medical Area
University of Udine
Udine, Italy

Cesar Rodriguez-Diaz, MD
Assistant Professor of Anesthesiology
Department of Anesthesiology Perioperative, and Pain Medicine
Icahn School of Medicine at Mount Sinai Hospital
New York, New York

Benjamin S. Salter, DO
Assistant Professor of Anesthesiology
Anesthesiology, Perioperative and Pain Medicine
Icahn School of Medicine at Mount Sinai
New York, New York

Kei Satoh, MD
Cardiothoracic Anesthesia Fellow
Department of Anesthesiology
Yale University School of Medicine
New Haven, Connecticut

Thomas Schilling, MD, PhD, DEAA
Professor of Anesthesia
Department of Anesthesiology and Intensive Care Medicine
Otto-von-Guericke-University
Magdeburg, Germany

Travis Schisler, MD, FRCPC
Clinical Assistant Professor
Department of Anesthesiology, Pharmacology and Therapeutics
University of British Columbia
Vancouver, Canada

Eric S. Schwenk, MD, FASA
Associate Professor of Anesthesiology and Orthopedic Surgery
Department of Anesthesiology
Sidney Kimmel Medical College at Thomas Jefferson University
Philadelphia, Pennsylvania

Evren Şentürk, MD, EDIC
Assistant Professor of Anesthesiology and Critical Care
Anesthesiology and Reanimation
School of Medicine
Koc University
Istanbul, Turkey

Mert Şentürk, MD
Professor of Anesthesiology
Anesthesiology and Reanimation
Istanbul University, Istanbul Faculty of Medicine
Istanbul, Turkey

David M. Shapiro, MD
Associate Attending Anesthesiologist
Department of Anesthesiology
Greenwich Hospital, Yale New Haven Health
Greenwich, Connecticut

Archit Sharma, MD, MBA
Clinical Assistant Professor in Anesthesia
University of Iowa Carver College of Medicine
Iowa City, Iowa

George Silvay, MD, PhD
Professor of Anesthesiology
Department of Anesthesiology, Perioperative, and Pain Medicine
Icahn School of Medicine at Mount Sinai
New York, New York

Theodore C. Smith, MD
Professor Emeritus of Anesthesiology
Department of Anesthesia
Loyola University Stritch School of Medicine
Maywood Illinois

Jamie L. Sparling, MD
Anesthesiology and Critical Care Medicine
Harvard Medical School
Massachusetts General Hospital
Boston, Massachusetts

Jessica Spellman, MD, FASE
Associate Professor of Anesthesiology
Columbia University Irving Medical Center
New York New York

Andrew C. Steel, BSc., MBBS, MRCP, FRCA, EDIC, FRCPC, FFICM
Interdepartmental Division of Critical Care Medicine
Department of Anesthesiology and Pain Medicine
Faculty of Medicine
University of Toronto;
Department of Anesthesiology and Pain Medicine
Toronto General Hospital
Ontario, Canada

Breandan Sullivan, MD
Associate Professor of Anesthesiology
Department of Anesthesiology and Critical Care Medicine
University of Colorado School of Medicine
Aurora, Colorado

Zerrin Sungur, MD
Professor of Anesthesiology
Anesthesiology and Reanimation
Istanbul University, Istanbul Medical Faculty
Istanbul, Turkey

Lauren Sutherland, MD
Assistant Professor of Anesthesiology
Columbia University Irving Medical Center
New York, New York

Laszlo L. Szegedi, MD, PhD
Professor of Anesthesiology
Department of Anesthesiology
C.U.B. Hospital Erasme, Université Libre de Bruxelles (U.L.B.)
Brussels, Belgium

Emily G. Teeter, MD, FASE
Associate Professor of Anesthesiology
Department of Anesthesiology
University of North Carolina at Chapel Hill
Chapel Hill, North Carolina

Richard Templeton, MBChB, FRCA, FFICM
Consultant
Department of Cardiothoracic Anaesthesia
Critical Care and ECMO
Wythenshawe Hospital, Manchester University
NHS Foundation Trust
Manchester, United Kingdom

Robert H. Thiele, MD
Associate Professor
Anesthesiology and Biomedical Engineering
University of Virginia
Charlottesville Virginia

Stefan van der Heide, MD
Cardiothoracic Surgeon
Cardiothoracic Surgery
Radboud University Medical Centre
Nijmegen, Netherlands

Marcos F. Vidal Melo, MD
Professor of Anaesthesia
Harvard Medical School
Massachusetts General Hospital
Boston, Massachusetts

Eugene R. Viscusi, MD
Professor of Anesthesiology
Chief of Pain Medicine
Department of Anesthesiology
Director, Acute Pain Management
Sidney Kimmel Medical College of Thomas Jefferson University
Philadelphia, Pennsylvania

Elizabeth May Vue, MD
Assistant Program Director of Adult Cardiothoracic Anesthesiology Fellowship
Montefiore Medical Center;
Assistant Professor
Anesthesiology
Albert Einstein College of Medicine
Bronx, New York

Spencer P. Walsh, MD
Instructor in Anesthesiology
Weill Cornell Medical College
New York, New York

Menachem M. Weiner, MD
Professor of Anesthesiology
Department of Anesthesiology, Perioperative and Pain medicine
Director of Cardiac Anesthesia
Icahn School of Medicine at Mount Sinai
New York, New York

Alexander White, MD, FRCPC
Interdepartmental Division of Critical Care Medicine
Department of Anesthesiology and Pain Medicine
Faculty of Medicine
University of Toronto;
Department of Anesthesiology and Pain Medicine
Toronto General Hospital
Toronto, Ontario
Canada

Roger S. Wilson, MD
Chairman, Emeritus
Department of Anesthesiology and Critical Care Medicine
Memorial Sloan Kettering Cancer Center
New York, New York

Jakob Wittenstein, MD
Department of Anaesthesiology and Intensive Care Medicine
Pulmonary Engineering Group
University Hospital Carl Gustav Carus at Technische Universität Dresden
Dresden, Germany

Uzung Yoon, MD, MPH
Assistant Professor of Anesthesiology
Co-Director of Liver Transplantation Anesthesiology
Department of Anaesthesiology
Thomas Jefferson University Hospital
Philadelphia, Pennsylvania

Contents

Section 1 Preoperative Assessment

1 **The Development of Thoracic Anesthesia and Surgery, 1**
Marcelle Blessing, Kei Satoh, Edmond Cohen

2 **Anatomic Correlates of Physiologic Function, 17**
Theodore C. Smith, Edmond Cohen

3 **Radiology of the Thorax, 33**
Javier H. Campos, Archit Sharma

4 **Intrathoracic Tumors: Current Status and Classification, 52**
Dong-Seok Lee, Raja Flores

5 **Pulmonary Pathophysiology and Lung Mechanics in Anesthesiology, 66**
Jamie L. Sparling, Marcos F. Vidal Melo

6 **Physiology of the Lateral Position and One-Lung Ventilation, 88**
Edmond Cohen

7 **Modulating the Pulmonary Circulation: Nitric Oxide and Beyond, 105**
Thomas Schilling, Astrid Bergmann

Section 2 Preoperative Preparation

8 **Preoperative Evaluation: Assessment of Preoperative Risk, 115**
Allen Ninh, David Bronheim

9 **Prehabilitation for Thoracic Surgery, 125**
Michael Charlesworth, Richard Templeton

Section 3 Intraoperative Preparation

10 **Positioning in Thoracic Surgery, 133**
Alessia Pedoto, Nicole Ginsberg

11 **Monitoring of Oxygenation and Ventilation, 143**
Benjamin M. Hyers, James B. Eisenkraft

12 **Hemodynamic Monitoring in Thoracic Surgical Patients, 154**
Karl D. Hillenbrand, Robert H. Thiele

13 **Flexible and Rigid Bronchoscopy in Thoracic Anesthesia, 171**
Manuel Granell Gil, Elena Biosca Pérez, Ruth Martínez Plumed

14 **High-Frequency Ventilation: Applications in Thoracic Anesthesia, 182**
Jakob Wittenstein, Marcelo Gama de Abreu

Section 4 Intraoperative Management

15 **Anesthesia, Mechanical Ventilation, and Hypoxic Pulmonary Vasoconstriction, 193**
Andres Hagerman, Marc Licker

16 **Separation of the Lung: Double-Lumen Endotracheal Tubes and Endobronchial Blockers, 213**
Javier H. Campos

17 **Lung Isolation in Patients With a Difficult Airway in Thoracic Anesthesia, 240**
Javier H. Campos

18 **Pathophysiology of Perioperative Lung Injury, 249**
Alexander White, Andrew C. Steel

19 **Intraoperative Lung Injury During One-Lung Ventilation: Causes and Prevention, 260**
Waheedullah Karzai

20 **Management of One-Lung Ventilation: Protective Lung Ventilation, 279**
Marcelo Gama de Abreu, Jakob Wittenstein

21 **Fluid Management During Lung Resection, 293**
Felice Eugenio Agrò, Chiara Piliego

22 Perioperative Arrhythmias During Thoracic Surgery, 308
Spencer P. Walsh, David Amar

23 Anesthesia for Pediatric Thoracic Surgery, 318
Cesar Rodriguez-Diaz

Section 5 Postoperative Management

24 Postoperative Management of Acute Pain, 328
Jeffrey J. Mojica, Eric S. Schwenk, Uzung Yoon, Mark S. Kim, Omar Ben Amer, Eugene R. Viscusi

25 Postthoracotomy Chronic Pain, 345
Paul Ryan Haffey, Neal Rakesh, Grant H. Chen, Amitabh Gulati

26 Postoperative Care of the Thoracic Patient, 353
Evren Şentürk, Funda Gök, Mert Şentürk

27 Postthoracotomy Complications, 376
Thomas Hachenberg, Torsten Loop

28 Extracorporeal Ventilatory Therapies, 392
Steven P. Keller

Section 6 Specific Anesthetic Considerations

29 Lung Volume Reduction Surgery, 410
Edmond Cohen

30 The Patient With Cardiovascular Disease for Lung Resection Surgery, 423
Anahita Dabo-Trubelja, Gregory W. Fischer

31 Video-Assisted Thoracoscopy: Multiportal Uniportal, 438
Zerrin Sungur, Mert Şentürk

32 Endoscopic Treatment of Chronic Obstructive Pulmonary Disease, 468
Timothy J. Harkin, John Pawlowski

33 Thoracic Trauma, 488
Alf Kozian, Moritz A. Kretzschmar

34 Mediastinal Mass and Superior Vena Cava Syndrome, 501
Daniel Kalowitz, Menachem M. Weiner

35 Mediastinoscopy, 516
Elizabeth May Vue, Nicole Morikawa, Jonathan Leff

36 Lung Resection and Pulmonary Hypertension, 523
Leila Hosseinian, Benjamin S. Salter

37 Tubeless Thoracic Procedures, 533
Jiaxi HE, Diego Gonzalez-RIVAS, Hui Liu, Qinglong Dong, Lixia Liang, Jianxing He, Shuben Li, Edmond Cohen

38 Thoracic Anesthesia for the Geriatric Patient, 544
Maria Castillo

39 Thoracic Aortic Aneurysm Resection, 557
George Silvay, Jacob Michael Lurie

40 Wedge Resection, Lobectomy, Pneumonectomy, 579
Travis Schisler, Patrick Hecht, Jens Lohser

41 Repair of Pectus Excavatum, 597
Jo Mourisse, Stefan van der Heide

42 Tracheal Resection and Reconstruction, 609
Elizabeth Cordes Behringer, Roger S. Wilson

43 Lung Transplantation, 623
Jessica Spellman, Lauren Sutherland

44 Esophageal Procedures, 649
Wolfgang Baar, Johannes Hell, Torsten Loop

45 Airway Fistulas in Adults, 669
Dawn P. Desiderio, Jacob C. Jackson

46 Thoracic Approach to Spine Procedures, 678
David M. Shapiro, Baron Lonner, Lily Eaker, Jonathan Gal

47 Myasthenia Gravis and Thymectomy, 688
Daniel Blech, James B. Eisenkraft

48 Hemoptysis, Empyema, 696
Mohamed R. El Tahan

49 Thoracic Anesthesia in the Morbidly Obese Patient: Obstructive Sleep Apnea, 713
George W. Kanellakos, Jay B. Brodsky

50 Cystic Fibrosis, 729
Giorgio Della Rocca, Alessandra Della Rocca

51 Tracheal Stents, 741
Karen McRae

52 Robotic Thoracic Surgery, 757
Laszlo L. Szegedi

53 Enhanced Recovery After Thoracic Surgery, 766
Emily G. Teeter, Anoushka M. Afonso, Wanda M. Popescu

54 Ultrasound of the Lung: Clinical Applications, 775
Massimiliano Meineri

55 Transesophageal Echocardiography in Noncardiac Thoracic Surgery, 785
Breandan Sullivan, Eric Leiendecker

Index, 813

1 The Development of Thoracic Anesthesia and Surgery

MARCELLE BLESSING, KEI SATOH, EDMOND COHEN

Introduction

The history of anesthesia for thoracic surgery incorporates much of the history of anesthesia because contemporary thoracic anesthesia is a culmination of advances in all aspects of anesthesia. Knowledge and expertise with preoperative evaluation, airway management, intraoperative monitoring, pharmacologic agents, regional anesthesia, and intensive care management are all crucial for the thoracic anesthesiologist. Anesthesia for thoracic surgery encompasses over 100 years of advances in anesthesia techniques, and these techniques are still evolving and improving. Complex thoracic procedures are now routinely performed on frail patients with associated comorbidities, who may not have been considered candidates in the past, thanks to improvements in anesthesia and surgical techniques.

Before advances in general anesthesia techniques, specifically positive pressure ventilation and controlled respiration with endotracheal intubation, surgery that trespassed the chest wall was performed very rarely because it was both dangerous to patients and very difficult for surgeons. Because of the unique challenges of performing surgery on an open thorax safely, the delivery of thoracic anesthesia is a relatively late development in the history of anesthesia. During the early 20th century, thoracic surgery procedures were frequently attempted through local anesthesia. The pneumothorax created after opening of the chest wall was viewed as invariably fatal. That was changed based on the observation that, during World War I, soldiers with large chest openings could survive.

Inhalational anesthesia was introduced in the 1840s, but it took another 100 years before much headway was made in anesthesia for thoracic surgery. Thoracic surgery could only flourish as a specialty once progress was made in thoracic anesthesia; the development of no other surgical subspecialty relied so heavily on the refinement of anesthesia techniques. Although intrathoracic procedures have become routine, thoracic surgeons and anesthesiologists retain a unique relationship; coordination between surgeon and anesthesiologist is especially critical in thoracic surgery.

Today, knowledge of thoracic anesthesia is more important than ever; as the scope of thoracic surgery has broadened, so has the range of anesthesia practice for it. One-lung ventilation (OLV), critical to thoracic anesthesia, is essential for more and more thoracic approaches to lung, esophageal, mediastinal, spinal, and cardiac procedures. Minimally invasive approaches to intrathoracic procedures rely heavily on OLV for adequate, still surgical exposure. Because of the wide variety of double lumen endotracheal tubes and endobronchial blockers that are currently available, OLV can be provided safely and reliably for virtually all patients. With mastering lung separation, in addition to being knowledgeable about the tools needed, it behooves the thoracic anesthesiologist to have a sound understanding of the physiology of OLV for preventing hypoxemia owing to the transpulmonary shunt.

Early History of Thoracic Anesthesia

John W. Strieder, a seasoned thoracic surgeon of the early 20th century, described "the good old days" of thoracic anesthesia colorfully: "the period of operation was, with dismaying frequency, a race between the surgeon and the impending asphyxia of the patient."[1] Aurelius Cornelius Celsus (25 BC–AD 50), the Roman encyclopedist, knew 2000 years ago that entering the thorax posed unique dangers to the patient. In *De Medicina*, Celsus describes "for the belly indeed, which is of less importance, can be laid open with the man still breathing; but as soon as the knife really penetrates to the chest…the man loses his life at once."[2] This is an early description of the "pneumothorax problem": opening the chest immediately causes an open pneumothorax. When the lung is exposed directly to the atmosphere, it will rapidly collapse because of the loss of the normally negative intrapleural pressure. In addition, air would be transferred between the two lungs known as "pendulluft," and the collapsed lung would paradoxically expand during expiration and collapse during inspiration. To further terrify the surgeon, vigorous side-to-side movement of the mediastinum could occur, known as "mediastinal flapping," that could compress the nonoperative lung. In the lateral decubitus position, it would result in "mediastinal shift" and hypotension. Not surprisingly, respiratory and hemodynamic compromise would ensue as the patient would struggle to breathe spontaneously. Hence most thoracic procedures were limited to the extrathoracic chest wall until the 1930s. Only very brief intrathoracic procedures were possible without patient asphyxiation.

Most areas of surgery flourished after the discovery of inhalational anesthesia in the 1840s, and the delivery of general anesthesia became routine. Until the 1930s, delivery of inhalational anesthesia was typically by mask or open drop administration, using ether or chloroform with or without nitrous oxide. Because patients would typically breathe spontaneously, they could control their own depth of anesthesia with their own respirations. Muscle relaxants were not developed yet, and endotracheal intubation was considered an invasive procedure and only rarely used by a few experts. Most thoracic procedures performed were the same pathology that concerned Celsus 2000 years ago: management of empyema, pulmonary abscess, and tuberculosis. Without antibiotics, patients would frequently present for surgery with copious secretions and formidable coughs. It was common to keep a patient only lightly anesthetized to keep the cough reflex intact to protect the lungs from gastric aspiration and to allow the patient to clear their own copious secretions. Envisioning a harrowing scene of a lightly anesthetized patient choking on their secretions with an unprotected airway, it is hardly surprising that thoracic surgery remained in its infancy well into the 20th century. Better operating conditions and improved anesthesia techniques were needed to allow thoracic surgery to flourish.

Before the discovery of antibiotics, most thoracic procedures were performed to treat infection, opening the pleural cavity did not always result in an open pneumothorax because prolonged infections often resulted in adhesions between the lung and chest wall with a loculated empyema. The utility of these adhesions was known, and repeated aspirations were sometimes attempted to promote adhesion formation before surgery. Alternatively, air or water could be injected into the pleural space as an irritant to promote adhesion formation preoperatively.[3,4] "Muller's handgrip" was another primitive method used to cope with the pneumothorax problem: while the chest was open, the surgeon would pull the lung into the wound to plug the thoracotomy incision.[5] Pulmonary resections were frequently performed in a staged manner and had a very high mortality. A snare or tourniquet technique would be used to facilitate a quick resection, and then a reoperation would be needed to remove necrotic tissue later. It is not surprising that sepsis was not uncommon from the remaining necrotic tissue. A review from 1922 reported a mortality rate of 42% for lobectomy, and as high as 70% for cases that involved more than one lobe.[6] Clearly, surgeons and patients needed safer, less harmful solutions.

Differential Pressure Breathing

The German surgeon Ernst Ferdinand Sauerbruch developed the first promising solution to the "pneumothorax problem." In 1893, his mentor, Johann von Mikulicz-Radecki, urged him to address the difficulty of operating with an open pneumothorax. His solution, differential pressure breathing, became the principal method for management of ventilation in thoracic surgery until World War II. In Sauerbruch's experiments on dogs, he found that, during thoracotomy, spontaneous ventilation was maintained and the lung did not collapse if it was exposed to a pressure 10 cm H_2O below atmospheric pressure.[7] After his experimental thoracotomies on dogs, he applied the technique to humans (Fig. 1.1). To maintain the negative pressure, a large negative pressure chamber was needed that would maintain the normal negative intrapleural pressure. The patient and surgical team were placed within the steel negative pressure chamber while the patient's head protruded from the chamber and was exposed to atmospheric pressure. With the negative pressure applied directly to the lung, the patient could breathe spontaneously and the lung would remain inflated.

Sauerbruch championed his pneumatic chamber technique as a physiologic method, and differential pressure breathing was widely adapted. However, Sauerbruch's method was very impractical because of the large, expensive, negative pressure chamber that was needed. Operating conditions were less than ideal. Rudolph Nissen described the limitations of this operating suite: "the surgeon and his assistants had very little room to move; the heat was almost unbearable; and, finally, it was extremely difficult to communicate satisfactorily with the anesthetist outside the chamber."[8] An anesthetist would be outside the chamber at the patient's airway and could only communicate with the

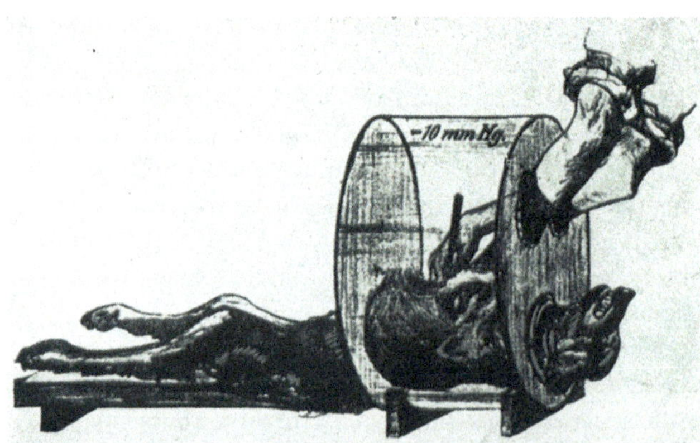

• **Fig. 1.1** Sauerbruch's experimental negative pressure box for performing thoracotomies on dogs. The dog's chest is enclosed in the box, in which the pressure is −10 mm Hg (1904). (From Mushin WW, Rendell-Baker L, eds. *The Principles of Thoracic Anesthesia*. Springfield, IL: Charles C Thomas; 1953. Copyright Wiley-Blackwell.)

surgeon within the chamber by phone over the loud whirring of pumps.

A more practical alternative method for using differential pressure to maintain lung inflation was developed in parallel by a colleague of Sauerbruch's, Ludolph Brauer. His alternative method for using differential pressure breathing was published alongside Sauerbruch's. Brauer's method used a positive pressure chamber to increase the intrapulmonary pressure. Brauer's chamber was simply a large box and the patient's head was placed within it after the induction of anesthesia, and anesthesia was maintained with the patient breathing oxygen and chloroform spontaneously. Before the chest was opened, compressed air would be added to the chamber to raise the pressure above atmospheric pressure, and this would prevent the development of an open pneumothorax. The anesthetist would have no access to the head during the procedure.[7] Brauer's design resembles specialized helmets developed for delivering continuous positive airway pressure (CPAP) or for noninvasive ventilation that could be used for treating respiratory failure.[9]

Although Brauer's positive pressure technique was simpler than Sauerbruch's, Sauerbruch had his devotees in Europe and the United States. In 1909, the American surgeon Willy Meyer created his own "universal differential pressure chamber," a modified version of Sauerbruch's negative pressure chamber.[10] Meyer's chamber was even more complicated than Sauerbruch's; it included both a positive and negative pressure chamber. The overall chamber was 1000 cubic feet in volume and could contain up to 17 people. The patient, anesthetist, and an assistant could be enclosed in the positive pressure chamber within the negative pressure room. By using both chambers, the normal negative intrapleural pressure gradient could be maintained, either by applying positive pressure to the head, negative pressure to the open chest, or both. Meyer described "if the differential pressure in the universal pressure is composed of part vacuum and part pressure, only the patient is exposed to the full differential, while all others are exposed only to the component… the anesthetizer to the positive fraction and the surgeon… to the negative fraction, which still more reduces any possibility of detrimental effects on the users of the chamber." This was the only negative pressure chamber built for this purpose in America, and Meyer also used it for improving wound drainage and lung expansion postoperatively.[11]

Both the positive pressure and negative pressure methods relied on maintaining a pressure gradient between the air outside and within the lungs, otherwise known as differential pressure breathing. Differential pressure breathing was successful at preventing the formerly inevitable open pneumothorax after thoracotomy; however, it was doomed to become a historical relic because it provided dangerously inadequate ventilation. Hypoventilation, hypercarbia, hypoxemia, and impaired venous return were significant problems during prolonged cases and clinical deterioration was not uncommon. Meyer attributed the cause of unexplained shock to hypercarbia, and he recommended applying rhythmic variations in pressure coordinated with spontaneous respirations to assist with ventilation. Remarkably, although this method of preserving respiration with an open chest seems so cumbersome to modern readers, Sauerbruch and his followers felt it was endotracheal intubation that was impractical and unsafe. Meyer felt "combining intubation and masks appears so manifestly inadequate and dangerous for everyday surgery that it cannot deserve preference over apparatus leaving the mouth of the patient unincumbered [sic]."[10]

Tracheal Insufflation and Endotracheal Anesthesia

Tracheal insufflation anesthesia, an alternative method for preventing the development of the open pneumothorax, became popular in America in the early 20th century. This new method is the clear precursor to the endotracheal anesthesia we use today. Because of widespread skepticism about the routine use of tracheal intubation, the development did not follow a smooth path. Tracheal intubation and mechanical ventilation were not new discoveries; many pioneers deserve credit in the development of intubation, laryngoscopy, and positive pressure ventilation, especially considering how much skepticism they faced.

Andreas Vesalius used tracheal intubation for positive pressure ventilation of a pig in 1543. He performed a tracheotomy and passed a reed into the trachea of a pig and blew into the tube to provide artificial ventilation during a thoracotomy and thus prevented a potentially fatal open pneumothorax. His findings went unnoticed and were only later rediscovered. In 1788, Charles Kite resuscitated victims of drowning from the River Thames using curved metal cannulas that he placed blindly in the trachea. Soon after the development of inhalational anesthesia, there were early enthusiasts trying to apply these resuscitation techniques to anesthesia delivery. In 1869, Friedrich Trendelenburg used a tracheostomy tube with an inflatable cuff to administer chloroform during head and neck surgery. William MacEwan, a Scottish surgeon, is credited with the first use of oral endotracheal intubation for an anesthetic. On July 5, 1878, MacEwan placed a flexible metal tube in the larynx of an awake patient who was to have an oral tumor removed at the Glasgow Royal Infirmary.[12] In 1885, Joseph O'Dwyer, a pediatrician unaware of earlier uses of intubation, performed blind oral tracheal intubations on children suffering from diphtheria.[13] O'Dwyer designed a rigid tube with a conical tip that could occlude the larynx to facilitate positive-pressure ventilation. In 1893, George Fell attached O'Dwyer's metal tube to a bellows and T-piece, creating the Fell-O'Dwyer apparatus. Fell used the apparatus to provide ventilatory support for opiate-induced respiratory depression (Fig. 1.2).

By the 1890s, there was interest in applying endotracheal anesthesia technique to thoracic surgery in an attempt to prevent the pneumothorax problem. In 1896, the French surgeons Tuffier and Hallion reported on their use of tracheal

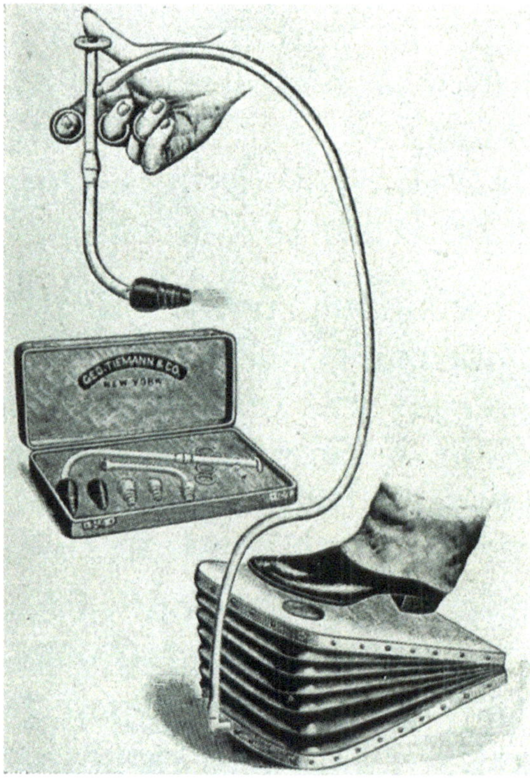

• **Fig. 1.2** The Fell-O'Dwyer Apparatus (c. 1888). O'Dwyer's laryngeal tube has a curved right angle and uses fitted, interchangeable, conical heads of different sizes designed to fit securely into the larynx. Rings were provided for the operator's fingers and the operator's thumb was placed over the expiratory orifice during inflation. (From Mushin WW, Rendell-Baker L, eds. *The Principles of Thoracic Anesthesia*. Springfield, IL: Charles C Thomas; 1953. Copyright Wiley-Blackwell.)

intubation with artificial ventilation to perform thoracotomies on animals.[12] They used a device with a bellows for the rhythmic inflation of the lungs, and a water valve that could control the degree of resistance to expiration, a precursor to the modern use of positive end-expiratory pressure (PEEP). Inspired by Tuffier and Hallion, Rudolph Matas made modifications to the Fell-O'Dwyer apparatus to make it appropriate for use during surgery. Matas was convinced that such a device would be ideal for thoracic cases. His modifications included adding a graduated cylinder for delivery of precise volumes of gases and a mercurial manometer for the measurement of intrapulmonary pressures. He also modified it to be a simple anesthesia machine by adding an intralaryngeal cannula connected by a stopcock to a rubber tube and funnel that could be used for administering chloroform.[14]

These early pioneers of endotracheal techniques were using endotracheal tubes that were similar in size to the trachea, through which inspiration and exhalation occurred. In 1907, Barthélemy and Dufour used a new method called "tracheal insufflation."[12] A thin tube was placed in the trachea and gases were continuously insufflated under positive pressure into the lower portion of the trachea. Expired gases exited between the tracheal tube and the tracheal wall. Meltzer and Auer, American physiologists, used this technique extensively in animal studies and showed that curarized dogs could be anesthetized and kept alive by blowing air and ether continuously into a tube inserted into the trachea. Gas exchange would still occur "without any normal or artificial rhythmical respiratory movements whatever" because expired gases could escape around the tracheal tube.[15] This was essentially an improvement of Brauer's method of continuously applying positive pressure; however, because dead space was decreased significantly by the placement of the cannula in the trachea, gas exchange was improved although still not optimized.

Charles Elsberg, a thoracic surgeon in New York City, was familiar with Meltzer and Auer's research and applied this method to thoracic surgery. He first used tracheal insufflation to resuscitate a myasthenic patient who had become cyanotic and pulseless. The technique was successful in that she regained spontaneous circulation; however, she did not regain consciousness so the resuscitation was eventually discontinued. Elsberg modified Meltzer and Auer's apparatus by replacing the bellows with an electric motor. He also placed the tracheal cannula under visualization after topicalization of the larynx with cocaine by using either a Killian bronchoscope or a Chevalier Jackson laryngoscope.[16] In February 1910, Elsberg presided over the historical first use of tracheal insufflation anesthesia for thoracotomy.[17] The thoracic surgeon Howard Lilienthal recruited Elsberg to help him treat a butcher with a 13-month history of productive cough. The presumptive diagnosis was lung abscess, and Lilienthal wanted to attempt an operative cure. When the pleura was opened, 15 mm Hg was applied intratracheally, and the lung was noted to be "two-thirds of its capacity, mottled, and rosy pink in color." Different pressures were applied and the lung collapsed and swelled. Elsberg periodically interrupted the insufflation every 2 to 3 minutes, to allow the lungs to collapse and facilitate carbon dioxide elimination, thus resembling modern positive-pressure ventilation. After his success in this landmark surgery, Elsberg promoted tracheal insufflation for all surgeries requiring general anesthesia. Only 1 year later, he published on his experiences using this technique to anesthetize over 200 patients.[18] Elsberg's method of tracheal insufflation is very similar to the modern practice of oxygen insufflation during rigid bronchoscopy that was first introduced by Sanders in 1968.[19]

Endotracheal Intubation and Laryngoscopy

After Elsberg's triumph, tracheal insufflation anesthesia became the most popular anesthetic method for thoracic surgery in the United Sates in the 1920s and 1930s. Differential pressure anesthesia was still preferred in Europe for thoracic procedures. Tracheal insufflations remain popular in Europe only for head and neck procedures where mask or hand drop techniques could interfere with the surgical field. A major reason for the reluctance to widely adopt the tracheal insufflation technique in Europe was the dominance of Sauerbruch and his unwillingness to adopt any other method. Sauerbruch's own assistant, Giertz, performed experiments on animals that showed that rhythmic inflation of the lungs was superior to differential pressure breathing. He also showed that differential pressure anesthesia resulted in inadequate ventilation, hypercarbia, impaired venous return, and circulatory collapse.[7] Although better than the alternative, tracheal insufflation was far from perfect. Carbon dioxide accumulation would occur if gas flow was interrupted. This was addressed with modifications to Elsberg's apparatus that periodically stopped airflow to allow the lungs to collapse. Also, barotrauma was possible when dangerously high intrapulmonary pressure occurred when the return of gas was impeded. Alveolar rupture and surgical emphysema could occur and were called "wind-tumor," likely caused by an interruption in the exit of expired gases when laryngospasm occurred around thin tracheal insufflation catheters.[12]

Another impediment to the routine use of endotracheal techniques was that blind placement of endotracheal tubes was the norm. Instruments for direct laryngoscopy existed by the 1920s, but were infrequently used. Blind placement required considerable skill and could be traumatic and cause airway laceration from the rigid tube. Alfred Kirstein, a physician in Berlin, is credited with inventing the first direct laryngoscope in 1895; before 1895, direct visualization of the larynx was considered impossible. Kirstein's "autoscope" was not used for anesthesia, but it was the prototype for many laryngoscopes to follow.[20] In 1913, Chevalier Jackson developed his own laryngoscope and described proper positioning and technique for laryngoscopy in a landmark paper.[21] In 1941, Robert Miller created the still familiar Miller blade, its origins clearly rooted in the laryngoscopes of Kirstein and Jackson. Sir Robert Macintosh released his curved blade in 1943, that remains until today the most popular laryngoscope blade in the world because of its ease of use.

Improvements in endotracheal tubes occurred alongside these developments in direct laryngoscopy. World War I produced many wounded warriors requiring reconstructive surgery for head and neck injuries. In 1919, the British anesthetists Ivan Magill and Stanley Rowbotham were assigned to work with the British army plastics unit. Under pressure to provide unhindered access to the face and airway, they became experts in blind nasal intubations. They rejected the popular insufflation technique and used larger tubes that permitted inhalation and exhalation to occur through the tube. Magill's wide-bore red rubber tubes resisted kinking and adjusted to the contours of the upper airway. They remained the standard endotracheal tube until plastic tubes were introduced.

The next step was the development of the cuffed tracheal tube. Without this, controlled positive-pressure would not be effective. In the 19th century, there were sporadic attempts at using cuffed tubes. In 1871, Trendelenburg used a cuffed tracheotomy tube, as did Eisenmenger in 1893, and Dorrance in 1910.[22] None of these attempts sparked much interest in cuffed endotracheal tubes. In 1928, Guedel and

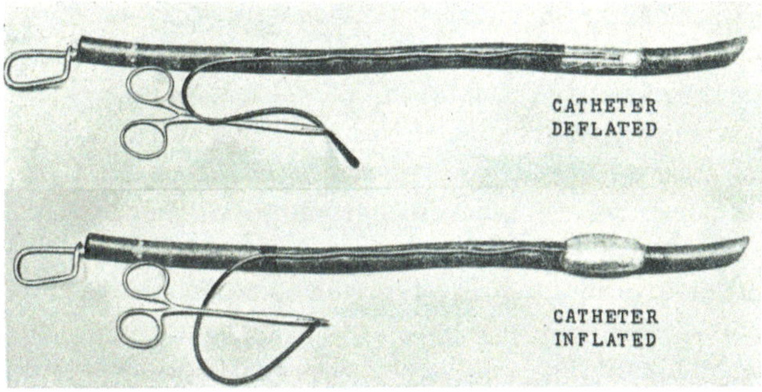

• **Fig. 1.3** Guedel and Waters "new intratracheal catheter" (1928). The catheter is shown deflated, and then inflated. The tube was 14 inches along, and made of rubber. (From Mushin WW, Rendell-Baker L, eds. *The Principles of Thoracic Anesthesia*. Springfield, IL: Charles C Thomas; 1953. Copyright Wiley-Blackwell.)

Ralph Waters introduced their endotracheal tube with a detachable inflatable cuff, and became strong advocates for the routine use of cuffed endotracheal tubes (Fig. 1.3).[23] Guedel performed his famous "dunked dog" demonstrations to show the effectiveness of the tube's seal. He submerged his intubated and sedated dog in an aquarium, from which he emerged unscathed.[24] Not only would this tube facilitate the use of controlled positive-pressure ventilation, it could prevent aspiration of gastric contents, no longer making it necessary for patients to be kept lightly anesthetized to preserve the cough reflex. With deeper planes of anesthesia, the trachea could be suctioned and operating conditions improved. Through hyperventilation, it was often possible to suppress respiratory efforts even without muscle relaxation. Control of ventilation and protection from aspiration of gastric contents represent an historic milestone in patient ventilation strategy.

Even though all of the components of airway management necessary to conquer the "pneumothorax problem" existed by 1930, unfortunately, these methods did not immediately gain widespread use. Sauerbruch's differential pressure breathing was still commonly used in Europe until World War II. Cuffed endotracheal tubes were not initially deemed necessary and took many years to gain widespread approval. In 1948, a review of 309 anesthetics for thoracic cases still advocated routine use of steep Trendelenburg to promote drainage of secretions around uncuffed endotracheal tubes and still did not recommend routine use of controlled positive-pressure ventilation.[25]

Milestones in Thoracic Surgery

Thoracic surgery progressed at a snail's pace in the 1920s. Improvements in anesthetic techniques in the 1930s made several advances in thoracic surgery possible. In 1929, Harold Brunn used the individual-structure ligation technique to replace the two-stage snare or tourniquet technique for lung resection. This new technique reduced complications, such as air leak, tension pneumothorax, hemorrhage, and infection from necrotic residual tissue.[26] Rudolph Nissen performed the first two-stage pneumonectomy in 1931, soon followed by Evarts Graham's one-stage total pneumonectomy for lung cancer in 1933.[27,28] The trajectory of thoracic surgery was changing; opening the chest had been so risky that it had been reserved only for refractory infections, but now the role of thoracic surgery for treating malignancy could flourish and overshadow its use for the treatment of infection. The addition of routine postoperative pleural drainage in the 1930s by closed chest thoracostomy also aided surgical progress. Advances in esophageal surgery also occurred in the 1930s. The first transthoracic esophagectomy with an intrathoracic esophagogastric anastomosis was performed successfully in Japan in 1933.[29] Thoracic surgery was starting to flourish as thoracic anesthesia improved.

Thoracic Surgery Under Regional Anesthesia

Regional anesthesia for thoracic surgery had its advocates before the 1940s. Proponents of regional anesthesia claimed its safety because it kept the cough reflex intact and maintained spontaneous ventilation. These are still valuable attributes of regional anesthesia. In a 1936 review of thoracic anesthesia, Magill describes spinal anesthesia as an excellent technique for a wide range of thoracic procedures, even pneumonectomy! He recognized that regional anesthesia is best for cooperative patients, as it still is today. The awake patient could assist more easily with breath-holding because controlled ventilation was not routine during general anesthesia.[30] Not everyone was so enamored with spinal anesthesia for thoracic surgery. Nosworthy declared, "I like my anesthetic technique to be such that I have the whole situation under control. I do not feel that I am in a position to cope with any emergency when chest surgery is performed under spinal anesthesia."[31] Nosworthy went on to describe an inadequate cough reflex and frequent dyspnea during open chest procedures under spinal anesthesia. It is interesting that tubeless thoracic procedures are presently gaining widespread popularity because of concerns that positive pressure ventilation has the potential to injure the lung parenchyma.

Emergence of One-Lung Ventilation

The union of direct laryngoscopy, tracheal intubation, cuffed endotracheal tubes, and controlled ventilation set the stage for the development of OLV in the 1930s. Lung separation for prevention of contamination or for surgical exposure was the next frontier. Lung surgery was still frequently performed for infection, and spillage from the infected lung was a frequent problem in the setting of copious secretions. Gale and Waters published the first use of OLV for thoracic surgery in 1931.[32] They used a long standard rubber Guedel-Waters tube that was softened with hot water to have a lateral bend. It was placed in the trachea, and then blindly advanced into either bronchus until resistance was met. In addition to preventing the "pneumothorax problem" by isolating the lung exposed to ambient pressure, this lung isolation technique also provided the advantage of an immobile lung and a quiet surgical field. Their technique was elegant in its simplicity, but not widely practiced because blind placement was difficult and tube positioning could be unstable.

Rovenstine tried to improve upon Gale and Waters' endobronchial technique. In 1936, he described the use of a single lumen endobronchial tube with two cuffs that could ventilate either one lung or both.[33] The endobronchial tube was made of woven silk and would be molded in hot water to have a lateral curve, and then advanced blindly into either bronchus as Gale and Waters described. If only the upper cuff was inflated above the carina, both lungs could be ventilated. The endobronchial cuff would occlude the other mainstem bronchus when inflated, thus enabling OLV. This tube also did not gain wide popularity because of the difficulty and instability of placement.

Bronchial Blockade

The initial use of bronchial blockers also began in the 1930s. By placing a foreign body to obstruct ventilation in the intended bronchus to a lung or lobe, ventilation is interrupted, and the unventilated lung distal to the obstruction will collapse. Archibald described the first use of a bronchial blocker in 1935; he used an inflatable balloon attached to the end of a rubber catheter to occlude the main bronchus of the affected lung during lobectomy and prevent contamination by spillage of pus to the healthy lung. He used x-ray films to confirm appropriate placement.[34] Because of its complexity, this particular technique with x-ray guidance did not gain popularity, however, the use of a balloon for bronchial blockade had significant potential and would undergo several refinements and is still used today.

Magill improved Archibald's design. In 1936, he used a similar bronchial blocker but placed it under direct vision using a tracheoscope, thus eliminating the need for x-ray guidance. His bronchial blocker was a long tube with a balloon at the distal end and was inserted alongside an endotracheal tube. Magill recommended the use of the blocker for the control of secretions, and it had a suction catheter for the blocked lung. Magill realized the blocker could improve surgical exposure by causing atelectasis of the operative lung. He recommended placement after topicalizing the larynx but before induction of general anesthesia, so that secretions could be suctioned during induction. In addition, Magill designed an endobronchial tube for lung separation; his endobronchial tube was also placed under direct vision using an endoscope through its lumen.[30] Many other instruments were used to provide bronchial blockade before the development of the plastic bronchial blockers that are currently used. In 1938, Crafoord used a ribbon gauze tampon for the control of secretions for "bronchial tamponage." The tampon was inserted using a rigid bronchoscope into the selected bronchus, while the healthy lung was ventilated by an endotracheal tube at the carina.[35] None of these techniques were commonly used because they required considerable skill and expertise. Thompson's bronchial blocker was introduced in 1943 and is the prototype for all the blockers to follow. It had a stylet and was placed through a rigid bronchoscope, and it consisted of two tubes fused together. One tube inflated a gauze-covered balloon, and the other was for applying suction to the blocked bronchus.[36]

In the 1950s, several single-lumen endotracheal tubes were developed with incorporated bronchial blockers: Steurtzbecher in 1953, Vellacott in 1954, Macintosh and Leatherdale in 1955, and Green in 1958.[37–39] These are the predecessors of the Uninvent tube, which was the first modern endotracheal tube with incorporated bronchial blockade. The Univent tube is a large endotracheal tube with a small internal lumen that contains a retractable cuffed bronchial blocker.[40] At the end of the procedure, once OLV is no longer needed, the blocker can be retracted to its internal lumen, and the tube functions as a conventional single lumen tube. Although this design is convenient, the Univent tube has a larger external diameter than a single-lumen tube of the same internal diameter, making it more traumatic to place and potentially causing increased air-flow resistance.[41]

Fogarty embolectomy catheters, Swann-Ganz catheters, and Foley catheters have all been attempted to be used as bronchial blockers. Fogarty catheters, mainly designed for vascular surgery, are described as providing successful bronchial blockade in numerous case reports.[42] However, because they were not designed for this use, they have limitations for this purpose. Their low-volume, high-pressure spheric shaped cuffs could damage bronchial mucosa, and there is no communicating channel for suction or oxygen insufflation. Positioning may be difficult, especially in the left main bronchus, because there is no steering mechanism for guiding it. All the modern balloon-tipped bronchial blockers used in clinical practice address these design flaws.[43–45] All use balloons with low-pressure, high-volume cuffs to decrease bronchial trauma, and all are intended to be placed with guidance by a 4.0-mm flexible fiberoptic bronchoscopy.

Double-Lumen Endobronchial Tubes

The first known description of a double-lumen tube (DLT) dates back to 1889 when Head used a tube with two lumens to study respiratory physiology in dogs. In 1949, Bjork and Carlens designed the first DLT for thoracic surgery, although it was originally intended for use in differential bronchospirometry to evaluate the predicted residual lung capacity post-pneumonectomy.[46] Carlens tube was designed for intubation of the left main bronchus; because endobronchial placement was performed blindly, a carinal hook was included in the design to grip the carina and to aid placement (Fig. 1.4). Bryce-Smith modified the Carlens tube in 1959 by eliminating the carinal hook because it did not in practice aid with the placement.[47] Both of these tubes could be used for right or left-sided procedures with few exceptions because ventilation could occur through either the tracheal or bronchial lumen, depending on what was needed for surgical exposure.

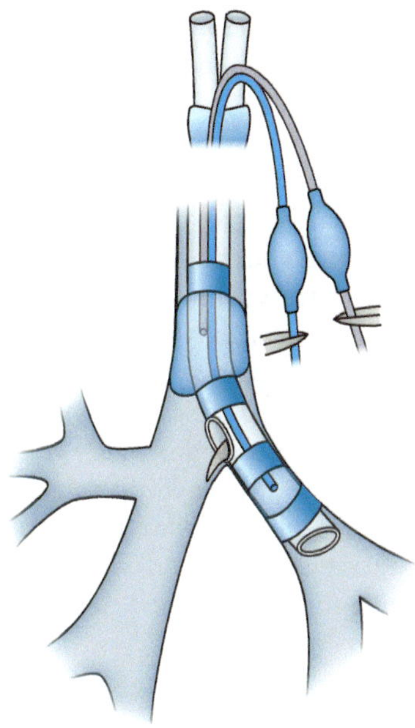

• **Fig. 1.4** Bjork and Carlens Double Lumen Catheter (1949). This is the first double-lumen endobronchial tube intended for intubation of the left mainstem bronchus. Note the presence of the carinal hook. (From Mushin WW, Rendell-Baker L, eds. *The Principles of Thoracic Anesthesia*. Springfield, IL: Charles C Thomas; 1953. Copyright Wiley-Blackwell.)

Because left-sided DLTs could not be used for left pneumonectomy, where the left main bronchus is cut close to the carina, a right-sided DLT was sought. Early DLTs were all left-sided because intubating the right main bronchus with an endobronchial lumen without occluding the opening of the right upper lobe bronchus was challenging. In 1960, Bryce-Smith and Salt described a right-sided DLT that included a slit in the endobronchial cuff for ventilation of the right upper lobe, and White designed a right-sided version of the Carlens tube with a ventilating orifice in the endobronchial cuff.[48,49]

Early DLTs were bulky, difficult to use, and potentially dangerous. Occlusion by kinking, trauma from carinal hooks, high airway resistance during OLV, and difficult blind placement were common. In 1962, Robertshaw introduced a new DLT that closely resembles those in use today.[50] He removed the carinal hook, and he introduced the novel cross-section D-shaped lumens that provided a larger cross-sectional area and reduced resistance to airflow compared with the older round lumens. Disposable plastic DLTs have replaced the older red rubber tubes, but red rubber reusable tubes are still used in many parts of the world where resources are scarce. Of interest, a European company (P3 Medical, Bristol UK) is currently manufacturing a single-use red rubber Robertshaw design DLT.

It was not until the 1980s that flexible fiberoptic bronchoscopy became available for precise positioning DLTs in the operating room (OR). Remarkably, DLTs were in use for 30 years before this development of flexible bronchoscopy, and placement was essentially blind and relied on clinical examination. The use of small flexible bronchoscopes (4.0 mm) for precise evaluation of the positioning of DLTs or endobronchial blockers is now a common practice. Newer video bronchoscopes have replaced fiberoptic bundles with video cameras that project higher quality video images on an external monitor. In fact, almost all endobronchial blockers rely on bronchoscopy for proper positioning. With flexible bronchoscopy, positioning can be reconfirmed after positioning in lateral decubitus position and can be reassessed mid-operation. Also, bronchoscopy can be used for evaluation of unusual airway anatomy, laryngoscopy of the difficult airway, and for guided pulmonary toilet. For all these reasons, flexible bronchoscopy has become routine in thoracic anesthesia and is widely considered crucial for placement of DLTs safely and effectively.[51,52] At present, there are several companies that have introduced a variety of disposable fiberoptic bronchoscopy that eliminate the need for equipment cleaning and maintenance.

Mechanical Ventilation

Although the "pneumothorax problem" was solved by the application of positive pressure to the lungs, the routine use of intermittent positive pressure ventilation was impractical before the development of mechanical ventilation and muscle relaxation. Mechanical ventilators were not routinely used in the OR until the 1960s to 1970s, only after their acceptance in the intensive care unit. Meltzer and Auer used curare in their animal studies of tracheal insufflation, but it was not used as part of general anesthetic in a human until 1942 when Griffith and Johnson used it for an appendectomy.[53] Harroun used curare with nitrous oxide and morphine as a general anesthetic for thoracic surgery, a useful new technique because it included a nonflammable agent that permitted the use of electrocautery.[54] Curare was soon replaced by safer neuromuscular agents, and neuromuscular blockade became a routine component of general anesthesia. Muscle relaxants facilitate the use of controlled ventilation by suppressing spontaneous respiratory efforts, essentially replacing the hyperventilation method that was used in the past.

Examples of early ventilators have already been mentioned here, such as the Fell-O'Dwyer apparatus from 1892, and Matas' modification of the Fell-O'Dwyer apparatus into a primitive anesthesia machine by incorporating manometry and the delivery of inhalational anesthesia. Innovations by Scandinavian surgeons and anesthesiologists bridged the gap between these early ventilators and the modern ones. Giertz, the student of Sauerbruch's who proved the superiority of intermittent ventilation over constant tracheal insufflation, inspired Frenckner, a Swedish otolaryngologist, to develop the "Spiropulsator" in 1934 for intermittent inflation of the lungs. Frenckner's colleague, Crafoord, included a reservoir bag to permit spontaneous respirations, to prevent the patient from "fighting" the ventilator because muscle relaxation was not yet available.[55] After intubation under local anesthesia, Crafoord and Frenckner's patients were ventilated by the "Spiropulsator" during thoracic surgery. Use of this ventilator was common in Scandinavia, but there was limited interest in controlled ventilation elsewhere in the 1930s and 1940s (Fig. 1.5).

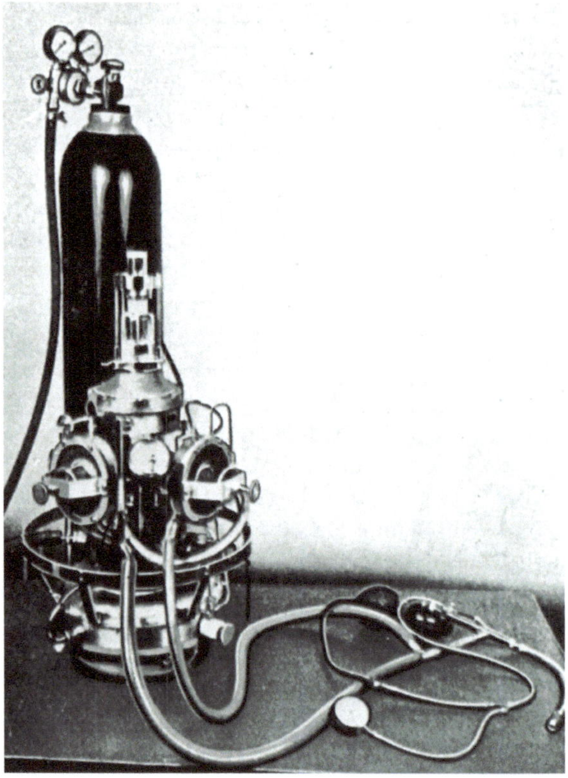

• **Fig. 1.5** The Frenckner Spiropulsator (1934). Note the endotracheal tube with cuff lying to the right. (From Mushin WW, Rendell-Baker L, eds. *The Principles of Thoracic Anesthesia*. Springfield, IL: Charles C Thomas; 1953. Copyright Wiley-Blackwell.)

In 1952, an epidemic of poliomyelitis in Copenhagen inundated Blegdam's hospital where 3000 patients presented with polio, one-third of them presented with paralysis. Faced with so many patients in need of respiratory support, the hospital sought help from Bjorn Ibsen, an anesthesiologist. Ibsen advocated for performing tracheostomies and providing controlled ventilation to weak children to increase their survival.[56] At first the hospital had few mechanical ventilators, so medical students squeezed breathing bags in shifts until more ventilators were acquired. Ibsen's aggressive treatment was a success; survival rates increased dramatically, and the modern intensive care unit was born and the iron lung abandoned. Once the ventilator could be used inside and outside the OR, postoperative ventilatory support was inevitable. In 1955, Björk and Engstrom used postoperative mechanical ventilation for their frailest thoracic surgical patients.[57] After acceptance outside the OR, mechanical ventilators finally gained acceptance in ORs in the 1960s.

Improvements in Intraoperative Monitoring

Complex intraoperative patient monitors are ubiquitous today and mandated by the American Society of Anesthesiologists; however, before the 1960s, intraoperative monitoring consisted of merely observation of color, palpation, and auscultation. An anesthesiologist had only a blood pressure cuff, electrocardiogram, and esophageal stethoscope to rely on. Hypoxemia was only detected by the presence of peripheral cyanosis, frequently, a late, subjective, and unreliable sign. Although the development of accurate invasive monitoring of peripheral arterial, pulmonary arterial, and central venous pressures have helped guide care in the OR, it is the development of noninvasive monitors of oxygenation and ventilation that have become crucial elements of providing safe anesthesia for all types of surgery, and for OLV especially. In 1942, Glen Millikan developed the first oximeter for the ear, intended for use by pilots in World War II to warn them of hypoxia from an oxygen supply failure. In 1972, Takuo Aoyagi, a Japanese engineer, invented the first pulse oximeter that could measure pulse in addition to oximetry.[58] Pulse oximetry gained acceptance in the ORs in the 1980s. Severinghaus declared, "Pulse oximetry is arguably the most important technologic advance ever made in monitoring the well-being and safety of patients during anesthesia, recovery and critical care."[59] Needless to say, pulse oximetry has become the most important monitoring device during OLV. The recognition of potential hypoxemia caused by the transpulmonary shunt can be closely and continuously monitored.

The history of capnography mirrors the development of pulse oximetry. The initial application of infrared absorption to measure expired carbon dioxide occurred in 1943, but capnography was not used widely intraoperatively until the 1980s.[60] It practically eliminated the incidence of accidental esophageal intubation. With good noninvasive monitors of oxygenation and ventilation, the need for the direct measurement of arterial blood gases has decreased but has not been eliminated. Both provide rapid and continuous guides to gas exchange and help guide when direct blood gas measurements are needed.

Additional monitors continue to be developed. With the declining popularity of pulmonary catheters, several noninvasive methods for assessing cardiac output have been developed using a variety of techniques: transthoracic bioimpedance monitors, esophageal dopplers, and monitors of arterial pulse wave analysis. Each of these techniques has its own limitations, and only time will tell whether they will gain popularity for monitoring the thoracic surgical patient.

Improvements in Ventilation

In 1956, halothane was introduced in England, and it rapidly replaced ether and cyclopropane for several reasons. Its favorable safety profile, high potency, less noxious odor, nonflammability, and favorable kinetics with rapid induction and emergence made it preferable to its predecessors.[61] Halothane's potency eliminated the need for supplemental nitrous oxide during OLV. Without nitrous oxide, hypoxemia was less likely. Because of halothane's ability to cause hepatotoxicity and cardiac arrhythmias, it has largely been replaced by newer potent volatile agents, such as isoflurane, sevoflurane, and desflurane. The practices of using potent inhaled agents without nitrous oxide remains common during OLV.

Even with 100% oxygen delivery during OLV, hypoxemia was still common because of blood shunted through the nonventilated lung. CPAP and PEEP are two ventilatory maneuvers for respiratory support outside the OR, and have both been applied to improve oxygenation in OLV. In 1971, CPAP was first described for use in infants with idiopathic respiratory distress syndrome.[62] CPAP can be applied to the nonventilated lung to improve oxygenation by apneic oxygenation, and it has been used for this purpose since the 1980s. Its limitation is that it may interfere with surgical exposure, so it has a limited use during thoracoscopic procedures.[63] PEEP is typically applied to the ventilated lung to improve oxygenation and to prevent atelectasis during OLV.[64] High-frequency jet ventilation (HFJV) with oxygen to the nondependent lung has also been used during OLV to improve oxygenation.[65] HFJV uses a jet of fresh gas delivered from a high-pressure source into the airway at a high rate (100–150 breaths per minute) either through a small catheter or a rigid bronchoscope. Because the tidal volumes are so small, the lung remains collapsed in the surgical field. HFJV is useful in many situations, such as ventilating patients with bronchopleural fistulas, for patients with tracheal stenosis, or for those undergoing tracheal surgery. Today, the use of HFJV has extended outside of the OR, finding a role in procedures where minimization of chest wall movement is desirable, such as cardiac ablations, stereotactic tumor ablations, and extracorporeal shockwave lithotripsy.[66]

Development of Postoperative Analgesia

Advances in pain management have improved care for patients undergoing thoracic surgery. Severe pain results from thoracotomy incisions, and postthoracotomy pain has a profound impact on recovery after surgery by interfering with the return of pulmonary function. Also, inadequate treatment of acute pain following thoracic surgery can contribute to the development of disabling chronic pain. Awareness by anesthesiologists and thoracic surgeons of the impact of inadequately managed acute pain on morbidity has sparked the development of multiple modalities of pain management. Before the 1980s, the only option for patients was systemic opioids, frequently administered intramuscularly. Today, options include systemic opioids, nonopioid analgesics, regional nerve blocks, and epidural local anesthesia and epidural opioids. All can be delivered using patient-controlled analgesia. Recently, emphasis has steered toward nonopioid analgesics and nonepidural regional anesthesia to try to optimize postoperative analgesia but minimize side effects. Between the variety of pharmacologic agents available and the possibility of multimodal analgesia, the options for patients are numerous, and analgesic regimens can be individually tailored to patient needs.

The introduction of neuraxial opioids to the analgesic armamentarium was an early improvement in regional anesthesia. Thoracic epidural analgesia had been attempted for postthoracotomy pain, but when limited to local anesthetics, hypotension was frequently encountered, so this method was not considered viable for routine use.[67] The first advocate for the use of neuraxial opioids was Rudolf Matas himself, who, in 1900, combined morphine with cocaine for spinal anesthesia to reduce the excitatory effect on the central nervous system caused by cocaine.[68] Interest in neuraxial opioid use remained dormant until the 1970s. In 1979, Behar et al., first described the use of epidural morphine for the treatment of pain, and noted its long duration of action.[69] Numerous studies have demonstrated the advantages of epidural over intravenous opioid analgesia. Because of this, thoracic epidural analgesia using opioids combined with low dose local anesthetics became the gold standard for postthoracotomy patients, and the use of epidural catheters for postoperative pain management has contributed to the development of acute pain services and expanded the perioperative role of anesthesiologists.[70,71] The trend of less invasive surgical techniques are currently frequently used, therefore, there has been a focus on less invasive analgesia. Paravertebral blockade has received attention as an alternative to thoracic epidural analgesia. Many studies have demonstrated the analgesic equivalence between the two techniques, whereas paravertebral blocks consistently have fewer side effects.[72]

However, although paravertebral blockade has become a popular alternative to thoracic epidural analgesia, it is still a deep block with many of the same limitations and contraindications as neuraxial blockade, with the added risk of pneumothorax. This has ushered a new interest in fascial plane blocks that are easier to perform with good efficacy and an improved safety profile. Routine use of ultrasound for regional anesthesia has helped spur the development of these fascial plane blocks. Fascial plane blocks that have been used for thoracic surgery include serratus anterior, erector spinae, and pectoralis blocks. Further investigation is warranted, however, studies have suggested that serratus anterior blockade provides improved analgesia for patients undergoing both thoracotomy and video-assisted thoracoscopic surgery (VATS), and may be comparable to paravertebral blockade in certain situations.[73–75] Evidence for the efficacy of erector spinae blockade for thoracic surgery is still limited to case studies and small trials; however, the majority of reports indicate that it is effective with a low risk of complications.[76] Pectoralis blocks are less applicable for thoracic surgery than for breast surgery, however, they have been used as an adjuvant to other analgesic modalities.[77] Intercostal blocks can also be performed before or after thoracic procedures for postoperative analgesia, often performed by the surgeon from within the thorax. These regional block modalities are gaining new interest for the procedures that are performed tubeless with the spontaneously breathing patient.

Broadened Horizons: The Current Scope of Anesthesia for Thoracic Surgery

Thoracic surgical procedures have increased in both number and complexity, and the increased quality and diversity of anesthetic methods for caring for these patients has contributed to this development. Lung cancer continues to be a major public health problem, with 228,150 estimated new cases of lung cancer in the United States in 2019.[78] Since the development of antibiotics, malignancy has been the most common indication for pulmonary surgery. However, important procedures for nonmalignant disease, such as lung transplantation and lung volume reduction surgery (LVRS), are now performed routinely at academic centers, thus making the frailest patients surgical candidates. Lung transplantation has increased from 33 transplants performed in the United States in 1988 to 2501 in 2019.[79] The most common indications for transplantation are severe chronic obstructive respiratory disease (COPD), followed by idiopathic pulmonary fibrosis, cystic fibrosis, alpha 1-antitrypsin deficiency, and primary pulmonary hypertension. LVRS is an option for patients with COPD to try and decrease the frequency and severity of debilitating symptoms; however, the surgery remains controversial because of the high cost of the surgery and rehabilitation, limited improvement, and the high morbidity and mortality postoperatively. Alternative, nonsurgical approaches includes Endoscopic lung volume reduction which encompasses endobronchial insertion of bronchial valves, injection of tissue fibrin glue, endobronchial stents insertion, or coils insertion are nonsurgical approaches to treat end stage emphysema.

Progress in surgical treatment of patients with such compromised pulmonary function has increased the need for anesthesiologists to be involved as perioperative and pain physicians, in addition to their role intraoperatively. Careful preoperative evaluation of patients for thoracic surgery is crucial so that anesthetic management can be tailored appropriately, and that often includes making appropriate plans for postoperative management. Anesthesiologists are increasingly involved in pain management, as well as management of the sickest patients who require intensive care unit stays postoperatively. Because of the variety of roles anesthesiologists fill when caring for patients undergoing thoracic surgery, care for these patients exemplifies the expanded role of anesthesiologists as perioperative physicians.

As the major hurdles of providing safe and effective thoracic anesthesia have been overcome, anesthesiologists are now able to better refine their anesthetic management with the goal of improving short- and long-term outcomes. The development of enhanced recovery after surgery (ERAS) protocols for thoracic surgery is another example of the expanded role of the anesthesiologist in optimizing all phases of care. In ERAS protocols, emphasis includes not only intraoperative management, but also preoperative optimization, postoperative pain management, and anesthetic implications for postoperative recovery, healing, and outcomes. ERAS protocols, already well established in other surgical specialties, aim to reduce postoperative complications and facilitate faster recovery through multidisciplinary implementation of multiple evidence-based measures.

ERAS guidelines for thoracic surgery typically include measures for the prevention of acute lung injury. As the anesthetic management of OLV has improved, the incidence of intraoperative hypoxemia during OLV has dramatically decreased; however, despite improvements in surgical mortality, the rate of acute lung injury was not accompanied by a similar improvement. The ideal ventilation strategy for OLV continues to be controversial, but common components of protective lung ventilation strategies, which most practitioners agree, are low tidal volumes, the use of PEEP, and recruitment maneuvers to limit the parenchymal damage and mitigate the proinflammatory effects of mechanical ventilation. In the past, applying tidal volumes up to 10 to 12 mL/kg during OLV to compensate for the nonventilated lung used to be a common practice. Current understanding of the risks of large tidal volumes favor the use of smaller tidal volumes in the range of 5 to 6 mL/kg.[80] Optimizing fraction of inspired oxygen (FiO2) is another area of interest. It was once standard to use 100% FiO2 for all patients undergoing thoracic surgery. Since hypoxemia has become more preventable during OLV, there has been more interest in decreasing FiO2 levels, with research suggesting that high FiO2 levels may result in more arrhythmia, respiratory failure, and pulmonary hypertension.[81]

There has been longstanding debate about the merits of volatile versus total intravenous anesthesia in thoracic surgery. Although some studies have shown a protective role of volatile anesthetics on the proinflammatory effects of surgery, others have shown no difference between propofol and volatile agents in major postoperative complications.[82–84] There has also been growing interest in the effect of anesthetic management on tumor recurrence, which is thought to be mediated in part by anesthetic modulation of immune response. For example, limited preclinical studies have reported that propofol may help antitumor activation of T-helper cells.[85] Also, because mu opioid receptors exist on lung cancer cells, the use of opioids may promote lung cancer progression.[86] Regional anesthesia may be protective against cancer recurrence, also through immune modulation. At the present time, to conclusively assess the impact of these anesthetic factors on cancer progression will require more research and no clear recommendations can be offered.

A major advance in thoracic surgery has been the development of minimally invasive techniques. The success of laparoscopy for minimally invasive abdominal surgery in the 1980s, alongside improvements in endoscopic video systems and instruments, spurred thoracic surgeons to develop minimally invasive techniques of their own procedures. VATS has been widely performed since the early 1990s and is increasingly replacing traditional open approaches for more complex procedures. VATS requires optimum lung separation with OLV for adequate surgical exposure because retraction of the operative lung by the surgeon is limited. The benefits of VATS over open techniques include less postoperative pain and shorter hospital stays with faster recovery of preoperative function and increased patient satisfaction.[87] The increase in patient demand for minimally invasive surgery forces surgeons to become more agile with these techniques. Available data confirm that the survival rate following VATS lobectomy for early-stage lung cancer is equivalent to an open thoracotomy.[88] Minimally invasive esophagectomies and mediastinal procedures are routinely performed by VATS. Improvements in camera technology and new, specialized instruments have allowed surgeons to push the boundaries of traditional VATS procedures and begin performing uniportal surgeries. Robotic-assisted techniques for thoracic procedures are also increasingly common, but the benefits and utility of these minimally invasive techniques need to be further defined (Fig. 1.6).

All of these minimally invasive surgical techniques rely heavily on OLV, thus spurring the development of new techniques for lung separation, especially the proliferation of bronchial blockers. The Arndt blocker (Cook Critical Care, Bloomington, IN), introduced in 1994, is wire-enabled and requires coaxial placement for fiberoptic bronchoscopic guided placement. In 2004, the Cohen Tip Deflecting Endobronchial Blocker (Cook Critical Care) was introduced. It possesses a rotating wheel for flexing the tip of the blocker and can be placed under either coaxial or parallel bronchoscopic guidance. Fuji Systems now also manufactures a bronchial blocker, the Uniblocker that is essentially the bronchial blocker from the Univent tube sold separately. The EZ blocker (EZ blocker bv, Rotterdam, The Netherlands) has a novel design featuring a bifurcated distal end that allows for alternating lung isolation and can be positioned without the need of fiberoptic bronchoscopy. The newest developments in the management of bronchial blockers include the VivaSight SL (Ambu Inc Columbia, MO USA) single lumen tube with a distal camera that allows for a bronchial blocker to be placed under direct vision without the need for flexible bronchoscopy.[89]

The search for the ideal DLT continues to be refined. At least five different manufacturers now produce DLTs for either the right or the left bronchus in a variety of sizes. The Silbroncho, is a left-sided DLT made of silicone rubber with a wire-reinforced tip. Proposed advantages of the Silbroncho include a smaller cuff to prevent left upper lobe occlusion, and the flexible, reinforced tip is intended to prevent bronchial lumen kinking or occlusion from compression.[90] The VivaSight DL, similar to the single lumen and bronchial blocker version, offers a high-resolution camera at the end of the tracheal lumen for confirmation of placement by providing a real-time view of the tube at the carinal level and reduces the need for flexible bronchoscopy. It may be useful in cases where the anesthesiologist is away from the patient's head and continued view of the correct position of the DLT is helpful (Fig. 1.7).

Improvement in video technology has resulted in the proliferation of new video integrated airway devices. Flexible video bronchoscopes, which continue to improve in image quality and resolution, are now available as single-use disposable devices by several companies in an effort to decrease the cost and the maintenance associated with reusable scopes. In many situations, video laryngoscopy has replaced flexible bronchoscopy for intubation of the difficult airway, and has been adopted for use for placement of DLTs. Video laryngoscopy allows the patient's airway to be secured from

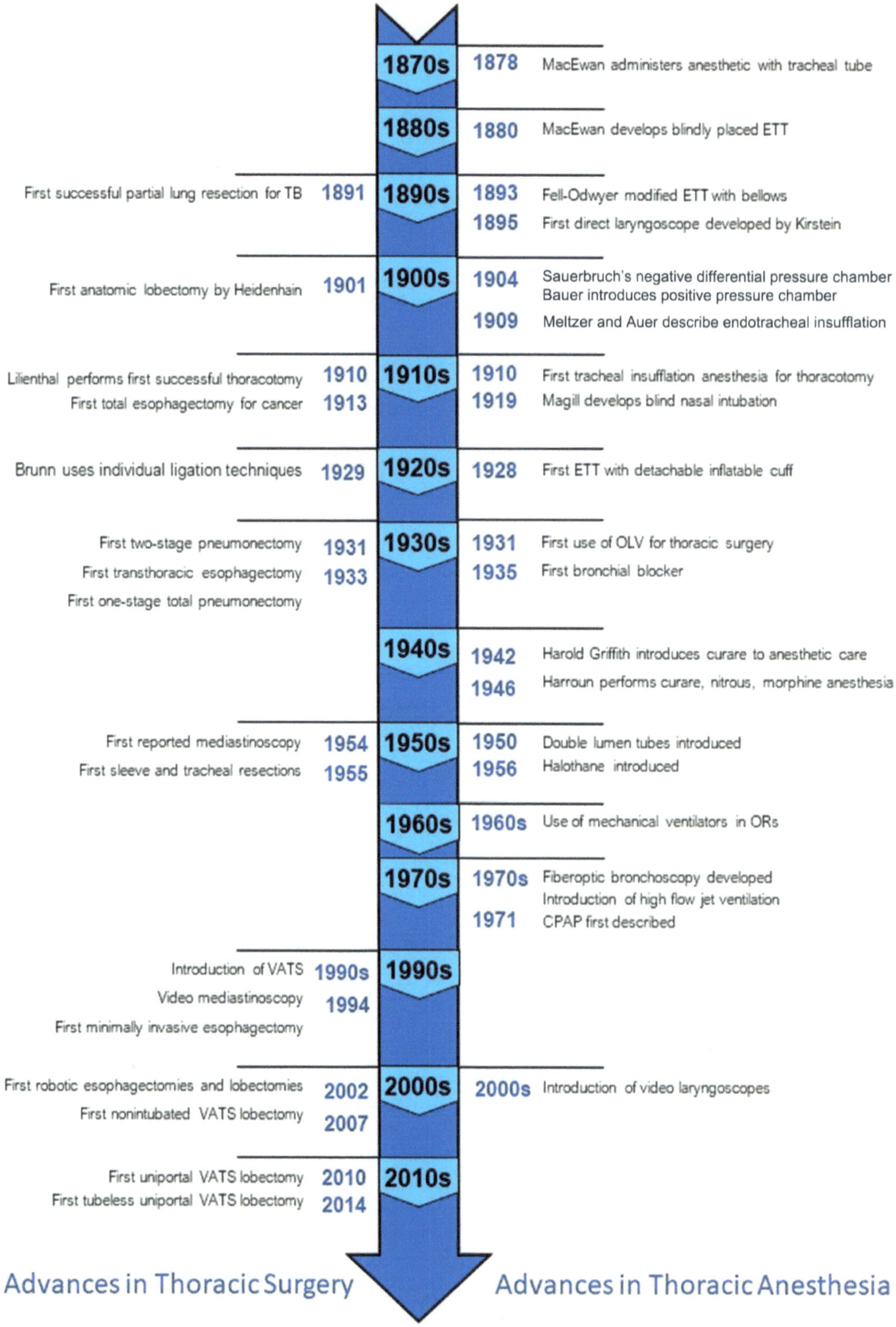

• **Fig. 1.6** Milestones in the development of thoracic surgery and anesthesia. *CPAP*, Continuous positive airway pressure; *ETT*, Endotracheal tube; *OLV*, One-lung ventilation; *OR*, operating room; *VATS*, video-assisted thoracoscopic surgery.

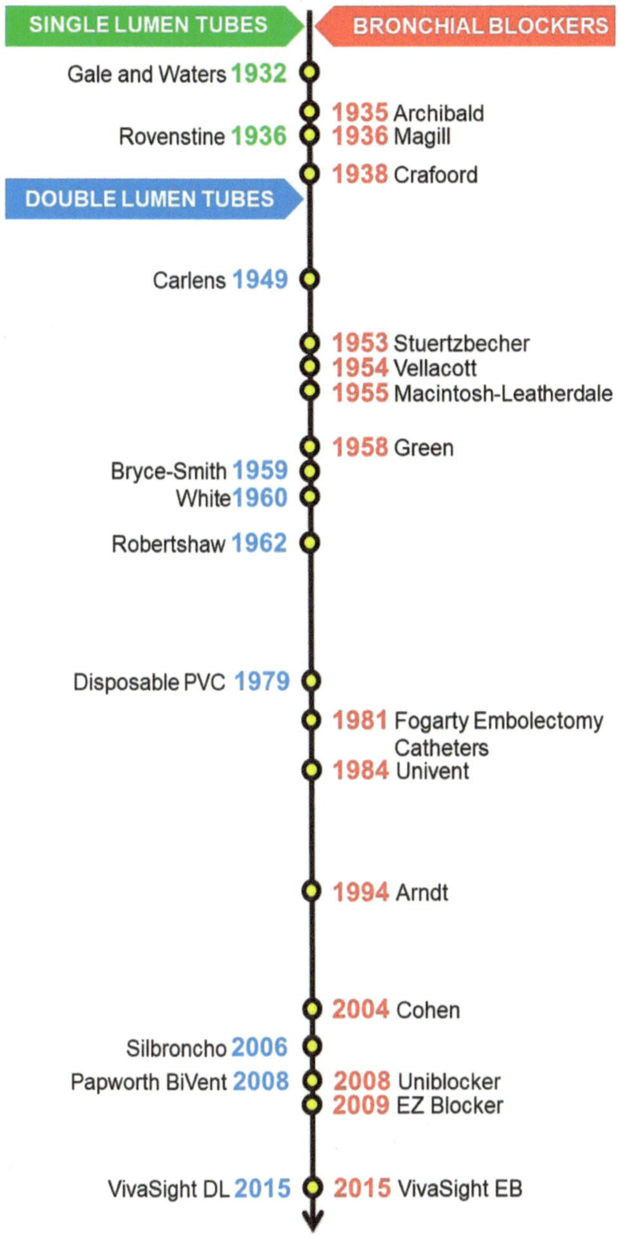

• **Fig. 1.7** Developments in the history of lung separation techniques. *PVC*: Polyvinyl chloride.

a greater distance, potentially decreasing the spread of infection. For this reason, video laryngoscopy has been widely used during the COVID-19 pandemic.

With the array of bronchial blockers and DLTs now available, providing OLV is easier, safer, and more versatile than ever. Today, single lumen endotracheal tubes are only rarely used for OLV for adults because of the availability of DLTs and the variety of endobronchial blockers that are better suited for lung separation. However, they are still used frequently for children because the relatively small airways of infants and small children cannot accommodate DLTs. The smallest size DLT is 28F that can accommodate adolescent patients. For the pediatric patients that can be managed by 5.0F, the Arndt (Cook Medical, Bloomington IN) or Uniblocker (Fuji Medical, Japan) endobronchial blocker is available. The proliferation of tools and techniques for OLV has also been spurred by increased use of thoracic approaches to spinal, cardiac, esophageal, and vascular procedures. Robotic-assisted techniques for cardiac surgery, including robotic mitral valve repairs, atrial septal defect repairs, and pericardial procedures increasingly use OLV.[91] Such a wide range of procedures requiring OLV has made facility with these techniques a necessity for most anesthesiologists because these surgical techniques may not be possible without adequate lung separation for exposure.

Today, the reliance on OLV has been put to the challenge with the introduction of tubeless thoracic surgery. The definition of tubeless surgery can range from avoidance of endotracheal intubation to the avoidance of all catheters and tubes, including chest tubes and urinary catheters. The procedures are performed with a spontaneously ventilating patient or with an airway laryngeal mask (LMA) or under regional anesthesia. The cough reflex, which was once a hindrance to thoracic surgeons before the invention of endotracheal tubes and muscle relaxation is blunted by aerosolized lidocaine or nerve block. Combining multiple novel minimally invasive techniques, the first uniportal VATS lobectomy was performed on a nonintubated patient in 2014, recalling regional anesthesia used for open thoracic anesthesia in the first half of the 20th century.[92] As thoracic surgery advances, we have started to see echoes of the past, with new technologies and techniques overcoming the problems that made the procedures so dangerous in the past complemented by a return to older techniques. Certainly, history is repeating itself!

Anesthesiologists are also frequently involved in other types of thoracic procedures. Tumors of the bronchi and trachea are frequently treated with stents and/or laser therapy. Airway stenting to palliate patients with severe airway obstructions, usually because of malignant causes, has become increasingly common. These procedures may require special ventilatory techniques, such as HFJV or the Sanders injection system. Also, stents are now frequently placed by interventional pulmonologists outside of the OR, posing unique challenges to the anesthesiologist. When performed under general anesthesia, tracheal resection required cross-field intubation with intermittent ventilation. However, as part of the recent tubeless era, there are recent reports of tracheal resections being performed under regional and neuraxial anesthesia, including cervical epidurals.[93] The improvement in extracorporeal membrane oxygenation (ECMO) technology has made it a more accessible option for these difficult tumors, allowing for better operating conditions, while maintaining oxygenation and hemodynamic support as needed. Novalung, a pumpless lung assistance device can be used to remove carbon dioxide with greater ease, although its oxygenation capacity is poor compared with traditional ECMO.[94]

Anterior mediastinal masses are also particularly challenging for anesthesiologists because of their potential to cause extrinsic compression of the airway and critical obstructions. Patients with anterior mediastinal masses may need anesthesia for diagnostic or therapeutic procedures, and anesthetic management needs to be based on careful preoperative assessment of the potential for airway compression and requires a close collaboration with the thoracic surgeon. As ECMO has become more accessible, precannulation for ECMO is now recommended for those patients at highest risk of cardiovascular and respiratory collapse on induction of anesthesia.

Conclusion

The variety and complexity of procedures now routinely performed by thoracic surgeons would not be possible without the improvements in anesthetic techniques described here. Anesthesiologists over the past 100 years have refined methods of securing the airway, lung isolation, physiologic monitoring, and ventilatory techniques to the point where anesthetizing frail patients for complex procedures appears deceptively easy. Thoracic surgery has flourished with the support of improved anesthesia techniques. The thoracic anesthesiologist of the future will be able to provide the safest anesthesia that will not only facilitate surgery but also optimize short-term recovery and long-term outcomes.

References

1. Strieder JW. Anesthesia from the viewpoint of the thoracic surgeon. *Anesthesiology*. 1950;11(1):60–64.
2. Celsus A. *De Medicina*. Loeb Classical Library; 1938 http://penelope.uchicago.edu/Thayer/E/Roman/Texts/Celsus/Prooemium*.html. Accessed December 23, 2019.
3. Souttar HS. A British Medical Association lecture on recent advances in the surgery of the chest. *Br Med J*. 1926;1(3413):933–936.
4. Matas R. On the management of acute traumatic pneumothorax. *Ann Surg*. 1899;29(4):409–434.
5. Barry JE, Adams AP. The development of thoracic anesthesia. In: Hurt R, ed. *The History of Cardiothoracic Surgery From Early Times*. New York: Parthenon; 1996.
6. Lilienthal H. Resection of the lung for suppurative infections with a report based on 31 operative cases in which resection was done or intended. *Ann Surg*. 1922;75(3):257–320.
7. Mushin WM, Rendell-Baker L. The current practice of anesthesia for thoracic surgery represents a culmination. In: *The Principles of Thoracic Anaesthesia: Past and Present*. Springfield, IL: Charles C Thomas; 1953.
8. Nissen R. Historical development of pulmonary surgery. *Am J Surg*. 1955;89(1):9–15.
9. Bellani G, Patroniti N, Greco M, et al. The use of helmets to deliver non-invasive continuous positive airway pressure in hypoxemic respiratory failure. *Minerva Anestesiol.* 2008;74(11):651–656.
10. Meyer W. Pneumectomy with the aid of differential air pressure: an experimental study: the new type of apparatus used. *JAMA*. 1909;53(24):1978–1987.
11. Meyer W. Some observations regarding thoracic surgery on human beings. *Ann Surg*. 1910;52(1):34–58.
12. Gillespie NA. The evolution of endotracheal anaesthesia. *J Hist Med Allied Sci*. 1946;1(4):583–594.
13. O'Dwyer J. Fifty cases of croup in private practice treated by intubation of the larynx. *Med Rec*. 1887;32:557–561.
14. Matas R. Intralaryngeal insufflation. *JAMA*. 1900;34(23):1468–1473.
15. Meltzer SJ, Auer J. Continuous respiration without respiratory movements. *J Exp Med*. 1909;11(4):622–625.
16. Elsberg CA. Clinical experiences with intratracheal insufflation (Meltzer), with remarks upon the value of the method for thoracic surgery. *Ann Surg*. 1910;52(1):23–29.
17. Lilienthal H. The first case of thoracotomy in a human being under anaesthesia by intratracheal insufflation. *Ann Surg*. 1910; 52(1):58–66.
18. Elsberg CA. Experiences in thoracic surgery under anaesthesia by the intratracheal insufflation of air and ether. *Ann Surg*. 1911;54(6):749–757.
19. Mette PJ, Sanders RD. Ventilation bronchoscopy: a new technic. *Anaesthesist*. 1968;17(10):316–321.
20. Kirstein A. Autoskopie des larynx und der trachea. *Berl Klin Woch*. 1895;32:476–478.
21. Jackson C. The technique of insertion of intratracheal insufflation tubes. *Surg Gyn Obst*. 1913(17):507–509.
22. White GM. Evolution of endotracheal and endobronchial intubation. *Brit J Anaesth*. 1960;32(5):235–246.
23. Guedel AE, Waters RM. A new intratracheal catheter. *Curr Res Anesth Analg*. 1928(7):238–239.
24. Waters RM, Arthur E. Guedel. *Brit J Anaesth*. 1952;24(4):292–299.
25. Fisher K, Lee LD, Stegeman DE, et al. Anesthetic management for surgery with the thorax: a report of 309 cases. *Anesthesiology*. 1948;9(6):623–636.
26. Brunn H. Surgical principles underlying one-stage lobectomy. *Arch Surg*. 1929;18(1):490–515.
27. Herbsman H. Early history of pulmonary surgery. *J Hist Med Allied Sci*. 1958;13(3):329–348.
28. Graham AE, Singer JJ. Successful removal of an entire lung for carcinoma of the bronchus. *JAMA*. 1933;101(18):1371–1374.
29. Ohsawa T. Surgery of the esophagus. *Arch Jpn Chir*. 1933(10): 605–608.
30. Magill IW. Anaesthesia in thoracic surgery with special reference to lobectomy. *Proc Roy Soc Med*. 1936;29(6):643–653.
31. Nosworthy MD. Anesthesia in chest surgery. *Proc Roy Soc Med*. 1941;34(8):479–506.
32. Gale JW, Waters RM. Closed endobronchial anesthesia in thoracic surgery. *J Thorac Surg*. 1931(1):432–437.
33. Rovenstine EA. Anaesthesia for intrathoracic surgery: the endotracheal and endobronchial techniques. *Surg Gyn Obst*. 1936(63):325–330.
34. Archibald E. A consideration of the dangers of lobectomy. *J Thorac Surg*. 1935(4):335–351.
35. Crafoord C. On the technique of pneumonectomy in man. *Acta Chir Scand*. 1938(81):5–142.
36. Rusby NL, Thompson VC. Carcinoma of the lung: diagnosis and surgical treatment. *Postgrad Med J*. 1943;19(207):44–53.
37. Vellacott WN. A new endobronchial tube for broncho-pleural fistula repair. *Brit J Anaesth*. 1954;26(6):442–444.
38. Macintosh R, Leatherdale RA. Bronchus tube and bronchus blocker. *Brit J Anaesth*. 1955;27(11):556–557.
39. Gordon W, Green R. Right lung anaesthesia: anaesthesia for left lung surgery using a new right endobronchial tube. *Anaesthesia*. 1957;12(1):86–93.
40. Kamaya H, Krisha PR. New endotracheal tube (Univent tube) for selective blockade of one lung. *Anethesiology*. 1985;63(3):342–343.

41. Slinger PD, Lesiuk L. Flow resistances of disposable double-lumen, single-lumen and Univent tubes. *J Cardiothorac Vasc Anesth.* 1998;12(2):142–144.
42. Ginsberg RJ. New technique for one-lung anesthesia using an endobronchial blocker. *J Thorac Cardiovsc Surg.* 1981;82(4):542–546.
43. Arndt GA, Buchika S, Kranner PW, DeLessio ST. Wire-guided endobronchial blockade in a patient with a limited mouth opening. *Can J Anaesth.* 1999;46(1):87–89.
44. Cohen E. The Cohen flexitip endobronchial blocker: an alternative to a double lumen tube. *Aneth Analg.* 2005;101(6):1877–1879.
45. Mungroop HE, Mijzen L, Woltersom B, et al. Feasibility of a new Y shaped bronchial blocking device and comparison with a DLT: A Manikin Study. 2009 ASA meeting. Abstract A541.
46. Bjork VO, Carlens E. The prevention of spread during pulmonary resection by the use of a double lumen catheter. *J Thorac Surg.* 1950;20(1):151–157.
47. Bryce-Smith R. A double-lumen endobronchial tube. *Brit J Anaesth.* 1959(31):274–275.
48. Bryce-Smith R, Salt R. A right-sided double lumen tube. *Brit J Anaesth.* 1960(32):230–231.
49. White GM. A new double lumen tube. *Brit J Anaesth.* 1960(32): 232–234.
50. Robertshaw FL. Low resistance double-lumen endobronchial tubes. *Brit J Anaesth.* 1962(34):576–579.
51. Ehrenwerth J. Pro: proper positioning of a double-lumen endobronchial tube can only be accomplished with endoscopy. *J Cardiothoracic Anesth.* 1988;2(1):101–104.
52. Campos JH. Current techniques for perioperative lung isolation in adults. *Anesthesiology.* 2002;97(5):1295–1301.
53. Griffith HR, Johnson GE. The use of curare in general anesthesia. *Anesthesiology.* 1942;3(4):418–420.
54. Harroun P, Beckert FE, Hathaway HR. Curare and nitrous oxide anesthesia for lengthy operations. *Anesthesiology.* 1946;7(1):24–28.
55. Anderson E, Crafoord C, Frenckner P. A new and practical method of producing rhythmic ventilation during positive pressure anaesthesia with description of apparatus. *Acta Oto-laryngolica.* 1940;28(1):95–102.
56. Ibsen B. The anaesthetist's viewpoint on the treatment of respiratory complications in poliomyelitis during the epidemic in Copenhagen, 1952. *Proc Roy Soc Med.* 1954;47(1):72–74.
57. Bjork VO, Engstrom CG. The treatment of ventilatory insufficiency after pulmonary resection with tracheotomy and prolonged artificial ventilation. *J Thorac Surg.* 1955;30(3):356–367.
58. Severinghaus JW. Takuo Aoyagi: discovery of pulse oximetry. *Anesth Analg.* 2007;105(6 suppl):S1–S4.
59. Severinghaus JW, Honda Y. Pulse oximetry. *Int Anesthesiol Clin.* 1987;25(4):205–214.
60. Luft K. Method der registrieren gas analyse mit hilfe der absorption ultraroten Strahlen ohne spectrale Zerlegung. *Z Tech Phys.* 1943(24):97.
61. Raventos J. The action of fluothane—a new volatile anaesthetic. *Br J Pharmacol.* 1956;11(4):394–410.
62. Gregory GA, Kitterman JA, Phibbs RH, et al. Treatment of the idiopathic respiratory distress syndrome with continuous positive airway pressure. *NEJM.* 1971;284(24):1333–1340.
63. Capan LM, Turndorf H, Patel C, et al. Optimization of arterial oxygenation during one-lung anesthesia. *Anesth Analg.* 1980; 59(11):847–851.
64. Cohen E, Eisenkraft JB. Positive end-expiratory pressure during one-lung ventilation improves oxygenation in patients with low arterial oxygen tensions. *J Cardiothorac Vasc Anesth.* 1996;10(5):578–582.
65. Godet G, Bertrand M, Ben Ammeur M, et al. Comparison of HFJV vs CPAP for separate lung ventilation in patients surgically treated aneurysm of the thoracic aorta. *Ann Fr Anesth Reanim.* 1989(8 Suppl):R266.
66. Raiten J, Elkassabany N, Mandel JE. The use of high-frequency jet ventilation for out of operating room anesthesia. *Curr Opin Anaesthesiol.* 2012;25(4):482–485.
67. Shuman RL, Peters RM. Epidural anesthesia following thoracotomy in patients with chronic obstructive airway disease. *J Thorac Cardiovasc Surg.* 1976;71(1):82–88.
68. Matas R. Local and regional anesthesia with cocaine and other analgesic drugs, including the subarachnoid method, as applied in general surgical practice. *Philadelph Med J.* 1900(6):820–843.
69. Behar M, Magora F, Olshwang D, Davidson JT. Epidural morphine in treatment of pain. *Lancet.* 1979;1(8115):527–529.
70. Slinger PD. Pro: every postthoracotomy patient deserves thoracic epidural analgesia. *J Cardiothorac Vasc Anesth.* 1999;13(3):350–354.
71. Ready LB, Oden R, Chadwick HS, et al. Development of an anesthesiology-based postoperative pain management service. *Anesthesiology.* 1988;68(1):100–106.
72. Joshi GP, Bonnet F, Shah R, et al. A systematic review of randomized trials evaluating regional techniques for postthoracotomy analgesia. *Anesth Analg.* 2008;107(3):1026–1040.
73. Viti A, Bertoglio P, Zamperini M, et al. Serratus plane block for video-assisted thoracoscopic surgery major lung resection: a randomized controlled trial. *Interac Cardiovasc Thorac Surg.* 2019(1): 1–7.
74. Semyonov M, Fedorina E, Grinshpun J, et al. Ultrasound-guided serratus anterior plane block for analgesia after thoracic surgery. *J Pain Res.* 2019;12:953–960.
75. Khalil AE, Abdallah NM, Bashandy GM, Kaddah TA. Ultrasound-guided serratus anterior plane block versus thoracic epidural analgesia for thoracotomy pain. *J Cardiothorac Vasc Anesth.* 2017;31(1):152–158.
76. Kot P, Rodriguez P, Granell M, et al. The erector spinae plane block: a narrative review. *Korean J Anesthesiol.* 2019;72(3):209–220.
77. Marciniak D, Kelava M, Hargrave J. Fascial plane blocks in thoracic surgery: a new era or plain painful. *Curr Opin Anaesthesiol.* 2020;33(1):1–9.
78. National Cancer Institute. Surveillance epidemiology and end results. http://seer.cancer.gov/statfacts/html/lungb.html. Accessed January 3, 2020.
79. Organ procurement and transplant network data reports. http://optn.transplant.hrsa.gov/latestData/viewDataReports.asp. Accessed January 3, 2020.
80. Batchelor TJP, Rasburn NI, Abdelnour-Berchtold E, et al. Guidelines for enhanced recovery after lung surgery: recommendations of the Enhanced Recovery after Surgery (ERAS) Society and the European Society of Thoracic Surgeons (ESTS). *Eur J Cardiothoracic Surg.* 2019;55(1):91–115.
81. Misthos P, Katsaragakis S, Theodorou D, Milingos N, Skottis I. The degree of oxidative stress is associated with major adverse effects after lung resection: a prospective study. *Eur J Cardiothorac Surg.* 2006;29(4):591–595.
82. Beck-Schimmer B, Bonvini JM, Braun J, et al. Which anesthesia regimen is best to reduce morbidity and mortality in lung surgery. *Anesthesiology.* 2016;125(2):313–321.
83. Schilling T, Kozian A, Senturk M, et al. Effects of volatile and intravenous anesthesia on the alveolar and systemic inflammatory response in thoracic surgical patients. *Anesthesiology.* 2011;115(1):65–74.

84. De Conno E, Steurer MP, Wittinger M, et al. Anesthetic-induced improvement of the inflammatory response to one-lung ventilation. *Anesthesiology*. 2009;110(6):1316–1326.
85. Ren XF, Li WZ, Meng FY, Lin CF. Differential effects of propofol and isoflurane on the activation of T-helper cells in lung cancer patients. *Anaesthesia*. 2010;65(5):478–482.
86. Mathew B, Lennon FE, Siegler J, et al. The novel role of the mu opioid receptor in lung cancer progression: a laboratory investigation. *Anesth Analg*. 2011;112(3):558–567.
87. Demmy TL, Nwogu C. Is video-assisted thoracic surgery lobectomy better? Quality of life considerations. *Ann Thorac Surg*. 2008; 85(2):719–728.
88. Flores RM, Alam N. Video-assisted thoracic surgery lobectomy (VATS), open thoracotomy, and the robot for lung cancer. *Ann Thorac Surg*. 2008;85(2):710–715.
89. Saracoglu A, Saracoglu KT. VivaSight: a new era in the evolution of tracheal tubes. *J Clin. Anesth*. 2016;33:442–449.
90. Lohser J, Brodsky JB. Silbroncho double-lumen tube. *J Cardiothorac Vasc Anesth*. 2006;20(1):129–131.
91. Grocott HP, Darrow TR, Whiteheart DL, et al. Lung isolation during port-access cardiac surgery: double-lumen endotracheal tube versus single-lumen endotracheal tube with a bronchial blocker. *J Cardiothorac Vasc Anesth*. 2003;17(6):725–727.
92. Tamburrini A, Mineo TC. A glimpse of history: non-intubated thoracic surgery. *Video-Assisted Thorac Surg*. 2017;2(9):52.
93. Macchiarini P, Rovira I, Ferrarello S. Awake upper airway surgery. *Ann Thorac Surg*. 2010;89(2):387–391.
94. Schieren M, Böhmer A, Dusse F, et al. New approaches to airway management in tracheal resections—a systematic review and meta-analysis. *J Cardiothorac Vasc Anesth*. 2017;31(4):1351–1358.

2

Anatomic Correlates of Physiologic Function

THEODORE C. SMITH, EDMOND COHEN

The respiratory and circulatory systems play a major role in the transportation of oxygen from the atmosphere to mitochondria and transportation of carbon dioxide from cells to the atmosphere. They accomplish these tasks by alternate steps of convection and diffusion. The respiratory system provides for the first two steps for oxygen, convection from the atmosphere and diffusion into the blood stream. Anatomic features are best understood by appreciation of their role in the several functions, as outlined in Table 2.1. The structures include an air-conditioning subsystem, a pump, and a marvelously fractile convective system, terminating in well-perfused, close-packed, polyhedral air spaces that ingeniously incorporate a very large area with the thinnest possible barrier between blood and gas, and an energy storage device to power the usually passive exhalation.

This chapter stresses that form and function are interrelated. Therefore it does not follow a distinctly anatomic organization.

The Muscle-Powered Air Pump

The work of breathing is supplied by two groups of muscles (three sets are inspiratory and three are expiratory) that act on skeletal and soft tissue structures of the trunk (chest plus abdomen or, in the classic Greek sense, the thorax). The thorax is bounded by the sternum, ribs, spine, intercostal muscles, abdominal wall muscles, clavicle and strap muscles superiorly, and the pelvic floor inferiorly. The actions of the muscles on the skeletal and soft tissue organs provide active inspiration, store energy in the parenchyma and thorax for passive exhalation, and provide active exhalation when required (see Table 2.1).

The inspiratory muscles consist of the diaphragm; the external intercostals; and the accessory muscles, including the strap muscles of the neck and the erector spini (Fig. 2.1).[1,2]

The diaphragm is a dome-shaped structure consisting of a central tendon with muscle fibers radiating outward to attach on the xiphoid, on the seventh to twelfth ribs, and on the vertebral bodies. Contraction under phrenic nerve control flattens the dome shape, increasing the cephalocaudal (CC) dimension of the lung. Simultaneously, it displaces the liver, spleen, and stomach both anteriorly and laterally, increasing the anterior-posterior (AP) and the side-to-side (S-S) or lateral dimension of the chest through passive movement of the rib cage (Fig. 2.2).

The rib cage volume is also increased by the action of the external (oblique) intercostal muscles. The fibers of these muscles run diagonally upward and backward from the top of one rib to the bottom of the next above. Three types of motion result from the slightly different articulation of: (1) the first two or three ribs, (2) the middle ribs, and (3) the lowermost two pairs of ribs: pump handle, bucket handle, and caliper motion. The first three or four ribs lie in planes that slope primarily from back to front. When they move upward, they increase the AP and CC diameters. This movement is like a pump handle. The next six or seven ribs lie in planes that are increasingly tilted to the side. When they move, the S-S diameter increases by the bucket handle motion induced by the articulation of these ribs at the sternum, as well as at the vertebral column. The eleventh and twelfth ribs move primarily outward, aided by pressure of the viscera, as well as upward, like the jaws of a caliper or tongs, primarily increasing the S-S diameter.[3]

Although the diaphragm or the external intercostals are independently able to supply the tidal volume and about half of the vital capacity, the accessory muscles most often play an accessory role. The paravertebral muscles can straighten the spinal kyphosis, and the strap muscles of the neck lift the thoracic inlet. The strap muscles of the neck, including most importantly the sternocleidomastoid, and also those muscles from tongue to hyoid to thyroid to cricoid to sternum, generally referred to as the accessory muscles of inspiration, are capable of adding perhaps 10% to the inspiratory capacity on their own. Normally, during inspiration, they have a phasic increase in tone with each breath (i.e., isometric contraction), which serves to stabilize the thoracic inlet. This permits the external intercostals to increase the S-S diameter, each lifting the rib below. When the clavicle and first rib can be seen to move up and out, in

TABLE 2.1 Anatomy and Physiology Related to Pulmonary Function Tests

Major Function	Testable Physiology	Anatomic Feature	Applicable Tests
Ventilation	Pump	Skeleton	Inspection, radiography
	Conduits	Muscles	PI_{max}, PE_{max}, vital capacity
	Expandable tissue	Airways	Airway resistance, forced expiratory flow
		Small airways	Flow-volume loops
		Alveolar ducts	Lung compliance, Closing capacity
Perfusion	Pump	Right ventricle	Pre- and afterloads, ejection fraction, wall fraction, wall motion, cardiac output
Exchange	Distribution:		
	gas	Alveolar interdependence	Chest radiograph
	blood	Airways morphology	A-a differences/O_2, CO_2
	surface	Hydrostatic gradient	DL carbon monoxide
		Vessel potency	
		Alveolar Facet	Capillary volume
			Inert gas ventilation-perfusion distribution
Defense	Filtering	Nose and pharynx	Inspection
	Humidification	Epithelium	Tantalum transport
	Mucociliary transport	Larynx	Cough reflex
	Separation from gut	Cell types	Bronchial brushing, lavage
	Immune mechanism		
Control	Sensors	Carotid body	Doxapram
		Aortic body	
		Medulla:	Ventilatory response:
		respiratory centers	to CO_2
		ventrolateral surface	to hypoxia
		Irritant and J receptors	
	Reflexes	Vagus nerve	Breathing pattern
		Central connections	Response to loading

DL, Diffusing capacity of the lungs; PE_{max}, maximal expiratory pressure; PI_{max}, maximal inspiratory pressure.

either spontaneous or mechanical ventilation, one can be sure it represents an augmented tidal volume.[4]

The inspiratory muscles have expiratory functions as well. First, by stretching the expiratory muscles, they increase their contractility when activated. Second, they stretch the lung, and with large tidal volumes the rib cage as well, storing elastic energy for exhalation. Finally, their tone is decreased slowly and progressively during expiration, providing a braking effect on expiratory flow, minimizing expiratory flow problems, and tending to increase average lung volume (Fig. 2.3).

The expiratory muscles consist of the muscles of the abdominal wall, the internal intercostals muscles, and a number of other muscles of the upper limb and thorax. The expiratory muscles are not ordinarily involved in quiet expiration. They markedly increase expiratory flow in the sneeze or cough, and can decrease lung volume below functional residual capacity, to residual volume. The muscles involved in active expiration are, most importantly, those of the abdominal wall (external obliques, internal obliques, rectus abdominis, and transversus abdominis); the internal intercostals (whose fibers run more vertically than the external obliques); and to a very small

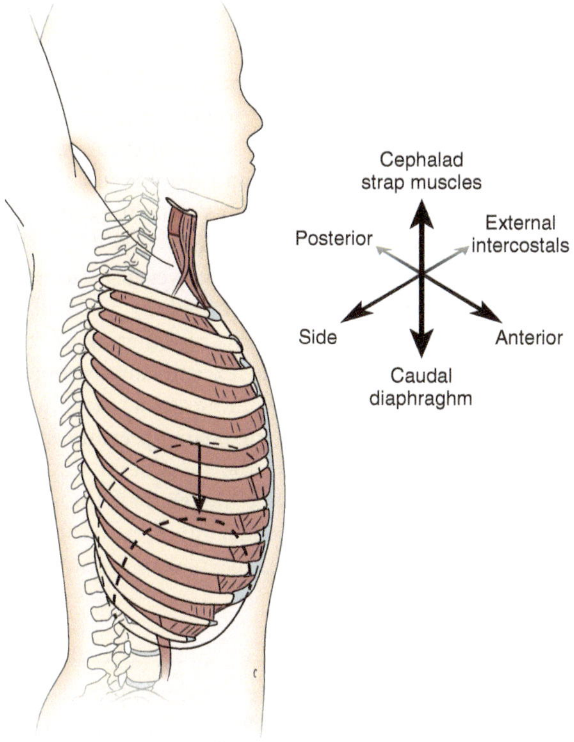

• **Fig. 2.1 Inspiratory muscles.** The major inspiratory muscles are the diaphragm, the external intercostals, and to a lesser extent, the strap muscles of the neck, particularly the sternocleidomastoid and three scalenes. Muscles of the shoulder girdle and spinal erectors may play a minor role at the end of a deep inspiration.

degree, the muscles of the thoracic girdle and spine, which pull the shoulders forward and flex the vertebral column (and might be called the accessory muscles of expiration). These muscles ordinarily have little tone during anesthesia but come into play with cough. On emergence or in very light anesthesia, the abdominal components may be activated at the end of expiration. This end-expiratory tightening of the oblique abdominals thrusts the abdominal wall forward and may be mistaken for an inspiratory effort. Attendants trying to assist breathing with resuscitation bags (Ambu-bags or equivalent) may thus be out of synchronization, and their efforts may be counterproductive.

Lung Volumes: Anatomic Determinants

The nomenclature of the lung volumes was originally based on four independent volumes: residual volume (RV), expiratory reserves volume (ERV), tidal volume (V_T), and inspiratory reserve volume (IRV). A fifth, overlapping lung volume closing volume (CV) has been added. Two or more volumes may be added to obtain a capacity.

Functional residual capacity (FRC) = RV + ERV
Inspiratory capacity (IC) = V_T + IRV
Vital capacity (VC) = ERV + V_T + IRV
Total lung capacity (TLC) = RV + ERV + V_T + IRV
Closing capacity (CC) = CV + RV

When the lungs and viscera are removed from the body and all muscles are relaxed or paralyzed, the volume of the thoracic cage is several hundred milliliters larger than the

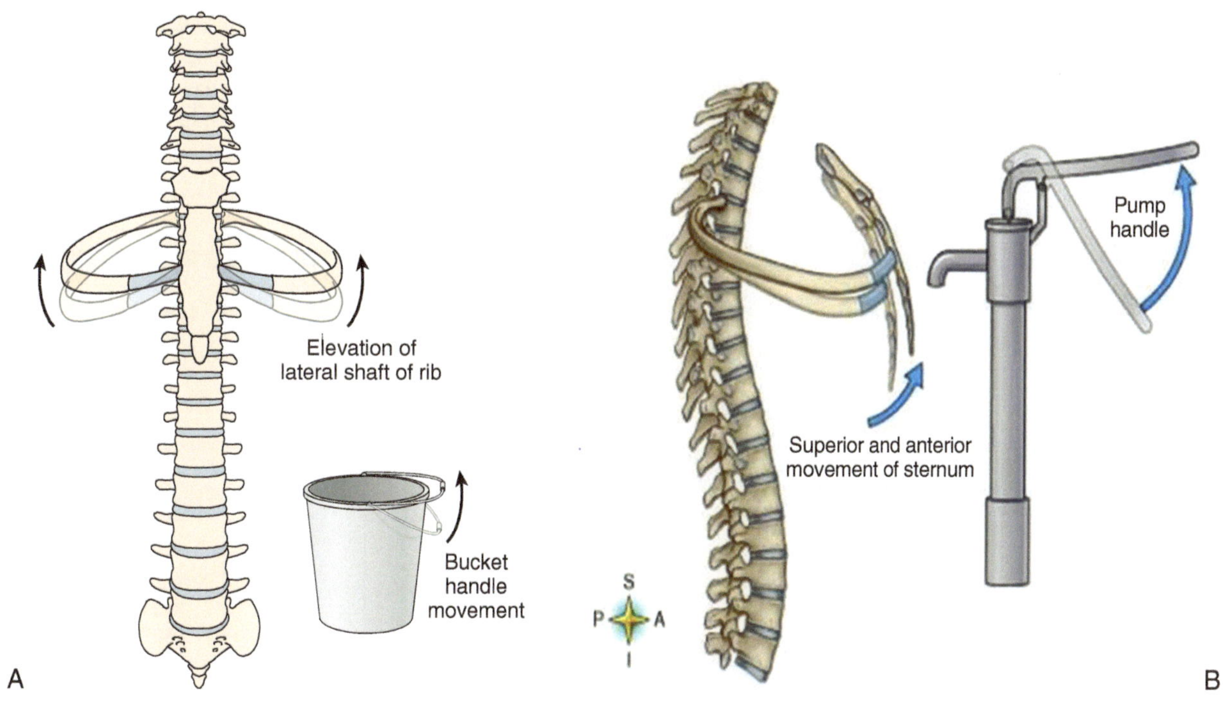

• **Fig. 2.2** Motions of the ribs. **A.** The scalene muscles, inserting on the first two ribs, the sternocleidomastoid inserting on the sternum and clavicle, and the other strap muscles of the neck lift the thoracic inlet, expanding the craniocaudal diameter like a pump handle. External intercostal muscles lift the middle ribs like a bucket handle, expanding both the side-to-side and anterior-posterior diameters. **B.** Lower intercostals and the insertion of the diaphragm on the ribs lift the ribs and push them upward and outward, aided by pressure from the organs just below the diaphragm, notably the liver, stomach, and spleen.

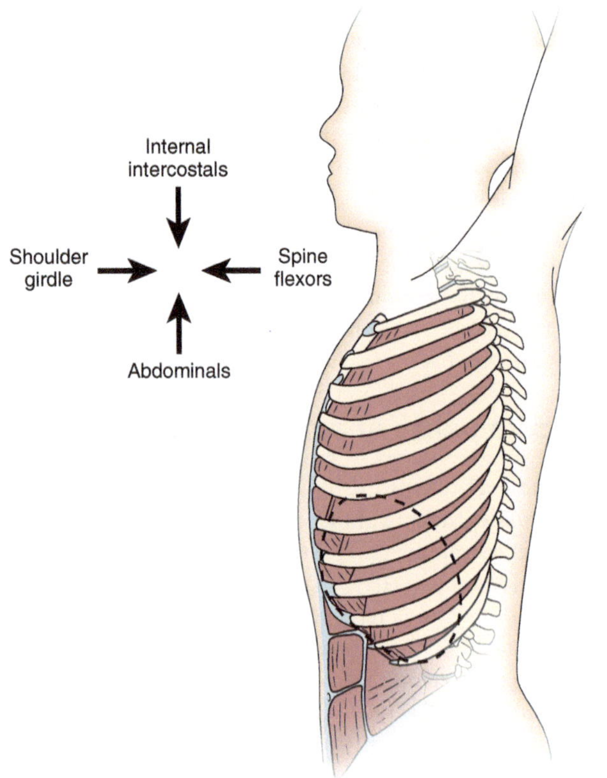

• **Fig. 2.3 Expiratory muscles.** The major expiratory muscles are the external intercostals which pull ribs down and in, the abdominal wall muscles which push viscera up against the diaphragm, elevating it, and to a minor extent at the extreme of expiration, the shoulder girdle and spinal muscles which flex the spine. Elastic recoil energy stored during inspiratory muscle effort supplies a major portion of expiratory force.

FRC. Similarly, when the lungs are removed from the thoracic cavity and opened to the atmosphere, they decrease their volume by up to several hundred milliliters.

The resting position, the FRC, is set by equating the forces of the parenchyma to further collapse, with the force of the thorax tending to reexpand. At this point, the expiratory muscles are stretched slightly beyond their rest length and can contract to decrease the gas volume in the chest from the FRC to the RV, but the limit of this contraction differs somewhat in children and youths from older adults (see later) (Fig. 2.4).

The VC is determined by the maximal excursion of the thoracic girdle, rib cage, spine, and diaphragm. From the FRC, the IC is limited by muscle shortening and rib excursion, not by lung compliance. The ERV and the RV are limited differently at different ages, however. In adults, the RV represents the volume of gas in the lung when all small airways have closed because of loss of tethering effect (see later). In children, the RV of the excised lung is somewhat smaller than the pleural cavity volume during maximum expiratory effort. Consequently, the pleural pressure is always negative. With increasing age, the increase of the closing capacity of lung tissue makes it higher than the minimal volume of the bony thorax at maximum expiration. Now expiratory effort produces a positive pleural pressure.[5,6]

The Upper Airway

The conducting passages from the nares and lips to the larynx serve not only as a simple conducting function, but as an important defensive function as well. They filter, warm, and humidify inspired gas and serve as a buffer against entry of irritating material to the more delicate lung parenchyma. During quiet breathing, maximal conservation of heat and humidity are obtained by nasal breathing. With hyperpnea, minimal work of breathing dictates mouth breathing, sacrificing supralaryngeal air conditioning. Bony, muscular, and mucosal structures provide for these optimizations and for the switch-over.

The nasal portion of the airway has a framework of cartilage and bone covered internally with hair-bearing, squamous epithelium in the funnel-shaped vestibule and ciliated, pseudostratified respiratory epithelium in the deeper cavum. The

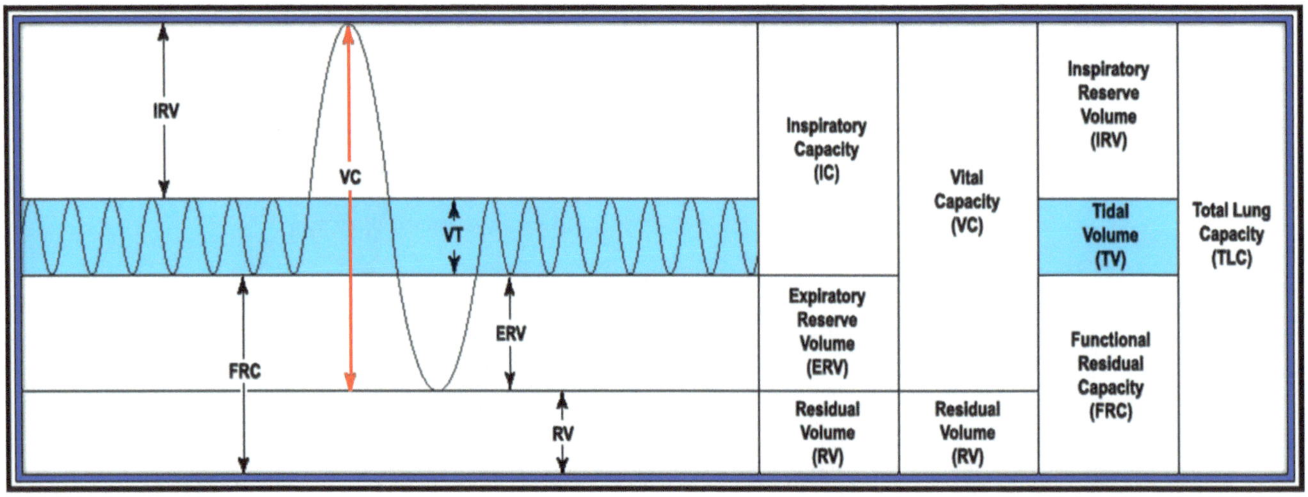

• **Fig. 2.4** The building blocks of lung volumes. The lung gas space is divided into four independent volumes: residual volume, expiratory reserve volume (*ERV*), tidal volume (TV), and inspiratory reserve volume. A fifth volume, the closing volume, is normally a portion of the ERV, but with age, recumbancy, and disease, may enlarge to include a portion of the TV. A capacity is the sum of two or more volumes.

entrance is a pair of oval openings framed by the alar cartilages and the anterior border of the septal cartilage. Hairs called vibrissae form a coarse net across the openings to filter large particles. They can elicit a sneeze when moved lightly. Slips of striated muscle (the nasalis muscle under facial, cranial nerve VII control) dilate the entrance somewhat in hyperpnea. The nares can be narrowed, as in a sniff, when the decreasing pressure attendant on increased inspiratory air flow causes the lateral (cartilaginous) walls to move inward, narrowing the passageway and creating a jet directing the gas flow into the roof of the cavum in greater part. This has several functions: improving olfaction, clearing secretions into the pharynx, and directing dry cold gas over moist, warm surfaces (Fig. 2.5).

Beyond the vestibule, the cavum opens up into two bilaterally symmetric chambers with a floor provided by the hard palate, a medial wall by the nasal septum and a lateral wall by the maxilla with three curved, bony protuberances called turbinates or conchae. In the cavum the direction of the airstream is bent, and the flow further broken up by the turbinates. The medial-lateral surfaces, about 150 square centimeters in area, are rarely more than a few millimeters apart, except along the floor of the cavum, where there may be as much as a centimeter between medial, lateral, and inferior borders. Thus the floor is the obvious route of choice for advancing fiberoptic endoscopes and airways. The submucosa is so rich in blood vessels that it resembles erectile tissue. These vessels provide the heat and water necessary for

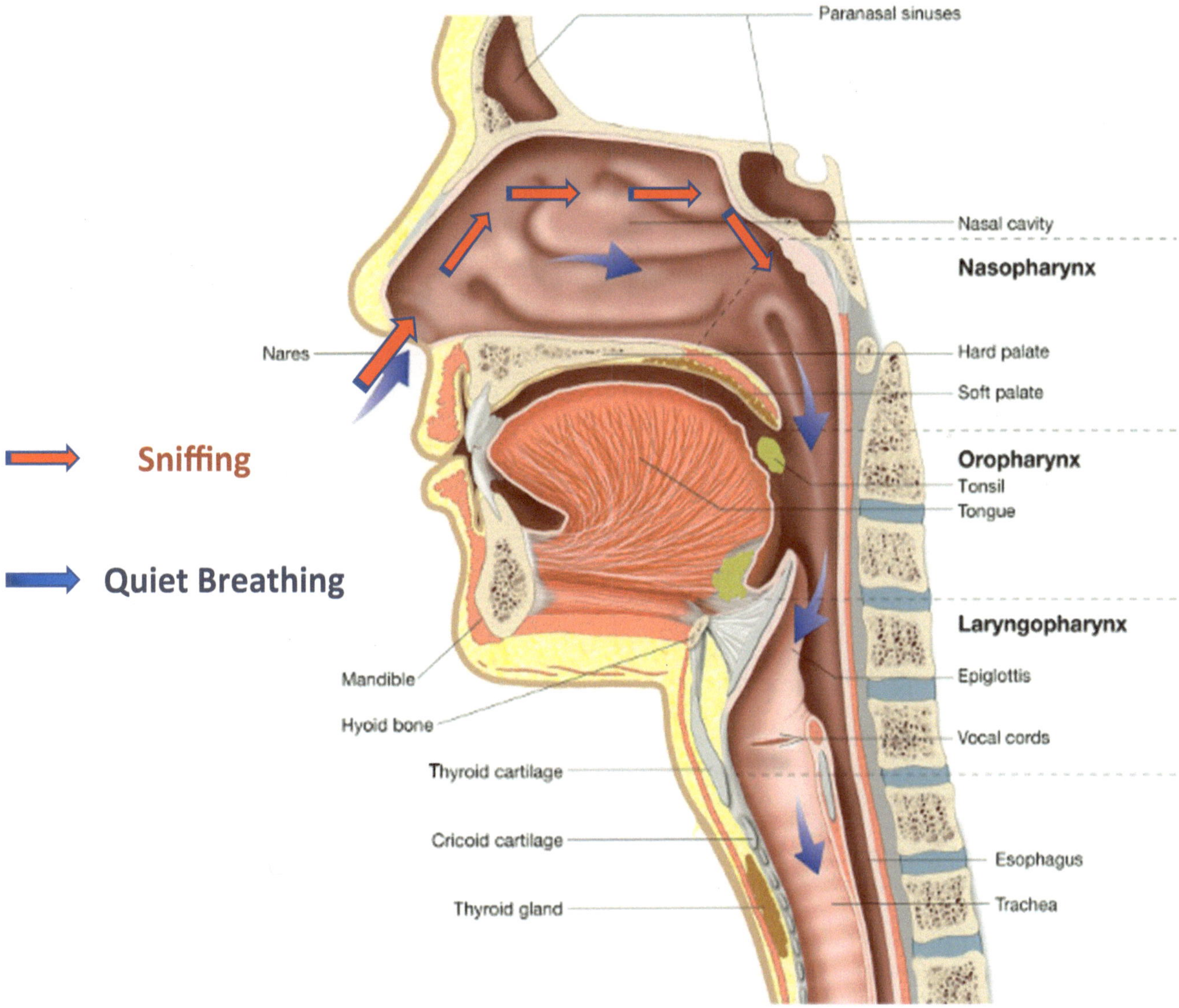

• **Fig. 2.5 The nose.** In quiet breathing, the inspiratory airstream flows over and around the turbinates (promoting humidification), bends sharply at the pharynx (impacting large suspended particles on mucosa underlaid by lymphoid tissue of Waldeyer's ring), and enters the hypopharynx nearly fully humidified at body temperature and cleansed of large particulates. A sniff directs a jet of inspirate to the attic where olfactory nerves originate. The surface coiling attendant on inspiratory humidification promotes condensation of a major fraction of the humidity of alveolar expirate, thus conserving water.

the air-conditioning function of the nose. The nasolacrimal duct and orifices to the paranasal sinuses are found under the turbinates.

Innervation for olfaction is provided in the attic of the cavum by bipolar neurons in the epithelium, whose axons pass through the cribriform plate to the olfactory bulb and synapse there with axons of the olfactory cranial nerve I. Sensation is provided by the first two branches of the trigeminal cranial nerve V, which have broadly arborized before entering the mucosa. Motor innervation for facial expression and emotion comes from the facial cranial nerve VII. Autonomic innervation comes from the cervical (sympathetic) ganglia following the arterial supply (branches of the external carotid and parasympathetics) from cranial nerve V. Through autonomic reflexes, cold, dry inspirate increases both the flow and volume of blood in the mucosa, supplying calories and water to gas.

The nasopharynx begins at the posterior choanae with another sharp bend in the air stream. Inertia carries suspended particles into the posterior mucosal blanket where the rich supply of lymphoid tissue (Waldeyer's ring) promotes defense. The eustachian tubes draining the middle ear open into the lateral wall. The nasopharynx is bounded superiorly by the base of the skull and posteriorly by the vertebral column. When the soft palate and tongue are relaxed, the nasopharynx is a widely patent part of the airway with a cross-sectional area 2 to 3 times as large as the trachea.

The resistance to air flow provided by the nose is nearly half of the resting resistance of the total airway. Major components are the turbulent flow pattern and narrow spaces created by the conchae. Resistance provided by the vestibule is variable, as noted earlier, however, with decreased air flow as the result of valving collapse of the lateral nasal cartilages during a sniff. Alar flaring opposes this collapse, decreasing resistance, as well as conveying emotion. In contrast, the air flow resistance from the choanae through the nasopharynx is either negligible (nose breathing) or infinite (i.e., closed). This valve-like function is caused by the effect of the soft palate: when elevated it seals the nasopharynx, and gas transverses the oral cavity and pharynx with very little resistance to flow.

The oropharynx is simply the vertical continuation of the nasopharynx when the soft palate is relaxed in quiet breathing. With the switch to oral breathing and anterior movement of the base of the tongue, it becomes the segment of the airway with the lowest resistance and the largest cross-sectional area. It acts as a gentle curve directing gas flow into the larynx.

The hypopharynx consists of two funnel-shaped cavities, the pyriform sinuses, on either side of the larynx. The entrance to the esophagus is normally closed by the cricopharyngeal muscle. The superior laryngeal nerves are just submucosal in the anterolateral wall of the sinuses and may be blocked by two local anesthetic-soaked pledgets held at this spot. This is in contrast to the rest of the sensory innervation: no one other anatomically identifiable spot serves as a landmark for a nerve supplying a large area of mucosa. Hence topical anesthesia with several local anesthetic-soaked cotton swabs placed in the nose or throat do not produce satisfactorily topical anesthesia.[7]

Secondary functions of the nasal, oral, and pharyngeal anatomy are to give rich quality and variety to speech and song and to seal off the airway during deglutition. The details of these structure-function relations may be found elsewhere. With regret, the author notes that the newborn can do both simultaneously, that is, to suck and sing, or at least breathe and swallow. The neonate has a very curved and relatively long epiglottis that extends up to the soft palate to provide a sealed transit for gas to and from the nose through the oropharynx and to deflect liquid laterally around the larynx to the esophagus. This ability is lost in infancy. Worse still, throughout the rest of life, the loss of those reflexes that make the separation of inspirate and alimentation less and less certain slowly accelerates (Fig. 2.6).

The functional anatomy up to this point may be diagrammed by a capital letter F, in which are embedded four valves. The lateral alar cartilages move inward with increasing air flow through the nostrils to accelerate the airstream velocity and direct it upward in the nasal attic (V1). This is partially prevented by the facial muscles, which stiffen and flare the external nares. The soft palate and base of the tongue, which move together to open the nasopharynx to breathing, move apart to promote oropharyngeal

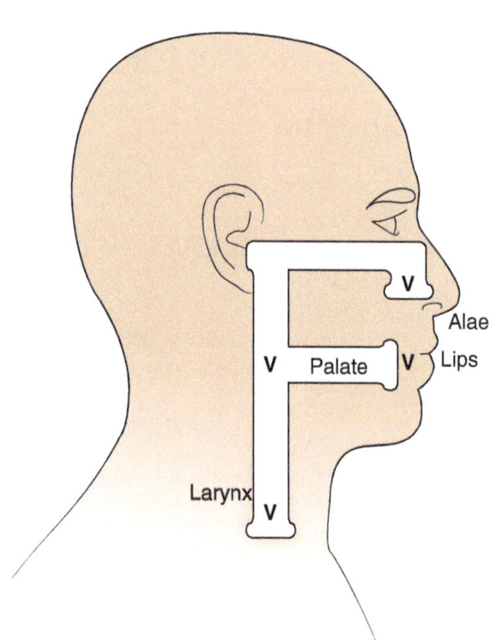

• **Fig. 2.6 The airway valves.** At four separate sites the airway can be narrowed or closed. At the nose, relaxation of the dilator naris and aerodynamic force associated with rapid inspiratory flow narrow the aperture by inward movement of the alar cartilages. At the lips, the orbicularis oris can close the mouth even with the mandible partly open. The soft palate can be elevated to seal off the nasopharynx (as when blowing up a closed balloon) or pulled down to seal off the oral cavity during nose breathing. The larynx is a complex valve with three separate mechanisms.

breathing (V2). The lips and teeth govern the entrance to the mouth (V3). The larynx is the fourth valve, which is described in the next section. These valves are the first line of pulmonary defenses.

The volume of this section of the airway is about 1 mL/kg during mouth breathing, and 1.5 mL/kg during nasal breathing. These numbers represent the reduction in dead space achieved by tracheostomy. The upper airway offers about one-half of the airway resistance at rest and one-third or less with hyperpnea and mouth breathing. Work of breathing overcoming this resistance normally represents about 1% of the basal metabolic oxygen demand. Bypassing the upper airway via tracheostomy or translaryngeal airways does not usually, by itself, provide an appreciable therapeutic effect. It does shift the burden of warming and humidifying the inspired gas and conserving calories and water on exhalation to another less elegantly designed site.

In summary, the upper airway is an active conduit with air-conditioning functions (heat, humidification, and filtration), defensive functions (coughing, sneezing, and swallowing), and certain advanced functions of civilization (including oration, singing, and emotional expressions such as crying and laughing). It offers minor compensation for some disease processes. Paradoxically, it can increase airway resistance, thereby controlling lung volume and shifting the equal pressure point oral (pursed lip breathing). In the practice of thoracic anesthesia, understanding these anatomic correlates aids in the diagnosis and evaluation of dyspnea, in fiberoptic bronchoscopy for both diagnostic indications and as an aid in intubation, and in the management of emerging and postoperative patients.

The Larynx

Although it may be more common to view the rima glottidis as the dividing section between upper and lower airway, this chapter will consider the larynx as a whole as separating the upper and lower airway and will include the hyoid as a laryngeal structure. The larynx is most simply a valve, which is opened during respiration, closed during deglutition, and intermediate during phonation. It plays a minor but crucial role when increased intraabdominal pressure is required (e.g., defecating, lifting). Because this structure is required to move, to open, and to close, it has the requisite structure and power. Most notably, it has three manners of closure, each more secure: the vocal cords close the larynx like a shutter, the epiglottis folds over the glottis, and the structures around the base of the epiglottis ball up and push the vestibular folds (false vocal cords) down onto the true vocal cords. This is rather like the box lock, the grille, and the massive vault door in a safe deposit box facility.

The larynx consists of one bone, three unpaired and three paired cartilages, nine intrinsic muscles, a variety of extrinsic muscles whose number depends on just how far afield one goes, ligaments that interconnect these, and appropriate nerves and vessels. Its movement is both intrinsic (motion in respect to other parts of the larynx) and extrinsic (motion as a whole in relation to adjacent structures).

The hyoid bone is extrinsic to the usual description of the larynx. However, it is as securely attached to the upper border of the thyroid cartilage as the cricoid is attached to the lower border by a tough membranous ligament. There is an aperture in each side, through which pass the superior laryngeal nerves and vessels. This provides a second site for neural blockade, a centimeter below and a centimeter anterior to the (posterior) greater comer of the hyoid, at a depth just subcutaneous. A tough ligament is perceived by an advancing needle at greater depths. Several muscles, extrinsic to the larynx, originate or insert on the hyoid, and are easily identified by the "hyo" in their name (e.g., omohyoid, hyothyroid, etc). They are part of the accessory muscles of respiration and partake in the swallowing mechanism. There is also a small but constant ligament from the center of the hyoid to the center of the epiglottis. In some reconstructions it would seem to prevent the epiglottis from backward and downward rotation to cover the glottis, but it is either just long enough or just low enough to permit the epiglottis to fold over the larynx in one of the three mechanisms of laryngeal closure (Fig. 2.7).[8]

The epiglottis is a spoon-shaped cartilage of compound curvature, that is, it is concave inward in horizontal section and concave backward vertically. It is one of the three unpaired cartilages; the thyroid and cricoid are the other two. Fink has pointed out that the action of extrinsic muscles on this compound curvature causes a folding motion, which brings the free top of the epiglottis down over the vestibule of the larynx like a hinged lid on a German beer stein.[9] This action is further promoted by the elevation of the larynx in the neck during swallowing, a motion that results from the collective effort of the strap muscles above the larynx (the genio-, glosso-, hyo-, stylo-, omothyroid, and other thyroid muscles). Because these motions are programmed into the motor cortex as part of the swallowing action, they are a regular and reliable valving mechanism. With maximum voluntary effort, they ball up tissue at the root of the epiglottis. This ball valve is the strongest of the three closing mechanisms. The inferior surface of the epiglottis is inverted by the vagus cranial nerve X, which also supplies muscles closing the glottis intrinsically by rotation of the aryteroids adducting the vocal cords (the least strong valve mechanism). The superior surface on the other hand is by innervated branches of the glossopharyngeal cranial nerve IX. Macintosh conjectured that stimulation of the inferior surface (X nerve) by a straight blade laryngoscope would be more likely to cause laryngospasm via motor fibers in the vagus than stimulation of the hypopharyngeal mucosa innervated by the IX nerve. Anesthesia would more likely block a reflex that requires neuronal connection between two different cranial nuclei than a simple reflex involving one nucleus. This reasoning led to the design of the MacIntosh blade, but there are no published data confirming the conjecture.

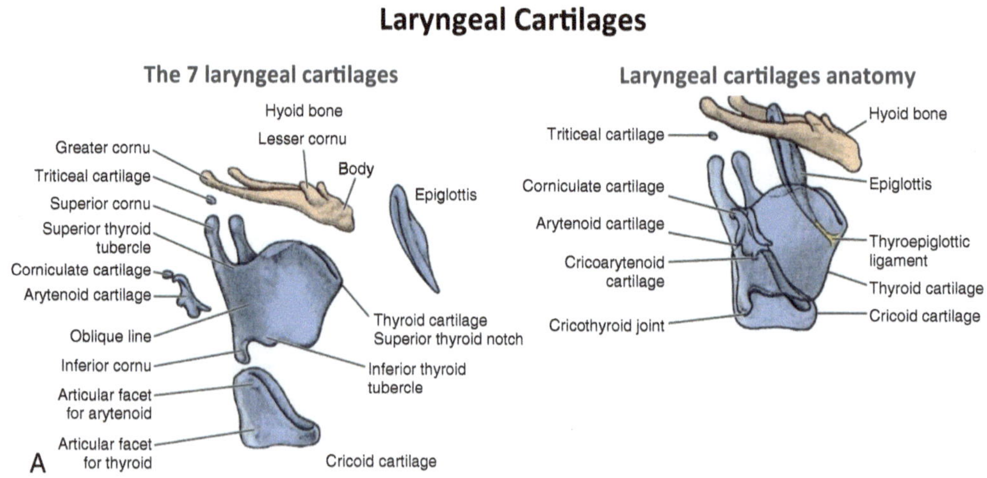

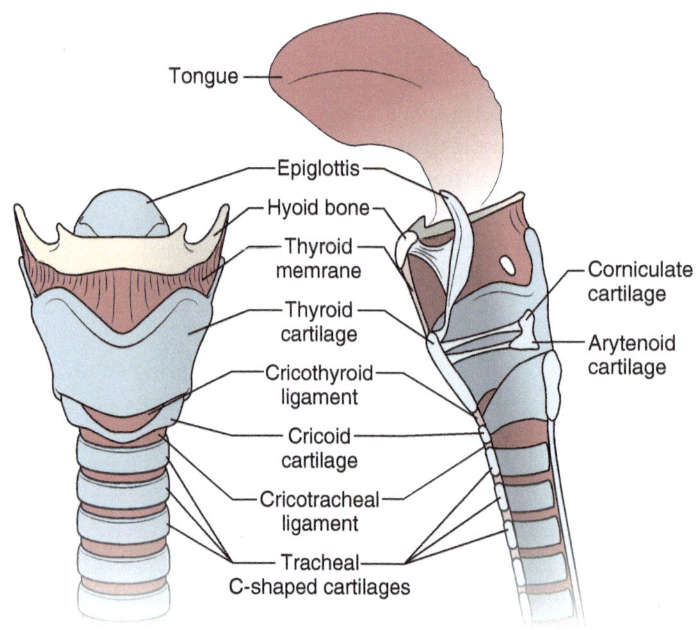

B

• **Fig. 2.7** The anterior and the lateral views of the larynx. (From Hicks GH. *Cardiopulmonary Anatomy and Physiology*. Philadelphia: WB Sanders; 2000.)

The thyroid cartilage, the second of the unpaired cartilages, is a roughly hemicylindrical structure forming the major part of the anterior and lateral walls of the larynx. Its size and the prominent notch at the top front provide an easily observable or palpable landmark. The base of the epiglottis is tightly bound to its intern surface in the midline by a tough ligament just above the origin of the vocal cords from the midline of the thyroid cartilage. The thyroid is articulated to the cricoid by a paired set of true joints that permit rotation, rather like how the visor of a medieval knight's headgear rotates on the helmet. This changes the tension on the cords and hence vocal pitch.[10]

The cricoid is the last unpaired cartilage, and the only completely circular cartilage in the airway. When its anterior arc (just below the thyroid) is identified and pressed posteriorly, the broad posterior arc compresses and seals the esophagus against the lower cervical vertebral bodies. Sellick demonstrated competency to over 100 mm Hg pressure with this maneuver.

The cricothyroid membrane is a midline, nearly avascular fibrous layer between the thyroid above, the cricoid below, and the cricothyroid muscles laterally. It is rarely covered with thyroid tissue as may be found below the cricoid. Just subcutaneous, it is easily located by palpation of the thyroid notch and the rounded cricoid cartilage as landmarks. This membrane is useful for emergency surgical airway provision, jet ventilation, retrograde tracheal intubation techniques, and topical anesthesia of the larynx and trachea.

The Lower Airway

The trachea, bronchi, and bronchioles are primarily conducting passages that do not participate in the gas exchange. They also serve as a backup heat and humidity exchanger (during hyperpnea or when tracheal intubation bypasses the upper airway) and as part of the pulmonary defense against inhaled particulates. The terminal bronchioles, the respiratory bronchioles, and the alveolar sacs are where the gas exchange takes place. Anatomic details contribute to their patency differently at different levels. Their design minimizes work of breathing. Recognition of certain features permits orientation of the image in bronchoscopy (Fig. 2.8).

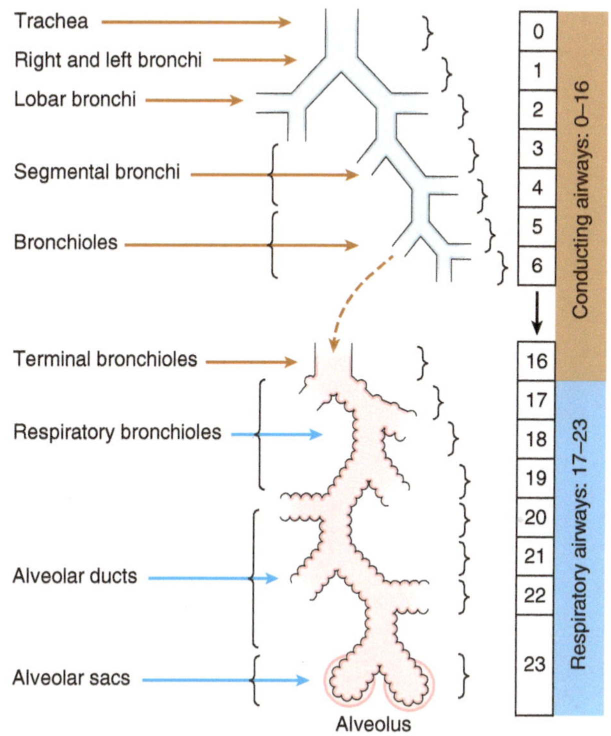

• **Fig. 2.8 The trachea, bronchi, and bronchioles** are primarily conducting passages that do not participate in the gas exchange. It also serves as a backup heat and humidity exchanger (during hyperpnea or when tracheal intubation bypasses the upper airway) and as part of the pulmonary defense against inhaled particulates. The terminal bronchioles, the respiratory bronchioles, and the alveolar sacs are where the gas exchange takes place. Anatomic details contribute to its patency differently at different levels. Their design minimizes work of breathing. Recognition of certain features permits orientation of the image in bronchoscopy.

The basic arrangement of the bronchial wall comprises mucosa, basement membrane, submucous layer of elastic tissue, nonstriated bronchial muscle and, finally, an outer fibrous coat containing cartilage. The lining epithelium of the trachea and larger bronchi is in several layers: a basal layer, which rests on a well-defined basal membrane, an intermediate zone of spindle-shaped cells, and a superficial sheet of columnar ciliated cells that are interspersed with mucus-secreting goblet cells. In the finer bronchi, the epithelium becomes cuboidal and ciliated, with far fewer goblet cells. The alveoli are lined with a layer of epithelium which is so thin that, except where nuclei are present, it is often invisible in conventionally prepared histologic material. Electron microscopy and special staining techniques have shown that the epithelium is, in fact, intact, although with a thickness of only 0.2 μm away from the cell nuclei, and rests on a fine basement membrane. Alveolar air is thus separated from blood in the pulmonary capillary tree by an extremely fine membrane which, nevertheless, consists of four layers: capillary wall, capillary basement membrane, alveolar basement membrane, and alveolar epithelium (Fig. 2.9).

Patency of the trachea is primarily maintained by the C-shaped cartilaginous rings that resist most physiologic forces, tending to collapse the extrathoracic trachea on inspiration and the intrathoracic trachea on forced expiration. The wall of the trachea is completed posteriorly by horizontally arranged smooth muscle, the cholinergically innervated trachealis muscle which is inserted not on the ends of the cartilages but higher up. When maximally contracted, the ends of the cartilage are pulled into a slightly overlapping arrangement, but when relaxed, the mucosa and trachealis can be pushed into the lumen of the intrathoracic trachea by a transtracheal pressure, such as is generated just after the glottic opening of a hard cough. It moves inward not as a piston nor symmetrically, but more on one side than the other, producing a yin-yang-like figure that pushes any mucus and entrapped mucosal particulates into a glob, as does a squeegee. The combination of accelerating air flow and decreasing cross-sectional area creates sufficient aerodynamic force to lift balled up drops of mucus into the airstream and expel them. During quiet breathing, the coordinated action of cilia of the pseudostratified mucosa move the blanket of mucus and impacted debris toward the larynx at a rate of a few centimeters per hour. Inhalation anesthetics stop this action (Fig. 2.10).[11,12]

Patency of the bronchi is achieved by a combination of plates and arcs of cartilage that are connected by thicker encircling smooth muscle (as compared with the trachea). Although lying within the lung parenchyma, there is little or no connection of fibrous or elastic strands between lung tissue and bronchi. There is a network of lymph capillaries in the potential space around airways and vessels that may be compared with the network of

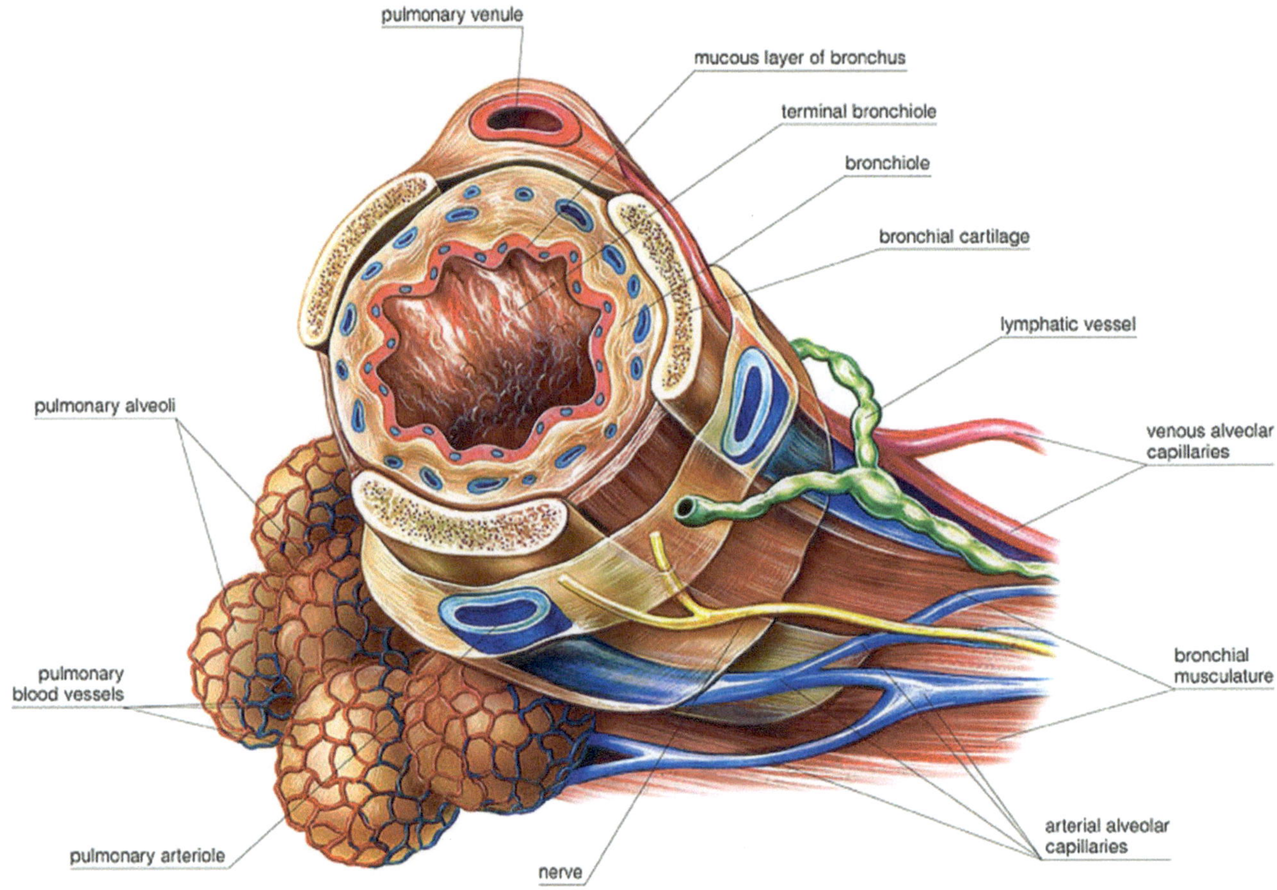

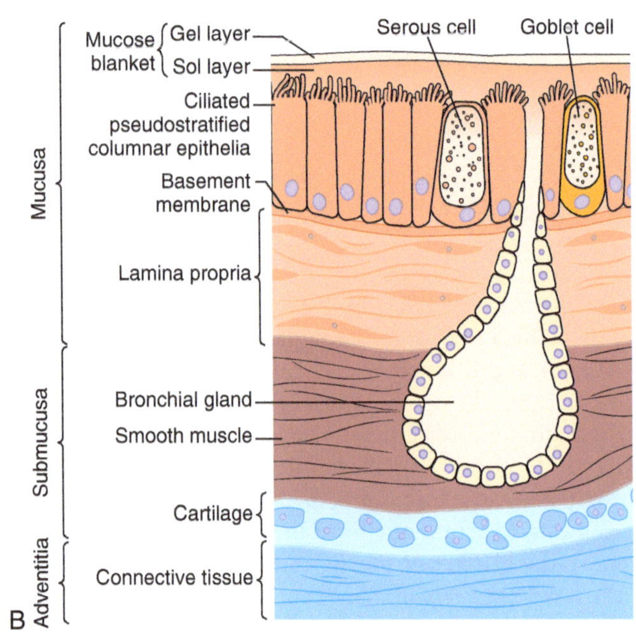

• **Fig. 2.9** A and **B.** The basic arrangement of the bronchial wall comprises mucosa, basement membrane, submucous layer of elastic tissue, nonstriated bronchial muscle and, finally, an outer fibrous coat containing cartilage. The lining epithelium of the trachea and larger bronchi is in several layers: a basal layer, which rests on a well-defined basal membrane, an intermediate zone of spindle-shaped cells and a superficial sheet of columnar ciliated cells which are interspersed with mucus-secreting goblet cells. In the finer bronchi, the epithelium becomes cuboidal and ciliated, with far fewer goblet cells. The alveoli are lined with a layer of epithelium which is so thin that, except where nuclei are present, it is often invisible in conventionally prepared histologic material. (Fig. 2.9A, From Lung Anatomy, a photograph by Asklepios Medical Atlas Fig. 2.9B, From Hicks GH. *Cardiopulmonary Anatomy and Physiology*. Philadelphia: WB Saunders; 2000.)

vines encasing an oak in an old forest. As lymph moves from parenchyma toward the hilum, the total cross-sectional area of these capillaries decreases. As a result, increased lymph flow meets an effective choke-point at the hilum. In the genesis of pulmonary edema, the first effect is distension of lymph vessels at or near the hilum producing perivascular and peribronchial cuffs of edema fluid. Transudation from the lymph capillaries begins at or near the hilum. Continued progression of the process causes an alveolar spread of irregular edema around the airway and vessels, both arterial and venous, with variable compression. The effect of airway compression is

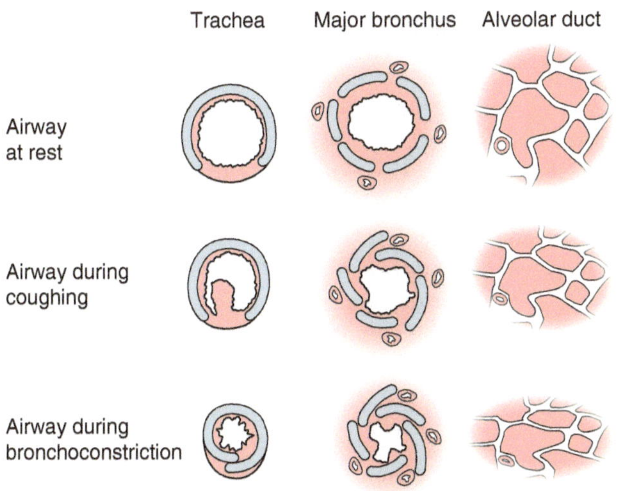

• **Fig. 2.10 Schematic cross-section of the airway:** at rest *(top row)*, during cough *(middle row)*, and during bronchoconstriction *(bottom row)*. The rows show, left to right, the trachea, a major bronchus, and alveolar duct, drawn to quite different scales! The tracheal lumen may be briefly invaginated by the trachealis muscle during the early moments of cough if the muscle is relatively flaccid. But if constricted, the tracheal lumen becomes totally enclosed by its cartilage. In bronchi the plates of cartilage are normally separated but may partially overlap because of aerodynamic forces in coughing, or may be jammed close together in bronchoconstriction. The alveolar duct diameter is largely set by current lung volume, widely open at total lung capacity by tethering action of adjacent alveolar facets, but capable of being pulled nearly closed by pneumoconstriction as with hypoxia or pulmonary emboli.

wheezing; the effect of vascular compression is spreading maldistribution of gas and blood.

Patency of bronchioles is maintained by anatomically different means. Bronchioles have no cartilage and less circular smooth muscle in their relatively thinner walls. There is no potential space around them, however. Fibers of collagen and elastin in the walls merge with the connective tissue of the parenchyma structure, alveolar ducts, and alveoli. These tissue strands are arranged radial to the bronchioles. They stretch as the lung gets larger and relax as the lung gets smaller. In fact, the closing capacity of a lung region is that volume where this radial tethering is so relaxed that there is no support to the thin bronchioles wall. The bronchioles then collapse (close) under small forces, such as decreased luminal pressure associated with the airflow (Venturi effect) or positive pressure in adjacent alveoli.

Patency of the alveolar gas spaces is maintained by the normal recoil of the chest wall below FRC, by ventilation that brings more gas to the alveoli than the blood removes in uptake of oxygen and anesthetic agents, by the presence of inert gas, such as nitrogen, and by the pull of adjacent air spaces in all directions. If the airway to a lung unit is closed (by collapse, tumor, secretion, or foreign body), continued perfusion of the distal air space continues to remove oxygen. Diffusion of carbon dioxide into the space stops when alveolar carbon dioxide tension equals that of mixed venous blood; this usually occurs within less than a minute of the cessation of ventilation. An inert gas, such as nitrogen (or even nitrous oxide at a concentration equal to that in mixed venous blood), may slow the rate of collapse markedly, so that it takes many hours, but atelectasis is still the eventual outcome. High concentrations of oxygen and anesthetic gas, especially nitrous oxide at a partial pressure well above the concurrent mixed venous level, speed the rate of collapse. With 100% oxygen, total atelectasis occurs in 8 to 10 minutes. The pull of adjacent alveoli tending to hold lung air spaces open, which is analogous to stretching a spring, is called "interdependence." The total force applied to the spring is shared by each loop and is not concentrated near the end. Protection of the air spaces against flooding with fluid is described later (Fig. 2.11).[13,14]

The airway design is basically dichotomous branching, although this sometimes varies. Not all of the branches are equal. At each branching, the sum of the areas of the daughter limbs exceeds that of the parent, although together they conduct the same gas flow. Thus the linear speed of air flow decreases progressively from trachea to alveoli. From basic

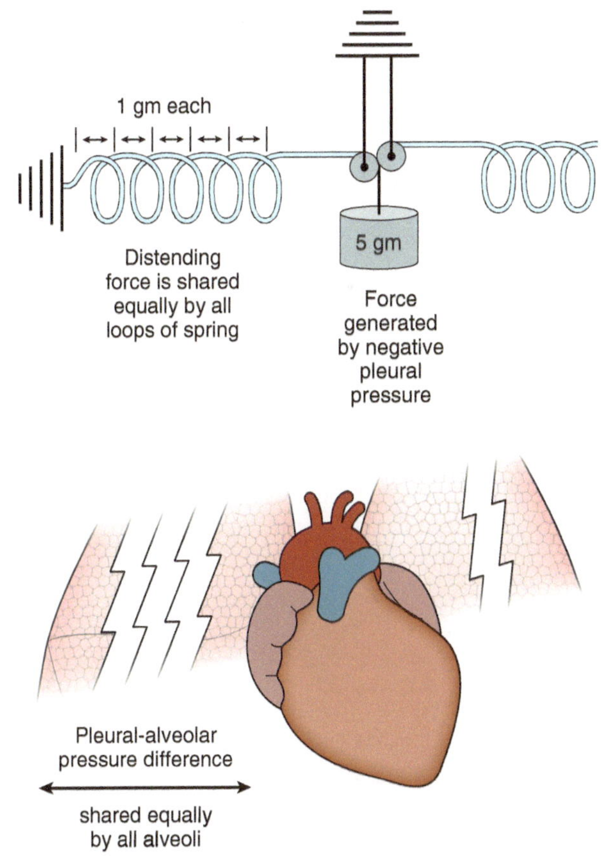

• **Fig. 2.11 Pulmonary interdependence.** The expansion of the lung is fairly uniform throughout the parenchyma even though the force is applied only at the pleural surfaces. It can be visualized as two springs stretched by forces analogous to the moving thoracic boundaries (diaphragm and rib cage). If the links are of uniform construction each will expand equally, distributing the distending force among all loops. Of course, if one loop is stiffer (analogous to local disease or scar) the equally shared force would cause less expansion.

aerodynamic analysis, the least work of breathing results when the two branches of a parent airway are equal in size and branch at a 60-degree angle. If the two branches are unequal, however, the larger should be a more direct continuation of the parent axis. This relation is actually found, starting at the carina. The right bronchus is both larger and less angled from the tracheal axis (20–25 degrees away from the midline, as opposed to 40–50 degrees for the left bronchus). The length of the bronchi is governed by the distance from the hilum of the gas spaces it supplies. The lower lobe bronchi, for example, give rise to a superior segmental bronchus almost immediately after the minor carina at the middle lobe (on the right) or upper lobe-cum-lingula (on the left). They then descend 4 to 6 cm to the basal segmental bronchi, which proliferate almost immediately in all directions. They give rise to subsegmental bronchi within a centimeter. Altogether there are about two dozen branch points from the major carina to the distal alveolar ducts, with an exponential increase in cross-sectional area and decrease in convective flow rate (Fig. 2.12).[15]

Thus the parenchyma of the lung can be divided into portions served by identifiable, named airways. The right

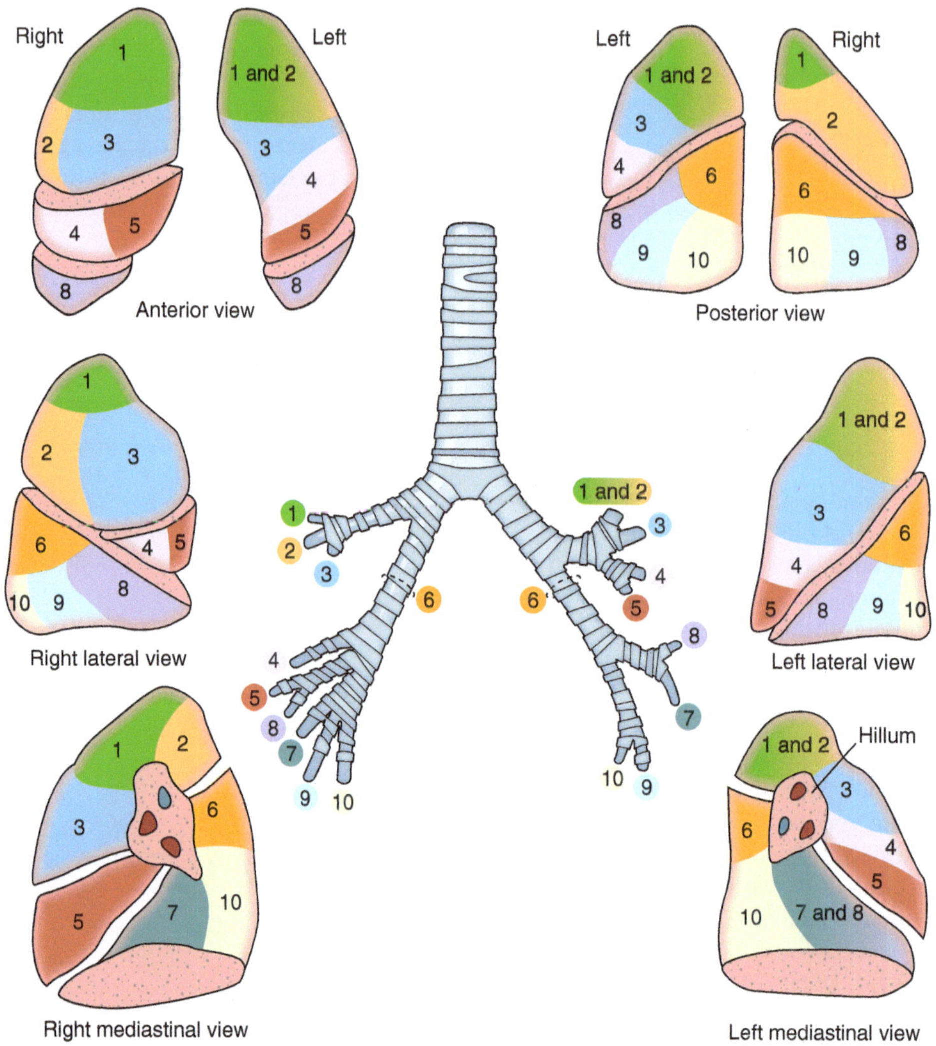

• **Fig. 2.12 The tracheobronchial tree.** The trachea divides into a right and left main bronchus, which further divide into upper lobes, a middle lobe on the right (for which the left lung has the analogous lingular portion of the upper lobe) and a lower lobe. Each lobe then divides into two or more segments with segmental bronchi that are numbered and named. Thus 1-apical, 2-posterior (usually fused with 1 on the left), and 3-anterior form the upper lobe. On the right 4-lateral, 5-medial form the middle lobe, whereas on the left these are called superior and inferior lingular segments of the upper lobe. There is usually not a clear fissure separating the lingula from the rest of the left upper lobe. The lower lobe consists of a superior segment numbered 6, and medial, anterior, lateral and posterior segments labeled 7, 8, 9, and 10 on the right. On the left, there is no clear 7-medial segment, the volume occupied by either expansion of 10 forward or 8 medially. Thus there are 18 segments, 10 on the right and eight on the left (because 1 and 2, and 7 and 8, are fused on the left into one segment each). (From Hicks GH. *Cardiopulmonary Anatomy and Physiology*. Philadelphia: WB Saunders; 2000.)

and left lungs are served by main bronchi. Each side is divided into lobes: upper middle and lower lobes on the right, and upper and lower on the left (the lingula of the left upper lobe is analogous to the right middle lobe). The lobes are separated by complete or nearly complete fissures that are externally visible. This scheme varies considerably in other species. For example, in dogs, there are usually four lobes on the right and two or three on the left depending on how completely the lingula is separated. This is of importance to the anesthesiologist only if they practice bronchoscopy in an animal laboratory.

The lobes of the lung are divided into segments, each with a named (and often numbered) segmental bronchus. There are no fissures nor even fascial planes, however. Instead, the major venous drainage from two adjacent segments is the anatomic feature separating the segments. The surgeon follows these veins in segmental resection of the lung; this accounts for the usually higher blood loss and greater initial loss of lung function in these operations as opposed to lobar resections. The names and numbers of the segmental bronchi are given in Fig. 2.12. Subsegmental bronchi may be identified and given a lower-case letter to identify them. Thus the three subsegmental bronchi to the posterior basal segment of the right lower lobe would be identified as rt B^{10}a, b, and c.

As the thoracic cage enlarges on inspiration, unfolding of the alveolar ducts accommodates most of the increased gas volume. Alveoli also increase in volume. Consequently, there is little convective flow through distal alveolar ducts and into alveoli. The dimensions are so small (tens of microns), however, that the physical process of diffusion can mix the gas in the volume of alveolar ducts and alveoli that is distal to a single terminal bronchiole within the period of one breath. Phenomena of convection of gas and airway resistance are thus confined to the passages from terminal bronchioles to larger airways.

The Gas Spaces and Gas Exchange

Gas exchange begins at the respiratory bronchioles, daughters and granddaughters of a terminal bronchiole (Fig. 2.13A). They are lined with ciliated, pseudostratified columnar epithelium, mucus secreting goblet cells, mucous, and Clara cells of unidentified function. Circular smooth muscle fibers are few. Bronchioles also have one or more true alveoli opening directly into the lumen. Distally, as each respiratory bronchiole branches into others, there are progressively more and more such openings into alveoli into further branching of passages having alveolar walls for their boundaries. Eventually, the openings are so numerous that there is no longer room for bronchial epithelium between them. These passages are termed alveolar ducts. The edges of alveolar facets bordering alveolar ducts have a few strands of smooth muscle encircling them as a geodesic framework. There is very scant intervention and little resting tone. However, this three-dimensional cage of smooth muscle can contract, pull on the attached gossamer alveolar walls, reduce the cross-sectional area and compliance of the alveolar ducts, and hence reduce the gas volume and ventilation of air spaces beyond. Stimuli for such contraction include hypoxia, hypercarbia, cholinergic stimuli, aerosols, allergins, and hypoperfusion of the adjacent parenchyma (by an unsettled mechanism). Alkalosis blunts the response: a respiratory alkalosis of 7.6 cuts it in half (carbon dioxide partial pressure [PCO_2] = 20), and 7.8 abolishes it entirely (PCO_2 = 10).

The alveoli are polygonal spaces with almost planar walls of (usually) five- to seven-sided facets. The walls are covered with very flattened cells called type I pneumocytes resting on a basement membrane. Typically, each alveolar facet borders two adjacent alveoli. The epithelium sandwiches an interstitial space a few microns in width. This space contains a network of elastin and collagen fibers that give it its tensile strength but contribute little to elasticity. Woven into the network are the pulmonary capillaries, which scanning electron microscopy indicates occupy about half of the area of each facet. On cross-section they appear to lie not symmetrically in the center of the interstitium, but to weave from side-to-side and protrude somewhat into the alveolar spaces. The best analogy is a sort of three-dimensional fisherman's net, with long strands of kelp weaving in and out of the net (the capillaries). The entire "net" is covered with an attenuated film like a shrink-wrapped package of small items in a discount hardware display. This film is the lipid-lining layer of the lung, which when stretched by inspiration, stores most of the energy for exhalation as increased surface forces. The film contains degenerating lamellar bodies and their lipid content, produced by occasional type II pneumocytes among the type I cells.[16,17]

There is an important element of asymmetry in the alveolar wall, which is enhanced by a sharing of the basement membrane between the type I pneumocyte and the capillary endothelial cell where it bulges into the alveolar lumen. This is called the "thin side." The majority of gas exchange diffuses through this side (Fig. 2.13B and C).

The other side of the capillary is within the interstitial space, where it has its own basement membrane separate from that of the alveolar pneumocyte on that side. In the interstitial space are found occasional wandering white blood cells, elastin and collagen fibers, and interstitial fluid. The latter is derived in part from capillary endothelial cells by pinocytotic extrusion, in smaller part from leakage between the endothelial cells and their tight junctions, in part by diffusion of water through cells, and in edema, from capillary leakage. The fluid flows along the interstitium on the thick side of the capillaries to the T- or Y-shaped mergers of alveolar walls that contain the smallest airways, arterioles, or venules. There, open-ended lymph capillaries are found that accompany the gas and blood conduits toward the hilum.

Although there are "elastic" fibers in the parenchyma, stretch of these fibers contributes little to elastic recoil of the lung except at very large lung volume. These fibers are quite

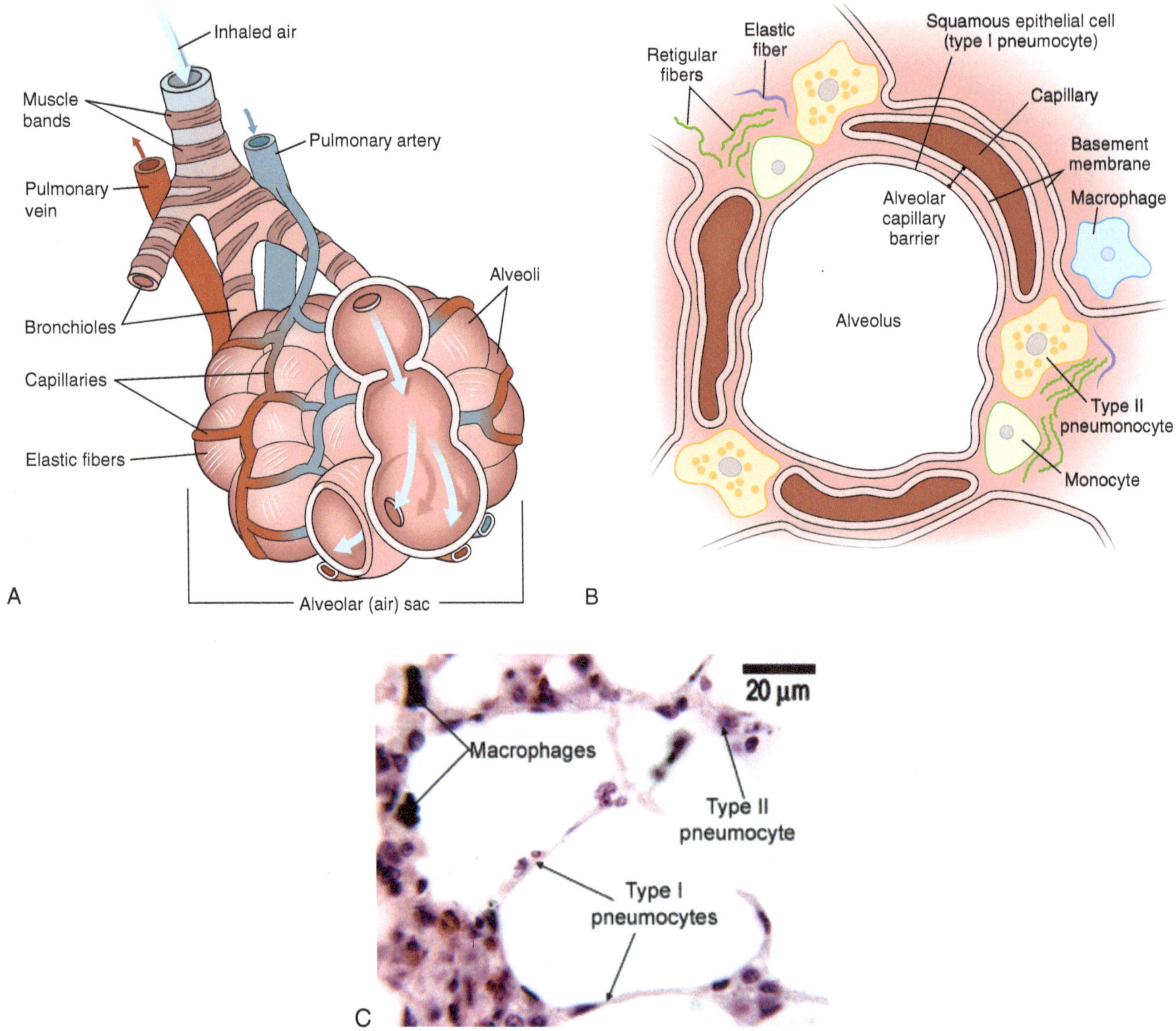

• **Fig. 2.13** (**A**) The junction of three alveolar facets in cross-section. (**B**) The walls of the delicate alveolar membrane are composed of a core of elastin and collagen fibers with a few wandering white blood cells supporting a mesh of capillaries eccentric to the axis of the facets with very thin walls at the air spaces for gas exchange, and thicker walls on their other side. (**C**) Thin endothelial cells pave the capillary lumen, and equally thin type I alveolar epithelial cells pave the alveolar surface forcing the air space. These thinner cells share a common basement membrane. Type II pneumocytes produce a surface-active material that causes retractile force at areas of curvature. (B, From © Dave Carlson. C, From Histology Guide © Faculty of Biological Sciences, University of Leeds.)

stiff and they unfold like a concertina more than stretch like a rubber band. A large part of the elastic recoil of the lung is attributable to the thin film of fluid, containing surface active molecules of a lipid called surfactant, which is primarily phosphatidyl inositol. Surfactant does lower the surface tension of the air-fluid interface, but it is more important to understand that surfactant produces a variable tension that is smaller at low lung volume. The lipid is produced by type II pneumocytes. Without its normal surface tension at the air-water (tissue) interface, the lung would retract to a very small volume and become atelectatic. Although this "lipid-lining layer of the lung" reduces the surface tension from 72 to 20 dynecm or less, it is still this surface tension of the curved surface, where two alveolar facets meet, that provides a major part of the elastic recoil of lung.

Pulmonary Vasculature

The lung has two entirely separate large vascular arborizations, the pulmonary arterial and pulmonary venous trees, and a third much smaller understory structure, the bronchial arterial circulation. There are no bronchial veins; bronchial

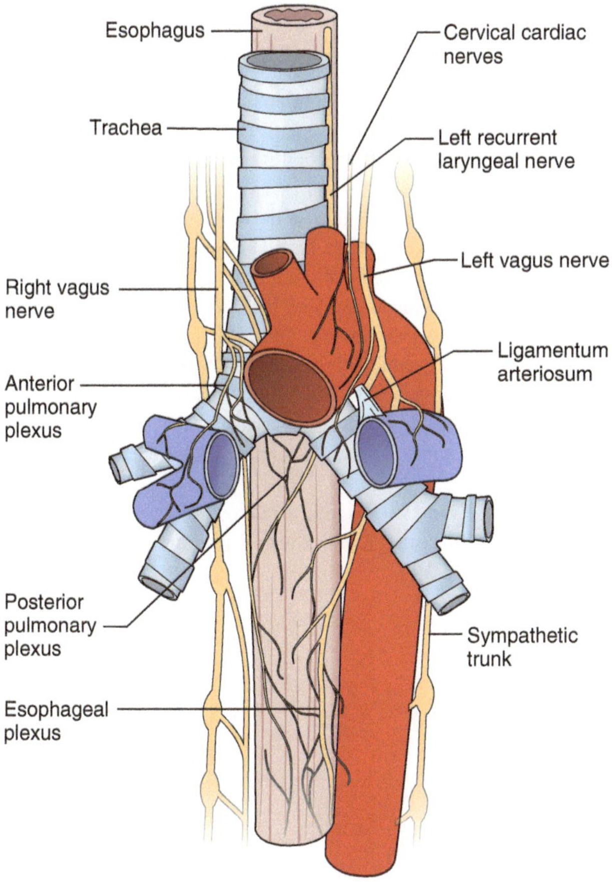

• **Fig. 2.14** Somatic sensory, autonomic sympathetic, and parasympathetic innervation of the lung. (Modified from Netter RH: Atlas of Human Anatomy. Netter Basic Science 7th Edition.)

capillary blood flows into pulmonary veins. Embryologically, the lung bud begins as a ventral outpouching of the foregut epithelium; it is encased in mesenchymal tissue that is derived from the sixth branchial arch and provides the bronchial arteries. It grows caudad into the thorax and splits into right-left buds along with the major vessel in the sixth arch, which eventually becomes the pulmonary artery. In contrast, the pulmonary veins arise from outpouching of the anlage of the cardiac atria as the primitive ventral blood vessel folds into an S-shaped structure that becomes the heart.[18] The venous vasculature grows laterally into the thoracic portion of the lung bud, and eventually capillaries form to unite the disparate arterial and venous vessels. The result is a pairing of artery and airway, starting at the hilum, branching together as the three-dimensional fractal arborization proceeds distally, as in the mature lung. The veins take an entirely separate path to the gas exchange spaces. Only at the hilum are the triad of artery, vein, and airway seen. The surgeon uses the segmental veins as landmarks in dissection of segmental and subsegmental resections. Except at the lobar level, there are no clear fascial planes in the human lung.[19,20]

Although the pulmonary arteries do have thicker walls with more smooth muscle than the pulmonary veins, both are relatively amuscular and thin-walled compared with systemic vessels. Both are wrapped in a network of lymph vessels little bigger than capillaries. They are relatively free of collagenous attachment to the parenchyma through which they course, down to the primary lung unit level beyond terminal bronchioles.

Innervation

Somatic sensory, autonomic sympathetic, and parasympathetic innervation are all represented in the lung, but all three are relatively sparse. Somatic sensation is largely confined to the trachea and carina. Thus there is major retention of airway-clearing cough reflexes after bilateral, single-lung transplantation as two separate lungs, as opposed to a two-lungcum-tracheal transplant. Below lobar bronchi are few irritant receptor-mediating nerves in the mucosa. Few sympathetic nerves are traceable from the third and fourth segments of the cord through sympathetic ganglia. Alpha-adrenergic impulses do dilate smooth muscle of the tracheobronchial tree, but there is little demonstrable function of the sympathetic nerve in the vasculature. This is partly attributable to the relatively small amount of vascular smooth muscle (Fig. 2.14).

The parasympathetic nervous system contains both efferent and afferent vagal fibers to the lung parenchyma; the latter predominate. Juxtacapillary receptors are responsive to both blood and airborne irritants, as well as interstitial water volume. Both inflation (stretch) and deflation receptors, which fire synchronously with breathing, serve minor roles in modulating the pattern of breathing. There is little demonstrable central nervous system integration of these afferent activities in normal humans. Such reflexes (Hering-Breuer reflexes) are much more prominent in animals, especially rodents.

References

1. Agostini E. Kinematics. In: Campbell EJM, Davis JM. *The Respiratory Muscles: Mechanics and Neural Controls*. London: WB Saunders; 1970:23.
2. Sharp JT. Organization of chest wall and diaphragm for coordinated interplay. In: Fisherman AP, ed. *Pulmonary Diseases and Disorders*. New York: McGraw-Hill; 1980:1525.
3. Agostoni E, Mead J. Statics of the respiratory system. In: Ferin WO, Rahn H, eds. *Handbook of Physiology, Section 3. Respiration*. Washington, DC: American Physiological Society; 1964:38.
4. Agostoni E, Hyatt RE. Static behavior of the respiratory system. In: Fishman AP, Macklem PT, Mead J (eds). *Handbook of Physiology, Section 3. The Respiratory System, Volume 3: Mechanics of Breathing, Part 1*. Bethesda: American Physiological Society; 1986.

5. Miller A, ed. *Pulmonary Function Tests in Clinical and Occupational Lung Disease.* New York: Grune & Stratton; 1986:15.
6. Wanner. Interpretation of pulmonary function tests. In: Sackner MA, ed. *Diagnostic Techniques in Pulmonary Disease, Part I.* New York: Marcel Dekker; 1980.
7. Ellis H, Feldman S. *Anatomy for the Anaesthetists.* 4th ed. Oxford: Blackwell Scientific Publications; 1983:16.
8. Fink BR. *The Human Larynx: A Functional Study.* New York: Raven Press; 1975.
9. Fink BR, Demarest RJ. *Laryngeal Biomechanics.* Cambridge, MA: Harvard University Press; 1978.
10. Collins VJ. Endotracheal anesthesia: I. Basic considerations. In: Collins VJ. *Principles of Anesthesiology.* Philadelphia: Lea & Febiger; 1976.
11. Staub NC. The interdependence of pulmonary structure and function. *Anesthesiology.* 1963;24:831.
12. Staub NC. Basics of RD: lung structure and function. *Am Thorac Soc.* 1982;10:1.
13. Weibel ER. Functional morphology of lung parenchyma. In: Fishman AP, Macklem PT, Mead J, eds. *Handbook of Physiology, Section 3: The Respiratory System, Vol. 3: Mechanics of Breathing.* Bethesda: American Physiological Society; 1986.
14. Horsfield K, Cumming G. Angels of branching and diameters of branches in the human bronchial tree. *Bull Math Biophys.* 1967;29:245.
15. Tompset DH. The bronchpulmonary segments. *Med Hist.* 1965:9177.
16. Shields TW. Surgical anatomy of the lung. In: Shields TW ed. *General Thoracic Surgery.* 2nd ed. Philadelphia: Lea & Febiger; 1983:61.
17. Weibel ER. Anatomical distribution of air channels, blood vessels, and issue in the lung. In: Arangeli P, ed. *Normal Values for Respiratory Function in Man.* Milano, Italy: Panminerva Medica; 1970:242.
18. Fishman AP. Dynamics of the pulmonary circulation. In: Hamilton WF, ed. *Handbook of Physiology, Section 2: Circulation.* Baltimore: Williams & Wilkins; 1963:1667.
19. Heath D, Smith P. The pulmonary endothelial cell. *Thorax.* 1979;34:200.
20. Smith U, Ryan JW. Electron d microscopy of endothelial components of the lung: correlations of structure and function. *Fed Proc.* 1973;32:1957.

3

Radiology of the Thorax

JAVIER H. CAMPOS, ARCHIT SHARMA

Introduction

Radiologic images play an important role in the preoperative, intraoperative, and postoperative evaluation, and diagnosis of patients undergoing thoracic surgery. During the preoperative visit for evaluation of the thoracic surgical patient, the clinician must have an understanding of the disease and also become familiar with radiologic studies to be able to identify abnormal airway anatomy or compromises to the airway or to use caliper measurements in the tracheobronchial tree if necessary when selecting lung isolation devices. An important component of a successful preoperative evaluation is an understanding of normal tracheobronchial anatomy.[1] This chapter will be focused on reviewing normal tracheobronchial anatomy, radiologic images, and thoracic ultrasound with special interest for anesthesiologists involved in the care of the thoracic surgical patient.

Normal Tracheobronchial Anatomy

The trachea is a cartilaginous and fibromuscular structure that extends from the inferior aspect of the cricoid cartilage to the level of the carina.[2] The adult trachea is, on average, 15 cm long. The trachea is composed of 16 to 22 C-shaped rings of cartilage that form the anterior and lateral walls and are connected posteriorly by the membranous wall of the trachea, which lacks cartilage and is supported by the trachealis muscle.

The average diameter of a normal trachea is 22 mm in men and 19 mm in women. In men, the coronal diameter ranges from 13 to 22 mm and the sagittal diameter ranges from 13 to 27 mm. In women, the average coronal diameter is 10 to 21 mm and the sagittal is 10 to 23 mm.[3] The tracheal wall is about 3 mm in thickness in both men and women, with a tracheal lumen that is often ovoid shape.

The trachea is located in the midline position, but often can be deviated to the right at the level of the aortic arch, with a greater degree of displacement in the setting of an atherosclerotic aorta, advanced age, or in the presence of severe chronic obstructive pulmonary disease (COPD). With COPD or aging, the lateral diameter of the trachea may decrease, with a corresponding increase in the anteroposterior diameter. Conversely, COPD may also lead to softening of the tracheal rings with a decrease in the anteroposterior diameter of the trachea.[4] The cricoid cartilage is the narrowest part of the trachea, with an average diameter of 17 mm in men and 13 mm in women.

The trachea bifurcates at the carina into the right and left mainstem bronchi. An important fact is that the tracheal lumen narrows slightly as it progresses toward the carina. The tracheal bifurcation is located at the level of the sternal angle anteriorly and the fifth thoracic vertebra posteriorly. The right mainstem bronchus continues as the bronchus intermedius after the branching point from the right upper lobe bronchus. In men, the average distance from the tracheal carina to the branching point from the right upper lobe bronchus is 2.0 cm, whereas it is approximately 1.5 cm in women. One in every 250 individuals from the general population may have an abnormal branching point from the right upper lobe bronchus emerging from above the tracheal carina on the right side.[5] The diameter of the right mainstem bronchus is an average of 17.5 mm in men and 14.0 mm in women. The trifurcation of the right upper lobe bronchus consists of the apical, anterior, and posterior divisions. The average distance from the tracheal carina to the bifurcation of the left upper and left lower lobes is approximately 5.0 cm in men and 4.5 cm in women. The left mainstem bronchus is longer than the right mainstem bronchus, and it divides into the left upper and the left lower lobe bronchus. The left upper lobe bronchus has a superior and inferior division.[6]

Chest Radiographs

The most common study in the patient undergoing thoracic, esophageal, or cardiac surgery is the chest x-radiograph (x-ray). The standard routine for chest radiography consists of an erect radiograph in the posterior-anterior (PA) projection and a left lateral radiograph, both obtained at full inspiration. The normal chest cavity contains four radiographic densities that are easily identified: air, fat, water, and calcium and other metals, including bones, granulomas, and vascular calcification. The lungs, which are mostly air and contain some water, blood vessels, bronchi, nerves, lymphatics, alveolar walls, and interstitial tissues, provide a natural contrast that is the basis of chest radiology. Evaluating a chest x-ray involves checking for any changes in these densities.

Radiologists generally consider two features in chest x-radiographs: the silhouette sign and summation. Depending on the part or parts of the lungs that are involved, a change in the absorption of x-rays is seen by the effect on the normal surface of the hemidiaphragm, for example. If the descending aorta cannot be seen, then this is an indication that an unusual amount of aerated lung no longer touches the anatomic part. This occurs in part because the alveolar spaces are wholly or partially filled with fluid, usually blood, pus, or water, or in part because the lung has collapsed and decreased the normal ratio of air and soft tissue. The end result in the latter case would be an increase in opacity which is what the x-ray beam reveals. The heart border and the diaphragm are normally seen because of their interface with aerated lung. When the adjoining lung is not aerated, the opaque tissue of the affected lung blends visually with the soft-tissue opacity of the heart, and the heart border is no longer visible. This is what is termed the silhouette sign. Summation by definition is the result of superimposition of many layers of lung tissue, so that the final visual effect is that of a greater amount of tissue in the path of a particular part of the x-ray beam. This is observed when the opacity of fluid in the pleural space, interstitial space, or even lung parenchyma has an additive effect on the normal structure of the lung.[7] The most important skill for evaluating a chest x-ray is knowledge of normal anatomic variants, specific patterns with pathologic changes, and the common signs of abnormal states. Lateral decubitus radiographs are commonly used to determine the presence or mobility of pleural effusions. These views can also be obtained to detect small pneumothoraces, particularly in patients who are confined to bed and unable to sit or stand erect. A new generation of digital x-ray systems based on flat panel detectors is now emerging, and these provide good image quality and very rapid direct access to digital images.

Chest Radiographs and Pulmonary Disease

The basic underlying change in a chest film that allows the detection and diagnosis of abnormalities is usually an alteration in lung opacity. This can be caused by technical factors, physiologic variation, or pathologic mechanisms.[8] Diseases that affect the chest can be thought of as either those that make the film lighter (increase opacity) or those that make it darker (increase lucency).

For chest disease with increased opacity on radiographs, conditions that are marked by a focal or global increase in the opacity of the film are first examined. These conditions include atelectasis, pulmonary edema, acute respiratory distress syndrome, and so on.

Lung Mass and Chest X-Rays

Pulmonary neoplasia presents as opacity on films, although usually as a more focal area with varying contours. However, smaller lesions may be very difficult to visualize, particularly when there are overlying bones or other soft tissue. Fig. 3.1A shows a PA chest radiograph of a 68-year-old male with a lung neoplasm on the right lower lobe. The mass is clearly visible between the eighth and ninth ribs on the right hemithorax. Fig. 3.1B shows a lateral chest radiograph with a round mass on the right hemithorax.

A 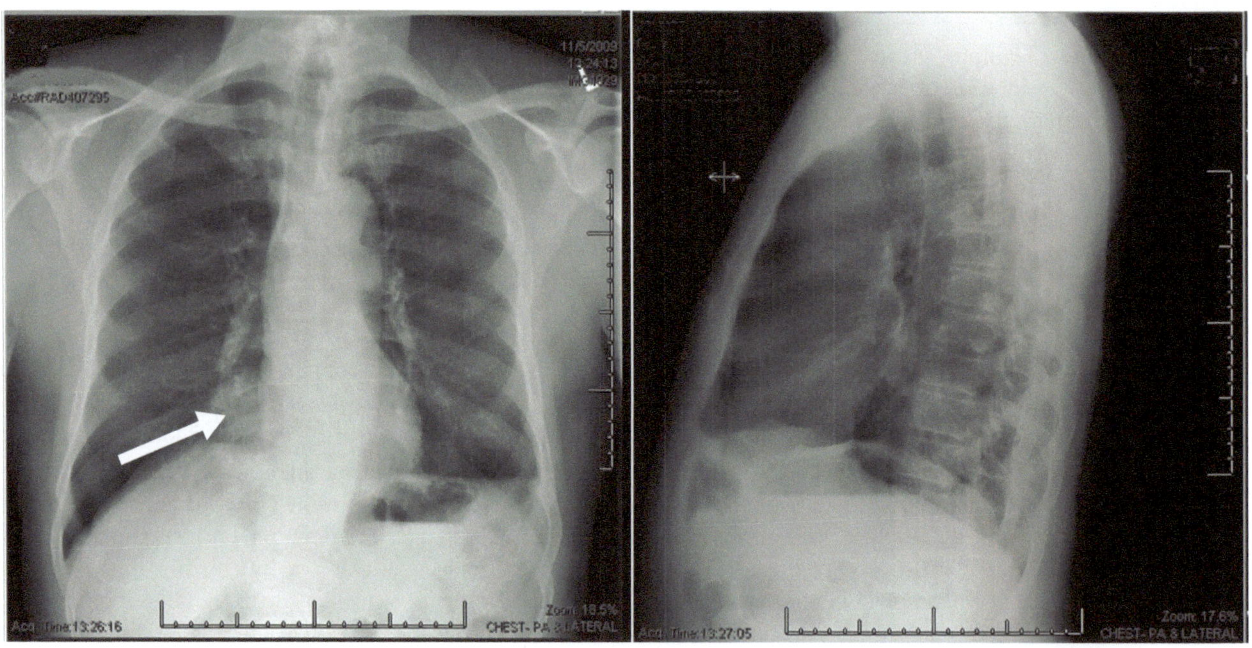 B

• **Fig. 3.1** (**A**) Posteroanterior chest radiograph of a 68-year-old male with a lung neoplasm (*arrow*) in the right lower lobe. The mass is visible between the eighth and ninth ribs on the right hemithorax. (**B**) Lateral chest radiograph showing a round mass on the right hemithorax.

Mediastinal Mass and Chest X-Rays

To understand mediastinal masses and radiologic images, it is important to be familiar with the anatomy of the mediastinum. The mediastinum is situated between the two pleural cavities (see Chapter 53). It extends superiorly from the root of the neck and the thoracic inlet to the hemidiaphragm inferiorly. It is divided into the superior and inferior mediastinum by the transverse thoracic plane, which is an imaginary plane extending horizontally from the sternal angle anteriorly to the border of the fourth thoracic vertebra posteriorly. The inferior mediastinum is subdivided into anterior, middle, and posterior compartments. The anterior mediastinum contains the thymus, trachea, esophagus, vessels, and arteries, as well as lymph nodes; any abnormal growth in this region will affect the adjacent area. A mass in this area may compress the tracheobronchial tree and/or major vessels (superior vena cava and pulmonary vessels). The middle mediastinum is the space occupied by the heart and pericardium.[9,10] Fig. 3.2A shows a schematic representation of the mediastinal anatomy and Fig. 3.2B a lateral normal radiograph of the chest showing the potential location of a mediastinal mass. A variety of neoplasms and other lesions present with anterior mediastinal involvement. Thymoma is the most common primary neoplasm of the anterior mediastinum.[11]

Regarding radiologic studies in patients with a suspected anterior mediastinal mass, the initial study generally is a standard biplane chest radiograph, which will identify up to 97% of mediastinal tumors. The chest x-ray also provides important information regarding the size and the location of the mass.[12]

In addition, in this patient group in particular, special attention must be paid to lateral radiographs of the chest to determine the overall extent of the mass and potential involvement of adjacent structures in this patient group. A barium contrast esophagogram may help to determine whether there is esophageal or tracheobronchial involvement. Fig. 3.3A shows an anterior mediastinal mass in the left hemithorax of the PA chest radiograph. Fig. 3.3B shows a lateral radiograph with esophageal contrast where there is a mediastinal mass without compromise to the tracheobronchial tree. Fig. 3.4A shows a posterior mediastinal mass in the right hemithorax of the PA chest radiograph in a female with severe kyphoscoliosis; Fig. 3.4B shows the corresponding lateral radiograph and Fig. 3.4C a portable PA chest radiograph after removal of the tumor.

Bullae

Emphysema is characterized by a permanent increase in air spaces distal to the terminal bronchiole beyond the normal size. There is destruction of tissue, leading to a loss of alveolar surface available to participate in air exchange and, sometimes, severe displacement of the adjacent normal lung. Many cases of emphysema seen in adult patients are strongly associated with cigarette smoking. The most striking image in a patient with advanced emphysema is marked hyperinflation with an increase in the anteroposterior diameter of the chest, flattening of the diaphragmatic surfaces,

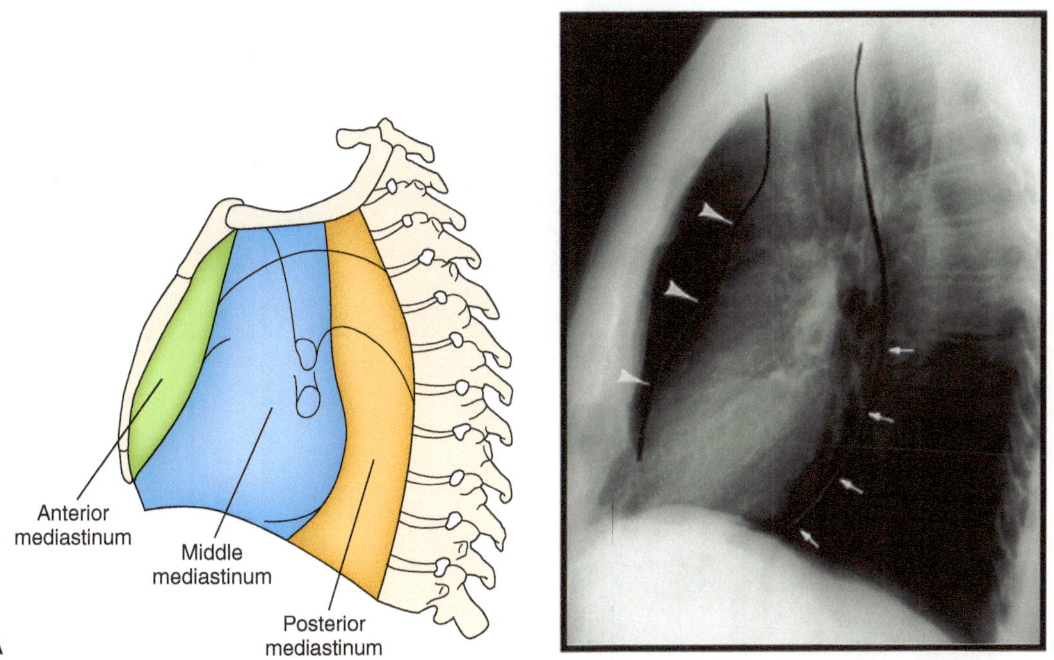

• **Fig. 3.2** (**A**) Schematic representation of the mediastinal anatomy and (**B**) a lateral normal radiograph of the chest showing the potential location of a mediastinal mass. The arrows to the left indicate potential areas of mediastinal mass growth. Arrows to the right indicate potential areas of posterior mediastinal mass growth. (From Campos JH. Managing the patient with an anterior mediastinal mass. In: Cohen NH, ed. *Medically Challenging Patients Undergoing Cardiothoracic Surgery*. Baltimore: Lippincott Williams & Wilkins; 2009:285–302. With permission.)

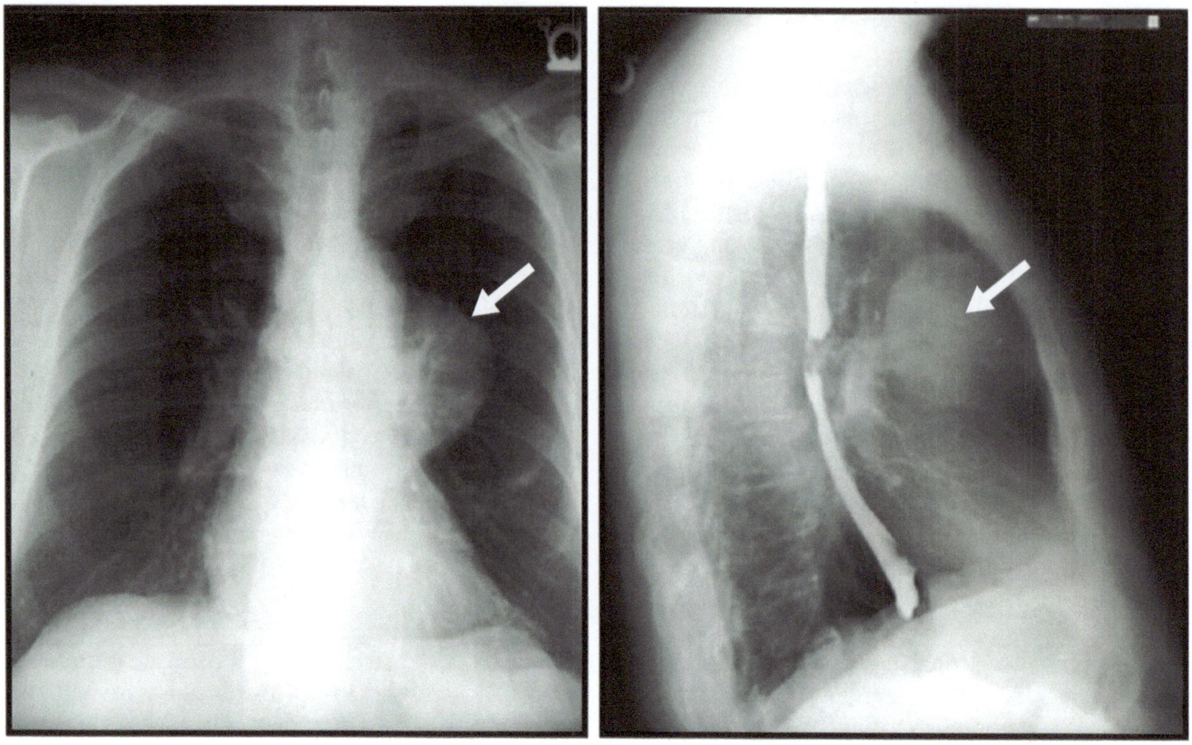

• **Fig. 3.3** (**A**) An anterior mediastinal mass (*arrow*) in the left hemithorax on a posteroanterior chest radiograph. (**B**) Lateral radiograph with esophageal contrast revealing a mediastinal mass (*arrow*) without compromise to the tracheobronchial tree.

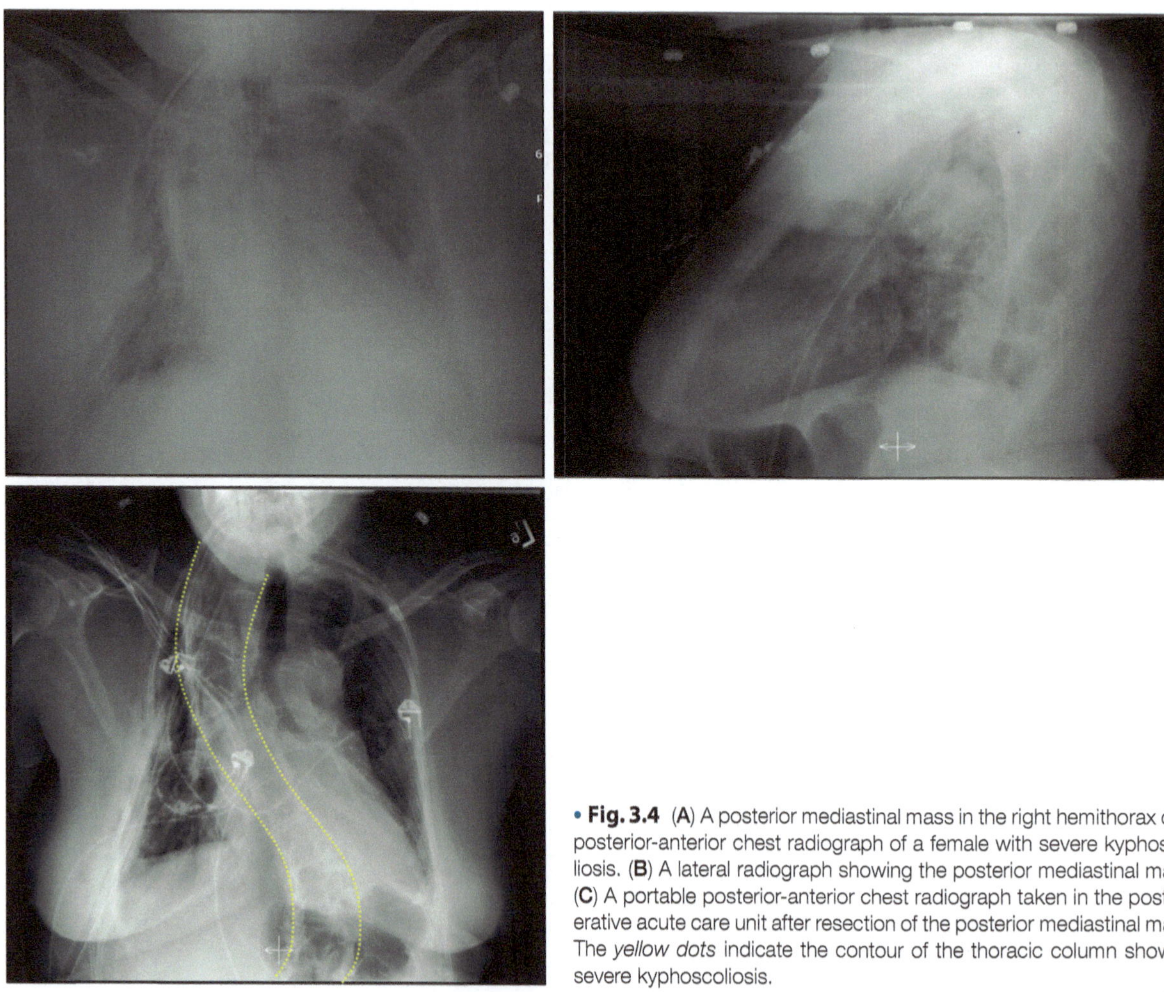

• **Fig. 3.4** (**A**) A posterior mediastinal mass in the right hemithorax on a posterior-anterior chest radiograph of a female with severe kyphoscoliosis. (**B**) A lateral radiograph showing the posterior mediastinal mass. (**C**) A portable posterior-anterior chest radiograph taken in the postoperative acute care unit after resection of the posterior mediastinal mass. The *yellow dots* indicate the contour of the thoracic column showing severe kyphoscoliosis.

A 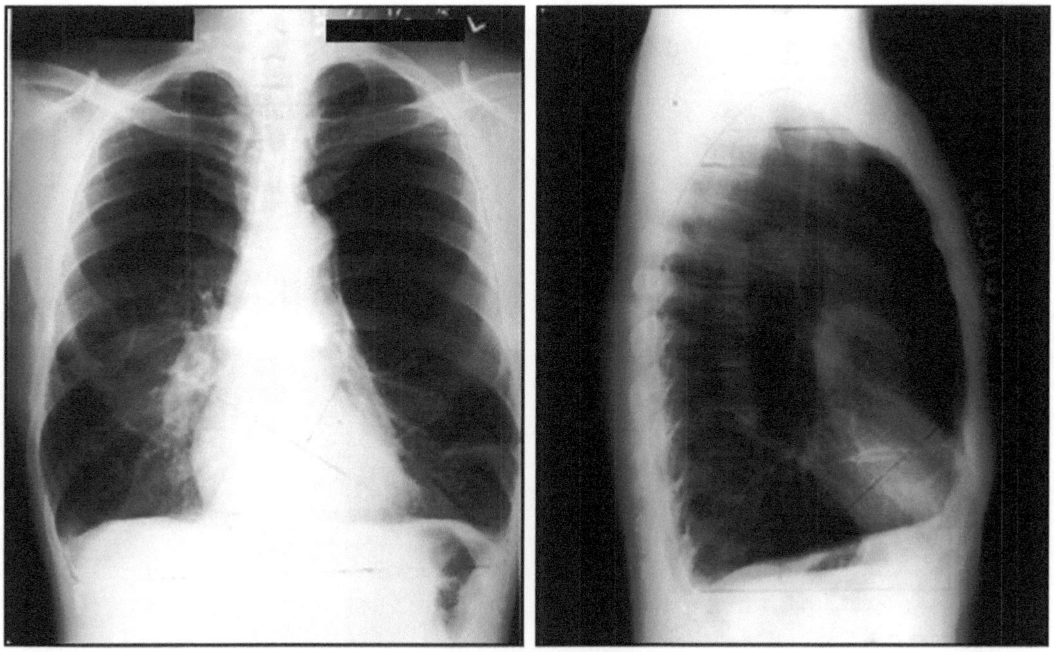 B

• **Fig. 3.5** (**A**) Posterior-anterior chest x-ray of a patient with emphysema. There is marked hyperinflation with an increase in the anterior-posterior diameter of the chest, as well as flattening of the diaphragm bilaterally and a general increase in the blackness of the film. (**B**) Lateral chest x-ray of the same patient.

A 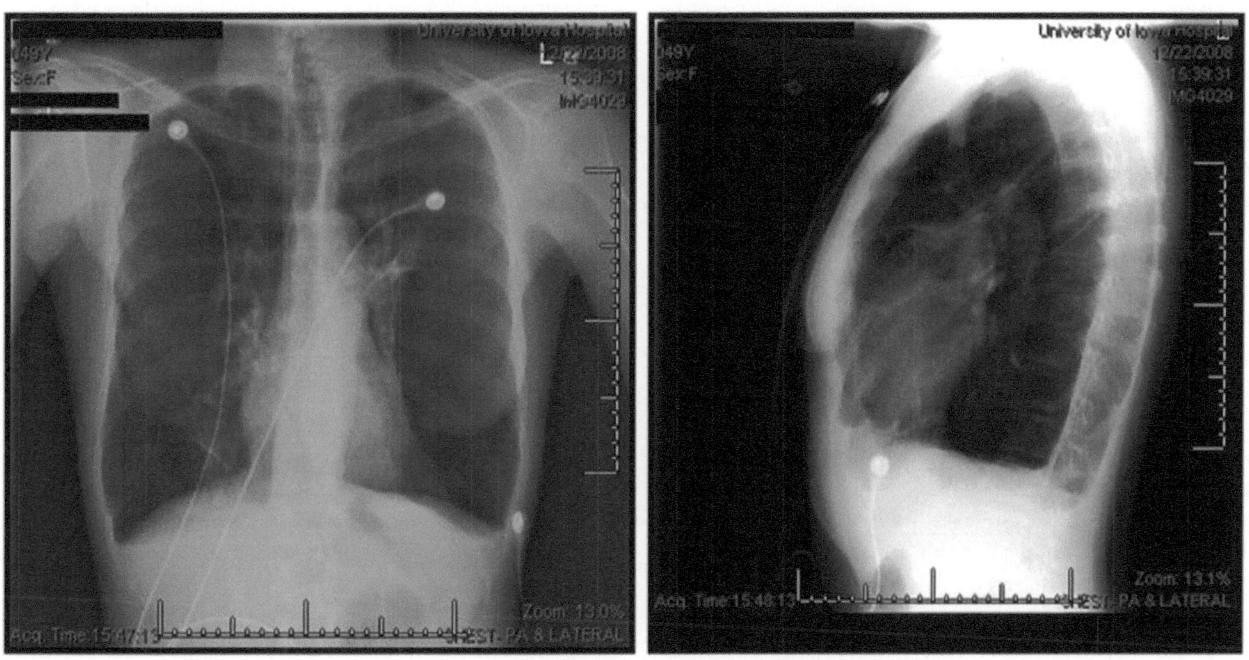 B

• **Fig. 3.6** (**A**) Posterior-anterior chest x-radiograph of a patient with a bulla in the left hemithorax. (**B**) Lateral radiograph of the same patient.

and a general increase in the blackness of the film. There is also a change in the vascular pattern, with attenuated vessels thinned and spread apart.

Often bullous areas are noted as large, thin-walled air cysts, especially the apices. A bulla is defined as an air-filled space of 1 cm or greater in diameter within the lung parenchyma that forms as a result of a destructive process. Rarely, one or more bullae enlarge to such a degree that they occupy more than one-third of the hemithorax. The term giant bullae is then applied. These easily distensible reservoirs are preferentially filled during inspiration, causing the collapse of adjacent, more normal lung parenchyma.[13,14] Fig. 3.5A shows a patient with emphysema, and Fig. 3.5B shows a lateral chest radiograph of the same patient. Fig. 3.6 shows a PA chest x-ray and lateral radiograph of a patient with bullae. Fig. 3.7 displays the chest x-ray showing a giant bulla occupying more than

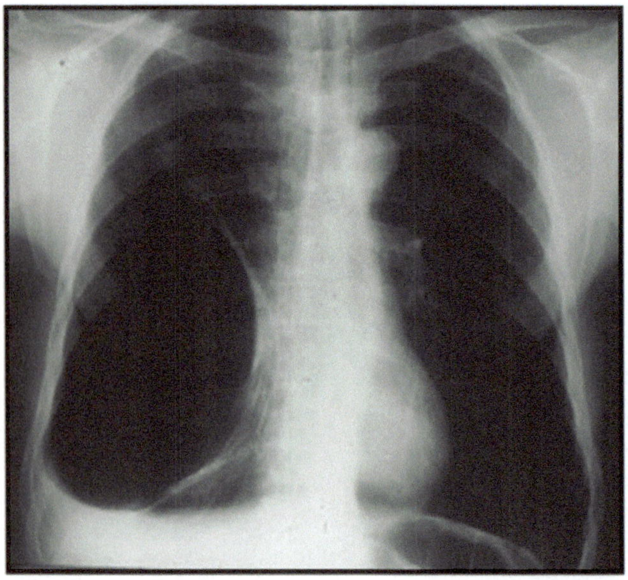

• **Fig. 3.7** Chest x-ray showing a giant bulla occupying more than two-thirds of the right hemithorax and compressing the underlying lung.

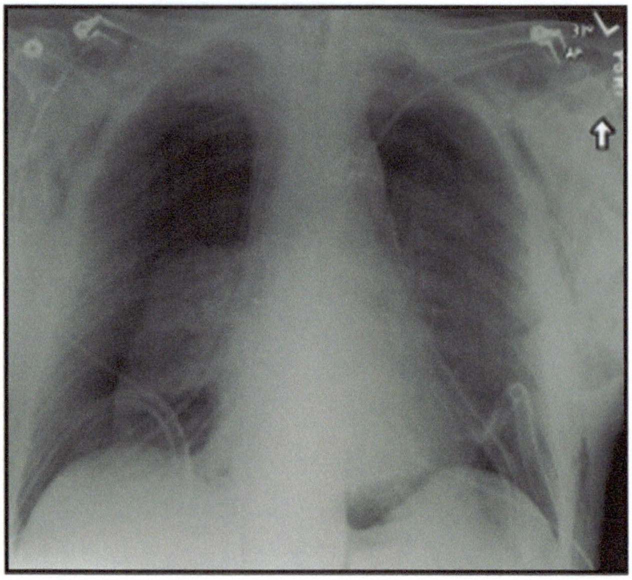

• **Fig. 3.8** Chest radiograph of a patient with a right-sided pneumothorax and bilateral chest tubes.

two-thirds of the right hemithorax and compressing the underlying lung.

Pneumothorax

Pneumothorax is the presence of air in the pleural space between the lung and the chest wall. Primary pneumothoraces arise in otherwise healthy people without any lung disease. Secondary pneumothoraces arise in subjects with underlying lung disease. Despite the absence of underlying pulmonary disease in patients with primary pneumothorax, subpleural blebs and bullae are likely to play a role in the pathogenesis. It is frequently the result of trauma, although sometimes the source of the air leak cannot be readily detected.

The radiographic diagnosis of pneumothorax is usually straightforward. A visceral pleural line is seen without distal lung markings. On standard lateral views, a visceral pleural line may be seen in the retrosternal position or overlying the vertebrae, parallel to the chest wall.[15,16]

Pneumothoraces can be seen on lateral chest radiographs; although the value of expiratory views is controversial, many clinicians still find them useful in the detection of small pneumothoraces when clinical suspicion is high and an inspiratory radiograph appears normal. The British Thoracic Society guidelines divide pneumothoraces into small and large based on the distance from visceral pleural surface (lung edge) to the chest wall: less than 2 cm is classified as small and more than 2 cm as large.[17] A small rim of air around the lung actually translates into a relatively large loss of lung volume, with a 2-cm-deep pneumothorax occupying about 50% of the hemithorax.

In the supine position, air in the pleural space will usually be most readily visible at the lung bases in the cardiophrenic recess and may enlarge the costophrenic angle. Fig. 3.8 shows a chest radiograph of a patient with right-sided pneumothorax.

Several well-known artifactual appearances can mimic the presence of a pneumothorax and should always be borne in mind during evaluation of chest radiography. The medial border of the scapula can imitate a lung edge, but once considered can be traced in continuity with the rest of the bone, revealing its true nature. Skin folds overlying the chest wall can simulate a visceral pleural line and, with the relative lack of lung markings in the upper zones, can lead to erroneous diagnosis. Once considered, however, the true nature of the image is readily apparent. Skin folds are usually seen to pass outside the chest cavity, are straight or only minimally curved, and do not run parallel to the chest wall as with a true visceral pleural line. Skin folds also form a dense line that is sharp on one side and blurred on the other, in contrast to the less dense visceral pleural line. Also radioopaque lines are often seen accompanying the inferior margins of ribs, which may simulate a visceral pleural line. These are often called companion shadows, although some restrict this term to densities accompanying the first and second ribs. They are caused by protruding extrapleural fat or the subcostal grove.

Tension pneumothorax occurs when the intrapleural pressure exceeds the atmospheric pressure throughout inspiration, as well as expiration. It is thought to result from the operation of a one-way valve system, drawing air into the pleural space during inspiration and not allowing it out during expiration. The development of tension pneumothorax is often, but not always, heralded by a sudden deterioration in the cardiopulmonary status of the patient related to impaired venous return, reduced cardiac output, and hypoxemia. The development of tension in a pneumothorax is not dependent on the size of the pneumothorax and the clinical scenario of tension pneumothorax may correlate poorly with chest radiographic findings.[18,19] In extreme cases of tension

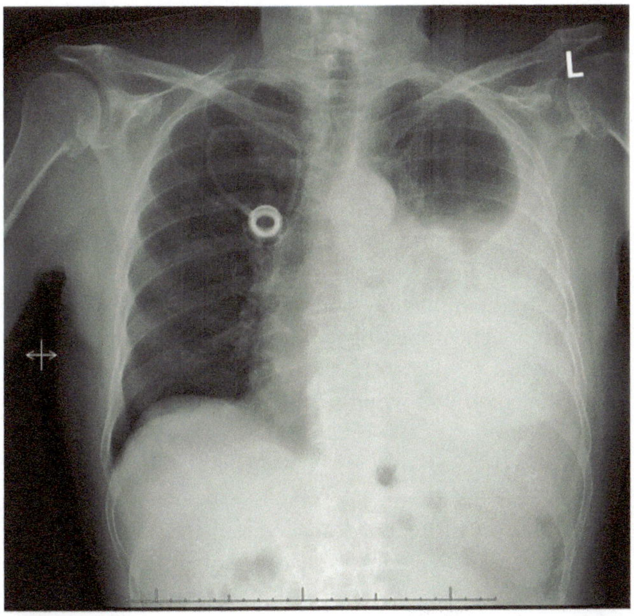

• **Fig. 3.9** Chest x-ray of a male patient with a large pleural effusion in the left hemithorax occupying two-thirds of the chest cavity on the left side. An infusion port device in the right hemithorax is also evident.

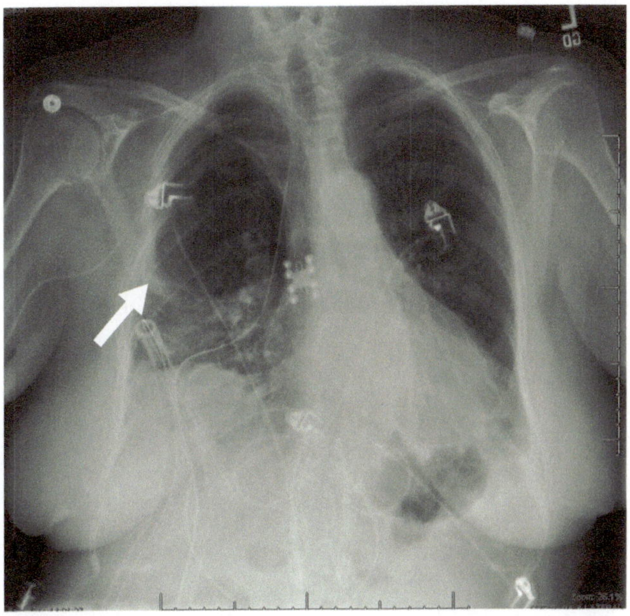

• **Fig. 3.10** Chest x-ray showing a chest tube in the right hemithorax. The tip of the tube can be clearly seen at the level of the sixth intercostal space (*arrow*). There is also a peripherally inserted central catheter (Picc) line going from a vein in the right arm to the entrance of the superior vena cava.

pneumothorax, the air leak leads to significant displacement of the mediastinum and contralateral lung into the opposite hemithorax, causing significant hemodynamic instability.

Pleural Effusion

Pleural effusion does not involve the lung parenchyma; it can be the source of a significant amount of absorbing material in the path of the x-ray beam, causing opacity on the films. Large pleural effusions are easy to spot on a chest radiograph, but small pleural effusions can be overlooked easily, especially on portable films because the patients are almost always supine or semierect, and the fluid can collect either in a subpulmonic location or deep in the posterior costophrenic sulcus where it is hidden from view. Most often smaller effusions are seen as a veil-like opacity that is most pronounced at the base and tapers toward the lung apex. Fig. 3.9 shows a male patient with a large pleural effusion of the left hemithorax occupying two-thirds of the chest cavity on the left side.

Chest Tube Placement

In general, appropriate use of chest tubes results in complete drainage of the collected air and fluid in the pleural space and allows full expansion and occupation of the entire pleural space by the lung, thus protecting the lung and pleural space from subsequent complications. Chest tubes are used routinely in the thoracic surgical patient. In practice, three main types are used: (1) large-caliber chest tubes of 20F to 30F in size; (2) small-caliber chest tubes; and (3) pigtail catheters. The typical and most common tubes have a side hole and end hole and an opaque marker that can be clearly seen on a chest x-radiograph. Chest tubes can be inadvertently placed either in the major fissure, lung parenchyma, or too high in the apex, and this can cause severe pain or damage to the lung.

To evaluate the position of a chest tube, an anterior–posterior chest radiograph or lateral film is useful.[20] In some circumstances, computed tomography (CT) scans of the chest are valuable for assessing chest tube position; for example, when misplacement is suspected but not confirmed on a plain radiograph.[21] Fig. 3.10 shows a chest tube in a female patient placed in the right hemithorax.

Surgical emphysema is a well-known complication of intercostal tube drainage.[22] The development of surgical emphysema associated with pneumothorax involves an air-filled space in subcutaneous tissue. This may occur in the presence of a malpositioned, kinked, blocked, or clamped tube. Likewise, a small tube in the presence of a very large leak may potentially cause surgical emphysema. Any malpositioned chest tube should be visible on a chest radiograph. If the emphysema results in airway obstruction or thoracic compression, it may lead to severe respiratory insufficiency. The treatment is usually conservative, but in life-threatening situations, skin incision decompression and insertions of large-bore modified subcutaneous chest drain have all been used successfully.

Previous Lobectomy

Resection of a segment of the lung will produce changes somewhat similar to segmental atelectasis in that a portion of the lung is no longer present, and the remaining segments of the lobe, and other lobes on that side, will expand to fill the space. A chest radiograph will show displacement of the interlobar fissure and elevation of the diaphragm. There might be displacement of the hilum. Often the most common sign of surgery in the chest is the presence of fine metallic sutures on the pleural surface at the site of the resection. If a chest tube is present after an acute resection, it will be visible on a chest radiograph, as will any rib osteotomy.

The post-lobectomy patient will often present with a greater initial deformity of the involved hemithorax and some shift of the midline structures. As in cases of atelectasis, there should be compensatory overinflation of the noninvolved lobes. Fig. 3.11 shows a chest x-ray of a female patient who had a left lower lobe lobectomy.

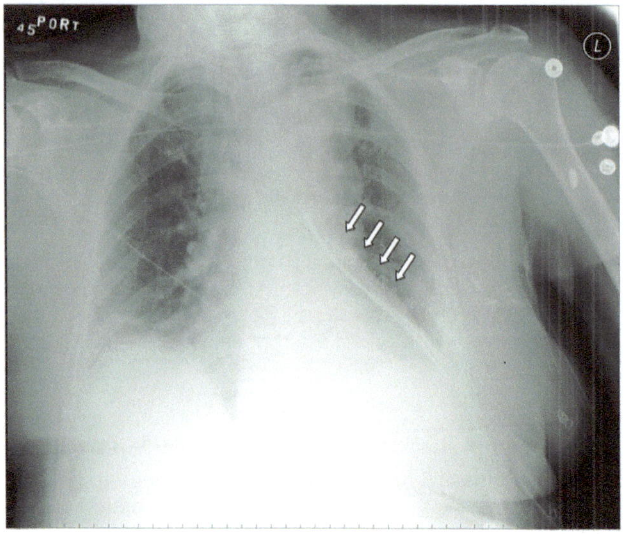

• **Fig. 3.11** Chest x-ray of a female patient who had a left lower lobe lobectomy. The *arrows* denote the stapling line. Bilateral postlobectomy infiltrates are also evident.

An important piece of information after lobectomy is the juxtaphrenic peak sign indicating upper lobe collapse. This is a common finding on chest radiographs of patients after upper lobectomy. It is more frequently seen after right upper lobectomy than after left upper lobectomy, and it is more often seen on erect than on supine radiographs. A study has shown that a juxtaphrenic peak can be expected to appear on chest radiographs in about 70% of patients 1 month or more after right upper lobectomy and in 50% after left upper lobectomy.[23] Fig. 3.12 shows a patient who had a right upper lobectomy showing a thin juxtaphrenic peak.

Pneumonectomy

Removal of an entire lung leads to more drastic radiographic changes that evolve with the passage of time. Initially, the affected side shows expected postoperative changes at the hilum and chest wall with a complete absence of lung tissue, leaving a very stark, air-filled cavity with extremely sharp margins of the heart and diaphragm. After pneumonectomy, air in the operated hemithorax is gradually reabsorbed and replaced by fluid, with a net volume loss. As a result, the trachea and mediastinum gradually shift toward the surgical side. In the immediate postoperative period, a mediastinal shift away from the surgical side indicates atelectasis of the contralateral lung or an abnormal accumulation of air or fluid on the surgical side.[24] A rapid mediastinal shift can signify the presence of an air leak with a "ball-valve" effect, leading to a tension pneumothorax. There is usually some

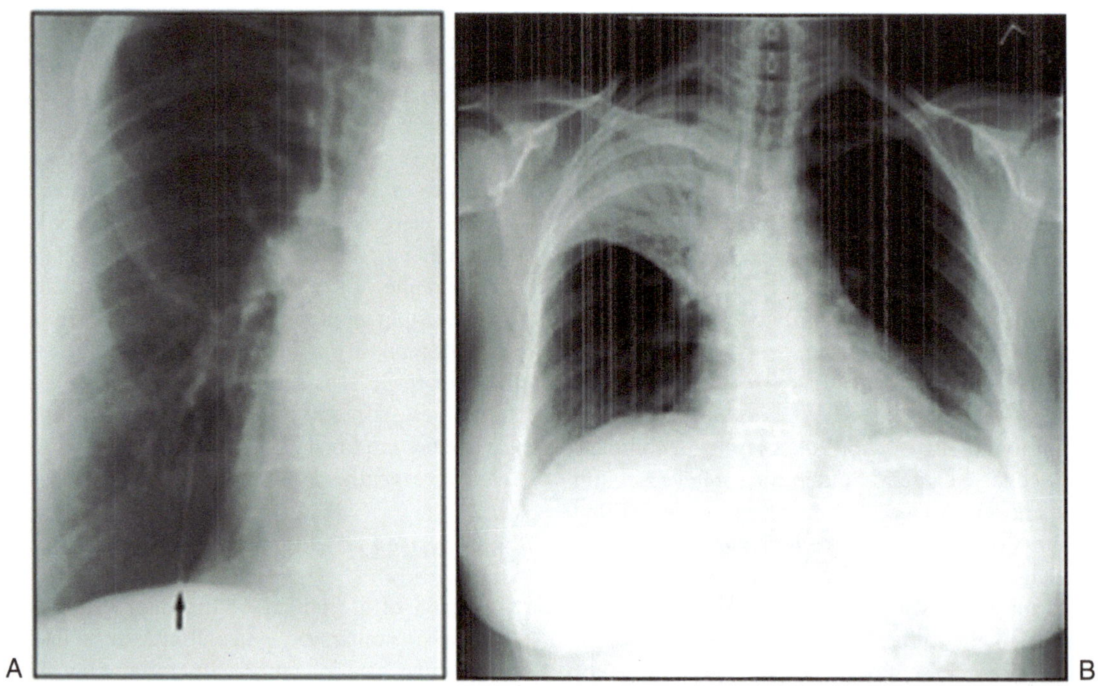

• **Fig. 3.12** (**A**) Chest x-ray of a patient who had a right upper lobectomy showing a thin juxtaphrenic peak, as indicated by the arrow. (**B**) Chest x-ray after a right upper lobectomy without the juxtaphrenic line.

elevation of the hemidiaphragm and a shift of the heart and other midline structures toward the operated side, as the remaining lung expands to take some of the space. Gradually the hemithorax fills with fluid, showing a distinct air fluid level if the patient is upright or a more subtle increase in opacity if the patient is in the supine position. Fig. 3.13 shows anterior-posterior and lateral chest radiographs of a patient with a left-sided pneumonectomy.

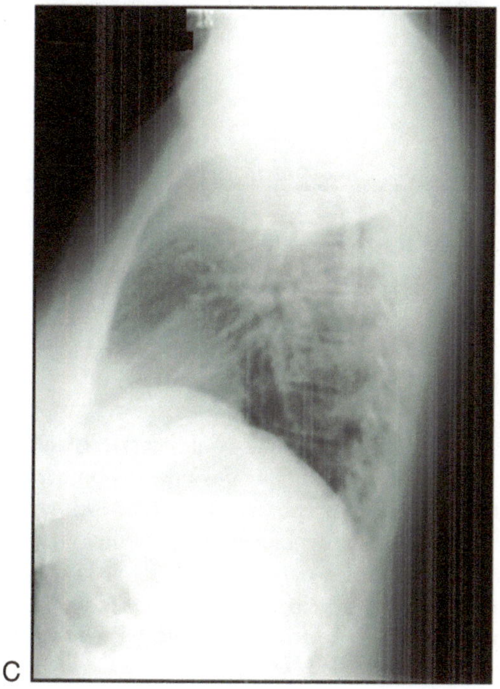

• **Fig. 3.12** *(Continued)* (**C**) Lateral chest radiograph of the same patient.

Single-Lumen Endotracheal Tubes

After a thoracic surgical procedure, a chest radiograph is required to assess lung expansion, chest tube placement, and, if the patient remains intubated, proper placement of the endotracheal tube. The proper position of a single-lumen endotracheal tube, as seen on a chest radiograph, is with the distal tip of the tube located approximately 3 cm above the tracheal carina. All endotracheal tubes have opaque markers that can be clearly identified on radiographs. Fig. 3.14A shows a male patient who underwent a right upper lobectomy and remained intubated in the postoperative period with a single-lumen endotracheal tube. Fig. 3.14B shows the same patient with a reconstruction of the single-lumen endotracheal tube.

Double-Lumen Endotracheal Tubes

With any thoracic surgical procedure involving lung isolation devices, the anesthesiologist must review the tracheobronchial anatomy at the preoperative visit to determine whether or not abnormal anatomy exists. A PA chest radiograph will allow assessment of the shadow of the tracheobronchial anatomy along with the bronchial bifurcation. It is estimated that in 75% of the films, the left mainstem bronchus shadow is seen. In addition, a chest radiograph can be useful to determine the proper size of a left-sided double-lumen tube (DLT). Brodsky et al.[25] reported that measurement of the tracheal diameter at the level of the clavicle on a

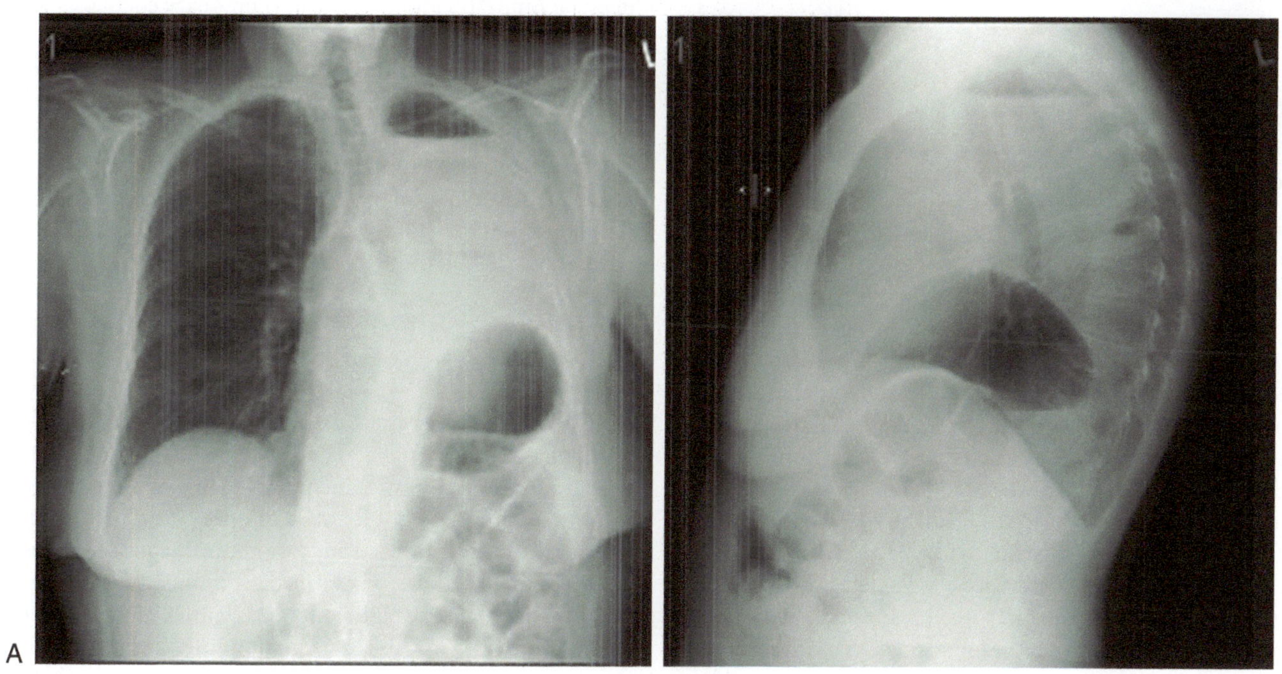

• **Fig. 3.13** (**A**) Anterior-posterior and (**B**) lateral chest radiographs of a patient post left-sided pneumonectomy. The white image in the left hemithorax corresponds to fluid.

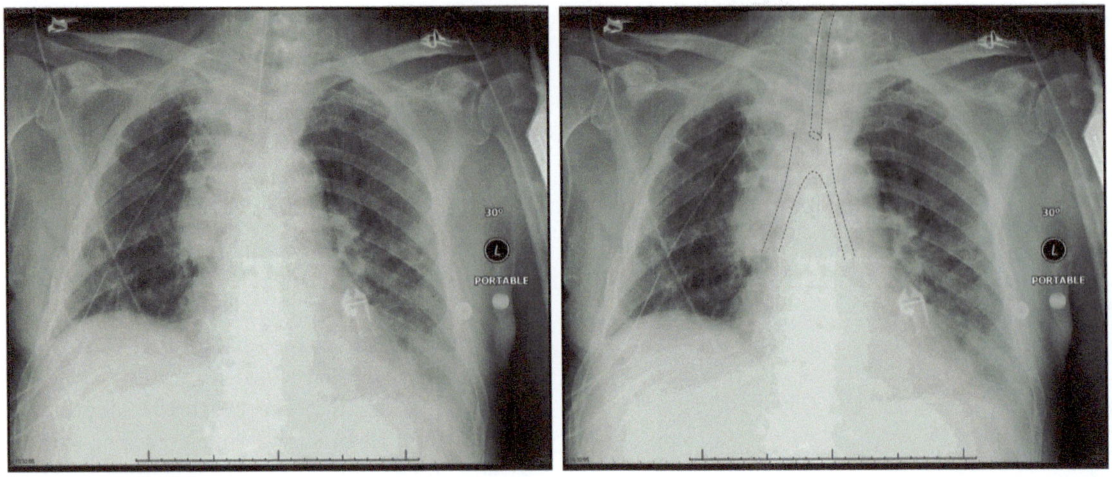

A B

• **Fig. 3.14** (**A**) Chest radiograph of a male patient who underwent a right upper lobectomy and remained intubated in the postoperative period with a single-lumen endotracheal tube. (**B**) Reconstruction of the single-lumen endotracheal tube in the same patient. Notice that the tip of the single-lumen endotracheal tube should be placed 3 cm above the tracheal carina.

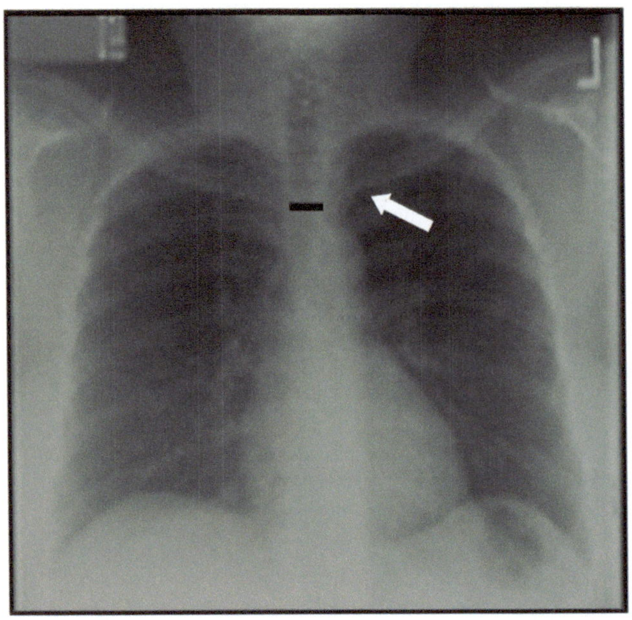

• **Fig. 3.15** Measurement of the tracheal width at the level of the clavicles to estimate the proper size of a left-sided double-lumen tube from a chest radiograph. The arrow points to the shadow of the trachea.

preoperative PA chest radiograph can be used to determine the proper left-sided DLT size. Fig. 3.15 shows the measurement of the tracheal width at the level of the clavicles to estimate the proper size of a left-sided DLT from a chest radiograph. In addition, a chest radiograph will allow visualization of the already placed DLT. The tip of each lumen is identified with a radiopaque marker. Fig. 3.16A shows a chest radiograph of a patient with a left-sided DLT in place. Notice that the endobronchial lumen is approximately 2 cm below the tracheal carina in the left mainstem bronchus. Fig. 3.16B shows a reconstruction of the DLT, which is marked in the chest radiograph.

Postoperative Acute Lung Injury

Acute lung injury (ALI) may complicate thoracic surgery and is a major contributor to postoperative mortality. The incidence of ALI after thoracic surgery is estimated to be 4.2%.[26,27] In a study by Licker et al.,[26] the authors found a biphasic distribution pattern of ALI after lung resection. The primary form developed within the first 3 days after surgery, while the onset of the secondary form of ALI was after the third postoperative day.

The clinical presentation is a severe respiratory insufficiency with progressive hypoxemia that does not respond to conventional treatment, including O_2 therapy. A chest radiograph of a patient with ALI shows patchy unilateral or bilateral infiltrates and dependent pulmonary edema, as well as zones of atelectasis. Fig. 3.17 shows a chest radiograph of a 60-year-old female taken 72 hours after a left lower lobectomy. The patient developed ALI, with progression of interstitial edema. The radiograph shows a single-lumen endotracheal tube and a pulmonary artery catheter introduced via the left internal jugular vein, as well as bilateral diffuse fluffy opacities that are typical signs of interstitial pulmonary edema due to ALI after lobectomy.

Computed Tomography Scan and Pulmonary Disease

A CT scan of the chest is used as a diagnostic study, after abnormal findings on a standard chest radiograph.[28] Common indications for CT include: staging of lung cancer, solitary pulmonary nodule, mass or opacity, diffuse infiltrative lung disease, widened mediastinum, mediastinal mass, or other abnormalities of the mediastinum, such as pleural abnormalities, chest wall lesions, and trauma, among others. CT also provides valuable information for the clinician with regard to airway compression at any level of the tracheobronchial tree, as well as vascular compression diagnosis.[29–32]

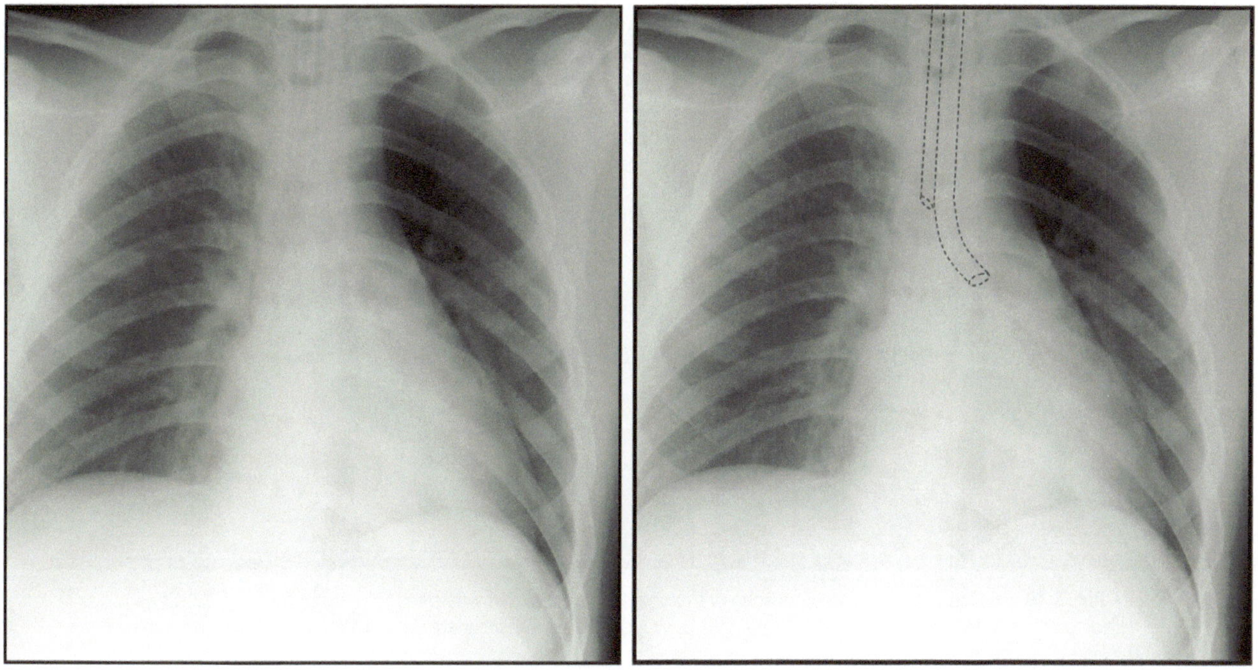

A B

• **Fig. 3.16** (**A**) Chest radiograph of a patient with a left-sided double-lumen tube (DLT) in place. Notice that the endobronchial lumen is approximately 2 cm below the tracheal carina in the left mainstem bronchus. (**B**) Reconstruction of the DLT, which is denoted by the *dotted lines*.

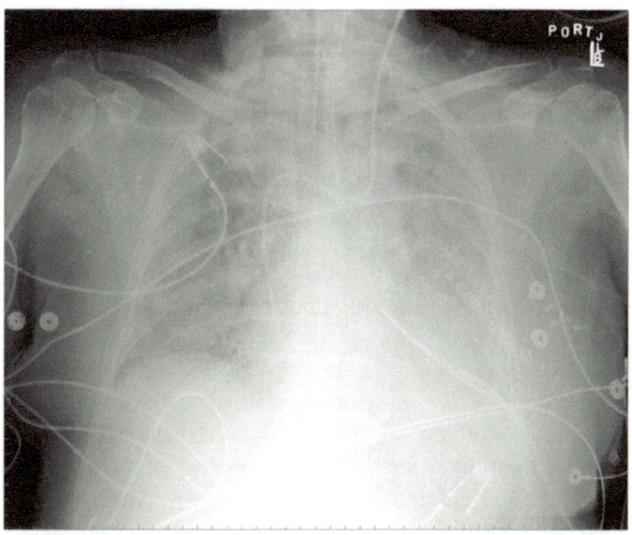

• **Fig. 3.17** Chest radiograph of a patient with an acute lung injury 72 hours after interstitial edema had progressed. There is a single-lumen endotracheal tube in place and a pulmonary artery catheter introduced via the left internal jugular vein is visible. The chest radiograph also shows bilateral diffuse fluffy opacities typical of interstitial pulmonary edema after lobectomy.

CT scans are performed in deep inspiration and at total lung capacity. For a routine helical CT scan of the chest, 2.5- to 5-mm sections are usually recommended. Thinner (1–2.5 mm) sections can be used to study fine details of the lung parenchyma. On routine studies, the field of view is adjusted to the size of the thorax, but small fields of view may be selected for smaller anatomic parts that require closer inspection. In addition, a contrast CT scan is useful in suspected vascular abnormalities, such as pulmonary embolism. Recent improvements in scanner technology have led to the introduction of spiral or helical volumetric CT.

Computed Tomography Scan and Lung Mass, Mediastinal Mass, Pleural Effusion, and Pericardial Effusion

A CT scan of the chest will confirm the presence of a mass in the chest and in many instances the specific location. Fig. 3.18A shows a CT scan of the chest for a female patient with a mass in the right lung. Fig. 3.18B shows the corresponding chest radiograph, with the lung mass visible in the right upper lobe. In addition, a CT scan of the chest will define the precise size and location of a mediastinal mass, any involvement of adjacent structures, and the degree of compression of the airway (trachea and/or bronchi). It is important during assessment of the CT scan to identify the location of the mass, define its relationship to adjacent structures, assess the extent and degree of tracheal and/or vascular compression, and assess the patency of the airway at the tracheal and bronchial levels. A CT scan also will permit accurate measurement of the airway diameter and the precise level and extent of compression of the trachea. The average cross-sectional diameter of the trachea in a 70-kg, 170-cm-tall person is approximately 18 to 23 mm. A tracheal diameter narrowing of 10 mm on CT corresponds to a 50% reduction in the tracheal cross-sectional area at that level. Fig. 3.19 shows a CT scan of the chest for a patient with a large anterior mediastinal mass in the left hemithorax. Fig. 3.20 shows a CT scan

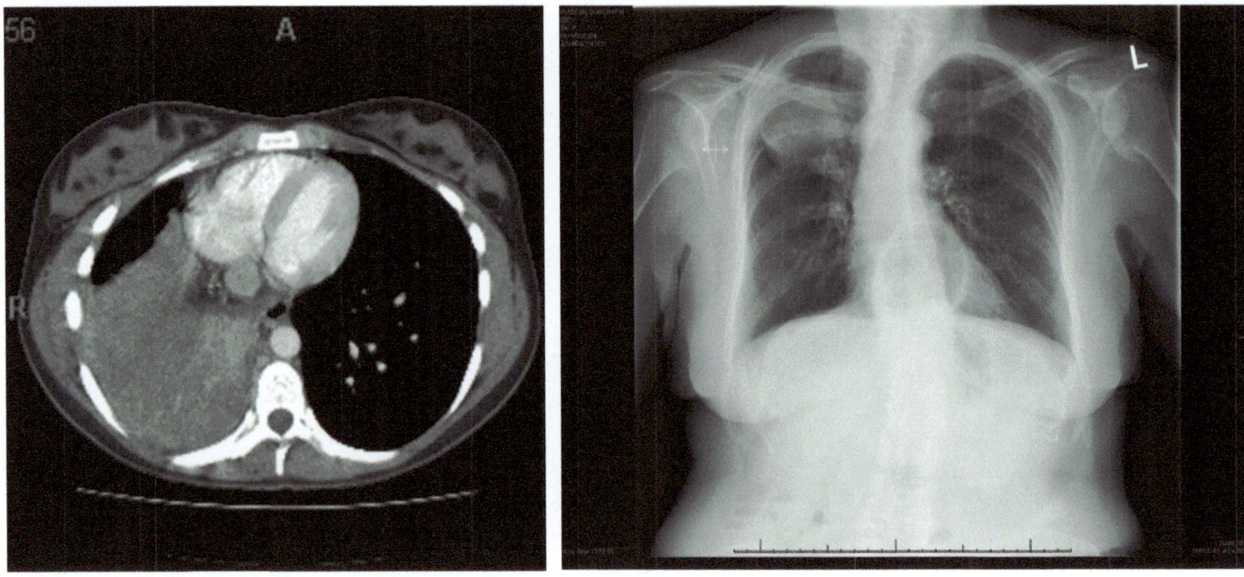

• **Fig. 3.18** (**A**) Computed tomography scan of the chest. The diagnosis was pseudotumor of the lung. (**B**) Chest radiograph showing the lung mass in the right upper lobe in the same patient. The diagnosis was a right upper lobe adenocarcinoma.

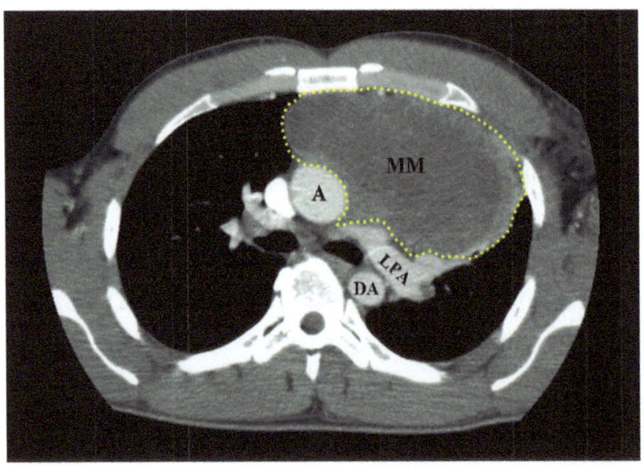

• **Fig. 3.19** A computed tomography scan of the chest with a large anterior mediastinal mass on the left hemithorax (the *dotted line* is surrounding the mass). This patient had a diagnosis of a mediastinal mass, classified as diffuse B-cell lymphoma. *A*, ascending aorta; *DA*, descending aorta; *L*, left; *LPA*, left pulmonary artery; *MM*, mediastinal mass; *R*, right.

of the chest for a patient with a large anterior mediastinal mass on the left side causing compression of the entrance of the left mainstem bronchus.

A CT scan of the chest allows precise identification of the location of any extrapulmonary fluid, whether in the peripheral pleural space or the interlobar fissure. Fig. 3.21 shows a CT scan of the chest for a patient with a large pleural effusion on the left hemithorax. A CT scan is also very useful for the diagnosis of pericardial effusions, because the precise location can be identified with this method. Fig. 3.22 shows a pericardial effusion; notice the fluid in the pericardial sac.

A three-dimensional (3D) reconstruction of the airway using a workstation connected to a multidetector CT (MDCT) scanner can provide further information in assessing the airway. MDCT provides high spatial resolution images of the whole lung without any anatomical gap. The technique consists of projecting the voxels with the lowest change in value in every view through the volume explored, at various angles, depending on the airway involved. If a tracheobronchial injury is suspected, 3D extraction of the airways may be useful by focusing the 3D volume-rendering technique on the tracheobronchial tree.[33] This technique is used for analyzing stenosis or distortion of the tracheobronchial tree but also may allow the diagnosis of tracheobronchial injury by demonstrating a wall defect and/or abnormal position of the lobar and segmental bronchi.[34,35]

A 3D scan of the chest can also be used to identify lymph nodes. The development of virtual bronchoscopy has led to interest in introducing CT-based computer-graphic techniques for lung cancer staging. In virtual bronchoscopy, 3D CT image serves as a high-resolution digital image replica of the chest.[36] Endoluminal renderings of the airways can be generated along paths following the central axes for offline simulation of video bronchoscopy as virtual endoscopy, with interior views computer-generated from radiologic images.

Imaging of the tracheobronchial tree has improved recently, in large part because of advances in CT that allow volumetric isotropic voxel imaging and associated improvements in postprocessing software for advanced 3D visualization.[37] Thus airway imaging has become a tool that physicians can use to plan interventional procedures, such as stent placement, surgery, and subsequent follow-up.

Patients undergoing thoracic surgical procedures who have large mediastinal masses with severe compromise of the airway require placement of an airway stent; therefore it

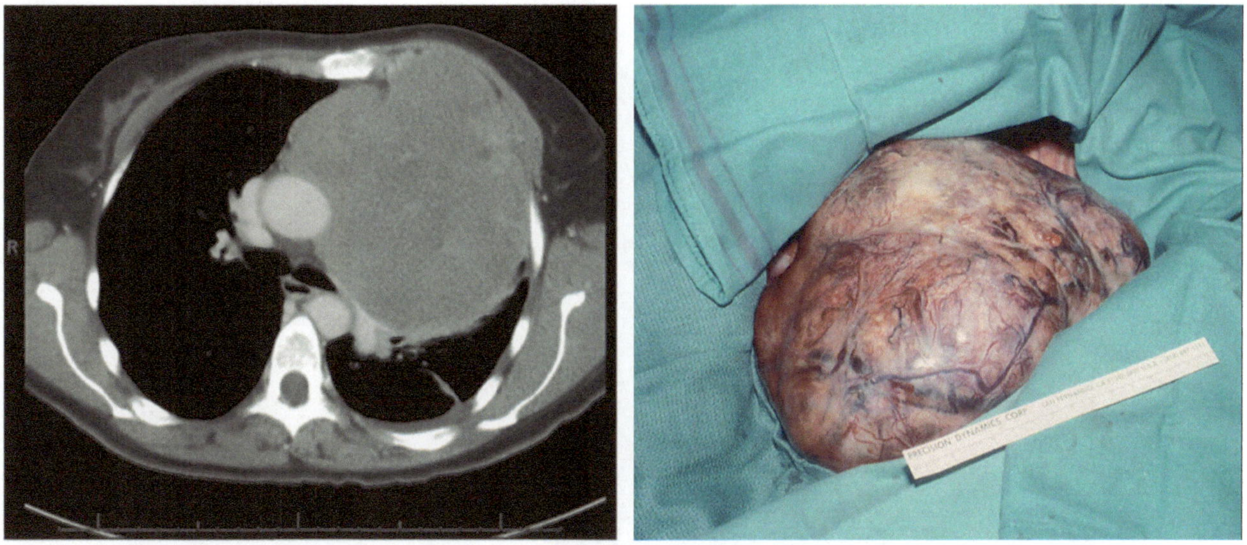

A B

R L

• **Fig. 3.20** (**A**) A computed tomography scan of the chest showing a large anterior mediastinal mass on the left side causing compression of the entrance of the left mainstem bronchus. The diagnosis for this patient was a germ cell tumor. (**B**) Large mediastinal mass in the left hemithorax.

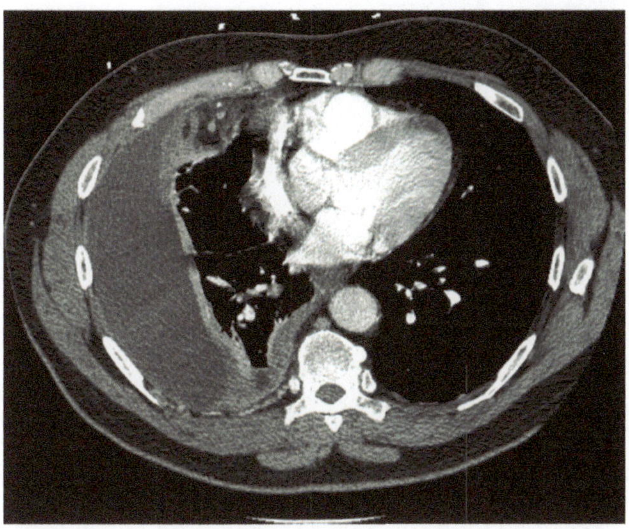

• **Fig. 3.21** Computed tomography (CT) scan of the chest showing a large pleural effusion on the left hemithorax.

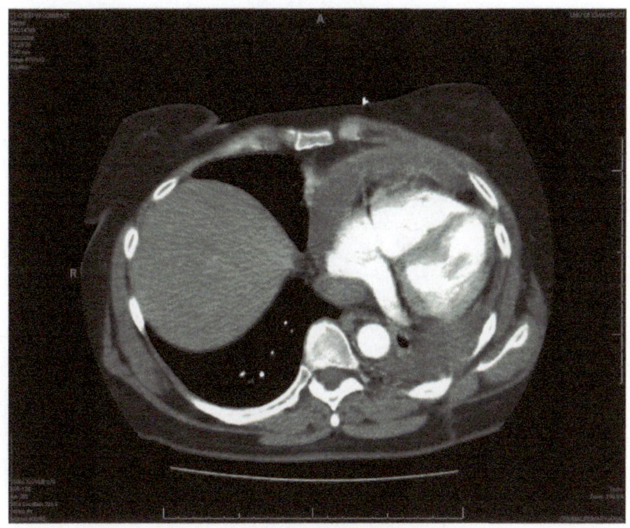

• **Fig. 3.22** Computed tomography scan showing a pericardial effusion; notice the fluid in the pericardial sac.

is crucial to review a CT scan for patients who have a stent in place before surgery to assess the patency of the airway.[38] Fig. 3.23 shows a tracheal stent in a patient with a mediastinal mass.

Multidetector Computed Tomography Scan of the Chest

Modern MDCT scanners readily provide very large, high-resolution 3D volumetric images of the chest. Many 3D visualization techniques have been devised for more exhaustive viewing of the information contained in 3D MDCT chest images. A 3D MDCT image provides views of the segments of the airway tree, computes the central axes of the extracted airways, and defines the endoluminal and exterior surfaces of the segmented airway tree and the exterior surfaces of the regions of interest for rendering.[39]

One of the advantages of MDCT and 3D reconstruction of the tracheobronchial tree is that it allows us to appreciate distorted tracheobronchial anatomy or changes in the airway with age. Fig. 3.24 shows an MDCT scan of the chest on a male patient.

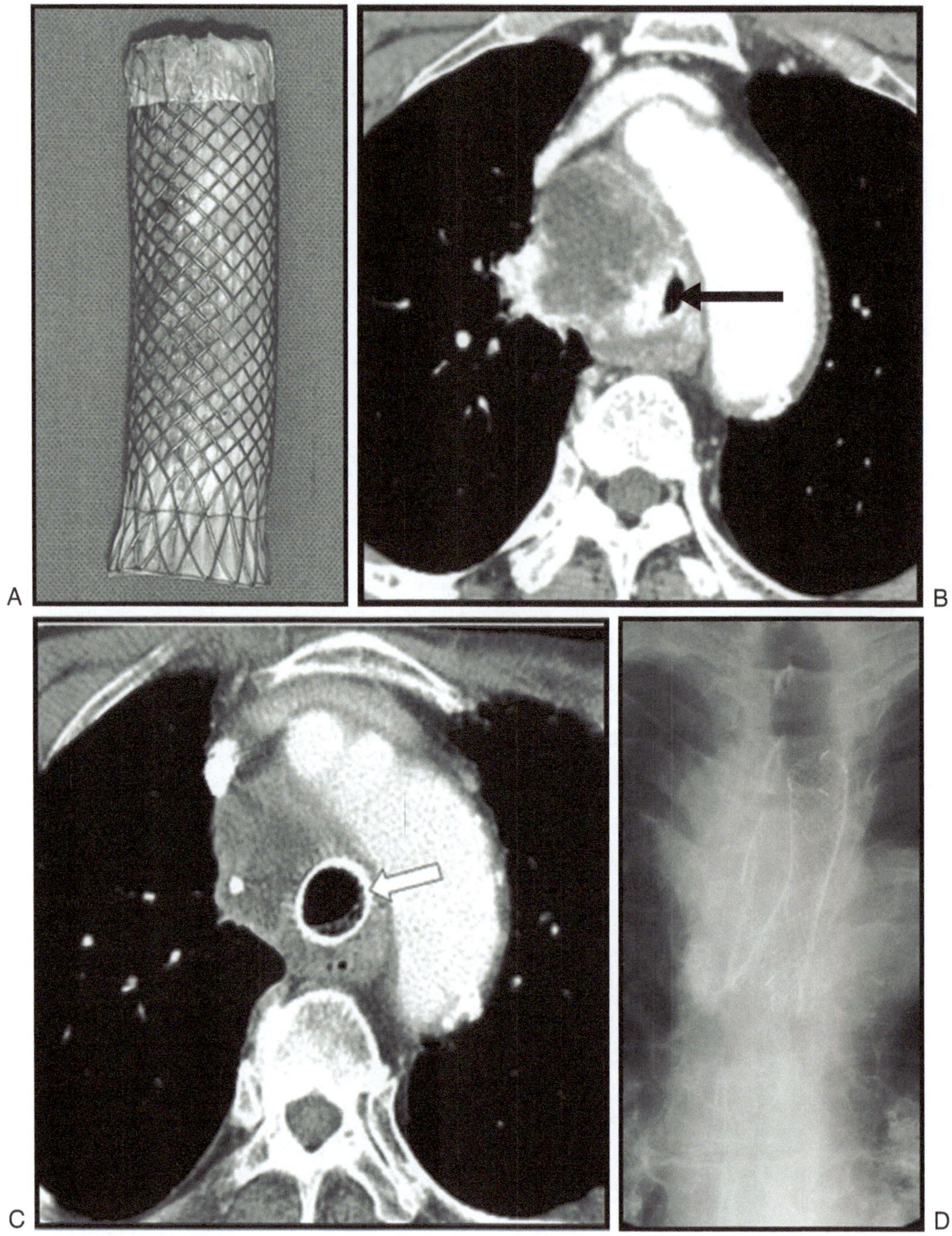

• **Fig. 3.23** Images showing a tracheal stent in a patient with a mediastinal mass. (**A**) Metallic expandable stent; (**B**) computed tomography (CT) scan showing a mediastinal mass compressing the trachea (*arrow*); (**C**) airway stent in place in the trachea (*arrow*) as seen on CT; and (**D**) a chest x-ray showing the stent in place. (From Shin JH, Song HY, Ko GY, et al. Treatment of tracheobronchial obstruction with a polytetrafluoroethylene-covered retrievable expandable nitinol stent. *J Vasc Interv Radiol*. 2006;17:657–663. With permission.)

Magnetic Resonance Imaging and Pulmonary Disease

MRI produces images that superficially appear similar to CT scans. MRI provides greater contrast resolution than CT scans and offers the potential for tissue characterization.[40] In addition, MRI of pulmonary parenchymal disease using a modified breath-hold 3D gradient echo technique allows imaging of a wide spectrum of solid and nonsolid pulmonary parenchymal diseases with reproducible high image quality, effective suppression of artifacts, high resolution, and visualization.[41] The 3D gradient echo technique allows better visualization of the peripheral and central parenchyma, pulmonary arteries, heart, and esophagus.

MRI yields computer-generated images, usually in cross-sectional orientation but also with direct sagittal or coronal views, with tissues displayed in varying shades of black, white, and gray. MRI scans rely primarily on the evaluation of the amount of protons (water) in different tissues. Imaging is performed by placing the patient in a powerful magnetic field and interrogating the body with radio waves of a specific frequency; then listening for the response. By varying the frequency of the radio wave, the body can be imaged in multiple planes, not just in axial sections. Direct sagittal and coronal images enable the radiologist to evaluate involvement of the lung parenchyma,[42] mediastinal structures, and the chest wall with greater clarity than with a CT scan. In addition, MRI is an adjunct to CT scan evaluation for patients for whom CT scans did not resolve the anatomic issues or for whom additional information about a mediastinal mass and its relationship to other vital organs is required, including invasion of the heart or great vessels.[31,43,44] Fig. 3.25 shows MRI scans of the chest in a patient with a mediastinal mass.

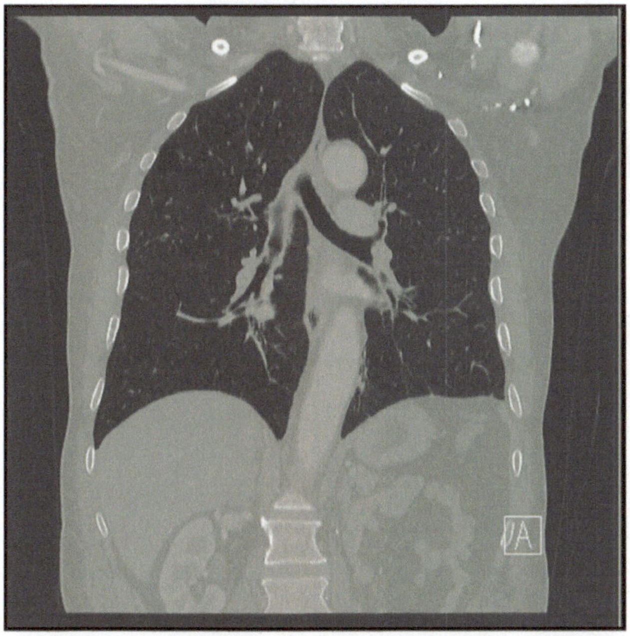

• **Fig. 3.24** Multidetector computed tomography scan of the chest on a male patient.

Thoracic Ultrasound

Ultrasound imaging has become a valuable tool in the assessment and diagnosis of pulmonary conditions, with the benefit of being able to be performed at the patient's bedside in a noninvasive manner and without exposing the patient to any radiation. Ultrasonography has been shown to be fairly sensitive for the detection of pleural effusion, pulmonary parenchymal disease, and pneumothorax. Lichtenstein et al.[45] described two protocols for lung ultrasound scans: bed-side lung ultrasound in emergency (BLUE) for the rapid diagnosis of life-threatening respiratory failure, and the FALLS (fluid administration limited by lung sonograph) protocol.[45] Most protocols suggest imaging of the hemithorax in different zones for a thorough and expedited examination.

The normal anatomy of the pleural cavity consists of two pleural layers: the visceral and the parietal pleura. During normal respiration, these two layers slide over each other, which can be appreciated as lung sliding.[46] The resulting image is commonly described as a line of "marching ants," seen as a line of black and white dots moving to and fro. The absence of lung sliding can occur in cases of pneumothorax,

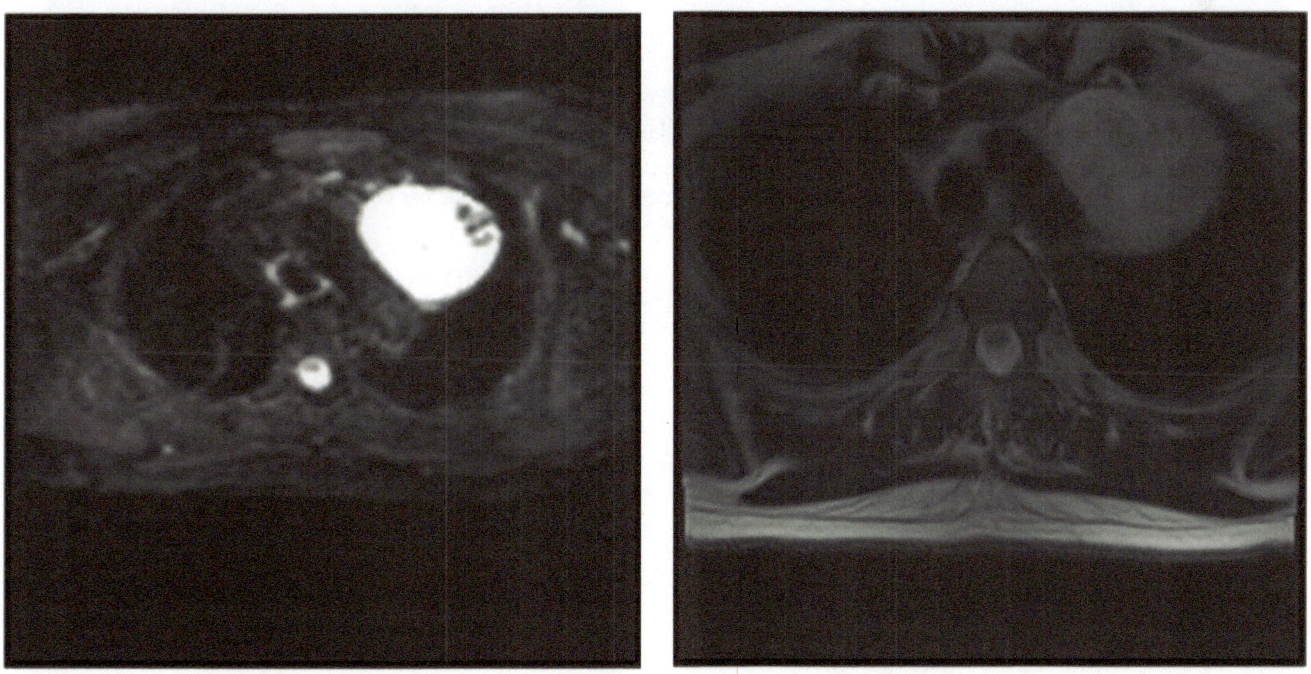

• **Fig. 3.25** Magnetic resonance imaging of the chest in a patient with a mediastinal mass. The patient had a diagnosis of schwannoma.

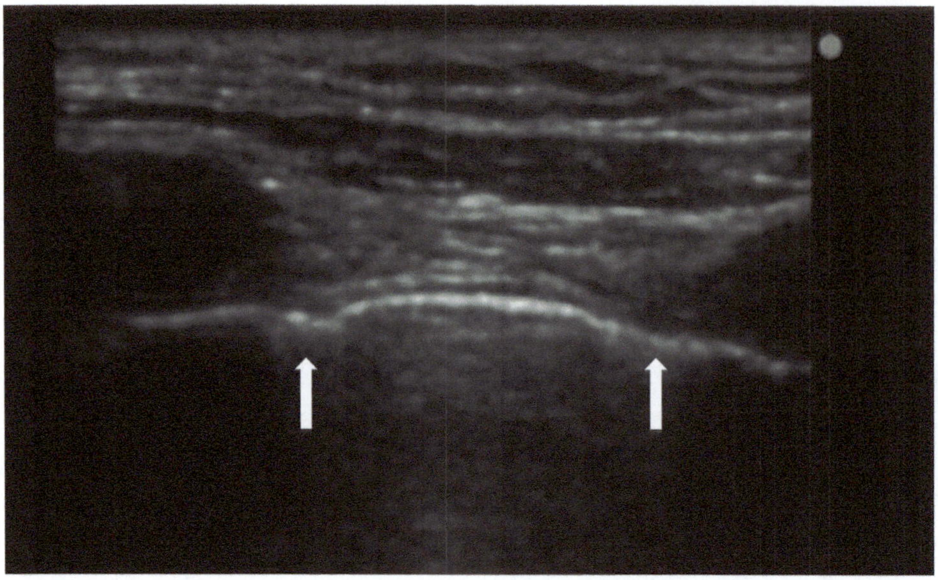

• **Fig. 3.26** Chest Ultrasound: The arrows point to the lung sliding visible at the pleural interface between two ribs.

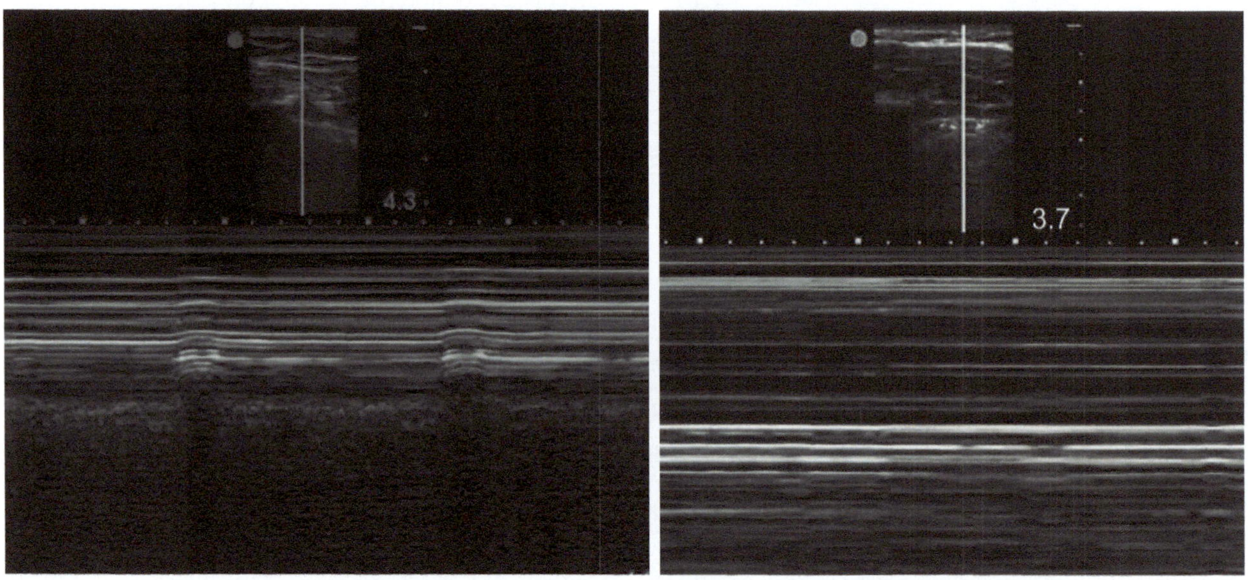

A B

• **Fig. 3.27** Chest ultrasound images demonstrating: (**A**) the **seashore sign**, with an appearance resembling sand and waves, because of the presence of pleural sliding; and (**B**) the **bar-code sign** in the absence of lung sliding after disruption of the pleural surfaces from a pneumothorax.

pleural effusion, pleurectomy/pleurodesis, and endobronchial intubation; all of these conditions prevent sliding between the pleural surfaces. Fig. 3.26 shows the lung sliding visible at the pleural interface between two ribs on the ultrasound image.

The absence of lung sliding is the hallmark for detection of a pneumothorax; motion mode (M-mode) assessment of the change in pleural movement is commonly used for diagnosis. Ultrasonography has a higher sensitivity than chest radiography for the detection of a pneumothorax.[47] A pneumothorax causes air entry between the two pleural layers, causing the absence of pleural sliding (Fig. 3.27). This absence of sliding creates a series of black and white horizontal lines on ultrasound images, called the "barcode sign" or "stratospheric sign." A normal lung with intact pleural sliding exhibits the "seashore sign", whereby pleural sliding gives the appearance of sand and subcutaneous tissues give the appearance of the sea/waves. Fig. 3.27 shows chest ultrasound images demonstrating the seashore sign and the barcode sign.

A-lines (Fig. 3.28A) are multiple horizontal, equidistant lines visible below the pleural line and depict reverberation artefacts in a normal lung when the ultrasound beam interacts with the pleural surface. B-lines (Fig. 3.28B) are hyperechoic reverberation artefacts formed because of the presence of fluid in the interstitial space. Unlike A-lines, they are vertical in nature, start at the pleural line, and span the entire depth of the image, giving the

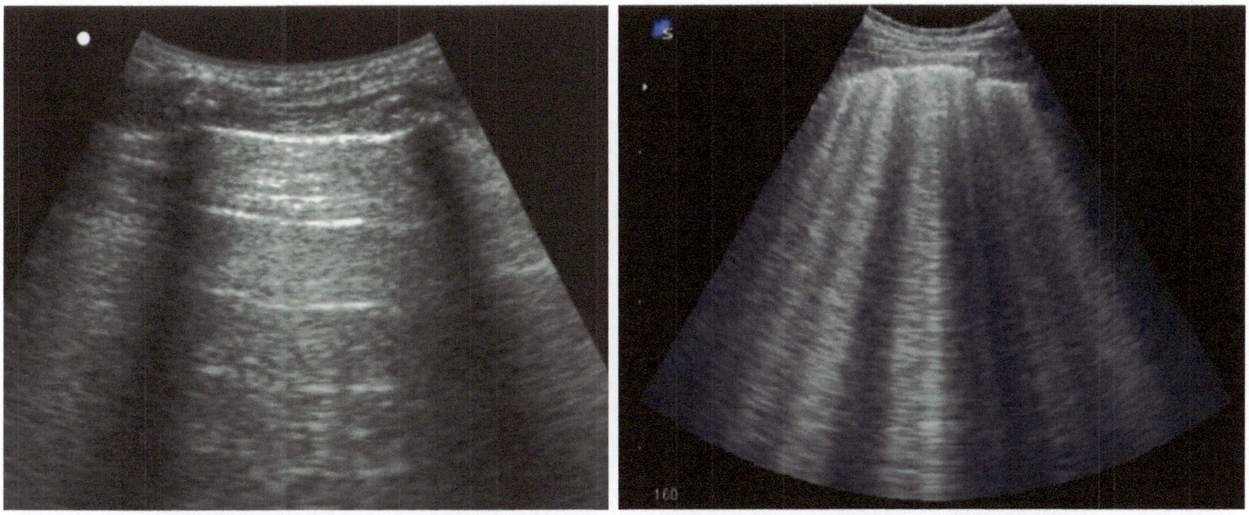
A B

• **Fig. 3.28** Pulmonary ultrasound images depicting: (**A**) **A-lines**, which are parallel, equidistant, and horizontal and depict normal lung; and (**B**) **B-lines**, which are vertical, give the appearance of a *comet tail*, and depict pulmonary edema.

appearance of "comet tails" or "lung rockets." The presence of more than three B-lines in more than two zones per anatomic side defines the diagnosis of pulmonary interstitial syndrome and increased fluid content in the lung interstitium.[48] Fig. 3.28 shows pulmonary ultrasound images depicting: (1) A-lines, which are parallel, equidistant and horizontal and depict normal lung; and (2) B-lines, which are vertical, give the appearance of a comet tail, and depict pulmonary edema.

Ultrasound is a highly sensitive tool for detecting the presence of pleural effusion and is able to detect as little as 5 to 15 mL of fluid in the pleural space, compared with a chest radiograph, which requires at least 250 mL of fluid to obliterate the costophrenic angle.[49] In a supine patient, ultrasound examination should be performed in the middle or posterior axillary line to view the interface between the diaphragm and the lung. Because fluid gravitates to the bottom, the examination should preferably be performed in the dependent part of the lung. Fig. 3.29 depicts the different structures that are visualized on ultrasound examination; part of the lung is also visible through the fluid.

Thoracic and lung ultrasound is very useful in the diagnosis and management of patients with hypoxia. It has distinct advantages over chest radiography, given its ease of access, mobility, rapidity, reproducibility, and lack of radiation. It does remain operator dependent, and a structured formation, such as the one proposed by the American College of Chest Physicians, is needed.[49] In addition, transthoracic ultrasound for diagnosis of pneumothorax is now feasible in the intraoperative period.[50,51]

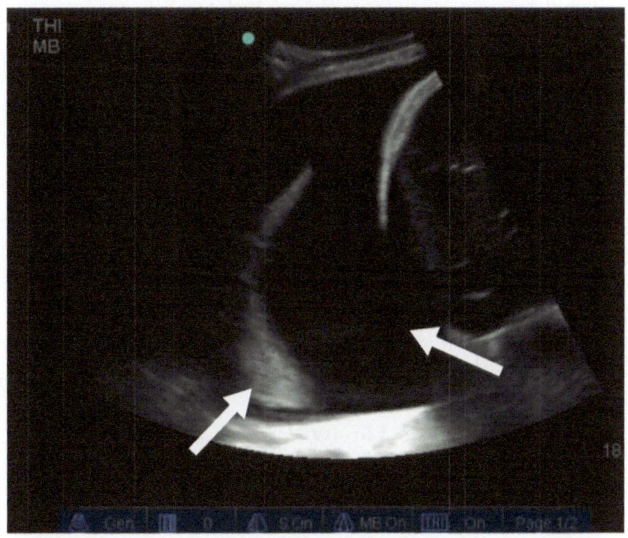

• **Fig. 3.29** Right upper quadrant ultrasound examination, depicting a large pleural effusion above the diaphragm (*right arrow*). The collapsed lung visible on the left (*left arrow*).

Conclusion

Radiologic studies play an important role in the diagnosis and treatment of candidates for thoracic surgery. Chest radiographs can identify distorted tracheobronchial anatomy, and the presence of lung masses or lung collapse, can aid in the placement of chest tobes and endotracheal tubes, and can reveal lung expansion or shifting of the mediastinum in cases of tension pneumothorax. CT scans of the chest permit identification and precise location of lung masses, mediastinal masses, or the presence of fluid and compromised adjacent structures, as well as the precise location of airway stents.[52]

MDCT imaging and 3D reconstruction allow identification of the tracheobronchial anatomy in a more precise form. All radiologic studies must be reviewed during preoperative evaluation of thoracic surgical patients. In cases where the diagnosis or anatomy is unclear, these studies must be reviewed in conjunction with a thoracic surgeon or a radiologist.[53]

References

1. Campos J, Parekh KR. Thoracic imaging. In: Slinger P, ed. *Principles and Practice of Anesthesia for Thoracic Surgery.* 2nd edition Cham: Springer 2019:43–61.
2. Boiselle PM. Imaging of the large airways. *Clin Chest Med.* 2008; 29:181–189.
3. Seymour AH. The relationship between the diameters of the adult cricoid ring and main tracheobronchial tree: a cadaver study to investigate the basis for double-lumen tube selection. *J Cardiothorac Vasc Anesth.* 2003;17:299–301.
4. Minnich DJ, Mathisen DJ. Anatomy of the trachea, carina and bronchi. *Thorac Surg Clin.* 2007;17:571–585.
5. Stene R, Rose M, Weigner MB, et al. Bronchial trifurcation at the carina complicating use of a double-lumen tracheal tube. *Anesthesiology.* 1994;80:1162–1164.
6. Campos JH. Update on tracheobronchial anatomy and flexible fiberoptic bronchoscopy in thoracic anesthesia. *Curr Opin Anaesthesiol.* 2009;22:4–10.
7. Goldwin RL, Reed JC. Radiology of the chest. In: Kaplan J, Slinger P, eds. *Thoracic Anesthesia.* 3rd ed. New York: Churchill Livingstone; 2003:24–56.
8. Fraser RS, Pare' JA, Fraser RG, et al. *Synopsis of Diseases of the Chest.* 2nd ed. Philadelphia: WB Saunders; 1994.
9. Datt V, Tempe DK. Airway management in patients with mediastinal masses. *Indian J Anaesth.* 2005;49:344–352.
10. Ahmed-Nusrath A, Swanevelder J. Anesthesia for mediastinoscopy. *Contin Educ Anaesth Crit Care Pain.* 2007;7:6–9.
11. Campos JH. Managing the patient with an anterior mediastinal mass. In: Cohen NH, ed. *Medically Challenging Patients Undergoing Cardiothoracic Surgery.* Baltimore: Lippincott Williams & Wilkins; 2009:285–302.
12. Harris GJ, Harman PK, Trinkle JK, et al. Standard biplane roentgenography is highly sensitive in documenting mediastinal masses. *Ann Thorac Surg.* 1987;44:238–241.
13. Morgan MDL, Edward CW, Morris J, et al. Origin and behavior of emphysematous bullae. *Thorax.* 1989;44:533–538.
14. Schipper PH, Meyers BF, Battafarano RJ, et al. Outcomes after resection of giant emphysematous bullae. *Ann Thorac Surg.* 2004; 78:976–982.
15. O'Connor AR, Morgan WE. Radiological review of pneumothorax. *BMJ.* 2005;330:1493–1497.
16. Glazer H, Anderson DJ, Wilson BS, et al. Pneumothorax: appearances on lateral chest radiographs. *Radiology.* 1989;173:707–711.
17. Henry M, Arnold T, Harvey J. BTS guidelines for the management of spontaneous pneumothorax. *Thorax.* 2003;58 (suppl 2): ii39–ii52.
18. Light RW. Tension pneumothorax. *Intens Care Med.* 1994;20: 468–469.
19. Baumann MH, Sahn SA. Tension pneumothorax: diagnostic and therapeutic pitfalls. *Crit Care Med.* 1994;22:896.
20. Symbas PN. Chest drainage tubes. *Surg Clin North Am.* 1989; 69:41–46.
21. Baldt MM, Bankier AA, Germann PS, et al. Complications after emergency tube thoracostomy: assessment with CT. *Radiology.* 1995;195:534–539.
22. Maunder RJ, Pierson DJ, Hudson LD. Subcutaneous and mediastinal emphysema. Pathophysiology, diagnosis, and management. *Arch Intern Med.* 1984;144:1447–1455.
23. Konen E, Rozenman J, Simansky DA, et al. Prevalence of the juxtaphrenic peak after upper lobectomy. *Am J Roentgenol.* 2001; 177:869–877.
24. Wechsler RJ, Goodman LR. Mediastinal position and air-fluid height after pneumonectomy: the effect of the respiratory cycle. *Am J Roentgenol.* 1985;145:1173–1176.
25. Brodsky JB, Macario A, Mark JB. Tracheal diameter predicts double-lumen tube size: a method for selecting left double-lumen tubes. *Anesth Analg.* 1996;82:861–864.
26. Licker M, de Perrot M, Spiliopoulos A, et al. Risk factors for acute lung injury after thoracic surgery for lung cancer. *Anesth Analg.* 2003;97:1558–1565.
27. Hayes JP, Williams EA, Goldstraw P, et al. Lung injury in patients following thoracotomy. *Thorax.* 1995;50:990–991.
28. McLoud T. Imaging the lungs. In: Patterson AG, Cooper JD, Deslauriers J, et al., eds. *Pearson's Thoracic and Esophageal Surgery.* 3rd ed. New York: Churchill Livingstone; 2008:415–428.
29. Harte BH, Jaklitsch MT, McKenna SS, et al. Use of a modified single-lumen endobronchial tube in severe tracheobronchial compression. *Anesthesiology.* 2002;96:510–511.
30. Slinger P, Karsli C. Management of the patient with a large anterior mediastinal mass: recurring myths. *Curr Opin Anaesthesiol.* 2007;20:1–3.
31. Chiles C, Woodard PK, Gutierrez FR, et al. Metastatic involvement of the heart and pericardium: CT and MR imaging. *Radiographics.* 2001;21:439–449.
32. Shepard JA, Grillo HC, McLoud TC, et al. Right-pneumonectomy syndrome: radiologic findings and CT correlation. *Radiology.* 1986;161:661–664.
33. Le Guen M, Beigelman C, Bouhemad B, et al. Chest computed tomography with multiplanar reformatted images for diagnosing traumatic bronchial rupture: a case report. *Crit Care.* 2007;11:1–8.
34. Rubin GD, Beaulieu CF, Argiro V, et al. Perspective volume rendering of CT and MR images: applications for endoscopic imaging. *Radiology.* 1996;199:321–330.
35. Boiselle PM, Reynolds KF, Ernst A. Multiplanar and three-dimensional imaging of the central airways with multidetector CT. *Am J Roentgenol.* 2002;179:301–308.
36. Higgins WE, Ramaswamy K, Swift RD, et al. Virtual bronchoscopy for three-dimensional pulmonary image assessment: state of the art and future needs. *Radiographics.* 1998;18:761–778.
37. Laroia AT, Thompson BH, Laroia ST, et al. Modern imaging of the tracheo-bronchial tree. *World J Radiol.* 2010;2:237–248.
38. Shin JH, Song HY, Ko GY, et al. Treatment of tracheobronchial obstruction with a polytetrafluoroethylene-covered retrievable expandable nitinol stent. *J Vasc Interv Radiol.* 2006;17:657–663.
39. Higgins WE, Helferty JP, Lu K, et al. 3D CT-video fusion for image-guided bronchoscopy. *Comput Med Imaging Graph.* 2008; 32:157–159.
40. Moore EH, Webb WR, Muller N, et al. MRI of pulmonary airspace disease: experimental model and preliminary clinical results. *Am J Roentgenol.* 1986;146:1123–1128.
41. Bader TR, Semelka RC, Pedro MS, et al. Magnetic resonance imaging of pulmonary parenchymal disease using a modified breath-hold 3D gradient-echo technique: initial observations. *J Magn Reson Imaging.* 2002;15:31–38.
42. Bergin CJ, Glover GH, Pauly JM. Lung parenchyma: magnetic susceptibility in MR imaging. *Radiology.* 1991;180:845–848.

43. Bremerich J, Roberts TP, Wendland MF, et al. Three-dimensional MR imaging of pulmonary vessels and parenchyma with NC100150 injection (Clariscan). *J Magn Reson Imaging*. 2000;11: 622–628.
44. Bittner RC, Felix R. Magnetic resonance (RM) imaging of the chest: state-of-the-art. *Eur Respir J*. 1998;11:1392–1404.
45. Lichtenstein DA. BLUE-protocol and FALLS-protocol: two applications of lung ultrasound in the critically ill. *Chest*. 2005; 147:1659–1670.
46. Lichtenstein DA, Menu Y. A bedside ultrasound sign ruling out pneumothorax in the critically ill: lung sliding. *Chest*. 1995;108:1345–1348.
47. Soldati G, Testa A, Sher S, et al. Occult traumatic pneumothorax: diagnostic accuracy of lung ultrasonography in the emergency department. *Chest*. 2008;133:204–211.
48. Capper SJ, Ross JJ, Sandström E, et al. Transoesophageal echocardiography for the detection and quantification of pleural fluid in cardiac surgical patients. *Br J Anaesth*. 2007;98: 442–446.
49. Mayo PH, Beaulieu Y, Doelken P, et al. American College of Chest Physicians/La Societe de Reanimation de Langue Francaise statement on competence in critical care ultrasonography. *Chest*. 2009;135:1050–1060.
50. Ueda K, Ahmed W, Ross AF. Intraoperative pneumothorax identified with transthoracic ultrasound. *Anesthesiology*. 2011;115:653–655.
51. Krishnan S, Kuhl T, Ahmed W, et al. Efficacy of an online education program for ultrasound diagnosis of pneumothorax. *Anesthesiology*. 2013;118:715–721.
52. Marchese R, Poidomani G, Paglino G, et al. Fully covered self-expandable metal stent in tracheobronchial disorders: clinical experience. *Respiration*. 2015;89:49–56.
53. Campos J, Parekh KR. Thoracic imaging. In: Slinger P, ed. *Principles and Practice of Anesthesia for Thoracic Surgery.* 1st edition. Cham: Springer; 2011:35–48.

NON-PRINT ITEMS

Abstract

Radiologic images play an important role during evaluation of patients undergoing thoracic surgery. Radiologic studies must be reviewed, including a posterior-anterior chest radiograph and computed tomography (CT) scan of the chest. There should be a special emphasis on reviewing CT scans for the presence of a mediastinal mass that compromises the airway or great vessels. Multidetector CT imaging and tracheobronchial reconstruction are more specific studies that allow measurements of the airway. Magnetic resonance imaging (MRI) provides greater contrast resolution than CT scans and offers the potential for tissue characterization. MRI is indicated in cases with a mediastinal mass with invasion of the superior vena cava.

Keywords

trachea bifurcation, chest radiograph, ultrasonography, mediastinal mass, computed tomography scan

4

Intrathoracic Tumors: Current Status and Classification

DONG-SEOK LEE, RAJA FLORES

Introduction

Thoracic oncology encompasses a large spectrum of diseases. Between the various anatomic spaces and the different organ systems, there are a large variety of benign and malignant tumors that can develop within the chest. This chapter will focus primarily on the surgical management of the most commonly encountered thoracic malignancies.

General Diagnostic Principles

Aside from a thorough history and examination, certain radiographic studies are essential tools for the thoracic surgeon. A standard chest x-ray provides a good overview—it can show larger lesions and may even show sequelae of smaller lesions such as effusions or postobstructive atelectasis. Different projections can offer additional information. Computed tomography (CT) enables visualization of smaller lesions and helps determine size, location, depth, and relation to other structures. Magnetic resonance imaging (MRI) is limited to assessing neural involvement or differentiating mediastinal structures; it does not usually offer more information than a CT. It is more often used for the evaluation of brain metastases. Positron emission tomography (PET) has become the standard for staging thoracic malignancies because it is more accurate than conventional imaging in detecting metastatic disease.[1]

Lung Cancer

Tumors within the lung parenchyma may arise from primary lung etiologies or because of metastatic disease. The focus of this section will remain on primary lung cancers, for which nonsmall cell and small cell cancers account for over 90%. Smoking remains the single most important risk factor for the development of lung cancer, increasing risk 20-fold compared with nonsmokers. Other risk factors include radiation, other environmental toxins, and pulmonary fibrosis that have synergistic effects.[2]

Most patients are asymptomatic and develop symptoms once locally advanced or metastatic disease is present. Typical symptoms can include cough, hemoptysis, chest pain, or dyspnea. Involvement of local structures can result in specific symptoms, such as hoarseness (because of recurrent laryngeal nerve invasion), superior vena cava (SVC) syndrome (facial and upper extremity swelling because of SVC obstruction), and Pancoast syndrome (shoulder pain and Horner syndrome because of superior sulcus tumor invasion).

CT imaging has revolutionized the detection of lung cancer, allowing the discovery of smaller tumors and, consequently, enabling the treatment of earlier stage disease. The International Early Lung Cancer Action Program showed that 85% of patients diagnosed with lung cancer during screening were clinical stage I disease, and that those patients who underwent surgical resection within 1 month of diagnosis had an estimated 10-year survival of 92%.[3] As a result, lung cancer screening has been deemed essential in the diagnosis and treatment of lung cancers such that it is recommended for patients aged 55 to 80 years with a 30-pack-year smoking history by the U.S. Preventive Services Task Force.

Diagnosis can only be confirmed with a tissue biopsy. Surgical biopsy has historically been performed, but, in more recent times, an initial biopsy is performed less invasively with a needle via either a transbronchial or transthoracic approach. Once a malignant diagnosis is obtained, decision on appropriate therapy is driven by the clinical stage. Lung cancer staging is based on the tumor node metastasis (TNM) classification (Table 4.1). In addition to PET imaging and MRI when clinically indicated to evaluate the presence of tumor spread, mediastinal staging may be necessary. This has classically been achieved with mediastinoscopy, but endobronchial ultrasound has seen increased utilization because of its less invasiveness and its ability to assess N1 nodes as well.

Surgery offers the best chance for cure in patients with resectable nonsmall cell lung cancer. For patients who are not surgical candidates or who refuse surgery, local therapy such as stereotactic body radiation therapy can be offered. It is important to differentiate between operability and resectability. Operability refers to the patient's comorbidities and ability to

TABLE 4.1 Lung Cancer Staging Tumor Node Metastasis Classification (8th Edition)

4.1A
T/N/M Classification

T (Primary Tumor)	
T0	No primary tumor
Tis	Carcinoma in situ (squamous or adenocarcinoma)
T1	Tumor ≤3 cm
T1mi	Minimally invasive adenocarcinoma
T1a	Superficial spreading tumor in central airways[a]
T1a	Tumor ≤1 cm
T1b	Tumor >1 but ≤2 cm
T1c	Tumor >2 but ≤3 cm
T2	Tumor >3 but ≤5 cm or tumor involving: visceral pleura,[b] main bronchus (not carina), atelectasis to hilum[b]
T2a	Tumor >3 but ≤4 cm
T2b	Tumor >4 but ≤5 cm
T3	Tumor >5 but ≤7 cm or invading chest wall, pericardium, phrenic nerve; or separate tumor nodule(s) in the same lobe
T4	Tumor >7 cm or tumor invading: mediastinum, diaphragm, heart, great vessels, recurrent laryngeal nerve, carina, trachea, esophagus, spine; or tumor nodule(s) in a different ipsilateral lobe
N (Regional Lymph Nodes)	
N0	No regional node metastasis
N1	Metastasis in ipsilateral pulmonary or hilar nodes
N2	Metastasis in ipsilateral mediastinal or subcarinal nodes
N3	Metastasis in contralateral mediastinal, hilar, or supraclavicular nodes
M (Distant Metastasis)	
M0	No distant metastasis
M1a	Malignant pleural or pericardial effusion‡ or pleural or pericardial nodules or separate tumor nodule(s) in a contralateral lobe
M1b	Single extrathoracic metastasis
M1c	Multiple extrathoracic metastases (1 or >1 organ)

4.1B
Subcategories

T/M	Subcategory	N0	N1	N2	N3
T1	T1a	IA1	IIB	IIIA	IIIB
	T1b	IA2	IIB	IIIA	IIIB
	T1c	IA3	IIB	IIIA	IIIB
T2	T2a	IB	IIB	IIIA	IIIB
	T2b	IIA	IIB	IIIA	IIIB
T3	T3	IIB	IIIA	IIIB	IIIC
T4	T4	IIIA	IIIA	IIIB	IIIC
M1	M1a	IVA	IVA	IVA	IVA
	M1b	IVA	IVA	IVA	IVA
	M1c	IVB	IVB	IVB	IVB

[a]Superficial spreading tumor of any size but confined to the tracheal or bronchial wall. ‡Atelectasis or obstructive pneumonitis extending to hilum; such tumors are classified as T2a if >3 and ≤4 cm, T2b if >4 and ≤5 cm.

[b]Pleural effusions are excluded that are cytologically negative, nonbloody, transudative, and clinically judged not to be because of cancer.

From Detterbeck FC. The eighth edition TNM stage classification for lung cancer: what does it mean on main street? *J Thorac Cardiovasc Surg*. 2018;155(1):356–359.

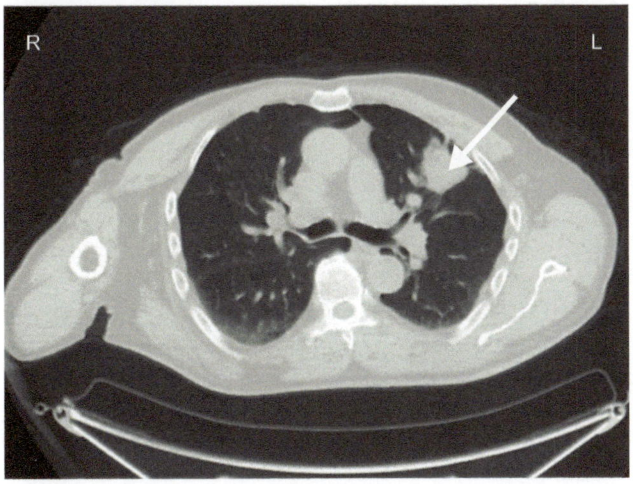

• **Fig. 4.1** A 70-year-old male with 3-cm left upper lobe mass. He underwent left upper lobectomy. Pathology was a 4-cm T2aN0 adenosquamous carcinoma.

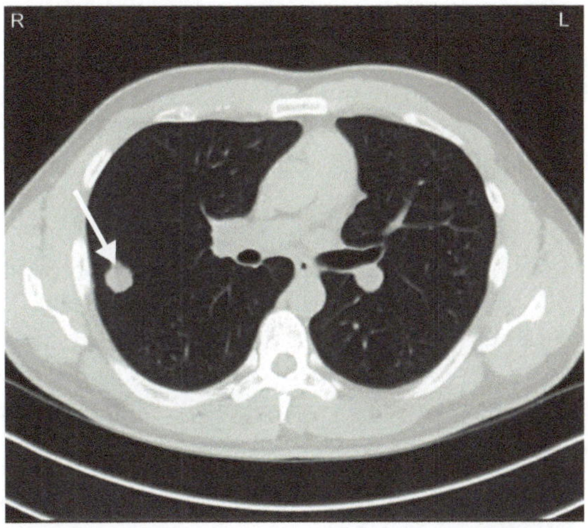

• **Fig. 4.2** A 37-year-old male with a 2-cm right upper lobe mass. He underwent video-assisted thoracoscopic surgery right upper lobe posterior segmentectomy. Pathology was a 1.7-cm pT1bN0 adenocarcinoma.

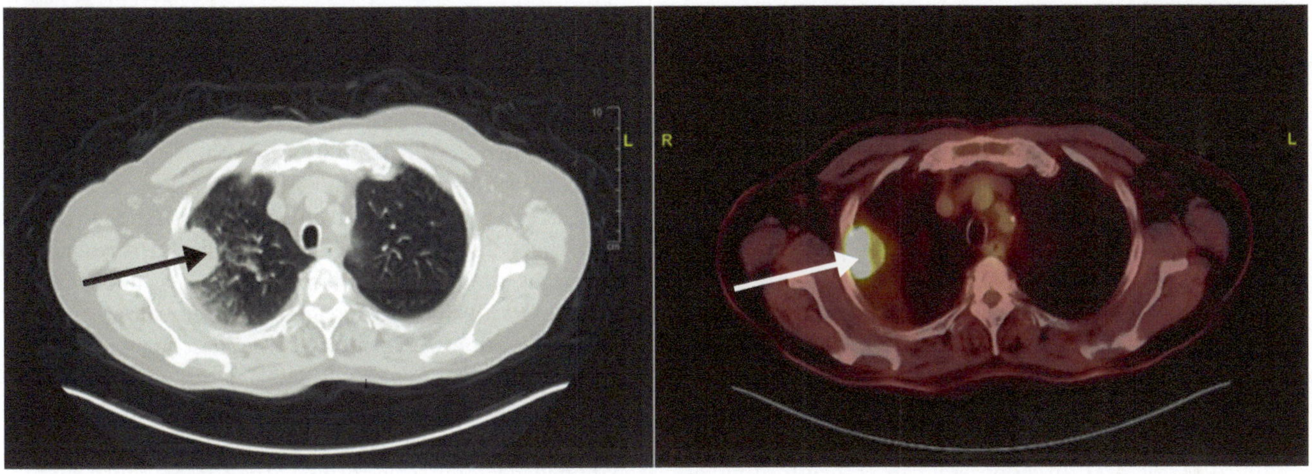

• **Fig. 4.3** A CT scan of a 73 years-old male (left) with hypermetabolic 4.2 cm right upper lobe on PET scan (right). Chest wall invasion was noted, and he underwent right upper lobectomy with chest wall resection and reconstruction. Pathology was a 7-cm T3N0 pleomorphic carcinoma.

undergo surgery. Resectability refers to the extent of parenchymal resection required and the patient's ability to tolerate it in light of their pulmonary functional status. For example, the patient may have a relatively small cancer centrally located such that a pneumonectomy would be required, but the patient would only be able to tolerate a lobectomy.

Clinical stage 1 and stage 2 cancers should proceed directly to surgery. Stage 3 cancers encompass a wide spectrum. N3 disease stage 3 cancers are not surgical candidates. A multidisciplinary approach is the best strategy for non-N3 disease stage 3 cancers and treatment can range from prompt surgery to induction therapy, followed by surgery to definitive chemotherapy with or without radiation therapy. Induction therapy may consist of either chemotherapy alone or chemoradiation therapy and is usually determined by institutional or surgeon practices. There are currently investigations in the role of immunotherapy into the neoadjuvant setting. Pembrolizumab (KEYTRUDA) recently approved by the FDA, is a sample of a drug that presumably stimulates the immune system to attack the cancer cells. Stage 4 cancers are referred for systemic therapy, and surgery is reserved for palliation of symptoms.

Once the decision to proceed with surgery has been made, the extent of resection and surgical approach must be considered. Lobectomy has been considered the gold standard technique for resection. The Lung Cancer Study Group reported increased locoregional recurrence rate and a trend toward decreased survival with limited resection versus lobectomy in 1995[4] (Fig. 4.1). However, with the advent of lung cancer screening and the discovery of smaller cancers, this is being challenged, as more recent studies suggest no significant differences in recurrence rates and overall survival.[5] The authors consider performing a sublobar resections in patients with small (<2 cm), anatomically feasible cancers with low standardized uptake value (Fig. 4.2). Extended resections may be required in the setting of locally advanced disease, such as chest wall invasion (Fig. 4.3) or invasion of the great vessels.

Thoracotomy is the standard approach for lung resection. However, minimally invasive techniques such as video-assisted thoracoscopic surgery (VATS) and robotic surgery are increasingly being used. Minimally invasive surgery offers short-term benefits, such as less pain, shorter hospital stays, and fewer complications.[6,7] VATS also appears to offer improved long-term outcomes.[8]

Morbidity after lung cancer surgery is approximately 35%,[9,10] with the risk of major adverse events 9.1%.[11] Cardiac and pulmonary events are the predominant complications seen. Several risk models have been developed to try to predict perioperative risk for patients.[12] Perioperative mortality is 1.5% to 2.5%.

Esophageal Cancer

Esophageal cancer is the most common primary esophageal malignancy. Squamous cell carcinoma is more prevalent worldwide, with its strong association with smoking and alcohol, but adenocarcinoma is more common in the United States, with the rise of obesity, gastroesophageal reflux disease, and Barrett metaplasia. Because the esophagus traverses through three anatomic domains—the neck, chest, and abdomen—determining the location of the cancer is essential in guiding treatment. Cervical esophageal cancers are primarily treated with chemotherapy and radiation. Middle and lower esophageal cancers are offered multimodality therapy consisting of surgery, chemotherapy, and radiation.

Patients commonly present with dysphagia and weight loss. Diagnosis is obtained with endoscopy. Direct visualization provides information, such as size and location of the mass, and tissue diagnosis is obtained with biopsy forceps. Once the diagnosis is confirmed, clinical stage must be determined (Table 4.2). In esophageal cancer, depth of radial invasion is more important than size in staging. Therefore determining T and N staging is best achieved with endoscopic ultrasound (EUS). Tissue biopsy via ultrasound-guided fine needle aspiration (FNA) can also be performed on suspicious lymph nodes. EUS and EUS-FNA have high sensitivity and specificity in accurately diagnosing T stage and N stage, respectively.[13] However, T2 lesions remain notoriously challenging with an accuracy of approximately 30% because both tumor upstaging and downstaging can occur[14] (Fig. 4.4). Bronchoscopy may be necessary to rule out airway invasion.

Small cancers limited to the mucosa (T1a) can be treated with endomucosal resection, but surgical resection remains the standard therapy for early stage esophageal cancer. Patients with clinical T1 cancers should proceed directly to surgery. Given the level of uncertainty regarding T2 lesions on EUS, it is reasonable to proceed with either surgery or induction therapy for clinical T2 cancers. The authors prefer to proceed directly to surgery. More locally advanced resectable cancers should undergo neoadjuvant chemoradiotherapy with carboplatin and paclitaxel and 41 Gy of radiation, as the Dutch ChemoRadiotherapy for Oesophageal cancer followed by Surgery Study (CROSS) trial showed improved complete resection rates and overall survival with induction therapy. The authors randomly assigned patients with resectable tumors to receive surgery alone or weekly administration of carboplatin and paclitaxel for 5 weeks, followed by surgery. They prospectively enrolled a total of 366 patients, 178 were randomly assigned to chemoradiotherapy followed by surgery, and 188 to surgery alone. Complete resection with no tumor within 1 mm of the resection margins (R0) was achieved in 92% of patients in the chemoradiotherapy-surgery group versus 69% in the surgery group ($P < .001$). Overall survival was significantly better in the chemoradiotherapy-surgery group.[15]

Surgical oncologic principles dictate R0 resection with adequate margins over 10 cm and locoregional clearance of metastatic lymph nodes. Surgeon preference, tumor location, patient factors, and ability to adhere to oncologic principles determine the type of approach. Mid- and distal esophageal cancers can be resected via total thoracic esophagectomy with the creation of a neck anastomosis. This is achieved with either a triincisional (McKeown) approach or a transhiatal approach. Distal esophageal cancers can be resected via partial thoracic esophagectomy with the creation of an intrathoracic anastomosis. The neoesophagus is typically recreated using the stomach as the first choice for the conduit but the colon or jejunum may also be used if the stomach is unusable.

McKeown esophagectomy begins in the left lateral decubitus position. A thoractomy is performed, and the right chest is entered in the fifth intercostal space. The inferior pulmonary ligament and the azygos vein are divided. The esophagus is then mobilized from the thoracic inlet down to the hiatus with all periesophageal tissue. A regional thoracic lymphadenectomy is performed. The chest is closed, and the patient placed supine. A midline laparotomy is performed and the stomach is mobilized in its entirety, taking care to preserve the gastroepiploic vessels. A regional abdominal lymphadenectomy is performed. The authors routinely perform a pyloroplasty as a gastric drainage procedure, and the stomach is tubularized into a conduit. A feeding jejeunostomy tube is placed for nutrition. A left cervical incision is then made and dissected down to the esophagus. Once the cervical esophagus is mobilized, the thoracic esophagus and the tubularized stomach is pulled up into the neck. The esophagus is resected and a hand-sewn anastomosis is performed between the cervical esophagus and the stomach.

Transhiatal esophagectomy allows for the resection of the thoracic esophagus without the morbidity of a thoracotomy. This is achieved by performing a laparotomy and a left cervical neck incision and mobilizing the esophagus bluntly by finger dissection from the neck and abdomen. Therefore this may be more advantageous for surgical candidates who are frailer and less likely to tolerate single lung ventilation. However, the main disadvantage of this technique is the inability to perform regional lymphadenectomy, which may be of some prognostic value.

The conventional less invasive **Ivor Lewis esophagectomy** consists of a laparotomy and a right thoracotomy for esophageal resection, followed by an intrathoracic anastomosis of the gastric conduit, with the proximal esophagus at the level of the proximal mediastinum.

TABLE 4.2 Esophageal Cancer Staging TNM Classification (8th Edition)

4.2A Category	Criteria
T category	
TX	Tumor cannot be assessed
T0	No evidence of primary tumor
Tis	High-grade dysplasia, defined as malignant cells confined by the basement membrane
T1	Tumor invades the lamina propria, muscularis mucosae, or submucosa
T1a[a]	Tumor invades the lamina propria or muscularis mucosae
T1b[a]	Tumor invades the submucosa
T2	Tumor invades the muscularis propria
T3	Tumor invades adventitia
T4	Tumor invades adjacent structures
T4a[a]	Tumor invades the pleura, pericardium, azygos vein, diaphragm, or peritoneum
T4b[a]	Tumor invades other adjacent structures, such as aorta, vertebral body, or trachea
N category	
NX	Regional lymph nodes cannot be assessed
N0	No regional lymph node metastasis
N1	Metastasis in 1–2 regional lymph nodes
N2	Metastasis in 3–6 regional lymph nodes
N3	Metastasis in 7 or more regional lymph nodes
M category	
M0	No distant metastasis
M1	Distant metastasis
Adenocarcinoma G Category	
GX	Differentiation cannot be assessed
G1	Well differentiated, >95% of tumor is composed of well-formed glands
G2	Moderately differentiated, 50% to 95% of tumor shows gland formation
G3[b]	Poorly differentiated. Tumors composed of nest and sheets of cells with <50% of tumor demonstrating glandular formation.
Squamous cell carcinoma G category	
GX	Differentiation cannot be assessed
G1	Well differentiated. Prominent keratinization with pearl formation and a minor component of nonkeratinizing basal-like cells. Tumor cells are arranged in sheets, and mitotic counts are low.
G2	Moderately differentiated. Variable histologic features, ranging from parakeratotic to poorly keratinizing lesions. In general, pearl formation is absent.
G3[c]	Poorly differentiated. Consist predominantly of basal-like cells forming large and small nests with frequent central necrosis. The nests consist of sheets or pavement-like arrangements of tumor cells, and occasionally are punctuated by small numbers of parakeratotic or keratinizing cells.
Squamous cell carcinoma L category[d]	
LX	Location unknown
Upper	Cervical esophagus to lower border of azygos vein
Middle	Lower border of azygos vein to lower border of inferior pulmonary vein
Lower	Lower border of inferior pulmonary vein to stomach, including esophagogastric junction

Continued

TABLE 4.2 Esophageal Cancer Staging TNM Classification (8th Edition) (*Continued*)

4.2B

cStage Group	cT	cN	cM
Squamous cell carcinoma			
0	Tis	N0	M0
I	T1	N0-1	M0
II	T2	N0-1	M0
	T3	N0	M0
III	T3	N1	M0
	T1–3	N2	M0
IVA	T4	N0–2	M0
	T1–4	N3	M0
IVB	T1–4	N0–3	M1
Adenocarcinoma			
0	Tis	N0	M0
I	T1	N0	M0
IIA	T1	N1	M0
IIB	T2	N0	M0
III	T2	N1	M0
	T3–4a	N0–1	M0
IVA	T1–4a	N2	M0
	T4b	N0–2	M0
	T1–4	N3	M0
IVB	T1–4	N0–3	M1

[a]Subcategories.
[b]If further testing of "undifferentiated" cancers reveals glandular components, categorize as adenocarcinoma G3.
[c]If further testing of "undifferentiated" cancers reveals squamous cell components, or if after further testing they remain undifferentiated, categorize as squamous cell carcinoma G3.
[d]Location is defined by epicenter of esophageal tumor.

From Rice TW, Patil DT, Blackstone EH. 8th edition AJCC/UICC staging of cancers of the esophagus and esophagogastric junction: application to clinical practice. *Ann Cardiothorac Surg*. 2017;6(2):119–130.

Ivor-Lewis esophagectomy begins in the supine position. A laparotomy is performed, and the stomach is mobilized as earlier. The authors do not tubularize the stomach in the abdomen or place a feeding jejunostomy tube when performing an Ivor-Lewis esophagectomy. The patient is then turned to the left lateral decubitus position, and a right thoracotomy is performed. The chest is entered through the fifth intercostal space, and the thoracic esophagus is mobilized up to the level of the azygos vein. The stomach is brought up in its entirety into the chest, and it is anastomosed to the esophagus.

Perioperative 30-day morbidity and mortality of esophagectomy is 33.1% and 3.1% respectively.[11] Pulmonary complications are most commonly encountered, but the most dreaded complications are anastomotic leak and conduit ischemia. Anastomotic leaks have been reported as high as 30% and are likely related to anastomotic tension and a poorly perfused conduit. Therefore it is not surprising that cervical anastomoses have a higher rate of anastomotic leaks compared with thoracic anastomoses (12.9% vs. 9.3%).[16] However, cervical leaks are easily managed by draining the neck wound and providing local wound control. Thoracic leaks, in contrast, require more invasive interventions with either reoperation for local control or placement of an esophageal stent. Conduit ischemia occurs in 9% of patients[17] and can present as an anastomotic leak or total ischemia. Patients with total ischemia are extremely ill with signs of septic shock. A high degree of suspicion is necessary, and a prompt endoscopy confirms the diagnosis. Emergent surgical removal of the conduit and proximal esophageal diversion is necessary.

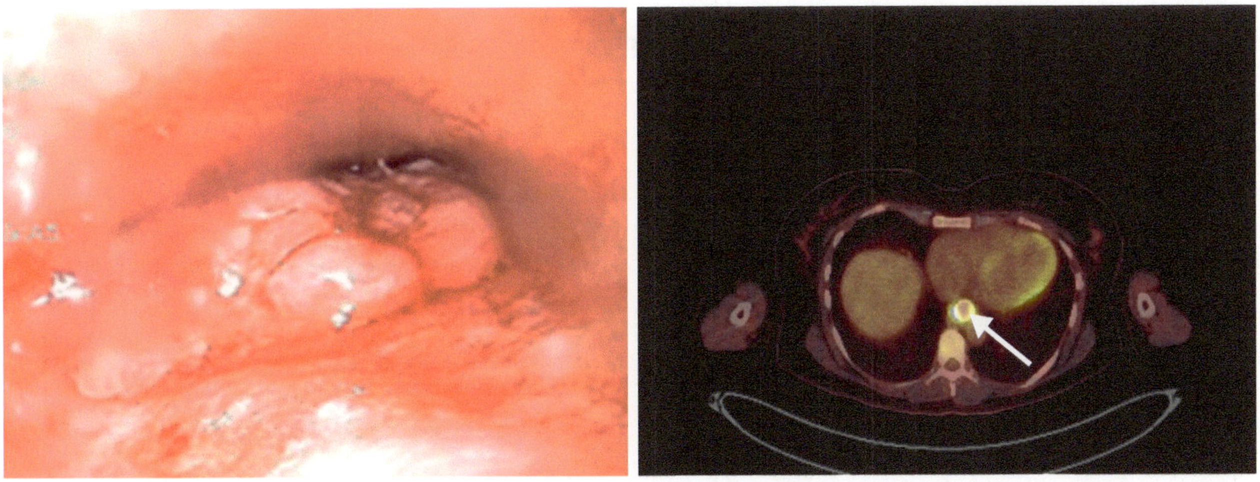

• **Fig. 4.4** A 35-year-old female diagnosed with a lower esophageal clinical T2N0 adenocarcinoma. She underwent hybrid Ivor-Lewis esophagectomy. Pathology was pT3N2 adenocarcinoma. She subsequently underwent adjuvant chemoradiation (**A** and **B**). **B**, PET scan image.

Mediastinal Tumors

It is important to be cognizant of mediastinal anatomy in the assessment of mediastinal tumors (see Chapter 34). This is the case as certain tumors have a propensity to present in specific mediastinal compartments. The posterior mediastinal space commonly presents with neurogenic tumors, usually benign schwannomas. The middle mediastinal space presents with cysts, lymphoma, or esophageal lesions. The anterior mediastinal space, the most common location of mediastinal masses, typically presents with thymic lesions, lymphoma, germ cell tumors, or thyroid lesions.

Mediastinal lesions may be incidentally found or patients may present with symptoms related to mass effect (dyspnea, stridor, dysphagia, pain) or systemic symptoms. A physical examination may reveal a testicular mass. CT imaging reveals the exact location of the mass and may even suggest specific diagnoses with its radiographic appearance. Laboratory values may provide value, as certain anterior mediastinal masses may have tumor markers—alpha fetoprotein and beta-human chorionic gonadotropin in germ cell tumors, antiacetylcholine receptor antibodies in thymic tumors, and lactate dehydrogenase in lymphoma.

Tissue diagnosis can be achieved with biopsy or surgical resection. Biopsy is usually performed if there is uncertainty whether the mass is a lymphoma, in which case surgery is not indicated. Core needle biopsy should be performed and, if inadequate, an anterior mediastinotomy can be performed for more tissue. FNA is inadequate in assessing lymph node architecture to determine the lymphoma subtype. Positive tumor markers for germ cell tumors are adequate for diagnosis and often help drive therapy. Lesions that are well-encapsulated with a typical appearance for thymoma are taken straight for surgical resection.

Surgical approaches depend on the size and location of the lesion. Most tumors in the anterior mediastinum are approached via a sternotomy. However, a hemi-clamshell or clamshell thoracotomy may even be necessary. Middle and posterior mediastinal tumors are more commonly approached with a thoracotomy. Minimally invasive approaches may be considered in all spaces with smaller lesions.

Thymic Tumors

Thymic tumors are the most common masses found in the anterior mediastinum. In addition to the previously mentioned symptoms, patients with thymic lesions may also present with paraneoplastic syndromes, such as myasthenia gravis. Thymomas are typically homogeneous, well-circumscribed lesions on a CT scan (Fig. 4.5). The more rare

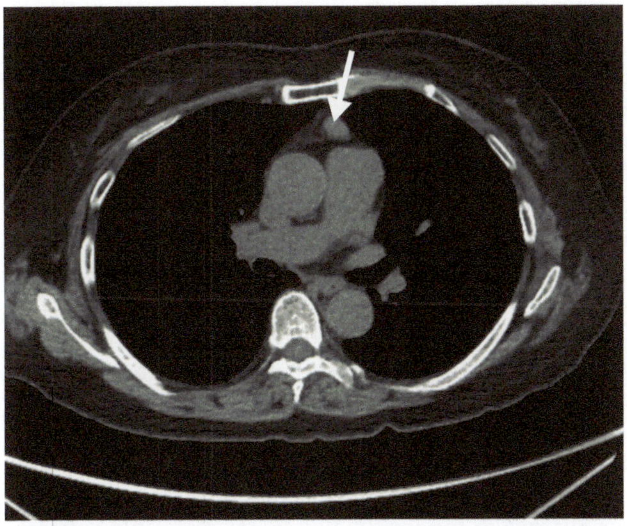

• **Fig. 4.5** A 63-year-old female with 1.5-cm anterior mediastinal mass suspicious for thymoma. She underwent video-assisted thoracoscopic surgery thymectomy. Pathology showed World Health Organization B2 thymoma.

TABLE 4.3 **World Health Organization Classification for Thymoma**

Thymoma Subtype		
A		Sparse or no immature lymphocytes
AB	Spindled epithelial cells	± Epithelioid/polygonal tumor cells, focal or diffuse abundance of immature lymphocytes
B1	Thymus-like architecture with distinct cortical areas and medullary islands (required), dispersed epithelial cells, dense immature lymphocytic population, low power "blue" appearance	
B2	Increased density of dispersed or clustered epithelial cells (≥3 adjacent cells), moderately dense immature lymphocytic population, low power "blue" appearance	
B3	Sheets of epithelial cells, sparse or (rarely) absent immature lymphocytic population, low power "pink" appearance	

From den Bakker MA, Roden AC, Marx A, et al. Histologic classification of thymoma: a practical guide for routine cases. *J Thorac Oncol*. 2014;9:S125–S130.

TABLE 4.4 **Masaoka Staging System for Thymoma**

Stage I	No capsular invasion
Stage II	A: microscopic capsular invasion
	B: macroscopic capsular invasion
Stage III	Invasion into neighboring organs
Stage IV	A: pleural and/or pericardial dissemination
	B: lymphatic or hematogenous spread

thymic carcinomas appear as heterogeneous, irregular masses that may be invading into surrounding tissues.

Thymoma are relatively bland tumors that are classified by histology. The World Health Organization (WHO) classification includes five subtypes for thymoma based on histopathology and is of prognostic significance as the patients with type A have the best prognosis whereas B3 patients have the worst (Table 4.3). Staging of thymic tumors is based on TNM classification. However, the Masaoka-Koga staging system (Table 4.4) retains significant clinical and prognostic significance, so it is routinely used.[18,19]

Surgery should be the initial treatment for patients in whom an R0 resection is deemed feasible preoperatively. It is important to rule out the presence of myasthenia gravis, as vigilant care must be taken in the perioperative setting to avoid respiratory failure in these patients. These patients may even require plasmapheresis or intravenous immune globulin preoperatively and will require monitoring postoperatively in intensive care. In the absence of metastatic disease, for resectable patients in whom R0 resection is not deemed feasible, surgery is offered after induction chemotherapy has been given. Postoperative radiation therapy is offered in patients with thymomas with transcapsular invasion and thymic carcinoma (Fig. 4.6).

Germ Cell Tumors

Germ cell tumors include teratomas (mature and immature), seminomas, and nonseminomatous germ cell tumors. Seminomas usually present with bulky metastatic disease and are usually not amenable to surgery. Mature teratomas do not present with tumor markers. These cancers are treated with prompt surgical resection. Immature teratomas and nonseminomatous germ cell tumors often present with abnormal tumor markers. These are best treated with platinum-based chemotherapy. Residual masses are surgically resected after treatment and normalization of tumor markers (Fig. 4.7).

Malignant Pleural Mesothelioma

Malignant pleural mesothelioma (MPM) is the most common primary pleural malignancy. It is a rare but aggressive disease. According to data from the U.S. Centers for Disease Control and Prevention, mesothelioma incidence among the 50 US states ranged from 0.58 to 1.65 per 100,000 people. It is primarily caused by the inhalation of asbestos fibers, but there is a long latency period of several decades from exposure to the development of malignancy. Patients are often asymptomatic but can present with cough and shortness of breath and symptoms of restrictive pulmonary disease.

Diagnosis is usually suspected incidentally. Chest x-ray may show the presence of a pleural effusion or evidence of pleural thickening and/or volume loss. Chest tomography offers better visualization of the extent of disease. Integrated PET-CT allows for clinical staging of the disease and may also offer prognostic value.[20] Although there is no universally accepted staging system for MPM, the TNM classification

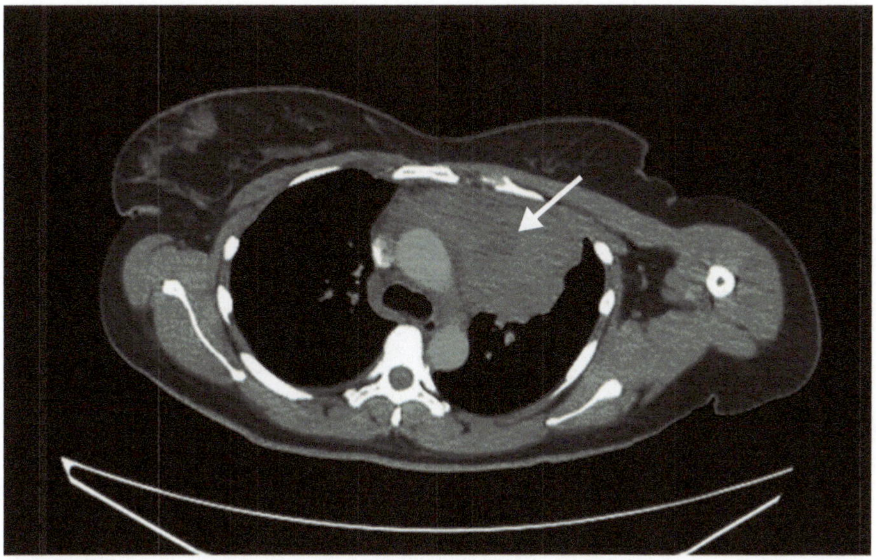

• **Fig. 4.6** A 40-year-old female who presented with 9.2-cm anterior mediastinal mass. Biopsy showed World Health Organization (WHO) B1 thymoma. She underwent resection via left hemiclamshell thoracotomy. Pathology showed WHO B3 thymoma. She was further treated with chemotherapy and radiation.

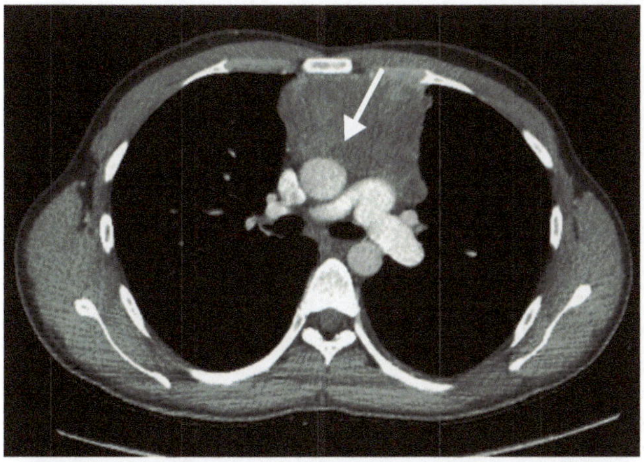

• **Fig. 4.7** A 25-year-old male with a nonseminomatous yolk sac tumor with elevated serum alpha fetoprotein (AFP). He underwent four cycles of chemotherapy with normalization of AFP. Residual mass persisted for which he underwent surgical resection via sternotomy.

is most commonly used. Fig. 4.8 illustrates the various stages of mesothelioma. A thoracentesis is often performed, but the diagnostic yield of fluid cytology is fairly unhelpful because tissue biopsy is ultimately required to confirm the diagnosis of MPM. This is achieved with minimal patient discomfort via surgical thoracoscopy. A single 10-mm incision is made in the lateral chest wall in the same line as future thoracotomy because MPM has a high probability of seeding surgical sites.

Although the goal of any oncologic resection is the complete removal of malignancy—both macroscopic and microscopic—this is usually not possible with MPM. Because of the diffuse nature of the disease, microscopic disease is invariably left behind. Consequently, there is some measure of uncertainty regarding the role of surgical resection in the treatment of MPM, and there remains much controversy regarding the optimal treatment strategy. A review of the Surveillance, Epidemiology, and End Results database showed only 22% of patient proceeded to cancer-directed surgery, and there was a wide spectrum of procedures performed.[21] However, surgery, like chemotherapy and radiotherapy, should be considered a useful adjunct in the treatment of MPM. Palliative surgery, such as pleurodesis or a long-term in-dwelling catheter placement may provide some temporary symptomatic benefit for these patients. If surgical resection is planned, preoperative workup must be meticulously performed after confirming the disease is limited to one hemithorax without mediastinal or transdiaphragmatic involvement (Fig. 4.9). In addition to imaging, the patient should undergo extensive cardiopulmonary evaluation.[22]

Extrapleural pneumonectomy (EPP) and pleurectomy/decortication (P/D) are the two primary resection strategies for mesothelioma. Preoperative evaluation may help elucidate which strategy is preferred. Patients with poor pulmonary function tests are likely not appropriate candidates for EPP but may tolerate P/D. Radiographic studies which reveal bulky disease may suggest that EPP is preferable, but the ultimate decision for EPP versus P/D remains a clinical one made in the operating room at the surgeon's discretion under direct visualization, as the extent of gross disease does not always correlate with the radiographic findings. Patients with stage I disease are ideal for P/D—parietal pleural disease with limited involvement of the visceral pleura. Stage II patients receive more benefit from EPP because it is characterized by bulky disease with invasion of the lung parenchyma.[23] The extent of disease and, consequently, the ideal operation may even be difficult for some inexperienced surgeons to differentiate.

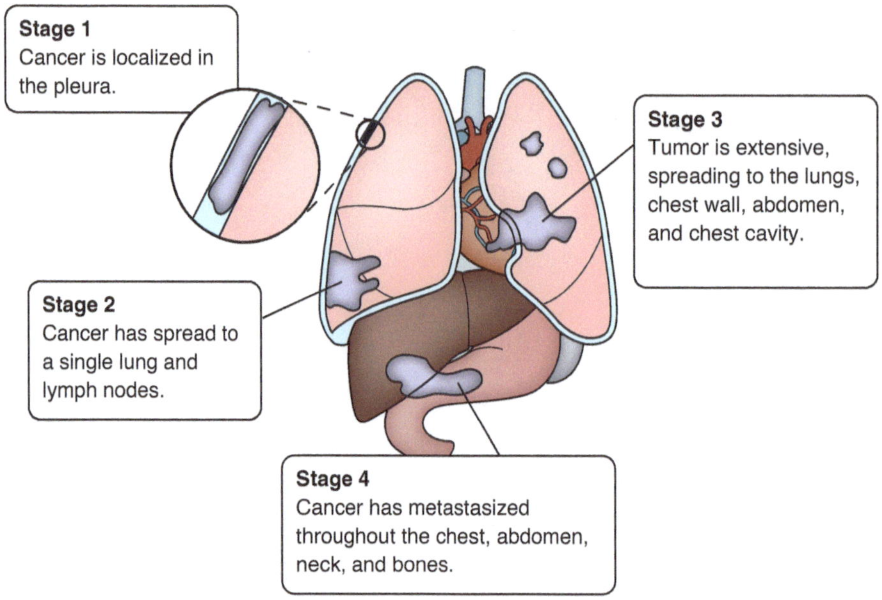

• **Fig. 4.8** Mesothelioma staging. (From Mesothelioma.com).

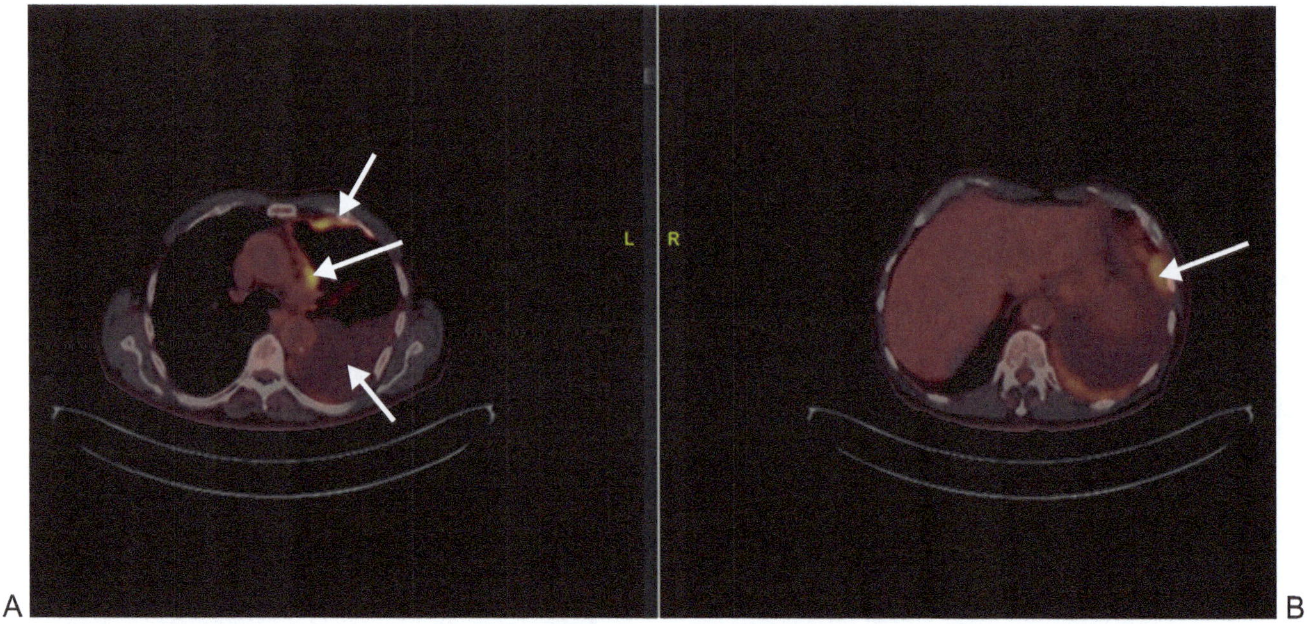

• **Fig. 4.9** **A.** A 77-year-old male who presented with dyspnea and left pleural effusion. Hypermetabolic pleural masses are noted on positron emission tomography (PET). Pleural biopsy revealed malignant pleural mesothelioma. **B.** PET revealed a suspicious celiac lymph node, which was confirmed to be metastatic on biopsy.

EPP is performed via an extended posterolateral thoracotomy through the sixth interspace. The sixth rib is removed. Any prior biopsy sites are excised within the line of the thoracotomy because of the risk of port site recurrence. Blunt finger dissection is performed and an en-bloc resection of the parietal pleura, lung, diaphragm, and pericardium is achieved. The diaphragm and pericardium are reconstructed with a patch.

Pleurectomy and decortication is an effective option in patients who would not otherwise tolerate a pneumonectomy. Similar to EPP, the chest is entered through an extended posterolateral thoracotomy in the sixth intercostal space, and the sixth rib is excised. Blunt dissection is performed to achieve an en-bloc resection of the parietal pleura, diaphragm, and pericardium. A combination of blunt and sharp dissection is used to remove the visceral pleura and the underlying lung is left in place. This may result in a prolonged air leak in the postoperative period. The diaphragm and pericardium are reconstructed using prosthetic patches.

Advocates of EPP believe that it offers a more complete cytoreduction, while allowing for high-dose radiotherapy without risk of lung injury to the affected hemithorax. Meanwhile, advocates of P/D believe that it is associated with lower morbidity and mortality, while offering adequate cytoreduction. There are limited data regarding the superiority of either technique. One prospective study showed median survival was almost double in patients who underwent

P/D, as opposed to those who underwent EPP, with a 5-year survival of 30% in P/D patients and 9% in EPP patients.[24] As previously mentioned, the characteristics of MPM render it difficult to treat with surgery alone. Therefore a multimodality approach must be taken. Chemotherapy regimens are predominantly platinum-based. Radiation therapy is dose-limited by the intrathoracic structures but can reach up to 45 Gy with EPP. Several other adjuncts are being investigated and include hyperthermic intrapleural chemotherapy, photodynamic therapy, and gene therapy.

With improvements in operative techniques and perioperative care, the initial high mortality rates of EPP have fallen to under 5% at experienced centers.[25] Perioperative mortality for P/D is generally better than EPP. Atrial arrhythmias are the most common complication, occurring in up to 44% of patients. Technical complications usually involve issues with patch reconstruction, such as cardiac tamponade or cardiac or gastric herniation. Postoperative empyema occurs infrequently, but the presence of prosthetic patches complicates their management. Bronchopleural fistulae develop rarely.[26]

Patterns of recurrence differ between the two surgical modalities. P/D patients tend to have recurrence locally in the ipsilateral hemithorax, whereas EPP patients develop distant recurrence. A multimodality approach improves median survival up to 38 months, and overall, 5-year survival is 12%,[27] and patients with complete resection margins, negative extrapleural lymph nodes, and epithelioid histology have improved long-term survival.[28]

Airway Tumors (see Chapter 42)

Airway malignancies are rare and symptoms may be mistaken for other etiologies. Most common symptoms include cough, dyspnea, wheezing, and hemoptysis. CT imaging may show the lesion itself or postobstructive atelectasis. Proximal airway tumors should undergo CT imaging with 1-mm slices to best evaluate the length and size of the lesion. Definitive diagnosis is achieved via bronchoscopy, which will provide visualization confirmation of the lesion, as well as tissue biopsy. The most common etiologies are squamous cell carcinoma and adenoid cystic carcinoma. Squamous cell carcinoma is aggressive, invading into structures beyond the tracheal wall and metastasizing early. Adenoid cystic carcinoma is more insidious, infiltrating and spreading along nerves.

Early diagnosis is key to management. Ideal treatment is surgical resection, but this may not be possible. For those patients who are not surgical candidates, radiation therapy and local ablative endoscopic therapies are offered. The principle of tracheal resection is segmental resection with reconstruction. Adequate length must remain after resection for successful reconstruction. Up to half the tracheal length can be safely removed and reconstructed.

Approach depends on the location of the cancer. Higher lesions involving the upper trachea are approached via a cervical collar incision, whereas lower tracheal lesions are approached via a right thoracotomy or a sternotomy. Communication between the surgical and anesthesia teams is especially essential as transection of the airway requires cross-field ventilation. Once the cancer has been resected, the trachea must be adequately mobilized to achieve a tension-free anastomosis. If inadequate, more length can be attained with release maneuvers, such as supra- or infrahyoid release for upper lesions and hilar release for lower lesions.

Complications are usually respiratory, but the most dreaded complication is anastomotic dehiscence. Attempts to minimize this risk are performed through careful patient selection, meticulous handling of peritracheal tissue and preservation of tracheal blood supply, tension-free anastomosis, and placement of a stitch from the patient's chin to the chest to keep the neck flexed and tension off the anastomosis in the early postoperative setting. Risk of anastomotic dehiscence has been reported as low as 5%, with perioperative mortality 1%.[29]

Chest Wall Tumors

Malignant chest wall tumors are either bony sarcomas (chondrosarcoma, osteosarcoma) or soft tissue sarcomas. These lesions present as either an asymptomatic or painful chest wall mass. A thorough history and physical may provide clues as to whether the mass is benign or malignant. A history of malignancy may suggest a metastatic lesion, and a firm, immobile mass may suggest a malignant mass with bony involvement (Fig. 4.10).

A CT scan offers a wealth of information regarding these tumors. It can provide measurements of size, location, depth of invasion, relation, and potential involvement of adjacent structures, and an evaluation of the underlying lung parenchyma for metastatic lesions. MRI is used only selectively in the evaluation of posterior lesions to assess spinal cord involvement and apical lesions to assess for brachial plexus or subclavian vessel involvement. Diagnosis is ultimately obtained with a tissue

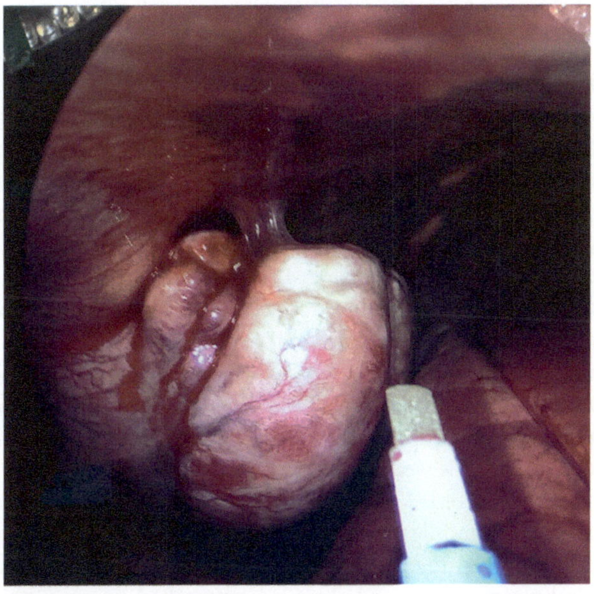

• **Fig. 4.10** A 41-year-old female with a 6.1 × 5.1 × 3.9 cm large, pleural-based mass solitary fibrous tumor within right chest associated with erosion and remodeling of the inner aspect of the adjacent right seventh rib.

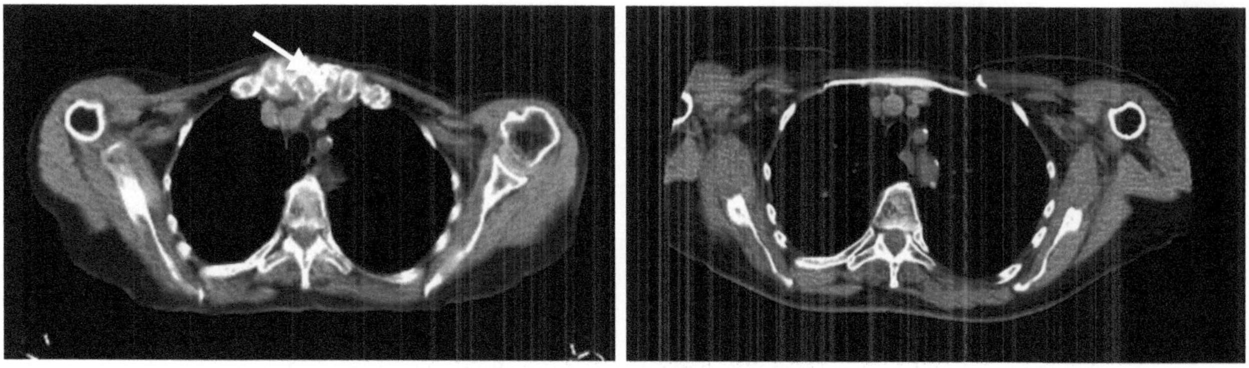

• **Fig. 4.11** An 80-year-old patient with sternoclavicular chondrosarcoma (**A**). Follow-up scan 4 years after resection and reconstruction with methyl methacrylate mesh (**B**).

biopsy. This is initially attempted with a CT-guided needle biopsy. If this is inconclusive, a surgical incisional biopsy is performed. For small lesions under 4 cm in diameter, an excisional biopsy with 2-cm margins can be performed.

Although chest wall sarcomas are predominantly resistant to chemotherapy and radiation, some surgeons prefer to give induction therapy in the hope that it will decrease tumor size. Ideally, this would allow for a more complete resection and provide immediate systemic therapy for micrometastatic disease. Unless the tumor involves vital structures, the authors favor proceeding with prompt surgical resection, followed by adjuvant therapy, as induction therapy is of limited benefit and a potential cure is best achieved by complete resection followed by adjuvant therapy for micrometastatic disease. Although prompt surgical resection is the standard-of-care treatment for primary chest wall tumors, there are a few that are first treated medically. Plasmacytomas usually respond to radiation, and surgery is offered as second-line therapy. Ewing sarcoma is chemosensitive, so these patients receive induction chemotherapy before surgical resection.

The tenets of surgical resection of chest wall tumors are complete resection, restoration of chest wall rigidity to maintain respiratory mechanics and to protect underlying structures, sealing of the pleural space, and placement of adequate soft tissue coverage. The surgical approach depends on the location of the lesion. Lateral or posterior lesions are approached from the lateral decubitus position. If the tumor appears to involve the spinal canal, the patient is first approached in the prone position by a spine surgeon to mobilize the tumor free from the spinal cord. A standard posterolateral thoracotomy is performed. If the muscles are not involved, the latissimus muscle is divided, and the serratus is mobilized anteriorly and spared. If these are involved, they are taken en-masse with the specimen. The pleural cavity is entered one rib away from the inferior margin of the tumor and inspected for pleural disease. Any lung adherent to the tumor is wedged free from the remaining lung with a stapler. The borders of the mass are identified, and care is taken to identify and ligate each intercostal bundle before dividing the ribs. The tumor is thus freed en-bloc with a sufficient surgical margin. Anterior lesions are approached via an anterior thoracotomy, with the patient in the prone position. Involvement of the sternum necessitates a sternotomy. If the skin is not involved, an incision is made over the lesion, and a skin flap is raised. If the skin is involved, an elliptical incision around the mass is made. All attempts are made to achieve a 4-cm surgical margin, but this may not be possible.

Chest wall defects underneath the body of the scapula can be left alone. Otherwise, any defect over 5 cm or a defect over vital structures (heart, great vessels) needs to be reconstructed. A defect of any size at the tip of the scapula is also reconstructed to prevent scapular tip entrapment. Defects are closed with a 2-mm polytetrafluoroethylene (Gore-Tex) patch by securing it to the surrounding ribs and soft tissue with Prolene stitches. Small perforations are cut into the patch to minimize the chance of seroma formation. If there is an anterior defect over vital structures, reconstruction is performed with a polypropylene (Marlex)-methyl methacrylate sandwich. This "sandwich" is created by applying a layer of methyl methacrylate in between two sheets of Marlex mesh and gently contouring it as it hardens. This is secured to the surrounding soft tissue and bony structures with Prolene stitches (Fig. 4.11). Posterior defects largely do not require a soft tissue flap to cover the mesh. This is most commonly needed for anterior lesions. There are several options for flap coverage and range from a simple local cutaneous advancement flap to a pedicled myocutaneous flap or a myocutaneous free flap with the assistance of a plastic surgeon. Skin flaps placed directly over the patch will invariably necrose. Muscle groups most commonly used are pectoralis and latissimus flaps. Less commonly, the rectus and external oblique muscles are used for soft tissue coverage of the chest wall.

Intraoperative complications are best avoided with knowledge of the anatomy from preoperative imaging. If the tumor appears closely related to the subclavian vessels on imaging, it is imperative to attain proximal and distal control during the operation. Postoperative complications are predominantly respiratory and can be minimized with effective pain control and aggressive chest physiotherapy. Infectious complications are particularly concerning given the presence of mesh. This can be minimized during the initial operation by debriding all nonviable tissue and ensuring good blood supply to the overlying soft tissue flap. Drainage of any collections, appropriate administration of intravenous antibiotics, and debridement of necrotic tissue are necessary and may obviate the need to remove the mesh, but, unfortunately, mesh removal is often required. Prognostic factors include adequacy of the surgical margin, the histology, and the histologic grade of the tumor.[30,31] Five-year overall survival exceeds 60%, and 5-year disease-free survival exceeds 45%.[31,32]

Conclusion

The quantity of intrathoracic tumors vastly outnumbers those mentioned within this chapter, from benign tumors to malignant cancers. However, diagnostic workup remains the same. Before definitive management, tissue biopsy and clinical staging are necessary to determine optimal therapy. In addition, despite this diverse variety, surgical principles remain the same and expert knowledge of the pertinent anatomy is important in surgical planning. A multidisciplinary approach is often required with involvement of thoracic surgery, medical oncology, and radiation oncology.

Acknowledgments

The authors have no conflicts of interest to disclose.

References

1. Marom EM, McAdams HP, Erasmus JJ, et al. Staging non-small cell lung cancer with whole-body PET. *Radiology.* 1999;212:803–809.
2. Alberg AJ, Samet JM. Epidemiology of lung cancer. *Chest.* 2003;123:21S–49S.
3. International Early Lung Cancer Investigators. Survival of patients with stage I lung cancer detected on CT screening. *N Engl J Med.* 2006;355:1763–1771.
4. Ginsberg RJ, Rubinstein LV. Randomized trial of lobectomy versus limited resection T1 N0 non-small cell lung cancer. Lung Cancer Study Group. *Ann Thorac Surg.* 1995;60:615–622.
5. Altorki NK, Yip R, Hanaoka T, et al. Sublobar resection is equivalent to lobectomy for clinical Stage 1A lung cancer in solid nodules. *J Thorac Cardiovasc Surg.* 2014;147:754–762.
6. Paul S, Altorki NK, Sheng S, et al. Thoracoscopic lobectomy is associated with lower morbidity than open lobectomy: a propensity-matched analysis from the STS database. *J Thorac Cardiovasc Surg.* 2010;139:366–378.
7. Nwogu CE, D'Cunha J, Pang H, et al. VATS lobectomy has better perioperative outcomes than open lobectomy: CALGB 31001, an ancillary analysis of CALGB 140202 (Alliance). *Ann Thorac Surg.* 2015;99:399–405.
8. Taioli E, Lee D, Lesser M, et al. Long-term survival in video-assisted thoracoscopic lobectomy vs open lobectomy in lung cancer patients: a meta-analysis. *Eur J Cardiothorac Surg.* 2013;44:591–597.
9. Allen MS, Darling GE, Pechet TT, et al. Morbidity and mortality of major pulmonary resections in patients with early stage lung cancer: initial results of the randomized, prospective ACOSOG Z0030 trial. *Ann Thorac Surg.* 2006;81:1013–1019.
10. Boffa DJ, Allen MS, Grab JD, et al. Data from The Society of Thoracic Surgeons General Thoracic Surgery Database: the surgical management of primary lung tumors. *J Thorac Cardiovasc Surg.* 2008;135:247–254.
11. Seder CW, Raymond DP, Wright CD, et al. The Society of Thoracic Surgeons General Thoracic Surgery Database 2017 update on outcomes and quality. *Ann Thorac Surg.* 2017;103:1378–1383.
12. Fernandez FG, Kosinski AS, Burfeind W, et al. The Society of Thoracic Surgeons lung cancer resection risk model: higher quality data and superior outcomes. *Ann Thorac Surg.* 2016;102:370–377.
13. Puli SR, Reddy JB, Bechtold ML, et al. Staging accuracy of esophageal cancer by endoscopic ultrasound: a meta-analysis and systematic review. *World J Gastroenterol.* 2008;14:1479–1490.
14. Shridhar R, Huston J, Meredith KL. Accuracy of endoscopic ultrasound staging for T2N0 esophageal cancer: A National Cancer Database analysis. *J Gastrointest Oncol.* 2018;9:887–893.
15. van Hagen P, Hulshof MC, van Lanschot JJ, et al. Preoperative chemoradiotherapy for esophageal or junctional cancer. *N Engl J Med.* 2012;366:2074–2084.
16. Kassis ES, Kosinski AS, Ross P, et al. Predictors of anastomotic leak after esophagectomy: an analysis of The Society of Thoracic Surgeons General Thoracic Surgery Database. *Ann Thorac Surg.* 2013;96:1919–1926.
17. Briel JW, Tamhankar AP, Hagen JA, et al. Prevalence and risk factors for ischemia, leak, and stricture of esophageal anastomosis: gastric pull-up versus colon interposition. *J Am Coll Surg.* 2004;198:536–541.
18. Masaoka A. Staging system of thymoma. *J Thorac Oncol.* 2010;5:S304–S312.
19. Roden AC, Yi ES, Jenkins S, et al. Modified Masaoka stage and size are independent prognostic predictors in thymoma and modified Masaoka stage is superior to histopathologic classifications. *J Thorac Oncol.* 2015;10:691–700.
20. Flores RM, Akhurst T, Gonen M, et al. Positron emission tomography predicts survival in malignant pleural mesothelioma. *J Thorac Cardiovasc Surg.* 2006;132:763–768.
21. Flores RM, Riedel E, Donington JS, et al. Frequency of use and predictors of cancer surgery in the management of malignant pleural mesothelioma in a community-based (Surveillance, Epidemiology, and End Results [SEER]) population. *J Thorac Oncol.* 2010;5:1649–1654.
22. Sugarbaker DJ, Norberto JJ. Multimodality management of malignant pleural mesothelioma. *Chest.* 1998;113:61S–65S.
23. Flores RF. Surgical options in malignant pleural mesothelioma: extrapleural pneumonectomy or pleurectomy/decortication. *Semin Thorac Cardiovasc Surg.* 2009;21:149–153.
24. Lang-Lazdunski L, Bille A, Lal R, et al. Pleurectomy/decortication is superior to extrapleural pneumonectomy in the multimodality management of patients with malignant pleural mesothelioma. *J Thorac Oncol.* 2012;7:737–743.
25. Flores RM, Krug LM, Rosenzweig KE, et al. Induction chemotherapy, extrapleural pneumonectomy, and postoperative high-dose radiotherapy for locally advanced malignant pleural mesothelioma: a phase II trial. *J Thorac Oncol.* 2006;1:289–295.
26. Sugarbacker DJ, Jaklitsch MT, Bueno R, et al. Prevention, early detection, and management of complications after 328 consecutive extrapleural pneumonectomies. *J Thorac Cardiovasc Surg.* 2004;128:138–146.
27. Flores RM, Pass HI, Sesha VE, et al. Extrapleural pneumonectomy versus pleurectomy/decortications in the surgical management of malignant pleural mesothelioma: results in 663 patients. *J Thorac Cardiovasc Surg.* 2008;135:620–626.
28. Sugarbaker DJ, Flores RM, Jaklitsch MT, et al. Resection margins, extrapleural nodal status, and cell type determine postoperative long-term survival in trimodality therapy of malignant

pleural mesothelioma: results in 183 patients. *J Thorac Cardiovasc Surg*. 1999;117:54–65.

29. Wright CD, Grillo HC, Wain JC, et al. Anastomotic complications after tracheal resection: prognostic factors and management. *J Thorac Cardiovasc Surg*. 2004;128:731–739.
30. Gross JL, Younes RN, Haddad FJ, et al. Soft-tissue sarcomas of the chest wall: prognostic factors. *Chest*. 2005;127:902–908.
31. Walsh GL, Davis BM, Swisher SG, et al. A single-institutional multidisciplinary approach to primary sarcomas involving the chest wall requiring full-thickness resections. *J Thorac Cardiovasc Surg*. 2001;121:48–60.
32. Kachroo P, Pak PS, Sandha HS, et al. Single-institution, multidisciplinary experience with surgical resection of primary chest wall sarcomas. *J Thorac Oncol*. 2012;7:552–558.

NON-PRINT ITEMS

Abstract

Thoracic oncology encompasses a large spectrum of diseases. Between the various anatomic spaces and the different organ systems, there are a large variety of benign and malignant tumors that can develop within the chest. This chapter will focus primarily on the surgical management of the most commonly encountered thoracic malignancies.

Keywords

common thoracic malignancies, surgical management, lung cancer, esophageal cancer, mesothelioma, thymoma

5 Pulmonary Pathophysiology and Lung Mechanics in Anesthesiology

JAMIE L. SPARLING, MARCOS F. VIDAL MELO

Introduction

The practice of thoracic anesthesia, in addition to involving patients with impaired pulmonary function, also necessitates dynamic changes in ventilation that impact perfusion and ventilation/perfusion matching. Thus it is imperative that the thoracic anesthesiologist has a thorough understanding of normal pulmonary physiology, as well as states of pathophysiology. Further, the practitioner must have an intimate familiarity with the impact of mechanical ventilation on both normal and injured lungs, to be able to manipulate the ventilation in response to the dynamic needs of thoracic surgery, as well as the evolution of lung injury. Lung mechanics is the expression of lung function through measures of pressure and flow.[1] In this chapter, we review normal lung structure and physiology, an overview of lung mechanics, clinical testing of lung function, and the implications and effects of anesthetics on these factors.

Essentials of Lung Structure

Tracheobronchial Structure

The trachea extends from the cricoid cartilage at the level of C6 to the carina at approximately the level of T4/5, at which point it branches into the right and left mainstem bronchi. The trachea is approximately 12 cm in women and 14 cm in men, and ranges from a mean of 19 ± 1.5 mm in diameter in women to 22 ± 1.5 mm in men. The right mainstem bronchus is shorter, wider, and more vertical than the left mainstem bronchus. Its length is approximately 1.4 to 1.8 cm compared with 4.4 to 4.9 cm on the left; thus the right lung is generally more susceptible to aspiration.

There are three right-sided lobes: the upper, middle, and lower lobes. On the left, there are two lobes, the upper and lower lobes, with the lingula being a "tongue-like" extension of the left upper lobe. The lobes are covered with visceral pleura and are separated by folds of pleura known as the horizontal and oblique fissures on the right, and by the oblique fissure on the left. Each lobe has a lobar, or secondary bronchus, as well as lobar blood supply. The lobes are further divided into bronchopulmonary segments, which again have dedicated named bronchi and blood supply. The right and left lungs each have 10 segments, although nomenclature for these segments may vary slightly in the literature (Fig. 5.1).[2,3]

The primary, or mainstem, bronchi branch from the trachea at the carina, then further branch into the lobar bronchi, and the segmental bronchi. These airways contain rings of cartilage that help keep them open. Once the airways branch into bronchioles, the walls are made of smooth muscle, and at the level of the respiratory bronchioles, the walls are made of only epithelium. This marks the transition from the conducting airways, encompassing the oropharynx and nasopharynx through bronchioles, to the respiratory airways, which participate in gas exchange and include the respiratory bronchioles and the alveoli.[2] On average, the lungs have 23 generations of dichotomous branching, as shown in Fig. 5.2.[4]

Respiratory Airways

The respiratory bronchioles end in the acinus, which is the functional unit of the lung, and consists of the alveolar ducts and alveolar sacs. The acinus appears as a cluster of grapes, each of which may contain up to 2000 alveoli. In total, the human lung consists of approximately 300 million alveoli creating a surface area for gas exchange of 40 to 80 m.[2,4] The alveoli contain alveolar type I cells, alveolar type II cells, and alveolar macrophages. Type I cells are squamous cells, comprising the very thin alveolar walls to facilitate gas exchange, and they cover up to 95% of the surface area of the alveoli. Type II cells are cuboidal and contain lamellar bodies, which secrete pulmonary surfactant, a film of phospholipids which reduces alveolar surface tension to facilitate lung expansion. Alveolar macrophages are scavengers that engulf foreign particles throughout the lungs, playing a key immunologic role.[2,3]

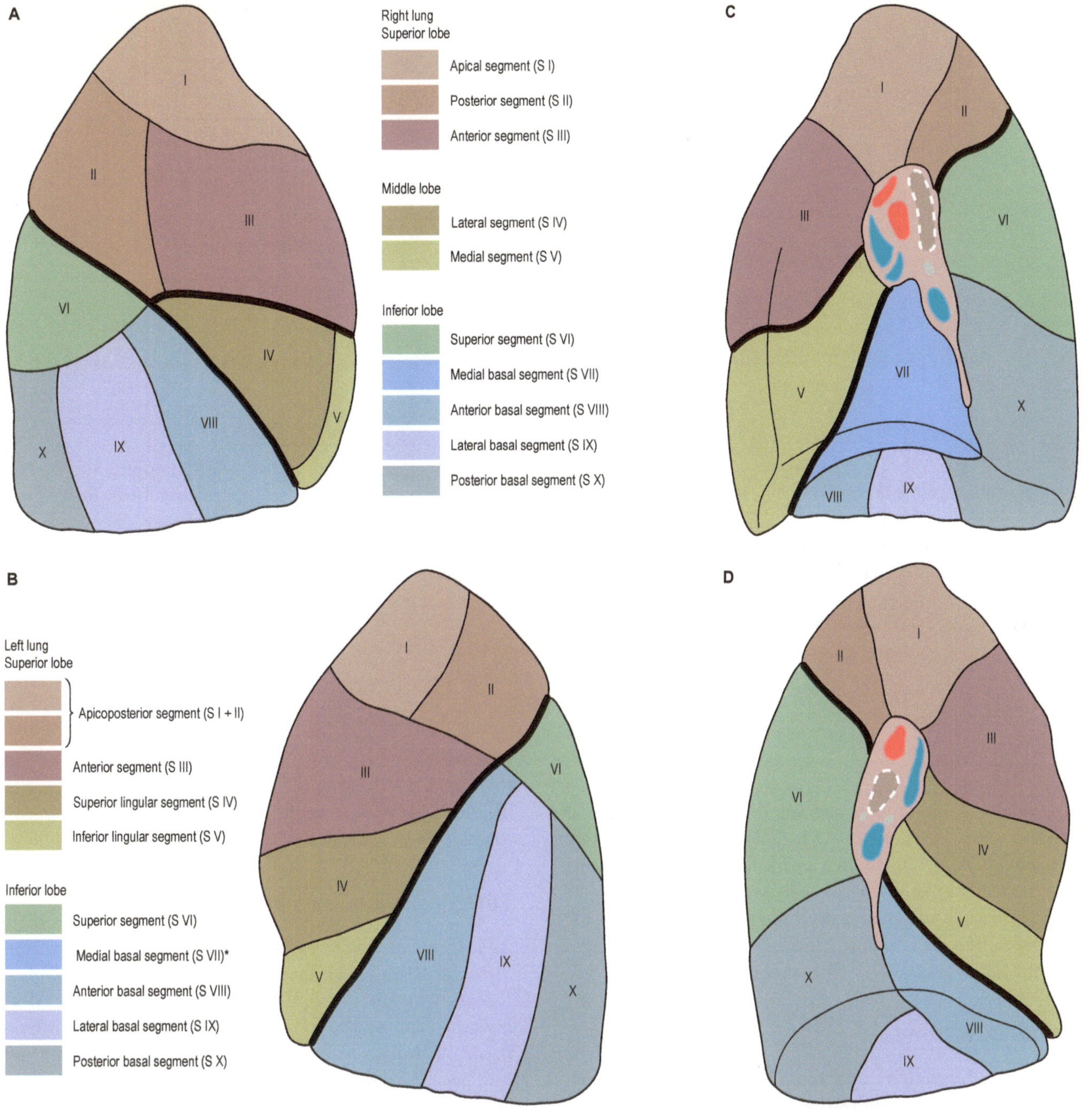

• **Fig. 5.1** Pleura, lungs, trachea, and bronchi. Bronchopulmonary segments of the right and left lungs, colored to indicate the different territories. (**A**) Right lung, lateral aspect. (**B**) Left lung, lateral aspect. (**C**) Right lung, medial aspect. (**D**) Left lung, medial aspect. (From Standring S, Anand N, Birch R, et al. *Gray's Anatomy: The Anatomical Basis of Clinical Practice*. 41st ed. New York: Elsevier; 2016: Fig. 54.6.)

Lung Volumes

Nomenclature

Lung volume at any given point in time depends upon lung and chest wall mechanics, the activity of the diaphragm and accessory muscles of respiration, and the size of the individual, as well as the ambient conditions (temperature, pressure, humidity) in which such volumes are measured. The standard lung volumes and capacities measured by spirometry are expressed at body temperature, atmospheric pressure, saturated with water vapor (BTPS), and are compared with volumes predicted by the individual's age, sex, and body size.[5] Measures of lung volume are denoted as either "volumes" or "capacities," where volumes are not subdivided, whereas capacities are the sum of two or more standard lung volumes. Of note, lung volumes correlate better with impairment of patient functional capabilities than respiratory function measurements related to airflow.[6]

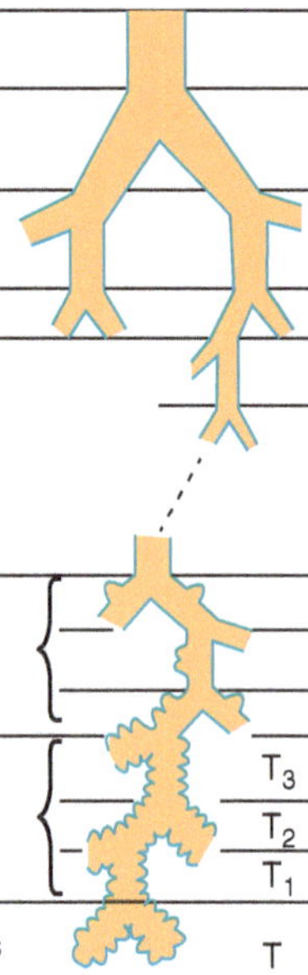

Zone	Generation		Diameter, cm	Length, cm	Number	Total cross-sectional area, cm^2
Conducting zone	Trachea	0	1.80	12.0	1	2.54
	Bronchi	1	1.22	4.8	2	2.33
	↓	2	0.83	1.9	4	2.13
		3	0.56	0.8	8	2.00
	Bronchioles	4	0.45	1.3	16	2.48
	↓	5	0.35	1.07	32	3.11
		↓	↓	↓	↓	↓
	Terminal bronchioles	16	0.06	0.17	6×10^4	180.0
Transitional and respiratory zones	Respiratory bronchioles	17	↓	↓	↓	↓
		18				
		19	0.05	0.10	5×10^5	10^3
	Alveolar ducts T_3	20	↓	↓	↓	↓
	T_2	21				
	T_1	22				
	Alveolar sacs T	23	0.04	0.05	8×10^6	10^4

Source: Michael G. Levitzky: *Pulmonary Physiology*, 9e

• **Fig. 5.2** Schematic representation of airway branching in the human lung with approximate dimensions. (From Levitzky MG. *Alveolar Ventilation. Pulmonary Physiology*. 9th ed. New York, NY: McGraw-Hill Education; 2017.)

Tidal Volume

The tidal volume (V_T) is the volume of gas inhaled and exhaled with each breath. With quiet breathing at rest, it is approximately 500 mL per breath for a 70-kg adult, that is, 5 to 7 mL/kg of predicted body weight. The V_T may be augmented considerably in several conditions (e.g., during exercise) and is achieved by increased work of the diaphragm and the accessory muscles of respiration.[5]

Residual Volume

The amount of gas left in the lungs following a forced maximal exhalation is known as the residual volume (RV). It is determined by the balance between the outward expansion of the chest wall opposing the inward recoil of the lungs with the force generated by the muscles of expiration. Normal RV for a 70-kg adult is around 1.5 L, but because of dynamic airway collapse with forced expiratory effort, gas may become trapped in the alveoli. Thus the RV can become much larger in emphysema, where the lungs' inward recoil is diminished and amount of gas trapping increases.[5]

Expiratory and Inspiratory Reserve Volumes

The expiratory reserve volume (ERV) is the difference between the functional residual capacity (FRC) and the RV, or the amount of gas that can be forcibly exhaled at the end of a normal tidal exhalation. Similarly, the inspiratory reserve volume (IRV) is the volume of gas that can be forcibly inhaled starting at the end of a normal tidal inhalation. The ERV is approximately 1.5 L, while the IRV is approximately 2.5 L in a healthy 70-kg adult.[5]

Functional Residual Capacity

FRC is the volume of gas remaining in the lungs at the end of a normal tidal exhalation; therefore it is the sum of the RV and the ERV. It is determined by the balance of the inward recoil of the lungs and the outward expansion of the chest wall, as well as the level of tone of the respiratory muscles. The FRC is approximately 3 L in a healthy 70-kg adult.[5] The point at which the inward recoil is exactly balanced by the outward expansion is known as the relaxation volume (V_r). FRC may be equal to, greater than, or less than the V_r, depending on the circumstances. For instance, in obstructive lung disease, relaxed exhalation can be incomplete as the next inspiratory effort starts resulting in FRC greater than V_r.[7]

Lung hyperinflation results in increased RV and FRC. Static hyperinflation is produced by the reduction in lung elasticity because of emphysema. It can also be caused by excessive positive end-expiratory pressure (PEEP). Dynamic hyperinflation results from air trapping from incomplete exhalation of inhaled gas. Interestingly, during mechanical ventilation, while PEEP adds to the risk of hyperinflation in chronic obstructive pulmonary disease (COPD) patients, it can also result in reduced hyperinflation in a subset of

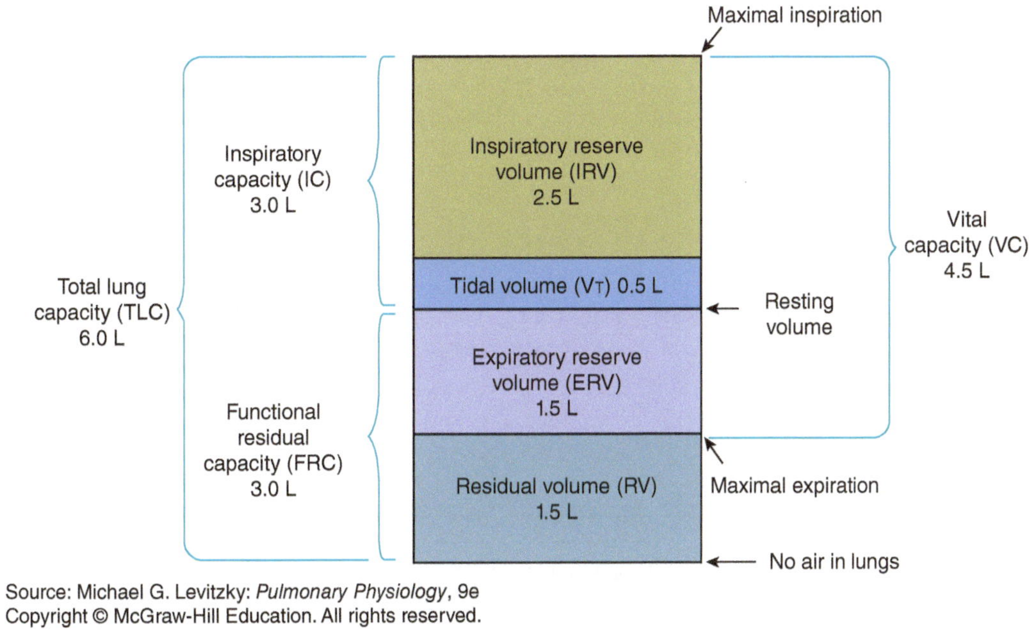

• **Fig. 5.3** The standard lung volumes and capacities. Typical values for a 70-kg adult (standing or sitting upright) are shown. (From Levitzky MG. *Alveolar Ventilation. Pulmonary Physiology*. 9th ed. New York, NY: McGraw-Hill Education; 2017.)

COPD patients because of airways being "stented open" by its application.[8]

Total Lung Capacity

The total lung capacity (TLC) is the maximal volume of gas in the lungs after a maximal inhalation; thus it is the sum of the RV, ERV, V_T, and IRV. TLC is approximately 6 L for a healthy 70-kg adult. The vital capacity (VC) is the maximal volume of gas exhaled during a forced exhalation after a forced inhalation. Thus VC is the sum of the V_T, IRV, and ERV. The VC is approximately 4.5 L in a healthy 70-kg adult.[5]

Fig. 5.3 shows a summary of how the standard lung volumes and capacities relate, along with average values for a 70-kg adult.

Closing Capacity and Closing Volume

Closing capacity (CC) is the lung volume at which small airway closure begins to occur. CC is the sum of the closing volume (CV) and RV.[9] Usually, the CC is smaller than FRC, so airways do not close with normal tidal breathing. However, age,[10] supine positioning, pregnancy,[11] and obesity,[12] among other conditions, all increase CC. Airway closure at a larger CC increases the likelihood of hypoxemia. CV is measured using the nitrogen washout test, as illustrated in Fig. 5.4.[13] In this method, the subject takes a breath of 100% oxygen and exhales through a one-way valve measuring nitrogen content and volume of the gas exhaled. The initial portion of the curve where the nitrogen content is zero is the dead space, where no gas exchange has occurred. The nitrogen content increases as the patient breathes a VC breath to RV. The CV is the volume between the terminal point of slope change and the RV. CC is the sum of the CV measured and the RV.[14] As CC increases with age, CC exceeds FRC, resulting in small airway closure during normal tidal breathing. This transition occurs at a younger age in the supine patient (approximately 44 years) compared with the upright patient (approximately 66 years), whereas FRC does not change with age (Fig. 5.5).

Effects of Anesthesia

It is well accepted that supine positioning and subsequent induction of general anesthesia with neuromuscular blockade reduces FRC, with reports of as much as a 9% decrease.[15] This reduction of FRC occurs consistently following induction, and progresses at a slower rate throughout the duration of anesthesia; it is further accentuated in obese patients.[16] The sitting position, as compared with supine, invariably increases FRC, even in patients under general anesthesia, as it favors the caudad displacement of the diaphragm.[17]

Importantly, recruitment breaths and increased V_T may temporarily recruit consolidated lung volume under anesthesia, but they are insufficient to keep an atelectatic lung open. This concept has been demonstrated both experimentally and in humans. In a study of pigs undergoing one lung ventilation, the ventilated lung experienced substantial $\dot{V}/\dot{Q}$ mismatch, hyperperfusion, and alveolar damage on histologic examination.[18] Further, tidal recruitment with a V_T of 10 mL/kg increased the volume of the ventilated lung that was normally aerated (versus consolidated), but applied cyclic recruitment was associated with the initiation of an injurious immune response.[19,20] Similarly, in a rabbit model, one lung ventilation with high

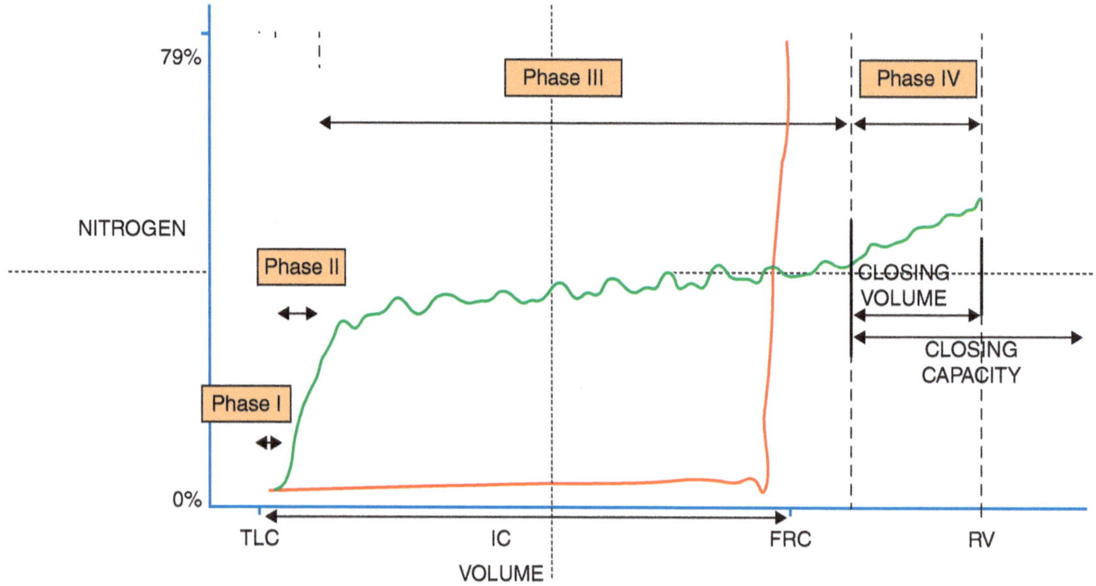

• **Fig. 5.4 Measurement of closing capacity and closing volume using the single nitrogen breath washout technique.** Tracing obtained during single breath nitrogen washout technique, in which 100% oxygen inspiration generally begins at residual volume (*RV*). Subject breathes room air until switched onto oxygen source at RV, inspires to total lung capacity (*TLC*), then expires a volume equivalent to vital capacity (VC) down to RV. **Phase I** is represented by the volume of gas exhaled with nitrogen = 0%, indicating air originated from conducting airways where no gas exchange takes place. This represents a portion of anatomic dead space. **Phase II** is the transition between the conducting airways and the alveolar gas. Phase III, the alveolar plateau, nearly a plateau in normal subjects, reflects exhalation of alveolar gas. Cardiogenic oscillations indicate changes in composition of exhaled air because of compression of lung tissue by the heart. A change in slope at the end of **phase III** indicates the onset of phase IV, which marks the closing volume. Such change in slope is caused by either closure or increased narrowing of small airways preceding alveolar units with diluted nitrogen (dependent lung regions). The anatomic dead space is determined by the volume that leads to area A = area B. Closing volume (CV) is the volume between the point of slope change from phase III to **phase IV** and RV. CC = CV + RV. RV must be determined independently. *FRC,* Functional residual capacity; *IC,* inspiratory capacity. (From Gilmour I, Burnham M, Craig DB. Closing capacity measurement during general anesthesia. *Anesthesiology*. 1976;45(5):477–482.)

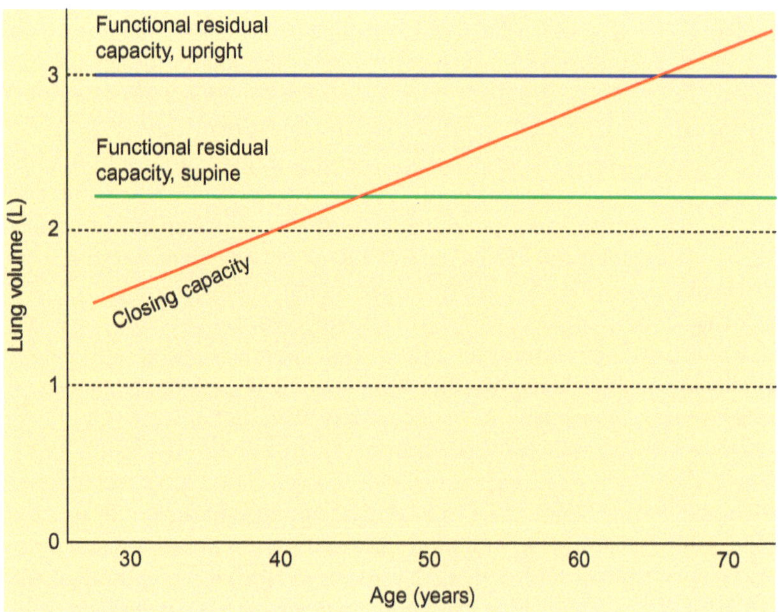

Source: Butterworth JF, Mackey DC, Wasnick JD. *Morgan & Mikhail's Clinical Anesthesiology*. 5th ed. www.accessmedicine.com.

• **Fig. 5.5 The effect of age and position on closing capacity, and its relationship to functional residual capacity.** Closing capacity increases with age. Although it is lower than functional capacity at younger ages, later in life it exceeds that. This implies increased susceptibility to small airway closure, which is more likely in the supine than in the upright position. (From Butterworth JF, Mackey DC, Wasnick JD. *Morgan & Mikhail's Clinical Anesthesiology*. 5th ed. www.accessmedicine.com.)

V_Ts and zero PEEP resulted in higher mean pulmonary artery pressure (MPAP), greater lung weight, and higher levels of thromboxane B_2, all suggestive of acute lung injury (ALI).[21] In morbidly obese patients, the effect of increased PEEP alone, a recruitment maneuver alone, and a recruitment maneuver followed by increased PEEP were compared using computed tomography (CT) scans and arterial partial pressure of oxygen (PaO_2)/inspired oxygen fraction (FiO_2) ratios. Similar to animal studies, the recruitment maneuver only transiently improved respiratory function, and PEEP by itself could not recruit the lungs, whereas the combination of the recruitment maneuver with the increased PEEP improved PaO_2/FiO_2 ratios and reduced atelectasis on CT.[22]

Respiratory Mechanics

Transpulmonary Pressure

The transpulmonary pressure, P_L, represents the distending pressure across the lungs, which is the difference between the airway pressure and the pleural pressure. It is an essential concept because it represents the pressure that effectively promotes air flow and distends the lungs. At end-inspiration, if respiratory flow equals zero and there is a clear plateau of the airway pressure, end-inspiratory $P_L = P_{plateau}$ − end-inspiratory $P_{pleural}$ represents the pressure acting across the alveolar units. At end exhalation, that pressure would be represented, in the absence of auto-PEEP, by end-expiratory P_L = PEEP − end-expiratory $P_{pleural}$. The importance of the concept of P_L becomes clear as the inspiratory P_L is the pressure which provides tidal ventilation at the same time that could produce stretch lung injury; and the end-expiratory P_L is that required to prevent lung collapse at end-exhalation by being kept positive.

Unfortunately, the assessment of P_L is not usual in clinical practice because measurement of pleural pressure is not simple, in contrast to measurement of airway pressure. Yet, pleural pressure may be estimated using an esophageal balloon, which is either standalone or attached to an esophagogastric tube and positioned in the lowest third of the esophagus[23–25] (Fig. 5.6). These esophagogastric tubes are generally 100 cm long, and the average depth for a correctly positioned balloon is approximately 35 to 45 cm. The catheter is connected to a pressure transducer via a three-way stopcock, and the balloon is inflated to a standard volume depending on the device, which is necessary to prevent artifact because of passive recoil of the balloon walls. Further, the balloon should be long enough to avoid regional variability, providing an average measurement of esophageal pressure to estimate pleural pressure. Although use of an esophageal balloon represents an improvement in the accuracy of pulmonary pressure monitoring, it is not without its limitations. Artifact may arise from mediastinal weight, gravitational gradients in pleural pressure, and airway closure at end exhalation.[23] Furthermore, there is considerable controversy in the literature on whether the esophageal pressure measurements should be directly taken as absolute estimates of pleural pressures for PEEP adjustments,[26] or whether changes in esophageal pressures should be used to compute chest wall and lung elastances, which are then used to set the level of the administered PEEP.[27] Although a ventilator strategy guided by the transpulmonary pressure measured with esophageal balloons improved

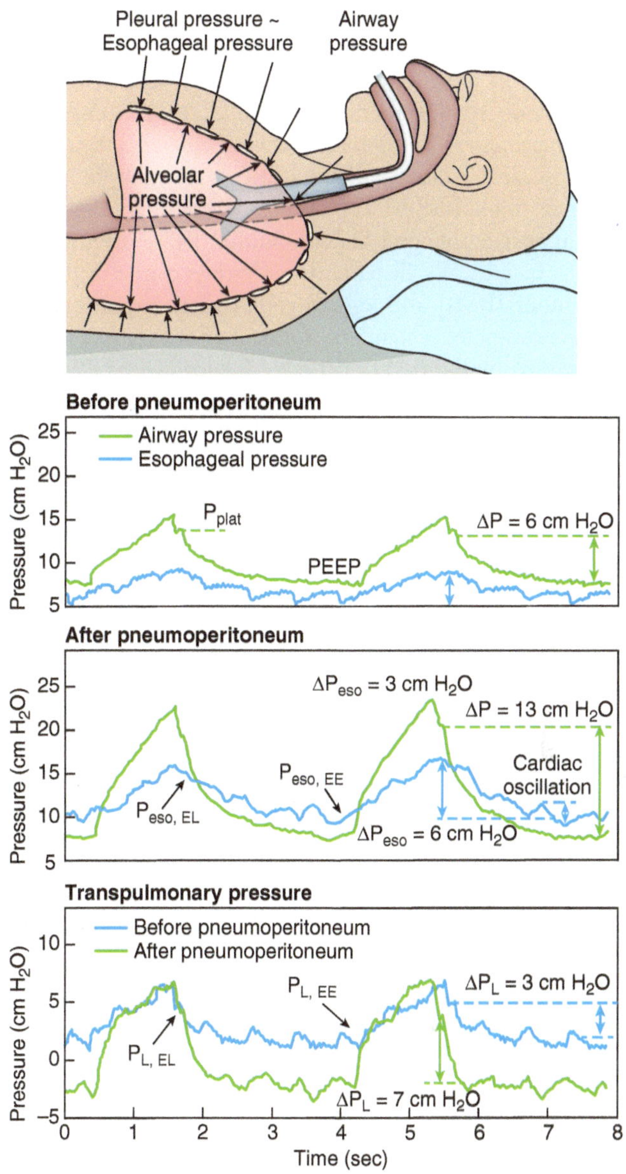

• **Fig. 5.6 Measurement of transpulmonary pressure using an esophageal balloon.** The balloon is positioned in the lower third of the esophagus. Transpulmonary pressure, P_L, is the difference between airway opening pressure (*blue lines*) and pleural pressure, estimated using the esophageal balloon pressure measurements (P_{eso}, *green lines*). In this case, the establishment of pneumoperitoneum produces a marked change in driving pressures (ΔP = plateau pressure, P_{Plat}, minus positive end-expiratory pressure, PEEP) of 7 cm H_2O, while ΔP_L increased by only 4 cm H_2O. This illustrates the fact that changes in airway pressures are not entirely transmitted to the lungs. Instead, they are also distributed to the chest wall. *EE*, End expiration; *EI*, end inspiration. (From Williams EC, Motta-Ribeiro GC, Vidal Melo MF. Driving pressure and transpulmonary pressure: how do we guide safe mechanical ventilation? *Anesthesiology*. 2019;131(1):155–163.)

oxygenation and compliance in a small group of acute respiratory distress syndrome (ARDS) patients,[28] a subsequent large trial on patients with moderate to severe ARDS resulted in no significant difference in death and days free from mechanical ventilation between patients receiving an esophageal balloon-guided PEEP and those receiving empirical high PEEP-FiO_2 settings.[29] Those findings did not support esophageal balloon-guided PEEP titration in ARDS. In critically ill patients with class 3 obesity (body mass index [BMI] ≥40 kg/m^2) and ARDS, a retrospective analysis compared a standard protocol of ventilator settings determined by the ARDS net table for lower PEEP/higher FiO_2 with a "lung rescue" management strategy with settings determined by an individualized protocol based on lung recruitment maneuvers, esophageal manometry, and hemodynamic monitoring.[29] Patients receiving the standard protocol had almost double the 28-day mortality compared with the lung rescue cohort (31% vs. 16%, P=.012; hazard ratio [HR], 0.32; 95% confidence interval [CI] 95%, 0.13–0.78).

In robotic-assisted laparoscopic surgery, esophageal manometry can help delineate the portion of increased driving pressure, which is applied to the lungs versus that applied to the chest wall; the increase in elastance associated with pneumoperitoneum is substantially greater for the chest wall (E_{CW}) than for the lungs (E_{LS}).[30] This may improve the ability to maintain open lung by appropriately titrating PEEP in this and other perioperative conditions with high susceptibility to lung derecruitment.

Driving Pressure

Driving pressure (ΔP) is the difference between the plateau pressure (P_{plat}) and PEEP (Fig. 5.7). The driving pressure can also be expressed as the V_T normalized by respiratory system compliance (C_{rs})—that is, the ΔP is proportional to the change in volume of the lung in a breath (V_T) divided by its initial volume, to the extent that C_{rs} changes in proportion to lung volume. Change in volume divided by initial volume is, by definition, the volumetric strain. Thus physiologically, the reason why ΔP may be important is because it provides a rough measure of the global volumetric strain of the lungs.[31–33]

Recent studies suggest that such physiologic considerations may be very important in the clinical setting. Driving pressures have been shown to be better associated with relevant clinical outcomes in ARDS[32,34] and surgical patients[33,35,36] than V_Ts. Indeed, a direct association of increased intraoperative ΔP with increased risk of significant postoperative pulmonary complications has been shown in patients undergoing noncardiothoracic surgery, in the absence of a corresponding association with V_T[33,35], in addition the relative risk of in-hospital death in relation to plateau pressure and driving pressure is depicted in Fig. 5.8. Such a relationship was also found in ARDS patients, with a greater association between increased ΔP and mortality compared with that of V_T[32] (Fig. 5.9). This finding was reinforced in a secondary analysis of observational data on patients with moderate to severe ARDS ventilated with standard lung-protective ventilation.[37] Variation in V_T or PEEP had no impact on mortality. In contrast, above a plateau pressure of 29 cm H_2O or a driving pressure of 19 cm H_2O, there was an ordinal increment in risk of death.[37]

In thoracic anesthesia, comparison of conventional lung-protective ventilation (one-lung ventilation [OLV] with V_T = 6 mL/kg ideal body weight, PEEP 5 cm H_2O, and recruitment maneuvers) with ΔP-guided ventilation (same VTs and recruitment, individualized PEEP to produce the lowest ΔP during OLV) showed a smaller incidence of pneumonia or ARDS in the ΔP-guided group.[38] A retrospective analysis of data of patients undergoing OLV for thoracic surgery (hospital electronic medical records and the

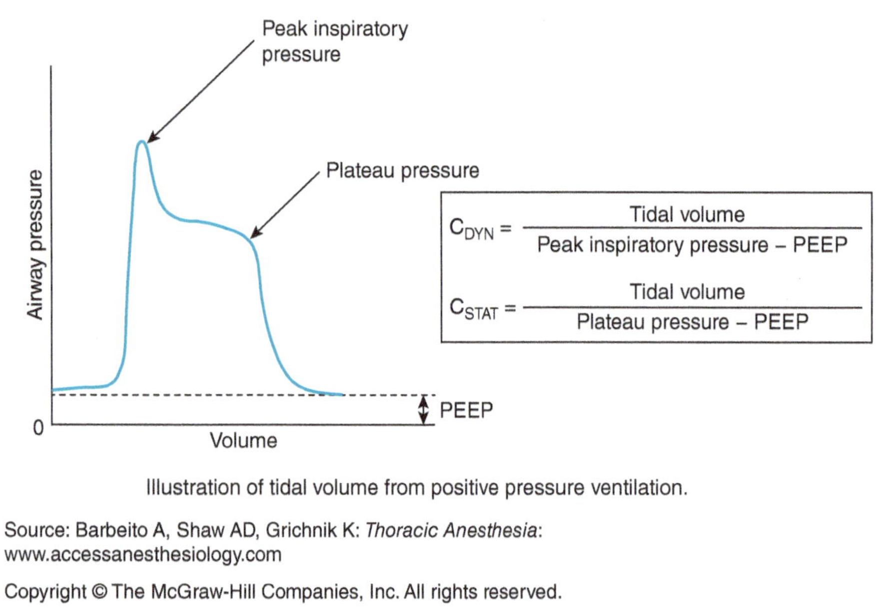

• **Fig. 5.7 Illustration of plateau pressure during volume control ventilation.** The plateau pressure (P_{plat}) is the airway pressure measured at the end of an inspiratory pause during volume control ventilation. The driving pressure (ΔP) is the difference between P_{plat} and positive end-expiratory pressure (*PEEP*). The dynamic compliance (C_{dyn}) is computed by normalizing the tidal volume (V_T) by the difference between the peak inspiratory pressure (PIP) and PEEP. The static compliance (C_{stat}) is computed by normalizing V_T by the difference between the P_{plat} and PEEP.

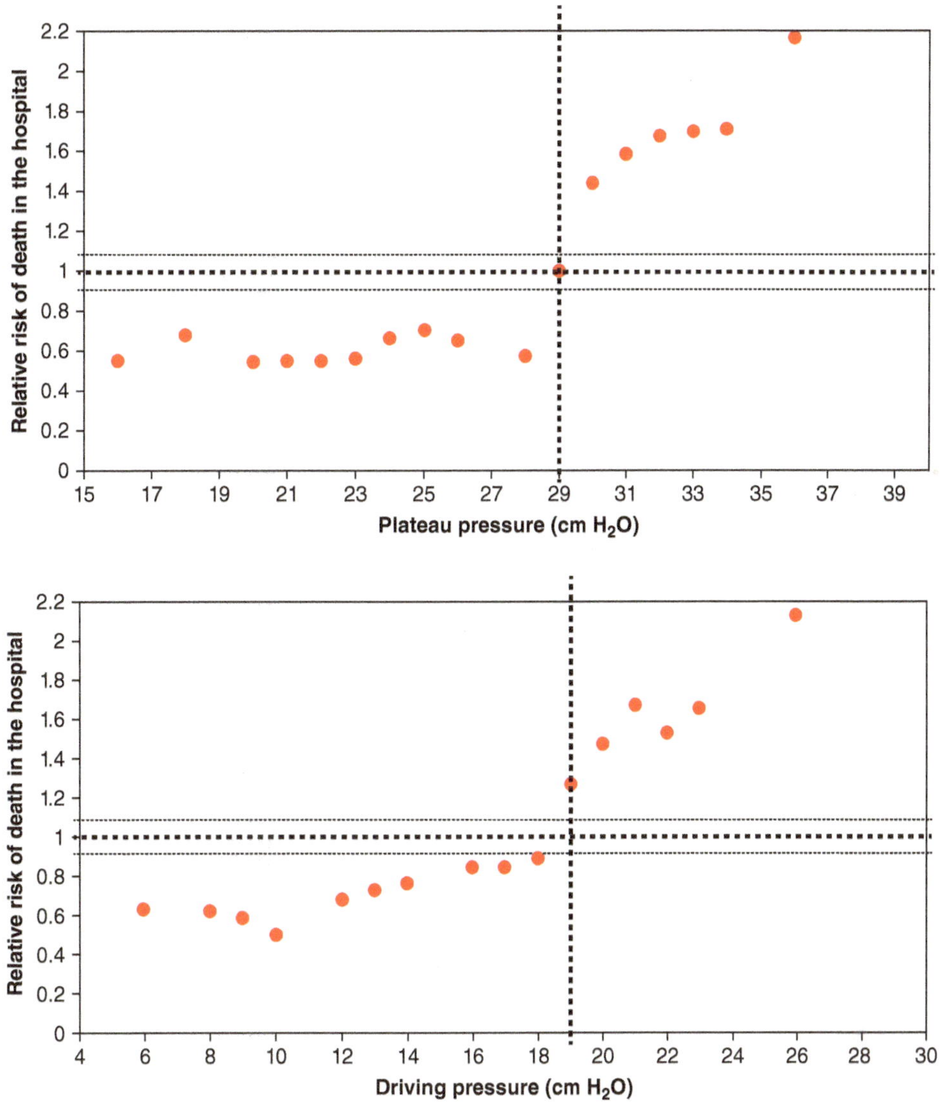

Fig. 5.8 Relative risk of death in hospital by plateau pressure and driving pressure quantile. 478 patients across a network of intensive care units were assessed based on quantiles of tidal volume (not shown), positive end-expiratory pressure (PEEP; not shown), plateau pressure, and driving pressure evaluated at 24 hours after the diagnosis of acute respiratory distress syndrome. Tidal volume and PEEP had no impact on mortality. **A plateau pressure cut-off value of 29 cm H_2O and a driving pressure cut-off value of 19 cm H_2O were found, above which an incrementally higher pressure was associated with a higher in-hospital risk of death.** (From Villar J, Martin-Rodriguez C, Dominguez-Berrot AM, et al. A quantile analysis of plateau and driving pressures: effects on mortality in patients with acute respiratory distress syndrome receiving lung-protective ventilation. *Crit Care Med*. 2017;45(5):843–850.)

Society of Thoracic Surgeons database) indicated that ΔP, when modeled together with V_T, predicted major morbidity, whereas V_T alone inversely correlated with respiratory complications.[39] This implied that low V_T by itself was not associated with less postoperative pulmonary complications, whereas low V_T taken together with strategies to minimize ΔP may be.[39]

Elastance and Compliance

The lungs and the chest wall have elastic properties that tend to restore them to their combined equilibrium configuration when they are displaced from baseline by spontaneous or mechanical ventilation. Thus if the pleural space is open at FRC, the lungs would recoil inward toward collapse, while the chest wall would recoil outward, toward expansion. **Elastance** is the change in distending pressure for a given change in volume ($E = \Delta P/\Delta V$). The elastance of the total respiratory system (E_{RS}) is the sum of the lung (E_L) and the chest wall (E_{CW}) elastances:

$$E_{RS} = E_L + E_{CW}$$

Compliance is the reciprocal of the elastance ($C = \Delta V/\Delta P$); that is, the change in volume for a given change in distending pressure. Compliance tends to be more frequently used

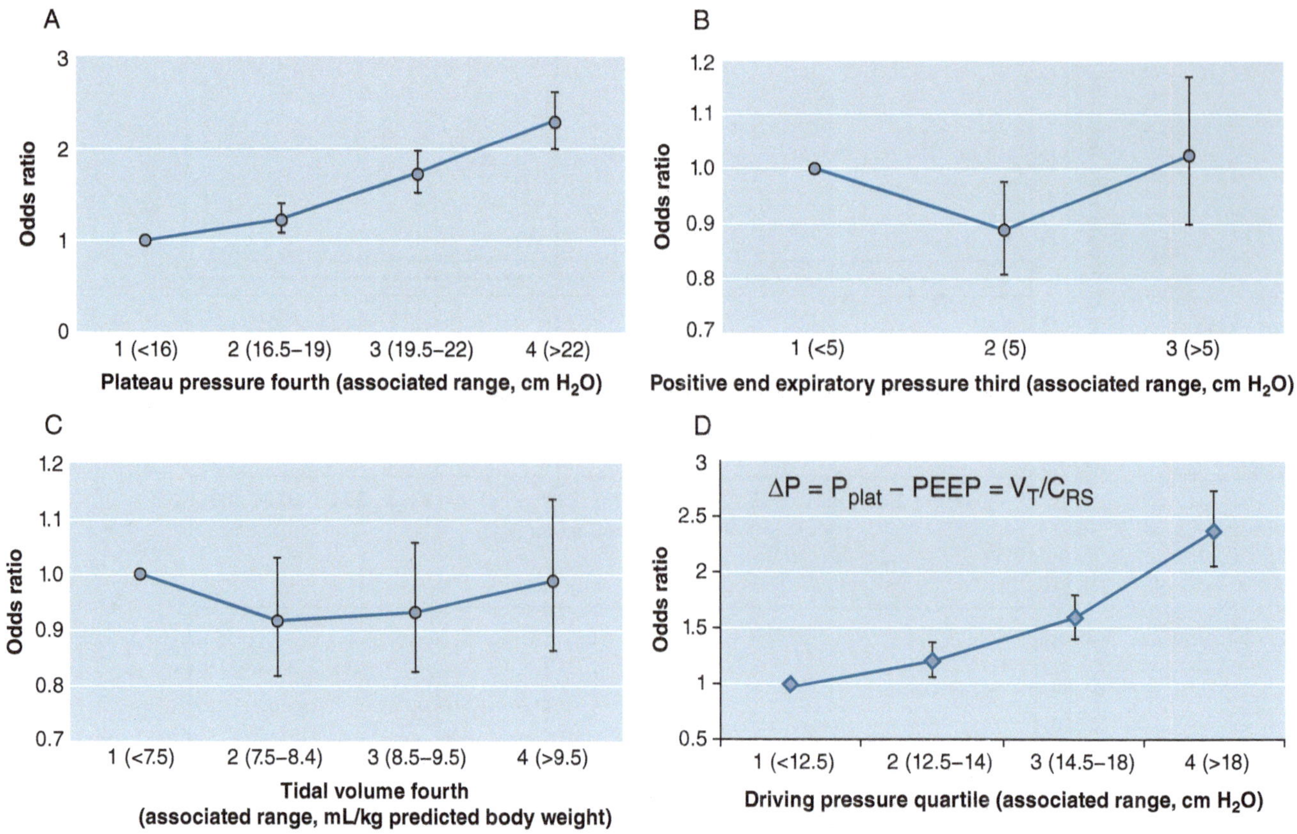

• **Fig. 5.9 Multivariate logistic regression analysis examining the impact of intraoperative ventilation parameters and risk of postoperative pulmonary complications.** Some 69,265 consecutively enrolled patients undergoing noncardiac surgery under general, endotracheal anesthesia were stratified by plateau pressure (quartiles, panel **A**), positive end-expiratory pressure (*PEEP*; tertiles, panel **B**), tidal volume (quartiles, panel **C**, and driving pressure quartiles, panel **D**). Odds ratio of postoperative pulmonary complication (composite of pulmonary edema, respiratory failure, pneumonia, and reintubation) increased with increased plateau pressure and driving pressure. (From Ladha K, Vidal Melo MF, McLean DJ, et al. Intraoperative protective mechanical ventilation and risk of postoperative respiratory complications: hospital based registry study. *BMJ*. 2015;351:h3646.)

clinically. Thus the earlier equation can be alternatively expressed as:

$$\frac{1}{C_{RS}} = \frac{1}{C_L} + \frac{1}{C_{CW}}$$

where C_{RS}, C_L, and C_{CW} are the compliances of the respiratory system, lung, and chest wall, respectively.

During mechanical ventilation with volume control, a peak inspiratory pressure (PIP) is usually seen, which is followed by a plateau pressure (P_{plat}) if an inspiratory pause (i.e., a period of no flow at end of inspiration) is provided (see Fig. 5.7). The difference between peak and plateau pressures is caused by dynamic factors, particularly airway resistance. Dynamic compliance (C_{dyn}) is defined as the compliance calculated using the PIP:

$$C_{dyn} = \frac{V_T}{PIP - PEEP}$$

where *PEEP* is the positive end-expiratory pressure (see Fig. 5.7). C_{dyn}, thus, conflates the distensibility of the lungs themselves with the resistance of the airways, in addition to the properties of the chest wall, to the overall quantification of compliance. Static compliance (C_{stat}) aims to eliminate the dynamic airflow-dependent component from the computation of compliance by using P_{plat}:

$$C_{Stat} = \frac{V_T}{P_{Plat} - PEEP}$$

Lung compliance represents the distensibility of the lung parenchyma; it is altered in various disease states. Compliance is decreased with consolidation, atelectasis, pulmonary edema, interstitial disease or fibrosis, pneumothorax, surgical resection, large effusion, and mainstem intubation. It is increased in emphysema because of loss of elastic tissue. In addition, lung compliance depends upon the lung volume in a nonlinear manner. The highest lung compliance is observed when lungs are at moderate volumes, and lowest at the extremes of low or high lung volumes. Such relationships are expressed in the pressure-volume curve of the lung (Fig. 5.10). That curve also shows that the pressure-volume relationship

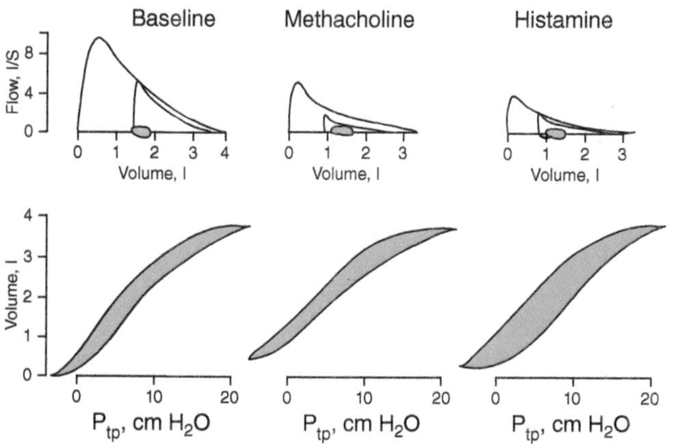

• **Fig. 5.10 Pressure-volume curve of the lung.** In a healthy human, the transpulmonary pressure-volume curve is sigmoidal, with lower compliances (ΔV/ΔP) at the low and high extremes of volume and pressure, and with a more linear intermediate region. **Baseline** (*B*). Use of **methacholine** does not change the properties of the pressure-volume curve (*MCh*). Yet, **histamine** increases the area of hysteresis, suggesting an effect on lung tissue properties (*His*). (From Pellegrino R, Violante B, Crimi E, Brusasco V. Effects of aerosol methacholine and histamine on airways and lung parenchyma in healthy humans. *J Appl Physiol* (1985). 1993;74(6):2681–2686.)

and the compliance for the same volume (or pressure) on inhalation differs from that on exhalation, a phenomenon known as *hysteresis.*

To compute the compliance of the lungs, the contribution of the chest wall needs to be subtracted. Accordingly, lung compliance ($C_L = \Delta V_L \Delta P_L$) can be estimated as:

$$C_L = \frac{V_T}{\left[\left(P_{awEI} - P_{esEI}\right)\right] - \left[\left(P_{awEE} - P_{esEE}\right)\right]},$$

where P_{awEI} is the airway pressure at end inhalation, P_{esEI} is the esophageal pressure at end inhalation, P_{awEE} is the airway pressure at end exhalation, and P_{esEE} is the esophageal pressure at end exhalation, measured using esophageal manometry, as explained earlier.

Chest wall compliance reflects the distensibility of the muscles, bones, and soft tissue that comprise the chest wall. Chest wall compliance is reduced with increased abdominal pressure (e.g., insufflation, abdominal compartment syndrome), chest wall edema, thoracic deformity, muscle tone, extensive thoracic/abdominal scar, supine positioning, and obesity. Chest wall compliance is *increased* with flail chest, muscle relaxation, and upright positioning. Using estimates of pleural pressure, the compliance of the chest wall (C_{CW}) can be calculated as:

$$C_{CW} = V_T / \left(P_{esEI} - O_{esEE}\right)$$

with variables that have been defined earlier.

Resistance

Resistance is the opposition to fluid flow because of friction and may be calculated as the ratio of the driving pressure to air flow ($R_{aw} = \Delta P / \dot{V}$). Airway resistance is determined by the dimensions of the airway, the viscosity of the gas, and whether the flow is laminar or turbulent, which in turn is predicted by the Reynold's number, Re:

$$Re = \frac{\rho u L}{\mu}$$

where ρ is the fluid/gas density (kg/m^3), u is the velocity (m/s), L is the length (m), and μ is the viscosity (kg/ms). Laminar flow dominates at Re less than 2300, while turbulent flow dominates at Re greater than 2900.

Laminar flow through a long cylindric pipe is governed by Poiseuille's Law, which is appropriately applied to conducting airways. Resistance is relatively low in laminar flow, and is calculated as follows:

$$R = \frac{8Lu}{\pi r^4}$$

where L is the length, u is the velocity, and r is the radius. Thus the airway radius is especially important in determining the resistance; if the radius is halved, the resistance increases by a factor of 16. Pathologic states, such as tracheal stenosis and bronchospasm, raise the resistance and increase the work of breathing. Reducing the density of the gas mixture (e.g., through mixing with helium, "Heliox") can improve resistance and lead to decreased work of breathing.

Because of the dependence on radius, an individual small airway has a higher resistance than a large airway. However, because the airways branch so prolifically, the overall resistance depends on the number of parallel pathways present, and it is the medium-sized airways that have the overall greatest resistance (see Fig. 5.2).

Stress and Strain

Stress is defined as force divided by the area over which it is applied.[31] Lung stress can be estimated through the transpulmonary pressure (P_L). This will be larger at end-inspiration and lower at end-exhalation, in the absence of patient effort. Strain is the change in dimension relative to the material's initial dimension. Based on this definition, lung volumetric strain can be calculated as the ratio of the change in lung volume (dV) to the resting lung volume (V_0), that is, dV/V_0.[40] Assuming a linear relationship, lung stress and strain are related to one another by the specific lung elastance, K.

$$\text{stress}\left(P_L\right) = K \cdot \text{strain}\left(\frac{dV}{V_0}\right).$$

Experimental studies indicate that when stress and strain are outside the normal physiologic limits, the lung releases inflammatory cytokines and mediators, which indicate, produce, and exacerbate lung injury. Very large V_Ts conducive to large strains, either through spontaneous or mechanical ventilation, can produce lung injury.[41,42] When mechanical ventilation is applied for more than 48 hours in initially normal animal lungs, injury occurs when lung expansion reaches approximately the TLC, that is when strain would be (TLC − FRC)/FRC.[40,43,44] In experiments representing usual clinical conditions, those large values are not present.[45] This suggests an increased susceptibility of lung tissue to strain in the presence of an additional injurious trigger (i.e., systemic inflammation).[46,47] A large animal study modeled moderate–severe ARDS (respiratory system compliance = 14.0 ± 4.9 mL/cm H_2O; PaO_2/FiO_2 = 92 ± 59) with surfactant depletion and ventilator-induced lung injury (VILI) and quantified volumetric strain using CT to support a relationship between strain and local inflammation assessed with positron emission tomography (PET) in those extreme lung injury cases.[48]

Stress is approximated by the transpulmonary pressure distending the airspaces, but the regional stress of the lung will vary because of gravity and other factors producing heterogeneous lung expansion. This will produce a distribution of stress throughout the lungs. For example, in uniformly expanded lungs, alveolar pressure is the same across the whole lung, but when the lung is not uniformly expanded (such as when air spaces are isolated from one another because of obstruction or closure), alveolar pressures will not be uniform throughout.[49] The presence of such heterogeneity leads to regional stress values substantially larger than those present at the global level.[45] This means that even when global transpulmonary pressures are low, local stresses can be high, even to the limit of being injurious.[45,50]

Mechanical Power

Stress and strain have been used for more than a century as criteria to determine material failure. Another variable used is energy.[51] In line with these traditional approaches, there has been recent interest in quantifying the power delivered to the lungs during mechanical ventilation as a means to measure risk of lung injury because of mechanical ventilation. Mechanical power is the energy delivered from the ventilator to the respiratory system per unit of time and is expressed in J · minute−1. The proposed equation for a mechanically ventilated lung with respiratory rate (RR), I:E ratio, and tidal volume V_T is:

$$\mathbf{MP = 0.098 \cdot RR \cdot Vt \cdot [Peak\ inspiratory\ pressure \\ -12(Plateau\ pressure\ \ PEEP)]}$$

(where 0.098 is a conversion factor from cm H_2O l min−1in J/min, RR is the respiratory rate, and Vt is the tidal volume in liters. The term (Plateau pressure − PEEP) is the driving pressure).

The interest in this equation is that it incorporates the known ventilator-generated causes of VILI (e.g., V_T, ΔP, flow, PEEP, RR), and thus may be used as a single quantity to predict the risk of VILI.[52] The power may be measured continuously using software on the ventilator, which agrees well with the earlier computed quantity in both normal subjects and in patients with ARDS.[52] Clinical validation of the concept is still pending.

Measures of Derecruitment and Overdistension

Just as atelectasis (derecruitment) is deleterious to the lung, alveolar overdistension places the lung at risk of ALI and overt barotrauma (Fig. 5.11). As detailed earlier, in injured lungs, regional lung inflation is heterogeneous, so regions of atelectasis may coexist with regions of normal ventilation and even overdistension.[53,54] Alveolar derecruitment and overdistension may be modeled by partitioning the dynamic respiratory system elastance ($E_{rs,dyn}$) into volume-dependent (E_1) and volume-independent (E_2) components and calculating the $\%E_2$ via the later formula.

$$\%\mathbf{E_2} = \frac{(100E_2V_T)}{(E_1 + E_2V_T)}.$$

A $\%E_2$ value greater than 30% represents overdistension, and was common, occurring at 40% of clinically set PEEP levels in one study of patients with ALI.[55] Conversely, a negative $\%E_2$ value represents atelectasis, and was found in all patients with abdominal distension when measured at a PEEP of 5 cm H_2O.[55]

An alternative measure of lung distension is the **stress index**, which measures the dynamic change in compliance during inspiration using the pressure-time curve of the ventilator.[1] Thus the stress index, gives information about both alveolar collapse and recruitment which help to prevent the deleterious effects of mechanical ventilation. The

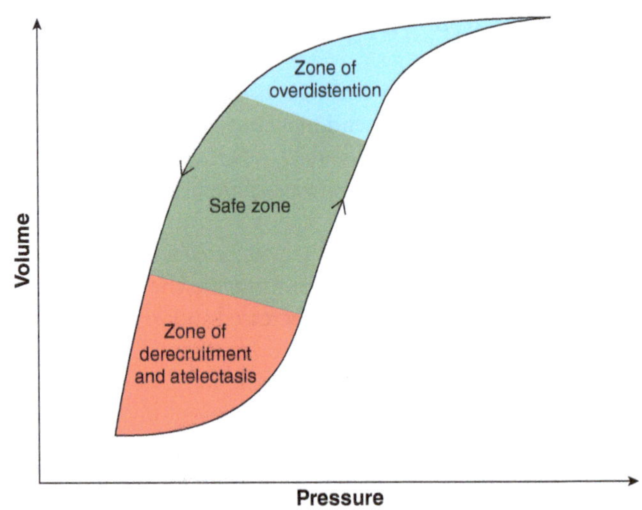

• **Fig. 5.11 Regions of risk for ventilator-induced lung injury as a function of lung pressure and volume.** Ventilator-induced lung injury occurs at both high and low extremes of lung volume. In the **zone of overdistension**, damage arises from fluid accumulation, surfactant degradation, and mechanical disruption. In the **zone of derecruitment** and atelectasis, lung injury arises from the trauma of repeated closure and reexpansion, through activation of the inflammatory cascade, and through local hypoxemia. High positive end-expiratory pressure (PEEP) and small tidal volumes enable ventilation to occur within the safe zone. (From Froese AB. High-frequency oscillatory ventilation for adult respiratory distress syndrome: let's get it right this time. *Crit Care Med*. 1997;25:906–908.)

stress index is determined by fitting the pressure-time curve during volume control ventilation with constant inspiratory flow to the following power equation:

$$P_{TP} = a \times time^{b} + c$$

where the coefficient a represents the slope of the pressure-time relationship in the time 0 to time 1 interval, and the coefficient c is the value of pressure at time 0 (P_{TP}: transpulmonary pressure).

Coefficient *b* is the stress index describing the shape of the curve (*b* = 1 indicates a straight curve, *b* < 1 indicates a progressive increase in compliance over time, and *b* > 1 indicates a progressive decrease in compliance with time). An application of this concept has been applied to choose the best PEEP as the titrated PEEP value, leading to a b = 0.9 − 1.1 (i.e., an approximately homogeneously expanding respiratory system).[56,57] The amount of lung subjected to hyperinflation increases with a stress index greater than 1.1, whereas values less than 0.9 correspond with atelectasis. Values less than 0.9 or greater than 1.1 correlate with a worsened VILI and release of inflammatory factors (e.g., interleukin-6, macrophage inflammatory protein-2).[58]

An application of such concepts was done in an investigation on the effects of stress index-guided PEEP titration on pulmonary mechanics and hemodynamics in the prone position that addressed severe lavage-induced lung injury in a piglet model.[56] Piglets underwent a decremental PEEP trial after full lung recruitment in the prone position. Stress-index PEEP was the level at which the airway pressure stress index was 1, and open-lung PEEP was the level which was required to keep the lung open according to CT scans. The authors found that the respiratory system elastance and lung elastance were improved in the prone position, but that the ratio of chest wall elastance to respiratory system elastance was higher in the prone position. There were no significant differences between the open-lung and stress index-guided groups in PEEP, collapsed lung volume, hyperinflation lung volume, oxygenation index, or arterial carbon dioxide partial pressure ($PaCO_2$). The authors concluded that the stress index can be used to titrate PEEP in the prone position in the studied model.

Effects of Anesthesia

The induction of general anesthesia decreases compliance because of the loss of muscle tone and the decrease in the FRC.[59] Reports differ on the effect of muscle relaxants on the overall respiratory system compliance. Some studies have found paralysis decreases the compliance for similar reasons,[60] but certainly compliance is increased in situations where paralytics promote improved ventilator synchrony.[61] Further, positioning while under anesthesia affects compliance, with prone positioning improving compliance, assuming that the lower body is at the same level as the chest.[59] Lateral decubitus positioning can worsen compliance because of the weight of the mediastinum and the abdominal contents on the dependent lung.[59] Certain surgical maneuvers may also affect compliance, with abdominal retraction and pneumoperitoneum worsening compliance, while abdominal wall lift, sternal splitting, and sternal lift all improve compliance.[62]

Pulmonary Gas Exchange

Ventilation

Ventilation is the bulk movement of gas into the lungs during inhalation and out of the lungs during exhalation, allowing the transport of oxygen into the lungs and removal of carbon dioxide from the lungs. Perfusion is the circulation of mixed venous blood through the pulmonary vascular bed. Therefore the PaO_2 and $PaCO_2$ are determined by the balance between alveolar ventilation and perfusion; this ratio is known as the $\dot{V}/\dot{Q}$. Both the overall ventilation ($\dot{V}$) and the overall perfusion ($\dot{Q}$) range approximately 4 to 6 L/min in an average-sized individual, so the overall $\dot{V}/\dot{Q}$ for the entire lung is approximately 0.8 to 1.2.[5] However, beyond average whole-lung values, the existence of a large number of alveolar units implies that optimal gas exchange depends on the matching of $\dot{V}$ and $\dot{Q}$ in each of these individual alveolar units.

Even in healthy conditions, there is a degree of heterogeneity in the $\dot{V}/\dot{Q}$ throughout the lungs. Ventilation per unit volume is greater in the more dependent regions of the lung in normal humans.[63] At rest, there is higher (less negative) pleural pressure in dependent regions because of gravity, resulting in lower transpulmonary pressure, less distention, greater compliance, and lower alveolar volumes.[64] Conversely, at lung volumes above FRC, that vertical gradient in pleural pressure results in dependent portions of the lung being more distended and less compliant than nondependent portions with inspiration, that is, larger dependent than nondependent ventilation, as airway pressure changes by a comparable amount in all areas.[65] Of note, differences in ventilation along the vertical axis are constant irrespective of body position (supine, lateral decubitus) in healthy humans.[65] At lung volumes between RV and FRC, expansion is larger in nondependent than dependent lung because of reasons beyond gravitational effects, that is, not only lower dependent compliances but also airway closure. Therefore most of the V_T during normal breathing will be delivered to the dependent part of the lung where the alveoli are less distended and more compliant.[65]

Perfusion

Perfusion per unit volume is also greater in more dependent areas of the lung. This is caused by hydrostatic effects, with higher hydrostatic pressure causing more alveolar capillary recruitment and distension, lower vessel resistance, and resulting in greater blood flow. On the other hand, nondependent areas of the lung have lower hydrostatic pressure, resulting in less recruitment and distension, a higher resistance to flow, and therefore less perfusion.[5,66] Fig. 5.12 illustrates the effect of gravity on both ventilation and perfusion in the upright lung.

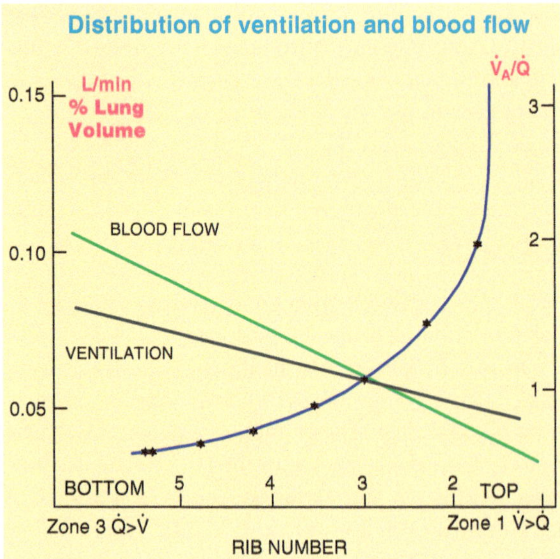

• **Fig. 5.12** Distribution of ventilation and perfusion and ventilation-perfusion ratio down the upright dog lung. (From West JB. *Ventilation/Blood Flow and Gas Exchange*. 5th ed. Oxford: Blackwell; 1990.)

Ventilation Perfusion Matching

Alterations in the relationship of ventilation and perfusion result in $\dot{V}/\dot{Q}$ mismatch. At one extreme, ventilation in the absence of perfusion is known as *alveolar dead space*. Without blood flow through the alveolar capillary, no gas exchange takes place, so the gas content of the alveolus is the same as the inspired gas. Alveolar dead space occurs in the upper (least dependent) part of the lung by a balance of airway and local vascular pressures. Other scenarios where perfusion is blocked, for example, pulmonary thromboembolism, air embolus, clamping or ligation of a pulmonary vessel intraoperatively will also result in dead space.

At the other extreme, perfusion in the absence of ventilation is known as *shunt*. If the ventilation to alveolar units is blocked (most frequently during OLV, mucus plugging, or atelectasis), the gas content of the mixed venous blood will equilibrate with that of the gas in the alveoli of the unventilated units. Once equilibrium is reached, no further gas exchange can take place, and the alveolar could eventually collapse depending on the local pressures and gas content. Higher FiO_2 may accelerate this collapse. The nonoxygenated mixed venous blood, derived from the right side of the heart, will mix with oxygenated blood transported to the left heart because of intrapulmonary right-to-left-shunt.

Fig. 5.13 illustrates how regions of different $\dot{V}/\dot{Q}$ affect the PaO_2.

Pulmonary Blood Flow

The pulmonary blood flow (PBF) consists of the entirety of the mixed venous blood pumped from the right ventricle in the absence of significant intracardiac shunts. The PBF is similar to the cardiac output (CO), which is approximately 3.5 to 4.0 L/min/m^2. The lung is also supplied by the bronchial circulation, which consists of oxygenated blood carried via the bronchial arteries, arising variably either from

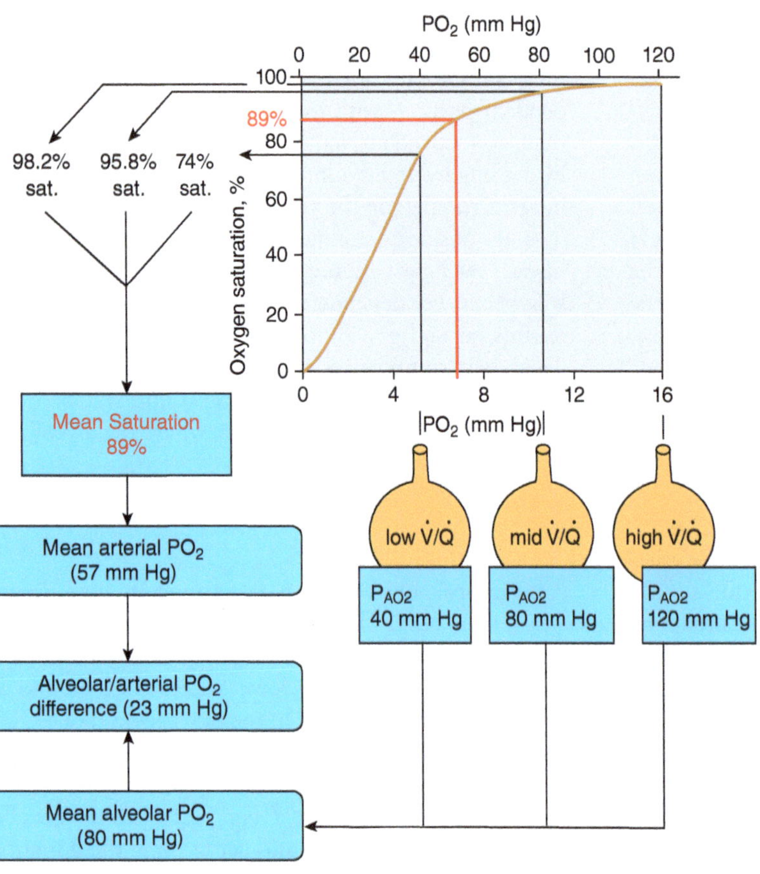

• **Fig. 5.13 Effect of different ventilation-perfusion ($\dot{V}/\dot{Q}$) regions on partial pressure of arterial oxygen (SaO_2).** In this example, the lung is composed by three regions of low, mid, and high $\dot{V}/\dot{Q}$, with equal perfusion to each of them. The consequent mean arterial saturation results approximately from the average of the saturations (strictly, the weighted mean of the oxygen contents). Because of the nonlinear shape of the oxygen dissociation curve, the corresponding arterial partial pressure of oxygen is not the mean of the partial pressures. Instead, it is a lower arterial partial pressure of oxygen (PaO_2) that corresponds to the mean arterial saturation of circulating hemoglobin (SaO_2) = 89%. (Modified from Lumb AB. *Nunn's Applied Respiratory Physiology*. 6th ed. Philadelphia, PA: Elsevier/Butterworth Heinemann; 2005: Fig. 8.13.)

the thoracic aorta or the intercostal arteries and representing a minor portion of the CO (approximately 2%). The bronchial circulation supports the tracheobronchial tree and extends down to the level of the terminal bronchioles.[5] More distal structures are supplied with oxygen through direct diffusion through intimate contact with the alveolus.

The PBF passes through the pulmonary arteries, which undergo approximately 28 dichotomous branchings, up until the pulmonary capillaries.[4] Pulmonary capillaries are approximately 6 µm in diameter, so erythrocytes must be deformed slightly from their normal diameter of approximately 8 µm to pass, which will increase the contact surface. A single erythrocyte will pass through several capillaries during its progress through the lung. Together, the pulmonary capillaries comprise of 50 to 100 m^2 of surface area for gas exchange.

Pulmonary Vascular Resistance

Pulmonary vascular resistance (PVR) is the resistance to flow across the pulmonary vasculature bed and is calculated as follows:

$$PVR = \left(\frac{MPAP - MLAP}{CO}\right) \times 80$$

where MPAP is the mean pulmonary artery pressure (mm Hg), mean left atrial pressure (MLAP) is the mean left atrial pressure (mm Hg), and CO is the cardiac output (L/min). PVR is most commonly expressed in dyn · s/cm.[5]

PVR is determined both by the tone of the vascular smooth muscle in the pulmonary circulation, as well as by a number of external factors. The volume of the lung affects alveolar and extraalveolar vessels differently. Alveolar vessels are stretched (that is, their length is increased and diameter decreased) at higher lung volumes, resulting in higher resistance to flow. Conversely, extraalveolar vessels are distended by more negative intrapleural pressure and by radial traction, so resistance in these vessels is decreased at higher lung volumes. The net effect on total PVR is a U-shaped curve relating PVR and lung volume with the lowest PVR near FRC (Fig. 5.14).

PBF affects PVR as well; increased blood flow decreases PVR. This can be explained by two mechanisms: distension and recruitment. Distension: as transmural pressure increases with increased PBF, vessels are distended, so their radius increases, and resistance to flow decreases. Recruitment: as PBF increases, the MPAP exceeds the opening

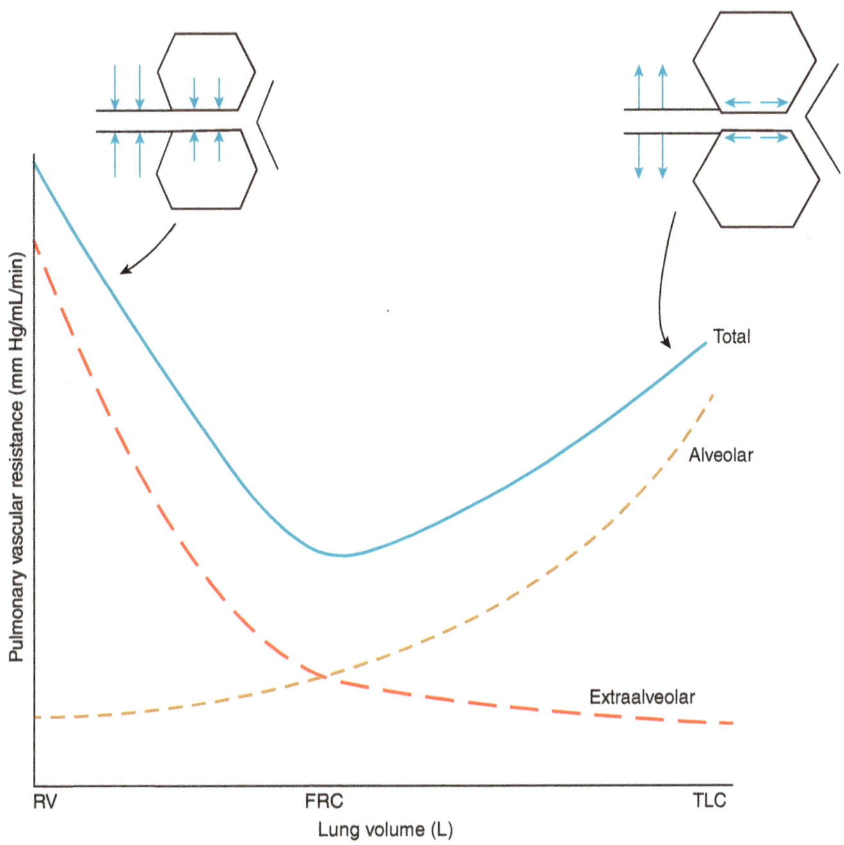

• **Fig. 5.14 The effects of lung volume on pulmonary vascular resistance (PVR).** A minimum PVR is present at intermediate lung volumes, where a balance is reached between compression of extraalveolar vessels and stretching and compression of alveolar vessels. *FRC,* Functional residual capacity; *RV,* residual volume; *TLC,* total lung capacity. (From Levitzky MG. *Alveolar Ventilation. Pulmonary Physiology*. Chapter 3, 9th ed. New York, NY: McGraw-Hill Education; 2017. All rights reserved.)

pressure for previously unperfused pulmonary capillaries, creating additional, parallel, pathways for PBF and decreasing the PVR. Similarly, more gravity-dependent areas of the lung will experience greater distension and recruitment, decreasing the regional PVR. Conversely, increased interstitial pressure compresses the pulmonary capillaries and increases PVR. Other factors which increase PVR include increased blood viscosity, such as polycythemia, which increases resistance in all vascular beds.

A number of humoral factors also affect the PVR. Norepinephrine,[67] epinephrine,[68] α-adrenergic agonists (e.g., phenylephrine),[69] prostaglandin (PG)$F_{2\alpha}$,[70,71] PGE_2,[72] thromboxane,[73] endothelin,[74] angiotensin,[74] and histamine[75] all have been empirically shown to increase the PVR. Acetylcholine,[76] β-adrenergic agonists,[77] PGE_1,[71] PGI_2,[78] nitric oxide,[79] and bradykinin[80] have been shown to decrease the PVR. In addition, hypoxia, hypercarbia, and acidosis increase PVR,[81] which will be further discussed in Chapters 15 on hypoxic pulmonary vasoconstriction.

Measurement of Ventilation-Perfusion Matching

Ventilation-Perfusion Scans

$\dot{V}/\dot{Q}$ scans have been used since the 1960s to assess the overall distribution of patients' ventilation and perfusion. The scan is obtained by having the patient inhale a radioactive gas (e.g., Xe-133, Krypton-81m, Tc99m), and an image is captured using a gamma camera. Similarly, albumin with a radioactive-tracer (Tc99m-macroaggregated albumin [MAA]) is injected into the bloodstream and the perfusion image is captured using the gamma camera. These images are overlaid, often with a chest x-ray to inform the interpretation of any anatomic abnormalities. The $\dot{V}/\dot{Q}$ scan can identify regions of mismatched ventilation and perfusion, classically, for the identification of pulmonary thromboembolism. $\dot{V}/\dot{Q}$ scans may also be used in planning lung resection by allowing the preoperative contribution to ventilation and perfusion to be estimated for the region to be resected, ensuring that the remaining VC postlung resection will maintain the capacity to eliminate CO_2.[82]

Diffusion

Diffusion is the net movement of a substance from a region of higher concentration to one of lower concentration. Diffusion is governed by Fick's first law:

$$J = -D\frac{d\varphi}{dx}$$

where J is the diffusion flux (amount of substance flowing through a unit area during a set time period), D is the diffusion coefficient, ϕ is the concentration, and x is the length.

Diffusion of oxygen, carbon dioxide, and other gases (e.g., anesthetic agents) across the alveolar-capillary membrane may be "diffusion-limited" in conditions which thicken the alveolar-capillary barrier, such as in interstitial lung disease or pulmonary edema.

Measurement of Hypoxemia and Hypercapnia

Hypoxemia may be caused by any of the following five physiologic conditions: (1) hypoventilation, (2) $\dot{V}/\dot{Q}$ mismatching, (3) right-to-left shunt, (4) diffusion limitation, and (5) diffusion-perfusion mismatch. Hypoxemia can be assessed by several different methods.

Oxygen Saturation (SpO_2)

SpO_2 refers to the peripheral arterial oxygen saturation, as measured by pulse oximetry. Pulse oximetry takes advantage of the differential absorption of light by oxygenated and deoxygenated hemoglobin. Most pulse oximeters emit light at 660 and 940 nm, where 660 nm is better absorbed by deoxygenated hemoglobin, whereas 940 nm is better absorbed by oxygenated hemoglobin. The ratio of the absorption of these two wavelengths is empirically calibrated to the arterial oxygen saturation based on each pulse oximeter. These devices are generally reliable to a standard deviation of ± 2% over a range of 70% to 100% SpO_2.[83] Pulse oximetry has been a standard American Society of Anesthesiologists monitor since 1986, and now is also part of the International Standards for a Safe Practice of Anesthesia,[84] as well as part of the World Health Organization safe surgery checklist.[85] Note that the measured SpO_2 corresponds to an estimate of the arterial saturation of circulating hemoglobin (SaO_2). More specifically, an estimate related to the properties of the blood within the field covered by the light absorbed by the transducer. Accordingly, the information refers to blood within that field, not to tissue oxygenation.

Shunt

A major cause of hypoxemia in the perioperative setting is right-to-left shunt. This occurs when mixed-venous blood from the right heart circulation passes to the left heart circulation without undergoing oxygenation. Right-to-left shunt can occur at the cardiac and the pulmonary levels, and may be caused by anatomic factors, such as intracardiac shunt, pulmonary arteriovenous malformations, and pulmonary vascular dilation as during the hepatopulmonary syndrome. In spontaneously breathing normal humans, intrapulmonary right-to-left shunt is negligible. A small component is caused by drainage from the bronchial and thebesian veins.[86] This increases to approximately 2% to 5% of the CO when measured with 100% FiO_2 because of oxygen absorption atelectasis.[87,88] As mentioned previously, shunt of pulmonary origin occurs because of regions of the lungs that are perfused, but not ventilated, that is, because of collapse of alveolar units or to gas trapping, resulting in the absence of alveolar-capillary gas exchange. Using oxygen as the measurement gas, the shunt fraction can be estimated by the following equation, while breathing an FiO_2 of 1.0:

$$\frac{Q_s}{Q_t} = \frac{(C_CO2 - C_aO2)}{(C_CO2 - C_vO2)}$$

where Q_s is the physiologic shunt, Q_t is the cardiac output, CcO_2 is the end-pulmonary capillary oxygen content, C_aO_2 is the arterial oxygen content, and CvO_2 is the mixed venous oxygen content. The reason that the shunt equation required the breathing of FiO_2 of 1.0 is that the capillary saturation cannot be measured and is assumed to be 100% saturated when FiO_2 of 1.0 is used.[89]

Venous admixture is a concept that is related to shunt; it represents the calculated volume of mixed venous blood that would need to be added to explain an observed difference between pulmonary end-capillary PO_2 and arterial PaO_2. Venous admixture arises from regions of the lung that participate in inefficient gas exchange, but where some degree of gas exchange still occurs.

PaO_2/FiO_2 Ratios

Another way to quantify the degree of hypoxemia is through expressing the PaO_2/FiO_2 ratio—that is the ratio of the arterial partial pressure of oxygen, PaO_2, normalized to the inspired oxygen concentration, FiO_2. The PaO_2/FiO_2 ratio depends on shunt, dead space, and FiO_2, but assuming an FiO_2 of 0.21, a normal PaO_2/FiO_2 ratio is approximately 475 mm Hg. PaO_2/FiO_2 cutoffs are used according to the Berlin criteria to rate the severity of ARDS: mild (200 mm Hg $< PaO_2/FiO_2 \leq$ 300 mm Hg), moderate (100 mm Hg $< PaO_2/FiO_2 \leq$ 200 mm Hg), and severe ($PaO_2/FiO_2 \leq$ 100 mm Hg).[90–92]

SpO_2/FiO_2 ratios have been recently proposed as noninvasive surrogates of PaO_2/FiO_2 ratios. In patients with ARDS, PaO_2 measurements imputed from SpO_2 measurements using nonlinear equations to describe the oxygen dissociation curve better approximated PaO_2 compared with linear or log-linear equations.[93,94] Yet, SpO_2 estimates were affected by use of vasopressors and better clinical validation is awaited.

A-a Gradient

The alveolar-to-arterial oxygen gradient, or A-a gradient, is another commonly used measure to describe impairment in oxygenation. It is expressed as the following:

$$\text{A} - \text{a gradient} = P_AO2 - P_aO2$$

where P_AO_2 is the alveolar partial pressure of oxygen, and the PaO_2 is the arterial partial pressure of oxygen. P_AO_2 can be calculated using the alveolar gas equation:

$$P_AO2 = \left(F_iO2\left[P_{atm} - P_H2O\right]\right) - \frac{P_aCO2}{R}$$

where FiO_2 is the inhaled fraction of oxygen, P_{atm} is the ambient barometric pressure, P_H2O is the partial pressure of water in the atmosphere, $PaCO_2$ is the arterial partial pressure of carbon dioxide, and R is the respiratory quotient (a dimensionless number that relates the amount of CO_2 produced by the body to the amount of O_2 consumed in the same unit of time). A normal A-a gradient can be estimated for a subject breathing ambient air using the following equation[95]:

$$\text{A} - \text{a gradient} = 2.5 + 0.21 \times (\text{age in years})$$

Dead Space

As discussed earlier, dead space represents the regions of the respiratory system that are ventilated but do not participate in gas exchange. Dead space can be conceptualized as anatomic dead space and physiologic dead space. The anatomic dead space corresponds to the gas volume of the conducting portions of the respiratory system which do not physiologically participate in the gas exchange (nose, pharynx, trachea, and bronchi). Normal anatomic dead space is approximately 30% of the normal V_T (approximately 150 cc for a 500 cc breath). The physiologic dead space is composed by the sum of the anatomic and the alveolar dead space. The alveolar dead space is the gas volume in alveolar regions that receive ventilation but do not exchange gas because of absent or mismatched alveolar perfusion, a concept implying wasted ventilation. Complete absence of blood flow would represent wasted ventilation corresponding to a condition of $\dot{V}/\dot{Q} = \infty$; alternatively, there could be alveolar units of excessive ventilation in relation to perfusion, that is, wasted ventilation in the form of high ventilation/perfusion ratio. In both of these cases, the regions of wasted ventilation would produce gas with low values of alveolar CO_2 partial pressure ($PACO_2$), ultimately lowering the value of the mean expired CO_2 partial pressure ($PeCO_2$). Quantitatively, these effects allow for the estimation of the physiologic dead space, such as by the Bohr equation:

$$\frac{V_D}{V_T} = \left(\frac{P_aCO2 - P_eCO2}{P_aCO2}\right),$$

where V_D is the physiologic dead space, V_T is the tidal volume, and $PaCO_2$ is the arterial carbon dioxide partial pressure.[96] The V_D/V_T ratio is a measure of ventilation efficiency. The normal value is approximately 0.33, and higher values indicate ventilation inefficiency. During mechanical ventilation, V_D/V_T increases because of increased $\dot{V}/\dot{Q}$ mismatch and potential distension of conducting airways. It is also increased in diseases, such as COPD[97] and ARDS.[98] In the latter, it has been suggested as a marker of poor outcome.[99,100]

Pulmonary Function Tests

Forced Expiratory Volume in 1 Second

The forced expiratory volume in one second (FEV_1) is the time period during which expiratory flow is most sensitive to changes in airway resistance. FEV_1 is also expressed as a fraction of the value predicted or as a ratio to the forced vital capacity (FVC). FEV_1 is a predictor of cardiopulmonary morbidity after surgery for lung resection. FEV_1 less than 60% of predicted has been shown to predict perioperative mortality and respiratory morbidity in patients undergoing surgery for lung cancer.[101]

The predicted postoperative FEV_1 ($ppoFEV_1$) is used to provide such a peroperative predictor. It is calculated as the product of the preoperative FEV_1 by a factor representing the expected reduction in lung function from surgery ($ppoFEV_1 = FEV_1 \times f$). This factor f can be computed from an expectation of the anatomic contribution of each lobe to FEV_1 or from measurements of regional ventilation and perfusion. The anatomic contribution can be calculated as $f = (1-y/z)$, where y is the number of functional lung segments to be resected and z is the total number of functional segments. In the intact lung, z = 20, as depicted in Fig. 5.1, which shows the z values for each lobe: right upper lobe = 3, right middle lobe = 2, right lower lobe = 5, left upper lobe = 5, left lower lobe = 5.[102,103]

There is a low correlation between $ppoFEV_1$ and FEV_1 measured the days after pulmonary resection, when most complications develop. In a prospective analysis of patients undergoing lobectomy or pneumonectomy with overall cardiorespiratory morbidity of 22%, $ppoFEV_1$ had a similar predictive value as postoperative pain score and type of analgesia. The FEV_1 measured on postoperative day 1 was the most important variable in predicting cardiorespiratory complications, followed by patient age and $ppoFEV_1$. However, such postoperative FEV_1 cannot be used to inform surgical decision making, as it is not available preoperatively.[104]

Although these relationships with outcomes have been observed, guidelines have a limited ability to select patients for surgery. This is caused by the limited performance of these parameters in predicting postoperative complications in COPD patients, probably related to the lung volume reduction effect.[105,106] For instance, in a retrospective analysis of over 500 patients who underwent lobectomy or pneumonectomy, the morbidity rate was not significantly different between patients with FEV_1 of 70% or more predicted versus those with FEV_1 under 70% predicted. Thus the role of FEV_1 as a selection criteria for high-risk patient is brought into question.[105]

Forced Vital Capacity

The FVC is the forced vital capacity. It requires that the subject make a maximal inspiration to TLC, then make a maximal forced expiratory effort, leaving only the RV.

In a normal subject, the FEV_1/FVC is greater than 0.8; patients with obstructive lung disease, such as asthma or COPD, show a decreased FEV_1/FVC. The FEV_1/FVC is thought to represent resistance from larger airways. Reduced FEV_1/FVC (<70%) is predictive of postoperative respiratory complication including long-term oxygen therapy and atelectasis after lung resection surgery.[107] More recently, preoperative FEV_1/FVC ratio below the lower limit of normal (LLN) was shown to provide a more accurate risk stratification than FEV_1/FVC less than 0.70, resulting in a 3-fold increase in prolonged oxygen therapy and a 50% increase in prolonged postoperative stay (compared with subjects with an FEV_1/FVC between the LLN and 0.70).[108] Furthermore, preoperative FEV_1/FVC below the LLN predicts an overall worse overall survival and disease-free survival than that observed in subjects with an FEV_1/FVC between the LLN and 0.70.[109]

Forced Vital $Capacity_{25\%-75\%}$

$FEV_{25\%-75\%}$, or the forced (mid) expiratory flow rate, is an alternate quantity to measure airway resistance. The $FEV_{25\%-75\%}$ is measured as the slope of the line drawn between the 25% and 75% points of maximal exhalation on the FVC curve. The slope will be shallower in patients with increased resistance because of obstructive disease. $FEV_{25\%-75\%}$ is thought to represent resistance from the small- to medium-sized airways. $FEV_{25\%-75\%}$ has not yet been validated as a predictor of patient outcomes in thoracic surgery. However, at least one study showed forced (mid) expiratory flow rate (defined as $FEV_{50\%-75\%}$ in this study) predicted prolonged ventilator support in cardiac surgery patients.[110]

Diffusing Capacity of Carbon Monoxide

The pulmonary diffusing capacity for substance x (DL_x) is the rate at which it is absorbed by the lungs, per unit partial pressure difference between the alveoli and the pulmonary capillaries:

$$DL_x = \frac{\dot{V}_x}{P_{Ax} - P_{\bar{C}x}}$$

where $\dot{V}_x$ is the uptake of gas x (mL/min), P_{Ax} is the partial pressure of x in the alveoli (mm Hg), and $P_{\bar{C}x}$ is the mean partial pressure of x in the pulmonary capillaries (mm Hg).

Clinically, carbon monoxide is the gas used to measure the pulmonary diffusing capacity, as it presents high solubility in blood. In this way, when carbon monoxide is administered through inhalation, it is quickly taken up by hemoglobin and its partial pressure in blood remains low, so that the partial pressure difference between the alveolus and the pulmonary capillary is well-maintained throughout the time blood spends in the pulmonary capillary. In this manner, the diffusion is presumed to be limited by the diffusivity of the alveolar-capillary barrier. That is, the pulmonary diffusion capacity of carbon monoxide (DLCO) is diffusion-limited, rather than perfusion-limited. DLCO may be measured using either a single-breath or a steady-state technique. DLCO is decreased in interstitial lung disease (e.g., idiopathic pulmonary fibrosis, sarcoidosis, systemic sclerosis), conditions that decrease the surface area for diffusion (emphysema, tumors, low cardiac output states), and in states of $\dot{V}/\dot{Q}$ mismatch. In this latter case, the reduction of DLCO is not only affected by the properties of the alveolar-capillary membrane in itself, but by $\dot{V}/\dot{Q}$ mismatch producing heterogeneous distribution of inhaled carbon monoxide throughout the lungs, with regions of low alveolar partial pressure of carbon monoxide resulting in lower carbon monoxide absorption and global DLCO measurement.[111]

DLCO is associated with postoperative mortality and pulmonary morbidity,[112–114] as well as with long-term survival[115] and residual quality of life.[116] Values of 60% of predicted have been used as the cutoff for postoperative risk. Predicted postoperative DLCO (ppoDLCO) is computed similarly to the ppoFEV_1 and is similarly relevant to outcomes. The predictive value of DLCO is exemplified by a large retrospective analysis in video-assisted thoracoscopic surgery (VATS) lobectomies or segmentectomies demonstrating an association of male sex, DLCO under 60% predicted, and operative time greater than 150 minutes with 90-day mortality.[117]

Robotic-assisted thoracoscopic lobectomy: Of note, clinical data are still limited for patients undergoing this new surgical modality. A recent study indicated a low incidence of pulmonary complications (13%).[118] Pulmonary function tests (PFTs) remained useful in patients undergoing robotic lobectomy and were particularly valuable in patients with poorer pulmonary function. Postoperative pulmonary complications were increased when the predicted FEV_1 was less than 60% and DLCO less than 50%, the ppoFEV_1 is under 50% or ppoDLCO under 50%.[118]

Cardiopulmonary Exercise Testing

Preoperative risk for lung resection is also assessed by exercise capacity. This is determined by three components: pulmonary, cardiovascular, and skeletal muscle. Subjects exercise using a treadmill or stationary bike, while their inspired and expired gas contents are measured via transducers connected to a facemask. In cardiopulmonary exercise testing (CPET), the maximal oxygen uptake ($\dot{V}O_{2max}$, expressed as mL O_2/kg/min consumed) is measured during incremental exercise as measured $\dot{V}O_2$ plateaus despite increased workload. $\dot{V}O_{2max}$ is correlated with CO and skeletal muscle blood flow.[119] Multiple studies have been performed using different cutoffs predictive of postlung resection morbidity and mortality. $\dot{V}O_2$ less than 65% or $\dot{V}O_{2max}$ less than 16 mL/min/kg are predictive of cardiorespiratory complications after lung resection surgery.[120]

The association between $\dot{V}O_2$ and postoperative outcomes has led to the implementation of interventions to improve $\dot{V}O_{2max}$, with the expectation that these would improve outcomes. Prehabilitation is a term used to describe such programs undertaken by the patient before surgery to improve postoperative outcomes. Prehabilitation includes lifestyle interventions, such as exercise, stress reduction, cognitive training, smoking cessation, and nutritional supplementation. Implementation of these interventions could optimize patients' physical capacity before surgery, improve outcomes, and enhance recovery. CPET is the gold standard technique to predict postoperative morbidity and mortality and may be used to measure the improvement in cardiopulmonary function effected by prehabilitation exercise programs. Prehabilitation has demonstrated reduction of morbidity and mortality in other surgeries, but continues to be under evaluation for thoracic surgery. Increased $\dot{V}O_2$ has been demonstrated for high-intensity interval training conducted before elective liver metastasis resection and major abdominal surgery.[121,122] In lung resection surgery, prehabilitation is also shown to improve $\dot{V}O_2$ and other CPET measures but may not improve ventilatory efficiency.[123]

Because CPET is both time- and resource-intensive, an alternative method to assess exercise capacity is the 6-minute walk distance (6MWD), which measures the distance a subject can walk in 6 minutes and is an indicator of both aerobic capacity and endurance.[124] A 2 week multimodal prehabilitation program in patients scheduled for thorascopic lobectomy improved the 6MWD by over 60 meters.[125] To date, however, while aerobic performance and physiologic endpoints have improved, the impact of prehabilitation programs on patient outcomes has been mixed. One retrospective study examined patients undergoing VATS lobectomy who had received prehabilitation versus those who had not over a 13-month period and showed the cohort of patients undergoing prehabilitation had fewer postoperative pulmonary complications (42% vs. 80%, $P = .04$).[126,127] Conversely, a prospective study randomizing patients to a high-intensity interval training program during the preoperative waiting period (mean = 25 days) did not show a statistically significant difference in the study's primary endpoint, a composite of mortality and in-hospital pulmonary mortality (35.5% vs. 50.6%, $P = .08$), although a trend toward such was noted.[127,128] In the same study, pulmonary complications were reduced in the prehabilitation group, driven primarily by reduction in the rates of atelectasis.[128]

Recommendations for Preoperative Assessment

Relevant current recommendations from the American College of Chest Physicians related to PFTs state the following. The strength of evidence backing the recommendation is included following each statement.[102]

- In patients with lung cancer being considered for surgery, it is recommended that both FEV_1 and DLCO be measured in all patients, and that both predicted postoperative ppoFEV_1 and ppoDLCO are calculated (grade 1B).
- In patients with lung cancer being considered for surgery, if both ppoFEV_1 and ppoDLCO are over 60% predicted, no further tests are recommended (grade 1C).
- In patients with lung cancer being considered for surgery, if either the ppoFEV_1 or ppoDLCO are less than 60% predicted and both are above 30% predicted, it is recommended that a low technology exercise test (stair climb or shuttle walk test [SWT]) is performed (grade 1C).
- In patients with lung cancer being considered for surgery, with either a ppoFEV_1 under 30% predicted or a ppoDLCO under 30% predicted, performance of a formal CPET with measurement of maximal oxygen consumption ($\dot{V}O_{2max}$) is recommended (grade 1B).

- In patients with lung cancer being considered for surgery, who walk less than 25 shuttles (or < 400 m) on the SWT or climb less than 22 m at symptom limited stair climbing test, performance of a formal CPET with measurement of $\dot{V}O_{2max}$ is recommended (grade 1C).
- In patients with lung cancer being considered for surgery, and a $\dot{V}O_{2max}$ less than 10 mL/kg/min or less than 35% predicted, it is recommended that they are counseled about minimally invasive surgery, sublobar resections, or nonoperative treatment options for their lung cancer (grade 1C).
- In patients with lung cancer being considered for surgery, and deemed at high risk (as defined by the proposed functional algorithm, that is, $ppoFEV_1$ or ppoDLCO < 60% predicted and $\dot{V}O_{2max}$ < 10 mL/kg/min or < 35% predicted), preoperative or postoperative pulmonary rehabilitation is recommended (grade 1C).

Use of these guidelines for FEV_1 and DLCO measurements seems to be fairly consistent in current clinical practice. Yet, despite such guidelines, there is substantial variation in preoperative cardiopulmonary assessment practices.[129] The effect of such lack of adherence on outcomes is unknown.

Conclusion

In this chapter, we reviewed a number of important concepts essential to the safe care of patients undergoing mechanical ventilation during thoracic surgery. Knowledge of normal lung structure and function informs decisions regarding appropriate ventilation parameters pre- and postoperatively, depending on the extent of resection. The vocabulary of lung volumes gives a standard nomenclature to characterize patients' baseline impairment in lung function. An overview of respiratory mechanics, which are readily assessed in mechanically ventilated patients helps to elucidate patients' underlying pathophysiology, protect patients against iatrogenic lung injury, and adjust to the dynamic needs of thoracic surgery. A thorough understanding of pulmonary gas exchange allows for the perioperative assessment of and differential diagnosis of hypoxemia and hypercarbia. Finally, review of pulmonary function testing, its role in predicting pulmonary outcomes following thoracic surgery, and evidence-based guidelines inform decision-making for lung resection in patients presenting with lung cancer.

References

1. Hess DR. Respiratory mechanics in mechanically ventilated patients. *Respir Care.* 2014;59(11):1773–1794.
2. Standring S, Anand N, Birch R, et al. *Gray's Anatomy: The Anatomical Basis of Clinical Practice.* 41st ed. New York: Elsevier Limited; 2016.
3. Barash PG, Cullen BF, Stoelting RK, et al. *Clinical Anesthesia.* 8th ed.: EBook Without Multimedia. Philadelphia, PA: Wolters Kluwer Health; 2017.
4. Weibel ER, Gomez DM. Architecture of the human lung. Use of quantitative methods establishes fundamental relations between size and number of lung structures. *Science* (New York, NY). 1962;137(3530):577–585.
5. Levitzky MG. *Alveolar Ventilation. Pulmonary Physiology.* 9th ed. New York, NY: McGraw-Hill Education; 2017.
6. Ferguson GT. Why does the lung hyperinflate? *Proc Am Thorac Soc.* 2006;3(2):176–179.
7. Leith DE, Brown R. Human lung volumes and the mechanisms that set them. *Eur Respir J.* 1999;13(2):468–472.
8. Caramez MP, Borges JB, Tucci MR, et al. Paradoxical responses to positive end-expiratory pressure in patients with airway obstruction during controlled ventilation. *Crit Care Med.* 2005; 33(7):1519–1528.
9. Drummond GB, Milic-Emili J. Forty years of closing volume. *Brit J Anaesth.* 2007;99(6):772–774.
10. Buist AS, Ross BB. Predicted values for closing volumes using a modified single breath nitrogen test. *Am Rev Respir Dis.* 1973; 107(5):744–752.
11. Garrard GS, Littler WA, Redman CW. Closing volume during normal pregnancy. *Thorax.* 1978;33(4):488–492.
12. Farebrother MJ, McHardy GJ, Munro JF. Relation between pulmonary gas exchange and closing volume before and after substantial weight loss in obese subjects. *Br Med J.* 1974;3(5927): 391–393.
13. Weygandt GR. A sensitive five-breath N2 washout test of distribution of ventilation. *J Appl Physiol.* 1976;40(3):464–467.
14. Gilmour I, Burnham M, Craig DB. Closing capacity measurement during general anesthesia. *Anesthesiology.* 1976;45(5):477–482.
15. Laws AK. Effects of induction of anaesthesia and muscle paralysis on functional residual capacity of the lungs. *Can Anaesthet Soc J.* 1968;15(4):325–331.
16. Don HF, Wahba M, Cuadrado L, Kelkar K. The effects of anesthesia and 100 per cent oxygen on the functional residual capacity of the lungs. *Anesthesiology.* 1970;32(6):521–529.
17. Don HF, Craig DB, Wahba WM, Couture JG. The measurement of gas trapped in the lungs at functional residual capacity and the effects of posture. *Anesthesiology.* 1971;35(6):582–590.
18. Kozian A, Schilling T, Freden F, et al. One-lung ventilation induces hyperperfusion and alveolar damage in the ventilated lung: an experimental study. *Br J Anaesth.* 2008;100(4):549–559.
19. Kozian A, Schilling T, Schutze H, Heres F, Hachenberg T, Hedenstierna G. Lung computed tomography density distribution in a porcine model of one-lung ventilation. *Br J Anaesth.* 2009;102(4):551–560.
20. Oudin S, Pugin J. Role of MAP kinase activation in interleukin-8 production by human BEAS-2B bronchial epithelial cells submitted to cyclic stretch. *Am J Respir Cell Mol Biol.* 2002;27(1): 107–114.
21. Gama de Abreu M, Heintz M, Heller A, Szechenyi R, Albrecht DM, Koch T. One-lung ventilation with high tidal volumes and zero positive end-expiratory pressure is injurious in the isolated rabbit lung model. *Anesth Analg.* 2003;96(1):220–228, Table of contents.
22. Reinius H, Jonsson L, Gustafsson S, et al. Prevention of atelectasis in morbidly obese patients during general anesthesia and

paralysis: a computerized tomography study. *Anesthesiology.* 2009;111(5):979–987.
23. Loring SH, O'Donnell CR, Behazin N, et al. Esophageal pressures in acute lung injury: do they represent artifact or useful information about transpulmonary pressure, chest wall mechanics, and lung stress? *J Appl Physiol (Bethesda, Md: 1985).* 2010;108(3): 515–522.
24. Mietto C, Malbrain ML, Chiumello D. Transpulmonary pressure monitoring during mechanical ventilation: a bench-to-bedside review. *Anaesthesiol Intens Ther.* 2015;47 Spec No:s27–s37.
25. Akoumianaki E, Maggiore SM, Valenza F, et al. The application of esophageal pressure measurement in patients with respiratory failure. *Am J Respir Crit Care Med.* 2014;189(5):520–531.
26. Loring SH, Topulos GP, Hubmayr RD. Transpulmonary pressure: the importance of precise definitions and limiting assumptions. *Am J Respir Crit Care Med.* 2016;194(12):1452–1457.
27. Gattinoni L, Carlesso E, Cressoni M. Selecting the 'right' positive end-expiratory pressure level. *Curr Opin Crit Care.* 2015; 21(1):50–57.
28. Talmor D, Sarge T, Malhotra A, et al. Mechanical ventilation guided by esophageal pressure in acute lung injury. *N Engl J Med.* 2008;359(20):2095–2104.
29. Beitler JR, Sarge T, Banner-Goodspeed VM, et al. Effect of titrating positive end-expiratory pressure (PEEP) with an esophageal pressure-guided strategy vs an empirical high PEEP-fio2 strategy on death and days free from mechanical ventilation among patients with acute respiratory distress syndrome: a randomized clinical trial. *JAMA.* 2019;321(9):846–857.
30. Brandao JC, Lessa MA, Motta-Ribeiro G, et al. Global and regional respiratory mechanics during robotic-assisted laparoscopic surgery: a randomized study. *Anesth Analg.* 2019;129(6): 1564–1573.
31. Williams EC, Motta-Ribeiro GC, Vidal Melo MF. Driving pressure and transpulmonary pressure: how do we guide safe mechanical ventilation? *Anesthesiology.* 2019;131(1): 155–163.
32. Amato MB, Meade MO, Slutsky AS, et al. Driving pressure and survival in the acute respiratory distress syndrome. *N Engl J Med.* 2015;372(8):747–755.
33. Ladha K, Vidal Melo MF, McLean DJ, et al. Intraoperative protective mechanical ventilation and risk of postoperative respiratory complications: hospital based registry study. *BMJ.* 2015; 351:h3646.
34. Bugedo G, Retamal J, Bruhn A. Driving pressure: a marker of severity, a safety limit, or a goal for mechanical ventilation? *Crit Care (London, England).* 2017;21(1):199.
35. Neto AS, Hemmes SN, Barbas CS, et al. Association between driving pressure and development of postoperative pulmonary complications in patients undergoing mechanical ventilation for general anaesthesia: a meta-analysis of individual patient data. *Lancet Respir Med.* 2016;4(4):272–280.
36. Florio G, Ferrari M, Bittner EA, et al. A lung rescue team improves survival in obesity with acute respiratory distress syndrome. *Crit Care (London, England).* 2020;24(1):4.
37. Villar J, Martin-Rodriguez C, Dominguez-Berrot AM, et al. A quantile analysis of plateau and driving pressures: effects on mortality in patients with acute respiratory distress syndrome receiving lung-protective ventilation. *Crit Care Med.* 2017;45(5): 843–850.
38. Park M, Ahn HJ, Kim JA, et al. Driving pressure during thoracic surgery: a randomized clinical trial. *Anesthesiology.* 2019; 130(3):385–393.
39. Blank RS, Colquhoun DA, Durieux ME, et al. Management of one-lung ventilation: impact of tidal volume on complications after thoracic surgery. *Anesthesiology.* 2016;124(6):1286–1295.
40. Gattinoni L, Carlesso E, Caironi P. Stress and strain within the lung. *Curr Opin Crit Care.* 2012;18(1):42–47.
41. D'Angelo E, Koutsoukou A, Della Valle P, Gentile G, Pecchiari M. The development of various forms of lung injury with increasing tidal volume in normal rats. *Respir Physiol Neurobiol.* 2020;274:103369.
42. Ziaka M, Makris D, Fotakopoulos G, et al. High-tidal-volume mechanical ventilation and lung inflammation in intensive care patients with normal lungs. *Am J Crit Care.* 2020;29(1):15–21.
43. Protti A, Cressoni M, Santini A, et al. Lung stress and strain during mechanical ventilation: any safe threshold? *Am J Respir Crit Care Med.* 2011;183(10):1354–1362.
44. Mandava S, Kolobow T, Vitale G, et al. Lethal systemic capillary leak syndrome associated with severe ventilator-induced lung injury: an experimental study. *Crit Care Med.* 2003;31(3):885–892.
45. Motta-Ribeiro G, Winkler T, Hashimoto S, Vidal Melo MF. Spatial heterogeneity of lung strain and aeration and regional inflammation during early lung injury assessed with PET/CT. *Acad Radiol.* 2019;26(3):313–325.
46. Wellman TJ, Winkler T, Costa EL, et al. Effect of local tidal lung strain on inflammation in normal and lipopolysaccharide-exposed sheep. *Crit Care Med.* 2014;42(7):e491–e500.
47. Motta-Ribeiro GC, Hashimoto S, Winkler T, et al. Deterioration of regional lung strain and inflammation during early lung injury. *Am J Respir Crit Care Med.* 2018;198(7):891–902.
48. Retamal J, Hurtado D, Villarroel N, et al. Does regional lung strain correlate with regional inflammation in acute respiratory distress syndrome during nonprotective ventilation? An experimental porcine study. *Crit Care Med.* 2018;46(6):e591–e599.
49. Mead J, Takishima T, Leith D. Stress distribution in lungs: a model of pulmonary elasticity. *J Appl Physiol.* 1970;28(5):596–608.
50. Paula LF, Wellman TJ, Winkler T, et al. Regional tidal lung strain in mechanically ventilated normal lungs. *J Appl Physiol (Bethesda, Md: 1985).* 2016;121(6):1335–1347.
51. Mittemeijer EJ. *Mechanical Strength of Materials Fundamentals of Materials Science: The Microstructure–Property Relationship Using Metals as Model Systems.* Berlin, Heidelberg: Springer; 2011:497–581.
52. Gattinoni L, Tonetti T, Cressoni M, et al. Ventilator-related causes of lung injury: the mechanical power. *Intens Care Med.* 2016;42(10):1567–1575.
53. Gattinoni L, Pesenti A, Bombino M, et al. Relationships between lung computed tomographic density, gas exchange, and PEEP in acute respiratory failure. *Anesthesiology.* 1988;69(6):824–832.
54. Maunder RJ, Shuman WP, McHugh JW, Marglin SI, Butler J. Preservation of normal lung regions in the adult respiratory distress syndrome. Analysis by computed tomography. *JAMA.* 1986;255(18):2463–2465.
55. Bersten AD. Measurement of overinflation by multiple linear regression analysis in patients with acute lung injury. *Eur Respir J.* 1998;12(3):526–532.
56. Pan C, Tang R, Xie J, et al. Stress index for positive end-expiratory pressure titration in prone position: a piglet study. *Acta Anaesthesiol Scand.* 2015;59(9):1170–1178.
57. Huang Y, Yang Y, Chen Q, et al. Pulmonary acute respiratory distress syndrome: positive end-expiratory pressure titration needs stress index. *J Surg Res.* 2013;185(1):347–352.

58. Ranieri VM, Zhang H, Mascia L, et al. Pressure-time curve predicts minimally injurious ventilatory strategy in an isolated rat lung model. *Anesthesiology.* 2000;93(5):1320–1328.
59. Saraswat V. Effects of anaesthesia techniques and drugs on pulmonary function. *Indian J Anaesth.* 2015;59(9):557–564.
60. Schindler MB, Bohn DJ, Bryan AC. The effect of single-dose and continuous skeletal muscle paralysis on respiratory system compliance in paediatric intensive care patients. *Intens Care Med.* 1996;22(5):486–491.
61. Fletcher ME, Stack C, Ewart M, et al. Respiratory compliance during sedation, anesthesia, and paralysis in infants and young children. *J Appl Physiol (Bethesda, Md: 1985).* 1991;70(5): 1977–1982.
62. Matsumoto K. [Changes in thorax-lung compliance during general anesthesia with mechanical ventilation in response to various intraoperative maneuvers.] *Masui Jap J Anesthesiol.* 2006; 55(6):704–707.
63. Bryan AC, Bentivoglio LG, Beerel F, Macleish H, Zidulka A, Bates DV. Factors affecting regional distribution of ventilation and perfusion in the lung. *J Appl Physiol.* 1964;19:395–402.
64. Rhodes CG, Valind SO, Brudin LH, Wollmer PE, Jones T, Hughes JM. Quantification of regional V/Q ratios in humans by use of PET. I. Theory. *J Appl Physiol (Bethesda, Md: 1985).* 1989;66(4):1896–1904.
65. Kaneko K, Milic-Emili J, Dolovich MB, Dawson A, Bates DV. Regional distribution of ventilation and perfusion as a function of body position. *J Appl Physiol.* 1966;21(3):767–777.
66. West JB, Dollery CT, Naimark A. Distribution of blood flow in isolated lung; relation to vascular and alveolar pressures. *J Appl Physiol.* 1964;19:713–724.
67. Shebuski RJ, Smith JM Jr, Ruffolo RR Jr. Comparison of the renal and pulmonary hemodynamic effects of fenoldopam, dobutamine, dopamine and norepinephrine in the anesthetized dog. *Pharmacology.* 1988;36(1):35–43.
68. Cheung PY, Barrington KJ, Pearson RJ, Bigam DL, Finer NN, Van Aerde JE. Systemic, pulmonary and mesenteric perfusion and oxygenation effects of dopamine and epinephrine. *Am J Respir Crit Care Med.* 1997;155(1):32–37.
69. Wodack KH, Graessler MF, Nishimoto SA, et al. Assessment of central hemodynamic effects of phenylephrine: an animal experiment. *J Clin Monitor Comput.* 2019;33(3):377–384.
70. Leffler CW, Passmore JC. Contribution of prostaglandins to the regulation of pulmonary vascular resistance in adult cats and dogs. *Prostaglandins Med.* 1979;3(6):343–360.
71. Dagher E, Dumont L, Chartrand C, Blaise G. Effects of PGE1 in experimental vasoconstrictive pulmonary hypertension. *Eur Surg Res Eur Chirurg Forsch Rec Chirurg Eur.* 1993;25(2):65–73.
72. Kadowitz PJ, Gruetter CA, Spannhake EW, Hyman AL. Pulmonary vascular responses to prostaglandins. *Fed Proc.* 1981;40(7):1991–1996.
73. Santillan-Doherty P, Sotres-Vega A, Jasso-Victoria R, Olmos-Zuniga R, Arreola-Ramirez L, Cedillo-Ley I. Plasma thromboxane B2 concentrations and pulmonary vascular resistance during lung reperfusion. *J Invest Surg.* 1997;10(4):165–171.
74. Wang M, Shibamoto T, Shinomiya S, et al. Pulmonary vascular and airway responses to systemic vasoconstrictors in anesthetized BALB/c mice. *J Cardiovasc Pharmacol.* 2015;65(4):325–334.
75. Barman SA, Taylor AE. Histamine's effect on pulmonary vascular resistance and compliance at elevated tone. *Am J Physiol.* 1989;257(2 Pt 2):H618–H625.
76. Barman SA, Senteno E, Smith S, Taylor AE. Acetylcholine's effect on vascular resistance and compliance in the pulmonary circulation. *J Appl Physiol.* (Bethesda, Md: 1985). 1989;67(4): 1495–1503.
77. Takashio T, Yamashita H, Onodera S. Effects of beta-agonist and antagonist on the pulmonary circulation and the pulmonary pressor response to 5-HT. *Eur J Pharmacol.* 1989;169(1):179–182.
78. Nair J, Lakshminrusimha S. Update on PPHN: mechanisms and treatment. *Semin Perinatol.* 2014;38(2):78–91.
79. Stamler JS, Loh E, Roddy MA, Currie KE, Creager MA. Nitric oxide regulates basal systemic and pulmonary vascular resistance in healthy humans. *Circulation.* 1994;89(5):2035–2040.
80. Bonner G, Preis S, Schunk U, Wagmann M, Chrosch R, Toussaint C. Effect of bradykinin on arteries and veins in systemic and pulmonary circulation. *J Cardiovasc Pharmacol.* 1992; 20(Suppl 9):S21–S27.
81. Rudolph AM, Yuan S. Response of the pulmonary vasculature to hypoxia and H+ ion concentration changes. *J Clin Invest.* 1966;45(3):399–411.
82. Bailey DL, Roach PJ. A brief history of lung ventilation and perfusion imaging over the 50-year tenure of the editors of seminars in nuclear medicine. *Semin Nucl Med.* 2020;50(1):75–86.
83. Nitzan M, Romem A, Koppel R. Pulse oximetry: fundamentals and technology update. *Med Devices* (Auckland, NZ). 2014; 7:231–239.
84. Merry AF, Cooper JB, Soyannwo O, Wilson IH, Eichhorn JH. International standards for a safe practice of anesthesia 2010. *Can J Anaesth.* 2010;57(11):1027–1034.
85. Haynes AB, Weiser TG, Berry WR, et al. A surgical safety checklist to reduce morbidity and mortality in a global population. *N Engl J Med.* 2009;360(5):491–499.
86. Ravin MB, Epstein RM, Malm JR. Contribution of thebesian veins to the physiologic shunt in anesthetized man. *J Appl Physiol.* 1965;20(6):1148–1152.
87. Ming DK, Patel MS, Hopkinson NS, Ward S, Polkey MI. The 'anatomic shunt test' in clinical practice; contemporary description of test and in-service evaluation. *Thorax.* 2014;69(8):773–775.
88. Berg SM BM. The postanesthesia care unit. Editors: Michael Gropper, Lars Eriksson, Lee Fleisher, Jeanine Wiener-Kronish, Neal Cohen, Kate Leslie. *Miller's Anesthesia.* 9th ed. Elsevier; 2019:2586–2613.
89. Cruz JC, Metting PJ. Understanding the meaning of the shunt fraction calculation. *J Clin Monitor.* 1987;3(2):124–134.
90. Covelli HD, Nessan VJ, Tuttle WK 3rd. Oxygen derived variables in acute respiratory failure. *Crit Care Med.* 1983;11(8):646–649.
91. Ranieri VM, Rubenfeld GD, Thompson BT, et al. Acute respiratory distress syndrome: the Berlin Definition. *JAMA.* 2012;307(23):2526–2533.
92. Ferguson ND, Fan E, Camporota L, et al. The Berlin Definition of ARDS: an expanded rationale, justification, and supplementary material. *Intens Care Med.* 2012;38(10):1573–1582.
93. Brown SM, Grissom CK, Moss M, et al. Nonlinear imputation of Pao2/Fio2 from Spo2/Fio2 among patients with acute respiratory distress syndrome. *Chest.* 2016;150(2):307–313.
94. Severinghaus JW. Simple, accurate equations for human blood O_2 dissociation computations. *J Appl Physiol: Respir Environment Exe Physiol.* 1979;46(3):599–602.
95. Mellemgaard K. The alveolar-arterial oxygen difference: its size and components in normal man. *Acta Physiol Scand.* 1966; 67(1):10–20.
96. Intagliata SRA, Gossman WG. Physiology, Lung Dead Space. StatPearls [Internet]: Treasure Island (FL): StatPearls Publishing; updated 2019 May 15. Available from: https://www.ncbi.nlm.nih.gov/books/NBK482501/.

97. O'Donnell DE, Parker CM. COPD exacerbations: pathophysiology. *Thorax.* 2006;61(4):354–361.
98. Ferluga M, Lucangelo U, Blanch L. Dead space in acute respiratory distress syndrome. *Ann Transl Med.* 2018;6(19):388.
99. Kallet RH, Zhuo H, Ho K, Lipnick MS, Gomez A, Matthay MA. Lung injury etiology and other factors influencing the relationship between dead-space fraction and mortality in ARDS. *Respir Care.* 2017;62(10):1241–1248.
100. Nuckton TJ, Alonso JA, Kallet RH, et al. Pulmonary dead-space fraction as a risk factor for death in the acute respiratory distress syndrome. *N Engl J Med.* 2002;346(17):1281–1286.
101. Licker MJ, Widikker I, Robert J, et al. Operative mortality and respiratory complications after lung resection for cancer: impact of chronic obstructive pulmonary disease and time trends. *Ann Thorac Surg.* 2006;81(5):1830–1837.
102. Brunelli A, Kim AW, Berger KI, Addrizzo-Harris DJ. Physiologic evaluation of the patient with lung cancer being considered for resectional surgery: diagnosis and management of lung cancer, 3rd ed: American College of Chest Physicians evidence-based clinical practice guidelines. *Chest.* 2013;143(5 suppl):e166S–e190S.
103. Bolliger CT, Guckel C, Engel H, et al. Prediction of functional reserves after lung resection: comparison between quantitative computed tomography, scintigraphy, and anatomy. *Respiration.* 2002;69(6):482–489.
104. Varela G, Brunelli A, Rocco G, et al. Measured FEV1 in the first postoperative day, and not ppoFEV1, is the best predictor of cardio-respiratory morbidity after lung resection. *Eur J Cardiothorac Surg.* 2007;31(3):518–521.
105. Brunelli A, Al Refai M, Monteverde M, Sabbatini A, Xiume F, Fianchini A. Predictors of early morbidity after major lung resection in patients with and without airflow limitation. *Ann Thorac Surg.* 2002;74(4):999–1003.
106. Linden PA, Bueno R, Colson YL, et al. Lung resection in patients with preoperative FEV1 < 35% predicted. *Chest.* 2005; 127(6):1984–1990.
107. Yoshimi K, Oh S, Suzuki K, et al. Impact of airflow limitation on comorbidities and postoperative complications in patients undergoing thoracic surgery: a retrospective observational study. *Ann Thorac Cardiovasc Surg.* 2016;22(3):146–152.
108. Osuka S, Hashimoto N, Sakamoto K, Wakai K, Yokoi K, Hasegawa Y. Risk stratification by the lower limit of normal of FEV1/FVC for postoperative outcomes in patients with COPD undergoing thoracic surgery. *Respir Invest.* 2015;53(3):117–123.
109. Matsuzaki A, Hashimoto N, Okachi S, et al. Clinical impact of the lower limit of normal of FEV1/FVC on survival in lung cancer patients undergoing thoracic surgery. *Respir Invest.* 2016;54(3): 184–192.
110. Peters RM, Brimm JE, Utley JR. Predicting the need for prolonged ventilatory support in adult cardiac patients. *J Thorac Cardiovasc Surg.* 1979;77(2):175–182.
111. Prisk GK, McKinnon AE. A modeling approach to the estimation of CO diffusing capacity. *J Appl Physiol (Bethesda, Md: 1985).* 1987;62(1):373–380.
112. Ferguson MK, Little L, Rizzo L, Popovich KJ, Glonek GF, Leff A, et al. Diffusing capacity predicts morbidity and mortality after pulmonary resection. *J Thorac Cardiovasc Surg.* 1988; 96(6):894–900.
113. Cerfolio RJ, Bryant AS. Different diffusing capacity of the lung for carbon monoxide as predictors of respiratory morbidity. *Ann Thorac Surg.* 2009;88(2):405–410; discussion 10-1.
114. Ferguson MK, Siddique J, Karrison T. Modeling major lung resection outcomes using classification trees and multiple imputation techniques. *Eur J Cardiothorac Surg.* 2008;34(5):1085–1089.
115. Ferguson MK, Dignam JJ, Siddique J, Vigneswaran WT, Celauro AD. Diffusing capacity predicts long-term survival after lung resection for cancer†. *Eur J Cardiothorac Surg.* 2012;41(5): e81–e86.
116. Handy JR Jr, Asaph JW, Skokan L, et al. What happens to patients undergoing lung cancer surgery? Outcomes and quality of life before and after surgery. *Chest.* 2002;122(1):21–30.
117. Brunelli A, Dinesh P, Woodcock-Shaw J, Littlechild D, Pompili C. Ninety-day mortality after video-assisted thoracoscopic lobectomy: Incidence and risk factors. *Ann Thorac Surg.* 2017; 104(3):1020–1026.
118. Cao C, Louie BE, Melfi F, et al. Impact of pulmonary function on pulmonary complications after robotic-assisted thoracoscopic lobectomy. *Eur J Cardiothorac Surg.* 2020;57(2):338–342.
119. Reddy HK, Weber KT, Janicki JS, McElroy PA. Hemodynamic, ventilatory and metabolic effects of light isometric exercise in patients with chronic heart failure. *J Am Coll Cardiol.* 1988; 12(2):353–358.
120. Loewen GM, Watson D, Kohman L, et al. Preoperative exercise Vo2 measurement for lung resection candidates: results of Cancer and Leukemia Group B Protocol 9238. *J Thorac Oncol.* 2007;2(7):619–625.
121. Dunne DF, Jack S, Jones RP, et al. Randomized clinical trial of prehabilitation before planned liver resection. *Br J Surg.* 2016;103(5):504–512.
122. Barberan-Garcia A, Ubre M, Roca J, et al. Personalised prehabilitation in high-risk patients undergoing elective major abdominal surgery: a randomized blinded controlled trial. *Ann Surg.* 2018;267(1):50–56.
123. Gravier FE, Bonnevie T, Boujibar F, et al. Effect of prehabilitation on ventilatory efficiency in non-small cell lung cancer patients: A cohort study. *J Thorac Cardiovasc Surg.* 2019;157(6):2504–2512.e1.
124. ATS statement: guidelines for the six-minute walk test. *Am J Respir Crit Care Med.* 2002;166(1):111–117.
125. Liu Z, Qiu T, Pei L, et al. Two-week multimodal prehabilitation program improves perioperative functional capability in patients undergoing thoracoscopic lobectomy for lung cancer: a randomized controlled trial. *Anesth Analg.* 2019. doi:10.1213/ANE.0000000000004342.
126. Boujibar F, Bonnevie T, Debeaumont D, et al. Impact of prehabilitation on morbidity and mortality after pulmonary lobectomy by minimally invasive surgery: a cohort study. *J Thorac Dis.* 2018;10(4):2240–2248.
127. Sanchez-Lorente D, Navarro-Ripoll R, Guzman R, et al. Prehabilitation in thoracic surgery. *J Thorac Dis.* 2018;10(suppl 22): S2593–s2600.
128. Licker M, Karenovics W, Diaper J, et al. Short-term preoperative high-intensity interval training in patients awaiting lung cancer surgery: a randomized controlled trial. *J Thorac Oncol.* 2017; 12(2):323–333.
129. Clark JM, Marrufo AS, Kozower BD, et al. Cardiopulmonary testing before lung resection: What are thoracic surgeons doing? *Ann Thorac Surg.* 2019;108(4):1006–1012.

6

Physiology of the Lateral Position and One-Lung Ventilation

EDMOND COHEN

Introduction

Thoracic procedures are usually performed with the patient in the lateral decubitus position. To understand the distribution of ventilation and perfusion in the lateral decubitus position and the degree of venous admixture of shunt (Qs/Qt) is expressed as a percentage. Alveolar ventilation/perfusion ratio distributions are plots of the total amounts of ventilation and total amounts of perfusion that are supplying each collection of lung units operating at a specific VA/Q ratio.[1,2] This chapter will discuss the distribution of perfusion and ventilation in the upright and in the lateral position and the ventilation-perfusion ratio and will focus on issues relevant to thoracic surgery and one-lung ventilation (OLV). The information regarding the lung physiology can be found in Chapters 5 and 7, while a detailed discussion of the hypoxic pulmonary vasoconstriction (HPV) is available in Chapter 15.

Hypoxemia

There are several reasons for hypoxemia:

- Equipment malfunction
- Hypoventilation
- Decreased functional residual capacity (FRC)
- Decreased cardiac output (CO)
- Inhibition of HPV
- Increased right to left shunt

The causes of hypoventilation are depicted in Fig. 6.1. Following shunt, hypoventilation is the second cause of hypoxemia. One of the determinants of alveolar partial pressure of oxygen (PaO_2) is the balance or ratio between ventilation and blood flow. In the patient with hypoventilation and normal blood flow results in a less oxygen delivery and unchanged removal of O_2, which lowers PaO_2. In an awake patient breathing room air, hypoventilation may result in severe hypoxemia because arterial partial pressure of carbon dioxide ($PaCO_2$) increases to dangerously high levels. Whereas during anesthesia, providing supplemental O_2 above 21%, will increase the PAO_2 and arterial oxygenation will be maintained.

The oxygen cascade is illustrated in Fig. 6.2. There are several factors that are essential for adequate gas exchange that must be considered as a cause of hypoxemia: diffusion block, shunt fraction, HPV and V/Q matching.

Diffusion block: Alveolar fresh gases and capillary venous blood exchange oxygen and CO_2 through a surface area of about 140 m^2, roughly the size of a tennis court. The pulmonary vascular tree bifurcates from the main pulmonary artery into arterioles and capillaries that cover 85% to 95% of the alveolar surface, an exceptionally thin membrane of only 1.0 mm separates the alveolar gas and blood compartments, allowing gases to diffuse rapidly between them.[3] As depicted in Fig. 6.3, normally a red cell passes through a capillary within 0.25 to 0.75 second, to complete the gas exchange. Diffusion block can typically present in patients with interstitial lung

Causes of hypoventilation

Respiratory system
- airway obstruction (upper or lower)
- decreased lung, pleural or chest wall compliance

Brainstem
- brainstem injury arising from trauma, hemorrhage, hypoxia, infarction, infection
- metabolic encephalopathy
- depressant drugs (anesthesia)

Spinal cord
- high spinal/epidural
- trauma, tumor, transverse myelitis

Nerve root injury

Nerve
- trauma
- neuropathy (Guillain Barré)
- motor neuron disease

Neuromuscular junction
- myasthenia gravis
- neuromuscular blockers

Respiratory muscles
- fatigue
- disuse atrophy
- myopathy
- malnutrition

• **Fig. 6.1** Causes of hypoventilation.

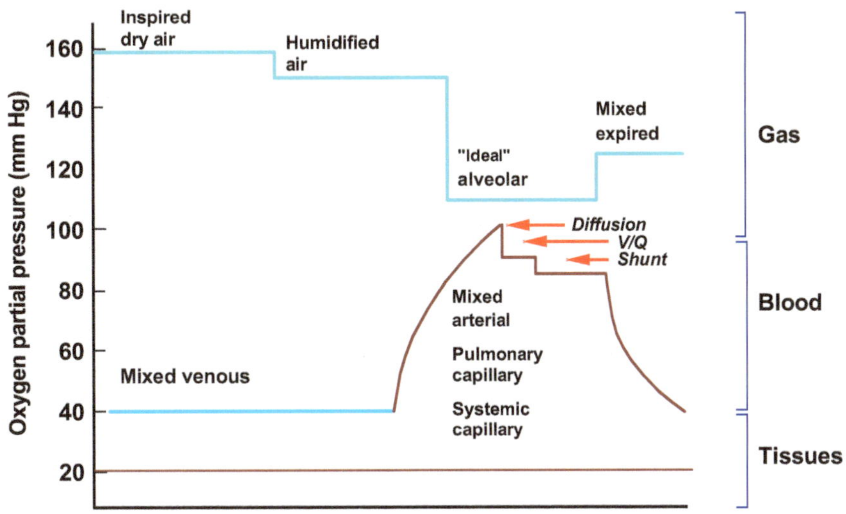

• **Fig. 6.2** Oxygen cascade.

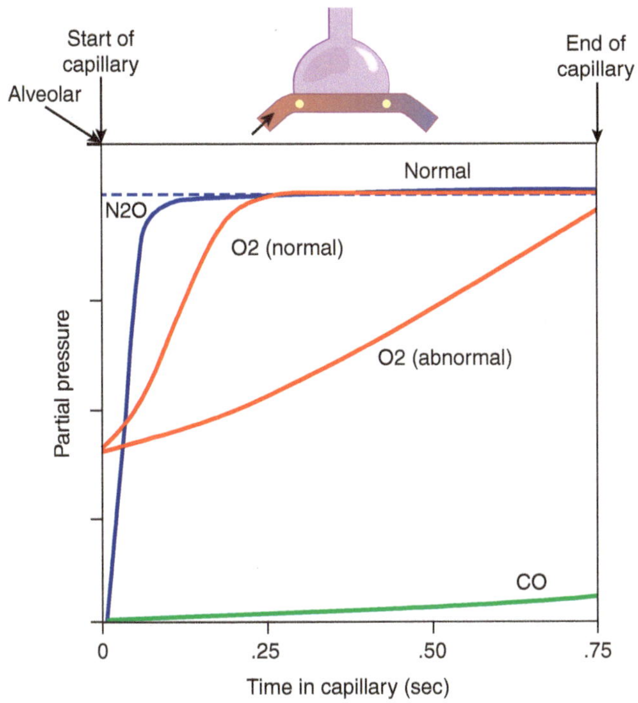

• **Fig. 6.3** Normally a red cell passes through a capillary within 0.25 to 0.75 second, to complete the gas exchange. Diffusion block can typically present in patients with interstitial lung diseases because of thickening of the alveolar–capillary membrane with increase resistance to diffusion.

diseases because of thickening of the alveolar–capillary membrane with increase resistance to diffusion. Patients with these diseases might have a normal arterial partial pressure of oxygen (PaO_2) at rest but develop hypoxemia during exercise. The lack of equilibration between PAO_2 and $PeCO_2$ creates an increased $PA–aO_2$. Hypoxemia in these patients, as a rule, responds positively to supplemental O_2. Although this does not correct the pathology of the diffusion limitation, it raises the PAO_2.

Shunt fraction: An extensive discussion of shunt can be found in Chapters 5 and 7. In brief, shunt is the fraction of CO (Qs/Qt) distributed to nonventilated units. A typical example is during OLV in which blood flow continue to perfuse the nonventilated lung to result in transpulmonary shunt.[4,5] As depicted in the shunt formula (Fig. 6.4), the effect on arterial oxygenation depends on this fraction and the O_2 content of mixed venous blood ($Cv\text{-}O_2$). Interventions aimed to increase oxygen content or mixed venous O_2 saturation ($Sv\text{-}O_2$) and raising the capillary oxygen content (CaO_2) through increased hemoglobin concentration, decreasing O_2 consumption or increasing CO would improve hypoxemia caused by a large shunt.[6]

The shunt equation quantifies the amount of blood in the three-compartment model that reaches the left heart without exchanging any gases. The equation quantitates venous admixture as a fraction of total lung blood flow. Arterial oxygen content (CAO_2) and mixed venous oxygen content $Cv\text{-}O_2$ are sampled from arterial and mixed venous blood from the pulmonary artery (through a pulmonary artery [PA] catheter), respectively. The CaO_2 is assumed that the capillary saturation is 100% (equals that of ideal alveolar gas equation).

Of interest, the shunt is essentially a ratio between the blood flow of a ventilated alveolar and the nonventilated alveoli. The equation for dead space displays a simple concept of a ratio. The shunt equation refers to oxygen in the capillary blood whereas the dead space equation refers to CO_2 in the aerated alveoli.

Ventilation Prefusion Upright Position

Distribution of Perfusion[7,8]

The reader should be familiar with the physiology of the upright position (Fig. 6.5).

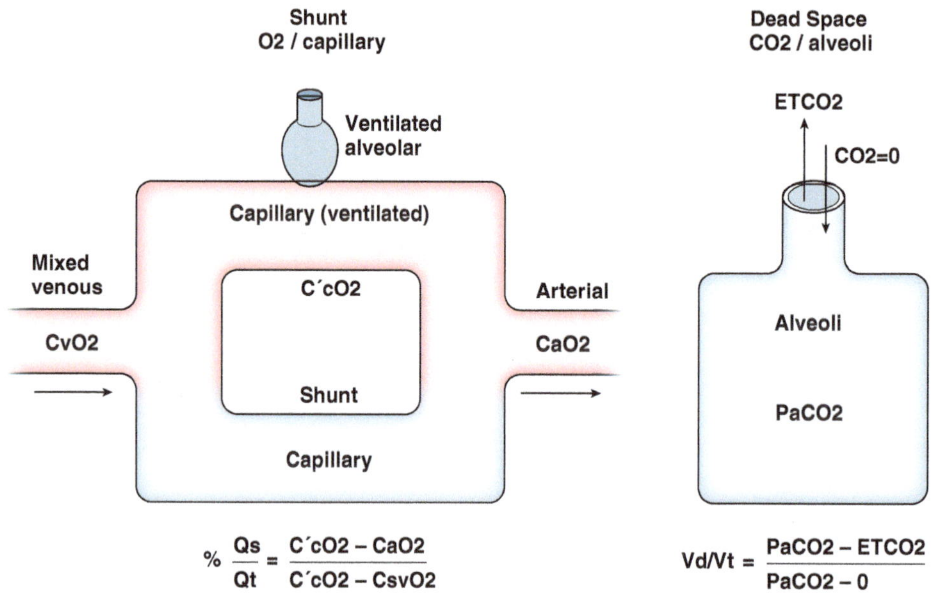

• **Fig. 6.4** The shunt is essentially a ratio between the blood flow of a ventilated alveoli and the nonventilated alveoli. The equation for dead space displays a simple concept of a ratio. The shunt equation refers to oxygen in the capillary blood whereas the dead space equation refers to CO2 in the aerated alveoli. (*ETCO2,* End-tidal carbon dioxide; *PaCO2,* arterial partial pressure of carbon dioxide.)

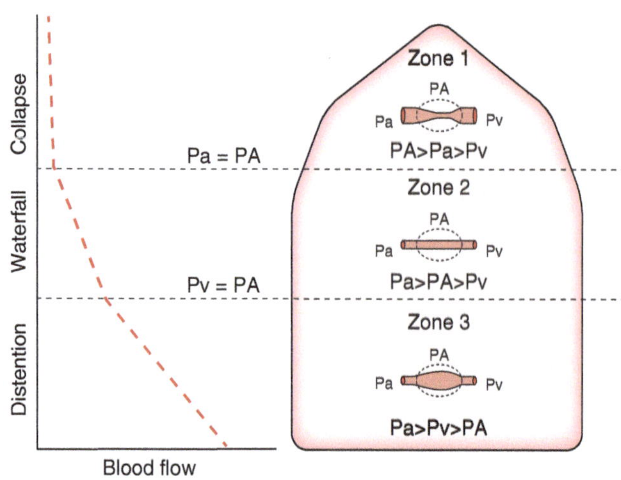

• **Fig. 6.5** Schematic diagram showing the distribution of the lung blood flow in the upright position. Because blood flow distribution to the lung is gravity-dependent and therefore is primarily directed to the dependent portion of the lung, **Zone 1:** $P_A > P_a > P_V$: in the apex of the lung the pressures in the alveolar vessel, both the Pa and the Pv, are lower than the pressure in the P_A which results in collapse vessel and poor perfusion. **Zone 2:** $P_a > P_A > P_v$: in the more dependent area of the lung with the increment in pressure in the pulmonary artery and vein, the flow is intermittent. As in an analogy to a waterfall, the upstream river (Pa) is flowing over a dam (P_A) to the downstream river (Pv). The P_A is intermittently obstructing the blood flow between the pulmonary artery and the veins. **Zone 3:** $P_a > P_v > P_A$, is the most dependent part of the lung where most of the perfusion is directed and the vessels therefor are most distended in this zone. The pressure in the pulmonary veins exceeds that of the alveolar pressure, which does not play any significant role in obstructing the blood flow because the mean P_a and P_v pressures are so high that they both exceed P_A. (*Pa,* Pulmonary artery pressure; P_A, alveolar pressure; (*Pv,* pulmonary venous pressure.)

The blood flow is directly dependent upon the relationship between the alveolar (PA) pressure, the pulmonary artery (Pa) pressure, and the pulmonary venous (Pv) pressure. There are several facts that should be highlighted:

- **Blood flow is gravity dependent**
- **The PA pressure is equal throughout the lung**
- **The absolute pressure in the pulmonary artery and the pulmonary veins is greater in the dependent part because of the vertical hydrostatic gradient; the pressure in a column of liquid is greatest at the base.**
- **The Pa pressure is always higher than the Pv pressure.**

Because blood flow distribution to the lung is gravity-dependent and therefore is primarily directed to the dependent portion of the lung. The amount of blood flow depends on the pressure difference between the Pa and the Pv. There are several factors that influence the distribution of perfusion:

Zone 1: PA > Pa > Pv: In the apex of the lung the pressures in the alveolar vessel, both the Pa and the Pv, are lower than the pressure in the PA which results in collapsed vessel and poor perfusion. As we move upward closer to the apex of an upright lung, the actual pressures in the lumens of pulmonary arterioles and venules fall by 1.0 cm H_2O for each 1 cm of vertical ascent. In the hypothetical case in which alveoli at the lung apex are 20 cm above the level of the left atrium, the mean PA of these alveoli would be 0 cm H_2O. A collapsed alveolus is considered to be a dead space.

Zone 2: Pa > PA > Pv. In the more dependent area of the lung with the increment in pressure in the pulmonary artery and vein, the flow is intermittent. As in an analogy to a waterfall, the upstream river (Pa) is flowing over a dam (PA) to the downstream river (Pv). The PA is intermittently obstructing the blood flow between the pulmonary artery and the veins. The blood flow, in addition to the pressure in the pulmonary artery and veins depends on the respiratory and the cardiac cycle. Downward in zone 2, the crushing force of the alveolar pressure proportionally decreases because the hydrostatic pressures in the arteriole, capillary, and venule all rise in parallel by 1 cm H_2O for each 1.0 cm of descent.

Zone 3: Pa > Pv > PA, is the most dependent part of the lung where most of the perfusion is directed and the vessels therefore are most distended in this zone. The pressure in the pulmonary veins exceeds that of the alveolar pressure, which does not play any significant role in obstructing the blood flow because the mean Pa and Pv pressures are so high that they both exceed PA. Thus transmural pressure gradient (P_{TM}) is positive along the entire length of the alveolar vessel, tending to dilate it. As we move downward in zone 3, the hydrostatic pressures in the arteriole, capillary, and venule all continue to rise by 1.0 cm H_2O for each 1 cm of descent. Because PA between breaths does not vary with height in the lung, the gradually increasing pressure of the alveolar vessel produces a greater and greater P_{TM}, causing the vessel to dilate more and more—an example of distention.

It is important to highlight that these lung zones are physiologic, not anatomic. The boundaries between the zones are neither fixed nor anatomically defined. These boundaries can move downward with positive-pressure ventilation which increases PA pressure or upward with exercise which increases Pa pressure.

Other Factors That Influence the Distribution of Blood Flow

Changes in CO and lung volumes can have significant effects on the distribution of pulmonary blood flow either independently or by modulating the determinants of flow mentioned earlier. An increase in CO results in greater uniformity of blood flow throughout all of the lung fields. The mechanisms proposed were an attenuation of HPV because of an increase in pulmonary arterial pressure and a lessening of the gravitational gradient.

Changes in lung volumes can alter the distribution of blood flow. The lung volume at which the pulmonary vascular resistance (PVR) is lowest is at FRC. When the lung volume is lower than FRC, the resistance of the pulmonary vascular system is increased because of decreased caliber of the extraalveolar vessels. This may be caused in part by the loss of radial traction supporting these vessels at low lung volumes. At lung volumes above FRC, PVR increases because of the stretch of the capillaries.

Distribution of Ventilation[1,2,7,8]

Alveolar ventilation in the upright position gradually falls from the base to the apex of the lung because of posture and gravity. The lung is a visceral elastic organ and because of the lung's weight, it tends to assume a bell shape in the chest cavity. Because the chest cavity is a closed space, the distance between the pleural lung and the parietal lung is greater at the apex of the lung. As a consequence, the intrapleural pressure (P_{IP}) is more negative at the apex than at the base when the subject is upright. The intrinsic mechanical properties of the airways are the same, regardless of whether the tissue is at the base or at the apex. At the base, where P_{IP} might be only −2.5 cm H_2O at FRC, the alveoli are relatively underinflated compared with tissues at the apex, where P_{IP} might be −10 cm H_2O and the alveoli are relatively overinflated. However, because the base of the lung is underinflated at FRC, it is on a steeper part of the pressure-volume curve (Fig. 6.6).

Ventilation is distributed mainly to the more compliant regions at the base of the lung. Because the alveoli at the apex of the lung in zone 1 are already distended by the negative intrapleural pressure at the apex, they are less compliant. In contrast, the alveoli at the base of the lung are less distended but more compliant. Therefore for the same increment in intraalveolar pressure, the alveoli at the base of the lung receive the major portion of the tidal volume. Because both perfusion and ventilation are primarily directed to the dependent portion of the lung, it would preserve the good ventilation/perfusion matching.[9]

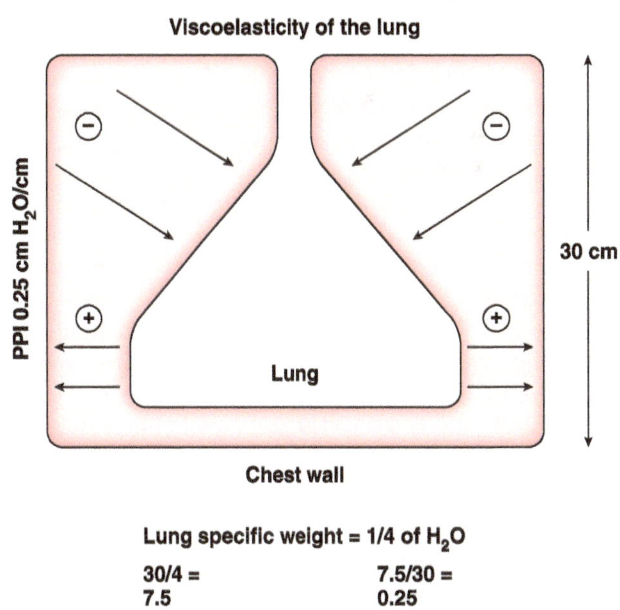

• **Fig. 6.6** Distribution of ventilation. The lung is a visceral elastic organ and because of the lung's weight, it tends to assume a bell shape in the chest cavity. Because the chest cavity is a close space, the distance between the pleural lung and the parietal lung is greater at the apex of the lung. As a consequence, the intrapleural pressure (P_{IP}) is more negative at the apex than at the base when the subject is upright. At the base, where P_{IP} might be only −2.5 cm H_2O at functional residual capacity (FRC), the alveoli are relatively underinflated compared with tissues at the apex, where P_{IP} might be −10 cm H_2O and the alveoli are relatively overinflated.

Ventilation-Perfusion Matching

V/Q matching is essential for normal gas exchange in the lungs. For normal gas exchange, alveoli must be in close proximity to pulmonary capillaries ventilation, which must be close to blood flow. The V/Q ratio expresses the matching of ventilation (V in L/min) to perfusion or blood flow (Q in L/min). It is useless if ventilated alveoli are not near perfused capillaries, or if perfused capillaries are not near ventilated alveoli. For the entire lung, the average normal value of V/Q is 0.8. This means for the whole lung, ventilation (L/min) is 80% of the lung perfusion (L/min). However, V/Q is not uniformly 0.8 throughout the entire normal lung; the regions above the level of the third ribs will have higher V/Q and some regions have lower V/Q. An average V/Q of 0.8 results in an arterial PaO_2 of 100 mm Hg and arterial $PaCO_2$ of 40 mm Hg, the normal values.

A maldistribution of ventilation and perfusion causes a defect in gas exchange. Alveoli that are ventilated and not perfused are considered a "dead space" while the perfused capillaries that are not ventilated represent a "shunt." A distribution of every possibility in between, high V/low Q = high V/Q and low V/high Q = low V/Q will be present, depending upon the lung zone. These regional variations in the upright position in both ventilation and blood flow are depended on the gravitational effects that cause blood flow to be highest at the base and lowest at the apex. The regional variations in ventilation occur in the same direction as those for blood flow; thus ventilation is highest at the base and lowest at the apex. However, and importantly, the variations in blood flow are greater than the variations for ventilation.[9]

The apex (zone 1) has the highest V/Q with the lowest blood flow, the lowest ventilation, but higher the ventilation relative to perfusion, the higher PaO_2 and a lower $PaCO_2$.

The base (zone 3) has a lower V/Q, the highest blood flow, the highest ventilation, but lower the ventilation relative to perfusion, lower PaO_2 and a higher $PaCO_2$. It is the main site of gas exchange. In zone 2, the V/Q ratio is in between (Fig. 6.7).

Fig. 6.8 shows a plot of the blood flow, ventilation, and V/Q ratio, the blood flow and ventilation lines cross at about the third rib in the diagram (ratio = 1). Below that rib the V/Q ratio is below 1.0 and rapidly increases above the third rib (>3).[1,2,10,11]

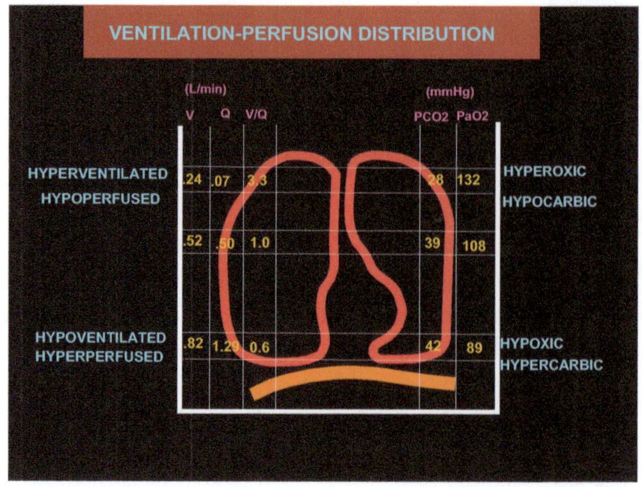

• **Fig. 6.7** The apex (**zone 1**) has the highest ventilation-perfusion (V/Q) with the lowest blood flow, the lowest ventilation, but higher the ventilation relative to perfusion, the higher PaO_2 and a lower PaCO2. The base (**zone 3**) has a lower V/Q, the highest blood flow, the highest ventilation, but lower the ventilation relative to perfusion, lower PaO_2 and a higher PaCO2. It is the main site of gas exchange. In **zone 2** V/Q ratio is in between. *PaCO2*, Arterial partial pressure of carbon dioxide; *PaO_2*, arterial partial pressure of oxygen.

Fractal Distribution of Perfusion and Ventilation

Fractal Distribution of Perfusion

The distribution of blood flow in the lung as being gravity-depended, as described in the chapter, has been challenged by the model of fractal distribution of both perfusion and ventilation.

In a human, approximately 5 L of blood per minute are distributed into a single red blood cell layer surrounding approximately 300 million alveoli. The highly complex structure of the pulmonary vascular network accomplishing this may easily be understood if the single vascular bifurcation is considered. The pulmonary vascular tree consists of a multitude of bifurcations, all having a similar structure but different sizes. This concept of self-similarity is also termed fractal (Latin *frangere*, to break; *fractus*, broken). It emphasizes the possibility that in contrast to objects in Euclidian geometry (lines, triangles), in which dimensions are integer numbers, natural objects may have fractional dimensions (e.g., 1.5 or 2.3).[12,13]

The pulmonary vasculature, by virtue of its tree-like structure, is a fractal object. At each bifurcation, a minimally

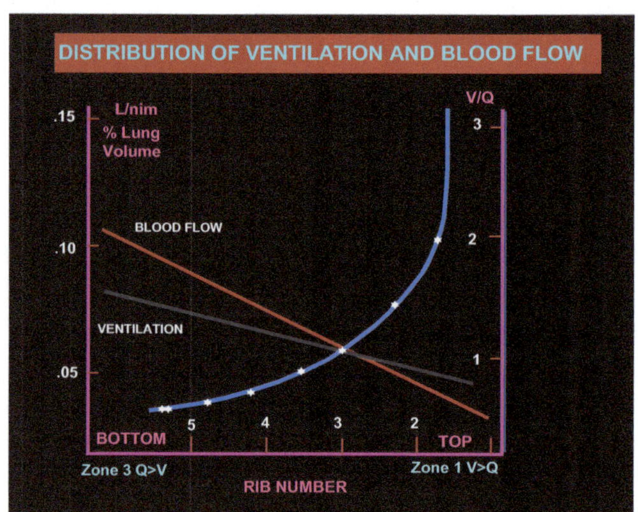

• **Fig. 6.8** Plot of the blood flow, ventilation, and ventilation-perfusion (V/Q) ratio: the blood flow and ventilation lines cross at about the third rib in the diagram (ratio = 1). Below that rib the V/Q ratio is below 1.0 and is rapidly increases above the third rib (>3).

uneven distribution of blood flow occurs. Heterogeneity is amplified by the many bifurcations in series. The function of the vascular tree is the distribution of blood to the pulmonary parenchyma. It is therefore logical to assume that the result of this distribution, perfusion heterogeneity, is also fractal. Therefore statistical measures of heterogeneity are also self-similar at different scales of magnification (i.e., fractal). Heterogeneity of pulmonary perfusion depends on the resolution of the measurement technique. Intuitively, this can be grasped by considering that low resolution hides more bifurcations (which are sources of heterogeneity) than high resolution.

Efficient gas exchange is dependent on the close matching of regional ventilation and perfusion. Given the high degree of heterogeneity observed at small regional volumes in this study, ventilation and perfusion must be closely correlated to achieve this matching. In the normal lung, this must occur by one of the following three mechanisms: (1) active matching of regional perfusion to ventilation, (2) active matching of regional ventilation to perfusion, or (3) passive matching of ventilation and perfusion by innate pulmonary structure. In the normal lung, basal pulmonary vascular tone is minimal, suggesting that vasoregulation is of minor importance for maintaining close V/Q matching in uninjured lungs. Passive matching of ventilation and perfusion by pulmonary structure is appealing because it requires the least amount of energy. An optimally engineered system requires no active feedback mechanisms during normal function.

Fractal distribution networks for ventilation and perfusion provide several inherent advantages. Fractal structures are the most efficient way to fill a three-dimensional structure and provide the most energy efficient substrate transport.

Studies that evaluated the effect of gravity on blood flow used animal models that were exposed to three or more G forces (using centrifuge) while tracing the blood flow distribution with fluorescent microsphere. Chornuk et al.[14] assessed the influence of cranial-to-caudal inertial force (+G) during positive pressure breathing during G (PBG) on regional pulmonary blood flow distribution. Unanesthetized swine were exposed randomly to a variety of G forces: from 0 G (resting), +3 G, +6 G, up to +9 G, with and without anti-G suit and PBG with the use of the Air Force Research Laboratory centrifuge. Fluorescent microspheres were injected into the pulmonary vasculature as a marker of regional pulmonary blood flow. Lungs were excised, dried, and diced into around 2-cm^3 pieces, and the fluorescence of each piece was measured. As =G was increased from 0 to +3 G, blood flow shifted from cranial and hilar regions toward caudal and peripheral regions of the lung. This redistribution shifted back toward cranial and hilar regions as anti-G suit inflation pressure increased at +6 and +9 G. Perfusion heterogeneity increased with +G stress and decreased at the higher anti-G suit pressures. The distribution of pulmonary blood flow was not affected by PBG. Of interest, as depicted in Fig. 6.9, the blood flow distribution within the lung was similar when the animal was exposed to 1 G or 3 G. That lead to the conclusion that almost 60% of the blood flow distribution was caused by anatomic fractal structure of the lung rather than gravity depended. The anatomic structure is the major determinant of pulmonary blood flow. Analysis of the variability of blood flow within individual regions shows that more than 60% of flow variation is caused by pulmonary vascular structure. Inertial force and anti-G suit account for less than 20% of the flow variation.

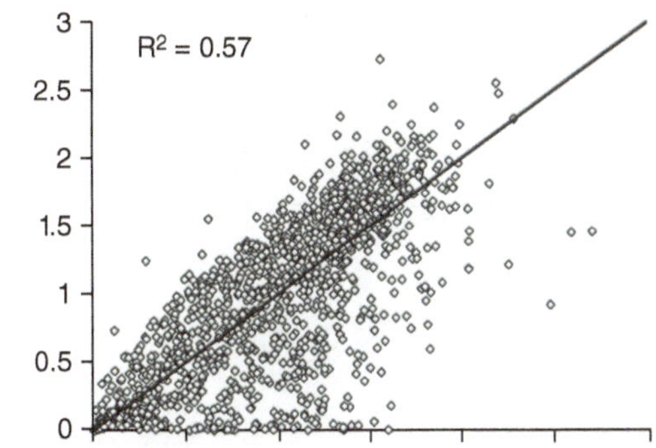

• **Fig. 6.9** Blood flow distribution within the lung was similar when the animal was exposed to 1 G or to three G. That lead to the conclusion that almost 60% of the blood flow distribution was caused by anatomic fractal structure of the lung rather than gravity depended. The anatomic structure is the major determinant of pulmonary blood flow. (Adapted from Chornuk MA, Bernard SL, Burns JW, et al. Effects of inertial load and countermeasures on the distribution of pulmonary blood flow. *J Appl Physiol.* 2000;89(2):445–457.)

Altemeier et al.[15] evaluated the fractal distribution of the ventilation. High-resolution measurements of pulmonary perfusion reveal substantial spatial heterogeneity that is fractally distributed and the vascular tree is the principal determinant of regional blood flow. Recent studies using aerosol deposition show similar ventilation heterogeneity that is closely correlated with perfusion. The authors hypothesized that ventilation has fractal characteristics similar to blood flow. They measured regional ventilation and perfusion with aerosolized and injected fluorescent microspheres in anesthetized, mechanically ventilated pigs in both prone and supine postures. Coefficients of variation were calculated for each cluster size to determine fractal dimensions. At the smallest size lung piece, local ventilation and perfusion are highly correlated, with no significant difference between ventilation and perfusion heterogeneity (Fig. 6.10). Ventilation has fractal properties similar to perfusion. Efficient gas exchange is preserved, despite ventilation and perfusion heterogeneity, through close correlation. They concluded that one potential explanation is the similar geometry of bronchial and vascular structures.

The Lateral Decubitus Position

Thoracic anesthesia is associated with the lateral decubitus position because, with the exception of mediastinal mass resection or tracheal resection, surgery is usually performed in that position. Several factors influence the distribution of ventilation and perfusion in the lateral decubitus position. The induction of general anesthesia, paralysis, and opening

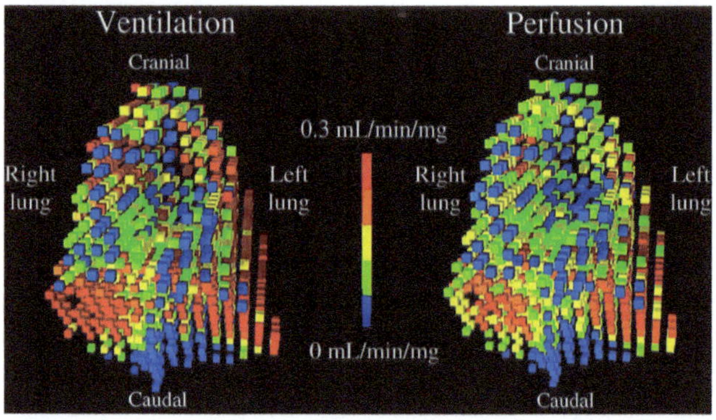

• **Fig. 6.10** The fractal distribution of the ventilation. High-resolution measurements of pulmonary perfusion reveal substantial spatial heterogeneity that is fractally distributed and the vascular tree is the principal determinant of regional blood flow. Recent studies using aerosol deposition show similar ventilation heterogeneity that has fractal properties similar to perfusion. Efficient gas exchange is preserved, despite ventilation and perfusion heterogeneity, through close correlation. (Adapted from WA Altemeir, Mckinney SI, Glenny RW. Fractal nature of regional ventilation distribution. *Appl Physiol.* 2000;88:1551–1557.)

the chest, cause major alterations in the distribution of perfusion (Q), ventilation (V), and the ventilation/perfusion ratio (V/Q ratio) when both lungs are being ventilated. The effect of the lateral position on the distribution of perfusion and ventilation will be considered before exploring each of these specific situations is discussed.

Distribution of Perfusion in the Lateral Position

The blood flow in the lateral position is similar to that of the upright position and is gravity-dependent. The relationship between PA, Pa, and Pv that exists in the lateral position is similar to that of the upright position. Blood flow distribution in the lateral position is essentially unchanged whether the patient is awake, anesthetized, or paralyzed. Pulmonary blood flow increases with lung dependency; it is greater in the dependent lung than in the nondependent lung. Therefore when considering the V/Q relationships in a variety of clinical situations, the distribution of the perfusion is primarily toward the dependent part of the lung. It is the distribution of the ventilation that changes during the various clinical situations.

Two important concepts affect the distribution of blood flow in the lateral position as compared with upright. First, because perfusion is gravity-dependent, the vertical hydrostatic gradient is smaller in the lateral position as compared with the upright position (Fig. 6.11). Consequently, in the lateral position, there is less of zone 1 and more of zones 2 and 3. The decrease in zone 1 reduces the extent of the patient dead space.[16,17]

In the upright position, the blood distribution to the lung is split; 55% goes to the right lung, which has three

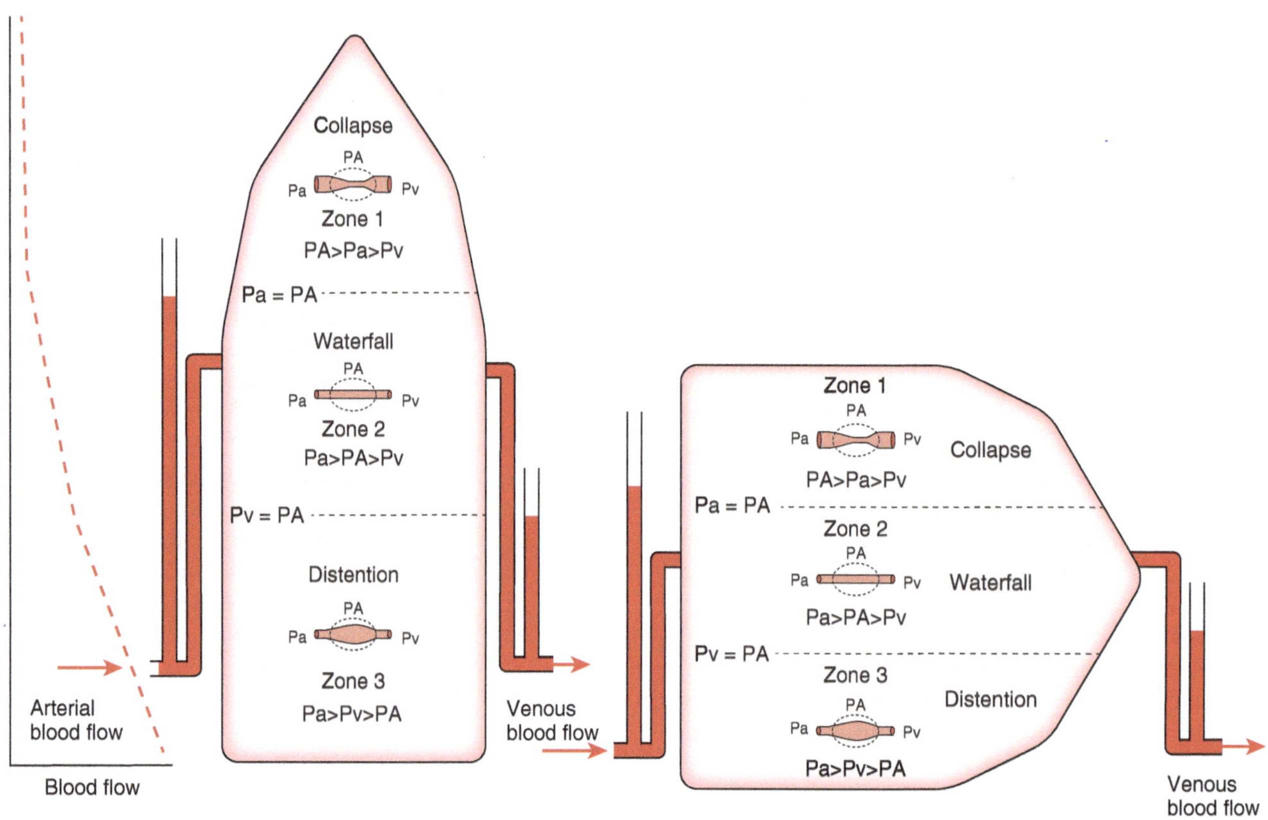

• **Fig. 6.11** Schematic diagram showing the distribution of blood flow in the lateral position. Because perfusion is gravity-dependent, the vertical hydrostatic gradient is smaller in the lateral position as compared with the upright position. Consequently, in the lateral position, there is less of zone 1 and more of zones 2 and 3. The decrease in zone 1 reduces the extent of the patient's dead space. (*Pa*, Pulmonary artery pressure; P_A, alveolar pressure; *Pv*, pulmonary venous pressure.)

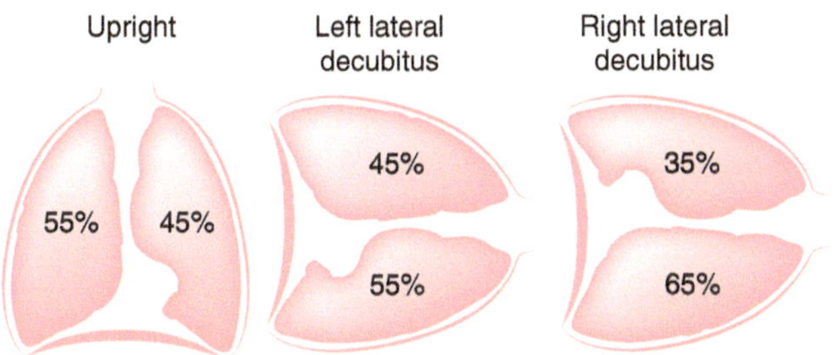

• **Fig. 6.12** Schematic representation of the blood flow distribution in the upright and the lateral position. In the upright position, the blood distribution to the lung is split; 55% goes to the right lung, which has three lobes, and 45% goes to the left lung, which has two lobes. In the right decubitus position the split is approximately 65% to the right dependent lung and 35% to the left lung. In the left lateral position, the dependent left lung receives 55% of the total blood flow, whereas the right lung receives 45%. It is reasonable to average blood flow regardless of which side is dependent; it can be assumed that 60% flows to the dependent lung and 40% flows to the nondependent lung.

lobes, and 45% goes to the left lung, which has two lobes. In the right decubitus position, the split is approximately 65% to the right dependent lung and 35% to the left lung. In the left lateral position, the dependent left lung receives 55% of the total blood flow, whereas the right lung receives 45% (Fig. 6.12). It is reasonable to average blood flow regardless of which side is dependent; it can be assumed that 60% flows to the dependent lung and 40% flows to the nondependent lung.

Distribution of Ventilation in the Supine and Lateral Positions

An in-depth evaluation of the influence of position and paralysis on diaphragmatic movement and the changes in lung volumes was reported by Froese et al.[18] The position and the pattern of the diaphragm movements during both supine and lateral decubitus positions were assessed by fluoroscopy in healthy volunteers. The patients were studied while awake, supine, breathing spontaneously in the lateral position, or paralyzed. Two components, the change in diaphragmatic position and the change in pattern of displacement, have been evaluated in particular.

Fig. 6.13 shows the regional diaphragm displacements during spontaneous breathing and paralysis in the supine position. Spontaneous ventilation in the awake subject is characterized predominantly by movement of the dependent part of the diaphragm. Anesthesia induces a cephalad shift during end-expiratory breathing in the diaphragmatic position that is most pronounced in the dependent areas. In spite of this shift, diaphragmatic movement remains greatest in the dependent diaphragm. Two mechanisms enable the actively contracting diaphragm to generate more force in the dependent diaphragm. One, the dependent part of the diaphragm has a smaller radius of curvature both in the supine and lateral positions. Therefore for the same diaphragmatic tension, more pressure is generated across the dependent part (Laplace Law). Two, the isometric force developed

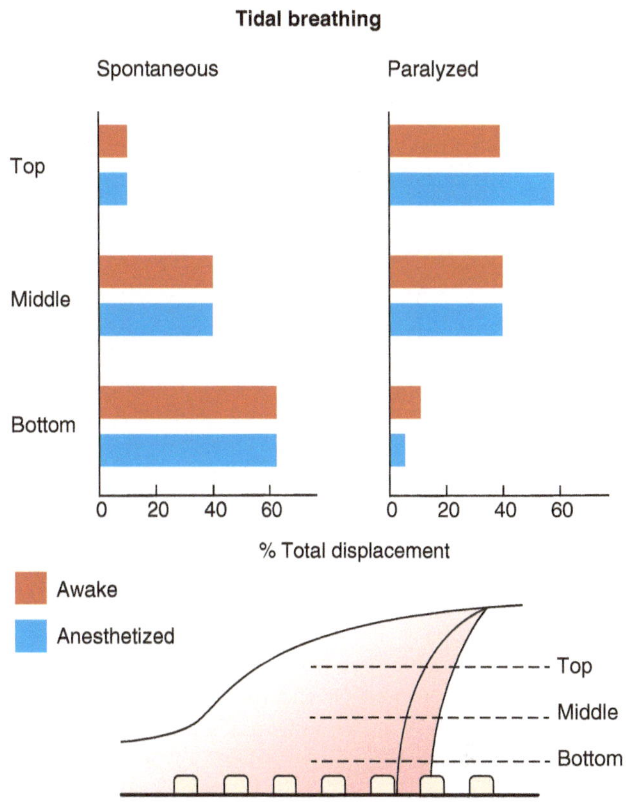

• **Fig. 6.13** Shows the regional diaphragm displacements during spontaneously breathing and paralysis in the supine position. Diaphragmatic displacement was analyzed in 3 levels: top, middle, and bottom. Spontaneous ventilation in the awake subject is characterized predominantly by movement of the dependent part of the diaphragm. Anesthesia induces a cephalad shift during end-expiratory breathing in the diaphragmatic position that is most pronounced in the dependent areas. In spite of this shift, diaphragmatic movement remains greatest in the dependent diaphragm. (Reproduced from Froese AB, Bryan AC. Effects of anesthesia and paralysis on diaphragmatic mechanics in man. *Anesthesiology*. 1974;42:242.)

by a muscle increases as its resting length increases. Not only is the dependent part of the diaphragm more curved, but it is also more stretched and therefore develops greater force because of the length/tension relationship. In paralyzed subjects, most of the cephalad displacement occurs in the nondependent areas, with minimal movement of the most dependent level.

Fig. 6.14 shows the regional diaphragmatic displacement during the lateral decubitus position in patients who are awake, anesthetized and spontaneously breathing, or paralyzed. In this position three levels of the diaphragm, upper, middle, and lower, were assessed in terms of percent of total displacement. Although the weight of the abdominal contents pushes the lower dependent part of the diaphragm, it still has the greatest displacement during spontaneous ventilation, whether in the awake or anesthetized state. In paralysis, the pattern of displacement is reversed, however, and displacement of the upper diaphragm is greater than that of the lower part. When the diaphragm is paralyzed, its motion is no longer determined by active contraction. The relatively uniform pressure that is applied to the thoracic side of the diaphragm is opposed by the hydrostatic pressure gradient of

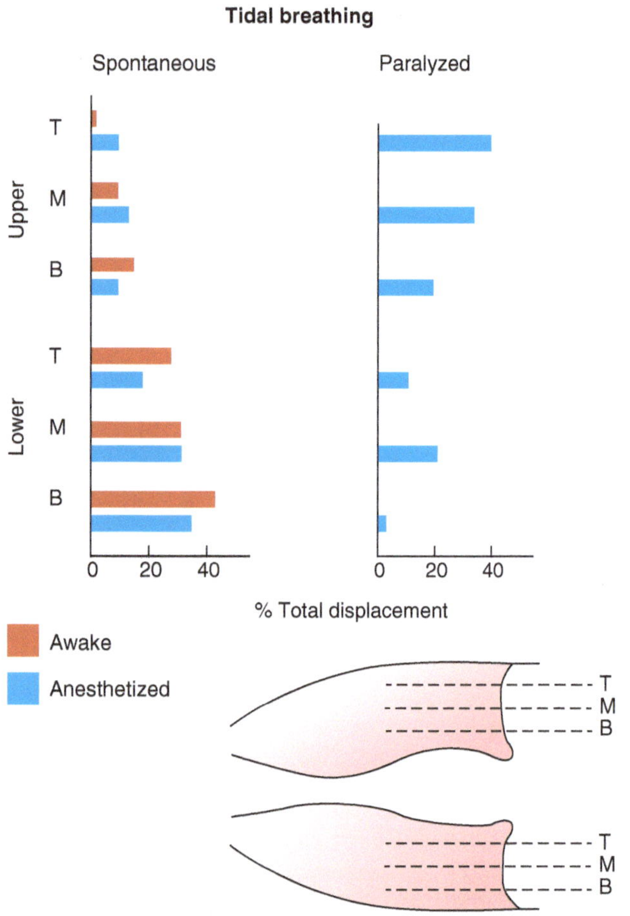

• **Fig. 6.14** Shows the regional diaphragmatic displacement during the lateral decubitus position in patients who are awake, anesthetized and spontaneously breathing, or paralyzed. Diaphragmatic displacement was analyzed in 3 levels: top (*T*) middle (*M*), and bottom (*B*). Although the weight of the abdominal contents pushes the lower dependent part of the diaphragm, still has the greatest displacement during spontaneous ventilation, whether in the awake or anesthetized state. In paralysis, the pattern of displacement is reversed, however, and displacement of the upper diaphragm is greater than that of lower part. When the diaphragm is paralyzed, its motion is no longer determined by active contraction. (From Froese AB, Bryan AC. Effects of anesthesia and paralysis on diaphragmatic mechanics in man. *Anesthesiology*. 1974;42:242.)

the abdominal content. Therefore the applied positive pressure ventilation displaces the diaphragm preferentially where abdominal pressure is least, that is, in the nondependent part.

In conclusion, the distribution of diaphragmatic displacement depends on whether the force develops as a result of active contraction of the diaphragm as a consequence of an external force acting on passive diaphragm.

The Lateral Decubitus Position, Awake, Spontaneously Breathing Patients

Chest Closed

The lateral position conserves adequate V/Q matching because most of the gravity-dependent blood flow is directed into the dependent lung, and ventilation continues primarily to the dependent lung. The distribution of blood flow and ventilation is similar to that in the upright position (see earlier) but it varies by 90 degrees.

The nonparalyzed, dependent diaphragm retains the ability to contact and maintains an adequate volume of the dependent lung. The abdominal contents push the dependent hemidiaphragm further into the chest, as compared with the nondependent hemidiaphragm (Fig. 6.15).

Fig. 6.16 shows the movement of each hemidiaphragm in the supine and in the lateral nonparalyzed and paralyzed patient. In the nonparalyzed patient, active and efficient contraction of the diaphragm keep the dependent lung from reducing the functional residual capacity. The more sharply curved dependent lung hemidiaphragm contracts more efficiently to maintain volume exchange to the dependent lung as a result of an increase in the pressure of the abdominal contents. In the lateral position, as in the upright position, gravity causes pleural pressure gradients that affect the distribution of ventilation. The dependent lung lies on a relatively steep portion of the pressure-volume curve, whereas the nondependent lung is on a relatively flat portion of the curve. Thus for an equal change in transpulmonary pressure, the dependent lung receives the vast majority of the delivered tidal volume.[18–21]

In conclusion, in the awake, spontaneously breathing patient in the lateral position, the tidal volume is preferentially delivered into the dependent lung where the gravity-dependent blood flow is primarily directed. The distribution of ventilation/perfusion ratios of the two lungs is not altered and is similar to that for a patient in the upright or supine position. The degree of shunt is not greatly affected; it depends on the age of the patient and the relationship between the closing capacity (CC) and the FRC.

Chest Open

Controlled positive pressure ventilation is the most common method used: (1) to provide adequate ventilation and (2) ensure gas exchange during open chest procedures. In most circumstances, thoracic procedures are carried out under general anesthesia with a double lumen tube or endobronchial blockers. In recent years however, several diagnostic and therapeutic procedures are being performed using thoracoscopy in spontaneously breathing patients with an open chest. Procedures such as lung biopsy, plural exploration and biopsy, random wedge resection, resection of a solitary lung lesion, and talc insufflation or pleuroabrasion, can be performed with video-assisted thoracoscopy. This has become increasingly popular in recent years and is performed while the patient is breathing spontaneously without endotracheal intubation, so called "tubeless procedures." In most cases a laryngeal airway mask (LMA) is used to manage the airway. The advantages of tubeless procedures are that the patient is not subjected to positive pressure ventilation. Mechanical ventilation has a number of potential side-effects, such as pressure-induced injury, lung overdistension from volutrauma, the release of a variety of

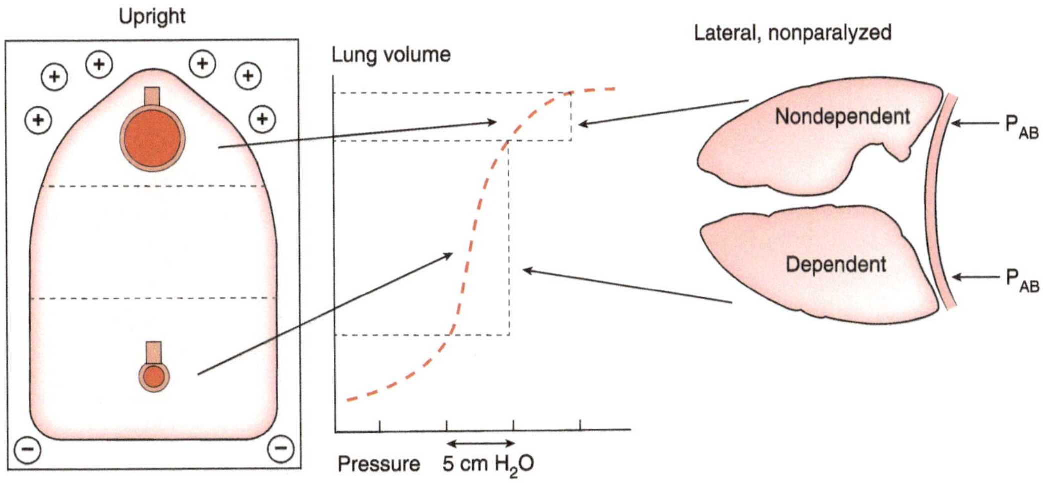

• **Fig. 6.15** Plural pressure (P_{pl}) in the awake, upright patient is most positive in the dependent portion of the lung, and therefore alveoli in this region are most compressed and have the lowest volume. In contrast, P_{pl} is most negative at the apex of the lung; here the alveoli are least compressed and have the largest volume. When these regional difference in alveolar volume are translated to a regional transpulmonary pressure-alveolar volume curve, the small, dependent alveoli lie on the steep portion of the curve (large slope), and the large nondependent alveoli are on a flat part (small slope). In this diagram, regional slope equals regional compliance. Thus for a given and equal change in transpulmonary pressure, the dependent part of the lung receives a much larger share of the tidal volume than the nondependent part. In the lateral decubitus position, gravity also causes pleural pressure gradients and therefore similarly affects the distribution of ventilation. The dependent lung lies on a relatively steep portion of the pressure-volume curve, and the nondependent lung lies on a relatively flat part. Thus in the lateral decubitus position, the dependent lung receives the majority of the tidal ventilation. *P*, Transpulmonary pressure; P_{AB}, pressure from abdominal content; *V*, alveolar volume. (Modified with permission from Benumof JL. Physiology of the open chest and one-lung ventilation. In: Kaplan JA, ed. *Thoracic Anesthesia*. 2nd ed. New York: Churchill Livingstone; 1991.)

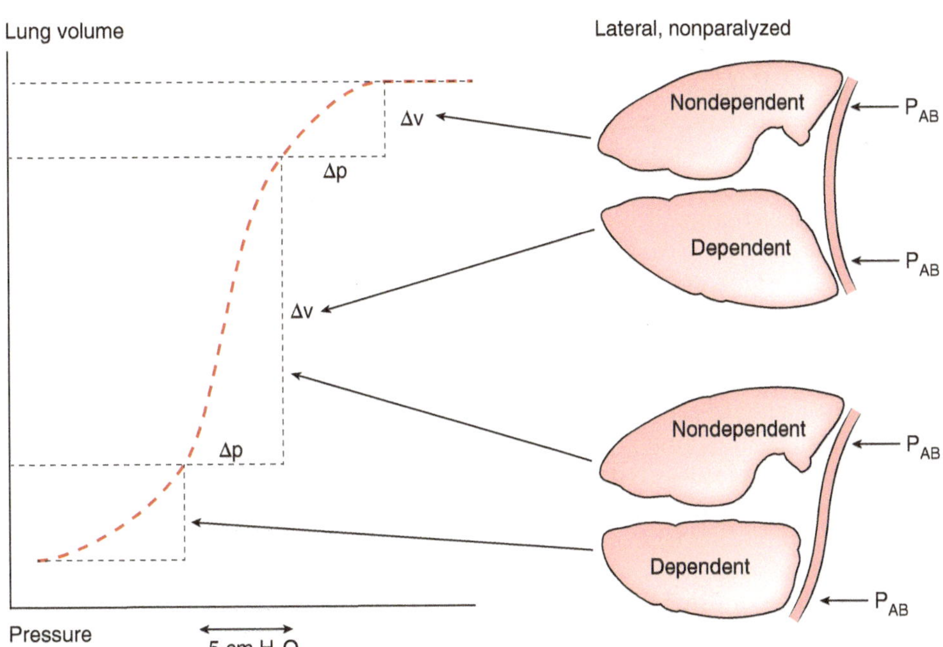

• **Fig. 6.16** Schematic diagram showing the distribution of ventilation in the anesthetized nonparalyzed patient in the lateral decubitus position (top right) and in the anesthetized paralyzed patient in the same position (bottom right). Paralysis causes a loss of lung volume in both lungs; the nondependent lung moves from a flat, noncompliant portion to the steep, compliant part of the pressure-volume curve, and the dependent lung moves from a steep, compliant part to a flat, noncompliant part. Thus the anesthetized patient in a lateral decubitus position has the majority of the tidal ventilation in the nondependent lung (where perfusion is least) and the minority of the tidal ventilation in the dependent lung (where perfusion is greatest). *P*, Transpulmonary pressure; P_{AB}, pressure from abdominal content; *V*, alveolar volume. (Modified with permission from Benumof JL. Physiology of the open chest and one-lung ventilation. In: Kaplan JA, ed. *Thoracic Anesthesia*. 2nd ed. New York: Churchill Livingstone; 1991.)

proinflammatory mediators, atelectasis, and potential laryngeal or tracheal injuries. In addition, the avoidance of using muscle relaxants will reduce the degree of atelectasis in the dependent zone of the lung from diaphragmatic dysfunction, will keep the V/Q matching, eliminate the potential for residual neuromuscular blockade, and decrease postoperative nausea and vomiting). They can be performed using an intercostal block or a thoracic epidural. In such a case, the patient breathes spontaneously to allow proper lung examination. With an open chest, once the lung is exposed to atmospheric pressure, the lungs will be collapsed in absence of positive pressure ventilation. The benefits and risk of general versus regional anesthesia should be carefully considered for each patient and patient-selection criteria should be carefully considered. The thoracoscope provides an adequate seal of the open chest to prevent a free, open-chest situation. In most cases, however, the surgeon often releases the seal intentionally to develop a pneumothorax and a collapsed lung and obtain an adequate surgical field. (Tubeless procedures are described in detail in Chapter. 37)

Two important complications, mediastinal shift and paradoxic respiration, may occur in a patient breathing spontaneously with an open chest.

Mediastinal shift: When the chest is closed, the inward recoil of the lung is balanced by the outward recoil of the chest wall. This results in equal negative pressures in each hemithorax. Only the weight of the mediastinum may cause some compression of the lower lung. When the chest is open, the negative pressure in the intact hemithorax compares relatively to the positive pressure in the open hemithorax, and causes the mediastinum to move downward and push into the dependent hemithorax. During inspiration, the caudad movement of the dependent lung further increases the negative pressure, resulting in additional downward displacement of the mediastinum. During expiration, the cephalad movement of the dependent lung diaphragm creates a relative positive pressure in the dependent hemithorax, which pushes the mediastinum upward (Fig. 6.17)[22,23] in the open chest, as the tidal volume in the dependent lung decreases by an amount equal to the resulting inspiratory displacement. In a young patient the mediastinal shift is marked, because the mobilit of the mediastinal structure diminishes with age. Mediastinal movements are minimal during quiet respiration, whereas they are significant with increase respiratory effort; this may interfere with cardiac filling and cause hypotension. In fact, the clinical presentation is similar to shock. The patient may develop hypotension and tachycardia, and be diaphoreic. Assisting patient's breathing by applying positive ventilation by continuous positive airway pressure, or in severe circumstances, by the LMA or endotracheal intubation, eliminates the ventilatory and circulatory changes associated with mediastinal shift.

The mechanism involved in the mediastinal shift is believed to be reflex mediated. Manipulation of the mediastinum and dissection around the lung hilum provoke vagally mediated bradycardia, hypotension, and bronchoconstriction, with increased bronchial secretion. Infiltration of local anesthetic at the pulmonary plexus at the hilum, vagal nerve block at the neck, or the use of atropine can reduce the severity of these reactions.

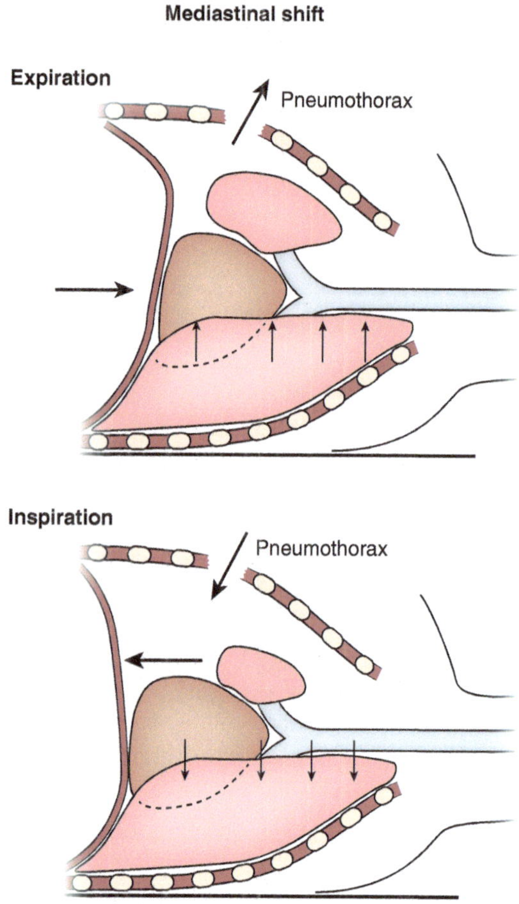

• **Fig. 6.17** Schematic representation of mediastinal shift in the spontaneously ventilating patient in the lateral decubitus position with an open chest. The open chest is always exposed to atmospheric pressure. **During inspiration**, negative pressure in the intact hemithorax causes the mediastinum to move downward. **During expiration**, relative positive pressure in the closed hemithorax causes the mediastinum to move upward (mediastinal shift). (Modified with permission from Tarhan S, Moffitt EA. Principles of thoracic anesthesia. *Surg Clin North Am*. 1973;53:813.)

Paradoxic respiration: When one hemithorax is exposed to atmospheric pressure, an inspiratory effort increases the negative pressure only of the dependent intact hemithorax. Gas is drawn into the trachea and then into the lung on the intact hemithorax. In contrast, during expiration, the ascendant hemidiaphragm creates a positive pressure in the intact dependent hemithorax relative to the atmospheric pressure of the exposed, nondependent hemithorax. Gas is then displaced from the dependent lung into the nondependent lung, which paradoxically expands during expiration. This reverse gas flow into the nondependent lung is termed "paradoxic respiration." The gas, so-called "pendulum air," represents wasted ventilation and may compromise the adequacy of gas exchange, resulting in hypercarbia and hypoxemia (Fig. 6.18).[24] The experience has shown that these changes are evident when spontaneous breathing occurs for more than 1 hour. As described earlier, a patient's paradoxic breathing can be controlled by giving positive pressure by face mask or by assisting with gentle ventilation if a laryngeal mask is in place.

Lateral Position, Anesthetized Patients

Chest Closed

The induction of general anesthesia and paralysis does not significantly change the distribution of blood flow but does have an important impact on ventilation. In the anesthetized paralyzed patient, the dependent lung continues to receive most of the blood perfusion. The distribution of ventilation is altered because most of the tidal volume switches to the nondependent lung; this results in a significant V/Q mismatch. With the induction of general anesthesia, FRC decreases. In the lateral position, this reduction is more pronounced in the dependent lung for several reasons.

1. The loss of lung volume induced by anesthesia results in a lower volume on the pressure-volume curve in each lung. The dependent lung is no longer on the initially steep portion of the pressure-volume curve but on the lower, flatter part of the curve. Instead, the nondependent lung has a steeper position on the compliance curve and receives most of the tidal volume.[25,26]
2. If anesthesia is associated with paralysis and mechanical ventilation, the diaphragm is no longer actively contracting and no longer offers any advantage to ventilation.
3. The mediastinum shifts downward and prevents the dependent lung from expanding.
4. The pressure of the abdominal content is larger in the dependent lung and interferes with expansion of that lung.

This reduction of volume of the dependent lung will have an impact on the V/Q relationship and results in significant increase in shunting because the nondependent lung is well ventilated but poorly perfused (V/Q ratio >1), whereas the dependent lung is well perfused but poorly ventilated (V/Q ratio <1).

Chest Open

The dependent lung continues to receive the vast majority of the perfusion, and opening of the chest wall causes further V/Q mismatch. Hypoxemia may result because of the upper lung being no longer restricted by the chest; it expands more freely than the dependent lung. Therefore the nondependent lung is hyperventilated but underperfused.

Paralysis affects the V/Q ratio during two-lung ventilation most unfavorably. Surgical retraction and compression

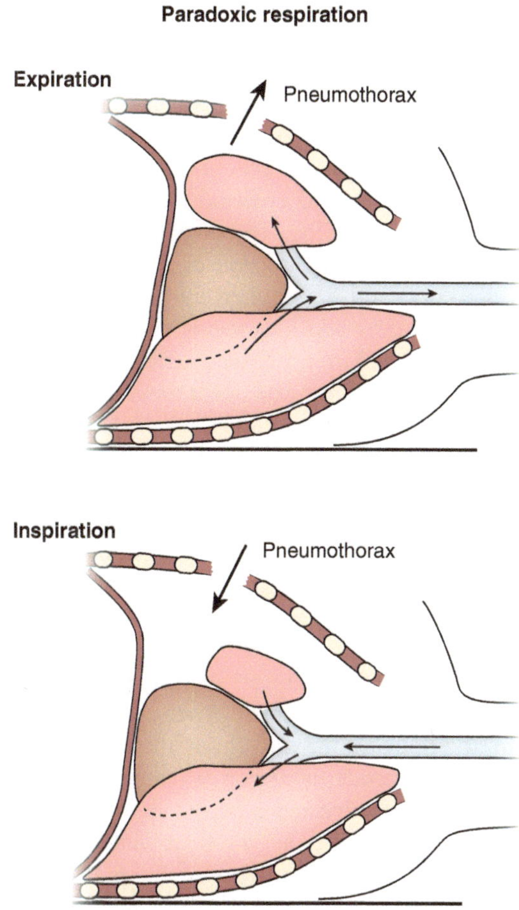

• **Fig. 6.18** Schematic representation of paradoxic respiration in the spontaneously ventilating patient in the lateral decubitus position with an open chest. The open chest is always exposed to atmospheric pressure. During inspiration, gas moves from the nondependent lung in the open hemithorax into the dependent lung in the closed hemithorax, and air that moves from the environment into the open hemithorax causes the lung in the open hemithorax to collapse (paradoxic respiration). During expiration, the gas passes from the dependent lung to the nondependent lung and from the open hemithorax to the environment. Consequently, the nondependent lung expands during expiration. (Modified from Tarhan S, Moffitt EA. Principles of thoracic anesthesia. *Surg Clin North Am*. 1973;53:813.)

of the nondependent lung may provide partial protection from hypoxemia by directing more blood to the dependent lung. The induction of general anesthesia and muscle relaxation results in a reduction in FRC, however. Diaphragmatic paralysis with a cephalad displacement of the diaphragm by pressure from the abdominal contents is more pronounced over the dependent part of the lung that will shift the ventilation toward the upper part of the lung. Because blood flow continues to be directed for the most part to the depended parts of the lung, paralysis will result in increase in V/Q mismatch. Both lungs are displaced to a lower resting volume on the sigmoid-shaped pressure-volume curve. The nondependent lung then lies on a more compliant portion of the curve and receives most of the tidal volume.[21,27] In addition, the mediastinal structures that press on the dependent hemithorax and the suboptimal positioning of the dependent lung on the operating table both contribute to a reduction in FRC.

Physiology of One-Lung Ventilation

In the lateral position general anesthesia, paralysis, and compression by abdominal contents and mediastinal structures results in reduction of FRC. Therefore the dependent lung is no longer on the steep portion of the pressure-volume compliance curve and does not receive the majority of the tidal volume. During one-lung ventilation, the nondependent lung is excluded from the ventilation, and all the tidal volume is directed into the dependent lung. In this case, the distribution of perfusion is a significant determinant of the degree of shunting. The blood flow through the nondependent lung becomes a right-to-left shunt, which will add to that in the dependent lung.[28,29] OLV results in an increased V/Q mismatch and a larger alveolar-arterial oxygen tension gradient.

In estimating the degree of shunt that is created by OLV, it should be kept in mind that in the lateral position, an average of 40% of CO perfuses the nondependent, nonventilated lung; the remaining 60% perfuses the dependent lung. In addition, the percent shunt through the nondependent lung depends on the HPV response. The HPV response is a protective reflex in which vasoconstriction diverts blood away from the nondependent hypoxic lung to the ventilated lung and therefore reduces the degree of venous admixture.[18] When the HPV response is intact, the transpulmonary shunt through the nondependent lung is approximately about 23% of the CO.[21] The Q_S/Q_T during two-lung ventilation is assumed to be distributed equally between the two lungs (5% in each lung). In addition, uninhibited HPV is believed to reduce 35% of the total blood flow of the nondependent lung by 50%. OLV at a given inspired FiO_2 (1) concentration results in a much larger alveolar-to-arterial tension difference with a low PAO_2 as compared with two-lung ventilation. This has been demonstrated in many studies where each patient served as his or her own control.[23,30–36]

Several factors affect the distribution of perfusion and ventilation, resulting in a wide variety of alveolar to arterial O_2 partial pressure difference (1) P (A – a) O_2 because of the transpulmonary shunt.

Schematic representation of two-lung ventilation versus OLV (Fig. 6.19). Typical values for fractional blood flow to the nondependent and dependent lungs, as well as PaO_2 and Q · S/Q · t for the two conditions, are shown. The Q · S/Q · t during two-lung ventilation is assumed to be distributed equally between the two lungs (5% to each lung). OLV creates an obligatory right-to-left transpulmonary shunt through the nonventilated, nondependent lung, which is not present during two-lung ventilation. The 35% of total flow perfusing the nondependent lung, which was not shunt flow, was assumed to be able to reduce its blood flow by 50% by HPV. Therefore it is (35/2) = 17.5%. To this, 5% must be added, which is the obligatory shunt

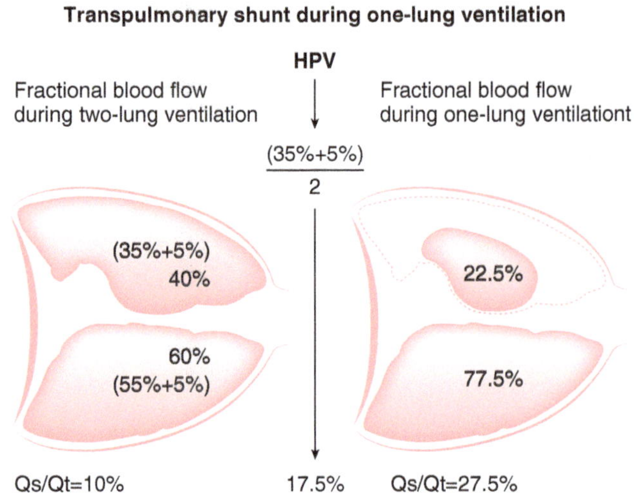

• **Fig. 6.19** Schematic representation of two-lung ventilation versus one-lung ventilation. The Qs/Qt during two-lung ventilation is assumed to be distributed equally between the two lungs (5% to each lung). Hypoxic pulmonary vasoconstriction (*HPV*) is assumed to reduce the 35% of the total flow perfusing the nondependent lung that is not shunt flow during two-lung ventilation by half to 17.5%. The total blood flow (obligatory shunt) through the nondependent lung is therefore 22.5%. (From Benumof JL. Special physiology of the lateral decubitus position, the open chest, and one-lung ventilation. In: Benumof JL, ed. *Anesthesia for Thoracic Surgery*. Philadelphia: WB Saunders; 1987:112.)

through the nondependent lung. The shunt through the nondependent lung is therefore 22.5%. Together with the 5% shunt in the dependent lung, total shunt during OLV is 22.5% + 5% = 27.5%. This results in a PaO_2 of approximately 150 mm Hg (FiO_2 = 1).[21]

Dependent Lung Atelectasis

Atelectasis of the dependent lung during OLV is one of the many factors that can contribute to hypoxemia during anesthesia. The formation of an atelectatic area in the dependent lung has several causes.[37]

1. The increment of systemic vascular resistance resulting from the existence of a significant hypoxic compartment within the dependent lung interferes with the ability to ventilate the lung. That results in decreasing blood flow to the dependent lung; this blood is directed into the nondependent lung. The extent of disease in the lung determines the PVR and the degree of Q_S/Q_T.[38,39]
2. Absorption atelectasis may occur in the dependent area of the lung that has a low V/Q ratio when exposed to high inspired oxygen concentration.[39,41]
3. Loss of dependent lung volume because of the induction of general anesthesia and paralysis, compression from the mediastinal weight, and lung secretion.[17–19]
4. Finally, prolonged stat lateral decubitus position may cause fluid to transudate in the dependent lung; this leads to reduction in FRC and increased airway closure in the dependent lung.

Hypoxic Pulmonary Vasoconstriction (See Chapter 15) (Fig. 6.20)

HPV is a protective autoregulatory mechanism that diverts blood flow away from the atelectatic portion of the lung by active contraction.[29,42–44] HPV is discussed in-depth in Chapter 15. It is a reflex contraction of vascular smooth muscle in the pulmonary circulation in response to low regional PaO_2. This vasoconstriction by the pulmonary vasculature represents its fundamental difference from the systemic circulation, which typically vasodilates in response to hypoxia. Studies using pulmonary arterial smooth muscle cells confirm that HPV occurs in these cells even when isolated.

The relationship between PaO_2 and the size of the hypoxic segment shows that, when a small part of the lung is hypoxic, HPV has little effect on PaO_2 because shunt is small in this situation. When most of the lung is hypoxic, there is no significant normoxic region to which the hypoxic region can divert flow, and then it does not matter, in terms of PaO_2, whether the hypoxic region has active HPV. When the amount of lung made hypoxic is 30% to 70%, such as occurs during OLV, there may be a large difference between the PaO_2 to be expected with normal HPV compared with that expected in its absence.

Several factors listed later may inhibit HPV and thus lead to a further deterioration in arterial oxygenation:

Low V/Q ration or nitrogen-ventilated lung. Most of the blood flow reduction in the acutely atelectatic lung is caused by HPV. Reexpansion and ventilation of a collapsed lung with nitrogen does not increase the blood flow to the lung, whereas ventilation with oxygen restores all blood flow to the precollapsed value.[45–47]

Systemic vasodilators, such as nitroglycerin,[48–50] nitroprusside,[51–53] calcium antagonist, and beta$_2$-agonist,[54–56] inhibit HPV.

Vasoconstricting drugs, preferably those that constrict the normoxic lung vessels.

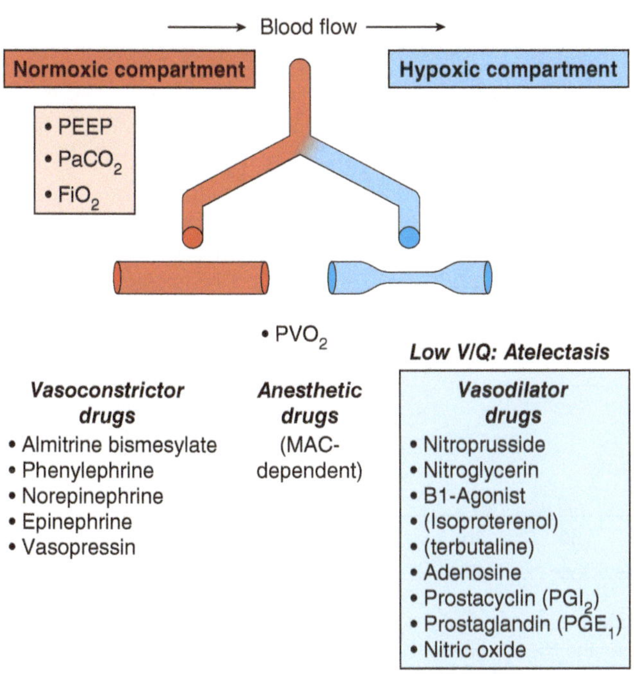

• **Fig. 6.20** Hypoxic pulmonary vasoconstriction (*HPV*): factors influencing the degree of HPV response. *FiO2*, Fraction of inspired oxygen; *MAC*, minimal alveolar concentration; *PaCO2*, arterial partial pressure of carbon dioxide; *PEEP*, positive end-expiratory pressure; *PvO2*, mixed venous oxygen tension.

High pulmonary vascular pressure (smooth muscle cannot constrict to counter high vascular pressure) or low resistance (more areas of the lung are in zone 1 condition with a resultant increase in PVR). HPV is maximal when pulmonary vascular pressure is normal.

Either with low or high SvO_2, HPV is maximal when SvO_2 is normal. With high SvO_2, reverse diffusion of oxygen occurs, which increases the oxygen tension above the HPV threshold. Low SvO_2 decreases alveolar oxygen tension in the normoxic ventilated lung to raise HPV. This offsets the blood flow diversion that results from the HPV in the collapsed lung.[57–59]

Normocarbia has the least influence on HPV. Hypercarbia increases PVR and decreases HPV. Hypocarbia is achieved by hyperventilation of the dependent lung, therefore an increases in the period of positive pressure in that lung raises PVR and lowers HPV.

The choice of anesthetic technique for OLV must take into consideration the effects on oxygenation and therefore on HPV. Normally, collapse of the nonventilated, nondependent lung results in activation of reflex HPV in this lung. This causes local increases in PVR and diversion of blood flow to other, better oxygenated parts of the pulmonary vascular bed.

Inhaled anesthetic and HPV:[59–66] The average effect of a minimal alveolar concentration (1) (1-MAC) dose of inhalational anesthetic is to reduce HPV response in 20% to 30% of cases (Fig. 6.21). According to Domino et al.,[67] administration of 1-MAC isoflurane anesthesia should cause a 21% decrease in HPV response, which would increase the expected blood flow through the nondependent lung from 20% to 24%. Fig. 6.22 shows the percent pulmonary shunt and the proportion of atelectatic lung in humans undergoing anesthesia for thoracic surgery. In (1), the lateral position, the shunt is less than 5%; in (2), when the chest is open, it is slightly increased; in (3) when the upper lung is collapsed, the pulmonary shunt is not along the ling of identity, and flow diversion is caused by HPV response; and in (4), with the ligation of the pulmonary artery of the nondependent lung, the shunt returns to the expected value for the dependent lung.

Surgical Manipulation

Nondependent lung compression or retraction inhibits HPV response. Recent evidence shows that lung trauma may release the vasodilator prostaglandin, which inhibits HPV. Therefore surgical manipulation and lung dissection reduce the effectiveness of the HPV response.

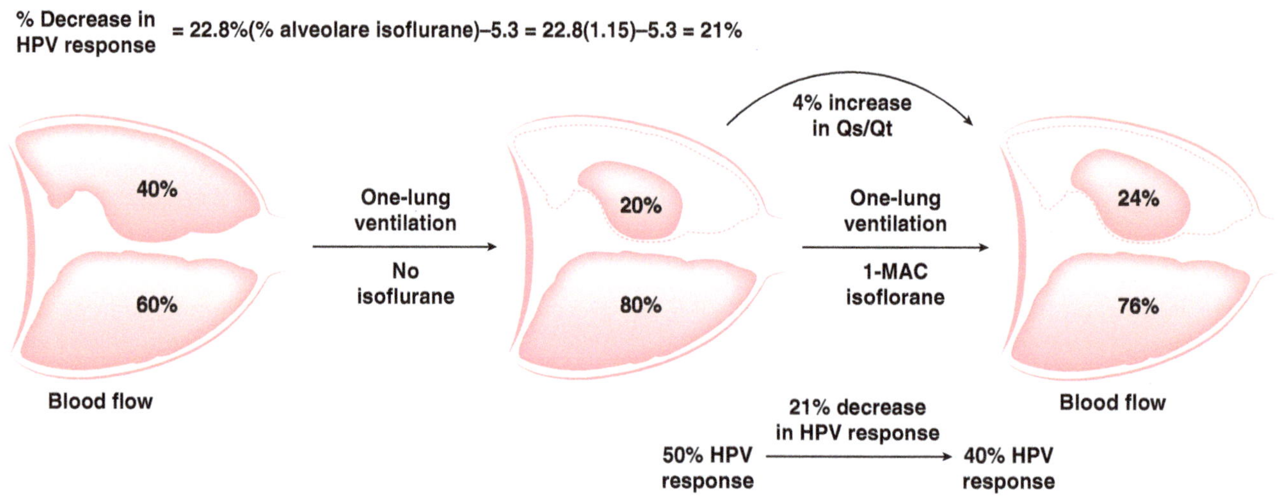

• **Fig. 6.21** Schematic diagram showing the effect of 1-MAC isoflurane on shunt during one-lung ventilation (OLV) of normal lungs. The two-lung ventilation, nondependent/dependent lung blood flow ratio is 40%/60% (left). When two-lung ventilation is converted to OLV (as indicated by atelectasis of the nondependent lung), the hypoxic pulmonary vasoconstriction (*HPV*) response decreases the blood flow to the nondependent lung by 50%. The nondependent/dependent lung blood flow ratio is now 20%/80% (middle). According to Domino et al., administration of 1-MAC isoflurane should cause a 21% decrease in the HPV response. Consequently, the nondependent/dependent lung blood flow ration would become 24%/76%, which represents a 4% increase in the total shunt across the lungs (right). *MAC*, Minimal alveolar concentration.

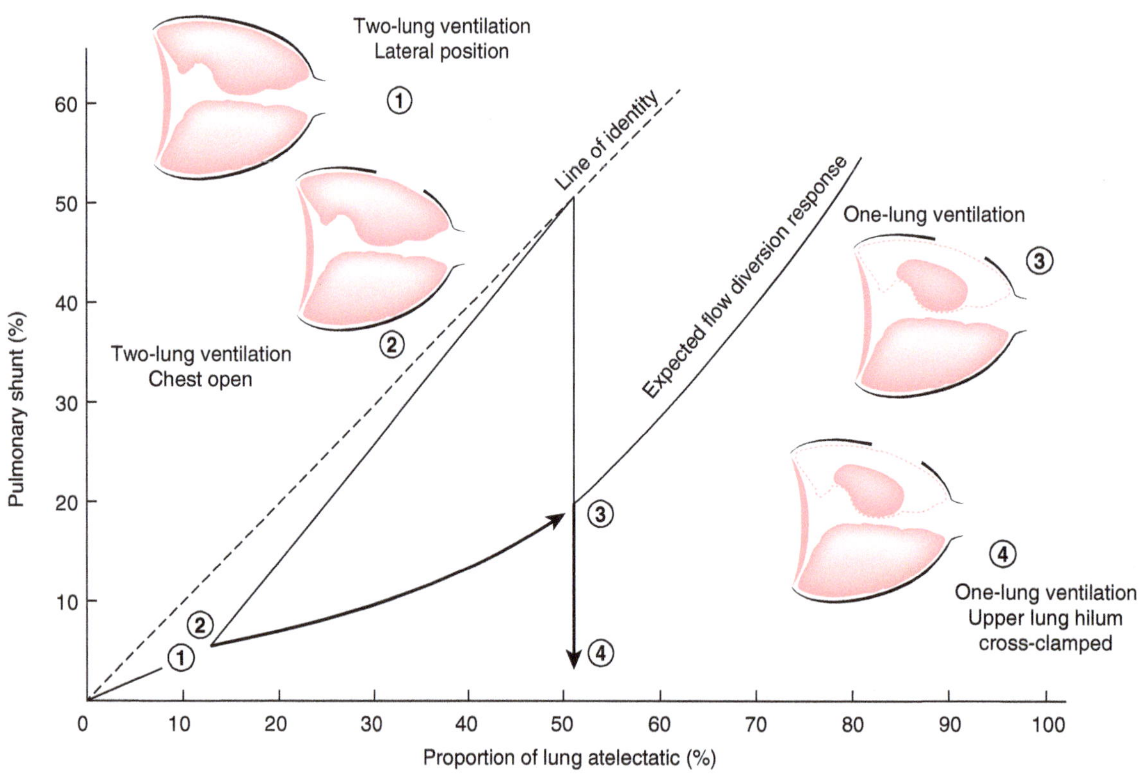

• **Fig. 6.22** Pulmonary shunt measured in patient undergoing anesthesia for the thoracic surgery. In 1, the shunt is less than 5%, and the patient is in lateral position with two-lung ventilation. In 2, this increases only slightly when the chest is opened. In 3, the lung is collapsed, and the ventilatory exchange is maintained only through the dependent lung. The pulmonary shunt increases but not along the 45-degree line of identity that is expected in the absence of hypoxic pulmonary vasoconstriction (*HPV*). In 4, the upper lung hilum is cross-clamped, and the shunt returns to the value expected for the dependent lung. (From Kerr LH, Smith AC, Prys-Roberts C, Meloche R. Observation during endobronchial anesthesia. II. Oxygenation. *Br J Anaesth.* 1974;46;84.)

Carbon Dioxide During One-Lung Ventilation

OLV has less impact on $PaCO_2$ than it does on arterial oxygenation. Blood flow through the nondependent lung retains CO_2, because it does not take part in the gas exchange. Blood that flows through the overventilated, dependent lung compensates by giving up additional CO_2. In addition, the arterial-venous gradient in very small. The $PaCO_2$ is approximately 40 mm Hg, whereas the $PvCO_2$ is 45 mm Hg; this difference is only 5 mm Hg. Thus venous admixture caused by increased shunt affects arterial oxygen more than arterial carbon dioxide. The ventilated lung cannot take up enough oxygen to compensate for the nonventilated lung, and therefore the difference between PAO_2 and PaO_2 is large.

The lung is a wonder and the most complex organ with a variety of functions. After many years of research, there are still unexplored parts and functions of this organ.

References

1. West JB. *Ventilation/Blood Flow and Gas Exchange*. 3rd ed. Oxford: Blackwell Scientific Publication; 1985.
2. West JB, Ct Dollery, Naimark A. Distribution of blood flow in isolated lung: relation to vascular and alveolar pressures. *J Appl Physiol*. 1964;19:713.
3. Knudsen L, Ochs M. The micromechanics of lung alveoli: structure and function of surfactant and tissue components. *Histochem Cell Biol*. 2018;150(6):661–676.
4. Rodríguez-Roisin R, Roca J. Mechanisms of hypoxemia. *Intensive Care Med*. 2005;31:1017.
5. Cruz JC, Metting PJ. Understanding the meaning of the shunt fraction calculation. *J Clin Monit*. 1987;3(2):124–134.
6. Chang EM, Bretherick A, Drummond GB, Baillie JK. Predictive validity of a novel non-invasive estimation of effective shunt fraction in critically ill patients. *Intensive Care Med Exp*. 2019(7):49.
7. West JB. Blood flow to the lung and gas exchange. *Anesthesiology*. 1974;41:124.
8. Hoppin Jr FG, Green ID, Mead J. Distribution of pleural surface pressure. *J Appl Physiol*. 1969;127:863.
9. West JB. Regional differences in gas exchange in the lung of erect man. *J Appl Physiol*. 1962;17:893.
10. Milic-Emili J, Henderson JAM, Dolovich MB, et al. Regional distribution of inspired gas exchange in the lung. *J Appl Physiol*. 1966;21:749.
11. Wagner PD, Saltzman HA, West JB. Measurement of continuous distribution of ventilation-perfusion ratios: theory. *J Appl Physiol*. 1974;36:588.
12. Kleen M, Zwissler B. Physiology of pulmonary perfusion: new concepts. *Curr Opin Anaesthesiol*. 2001;14(1):51–57.
13. Glenny RW, Bernard SL, Robertson HT. Pulmonary blood flow remains fractal down to the level of gas exchange. *J Appl Physiol*. 2000;89(2):742–748.
14. Chornuk MA, Bernard SL, Burns JW, et al. Effects of inertial load and countermeasures on the distribution of pulmonary blood flow. *J Appl Physiol*. 2000;89(2):445–457.
15. WA Altemeir, Mckinney SI, Glenny RW. Fractal nature of regional ventilation distribution. *Appl Physiol*. 2000;88:1551–1557.
16. Svanberg L. Influence of posture on lung volumes, ventilation and circulation in normal. *Scan J Clin Lab Invest*. 1957;9(25):1–195.
17. Rehder K, Sessler AD. Function of each lung in spontaneously breathing man anesthetized with thiopental-meperidine. *Anesthesiology*. 1973;38:320.
18. Froese AB, Bryan AC. Effects of anesthesia and paralysis on diaphragmatic mechanics in man. *Anesthesiology*. 1974;42:242.
19. Wulff KE, Aulin I. The regional lung function in the lateral decubitus position during anesthesia and operation. *Acta Anaesthesiol Scand*. 1972;16:195.
20. Rehder K, Wenthe FM, Sessler AD. Function of each lung during mechanical ventilation with ZEEP and with PEEP in man anesthetized with thiopental meperidine. *Anesthesiology*. 1973;39:597.
21. Benumof JL, ed. *Anesthesia for Thoracic Surgery*. Philadelphia: WB Saunders; 1987.
22. Guz A, Noble MIM, Eislele JH, et al. The effect of lung deflation on breathing man. *Clin Sci*. 1971;40:451.
23. Tarhan S, Moffitt EA. Principles of thoracic anesthesia. *Surg Clin North Am*. 1973;l53:813.
24. Maloney JV, Schmutzer KJ, Raschke E. Paradoxical respiration and "pendelluft". *Thorac Cardiovasc Surg*. 1961;41:291.
25. Werner O, Malmkvist G, Beckman A, et al. Gas exchange and haemodynamics during thoracotomy. *Br J Anaesth*. 1984;56:1343.
26. Rehder K, Hatch DJ, Sessler AD, et al. The function of each lung of anesthetized and paralyzed man during mechanical ventilation. *Anesthesiology*. 1972;37:16.
27. Nunn JF. The distribution of inspired gas during thoracic surgery. *Ann R Coll Surg Engl*. 1961;28:223.
28. Tarhan S, Lungborg RO. Carlens endotracheal catheter versus regular endotracheal tube during thoracic surgery: a comparison of blood tensions and pulmonary shunting. *Cam J Anaesth*. 1971;18:594.
29. Marshall BE, Marshall C. Continuity of response to hypoxic pulmonary vasoconstriction. *J Appl Physiol*. 1980;59:189.
30. Benumof JL. One-lung ventilation and hypoxic pulmonary vasoconstriction: implications for anesthetic management. *Anesth Analg*. 1985;64:821.
31. Capan L, Turndorf H, Chandrakant P, et al. Optimization of arterial oxygenation during one-lung anesthesia. *Anesth Analg*. 1980;59:847.
32. Cohen E, Eisenkraft JB, Thys DM, et al. Oxygenation and hemodynamic changes during one-lung ventilation: effects of $CPAP_{10}$, $PEEP_{10,}$ an $CPAP_{10}/PEEp_{10}$. *J Cardiothorac Anesth*. 1988;2:34.
33. Aalto-Setala M, Heinonen J, Salorinne Y. Cardiorespiratory function during thoracic anesthesia: comparison of two-lung ventilation and one-lung ventilation with and without PEEP. *Acta Anaesthesiol Scand*. 1974;19:287.
34. Katz JA, Laverne RG, Fairley HB. Pulmonary oxygen exchange during endobronchial anesthesia. *Anesthesiology*. 1982;56:164.
35. Tarhan S, Lundborg RO. Effects of increased respiratory pressure on blood gas tensions and pulmonary shunting during thoracotomy with use of the Carlens catheter. *Can J Anaesth*. 1970;17:4.
36. Slinger PD, Hickey D, Gottfried S. Intrinsic PEEP during one-lung ventilation. *Anesth Analg*. 1989;68:S269.
37. Benumof JL, ed. *Anesthesia for Thoracic Surgery*. Philadelphia: WB Saunders; 1987:120.
38. Craig JOC, Bromley LL, Williams R. Thoracotomy and contralateral lung. A study of the changes occurring in the dependent and contralateral lung during and after thoracotomy in the lateral decubitus position. *Thorax*. 1962;17:9.
39. Kerr JH. Physiological aspects of one lung (endobronchial) anesthesia. *Int Anesthesiol Clin*. 1972;10:61.

40. Benumof JL. Respiratory physiology and respiratory function during anesthesia. In: Miller R, ed. *Anesthesia*. New York: Churchill Livingstone; 1986:1115.
41. Dantzker DR, Wagner PD, West JB. Instability of lung units with low V/Q ratios during O_2 breathing. *J Appl Physiol.* 1975;38:886.
42. Benumof JL. Mechanism of decreased blood flow to atelectatic lung. *J App Physiol.* 1979;46:1047.
43. Benumof JL. One-lung ventilation and hypoxic pulmonary vasoconstriction: implication for anesthetic management. *Anesth Analg.* 1985;64:821.
44. Bjertanes LJ, Mundal R, Huage A, et al. Vascular resistance in atelectatic lungs: effect of inhalation anesthetics. *Acta Anaesthesiol Scand.* 1980;24:109.
45. Prilo AF, Benumof JL, Trousdale FR. Atelectatic lung lobe blood flow: open versus closed chest, positive pressure versus spontaneous ventilation. *J Appl Physiol.* 1981;50:1022.
46. Glasser SA, Domino KB, Lindgren L, et al. Pulmonary pressure and flow during atelectasis. *Anesthesiology.* 1982;57:A504.
47. Carlsson AJ, Bindslev L, Santesson J, et al. Hypoxic pulmonary vasoconstriction in the human lung: the effect of prolonged unilateral hypoxic challenge during anesthesia. *Acta Anaesthesiol Scand.* 1985;29:346.
48. Hill NS, Antman EM, Green LH, et al. Intravenous nitroglycerin. A review of pharmacology, therapeutic effects and indications. *Chest.* 1981;79:69.
49. Kadowithz PJ, Nandiwada P, Grueter CA, et al. Pulmonary vasodilator responses to nitroprusside and nitroglycerin in the dog. *J Clin Invest.* 1981;67:893.
50. Anjou-Lindskog E, Broman L, Holmgren A. Effects of nitroglycerin on central hemodynamics and V_A/Q distribution early after coronary bypass surgery. *Acta Anaesthesiol Scand.* 1982;26:489.
51. Parsons GH, Leventhal JP, Hansen MM, et al. Effect of sodium nitroprusside on hypoxic pulmonary vasoconstriction in the dog. *J Appl Physiol.* 1981;51:288.
52. Sivak ED, Gray BA, McCurdy TH, et al. Pulmonary vascular response to nitroprusside in dogs. *Circ res.* 1979;45:360.
53. Hills AB, Sykes MK, Reyes A. Hypoxic pulmonary vasoconstrictor response in dogs and after sodium nitroprusside infusion. *Anesthesiology.* 1979;50:484.
54. McFarlane PA, Mortimer AJ, Ryder WA, et al. Effects of dopamine and dobutamine on the distribution of pulmonary blood flow during lobar ventilation hypoxia and lobar collapse in dogs. *Eur J Clin Invest.* 1985;15:53.
55. Furman WR, Summer WR, Kennedy PP, et al. Comparison of the effects of dobutamine, dopamine and isoproterenol on hypoxic pulmonary vasoconstriction in the pig. *Crit Care Med.* 1982;10:371.
56. Bishop MJ, Cheney FW. Minoxidil and nifedipine inhibit hypoxic pulmonary vasoconstriction. *J Cardiovasc Pharmacol.* 1983;5:184.
57. Domino KB, Glasses SA, Wetstein L, et al. Influence of P_VO_2 on blood flow to atelectatic lung. *Anesthesiology.* 1982;57:A471.
58. Benumof JL, Pirlo AF, Trousdale FR. Inhibition of hypoxic pulmonary vasoconstriction by decreased P_VO_2: a new indirect mechanism. *J Appl Physiol.* 1981:51871.
59. Pease RD, Benumof JL. P_AO_2 and P_VO_2 interaction on hypoxic pulmonary vasoconstriction. *J Appl Physiol.* 1982;53:134.
60. Benumof JL. Choice of anesthetic drugs and techniques. In: Benumof JL, ed. *Anesthesia for Thoracic Surgery.* Philadelphia: WB: Saunders; 1987:209.
61. Lawler PGP, Nunn JF. A reassessment of the validity of the isoshunt graph. *Br J Anaesth.* 1984;56:1325.
62. Benumof JL. Special physiology of the lateral decubitus position, the open chest, and one-lung ventilation. In: Benumof JL, ed. *Anesthesia for Thoracic Surgery.* Philadelphia: WB Saunders; 1987:113.
63. Benumof JL, Augustine SD, Gibbins J. Halothane and isoflurane only slightly impair arterial oxygenation during one-lung in patient undergoing thoracotomy. *Anesthesiology.* 1987;67:910.
64. Carlsson AJ, Bindslev L, Hedenstierna G. Hypoxia pulmonary vasoconstriction in the lung. *Anesthesiology.* 1987;66:312.
65. Carlsson AJ, Hedenstierna G, Bindslev L. Hypoxiainduced vasoconstriction in human lung exposed to enflurane anaesthesia. *Acta Anaesthesiol Scand.* 1987;31:57.
66. Eisenkraft JB. Effects of anaesthesia on the pulmonary circulation. *Br J Anaesth.* 1990;65:63–78.
67. Domino KB, Borowec L, Alexander CM, et al. Influence of isoflurane on hypoxic pulmonary vasoconstriction in dogs. *Anesthesiology.* 1986;65:423.

7

Modulating the Pulmonary Circulation: Nitric Oxide and Beyond

THOMAS SCHILLING, ASTRID BERGMANN

Introduction

Thoracic surgery commonly requires the separation of the patient's airway, followed by exclusion of one lung from ventilation (i.e., one-lung ventilation [OLV]) to facilitate surgical interventions.[1] However, ventilation of one lung will result in an increased intrapulmonary shunt because of continuous perfusion in the nonventilated collapsed lung. In addition, insufficient oxygenation of pulmonary blood through the atelectatic regions of the ventilated lung will increase venous admixture and ventilation/perfusion (V_A/Q) mismatching.[2] In fact, in the lateral position, the blood flow that is delivered to the ventilated lung can comprise more than 60% of the cardiac output as compared with less than 40% in the nonventilated collapsed lung.

During OLV in lateral position, because of the absence of any ventilation in the nondependent lung, accompanied by persistent perfusion in the collapsed region, the percentage of cardiac output that will participate in gas exchange becomes even less, and an increase in total intrapulmonary shunt of 30% to 35% can occur.

Other factors may disturb the distribution of pulmonary perfusion, resulting in a more pronounced V_A/Q mismatch. These may include a decrease in cardiac output and an increase in pulmonary vascular resistance (PVR), augmented by the effects of different volatile or intravenously administered anesthetics. In addition, blood loss, or an impaired alveolar ventilation (e.g., because of double-lumen-tube misplacement or bronchial blocker malposition), development of pulmonary edema, or absorption atelectasis may increase the transpulmonary shunt.[3]

As a result, hypoxemia, reported in about 10% of patients undergoing thoracic surgery, is defined as a decline of arterial oxygen saturation below 90%, despite the use of high inspiratory fractions of oxygen (FiO_2) during OLV.[4] The hypoxemia during OLV is usually not severe; however, in some cases, life-threatening conditions may occur that respond poorly to corrective maneuvers.[5] These therapeutic approaches may include application of positive end-expiratory pressure (PEEP) to the ventilated lung, continuous positive airway pressure (CPAP), as well as pure oxygen insufflation/apneic oxygenation[6] into the nonventilated lung. Besides, the use of relatively high tidal volumes (6–8 mL/kg) and assurance of normal blood hemoglobin concentrations are advised.[3]

In addition, alveolar recruitment maneuvers are recommended to recruit poorly aerated alveoli in the ventilated lung and to minimize blood shift to the nondependent lung during OLV.[7,8] However, this strategy may reinforce mechanical stress applied to the lungs, including higher driving pressures, alveolar stretching, and shear stress secondary to cyclic recruitment/derecruitment of alveoli.[9] Subsequently, OLV can result in significant diffuse parenchymal injury.[10]

The simple manipulation of respiratory parameters often fails to improve oxygenation, especially in patients who additionally suffer from obstructive or restrictive pulmonary diseases[11] or pulmonary hypertension.[12] Different attempts have therefore been made to manage life-threatening complications of OLV intraoperatively and have encouraged the search for coadjuvant or alternative pharmacologic treatments.

An important concept seems to accelerate the onset of hypoxic pulmonary vasoconstriction (HPV) by reduction of perfusion in the nonventilated lung and to increase distribution of perfusion to the dependent, ventilated lung regions,[13] thereby improving V_A/Q matching and to decrease hypoxemia. HPV is an important physiologic defensive mechanism by which pulmonary blood flow is diverted from nonventilated hypoxemic areas toward better ventilated regions. Accordingly, HPV decreases blood flow to the collapsed lung regions during OLV, controlled by alveolar PO_2 (Fig. 7.1).

However, many anesthetics, such as volatiles in concentrations above 1 MAC, and different procedures can impair beneficial effects of HPV during OLV with subsequently impaired arterial oxygenation and hypoxemia.[14,15] Therefore the anesthesiologist makes an effort to increase HPV response with various drugs and techniques to reduce the intrapulmonary shunt.

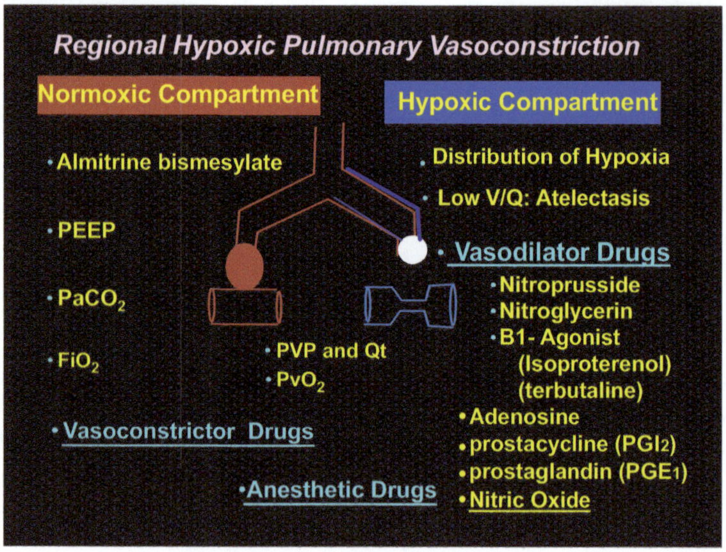

• **Fig. 7.1** Overview of the hypoxic vasoconstriction, its effects on the lung, and how it can be influenced to end in physiologic or pathophysiologic settings. *FiO_2*, Fraction of inspired oxygen; *PEEP*, positive end-expiratory pressure; *V_A/Q*, ventilation/perfusion relation; *PVP*, pulmonary vascular pressure; *PvO_2*, venous partial pressure of oxygen; *$PaCO_2$*, arterial partial pressure of carbon dioxide; *PGI2*, Prostaglandi I2; *PGE1*, Prostaglandin E1; *Qt*, intrapulmonary shunt. (Courtesy of Edmond Cohen M.D.)

A number of clinical studies have evaluated the possibility to increase perfusion distribution to the ventilated regions by administration of a vasodilator, that is, inhalation of nitric oxide (NO) or aerosolized prostacyclin (PGI2, Iloprost) to the dependent lung with a combination of vasoconstriction agents, such as almitrine or phenylephrine, to diminish the perfusion in the nonventilated regions.[13]

As an example, dexmedetomidine as a highly selective α_2-adrenergic receptor agonist with sedative, analgesic, anti-inflammatory, and organ protection side effects was accordingly evaluated during OLV.[16] The drug diminishes high sympathetic activation and results in lower heart rates, decreased blood pressure, and myocardial oxygen consumption.

Applied Physiology of Pulmonary Circulation

General Considerations

The primary mission of the coordinated interplay of respiration and circulation is to deliver oxygen to peripheral organs and tissues with relation to their metabolic requirements, and to eliminate the carbon dioxide that is generated during metabolism. For the purpose of gas exchange, the pulmonary circulation transports the blood to and from the alveoli.

The normal pulmonary circulation uses a low-resistance, highly compliant vascular bed, which is interposed between the two ventricles of the heart that function in synchrony. As a consequence, another important function of pulmonary circulation is to serve as a major reservoir for blood volume.

The pulmonary circulation operates in close relation with the alveolar ventilation to ensure optimal gas exchange. For this interchange, the lungs receive the entire cardiac output, and the pulmonary blood flow is about the match of the alveolar ventilation. Although the respiratory and circulatory cycles are phasic, their rates are entirely different (i.e., about 15 breaths and 80 heartbeats per minute at rest). Therefore the matching of respiration and perfusion for optimal arterialization of mixed venous blood requires subtle tuning of operations that are not in phase, at rest, during exercise, or during general anesthesia.

The outputs of the two cardiac ventricles are approximately the same when calculated over many respiratory cycles, although the left ventricle delivers slightly more blood than the right one, because of venous admixture of bronchial to pulmonary venous blood. This anatomic shunt comprises less than 2% of the total left cardiac output. However, even a doubling of total cardiac output can be accommodated in the capacious pulmonary vessels with virtually no increase in the mean pulmonary arterial pressure (MPAP).

Thus the lungs have a remarkable ability to maintain their PVR even as their vascular pressures, raised through the mechanisms of recruitment and distension. These mechanisms allow the lungs to increase their blood volume capacity with relatively small increases in pulmonary arterial and venous pressure. This may also be observed when a subject lies down after standing or when a patient is placed from supine to lateral position, for example, for thoracic surgery. The blood is then diverted from both lungs into the more dependent parts.

The pulmonary circulation has a relatively poor autoregulation. Consequently, it is important to monitor and control vascular pressures. A change in mechanical ventilation pattern or in cardiac performance as it may occur during the shift from two-lung ventilation (TLV) to OLV can passively affect the partition between the stored and pass-through components of the stroke volume, as well as modify the peripheral transmission of the pressure and flow pulses.

Intraoperative Monitoring of Pulmonary Circulation

The key to intraoperative management of thoracic surgery patients is to limit dangerous increases in PVR or myocardial oxygen demand to preserve myocardial perfusion and oxygen delivery. The induction of anesthesia, mechanical ventilation, lateral positioning, OLV, pulmonary artery clamping, blood loss, and emergence from general anesthesia are the most critical periods. It is necessary to avoid hypoxemia, hypercarbia, acidosis, hypervolemia, hypothermia, and unnecessary sympathetic stimulation because each of them can induce maldistribution of pulmonary perfusion.

The standard monitoring in patients undergoing thoracic surgery usually comprises an electrocardiogram (ECG) with automated ST-segment analysis, temperature monitoring, pulse oximetry (SpO_2), and continuous end-tidal carbon dioxide ($EtCO_2$) measurement (Table 7.1).

The majority of patients scheduled for thoracic surgery with OLV in lateral position requires an intraarterial catheter for blood pressure monitoring and blood sampling for blood-gas-analysis. However, the insertion of a central venous, as well as a pulmonary artery catheter (PAC) is disputed and is for the most part not routinely inserted for thoracic procedures. In patients with significant cardiac debased or with known pulmonary hypertension, the PAC can provide simultaneous measurement of central venous pressure (CVP), pulmonary artery pressure (PAP), cardiac output, and mixed venous oxygen saturation (SvO_2); all of them represent very useful variables in assessing pulmonary circulation and possible effects of short-acting pulmonary vasodilators on HPV.

However, it should be noted that PAC usage did not result in decrease in patients mortality, hospital length of stay, or cost in intensive care unit.[17] On the contrary, a retrospective data analysis has demonstrated an association of PAC with increased mortality in patients submitted to cardiac surgery.[18] Nevertheless, PAC usage can be very helpful and should be limited for the management of hemodynamic therapy in selected high-risk patients undergoing thoracic surgery.

A modern approach to pressure load of the right ventricle, PAP, and volume status assessment is the use of transesophageal echocardiography (TEE), which is especially indicated in lung transplantation and other high-risk thoracic interventions.[19,20] The echocardiographic evaluation of these physiologic factors appears important because right heart hypertrophy or dilation and decreased left ventricular filling of the coronary arteries may result in dangerously restricted perfusion and ischemia. As a consequence, intraoperative ischemia can lead to right heart failure.

TABLE 7.1 Representative Hemodynamic Values for Normal Adults at Rest

Cardiac output (L/min)	4–6
Heart rate (beats/min)	80
Right atrial pressure (mm Hg)	4–6
Pulmonary artery pressures (mm Hg)	
Systolic	20–25
Diastolic	10–12
Mean	14–18
Pulmonary wedge pressure (mm Hg)	6–9
Systemic arterial pressure (mm Hg)	120/80
Mean	90–100
Pulmonary vascular resistance (units)	0.70–0.95

Pulmonary Vascular Resistance

In daily anesthetic practice, the rationale about the regulation of the pulmonary circulation follows the concept of PVR that can be described as a normal vascular muscle tone, as vasoconstriction or vasodilation. The small precapillary pulmonary muscular arteries and arterioles act as resistance vessels and are considered as the principal sites of pulmonary vasomotor activity. Several factors interact with pulmonary circulation and subsequently with right heart function by increasing PVR, especially during OLV. Mechanical ventilation, in particular, the effects of high tidal volume (V_T), driving pressures and PEEP, hypoventilation, hypoxia, hypercapnia, nitrous oxide (N_2O), isoflurane, and desflurane. In contrast, high FiO_2, hypocapnia, and intravenous anesthetics may act as pulmonary vasodilators.

The PVR can be calculated by $R = (P_{PA} - P_{LA})/Q_T$, where R represents PVR and $P_{PA} - P_{LA}$ gives the drop in mean pressure between the pulmonary artery and left atrium (mm Hg). Commonly, pulmonary wedge pressure (P_{PW}) is substituted for P_{LA}, Q_T is the mean pulmonary blood flow (mL/s). The formula expresses PVR in R (resistance) units. For normal pulmonary circulation, the value for R is about 0.1 mm Hg/L/min. PVR can also be displayed in dynes·s·cm^{-5}. For this, the numerator of the equation is multiplied by 1332. The normal value is around 100.

Ventilation-Induced Changes in Pulmonary Hemodynamics

In comparison with systemic blood pressures, pulmonary vascular pressures are rather low. The thin-walled pulmonary vessels are in close contact with the air-containing alveoli of the lungs; therefore marginal changes in external forces can exert rather large hemodynamic effects. This can be observed during mechanical positive pressure ventilation, and the effect is more pronounced during OLV, with application of much higher driving pressures.

From a hemodynamic point of view, the best-analyzed features of mechanical ventilation are positive-pressure ventilation (PPV) and PEEP. During PPV, airway pressures increase with inflation and return promptly to PEEP (or atmospheric pressure) during expiration.

In healthy humans, the imposition of high PEEP has several hemodynamic consequences: stroke volume, cardiac output, and central blood volume decrease, while heart rate remains unaffected. Pulmonary arterial pressures increase, and the increase in alveolar pressure may cause the P_{PW}s to exceed the left atrial pressures. The stiffening of the lungs by higher transpulmonary pressures or during pulmonary edema requires higher levels of PEEP to achieve a beneficial effect. At higher levels, however, the risk of barotrauma to the lungs markedly increased.

The cardiac output decreases when normal lungs are subjected to PEEP because of a reduction in venous

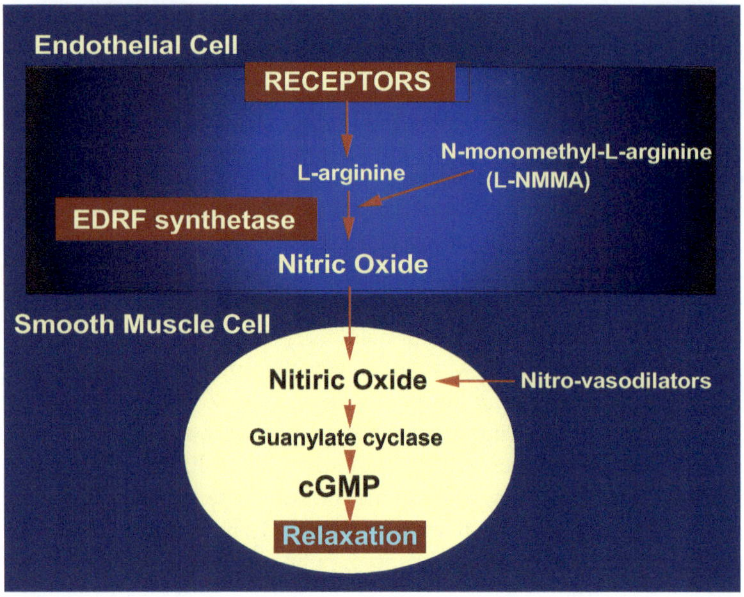

• **Fig. 7.2** The nitric oxide pathway from its synthesis in the endothelial cell to its effect in the smooth muscle cell. *cGMPm,* cyclic guanosine monophosphate; *EDRF,* endothelium derived relaxing factor; *L-NMMA,* N-monomethyl-L-arginine. (Courtesy of Edmond Cohen M.D.)

return (preload) to the right ventricle, a decrease in left ventricular preload, or from impairment of both right and left ventricular performance. In addition, cardiovascular inhibitory mechanisms in the brain and the local release of prostaglandins may contribute to this.

Regulation of Pulmonary Vascular Resistance

PVR is physiologically regulated by substances released by vascular endothelium: pulmonary vasodilators such as NO (Fig. 7.2) and endogenous prostacyclin, and by pulmonary vasoconstrictors such as endothelin-1 and thromboxane. Because of the balance in favor of vasodilation, vascular tone is predominantly low in normal pulmonary circulation. The vasodilators are released promptly in response to shear stresses, whereas endothelin-1 is released slowly and controls the vascular tone in a prolonged manner. It is believed that the pulmonary circulation is in a constant state of contraction and dilatation, which is controlled by the secretion of endogenous NO.

Administration of Pulmonary Vasodilators (See Chapter 36)

The application of pulmonary vasodilators by inhalation is basically preferable to the intravenous (IV) administration because the latter is usually accompanied by a decrease of systemic resistance (Table 7.2).

In human subjects, acute hypoxia, such as during OLV, causes an increase in pulmonary arterial pressure. Because cardiac output is marginally affected, the pulmonary perfusion would be differently distributed. The pressor response to hypoxemia would start within seconds and generally reach its peak by 3 minutes and attenuates gradually as hypoxia continues. Severe acidosis can augment the hypoxic pressor response.

Experimentally, increase in partial arterial pressure of oxygen (PaO_2) during OLV can be established by pharmacologic manipulation of pulmonary blood flow: vasodilatation in the dependent ventilated lung and vasoconstriction of the nondependent, collapsed lung.[21]

The site of pulmonary vasoconstriction in response to acute hypoxia is predominantly at the precapillary level, involving the small muscular arterioles. Acute hypoxic vasoconstriction can be inhibited by a variety of bronchodilators and vasodilators drugs, such as inhalational anesthetics nitroglycerin or nitroprusside. Endothelial-derived vasodilators such as prostacyclin administered intravenously can blunt or abolish the hypoxic pressor response. Similarly, inhalation of NO inhibits hypoxic vasoconstriction, whereas inhibitors of NO synthase (NOS) augment the hypoxic pressor response by blocking the endogenous synthesis of NO.[22]

Prostacyclins

Prostacyclin, a metabolic product of arachidonic acid metabolism, has been identified as a major determinant of regular tone in the pulmonary circulation. Prostacyclin (PGI2) is both a potent pulmonary and systemic vasodilator and an antithrombogenic agent. It is formed in pulmonary vascular endothelium by the action of prostacyclin synthetase on the prostaglandin endoperoxide PGH2. Shear stress of the endothelium and bradykinin seem to be powerful stimuli for the release of prostacyclin from endothelium. Prostacyclin antagonizes the effects of thromboxane A2, which is a potent pulmonary vasoconstrictor and stimulates platelet aggregation. An imbalance between the excretion of thromboxane and of prostacyclin metabolites may lead to pulmonary hypertension.

Prostacyclins stimulate cellular adenylate cyclase, thereby increasing the intracellular concentration of cyclic adenosine monophosphate (cAMP). This leads to a dilation of the pulmonary vasculature and reduction in PAP, and would improve arterial oxygenation. It also results in increased cardiac contractility, and to inhibition of platelet activation.[23]

TABLE 7.2 **Clinically Used Pulmonary Vasodilators**

Substance	Administration	Dosage	Effect on PVR	Effect on SVR
Nitric oxide (NO)	Inhalation	20–80 ppm	↓	0
Iloprost	Inhalation	20–25 mg	↓	(0)
Iloprost	IV	1.25–2.5 ng/kg/min	↓	↓
Sildenafil	p.o.	20 mg	↓	(↓)
Sildenafil	IV	10 mg	↓	(↓)

PVR, Pulmonary vascular resistance; *SVR*, systemic vascular resistance.

The prostacyclin analog iloprost is probably the most largely evaluated representative of this group of substances in thoracic surgery. It is available in IV (epoprostenol and veletri), subcutaneous (treprostinil), and oral (selexipag) formulations. Treprostinil can be administered in different ways, but its use is limited by severe side effects when not given intravenously.[24,25]

Iloprost can be administered by a nebulizer system by inhalation, as well as intravenously. The half-life time is rather short (about 5–25 minutes); therefore iloprost is administered 6 to 8 times a day. The drug effectively lowers the PVR, and there is only a slight rebound effect after discontinuation of administration.

In thoracic surgery, the substance induces selective vasodilation of the pulmonary vascular bed and can improve the arterial oxygenation during OLV, thereby ameliorating the ventilation–perfusion ratio.[13] In video-assisted thoracoscopic surgery, after initial desaturation to below 80% during OLV, administration of inhaled epoprostenol to the ventilated lung achieved an increase in oxygen saturation to above 92% for the remainder of OLV.[26]

Choi et al. evaluated the effects of off-label inhaled iloprost on oxygenation during OLV. Seventy-two patients who were scheduled for elective video-assisted thoracoscopic lobectomy were assigned to receive an inhaled nebulizer of distilled water (control group), 10 mcg iloprost (IL10 group), or 20 mcg iloprost (IL20 group). Arterial and venous blood gas and hemodynamic analyses were obtained. The changes in PaO_2, after the initiation of OLV and the resumption TLV, were similar in all three groups. However, PaO_2 in the IL10 group was comparable to that in the control group, whereas PaO_2 in the IL20 group was significantly higher than that in the control group at 10, 20, and 30 minutes after administration of iloprost.[27]

The present studies recommend the use of nebulized iloprost by inhalation to reduce the incidence of hypoxemia during OLV. Iloprost, in a correct dose, would vasodilate the pulmonary circulation and reduce the pulmonary arterial pressure and increase perfusion to the dilated lung regions without systemic hypotension or other major deleterious hemodynamic effects. Therefore its use is extremely favorable in patients with decompensated pulmonary hypertension with right heart failure during OLV.

Iloprost can be combined with inhaled NO to achieve additive effects.[28] In contrast to the data on selective NO administration, which exert controversial unpredictable effects on arterial oxygenation, iloprost consistently improved arterial oxygenation,[29,30] even in patients with acute respiratory failure.[31]

Inhaled Nitric Oxide

NO exerts an endogenous ubiquitous biologic role as a critical intercellular messenger in signal transduction in a wide variety of mammalian cells, in wide-ranging physiologic processes, including regulation of blood pressure and perfusion distribution. It is short-lived, only for a few seconds, because of its interactions with oxygen to form nitrogen dioxide. NO also reacts with superoxide radical (O_2^-) and with ferrous hemoproteins, such as guanylate cyclase and hemoglobin.

Endogenous NO is synthesized in endothelial cells by the action of endothelial NO synthase (eNOS) from one of the guanidium nitrogens (L-arginine) to yield L-citrulline and NO. Endothelial NO synthase is activated because of the dislodgement of the inhibitor caveolin from calmodulin in response to vasodilator agonists or shear stress.

NO diffuses to vascular smooth muscle and produces relaxation by activating guanylate cyclase and increasing cyclic guanosine monophosphate (cGMP), which triggers vasodilation and decreases in platelet aggregation (see Fig. 7.2).

Synthetic NO is delivered as a continuously inhaled gas that selectively dilates the pulmonary vasculature, thereby improving V_A/Q mismatch and increases oxygenation from reduced intrapulmonary shunt. The advantage of inhalation application is based on the specific effect on pulmonary vessels. When entering the capillary system, inhaled NO (iNO) is rapidly inactivated by binding hemoglobin; therefore the systemic side effects are essentially absent. Because of the rapid inactivation and the short half-life of NO, it requires a continuous form of application by a special delivery system.

The beneficial effect of NO during OLV is that iNO only accesses the ventilated alveoli where it causes localized vasodilation in ventilated lung areas, shifting the pulmonary blood flow toward these zones. This is the same effect during hypoxic pulmonary vasoconstriction that enhances the blood flow to the well-ventilated alveoli.[32] However, in most studies, administration of iNO alone during OLV was found to be ineffective.[30,33] On the other hand, it has been demonstrated that iNO administration in combination with intravenous almitrine limits the decline of PaO_2 during OLV.[34] In patients undergoing elective thoracic surgery, iNO administration neither significantly decreased mean pulmonary arterial pressure in patients with normal PAP nor improved oxygenation in the absence of hypoxia. Nevertheless, iNO is effective in patients with pulmonary hypertension and hypoxemia during OLV.[29] Not all patients benefit from a reduction in pulmonary vascular pressure with subsequent redistribution of perfusion. Some have no benefit or have minimal response ("nonresponder"). In addition, there is the risk of iNO rebound phenomena, with increased PVR, when administration is interrupted.[35,36]

iNO has currently only U.S. Food and Drug Administration approval for the use in neonates with hypoxic respiratory failure associated with pulmonary hypertension, but many institutions "off label" iNO to treat severely ill adult patients with compromised right heart and pulmonary function.[37] Despite the statement of a European board of experts[38] regarding the use of iNO that there is no evidence to support the routine use of iNO for the prevention or reversal of hypoxemia during OLV, some patients with severe hypoxemia may benefit from this drug.[38] The data regarding the use of iNO and PEEP have mixed messages: previous data suggest that iNO oxide affects hypoxemia only when it is used with high PEEP,[39] while others suggest that it was also helpful when administered without PEEP in patients with severe hypoxemia.[29]

Almitrine

Almitrine bismesylate is a diphenylmethylpiperazine derivative that acts as an agonist of peripheral chemoreceptor located on the carotid bodies classified as a respiratory stimulant that potentiates HPV (Fig. 7.3). The drug increases arterial oxygenation while decreasing arterial carbon dioxide partial pressure in patients with chronic obstructive pulmonary disease (COPD) by improving the ventilation perfusion matching. Accordingly, the substance was first used orally in patients with COPD to delay, discontinue, or even avoid long-term oxygen therapy. Almitrine treatment of patients with severe COPD and moderate hypoxemia resulted in a small but significant improvement in PaO_2 over 12 months. A clinically important improvement in gas exchange was observed in 33% of treated patients.[40]

Almitrine may improve oxygenation by correcting the V_A/Q mismatch because of OLV[41–45] by enhancing the HPV mechanism in nonventilated areas. The hemodynamic effects of almitrine on the pulmonary circulation are dose-related,[45,46] and severe pulmonary hypertension is not expected if a lower dose combined with iNO is used during OLV.[45] Nevertheless, an adverse effect of almitrine is the elevation of PVR, which, if excessive and prolonged, could potentially induce right ventricular dysfunction.

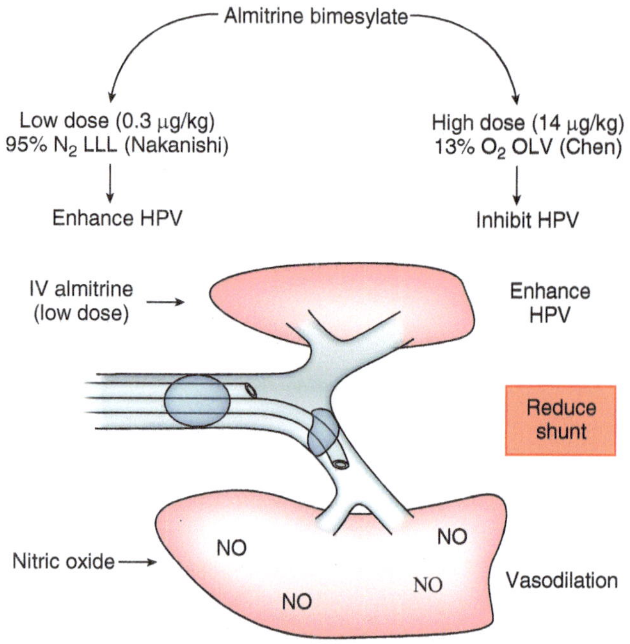

• **Fig. 7.3** The administration of different doses of almitrine and its effects on the lung. *HPV,* Hypoxic pulmonary vasoconstriction; *NO,* nitric oxide; *OLV,* one-lung ventilation; *LLL,* left lower lobe. (From Payen D, Muret J, Beloucif S, et al. Inhaled nitric oxide, almitrine infusion, or their coadministration as a treatment of severe hypoxemic focal lung lesions. *Anesthesiology* 1998;89(5):1157–1165.)

The drug was introduced in Europe in the 1980s, but its use in clinical practice has been limited by significant side effects, such as peripheral neuropathy and dyspnea. The severity of almitrine side effects seems to be dose-dependent, and several studies have demonstrated that the treatment may retain its ability to improve oxygenation even at lower dosages, which decrease the incidence of side effects. A long-term evaluation of the therapeutic efficacy and safety of oral almitrine bismesylate (50 mg twice daily) was made on 25 patients with COPD and moderate hypoxemia residing at an altitude of 1500 m in a double-blind placebo-controlled study. Thirteen patients receiving almitrine (baseline PaO_2, 54.3 ± 4.9 mm Hg) and 12 patients receiving placebo (baseline PaO_2, 53.0 ± 4.1 mm Hg), were periodically followed by arterial blood gas measurements. The authors concluded that almitrine causes a long-term improvement in arterial oxygenation in hypoxemic patients with COPD residing at an altitude of 1500 m and suggested that lower doses of almitrine might produce the same effect on PaO_2 with less adverse associated effects.[47] In contrast, almitrine failed to improve arterial oxygenation in patients anesthetized with sevoflurane during open-chest OLV.[48]

Despite the promising beneficial effects previously published with lower doses of this drug, almitrine is only little used in clinical practice. Nevertheless, there is an interest regarding the effects of this drug combined with NO to enhance HPV as a means of improving V_A/Q matching to treat acute hypoxemia during thoracic surgery.

Phosphodiesterase-5 Inhibitors

Phosphodiesterase inhibitors increase cardiac contractility and induce vasodilation, while inhibiting platelet aggregation. The phosphodiesterase-3 inhibitors milrinone, enoximone, and inamrinone effects are achieved by suppressing the breakdown of cAMP.

Like iNO, the phosphodiesterase-5 inhibitors sildenafil, tadalafil, and vardenafil act by suppression of the cGMP degradation pathway resulting in vasodilation. In particular, sildenafil is widely used to treat episodes of pulmonary hypertension. Despite an IV or oral application route, phosphodiesterase-5 inhibitors affect predominantly the lungs because of target receptor distribution that causes limited systemic vasodilation. Although their vasodilating effect is more pronounced in the pulmonary pathway than in systemic circulation, caution is strongly advised in hypotensive patients.[49] The administration of sildenafil can treat an unwanted rebound effect during the weaning from iNO therapy, and it can be administered before the discontinuation of the therapy.[50]

Endothelin Receptor Antagonists

The endothelin-receptor antagonists bosentan, ambrisentan, and macitentan are the most clinically used endothelin receptor blockers. They competitively inhibit the binding of endothelin to receptors A and B of the endothelin system, which decreases pulmonary vasoconstriction. In general, they are administered over weeks until a desired plasma level is reached. In addition to reducing the PVR, they exert antiproliferative and antifibrotic effects.

Therefore endothelin receptor antagonists are not suitable for acute perioperative therapy. However, this group of substances can be found regularly as concomitant medication in patients with pulmonary hypertension.

Calcium Channel Blockers

In certain conditions, the calcium channel blockers nifedipine, diltiazem, and amlodipine, are commonly prescribed for systemic hypertension and coronary artery disease (comorbidities of COPD), and have become useful in patients with pulmonary hypertension who are responders to pulmonary vasodilators such as iNO or prostacyclin.[51] The major disadvantage of calcium channel blockers is the nonselective vasodilation, which, intraoperatively, may result in significant systemic hypotension associated with a decreased cardiac output. Consequently, its use during thoracic surgery is limited.

Administration of Different Vasoactive Substances

A variety of endogenous and exogenous substances have been used to modify the tone of the pulmonary resistance vessels, predominantly, the small pulmonary arteries and arterioles in which the route of administration determines the effects of pulmonary vasodilators on HPV. These drugs comprise different vasodilators, such as acetylcholine, bradykinin, or isoproterenol, as well as vasoconstrictors like catecholamines, angiotensin II, histamine, or serotonin.

Although they are consistently powerful systemic vasoactive drugs, they are not as predictable as pulmonary vasodilators.

Drugs to Improve Right Heart Function That May Affect Pulmonary Circulation

During OLV, the acute increase in right heart afterload that can be accompanied by chronic pulmonary hypertension, right heart hypertrophy, or dilatation and cardiac dysfunction,[52] may require pharmacologic support. It should be directed on lowering the PAP, maintenance of sufficient coronary perfusion, and right ventricular ejection performance.

For this objective, adrenoreceptor (α_1-receptor agonist noradrenaline, β_1-receptor agonist dobutamine) and vasopressin receptor agonists, phosphodiesterase-3-inhibitors (enoximone and milrinone), as well as calcium sensitizer (levosimendan) can be helpful. The vasopressors selectively increase the systemic resistance, while marginally influencing the PVR.[53] It should be noted that administration of these drugs requires direct arterial blood pressure monitoring to anticipate abrupt changes in blood pressure.

Phosphodiesterase-3-inhibitors increase the cardiac contractility and decrease the pulmonary vascular tone at the same time. The negative effect from the decrease in the systemic vascular resistance can be compensated by the administration of vasoconstrictor drugs. Milrinone, which is the most used representative of phosphodiesterase-3-inhibitors, is available in an intravenous as well as an inhalation form.[54]

Levosimendan increases calcium sensitivity and results in an increase of cardiac contractility and output, as well as in systemic vasodilation with reduction of the PVR without affecting myocardial oxygen consumption. Although the right ventricular function may be improved, the concomitant systemic hypotension can be of concern.[55]

Conclusion

In addition to the effects of anesthetic drugs on pulmonary circulation, there is a number of clinically used substances that may influence distribution of pulmonary perfusion, PVR, and V_A/Q matching, several of which have been demonstrated to modify directly the HPV response. However, comprehensive pharmacodynamic data are missing for many of these drugs regarding their effects in thoracic anesthesia. As a consequence, it is quite difficult to extrapolate from their ordinary effects to the intraoperative setting. Especially in thoracic surgery, the potential effects of different vasoactive drugs on HPV can be deleterious. For example, angiotensin II receptor blockers and angiotensin converting enzyme inhibitors may attenuate HPV response in acute hypoxia.

Inhaled pulmonary vasodilators are selective and are distributed to well-ventilated lung regions with subsequently enhanced pulmonary blood flow. The intention is to enhance the HPV response in the poorly ventilated regions. Inhaled NO, inhaled PGI2, and sildenafil control the pulmonary hypertension and improve the right ventricular afterload by modulating the HPV response.[56,57] iNO can inhibit the HPV response in patients with COPD, but during OLV, it vasodilates ventilated lung regions to shift the pulmonary blood flow toward these zones without modifying HPV response. However, a downregulation of the HPV mechanisms occurs in diseases accompanied with chronic hypoxia; therefore interventions, such as the administration of iNO, would have a limited beneficial effect.

Almitrine and iNO are not used routinely but their combined administration can dramatically improve oxygenation during OLV,[58,59] and thus might be considered as alternative treatments when other strategies fail to improve hypoxemia.

There are some pitfalls in the attempts to modify HPV by improving the inotropic state of the heart, especially of the right ventricle,[52] with phosphodiesterase inhibitors like milrinone that will concurrently vasodilate the pulmonary vasculature.[60] Different potent vasodilators (e.g., sodium nitroprusside, nitroglycerin, and hydralazine) can worsen PaO_2 rapidly by inhibiting the protective HPV response. However, improvement in cardiac output may enhance systemic oxygen delivery and mixed venous PO_2 so that the overall effect on V_A/Q matching could be beneficial.

The disturbance of gas exchange in the patient undergoing thoracic surgery is of complex etiology, highly variable, and may change throughout the course of surgery. Certain aspects of the effect of pulmonary mechanics and control of pulmonary blood flow distribution have been already established, but the interaction between mechanical ventilation, especially during OLV, is poorly understood. The impact of both, acute and chronic pharmacologic interventions, have yet to be satisfactorily defined. Until more details are known, it will be rather difficult to define their exact role in thoracic anesthesia.

Acknowledgments

The work was supported by institutional sources of the Otto-von-Guericke University Magdeburg, Magdeburg, Germany. The authors declare no conflict of interest.

References

1. Cohen E. Recommendations for airway control and difficult airway management in thoracic anesthesia and lung separation procedures. Are we ready for the challenge. *Minerva Anestesiol.* 2009;75(1–2):3–5.
2. Hedenstierna G, Tokics L, Strandberg A, et al. Correlation of gas exchange impairment to development of atelectasis during anaesthesia and muscle paralysis. *Acta Anaesthesiol Scand.* 1986;30(2):183–191.
3. Campos JH, Feider A. Hypoxia during one-lung ventilation-a review and update. *J Cardiothorac Vasc Anesth.* 2018;32(5):2330–2338.
4. Karzai W, Schwarzkopf K. Hypoxemia during one-lung ventilation: prediction, prevention, and treatment. *Anesthesiology.* 2009;110(6):1402–1411.
5. Ishikawa S, Lohser J. One-lung ventilation and arterial oxygenation. *Curr Opin Anaesthesiol.* 2011;24(1):24–31.
6. Lyons C, Callaghan M. Uses and mechanisms of apnoeic oxygenation: a narrative review. *Anaesthesia.* 2019;74(4):497–507.
7. Unzueta C, Tusman G, Suarez-Sipmann F, et al. Alveolar recruitment improves ventilation during thoracic surgery: a randomized controlled trial. *Br J Anaesth.* 2012;108(3):517–524.
8. Tusman G, Bohm SH, Warner DO, et al. Atelectasis and perioperative pulmonary complications in high-risk patients. *Curr Opin Anaesthesiol.* 2012;25(1):1–10.
9. Kozian A, Schilling T, Schutze H, et al. Ventilatory protective strategies during thoracic surgery: effects of alveolar recruitment maneuver and low-tidal volume ventilation on lung density distribution. *Anesthesiology.* 2011;114(5):1025–1035.
10. Kozian A, Schilling T, Rocken C, et al. Increased alveolar damage after mechanical ventilation in a porcine model of thoracic surgery. *J Cardiothorac Vasc Anesth.* 2010;24(4):617–623.
11. Fernandez FG, Kosinski AS, Furnary AP, et al. Differential effects of operative complications on survival after surgery for primary lung cancer. *J Thorac Cardiovasc Surg.* 2018;155(3):1254–1264 e1.
12. Francis LWS, McKinnon J, Whitener G. Pulmonary hypertension and thoracic surgery: impact and treatment options. *Curr Anesthesiol Rep.* 2019;9:436–445.
13. Lumb AB, Slinger P. Hypoxic pulmonary vasoconstriction: physiology and anesthetic implications. *Anesthesiology.* 2015;122(4):932–946.
14. Schwarzkopf K, Schreiber T, Preussler NP, et al. Lung perfusion, shunt fraction, and oxygenation during one-lung ventilation in pigs: the effects of desflurane, isoflurane, and propofol. *J Cardiothorac Vasc Anesth.* 2003;17(1):73–75.
15. Pruszkowski O, Dalibon N, Moutafis M, et al. Effects of propofol vs sevoflurane on arterial oxygenation during one-lung ventilation. *Br J Anaesth.* 2007;98(4):539–544.
16. Xia R, Yin H, Xia ZY, et al. Effect of intravenous infusion of dexmedetomidine combined with inhalation of isoflurane on arterial oxygenation and intrapulmonary shunt during single-lung ventilation. *Cell Biochem Biophys.* 2013;67(3):1547–1550.
17. Rajaram SS, Desai NK, Kalra A, et al. Pulmonary artery catheters for adult patients in intensive care. *Cochrane Database Syst Rev.* 2013;2013(2):CD003408.
18. Schwann NM, Hillel Z, Hoeft A, et al. Lack of effectiveness of the pulmonary artery catheter in cardiac surgery. *Anesth Analg.* 2011;113(5):994–1002.

19. Ashes C, Roscoe A. Transesophageal echocardiography in thoracic anesthesia: pulmonary hypertension and right ventricular function. *Curr Opin Anaesthesiol.* 2015;28(1):38–44.
20. Strumpher J, Jacobsohn E. Pulmonary hypertension and right ventricular dysfunction: physiology and perioperative management. *J Cardiothorac Vasc Anesth.* 2011;25(4):687–704.
21. Hedenstierna G, Reber A. Manipulating pulmonary blood flow during one-lung anesthesia. *Acta Anaesthesiol Scand.* 1996;40(1):2–4.
22. Hill NS, Preston IR, Roberts KE. Inhaled therapies for pulmonary hypertension. *Respir Care.* 2015;60(6):794–802; discussion 02-5.
23. Mubarak KK. A review of prostaglandin analogs in the management of patients with pulmonary arterial hypertension. *Respir Med.* 2010;104(1):9–21.
24. Mitchell JA, Ahmetaj-Shala B, Kirkby NS, et al. Role of prostacyclin in pulmonary hypertension. *Glob Cardiol Sci Pract.* 2014;2014(4):382–393.
25. Safdar Z. Treatment of pulmonary arterial hypertension: the role of prostacyclin and prostaglandin analogs. *Respir Med.* 2011;105(6):818–827.
26. Raghunathan K, Connelly NR, Robbins LD, et al. Inhaled epoprostenol during one-lung ventilation. *Ann Thorac Surg.* 2010;89(3):981–983.
27. Choi H, Jeon J, Huh J, et al. The effects of iloprost on oxygenation during one-lung ventilation for lung surgery: a randomized controlled trial. *J Clin Med.* 2019;8(7):982.
28. Antoniou T, Koletsis EN, Prokakis C, et al. Hemodynamic effects of combination therapy with inhaled nitric oxide and iloprost in patients with pulmonary hypertension and right ventricular dysfunction after high-risk cardiac surgery. *J Cardiothorac Vasc Anesth.* 2013;27(3):459–466.
29. Rocca GD, Passariello M, Coccia C, et al. Inhaled nitric oxide administration during one-lung ventilation in patients undergoing thoracic surgery. *J Cardiothorac Vasc Anesth.* 2001;15(2):218–223.
30. Schwarzkopf K, Klein U, Schreiber T, et al. Oxygenation during one-lung ventilation: the effects of inhaled nitric oxide and increasing levels of inspired fraction of oxygen. *Anesth Analg.* 2001;92(4):842–847.
31. Sawheny E, Ellis AL, Kinasewitz GT. Iloprost improves gas exchange in patients with pulmonary hypertension and ARDS. *Chest.* 2013;144(1):55–62.
32. Gallart L, Rouby JJ, Puig MM. [Pharmacologic treatment of hypoxemia in adult respiratory distress syndrome]. *Rev Esp Anestesiol Reanim.* 1997;44(7):273–283.
33. Karzai W, Schwarzkopf K, Bloos F, et al. Inhaled nitric oxide does not improve oxygenation nor reduce rate of desaturation during one-lung ventilation. *Anesthesiology.* 2000;93(3A):A1326.
34. Moutafis M, Liu N, Dalibon N, et al. the effects of inhaled nitric oxide and its combination with intravenous almitrine on PaO_2 during one-lung ventilation in patients undergoing thoracoscopic procedures. *Anesth Analg.* 1997;85(5):1130–1135.
35. Griffiths MJ, Evans TW. Inhaled nitric oxide therapy in adults. *N Engl J Med.* 2005;353(25):2683–2695.
36. Bigatello LM, Stelfox HT, Hess D. Inhaled nitric oxide therapy in adults–opinions and evidence. *Intensive Care Med.* 2005;31(8):1014–1016.
37. Bhatraju P, Crawford J, Hall M. et al. Inhaled nitric oxide: current clinical concepts. *Nitric Oxide.* 2015;50:114–128.
38. Germann P, Braschi A, Della Rocca G, et al. Inhaled nitric oxide therapy in adults: European expert recommendations. *Intensive Care Med.* 2005;31(8):1029–1041.
39. Michelet P, Roch A, Brousse D, et al. Effects of PEEP on oxygenation and respiratory mechanics during one-lung ventilation. *Br J Anaesth.* 2005;95(2):267–273.
40. Gorecka D, Sliwinski P, Palasiewicz G, et al. Effects of almitrine bismesylate on arterial blood gases in patients with chronic obstructive pulmonary disease and moderate hypoxaemia: a multicentre, randomised, double-blind, placebo-controlled study. *Respiration.* 2003;70(3):275–283.
41. Moutafis M, Dalibon N, Liu N, et al. The effects of intravenous almitrine on PaO_2 during one-lung ventilation (OLV). *Anesthesiology.* 2000;93(3A):A1330.
42. Dalibon N, Liu N, Moutafis M, et al. Treatment of hypoxaemia during one-lung ventilation with almitrine. *Lancet.* 2002;359(9314):1347–1348.
43. Moutafis M, Dalibon N, Liu N, et al. The effects of intravenous almitrine on oxygenation and hemodynamics during one-lung ventilation. *Anesth Analg.* 2002;94(4):830–834.
44. Richard JC, Janier M, Lavenne F, et al. Effect of position, nitric oxide, and almitrine on lung perfusion in a porcine model of acute lung injury. *J Appl Physiol (1985).* 2002;93(6):2181–2191.
45. Silva-Costa-Gomes T, Gallart L, Valles J, et al. Low- vs high-dose almitrine combined with nitric oxide to prevent hypoxia during open-chest one-lung ventilation. *Br J Anaesth.* 2005;95(3):410–416.
46. Gallart L, Lu Q, Puybasset L, et al. Intravenous almitrine combined with inhaled nitric oxide for acute respiratory distress syndrome. The No Almitrine Study Group. *Am J Respir Crit Care Med.* 1998;158(6):1770–1777.
47. Watanabe S, Kanner RE, Cutillo AG, et al. Long-term effect of almitrine bismesylate in patients with hypoxemic chronic obstructive pulmonary disease. *Am Rev Respir Dis.* 1989;140(5):1269–1273.
48. Bermejo S, Gallart L, Silva-Costa-Gomes T, et al. Almitrine fails to improve oxygenation during one-lung ventilation with sevoflurane anesthesia. *J Cardiothorac Vasc Anesth.* 2014;28(4):919–924.
49. Buckley MS, Staib RL, Wicks LM, et al. Phosphodiesterase-5 inhibitors in management of pulmonary hypertension: safety, tolerability, and efficacy. *Drug Healthc Patient Saf.* 2010;2:151–161.
50. Lee JE, Hillier SC, Knoderer CA. Use of sildenafil to facilitate weaning from inhaled nitric oxide in children with pulmonary hypertension following surgery for congenital heart disease. *J Intensive Care Med.* 2008;23(5):329–334.
51. Pilkington SA, Taboada D, Martinez G. Pulmonary hypertension and its management in patients undergoing non-cardiac surgery. *Anaesthesia.* 2015;70(1):56–70.
52. Cheng JW, Tonelli AR, Pettersson G, et al. Pharmacologic management of perioperative pulmonary hypertension. *J Cardiovasc Pharmacol.* 2014;63(4):375–384.
53. Jeon Y, Ryu JH, Lim YJ, et al. Comparative hemodynamic effects of vasopressin and norepinephrine after milrinone-induced hypotension in off-pump coronary artery bypass surgical patients. *Eur J Cardiothorac Surg.* 2006;29(6):952–956.
54. Wang H, Gong M, Zhou B, et al. Comparison of inhaled and intravenous milrinone in patients with pulmonary hypertension undergoing mitral valve surgery. *Adv Ther.* 2009;26(4):462–468.
55. Papp Z, Edes I, Fruhwald S, et al. Levosimendan: molecular mechanisms and clinical implications: consensus of experts

on the mechanisms of action of levosimendan. *Int J Cardiol.* 2012;159(2):82–87.

56. Weissmann N, Gerigk B, Kocer O, et al. Hypoxia-induced pulmonary hypertension: different impact of iloprost, sildenafil, and nitric oxide. *Respir Med.* 2007;101(10):2125–2132.
57. Reichenberger F, Kohstall MG, Seeger T, et al. Effect of sildenafil on hypoxia-induced changes in pulmonary circulation and right ventricular function. *Respir Physiol Neurobiol.* 2007;159(2):196–201.
58. Dalibon N, Moutafis M, Liu N, et al. Treatment of hypoxemia during one-lung ventilation using intravenous almitrine. *Anesth Analg.* 2004;98(3):590–594.
59. Moutafis M, Dalibon N, Colchen A, et al. Improving oxygenation during bronchopulmonary lavage using nitric oxide inhalation and almitrine infusion. *Anesth Analg.* 1999;89(2):302–304.
60. Kato R, Sato J, Nishino T. Milrinone decreases both pulmonary arterial and venous resistances in the hypoxic dog. *Br J Anaesth.* 1998;81(6):920–924.

NON-PRINT ITEMS

Abstract

One-lung ventilation is required for thoracic surgery interventions; however, it can impair ventilation/perfusion (V_A/Q) matching, thus putting the patient at increased risk for hypoxemia that might compromise the overall outcome. Both anesthetic and surgical management may influence the pulmonary and systemic reaction. Concerning the anesthetic management, plenty of research has been undertaken to highlight the impact of anesthetic drugs and ventilatory settings, especially the use of pressures and volumes.

Intraoperative hypoxia and its consequences have been widely elucidated, opening the way for V_A/Q matching to reach the focus of interest. Several drugs that affect the vasculature and/or the respiratory system have been analyzed, as they might lead to dilation or constriction within the pulmonary vessels and therefore impact on V_A/Q relation.

One of the key issues in anesthetic management is to impede a rise in pulmonary vascular resistance and a rise in cardiac oxygen demand. Inhalational agents, such as nitric oxide or prostacyclin analogs, act as potent vasodilators that do not compromise systemic vascular resistance, as they act locally in the ventilated areas. Phosphodiesterase inhibitors have promising effects on V_A/Q matching, as well as the chemoreceptor agonist almitrine. Even though calcium channel blockers and endothelin receptor antagonists do not play a role within the intraoperative setting, they will be frequently encountered in patients suffering from pulmonary hypertension.

Pulmonary vasculature and perfusion distribution are also affected by several vasoconstricting agents, such as catecholamines or by different vasodilators and inotropes. All of them impact on V_A/Q relation depending on their site of action and can thus influence management in thoracic anesthesia.

Keywords

one-lung ventilation, hypoxemia, pulmonary circulation, pharmacologic intervention, nitric oxide, prostacyclin, phosphodiesterase inhibitors

8

Preoperative Evaluation: Assessment of Preoperative Risk

ALLEN NINH, DAVID BRONHEIM

Introduction

The main purposes of a comprehensive preoperative evaluation before thoracic surgery are to assess the risk associated with anesthesia and surgery throughout the perioperative period; to identify, modify, and optimize the treatment of comorbidities that may affect perioperative outcome; and to provide the basis for the design of an appropriate, individually tailored, anesthetic plan. Additional advantages include patient education and consent, providing advanced knowledge to clinicians when preparation needs vary from the usual routine, and avoiding delay or cancellation on the day of surgery. All patients undergoing thoracic surgery, regardless of age, type of planned surgery, or extent of underlying disease, should be thoroughly evaluated for comorbid risk factors. These include but are not limited to the severity of their underlying pulmonary disease, the presence of cardiovascular disease, nutritional status, and any or all medical conditions whose modification could potentially improve outcome.

For the anesthesiologist, the preoperative evaluation should include the patient's American Society of Anesthesiologists (ASA) classification, a primary anesthetic plan and potential adjunctive measures, considerations for special monitoring (i.e., arterial catheter, central line, pulmonary artery catheter, intraoperative esophageal echocardiography, neuromonitoring), and likelihood of requiring continued postoperative mechanical ventilation or additional critical care monitoring.[1] The use of the Revised Cardiac Risk Index (RCRI) and a frailty index may further aid in risk stratification. This chapter will serve to highlight the preoperative assessment and independent risk factors of patients planned for thoracic surgery, and the tools used to evaluate surgical risk. The preoperative rehabilitation of these patients will be discussed in a following chapter (see Chapter 9).

Preoperative Medical Assessment

A focused medical history that includes past surgical and anesthetic experiences is the foundation of the preoperative medical assessment. Patients should be evaluated for the history of the present illness resulting in the need for surgery, significant past medical history, with an emphasis on all the past and current medical problems. Specific attention should be paid to exercise tolerance, surgical and anesthetic history, current medications, drug allergies, and social history, including tobacco, alcohol, and drug use. This must be followed by a thorough physical examination, which includes meticulous airway assessment in particular in anticipation of the need to provide lung separation. Relevant preoperative testing (i.e., electrocardiogram, echocardiography, myocardial stress testing, pulmonary function testing [PFT], exercise testing) should be based on the history and physical, and reviewed before surgery. An impression of the patient's overall medical condition can then be summarized and be applied to various patient preoperative risk assessment tools to stratify a patient's overall surgical risk, such as the ASA physical status classification system (Table 8.1), the RCRI, and in patients undergoing thoracic surgery, the ThRCRI.

Age (see Chapter 38)

Geriatric patients are a major growing segment of the surgical population.[2] Age has repeatedly been shown to be an independent predictor of operative risk and postoperative complications, resulting in increased morbidity and mortality.[3–5] In addition, age is one of the more prominent risk factors for the development of atrial fibrillation in the postoperative period. Pulmonary complications following surgery increase after the fifth decade of life.[6] Lung cancer is predominately a disease of the elderly. In the United States, up to two-thirds of new diagnoses are made in patients

TABLE 8.1 American Society of Anesthesiology Physical Classification System

American Society of Anesthesiology Physical Status Classification	Definition
ASA I	Normal healthy patient
ASA II	Patient with mild systemic disease
ASA III	Patient with severe systematic disease
ASA IV	Patient with severe systemic disease that is a constant threat to life
ASA V	Moribund patient who is not expected to survive without the operation
ASA VI	Declared brain-dead patient whose organs are being removed for donor purposes

Addition of "E" to the ASA physical classification denotes emergency surgery where delay in treatment would be a significant threat to life or body part.

(From ASA Physical Status Classification System. | American Society of Anesthesiologists (ASA) at https://www.asahq.org/standards-and-guidelines/asa-physical-status-classification-system. With permission.)

age 65 years and above, with a median age of 71 years.[7] Aging patients with pulmonary malignancies are disproportionately at increased risk because of inherent unmodifiable risk factors. Although there is no upper age limit that precludes a patient from surgery, physiologic age is likely a better predictor of outcome than chronologic age. Elderly patients with adequate cardiopulmonary reserve and without additional significant risk factors may still have an acceptable level of risk for surgery.

Cardiovascular Disease

Cardiac complications are the second most common cause of perioperative morbidity and mortality after pulmonary morbidity in patients undergoing thoracic surgery.[8] The reported incidence of an adverse cardiac event following major pulmonary surgery is approximately 10% to 15%.[9] Because smoking both increases the incidences of cardiac disease by over 60% and causes lung cancer, this is not surprising.[10] Because intrathoracic surgery itself is associated with increased risk of cardiac complications, an electrocardiogram before surgery is appropriate even in otherwise asymptomatic individuals, and is recommended in all patients above the age of 65 years. Anginal symptoms, suspected valvular disease, arrhythmias, shortness of breath, or a history of cardiac disease warrant an appropriate evaluation and noninvasive cardiac testing.

The RCRI predicts major cardiac complications, such as cardiac arrest, complete heart block, acute myocardial infarction, pulmonary edema, and cardiac-related death following noncardiac surgery. It is useful in assessing patients for the following preoperative risk factors: ischemic heart disease, congestive heart failure, cerebrovascular disease, insulin dependence, and renal dysfunction, as well as the nature of the surgery (Tables 8.2 and 8.3).[11,12] It remains widely used to assess patients for thoracic surgery. Originally validated in a cohort with a limited number of thoracic surgery patients, the RCRI was subsequently demonstrated as able to stratify risk in this population. However, the ThRCRI, a modified and validated version of this tool, which uses only a four-point system that includes the presence of cerebrovascular disease, coronary ischemia, renal disease, and a pneumonectomy as the planned procedure, more effectively stratifies the cardiac risks of thoracic surgery (Tables 8.4 and 8.5).[13,14] Patients planned for lung resection with a ThRCRI score of 2 to 2.5 (class C risk) or more than 2.5 (class D risk) are at significantly higher risk with cardiac complications rates up to 23%.[13,15] Besides its use in stratifying risk, more recently, the ThRCRI has been used to select which thoracic surgery patients warrant formal cardiac evaluation preoperatively.

TABLE 8.2 Revised Cardiac Risk Index

Risk Factors	Points
High-risk surgery (intrathoracic, intraperitoneal, suprainguinal vascular)	1
History of ischemic heart disease	1
History of congestive heart failure	1
History of cerebrovascular disease	1
Insulin-dependent diabetes mellitus	1
Renal dysfunction (creatinine > 2 mg/dL)	1

(From Lee TH, Marcantonio ER, Mangione CM, Thomas EJ, Polanczyk CA, Cook EF, et al. Derivation and prospective validation of a simple index for prediction of cardiac risk of major noncardiac surgery. *Circulation*. 1999;100:1043–1049. With permission.)

TABLE 8.3 Revised Cardiac Risk Index Scoring System and Interpretation

RCRI Score	Risk of Major Adverse Cardiac Event
0	3.9%
1	6.0%
2	10.1%
≥3	15%

(From Duceppe E, Parlow J, MacDonald P, Lyons K, McMullen M, Srinathan S, et al. Canadian Cardiovascular Society Guidelines on perioperative cardiac risk assessment and management for patients who undergo noncardiac surgery. *Can J Cardiol*. 2017;33:17–32. With permission.)

TABLE 8.4 Thoracic-Revised Cardiac Risk Index

Risk Factors	Points
Pneumonectomy	1.5
History of ischemic heart disease	1.5
History of cerebrovascular disease	1.5
Renal dysfunction (creatinine > 2 mg/dL)	1

(From Brunelli A, Varela G, Salati M, et al. Recalibration of the Revised Cardiac Risk Index in lung resection candidates. *Ann Thorac Surg.* 2010;90:199–203. With permission.)

Assessment for Risk of Atrial Fibrillation (see Chapter 22)

Postoperative atrial fibrillation (POAF) is a very frequent complication following thoracic surgery, occurring most commonly 2 to 4 days postoperatively.[7,8,16] In the 2014 American Association for Thoracic Surgery Guidelines for the Prevention and Management of Perioperative Atrial Fibrillation and Flutter for Thoracic Surgical Procedures, the take home message was that "POAF is triggered by: age, ischemia, atrial dilation, volume overload, and history of heart failure. Standard rate and rhythm control approaches were listed to treat POAF. Hemodynamically unstable patients may require electrical cardioversion. Prevention of POAF included drugs, such as amiodarone, diltiazem, statins (for antiinflammatory actions), and magnesium supplementation. Digoxin prophylaxis is not helpful."[17] More recently, an improved brain natriuretic peptide-based prediction model, which incorporates the extent of surgery, a baseline elevation of brain natriuretic peptide, age, body mass index (BMI), and a history of atrial fibrillation to predict POAF has become available.[18] Either the brain natriuretic peptide or something similar may soon become a standard part of preoperative assessment for thoracic surgery to more clearly guide decisions on active prevention of POAF with medications, such as amiodarone, diltiazem, and beta blockers.

TABLE 8.5 Thoracic-Revised Cardiac Risk Index Risk Classes

Thoracic-Revised Cardiac Risk Index Score	Risk Class	Risk of Major Adverse Cardiac Event
0	A	1.5%
1–1.5	B	5.8%
2–2.5	C	19%
≥2.5	D	23%

(From Brunelli A, Varela G, Salati M, et al. Recalibration of the Revised Cardiac Risk Index in lung resection candidates. *Ann Thorac Surg.* 2010;90:199–203. With permission.)

Asthma

Severe asthma is predictive of an increase in postoperative pulmonary complications during the perioperative period, although no recent study specifically assesses its relative risk in thoracic surgery.[19] Thus a history that documents the frequency of exacerbation and bronchodilator administration, the need for inhaled or oral steroids, the number and frequency of emergency room visits, hospitalizations, and the need for intensive care and endotracheal intubation during exacerbations will help categorize the severity of the asthmatic's disease process and the likelihood of perioperative exacerbation and probability of postoperative pulmonary complications. Active wheezing at the time of preoperative evaluation in a patient whose symptoms are typically reversible, is a relative indication for deferring surgery because even an excellent acute response to bronchodilator therapy does not also reverse the inflammatory changes in the bronchial tree, which may persist for weeks. The risk of exacerbation of asthma during the perioperative period can be reduced by continuing an effective regimen of inhaled bronchodilators and steroids leading up to the day of surgery and continued throughout the perioperative period.[20]

Chronic Obstructive Pulmonary Disease

Chronic obstructive pulmonary disease (COPD) is the most common comorbid condition in the thoracic surgical population, and is the third leading cause of death in the United States. It is estimated that 3.8 million adults in the United States are currently diagnosed with COPD, and it is widespread in both the general and smoking population. It is associated with abnormal and permanent enlargement of the airspaces in the lung, with destruction of the alveolar walls resulting in loss of gas exchange surface area, air-trapping, and hyperinflation of the airspaces distal to the terminal bronchioles. This leads to compromised lung mechanics, hypercapnia, dyspnea, and hypoxia that often require oxygen therapy. It is a progressive and debilitating disease, which in its final stages, greatly impacts the patient's quality of life and increases healthcare utilization.

COPD is an overarching term that refers to two major lung disease states: (1) chronic bronchitis, and (2) emphysema, both of which are characterized by mucus hypersecretion and airway inflammation. COPD is most commonly caused by cigarette smoking, and more rarely by airborne pollutants or irritants. Although these two conditions may display similar symptoms, such as dyspnea, cough, increased sputum production, and rhonchorous breath sounds, they are distinctly different from one another. **Chronic bronchitis** results from the repeated inflammation of the airways and narrowing of the bronchial tree resulting in difficulty moving air. **Emphysema** primarily affects the alveolar sacs, where chronic inflammation leads to the alveolar membrane breakdown, impaired gas exchange, and increased air trapping. Unlike asthma, these conditions are not fully reversible by bronchodilators, and lung function does not return to normal between exacerbations because the alveolar destruction is permanent. In addition to patient history and physical examination findings, the severity of COPD can be categorized on the basis of the results of PFT predicted values by using the criteria established in the Global Initiative for Obstructive Lung Disease.[21] COPD is a major patient-related risk factor that is predictive of postoperative pulmonary complications, including postoperative pneumonia, prolonged mechanical ventilation, and respiratory failure requiring reintubation. Severe COPD may also result in right ventricular dysfunction or cor pulmonale, complicating intraoperative management. Nonpulmonary adverse outcomes, such as myocardial infarction or cardiac arrest are also more likely in patients with COPD.[22]

Obstructive Sleep Apnea

Obstructive sleep apnea (OSA) is characterized by episodes of hypopnea (slow shallow breathing) or apnea (cessation of breathing) during sleep as a direct result of collapsing upper airway tissues. This results in intermittent periods of hypoxia and hypercarbia. Factors that increase the likelihood of OSA include obesity (BMI > 35 kg/m^2), large neck circumference (>40 cm), age (>50 years), and male gender. Symptoms include loud snoring, daytime somnolence, episodes of apnea observed by a partner, and hypertension.[23] Patients with three or more of these features are at high risk for OSA as described by the STOP-BANG (**T**ired, **O**bserved, **P**ressure, **B**ody **M**ass Index, **A**ge, **N**eck size, **G**ender) score for OSA. The STOP-BANG questionnaire for OSA consists of eight dichotomous (yes/no) items related to the clinical features of sleep apnea as described earlier and was specifically developed to meet the need for a reliable, concise, and easy-to-use screening tool described in Table 8.6.[24] Patients with abnormal craniofacial features, such as an enlarged uvula, macroglossia, or mandibular micrognathia are also predisposed to pharyngeal airway collapse. The formal diagnosis of OSA is made by nocturnal polysomnography in a sleep laboratory, and patients are often prescribed a positive pressure airway device (bilevel positive airway pressure or continuous positive airway pressure) to be worn at home while asleep. The preoperative assessment visit is the ideal time to establish and record the usual settings on these devices, as their continuation postoperatively is usually indicated.

TABLE 8.6 STOP-BANG Questionnaire for Obstructive Sleep Apnea Screening

Three or More Features = High-Risk for Obstructive Sleep Apnea	
Do you snore loudly?	Yes / No
Do you often feel tired, fatigued, or sleepy during the daytime?	Yes / No
Has anyone observed you stop breathing while asleep?	Yes / No
Do you have (or are being treated for) high blood pressure?	Yes / No
BMI > 35 kg/m^2	Yes / No
Age ≥ 50 years	Yes / No
Neck circumference > 40 cm	Yes / No
Male gender	Yes / No

(From Chung F, Yegneswaran B, Liao P, Chung SA, Vairavanathan S, Islam S, et al. STOP questionnaire: a tool to screen patients for obstructive sleep apnea. *Anesthesiology.* 2008;108:812–821; Chung F, Subramanyam R, Liao P, Sasaki E, Shapiro C, Sun Y. High STOP-BANG score indicates a high probability of obstructive sleep apnoea. *Br J Anaesth*. 2012;108:768–775. With permission.)

Smoking

Smoking is a well-established risk factor for COPD and heart disease and dramatically increases, up to 20-fold the risk of lung and esophageal cancers.[25,26] Smokers have increased postoperative morbidity with a positive correlation between the frequency of postoperative pulmonary complications and the increasing number of pack-years. In a large retrospective study by Matsuoka et al., the relationship between preoperative smoking habits and postoperative pulmonary complications in 1248 thoracic surgical patients who underwent lobectomy was assessed. The incidence of postoperative complications was higher in smokers than in nonsmokers, and the frequency of respiratory-related complications increased along with the number of pack-years. However, there was no relationship between the length of the preoperative smoking cessation period and the frequency of postoperative complications.[27] Therefore while patients who have stopped smoking have a lower risk of postoperative respiratory-related complications when compared with patients that are actively smoking, the optimal duration of cessation is unclear.[28] Some thoracic surgeons require that their patients stop smoking for a minimum 2 weeks before surgery, but a majority of thoracic surgeons do not require smoking cessation at all, should that delay the procedure, as there are concerns about disease progression during the cessation period.[29]

Obesity

Obesity (BMI ≥ 30 kg/m^2), often accompanied by metabolic syndrome, results in physiologic changes that reduce lung volumes and aggravate ventilation/perfusion mismatch, both of which lead to hypoxemia.[30] This is magnified under general anesthesia and even more so in thoracic surgical patients requiring one-lung ventilation.[31] However, obesity does not appear to increase the risk of pulmonary complications following surgery.

Malnutrition

All nonemergent thoracic surgical patients should be assessed for nutritional risk before surgery. Because a vast majority of patients planned for thoracic surgery are patients with esophageal or lung cancer, BMI is a simple surrogate for malnutrition in the setting of cancer-related weight loss or cachexia. Patients who are underweight (BMI < 18.5 kg/m^2) are more likely to have pulmonary complications postoperatively, such as pulmonary leaks.[31,32] Preoperative serum albumin levels have also been established as an independent prognostic factor for patient outcomes following thoracic surgery. Low albumin levels can be seen in malnourished states, but are not diagnostic, as concomitant cirrhotic liver disease, chronic kidney disease, or nephrotic syndromes may result in low serum albumins. Hypoalbuminemia is however associated with decreased survival of patients with lung cancer following surgical resection.[33] In patients undergoing lobectomy for lung cancer, hypoalbuminemia is predictive of prolonged air leaks commonly caused by postoperative alveolar pleural fistulas.[34] Furthermore, patients with low preoperative serum albumin are more likely to develop bronchopleural fistulas and related complications following pneumonectomy.[35] Following surgical insult, adequate nutrition is vital for satisfactory wound healing. Patients who are at high nutritional risk would benefit from having their nutritional status optimized before surgery.

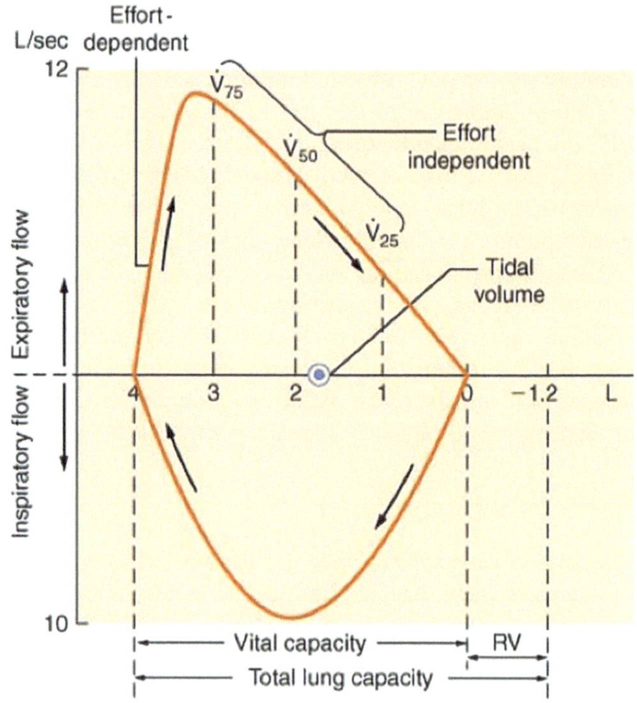

• **Fig. 8.1** Flow–volume loop in a normal subject. $\dot{V}_{75}$, $\dot{V}_{50}$, and $\dot{V}_{25}$ represent flow at 75%, 50%, and 25% of vital capacity, respectively. *RV*, Residual volume. (From Goudsouzian N, Karamanian A. *Physiology for the Anesthesiologist*. 2nd ed. Norwalk, CT: Appleton-Century-Crofts; 1984. With permission.)

Preoperative Evaluation of Patients Undergoing Lung Resection

Lung resections are commonly performed for the diagnosis and treatment of pulmonary malignancies, and less commonly to treat pulmonary bullae, bronchiectasis, complicated infectious lung disease, and traumatic lung injury. In patients with lung cancer, a detailed anatomic staging plan using computed tomography (CT), magnetic resonance (MR) imaging, bronchoscopy, or mediastinoscopy is crucial for defining the extent of disease. Before proceeding to lung resection surgery, a multidisciplinary assessment involving the medical specialists, surgeon, and anesthesiologist is appropriate, followed by discussion with the patient. The goal of lung resection surgery is to maximize the chance for cure, minimize the chance for recurrence, and maintain adequate residual pulmonary function postoperatively.

Pulmonary Function Testing: Spirometry and Diffusing Capacity

In preparation for surgery, candidates for pulmonary resection must undergo basic PFT. The role of PFT is to determine the risk for respiratory complications and mortality based on the patient's preoperative lung function and the predicted function of the residual lung. Spirometry is the most common and easily performed assessment of pulmonary function that is often done alongside lung volume measurements and submaximal exercise testing. Spirometry measures the volume of expired air over time during a forceful exhalation that is preceded by a maximum inhalation (Fig. 8.1). The total exhaled volume is known as the forced vital capacity (FVC), and volume exhaled in the first second is known as the forced expiratory volume in one second (FEV_1). The ratio FEV_1/FVC is reported as a percentage and is used as a key diagnostic test for common pulmonary diseases, such as asthma, COPD, and interstitial lung disease (Fig. 8.2). In healthy adults, FEV_1/FVC is approximately 70% to 80%, and declines with age. In patients undergoing major pulmonary surgery, FEV_1 has been shown to be

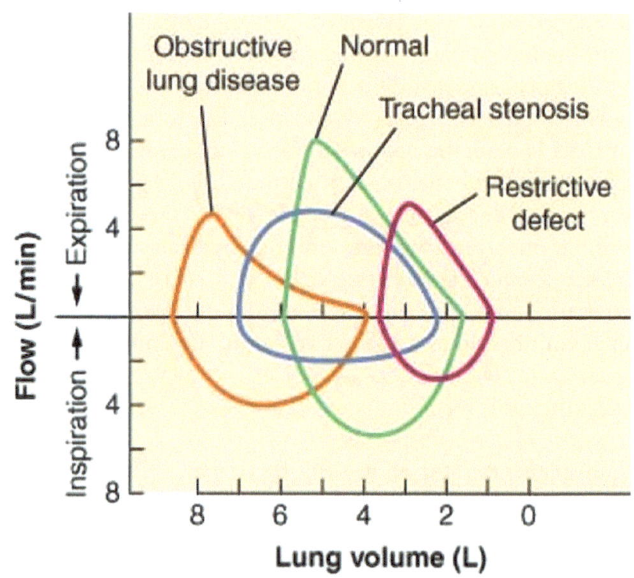

• **Fig. 8.2** Flow–volume loops relative to lung volumes in a normal subject, in a patient with chronic obstructive pulmonary disease (COPD), in a patient with fixed obstruction (i.e., tracheal stenosis), and in a patient with a restrictive defect (i.e., pulmonary fibrosis). Note the concave expiratory form in the patient with COPD and the flat inspiratory curve in the patient with a fixed obstruction. (From Goudsouzian N, Karamanian A. *Physiology for the Anesthesiologist*. 2nd ed. Norwalk, CT: Appleton-Century-Crofts; 1984.)

predictive of postoperative complications including mortality. Patients with an FEV_1 under 60% are more likely to experience postoperative respiratory morbidity.[36] Patients with an FEV_1 under 30% have a 43% morbidity rate, which decreases to approximately 12% when FEV_1 is over 60%.

In addition, the assessment of parenchymal lung function by measuring the diffusing capacity of the lungs for carbon monoxide (DLCO) is also clinically valuable when assessing patients for surgery. This test measures the ability of the lungs to transfer gas from inhaled air to the red blood cells in the pulmonary capillaries. DLCO is commonly used as an index of severity in numerous pulmonary conditions, and can aid in the diagnosis of restrictive lung diseases and pulmonary vascular disease. It is especially important in patients with emphysema, where there is often a significant reduction of gas exchange surface area because of alveolar destruction. During the preoperative evaluation, the DLCO is useful for risk stratification because it is predictive of poor patient outcomes following lung resection and lung volume reduction surgery.[37] In fact, DLCO has proven to be a stronger predictor of postoperative complications than FEV_1.[38,39] PFTs, including spirometry and DLCO, are performed as a part of baseline preoperative testing to maximize the amount of information available for shared decision making.[40]

Predicted Postoperative Lung Function

When applying PFT findings to practical presurgical planning, guidelines by the American College of Chest Physicians, the British Thoracic Society, and the European Respiratory Society/European Society of Thoracic Surgery have suggested the use of both absolute (single-cutoff) and percentage predicted values of FEV_1 and DLCO to assess preoperative risk. The current recommendations for the suitability of lobectomy and pneumonectomy is a preoperative post-bronchodilator FEV_1 cut-off value of more than 1.5 L and more than 2 L, respectively, or a preoperative FEV_1 over 80%.[40] However, percentage predicted values correlate better with outcome when compared with absolute values, as it is more likely to account for individual differences between patients, such as age, sex, and race.[41] Therefore percentage predicted values of pulmonary function are of more utility when used to assess patients planned for major pulmonary resection. Percentage predicted values can be calculated using one of two methods, which will be dependent on the extent of lung resection: (1) anatomic method for lobectomy or (2) perfusion method for pneumonectomy.

In the **anatomic method** for planned lobectomy, the percent predicted value of postoperative FEV_1 (PPO FEV_1) and percent predicted value of postoperative DLCO (PPO DLCO) are determined by the number of functional or unobstructed lung segments to be removed and the total number of functional lung segments. Functional or unobstructed lung segments are determined by preoperative CT scan or bronchoscopy. The lungs classically consist of 19 total segments; 10 segments make up the right lung, and nine segments make up the left lung (Table 8.7). Following spirometry and DLCO testing, percent predicted postoperative values can then be estimated using the following formulas, where y = the number of functional or unobstructed lung segments to be removed and z = the total number of functional lung segments.

TABLE 8.7 Lung Segments

Lung	Number of Lung Segments
Right lung	(10)
Right upper lobe	3
Right middle lobe	2
Right lower lobe	5
Left lung	(9)
Left upper lobe	5
Left lower lobe	4

$$\text{PPO FEV}_1 = \text{preoperative FEV}_1 \times (1 - y/z)$$

$$\text{PPO DLCO} = \text{preoperative DLCO} \times (1 - y/z)$$

In the **perfusion method** for planned pneumonectomy, radionuclide perfusion scintigraphy of the lung is performed to measure the fraction of total perfusion to the potential resected lung. A calculation of the percent predicted postoperative values is possible using the following formulas following spirometry and DLCO testing.

$$\text{PPO FEV}_1 = \text{preoperative FEV}_1 \times (1 - \text{fraction of total perfusion for lung to-be-resected})$$

$$\text{PPO DLCO} = \text{preoperative DLCO} \times (1 - \text{fraction of total perfusion for lung to-be-resected})$$

The PPO FEV_1 and PPO DLCO can then be expressed as a percentage, %PPO FEV_1 and %PPO DLCO by using the ratio of the calculated PPO FEV_1 or calculated PPO DLCO to the predicted normal FEV_1 or DLCO, respectively.

$$\%\text{PPO FEV}_1 = \text{PPO FEV}_1/\text{predicted normal FEV}_1 \times 100\%$$

$$\%\text{PPO DLCO} = \text{PPO DLCO}/\text{predicted normal DLCO} \times 100\%$$

Patients with %PPO FEV_1 or DLCO of 60% or higher in the absence of other cardiopulmonary conditions can undergo pulmonary resection with low risk and can proceed with surgery without further physiologic testing. Patients with %PPO values ranging from 30% to 60% make up an intermediate-risk group that warrants further evaluation by ergometric testing. Patients with %PPO values less than 30% are high risk and are required to undergo further cardiopulmonary exercise testing (CPET) (Fig. 8.3).[40]

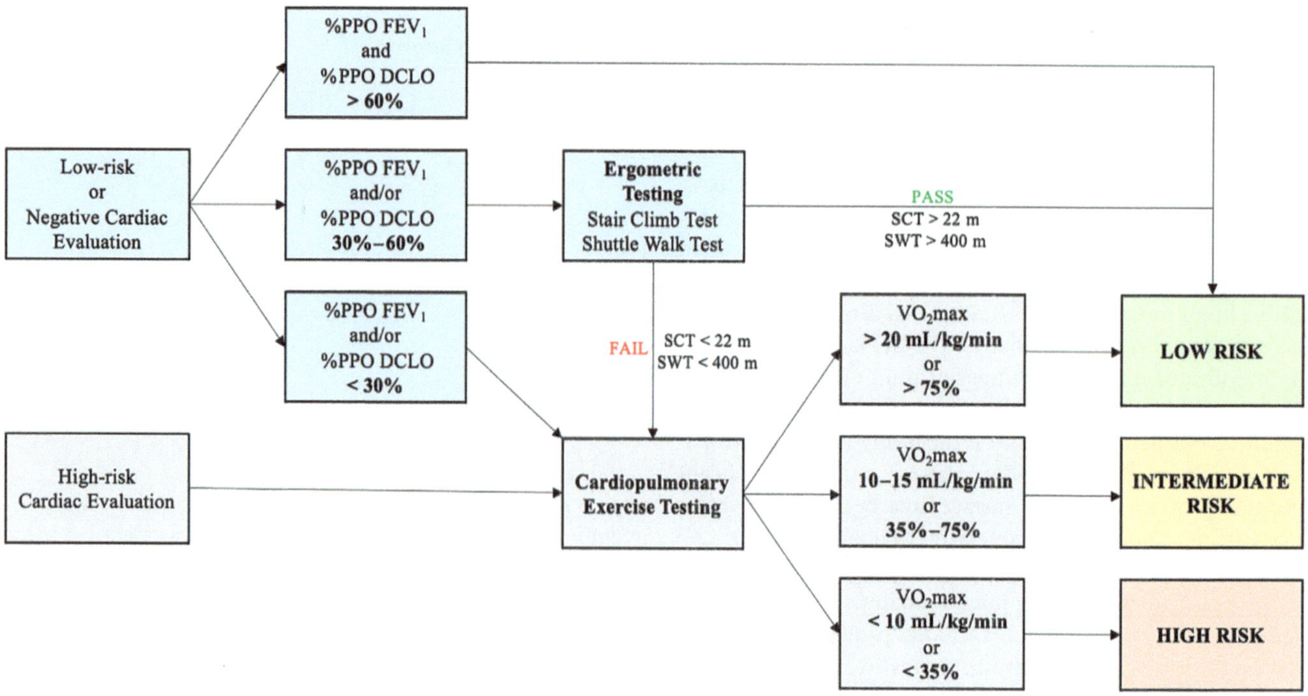

• **Fig. 8.3** Overview of the preoperative physiologic evaluation for lung resection: ACCP Evidence-Based Clinical Practice Guidelines (2013). *DLCO*, diffusing capacity of the lungs for carbon monoxide; *FEV_1*, forced expiratory volume in one second; *PPO*, percent predicted value of postoperative; *SCT*, stair climbing test; *SWT*, shuttle walk test; *VO_2max*, peak oxygen consumption. (From Brunelli A, Kim AW, Berger KI, Addrizzo-Harris DJ. Physiologic evaluation of the patient with lung cancer being considered for resectional surgery: diagnosis and management of lung cancer, 3rd ed: American College of Chest Physicians Evidence-Based Clinical Practice Guidelines. *Chest*. 2013;143. With permission.)

Ergometric Testing

Ergometric testing is composed of the stair climbing test (SCT) and the shuttle walk test (SWT). The SCT is the first-line functional screening test in the intermediate-risk group. Patients who can ascend more than 22 m without cardiopulmonary discomfort are considered fit for lung resection. In patients who are unable to climb at least 12 m, the risk of cardiopulmonary complications increases by 2-fold and mortality increases by 13-fold when compared with patients who can climb greater than 22 m.[42] The SWT is performed by having the patient walk back and forth between two markers, typically set 10 m apart, with increasing speed in a graded fashion. The ability to complete 400 m on the SWT is considered fit for surgery.[40] Failure of either of these functional examinations is an indication for additional CPET.

Cardiopulmonary Exercise Testing

CPET is a safe and reliable examination that objectively evaluates the function of both the heart and lungs under load. The inability to perform a preoperative CPET suggests that the patient has limited aerobic capacity and may not be suitable for thoracic surgery. Although there are numerous CPET indices, the most critical in assessing suitability for lung resection is the peak oxygen consumption (VO_2max), which is defined as the maximum oxygen uptake by the body despite increasing workload. Thus VO_2max reflects the upper limit of the cardiovascular response and overall cardiorespiratory fitness. In patients undergoing lung resection, perioperative complications have been associated with lower VO_2max, and risk stratification is defined by the following:

- **VO_2max greater than 20 mL/kg/min** or more than 75% predicted can safely undergo planned lung resection including pneumonectomy with good prognosis.[40,43]
- **VO_2max between 10 and 15 mL/kg/min** or between 35% and 75% predicted have increased risk of perioperative morbidity and mortality when compared with patients with VO_2max more than 75%.
- **VO_2max less than 10 mL/kg/min** or under 35% predicted are extremely high risk for postoperative morbidity and mortality and is often regarded as a relative contraindication to major anatomic resections. In such cases, a reduction of the originally planned resection may be required or a nonoperative treatment modality may need to be pursued.

Interestingly, it appears that it is possible that the risk of low VO_2max can be mitigated through carefully constructed exercise programs to optimize cardiorespiratory fitness before lung resection.[44]

Split Lung Function Testing

Quantitative Lung Perfusion Scintigraphy (Ventilation-Perfusion Scan)

The use of a ventilation (V) or perfusion (Q) scan to assess and predict postoperative lung function is currently recommended by society guidelines by the American College of Chest Physicians and the British Thoracic Society for patients with borderline pulmonary function tests (i.e., FEV_1 < 60%) planned for pneumonectomy.[45] However, there is no consensus for whether one scan is superior to the other or whether a combination of both scans should be performed to guide surgical decision making.[46,47] A **ventilation scan** is performed by having a patient inhale a nebulized radiolabeled aerosol, which often requires less radioactive material compared with a perfusion scan. A **perfusion scan** is performed by injecting a radiotracer intravenously over several respiratory cycles. The radiation emitted by the radiotracer from uptake by the alveoli (V-scan) or the pulmonary circulation (Q-scan) is then captured by a scintillation (gamma-γ) camera in anterior and posterior views. Sometimes a single-photon emission CT (SPECT-CT) image is also acquired. Regions of interest containing radiotracer are then grossly assessed (Fig. 8.4), and the amount of radiotracer uptake in various regions of the lung can be counted using software, generating a radiotracer uptake percentage.[48,49] The uptake percentage can then be applied to spirometry findings to predict postoperative FEV_1 and DLCO. Although both ventilation and perfusion scans underestimate actual postoperative lung function, predicted lung function by ventilation scan appears to better correlate with actual postoperative lung function when compared with a perfusion scan.[46]

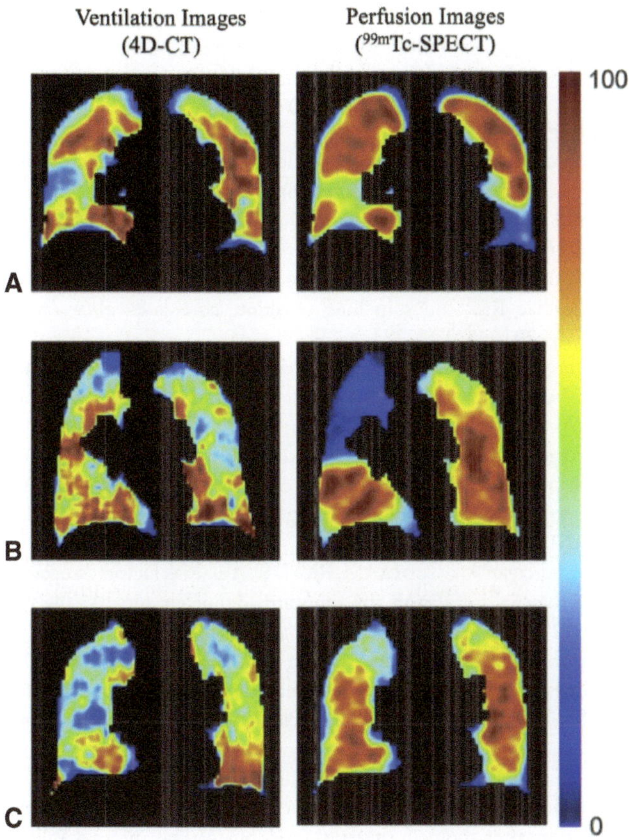

• **Fig. 8.4** **A.** Four-dimensional-computed tomography ventilation and single-photon emission computed tomography perfusion (^{99m}Tc-macroaggregated albumin). Agreement of dose-ventilation and dose-perfusion. **B.** Ventilation metrics greater than dose-perfusion. **C.** Perfusion metrics greater than dose-ventilation metrics. *SPECT-CT*, single-photon emission. (From Nakajima Y, Kadoya N, Kimura T, Hioki K, Jingu K, Yamamoto T. Variations between dose-ventilation and dose-perfusion metrics in radiation therapy planning for lung cancer. *Adv Radiat Oncol*. 2020;5:459-465. With permission.)

Unilateral Pulmonary Artery Occlusion

Unilateral pulmonary artery occlusion (UPAO) is rarely performed today, but it can be used as a preoperative predictor of postoperative cardiopulmonary function, particularly of the right ventricle, following lung resection. UPAO testing involves selectively blocking a lung or lobe artery using a pulmonary artery balloon catheter, which simulates a postoperative respiratory situation where a reduced pulmonary vascular bed is available for gas exchange, and measures the dynamic changes required of the right heart to accommodate the changes in pulmonary artery pressure following potential surgery. This allows for evaluation of the cardiopulmonary reserve of surgical candidates and their likelihood of experiencing potential life-threatening complications postoperatively, such as acute respiratory failure, pulmonary hypertension, and cor pulmonale. However, because it is an invasive test, it is not without risk. Misplacement of the pulmonary artery balloon catheter or inadvertent migration of the balloon catheter during the procedure can lead to procedure-related cardiac events, including arrythmia and cardiac arrest.[50] Pulmonary thrombosis has also been reported as a complication of this procedure.[51]

Prediction of Desaturation During One-lung Ventilation

One-lung ventilation (OLV) is required for a variety of thoracic surgical procedures involving the esophagus, lung, aorta, vena cava, mediastinum, and thoracic spine. When not absolutely required, OLV is often still preferred when it can be done safely, as it optimizes the view of the operating field by providing a still lung and maximizing access to the surgical target of interest. During OLV, only one lung is ventilated, but both lungs are being perfused. This invariably creates a V/Q mismatch through increased transpulmonary shunting, which results in varying degrees of hypoxemia. Furthermore, thoracic procedures often require a patient be placed in a lateral decubitus position. In the lateral decubitus position, the dependent lung is compressed by mediastinal and abdominal structures, leading to varying degrees of hypoventilation. Identification of patients who are at greater risk for desaturation during OLV is of significant importance, as it allows for a more informed discussion and preparation regarding the intraoperative plan-of-care between the anesthesiologist and surgeon. In patients who are at higher risk, prophylactic measures, such as individualized positive end-expiratory pressure, frequent lung recruitment maneuvers, or continuous positive airway pressure to the nonventilated lung can be used to reduce the risk of desaturation at the expense of reducing surgical field exposure.

The most important predictor of desaturation during OLV is the partial pressure of oxygen in arterial blood (PaO_2) during spontaneous two-lung ventilation. The PaO_2 during spontaneous two-lung ventilation is directly correlated with PaO_2 levels during OLV.[52] Therefore in patients with blood gas samples showing poor PaO_2 intraoperatively during two-lung ventilation, there is a higher likelihood for the patient to experience hypoxemia during OLV intraoperatively. The side of operation is also of significant importance when attempting to predict desaturation during OLV. Given that the right lung is larger than the left lung, oxygenation during OLV is better during left-sided thoracotomy, where the left lung is deflated and the right lung is the ventilated lung.[52,53] Patient positioning and the distribution of perfusion plays a role in oxygenation because of gravity-dependent perfusion of the ventilated lung. Patients in a lateral decubitus position oxygenate better than patients in supine during OLV because of improved ventilation-perfusion matching.[54] Patients who have had previous resection of the lung contralateral to the site of surgery are at higher risk for hypoxemia during OLV because less dependent lung tissue is available for gas exchange.[55] Obese patients are also more likely to experience hypoxemia intraoperatively during OLV because of the decreased functional residual capacity of the lungs.[31] Excessive adipose tissue in the abdomen and around the ribcage places an external load on the chest cavity that disrupts normal chest wall and respiratory mechanics.

Conclusion

The ideal preoperative assessment should be goal directed and evidence based. The preoperative evaluation should be individually tailored for each patient. Identifying high-risk patients allows for targeted optimization of comorbid conditions and assists with perioperative decision making by both the anesthesiologist and the surgeon. The anesthesiologist and surgeon must ensure thorough evaluation of each surgical patient to maximize patient safety, while minimizing patient morbidity and mortality.

References

1. ASA Physical Status Classification System. American Society of Anesthesiologists (ASA) at https://www.asahq.org/standards-and-guidelines/asa-physical-status-classification-system.
2. Fowler AJ, Abbott TEF, Prowle J, Pearse RM. Age of patients undergoing surgery. *BJS*. 2019;106:1012–1018.
3. Fernandez-Bustamante A, Frendl G, et al. Postoperative pulmonary complications, early mortality, and hospital stay following noncardiothoracic surgery: a multicenter study by the perioperative research network investigators. *JAMA Surg*. 2017;152:157–166.
4. Gupta S, Fernandes RJ, Rao JS, Dhanpal R. Perioperative risk factors for pulmonary complications after non-cardiac surgery. *J Anaesthesiol Clin Pharmacol*. 2020;36:88–93.
5. McAlister FA, Bertsch K, Man J, Bradley J, Jacka M. Incidence of and risk factors for pulmonary complications after nonthoracic surgery. *Am J Respir Crit Care Med*. 2005;171:514–517.
6. Smetana GW, Lawrence VA, Cornell JE. Preoperative pulmonary risk stratification for noncardiothoracic surgery: systematic review for the American College of Physicians. *Ann Intern Med*. 2006;144:581–595.
7. Frendl G, Sodickson AC, Chung MK, et al. 2014 AATS guidelines for the prevention and management of perioperative atrial fibrillation and flutter for thoracic surgical procedures. *J Thorac Cardiovasc Surg*. 2014;148:e153.
8. Ivanovic J, Seely AJE, Anstee C, et al. Measuring surgical quality: comparison of postoperative adverse events with the American College of Surgeons NSQIP and the thoracic morbidity and mortality classification system. *J Am Coll Surg*. 2014;218:1024–1031.
9. Kozower BD, Sheng S, O'Brien SM, et al. STS database risk models: predictors of mortality and major morbidity for lung cancer resection. *Ann Thorac Surg*. 2010;90:875–883.
10. Banks E, Joshy G, Korda RJ, et al. Tobacco smoking and risk of 36 cardiovascular disease subtypes: fatal and non-fatal outcomes in a large prospective Australian study. *BMC Med*. 2019;17:128.
11. Lee TH, Marcantonio ER, Mangione CM, et al. Derivation and prospective validation of a simple index for prediction of cardiac risk of major noncardiac surgery. *Circulation*. 1999;100:1043–1049.
12. Duceppe E, Parlow J, MacDonald P, et al. Canadian Cardiovascular Society Guidelines on perioperative cardiac risk assessment and management for patients who undergo noncardiac surgery. *Can J Cardiol*. 2017;33:17–32.
13. Brunelli A, Varela G, Salati M, et al. Recalibration of the Revised Cardiac Risk Index in lung resection candidates. *Ann Thorac Surg*. 2010;90:199–203.
14. Thomas DC, Blasberg JD, Arnold BN, et al. Validating the Thoracic Revised Cardiac Risk Index following lung resection. *Ann Thorac Surg*. 2017;104:389–394.
15. Ferguson MK, Saha-Chaudhuri P, Mitchell JD, Varela G, Brunelli A. Prediction of major cardiovascular events after lung resection using a modified scoring system. *Ann Thorac Surg*. 2014;97:1135–1140.
16. Vaporciyan AA, Correa AM, Rice DC, et al. Risk factors associated with atrial fibrillation after noncardiac thoracic surgery: analysis of 2588 patients. *J Thorac Cardiovasc Surg*. 2004;127:779–786.
17. Frendl G, Sodickson AC, Chung MK, et al. 2014 AATS guidelines for the prevention and management of perioperative atrial fibrillation and flutter for thoracic surgical procedures. *J Thorac Cardiovasc Surg*. 2014:148.
18. Amar D, Zhang H, Tan KS, Piening D, Rusch VW, Jones DR. A brain natriuretic peptide-based prediction model for atrial fibrillation after thoracic surgery: development and internal validation. *J Thorac Cardiovasc Surg*. 2019;157:2493–2499.e1.
19. Numata T, Nakayama K, Fujii S, et al. Risk factors of postoperative pulmonary complications in patients with asthma and COPD. *BMC Pulm Med*. 2018;18.
20. Mercado DL, Petty BG. Perioperative medication management. *Med Clin North Am*. 2003;87:41–57.
21. Vogelmeier CF, Criner GJ, Martinez FJ, et al. Global strategy for the diagnosis, management, and prevention of chronic

obstructive lung disease 2017 report. *Am J Respir Crit Care Med.* 2017;195:557–582.

22. Gupta H, Ramanan B, Gupta PK, et al. Impact of COPD on postoperative outcomes: results from a national database. *Chest.* 2013;143:1599–1606.
23. Chung F, Yegneswaran B, Liao P, et al. STOP questionnaire: a tool to screen patients for obstructive sleep apnea. *Anesthesiology.* 2008;108:812–821.
24. Chung F, Subramanyam R, Liao P, Sasaki E, Shapiro C, Sun Y. High STOP-BANG score indicates a high probability of obstructive sleep apnoea. *Br J Anaesth.* 2012;108:768–775.
25. Warren GW, Cummings KM. Tobacco and lung cancer: risks, trends, and outcomes in patients with cancer. *Am Soc Clin Oncol Educ B.* 2013:359–364.
26. Castro C, Peleteiro B, Lunet N. Modifiable factors and esophageal cancer: a systematic review of published meta-analyses. *J Gastroenterol.* 2018;53:37–51.
27. Matsuoka K, Yamada T, Matsuoka T, Nagai S, Ueda M, Miyamoto Y. Preoperative smoking cessation period is not related to postoperative respiratory complications in patients undergoing lung cancer surgery. *Ann Thorac Cardiovasc Surg.* 2019;25:304–310.
28. Lugg ST, Tikka T, Agostini PJ, et al. Smoking and timing of cessation on postoperative pulmonary complications after curative-intent lung cancer surgery. *J Cardiothorac Surg.* 2017:12.
29. Marrufo AS, Kozower BD, Tancredi DJ, et al. Thoracic surgeons' beliefs and practices on smoking cessation before lung resection. *Ann Thorac Surg.* 2019;107:1494–1499.
30. Littleton SW, Tulaimat A. The effects of obesity on lung volumes and oxygenation. *Respir Med.* 2017;124:15–20.
31. Suemitsu R, Sakoguchi T, Morikawa K, Yamaguchi M, Tanaka H, Takeo S. Effect of body mass index on perioperative complications in thoracic surgery. *Asian Cardiovasc Thorac Ann.* 2008; 16:463–467.
32. Sood A, Abdollah F, Sammon JD, et al. The effect of body mass index on perioperative outcomes after major surgery: results from the National Surgical Quality Improvement Program (ACS-NSQIP) 2005–2011. *World J Surg.* 2015;39:2376–2385.
33. Miura K, Hamanaka K, Koizumi T, et al. Clinical significance of preoperative serum albumin level for prognosis in surgically resected patients with non-small cell lung cancer: comparative study of normal lung, emphysema, and pulmonary fibrosis. *Lung Cancer.* 2017;111:88–95.
34. Okada S, Shimada J, Kato D, Tsunezuka H, Inoue M. Prolonged air leak following lobectomy can be predicted in lung cancer patients. *Surg Today.* 2017;47:973–979.
35. Matsuoka K, Misaki N, Sumitomo S. Preoperative hypoalbuminemia is a risk factor for late bronchopleural fistula after pneumonectomy. *Ann Thorac Cardiovasc Surg.* 2010;16:401–405.
36. Licker MJ, Widikker I, Robert J, Frey JG, Spiliopoulos A, Ellenberger C, et al. Operative mortality and respiratory complications after lung resection for cancer: impact of chronic obstructive pulmonary disease and time trends. *Ann Thorac Surg.* 2006;81:1830–1837.
37. Ferguson MK, Little L, Rizzo L, et al. Diffusing capacity predicts morbidity and mortality after pulmonary resection. *J Thorac Cardiovasc Surg.* 1988;96:894–900.
38. Cerfolio RJ, Bryant AS. Different diffusing capacity of the lung for carbon monoxide as predictors of respiratory morbidity. *Ann Thorac Surg.* 2009;88:405–411.
39. Ferguson MK, Vigneswaran WT. Diffusing capacity predicts morbidity after lung resection in patients without obstructive lung disease. *Ann Thorac Surg.* 2008;85:1158–1165.
40. Brunelli A, Kim AW, Berger KI, Addrizzo-Harris DJ. Physiologic evaluation of the patient with lung cancer being considered for resectional surgery: diagnosis and management of lung cancer 3rd edition. American College of Chest Physicians Evidence-Based Clinical Practice Guidelines. *Chest.* 2013:143.
41. Yuan N, Fraire JA, Margetis MM, Skaggs DL, Tolo VT, Keens TG. The effect of scoliosis surgery on lung function in the immediate postoperative period. *Spine (Phila Pa 1976).* 2005;30:2182–2185.
42. Brunelli A, Refai M, Xiumé F, et al. Performance at symptom-limited stair-climbing test is associated with increased cardiopulmonary complications, mortality, and costs after major lung resection. *Ann Thorac Surg.* 2008;86:240–248.
43. Bayram AS, Candan T, Gebitekin C. Preoperative maximal exercise oxygen consumption test predicts postoperative pulmonary morbidity following major lung resection. *Respirology.* 2007;12: 505–510.
44. Jones LW, Peddle CJ, Eves ND, et al. Effects of presurgical exercise training on cardiorespiratory fitness among patients undergoing thoracic surgery for malignant lung lesions. *Cancer.* 2007;110:590–598.
45. Detterbeck FC, Lewis SZ, Diekemper R, Addrizzo-Harris D, Alberts WM. Executive summary: diagnosis and management of lung cancer, 3rd edition. American College of Chest Physicians Evidence-Based Clinical Practice Guidelines. *Chest.* 2013;143:7S–37S.
46. Win T, Tasker AD, Groves AM, White C, Ritchie AJ, Wells FC, Laroche CM. Ventilation-perfusion scintigraphy to predict postoperative pulmonary function in lung cancer patients undergoing pneumonectomy. *Am J Roentgenol.* 2006;187:1260–1265.
47. Subramanyam P, Sundaram SP. Which is better—a standalone ventilation or perfusion scan or combined imaging to predict postoperative FEV1 in one seconds in patients posted for lung surgeries with borderline pulmonary reserve. *Indian J Nucl Med.* 2018;33:105–111.
48. Vinogradskiy Y, Castillo R, Castillo E, et al. Use of 4-dimensional computed tomography-based ventilation imaging to correlate lung dose and function with clinical outcomes. *Int J Radiat Oncol Biol Phys.* 2013;86:366–371.
49. Nakajima Y, Kadoya N, Kimura T, Hioki K, Jingu K, Yamamoto T. Variations between dose-ventilation and dose-perfusion metrics in radiation therapy planning for lung cancer. *Adv Radiat Oncol.* 2020;5:459–465.
50. Shimohira M, Hashizume T, Ohta K, et al. Unilateral pulmonary artery pre-operative occlusion test: technical feasibility and safety prior to pneumonectomy or pleuropneumonectomy for malignancy. *Br J Radiol.* 2018:91.
51. Kobayashi R, Nogimura H, Suzuki K, Harada Y, Horiguchi T, Sugimura H. A case of the pulmonary thrombosis caused by unilateral pulmonary artery occlusion test. *Jpn J Thorac Cardiovasc Surg.* 1998;46:491–495.
52. Slinger P, Suissa S, Triolet W. Predicting arterial oxygenation during one-lung anaesthesia. *Can J Anaesth.* 1992;39:1030–1035.
53. Katz Y, Zisman E, Isserles SA, Rozenberg B. Left, but not right, one-lung ventilation causes hypoxemia during endoscopic transthoracic sympathectomy. *J Cardiothorac Vasc Anesth.* 1996;10: 207–209.
54. Bardoczky GI, Szegedi LL, D'Hollander AA, Moures JM, De Francquen P, Yernault JC. Two-lung and one-lung ventilation in patients with chronic obstructive pulmonary disease: the effects of position and FIO2. *Anesth Analg.* 2000;90:35–41.
55. Ruiz P, Kovarik G. Lung mechanics and gas exchange in one-lung ventilation following contralateral resection. *Can J Anesth.* 2005;52:986–989.

9

Prehabilitation for Thoracic Surgery

MICHAEL CHARLESWORTH, RICHARD TEMPLETON

Introduction

Lung cancer accounts for 30% of all cancer cases, with outcomes for patients improving at a modest pace.[1] That said, 5-year survival for patients with stage IA to IIA cancer managed with a combination of chemotherapy and surgery exceeds 50%.[1] Lung cancer screening programs are increasingly used to identify patients at a stage where lung resection is possible.[2] Lung resection surgery is associated with a high incidence of postoperative pulmonary complications,[3] which are themselves associated with reduced survival, increased morbidity, and a prolonged intensive care and hospital length of stay.[4,5] Enhanced recovery after surgery protocols and postoperative pulmonary rehabilitation are now engrained in perioperative pathways,[6–8] but preoperative rehabilitation, or prehabilitation, is a relatively new concept. The aim of thoracic prehabilitation is to reduce perioperative risk for patients who are suitable for surgery, or in some cases, move a patient who was previously unfit for surgery into a group which is suitable for surgery. For both these cohorts, the chance of survival may be increased.[9] In this chapter, we discuss how that goal can be achieved using risk prediction, shared decision making, and a range of multimodal preoperative interventions that can be integrated into the preoperative pathway.

Risk Prediction

Patients presenting for thoracic surgery often have respiratory and/or cardiovascular comorbidities. The most widely used method for risk stratification are preoperative tests of pulmonary function.[10] Respiratory mechanics are assessed by measuring the forced expiratory volume in one second (FEV_1), which can directly reflect the incidence of postoperative pulmonary complications. The ability of the lungs to undertake gaseous exchange is measured with the diffusing capacity for the lung for carbon monoxide (DLCO), which is associated with postoperative mortality. Finally, cardiopulmonary reserve can be evaluated using functional tests, such as shuttle walking or formal cardiopulmonary exercise testing.

Preoperative tests of pulmonary function help guide the extent of operative management. In patients with a value of more than 80% for FEV_1 and DLCO, resection might be undertaken up to a pneumonectomy. If either one is below 80%, exercise testing is required to measure the peak oxygen consumption (VO_2). If the peak or predicted postoperative VO_2 is less than 35% or less than 10 mL/kg/min, a lobectomy or pneumonectomy are not recommended.[11] For palliative procedures, such as lung volume reduction surgery or airway stenting, the decision to proceed is based on a risk versus benefit judgment on a case by case basis, although guidance on patient selection does exist.[12] The decision to operate and the extent of the surgical resection are nevertheless decided following physiological evaluation of the patient. This is made in conjunction with risk prediction, consent, shared decision making, and prehabilitation.

There are a range of systems currently used to risk stratify patients before thoracic surgery.[13] Such systems have well-described flaws. Instead, a more holistic approach, considering patient factors beyond traditional measures of cardiorespiratory reserve, can provide a better understanding of perioperative risk. These additional measures can help highlight the presence of "red flags" to guide our decisions as to whether patients scheduled for surgery should fall into a high-risk category. These include, but are not limited to: low (and high) body mass index (>40 kg/m^2, BMI)[14]; low degree of functional independence; heavy nicotine dependence; heavy alcohol dependence; severe limitation of ability to walk short distances (unable to complete the 6 minutes walking test) or climb stairs; severe chronic cardiac disease, respiratory comorbidity and obstructive sleep apnea; and anemia; sarcopenia; and frailty. Risk assessment is integral to all prehabilitation programs, but prehabilitation should be for all patients, regardless of risk.

Shared Decision Making Versus Consent

Shared decision making can be defined as a process through which care is tailored to the values and choices of the patient and the expertise of the clinician.[15] Confusion usually arises when the concept of shared decision making is conflated with consent, risk assessment, and decision aids or protocols.[16] Despite general acceptance of its positive role in the perioperative period, the main barrier to its implementation is time. If the patient meets the anesthetist for the first time on the morning of surgery, the preoperative assessment will be more focused with information retrieval and navigating the choice of the safest anesthetic, long after the patient has agreed to surgery. For this reason, perioperative pathways must be reengineered toward contact with patient-anesthetists in the preoperative clinics, long before and after surgery, as shared decision making arguably extends into the postoperative period up to the time of discharge from the hospital. It is, therefore, integral to all prehabilitation programs.

Prehabilitation

The presurgical period is an ideal time for targeted interventions aimed at improving postoperative outcomes for all surgical patients. The aim is to restore physical and psychologic function following surgery. It is for all patients scheduled for surgery, and is not restricted to just those who are at high or low risk. It can be defined as "a process on the cancer continuum of care that occurs between the time of cancer diagnosis and the beginning of acute treatment and includes physical and psychologic assessments that establish a baseline functional level, identify impairments, and provide interventions that promote physical and psychologic health to reduce the incidence and/or severity of future impairments."[17] That said, it presents many challenges. Specifically, for thoracic surgical patients awaiting resection of cancer, there is limited time available between diagnosis and surgery, and other related hospital appointments or treatments might place a burden on the patient, both physically and psychologically. Prehabilitation must be multimodal. It is the sum of marginal gains from several interventions, which are themselves complementary.[18] It requires invested resources, infrastructure, organization, and an acceptance of the longer-term benefits for surgical outcomes, value for money, and public health.[19] Herein, we describe various components which might comprise a multimodal thoracic surgical prehabilitation program.

Exercise

Most published evidence in relation to thoracic prehabilitation focuses on data resulting from implementation of exercise programs.[9] Most programs include aerobic training, resistance training, and respiratory muscle training, which may or may not be supervised.[4] Although high-level evidence from two recent systematic reviews seems to suggest preoperative exercise programs in patients with lung cancer might be beneficial,[4,5] the included evidence was low to moderate. There are also questions about whether this evidence can be applied to lower risk populations and the resources required to implement these programs by organizations. Recently, guidelines on preoperative exercise training in patients awaiting major noncardiac surgery were published by Tew et al.[20] This provides a useful sample program of exercise aimed at reducing the incidence of postoperative complications in thoracic surgical patients. However, the authors concluded that successful implementation of prehabilitation programs may prove challenging. A range of institutionalized cultural and attitudinal barriers exist that could affect preoperative initiatives to varying degrees. Patient-related factors include motivation, time and financial worries, and limiting comorbidities. System-related barriers include lack of educational opportunities highlighting the benefits of exercise, insufficient infrastructure, and concerns about the feasibility of delivery and cost effectiveness of potential programs.

Nutrition

Low BMI is a known risk factor for patients undergoing lung resection surgery.[21] This is a modifiable risk factor, and there exists several scoring systems to detect malnutrition.[22] Every patient interaction is an opportunity to reinforce the importance of optimizing the nutritional state. Regarding perioperative malnutrition, there is no accepted definition, although this must account for under- and overnourished states. Although overnourished patients are at risk of postoperative complications, undernourished patients with lung cancer may be sarcopenic and have limited reserve to cope with the insult of surgery. Avoiding malnutrition and supporting anabolism are basic perioperative goals, and they can be met with screening, referral to dietetics, and nutritional prehabilitation.[23] This can take the form of oral nutritional supplements, vitamins, immunonutrition, protein, and carbohydrate loading.

Fig. 9.1 is reported by the American Society for Enhanced Recovery and Perioperative Quality Initiative Joint Consensus Statement on Nutrition Screening and Therapy Within a Surgical Enhanced Recovery Pathway. After literature

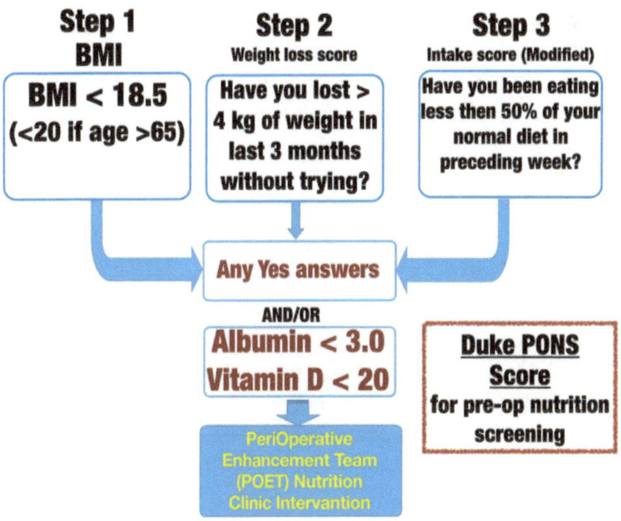

• **Fig. 9.1** Perioperative nutrition screen (*PONS*). The PONS determines the presence of nutrition risk based on a patient's body mass index, recent changes in weight, reported recent decrease in dietary intake, and preoperative albumin level. In addition, the PONS includes evaluation of a preoperative albumin level, as this is a predictor of postoperative complications, including morbidity/mortality. *BMI*, Body mass index. (From Gillis C, Wischmeyer PE. Pre-operative nutrition and the elective surgical patient: why, how and what? *Anaesthesia*. 2019;74:27–35.)

review, they developed and proposed the perioperative nutrition screen (PONS). The PONS is a modified version of the malnutrition universal screening tool (MUST) that has been altered for use perioperatively. The PONS determines the presence of nutrition risk based on a patient's BMI, recent changes in weight, reported recent decrease in dietary intake, and preoperative albumin level. In addition, the PONS includes evaluation of preoperative albumin level because this is a predictor of postoperative complications, including morbidity/mortality.[24]

Surgical nutrition guidelines, such as the European Society for Clinical Nutrition and Metabolism, American Society of Parenteral Enteral Nutrition, and the American Society for Enhanced Recovery with Perioperative Quality Initiative all provide details on selecting nutrition screening tools, malnutrition assessment tools, and treatment for malnourished and at-risk patients. A comprehensive nutrition assessment involves understanding the personal cause(s) of malnutrition and correcting barriers to adequate food intake. Patients identified as malnourished, or at risk, require individualized treatment plans that may include therapeutic diets or fortified foods.

The Duke University PeriOperative Enhancement Team (POET) program is shown in Fig. 9.2. Any patient assessed as being at malnutrition risk (PONS score ≥ 1) is referred for evaluation by a dietitian and receives nutrition care according to this pathway.

A meta-analysis of 15 randomized controlled trials, including 3831 malnourished patients undergoing a variety of surgical procedures, identified that perioperative nutritional support was significantly more effective than the control at decreasing the incidence of infectious and noninfectious complications, and shortening the length of hospital stay by approximately 2 days.[25]

A Cochrane review of 13 randomized control trials, including 548 patients, of preoperative nutritional therapy in gastrointestinal surgery, found that preoperative immune-enhancing nutrition compared with no or standard nutrition significantly reduced total postoperative complications. Collectively, these studies indicate that both nutritional deficiencies and nutritional repletion have an impact on surgical recovery.[23]

Psychology

Hitherto, we have focused on physical elements of a prehabilitation program, and preoperative psychologic prehabilitation is often overlooked.[26] Park et al. found that the incidence of postoperative psychologic distress and depression is high amongst patients with lung cancer, and increases after surgery. They prospectively enrolled 278 patients with a mean age of 62 years. Thoracoscopic resection was performed in 246 patients (89%). The prevalence rates of preoperative anxiety and depression were 8% ($n = 22$) and 12% ($n = 32$), and changed to 9% ($n = 26$) and 19% ($n = 54$) postoperatively ($P = .37$ and $< .001$, respectively). Gender, age, marital status, advanced clinical stage, alcohol abuse, smoking status, length of hospital stay, pulmonary function, and preoperative comorbidities were not associated with postoperative anxiety and depression. They concluded that postoperative psychologic distress and, in particular, depression increased after surgical treatment for lung cancer. Postoperative anxiety and depression were aggravated by residual symptoms after surgery.[27]

Despite the seemingly logical need for psychologic preparation and/or interventions before major surgery, there is currently insufficient evidence on whether this is of benefit.[28] This is currently an area where there is an urgent need for high-quality prospective trials that include baseline psychological evaluation data.

Smoking Cessation and Respiratory Optimization

Smoking status is strongly associated with long-term mortality and the incidence of postoperative pulmonary complications after lung resection.[29,30] Despite the potential of

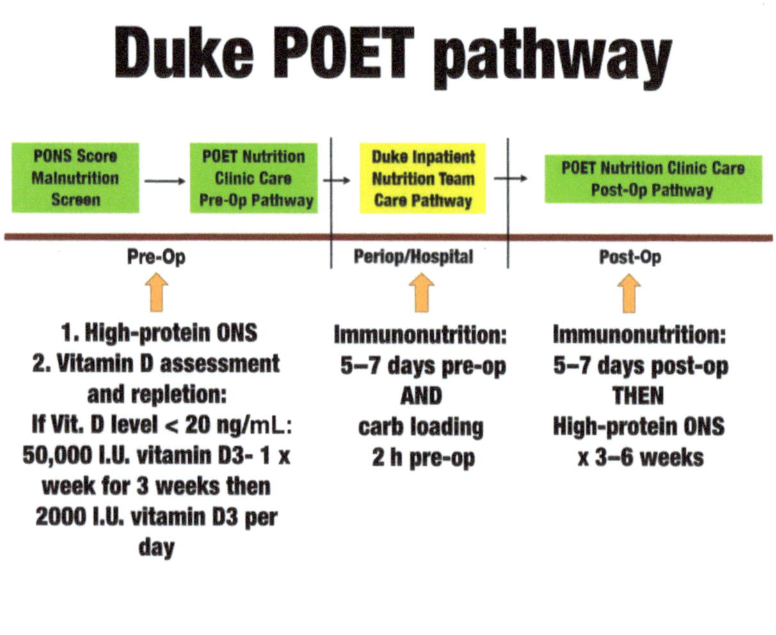

• **Fig. 9.2** Program for patients at risk of perioperative malnutrition at Duke University, the PeriOperative Enhancement Team (POET) clinic. Any patient assessed as being at malnutrition risk (perioperative nutrition screen score ≥ 1) is referred for evaluation by a dietitian and receives nutrition care according to this pathway. *ONS*, Oral nutritional supplements; *PONS*, perioperative nutrition screen. (From Gillis C, Wischmeyer PE. Pre-operative nutrition and the elective surgical patient: why, how and what? *Anaesthesia*. 2019;74:27–35.)

the preoperative surgical period as a "teachable moment," success rates of smoking cessation programs in this population of patients are low.[31,32] Lugg et al. evaluated 462 patients, which included 111 (24%) current smokers, 55 (12%) ex-smokers less than 6 weeks, 245 (53%) ex-smokers for 6 weeks or more, and 51 (11%) never smokers.[33] Postoperative pulmonary complications (PPC) occurred in 60 (13%) patients in total. Compared with never smokers, current smokers had a higher frequency of PPC (22% vs. 2%, P = .004), higher frequency of intensive care unit admission (14% vs. 0%; P = .001), and a longer median hospital stay (6^5 vs. 5^2; P = .001). However, there was no significant difference in long-term survival found between the groups of differing smoking status. They concluded that current smokers have higher postoperative morbidity, which can be reduced following smoking cessation.[33] Smoking cessation advice and support should nevertheless be offered to all smokers awaiting thoracic resection surgery. Discussion should focus on: the use of all patient contact to discuss smoking cessation; gaining an understanding of the patient's level of addiction; prescribing appropriate nicotine replacement therapy; and signposting to cessation services.[9] Other interventions might include deep breathing exercises and inspiratory muscle training programs.[34]

Anemia

There now exists multiple guidelines on the perioperative management and optimization of anaemia.[35–38] A large proportion of patients scheduled for major surgery are anemic. Perioperative anemia, which is more frequent in patients undergoing major elective surgical procedures than the general population, has been linked to increased rates of postoperative morbidity and mortality, as well as to longer stays in the hospital and higher 30-day mortality.[39]

Iron deficiency anemia is the most prevalent among patients considered for cancer surgery, and has a complex pathophysiology, which includes nutritional deficiency and chronic inflammation.[35] It is best diagnosed by a serum ferritin of less than 100 mcg/L, or a transferrin saturation of less than 20%.[35] Although the World Health Organization defines the threshold of anemia as 130 g/L for men and 120 g/L for women, women are more likely to be anemic, and more likely to require perioperative allogeneic blood transfusions. There have been calls for this threshold to be raised to less than 130 g/L for all patients at preoperative assessment,[40] which we fully support.

Whenever feasible, preoperative anemia should be detected and classified at least 4 weeks before the scheduled procedure, and appropriate pharmacologic treatment implemented, if possible. Blood transfusion should be reserved for patients with severe anemia, ongoing bleeding, and/or poor physiological reserve. Treatment of iron deficiency anemia is with iron supplementation.[41] Oral iron might be considered when there is adequate time before surgery, and usually takes around 6 weeks. If this is poorly tolerated or if there is more urgency, intravenous iron is indicated. It is our experience that, in patients with a hemoglobin of more than 130 g/L and either a ferritin less than 100 mcg/L or a transferrin saturation of less than 20%, intravenous iron should be considered. This has been shown to be safe and efficacious.[42] The routine use of erythropoietin is not recommended and is not licensed for use in the United Kingdom, and has been associated with adverse outcomes.[43] Iron clinics may be established in either primary or secondary care to provide this service. Finally, it must be borne in mind that the aim of performing major surgical procedures without the use of antibiotic therapy and without placing the patient at risk of complications may be better accomplished by combining several blood conservation strategies.

Diabetes

Diabetes mellitus is a multisystem disorder with an increasing prevalence. It is a modifiable risk factor and can be optimized before surgery, with demonstrable improvements in postoperative outcomes.[44] The prevalence of diabetes is increasing. The most recent estimates from the International Diabetes Federation suggest that the number of people worldwide who have diabetes mellitus is about 425 million, that is, one in 11 adults. This number is predicted to rise to almost 700 million by 2045. In a recently published single-center Australian prospective study of patients aged over 54 years undergoing inpatient surgery, it was demonstrated that of 7565 patients, 2047 (27%) had diabetes, as defined by hemoglobin A1c (HbA1c) more than 48 mmol/mol (6.5%); 2825 (37%) had prediabetes, as defined by HbA1c of 39 to 47 mmol/mol (5.7%–6.4%); and only 2457 (32%) patients were normoglycemic. Diabetes may be diagnosed or undiagnosed, but there is currently no screening program in the United Kingdom for diabetes in patients scheduled for surgery. Some have argued that this is a missed opportunity. The International Diabetes Federation currently estimates that worldwide just over 210 million people have undiagnosed diabetes.[45] People with diabetes (both diagnosed and undiagnosed) have a significantly longer hospital length of stay; more major complications; a higher requirement for postoperative critical care admission; a higher requirement for postoperative ventilation; and higher mortality rates and episode costs compared with people without diabetes admitted for the same conditions. In surgical patients, the length of hospital stay is up to 45% higher than those without diabetes. Strategies to optimize glycemic control in diabetic patients include: modification of normal glucose lowering medication; initiation of insulin therapy; and continuous subcutaneous insulin. That said, the best intervention is meticulous preoperative assessment and communication.[44] The referral letter to the surgical team should detail the relevant pathology and the current HbA1c, but there is evidence that this is not universally done.[46] If diabetes control is poor, early advice from a specialist diabetes team should be sought.

Cardiac

The prevalence of cardiac comorbidities in thoracic surgical patients is high, and there is evidence to suggest that it is among the most important of risk factors in this population.[47,48] It is estimated that around 200 million major operations are performed every year worldwide. Overall complication rates vary among different countries but are probably around 10%, with cardiac complications now one of the leading causes of all morbidity and mortality, accounting for 40% of postoperative mortality in one study using troponin levels. Major adverse cardiac events comprise: acute myocardial ischemia or infarction; angina; congestive heart failure; atrioventricular block; arrhythmias; and cardiac arrest. That said, most patients undergoing thoracic surgery should have a transthoracic echocardiogram performed before surgery, particularly if they have an abnormal electrocardiogram, and there are several conditions that are amenable to medical optimization.[49] This includes: hypertension; chronic heart failure; and the management of patients with a cardiac implantable electronic device.

Frailty and Comprehensive Geriatric Assessment

Frailty is to some extent a modifiable risk factor, but its assessment differs from those items discussed already because it is not organ specific. There is no accepted definition of frailty, but there exists a number of tools for its measurement including the Clinical Frailty Scale[50] the Edmonton Frailty Scale,[51] and others.[52] Its measurement allows more appropriate planning of a stratified perioperative package, such as a minimally invasive, staged, or "damage control" approach. There is an urgent need for high-quality perioperative trials of interventions aimed at attenuating or reversing frailty before surgery for any patient undergoing major surgery.[53]

In the past, major surgery was seldom performed on patients older than 80 years. With advancements in surgical techniques and perioperative care, surgery may be a viable treatment even at a very advanced age. Although chronologic age itself predicts surgical outcome poorly, age-related decline in physiological reserve and functional capacity are inevitable, and affect all organ systems. Comprehensive geriatric assessment involves collaboration between all members of the perioperative team, as well as geriatricians, nurses, therapists, and dieticians. Components include assessment of: comorbid conditions; medications; nutrition; mental health, including risk factors for delirium; functional capacity; social circumstances; and home environment. There is good evidence that it has a positive role in enhancing outcomes for elderly patients undergoing thoracic surgery.[54]

Oral Hygiene

Poor oral hygiene increases the risk of postoperative pulmonary complications, and there is reasonable evidence that improving oral hygiene reduces this risk in thoracic surgical patients. This cheap and effective patient-led intervention should form part of any prehabilitation pathway. In one study of 972 patients, there were 466 interventions with an instruction to follow an oral hygiene regime and 506 controls. Of the intervention patients, 405 (86.9%, 95% CI, 83.3–89.8%) reported that they had adhered to the oral hygiene recommendation. Sixty-four (12.6%) control patients and 36 (7.7%) in the intervention group ($P = .015$) were treated with antibiotics postoperatively. They concluded that it was feasible to involve patients in a program for oral hygiene and thereby reduce the number of patients needing antibiotics after open-heart surgery, and this might contribute to reducing costs.[55]

The Ideal Thoracic Perioperative Pathway

Traditionally, the perioperative pathway would focus on investigations and contemplation of surgery before the first formal physiological assessment much later in the process, and risk assessment just before surgery.[56] We propose a modern pathway, whereby prehabilitation and optimization begin at the point of hospital referral. This finishes at the point of preoperative assessment, which is just before surgery (Fig. 9.3).

Effectively caring for patients with lung cancer requires close and coordinated collaboration. Not just between healthcare providers (surgeons, anesthetists, physicians, nurses, physiotherapists, dieticians, and pharmacists all play

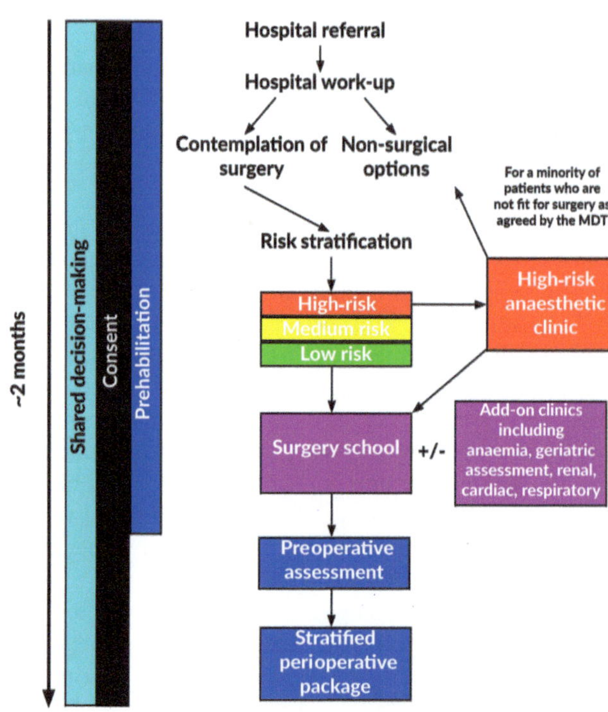

• **Fig. 9.3** An ideal pathway to facilitate prehabilitation of the thoracic surgical patient. The opportunity for multimodal prehabilitation extends from the moment of general practitioner referral to the point of preoperative assessment. It integrates with all aspects of shared decision-making, consent, risk stratification, and preoperative optimization. *MDT,* multidisciplinary team.

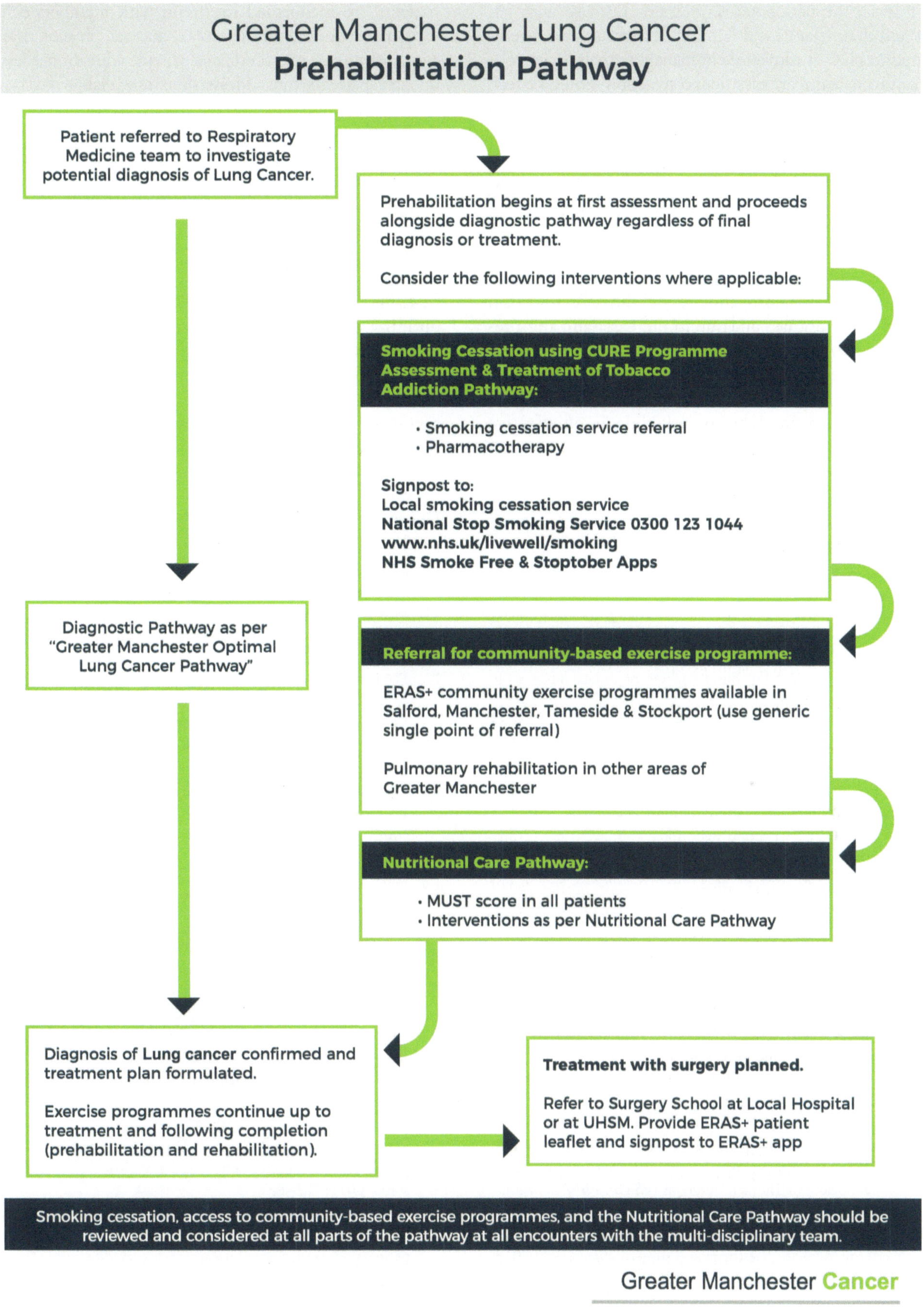

• **Fig. 9.4** The Greater Manchester Lung Cancer Prehabilitation Pathway. *CURE,* Conversation, Understand, Replace, Experts and evidence-based treatment; *ERAS,* Enhanced recovery after surgery; *UHSM,* University Hospital of South Manchester.

vital roles in the perioperative journey), but also with patients and their friends and families. Patients should be empowered to play an active role in managing their illness. For the healthcare team, every patient interaction should be seen as an opportunity for a "teachable moment," to support and guide patients in addressing their modifiable risk factors.

Within our center, we support the patient education and prehabilitation process through weekly "Surgery School" events (Fig. 9.4). These are consultant-led sessions that patients are encouraged to attend with members of their support network. At these events, doctors, physiotherapists, specialist nurses, and dieticians provide educational sessions on how patients can address their modifiable risk factors. Patients are also signposted toward collaborations with community fitness centers, where they can be supported through both pre- and postoperative fitness programs. Patients are also helped to access a bespoke website and app, that provides further educational materials.

Conclusion

The number of patients undergoing thoracic resection surgery will no doubt continue to increase, and the preoperative period offers an ideal opportunity to at once improve: underlying health issues, perioperative outcomes, the cost effectiveness of surgery, and more generally, public health. The key principle is of effective training and education, which will empower patients to optimize their condition before surgery and return to a level of health and function similar to their premorbid state. There remains a need for high-quality prospective data on the cumulative impact of such programs and the barriers to their implementation.

Acknowledgments

We acknowledged the department of cardiothoracic anaesthesia and critical care, Wythenshawe Hospital, Manchester University NHS Foundation Trust, Manchester, UK. No conflicts of interest or external funding.

References

1. Johnson DH, Schiller JH, Bunn PA. Recent clinical advances in lung cancer management. *J Clin Oncol.* 2014;32:973–982.
2. Oudkerk M, Devaraj A, Vliegenthart R, et al. European position statement on lung cancer screening. *Lancet Oncol.* 2017;18:e754–e766.
3. Charlesworth M, Glossop AJ. Strategies for the prevention of postoperative pulmonary complications. *Anaesthesia.* 2018;73:923–927.
4. Cavalheri V, Granger C. Preoperative exercise training for patients with non-small cell lung cancer. *Cochrane Database Syst Rev.* 2017;6:CD012020.
5. Steffens D, Beckenkamp PR, Hancock M, Solomon M, Young J. Preoperative exercise halves the postoperative complication rate in patients with lung cancer: a systematic review of the effect of exercise on complications, length of stay and quality of life in patients with cancer. *Br J Sports Med.* 2018;52:344.
6. Moore JA, Conway DH, Thomas N, Cummings D, Atkinson D. Impact of a peri-operative quality improvement programme on postoperative pulmonary complications. *Anaesthesia.* 2017;72:317–327.
7. Batchelor TJP, Rasburn NJ, Abdelnour-Berchtold E, et al. Guidelines for enhanced recovery after lung surgery: recommendations of the Enhanced Recovery After Surgery (ERAS®) Society and the European Society of Thoracic Surgeons (ESTS). *Eur J Cardiovasc Surg.* 2019;55:91–115.
8. Jones NL, Edmonds L, Ghosh S, Klein AA. A review of enhanced recovery for thoracic anaesthesia and surgery. *Anaesthesia.* 2013;68:179–189.
9. Templeton R, Greenhalgh D. Preoperative rehabilitation for thoracic surgery. *Curr Opin Anaesthesiol.* 2019;32:23–28.
10. Ntima NO, Lumb AB. Pulmonary function tests in anaesthetic practice. *BJA Educ.* 2019;19:206–211.
11. Lim E, Baldwin D, Beckles M, et al. Guidelines on the radical management of patients with lung cancer. *Thorax.* 2010;65:1–27, iii.
12. Fishman A, Martinez F, Naunheim K, et al. A randomized trial comparing lung-volume–reduction surgery with medical therapy for severe emphysema. *N Engl J Med.* 2003;348:2059–2073.
13. Salati M, Brunelli A. Risk stratification in lung resection. *Curr Surg Rep.* 2016:4.
14. Pichard C, Kyle UG, Morabia A, Perrier A, Vermeulen B, Unger P. Nutritional assessment: lean body mass depletion at hospital admission is associated with an increased length of stay. *Am J Clin Nutr.* 2004;79:613–618.
15. Barry MJ, Edgman-Levitan S. Shared decision making—The pinnacle of patient-centered care. *N Engl J Med.* 2012;366:780–781.
16. Sturgess J, Clapp JT, Fleisher LA. Shared decision-making in peri-operative medicine: a narrative review. *Anaesthesia.* 2019;74:13–19.
17. Silver J, Baima J. Cancer prehabilitation: an opportunity to decrease treatment-related morbidity, increase cancer treatment options, and improve physical and psychological health outcomes. *Am J Phys Med Rehabil.* 2013;92:715–727.
18. Carli F, Ferreira V. Prehabilitation: a new area of integration between geriatricians, anesthesiologists, and exercise therapists. *Aging Clin Exp Res.* 2018;30:241–244.
19. Levy N, Grocott MPW, Carli F. Patient optimisation before surgery: a clear and present challenge in peri-operative care. *Anaesthesia.* 2019;74:3–6.
20. Tew GA, Ayyash R, Durrand J, Danjoux GR. Clinical guideline and recommendations on pre-operative exercise training in patients awaiting major non-cardiac surgery. *Anaesthesia.* 2018;73:750–768.
21. Law H, Foden P, Evison M, et al. P107 Predictors of mortality in patients undergoing lung cancer surgery. *Thorax.* 2016;71:A141.
22. Vigano A, Kasvis P, Di Tomasso J, Gillis C, Kilgour R, Carli F. Pearls of optimizing nutrition and physical performance of older

adults undergoing cancer therapy. *J Geriatr Oncol.* 2017;8:428–436.
23. Gillis C, Wischmeyer PE. Pre-operative nutrition and the elective surgical patient: why, how and what? *Anaesthesia.* 2019;74:27–35.
24. Wischmeyer PE, Carli F, Evans DC, et al. American society for Enhanced Recovery and Perioperative Quality Initiative Joint Consensus Statement on Nutrition Screening and Therapy within a Surgical Enhanced Recovery Pathway. *Anesth Analg.* 2018;126: 1883–1895.
25. Zhong X-Z, Kang K, Shu X-L. Effect of nutritional support on clinical outcomes in perioperative malnourished patients: a meta-analysis. *Asia Pac J Clin Nutr.* 2015;24(3):367–378 367.
26. Wynter-Blyth V, Moorthy K. Prehabilitation: preparing patients for surgery. *BMJ.* 2017:358.
27. Park S, Kang CH, Hwang Y, et al. Risk factors for postoperative anxiety and depression after surgical treatment for lung cancer. *Eur J Cardiovasc Surg.* 2016;49:e16–e21.
28. Levett DZH, Grimmett C. Psychological factors, prehabilitation and surgical outcomes: evidence and future directions. *Anaesthesia.* 2019;74:36–42.
29. Agostini P, Cieslik H, Rathinam S, et al. Postoperative pulmonary complications following thoracic surgery: are there any modifiable risk factors? *Thorax.* 2010;65:815–818.
30. Maeda R, Yoshida J, Ishii G, Hishida T, Nishimura M, Nagai K. The prognostic impact of cigarette smoking on patients with non-small cell lung cancer. *J Thorac Oncol.* 2011;6:735–742.
31. Webb AR, Coward L, Soh L, et al. Smoking cessation in elective surgical patients offered free nicotine patches at listing: a pilot study. *Anaesthesia.* 2020:75.
30. McDonald S, Yates D, Durrand JW, et al. Exploring patient attitudes to behaviour change before surgery to reduce peri-operative risk: preferences for short- vs. long-term behaviour change. *Anaesthesia.* 2019;74:1580–1588.
33. Lugg ST, Tikka T, Agostini PJ, et al. Smoking and timing of cessation on postoperative pulmonary complications after curative-intent lung cancer surgery. *J Cardiothorac Surg.* 2017;12:52.
32. Lumb AB. Pre-operative respiratory optimisation: an expert review. *Anaesthesia.* 2019;74:43–48.
35. Muñoz M, Acheson AG, Auerbach M, et al. International consensus statement on the peri-operative management of anaemia and iron deficiency. *Anaesthesia.* 2017;72:233–247.
36. Meybohm P, Froessler B, Goodnough LT, et al. "Simplified International Recommendations for the Implementation of Patient Blood Management" (SIR4PBM). *Perioper Med.* 2017;6:5.
37. Klein AA, Bailey CR, Charlton AJ, et al. Association of Anaesthetists guidelines: cell salvage for peri-operative blood conservation. *Anaesthesia.* 2018;73:1141–1150.
38. Munting KE, Klein AA. Optimisation of pre-operative anaemia in patients before elective major surgery—why, who, when and how? *Anaesthesia.* 2019;74:49–57.
39. Muñoz M, Gómez-Ramírez S, Campos A, Ruiz J, Liumbruno GM. Pre-operative anaemia: prevalence, consequences and approaches to management. *Blood Transfus Trasfusione Del Sangue.* 2015;13:370–379.
40. Butcher A, Richards T, Stanworth SJ, Klein AA. Diagnostic criteria for pre-operative anaemia–time to end sex discrimination. *Anaesthesia.* 2017;72:811–814.
41. Auerbach M, Adamson JW. How we diagnose and treat iron deficiency anemia. *Am J Hematol.* 2016;91:31–38.
42. Avni T, Bieber A, Grossman A, Green H, Leibovici L, Gafter-Gvili A. The safety of intravenous iron preparations: systematic review and meta-analysis. *Mayo Clin Proc.* 2015;90:12–23.
43. Unger EF, Thompson AM, Blank MJ, Temple R. Erythropoiesis-stimulating agents—time for a reevaluation. *N Engl J Med.* 2010;362:189–192.
44. Levy N, Dhatariya K. Pre-operative optimisation of the surgical patient with diagnosed and undiagnosed diabetes: a practical review. *Anaesthesia.* 2019;74:58–66.
45. Dhatariya KK, Wiles MD. Pre-operative testing guidelines: a NICE try but not enough. *Anaesthesia.* 2016;71:1403–1407.
46. Pournaras DJ, Photi ES, Barnett N, et al. Assessing the quality of primary care referrals to surgery of patients with diabetes in the East of England: a multi-centre cross-sectional cohort study. *Int J Clin Pract.* 2017;71:e12971.
47. Mishra PK, Pandey R, Shackcloth MJ, et al. Cardiac comorbidity is not a risk factor for mortality and morbidity following surgery for primary non-small cell lung cancer. *Eur J Cardiovasc Surg.* 2009;35:439–443.
48. Takenaka T, Katsura M, Shikada Y, Tsukamoto S, Takeo S. The impact of cardiovascular comorbidities on the outcome of surgery for non-small-cell lung cancer. *Interact Cardiovasc Thorac Surg.* 2013;16:270–274.
49. Lee LKK, Tsai PNW, Ip KY, Irwin MG. Pre-operative cardiac optimisation: a directed review. *Anaesthesia.* 2019;74:67–79.
50. Rockwood K, Song X, MacKnight C, et al. A global clinical measure of fitness and frailty in elderly people. *CMAJ.* 2005;173: 489–495.
51. Rolfson DB, Majumdar SR, Tsuyuki RT, Tahir A, Rockwood K. Validity and reliability of the Edmonton Frail Scale. *Age Ageing.* 2006;35:526–529.
52. Theou O, Brothers TD, Mitnitski A, Rockwood K. Operationalization of frailty using eight commonly used scales and comparison of their ability to predict all-cause mortality. *J Am Geriatr Soc.* 2013;61:1537–1551.
53. Chan SP, Ip KY, Irwin MG. Peri-operative optimisation of elderly and frail patients: a narrative review. *Anaesthesia.* 2019;74: 80–89.
54. Partridge JSL, Harari D, Martin FC, Dhesi JK. The impact of pre-operative comprehensive geriatric assessment on postoperative outcomes in older patients undergoing scheduled surgery: a systematic review. *Anaesthesia.* 2014;69:8–16.
55. Pedersen PU, Tracey A, Sindby JE, Bjerrum M. Preoperative oral hygiene recommendation before open-heart surgery: patients' adherence and reduction of infections: a quality improvement study. *BMJ Open Qual.* 2019;8.
56. Grocott MPW, Edwards M, Mythen MG, Aronson S. Peri-operative care pathways: re-engineering care to achieve the 'triple aim'. *Anaesthesia.* 2019;74:90–99.

NON-PRINT ITEMS

Abstract

The presurgical period is an ideal time for targeted interventions aimed at improving postoperative outcomes for all surgical patients. The aim is to restore physical and psychologic function following surgery. It is for all patients, and is not restricted to just those who are high or low risk. It can be defined as "a process on the cancer continuum of care that occurs between the time of cancer diagnosis and the beginning of acute treatment and includes physical and psychologic assessments that establish a baseline functional level, identify impairments, and provide interventions that promote physical and psychologic health to reduce the incidence and/or severity of future impairments." That said, it presents many challenges. Specifically, for thoracic surgical patients awaiting resection of cancer, there is limited time available between diagnosis and surgery, and other related hospital appointments or treatments might place a burden on the patient, both physically and psychologically. Prehabilitation must be multimodal. It is the sum of marginal gains from several interventions, which are themselves complementary. It requires invested resources, infrastructure, organization, and an acceptance of the longer-term benefits for surgical outcomes, value for money, and public health. Herein, we describe various components which might comprise a multimodal thoracic surgical prehabilitation program.

Keywords

thoracic surgery, prehabilitation, exercise, smoking nutrition

10

Positioning in Thoracic Surgery

ALESSIA PEDOTO, NICOLE GINSBERG

Introduction

Adequate patient position is essential to facilitate surgical exposure. This in turn has direct consequence on the anesthetic management. In addition to providing best access to the patient, optimal position should minimize any potential harm and injuries, especially when positional changes occur during general anesthesia, because of lack of patient feedback. The anesthesiologist has a key role during the perioperative period as the person in charge for the safety of this task.

Ideally, patient position should facilitate both the performance of surgery by providing optimal access to the operative site and access to the patient for the anesthesiologist. Optimal position should not interfere with respiration or circulation or cause undue nerve pressure or muscular discomfort.

Common positions for thoracic surgery include supine, lateral, or prone, which can be modified by the addition of flexion or reverse Trendelenburg, usually while the patient is anesthetized. Preventing both long- and short-term damage requires careful planning, which should be implemented during the preoperative encounter. A meticulous evaluation and documentation of any preoperative neuropathy and limited range of motion should take place at this time. Unfortunately, a clear mechanism for positional injury can be recognized only in less than 10% of cases,[1] therefore patients deemed at risk for positional injury, such as the elderly, diabetics, or those with an extreme body mass index (BMI) should be carefully evaluated. In the presence of significant limitations of the range of motion, the final surgical position should be checked while the patient is awake, to avoid significant or permanent damage when changing position following the induction of general anesthesia. In addition, any concerns or limitations should prompt an alternative position in cooperation with the surgeon.

The aims of this chapter are to describe the most common positions used during thoracic noncardiac surgery, highlighting the challenges and physiologic changes associated with each one, and to discuss how to prevent possible complications.

Positions for Thoracic Noncardiac Surgery

Thoracic noncardiac surgery involves multiple positions often assumed after the patient is anesthetized.

Supine Position

General anesthesia is usually induced in the supine position. The neck is placed in the sniffing position to facilitate intubation with the arms alongside the body. The use of video laryngoscopes and the availability of the fiberoptic bronchoscope in the room has made intubation less dependent on optimal positioning. Nevertheless, the presence of neck stiffness or any preoperative neck injury should be addressed before induction. Special attention should be given when the patient is placed in the final surgical position, commonly being the lateral decubitus with the bed flexed. The double-lumen tube (DLT) or the bronchial blocker (BB) should be correctly positioned before turning the patient and rechecked in the final operating position. Intravascular lines, endotracheal tubes, and urinary catheters should be secured and have enough length to be safely moved.

Thoracic noncardiac cases that are performed in the supine position include resection of the esophagogastric tract, mediastinal tumors, or tracheal disease. In the supine position, the arms may be either abducted, tucked, or secured above the head ("hands up"). When abducted, they should be at less than a 90-degree angle and secured to prevent sliding off the arm boards, especially in cases that require reverse Trendelenburg. All pressure points should be padded and protected, and any source of direct skin pressure removed. If the arms are tucked alongside the patient, they should be in a neutral position, with the thumbs up and the palms inward.[2] They should be secured to prevent sliding without causing distal hypoperfusion. In addition, stopcocks on arterial or intravenous (IV) lines should be padded to prevent pressure injuries to the skin. The hands-up position (90 degrees flexion at the elbows, and 90 degrees abduction at the shoulder) can result in brachial plexus stretching, as observed in cadaveric studies.[3] In sternotomies, a shoulder

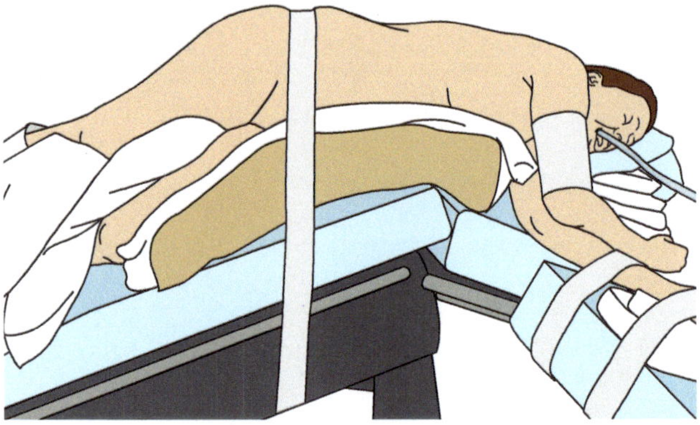

• **Fig. 10.1** Lateral decubitus with bed flexed and patient secured with tape. A sandbag is used to prevent lateral movements. The dependent lower extremity is slightly flexed, while the nondependent is straight, with a pillow placed between the knees to prevent common peroneal nerve compression.

roll is usually placed at the level of the scapula to open the clavicles and facilitate the sternal split. The head should be secured and not overextended or rotated to prevent brachial plexus injury.[4] Pillows or protective foam should be placed under the head for support and protection from contact pressure. Dangling of the head will apply pressure to the cervical spinal cord, which in turn could lead to postoperative neurologic injuries. Before prepping and draping the patient, all the IV lines should be checked to confirm a free flow. If an epidural catheter was inserted, access to the port should be ensured.

Lateral Decubitus

The lateral decubitus position is commonly used for most intrathoracic resections, with the patient being turned after induction of general anesthesia (Fig. 10.1). The anesthesia team should oversee the turning, to avoid displacement or loss of lines and airway devices. When in the lateral decubitus position, any unnatural positions that could cause injury to the patient, even if transient, should be avoided. The staff moving the patient should take precaution to prevent injuring themselves in the act of turning.[5–7] Once in the lateral decubitus, all pressure points should be padded, and the patient secured to prevent potential sliding or falls. Periodic intraoperative checks should be frequently done, and adjustments made in case of shifts from the original position. During thoracic procedures in the lateral position it is essential to have at least two IV accesses before placing the patients in the lateral position. Placing an IV line in the lateral position may present a significant challenge, and is time consuming.

Lower extremities (see Fig. 10.1): The dependent leg is slightly flexed with padding under the knee to avoid pressure on the common peroneal nerve. A pillow is placed in between the legs to decompress the common peroneal nerve of the nondependent leg, which is usually positioned straight. The saphenous nerve should be free of any compression. Vascular compression should be avoided because of the potential of ischemia, especially in patients with peripheral vascular disease. The hips are usually secured to the bed with tape or Velcro straps to prevent rotation and dislodgment, as well as distal hypoperfusion. Compartment syndrome has been reported in the lower extremities secondary to pressure of the dependent leg and decreased inguinal venous return.[8–10] A combination of risk factors, such as long duration of surgery (>5 hours), BMI higher than 40 kg/m^2,[11] low venous return and hypoperfusion have been suggested as contributing factors. The gluteal area is also at risk, because the gluteus muscle is compartmentalized.[8] Cases of gluteal compartment syndrome have been reported after prolonged lateral decubitus especially in young patients with high BMI.[12,13]

The upper extremities should be in a neutral position (Fig. 10.2).[14] The dependent arm should rest on a padded arm board and abducted to less than 90 degrees. Padding

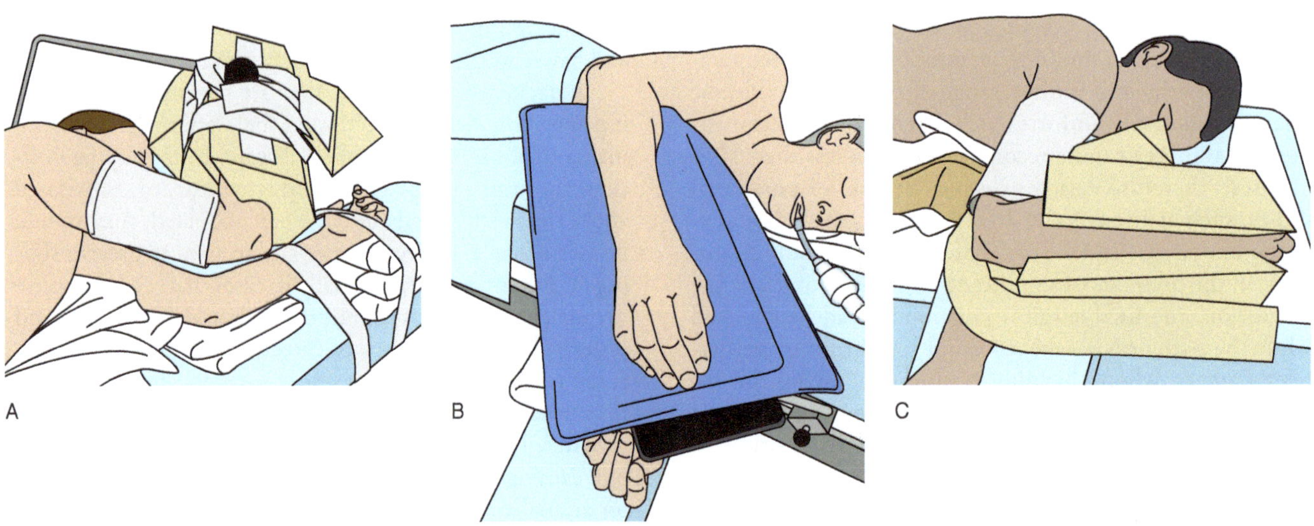

• **Fig. 10.2** The upper extremities are placed in a neutral position. The dependent arm is secured on an arm board in a neutral position with padding at the elbow and wrist. The nondependent arm can be placed on a sling (**A**), on a board (**B**), or close to the face on the bed (**C**). In all cases, padding should be used, and neutrality maintained.

under the elbows prevents ulnar nerve compression. The wrist should be in a neutral position to avoid radial nerve injury. An "axillary roll" is often placed under the axilla at the level of T4 to free the space, avoiding both brachial plexus injury and vascular compression.[15] After its placement and before draping, the provider should check that the roll did not migrate cephalad, especially if the position is readjusted. Placing the pulse oximeter on the dependent arm can be used as an indicator of adequate perfusion.[16] The nondependent arm can be suspended on a sling (see Fig. 10.2A) or rest on a board (see Fig. 10.2B). In both cases, extreme flexion at the elbow or stretch of the shoulder should be avoided to prevent brachial plexus or ulnar nerve injury.[3] Resting the upper extremity on a pillow placed on top of the dependent arm can potentially cause compression injuries and make intraoperative access to the patient and lines difficult. If not well secured, the pillow and the arm can slide into unnatural positions. If the tape is placed too tight over the elbow, it can cause direct pressure on the ulnar nerve, leading to postoperative neuropathy. Finally, the upper extremity can be placed on the operating room (OR) table close to the face (see Fig. 10.2C), but only if there is enough space available to maintain neutral position and avoid falls during surgery. Access to the chest will be difficult, making intraoperative checks challenging.

The neck should be neutral and supported by a gel or a foam pillow, as well as blankets or pillows when the bed is flexed. A careful evaluation of the cervical spine position should be done from the side before draping to confirm neutral positioning (Fig. 10.3). If the patient has any cervical spine limitation, extreme caution should be applied to keep the head in a neutral position. If commercially available devices are used to facilitate cervical spine neutrality, they should be of the appropriate size for the specific patient. Careful attention should be given to the dependent ear and eye to be free from compression. An increase in intraocular pressure has been reported while in the lateral decubitus, with values higher in the dependent eye, persisting until returning to the supine position[17] and worse with the use of sevoflurane. Yamada et al.[18] evaluated the intraocular pressure (IOP) in 28 patients undergoing surgery in the lateral position, randomly allocating them to either a sevoflurane or propofol group. IOP in both eyes was recorded and compared between the groups at several points during the procedure. In the sevoflurane group, IOP was significantly increased in both the dependent and nondependent eye 1 hour after changing to the lateral position. The number of patients in whom IOP increased to 28 mm Hg or higher was greater in the sevoflurane group than in the propofol group. The authors concluded that propofol may be better than sevoflurane for the maintenance of anesthesia in the lateral position.

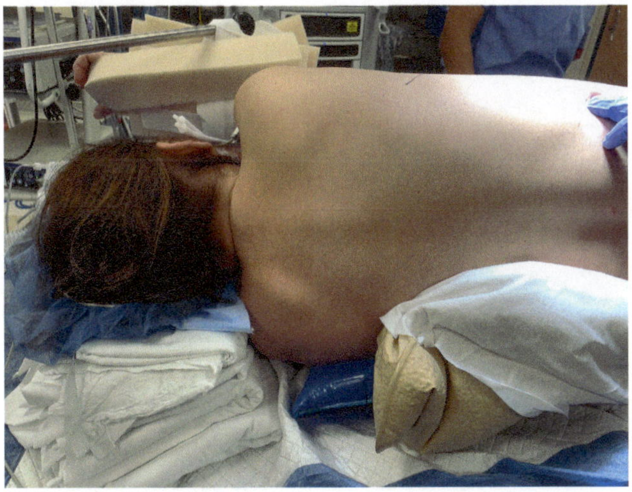

• **Fig. 10.3** The neck should be neutral and checked from the side.

Before extubation, the bed should be unflexed or even seated to facilitate spontaneous ventilation. If flexible bronchoscopy is needed before awakening, it should be done in the supine or semi-sitting position and the DLT (if used) exchanged to either a single-lumen tube (preferable in case of esophagectomy to avoid possible aspiration) or a supraglottic airway device, to accommodate the 6.0 mm fiberoptic bronchoscope. In cases of prolonged lateral decubitus, the face may be edematous because of decreased venous return. All precautions should be used when exchanging the DLT, starting with placing the patient in an optimal sniffing position. Strict extubation criteria should be met because reintubation may be difficult in such instance. If a BB was used to provide lung separation, flexible bronchoscopy can be performed following its removal.

Flexion

The goal of the bed flexion is to move the hips away from the chest and facilitate the opening of the spaces between the ribs. This is usually achieved by using the kidney rest or flexing the table (see Fig. 10.1). The flexion point should be at the level of the iliac crest, avoiding direct compression of the bony structures of the hip to prevent ischemia or necrosis, especially in elderly or cachectic patients. Protective foam or a gel pad is placed under the dependent iliac crest.[16] Flexion at the flank can cause compression of the abdominal organs and the inferior vena cava with hypotension from reduced venous return. Obese patients may be difficult to secure to the table because of their body habitus. Falls from the OR table may occur if the patient is not secured properly. A vacuumed sandbag or gel rolls properly placed and secured to the table are used to stabilize the patient and avoid potential disaster. All pressure points should be padded to avoid compression injury,[16] while avoiding distal ischemia secondary to tight straps.

Reverse Trendelenburg

This position is commonly used for surgery in the upper abdomen, such as minimally invasive esophagectomy, Nissen fundoplication, or Heller myotomy, because it facilitates organ exposure by displacing the abdominal content in a caudal direction (Fig. 10.4). Great care needs to be taken in preventing the patient from sliding off the table. Nonslip

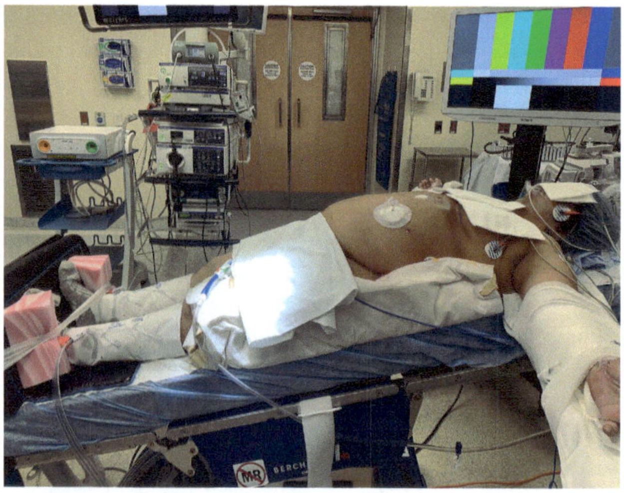

• **Fig. 10.4** Reverse Trendelenburg. The arms are neutral, padded, and secured. The feet are protected by foam crates and secured to the foot board to prevent sliding.

gel mattresses, chest and pelvic straps, as well as padded foot boards can be used for this purpose.[16] Independently from the device chosen to secure the patient, excessive pressure that could cause harm should be avoided at all times.[16] Significant hypotension can occur secondary to venous pooling in the lower extremities because of the additional use of pneumoperitoneum. Frequent blood pressure measurements are required, either via noninvasive or invasive monitors. Because the head is positioned above the heart, there is potential risk of cerebral hypoperfusion. This should be considered when managing the mean arterial pressure (MAP). For every 2.5 cm in vertical height, there is a 2 mm Hg decrease in MAP.[19]

Prone

The prone position is sometimes advocated for the thoracic dissection and reconstruction of the esophagus during minimally invasive surgery because of its posterior location,[20,21] offering the advantages of superior surgical ergonomics and physiologic benefits[22] when compared with other approaches.

The greatest challenge of turning the patient prone is to avoid loss of monitors, lines, and the endotracheal tube. A single lumen tube is often adequate because gravity facilitates the displacement of the lungs anteriorly, which is expedited by using insufflation. If lung isolation is required, a BB may be preferred to a DLT because maintaining proper position without kinks or dislodgment may be difficult, because of its shape and stiffness.[23] The head is usually placed on a soft foam molded facial mask or a commercial device (Proneview™, Mizuho OSI, Tokyo, Japan), with the eyes, the nose, and the chin free from compression and resting in the proper cutouts. Mirrors can be used for periodic checks during the procedure.[16] The face should be resting above the heart to avoid facial edema, which has been associated with devastating postoperative visual loss, especially when paired with high volumes of intravenous fluids.[14] The head should still be in a neutral position because rotation above 60 to 80 degrees has been associated with compression of the carotid and vertebral arteries.[14] The arms are placed to accommodate the surgeon and the instruments, usually with the left side tucked along the body and the right elevated above the head (90–100 degrees abduction). The shoulders and elbows should be flexed to less than 90 degrees, and the cervical spine kept neutral. The chest and the abdomen are held in place by gel bolsters that extend from the clavicles to the iliac crests, to alleviate the pressure on the chest.[14] Abdominal compression with secondary cephalad dislodgment of the diaphragm and decreased functional residual capacity (FRC) should be avoided. The breasts, iliac crests, and genitalia should be free of compression. The Foley catheter should be secured to avoid pulling on the genitalia. A dedicated stretcher should also be readily available for rapid turning to the supine position in case of emergency.

Robotic Surgery and Position

Robotic thoracic noncardiac surgery continues to gain popularity worldwide and in the United States[24] because of the ongoing reports of its advantages.[25,26] Patient position for these procedures should facilitate surgical access, enable docking, and access to the robot, as well as avoiding injuries.[26] In addition to confirming neutral position of the patient on the bed, it is imperative to avoid any direct compression of the face and shoulders by the robotic arms. In some institutions, the bed is rotated 90 degrees and moved away from the anesthesia station to accommodate the robot. In this case, extensions are needed for the anesthesia circuit and the IV tubing. After the patient is covered by the drapes and the robotic arms are docked, access may be extremely difficult (Fig. 10.5). All the necessary lines should be placed before turning the patient for ease and safety. Possible burns or fire can occur if the heated lights of the robotic camera get in touch with the drapes. Additional vigilance and periodic inspection of the head position and face appearance, the tube position, is required.

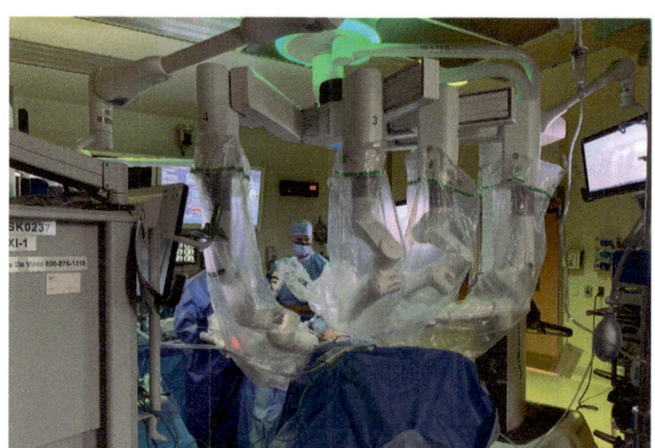

• **Fig. 10.5** The robot docked to the patient after prepping and draping.

Specific positions that are peculiar to robotic cases include:

Extreme flexion: This position may be necessary for lung or diaphragmatic surgery to allow docking of the robot and facilitate free arm movement while avoiding direct pressure on the patient. The table break should be at the flank to open the rib interspaces.

Steep reverse Trendelenburg: This position is adopted during the abdominal dissection of gastric structures. This position facilitates the caudad displacement of the abdominal organs, allowing exposure of the gastric structures. The combination of this position and the abdominal insufflation can cause significant hypotension, which requires frequent or continuous measurements. Volume resuscitation, or more commonly vasopressors are used for hemodynamic support until the supine position is regained.[27,28] Goal-directed fluid therapy has been proposed as a guiding tool for volume replacement during these cases, in particular to avoid upper airway edema.[29] However, the reliability of the data is still questioned by several providers, because of the positioning, the changes in intrathoracic pressures, and the effects of one lung ventilation.

Semi-lateral: This position is commonly used for minimally invasive thymectomy (Fig. 10.6A and B). The patient is positioned supine with a gel roll or a sandbag inflated under the chest at the level of the scapula to achieve a 30-degree elevation at the side the instruments are entering the chest. The ipsilateral arm is abducted, with the shoulder rolled back and secured to the bed on a plane below the body to facilitate the entry of the robotic arms into the chest.[30] This position can potentially cause brachial plexus damage from overstretching. Direct shoulder compression from the robotic arms should be recognized and excluded before the start of the procedure and necessary adjustments made. Periodic checks during the procedure should reconfirm that none of the robotic arms are in direct contact with the patient.

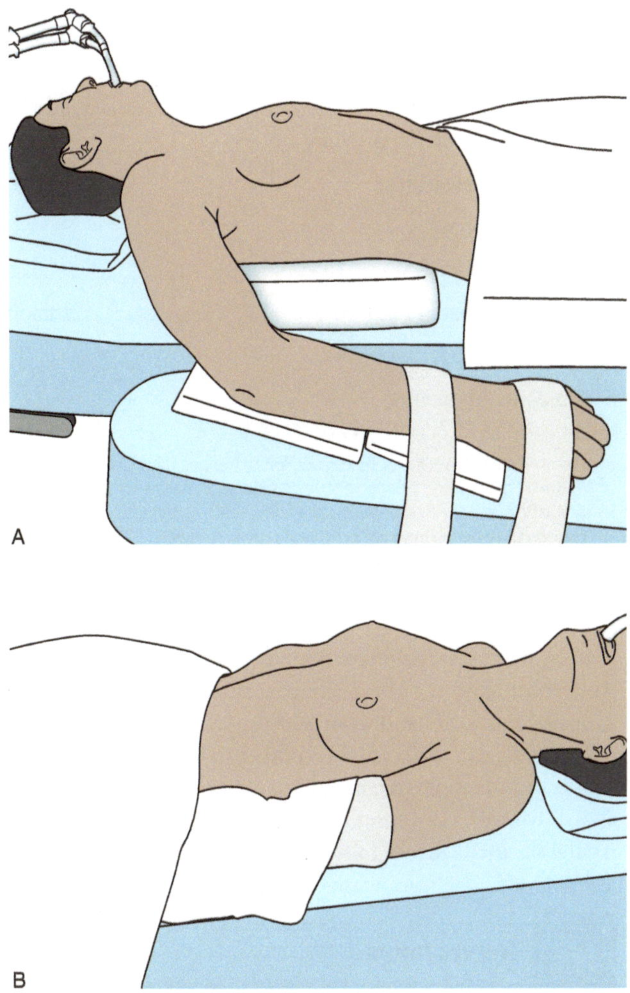

A

B

• **Fig. 10.6** Patient positioned for a minimally invasive thymectomy. (**A**) Semi-lateral decubitus with a gel roll placed vertically under the chest. The ipsilateral arm is placed neutral on the arm board, slightly bent and away from the chest to allow the robotic ports entry. (**B**) The contralateral arm is tucked. A shoulder roll is placed to open the clavicles. The field is marked, prepped, and draped for potential sternotomy.

Complications Related to Patient Positioning

Positional nerve injury (PNI) can have legal implications. PNI is still one of the most common causes of lawsuits for the anesthesiologist, secondary to potentially permanent consequences and disability for the injured party. Grant et al.[31] evaluated the data from the American Society of Anesthesiologists (ASA) Closed Claims database, looking at closed claims from 1996 to 2015 and identified 75 cases related to positional neuropathy after general anesthesia. Patient ages ranged from 23 to 94 years, and surgical procedures covered a variety of cases. The severity of nerve injury ranged from "insignificant" to "grave." Some 56% of cases involved the brachial plexus and occurred while in the supine position with the arms abducted, 76% resulted in permanent damage, which in 92% of cases was attributed to provider lack of knowledge. Some 24% of PNI claims were found to be temporary, whereas 76% were permanent. The ASA practice advisory update for prevention of positional neuropathy recommends a high focus on proper positioning and padding, as well as careful preoperative history and physical examination.[2]

Several factors have been proposed to contribute to position-related PNI (Table 10.1).[2] However, most of the data result from observational studies and identify orthopedic, gynecologic, general, and cardiac procedures as the highest risk. The most common nerves affected are summarized in Table 10.2.

Careful planning to prevent PNI should involve the entire care providers team and should start in the preoperative period with a detailed history, physical examination, and documentation of the affected nerve. In case of PNI, the

TABLE 10.1 Risk Factors Contributing to Peripheral Nerve Injury

Procedure Related	Patient	Physiologic
Wrongdoing by the provider	Hypertension	Hypotension
Documentation error	Diabetes mellitus	Hypoxemia
Delayed consult	Smoking	Dehydration
Surgical trauma	Preexisting radiculopathy	Hypothermia
Delayed/missing diagnosis	Anatomic abnormalities	Electrolyte imbalances
Bleeding or coagulopathy		
Fluids extravasation		

From Practice Advisory for the Prevention of Perioperative Peripheral Neuropathies 2018. An updated report by the American Society of Anesthesiologists Task Force on prevention of perioperative peripheral neuropathies. *Anesthesiology*. 2018;128(1):11–26; O'Connor D, Radcliffe J. Patient positioning in anaesthesia. *Anaesth Intens Care Med*. 2018;19(11):585–590; Grant I, Brovman EY, Kang D, Greenberg P, Saba R, Urman RD. A medicolegal analysis of positioning-related perioperative peripheral nerve injuries occurring between 1996 and 2015. *J Clin Anesth*. 2019;58:84–90.

patient may report symptoms 1 to 7 days after surgery.[14,16] Any complaint should be documented, investigated, and a neurologist's consultation should be requested. Electromyography can help in the differential diagnosis between single and multiple nerves injuries. Any subacute injury can evolve toward a complex regional pain syndrome (CRPS). Analgesic medications, splinting, and physical therapy are the initial recommended treatments, followed by neurolysis, sympathetic nerve blockade, or nerve grafting for more severe cases.[14]

Skin and tissue injury can occur secondary to breakdown from friction, pressure-induced injury, and ulceration, as well as compartment syndrome. Risk factors include old age, extreme BMI (high or low), long surgical times, hypotension, use of

TABLE 10.2 Nerves Injured

Nerve Injured	Nerve Affected	Mechanism	Risk Factors	Presentation
Ulnar nerve	C7, C8–T1	– Direct pressure at the medial condyle – Prolonged forearm flexion	Male Median age 50 years	Up to 28 days postop Tingle/paresthesia at the 5th finger Weakness at ab + adduction
Brachial plexus	C_5–T_1	– Direct pressure – Stretching – Direct injury (retractors during sternotomy)		Waiter tip position + claw hand + numbness in the ulnar distribution
Radial nerve	C_5–T_1	– Tourniquet, blood pressure cuff – Compression against ether screen – Uneven arm board		Wrist drop + posterior arm/hand numbness
Median nerve	C_5–T_1	Direct compression		Paresthesia in the palmar area of the hand and 3rd–5th fingers
Sciatic nerve (mostly as common peroneal nerve)	L_4–S_3	– Stretch – Compression – Direct damage	Lithotomy—frog legs – Men 45–50 years old – Diabetes mellitus	Weak knee flexion Foot drop
Superficial peroneal	S1–S2, L_4–L_5	Compression at the fibular head		Loss of foot dorsiflexion and eversion

From Lalkhen AG, Bhatia K. Perioperative peripheral nerve injuries. *Contin Educ Anaesth Crit Care Pain*. 2011;12(1):38–42.

vasopressors, and diabetes mellitus. Complications secondary to improper positioning include neuropathies and decubitus ulcers, where a reduction in perfusion leads to tissue ischemia and subsequent tissue breakdown.[16] Pressure redistribution seems to be the best way to prevent these injuries and therefore recommended along with frequent position changes when possible.[2] Areas at risk for injury include bony prominences (such as the ileum, ischial tuberosity, and the elbow), which should be adequately padded. Stopcocks, intravenous tubing connectors, and wires can also become potential point of pressure injuries and should be padded, especially when the arms are wrapped or tucked.[7] It is unclear if gel foam versus memory foam or any other material is better to prevent pressure ulcers. If possible, pressure points should be elevated and not touching hard surfaces. Any plastic surface should be covered to avoid intraoperative overheating and blistering.

Deep venous thrombosis can result from prolonged immobilization, which causes venous stasis and can lead to pulmonary embolism.[7] Prophylactic compression stockings, pneumatic compression boots, and subcutaneous low-molecular-weight heparin injections have been used to prevent this complication. Ahmed et al.[32] reported in 2018 the latest guidelines from the European Society of Anesthesia, which identify patients with lung cancer undergoing thoracic surgery at high risk of developing postoperative thromboembolism. Risk factors for perioperative venous thromboembolism included age over 70 years old, transfusion of more than 4 units of red blood cells/fresh frozen plasma/cryoprecipitate, mechanical ventilation lasting more than 24 hours, and postoperative complications, such as acute kidney injury, infection/sepsis, and neurologic events. Mechanical compression devices and low dose aspirin in adjunct to unfractionated heparin is recommended for a short period to avoid heparin-induced thrombocytopenia. Low-molecular-weight heparin should be used in case prophylaxis is needed for longer periods, with dose adjustments according to renal function. Patients undergoing thoracic surgery in the absence of cancer can be considered at low risk for venous thromboembolism. Patients undergoing thoracic surgery with a diagnosis of primary or metastatic cancer should be considered at high risk for venous thromboembolism. In **low-risk patients**, the use of mechanical prophylaxis using intermittent pneumatic compression is suggested, while in **high-risk patients**, pharmacologic prophylaxis should be added to intermittent pneumatic compression.[32]

Compartment syndrome is a rare occurrence in thoracic surgery but still possible in cases lasting longer than 5 hours. It has been described in the supine position,[10] and attributed possibly to the surgical staff leaning against the patient. In the lateral decubitus, pressure on the dependent lower extremity and venous obstruction at the inguinal area from leg flexion can cause ischemia and decreased venous drainage. Gluteal compartment syndrome has been described in the lateral decubitus after hip and renal surgery, when the flex is against the iliac crest.[33] Aggressive taping of the nondependent iliac crest to prevent falls in the lateral decubitus position can decrease perfusion and cause compartment syndrome, especially with prolonged duration of surgery.

Perioperative visual loss is a rare but devastating complication associated with the prone position. The two common causes are central retinal artery occlusion and ischemic optic neuropathy.[34] The former is usually secondary to direct external pressure on the eye with an increase in intraocular pressure and retinal ischemia. The latter seems to be related to lengthy procedures associated with significant blood loss, hypotension, and large volume resuscitation with crystalloids. In both cases, the best strategy to prevent these complications relies on proper position and frequent intraoperative checks.[35]

Special Considerations

Changes in Position During Emergency

Cardiac arrest in the flexed lateral decubitus requires the rapid return to the unflexed supine position to begin successful cardiopulmonary resuscitation (CPR). Unflexing the bed and turning the patient needs to be rapid, requiring a degree of coordination among providers. The use of the robot may delay this task by the additional step of "undocking" the robot. In addition, if a robotic OR table is used (Trumpf™ TruSystem, Saalfeld, Germany), it must be unpaired from the robot itself before being able to change position. This built-in safety step avoids accidental intraoperative changes in the bed position while the robot is docked, with the goal of preventing patient harm. However, in case of an emergency, undocking, unpairing, and changing position of the OR table add precious time that delays the start of CPR. As previously mentioned, if the patient is in the prone position, a bed or stretcher should be readily available to turn the patient supine.

Equipment malfunction may prevent rapid undocking of the robot or change in the OR table position. Both instances have been reported through the U.S. Food and Drug Administration MAUDE (Manufacturer And User Facility Device Experience) database as a cause of emergency and patient harm.[36] From 2000 to 2013, a total of 20 cases of malfunction were identified, with cardiothoracic surgery having the highest incidence of death (6.4%), conversion (16%), or rescheduling (2.8%) when compared with other cases.

Position for Extracorporeal Mechanical Oxygenation During Thoracic Cases (see Chapter 28)

Extracorporeal mechanical oxygenation (ECMO) has been used for thoracic cases as an aid to facilitate oxygenation during lung resection, transplantation,[37] and lavage,[38] as well as airway[39–41] or mediastinal mass resections.[42] Cannulation is usually done in the supine position either before or after induction of general anesthesia. When changing position, meticulous care must be taken to avoid cannula dislocation. Cannula dislodgment, bleeding, and air embolism are the major concerns when changing position during ECMO.[43]

Extensive data are available for the prone position,[43] while case reports on the use of venovenous ECMO in the lateral decubitus have been described.[44–46]

Position in Obese Patients (see Chapter 49)

In obese patients, general anesthesia should not be induced in the supine position, because of the cephalad shifting of the diaphragm and the abdominal contents causing a decrease in compliance, FRC, and an increase in work of breathing, with rapid desaturation and possible difficult mask ventilation. Ideally, patients should be positioned either in the semi-sitting[47–49] or in reverse Trendelenburg position[50,51] (Fig. 10.7A), being careful to avoid sliding and falls. The caudad fall of the pannus allows the unloading of the diaphragm, with an improvement in FRC and lung compliance. Ideally, the sternum should be aligned with the ear to allow optimal laryngoscopy,[52] especially when paired with manual caudad displacement of the lower cervical adipose tissue. The arms should be adequately supported to prevent brachial plexopathy (Fig. 10.7B). Long Velcro straps may be needed to secure the patient to the bed and prevent falls.

Changing position after induction of general anesthesia is particularly challenging, often requiring additional help and coordination. Safe patient positioning should not be at the expense of staff injuries.[4] Once in the lateral decubitus, an adequate size axillary roll is needed to free the pressure at the axilla. Securing the patient in the proper position may be difficult. The sandbag may not be large enough to prevent the patient from rolling or sliding. Gel rolls may not fit properly because of the patient body habitus and the dimensions of the OR table. Anterior and posterior pegs may be in the surgical field and therefore not an option. If additional tape or Velcro straps are used at the hip, it is imperative to make sure that they are not too tight to prevent distal ischemia or cause compartment syndrome. To maintain the head in a neutral position, extra blankets and foam pillows may be needed because of the short neck and torso (Fig. 10.7C). Additional arm boards may be necessary to properly secure the dependent

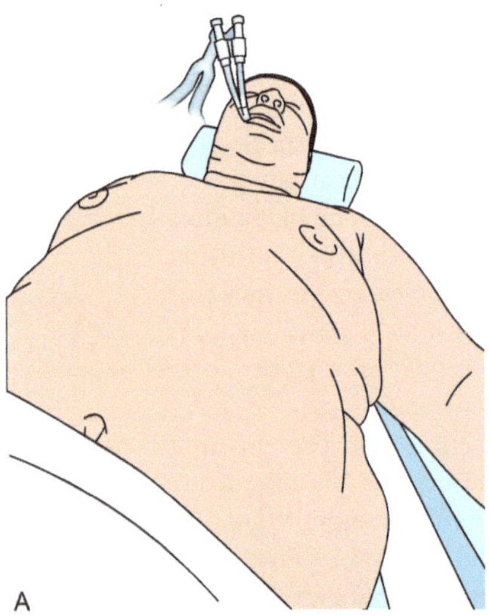
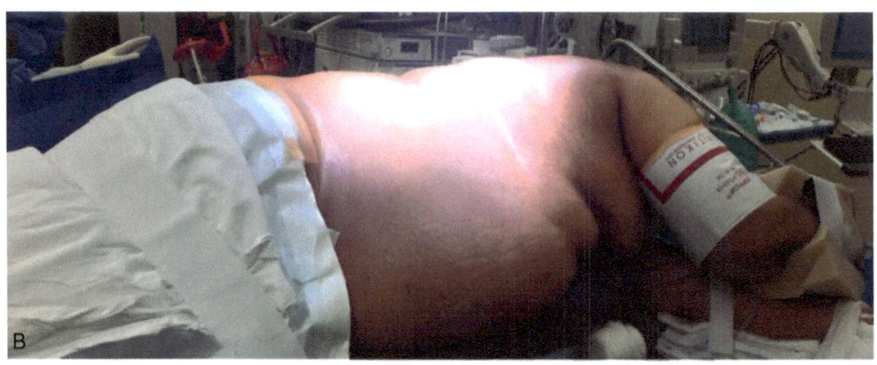
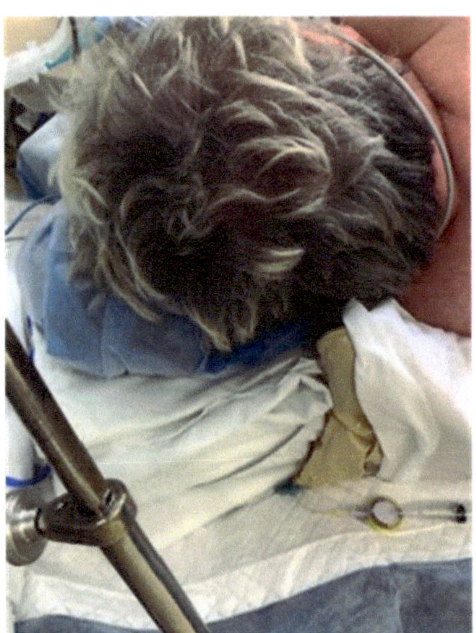

• **Fig. 10.7** Position in the obese. (**A**) Slight reverse Trendelenburg to facilitate intubation. The caudad displacement of the pannus improves the respiratory mechanics and the intubation conditions. (**B**) Lateral decubitus with the caudad displacement of the pannus; (**C**) head in neutral position with multiple blankets.

arm. Periodic intraoperative position checks are imperative to promptly recognize any shift in position that could cause PNI. Invasive monitors may be required for blood pressure management, since the noninvasive devices may not fit properly or become dislodged once the position is changed. Noninvasive blood pressure cuff reading at the forearm may not be accurate.[53,54] Continuous noninvasive blood pressure devices (e.g., ClearSight® Edwards Lifesciences Corporation, Irvine, CA) may be a viable alternative to arterial cannulation in this patient population, with promising results in bariatric surgery. Rogge et al.[55] recorded simultaneously noninvasive (ClearSight system, Edwards Lifesciences Corporation, Irvine, CA) and invasive arterial pressure measurements over a period of 45 minutes in 35 severely obese patients (median BMI, 47 kg/m^2) during laparoscopic bariatric surgery. They concluded that the accuracy and precision of the noninvasive technique (ClearSight system) was good for MAP and diastolic arterial pressure but only moderate for systolic arterial pressure. In the error grid analysis, more than 99% of vascular unloading technique-derived arterial pressure measurements were categorized into no- or low-risk zones.

Respiratory mechanics and hemodynamics may improve in the lateral decubitus when compared with the supine position because of the anterior displacement of the pannus, leading to better total respiratory compliance.[51] The weight of the mediastinum and the decreased excursion of the dependent lung, especially when protective lung ventilation is adopted, contribute to an increase in atelectasis formation. Positive end-expiratory pressure and recruitment maneuvers are recommended during this phase of surgery.[56]

The prone position is usually well tolerated in the obese patient if the abdomen and the chest are free, to avoid compression of the inferior vena cava, femoral vessels, and chest wall. Proper placement of the gel rolls may be challenging in addition to the logistics of turning a morbidly obese patient into the prone position.

Conclusion

Positioning for thoracic noncardiac surgery is a dynamic process, where the anesthesiologist's role is to facilitate and supervise the required steps to prevent injury. A detailed preoperative evaluation to exclude preexisting conditions, a thorough knowledge of the patient's limitations in range of motion and an active participation in guiding what is natural and what is not are paramount in preventing long-term sequelae. Positional nerve damage is still the number one cause of lawsuits according to the ASA Closed Claims database, with a significant percentage of patients developing permanent sequelae. Anesthesiologists are very knowledgeable and skilled providers when positioning patients. Our efforts should be focused in preventing such catastrophic outcomes as part of a multidisciplinary effort that begins in the preoperative area and continues during the perioperative period.

References

1. Knight DJ, Mahajan RP. Patient positioning in anaesthesia. *Contin Educ Anaesth Crit Care Pain*. 2004;4(5):160–163.
2. Practice Advisory for the Prevention of Perioperative Peripheral Neuropathies 2018. An Updated Report by the American Society of Anesthesiologists Task Force on prevention of perioperative peripheral neuropathies. *Anesthesiology*. 2018;128(1):11–26.
3. Winfree CJ, Kline DG. Intraoperative positioning nerve injuries. *Surg Neurol*. 2005;63(1):5–18.
4. Wanless S. Principles for safe moving and handling of patients. *Pielegniarstwo XXI Wieku*. 2016:66–69.
5. Pompeii LA, Lipscomb HL, Schoenfisch AL, Dement JM. Musculoskeletal injuries resulting from patient handling tasks among hospital workers. *Am J Ind Med*. 2009;52(7):571–578.
6. Hegewald J, Berge W, Heinrich P, et al. Do technical aids for patient handling prevent musculoskeletal complaints in health care workers?—a systematic review of intervention studies. *Int J Environ Res Public Health*. 2018;15:476–495.
7. Adedeji R, Oragui E, Khan W, Maruthainar N. The importance of correct patient positioning in theatres and implications of mal-positioning. *J Perioper Pract*. 2010;20(4):143–147.
8. Halvachizadeh S, Jensen KO, Pape H-C. Compartment syndrome due to patient positioning. In: Mauffrey C, Hak DJ, Martin MP III, eds. *Compartment Syndrome: A Guide to Diagnosis and Management*. Champaign, IL: Springer International Publishing; 2019: 113–123.
9. Cascio BM, Buchowski JM, Frassica FJ. Well-limb compartment syndrome after prolonged lateral decubitus positioning: a report of two cases. *J Bone Joint Surg*. 2004;86(9):2038–2040.
10. Garner MR, Taylor SA, Gausden E, Lyden JP. Compartment syndrome: diagnosis, management, and unique concerns in the twenty-first century. *HSS J*. 2014;10(2):143–152.
11. Jamil R, Boglia J, Chughtai B, et al. High body mass index in muscular patients and flank position are risk factors for rhabdomyolysis: case report after laparoscopic live-donor nephrectomy. *J Endourol*. 2006;20(9):646–650.
12. Mathes DD, Assimos DG, Donofrio PD. Rhabdomyolysis and myonecrosis in a patient in the lateral decubitus position. *Anesthesiology*. 1996;84(3):727–729.
13. Warner ME, LaMaster LM, Thoeming EK, Marienau ME, Warner MA. Compartment syndrome in surgical patients. *Anesthesiology*. 2001;94(4):705–708.
14. Schubert A. Positioning injuries in anesthesia: an update. *Adv Anesth*. 2008;26:31–65.
15. Li J, Wang W, Qian Q, Chen X, Hecheng L. Collaboration between the surgeon, assistants and nurses in robotic-assisted thoracic surgery. *AME Med J*. 2017;2(2).
16. O'Connor D, Radcliffe J. Patient positioning in anaesthesia. *Anaesth Intens Care Med*. 2018;19(11):585–590.
17. Park HP, Hwang JW, Jeon YT, Lee PB, Oh YS. The effect of the lateral decubitus position on the intraocular pressure in anesthetized patients undergoing lung surgery. *Acta Anaesthesiol Scand*. 2006;50(8):988–992.

18. Yamada MH, Takazawa T, Iriuchijima N, Horiuchi T, Saito S. Changes in intraocular pressure during surgery in the lateral decubitus position under sevoflurane and propofol anesthesia. *J Clin Monitor Comput.* 2016;30(6):869–874.
19. Drummond JC. Blood pressure and the brain: how low can you go? *Anesth Analg.* 2019;128(4):759–771.
20. Koyanagi K, Ozawa S, Tachimori Y. Minimally invasive esophagectomy performed with the patient in a prone position: a systematic review. *Surg Today.* 2016;46(3):275–284.
21. Souche R, Nayeri M, Chati R, et al. Thoracoscopy in prone position with two-lung ventilation compared to conventional thoracotomy during Ivor Lewis procedure: a multicenter case-control study. *Surg Endosc.* 2020;34(1):142–152.
22. Jarral OA, Nakamura T, Otowa Y, et al. Thoracoscopic esophagectomy in the prone position. *Surg Endosc.* 2012;26(8):2095–2103.
23. Reimer C, Slinger P. Intraoperative patient positioning and neurological injuries. In: Slinger P, ed. *Principles and Practice of Anesthesia for Thoracic Surgery.* Champaign, IL: Springer International Publishing; 2019:337–342.
24. Marshall MB, Wee JO. Robotic platform use in general thoracic surgery. *JAMA Surg.* 2019;154(11):1066–1067.
25. Ziarat CC, Romano G, Hung Key T, Davini F, Melfi F. The evolution of robotic thoracic surgery. *Ann Cardiothorac Surg.* 2019; 8(2):210–217.
26. Pauli H, Eladawy M, Park J. Anesthesia for robotic thoracic surgery. *Ann Cardiothorac Surg.* 2019;8(2):263–268.
27. Budacan A-M, Naidu B. Fluid management in the thoracic surgical patient: where is the balance? *J Thorac Dis.* 2019;11(6):2205–2207.
28. Assaad S, Popescu W, Perrino A. Fluid management in thoracic surgery. *Curr Opin Anaesthesiol.* 2013;26(1):31–39.
29. Haas S, Eichhorn V, Hasback T, et al. Goal-directed fluid therapy using stroke volume variation does not result in pulmonary fluid overload in thoracic surgery requiring one-lung ventilation. *Crit Care Res Pract.* 2012:687018.
30. Li F, Ismail M, Elsner A, et al. Surgical techniques for myasthenia gravis: robotic-assisted thoracoscopic surgery. *Thorac Surg Clin.* 2019;29(2):177–186.
31. Grant I, Brovman EY, Kang D, Greenberg P, Saba R, Urman RD. A medicolegal analysis of positioning-related perioperative peripheral nerve injuries occurring between 1996 and 2015. *J Clin Anesth.* 2019;58:84–90.
32. Ahmed AB, Koster A, Lance M, Faraoni D. for the ESA VTE Guidelines Task Force. European guidelines on perioperative venous thromboembolism prophylaxis: cardiovascular and thoracic surgery. *Eur J Anaesthesiol.* 2018;35(2):84–89.
33. Brown JA. Lateral gluteal myonecrosis in a patient undergoing partial nephrectomy in the modified flank position. *Urology.* 2003; 61(2):462.
34. Newman NJ. Perioperative visual loss after nonocular surgeries. *Am J Ophthalmol.* 2008;145(4):604–610.
35. Emery SE, Daffner S, France J, et al. Effect of head position on intraocular pressure during lumbar spine fusion: a randomized, prospective study. *J Bone Joint Surg Am.* 2015;97(22):1817–1823.
36. Alemzadeh H, Raman J, Leven N, Kalbarczyk Z, Iyer RK. Adverse events in robotic surgery: a retrospective study of 14 Years of FDA data. *PLoS One.* 2016;11(4):e0151470.
37. Ius F, Sommer W, Tudorache I, et al. Five-year experience with intraoperative extracorporeal membrane oxygenation in lung transplantation: indications and midterm results. *J Heart Lung Transplant.* 2016;35(1):49–58.
38. Awab A, Khan MS, Youness HA. Whole lung lavage-technical details, challenges and management of complications. *J Thorac Dis.* 2017;9(6):1697–1706.
39. Hoetzenecker K, Klepetko W, Keshavjee S, Cypel M. Extracorporeal support in airway surgery. *J Thorac Dis.* 2017;9(7):2108–2117.
40. Malpas G, Hung O, Gilchrist A, et al. The use of extracorporeal membrane oxygenation in the anticipated difficult airway: a case report and systematic review. *Can J Anaesth.* 2018;65(6):685–697.
41. Rosskopfova P, Perentes JY, Ris H-B, Gronchi F, Krueger T, Gonzalez M. Extracorporeal support for pulmonary resection: current indications and results. *World J Surg Oncol.* 2016;14(1):25.
42. Maurizi G, D'Andrilli A, Vanni C, et al. Salvage resection of advanced mediastinal tumors. *J Thorac Dis.* 2019;11(suppl 13): S1653–S1661.
43. Fierro MA, Daneshmand MA, Bartz RR. Perioperative management of the adult patient on venovenous extracorporeal membrane oxygenation requiring non-cardiac surgery. *Anesthesiology.* 2018;128(1):181–201.
44. Kocher GJ, Zehnder A, Erdoes G, Seidl C, Winkler B, Schmid RA. Single-cannula, single-incision thoracoscopic anatomic segmentectomy after pneumonectomy. *J Thorac Cardiovasc Surg.* 2017;154(2):e29–e31.
45. Gillon SA, Toufektzian L, Harrison-Phipps K, Meadows CIS, Wyncoll DLA, Barret NA. Perioperative extracorporeal membrane oxygenation to facilitate lung resection after contralateral pneumonectomy. *Ann Thorac Surg.* 2016;101(3):e71–e73.
46. Miyamoto Y, Nagamine Y, Goto T, Kurahashi K. Intraoperative venovenous extracorporeal membrane oxygenation during thoracic surgery that requires 1-lung ventilation: a case report. *A A Pract.* 2018;10(4):79–82.
47. Bluth T, Pelosi P, de Abreu MG. The obese patient undergoing nonbariatric surgery. *Curr Opin Anaesthesiol.* 2016;29(3):421–429.
48. Shah U, Wong J, Wong DT, Chung F. Preoxygenation and intraoperative ventilation strategies in obese patients: a comprehensive review. *Curr Opin Anaesthesiol.* 2016;29(1):109–118.
49. Bazurro S, Ball L, Pelosi P. Perioperative management of obese patient. *Curr Opin Crit Care.* 2018;24(6):560–567.
50. Couture EJ, Provencher S, Somma J, Lellouche F, Marceau S, Bussières JS. Effect of position and positive pressure ventilation on functional residual capacity in morbidly obese patients: a randomized trial. *Can J Anaesth.* 2018;65(5):522–528.
51. Liou DZ, Berry MF. Thoracic surgery considerations in obese patients. *Thorac Surg Clin.* 2018;28(1):27–41.
52. Sanaie S, Bilejani I, Mortazavi M, et al. Effect of manual caudal and downward displacement of lower cervical adipose tissue on laryngoscopic grade of patients with morbid obesity. *Anesthesiol Pain Med.* 2018;8(1):e63061.
53. Verkhovsky A, Smit M, Levin A, Coetzee JF. Blood pressure measurement in obese patients: non-invasive proximal forearm versus direct intra-arterial measurements. *SAJAA.* 2018;24(3):70–74.
54. Meidert AS, Saugel B. Techniques for non-invasive monitoring of arterial blood pressure. *Front Med.* 2018;4(231) doi: 10.3389/fmed.2017.00231. eCollection 2017.
55. Rogge DE, Nicklas JY, Haas SA, Reuter DA, Saugel B. Continuous noninvasive arterial pressure monitoring in obese patients during bariatric surgery: an evaluation of the vascular unloading technique (ClearSight system). *Anesth Analg.* 2019;128(3):477–483.
56. Fernandez-Bustamante A, Hashimoto S, Sherpa Neto A, Moine P, Vidal Melo M, Repine JE. Perioperative lung protective ventilation in obese patients. *BMC Anesthesiol.* 2015;15:56.
57. Lalkhen AG, Bhatia K. Perioperative peripheral nerve injuries. *Contin Educ Anaesth Crit Care Pain.* 2011;12(1):38–42.

NON-PRINT ITEMS

Abstract

Ideal position should facilitate surgical procedures and anesthesia management, without causing harm to patients and any involved personnel. The aim of this chapter is to describe the most common positions used during thoracic noncardiac surgery, highlighting the challenges and physiologic changes associated with each one, and how to prevent possible complications.

Keywords

position, thoracic noncardiac surgery, complications, nerve injury, compartment syndrome

11

Monitoring of Oxygenation and Ventilation

BENJAMIN M. HYERS, JAMES B. EISENKRAFT

Introduction

During anesthesia for a thoracic surgical procedure, many alterations in physiology occur, including changes in oxygenation and ventilation. Whether the patient is receiving monitored anesthesia care (MAC), regional anesthesia, or general anesthesia, it is essential that the anesthesiologist monitor each patient diligently to optimize management and avoid complications. ("Vigilance" is the motto of the American Society of Anesthesiologists [ASA]). Monitoring of oxygenation and ventilation are of vital importance, particularly in thoracic anesthesia, where one-lung ventilation (OLV) is necessary in most cases. The anesthesiologist should be familiar with the various methods available to monitor oxygenation and ventilation, and how to correctly interpret data.

American Society of Anesthesiologists Standards for Basic Anesthetic Monitoring

The ASA has adopted two standards for basic anesthetic monitoring.[1] **Standard I** requires that qualified anesthesia personnel be present in the procedural room over the entirety of all general anesthetics, regional anesthetics, and MAC. **Standard II** (Box 11.1) requires continual evaluation of a patient's oxygenation, ventilation, circulation, and temperature during all anesthetics. This chapter will explore the various methods of monitoring oxygenation and ventilation and will emphasize their importance during thoracic anesthesia.

Oxygenation

Oxygen Cascade

The oxygen cascade refers to the process and pathway of oxygen being delivered from the atmosphere to a cell's mitochondria. It consists of four steps: (1) mass transport of oxygen from the atmosphere (or breathing circuit) to the alveolar spaces; (2) diffusion of oxygen from the alveoli to the blood in the pulmonary capillaries; (3) transport of blood from the pulmonary system to the systemic circulation; (4) diffusion of oxygen from the systemic circulation to each target tissue cell. Pathology that interrupts this pathway at any of its steps can cause hypoxemia resulting in tissue and organ dysfunction.[2] Monitoring a patient's oxygenation can occur at several places in this pathway.

The partial pressure of oxygen in the alveoli (P_AO_2) is approximately 100 mm Hg in a healthy patient breathing room air. This can be calculated by using the alveolar gas equation:

$$P_AO_2 = F_iO_2 \times (P_{atm} - P_{water}) - (P_ACO_2/R) \quad \text{(Eq. 11.1)}$$

where F_iO_2 is the fractional concentration of inspired oxygen in air (21%), P_{atm} is atmospheric pressure (760 mm Hg at sea level), P_{water} is the saturated vapor pressure of water at body temperature (47 mm Hg at 37° C), P_ACO_2 is the partial pressure of carbon dioxide in arterial blood (40 mm Hg), and R is the respiratory quotient (usually 0.8).

Hypoxemia results when there is ventilation-perfusion (V/Q) mismatch in the lungs. Regions of the lung that are ventilated but not perfused are termed dead space, whereas regions of the lung that are perfused but not ventilated are termed shunts. Dead space and shunts are the extreme opposite ends of the V/Q spectrum. Pulmonary vasculature demonstrates a phenomenon known as hypoxic pulmonary vasoconstriction (HPV), a protective mechanism that diverts blood away from parts of the lung that are not well ventilated and are hypoxic, to parts that are well ventilated in an effort to minimize V/Q mismatch.[3] This is an important mechanism during thoracic surgery to reduce the transpulmonary shunt during OLV (see Ch. 15).

The approximate transit time for a red blood cell to travel through the pulmonary capillary bed is 0.7 seconds. Four lung characteristics ensure an efficient transfer of oxygen from the alveoli to the pulmonary capillaries: a large oxygen partial pressure (PO_2) gradient, a thin diffusion barrier with a large surface area for gas exchange, a high diffusion

• BOX 11.1 American Society of Anesthesiologists Standards for Basic Anesthetic Monitoring

2. STANDARD II

During all anesthetics, the patient's oxygenation, ventilation, circulation, and temperature shall be continually evaluated.

2.1 Oxygenation

2.1.1 Objective

To ensure adequate oxygen concentration in the inspired gas and the blood during all anesthetics.

2.2 Methods

2.2.1 Inspired gas: During every administration of general anesthesia using an anesthesia machine, the concentration of oxygen in the patient breathing system shall be measured by an oxygen analyzer with a low oxygen concentration limit alarm in use.[a]

2.2.2 Blood oxygenation: During all anesthetics, a quantitative method of assessing oxygenation, such as pulse oximetry, shall be used.[a] When the pulse oximeter is used, the variable pitch pulse tone and the low threshold alarm shall be audible to the anesthesiologist or the anesthesia care team personnel.[a] Adequate illumination and exposure of the patient are necessary to assess color.[a]

3. VENTILATION

3.1 Objective

To ensure adequate ventilation of the patient during all anesthetics.

3.2 Methods

3.2.1 Every patient receiving general anesthesia shall have the adequacy of ventilation continually evaluated. Qualitative clinical signs, such as chest excursion, observation of the reservoir breathing bag, and auscultation of breath sounds are useful. Continual monitoring for the presence of expired carbon dioxide shall be performed unless invalidated by the nature of the patient, procedure, or equipment. Quantitative monitoring of the volume of expired gas is strongly encouraged.[a]

3.2.2 When an endotracheal tube or laryngeal mask is inserted, its correct positioning must be verified by clinical assessment and by identification of carbon dioxide in the expired gas. Continual end-tidal carbon dioxide analysis, in use from the time of endotracheal tube/laryngeal mask placement, until extubation/removal or initiating transfer to a postoperative care location, shall be performed using a quantitative method, such as capnography, capnometry, or mass spectroscopy.[a] When capnography or capnometry is used, the end-tidal CO_2 alarm shall be audible to the anesthesiologist or the anesthesia care team personnel.[a]

3.2.3 When ventilation is controlled by a mechanical ventilator, there shall be in continuous use a device that is capable of detecting disconnection of components of the breathing system. The device must give an audible signal when its alarm threshold is exceeded.

[a]Under extenuating circumstances, the responsible anesthesiologist may waive the requirements marked ([a]); it is recommended that when this is done, it should be so stated (including the reasons) in a note in the patient's medical record.

coefficient for oxygen, and the rapid binding of oxygen to hemoglobin. As oxygen diffuses from the alveoli into the plasma, it immediately enters an erythrocyte and is bound by hemoglobin. This ensures that the PO_2 in the plasma remains low, which is essential for continued diffusion of oxygen from the alveoli into the plasma inadvertently.[3]

Oxygen Analyzers

Probably the most important monitor on the anesthesia workstation is the oxygen analyzer with a low oxygen concentration alarm because it continuously monitors the concentration of oxygen (F_iO_2) that the patient will inspire from the breathing circuit. This is essential and should alert the anesthesiologist if a hypoxic gas mixture is inadvertently being delivered to the patient. Before oxygen analyzers were in general use, a number of complications and adverse outcomes were reported because of patients unintentionally receiving hypoxic gas mixtures.[4] Such scenarios may be caused by a hypoxic gas (e.g., nitrogen, nitrous oxide) being delivered in the oxygen pipeline, failure of the "fail safe system", failure of the nitrous oxide-oxygen proportioning system, system leaks, or low-flow anesthesia with inadequate flow of oxygen into the breathing system. The oxygen analyzer must be calibrated, and, if not performed by the workstation automatically, it is important to set the low oxygen concentration alarm limit and audible volume. The patient's inspired gas mixture is always sampled downstream of the inspiratory unidirectional valve in the circle breathing circuit.

The two most commonly used oxygen analyzers are the fuel cell and the paramagnetic oxygen analyzer.[5] The **fuel cell oxygen analyzer** is essentially a galvanic cell that acts as an oxygen battery. Oxygen diffuses from the breathing circuit through an oxygen-permeable membrane that covers the sensor of the fuel cell. Oxygen is first reduced to negative hydroxyl ions at the cathode. The hydroxyl ions then oxidize the metal at the anode. The overall chemical reaction produces a current and creates a voltage potential that is directly proportional to the PO_2 in the breathing circuit. The result is displayed on the anesthesia monitor, usually as a percentage of total inspired gas mixture. The fuel cell analyzer is calibrated by exposing it to room air (21%) at sea level. The analyzer actually measures partial pressure and not percentage. If it is calibrated to 21% at sea level and then exposed to room air (still 21% by volume) at a lower ambient pressure (i.e., at higher altitude), it will read less than 21%. The standard fuel cell oxygen analyzers are slow responding (~30 seconds) and measure average oxygen concentrations.[5] Exposure to oxygen causes the fuel cell to wear out over time and periodically it must be replaced.

The **paramagnetic oxygen analyzer** has a very rapid response time to changing oxygen concentrations. By sampling gas at the patient's airway (i.e., in the vicinity of the Y-piece in a circle breathing system), it provides for breath-by-breath monitoring of inspired and end-tidal oxygen concentrations. Oxygen molecules are paramagnetic and attracted to a magnetic field.[6] These analyzers have two chambers, a sampling chamber and a reference chamber, separated by a sensitive pressure transducer. The reference chamber receives room air and the sampling chamber receives the gas that is being aspirated from the breathing circuit. An electromagnet rapidly switches on and off, creating a changing magnetic field that causes oxygen molecules to be attracted and agitated. This creates a pressure differential in the pressure transducer, which is directly proportional to the oxygen partial pressure difference between the sampled gas and reference gas (room air). The pressure differential is converted to a DC voltage that is directly proportional to the PO_2. Paramagnetic oxygen analyzers require an in-line water trap in the gas sampling pathway because their function can be compromised by the presence of water vapor. The rapid response time of the paramagnetic oxygen analyzer allows breath-by-breath monitoring of oxygen concentration, the graphical display of which is termed the oxygram. Because oxygen and carbon dioxide (CO_2) are moving in opposite directions during respiration, the oxygram is a mirror image of the capnogram. Monitoring of inspired and end-tidal oxygen concentrations is valuable in determining the efficacy of preoxygenation in a patient breathing 100% oxygen before induction of anesthesia. Ideal preoxygenation exists when the end-tidal oxygen concentration is 95% and end-tidal CO_2 is 5%.[6]

Monitoring Blood Oxygenation

Oxygen content in arterial blood (CaO_2) has two components: oxygen that is bound to hemoglobin and oxygen that is dissolved in the blood. It is represented by Eq. 11.2.

$$CaO_2 = [1.34 \times Hgb \times (SaO_2)] + (0.003 \times P_AO_2) \quad \text{(Eq. 11.2)}$$

1.34 is the oxygen combining capacity of hemoglobin (Hgb) with units of mL O_2/g Hgb, Hgb is the hemoglobin concentration in units of grams of Hgb/100 mL blood, SaO_2 is the percent saturation of arterial hemoglobin, 0.003 is the solubility coefficient of oxygen in units of mL O_2/100 mL blood/mm Hg, and P_AO_2 is the partial pressure of oxygen in arterial blood in units of mm Hg.

The first part of Eq. 11.2 [in the brackets] represents the oxygen that is bound to hemoglobin, and the second part of Eq. 11.2 represents oxygen dissolved in the blood. The major contributor to the total oxygen content is the oxygen bound to hemoglobin because the dissolved component has the 0.003 conversion factor. Eq. 11.2 can also be used to determine the mixed venous blood oxygen content (CvO_2). By disregarding the dissolved component and assuming an SaO_2 of 100%, an SvO_2 (mixed venous saturation) of 75%, and a hemoglobin concentration of 15 g Hgb/100 mL blood, CaO_2 is 20 mL O_2/100 mL blood and CvO_2 (venous oxygen content) is 15 mL O_2/100 mL blood.

Arterial oxygen content is directly proportional to hemoglobin concentration and hemoglobin saturation. Hemoglobin saturation and P_AO_2 are related by the oxygen-hemoglobin dissociation curve, which is sigmoid in shape. In adults, a P_AO_2 of 27 mm Hg, 40 mm Hg, and 60 mm Hg correspond to hemoglobin saturations of 50%, 75%, and 90%, respectively. Because the oxygen-hemoglobin dissociation curve is sigmoid in shape, saturations all approach 100% for P_AO_2 values of 90 mm Hg or higher. Certain physiologic conditions can shift the oxygen-hemoglobin dissociation curve to the right, which facilitates oxygen unloading at the tissues. These include acidosis, hypercarbia, increased 2,3-diphosphoglycerate (2,3-DPG) concentrations, and hyperthermia. The opposite of these physiologic conditions, as well as the presence of fetal hemoglobin, causes the curve to shift to the left, which increases hemoglobin's affinity for oxygen and decreases release to the tissues.

The quantity of oxygen delivered to peripheral tissues (oxygen flux) per minute can be calculated by multiplying the CaO_2 by the cardiac output:

$$O_{2del} = CaO_2 \times \text{cardiac output} \times 10 \quad \text{(Eq. 11.3)}$$

O_{2del} is the amount of oxygen delivered to tissues by the arterial blood in units of mL O_2/min. The 10 is a necessary conversion factor because CaO_2 has units of mL O_2/100 mL blood and cardiac output has units of liters of blood per minute. Replacing CaO_2 with CvO_2 in Eq. 11.3 gives mL O_2/min that returns to the heart. Oxygen consumption (VO_2) can be calculated by subtracting oxygen returning from oxygen delivery using this form of the Fick equation:

$$VO_2 = \text{cardiac output} \times (CaO_2 - CvO_2) \times 10 \quad \text{(Eq. 11.4)}$$

Eq. 11.4 relates oxygen consumption to cardiac output, total hemoglobin concentration, arterial hemoglobin saturation, and mixed venous saturation.

Oxygenation during thoracic surgical procedures where OLV is used is determined by a variety of elements, including blood pressure, oxygen consumption, anesthetic effects on HPV, airway mechanics and reactivity, preexisting pulmonary disease, V/Q matching, and cardiac output. Significant desaturations can occur during OLV despite a high F_iO_2. This is caused by an obligate shunt in the nonventilated lung added to the intrapulmonary shunts present in the ventilated lung. Patients are typically placed in the lateral decubitus position for thoracotomies and thoracoscopies. In this position, rapid changes in oxygen saturation can occur secondary to compression of the mediastinal great vessels and intrapulmonary shunting.[7]

Pulse Oximetry

The pulse oximeter, a noninvasive monitor that provides continuous real-time estimates of arterial hemoglobin saturation with oxygen, can be used to warn the anesthesiologist of significant hypoxemia. It is essentially risk free to the patient and has revolutionized the practice of anesthesiology. It monitors oxygen at the level of the arterial blood, which helps to confirm that the lungs are able to transfer oxygen from the alveoli to the blood. However, the pulse oximeter does not guarantee that adequate oxygen is being delivered to, and used by, body tissues.

Principles of Operation

The principles of operation of the pulse oximeter are optical plethysmography, whereby the pulsatile change in volume at the probe site is detected optically, and spectrophotometry, which determines the proportion of hemoglobin that is saturated with oxygen (oxyhemoglobin) in pulsatile arterial blood. The spectrophotometry is an application of the Beer-Lambert law, which relates solute concentrations (in this case oxygenated and deoxygenated hemoglobin) to the intensity of light transmitted through a solution (in this case, blood). The standard pulse oximeter probe contains two light emitting diodes (LEDs) and a photodetector that are typically positioned opposite each other, separated by the arterial bed being monitored (usually a fingertip or ear lobe). The LEDs emit light at 660 nm and 940 nm because deoxyhemoglobin maximally absorbs light in the 600 to 750 nm range (red band) and oxyhemoglobin maximally absorbs light in the 850 to 1000 nm range (infrared band). The LEDs are turned on and off hundreds of times per second and absorption values at each wavelength are measured by the photodetector during pulsatile flow (arterial systole) and nonpulsatile flow (diastole). The absorption values measured from pulsatile flow (the pulse-added absorbance) is considered as originating from arterial blood, whereas nonpulsatile flow is caused by venous blood and background tissue absorptions (Fig. 11.1). The photodetector measures the absorptions of light at the two wavelengths and the software divides the pulsatile flow absorption values at each wavelength by the nonpulsatile flow absorption values to produce a ratio, R. An empiric algorithm is used to relate the ratio of absorptions, R, to a saturation reading designated as SpO_2. The most common locations to place pulse oximeter probes include the fingers, toes, ear lobes, and nasal ala.[8]

Advantages and Disadvantages

Clear advantages of the pulse oximeter for monitoring oxygenation compared with direct arterial blood sampling and analysis in a laboratory cooximeter and/or blood gas analyzer include its ability to provide continuous data noninvasively and rapidly. This is especially important in thoracic procedures during OLV. Hypoxemia can occur suddenly without warning, even when the patient is breathing 100% oxygen. Analyzing a patient's arterial blood directly for the arterial hemoglobin oxygen saturation takes time and requires invasive techniques (i.e., an arterial line). Because the pulse oximeter provides immediate and reliable data on a patient's arterial hemoglobin oxygen saturation, particularly during OLV, the anesthesiologist is alerted and can attempt to correct hypoxemia early on, and optimize oxygenation by performing maneuvers such as applying positive end-expiratory pressure (PEEP) to the ventilated lung or continuous positive airway pressure (CPAP) to the nonventilated lung, or resuming two-lung ventilation.[9]

There are some limitations associated with the pulse oximeter. Because it estimates oxygen saturation based on the relative amounts of oxyhemoglobin and deoxyhemoglobin present, it is not able to measure arterial oxygen tension. This means it cannot detect hypoxemia until the P_AO_2 approaches the steep portion of the sigmoid oxygen-hemoglobin dissociation curve at values of about 60 to 70 mm Hg. Furthermore, the saturation value (SpO_2) that is displayed on the monitor is reflective of data averaged over the previous 3 to 6 seconds. This delay may result in the anesthesiologist responding to a hypoxemic event close to a minute after it has occurred.[10] The sigmoid shape of the oxygen-hemoglobin dissociation curve also prevents the pulse oximeter from detecting hyperoxemia because the curve is flat at saturations close to and greater than 100%. According to the manufacturers, the standard deviation (SD) of the SpO_2 reading is $\pm2\%$ for SpO_2 values between 70% and 100%. This means that if the SpO_2 reads 95%, there is a 68% likelihood that the SaO_2 (actual saturation of a simultaneously drawn arterial blood sample measured in a laboratory cooximeter) will be between 93% and 97% (i.e., ±1 SD), and a 95% likelihood that SaO_2 will be between 91% and 99% (i.e., ±2 SD). Pulse oximeters are calibrated empirically with SaO_2 data measured using cooximetry in healthy volunteers exposed to decreasing concentrations of oxygen to yield saturations down to approximately 70%. Pulse oximetry values below this are estimated based on the trends of these data and therefore less reliable.

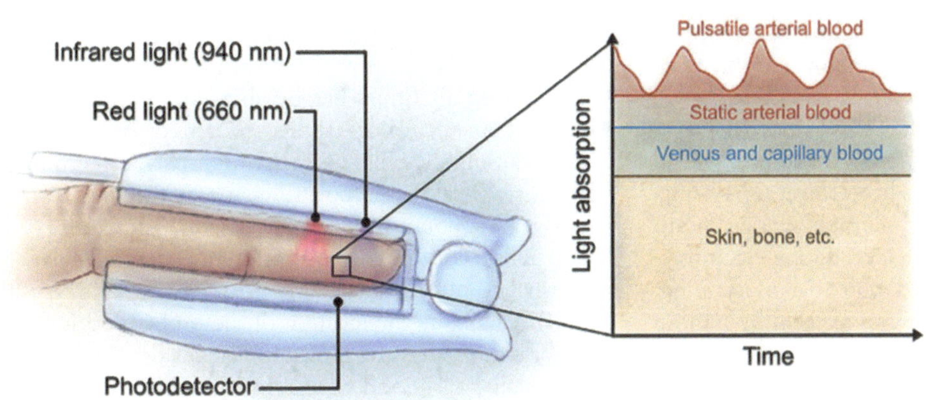

• **Fig. 11.1** Physical principle of pulse oximetry. Most of the tissue in the path of the light beam has a static pattern of absorption, but the volume of arterial blood (and therefore the absorption of light) varies in time with the pulse. (From ACE Question. *ASA Monitor.* 2020;84(8):12.)

Complications

Because the pulse oximeter is a noninvasive monitor, local complications are extremely uncommon. There have been reports of injury to digits on which the pulse oximeter probe was applied in critically ill patients. However, it is more likely that these injuries were caused by underlying pathology, such as hypoperfusion and vasopressor use.[11]

Spurious Readings and Sources of Error

There are many potential sources of error when using a pulse oximeter, which can lead to unreliable data. It is important for the anesthesiologist to have a high index of suspicion so that troubleshooting can occur sooner rather than later. A simple and quick first test to determine if the error is originating from the equipment is for the anesthesiologist to place the pulse oximeter probe on him or herself in the same location as on the patient.[12] Sources of error can essentially be broken down into three categories: inadequate waveform, spuriously normal or increased SpO_2 readings, and spuriously low SpO_2 readings.[13]

Inadequate Waveform. For the pulse oximeter to provide reliable data, there must be adequate pulsatile flow that produces an adequate optical plethysmographic waveform. The waveform is similar to that of the arterial pressure waveform, including a dicrotic notch. Improper probe placement, motion or noise artifact, hypoperfusion, and hypothermia can all lead to inadequate waveform. Usually the error that results is a spuriously low SpO_2 reading. During thoracic surgeries, cardiac arrythmias secondary to manipulation of lung parenchyma or the mediastinum can also disrupt pulse oximeter readings.

The pulse oximeter assumes that both wavelengths (660 and 940 nm) from the two LEDS are transmitted through the tissue so it can be detected by the photodetector on the other side of the tissue bed. Probe malpositioning or poor adherence to the patient's skin can prevent some of the light from passing through the tissue, rather bypassing it. This is called the penumbra effect and can lead to falsely high or low SpO_2 readings.[14] This can occur in patients with small fingers, such as children and infants. It is not recommended to place the pulse oximeter probe on the same side as the noninvasive blood pressure cuff because of the intermittent decrease in blood flow that occurs.[15] These issues can usually be solved by using a different digit or an ear probe to ensure that the LEDs and photodetector are aligned optimally.

A poor signal-to-noise ratio (i.e., amount of light from the LEDs reaching the photodetector vs. extraneous light) usually results in loss of the normal pulse oximeter waveform and leads to falsely low readings or no reading and an error message.[16] This can occur from shivering, seizing, and patient movement, and during neurophysiologic monitoring when the extremity is stimulated during electromyography or somatosensory evoked potential monitoring. Contemporary pulse oximeters are less affected by motion artifact.[17,18] Hypoperfusion and shivering can also lead to falsely low SpO_2 readings because the pulse oximeter is dependent on pulsatile blood flow. This is commonly seen in critically ill patients, patients with peripheral vascular disease, and patients on vasopressors. It was demonstrated that finger pulse oximeter SpO_2 measurements can be affected by peripheral vascular tone independent of temperature.[19] The accuracy of the pulse oximeter decreases significantly when the systolic blood pressure approaches 80 mm Hg.[20] In the case of hypothermia, warming the patient can remedy this problem. Another solution is switching to an ear probe.

Spuriously Normal and Increased Oxygen Saturation Readings. The pulse oximeter can display falsely normal or increased SpO_2 readings in a variety of situations, the most common cause being carbon monoxide (CO) poisoning. This can occur in patients exposed to fires or in chronic, heavy smokers. Carbon monoxide has a much greater affinity for hemoglobin compared with oxygen. In CO toxicity, the CO outcompetes the oxygen bound to hemoglobin. Because most oxygen content in the blood is contributed from the oxygen bound to hemoglobin, patients can suffer life-threatening arterial hypoxemia. CO absorbs light in the 660 nm wavelength range like oxyhemoglobin and is relatively transparent in the infrared region.[21] As a result, the pulse oximeter cannot distinguish between oxyhemoglobin and carboxyhemoglobin. Arterial oxygen tension will be normal on arterial blood gas monitoring because CO does not affect oxygen that is dissolved in blood. In this situation, laboratory cooximetry or pulse cooximetry (using a multiwavelength rather than a 2-wavelength pulse oximeter) should be used to measure carboxyhemoglobin levels.

Pulse oximetry theory predicts that skin pigment should not affect SpO_2, but SpO_2 tends to over-estimate SaO_2 in dark-skinned persons.[21] This positive bias (SpO_2-SaO_2) has been reported in one study as 3.56+2.45%, and increased in proportion to desaturation. The bias has been described as small at SaO_2 greater than 80% and probably of no general clinical significance but in darkly pigmented skin a bias of up to 8% was observed at lower SaO_2 levels. Monitoring oxygenation by SpO_2 in a dark-skinned patient may lead to "occult hypoxemia." When monitoring SpO_2 in a dark-skinned patient it may be prudent to increase the low SpO_2 alarm threshold to 94%, and draw an arterial blood sample for analysis if oxygenation is in doubt.

Spuriously Low Oxygen Saturation Readings. The pulse oximeter can also display falsely low SpO_2 readings for a variety of reasons. These include the presence of methemoglobin, severe anemia, venous congestion, skin pigmentation, black, green, or blue nail polish, and certain intravenous dyes. These abnormal hemoglobins and dyes absorb light in the 660 nm region (similar to deoxygenated hemoglobin), causing the pulse oximeter to display a spuriously low SpO_2 reading. In the operating room, the most common causes are suboptimal probe placement, the presence of dark nail polish, and the administration of intravenous dyes (i.e., methylene blue, indocyanine green, fluorescein, isosulfan blue). Changing the location of the probe, positioning the probe sideways so the transmitted light does not penetrate dark nail polish, and the rapid metabolism of most dyes used in the operating room address these problems.

Cooximetry

The conventional pulse oximeter uses only two wavelengths of light and assumes that only oxyhemoglobin and deoxyhemoglobin are present in the blood to determine the arterial saturation. When the presence of a dyshemoglobin is suspected, an arterial blood sample should be drawn and analyzed in a multiwavelength laboratory cooximeter (contemporary cooximeters use >100 wavelengths of light) to detect and accurately measure the species of hemoglobins that are present.

Oxygen Reserve Index

The oxygen reserve index (ORi) is a noninvasive and continuous monitor, like the pulse oximeter, that uses multiwavelength pulse cooximetry to display a number between one and zero. One indicates substantial oxygen reserve, whereas zero indicates no oxygen reserve. Its purpose is to provide insight into a patient's oxygenation status in the moderate hyperoxic range (P_AO_2 >100 ≤200 mm Hg), which is something the pulse oximeter is unable to do because the oxygen-hemoglobin dissociation curve flattens and approaches a SpO_2 value of 100% for P_AO_2 values more than 90 mm Hg (Fig. 11.2). Therefore the basic pulse oximeter can only provide insight into a patient's oxygenation status in the normoxic and hypoxic states. When supplemental oxygen is administered to a patient resulting in a hyperoxic state, arterial blood gas monitoring is necessary to measure P_AO_2 to assess the patient's oxygenation status. This takes time and provides only intermittent data. Monitoring a patient's oxygenation with both standard pulse oximetry and the ORi can widen the visibility of that patient's oxygen status.[13]

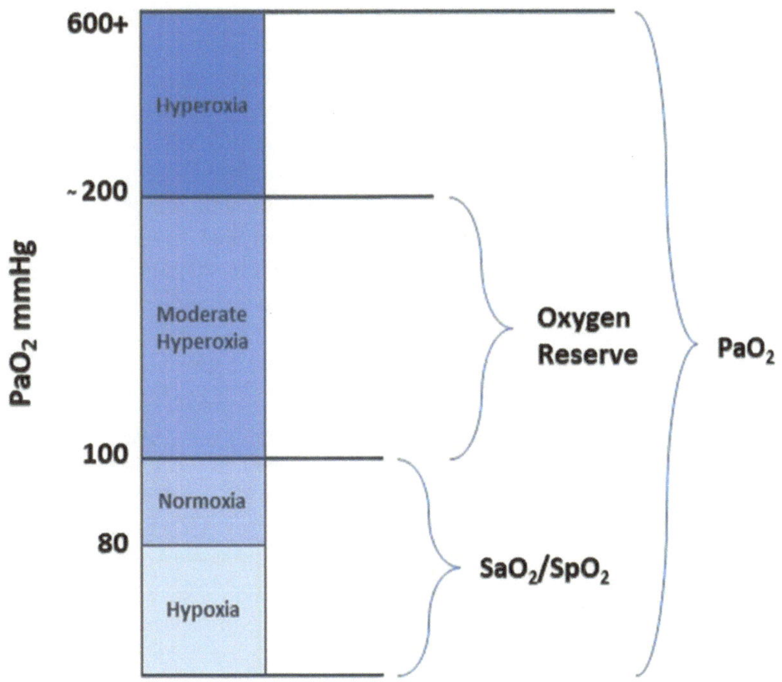

• **Fig. 11.2** Range of oxygenation states that can be assessed with the percent saturation of arterial hemoglobin (SaO_2)/oxygen saturation (SpO_2), oxygen reserve index, and arterial oxygen partial pressure (P_AO_2). (Modified with permission from Masimo).

Using the ORi with a pulse oximeter may be a better way of monitoring oxygenation in patients undergoing surgeries requiring OLV compared with using a standard pulse oximeter alone. Studies have shown that for P_AO_2 values less than 240 mm Hg, there is a positive correlation with ORi.[23] Studies have also shown that ORi decreases before SpO_2 when inducing anesthesia in adult and pediatric patients.[24,25] Koishi et al. showed that the ORi decreased significantly earlier than SpO_2 during OLV, with a mean response of 200 seconds; they also confirmed that ORi and P_AO_2 are highly correlated during OLV. Limitations in these studies included a variety of factors including small sample size and extreme exclusion criteria.[26] Although more research needs to be done, these preliminary studies suggest that ORi may be a very useful and beneficial monitor during thoracic surgeries.

Ventilation

Carbon Dioxide Cascade

The CO_2 cascade is essentially the opposite of the oxygen cascade. CO_2 is produced by cellular metabolism and diffuses into the blood down a concentration gradient. It is transported in the blood by three different mechanisms: (1) dissolved in plasma; (2) as bicarbonate (HCO_3^-); (3) bound to hemoglobin as carbaminohemoglobin. About 10% of CO_2 is dissolved in blood plasma to a partial pressure of about 45 mm Hg.[27] Another 10% of CO_2 is bound to hemoglobin as carbaminohemoglobin. The vast majority of CO_2 diffuses into capillary erythrocytes and is converted to carbonic acid (H_2CO_3) by the enzyme carbonic anhydrase. Carbonic acid then quickly dissociates into a hydrogen ion and bicarbonate. These species are all in equilibrium with each other, as represented by Eq. 11.5.

$$CO_2 + H_2O \leftrightarrow H_2CO_3 \leftrightarrow H^+ + HCO_3^- \quad \text{(Eq. 11.5)}$$

The constant production of CO_2 in tissues drives this reaction to the right according to Le Chatelier's principle. Hemoglobin acts as a buffer by binding the H^+ ions, and bicarbonate is transported out of the erythrocytes to the plasma by the HCO_3^-/Cl^- exchanger, further shifting this reaction to the right.

As blood is returned to the lungs, the reaction is reversed, allowing CO_2 to diffuse down its concentration gradient into the alveoli to be exhaled. This is known as the Haldane effect. Hemoglobin becomes more acidic as it binds oxygen, causing protons to dissociate. The increase in hydrogen ions promotes bicarbonate back into erythrocytes and forces the reaction to the left to produce CO_2. In addition, oxygen binding to hemoglobin decreases the affinity of CO_2 for hemoglobin, promoting its dissociation.[28]

Respiratory Rate and Volume Measurement

A patient's minute ventilation is the product of the respiratory rate and tidal volume. Direct observation of the respiratory rate can be used to monitor ventilation; however, this can be challenging for a number of reasons, such as interobserver variability, length of time needed for accurate measurements, and confounding effects (i.e., upper airway obstruction can cause chest wall movement). Therefore other means of monitoring the respiratory rate are more valuable to the anesthesiologist. Respiration can be measured directly, by means of airflow sensors, or indirectly by taking into account changes in thoracic dimension or breath sounds. In the operating room, the most practical way of monitoring respiration is with capnography, as discussed later.

Dead Space

Dead space is that part of tidal volume that does not participate in gas exchange. It corresponds to those areas of the lung that are well ventilated but not perfused.[29,30] Physiologic dead space comprises three components (Fig. 11.3): mechanical/apparatus, anatomic, and alveolar. **The mechanical component** consists of the artificial airways (i.e., tracheal tube, laryngeal mask airway, "goose neck" extension) and anything else that is located between the patient's airway and the Y-piece in the breathing circuit. **The anatomic component** consists of the volume of gas that fills the trachea, bronchi, and bronchioles where no gas exchange takes place. **The alveolar component** consists of the alveoli that are well ventilated but not perfused. Mechanical dead space can be increased, possibly up to 50 mL (depending on the manufacturer), in thoracic surgeries because typically extra connectors are placed between the double-lumen tube (DLT) and the Y-piece.[31] When this is combined with the shunting that occurs during OLV, significant impairment of gas exchange can occur.[32]

OLV can predispose a patient to ventilator-induced lung injury from volume overdistension (volutrauma). Tidal volumes can be decreased to minimize the risk of lung injury. However, as tidal volumes decrease, a greater fraction of each breath does not participate in gas exchange because apparatus and anatomic dead space remains constant and alveolar ventilation is decreased. Taking into consideration the effects of changes in ventilation on dead space during thoracic surgeries is important so the anesthesiologist can balance alveolar ventilation with lung protective ventilation settings to reduce the risk of lung injury.

Spirometry

Spirometry is used in the operating rooms and intensive care units to help assess ventilation and airway issues.[33] The spirometry display in the operating room is typically shown in graphic form (spirogram). Four variables can typically be at play: time, volume, flow, and pressure. Spirometry curves depict two of these variables in a visual format. Typically, time is shown on the x-axis and either volume, flow, or pressure on the y-axis. Volume-time curves show inhalation/inspiration as an upslope and exhalation as a downslope. Auto-PEEP, forced exhalation, expiratory limb leaks, and flow transducer miscalibration can all be identified using these curves.[34,35]

Flow-time curves can be depicted in many different shapes including square, decelerating, descending ramp, or sine flow patterns when controlled ventilation is used. The type of ventilation dictates the shape of these curves.

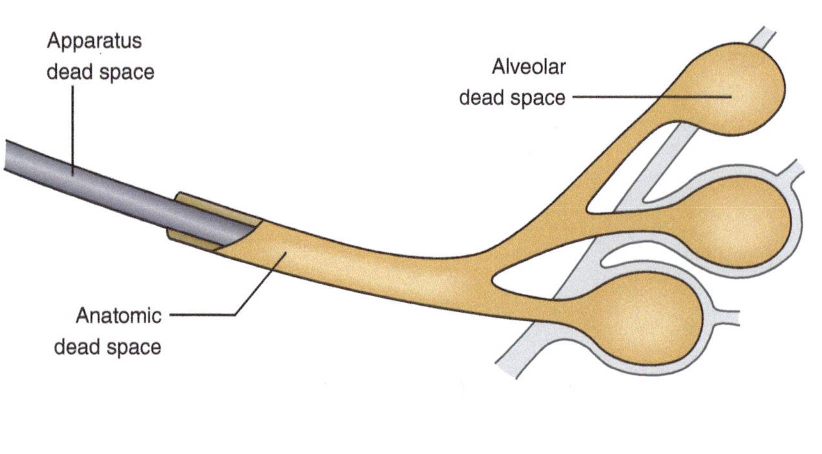

• **Fig. 11.3** The three components to an anesthetized patient's dead space: mechanical/apparatus, anatomic, and alveolar. (From Berry JM, Eisenkraft JB. Monitoring ventilation. In: Ehrenwerth J, Eisenkraft JB, Berry JM, eds. *Anesthesia Equipment: Principles and Applications*. 3rd ed. New York: Elsevier; 2021.)

For example, pressure control or pressure support ventilation yields a decelerating or descending pattern. Peak flow is delivered early in this case and decreases until the set pressure is reached. Volume control, on the other hand, yields a square flow pattern resulting in a shorter inspiratory time and longer expiratory time. High peak inspiratory pressure increases the risk of ventilator-associated lung injury. This is especially undesirable when OLV is used during thoracic surgeries.

Pressure-volume loops depict pressure on the x-axis and volume on the y-axis. Their shape and characteristics depend on the mode of ventilation used. Negative pressures will only be seen during spontaneous ventilation. Negative pressures seen during mechanical ventilation indicate equipment malfunction. The pressure-volume loops move counterclockwise during mechanical ventilation and clockwise during spontaneous ventilation.

Compliance is defined as the change in volume per unit change in pressure; resistance is defined as pressure per unit of flow. Secretions, kinking of the tracheal tube, and obstructions that decrease the diameter of the tube all act to increase airway resistance.[36] Increased resistance in the circuit causes bowing and widening of the pressure-volume loop, whereas low lung compliance causes the slope of the pressure-volume loop to decrease (Fig. 11.4). This happens during OLV or when unintentional endobronchial intubation occurs. A decrease in expiratory flow is also seen.

Airway Pressures

Measuring airway pressure is important when monitoring ventilation. Pressure sensors can detect mechanical problems, such as breathing circuit disconnection or tracheal tube occlusion, circuit leaks, inspiratory limb kinking, fresh gas flow line kinking or disconnection, low and high waste gas scavenging system pressure, high circuit pressure, and kinking of the circuit pressure-sensing hose.[4] Airway and alveolar pressures can also be monitored.

During mechanical ventilation, positive airway pressure provides a transpulmonary inflation gradient that delivers a tidal volume. This pressure may be constant or may vary during the inspiratory phase of the respiratory cycle. The airway pressure-time product divided by the total cycle time equals mean airway pressure. **Mean airway pressure** best approximates alveolar pressure and also correlates with alveolar ventilation, venous return, arterial oxygenation, and barotrauma risk. **Peak airway pressure** is the total airway pressure that includes work to overcome the flow resistance of tidal volume administration and the inherent properties (compliance) of the lungs. Lung and chest wall compliance, partial occlusions, secretions, and tracheal tube resistance all affect peak airway pressure. **Plateau pressure** is measured during the inspiratory pause when there is no gas flow and therefore no resistance.

Patient position and the different ventilatory modes used during mechanical ventilation can affect airway pressures. During thoracic surgeries, patients are often placed in the lateral decubitus position. Increased intraabdominal pressure and restricted lateral chest wall movement can both contribute to increased airway pressures because of decreases in compliance.[37] Volume control ventilation delivers the set tidal volume because pressure increases until this volume (or a pressure limit) is reached. Patients with acute respiratory distress syndrome or other low lung compliance conditions may require high airway pressures to deliver the desired volume. Pressure control ventilation involves setting a pressure, and the volume that is delivered is not only dependent on lung and chest wall compliance, but also airway resistance. Patients with low lung compliance may not receive adequate tidal volumes, resulting in hypoventilation. Pressure support ventilation applies a set positive pressure that is maintained throughout inspiration when a patient makes an inspiratory effort. The volume that is delivered depends on the pressure set, airway resistance and compliance, and inspiratory time and effort.

Capnography and Capnometry

Arguably the most important monitor of ventilation is capnometry. Capnometry measures the concentration of carbon dioxide in respired gases. The data can be displayed as a capnogram, which is the visual, continuous, time-based monitoring of carbon dioxide throughout the respiratory cycle in

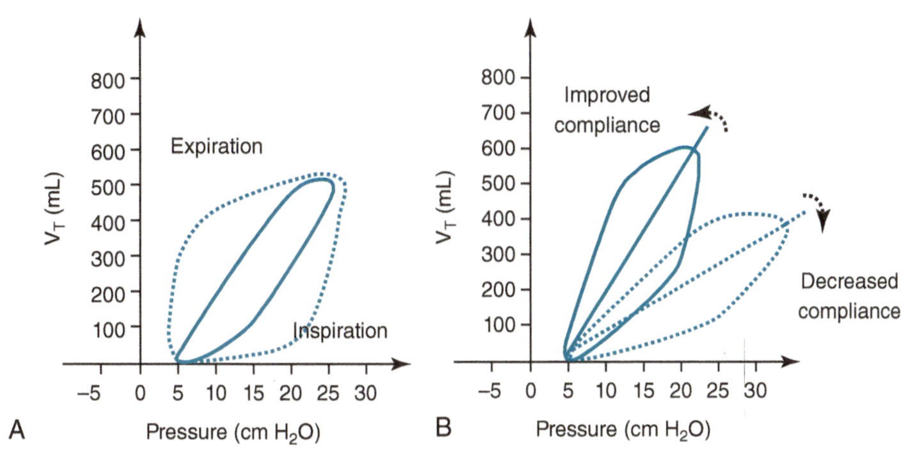

• **Fig. 11.4** Pressure-volume loops with tidal volume on the y-axis. *Solid lines* are normal loops. (**A**) Increased airway resistance indicated by bowing and widening of the dotted loop. (**B**) Decreased compliance indicated by a decreased slope of the *dotted loop*. (From Berry JM, Eisenkraft JB. Monitoring ventilation. In: Ehrenwerth J, Eisenkraft JB, Berry JM, eds. *Anesthesia Equipment: Principles and Applications*. 3rd ed. New York: Elsevier; 2021.)

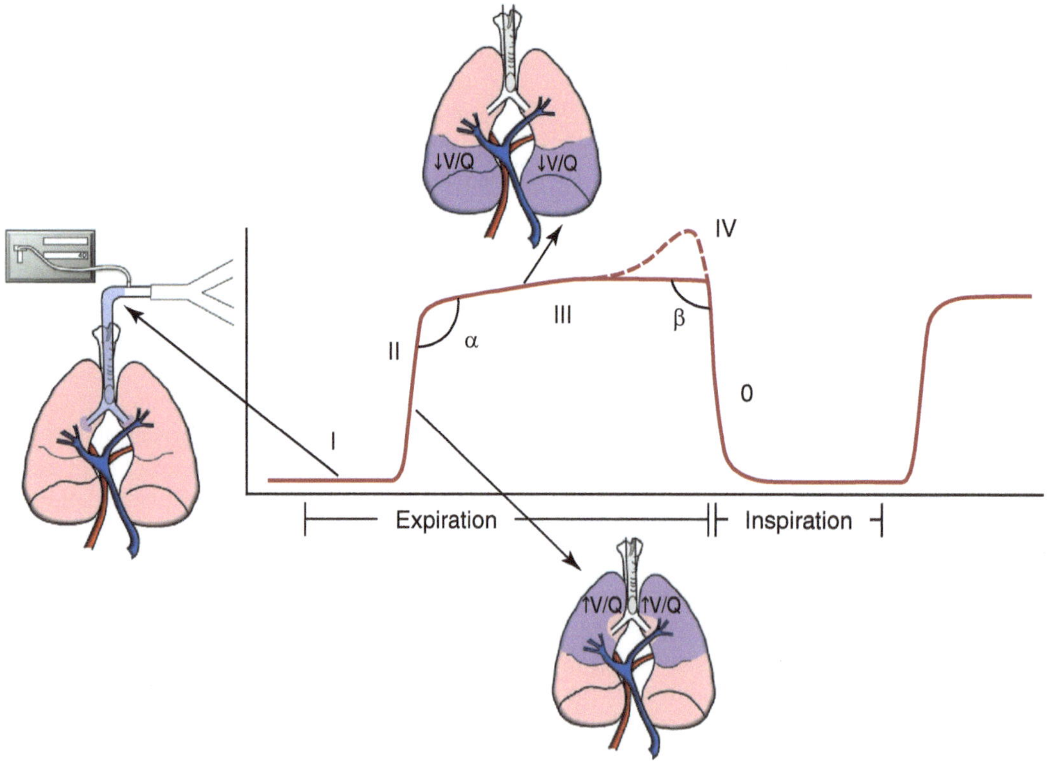

• **Fig. 11.5** A typical capnogram of the upright lung during controlled mechanical ventilation. (From Gravenstein N, Jaffe MB. In: Ehrenwerth J, Eisenkraft JB, Berry JM, eds. *Anesthesia Equipment: Principles and Applications*. 3rd ed. New York: Elsevier; 2021.)

graphic form.[38,39] The gold standard for carbon dioxide monitoring is arterial blood gas analysis, but this would require an invasive procedure (i.e., arterial line placement) and, importantly, time to process each sample.[40] Because CO_2 levels can fluctuate rapidly, the continuous nature of capnography with end-tidal CO_2 monitoring makes this monitor essential for monitoring ventilation in anesthetized patients.

CO_2 is measured by a CO_2 analyzer (capnometer), which can be located in the airway itself (mainstream) or nearby on the anesthesia workstation (sidestream sampling). Mainstream, or in-line, capnography positions the CO_2 analyzer in the airway so gas analysis occurs in situ. Sidestream capnography involves sampling respired gases at a rate of about 200 mL/min through a small tube that conducts these gases to the CO_2 analyzer. Although there are several methods by which CO_2 can be measured, the most common uses absorption of infrared (IR) radiation because CO_2 strongly absorbs IR light at a wavelength of 4.3 nm. The amount of IR light absorbed is directly proportional to the partial pressure of CO_2, which can be derived by comparing the measured absorbance to a known standard concentration of CO_2. Other CO_2 measurement techniques include mass spectroscopy, molecular correlation spectrography, Raman spectroscopy, and photoacoustic spectrography, but these are more expensive and are rarely used nowadays.[4]

The appearance of a normal capnogram is important to understand because variants from this normal shape may indicate pathology. This is especially important in thoracic anesthesia because the typical patient often has significant pulmonary pathology and a chronic smoking history that could produce an abnormal capnogram in the operating room. A typical capnogram (Fig. 11.5) has a characteristic shape with an inspiratory and expiratory segment that flow into each other. **Phase 0** occurs during inspiration with end-tidal CO_2 approaching zero. The expiratory segment is typically divided into three phases. **Phase I** occurs immediately after inspiration ceases. As the lungs recoil, gas from the apparatus and anatomic dead spaces pass by the CO_2 sampling point. **Phase II** is denoted by a sharp upstroke in the capnogram, which represents CO_2-rich alveolar gas replacing CO_2-free gas from the apparatus and anatomic dead spaces. The alpha angle separates phase II and phase III and it correlates with sequential emptying of the alveoli and V/Q matching. **Phase III** occurs when the capnogram plateaus with a slightly increasing slope and represents the exhalation of CO_2-rich gas from the gas-exchanging alveoli. CO_2 continues to rise very slightly during this phase because of steady excretion of CO_2 into the alveoli and also late emptying of alveoli with lower V/Q ratios (relatively higher PCO_2). The beta angle immediately follows phase III and is normally at a 90-degree angle. This represents the inspiratory phase when CO_2-free gas passes by the CO_2 sampling point.

The characteristic shape of the capnogram will change in certain conditions. End-tidal CO_2 above zero during phase 0 is suggestive of CO_2 rebreathing, which can be caused by an incompetent unidirectional (inspiratory

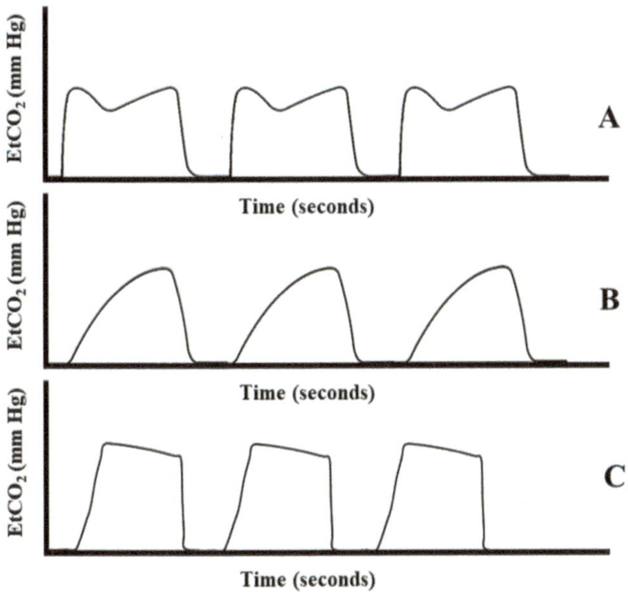

• **Fig. 11.6** Common capnograms seen during thoracic surgical procedures. **(A)** depicts a biphasic capnogram; **(B)** depicts a capnogram with increasing phase III slope; **(C)** depicts a capnogram with reverse phase III.

or expiratory) valve, exhausted CO_2 absorbent, gas channeling through the absorbent, or an imperfectly calibrated capnometer. When the upstroke of phase II becomes slanted or S-shaped, this suggests gas flow obstruction (e.g., a kinked tracheal tube, chronic obstructive pulmonary disease, acute bronchospasm). As V/Q mismatching worsens, the alpha angle and the slope in phase III increase. This could be caused by changes in airway resistance, functional residual capacity, CO_2 production, or cardiac output. The beta angle increases and the capnogram may not return to baseline if caused by a malfunctioning inspiratory valve, rebreathing, and a low tidal volume-high respiratory rate setting. Capnography can also detect esophageal intubation, breathing circuit disconnection, cardiac output changes, and pulmonary embolism.

Continuous end-tidal CO_2 monitoring is considered the most sensitive method to detect a breathing circuit disconnect, although low pressure alarms respond faster. This ensures the problem can be addressed before changes in SpO_2 and heart rate occur.

Fig. 11.6 depicts three capnograms that may be seen specifically during thoracic surgical procedures. "A" shows a biphasic capnogram. This occurs when the lungs have different V/Q matching and exhalation time constants. When patients are in the lateral decubitus position during two lung ventilation, the upper, nondependent lung has a high V/Q ratio, low airway resistance, and low CO_2 concentration, whereas the lower, dependent lung has a low V/Q ratio, higher airway resistance, and higher CO_2 concentration. Expired gases (with low CO_2) from the nondependent lung are responsible for the first part of this capnogram and expired gases (with higher CO_2) from the dependent lung are responsible for the second part of this capnogram. A biphasic capnogram can also be seen after a single lung transplant because two different populations of alveoli exist with different time constants. "B" shows a capnogram with increased phase III slopes which represents a large spread of V/Q ratios or obstruction. "C" shows a reverse phase III capnogram that could be seen in patients with emphysema.[41]

Gas for end-tidal CO_2 monitoring is typically sampled just proximal to the endotracheal tube. This ensures monitoring of the gas exhaled from both lungs. However, if one lung has significant pathology, this may not be as helpful as dual capnography, which can monitor end-tidal CO_2 from each lung separately as long as a DLT is in place. Bhavani-Shankar et al. suggest attaching each gas sampling line to a three-way stopcock connected to a line that connects to the capnometer. This allows the anesthesiologist to monitor end-tidal CO_2 simultaneously from both lungs or from each lung separately. Dual capnography is useful in patients who cannot tolerate OLV long enough to reach a steady state because then the ventilation-perfusion status can be determined for each lung individually.[42]

Conclusion

Anesthesiologists use a variety of monitors to assess a patient's oxygenation and ventilation status during surgery. These include pulse oximetry, spirometry, airway pressure, and capnometry. These real time, continuous monitors alert the anesthesiologist early on to dangerous situations, which helps ensure the safety of the patient. The changes in physiology that occur during OLV make these monitors especially important because life-threatening changes in oxygenation and ventilation can occur very quickly. Anesthesiologists should be familiar with these monitors, how to use them, and how to interpret their data correctly.

References

1. Standards for Basic Anesthetic Monitoring. American Society of Anesthesiologists. Last Amended: October 28, 2015 (original approval: October 21, 1986). Shaumburg, IL: The American Society of Anesthesiologists.
2. Biro GP. From the atmosphere to the mitochondrion: the oxygen cascade. In: Kim H, Greenburg A, eds. *Hemoglobin-Based Oxygen Carriers as Red Cell Substitutes and Oxygen Therapeutics*. Berlin, Heidelberg: Springer; 2013.
3. Lumb AB. *Nunn's Applied Respiratory Physiology*. 8th ed. New York: Elsevier; 2017.
4. Eisenkraft JB, Jaffe MB. Hazards of the anesthesia workstation. In: Ehrenwerth J, Eisenkraft JB, Berry JM, eds. *Anesthesia Equipment: Principles and Applications*. 3rd ed. New York: Elsevier; 2021.

5. Jaffe MB, Eisenkraft JB, Orr J. Respiratory gas monitoring. In: Ehrenwerth J, Eisenkraft JB, Berry JM, eds. *Anesthesia Equipment: Principles and Applications.* 3rd ed. New York: Elsevier; 2021.
6. Garg R, Gupta RC. Analysis of oxygen, anaesthesia agent and flows in anaesthesia machine. *Indian J Anaesth.* 2013;57(5):481–488.
7. Slinger PD, ed. *Principles and Practice of Anesthesia for Thoracic Surgery (Second)*: Springer; 2019.
8. Morey TE, Rice MJ, Vasilopoulos T, et al. Feasibility and accuracy of nasal alar pulse oximetry. *Br J Anaesth.* 2014;112:1109.
9. Brodsky JB, Shulman MS, Swan M, Mark JB. Pulse oximetry during one-lung ventilation. *Anesthesiology.* 1985;63(2):212–214.
10. Jubran A. Pulse oximetry. *Crit Care.* 2015;19:272.
11. Wille J, Braams R, van Haren WH, van der Werken C. Pulse oximeter-induced digital injury: frequency rate and possible causative factors. *Crit Care Med.* 2000;28:3555.
12. Ralston AC, Webb RK, Runciman WB. Potential errors in pulse oximetry. III: Effects of interferences, dyes, dyshaemoglobins and other pigments. *Anaesthesia.* 1991;46:291.
13. Barker SJ. Pulse oximetry. In: Ehrenwerth J, Eisenkraft JB, Berry JM, eds. *Anesthesia Equipment: Principles and Applications.* 3rd ed. New York: Elsevier; 2021.
14. Guan Z, Baker K, Sandberg WS. Misalignment of disposable pulse oximeter probes results in false saturation readings that influence anesthetic management. *Anesth Analg.* 2009;109:1530.
15. Mardirossian G, Schneider RE. Limitations of pulse oximetry. *Anesth Prog.* 1992;39:194.
16. Ortega R, Hansen CJ, Elterman K, Woo A. Videos in clinical medicine. Pulse oximetry. *N Engl J Med.* 2011;364:e33.
17. Barker SJ. Motion-resistant" pulse oximetry: a comparison of new and old models. *Anesth Analg.* 2002;95:967.
18. Gehring H, Hornberger C, Matz H, et al. The effects of motion artifact and low perfusion on the performance of a new generation of pulse oximeters in volunteers undergoing hypoxemia. *Respir Care.* 2002;47:48.
19. Talke P, Stapelfeldt C. Effect of peripheral vasoconstriction on pulse oximetry. *J Clin Monit Comput.* 2006;20:305.
20. Hinkelbein J, Genzwuerker HV, Fiedler F. Detection of a systolic pressure threshold for reliable readings in pulse oximetry. *Resuscitation.* 2005;64:315.
21. Sjoding MW, Dickson RP, Iwashyna TJ, Gay SE, Valley TS. Racial Bias in Pulse Oximetry Measurement. *New England Journal of Medicine.* 2020;383:2477–8.
22. Hampson NB. Pulse oximetry in severe carbon monoxide poisoning. *Chest.* 1998;114:1036.
23. Applegate RL 2nd, Dorotta IL, Wells B, Juma D, Applegate PM. The relationship between oxygen reserve index and arterial partial pressure of oxygen during surgery. *Anesth Analg.* 2016;123:626–633.
24. Yoshida K, Isosu T, Noji Y, Hasegawa M, Iseki Y, Oishi R, et al. Usefulness of oxygen reserve index (ORi™), a new parameter of oxygenation reserve potential, for rapid sequence induction of general anesthesia. *J Clin Monit Comput.* 2018;32(4):687–691.
25. Szmuk P, Steiner JW, Olomu PN, Ploski RP, Sessler DI, Ezri T. Oxygen reserve index: a novel noninvasive measure of oxygen reserve—a pilot study. *Anesthesiology.* 2016;124:779–784.
26. Koishi W, Kumagai M, Ogawa S, Hongo S, Suzuki K. Monitoring the oxygen reserve index can contribute to the early detection of deterioration in blood oxygenation during one-lung ventilation. *Minerva Anestesiol.* 2018;84(9):1063–1069.
27. Hsia CC. Respiratory function of hemoglobin. *N Engl J Med.* 1998;338(4):239–247.
28. Jensen FB. Red blood cell pH, the Bohr effect, and other oxygenation-linked phenomena in blood O_2 and CO_2 transport. *Acta Physiol Scand.* 2004;182(3):215–227.
29. Sinha P, Flower O, Soni N. Deadspace ventilation: a waste of breath!. *Intensive Care Med.* 2012;2:303–314.
30. Tusman G, Suarez Sipmann F, Böhm SH. Rationale of dead space measurement by volumetric capnography. *Anesth Analg.* 2012;114:866–874.
31. Tusman G, Böhm SH, Suarez-Sipmann F, et al. Lung recruitment improves the efficiency of ventilation and gas exchange during one-lung ventilation anesthesia. *Anesth Analg.* 2004;98:1604–1609.
32. Tusman G, Böhm SH, Suarez-Sipmann F. Dead space during one-lung ventilation. *Curr Opin Anaesthesiol.* 2015;28(1):10–17.
33. Pierce R. Spirometry: an essential clinical measurement. *Aust Fam Physician.* 2005;34:535–539.
34. Lian JX. Understanding ventilator waveforms and how to use them in patient care. *Nurs Crit Care.* 2009;4:43–55.
35. Berry JM, Eisenkraft JB. Monitoring ventilation*Anesthesia Equipment: Principles and Applications.* 3rd ed. New York: Elsevier; 2021.
36. Weissman C. Flow-volume relationships during spontaneous breathing through endotracheal tubes. *Crit Care Med.* 1992;20:615–620.
37. Iwasaka H, Itoh K, Miyakawa H, Kitano T, Taniguchi K, Honda N. Continuous monitoring of ventilatory mechanics during one-lung ventilation. *J Clin Monit.* 1996;12(2):161–164.
38. Cheifetz IM, Myers TR. Should every mechanically ventilated patient be monitored with capnography from intubation to extubation? *Respir Care.* 2007;52:423–438.
39. Gravenstein N, Jaffe MB. Capnography*Anesthesia Equipment: Principles and Applications.* 3rd ed. New York: Elsevier; 2021.
40. Eberhard P. The design, use, and results of transcutaneous carbon dioxide analysis: current and future directions. *Anesth Analg.* 2007;105:S48–S52.
41. Kodali Bhavani. Shankar. *Capnography.* 2019. Mar. www.capnography.com/.
42. Shankar KB, Moseley HSL, Kumar AY. Dual end tidal CO_2 monitoring and double lumen tubes. *Can J Anaesth.* 1992;39:100–101.

12

Hemodynamic Monitoring in Thoracic Surgical Patients

KARL D. HILLENBRAND, ROBERT H. THIELE

Introduction

Thoracic surgery is a rapidly changing surgical subspecialty that presents the anesthesiology community with a myriad of challenges, one of which is hemodynamic monitoring. Thoracic surgical patients range from relatively healthy adults with refractory gastroesophageal reflux in need of a laparoscopic Nissen fundoplication, to patients with severe atherosclerosis and chronic obstructive pulmonary disease needing a pneumonectomy for cancer resection, to patients in need of lung transplantation. The 30-day mortality for this population ranges from less than 1% for wedge resections, to almost 4% for pneumonectomies, and to 6% for lung transplantation.[1,2] By comparison, 30-day mortality for coronary artery bypass grafting is approximately 1%.[3] Complicating hemodynamic monitoring and management of this population is the deep interdependence between the cardiac and pulmonary systems. The combination of comorbidities, invasiveness of the procedure, impact of thoracic surgery on oxygenation and hemodynamics, and challenges associated with monitoring make thoracic surgical procedures some of the most challenging and rewarding procedures that an anesthesiologist will manage.

Blood Pressure Monitoring

Oscillometry

Oscillometric blood pressure measurement is by far the most popular method of measuring blood pressure in the operating room (OR) in developed countries—at academic medical centers in the United States, 84% of surgical patients receive oscillometry alone.[4] The engineering principles behind oscillometry were first described in 1876 by Marey.[5] With the oscillometric technique, a cuff is inflated to a pressure higher than the systolic blood pressure (SBP), which occludes all flow to the extremity. At this occlusion pressure, no (Korotkoff) sounds are produced on auscultation, and pulsatile pressure transmitted to the cuff is minimal (Fig. 12.1). Gradually (or stepwise), the cuff is deflated until the pressure is below the diastolic blood pressure (DBP). As the pressure within the cuff is deflated, blood begins to flow into the extremity, which produces oscillations in the cuff pressure, which can be measured and recorded. As noted by Posey et al., the pressure within the cuff at which oscillations are maximal is closely correlated with mean arterial pressure (MAP).[6] The algorithms used to determine SBP and DBP are propriety to each manufacturer.

The introduction of oscillometric blood pressure measurement offered to the anesthesiologists many advantages in an OR environment when compared with the classic auscultatory noninvasive method: it can be automated (freeing up the anesthesia provider to perform other tasks), it requires significantly less skill and training to use, it can be more forgiving in patient positions in which frequent access to a distal artery for auscultation would prove difficult or impossible, and it is easier to use in a noisy OR environment.

Unlike intra arterial catheters, which are site independent (measured blood pressure does not change with movement of the extremity as long as the level of the transducer is not changed), oscillometric cuffs measure blood pressure at a specific location, irrespective of its location relative to the right atrium. The anesthesiologist caring for the thoracic surgical patient must therefore take care to account for cuff position relative to the organ of interest when interpreting blood pressure values. Given the frequent use of lateral positioning during thoracic procedures, the extremity on which the blood pressure cuff is placed may be higher or lower than the heart and brain, which are the primary organs of interest for blood pressure management. The arterial system is valve-less, and the pressure within it will therefore fall linearly with increasing height against gravity. However, given that blood pressure is measured in mm Hg and mercury is far denser than blood, a correction factor (0.74 mm Hg lower for every 1 cm) must be applied to measure the impact of these changes. Moving the blood pressure cuff from the dependent to nondependent arm in a patient in the lateral position can significantly change the reported blood pressure because of hydrostatic effects,[7] despite the fact that

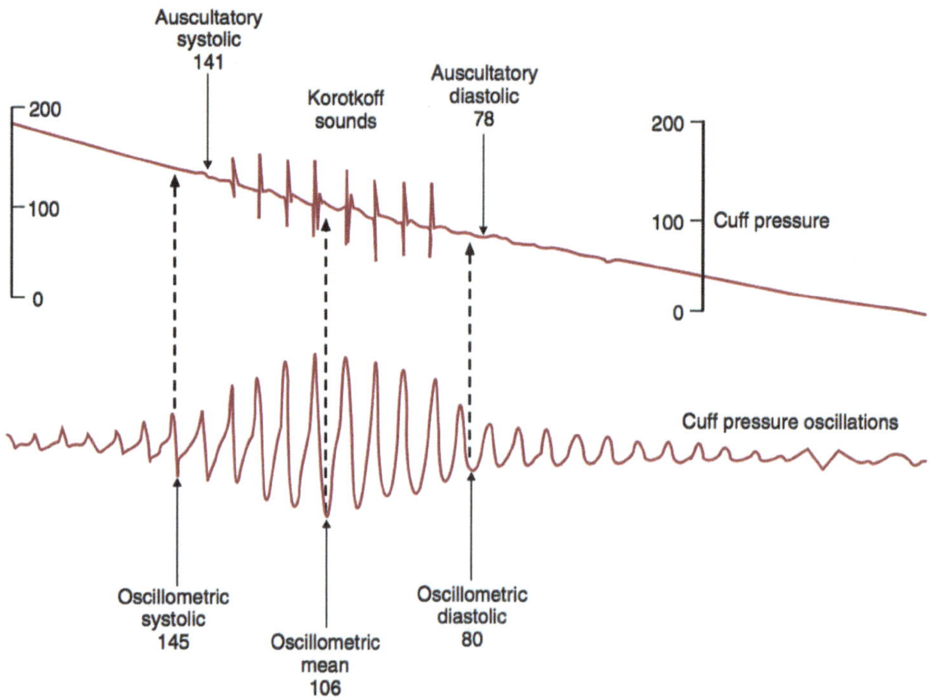

• **Fig. 12.1** Superimposed Korotkoff sounds (upper) and measured cuff pressure (lower) as a blood pressure cuff declines from 200 to 0 mm Hg. The point at which cuff oscillations are maximal closely approximates mean arterial pressure. (From Karsten Bartels, Stephen A Esper, Robert H Thiele. Blood Pressure Monitoring for the Anesthesiologist: A Practical Review. *Anesth Analg*. 2016;122(6):1866–1879 {John Wiley & Sons}.)

actual blood pressure in the areas of interest (brain, heart) has not changed at all (Fig. 12.2).

Oscillometry has been extensively compared with the gold standard of intraarterial catheterization. A single center, retrospective analysis of 15,310 noncardiac anesthetics in which the patient had both intraarterial catheters placed as well as oscillometry used found that the standard deviation of MAP was ± 12.5 mm Hg around a MAP of 75 mm Hg, when oscillometry was most accurate—this equates to 95% confidence intervals of approximately ± 25 mm Hg (Bland-Altman analysis). When MAP deviated substantially, the performance of the oscillometric technique decreased even further.[8]

Tonometry

In 1963, Pressman and Newgard published the first description of what would become artery applanation tonometry.[9] This was the first development of a continuous form of noninvasive blood pressure monitoring, and the concept was advanced by O'Rourke.[10] Applanation tonometry involves the flattening (applanation) of a superficial artery, most commonly the radial, with a pressure sensing device.[11] Only arteries that can be compressed (e.g., a radial artery) can be assessed. When the artery is compressed enough to reach a flattened state, the pressure sensed by the detector is similar to the intraarterial pressure, and the resulting pressure waveform closely mimics the true intraarterial pressure waveform.[12] Tonometers are incapable of making absolute pressure measurements and thus need to be calibrated against another device (e.g., blood pressure

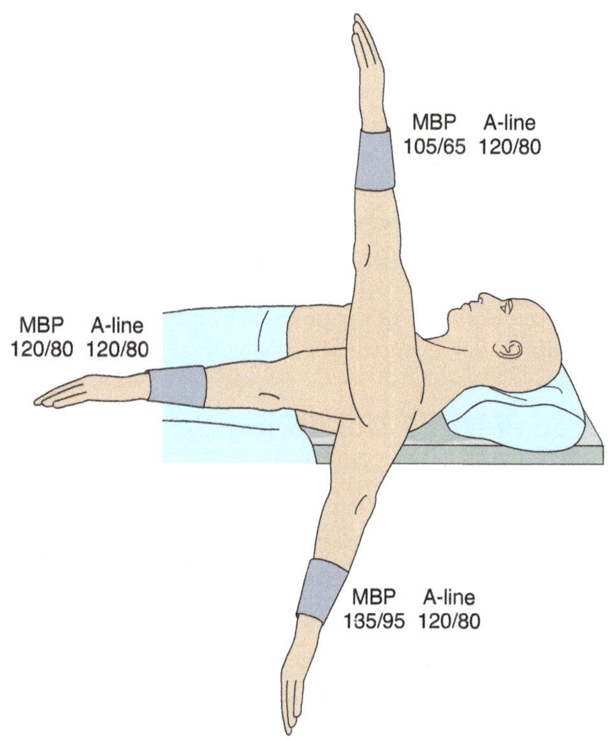

• **Fig. 12.2** Intraarterial pressure catheters are independent of extremity location and are accurate as long as the transducer height is even with the right atrium. In contrast, blood pressure cuffs measure blood pressure at a specific location, thus changes in positioning relative to the right atrium can affect the measurement. *MBP*, Mean blood pressure.

cuff).[12] The use of frequency domain mathematical analysis (e.g., fast Fourier transformation) allows a peripheral artery tracing to be "transformed" into an estimate of central arterial blood pressure using what is referred to as a transfer function.[13]

If measurements are taken at a "large" artery, applanation tonometry is relatively resistant to confounding variables that can disrupt other noninvasive continuous blood pressure measurement methodologies (see later) such as vasoconstriction. Applanation tonometry has been validated in over 1600 patients, including over 15,000 individual blood pressure measurements[14] but is clinically impractical in the OR because it requires unrestricted access to the wrist for placement of the pen-like "tonometer."

Because the underlying technology is sound, but the practical implementation is cumbersome, efforts have been made to miniaturize applanation tonometers for utility in the OR environment. Testing by multiple groups has revealed relatively low bias (6.3 mm Hg, range 4.8–12.6 mm Hg)[15–19] and limits of agreement (approximately ± 12.4 mm Hg, range ± 9.4 to ± 24.7 mm Hg) that are at least comparable, if not slightly better than noninvasive devices generally.[20] A recent large metaanalysis has cast some doubt onto the accuracy of tonometers in patients who have cardiovascular disease. "The results from this metaanalysis found that inaccuracy and imprecision of continuous noninvasive arterial pressure monitoring devices are larger than what was defined as acceptable. This may have implications for clinical situations where continuous noninvasive arterial pressure is being used for patient care decisions."[21]

Volume Clamp Technique

First described by Penaz in 1973, volume clamping is a method of noninvasive blood pressure measurement that can provide beat-to-beat information in real time.[22] It involves placement of an ultrafast, inflatable cuff upstream of a finger-based infrared sensor and emitter. By using a feedback loop between the cuff and the infrared sensor, the cuff is inflated and deflated cyclically such that the intensity of the infrared radiation is nearly constant (i.e., the blood volume of the finger is unchanged). In theory, if the pressure in the cuff exactly matches the arterial blood pressure, changes in finger blood volume (and absorbance of infrared light) are minimal. Thus the pressure waveform required to maintain minimal variation in infrared absorbance is thought to closely approximate arterial blood pressure (Fig. 12.3).

These devices need to be periodically calibrated by taking advantage of the fact that detected pulsatility distal to a cuff is maximal near MAP (discussed earlier during oscillometry). When external cuff pressure is close to blood pressure, the arterial wall experiences minimal tension and is said to exist in an "unloaded" state. Commercially available devices that use the volume-clamp technique differ in the algorithms used to achieve vascular unloading.

Given the dependence of the volume clamp technique on small vessel, distal extremity perfusion, it is susceptible to periods of hypoperfusion[6,7] and poor blood flow as can be seen in shock, and hypothermia[23] will impact the accuracy of the blood pressure measurements.

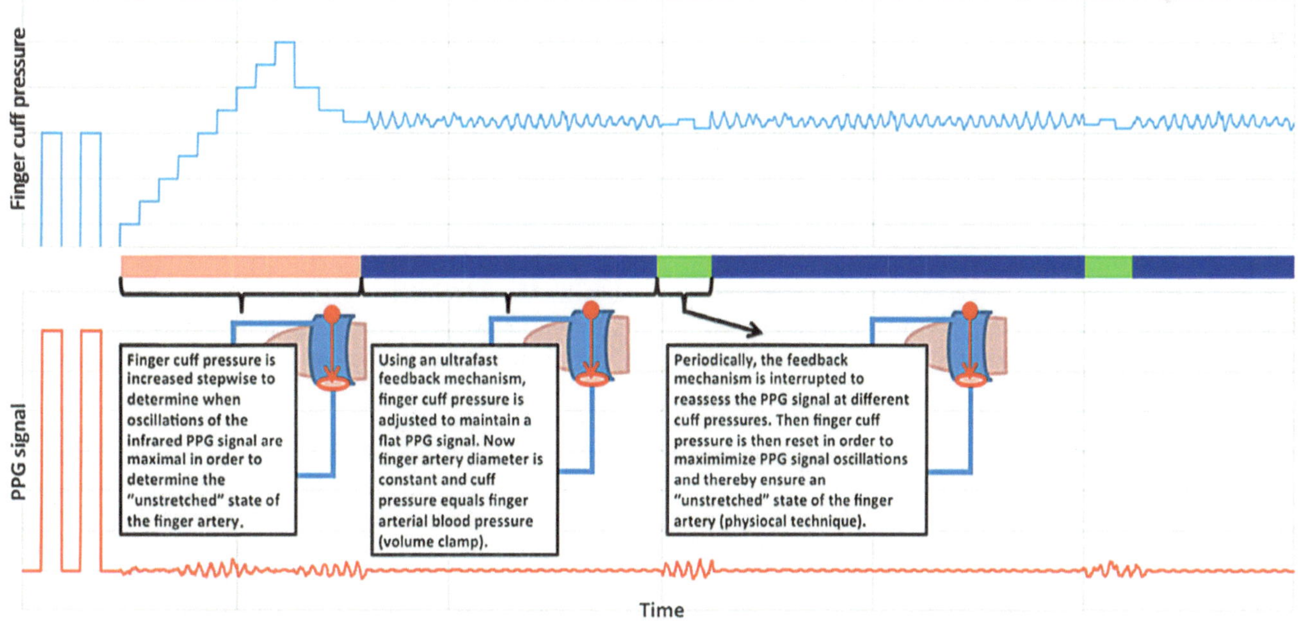

• **Fig. 12.3** Finger cuff (*blue*) and photoplethysmographic (*red*) signals during noninvasive measurement of blood pressure using the volume clamp technique. A feedback mechanism between the photoplethysmographic device and the finger cuff alters the finger pressure in an attempt to keep the photoplethysmographic signal flat—the resulting pressure waveform in the finger cuff closely approximates intraarterial blood pressure. Periodically, the finger cuff deflates in an effort to recalibrate. *PPG*, Photoplethysmogram. (From Bartels K, Thiele RH. Advances in photoplethysmography: beyond arterial oxygen saturation. *Can J Anaesth*. 2015;62(12):1313–1328. License Number 4722100482584.)

Individual studies looking at agreement between volume clamping and applanation tonometry in a variety of settings have been mixed; and in 2014, a metaanalysis of both of these techniques demonstrated an accuracy that was slightly worse than noninvasive technique overall.[20] Of course, this decrease in accuracy needs to be counterbalanced by the continuous measurements provided by these devices, which is an important advantage. As the technology improves, its potential to provide beat-to-beat blood pressure values noninvasively is tantalizing and has significant implications in large surgeries with significant fluid shifts and hemodynamic swings, such as thoracic surgery.

Intraarterial Catheterization

When continuous, accurate blood pressure monitoring is indicated, intraarterial catheterization is most widely used. This technique is particularly useful in thoracic surgery patients because it also permits sampling for arterial blood gas analysis. A detailed review of arterial physiology is beyond the scope of this chapter and is available elsewhere.[24] Three key points related to intraarterial blood pressure monitoring deserve mentioning.

First, a basic understanding of the engineering principles behind intraarterial blood pressure monitoring is necessary to use the technology properly. Intraarterial blood pressure monitors use a "Wheatstone bridge" strain gauge to estimate the intraarterial pressure. This pressure is transmitted through an uninterrupted column of fluid that begins with an intraarterial catheter and extends to the strain gauge, where the column terminates.[25,26] The physical characteristics (length, diameter, distensibility) of the tubing used to connect the catheter to the strain gauge impact the appearance of the pressure waveform.

To accurately measure relevant features of the waveform (systolic and diastolic pressure), it is essential that the measurement system has an appropriate dynamic response—this can be determined by measuring the natural frequency (f_n, the oscillating frequency after application of a pressure pulse) and the damping coefficient (ζ, the time it takes an oscillating waveform to decay). Both f_n and ζ can be measured using the "flush test"—f_n is the inverse of the time between two peaks (in s^{-1}), and ζ is the ratio of two successive amplitudes (A_2/A_1). By plotting f_n and ζ on a "dynamic response map," the adequacy of the measurement system can be ensured[27,28] (Fig. 12.4).

In general, clinicians should use rigid, short tubing systems to connect the pressure monitor to the intraarterial catheter, and take great care to avoid air bubbles. The compressible air bubbles results in damping of the arterial tracing. Of note, the MAP reading will not be affected by inadequate dynamic response, only the shape of the waveform and the resultant estimates of systolic and diastolic pressure.

Second, the shape of the blood pressure waveform is highly dependent on the physical characteristics of the cardiovascular system, as well as the measurement location (Fig. 12.5). Rigid, noncompliant vessels will alter the arterial waveform, which is a combination of forward and backwards (from reflection sites) traveling wavefronts.[24] A common clinical mistake is to see an extremely high systolic pressure and attribute it to "whip" (i.e., an underdamped system), when in reality the dynamic response of the arterial measurement system is fine. This is common in patients with significant cardiovascular disease and atherosclerosis, especially when pressure is measured at a peripheral site (e.g., radial artery).

Third, although the infection rate of intraarterial catheters is low (approximately 1.7 per 1000 catheter days), it is comparable to the infection rate of nontunneled, centrally inserted central venous catheters (2.7 per 1000 catheter days).[29–31] The risk of infection can be lowered through sterile insertion technique and the use of a chlorhexidine-impregnated dressing.[32]

Central Venous Pressure

Traditionally, central venous pressure (CVP) was thought to represent "preload" and has served as a guide for volume administration in various goal-directed therapy algorithms.[33] Rigorous physiologic research has subsequently demonstrated that there is no relationship between CVP and blood volume, no relationship between changes in CVP and changes in blood volume, and that CVP has no relationship with fluid responsiveness.[34] In addition to the complex chain of physiologic interactions linking the systemic venous system to left ventricular end diastolic volume (including left ventricular compliance, intrathoracic pressure, pulmonic and mitral valve function, pulmonary vascular resistance, and right ventricular function),[35,36] healthcare practitioners themselves show wide variation in transducer placement,[37] adding a component of technical error to an already complex measurement. Complicating matters in the thoracic surgery population is the impact of lateral positioning on CVP, which should be measured at the level of the right atrium—both clinical and imaging studies have confirmed that great attention must be paid to transducer height when moving to the lateral position.[38–40]

Given the growing emphasis on dynamic indicators of volume status (see "Fluid Responsiveness" later), and the known risks of central venous catheter placement, CVP is rarely used as a physiologic guide at the authors' institution. Unfortunately, large datasets on usage rates are not currently available.[41]

One relatively recent use of CVP monitoring that may be useful in particularly high risk thoracic surgical patients (e.g., lung transplantation) is the pulmonary artery pulsatility index (PAPi) (Fig. 12.6). The idea behind PAPi is that combining data from the systemic venous system and pulmonary arteries may give practitioners some insight into right ventricular function.[42] As described earlier, unlike the CVP alone, which is distantly related to left ventricular filling, the systemic venous system and pulmonary artery are separated by fewer anatomic structures. PAPi is defined as pulmonary artery systolic pressure—pulmonary artery diastolic pressure/CVP and essentially indexes the

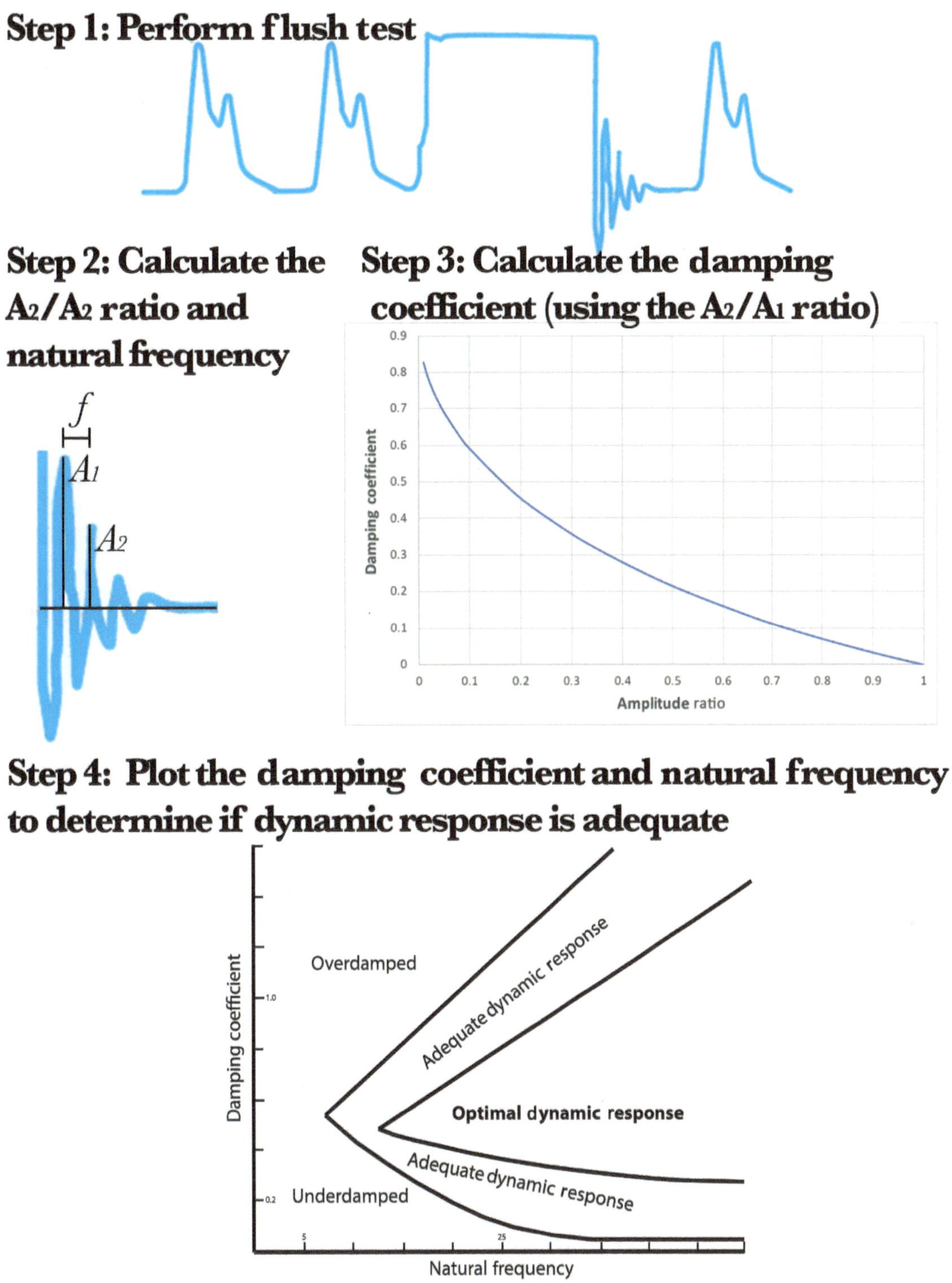

• **Fig. 12.4** To ensure that an intraarterial blood pressure tracing is accurate, the dynamic response needs to be measured. This is accomplished by performing a flush test and calculating both the natural frequency and the damping coefficient, and then locating the pressure monitoring system on a dynamic response map. (From Roach JK, Thiele RH. Perioperative blood pressure monitoring. *Best Pract Res Clin Anaesthesiol.* 2019;33(2):127–138 {Elsevier}.)

pulmonary artery pulse pressure (which is related to right ventricular stroke work) to CVP. A normally functioning right ventricle can produce adequate cardiac output without the need for high right atrial pressures. In contrast, a failing right ventricle requires higher and higher right atrial pressure to generate adequate cardiac output. Although use of this metric is still relatively new, it appears to predict right ventricular dysfunction in a variety of patient populations. These include after insertion of left ventricular assist device,[43] emergency transcatheter aortic valve replacement,[44] as well as predicting adverse events in advanced heart failure patients[45] and with right heart failure in particular,[46] and may be useful in select thoracic surgery patient populations.

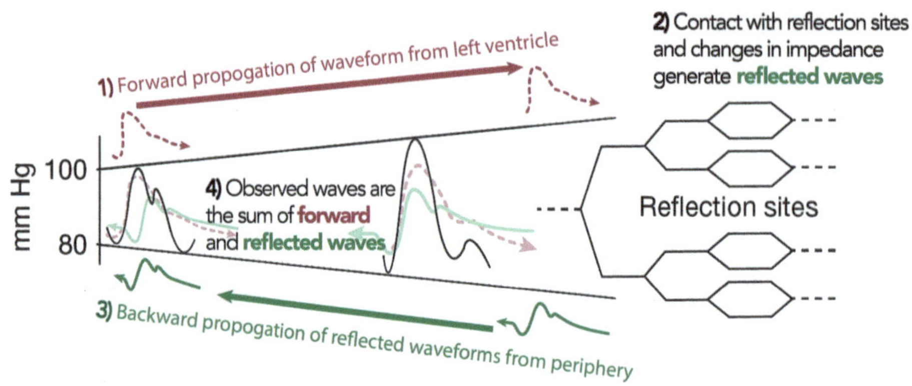

• **Fig. 12.5** The intraarterial blood pressure waveform is the sum of forward traveling and backwards traveling wave fronts, which are affected by branch points (reflection sites) and changes in compliance. (From Roach JK, Thiele RH. Perioperative blood pressure monitoring. *Best Pract Res Clin Anaesthesiol.* 2019;33(2):127–138 {Elsevier}.)

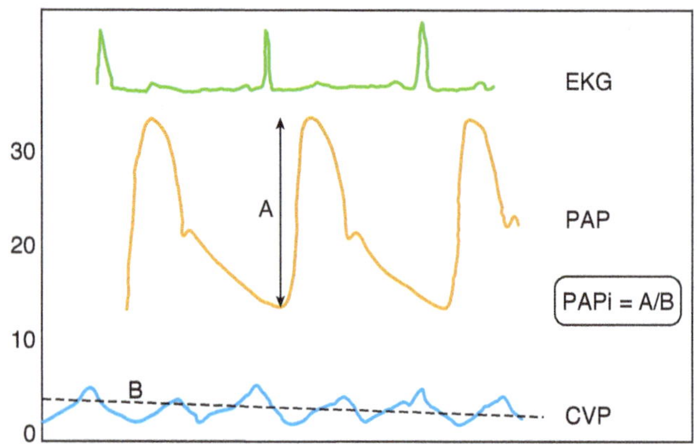

• **Fig. 12.6** Pulmonary artery pulsatility index (*PAPi*) is a relatively new metric that indexes the pressure output of the right ventricle to the central venous pressure (*CVP*). A, pulmonary artery systolic pressure—pulmonary artery diastolic pressure; B, central venous pressure; *EKG*, Electrocardiogram.

Pulmonary Artery Pressure

Pulmonary artery catheters (PACs), in addition to providing cardiac output (CO) information, can provide contentious real-time information on CVP and pulmonary arterial pressures. This can be especially important in the thoracic surgical patient who may present with, develop, or worsen intraoperatively pulmonary hypertension because of the pathology of their lung disease or during the intraoperative course. The data provided by a PAC can be interpreted to give some information regarding the function of the patient's right ventricle. A PAC may be especially valuable in the patient with pulmonary hypertension, as Doppler ultrasound can give inaccurate values for pulmonary artery pressure.[47,48] Any potential benefits to PAC placement must be balanced against its risks, including pulmonary artery rupture (especially in patients with pulmonary arterial hypertension), damage to cardiac valves, endocarditis, arrythmia, including ventricular fibrillation, catheter knotting, intravascular thrombosis, vascular stenosis, and catheter-related bloodstream infection. In addition, multiple studies[49–51] have failed to demonstrate a mortality benefit to PAC use in critically ill intensive care unit (ICU) patients, however, these studies did not focus on thoracic surgical patients specifically. Because of the lack of proven benefit and the continued improvement in noninvasive monitoring techniques, a sharp drop-off in the use of PACs has been seen in North American ICUs,[52,53] although this trend may be reversing.[54] More recent metaanalyses have demonstrated a mortality benefit with the use of PACs in critically ill patients undergoing major surgery.[55,56] Although the fate of the PAC has yet to be determined, it remains a valuable tool available to the anesthesiologist especially when supporting patients with pulmonary hypertension or right heart dysfunction. In thoracic surgical populations, common usage of the PAC is typically limited to lung transplantation.

Cardiac Output Monitoring

The measurement of blood pressure, discussed earlier, is to a large extent conducted in an effort to gauge delivery of oxygen (DO_2) to important organs, with blood pressure acting as a surrogate marker of end-organ perfusion. Blood pressure has the benefit of being easily and directly measurable, but it is an imperfect surrogate for oxygen delivery, which is of primary importance to the anesthesiologist. Although MAP is a critical component of global CO (and thus oxygen delivery globally) in the surgical setting, there is very little relationship between MAP and DO_2, likely because of differences in systemic vascular resistance[57] (Fig. 12.7). Thus an accurate measure of CO, which directly affects oxygen delivery, has long been a desired but elusive physiologic parameter for the anesthesiologist.

Pulmonary Artery and Transpulmonary Thermodilution

The de facto gold standard for CO monitoring is currently the pulmonary artery thermodilution method, which was first published by Fegler in 1954.[58] This technique is based on previous work using dilutional methods for monitoring CO involving dyes or other chemicals, such as lithium. An advantage of the thermodilution technique is its ability to be used repeatedly without concerns for increasing levels of

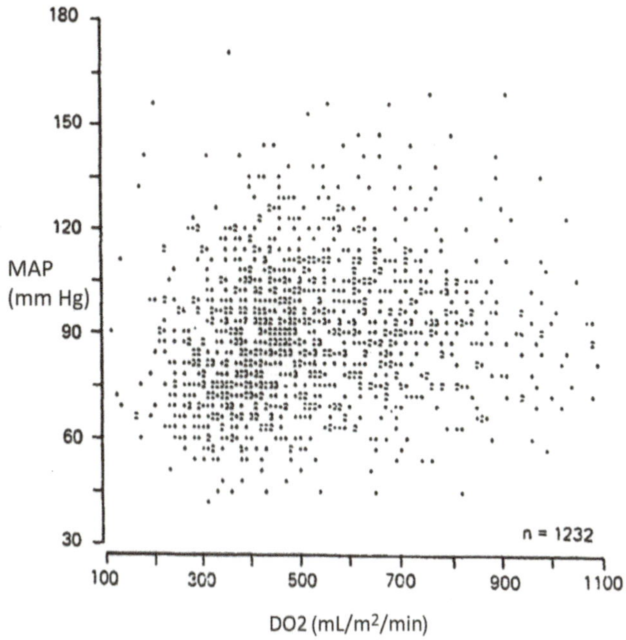

• **Fig. 12.7** In patients undergoing major vascular surgery, there is essentially no relationship between mean arterial pressure (*MAP*) and delivery of oxygen (*DO_2*). Thus, while blood pressure is essential to perfusion, mean arterial pressure is not a reliable surrogate. (From Karsten Bartels, Stephen A Esper, Robert H Thiele. Blood Pressure Monitoring for the Anesthesiologist: A Practical Review. *Anesth Analg.* 2016;122(6):1866–1879 {Wolters Kluwer -> Springer}.)

a foreign substance within the body. Pulmonary artery thermodilution requires the placement of a PAC, as an accurate measurement requires the ability to measure temperature before and after the right ventricular outflow tract. After pulmonary artery placement is complete and verified, a known volume of an injectate (typically crystalloid solution) at a known temperature is injected briskly and mixes with the patient's blood. A thermistor at the tip of PAC then measures the change in temperature over time, and the area under the curve is used to calculate the CO: the total thermal mass of the fluid bolus is known (based on temperature, volume, and specific heat of crystalloid solution), and a complex series of equations (known as the Stewart-Hamilton equations[59]) can be used to convert the temperature profile in the pulmonary artery to right ventricular output. From a qualitative sense, a high CO will produce a sharp but brief change in temperature as cold crystalloid races past the tip of the PAC, whereas in the setting of low CO, the temperature change will be more gradual and prolonged because the blood is moving more slowly and the cold fluid has more time to mix.

Pulmonary artery thermodilution has limitations. It assumes all blood flow is forward and in series, at least on the right side of the heart. Both tricuspid regurgitation and intracardiac shunts can give erroneous CO values by having some of the thermal mass of the injectate be delayed in its presentation to the thermistor or bypass it all together. Flow must not be so slow nor so fast such that adequate mixing of the injectate and patient's blood volume does not occur before the thermistor, and the temperature difference between the patient's blood and injectate must be sufficient enough to induce a measurable change in temperature at the thermistor. Although the temperature of the injectate does not seem to change CO values measured, using a colder injectate (i.e., 0°C) does reduce the variability of the values obtained compared with using room temperature injectate at the cost of additional equipment. Similarly, injecting a larger volume of injectate can improve the reliability of the results.[60]

For more continuous feedback, the practitioner can decide to place a continuous cardiac output (CCO) PAC. With this method, the PAC contains a filament midway along the catheter that is periodically heated, warming the blood. This change in temperature is then measured by the thermistor at the tip of the PAC, and CO is calculated in a similar manner to the intermittent thermodilution method described earlier. Because the "thermal mass" associated with these temperature changes is smaller than the thermal mass of a 10 mL bolus of room temperature (or cold) crystalloid, a substantial number of readings must be taken and averaged over time—thus CCO PACs typically have a time delay of as many as 5 minutes which limits its clinical use in an acute setting.[61–63]

Whether or not CO measurement improves clinical outcomes is a matter of fierce debate, initiated by a series of large, randomized controlled trials (RCTs) that failed to show improvements in mortality when PACs were used in critically ill patients.[51,64,65] Although questions about study design and protocol adherence plague these studies, the impact on PAC use is not debatable. By 2004, PAC insertions had fallen to 1.99 per 1000 medical admissions in the United States,[52] with even more recent Canadian data suggesting a similar decrease in PAC use.[53] There is some evidence that the trend toward decreasing PAC use is starting to reverse.[54]

Given the lack of high-quality data suggesting that PACs improve outcomes, and the increased appreciation for the risks and costs associated with their placement, substantial effort has been invested in the development of techniques to accurately measure CO without the need for the invasive use of a PAC. An obvious starting place would be to attempt to measure temperature changes somewhere other than the pulmonary artery, and transpulmonary thermodilution CO (TDCO) devices do just that. Room temperature crystalloid is injected into the right atrium, and temperature changes are measured in a large artery *after* the fluid bolus has travelled through the lungs and left atrium/ventricle. Transmission across these additional structures, as well as the fact that not all CO passes through the measurement site (e.g., femoral, axillary, or brachial artery) complicate the measurement. However, overall comparisons to both experimental gold standards, as well as thermodilution in animals and humans[66–79] suggest that transpulmonary thermodilution measurements are likely to be noninferior to that of pulmonary artery thermodilution.[80]

Still, TDCO devices require the placement of a central venous catheter, as well as catheterization of a large artery, therefore, there is intense interest in the development of CO monitors that require either a radial artery catheter (minimally invasive) or no catheterization at all (noninvasive). Although this chapter will review current technologies available at the time of this writing, the pace of change in this particular field is so rapid that the reader would be best served reviewing the latest literature to stay abreast of new developments.

Arterial Waveform Analysis

The majority of arterial waveform analysis devices, with the exception of FloTrac (Edwards Lifesciences, Irvine, CA), are based on the **Windkessel model** which was developed by Otto Frank.[81] Frank's model makes three assumptions that allow for mathematical modeling of flow—first, that at steady state, the amount of blood entering and leaving a vessel over one cardiac cycle must be the same (conservation of mass); second, that the vessels downstream of the left ventricle are compliant; and third, that blood flow travels in one direction. The simplest mathematical model contains only two elements—a resistor and a capacitor, but models, including additional elements such as aortic input impedance and inductance, have been proposed.[82] For additional details on the mathematical features of the Windkessel model, see more detailed reviews on the topic[83] (Fig. 12.8).

A key, common feature of arterial waveform analyzers is that they attempt to estimate features of the cardiovascular system (e.g., vascular resistance, often referred to as "k" in the underlying equations) based on the shape of the waveform. The reality is that these changes are not fully accounted for by the shape of the waveform. Arterial vascular resistance, compliance, and other descriptive features can change over time and devices that do not or cannot account for changes in *k* are referred to as **"uncalibrated" arterial waveform analyzers**. This category includes the LiDCO Rapid (LiDCO Rapid Group PLC, London, UK) and the ProAQT (Pulsion Medical Systems, Munich, Germany). FloTrac is similarly an uncalibrated arterial waveform analyzer but instead of using an analytical (Windkessel model) technique, uses an **empiric technique** in which specific features (e.g., kurtosis) of the arterial waveform are correlated to hemodynamic variables using very large datasets. The empiric technique is fundamentally different from the analytical techniques in that it does not seek to discover an equation based on underlying physiologic truths but rather focuses on real world performance.[84]

Unfortunately, because *k* does change with time, especially in hemodynamically unstable patients, the accuracy of uncalibrated waveform analysis devices (both analytical and empirical) can be unreliable.[71,85–91] Regarding thoracic surgical procedures specifically, there appears to be poor concordance between these devices and stable patients undergoing one-lung ventilation (OLV)[92] and lung transplantation.[93] Recently, Koichi Suehiro et al. compared the CO measured by the Vigileo™-FloTrac™ system with that estimated by the thermodilution PAC during OLV and determined the reliability of this system in tracking phenylephrine-induced CO changes during OLV in 16 patients. They concluded that the reliability of the Vigileo™-FloTrac™ system during OLV to estimate CO and track phenylephrine-induced CO changes was not acceptable.[92] Two additional techniques have been developed to measure stroke volume using the arterial blood pressure tracing—long time interval analysis[94–96] and the pressure recording analytic method.[97,98] Both techniques are in need of additional validation before they can be compared with more established techniques.

In an effort to improve accuracy, some arterial waveform analysis devices can be periodically recalibrated to a second, independent measure of CO. This allows the monitor to compensate for changes in arterial resistance and compliance which would in turn change *k*. The PulseCO (LiDCO Group PLC, London, UK) uses lithium dilution,[99] whereas the VolumeView (Edwards Lifesciences, Irvine, CA)[100] and PiCCO (Pulsion Medical Systems, Munich, Germany)[101] use transpulmonary thermodilution. A calibrated waveform analyzer results in significant improvements in accuracy when compared with the noncalibrated devices,[102] however, this benefit must be weighed against the requirement for additional invasive lines and/or increased expense and complexity. One benefit of the PulseCO system is that it may also allow relatively accurate calculations of extravascular lung water[103] (see later).

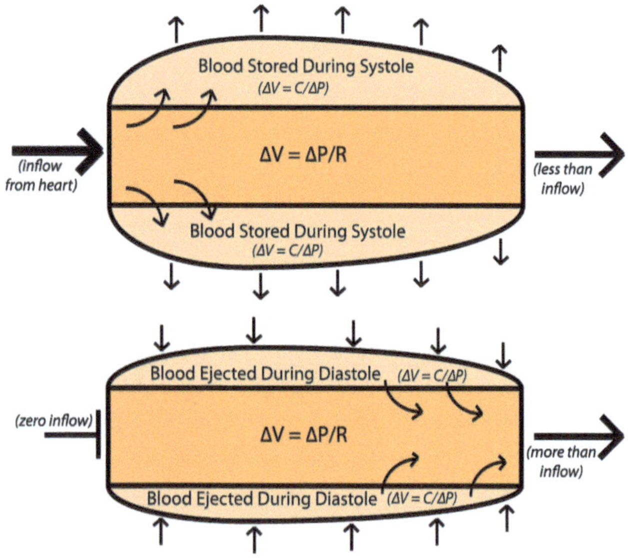

• **Fig. 12.8** Frank's Windkessel model assumes that the aorta functions as a capacitor and only allows unidirectional flow. During systole, the majority of blood passes through the aorta, but the increased blood pressure leads to aortic expansion and storage of blood in this "capacitance vessel." During diastole, the aortic valve closes, pressure drops, and the aorta contracts, ejecting blood downstream. (From License Number 4722101307490.)

Doppler-Based Techniques

Ultrasound has seen a large increase in its utility as a diagnostic tool, as well as physiologic monitor in recent decades. The Doppler principle serves as the foundation for ultrasound-based calculation of CO. Under the Doppler principle, when a moving object (i.e., red blood cells) encounters an incident wave (i.e., ultrasound beam), the frequency of the reflected wave is changed according to the formula:

$$v = c^{*}\Delta f/2f_0^{*}\cos(\theta)$$

where v is the calculated velocity, θ is the angle between the incident wave and motion of the object, c is the speed of the wave, Δf is the change in frequency, and f_0 is the frequency of the incident beam.[80]

Although this chapter will not discuss formal, two- (and three-) dimensional transesophageal echocardiography (TEE), there are commercially available ultrasound devices, such as the CardioQ (Deltex Medical, Chichester, UK) which can be placed into the esophagus and only perform Doppler measurements to determine blood flow in the descending aorta. Although not as robust as the full suite of options available with TEE (e.g., two-dimensional and color imaging), the CardioQ device allows continuous monitoring of CO with less expertise required by the practitioner.

Esophageal Doppler monitoring has been found to correlate well with Fick CO measurements in animals,[104,105] and humans,[105–107] as well as thermodilution in humans.[107–109] There are also limited data supporting the use of esophageal Doppler monitoring during OLV showing good concordance with thermodilution techniques.[110,111] Diaper et al. evaluated the accuracy of cardiac index (CI) as measured by echotransesophageal Doppler monitoring (echo-TDM) with CI measured by the transpulmonary thermodilution technique in patients scheduled for elective lung cancer resection. The device appears to be useful, safe, and fairly reliable in documenting absolute values and changes in CO. The agreement between the echo-TDM and thermodilution appears to lie within clinically acceptable limits. Other derived Doppler parameters may provide additional useful information regarding circulatory volume (corrected ejection time) and ventricular contractility (flow acceleration and peak velocity). As a substitute for a PAC, it may guide hemodynamic control and fluid infusion in patients undergoing lung resection.[110]

Esophageal Doppler monitoring has several limitations: first, it only measures blood flow in the descending aorta therefore potentially discounting changes in blood flow to the heart, brain, and upper extremities. Second, current commercially available probes measure only blood velocity over time. To obtain volumetric measurements (i.e., stroke volume and CO), one must know the diameter of the aorta at the site of Doppler measurement and presently, this is determined morphologically, potentially adding another source for error. Third, although an esophageal probe is less invasive than placement of a PAC, there is still the theoretical risk of complications seen in traditional TEE,[112] although the risk is likely lower given the smaller probe size. Last, the accuracy of Doppler measurements of velocity is highly dependent on the angle of incidence between the emitting beam and the velocity of the measured object (i.e., blood flow). The accuracy is highest when this angle is zero, but the velocity is rapidly underestimated with angles increasing beyond 20 degrees. Obviously, esophageal Doppler monitoring is impossible in surgery involving the esophagus, but its availability provides an additional tool to the anesthesiologist desiring to measure CO in a minimally invasive manner.

Bioimpedance and Bioreactance

A relatively newer development in noninvasive CO measurement involves bioreactance, which was developed as a modification of the much older bioimpedance technique. Bioimpedance is based on the thorax's natural resistance to electrical current when a voltage is placed across it. This resistance (referred to as impedance when an oscillating voltage potential is applied) changes with each heartbeat as the amount of air and fluid within the thorax changes. By measuring the changes in impedance to the flow of electrical current, devices relying on bioimpedance attempt to noninvasively estimate CO and stroke volume.[113–115] Although initially promising in animal models,[116–121] bioimpedance has not yet been acceptably accurate in the OR environment,[122–125] relying on too many assumptions and being too susceptible to artifact in a surgical setting that presents, among other sources of artifact, substantial electrical interference. In an effort to improve upon this, noninvasive cardiac output monitoring (NICOM, Cheetah Medical, Vancouver, WA) uses the phasic component of impedance rather than the amplitude component which is used in traditional bioimpedance monitors.[126] However, there have been very few clinical studies involving bioreactance, which limits the ability to draw conclusions regarding its accuracy.[126–129]

Fluid Responsiveness

As discussed elsewhere (see Chapter 21) fluid optimization is critical in the thoracic surgical patient. Fluid overload and pulmonary edema carries a high morbidity and mortality[130–133] and can be difficult to manage, especially in a patient who is newly dependent on reduced lung volumes. Consequently, there is great interest, both in the thoracic surgical world and beyond, in appropriate fluid management. In general, the anesthesiologist will aim to give intravenous fluid to the patient to place the cardiac function onto the plateau portion of the Frank-Starling curve with the goal of "optimizing" (not "maximizing") stroke volume, CO, and O_2 delivery—administration of fluid given beyond the point of optimization will result in minimal change in hemodynamic variables and put the patient at risk for fluid overload and pulmonary edema, particularly following lung resection. The key to proper fluid management is therefore to try to predict where on the Frank-Starling curve a patient is and if a fluid bolus will result in an improvement in stroke volume and CO, that is, whether or not the patient is "fluid responsive" (Fig. 12.9).

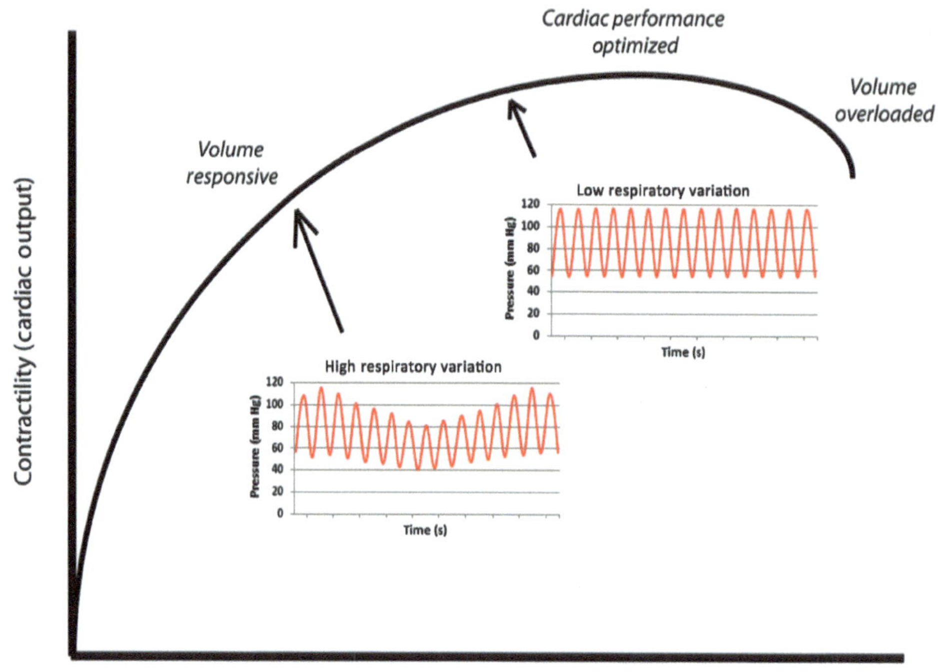

• **Fig. 12.9** Arterial respiratory variation provides some information on the relative location of a patient on the Frank-Starling curve. It is important to note that there are scenarios, for example, right ventricular failure, in which arterial respiratory variation is present, but the patient is not fluid responsive. (From License Number 4722100804187.)

Indeed, a series of RCTs from the 1990s and 2000s demonstrated that fluid resuscitation guided by esophageal Doppler to maximize stroke volume resulted in a reduced length of stay and complication rate in patients having major surgery[134–138] or admitted to the trauma ICU.[139] These benefits are not restricted to esophageal Doppler technology and similar benefits have been seen using arterial waveform analysis[140–145] and other indicators of fluid responsiveness which will be discussed later. Ultimately, metaanalytic data suggest that goal-directed fluid resuscitation appears to be associated with improvements in outcomes,[55,56,145] although no single, large, multicenter, RCT has demonstrated this definitively.

Respiratory Variation

One of the most common methods of predicting for fluid responsiveness involves analysis of the arterial waveform as it varies with respiration: designated systolic pressure variation, pulse pressure variation (PPV), or stroke volume variation (SVV). Many anesthesia monitors can perform this analysis and display the resultant value, although it appears that anesthesiologists are able to make accurate visual judgements via estimation as well.[146] PPV (or any of the other methods mentioned) is based on the concept that as intrathoracic pressure varies while a patient is being ventilated with positive pressure, venous return to the heart varies inversely with intrathoracic pressure. This effectively provides a "mock" fluid bolus with each breath predicting how a patient may respond to a fluid challenge.

However, thoracic surgery introduces a few complications for the provider attempting to use PPV to determine fluid responsiveness. First, PPV was validated using tidal volumes of generally above 8 mL/kg ideal body weight,[38,39] which is a much larger volume than is typically used during protective lung ventilation during OLV. Studies looking specifically at the predictiveness of respiratory variation on fluid responsiveness during OLV have varied in their conclusion, with some showing predictiveness at 8 mL/kg,[147,148] some showing the opposite,[149] and some showing predictiveness, with tidal volumes as low as 6 mL/kg.[150,151] Any utility of fluid responsiveness using respiratory variation while on OLV will be diminished by the decreased sensitivity and specificity compared with conventional ventilation strategies. Another limitation for the use of PPV during thoracic surgery is that the thoracic cavity is often open to the atmosphere, reducing the transmission of intrathoracic pressure changes to the vascular system, and further reducing the predictiveness of respiratory variation for fluid responsiveness. de Waal et al. evaluated the ability of PPV and SVV to predict fluid responsiveness under open- and closed-chest conditions in 22 patients scheduled for elective coronary artery bypass graft surgery. PPV and SVV (both obtained with the PiCCO system) were recorded. Fluid-responders were defined by an increase in stroke volume index of 12% or more subsequent to a volume load. They concluded that the dynamic preload indicators PPV and SVV are able to predict fluid responsiveness under closed-chest conditions, whereas all static and dynamic preload indicators fail to predict fluid responsiveness under open-chest conditions.[152]

Microbolus Technique

One potential opportunity to gauge fluid responsiveness in thoracic surgery patients is the "mini" or "micro" bolus technique, in which as little as 50 mL of intravenous fluid is given and the hemodynamic response measured. Although not validated in thoracic surgical patients specifically, the microbolus technique has been used in patients undergoing neurosurgery, liver transplant surgery, and cardiac surgery.[153–155] This technique is not continuous and requires administration of fluid, as well as operator intervention, but if performed every 10 minutes over a 3-hour period, requires the administration of as little as 900 mL of intravenous fluid.

Extravascular Lung Water

Extravascular lung water (EVLW) refers to a patient's lung fluid which is outside the vasculature, with a normal amount being 3 to 7 mL/kg. In the setting of pulmonary edema, this value can increase to over 10 mL/kg.[156] The etiology of EVLW includes increased capillary hydrostatic pressure (i.e., from left ventricular dysfunction or fluid overload) and increased capillary permeability as may be seen in acute respiratory distress syndrome.[157] There is considerable interest in accurate, inexpensive, and fast measurement of EVLW, given the potential for using EVLW as a marker and correlate for pulmonary edema and acute lung injury (ALI) in patients. In esophagectomy,[158,159] and other critically ill[160] patients, EVLW was found to be predictive of arterial partial pressure of oxygen/fraction of inspired oxygen (PaO_2/FiO_2) ratio, pulmonary compliance, lung injury scores,[158] and even mortality.[160] EVLW may also be useful in the early identification of patients with pulmonary graft dysfunction following lung transplantation.[161] With numerous studies demonstrating the association between fluid overload and ALI, and ALI's association with morbidity and mortality,[130–133,159,162–164] having an accurate measure of EVLW to guide fluid resuscitation may result in a significant improvement in current perioperative care of the thoracic surgical patient.

The gold standard for EVLW is **gravimetry** whereby the blood volume of the lungs is subtracted from the total water content of the lungs (taken postmortem).[165] Given that calculating the total water content of the lungs requires comparison between wet and desiccated lung weights, this method clearly cannot be applied clinically. The most common bedside technique used to determine EVLW is the **double indicator dilution technique.** With this, a freely diffusible indicator (e.g., heated or cooled saline) and nondiffusible indicator (e.g., an albumin bound dye) are both injected and transit the lung. While in the lung, the indicators have different volumes of distribution, as the diffusible indicator will equilibrate with all lung water (both vascular and extravascular) and the nondiffusible indicator will only equilibrate with the water in the vascular space. The indicator concentrations and transit times are detected by an arterial catheter and EVLW can then be calculated. Unfortunately, this technique is time consuming and expensive, and therefore it is infrequently performed. There are numerous other modalities that attempt to measure EVLW noninvasively with varying degrees of accuracy including chest x-ray, magnetic resonance imaging, computed tomography scan, and positron emission tomography scan. However, given the time, expense, radiation exposure, and/or lack of accuracy, these modalities are not in use clinically in any significant manner.[166]

In theory, bioimpedance can be used to determine EVLW, however, as stated earlier, refinement in the technology is still required.[167–169] An intriguing newer bedside technique for EVLW determination is the PiCCO (Pulsion Medical Systems, Munich, Germany) system, which is able to calculate EVLW using a single indicator (cold saline) via transpulmonary thermodilution. This system showed good correlation with gravimetry,[157] which is promising, however, it does suffer from a few shortcomings. First, using transpulmonary thermodilution is invasive requiring both a central venous and central arterial line. Second, because the system is based on blood flow through the lungs, it can only measure EVLW in areas of the lung which are perfused. High positive end-expiratory pressure, low CO, and obstructive disease such as pulmonary emboli may make the estimations inaccurate. Third, there are some concerns that transpulmonary thermodilution suffer from inaccuracy in the setting of lung resection.

There is some evidence that electrical impedance tomography (EIT) can measure EVLW.[170,171] EIT applies current to the chest from various electrodes (up to 32) located around the thorax, and in doing so is able to estimate electrical impedance in specific locations of the chest. Similarly to the manner in which bioimpedence devices use impedance data to estimate the flow of fluid in and out of the chest with each heartbeat, EIT devices are able to use bioimpedance measurements to estimate the amount of fluid that is extravascular (i.e., which does not change with each heart beat).[171] Although not a hemodynamic variable per se, EVLW may eventually be useful in making hemodynamic decisions related to fluid management, as well as the use of inotropes. Although not originally designed for intraoperative use, there are reports of EIT use to determine the individuality tittered PEEP and during thoracic surgery, including OLV.[172]

Conclusion

Hemodynamic monitoring is an important component of the management of thoracic surgery patients. Many of these patients have cardiovascular comorbidities that place them at high risk for perioperative complications and explain their single digit percentile 30-day mortality rates (depending on the procedure). Accurate blood pressure measurement is important in this population and traditionally required use of an intraarterial catheter with appropriate dynamic response. Noninvasive oscillometric cuffs produce errors of approximately ±25 mm Hg (95% confidence interval) when compared with arterial catheters and should not be depended upon when accurate blood pressure measurements are needed. In the future, advances in other noninvasive techniques such as the volume-clamp technique may provide a compromise solution between the oscillometric cuff and the intraarterial catheter. Central venous and pulmonary arterial pressure measurements are largely restricted to thoracic surgical patients undergoing lung transplantation, although the development of the PAPi may one day extend the utility of these measurements in patients with known right ventricular dysfunction undergoing thoracic surgery. CO monitoring is rarely performed in patients undergoing thoracic surgery, with the exception of lung transplantation; esophageal Doppler is accurate but complicated by lateral positioning and/or esophageal location; arterial waveform devices have difficulty handling changes in vascular resistance; newer algorithms may be able to handle these changes better, but further investigation is needed. Fluid responsiveness is increasingly recognized as an important hemodynamic variable, not as an endpoint in and of itself but as a fluid management guide, and is challenging in patients undergoing OLV, lung protective ventilation, or surgery on an open thorax. In this patient population, the microbolus technique, although not continuous, may be the most reliable. Measurements of extravascular lung water, either through transpulmonary thermodilution or EIT, although not a traditional hemodynamic endpoint, may help guide decisions on fluid management, as well as the use of inotropes.

References

1. Cantarutti A, Galeone C, Leuzzi G, et al. Thirty-day mortality and five-year survival in thoracic surgery: "real-world" assessment of outcomes from a single-institution audit. *Tumori*. 2018; 104:96–104.
2. Banga A, Mohanka M, Mullins J, et al. Incidence and variables associated with 30-day mortality after lung transplantation. *Clin Transplant*. 2019;33:e13468.
3. Nuru A, Weltzien JAH, Sandvik L, Tonnessen T, Bjornstad JL. Short- and long-term survival after isolated coronary artery bypass grafting, the impact of gender and age. *Scand Cardiovasc J*. 2019;53:342–347.
4. Maguire S, Rinehart J, Vakharia S, Cannesson M. Technical communication: respiratory variation in pulse pressure and plethysmographic waveforms: intraoperative applicability in a North American academic center. *Anesth Analg*. 2011;112:94–96.
5. Alpert BS, Quinn D, Gallick D. Oscillometric blood pressure: a review for clinicians. *J Am Soc Hypertens*. 2014;8:930–938.
6. Posey JA, Geddes LA, Williams H, Moore AG. The meaning of the point of maximum oscillations in cuff pressure in the indirect measurement of blood pressure. *Cardiovasc Res Cent Bull*. 1969;8:15–25.
7. Kinsella SM. Effect of blood pressure instrument and cuff side on blood pressure reading in pregnant women in the lateral recumbent position. *Int J Obstet Anesth*. 2006;15:290–293.
8. Wax DB, Lin HM, Leibowitz AB. Invasive and concomitant noninvasive intraoperative blood pressure monitoring: observed differences in measurements and associated therapeutic interventions. *Anesthesiology*. 2011;115:973–978.
9. Pressman GL, Newgard PM. A transducer for the continuous external measurement of arterial blood pressure. *IEEE Trans Biomed Eng*. 1963;10:73–81.
10. O'Rourke MF, Adji A. Basis for use of central blood pressure measurement in office clinical practice. *J Am Soc Hypertens*. 2008; 2:28–38.
11. Matthys K, Verdonck P. Development and modelling of arterial applanation tonometry: a review. *Technol Health Care*. 2002;10: 65–76.
12. Salvi P, Grillo A, Parati G. Noninvasive estimation of central blood pressure and analysis of pulse waves by applanation tonometry. *Hypertens Res*. 2015;38:646–648.
13. Laugesen E, Rossen NB, Peters CD, et al. Assessment of central blood pressure in patients with type 2 diabetes: a comparison between SphygmoCor and invasively measured values. *Am J Hypertens*. 2014;27:169–176.
14. Nelson MR, Stepanek J, Cevette M, Covalciuc M, Hurst RT, Tajik AJ. Noninvasive measurement of central vascular pressures with arterial tonometry: clinical revival of the pulse pressure waveform? *Mayo Clin Proc*. 2010;85:460–472.
15. Kemmotsu O, Ueda M, Otsuka H, Yamamura T, Winter DC, Eckerle JS. Arterial tonometry for noninvasive, continuous blood pressure monitoring during anesthesia. *Anesthesiology*. 1991; 75:333–340.
16. Janelle GM, Gravenstein N. An accuracy evaluation of the T-Line Tensymeter (continuous noninvasive blood pressure management device) versus conventional invasive radial artery monitoring in surgical patients. *Anesth Analg*. 2006;102:484–490.
17. Szmuk P, Pivalizza E, Warters RD, Ezri T, Gebhard R. An evaluation of the T-Line Tensymeter continuous noninvasive blood pressure device during induced hypotension. *Anaesthesia*. 2008;63:307–312.
18. Dueck R, Goedje O, Clopton P. Noninvasive continuous beat-to-beat radial artery pressure via TL-200 applanation tonometry. *J Clin Monit Comput*. 2012;26(2):75–83.
19. Colquhoun DA, Forkin KT, Dunn LK, Bogdonoff DL, Durieux ME, Thiele RH. Non-invasive, minute-to-minute estimates of systemic arterial pressure and pulse pressure variation using radial artery tonometry. *J Med Eng Technol*. 2013;37:197–202.
20. Kim SH, Lilot M, Sidhu KS, et al. Accuracy and precision of continuous noninvasive arterial pressure monitoring compared with invasive arterial pressure: a systematic review and meta-analysis. *Anesthesiology*. 2014;120:1080–1097.
21. Greiwe G, Hoffmann S, Herich L, et al. Comparison of blood pressure monitoring by applanation tonometry and invasively assessed blood pressure in cardiological patients. *J Clin Monit Comput*. 2018;32:817–823.
22. Penaz J. *Photoelectric measurement of blood pressure, volume and flow in the finger*. In: Proceedings of the Conference Committee of the 10th International Conference on Medicine and Biological Engineering, Dresden. 1973, p. 104.
23. Dorlas JC, Nijboer JA, Butijn WT, van der Hoeven GM, Settels JJ, Wesseling KH. Effects of peripheral vasoconstriction on the blood pressure in the finger, measured continuously by a new noninvasive method (the Finapres). *Anesthesiology*. 1985;62:342–345.

24. O'Rourke MF. The arterial pulse in health and disease. *Am Heart J.* 1971;82:687–702.
25. Bartels K, Esper SA, Thiele RH. Blood pressure monitoring for the anesthesiologist: a practical review. *Anesth Analg.* 2016;122: 1866–1879.
26. Roach JK, Thiele RH. Perioperative blood pressure monitoring. *Best Pract Res Clin Anaesthesiol.* 2019;33:127–138.
27. Gardner RM. Direct blood pressure measurement—dynamic response requirements. *Anesthesiology.* 1981;54:227–236.
28. Boutros A, Albert S. Effect of the dynamic response of transducer-tubing system on accuracy of direct blood pressure measurement in patients. *Crit Care Med.* 1983;11:124–127.
29. Handlogten KS, Wilson GA, Clifford L, Nuttall GA, Kor DJ. Brachial artery catheterization: an assessment of use patterns and associated complications. *Anesth Analg.* 2014;118:288–295.
30. Maki DG, Kluger DM, Crnich CJ. The risk of bloodstream infection in adults with different intravascular devices: a systematic review of 200 published prospective studies. *Mayo Clin Proc.* 2006;81:1159–1171.
31. Scheer B, Perel A, Pfeiffer UJ. Clinical review: complications and risk factors of peripheral arterial catheters used for haemodynamic monitoring in anaesthesia and intensive care medicine. *Crit Care.* 2002;6:199–204.
32. Timsit JF, Schwebel C, Bouadma L, et al. Dressing Study G. Chlorhexidine-impregnated sponges and less frequent dressing changes for prevention of catheter-related infections in critically ill adults: a randomized controlled trial. *JAMA.* 2009; 301:1231–1241.
33. Rivers E, Nguyen B, Havstad S, et al. Early goal-directed therapy in the treatment of severe sepsis and septic shock. *N Engl J Med.* 2001;345:1368–1377.
34. Marik PE, Baram M, Vahid B. Does central venous pressure predict fluid responsiveness? A systematic review of the literature and the tale of seven mares. *Chest.* 2008;134:172–178.
35. Magder S. Understanding central venous pressure: not a preload index? *Curr Opin Crit Care.* 2015;21:369–375.
36. De Backer D, Vincent JL. Should we measure the central venous pressure to guide fluid management? Ten answers to 10 questions. *Crit Care.* 2018;22:43.
37. Figg KK, Nemergut EC. Error in central venous pressure measurement. *Anesth Analg.* 2009;108:1209–1211.
38. Song IK, Ro S, Lee JH, Kim EH, Kim HS, Bahk JH, Kim JT. Reference levels for central venous pressure and pulmonary artery occlusion pressure monitoring in the lateral position. *J Cardiothorac Vasc Anesth.* 2017;31:939–943.
39. Potger KC, Elliott D. Reproducibility of central venous pressures in supine and lateral positions: a pilot evaluation of the phlebostatic axis in critically ill patients. *Heart Lung.* 1994;23:285–299.
40. Emerson RJ, Banasik JL. Effect of position on selected hemodynamic parameters in postoperative cardiac surgery patients. *Am J Crit Care.* 1994;3:289–299.
41. Adrian Vk Wong, Nitin Arora, Olusegun Olusanya, et al. First Intensive Care National Audit Project (ICNAP-1) group. Insertion rates and complications of central lines in the UK population: A pilot study. *J Intensive Care Soc.* 2018;19(1):19–25.
42. Lim HS, Gustafsson F. Pulmonary artery pulsatility index: physiological basis and clinical application. *Eur J Heart Fail.* 2019;22(1):32–38.
43. Gudejko MD, Gebhardt BR, Zahedi F, et al. Intraoperative hemodynamic and echocardiographic measurements associated with severe right ventricular failure after left ventricular assist device implantation. *Anesth Analg.* 2019;128:25–32.
44. Huang H, Kovach CP, Bell S, et al. Outcomes of emergency transcatheter aortic valve replacement. *J Interv Cardiol.* 2019;2019: 7598581.
45. Kochav SM, Flores RJ, Truby LK, Topkara VK. Prognostic impact of pulmonary artery pulsatility index (PAPi) in patients with advanced heart failure: insights from the ESCAPE trial. *J Card Fail.* 2018;24:453–459.
46. Mazimba S, Welch TS, Mwansa H, et al. Haemodynamically derived pulmonary artery pulsatility index predicts mortality in pulmonary arterial hypertension. *Heart Lung Circ.* 2019;28: 752–760.
47. Fisher MR, Forfia PR, Chamera E, et al. Accuracy of Doppler echocardiography in the hemodynamic assessment of pulmonary hypertension. *Am J Respir Crit Care Med.* 2009;179:615–621.
48. Rich JD, Shah SJ, Swamy RS, Kamp A, Rich S. Inaccuracy of Doppler echocardiographic estimates of pulmonary artery pressures in patients with pulmonary hypertension: implications for clinical practice. *Chest.* 2011;139:988–993.
49. Sandham JD, Hull RD, Brant RF, et al. Canadian Critical Care. Clinical Trials G. A randomized, controlled trial of the use of pulmonary-artery catheters in high-risk surgical patients. *N Engl J Med.* 2003;348:5–14.
50. Richard C, Warszawski J, Anguel N, et al. French Pulmonary Artery Catheter Study G. Early use of the pulmonary artery catheter and outcomes in patients with shock and acute respiratory distress syndrome: a randomized controlled trial. *JAMA.* 2003;290:2713–2720.
51. Harvey S, Harrison DA, Singer M, et al. Assessment of the clinical effectiveness of pulmonary artery catheters in management of patients in intensive care (PAC-Man): a randomised controlled trial. *Lancet.* 2005;366:472–477.
52. Wiener RS, Welch HG. Trends in the use of the pulmonary artery catheter in the United States, 1993-2004. *JAMA.* 2007;298: 423–429.
53. Koo KK, Sun JC, Zhou Q, Guyatt G, Cook DJ, Walter SD, Meade MO. Pulmonary artery catheters: evolving rates and reasons for use. *Crit Care Med.* 2011;39:1613–1618.
54. Pandey A, Khera R, Kumar N, Golwala H, Girotra S, Fonarow GC. Use of pulmonary artery catheterization in us patients with heart failure, 2001-2012. *JAMA Intern Med.* 2016;176:129–132.
55. Hamilton MA, Cecconi M, Rhodes A. A systematic review and meta-analysis on the use of preemptive hemodynamic intervention to improve postoperative outcomes in moderate and high-risk surgical patients. *Anesth Analg.* 2011;112:1392–1402.
56. Gurgel ST, do Nascimento P Jr. Maintaining tissue perfusion in high-risk surgical patients: a systematic review of randomized clinical trials. *Anesth Analg.* 2011;112:1384–1391.
57. Reinhart K, Kersting T, Fohring U, Schafer M. Can central-venous replace mixed-venous oxygen saturation measurements during anesthesia? *Adv Exp Med Biol.* 1986;200:67–72.
58. Fegler G. Measurement of cardiac output in anaesthetized animals by a thermodilution method. *Q J Exp Physiol Cogn Med Sci.* 1954;39:153–164.
59. Levett JM, Replogle RL. Thermodilution cardiac output: a critical analysis and review of the literature. *J Surg Res.* 1979;27: 392–404.
60. Pearl RG, Rosenthal MH, Nielson L, Ashton JP, Brown BW Jr. Effect of injectate volume and temperature on thermodilution cardiac output determination. *Anesthesiology.* 1986;64:798–801.
61. Philip JH, Long MC, Quinn MD, Newbower RS. Continuous thermal measurement of cardiac output. *IEEE Trans Biomed Eng.* 1984;31:393–400.

62. Aranda M, Mihm FG, Garrett S, Mihm MN, Pearl RG. Continuous cardiac output catheters: delay in in vitro response time after controlled flow changes. *Anesthesiology.* 1998;89:1592–1595.
63. Goldstein LJ. Response time of the Opti-Q continuous cardiac output pulmonary artery catheter in the urgent mode to a step change in cardiac output. *J Clin Monit Comput.* 1999;15:435–439.
64. Sandham JD, Hull RD, Brant RF, et al. A randomized, controlled trial of the use of pulmonary-artery catheters in high-risk surgical patients. *N Engl J Med.* 2003;348:5–14.
65. Richard C, Warszawski J, Anguel N, et al. Early use of the pulmonary artery catheter and outcomes in patients with shock and acute respiratory distress syndrome: a randomized controlled trial. *JAMA.* 2003;290:2713–2720.
66. Lopez-Herce J, Ruperez M, Sanchez C, Garcia C, Garcia E. Correlation between cardiac output measured by the femoral arterial thermodilution technique pulmonary arterial and that measured by contour pulse analysis in a paediatric animal model. *J Clin Monit Comput.* 2006;20:19–23.
67. Ruperez M, Lopez-Herce J, Garcia C, Sanchez C, Garcia E, Vigil D. Comparison between cardiac output measured by the pulmonary arterial thermodilution technique and that measured by the femoral arterial thermodilution technique in a pediatric animal model. *Pediatr Cardiol.* 2004;25:119–123.
68. Pauli C, Fakler U, Genz T, Hennig M, Lorenz HP, Hess J. Cardiac output determination in children: equivalence of the transpulmonary thermodilution method to the direct Fick principle. *Intensive Care Med.* 2002;28:947–952.
69. Goedje O, Hoeke K, Lichtwarck-Aschoff M, Faltchauser A, Lamm P, Reichart B. Continuous cardiac output by femoral arterial thermodilution calibrated pulse contour analysis: comparison with pulmonary arterial thermodilution. *Crit Care Med.* 1999;27:2407–2412.
70. Zollner C, Briegel J, Kilger E, Haller M. [Retrospective analysis of transpulmonary and pulmonary arterial measurement of cardiac output in ARDS patients]. *Anaesthesist.* 1998;47:912–917.
71. Zollner C, Haller M, Weis M, Morstedt K, Lamm P, Kilger E, Goetz AE. Beat-to-beat measurement of cardiac output by intravascular pulse contour analysis: a prospective criterion standard study in patients after cardiac surgery. *J Cardiothorac Vasc Anesth.* 2000;14:125–129.
72. Kuntscher MV, Blome-Eberwein S, Pelzer M, Erdmann D, Germann G. Transcardiopulmonary vs pulmonary arterial thermodilution methods for hemodynamic monitoring of burned patients. *J Burn Care Rehabil.* 2002;23:21–26.
73. Sakka SG, Kozieras J, Thuemer O, van Hout N. Measurement of cardiac output: a comparison between transpulmonary thermodilution and uncalibrated pulse contour analysis. *Br J Anaesth.* 2007;99:337–342.
74. Della Rocca G, Costa MG, Pompei L, Coccia C, Pietropaoli P. Continuous and intermittent cardiac output measurement: pulmonary artery catheter versus aortic transpulmonary technique. *Br J Anaesth.* 2002;88:350–356.
75. Hamzaoui O, Monnet X, Richard C, Osman D, Chemla D, Teboul JL. Effects of changes in vascular tone on the agreement between pulse contour and transpulmonary thermodilution cardiac output measurements within an up to 6-hour calibration-free period. *Crit Care Med.* 2008;36:434–440.
76. Buhre W, Weyland A, Kazmaier S, et al. Comparison of cardiac output assessed by pulse-contour analysis and thermodilution in patients undergoing minimally invasive direct coronary artery bypass grafting. *J Cardiothorac Vasc Anesth.* 1999;13:437–440.
77. Gust R, Gottschalk A, Bauer H, Bottiger BW, Bohrer H, Martin E. Cardiac output measurement by transpulmonary versus conventional thermodilution technique in intensive care patients after coronary artery bypass grafting. *J Cardiothorac Vasc Anesth.* 1998;12:519–522.
78. Godje O, Peyerl M, Seebauer T, Dewald O, Reichart B. Reproducibility of double indicator dilution measurements of intrathoracic blood volume compartments, extravascular lung water, and liver function. *Chest.* 1998;113:1070–1077.
79. Sander M, Spies CD, Grubitzsch H, Foer A, Muller M, von Heymann C. Comparison of uncalibrated arterial waveform analysis in cardiac surgery patients with thermodilution cardiac output measurements. *Crit Care.* 2006;10:R164.
80. Thiele RH, Bartels K, Gan TJ. Cardiac output monitoring: a contemporary assessment and review. *Crit Care Med.* 2015;43:177–185.
81. Frank O. Die Grundform des arteriellen Pulses. *Zeitung für Biol.* 1899;37:483–586.
82. Essler S, Schroeder MJ, Phaniraj V, Koenig SC, Latham RD, Ewert D. Fast estimation of arterial vascular parameters for transient and steady beats with application to hemodynamic state under variant gravitational conditions. *Ann Biomed Eng.* 1999;27:486–497.
83. Thiele RH, Durieux ME. Arterial waveform analysis for the anesthesiologist: past, present, and future concepts. *Anesth Analg.* 2011;113:766–776.
84. Pratt B, Roteliuk L, Hatib F, Frazier J, Wallen RD. Calculating arterial pressure-based cardiac output using a novel measurement and analysis method. *Biomed Instrum Technol.* 2007;41:403–411.
85. Cooper ES, Muir WW. Continuous cardiac output monitoring via arterial pressure waveform analysis following severe hemorrhagic shock in dogs. *Crit Care Med.* 2007;35:1724–1729.
86. Johansson A, Chew M. Reliability of continuous pulse contour cardiac output measurement during hemodynamic instability. *J Clin Monit Comput.* 2007;21:237–242.
87. Schuerholz T, Meyer MC, Friedrich L, Przemeck M, Sumpelmann R, Marx G. Reliability of continuous cardiac output determination by pulse-contour analysis in porcine septic shock. *Acta Anaesthesiol Scand.* 2006;50:407–413.
88. Hamm JB, Nguyen BV, Kiss G, et al. Assessment of a cardiac output device using arterial pulse waveform analysis, Vigileo, in cardiac surgery compared to pulmonary arterial thermodilution. *Anaesth Intensive Care*; 38:295–301.
89. Jeong YB, Kim TH, Roh YJ, Choi IC, Suh JH. Comparison of uncalibrated arterial pressure waveform analysis with continuous thermodilution cardiac output measurements in patients undergoing elective off-pump coronary artery bypass surgery. *J Cardiothorac Vasc Anesth*; 24:767–771.
90. Krejci V, Vannucci A, Abbas A, Chapman W, Kangrga IM. Comparison of calibrated and uncalibrated arterial pressure-based cardiac output monitors during orthotopic liver transplantation. *Liver Transplant.* 2010;16:773–782.
91. Bein B, Meybohm P, Cavus E, et al. The reliability of pulse contour-derived cardiac output during hemorrhage and after vasopressor administration. *Anesth Analg.* 2007;105:107–113.
92. Suehiro K, Tanaka K, Yamada T, et al. The ability of the Vigileo-FloTrac system to measure cardiac output and track cardiac output changes during one-lung ventilation. *J Clin Monit Comput.* 2015;29:333–339.
93. Tomasi R, Prueckner S, Czerner S, et al. Comparison of an advanced minimally invasive cardiac output monitoring with a continuous invasive cardiac output monitoring during lung transplantation. *J Clin Monit Comput.* 2016;30:475–480.

94. Xu D, Olivier NB, Mukkamala R. Continuous cardiac output and left atrial pressure monitoring by long time interval analysis of the pulmonary artery pressure waveform: proof of concept in dogs. *J Appl Physiol.* 2009;106:651–661.
95. Greiwe G, Peters V, Hapfelmeier A, Romagnoli S, Kubik M, Saugel B. Cardiac output estimation by multi-beat analysis of the radial arterial blood pressure waveform versus intermittent pulmonary artery thermodilution: a method comparison study in patients treated in the intensive care unit after off-pump coronary artery bypass surgery. *J Clin Monit Comput.* 2020;34(4):643–648.
96. Saugel B, Heeschen J, Hapfelmeier A, Romagnoli S, Greiwe G. Cardiac output estimation using multi-beat analysis of the radial arterial blood pressure waveform: a method comparison study in patients having off-pump coronary artery bypass surgery using intermittent pulmonary artery thermodilution as the reference method. *J Clin Monit Comput.* 2020;43(4):649–654.
97. Scolletta S, Romano SM, Biagioli B, Capannini G, Giomarelli P. Pressure recording analytical method (PRAM) for measurement of cardiac output during various haemodynamic states. *Br J Anaesth.* 2005;95:159–165.
98. Gopal S, Do T, Pooni JS, Martinelli G. Validation of cardiac output studies from the Mostcare compared to a pulmonary artery catheter in septic patients. *Minerva Anestesiol.* 2014;80: 314–323.
99. Linton NW, Linton RA. Estimation of changes in cardiac output from the arterial blood pressure waveform in the upper limb. *Br J Anaesth.* 2001;86:486–496.
100. D'Arrigo S, Sandroni C, Cacciola S, et al. Are peripherally inserted central catheters suitable for cardiac output assessment with transpulmonary thermodilution? *Crit Care Med.* 2019;47:1356–1361.
101. Orme RM, Pigott DW, Mihm FG. Measurement of cardiac output by transpulmonary arterial thermodilution using a long radial artery catheter. A comparison with intermittent pulmonary artery thermodilution. *Anaesthesia.* 2004;59:590–594.
102. Hadian M, Kim HK, Severyn DA, Pinsky MR. Cross-comparison of cardiac output trending accuracy of LiDCO, PiCCO, FloTrac and pulmonary artery catheters. *Crit Care.* 2010;14:R212.
103. Kiefer N, Hofer CK, Marx G, et al. Clinical validation of a new thermodilution system for the assessment of cardiac output and volumetric parameters. *Crit Care.* 2012;16:R98.
104. Kamal GD, Symreng T, Starr J. Inconsistent esophageal Doppler cardiac output during acute blood loss. *Anesthesiology.* 1990;72:95–99.
105. Smith HJ, Grottum P, Simonsen S. Doppler flowmetry in the lower thoracic aorta. An indirect estimation of cardiac output. *Acta Radiol Diagn* (Stockh). 1985;26:257–263.
106. Davies JN, Allen DR, Chant AD. Non-invasive Doppler-derived cardiac output: a validation study comparing this technique with thermodilution and Fick methods. *Eur J Vasc Surg.* 1991;5:497–500.
107. Valtier B, Cholley BP, Belot JP, de la Coussaye JE, Mateo J, Payen DM. Noninvasive monitoring of cardiac output in critically ill patients using transesophageal Doppler. *Am J Respir Crit Care Med.* 1998;158:77–83.
108. Knirsch W, Kretschmar O, Tomaske M, et al. Comparison of cardiac output measurement using the CardioQP oesophageal Doppler with cardiac output measurement using thermodilution technique in children during heart catheterisation. *Anaesthesia.* 2008;63:851–855.
109. Ferreira RM, do Amaral JL, Valiatti JL. [Comparison between two methods for hemodynamic measurement: thermodilution and oesophageal doppler]. *Rev Assoc Med Bras.* 2007;53:349–354.
110. Diaper J, Ellenberger C, Villiger Y, et al. Comparison of cardiac output as assessed by transesophageal echo-Doppler and transpulmonary thermodilution in patients undergoing thoracic surgery. *J Clin Anesth.* 2010;22:97–103.
111. Diaper J, Ellenberger C, Villiger Y, Robert J, Tschopp JM, Licker M. Transoesophageal Doppler monitoring for fluid and hemodynamic treatment during lung surgery. *J Clin Monit Comput.* 2008;22:367–374.
112. Kallmeyer IJ, Collard CD, Fox JA, Body SC, Shernan SK. The safety of intraoperative transesophageal echocardiography: a case series of 7200 cardiac surgical patients. *Anesth Analg.* 2001;92:1126–1130.
113. Nyboer J. Electrical impedance plethysmography; a physical and physiologic approach to peripheral vascular study. *Circulation.* 1950;2:811–821.
114. Bernstein DP. A new stroke volume equation for thoracic electrical bioimpedance: theory and rationale. *Crit Care Med.* 1986;14:904–909.
115. Kubicek WG, Kottke J, Ramos MU, et al. The Minnesota impedance cardiograph- theory and applications. *Biomed Eng.* 1974;9:410–416.
116. Patterson RP, Witsoe DA, From A. Impedance stroke volume compared with dye and electromagnetic flowmeter values during drug-induced inotropic and vascular changes in dogs. *Ann N Y Acad Sci.* 1999;873:143–148.
117. Wallace AW, Salahieh A, Lawrence A, Spector K, Owens C, Alonso D. Endotracheal cardiac output monitor. *Anesthesiology.* 2000;92:178–189.
118. Gotshall RW, Miles DS. Noninvasive assessment of cardiac output by impedance cardiography in the newborn canine. *Crit Care Med.* 1989;17:63–65.
119. Miles DS, Gotshall RW, Sexson WR. Evaluation of impedance cardiography in the canine pup. *J Appl Physiol.* 1986;60:260–265.
120. Pappas CG, Wang X, Connolly RJ, Schwaitzberg SD. Impedance cardiography in the measurement of cardiac output: studies in rabbits. *J Surg Res.* 1995;59:504–510.
121. Spinelli JC, Valentinuzzi ME. Stroke volume in the dog: measurements by the impedance technique and thermodilution. *Med Prog Technol.* 1983;10:45–53.
122. Ball TR, Culp BC, Patel V, Gloyna DF, Ciceri DP, Culp WC Jr. Comparison of the endotracheal cardiac output monitor to thermodilution in cardiac surgery patients. *J Cardiothorac Vasc Anesth.* 2010;24:762–766.
123. Maus TM, Reber B, Banks DA, Berry A, Guerrero E, Manecke GR. Cardiac output determination from endotracheally measured impedance cardiography: clinical evaluation of endotracheal cardiac output monitor. *J Cardiothorac Vasc Anesth.* 2011; 25:770–775.
124. Moller-Sorensen H, Hansen KL, Ostergaard M, Andersen LW, Moller K. Lack of agreement and trending ability of the endotracheal cardiac output monitor compared with thermodilution. *Acta Anaesthesiol Scand.* 2012;56:433–440.
125. van der Kleij SC, Koolen BB, Newhall DA, et al. Clinical evaluation of a new tracheal impedance cardiography method. *Anaesthesia.* 2012;67:729–733.
126. Keren H, Burkhoff D, Squara P. Evaluation of a noninvasive continuous cardiac output monitoring system based on thoracic bioreactance. *Am J Physiol Heart Circ Physiol.* 2007;293:H583–H589.
127. Weisz DE, Jain A, McNamara PJ, EL-Khuffash A. Non-invasive cardiac output monitoring in neonates using bioreactance: a comparison with echocardiography. *Neonatology.* 2012;102:61–67.

128. Raval NY, Squara P, Cleman M, Yalamanchili K, Winklmaier M, Burkhoff D. Multicenter evaluation of noninvasive cardiac output measurement by bioreactance technique. *J Clin Monit Comput*. 2008;22:113–119.
129. Marque S, Cariou A, Chiche JD, Squara P. Comparison between Flotrac-Vigileo and Bioreactance, a totally noninvasive method for cardiac output monitoring. *Crit Care*. 2009;13:R73.
130. Kutlu CA, Williams EA, Evans TW, Pastorino U, Goldstraw P. Acute lung injury and acute respiratory distress syndrome after pulmonary resection. *Ann Thorac Surg*. 2000;69:376–380.
131. Licker M, de Perrot M, Spiliopoulos A, et al. Risk factors for acute lung injury after thoracic surgery for lung cancer. *Anesth Analg*. 2003;97:1558–1565.
132. Alam N, Park BJ, Wilton A, et al. Incidence and risk factors for lung injury after lung cancer resection. *Ann Thorac Surg*. 2007;84:1085–1091; discussion 91.
133. Marret E, Miled F, Bazelly B, et al. Risk and protective factors for major complications after pneumonectomy for lung cancer. *Interact Cardiovasc Thorac Surg*. 2010;10:936–939.
134. Noblett SE, Snowden CP, Shenton BK, Horgan AF. Randomized clinical trial assessing the effect of Doppler-optimized fluid management on outcome after elective colorectal resection. *Br J Surg*. 2006;93:1069–1076.
135. Wakeling HG, McFall MR, Jenkins CS, et al. Intraoperative oesophageal Doppler guided fluid management shortens postoperative hospital stay after major bowel surgery. *Br J Anaesth*. 2005;95:634–642.
136. Venn R, Steele A, Richardson P, Poloniecki J, Grounds M, Newman P. Randomized controlled trial to investigate influence of the fluid challenge on duration of hospital stay and perioperative morbidity in patients with hip fractures. *Br J Anaesth*. 2002;88:65–71.
137. Gan TJ, Soppitt A, Maroof M, et al. Goal-directed intraoperative fluid administration reduces length of hospital stay after major surgery. *Anesthesiology*. 2002;97:820–826.
138. Sinclair S, James S, Singer M. Intraoperative intravascular volume optimisation and length of hospital stay after repair of proximal femoral fracture: randomised controlled trial. *BMJ*. 1997;315:909–912.
139. Chytra I, Pradl R, Bosman R, Pelnar P, Kasal E, Zidkova A. Esophageal Doppler-guided fluid management decreases blood lactate levels in multiple-trauma patients: a randomized controlled trial. *Crit Care*. 2007;11:R24.
140. Lopes MR, Oliveira MA, Pereira VO, Lemos IP, Auler JO Jr, Michard F. Goal-directed fluid management based on pulse pressure variation monitoring during high-risk surgery: a pilot randomized controlled trial. *Crit Care*. 2007;11:R100.
141. Benes J, Chytra I, Altmann P, et al. Intraoperative fluid optimization using stroke volume variation in high risk surgical patients: results of prospective randomized study. *Crit Care*. 2010;14:R118.
142. Jones C, Kelliher L, Dickinson M, et al. Randomized clinical trial on enhanced recovery versus standard care following open liver resection. *Br J Surg*. 2013;100:1015–1024.
143. Buettner M, Schummer W, Huettemann E, Schenke S, van Hout N, Sakka SG. Influence of systolic-pressure-variation-guided intraoperative fluid management on organ function and oxygen transport. *Br J Anaesth*. 2008;101:194–199.
144. Ramsingh DS, Sanghvi C, Gamboa J, Cannesson M, Applegate RL 2nd. Outcome impact of goal directed fluid therapy during high risk abdominal surgery in low to moderate risk patients: a randomized controlled trial. *J Clin Monit Comput*. 2013;27:249–257.
145. Pearse R, Dawson D, Fawcett J, Rhodes A, Grounds RM, Bennett ED. Early goal-directed therapy after major surgery reduces complications and duration of hospital stay. A randomised, controlled trial [ISRCTN38797445]. *Crit Care*. 2005;9:R687–R693.
146. Thiele RH, Colquhoun DA, Blum FE, Durieux ME. The ability of anesthesia providers to visually estimate systolic pressure variability using the "eyeball" technique. *Anesth Analg*. 2012;115:176–181.
147. Suehiro K, Okutani R. Influence of tidal volume for stroke volume variation to predict fluid responsiveness in patients undergoing one-lung ventilation. *J Anesth*. 2011;25:777–780.
148. Suehiro K, Okutani R. Stroke volume variation as a predictor of fluid responsiveness in patients undergoing one-lung ventilation. *J Cardiothorac Vasc Anesth*. 2010;24:772–775.
149. Fu Q, Zhao F, Mi W, Zhang H. Stroke volume variation fail to predict fluid responsiveness in patients undergoing pulmonary lobectomy with one-lung ventilation using thoracotomy. *Biosci Trends*. 2014;8:59–63.
150. Fu Q, Duan M, Zhao F, Mi W. Evaluation of stroke volume variation and pulse pressure variation as predictors of fluid responsiveness in patients undergoing protective one-lung ventilation. *Drug Discov Ther*. 2015;9:296–302.
151. Lee JH, Jeon Y, Bahk JH, et al. Pulse pressure variation as a predictor of fluid responsiveness during one-lung ventilation for lung surgery using thoracotomy: randomised controlled study. *Eur J Anaesthesiol*. 2011;28:39–44.
152. de Waal EE, Rex S, Kruitwagen CL, Kalkman CJ, Buhre WF. Dynamic preload indicators fail to predict fluid responsiveness in open-chest conditions. *Crit Care Med*. 2009;37:510–515.
153. Vistisen ST, Berg JM, Boekel MF, et al. Using extra systoles and the micro-fluid challenge to predict fluid responsiveness during cardiac surgery. *J Clin Monit Comput*. 2019;33:777–786.
154. Mukhtar A, Awad M, Elayashy M, et al. Validity of mini-fluid challenge for predicting fluid responsiveness following liver transplantation. *BMC Anesthesiol*. 2019;19:56.
155. Biais M, de Courson H, Lanchon R, et al. Mini-fluid challenge of 100 mL of crystalloid predicts fluid responsiveness in the operating room. *Anesthesiology*. 2017;127:450–456.
156. Bindels AJ, van der Hoeven JG, Meinders AE. Pulmonary artery wedge pressure and extravascular lung water in patients with acute cardiogenic pulmonary edema requiring mechanical ventilation. *Am J Cardiol*. 1999;84:1158–1163.
157. Brown LM, Liu KD, Matthay MA. Measurement of extravascular lung water using the single indicator method in patients: research and potential clinical value. *Am J Physiol Lung Cell Mol Physiol*. 2009;297:L547–L558.
158. Oshima K, Kunimoto F, Hinohara H, et al. Evaluation of respiratory status in patients after thoracic esophagectomy using PiCCO system. *Ann Thorac Cardiovasc Surg*. 2008;14:283–288.
159. Sato Y, Motoyama S, Maruyama K, et al. Extravascular lung water measured using single transpulmonary thermodilution reflects perioperative pulmonary edema induced by esophagectomy. *Eur Surg Res*. 2007;39:7–13.
160. Jozwiak M, Silva S, Persichini R, et al. Extravascular lung water is an independent prognostic factor in patients with acute respiratory distress syndrome. *Crit Care Med*. 2013;41:472–480.
161. Pottecher J, Roche AC, Degot T, et al. Groupe de Transplantation Pulmonaire des Hopitaux Universitaires de S. Increased extravascular lung water and plasma biomarkers of acute lung injury precede oxygenation impairment in primary graft dysfunction after lung transplantation. *Transplantation*. 2017;101:112–121.

162. Kim HJ, Cha SI, Kim CH, et al. Risk factors of postoperative acute lung injury following lobectomy for nonsmall cell lung cancer. *Medicine* (Baltimore). 2019;98:e15078.
163. Chau EH, Slinger P. Perioperative fluid management for pulmonary resection surgery and esophagectomy. *Semin Cardiothorac Vasc Anesth*. 2014;18:36–44.
164. Casado D, Lopez F, Marti R. Perioperative fluid management and major respiratory complications in patients undergoing esophagectomy. *Dis Esophagus*. 2010;23:523–528.
165. Michard F. Lung water assessment: from gravimetry to wearables. *J Clin Monit Comput*. 2019;33:1–4.
166. Lange NR, Schuster DP. The measurement of lung water. *Crit Care*. 1999;3:R19–R24.
167. Nierman DM, Eisen DI, Fein ED, Hannon E, Mechanick JI, Benjamin E. Transthoracic bioimpedance can measure extravascular lung water in acute lung injury. *J Surg Res*. 1996;65:101–108.
168. Zellner JL, Spinale FG, Crawford FA. Bioimpedance: a novel method for the determination of extravascular lung water. *J Surg Res*. 1990;48:454–459.
169. Spinale FG, Reines HD, Cook MC, Crawford FA. Noninvasive estimation of extravascular lung water using bioimpedance. *J Surg Res*. 1989;47:535–540.
170. Trepte CJ, Phillips CR, Sola J, et al. Electrical impedance tomography (EIT) for quantification of pulmonary edema in acute lung injury. *Crit Care*. 2016;20:18.
171. Tomicic V, Cornejo R. Lung monitoring with electrical impedance tomography: technical considerations and clinical applications. *J Thorac Dis*. 2019;11:3122–3135.
172. Pulletz S, Elke G, Zick G, Schadler D, Scholz J, Weiler N, Frerichs I. Performance of electrical impedance tomography in detecting regional tidal volumes during one-lung ventilation. *Acta Anaesthesiol Scand*. 2008;52:1131–1139.

NON-PRINT ITEMS

Abstract

Thoracic surgery is a rapidly changing surgical subspecialty that presents the anesthesiology community with a myriad of challenges, one of which is hemodynamic monitoring. Thoracic surgical patients range from relatively healthy adults with refractory gastroesophageal reflux in need of a laparoscopic Nissen fundoplication, to patients with severe atherosclerosis and chronic obstructive pulmonary disease needing a pneumonectomy for cancer resection, to patients in need of lung transplantation. The 30-day mortality for this population ranges from less than 1% for sublobar resections, to almost 4% for pneumonectomies, and to 6% for lung transplantation. Complicating hemodynamic monitoring and management of this population is the deep interdependence between the cardiac and pulmonary systems. The combination of comorbidities, invasiveness of the procedure, impact of thoracic surgery on hemodynamics, and challenges associated with monitoring make thoracic surgical procedures some of the most difficult and rewarding procedures that an anesthesiologist will manage. The purpose of this chapter is to review the hemodynamic monitoring devices available to assist in the management of this diverse population, with a particular focus on blood pressure monitoring, cardiac output, and fluid responsiveness. Also included are central venous pressure, pulmonary artery pressure, and extravascular lung water.

Keywords

blood pressure monitoring, central venous pressure, pulmonary artery pressure, cardiac output monitoring, fluid responsiveness, extravascular lung water

13

Flexible and Rigid Bronchoscopy in Thoracic Anesthesia

MANUEL GRANELL GIL, ELENA BIOSCA PÉREZ, RUTH MARTÍNEZ PLUMED

Introduction

The complex cardiopulmonary interactions, combined with abnormal secretion and surgical impairment of lung-chest wall dynamics makes hypoxemia, hypo- and hypertension, dysrhythmia, hypercapnia, and acidosis common threats in the perioperative period. Bronchoscopy by definition is a procedure that allows for the visualization and examination of the tracheobronchial tree. This discipline has been one of the most significant advances in respiratory disease diagnosis and treatment, and is considered an essential instrument in pneumonology.[1]

Bronchoscopy originated at the end of the 19th century. Before this, direct exploration of the distal respiratory tract was considered an overly dangerous procedure. Nevertheless, in 1887, Dr. Gustav Killian, otorhinolaryngology specialist of the University of Freiburg in Germany, carried out the first direct laryngoscopy on a patient suffering from dyspnea, cough, hemoptysis, and foreign body aspiration. Using a Kirstein laryngoscope, Killian was able to visually inspect the primary bronchi and observe the presence of a solid foreign mass in the patient's lungs. Through esophagoscopy and under a local anesthesia using cocaine, Killian was able to extract the foreign body successfully. History considers Killian as the father of modern bronchoscopy.

Sometime afterwards, Dr. Chevalier Jackson, a North American physician, offered an alternative without the need for a laryngoscope; the autonomous rigid bronchoscope. This self-illuminating instrument contains a small bulb at the distal extremity, providing the distinct advantage of visualizing endobronchial lesions. This can be considered one of the most significant advances in bronchoscopy, providing greater possibilities for visual diagnostics and providing possible treatments.

In 1966, Japanese physician Dr. Shigeto Ikeda, introduced the first flexible bronchoscope containing optical fibers, revolutionizing bronchial endoscopic procedures, following which, the use of rigid bronchoscopes diminished significantly. Nevertheless, toward the end of the 20th century, there was an increase in the variety of therapeutic techniques, including procedures using lasers, endobronchial implants, stents, and bronchial prosthetics, known as *interventional bronchoscopy*.

Anesthesiologists presently use flexible bronchoscopy (FB) in various clinical scenarios with regards to bronchoscopy, the most common of which incorporates the use of the guided insertion or optimal positioning of double-lumen tubes (DLTs) and/or endobronchial blockers for pulmonary isolation and/or separation. Moreover, bronchoscopy is useful and necessary in managing difficult airways, allowing for tracheal intubations by using FB. Other scenarios that implicate these types of instruments include the cardio thoracic surgery intensive care units (ICUs) and in procedures for interventional pneumology.

Rigid Bronchoscopy

Rigid bronchoscopy (RB) is an invasive procedure that allows for the simultaneous ventilation, oxygenation, inspection, and intervention on the airways

Composition

A rigid bronchoscope is composed of a hollow metallic tube with a bevelled distal extremity. In the proximal extremity, the "head" of the endoscope has three ports; one designated to an optic device, one for the instrument at work, and another for ventilation (lateral port). The lengths may vary between 33 cm (tracheoscope) and 43 cm (bronchoscope), while diameters may vary between 3 and 14 mm. Rigid bronchoscopes have fenestrations on the distal segment that allow for lateral ventilation when performing selective intubation.

Indications

These instruments are ideal for complex cases, allowing for greater control of the respiratory tract, respiration, blood, secretions, and obtaining large samples. RB is used to place rigid silicone tracheal stents that are used as primary treatment for lumen collapse or to stabilize a reconstructive effort of the larynx or trachea to prevent collapse.

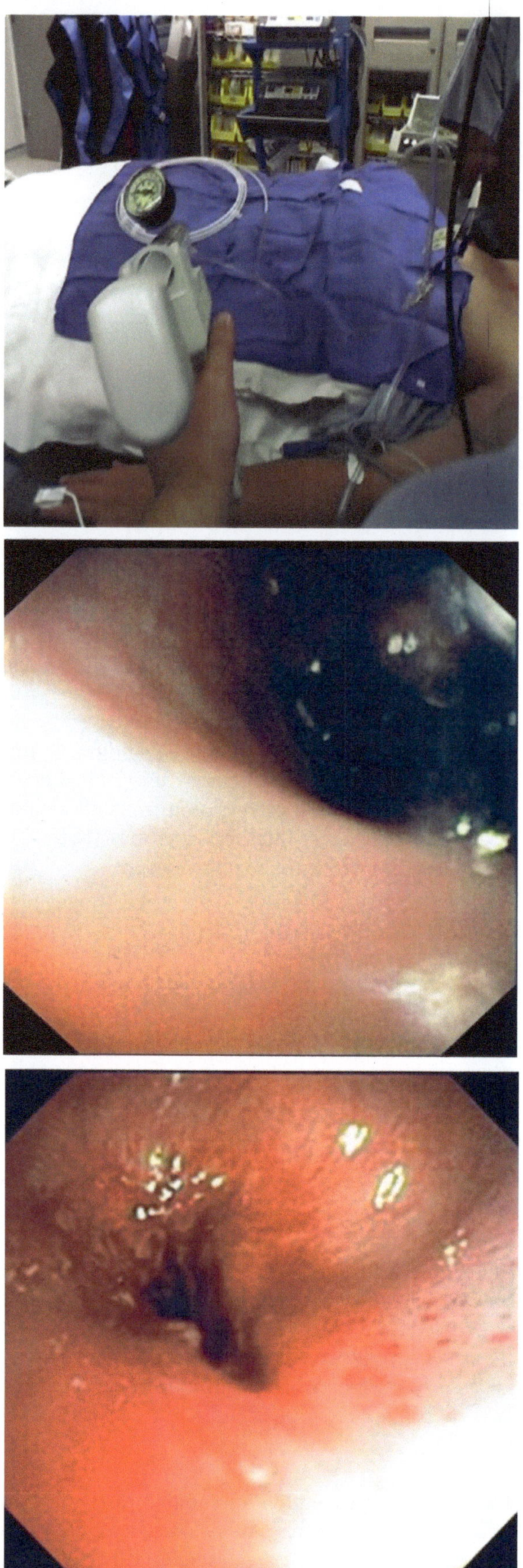

A
B
C

• **Fig. 13.1** Trachealstenosis dilation with balloon. (Courtesy of Edmond Cohen.)

They are frequently used for the extraction of foreign bodies and interventional pulmonary procedures such as the insertion of stents, dilation of tracheal and bronchial stenosis, as well as laser ablation. Such procedures are frequently performed under general anesthetic alongside neuromuscular blockades (Fig. 13.1).

Flexible Bronchoscopy

The flexible fiberoptic bronchoscope (FFB) has become an essential tool in the thoracic anesthesiologist's practice over the past 25 years. It was the logical successor to the rigid intubating bronchoscope as a tool for precise positioning of transthoracic echocardiography. It is used as an intubation guide, a directed suction catheter, a short-term airway, and a therapeutic instrument in a number of perianesthetic settings. Fiberoptic bronchoscopy is the most widely performed procedure, noninvasive, simple, and associated with a lower morbidity rate (0.1%–2.5%) and a practically null mortality rate (<0.05%).[2]

The development of FB, as described by Ikeda in 1968, revolutionized bronchology to allow visualization of airways down to the segmental bronchi and is used in guiding the pulmonary isolation and separation procedures. Furthermore, FB is used for diagnostics for a variety of pulmonary diseases.

Composition

FFB is a flexible instrument with the length measuring between 50 and 60 cm, made from fiberoptics, and encased in a vinyl covering. The interior contains a work canal, with the last 2.5 cm having a steerable angulation. The external diameter for adults is usually between 5.2 and 6 mm, with a work canal of 2.0 and 2.8 mm, respectively. Small size FFBs from 2.0 mm to 4.0 mm are available and recently introduced as disposable for single use. Flexible video-bronchoscopes have a digital chip in the distal extremity that transmits images to a video processer for external monitoring. A newer generation of FFBs, with improved optics, a larger working channel, greater stiffness, and a more slender profile, is more easily used to assess or position a device in optimal bronchial position or within small bronchopulmonary segments and is less likely to obstruct ventilation during use with consequent air trapping and barotrauma. It is logical that the thoracic anesthesiologist with knowledge of cardiorespiratory function and the pathology of pulmonary disease, should master the use of fiberoptic instruments as an adjunctive means for precise definition of the dynamics of airway pathology, for direct control of DLT, EET, or bronchial blocker (BB) placement.[3]

The FFB is connected to an external light source. Image processor connections allow for the adjustment of light intensity, color, and brightness, also having the ability to save images. The majority of anesthesiologists prefer to use an external monitor, which is more comfortable, allowing access to enlarged images and is useful as a teaching tool.

Portable FFB exists that include a small screen incorporated into the head, which uses a battery that economically powers the device and also helps adjust the intensity of light. This is especially useful for procedures outside of an endoscopic unit, such as in an ICU, emergency room, or in an operating theatre.

Indications

Among the indications for FB for the anesthesiologist during thoracic surgery intraoperatively are practices related to general airways and isolation and/or separation of lungs. The latter is additionally associated with requirements for one-lung ventilation (OLV) during thoracic surgery; for example, the insertion of DLTs or a BB. Moreover, FB is fundamental throughout the postoperative periods for the diagnostics and treatment of complications associated with thoracic surgery.

FB is also considered a diagnostic procedure and has been the focus of most basic therapeutic procedures in pneumology and is used to obtain biopsies from the mediastinum and the pulmonary parenchyma, among other anomalies in the respiratory tract. From this perspective, a large number of therapeutic techniques are available, including the use of cryotherapy (Fig. 13.2) and cryobiopsies using flexible probes, coagulation with argon plasma (Fig. 13.3), and electrocautery. In other cases, these may also include the implantation of prosthetics stents and devices that can be used to place a unidirectional airways valve for the treatment of pulmonary emphysema. Although many of these techniques can be successfully carried out under moderate sedation, the complexity and longer duration of these procedures combined with the necessity to guarantee the tolerance and comfort of the patient usually makes a deep general anesthetic necessary. The type of anesthetic will be dependent on the difficulty and approximate duration of the procedure, as well as the comorbidities and level of cooperation of the patient.[3]

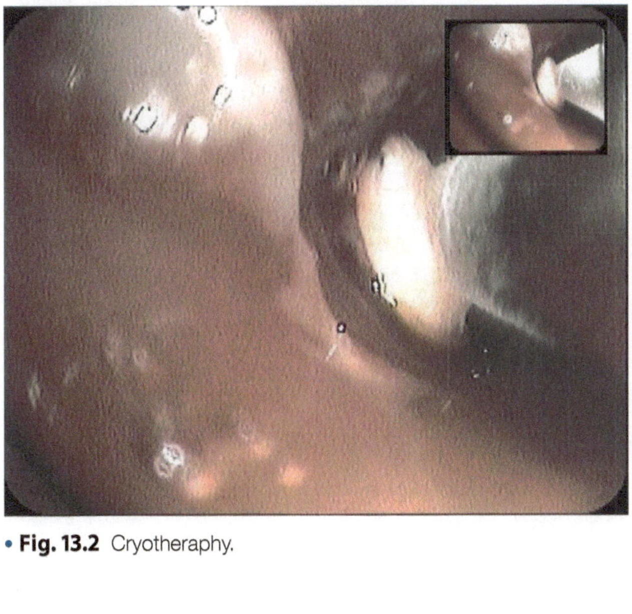

• **Fig. 13.2** Cryotheraphy.

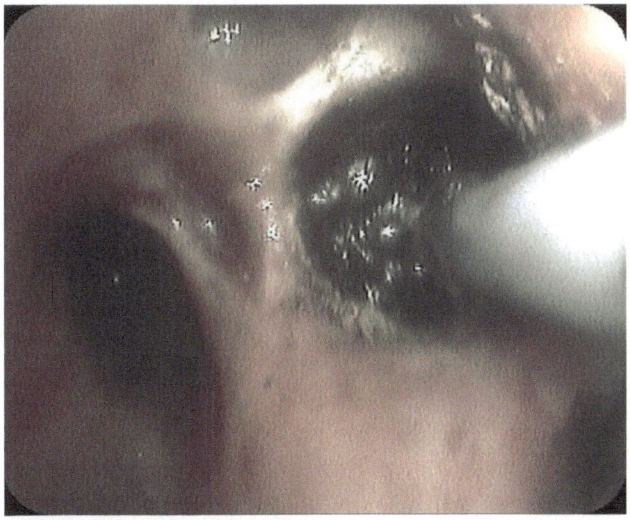

• **Fig. 13.3** Argon on tumor tissue.

Contraindications

Contraindications are few taking into consideration the risk-benefit ratio of each disease and the contraindications of the technique itself.

Some clinical situations are considered particularly high risk, such as severe arrhythmias during the 4 weeks after an acute myocardial infarction in a patient with unstable angina. Other cases include refractory hypoxemia and the existence of uncontrolled coagulopathies in severe cases of renal failure and in the patient objection.

Flexible Bronchoscopy in Thoracic Surgery

Presurgical Diagnostics

The advantage of a flexible instrument is that it can be steered and directed around the anatomic structures. The FFB is not rigid enough to force its way past obstructions and foreign bodies. Consequently, lifting or displacing tissues the way one does with rigid instruments should not be attempted. The tip is advanced and angled by both hands to follow the most convenient, least resistant path to reach its goal. Once there, it can provide information and be used to direct drug application or suction for pulmonary toilet. Fibrobronchoscopic diagnostics before surgery is a fundamental procedure to extensively evaluate the type of tumor, the possibility of resectability, or any tracheal or main stem pathology that could interfere with the placement of isolating devices to provide OLV.[4]

Once the lesion has been located, biopsy forceps can be used through the working channel to obtain histologic samples for analysis. A sample of a purely cytologic nature can be obtained through brushing the area. Furthermore, in cases where the lesion is difficult to locate with bronchoscopy, obtaining distal samples can be performed via blind brushing of the area, as well as bronchoalveolar lavage (BAL). In microbiologic diagnostic cases, BAL is of great importance, while brushes and biopsies are also viable resources.[5]

Following an evaluation of the airway, the possibility of placing a conventional endotracheal tube (ETT) can be assessed, as well as the size of the tube. Additionally, the possibility of ventilation using a laryngeal mask or ventilation jets through a cannula can be considered. The information provided by FB can thus be considered of great value in each of these cases.

Airway Management

The patients frequently subjected to thoracic surgery are more likely to present abnormalities of the superior and inferior airways in comparison to the rest of the general population. These patients therefore potentially present with a difficult airway (DA).[6] Despite the availability of other devices for airway management such as the videolaryngoscopes, FB can be considered the "gold standard" for endotracheal intubation in cases of DA.[6]

Use of Flexible Bronchoscopy in Difficult Airways

Handling of DAs in thoracic surgery and the need for separation can be a challenging. In high-risk situations such as hemorrhage, infection, and tracheobronchial fistulas among others, securing the airway will always be the priority.[7]

DA is the "gold standard" to perform awake intubation with FB. In cases where pulmonary isolations are absolutely necessary, tube exchangers can be used to place a DLT. Otherwise, a BB can be placed through the single lumen tube to provide lung separation. Only in those patients where mask ventilation is presumed easy, can the insertion of a DLT be performed with the aid of a videolaryngoscope as a main option.[6,8,9]

The direct insertion of a DLT through FB while the patient is awake is not an easy task because of the angled morphology of the distal extremity of the device, making the correct placement difficult as well as maneuvering the device through the vocal cords.

For the technique to be successful, the key is the adequate preparation of the patient before intervention. Unless specified as a contraindication, antisialogues are generally recommended, especially in cases of thoracic surgery because of the high percentage of patients who are smokers and/or chronic bronchial patients with increased basal secretions. Likewise, other common actions include a degree of sedation that allows for spontaneous ventilation and a correct topicalization of the airway with 1% lidocaine, allowing for the elimination of cough reflexes, as well as laryngospasms.[10]

Use of Flexible Bronchoscopy for the Correct Positioning of Double-Lumen Tubes (See Chapters 16 and 17)

To achieve an adequate OLV, two main devices are available, including BBs and DLTs. The FFB provides both diagnostic and therapeutic information when used for precise placement of lung isolation devices, selective tracheobronchial suction and lavage, and management of otherwise difficult airways. Surgical procedures in the thorax actively manipulate intrathoracic structures and may displace the tracheobronchial structure and secretion possibly requiring intraoperative bronchoscopy. Secretion obstruction, misalignment, and/or kinking of ETT and DLTs can present as clinical bronchospasm, with decreased tidal volume, air trapping, or increased intraoperative "shunt". For these reasons, hypoxemia during OLA requires repeat endoscopy for verification of EBT or BB position.

The incorrect positioning of DLTs are one of the most common causes of hypoxemia during OLV. This then requires checking the instrument positioning after blind insertion. Although this was traditionally performed through visual inspection and monitoring, a 35% rate of malpositioning had been reported, putting the reliability of these techniques into question. Current practice, if available, recommends using an FFB (Fig. 13.4).[11]

Right-sided DLTs are of particular relevance considering the increased rate of malpositioning caused by the potential obstruction of the right main bronchus orifice. With an entry of the right upper lobe of less than 2 cm from the carina, there is a narrow margin of safety for the correct position. This requires frequent monitoring. To check the position of a left DLT, an FFB is introduced through the tracheal lumen, observing the carina to certain that the semilunar rim of the bronchial cuff is viewed. That will ensure that the left upper lobe is not obstructed by the tip of the bronchial lumen of the DLT.

After positional changes or any alteration in gas exchanges, as well as increased airway pressures during the interoperative period, checking the position of the isolating device with FB is recommended.

Various sizes of FFB are available, with diameters of 6, 5, 4.9, and 3.9 mm. The latter is easily handled using a DLT of 37 Fr, however, it can be difficult for 35 Fr. In such

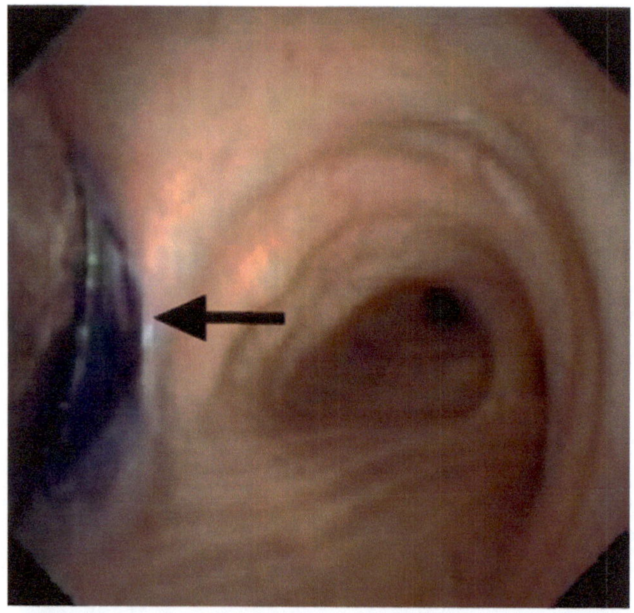

• **Fig. 13.4** Left double-lumen tube position checking using flexible bronchoscopy (the semi lunar view of the blue bronchial cuff is indicated by the *arrow*). (Courtesy of Edmond Cohen.)

a situation, an FFB of 2.2 mm without a suction channel can be used.

An additional notable device is the relatively recent introduction of DLTs with a built-in high-resolution camera, facilitating the correct positioning of the tube accompanied and aided with a continuous stream of video throughout the operation. This can also be performed without the need of a fibrobronchoscope.[12]

Use of Flexible Bronchoscopy With Bronchial Blockers

For BBs, FB has a fundamental role in their insertion and placement. FB is also important in ensuring correct position and efficient sealing after inflation of cuff under direct vision, thus preventing leakage. FFBs as well as BBs being introduced simultaneously through the single lumen tube should have a sufficient diameter of 7.5 to 8.0 mm.

BBs are equipped with a 3-port connection that allows coupling to the anesthesia circuit, introduction of the FFB, and also the handling of the BB itself. The insertion of each BB has some particular characteristics.

For the placement of other types of BB, it is recommended that the FFB remains about 2 to 4 cm from the carina (Fig. 13.5), allowing for the correct visualization of the final position of the BB obtained through external manipulation.[13]

Although an FB can be replaced in some situations by camera-equipped TETs, the appearance of secretions, such as blood, can cause the fogging of the tube chamber and may make FB necessary at some point.

Finally, as with the case of DLTs, in the event of changes in the patient's position, as well as alterations in the ventilation or a lack of optimal collapse conditions, the best position of the BB should be checked via FB.[14]

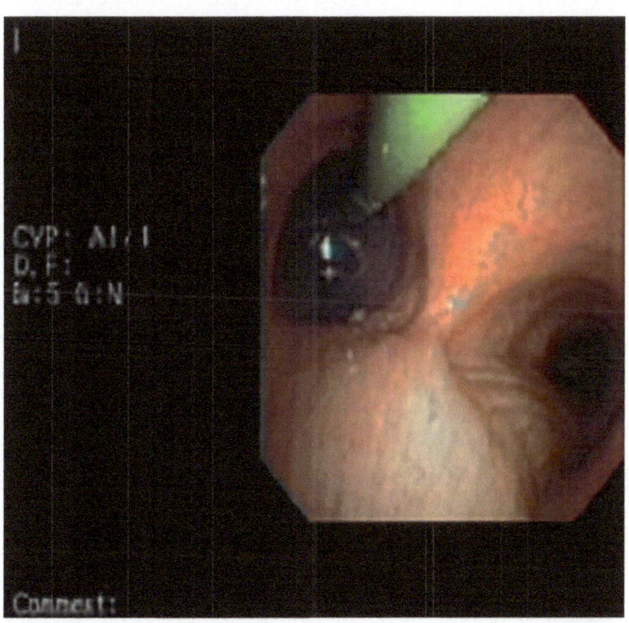

• **Fig. 13.5** Cohenbronchial blocker's position checking using flexible bronchoscopy. (Courtesy of Edmond Cohen.)

Postoperative Thoracic Surgery

Thoracic surgery includes procedures in which a high percentage of patients may develop serious complications in the postoperative period immediately following surgery, therefore requiring the use of ICUs, where FB is an important tool in the diagnosis and treatment of complications.

Hemoptysis

A small hemorrhage is relatively frequent during postoperative periods after thoracic surgery. Nevertheless, if hemorrhaging increases persist, bronchoscopy is necessary to determine, if possible, the location and quantity present. Airway bleeding presents a special problem to the endoscopist. Blood obscures the visual field, while it also causes airway obstruction and air trapping. Smaller FFBs that are less likely to exacerbate these problems during use have small, relatively ineffective suction channels, ultrathin instruments have no internal channel, whereas 4 mm intubating and portable instruments are only available with 1 to 1.5 mm channels.

In treating hemoptysis, either rigid or large caliber flexible bronchoscopes can be used to ensure proper suctioning of blood during this procedure. Hemorrhage makes FB difficult, unless lavage and suction are effective in clearing blood and clots. Despite these problems, the FB is the a most useful tool in this setting. It can establish whether the pulmonary source of bleeding is focal or diffuse when bilateral pulmonary injury is demonstrated by chest x-ray.

These cases can be initially treated by instilling cold physiologic serums with vasoconstrictors and coagulants. If the bleeding persists, then it may be necessary to block the affected bronchus. If the origin of bleeding can be determined and attributed to a segmental bronchus, then the bronchoscope should be placed in its light and used for continuous aspiration or laser photocoagulation. In cases where the origin cannot be located, the bronchial lumen can be blocked by means of an inflatable balloon of a BB or lung isolation established with a DLT or procoagulant material.[15] In cases where these measures are ineffective, a surgical revision would be necessary.

Atelectasis

Atelectasis are considered one of the most frequent complications during the postoperative period.

These are frequently observed ipsilateral to the operated lung and are usually caused by retained bronchial secretions.

Among the key risk factors, there is chronic obstructive pulmonary disease (COPD), poor pain control, neuromuscular relaxation, chest wall resection, abdominal distension, surfactant alterations, decreased mucociliary clearance, and diaphragmatic motility.

Using FB, even subsegmental bronchi are accessible for the extraction of secretions or a mucus plague that cause atelectasis. A microbiologic analysis can be performed for the administration of specific antibiotic treatments. This is especially important after resection surgery to clear the anastomosis from any remaining blood and secretions.[16]

Treatment of Air Leaks

Postoperative air leaks continue to be a common complication following surgical resection of the lung and a leading cause of increased hospitalization, morbidity, and cost. The use of endobronchial valves can be applied to the treatment of persistent tension pneumothorax, used to achieve the functional closure of the bronchus, and thus allowing for the closure and healing of the alveolar laceration that produces it.[17] The Spiration Valve is the only valve that is approved by the U.S. Food and Drug Administration for treatment of persistent air leak usually defined as more than 6 days. The Spiration Valve is a minimally invasive procedure that provides surgeons and pulmonologists a novel method for limiting distal airflow to a damaged lung (Fig. 13.6). It is a proactive option in the management of prolonged air leaks. The valve is an umbrella-shaped, one-way valve that is placed via a delivery catheter, introduced through the working channel of a flexible bronchoscope.

Treatment of Bronchopleural Fistulas (see Chapter 45)

Bronchopleural fistulas are one of the most serious postoperative complications in thoracic surgery. It occurs in between 0.8% and 15% of cases after pneumonectomy and in less than 1% after lobectomy. Anesthesia care of patients with large bronchopleural fistula (BPF) is technically difficult because ventilation, already impaired with spontaneously breathing ventilatory modes, may be impossible when spontaneous ventilation is lost. More commonly, a large BPF contributes to inadequate lung volume with hypoxemia because of ventilation perfusion mismatching as the underlying lung is partially collapsed and/or hypercapnia because of limited ventilation. Previous chemotherapy and radiotherapy treatments, treatment with corticoids, a small margin for tumor resections, long bronchial stumps, right-handed pneumonectomy, and prolonged postoperative mechanical ventilation have been described as factors favoring the appearance of bronchial fistulas.

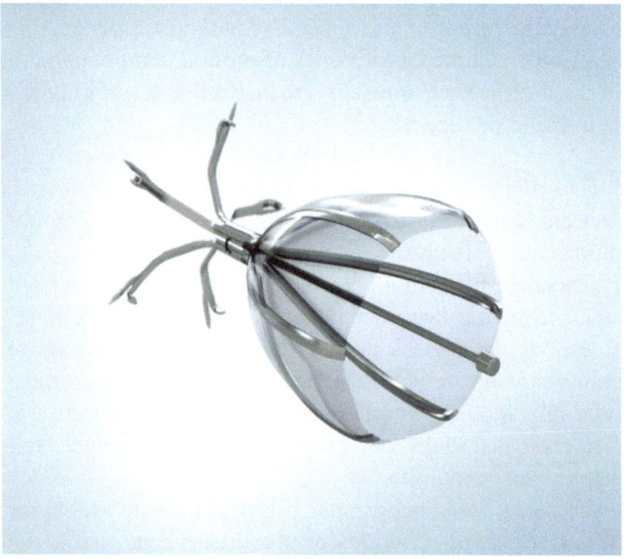

• **Fig. 13.6** SpirationValve. (Courtesy of Edmond Cohen and Spiration, Inc.)

Traditionally, the treatment of these fistulas was performed through the opening of a permanent thoracotomy and daily treatments helping in the secondary closure of the injury. Other options include highly aggressive surgical alternatives such as muscle or omentum interposition.

Nevertheless, in recent years, specialists have opted for endobronchial closure of this type of lesion. The possibilities for endoscopic treatment are diverse; repeated cauterizations, placement of tissue adhesives, stents, and placement of one-way valves. Adopting techniques used by interventional cardiology for ductus arteriosus closure, bronchoscopic placement of this device has been performed to achieve closure of bronchial fistulas.[18] Lung isolation is key to management of large, unilateral BPF. Thoracoscopic approaches with lung isolation facilitated by FB are common with smaller, persistent BPF. Alternatively, with large, open chest lesions, direct surgical tamponade can be established simultaneously with initiation of positive pressure ventilation and subsequent endobronchial control.

Empyema is a complication often associated with fistulas, especially those that are larger and appear later. Its presence increases the morbidity of patients, and some authors consider that it hides the success of endoscopic techniques, such as the treatment for fistulas. This therefore leads specialists to recommend surgical treatment.

Tracheal Lacerations

Tracheal lacerations are rarely associated with trauma related to orotracheal intubation maneuvers. Its occurrence is higher after intubations with DLTs, noted at approximately 1%. Ruptures normally occur in the first hours of the postoperative period, with clinical presentation of subcutaneous emphysema in the face, neck, and chest, as well as hemoptysis and cyanosis. Bronchoscopy together with computerized axial tomography can be considered the diagnostic methods of choice.

This pathology is rare; however, if not diagnosed or treated, it can produce a high risk of morbimortality. Bronchoscopy should be used as early as possible for its detection.

Although treatments may be considered controversial, modern day specialists are imposing the conservative and expectant use of medical treatment and radiologic control, as well as fibrobronchoscopy.[19,20]

When the injury is detected during thoracic surgery, immediate restorative surgery is the best option. Most adopt an expectant behavior in the case of lesions smaller than 2 cm, with a tendency to perform surgical treatment depending on the clinical evolution of the condition in cases larger than 2 cm.

Lobe or Lung Segment Torsions

Pulmonary torsion is defined as the rotation of the lung parenchyma on its vascular pedicle. This is a serious complication that often leads to the death of the patient, whatever the etiologic cause. Early diagnosis and treatment can prevent mortality and decrease the morbidity associated with this entity.

Most cases of pulmonary torsion affect the right middle lobe (ML) and are secondary to the lobectomy of the right upper lobe (RUL). During RUL surgery, the ML vascular pedicle is dissected, allowing the LM to move freely. To avoid this complication, surgeons routinely attach the medial lobe to the lower right lobe after lobectomy. Twisting of other lobes has also been noted, such as the right lower lobe after lobectomy and URL, the left lower lobe (LLL) after lobectomy of left upper lobe (LUL), and the LUL after the lobectomy of LLL and after lingulectomy.

Bronchoscopy is usually performed to exclude other alterations with pulmonary opacities, such as endobronchial obstruction because of retained secretions. Computed tomography (CT) scans provide high resolution data and are useful for their sensitivity to interstitial-alveolar changes with topographic location of the lesions.[21] Surgical intervention is the treatment of choice, and resection of the affected portion of the lung depends on whether or not necrosis has developed.

Interventional Pneumology

Diagnostic and Therapeutic Techniques

Bronchoscopy allows for the localization of lesions and obtaining material for anatomopathologic and microbiologic analyses. Some of these lesions are not macroscopically visible, such as preinvasive lesions of bronchial mucosa. In these cases, autofluorescence is used as a complement to the white light of bronchoscopy, with a relative sensitivity when compared with classic bronchoscopy with white light of up to 4.25 (95% confidence interval [CI], 2.00–16.00).[22]

The collection of samples external to the airway, especially adenopathy by puncture, has been classically done blindly, based on the knowledge of the location of adenopathy from an intrabronchial perspective. This has the added consequent risk of puncturing neighboring structures, less effectiveness, and a greater morbidity.[23]

Nevertheless, the possibility of incorporating ultrasound devices into endoscopes has allowed the development of techniques such as endobronchial ultrasound (EBUS). EBUS is a technique that permits the combined use of conventional bronchoscopy and ultrasound in the same flexible bronchoscope. This allows the evaluation of lesions close to the respiratory tract, as well as transbronchial needle aspiration (TBNA) guided by EBUS through a probe located at the end of the bronchoscope (EBUS-TBNA). Multiple studies recommend EBUS-TBNA as the main tool for the diagnosis and staging of lung cancer, according to international guidelines such as the American College of Chest Physicians (ACCP) and the European Society of Medical Oncology.[24,25]

This procedure is ambulatory and minimally invasive, however, it requires general anesthesia or deep sedation to perform.

For the case of therapeutic techniques, generally, a regional block is used systematically, although many of the interventions performed can be carried out with both rigid and flexible bronchoscopy, even though rigid bronchoscopy is poorly tolerated under RG.

Therapeutic bronchoscopic procedures are considered less invasive than their corresponding surgical procedures; however, the risks present should not be underestimated. These patients generally have multiple comorbidities and are at high anesthetic risk, therefore often excluded from being a surgical candidate. On the other hand, many of these interventions are urgent or in an emergency, in which the patients may not be optimized for the procedure. It is therefore a great challenge for the anesthesiologist to manage the anesthesia of these patients given the high morbidity and mortality associated with these procedures.[26]

Anesthesia Applied to the Use of a Bronchoscope

In accordance with the recommendations established by the ACCP, unless opposed by counterindications, all patients undergoing bronchoscopy should receive some degree of sedation to improve the tolerability and comfort of the procedure.[27–29]

Previous assessments of the patient are therefore required in preanesthetic visits, emphasizing the patient's comorbidities, baseline lung function, and possible DA either because of anatomic characteristics, presence of obstructive mass, previous radiotherapy, or narrowing of the airways.[30] The presence of stridor before the procedures is an indicator of possible narrowing of the airway or vocal cord involvement. A CT scan or magnetic resonance imaging in selected cases is helpful to highlight the patient's pathology. American Society of Anaesthesiologists (ASA) standard monitoring, such as oxygen fraction analyzer, pulse oximeter, capnography, pressure and flow sensors, electrocardiogram, noninvasive pressure, and temperature is usually sufficient.

The use of hypnosis monitoring is recommended whether general anesthesia (in the case of bispectral index monitoring [BIS] values 40–60) or sedation (BIS 60–85) is chosen, because it allows the dose of the sedative to be reduced for early recovery.[30]

In general, a total intravenous anesthesia (TIVA) is preferred to inhalation anesthesia despite the bronchodilator and antiinflammatory effects of inhaled anesthetics. These are attributed to the continuous leaks that are generated with an open airway procedure, which lead to difficulty in monitoring the fraction of anesthetic inhaled and therefore the depth of hypnosis, as well as air pollution, and spread of contaminated particells.[27,30]

The use of anticholinergics to decrease secretions (depending on the patient's cardiac comorbidity) may be assessed, although the ACCP does not routinely recommend it.[31] This could, however, have more of a role in the case of thermoplasty in asthmatic patients.[32]

Similarly, the use of corticosteroids (methylprednisone at 1 mg/kg or dexamethasone at 0.1 mg/kg) as prophylaxis of airway edema seems reasonable, although there is no clear recommendation on its implementations, and its systematic use can be considered controversial.[30]

Flexible Bronchoscopy

The use of one anesthetic modality or another will depend on the bronchoscopy techniques used, the complexity of the case, the patient's comorbidity, and the experience of both the bronchoscopist and the anesthesiologist. Relative contraindications could be considered for sedation, history of severe gastroesophageal reflux, risk of aspiration, respiratory failure, or extreme anxiety.[33]

Topical anesthesia of the airway (glottic and supraglottic area) has a complementary role to procedures performed under light or moderate sedation.[34] This includes the vocal cords, so the protective reflexes of the airway are abolished, and can last up to 2 to 4 hours. Sedative drugs doses can be adjusted to avoid coughing and nausea reflexes. Lidocaine is classically used because of its rapid effect and short duration.

The use of sedation in collaborative patients with a stable pulmonary function, and in the face of short and simple procedures, is considered a standard both to achieve comfort for the patient and a better tolerance of the technique.[27] Moreover, most sedative drugs attenuate the hemodynamic response to the introduction of the bronchoscope, achieving greater cardiovascular stability.

Sedation is best achieved with rapid onset of action and short duration drugs. Propofol appears to be the drug of choice if used alone,[35] although there is no clear recommendation for the ideal sedation schedule for these procedures. It appears that the combination of two or even three drugs, such as midazolam, fentanyl, remifentanil, dexmethomidine, or ketamine has advantages over the use of a single drug.[28] Interindividual variability is present when considering the necessary dose and metabolism of some of these drugs, therefore adjusting the doses and individualizing them is considered key to avoiding episodes of respiratory depression.[29] Dexmethomidine is a selective $\alpha 2$ agonist that provides conscious sedation and analgesia without respiratory depression. Dexmethomidine also has antisialagogue properties therefore it may be especially useful in those patients at high risk of respiratory depression. Moreover, this drug seems to have a greater effect in combination with other drugs (propofol, opioids) than its use alone.[36] Negative effects to be taken into account include bradycardia and a longer recovery time that could limit its use in ambulatory procedures.[35] Its use is limited by the increased secretions it produces, stimulation of the sympathetic nervous system, and the possible hallucinations that can be avoided by the use of benzodiazepines.[34]

Finally, the choice of one anesthetic method over another will depend fundamentally on the specific procedure to be performed, its duration, the patient's comorbidity and pulmonary reserve, as well as the preferences of the bronchoscopist and anesthesiologist.[27]

Rigid Bronchoscopy

For RB, the need for general anesthesia is routine because of the greater discomfort and the more intense stimulus that it generates on the airway as compared with FB.[27] It is also frequently included in addition to the use of neuromuscular blockers. If it must be performed under sedation, topicalization of supraglottic and glottic areas with local anesthesia is recommended, to tolerate the FB insertion and reduce the cardiovascular response.

TIVA is indicated when using jet ventilation as a ventilatory method. The most commonly used drug combination is propofol and remifentanil. The association of other drugs, such as dexmethomidine and ketamine is also valid, although they have a greater role in sedation. Inhalation anesthesia is mainly used in the event of tracheal stenosis or a foreign body as a method of induction, maintaining spontaneous ventilation, with sevoflurane being chosen until the airway are secured.

The reversal of neuromuscular blockade with the use of neuromuscular monitoring is considered paramount. Because of the cholinergic effect of neostigmine (increased secretions), the use of sugammadex is recommended as the reversal drug of choice, and therefore does not depolarize neuromuscular blockers of the steroid type.

Ventilation Techniques

The maintenance of an open airway and ventilation and sharing the airway with the endoscopist represents a challenge for the anesthesiologist, particularly with a limited pulmonary reserve. Because of the high risk of compromised gas exchange during these interventions, adequate preoxygenation is considered essential.

Flexible Bronchoscopy

During procedures performed under sedation, the use of supplemental oxygen is a standard component. This can be administered in a variety of ways; through nasal cannulas allowing flows between 2 and 5 L/min; connected to the bite block through which the bronchoscope is introduced allowing flows of up to 10 L/min; through high flow oxygen systems (between 30 and 70 L/min), with lower percentages of desaturation;[37] and the use of noninvasive mechanical ventilation with a specially designed mask.[38] The latter of which being particularly useful in patients with a previous respiratory failure, demonstrating superiority over other forms of oxygen therapy.[27,38,39]

If general anesthesia is used, the airway should be secured either by the use of a laryngeal mask (LMA) or an ETT. In both cases, to compensate for continuous leakage during ventilation, high flows of around 12 to 15 L/min and high fraction of inspired oxygen (FiO2) are recommended (provided no laser or electrocautery is being used during the procedure).

In general, and unless stated otherwise in contraindications, most bronchoscopists prefer the use of LMA (2nd generation) over ETT particularly if a lesion is located just below the vocal cords which excludes the placement of an ETT. These allow the aspiration of gastric content and easy access and inspection of the vocal cords and proximal trachea, and access the tracheal wall motion with respiration in case of tracheomalacia, which is not possible with the use of ETTs. It is also the method of choice in EBUS because it facilitates the access to the paratracheal lymph nodes.[27,30] Usually i-Gel® is preferred by some authors,[30] although others use indistinctly different LMAs, such as AuraGain®. The recommended sizes are No. 4–5, depending on the patient's anatomy. Except for EBUS, where the use of neuromuscular blockers is recommended to avoid all movement during the biopsy of a node, it can be avoided in the rest of the procedures.[30] Because of the increased risk of laryngospasm with respect to the use of ETT, local anesthesia of the glottic area is considered in conjunction with the use of LMA.

In the case of opting for the use of TET (e.g., high risk of broncho aspiration, very long procedure, or estimation of high ventilatory pressures), large size ETT allow passage of the bronchoscope and adequate ventilation. ETTs larger than 8.0 mm or 8.5 mm in diameter are recommended for EBUS. In addition, it appears that smaller calibers may favor autopositive end-expiratory pressure.[33] When glottal or tracheal stenosis is suspected, standard ETT or those with built-in cameras of smaller calibers than usual[40] can be used, along with smaller diameter bronchoscopes or the use of LMA.

Rigid Bronchoscopy

There are currently two possible ventilatory modes during the use of RB: positive pressure ventilation and jet ventilation. Traditionally, apneic oxygenation with preoxygenation, denitrogenation, and preventilation with 100% oxygen were used. When oxygen saturation was less than 92%, the bronchoscopist had to remove the rigid bronchoscope to manually ventilate the patient. Today, this practice is discouraged because of increased risk of acid-base and gas exchange alterations,[27,33] as well as increased irritation of the airway by successive introduction and removal of the bronchoscope.

Positive pressure ventilation is achieved by connecting the tubes to an external port of the rigid bronchoscope. Manual ventilation with periods of apnea is usually performed according to the requirements of the bronchoscopist. It is important to minimize leakage around the bronchoscope by using high fresh gas flows, plugging free ports, and placing saline soaked gauze in the mouth if necessary. A frequent complication is hypoventilation with hypercapnia and desaturation. This is the most common method used to ventilate these patients.[35]

The other alternative is jet ventilation. Based on Bernoulli's principle, this allows the insufflation of the airway with a release of gas at high pressure (0.3–3 bar) through a narrow catheter (12–16 G) connected to the bronchoscope. This can be manually implemented with frequencies around 15 to 30 breaths per minute (rpm) or mechanical with high frequency respiratory cycles between 60 to 120 rpm, low tidal volume (less than the anatomic dead space), and a passive aspiration system. Other parameters to be taken into account are the ventilator driving pressure (optimal conditions between 18 and 25 mm Hg; <35 mm Hg),[35] E:I ratio of 30% and FiO_2 (from 0.3 for laser procedures to 1 if hypoxemia is present). The main complications described are air entrapment and barotrauma, pneumothorax, pneumomediastinum, subcutaneous emphysema, and alterations in gas exchange. An electronic jet ventilation system (Monsoon Jet Ventilator, Acutronic Medical Systems), whose catheters measure pressures, blocking ventilation when these exceed the established threshold can be used, thus avoiding most of the complications associated with manual jet ventilation (see Chapter 14).

After finishing the process, the removal of the rigid bronchoscope with a deep hypnosis is preferred, replacing it with ETT or LMA or assisting with manual mask ventilation until the recovery of spontaneous ventilation. A reasonable approach and preparation for extubation is part of the difficult airway guideline. Urgent reintubation is not a benign procedure in this setting. Alternatively, a trial of extubation may be very appropriate in the acute setting. FB can be used as an oxygen insufflation or jet ventilation stylette over which reintubation can be performed when the patient fails an extubation trial. If there is any concern regarding the airway control following extubation, a "staged extubation" should be done. A vascular guidewire can be passed through the suction channel into a known area of the trachea as a placeholder for staged reintubation. Most adult patients will tolerate a small 3 to 4 mm catheter via the cords after extubation, especially if narcotics was part of the anesthetic technique.

Conclusion

RB is an essential part of thoracic procedure and is crucial in the management of a variety of airways and lung diseases. The natural introduction of FFBs as diagnostic and, later, therapeutic medical instruments opened a wide range of airway applications to anesthesiologists and other airway experts in the 1980s. Recognition of the potential uses for the FB in anesthesia practice later led to the marketing of both specialized smaller external diameter intubating and disposable FFBs by the major fiberoptic instrument manufacturing companies worldwide. Anesthesiologists have become adept in lung isolation and other specialized thoracic procedures with the wider availability of instruments for more precise management of both upper and lower airway problems. FB is widely used for lung isolation during various thoracic and nonthoracic procedures facilitated by DLTs, and a growing variety of BBs. FFBs are very useful in solving airway problems, such as lung separation in patients with difficult airways, control of BPFs, tamponade of endobronchial bleeding.

References

1. Ernst A, Herth FJF. *Principles and Practice of Interventional Pulmonology*. New York, NY: Springer; 2013.
2. Dooms C, Seijo L, Gasparini S, Trisolini R, Ninane V, Tournoy KG. Diagnostic bronchoscopy: state of the art. *Eur Respir Rev*. 2010;19:229–236.
3. Nadel JA, Murray JF. *Textbook of Respiratory Medicine*. 5th ed: Mason; 2010 Saunders (Elsevier, Philadelphia).
4. Du Rand IA, Blaikley J, Booton R, et al. British Thoracic Society guideline for diagnostic flexible bronchoscopy in adults: acredited by NICE. *Thorax*. 2013;68(suppl 1):i1–44.
5. Castro Otero MC, Torrego Fernández A. Optimización en la obtención y el manejo de las muestras tomadas por vía endoscópica en la broncoscopia estándar. En: SEPAR. *Manual SEPAR de Procedimientos*. Barcelona: Respira; 2013:9–28.
6. Granell M, Parra MJ, Jiménez MJ, et al. Review of difficult airway management in thoracic surgery. *Rev Esp Anestesiol Reanim*. 2018;65(1):31–40.
7. Collins SR, Titus BJ, Campos JH, Blank RS. Lung isolation in the patient with a difficult airway. *Anesth Analg*. 2018;126(6):1968–1978.
8. Liu TT, Li L, Wan L, Zhang CH, Yao WL. Videolaryngoscopy vs. Macintosh laryngoscopy for double-lumen tube intubation in thoracic surgery: a systematic review and meta-analysis. *Anaesthesia*. 2018;73(8):997–1007.
9. Granell M. Lung isolation/lung separation. Indications and specific devices. 2019: https://chguv.san.gva.es/servicios-salud/servicios-unidades/anestesia/sesiones-clinicas/sesiones-clinicas-2019-2020.
10. Rodrigues AJ, Scordamaglio PR, Palomino AM. Difficult airway intubation with flexible bronchoscope. *Brazilian J Anesthesiol* (Edicion en Esp). 2013;63(4):358–361.
11. Clayton-Smith A, Bennett K, Alston RP, et al. A comparison of the efficacy and adverse effects of double-lumen endobronchial tubes and bronchial blockers in thoracic surgery: a systematic review and meta-analysis of randomized controlled trials. *J Cardiothorac Vasc Anesth [Internet]*. 2015;29(4):955–966.
12. Heir JS, Guo SL, Purugganan R, et al. A randomized controlled study of the use of video double-lumen endobronchial tubes versus double-lumen endobronchial tubes in thoracic surgery. *J Cardiothorac Vasc Anesth [Internet]*. 2018;32(1):267–274.
13. Valencia O, Real MI, Cortés M, García AF, Marrón C, Pérez-Cerdá F. Lung isolation in patients with previous lung resections: selective sequential lobar blockade using a Fuji Uniblocker® endobronchial blocker. *Rev Esp Anestesiol Reanim [Internet]*. 2016;63(9): 539–543.
14. Cohen E. Recommendations for airway control and difficult airway management in thoracic anesthesia and lung separation procedures. Are we ready for the challenge? *Minerva Anestesiol*. 2009; 75(1–2):3–5.
15. Cordovilla R, Bollo de Miguel E, Nuñez Ares A. Diagnosis and treatment of hemoptysis. *Arch Bronconeumol*. 2016;52:368–737.
16. En Bolufer Nadal S, Morcillo Aixela A, Galvez Munõz C. Cuidados postoperatorios inmediatos. En: Martinez Hernández NJ, López Villalobos JL, eds. *Documento de Consenso SECT Sobre Cirugía Traqueal y Laringotraqueal*. Madrid: Panamericana; 2015:41–46.
17. Bakhos C, Doelken P, Pupovac S, Ata A, Fabian T. Management of prolonged pulmonary air leaks with endobronchial valve placement. *JSLS*. 2016;20(3) pii e2016.00055.
18. Galbis JM, Sanchez F, Estors M. Closure of a fistula in the main bronchus after pneumonectomy with an Occlutech Figulla Flex ASD. *Arch Bronconeumol*. 2012;48:137–140.
19. Fong PA, Seder CW, Chmielewski GW, Welsh RJ. Nonoperative management of postintubation tracheal injuries. *Ann Thorac Surg*. 2010;89(4):1265–1266.
20. Carretta A, Melloni G, Bandiera A, Negri G, Voci C, Zannini P. Conservative and surgical treatment of acute post-traumatic tracheobronchial injuries. *World J Surg*. 2011;35(11):2568–2574.
21. Mateo Cerdan CM, Garcia Verdun F, Cuartero del Pozo AB, de Capadocia Rosell J, Geronimo Pardo M. Pulmonary torsion complicating lobectomy: report of 2 cases. *Rev Esp Anestesiol Reanim*. 2010;57:245–249.
22. Edell E, Lam S, Pass H, et al. Detection and localization of intraepithelial neoplasia and invasive carcinoma using fluorescence-reflectance bronchoscopy: an international multi-center clinical trial. *J Thorac Oncol*. 2009;4:49–54.
23. Roth K, Eagan T, Hardie J. Expert opinion of mediastinal lymph node positions from an intrabronchial view. *BMC Pulm Med*. 2016;6:15.
24. Silvestri GA, Gonzalez AV, Jantz MA, et al. Methods for staging non-small cell lung cancer, 3rd edition: American College of Chest Physicians evidence-based clinical practice guidelines. *Chest*. 2013;143(5_suppl):e211S–e250S.
25. Vansteenkiste J, De Ruysscher D, Eberhardt WE, et al. ESMO Guidelines Working Group. Early and locally advanced non-small-cell lung cancer (NSCLC): ESMO Clinical Practice Guidelines for diagnosis, treatment and follow-up. *Ann Oncol*. 2013;24(suppl 6): vi89–vi98.
26. Ernst A, Simoff M, Ost D, Goldman Y, Herth FJF. Prospective risk-adjusted morbidity and mortality outcome analysis after therapeutic bronchoscopic procedures: results of a multiinstitutional outcomes database. *Chest*. 2008;134:514–519.
27. de Lima A, Kheir F, Majid A, Pawlowski J. Anesthesia for interventional pulmonology procedures: a review of advanced diagnostic and therapeutic bronchoscopy. *Can J Anesth* [Internet]. 2018; 65(7):822–836.
28. Müller T, Thümmel K, Cornelissen CG, Krüger S, Dreher M. Analogosedation during flexible bronchoscopy using a combination of midazolam, propofol and fentanyl—a retrospective analysis. *PLoS One*. 2017;12(4):1–11.
29. Mondoni M, Radovanovic D, Sotgiu G, et al. Interventional pulmonology techniques in elderly patients with comorbidities. *Eur J Intern Med* [Internet]. 2019;59:14–20.
30. Galway U, Zura A, Khanna S, Wang M, Turan A, Ruetzler K. Anesthetic considerations for bronchoscopic procedures: a narrative review based on the Cleveland clinic experience. *J Thorac Dis*. 2019;11(7):3156–3170.
31. Du Rand IA, Blaikley J, Booton R, et al. British Thoracic Society guideline for diagnostic flexible bronchoscopy in adults. *Thorax*. 2013;68(8):786–787.
32. Saran JS, Kreso M, Khurana S, Nead M, Larj M, Karan S. Anesthetic considerations for patients undergoing bronchial thermoplasty. *Anesth Analg*. 2018;126(5):1575–1579.
33. Paradis TJ, Dixon J, Tieu BH. The role of bronchoscopy in the diagnosis of airway disease. *J Thorac Dis*. 2016;8(12):3826–3837.
34. Chadha M, Kulshrestha M, Biyani A. Anaesthesia for bronchoscopy. *Indian J Anaesth*. 2015;59(9):565–573.
35. José RJ, Shaefi S, Navani N. Anesthesia for bronchoscopy. *Curr Opin Anaesthesiol*. 2014;27(4):453–457.
36. Yuan F, Fu H, Yang P, et al. Dexmedetomidine-fentanyl versus propofol-fentanyl in flexible bronchoscopy: a randomized study. *Exp Ther Med*. 2016;12(1):506–512.
37. Douglas N, Ng I, Nazeem F, et al. A randomised controlled trial comparing high-flow nasal oxygen with standard management for

conscious sedation during bronchoscopy. *Anaesthesia*. 2018;73(2): 169–176.
38. Pieri M, Landoni G, Cabrini L. Noninvasive ventilation during endoscopic procedures: rationale, clinical use, and devices. *J Cardiothorac Vasc Anesth* [Internet]. 2018;32(2):928–934.
39. Simon M, Braune S, Frings D, Wiontzek AK, Klose H, Kluge S. High-flow nasal cannula oxygen versus non-invasive ventilation in patients with acute hypoxaemic respiratory failure undergoing flexible bronchoscopy—a prospective randomised trial. *Crit Care*. 2014;18(1):1–9.
40. Granell M, Solís P, Córdova C, Cobo I, Guijarro R, de Andrés JA. Intubation in two patients with difficult airway management and tracheal tracheostomy in thoracic surgery. *Rev Esp Anestesiol Reanim*. 2018;65(6):347–350.

NON-PRINT ITEMS

Abstract

Bronchoscopy can be considered among the most significant advances in diagnostics and treatment of respiratory disease. There are several types of bronchoscopies, including rigid and flexible, each with their own particular characteristics and indications.

In the field of thoracic surgery, flexible bronchoscopy has a crucial importance. Flexible bronchoscopes are still a key element in the management of anesthesia for thoracic surgery, particularly in confirming the correct position of the isolation device used to achieve one lung ventilation.

Parallel to the traditional use of the flexible bronchoscope in thoracic surgery, its uses in the field of interventional pneumonology continues to expand and develop. More and more procedures are being performed with both the rigid and flexible bronchoscope, which require adequate levels of sedation for tolerability and patient comfort. This presents a challenge for the anesthesiologist both because of the comorbidity of the subsidiary patients and because of the difficulties involved in ventilation and maintenance of the permeable airway. This is when the anesthesiologist has to share the airway with the surgeon and must have a close communication with the surgical team.

This review describes the use of the bronchoscope in thoracic surgery and the anesthetic management of the main branches of interventional pneumology: diagnostic and therapeutic bronchoscopy.

Keywords

flexible bronchoscope, rigid bronchoscope, thoracic surgery, interventional bronchology, diagnostic bronchology

14

High-Frequency Ventilation: Applications in Thoracic Anesthesia

JAKOB WITTENSTEIN, MARCELO GAMA DE ABREU

Introduction

The term high-frequency ventilation (HFV) summarizes different techniques of ventilation with a ventilator frequency of more than 60 breaths per minute, tidal volumes (V_T) of equal or less than dead space, as well as lower peak airway pressure, lower transpulmonary pressure, and increased functional reserve capacity when compared with conventional mechanical ventilation.[1] There are four types of HFV: high-frequency jet ventilation (HFJV), high-frequency oscillatory ventilation (HFOV), high-frequency percussive ventilation (HFPV), and high-frequency positive pressure ventilation (HFPPV), (Table 14.1). This chapter will describe the different modes of HFV and their application in thoracic anesthesia procedures.

HFV shows several particularities because of the high respiratory rate and the small V_T. Importantly, the mechanisms of gas exchange differ from those during conventional mechanical ventilation. During HFV, gas exchange is determined by so-called Taylor dispersion, convective dispersion, cardiogenic mixing, molecular diffusion, pendelluft, and bulk flow.[2] A detailed description of the mechanisms of gas exchange during HFV is beyond the scope of this chapter and can be found elsewhere.[3]

In thoracic surgery, there are different indications for HFV, including rigid bronchoscopy, airway stenosis, imaging and stereotactic and catheter ablation, treatment of bronchopleural fistula, and respiratory therapy after cardiac surgery. Possible contraindications for HFV are extreme adiposity, severe obstructive pulmonary disease, and an increased risk of aspiration whenever an open ventilation system is used, such as during HFJV. For successful HFV application, careful patient selection, close monitoring, knowledge of the technique, and a well-trained team are essential. The particular HFV technique to be used should be chosen according to local expertise and equipment availability.

Types, Application, and Equipment of High-Frequency Ventilation

High-Frequency Jet Ventilation

HFJV delivers gas from a high-pressure source through a small-bore cannula or catheter in the airway, an airway device, or a bronchoscope, followed by a passive expiration. HFJV maintains oxygenation and ventilation by delivering V_T of 1 to 3 mL/kg of predicted body weight (pbw), equal to or less than anatomic dead space at a respiratory rate of 60 to 300 breaths per minute. A diagrammatic representation of airway pressure versus time recording is illustrated in Fig. 14.1. Because of the high pressure, a characteristic noise appears. To deliver the jet of gas from the ventilator, a small cannula (usually 14–16 gauge) or catheter is placed in the endotracheal tube or the trachea, leaving the airways open to the atmosphere. If the catheter is long enough, it can be positioned at distant sites within the bronchial tree, allowing proximal surgical procedures.[4] HFJV is contraindicated in patients who are not fasted because of the open system and lack of aspiration protection.[5] After passing a pressure regulator, the gas mixture reaches a manifold of four electromagnetic solenoid valves, which portion the applied gas volume.[6] The high flow and high pressure at the tip of the cannula result in air entrainment from the surrounding tissue. Therefore the set jet inspiratory oxygen fraction does not equal the tracheal inspiratory oxygen fraction. During initiation of HFJV, the driving pressure is set at around 25 to 30 pounds per square inch (psi). Thereby a V_T of 2 to 3 mL/kg pbw can be reached depending on the compliance of the respiratory system. Furthermore, the inspiratory fraction (defined as inspiratory time divided by the sum of the inspiratory and expiratory times) can be chosen and is mostly set initially at 30%. Usually, a respiratory rate of 100 to 150 breaths per minute is chosen. In the United States, HFJV is only approved up to 150 breaths per minute. Increasing the respiratory rate results in lower

TABLE 14.1 Different Types of High-Frequency Ventilation

Type	Technique	Settings
High-frequency jet ventilation	- High-pressure source - Small-bore cannula or catheter	- V_T = 1–3 mL/kg pbw - RR = 60–300/min - driving pressure = 35 psi
Superimposed high-frequency jet ventilation	- Combination of high- with low-frequency jet ventilation - Catheter with two lumens	- V_T = depending on peak airway pressure - High RR ≥ 600/min - Lower RR = 10–30/min
High-frequency oscillatory ventilation	- Oscillatory pump or membrane ventilator - Endotracheal tube	- V_T ≤ 2 mL/kg pbw - RR = 180–900/min
High-frequency percussive ventilation	- Pneumatically powered, time-cycled, pressure-limited ventilator with inspiratory and expiratory oscillation - Endotracheal tube	- V_T = depending on peak airway pressure - Oscillatory RR ≥ 900/min - pressure-controlled RR = 10–15/min

pbw, Predicted body weight; *psi*, pressure per square inch; *RR*, respiratory rate; V_T, tidal volume.

V_T because of the reduced inspiratory time. A positive end-expiratory pressure (PEEP) can be added if deemed necessary. Thereby, the diaphragmatic excursion is reduced, and the lungs remain nearly static. Expiration is a passive process, with a continuous wall-mounted air outflow, which can protect the airways from contamination. However, this outflow does not confer protection against aspiration.

Superimposed High-Frequency Jet Ventilation

Superimposed HFJV combines a high- with low-frequency jet ventilation using a double or twin-jet technique. A diagrammatic representation of airway pressure versus time recording is shown in Fig. 14.2. Thereby, minute ventilation is increased and carbon dioxide (CO_2) removal improved. Although the low frequency is responsible for CO_2 removal, the high frequency is important for oxygenation. The technique allows achieving an adequate gas exchange with lower airway pressures as during conventional ventilation.[7] Ventilation is usually delivered via two different lumens, whereby both ventilation modes can be adjusted separately.[7]

Sanders Jet Ventilation (Manual Jet Ventilation)

The Sanders jet ventilation introduced in 1967, uses a high-pressure gas source that is applied to an open airway in short bursts via a small-bore catheter. The technique uses a hand-operated valve (manual jet ventilation), as illustrated in Fig. 14.3, connected to 100% oxygen, and a pressure-limiting device to deliver gas to the patient at 50 psi or less with a respiratory rate usually in the range of 10 to 14 breaths per minute.[8] Respiratory rate and duration of breath are determined by the anesthesiologist, who monitors chest rise and oxygen (O_2) saturations to determine adequacy of oxygenation and ventilation during the procedure.[9]

High-Frequency Oscillatory Ventilation

HFOV is based on an oscillatory pump or membrane which delivers a respiratory rate of 180 to 900 breaths per minute through the endotracheal tube. A diagrammatic representation of airway pressure versus time recording is shown in Fig. 14.4. A piston pump or membrane driven by an electric motor is used to create a high-frequency sine wave.[2] The

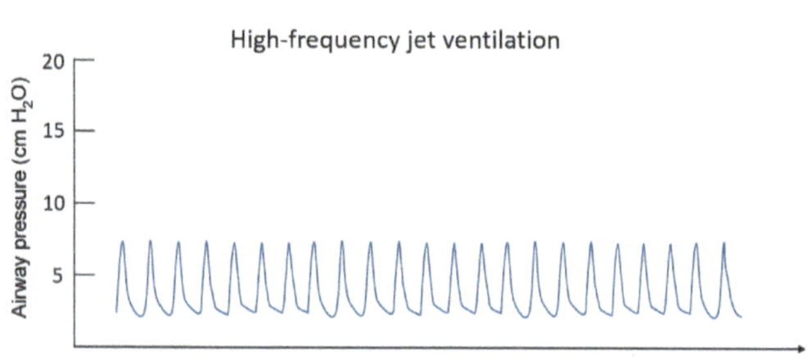

• **Fig. 14.1** Diagrammatic representation of airway pressure versus time recordings during high-frequency jet ventilation, which is defined as ventilation with small tidal volumes (of 1–3 mL/kg of predicted body weight) and a respiratory rate of 60 to 300 breaths per minute delivered from a high-pressure source through a small-bore cannula or catheter in the airway, followed by a passive expiration.

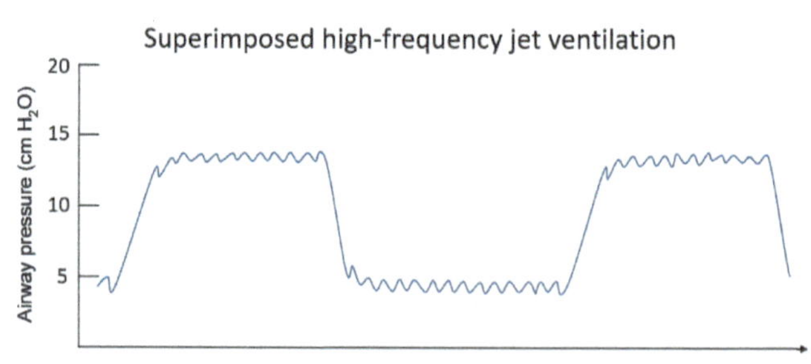

• **Fig. 14.2** Diagrammatic representation of airway pressure versus time recordings during superimposed high-frequency jet ventilation, which is defined as a combination of high-frequency jet ventilation with low-frequency jet ventilation using a double or twin-jet technique.

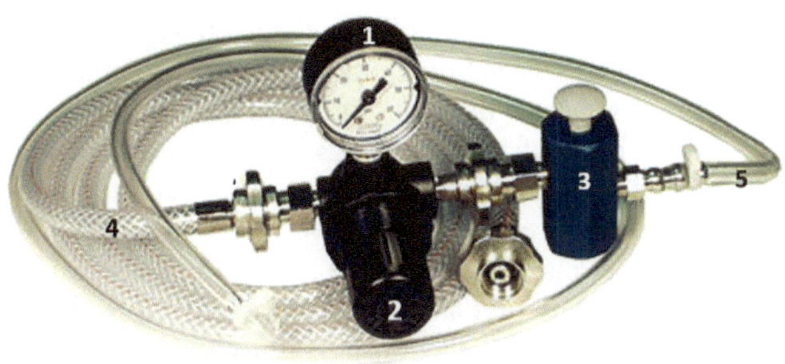

• **Fig. 14.3** Sanders jet ventilation 1. Pressure gauge. 2. Adjustable pressure-regulating valve. 3. Manual lever for delivering the pressurized gas. 4. Connection to the oxygen supply, pressure hose. 5. Noncompliant jet ventilation tubing.

deformation of the membrane is determined by the set working pressure. The generated V_T is usually less than anatomic dead space (≤2 mL/kg pbw). V_T is influenced by the respiratory rate with a higher rate allowing less inspiratory time and resulting in lower V_T. V_T size furthermore depends on the size of the endotracheal tube, and respiratory system resistance and compliance. The pressure amplitude or V_T size determines mainly CO_2 elimination.[10] Heated and humidified gas is continuously delivered at a flow rate of up to 60 L/min orthogonal to the membrane or pump, so-called bias flow. The airway pressure oscillates around a constant mean airway pressure determined by the expiratory valve and the bias flow. The oscillations are transmitted through the endotracheal tube and airways. However, oscillations are attenuated along the way with the smallest pressure swings in the alveoli. In contrast to HFJV and conventional ventilation, expiration is an active process. When the membrane/pump moves back, air is actively drawn out of the lungs. Thereby air trapping is less common during HFOV as compared with HFJV.

High-Frequency Percussive Ventilation

HFPV is an exceptionally pulsatile form of HFV that delivers small V_T at rates up to 900 breaths per minute. V_T is delivered by a pneumatically powered, time-cycled, pressure-limited ventilator with inspiratory and expiratory oscillation. A diagrammatic representation of airway pressure versus time recording is shown in Fig. 14.5. Basically, it is HFOV oscillating around two different pressure levels, which are the inspiratory and expiratory airway pressures. At the end of the endotracheal tube sits a sliding Venturi so-called phasitron, which acts as an inspiratory and expiratory valve and is driven by a high-pressure gas supply. The high frequency oscillatory subtidal volume breaths are superimposed on conventional inspiratory-expiratory pressure-controlled cycles, which are usually set at a rate of 10 to 15 breaths per minute. In the expiratory phase, the lungs empty passively until the preset PEEP. Although, during HFOV and HFJV, CO_2 elimination can be a problem, during HFPV, CO_2 removal is enhanced because of the increased minute ventilation. Further benefits include an increased clearance of secretions compared with other types of HFV.[1]

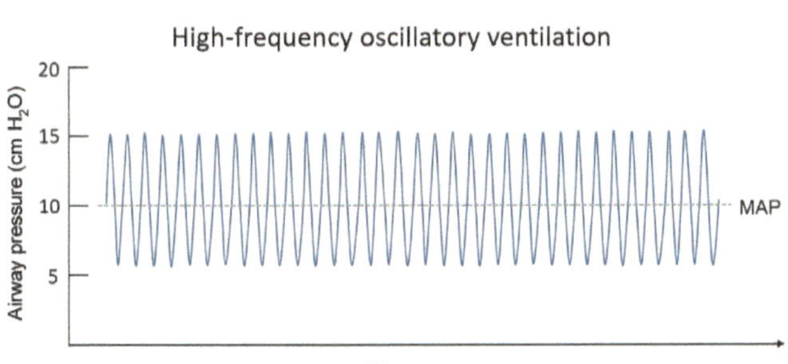

• **Fig. 14.4** Diagrammatic representation of airway pressure versus time recordings during high-frequency oscillatory ventilation, which is defined as ventilation with small tidal volumes (≤2 mL/kg predicted body weight) and a respiratory rate of 180 to 900 breaths per minute (high-frequency sine wave) delivered by a piston pump or membrane through the endotracheal tube. *MAP*, Mean airway pressure.

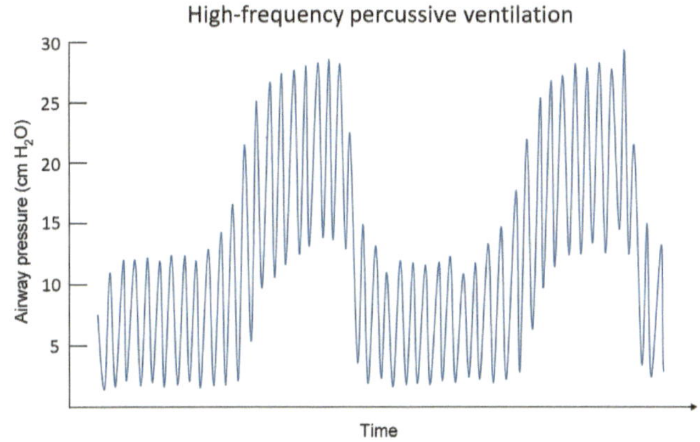

• **Fig. 14.5** Diagrammatic representation of airway pressure versus time recordings during high-frequency percussive ventilation, which is defined as ventilation with small tidal volumes and a respiratory rate of up to 900 breaths per minute delivered by a pneumatically powered, time-cycled, pressure-limited ventilator with inspiratory and expiratory oscillation through the endotracheal tube.

High-Frequency Positive Pressure Ventilation

HPPV is a rarely used form of HFV, which is delivered by a conventional ventilator with the respiratory rate set near the upper limits of the ventilator. A diagrammatic representation of airway pressure versus time recording is shown in Fig. 14.6. For HPPV, no special equipment is needed. However, the upper respiratory rate is limited.

Application

HFV can be administered supra- or infraglottic through a catheter (HFJV) or an endotracheal tube (HFOV and HFPV) or directly through a special laryngoscope or bronchoscope (HFJV) with an appropriate connector. The supraglottic airway access is usually established by the surgeon. Ventilation quality depends on the ability of the surgeon to align the gas flow with the airway, which is influenced by surgical priorities and anatomic abnormalities.[11]

The infraglottic approach is mostly used when direct laryngoscopy is difficult or an obscured surgical field is present.

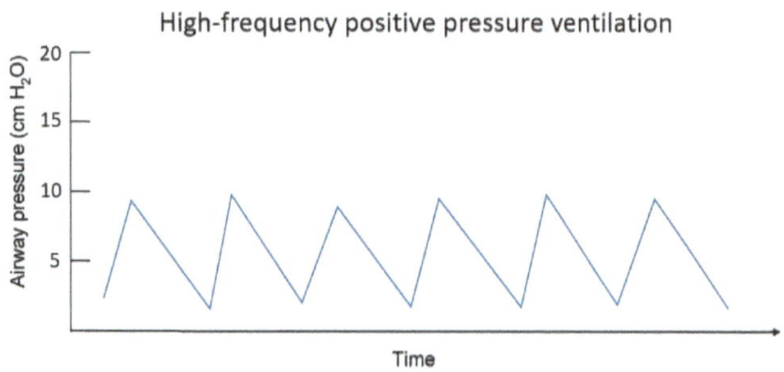

• **Fig. 14.6** Diagrammatic representation of airway pressure versus time recordings during high-frequency positive pressure ventilation, which is defined as ventilation with a conventional ventilator with the respiratory rate set near the upper limits of the respirator.

It may prevent contamination of the lungs from gastric contents and blood because of the continuous gas flow from the lungs protecting the distal airways.

The transtracheal airway access is used especially for patients with airway tumors that prevent the placement of an endotracheal tube, or condition after head and neck radiotherapy, with alterations of the trachea or as an emergency rescue maneuver. However, the transtracheal route is considered to be a higher risk strategy than supraglottic or subglottic HFV because establishing the airway is risky (e.g., tracheal trauma, pneumomediastinum).[11]

Equipment

HFOV and HFPV devices are connected to the endotracheal tube. For HFJV, the ventilator can be connected to a small-bore catheter or cannula, a bronchial blocker, or to a special laryngo- or bronchoscope. HFJV is dependent on the passive gas outflow from the lungs, in contrast to HFOV, where exhalation is an active process.

For HFJV, HFOV, and HFPV, a special ventilator is needed. There are several different jet ventilators available. Newer models have an internal or external gas climatization (heating and humidification of the gas) and can measure the airway pressure. If the pause pressure (pressure at the tip of the cannula measured between delivery of jet ventilation) exceeds a preset maximum, a safety alarm is activated, and the ventilator stops ventilation to avoid barotrauma. Furthermore, a jet catheter or jet cannula is necessary.

For HFOV, the ventilator generates the high respiratory rate with an electromagnetically driven membrane or an oscillatory pump. Newer HFOV ventilator models have a volume guarantee mode included. HFPV is generated by a phasitron which sits at the end of the endotracheal tube.

For the induction of anesthesia and at the end of the procedure until the complete reverse of anesthesia, it can be helpful to insert a laryngeal mask.[4]

Hunsaker Mon-Jet tube

The self-centering, laser-safe Hunsaker Mon-Jet tube, as illustrated in Fig. 14.7, was introduced in 1994 to provide subglottic automated jet ventilation.[12] The tube is approximately 35.5 cm long and has two lumens and is laser resistant. Through the smaller lumen, airway pressure can be measured continuously and end-tidal CO_2 intermittently, representing a safety feature of the Hunsaker tube. Therefore the risk of barotrauma can be minimized. The end of the tube has a green plastic cage that keeps the jet centered in the trachea to minimize any chance of the jet being directed against the wall of the trachea and dissecting through the mucosa causing a pneumomediastinum or pneumothorax. However, in case of laryngeal growths, especially vocal cord polyps, the cage of the Hunsaker tube might become trapped during intubation. Both the anesthetist and the operating surgeon should be

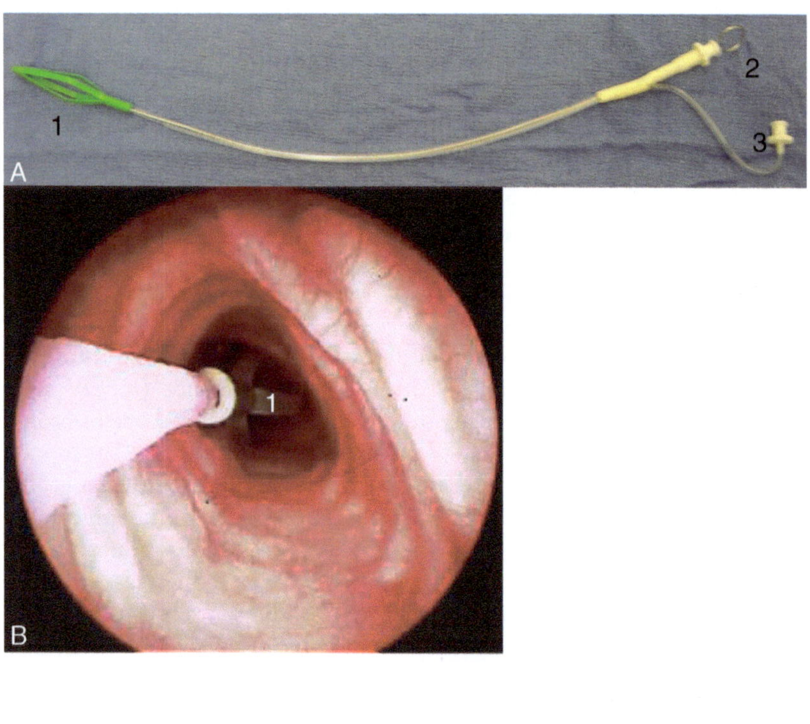

• **Fig. 14.7** **A.** Hunsaker Mon-Jet tube. 1. Basket at the distal end of the tube, which self-centers the tube within the trachea. Therefore contact of the jet port with the mucosa is prevented. 2. Metal stylet to allow tracheal intubation. 3. Monitoring port: continuous monitoring of airway pressure and intermittent monitoring of end-tidal carbon dioxide. **B.** Hunsaker tube in situ.

aware of this possible complication.[13] The tube itself is made of fluroplastic that is extremely resistant to combustion. Further details on use of laser and airway fire can be found in the package insert.

Indications for High-Frequency Ventilation in Thoracic Procedures

HFV offers many benefits such as increased visibility, decreased conflict of space within the airways, decreased gas leak because of lower peak airway pressure when a major bronchopleural fistula is present and minimizing movements associated with normal V_T for imaging purposes, and a quasi-static surgical field.[2] The reduced movement of the surgical field can reduce intervention time and harm to surrounding organs. Therefore HFV can be used for a wide range of indications during thoracic procedures, as summarized in Table 14.2.

Despite these benefits, use of HFV should be considered carefully or fully avoided in patients with severe obstructive lung disease. Because of the obstructed airways, expiration is prolonged. The high respiratory rate used for HFV shortens the expiratory time, which can cause end-expiratory air trapping with consecutive increasing auto-positive end-expiratory pressure (auto-PEEP) and increased risk for barotrauma.

TABLE 14.2 Indications for High-Frequency Ventilation

Rigid bronchoscopy
Surgery of airway obstructing tumor
Tracheal or carinal resection
Cannot ventilate cannot intubate situation
Ventilation of the nondependent lung
Imaging, stereotactic, and catheter ablation
Ventilation when a bronchopleural fistula is present
Ventilatory support after cardiac surgery

Rigid Bronchoscopy

Diagnostic and therapeutic rigid bronchoscopy is normally done under deep sedation or general anesthesia. The anesthetic technique mostly includes ultra-short acting intravenous sedatives, hypnotics, and neuromuscular blockade (e.g., propofol, remifentanil, vecuronium, or cisatracurium). Usually, HFV is used as ventilator support. HFJV can be connected to the bronchoscope and thereby gives room for the interventionist, as illustrated in Figs. 14.8 and 14.9. Alternative ventilation techniques are apneic oxygenation with intermittent positive pressure ventilation, spontaneous assisted ventilation, controlled ventilation, and manual jet ventilation. When general anesthesia is used, a laryngeal mask or endobronchial tube can be placed to allow proper weaning from the ventilator until the complete reversal of anesthesia.[9] Antagonization of neuromuscular blockade should be considered to allow fast recovery of the respiratory system. Factors that increase risk of the bronchoscopy are an unstable cervical spine and reduced range of motion of the cervical spine (for the placement of the bronchoscope, an extreme reclination is needed), reduced opening of the jaw, and pharyngeal diseases which prevent the safe passage of the bronchoscope.[9]

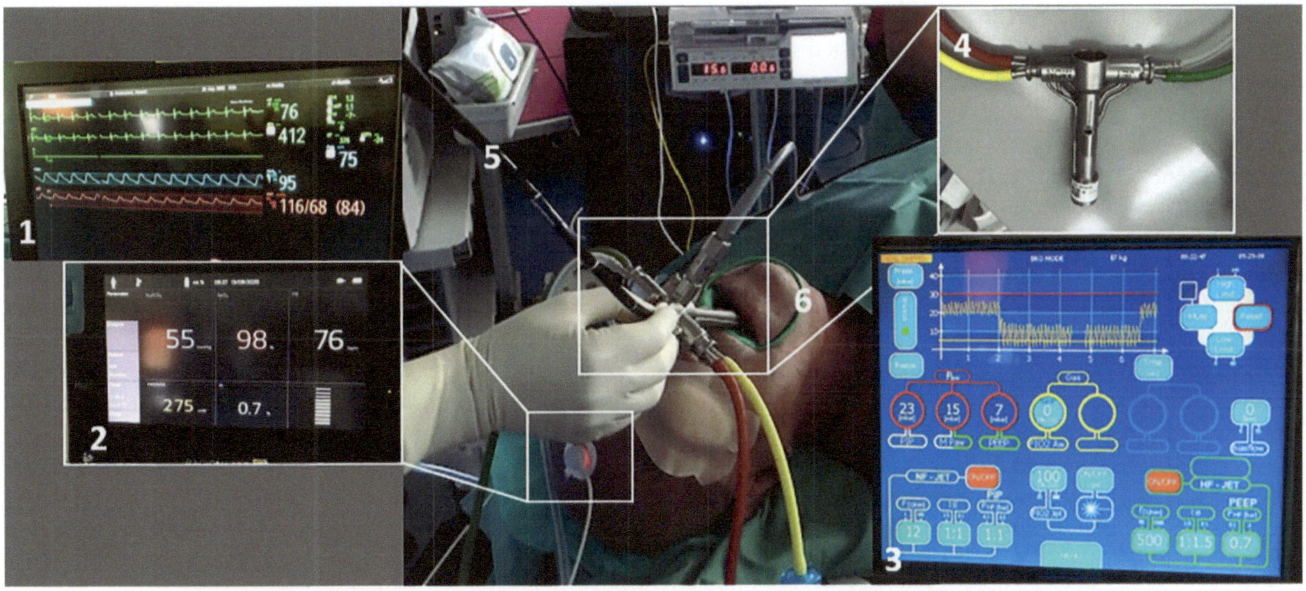

• **Fig. 14.8** Rigid bronchoscopy using superimposed high-frequency jet ventilation. 1. Monitoring (electrocardiogram, pulse-oximetry, invasive blood pressure). 2. Transcutaneous CO_2-monitoring. 3. Display of superimposed high-frequency jet ventilator. 4. Connector from the ventilator to the rigid bronchoscope. 5. Flexible bronchoscope. 6. Tooth protection.

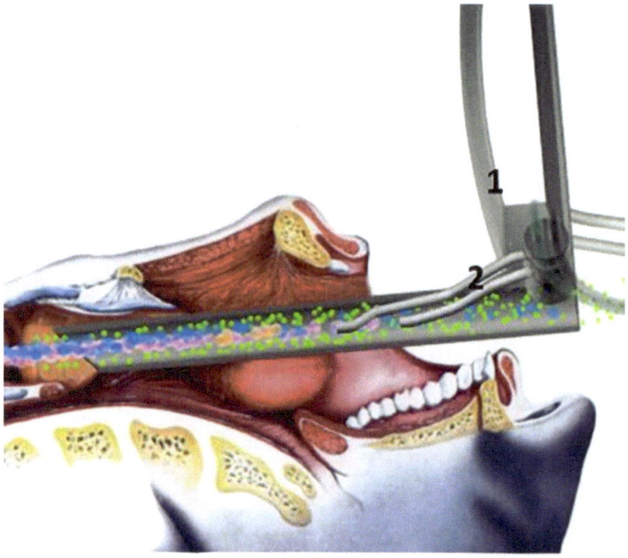

• **Fig. 14.9** Rigid bronchoscopy using superimposed high-frequency jet ventilation. 1. Rigid bronchoscope. 2. Low- and high-frequency jet ventilation. *Blue*, Entrainment of air from the upper airways; *green*, continuous expiration along the tracheal wall; *yellow and purple*, low- and high-frequency jet flow from the jet ventilator. (From CARL REINER GmbH, Wien. Bedienungsanleitung CTNI-910-D05 Stand: 2015.07.01 https://docplayer.org/19296349-Twinstream-bedienungsanleitung.html.)

Airway Obstructing Tumor

Infraglottic or tracheal stenosis can be approached endoscopically. Unimpaired vision is important while using microinstruments within the airway, which can be offered by HFJV. There are two possible approaches. For prestenotic ventilation, the catheter or tube is placed proximal to the stenosis. In this case, higher pressure and longer inspiratory times are necessary to secure ventilation through the stenosis. When the catheter or artificial airway is placed distal to the stenosis (poststenotic ventilation), the lumen is further reduced, limiting expiration through the stenosis even more. Therefore the I:E ratio should be adjusted so that the expiratory time is long enough to avoid air trapping, the buildup of auto-PEEP, and barotrauma.[14] Furthermore, the pause pressure alarm should be set low because the intrapulmonary pressure is usually higher than the end-expiratory intratracheal pressure measured by the ventilator.

For severe airway stenosis, the use of transtracheal HFJV should be considered, offering an alternative to operative tracheostomy. Decarboxylation can be a problem because of the reduced expiratory flow through the stenosis. In this case, superimposed HFJV can effectively increase lung volumes and maintain gas exchange and may be advantageous in severe airway obstruction.[15] Conventional intubation should be ready at any time as a backup option. Caution must be taken in most morbidly obese patients because of the weight of the adiposity on the chest wall further limiting the airways and the lung volume.[16] Nevertheless, in a small retrospective trial, complications were similar between obese patients and nonobese patients.[16] In all patients, use of the reverse Trendelenburg position can decrease abdominal pressure on the diaphragm and thereby improve ventilation.

Tracheal and Carinal Resection

For tracheal resection, HFJV offers a promising ventilation technique using a so-called tube-in-tube technique, with the jet catheter advanced through the endotracheal tube.[17] For one-lung ventilation (OLV) during carinal resection, HFJV with an unblocked bronchus blocker can be safely used.[18] Therefore a bronchial blocker can be advanced through an endobronchial tube and connected to a jet ventilator. The bronchial blocker has to be unblocked to allow passive expiration and avoid a potential pneumothorax. Alternative methods, in rare high-risk patients, are cardiopulmonary bypass, which, is associated with a high bleeding risk or placement of a long, single lumen tube, which may interfere with the surgical field and cause airway injury because of repeated insertion and removal.[18]

Cannot Ventilate Cannot Intubate Situation

A "cannot ventilate—cannot intubate" situation can be expected, especially when an infraglottic stenosis is present. Such situations may be handled successfully with transtracheal HFJV. Therefore a 14-gauge catheter is introduced through the cricothyroid membrane into the trachea using the Seldinger technique.[19] To optimize safety, the transtracheal catheter can be positioned before anesthetic induction under local anesthesia.[19]

Preoperative airway obstruction is a major factor that contributes to the difficulty of oxygenation. Transtracheal oxygenation using a jet ventilator equipped with a tracheal pressure control can be less iatrogenic compared with a tracheotomy in the emergency case, which has a high rate of complications.[19] However, personnel need to be well trained to perform safe placement of the cannula in an emergency situation.[20]

Ventilation of the Nondependent Lung

HFV can be used to ventilate the surgical lung during OLV.[21] The selective application of low driving pressure HFV to recruit the surgical lung during OLV improves arterial oxygenation, while only minimally limiting the surgical access during video-assisted thoracoscopy.[22] HFPV, when compared with continuous positive airway pressure (CPAP), applied to the surgical lung during partial pulmonary resection not only improved oxygenation, but also decreased the length of hospital stay.[23] Because of the pulsatile flow pattern during HFPV, mucostasis can be avoided. Furthermore, HFJV, when compared with CPAP of 2 and 5 cm H_2O applied to the surgical lung during open thoracotomy, could improve right ventricular function.[24] Alternatively, HFJV of both lungs might offer adequate surgical conditions not only for lung interventions, but also of the heart.[25] Compared with OLV with a double-lumen tube and conventional mechanical ventilation, HFJV procedures using a single-lumen tube resulted in a higher arterial partial pressure of oxygen with a lower peak inspiratory pressure in minimally invasive and total endoscopic coronary artery bypass procedures[25] and during thoracotomy.[26]

Imaging, Stereotactic Procedures, and Catheter Ablation

HFJV limits the movement of thoracic structures to a minimum[27] and therefore offers unique advantages for radiotherapy of lung lesions reducing both the exposure to radiation and dose itself, with less injury of the surrounding tissue. Accordingly, long-term radiation side effects can be reduced.[28] Nevertheless, because HFV usually requires tracheal intubation, it should be restricted to single-fraction or oligo fractionated treatment.[29] Furthermore, HFV may result in dorsal atelectasis, making lesions indistinguishable from normal lung tissue. HFJV can be used successfully for cryoablation, especially if the target tissue is close to the diaphragm and prone position is necessary. HFJV with a tube-in-tube technique can be the ventilation technique of choice for preserving gas exchange, while keeping the lungs almost static.[30]

To avoid general anesthesia, an unblocked nasal jet catheter (diameter < 2 mm, two channels, one for gas delivery and one for gas and pressure monitoring) can be advanced through the nose into the trachea while the patient is sedated and breathing spontaneously.[31]

During conventional mechanical ventilation, intrathoracic pressure swings during the respiratory cycle can dislodge the ablation catheter from its contact point during pulmonary vein isolation for atrial fibrillation. HFV minimizes the movement of the catheter from its contact site in the left atrium. Thereby, the number of radiofrequency applications can be reduced, as well as fluoroscopy time and the total ablation time.[32] In a prospective registry study, HFJV in patients undergoing pulmonary vein isolation for atrial fibrillation with radiofrequency, force-sensing catheters was associated with improved outcomes as compared with standard ventilation. Sivasambu et al. evaluated 84 HFJV patients and 84 matched control patients regarding 1-year outcome data. Atrial arrhythmia recurrence occurred in 26 of 84 HFJV patients (31%) and 42 of 84 control patients (50%; $P = .019$). In patients with paroxysmal atrial fibrillation, arrhythmia recurrence in HFJV and control patients was 27.3% and 47.3%, respectively ($P = .045$). Of note, vasopressor use during HFJV cases was significantly higher than during standard ventilation (79.7% vs. 22.4%; $P = .001$).[33] Complication rates attributable to HFJV were lower than those of the procedure itself.[32] Nevertheless, the high cost still prevents the widespread implementation of HFV during ablation.[34]

Bronchopleural Fistula

Bronchopleural fistula, a persistent communication between the tracheobronchial tree and the pleural cavity, may become challenging for the anesthesiologist if positive pressure ventilation is necessary. During conventional mechanical ventilation, airflow across the fistula must be minimized to avoid tension pneumothorax. Conventional mechanical ventilation can put patients at a risk because of high pressures and the resulting high air leak across the fistula. In such cases, HFV might be considered because, owing to the lower mean airway pressure and smaller V_T, alveolar distension is theoretically reduced and the air leak minimized.[35] However, this is not always the case.[36]

HFOV in combination with spontaneous breathing activity represents another promising approach during thoracic anesthesia.[37] Spontaneous breathing reduces the risk of tension pneumothorax, while optimizing ventilation and perfusion matching. HFOV combined with spontaneous breathing activity can increase minute ventilation, whereas the influence on mean tracheal pressure is relatively small, resulting in a proportionally low air leak across the fistula.[37]

Postcardiac Surgery Use

Postoperative respiratory failure is common following cardiac surgery.[38] HFPV provided significantly better gas exchange compared with conventional mechanical ventilation in this surgical population.[39] Furthermore, HFPV has the potential to improve not only oxygenation, but also hemodynamics following cardiac surgery.[40] Finally, HFPV might be used as rescue therapy for hypoxemia refractory to conventional mechanical ventilation in the postoperative period of cardiac surgery.[41]

Contraindications

A tracheal stenosis leading to more than an 80% reduction of the cross-section represents an absolute contraindication for HFV because of expiratory flow limitation with increased risk of barotrauma.[42] When HFJV is used with an open airway, it is important that patients have fasted and increased aspiration risk is excluded. Morbid obesity poses an increased risk of insufficient gas exchange during HFV because of higher thorax wall stiffness, but obesity itself does not represent an absolute contraindication. Also, restrictive and obstructive lung diseases are relative contraindications because of the limited expiration. Contraindications must be checked before the procedure and careful planning together with the surgeon or the interventionist is highly advisable.

Setup and Monitoring

During HFV, the thorax is almost static, obscuring clinical evaluation and increasing the value of auscultation. The jet sound should be equal on both hemi-thoraces. Standard monitoring should include pulse oximetry. Evaluation of ventilation (decarboxylation) is more difficult. When using an open system such as during HFJV, measurement of end-tidal CO_2 is possible if HFJV is paused, or, alternatively, a hybrid mode consisting of high- and low-frequency ventilation is used. Thus in most cases, placement of an arterial indwelling catheter for periodic arterial blood gas measurements is recommended. Alternatively, continuous transcutaneous capnography can be used,[9] as illustrated in Fig. 14.8.

Furthermore, ventilator parameters, such as V_T and compliance of the respiratory system cannot be measured directly during HFJV. Only airway pressure is measured, and pressure limits can be set. In addition, driving pressure, respiratory rate, inspiratory to expiratory time (I:E) or inspiratory fraction, FiO_2 (jet FiO_2), bias flow, mean airway pressure (HFOV), and PEEP can be set.

Driving Pressure

During HFJV, set driving pressure is higher compared with the pressure in the airways because of the open system. It can be titrated to arterial carbon dioxide tension ($PaCO_2$) and increased in increments of 5 psi to a maximum of 40 psi. During HFOV, the driving pressure determines the V_T and thereby ventilation. Increasing the driving pressure increases decarboxylation.

Peak inspiratory pressure, oscillatory continuous positive airway pressure: during HFPV the peak inspiratory pressure is usually set at approximately two-thirds the pressure used during conventional mechanical ventilation and oscillatory continuous positive airway pressure at 5 cm H_2O.

Tidal Volume

During HFOV, some ventilators allow a volume guarantee mode. Thereby, a predefined V_T can be set, the ventilator will adjust the delivered driving pressure as required to achieve the set V_T.

Respiratory Rate

During HFJV, respiratory rates of 90 to 150 breaths per minute are usually chosen[43] With an increased respiratory rate, V_T decreases. Increasing respiratory rates during HFV can result in a rise of $PaCO_2$ because of reduced gas elimination time and reduced V_T. During HFOV, the initial respiratory rate can be set at around 500 breaths per minute. For HFPV, pressure controlled respiratory rate can be initially set at 15 breaths per minute and the percussive frequency initially at 500 breaths per minute.

Fraction of Inspired Oxygen

For all modes of HFV during thoracic procedures, the initial FiO_2 should be set at 1.0 and adjusted according to oxygenation. During HFJV, the set FiO_2 does not equal the tracheal FiO_2 which is lower, because of the high flow and the resulting air entrainment from the supraglottic region.[42]

Inspiratory Fraction, I:E

Increasing inspiratory time and increasing V_T oxygenation and ventilation can be improved whereas increasing the expiration time will enhance the elimination of CO_2.[42] During HFJV, inspiratory fraction can be titrated to gas exchange, increasing inspiratory fraction in increments of 5% up to a maximum of 40%. During HFPV, I:E of both the oscillatory and pressure-controlled cycles is initially set at 1:1. During HFOV, I:E cannot be set and is determined by the ventilator.

Bias Flow

During HFOV, a bias flow of 20 L/min is set at the beginning of the intervention and can be increased as needed.

Mean Airway Pressure

The main principle of HFOV is to use a constant mean airway pressure keeping the lungs open. The initial mean airway pressure during HFOV can be set at 5 cm H_2O above the last mean airway pressure during conventional ventilation. During HFOV, mean airway pressure, which is important for oxygenation, is determined by the bias flow and the set end-expiratory pressure.

Anesthetic Considerations

For jet ventilation, total intravenous anesthetic technique is required because of the open circuit of the ventilation system.[9] To allow fast onset, but also fast offset of anesthesia, short- or ultrashort-acting anesthetic agents are required because HFV is used mainly for short procedures. To improve surgical conditions, the use of neuromuscular blockading agents can be considered. Rocuronium or cisatracurium should be used preferably because of their short half-life. However, whenever neuromuscular blockade is used, reversal of the blockade should be monitored using, for example, train of four measurement. In case of persisting paralysis at the end of the procedure, acetylcholinesterase inhibitors or antimuscarinic agents or sugammadex for rocuronium are highly recommended. For hypnosis and analgesia, propofol with remifentanil and alternatively etomidate or ketamine with fentanyl, alfentanil, or remifentanil can be used. According to a prospective clinical trial, the risk of awareness during total intravenous anesthesia was higher as compared with anesthesia with halogenated drugs.[44] Therefore electroencephalogram-based monitoring, for example, bispectral index (BIS) should be used to monitor depth of anesthesia and avoid awareness. At the end of the procedure, a laryngeal mask can be used to allow smooth reversal of anesthesia.[9]

Risks and Benefits

HFV offers several advantages, such as minimal movement of the thorax, greater surgical visibility, decreased conflict of space within the airways, and improved oxygenation and hemodynamics using lower airway pressure (Table 14.3). Furthermore, air leak through a bronchopleural fistula can be reduced.

Besides the positive effects, HFV also poses risks that should be known to the operator. Especially if supraglottic

TABLE 14.3 Advantages and Disadvantages of High-Frequency Ventilation Compared With Conventional Mechanical Ventilation

	Advantages	Disadvantages
Physiologic	• Reduced airway pressure • Less hemodynamic compromise	• Risk of barotrauma • Cooling and drying of conditioned inspiratory gases by expansion at nozzle • Efficacy of gas exchange less predictable • Increased dead space because of pendelluft
Surgical	• Minimal vocal cord/surgical field movement • Improved visibility and surgical access • Avoidance ETT ignition during LASER surgery	• Potential for lower airway soiling in ENT surgery • Contamination of expired gas flow by surgical debris
Anesthetic	• Good in low resistance large volume airway leak • Emergency transtracheal jet ventilation • Versatile application options during airway surgery	• Inhalational anesthesia often impractical • Contamination of operating room air if anesthetic gases are used • Delivered FiO_2 is multifactorial, cannot be set directly • Only intermittent end-tidal CO_2 monitoring • Pressure measurements may be unrepresentative • High gas flow required • Need for humidification

ENT, Ear, nose and throat; *ETT*, endotracheal tube; *FiO_2*, fraction of inspired oxygen.

Modified from Evans E, Biro P, Bedforth N. Jet ventilation. *BJA Educ.* 2007;7:2–5.

access is used, the catheter position should be monitored carefully. Intubation or dislocation into the esophagus can cause severe air entrapment and gastric perforation.[45] During HFJV, ventilation stops automatically as soon as the ventilator notices an obstruction. If it is not possible to reposition the jet catheter properly, alternative airway access should be ready immediately to avoid desaturation. Reintubation should be performed straight away using an airway exchange catheter with the Kleinsasser laryngoscope still in situ, during laryngeal or proximal tracheal interventions.[5]

Decarboxylation can be a problem during HFV because of the small V_T. Ventilation can be improved by decreasing respiratory rate and increasing driving pressure and inspiratory time. Alternatively, superimposed HFJV and HFPV offer higher minute ventilation.

Because of the high respiratory rate during HFV, the expiratory time is short, possibly leading to auto-PEEP with a consecutive risk of dynamic hyperinflation, barotrauma (cervical emphysema, tension pneumothorax), and hemodynamic instability. The risk further increases when stenosis of the airway is present.[46] Therefore stenosis with a narrowing of the cross-section under 20% represents a contraindication for HFJV. The high respiratory rate during HFV might result in increased mechanical power. Higher mechanical power was associated with worse clinical outcomes.[47] In fact, in acute respiratory distress syndrome patients, HFV was associated with higher mortality, when compared with conventional mechanical ventilation.[48] However, trials investigating the relationship between HFV and mechanical power are still missing.

A dreaded complication of HFJV is a necrotizing tracheobronchitis. However, the risk can be reduced if the gas is heated and humidified. In modern jet ventilators, there are built-in humidification systems. Overall, the number of complications is low directly related to the number of HFV cases performed.[11]

Conclusion

HFV during thoracic procedures offers several advantages compared with conventional mechanical ventilation. The complication rate is relatively low when patients are selected carefully, contraindications are excluded, the team is well-trained, and backup strategies are ready.

References

1. Salim A, Martin M. High-frequency percussive ventilation. *Crit Care Med.* 2005;33:S241–S245.
2. Galmen K, Harbut P, Freedman J, et al. The use of high-frequency ventilation during general anaesthesia: an update. *F1000Res.* 2017; 6:756.
3. Pillow JJ. High-frequency oscillatory ventilation: mechanisms of gas exchange and lung mechanics. *Crit Care Med.* 2005;3:S135–S141.
4. Dolan AM, Moore MF. Anaesthesia for tracheobronchial stent insertion using an laryngeal mask airway and high-frequency jet ventilation. *Case Rep Med.* 2013:950437.
5. Helmstaedter V, Tellkamp R, Schwab B, et al. High-frequency jet ventilation in otorhinolaryngology - surgical and anaesthesiologic issues. *Laryngorhinootologie.* 2014;93:455–460.

6. Putz L, Mayne A, Dincq AS. Jet ventilation during rigid bronchoscopy in adults: a focused review. *BioMed Res Int.* 2016: 4234861.
7. Sutterlin R, Priori R, Larsson A, et al. Frequency dependence of lung volume changes during superimposed high-frequency jet ventilation and high-frequency jet ventilation. *Br J Anaesth.* 2014; 112:141–149.
8. Sullivan MT, Neff WB. A modified Sanders ventilating system for rigid-wall bronchoscopy. *Anesthesiology.* 1979;50:473–474.
9. Pathak V, Welsby I, Mahmood K, et al. Ventilation and anesthetic approaches for rigid bronchoscopy. *Ann Am Thorac Soc.* 2014;11: 628–634.
10. Herrmann J, Lilitwat W, Tawhai MH, et al. High-frequency oscillatory ventilation and ventilator-induced lung injury: size does matter. *Crit Care Med.* 2019;48(1):66–73.
11. Ross-Anderson DJ, Ferguson C, Patel A. Transtracheal jet ventilation in 50 patients with severe airway compromise and stridor. *Br J Anaesth.* 2011;106:140–144.
12. Davies JM, Hillel AD, Maronian NC, et al. The Hunsaker Mon-Jet tube with jet ventilation is effective for microlaryngeal surgery. *Can J Anaesth.* 2009;56:284–290.
13. Khan I, Shakeel M, Nagaraja R, et al. A Hunsaker Mon-Jet tube trapped in the larynx. *J Laryngol Otol.* 2011;125:1204–1205.
14. Atkins JH, Mirza N, Mandel JE. Case report: respiratory inductance plethysmography as a monitor of ventilation during laser ablation and balloon dilatation of subglottic tracheal stenosis. *ORL J Otorhinolaryngol Relat Spec.* 2009;71:289–291.
15. Sutterlin R, Lomauro A, Gandolfi S, et al. Influence of tracheal obstruction on the efficacy of superimposed high-frequency jet ventilation and single-frequency jet ventilation. *Anesthesiology.* 2015; 123:799–809.
16. Philips R, Desilva B, Matrka L. Jet ventilation in obese patients undergoing airway surgery for subglottic and tracheal stenosis. *Laryngoscope.* 2018;128:1887–1892.
17. Kampe S, Rocha M, Darwiche K, et al. Sufficient high frequency jet ventilation during a period of 2.5 h—airway management during resection of a tracheaesophageal fistula and tracheal resection. *Anasthesiol Intensivmed Notfallmed Schmerzther.* 2016;51:368–371.
18. Chin JH, Lee EH, Choi DK, et al. High frequency jet ventilation of one lung using a bronchial blocker of Univent during carinal resection. *J Korean Med Sci.* 2010;25:1083–1085.
19. Bouroche G, Motamed C, De Guibert JM, et al. Rescue transtracheal jet ventilation during difficult intubation in patients with upper airway cancer. *Anaesth Crit Care Pain Med.* 2018;37:539–544.
20. Duggan LV, Ballantyne Scott B, Law JA, et al. Transtracheal jet ventilation in the 'can't intubate can't oxygenate' emergency: a systematic review. *Br J Anaesth.* 2016;117(suppl 1):i28–i38.
21. Shoman BM, Ragab HO, Mustafa A, et al. "High frequency/small tidal volume differential lung ventilation": a technique of ventilating the nondependent lung of one lung ventilation for robotically assisted thoracic surgery. *Case Rep Anesthesiol.* 2015:631450.
22. El-Tahan MR, El Ghoneimy YF, Regal MA, et al. Comparative study of the non-dependent continuous positive pressure ventilation and high-frequency positive-pressure ventilation during one-lung ventilation for video-assisted thoracoscopic surgery. *Interact Cardiovasc Thorac Surg.* 2011;12:899–902.
23. Lucangelo U, Antonaglia V, Zin WA, et al. High-frequency percussive ventilation improves perioperatively clinical evolution in pulmonary resection. *Crit Care Med.* 2011;37:1663–1669.
24. El Tahan MR, El Ghoneimy Y, Regal M, et al. Effects of non-dependent lung ventilation with continuous positive-pressure ventilation and high-frequency positive-pressure ventilation on right-ventricular function during 1-lung ventilation. *Semin Cardiothorac Vasc Anesth.* 2010;14:291–300.
25. Ender J, Brodowsky M, Falk V, et al. High-frequency jet ventilation as an alternative method compared to conventional one-lung ventilation using double-lumen tubes during minimally invasive coronary artery bypass graft surgery. *J Cardiothorac Vasc Anesth.* 2010;24:602–607.
26. Misiolek H, Knapik P, Swanevelder J, et al. Comparison of double-lung jet ventilation and one-lung ventilation for thoracotomy. *Eur J Anaesthesiol.* 2008;25:15–21.
27. Denys A, Lachenal Y, Duran R, et al. Use of high-frequency jet ventilation for percutaneous tumor ablation. *Cardiovasc Interv Radiol.* 2014;37:140–146.
28. Fritz P, Kraus HJ, Muhlnickel W, et al. High-frequency jet ventilation for complete target immobilization and reduction of planning target volume in stereotactic high single-dose irradiation of stage I non-small cell lung cancer and lung metastases. *Int J Radiat Oncol Biol Phys.* 2010;78:136–142.
29. Santiago A, Jelen U, Ammazzalorso F, et al. Reproducibility of target coverage in stereotactic spot scanning proton lung irradiation under high frequency jet ventilation. *Radiother Oncol.* 2013; 109:45–50.
30. Vazquez R, Beermann SL, Fintelmann FJ, et al. High-frequency jet ventilation in the prone position to facilitate cryoablation of a peridiaphragmatic pulmonary neoplasm: a case report. *A A Pract.* 2019;13:169–172.
31. Hohenforst-Schmidt W, Zarogoulidis P, Huang H, et al. A new and safe mode of ventilation for interventional pulmonary medicine: the ease of nasal superimposed high frequency jet ventilation. *J Cancer.* 2018;9:816–833.
32. Elkassabany N, Garcia F, Tschabrunn C, et al. Anesthetic management of patients undergoing pulmonary vein isolation for treatment of atrial fibrillation using high-frequency jet ventilation. *J Cardiothorac Vasc Anesth.* 2012;26:433–438.
33. Sivasambu B, Hakim JB, Barodka V, et al. Initiation of a high-frequency jet ventilation strategy for catheter ablation for atrial fibrillation: safety and outcomes data. *JACC Clin Electrophysiol.* 2018;4:1519–1525.
34. Raiten J, Elkassabany N, Mandel JE. The use of high-frequency jet ventilation for out of operating room anesthesia. *Curr Opin Anaesthesiol.* 2012;25:482–485.
35. Carlon GC, Ray C Jr, Klain M, et al. High-frequency positive-pressure ventilation in management of a patient with bronchopleural fistula. *Anesthesiology.* 1980;52:160–162.
36. Bishop MJ, Benson MS, Sato P, et al. Comparison of high-frequency jet ventilation with conventional mechanical ventilation for bronchopleural fistula. *Anesth Analg.* 1987;66:833–838.
37. Poulin V, Vaillancourt R, Somma J, et al. High frequency ventilation combined with spontaneous breathing during bronchopleural fistula repair: a case report. *Can J Anaesth.* 2009;56:52–56.
38. Thanavaro J, Taylor J, Vitt L, et al. Predictors and outcomes of postoperative respiratory failure after cardiac surgery. *J Eval Clin Pract.* 2020;26(5):1490–1497.
39. Oribabor C, Gulkarov I, Khusid F, et al. The use of high-frequency percussive ventilation after cardiac surgery significantly improves gas exchange without impairment of hemodynamics. *Can J Respir Ther.* 2018;54:58–61.
40. Forti A, Salandin V, Zanatta P, et al. Haemodynamics and oxygenation improvement induced by high frequency percussive ventilation in a patient with hypoxia following cardiac surgery: a case report. *J Med Case Rep.* 2010;4:339.

41. Wong I, Worku B, Weingarten JA, et al. High-frequency percussive ventilation in cardiac surgery patients failing mechanical conventional ventilation. *Interact Cardiovasc Thorac Surg*. 2017; 25:937–941.
42. Fritzsche K, Osmers A. Anesthetic management in laryngotracheal surgery. High-frequency jet ventilation as strategy for ventilation during general anesthesia. *HNO*. 2011;59:931–941 quiz 942–933.
43. Fritzsche K, Osmers A. [Anesthetic management in laryngotracheal surgery. High-frequency jet ventilation as strategy for ventilation during general anesthesia]. *Der Anaesth*. 2010;59:1051–1061, quiz 1062–1053.
44. Errando CL, Sigl JC, Robles M, et al. Awareness with recall during general anaesthesia: a prospective observational evaluation of 4001 patients. *Br J Anaesth*. 2008;101:178–185.
45. Kern M, Niemeyer D, Kerner T, et al. [Anesthesia in interventional pulmonology – bronchoscopy and jet ventilation]. *Anasthesiol Intensivmed Notfallmed Schmerzther*. 2015;50:8–18.
46. Ihra GC, Tsai CJ, Kimberger O. Intrinsic positive end-expiratory pressure at various frequencies of supraglottic jet ventilation in a model of dynamic upper airway obstruction. *Anesth Analg*. 2010; 111:703–706.
47. Serpa Neto A, Deliberato RO, Johnson AEW, et al. Mechanical power of ventilation is associated with mortality in critically ill patients: an analysis of patients in two observational cohorts. *Intensive Care Med*. 2018;44:1914–1922.
48. Ferguson ND, Cook DJ, Guyatt GH, et al. High-frequency oscillation in early acute respiratory distress syndrome. *N Engl J Med*. 2013;368:795–805.

15 Anesthesia, Mechanical Ventilation, and Hypoxic Pulmonary Vasoconstriction

ANDRES HAGERMAN, MARC LICKER

Introduction

One-lung ventilation (OLV) is a standard procedure required in thoracic surgery for cancer resection, treatment of bronchopulmonary fistula or bleeding, and lung transplantation, as well as for intrathoracic diagnostic investigations.[1] Over the past 3 decades, the incidence of intraoperative hypoxemia has decreased and clinical outcome after thoracic surgery has largely been improved owing to the mastering of lung isolation techniques, better understanding of physiology related to OLV, application of protective lung ventilation, and implementation of minimally invasive surgical techniques.[2]

Hypoxic pulmonary vasoconstriction (HPV) represents an intrinsic property of pulmonary vascular smooth muscle cells (VSMCs), and an important homeostatic mechanism that helps to ensure correct gas exchange during OLV. In 1946, von Euler and Liljestrand first described the opposing hypoxic responses in pulmonary and systemic circulations expressed by vasoconstriction and vasodilatation, respectively.[3] Ontogenetically, the HPV evolves in mammals from the need to ensure fetal oxygenation when the amniotic fluid-filled lungs are hypoxic.[4] Actually, sensing low oxygen (O_2) tension in pulmonary VSMC triggers HPV, which maintains high pulmonary vascular resistance (PVR) and diverts the oxygenated placental blood through the foramen ovale and the ductus arteriosus directly into the systemic arteries. Upon the first breath at birth, sensing the rising alveolar partial oxygen pressure (PO2) or PAO_2 in pulmonary VSMCs interrupts the HPV response, allowing the deoxygenated blood flow to be distributed to all ventilating lung areas through a low resistive pulmonary circulation, whereas the foramen ovale and the ductus arteriosus both obliterate to prevent right-left shunting.

Although exerting minimal effects in healthy lungs under normoxic conditions, HPV plays an important role during OLV in thoracic surgery and during pneumologic procedures to reduce intrapulmonary shunt and preserve blood oxygenation. In healthy volunteers undergoing awake fiberoptic bronchoscopy, the HPV response has been nicely demonstrated using lung scintigraphy and intravenous administration of 99mTc-labeled albumin.[5] After inflation of a balloon-tipped catheter in the left lower bronchus, P_AO_2 and alveolar carbon dioxide partial pressure (P_ACO_2) (distal to the tip of the occluding balloon) approached mixed venous levels within 80 to 300 seconds, and blood flow decreased by 50% in the lower lobe, with redistribution to other parts of the lungs.

In patients with pneumonia, atelectasis, asthma, chronic obstructive bronchopulmonary disease (COPD), and acute respiratory distress syndrome (ARDS), HPV represents a key homeostatic mechanism to attenuate hypoxemia by adapting ventilation to the perfusion (V/Q) ratio in various parts of the lungs.[6] In contrast, when the whole lung is exposed to hypoxia (e.g., high altitude, sleep apnea, pulmonary fibrosis), HPV can be detrimental, resulting in pulmonary hypertension and acute cor pulmonale owing to a progressive increase in right ventricular afterload.

Anesthesiologists should understand the basics of the HPV response, its role in various physiologic and pathologic conditions, including OLV, and the way perioperative drugs, including anesthetic agents, may interfere with this protective reflex.

Physiology of Hypoxic Pulmonary Vasoconstriction

The Hypoxic Signal in Different Tissues

Phylogenetically, the mammalian homeostatic O_2 sensing system (HOSS) has developed a multicomponent defense mechanism to hypoxic environments aimed to prevent cellular injuries, mitigate the decline in O_2 tension, and adjust the energetic metabolism. The HOSS implicates a synchronized transcriptional regulation of a variety of genes, and it is coordinated, in large part, by the hypoxic-inducible factor (HIF) and transcription factors such as nuclear factor-κB (NF-κB) and activated protein-1, which are "master regulators" for oxygen homeostasis and inflammatory processes.[7] The

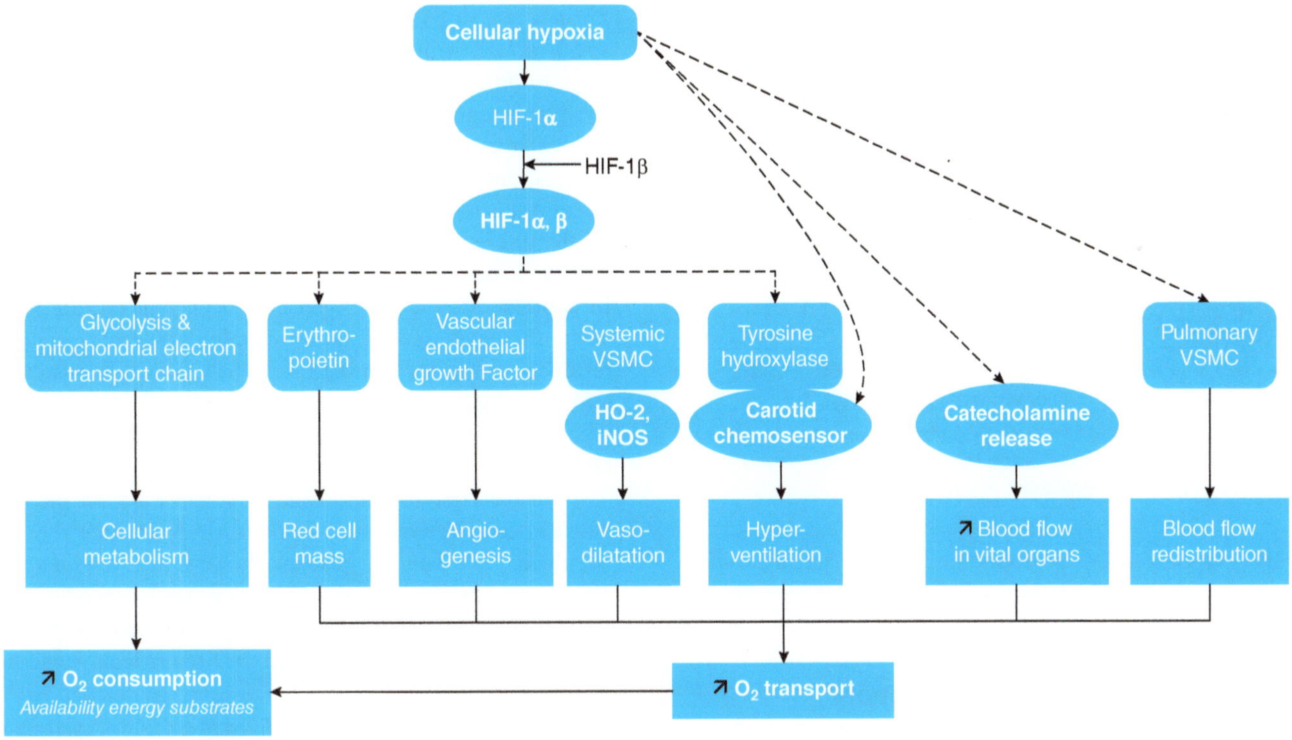

• **Fig. 15.1** Oxygen sensing and cellular response. *HIF*, Hypoxic inducible factor; *HO*, heme oxygenase; *iNOS*, inducible nitric oxide synthase; *VSMC*, vascular smooth muscle cell.

HOSS entails a network of specialized cells such as VSMCs (pulmonary and placental arteries, ductus arteriosus), endothelial cells (ECs), glomic cells in the carotid body, renal myofibroblasts, adrenomedullary chromaffin cells, and neuroepithelial bodies in the airways. When exposed to hypoxia, these specialized tissues detect low O_2 tension in their local environments through mitochondrial redox-based or cytoplasmic HIF, and they orchestrate coordinated responses to optimize oxygen uptake and delivery (Fig. 15.1).[8] In type I glomus cells from the carotid and aortic bodies, the low O_2 tension leads to inhibition of voltage-gated potassium channels (Kv), resulting in membrane depolarization and influx of extracellular Ca^{2+} via voltage-gated Ca^{2+} channels (VGCC), which triggers the release of neuromediators and a faster ventilatory drive. In the kidney, the low O_2 content (e.g., difference between O_2 delivery and O_2 utilization) leads to inhibition of prolyl-4-hydroxylase domain proteins, which activates HIF signaling to generate erythropoietin and in turn to enhance erythropoiesis. Hypoxia-mediated release of catecholamines, vascular endothelial growth factors, and erythropoietin all tend to enhance tissue O_2 delivery owing to increased cardiac output (CO), angiogenesis, and higher hemoglobin (Hb) concentrations.

The HPV response chiefly operates in arteriolar and venular pulmonary vessels (diameter < 900 µm), veins accounting for 20% of the total increase in PVR. By distorting the alveolar wall, contractile interstitial cells located within the alveolar septa slightly contribute to reduce capillary blood flow and to increase PVR.[9] The ECs modulate the HPV through the local release of vasodilators (nitric oxide [NO], prostacyclin [PGI2]) and vasoconstrictors (endothelin [ET], epoxyeicosatrienoic acid [EET], thromboxane A2 [TXA2], and platelet activating factor), with pulmonary veins exhibiting greater sensitivity to vasoconstrictor stimuli than arteries.[10,11]

From ex vivo ventilated/perfused lungs in which alveolar and blood O_2 tension were modified independently, Marshall et al. have demonstrated that acute elevation in PVR was predominantly triggered by sensing low P_AO_2 and less by sensing deoxygenated blood in mixed venous blood ($P_{mv}O_2$).[12,13] The stimulus of HPV (PO_2S) has been modeled according to the following equation: PO_2 stimulus = $P_AO_2{}^{0.62} + P_{mv}O_2{}^{0.38}$.

When pulmonary VSMCs or isolated lungs are exposed to decremental levels of local PO_2, the HPV develops at a threshold of 85 to 90 mm Hg, to reach a maximum at 65 to 70 mm Hg (about halfway between P_AO_2 and $P_{mv}O_2$) and declining thereafter to stop around 5 mm Hg (Fig. 15.2).[14]

The O_2 sensing area is thought to extend from precapillary arterioles to upstream pulmonary arteries with different vasoconstrictive responses according to the size of the vessels.[15] The small arteries (diameter < 0.5 mm) are closely exposed to P_AO_2 (from outside) and to $P_{mv}O_2$ (from inside), whereas larger arteries (diameter of 0.5–2 mm) that are supplied by systemic blood through the vasa vasorum are exposed to both $P_{mv}O_2$ (from inside) and to arterial O_2 pressure (P_aO_2 from outside). Hence, variable diffusion O_2 gradients are generated through the wall of pulmonary arteries that determine the true stimulus for HPV (PO_2S), being predominant in small arteries. In larger arteries, the

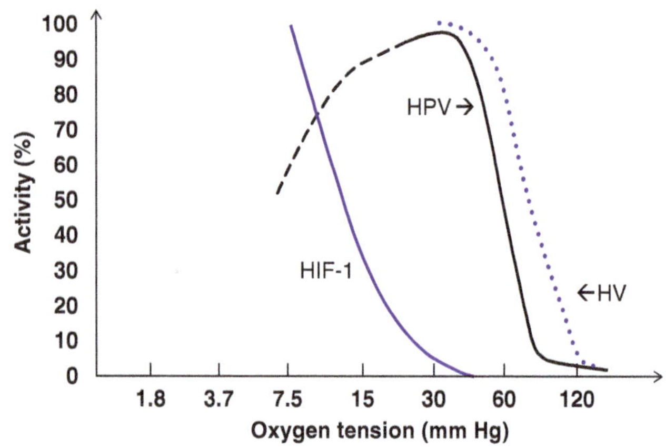

• **Fig. 15.2** Thresholds for physiologic responses to low oxygen tension. *HIF*, Hypoxic inducible factor; *HPV*, hypoxic pulmonary vasoconstriction; *HV*, hypoxic ventilation.

HPV response is less profound and mainly activated when systemic hypoxemia develops (P_aO_2 < 40–50 mm Hg), as bronchial arteries uniformly dilate like systemic vessels.

Time Course of Hypoxic Pulmonary Vasoconstriction

Hypoxic exposure of pulmonary VSMCs results in a biphasic vasoconstrictive response. The early phase starts immediately, peaking at 5 to 20 minutes and is associated with transient elevations of intracellular calcium concentrations. Phase 2 develops more gradually to reach a second peak at 60 to 120 minutes, as a result of myofibrillar calcium-sensitization coupled with enhanced release of vasoconstrictive compounds (ET-1 and EET) and decreased production of NO from the ECs (Fig. 15.3).[14] A sustained vasoconstrictive response may not persist in case of severe hypoxia. If normoxia is restored after or during the early hypoxic phase (<20 minutes), the HPV stops allowing normalization of PVR and pulmonary blood flow with improved V/Q ratios. In contrast, after a prolonged period of hypoxia, the HPV disappears over several hours despite full reoxygenation, resulting in greater ventilation-perfusion (V/Q) mismatch and consequently a larger alveolar-to-arterial O_2 pressure gradient (A-aPO_2). A second hypoxic challenge (in ipsilateral lung) will result in an enhanced HPV response.

Both atelectasis formation and persistent HPV are incriminated in causing hypoxemia in the early hours after thoracic anesthesia. Likewise, in bilateral thoracic interventions and after starting the second stage, a V/Q mismatch may develop in the dependent ventilated lung, which is attributed to the residual HPV response that lags behind the time of reoxygenation.

The Oxygen Sensing and Effector Mechanisms of Hypoxic Pulmonary Vasoconstriction

In eukaryotic cells, mitochondria are acting as powerhouses using mainly O_2 to convert nutrients into chemical energy in the form of adenosine triphosphate (ATP) that is used in

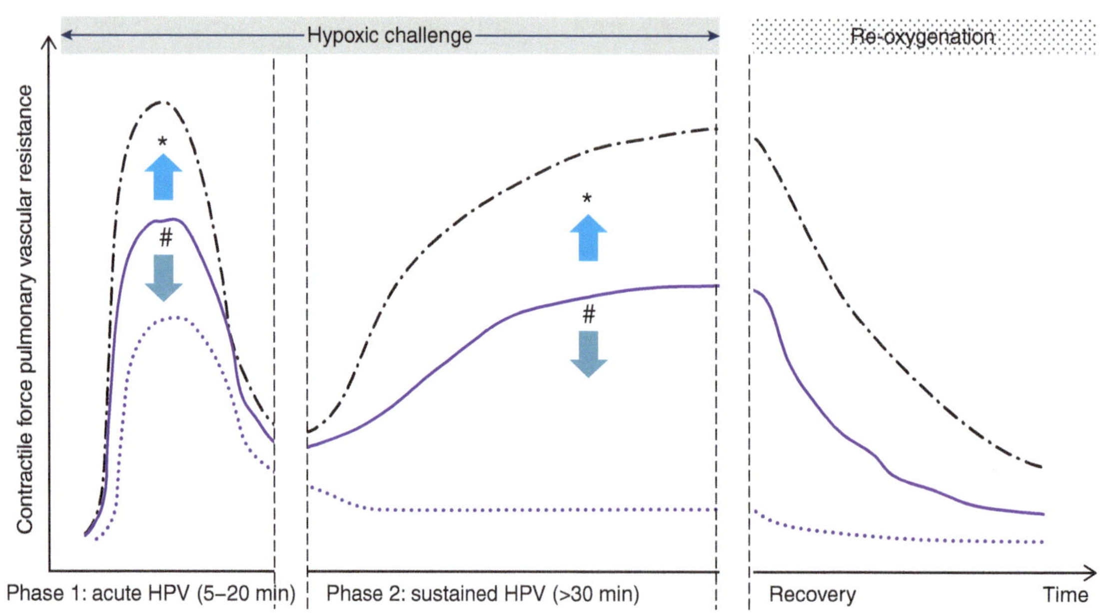

 # Conditions reducing HPV
- Injured endothelium
- Vessel distension (hypervolemia, pulmonary hypertension)
- Hyperthermia
- Alcalosis, hypocapnic alcalosis
- Sepsis, systemic inflammatory response syndrome
- >30% of lung volume exposed to hypoxia
- P_AO_2 < 40 mm Hg, lung units with a V/Q < 0.3

*** Conditions enhancing HPV**
- intact endothelium (phase 2)
- Age
- Hypothermia
- Acidosis, hypercapnic acidosis
- Red blood cell
- ≤30% of lung volume exposed to hypoxia
- P_AO_2 ~50–80 mm Hg, lung units with a V/Q ~ 0.4

• **Fig. 15.3** Time course and factors influencing hypoxic pulmonary vasoconstriction (*HPV*). *V/Q*, ventilation/perfusion.

processes including muscle contraction, ion transport, nerve impulse propagation, and chemical synthesis. A series of oxidation-reduction reactions involves the transfer of electrons from nicotinamide adenine dinucleotide (NADH) and flavin adenine dinucleotide (FADH2) across the electron transport chain (ETC). Because mitochondrial respiration continues even at very low O_2 levels (~7 mm Hg) to generate ATP, it is unlikely that variations in ATP concentrations trigger the hypoxic response.[16] Ultimately, in the process of oxidative phosphorylation, O_2 serves as the terminal electron acceptor of the ETC to form H_2O, while, at multiple sites along the ETC, some leaking electrons react with O_2, forming reactive oxygen species (ROSs), such as superoxide and hydrogen peroxide.

In pulmonary VSMCs, the most plausible mechanism to detect hypoxia is the mitochondrial PO_2-sensitive ability to vary the production of diffusible ROSs and/or to alter the cytosolic redox state. Although controversies surround the issue on whether ROSs generated by the ETC decrease or increase in response to hypoxia, there is strong evidence that HPV is triggered by mitochondrial signals that launch a coordinated response involving membranar and sarcolemnal potassium and calcium channel receptors to increase cytoplasmic calcium concentrations.[17] As proposed by Smith and Schumacker,[17] mitochondrial ROSs (see Fig. 15.4) move to the cytosol, where they activate several pathways leading to intracellular calcium mobilization: (1) inhibition of Kv channels causing membrane depolarization, which promotes the opening of VGCC; (2) activation of phospholipase C (PLC) to generate diacyl glycerol (DAG) and inositol 1,4,5-triphosphate (IP3) that stimulate calcium release, respectively, from membranal receptor-operating channels (ROCs) and sarcolemnal IP3 receptors; and (3) activation of ryanodine receptors (RyR) by oxidation of cysteine residues. In addition, by increasing the ratio of adenosine monophosphate (AMP) to ATP, low O_2 tension stimulates AMP-kinase (AMPK), resulting in activation of the RyRs and further Ca^{2+} release from the sarcoplasmic

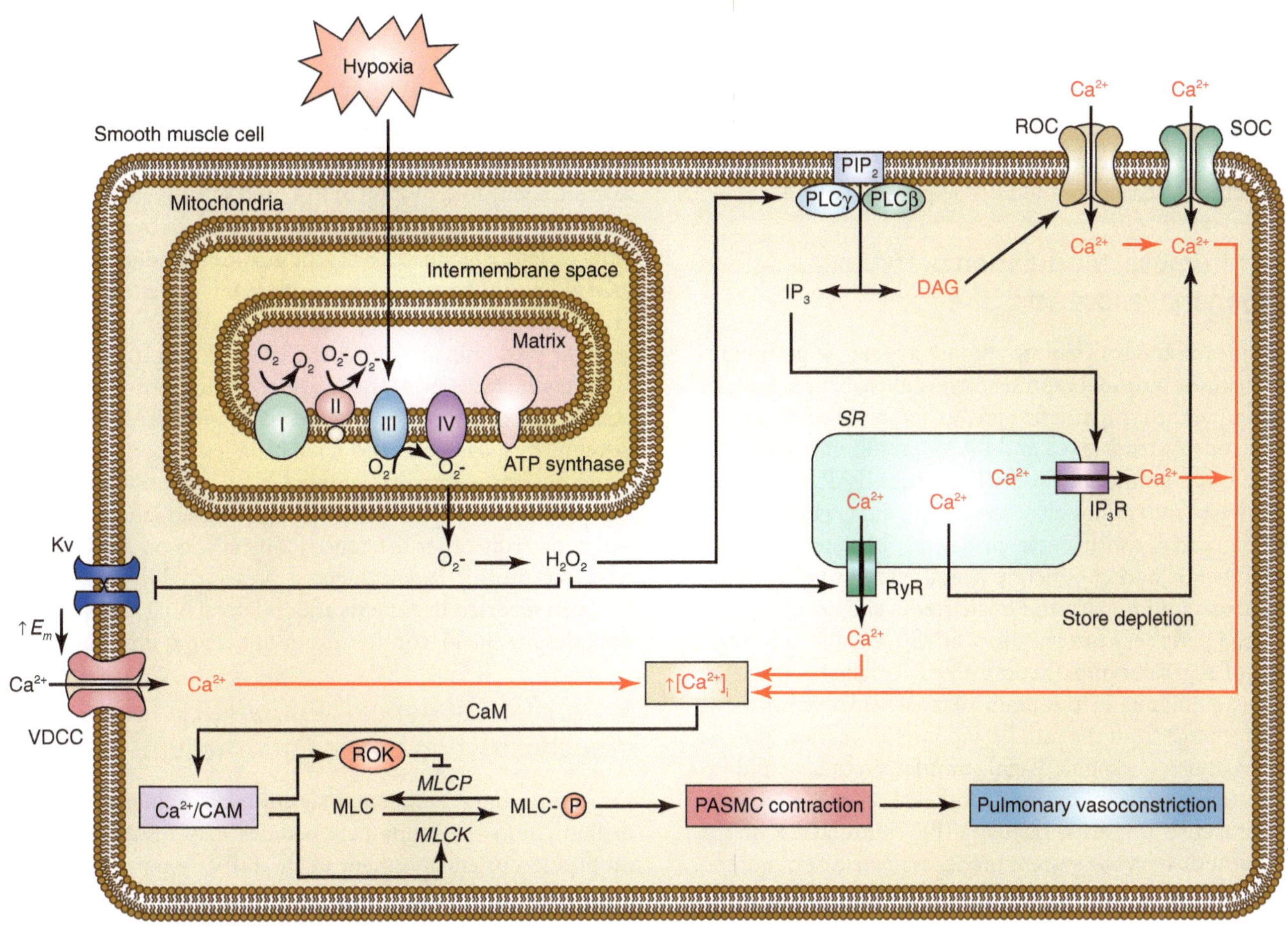

• **Fig. 15.4 Oxygen sensing and cellular response.** *ATP*, Adenosine triphosphate; *CaM*, calmodulin; *CRAC*, calcium release-activated Ca2; *DAG*, diacylglycerol; *IP_3*, inositol 1,4,5-trisphosphate; *K_V channels*, voltage gated-potassium channel; *MLC*, myosin light chain; *MLCK*, myosin light chain kinase; *PIP2*, phosphatidylinositol bisphosphate; *PLC*, phospholipase C; *ROCC*, receptor-operated Ca^{2+} channels; *ROS*, reactive oxygen species; *RyR*, ryanodine receptors; *SR*, sarcoplasmic reticulum; *VDCC*, voltage-dependent Ca^{2+} channels. (From Smith KA, Schumacker PT. Sensors and signals: the role of reactive oxygen species in hypoxic pulmonary vasoconstriction. *J Physiol*. 2019;597(4):1033–1043.)

reticulum (SR). Together, the elevation of intracellular Ca^{2+} concentrations induces calcium binding to calmodulin, subsequent activation of myosin light chain (MLC) kinase, myosin phosphorylation, and ultimately contractions of VSMCs.

After activation of Rho kinase and MLC phosphatase, myofibrillar proteins become more sensitized to the effects of calcium sensitization, resulting in sustained contractions of pulmonary VSMCs. Besides acting directly on calcium channels, ROSs influence the cytoplasmic redox state, namely, the ratio of oxidized to reduced proteins, glutathione (GSSG/GSH), and nicotinamide adenine dinucleotide (NAD/NADH). According to the redox hypothesis, hypoxic conditions are associated with lesser release of ROSs from the mitochondria that promotes a shift from an oxidized to reduced cellular redox state in the cytoplasm, which in turn triggers Ca^{2+} mobilization through inhibition of Kv channels and opening of VGCCs.

When exposed to hypoxia, both pulmonary and systemic VSMCs share the same effector mechanisms of calcium-mediated changes in vascular tone, whereas pulmonary VSMCs present the unique property to detect low levels of O_2 tension and transmit signals to mobilize Ca^{2+} close to myofibrillar proteins. Mitochondria are located closer to the plasmalemmal membrane in pulmonary VSMCs compared with systemic VSMCs.[18] Therefore a greater structural and functional coupling between mitochondria and Kv channels in pulmonary VSMCs could explain the specific O_2 sensitivity and HPV response.

Neurohumoral Modulation of Hypoxic Pulmonary Vasoconstriction

Exposures to intermittent or chronic hypoxia (e.g., pulmonary diseases, altitude) represent stressful challenges that, by stimulating the sympathetic nervous and renin-angiotensin-aldosterone systems (SNS and RAAS), result in elevation of systemic and pulmonary arterial pressures (PAPs).

Airways and pulmonary vessels are innervated by autonomic and sensory nerve fibers, the highest density of noradrenergic and cholinergic neural endings being found around extrapulmonary and hilar arteries and decreasing toward the periphery (artery size > 60–80 mcm).[19] The vagal nerve of the parasympathetic pathway originates from the nucleus ambiguus in the brain stem, whereas sympathetic nerves emerge from the middle and inferior cervical and the first five thoracic ganglia. **Vagal stimulation** causes mild vasorelaxation mediated by the endothelial release of NO and the vasoactive intestinal factor (VIP). **Stimulation of the sympathetic nervous system** produces the release of norepinephrine (NE) from sympathetic neural endings close to the arterial wall and of epinephrine from the adrenal medulla in the blood stream. **Stimulation of alpha-1–adrenergic-receptors** (AAR-1) with NE causes vasoconstriction, owing to the inhibition of adenylate cyclase and the combined activation of Gq/11-proteins and PLC, that produce IP3 and DAG, which in turn enhance the internal/external release of Ca^{2+}. In contrast, epinephrine causes potent vasodilatory effects by stimulation of beta-1 and beta-2 adrenergic receptors (BAR-1 and BAR-2) and consequent activation of the cAMP-dependent protein kinase pathway and the release of NO from ECs. Under normoxic and unstressed physiologic conditions, the sympathovagal systems play a negligible role in pulmonary vasomotor tone because PVR remains largely unchanged in animals subjected to a chemical, pharmacologic, or anesthetic sympathectomy. However, under hypoxic conditions, pulmonary BAR-mediated vasodilatation has been shown to predominate over AAR-1 vasoconstriction, partially blunting the potent acute HPV.[20] For instance, in patients with sleep apnea, BAR-mediated relaxation of pulmonary arteries offsets the HPV, mitigates the elevation of PVR which in turn alleviates the workload of the right ventricle. Lending support to these clinical findings, experimental data have demonstrated that the HPV response is attenuated with alpha-adrenergic blockers and enhanced with beta-adrenergic blockers.[21]

Hypoxic challenge has been shown to increase the activity of renal adrenergic receptors (AAR-1 and BAR-1) in juxtaglomerular cells, resulting in increased renin secretion and release of angiotensin II (Ang II) by the action of an angiotensin converting enzyme (ACE) largely present in the endothelium of pulmonary capillaries and in other tissues (e.g., brain, heart). In VSMCs, Ang II exerts dual effects on angiotensin receptors type 1 and 2 (AT-1 and AT-2): (1) vasoconstriction mediated by stimulation of the G-protein of AT-1, leading to Ca^{2+} mobilization, owing to activation of PLC and subsequent formation of IP3 and DAG; and (2) vasodilation mediated by stimulation of AT-2, leading to increased cyclic guanosine monophosphate (cGMP) and subsequent release of NO.[22] The attenuation of HPV in patients chronically treated with ACE inhibitors suggests the predominant constrictive effect of Ang II.[23]

Altogether, there is strong evidence supporting that hypoxia-induced stimulation of the SNS and RAAS results in systemic cardiovascular and renal changes (e.g., tachycardia, hypertension, oliguria), a blunted HPV response, owing to the predominant pulmonary BAR-2 vasodilatory effects, which partially offset the constricting effects on AAR-1 and AT-1 receptors.[24] Interestingly, a preserved HPV response has been reported in patients after bilateral lung transplantation, despite the loss of the autonomic neural innervation.[25]

Modulation of Hypoxic Pulmonary Vasoconstriction by the Endothelium

Depending on experimental settings, denuding the endothelium from the pulmonary arteries may result in either suppression or enhancement of the HPV response, and the reasons for these opposing effects still remain unclear.[26] Nevertheless, by sensing low O_2 tension and releasing active vasodilatory and vasoconstrictor compounds, ECs contribute to regulate vascular tone.

Real-time fluorescence imaging in intact lungs demonstrated that hypoxia induces membrane depolarization in capillary ECs that propagates retrogradely to the feeding arterioles via gap junctions and connexin proteins (C×40).

In parallel to this endothelial signal, a similar response is propagated upstream through precapillary VSMCs via other connexin proteins (Cx43).[27] A growing body of evidence indicates that the release of endothelial vasoactive compounds enhances the second phase of acute HPV, owing to decreased NO levels, increased ET-1 and EETs production, whereas the increased PG12-mediated relaxation is offset by the enhanced TXA2-mediated constriction of VSMCs.

During prolonged hypoxia, proliferation of ECs is associated with the release of mitogenic factors for VSMCs, and generation of ET-1 dose-dependently mediates the overexpression of Kv and transient receptor potential channels, thereby contributing to the development of pulmonary hypertension (PH).[28]

Physiologic Variations in Hypoxic Pulmonary Vasoconstriction Responses

In healthy individuals breathing air at sea level, pulmonary vessels are almost fully dilated, and inhalation of NO—a selective pulmonary vasodilator—does not improve oxygenation, suggesting that the HPV response is nonactivated under normoxic conditions.

Pulmonary Circulation

Compared with the systemic circulation, pulmonary vessels offer greater distensibility and recruitability to accommodate higher blood flow and volemia while blunting the elevation in pulmonary blood pressure. In contrast with the systemic circulation, the pressure-flow relationship in the pulmonary circulation is not linear because of the greater distensibility and potential recruitability of its vasculature. Therefore the pulmonary circulation may adapt to changing blood flow conditions, while minimizing the changes in PAP.[29] For instance, a reduction in CO (e.g., head-up position, blood loss) leads to a larger drop in pulmonary vascular driving pressure, even though the vasomotor tone remains per se unchanged.[30] Conversely, as pressure along the entire circuit increases, the pressure-flow curve becomes more linear because the fully distended vessels are by definition no longer distensible. Hence, when left atrial pressure increases with fluid loading or head-down position, the ability of hypoxic constriction to either redirect blood flow or reduce conductance is curtailed.

Lung volume also influences PVR, as described by a parabolic U-shaped curve. The PVR reaches a nadir at the functional residual capacity (FRC), and it increases at higher inflating pressures as alveolar capillaries are "squeezed" by elevated alveolar pressures, or when breathing operates below the FRC, as the extraalveolar vessels become distorted and partially obstructed, offering greater resistance to blood flow. Complete lung collapse, as occurs during OLV in thoracic surgery, results in mechanical vascular obstruction that contributes to blood flow diversion to the ventilated dependent lung.

Besides the P_AO_2 level, the strength of HPV also depends on the basal vascular tone and the volume of the lung exposed to hypoxia. A more potent HPV response is elicited when PVR is low (near FRC), and it decreases when the lung is overdistended or totally collapsed. From animal studies, we know that if exposure to hypoxia exceeds 40% of the whole lung, the redistribution of blood flow to nonhypoxic pulmonary areas is decreased, suggesting that the increased PAP tends to overcome the increased local arteriolar resistance generated by HPV.[31]

Physical Factors: Calcium, CO_2, pH, Temperature

Pulmonary arteries are minimally sensitive to changes in plasma calcium concentrations.[32] In the isolated blood perfused canine lung, severe hypocalcemia is required to induce vasodilation and fails to influence the HPV response. Conversely, acute hypercalcemia fails to modify the pressure-flow curves and PVR, suggesting that calcium chloride can be safely administered intraoperatively through a right-sided venous catheter.

With the development of whole body hypothermia (from 37°C –27°C), both systemic and PVR are increased mainly as a result of cardiac depression, lower CO, and enhanced vasomotor tone,[33] whereas the HPV decreases linearly with the drop in central temperature.[34] Blunting of HPV is also observed with hypocapnia and metabolic alkalosis. Conversely, hypercapnia has been associated with decreased exhaled NO and enhanced HPV response in isolated ventilated-perfused lungs.[35]

Senescence

With aging, oxidative stress and proinflammatory processes are the culprit mechanisms involved in atherogenesis, thickening and stiffening of systemic arteries that manifest clinically by hypertension, coronary artery disease, and heart failure. Likewise, the low pressure pulmonary circulation presents age-related reductions in arterial and venous distensibility, along with decreased left ventricle compliance leading to increased PAP. The reduction in antioxidant capacity with increased oxidative stress is incriminated in endothelial dysfunction and vascular extramatrix deposition of collagen.[36] Accordingly, PAP increases disproportionately more during exercise in older than in younger healthy humans, given lesser vasodilating mediators released from the ECs, stiffening of the vascular wall, and left ventricular diastolic dysfunction. In the elderly, the lesser increase in CO is associated with higher O_2 extraction in skeletal muscles, together with a greater fall in P_{mvO2} that may act as a stimulus for enhanced HPV and further elevation in PAP during intense aerobic exercise.

Middle-aged subjects exposed to moderate alveolar hypoxia (P_AO_2 ~50 mm Hg) over 20 minutes exhibit a greater increase in mean systolic PAP compared with younger individuals (+9 mm Hg) and similar changes in heart rate and in CO. These age-related enhanced HPV responses could be explained by the greater sensitivity of the O_2 sensing apparatus, greater propensity for Ca^{2+} cell entry, and greater activity of the calcium-calmodulin-dependent MLC kinase that contribute to sustained contractile response of pulmonary VSMCs.[37]

Altitude

In contrast with regional HPV acting in case of atelectasis or pneumonia, generalized HPV in response to hypobaric hypoxia causes various degrees of PH that may be associated with interstitial and alveolar edema in susceptible patients.[38] The so-called "high-altitude pulmonary edema" (HAPE) occurs in nonacclimatized healthy individuals within 1 to 5 days after arrival at altitudes higher than 2500 m but also in well-acclimatized high-landers returning from low altitudes.[39] Lung imaging in symptomatic HAPE shows a patchy peripheral and nodular distribution of edema, whereas bronchoalveolar lavage reveals a protein-rich exudate with mild hemorrhage, neutrophilia, and proinflammatory cytokines consistent with the heterogeneous distribution of HPV and the involvement of inflammation secondary to alveolar-capillary barrier disruption. In addition, the alveolar fluid clearance mechanisms are impaired by hypoxia, owing to the reduced expression and activity of epithelial sodium channels and sodium/potassium (Na^+/K^+) ATPase proteins linked to (BAR-2) signaling.

Genetics

Epidemiologic studies have shown an association between early hypoxic exposure and later development of hyperreactivity in pulmonary vascular response.[40] For instance, transient perinatal hypoxia was found to predispose to exaggerated HPV when low-altitude dwellers were exposed to acute hypobaric hypoxic conditions. Likewise, the occurrence of preeclampsia in Bolivian high-altitude dwellers was shown to predispose their offspring to greater sensitivity of HPV response, owing to augmented oxidative stress and impaired NO bioavailability.

Different adaptive phenotypes have been identified in populations living in high altitudes. Compared with Han Chinese low-landers, Tibetans high-landers show hyporesponsiveness of the HIF transcriptional system characterized by a blunted HPV response associated with high exhaled NO concentrations, few hypertrophic changes in pulmonary arteries, and minimal increase in Hb concentrations.[41] Andean highlanders exhibit other physiologic characteristics, namely, a blunted hypoxic ventilatory response, polycythemia, larger lung volumes, and better pulmonary diffusion compared with Tibetans. These variable adaptive solutions reflect different evolutionary pathways selected to survive in hypoxic environments.[42]

Variations of Hypoxic Pulmonary Vasoconstriction in Pathologic Conditions

In the clinical settings, the strength of the HPV response can be estimated by comparing physiologic markers under hypoxic versus normoxic/hyperoxic conditions: (1) the ratio of PAP under constant flow conditions, (2) the changes in PaO_2, (3) measurements or calculation of intrapulmonary shunt (Q_S/Q_T), and (4) the dispersion of the V/Q ratio before/after the administration of drugs affecting the HPV.

The multiple inert gas elimination technique (MIGET) uses the relationships between arterial, expired, and mixed venous concentrations of trace amounts of six marker gases dissolved in saline and infused intravenously.[43] The distribution of ventilation and perfusion is expressed as a function of V_A/Q ratio and provides an index of overall V_A/Q mismatch as characterized by the standard deviation of the distributions of ventilation and perfusion (LogSD Q and LogSD V). According to Riley and Cournand, the bell curve of V/Q scatter originally supported the theory of the three-lung units: one unit with ideal gas exchange (V/Q ratios close to 0.8–1), one consisting of true shunt (V/Q < 0.005), and one of "dead space ventilation" (V/Q > 100).[44] Currently, the MIGET model includes 50 units, each with a predefined V/Q ratio, and it provides a conceptually practical approach to understand the changes in pulmonary gas exchange, taking also into account participation of very low V/Q units in "venous admixture."

Chronic Lung Diseases

In chronic lung diseases (e.g., COPD, interstitial fibrosis, cystic fibrosis, bronchiectasis), hypoxic stress is known to induce pulmonary vascular cell proliferation (fibroblasts, VSMCs) and vascular remodeling (cellular hypertrophia, differentiation of fibroblast into myoblasts, extracellular deposits of collagen and elastin), resulting in eccentric wall thickening and the development of PH (~10% of COPD patients). The contribution of HPV to PH is greatest in the early disease stages of PH, when O_2 therapy alleviates the hypoxia-induced vasoconstriction, whereas at later stages, PH is resistant O_2 therapy because of structural "fixed" vascular remodeling.

The severity of airflow obstruction in COPD patients does not correlate with hypoxemia, which is largely determined by the heterogeneity of V/Q distribution (shunt and low V/Q units). In COPD patients, Melot et al.[45] demonstrated that almitrine besylate was associated with increased PaO_2 (+13%) and reduced V/Q inequalities, whereas nifedipine, a Ca^{2+} channel blocker, resulted in lower PaO_2 (−15%) by inhibition of HPV and consequent blood flow shifting from normal V/Q to low V/Q alveolar units.

Distinct phenotypes have been identified with regards to HPV that are linked to the expression of a regulatory subunit of NADPH oxidase (p22phox) in EC and in pulmonary VSMs.[46] In a small cohort of 71 patients with end-stage COPD, a positive correlation was found between the vascular expression of a regulatory subunit of NADPH oxidase (p22phox), mean pulmonary artery pressure, and the oxygenation index (PaO_2/FiO2 ratio).[47] These findings suggest distinct phenotypes: the low expression of p22phox was associated with diminished HPV and low PAP. In contrast, higher expression of p22phox was associated with preserved HPV that allowed better V/Q matching but at the cost of PH and later cor pulmonale.

Asthma

Studies using MIGET and positron emission tomographic/computed tomographic lung imaging in patients with asthma have shown that the uneven distribution of bronchoconstriction was paralleled by heterogeneous regional hypoxia and V/Q mismatch with consequent hypoxemia.[48] During methacholine-induced bronchoconstriction in patients breathing room air, blood flow was reduced by almost 30% in hypoventilating areas and increased by 10% in normal-/high-ventilated areas. In the same patients, breathing 80% O_2 was found to attenuate the averaged blood flow redistribution by 50%. Given the efficacy of HPV, blood flow was shifted from hypoxic low V/Q areas to normal and high V/Q areas. In addition, blood flow was also redistributed from nonhypoxic lung regions (low V/Q areas) as a result of mechanical and biologic interactions between the constricted airways, pulmonary vessels, and lung parenchyma.

Obstructive Sleep Apnea

In the absence of chronic cardiopulmonary diseases, about 30% of patients with obstructive sleep apnea (OSA) present PH.[49] Although presenting normal O_2 saturation while awake, these patients experience repeated short-lasting episodes of desaturation during sleep, often associated with arousals. The cumulative effects of these intermittent hypoxic/hypercapnic challenges result in activation of the SNS, polycythemia, and vascular remodeling in both systemic and pulmonary arteries. The mechanisms of PH are caused by an increased left ventricular preload (postcapillary PH), a sustained HPV response, and vascular changes characterized by proliferation of VSMCs and asymmetric neointimal hyperplasia (precapillary PH). Repeated short-lasting hypoxic episodes augment the pulmonary vasoconstrictor reactivity by triggering endothelial release of vasoconstrictor mediators (e.g., ET-1), as well as mitochondrial formation of ROSs with myofibrillar Ca^{2+} sensitization dependent on the protein kinase C-beta in VSMCs.

Acute Respiratory Distress Syndrome (ARDS)

Early or delayed forms of acute lung injury (ALI) or ARDS occur in 2% to 5% of patients after thoracic surgery and largely contribute to postoperative mortality.[50] The early form that develops within 3 days after surgery is mainly related to ventilator-induced lung injury (VILI) and preexisting morbidity factors, whereas the delayed form is linked to postoperative complications, such as sepsis (e.g., pneumonia, empyema) or massive transfusion. Excessive perioperative fluid overload represents an independent risk factor in both forms.[51]

Mild to moderate PH with variable degrees of right ventricular dysfunction is seen in the majority of these patients with ARDS. It correlates with the impairment in oxygenation (worsen PaO_2/FiO_2 ratio) and represents an independent risk factor of mortality.

The development of PH is linked to three main mechanisms[52]: (1) a disruption of the pulmonary capillary-alveolar barrier that is characterized by intercellular endothelial gaps, the release of tissue factor, and proinflammatory mediators causing interstitial and alveolar edema; (2) early mechanical obstruction of blood flow by formation of microthrombi, owing to enhanced procoagulant and antifibrinolytic activities; (3) the HPV response depending on the extent and distribution of a V/Q mismatch; and (4) delayed mechanical obstruction of blood vessels, owing to fibrocellular proliferation into the walls of pulmonary arteries, veins, and lymphatics.

In an experimental murine model of sepsis, the HPV response was attenuated by more than 50% compared with controls, and it was attributed to the enhanced activity of ATP-sensitive K^+ channels with a consequent increase in potassium efflux and decreased Ca^{2+} mobilization, whereas Kv channels and prostaglandin pathways were unaffected.[53] In sepsis, the generalized vasoplegia and poor responsiveness to vasopressors have been associated with the activation of the NF-κB and NO-dependent pathways, as well as the overexpression of K_{ATP}-channels in aortic, cerebral, coronary, mesenteric, and pulmonary VSMCs. The administration of 100% O_2 has been shown to decrease PAP by 10% to 15% in ARDS patients, and such treatment enables clinicians to unmask the importance of HPV in poorly ventilated units, not in those completely collapsed. In patients with severe ARDS ventilated with 100% O_2 and supported with extracorporeal membrane oxygenation, Benzing et al. observed a 29% reduction in PVR as PO_2mv increased from 46 to 84 mm Hg, clearly demonstrating the contribution of nonventilated units to HPV.[54] Interestingly, administration of inhaled vasodilators (NO or PGI_2) in some ARDS patients has also been shown to increase PaO_2 by redistributing blood flow to lung regions with the highest V/Q ratios, reducing, in turn, PAP and intrapulmonary shunts.[55]

Effects of Anesthesia and Mechanical Ventilation in Gas Exchange

Lung Perfusion (see Chapter 6)

Blood flow is not uniformly distributed across the lungs because the transmural vascular pressures are generated by variable opposing forces (Fig. 15.5): (1) intravascular pressures (pulmonary arterial and venous pressures [P_{pa} and P_{pv}], respectively), which are dependent on right ventricular pressure output, left ventricular preload, and gravitational forces varying with the distance from the middle part of the heart (baseline level or P = 0, P_{pa} increases by 1 mm Hg per cm of vertical distance) to the top and lower parts of the lung; (2) extravascular compressive forces represented by the alveolar pressure (P_{Alv}), the interstitial pressure (P_{Is}), and the weight of mediastinal and abdominal organs. Based on the interplay between these intra- and extravascular pressures, a lung

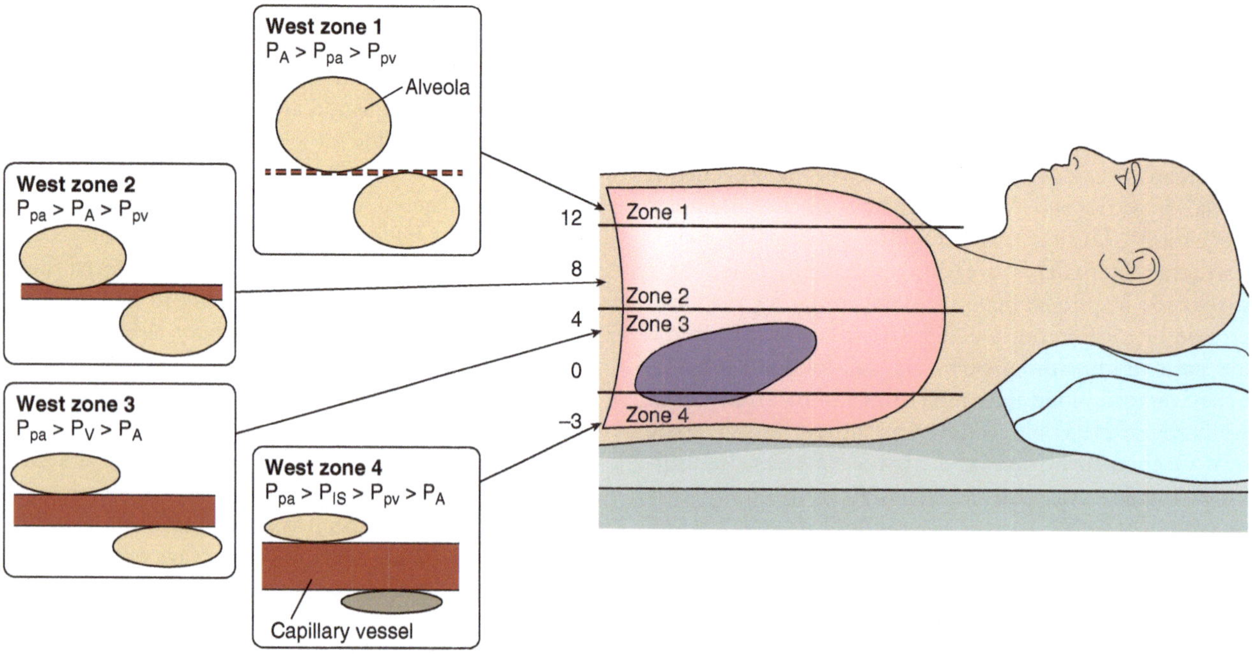

• **Fig. 15.5** Distribution of pulmonary blood flow in four zones depending on pulmonary artery pressure (P_{pa}), pulmonary venous pressure (P_{pv}), alveolar pressure (P_A), and interstitial pressure (P_{IS}) in a patient in supine position.

model with four distinct perfusion areas, called the West zones, has been described. In supine position, **zone 1** is located in the most ventral/upper lung areas and represents "dead-space," capillaries are nonperfused as P_A exceeds both P_{pa} and P_{pv}. When moving toward the middle lung areas, **zone 2** is characterized by increases in P_{pa} and P_{pv}, owing to gravitational forces, while P_A remains constant, capillary blood flow is therefore determined by the $P_{pa} - P_A$ gradient. In **zone 3**, further increases in gravitational forces result in blood flow being solely determined by the $P_{pa} - P_{pv}$ gradient, with no influence of PA. In **zone 4**, the extravascular compressive forces associated with interstitial lung edema result in a blood flow pattern, which is driven by the $P_{pa} - P_{Is}$ gradient.

Depending on patient positioning, fluid loading, cardiac function, and ventilatory mode, lung areas can move through different perfusion zones. For instance, with the initiation of mechanical ventilation (with high P_A), parts of zone 2 are converted in zone 1, particularly during the inspiratory phase and vice-versa following extubation and resumption of spontaneous ventilation with negative inspiratory pressure.

Lung Volume Ventilation

Following anesthesia induction in adults in supine position, the FRC decreases by 0.5 to 1.0 L as a result of a lower respiratory muscular tone, unopposed lung elastic recoil forces, and the weight of abdominal and mediastinal organs moving the diaphragm upwards (Fig. 15.6). The reduction in FRC is largely independent of the type of anesthetic agents or the use of neuromuscular blocking agents, but it is aggravated by pregnancy, morbid obesity, head-down position, and abdominal distension.

As the FRC approaches the closing capacity (CC) of the lungs, small airways progressively close in the most dependent parts of the lungs—over the whole respiratory cycle or during expiration—causing total or partial alveolar collapse. The "compression" atelectasis are formed within minutes after anesthesia induction, whereas "resorption" atelectasis arise more slowly in regions with a low V/Q ratio, particularly if an alveoli contains high inspired O_2 concentrations. During uneventful anesthesia, both partially/total collapsed alveola with venous admixture may extend up to 25% of lung volume.

The dead space of the respiratory system (V_D), which is the volume of gas that does not participate in O_2 and CO_2 exchange, tends to augment in anesthetized mechanically ventilated patients because of the addition of tubing from the ventilator, and overdistension of nondependent areas creating a greater V/Q mismatch.[56] Changes in physiologic dead space (V_{DPhys}) are assessed by volumetric capnography and application of the Enghoff's equation (Fig. 15.7):

$V_{DPhys}/V_T = (PaCO_2 - P_ECO_2)/PaCO_2$, where $PaCO_2$ = arterial C partial pressure; P_ECO_2 = mean expiratory CO_2 pressure.

Conversely, the efficiency of ventilation is better reflected by alveolar ventilation ($V_{Alv} = V_T - V_{DPhysiol}$), which is representative of the portion of a V_T that participates in gas exchange.

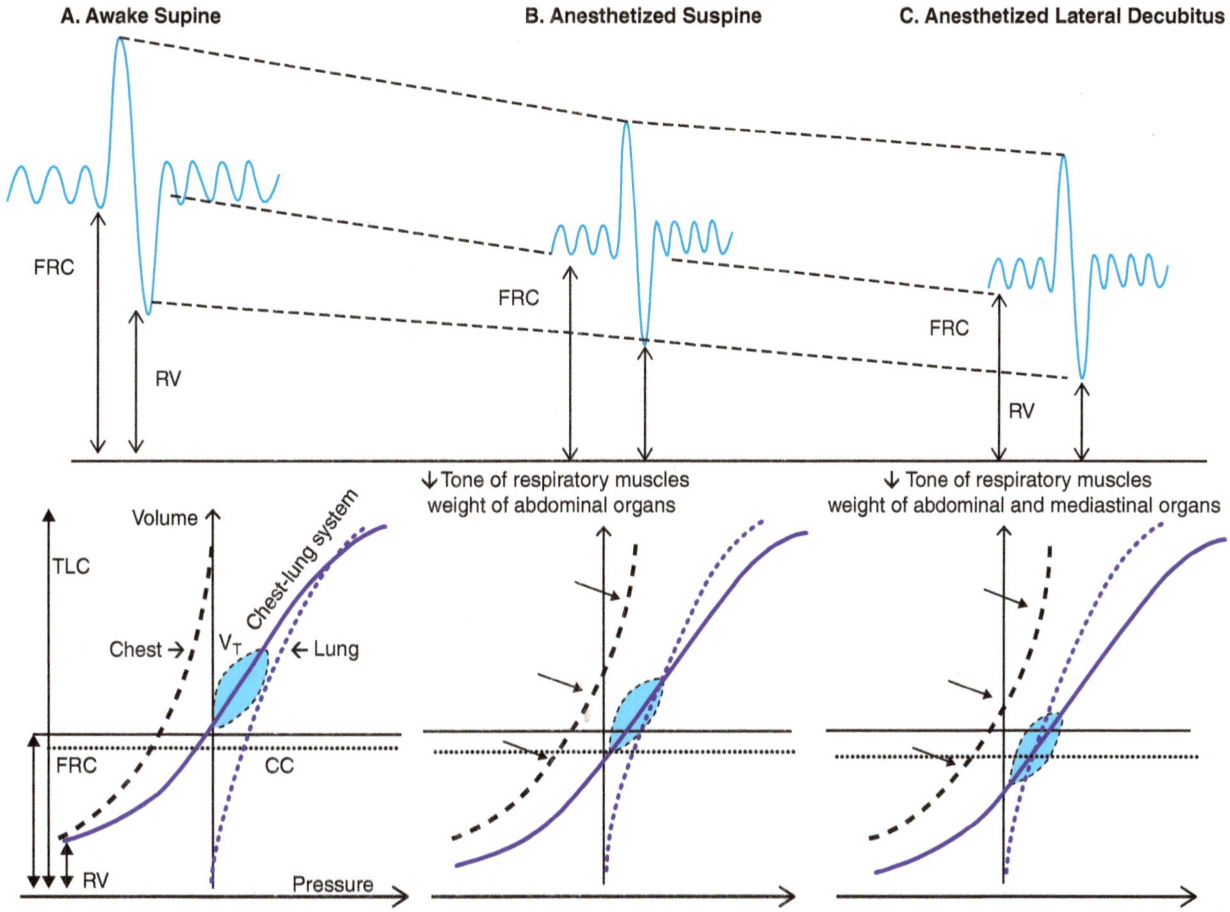

• **Fig. 15.6** Perioperative changes in pulmonary volumes. *CC*, Closing capacity; *FRC*, functional residual capacity; *RV*, residual volume; *VT*, tidal volume; *TLC*, total lung capacity.

Integrated Ventilatory and Perfusion Changes

Better understanding of pulmonary gas exchange has emerged from a comprehensive analysis of the distribution of V/Q ratios using MIGET, visualization of blood flow and gas movement by lung imaging (e.g., computed tomography, magnetic resonance, electrical impedance tomography), measurements of intrapulmonary shunt by thermodilution techniques (Q_S/Q_T ratio), and calculation of the $P_{A\text{-}a}O_2$ gradient, as well as dead space ventilation (V_D) by gas tonometry and volumetric capnometry.

In the multicompartment lung model, O_2 tension in each lung unit depends on a specific V/Q ratio (Fig. 15.8). As the strongest pulmonary vasoconstrictive effect occurs at a P_AO_2 around 65 to 70 mm Hg and given the slope of the Hb-O_2 dissociation curve, the effectiveness of HPV is greatest in lung units with a moderately reduced V/Q ratio (~0.4).[57] In contrast, the low P_AO_2 in collapsed lung areas produces a weaker stimulus, although the low $P_{mv}O_2$ values could partly compensate and activate the HPV response.

In spontaneously breathing volunteers, Nyren et al. using single photon emission computed tomography showed that sevoflurane anesthesia at 1 minimal alveolar concentration (MAC) resulted in similar ventral-to-dorsal distribution of ventilation with greater heterogeneity of V/Q ratios and a trend toward smaller median V/Q ratios compared with awake conditions.[58] Likewise, under mechanical positive pressure ventilation, there is a wider dispersion of V/Q ratios compared with spontaneous

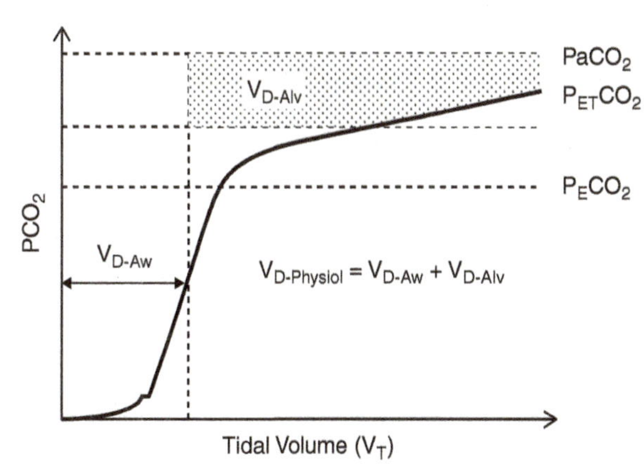

• **Fig. 15.7** Calculation of dead space volume (V_D) according to Enghoff's equation. *$PaCO_2$*, Arterial CO_2 pressure; *$P_{ET}CO_2$*, end-tidal CO_2 pressure; *P_ECO_2*, mean expiratory CO_2 pressure; *$V_{D\text{-}Aw}$*, airway (anatomic) dead space; *$V_{D\text{-}Alv}$*, alveolar dead space; *$V_{D\text{-}Phys}$*, physiologic dead space.

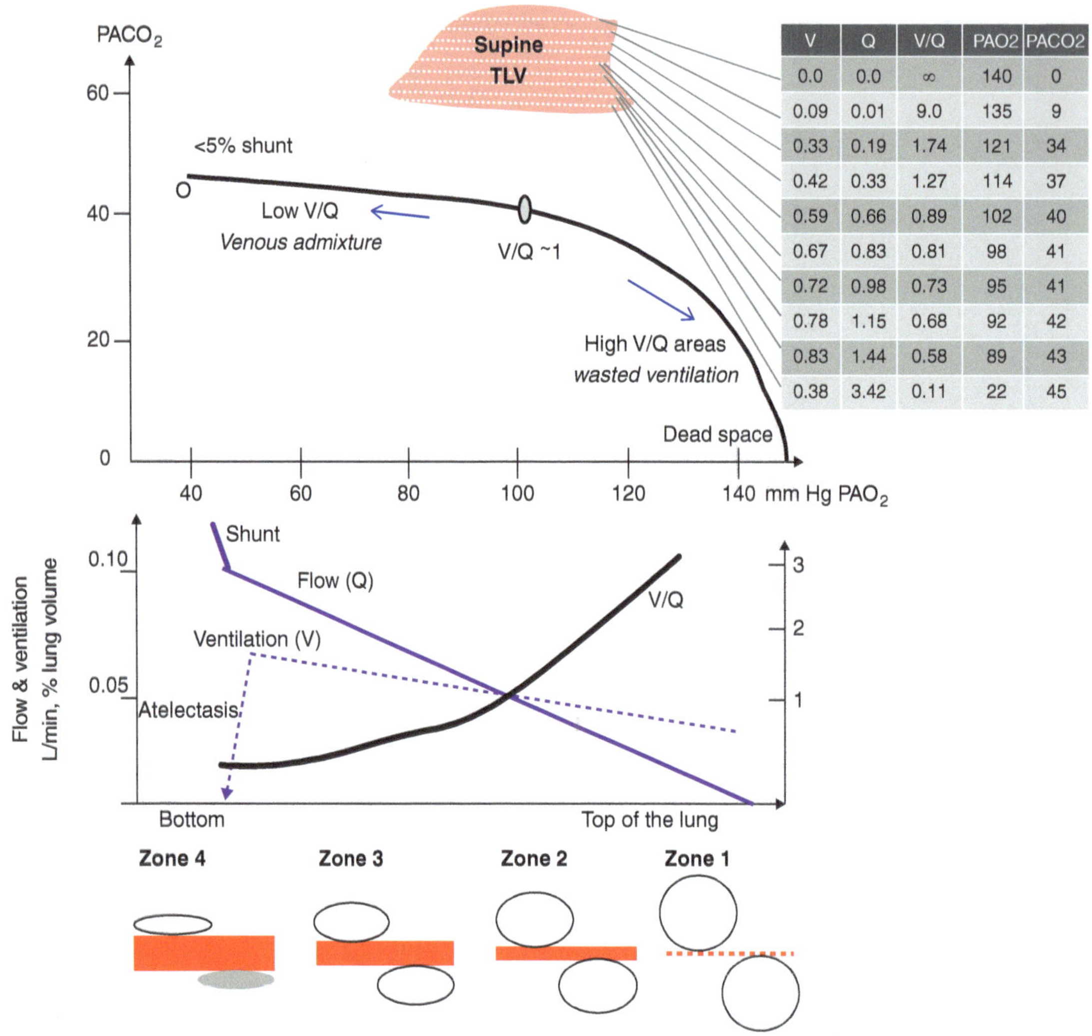

V	Q	V/Q	PAO2	PACO2
0.0	0.0	∞	140	0
0.09	0.01	9.0	135	9
0.33	0.19	1.74	121	34
0.42	0.33	1.27	114	37
0.59	0.66	0.89	102	40
0.67	0.83	0.81	98	41
0.72	0.98	0.73	95	41
0.78	1.15	0.68	92	42
0.83	1.44	0.58	89	43
0.38	3.42	0.11	22	45

• **Fig. 15.8** Distribution of blood flow (*Q*) and ventilation (*V*), V/Q ratio and alveolar partial pressure of oxygen (*PAO2*) and carbon dioxide (*PACO2*) through the lung in supine position. *TLV*, Two-lung ventilation.

breathing, with preferential distribution of ventilation toward ventral lung regions, whereas gravitational forces tend to direct blood flow in dorsal regions, except in the lowermost regions, where perfusion decreases because of interstitial compressive forces.[59]

After initiating anesthesia with mechanical ventilation, as FRC declines toward the lung CC, cyclic (or permanent) closure of small airways occurs in the dependent parts of the lungs, resulting in low V/Q areas and greater heterogeneity in V/Q distribution with increasing shear stress in lung tissue that are incriminated in VILI. During prolonged mechanical ventilation, such repetitive "cyclic" alveolar openings have been shown to generate an inflammatory response with the activation of neutrophils, the release of cytokines, ROSs, and procoagulant factors, as well as impaired surfactant formation.[60] These VILI result in variable degrees of postoperative restrictive pulmonary syndrome associated with increased work of breathing, paving the way for the development of atelectasis and pneūmonia, particularly in high-risk patients.

Ventilation modalities using oxygen-nitrogen mixture (FiO_2 < 80%) and positive end-expiratory pressure (PEEP) with recruitment maneuvers have been shown to minimize the importance of atelectasis and to improve respiratory compliance and blood oxygenation by attenuating the loss in FRC and optimizing V/Q ratios.[61] The extent of atelectasis and low V/Q lung areas have been shown to correlate with intrapulmonary shunt and impaired pulmonary oxygen uptake, both in healthy and diseased lungs, as reflected by an increased $P_{A\text{-}a}O_2$ gradient and low PaO_2.[62] Noteworthy, under normoxic or mild hypoxic conditions, the heterogeneity of pulmonary blood flow is likely not sufficient to stimulate the HPV response in patients with healthy lungs.[63]

One-Lung Ventilation in Thoracic Surgery and Gas Exchange

The effectiveness of blood oxygenation is largely determined by the homogeneous distribution of V/Q and the integrity of the alveolar-capillary layer (surface area, interstitial fluid, inflammation).

Switching from two-lung ventilation to OLV always causes a reduction in PaO_2 (–30% to 50%), owing to the

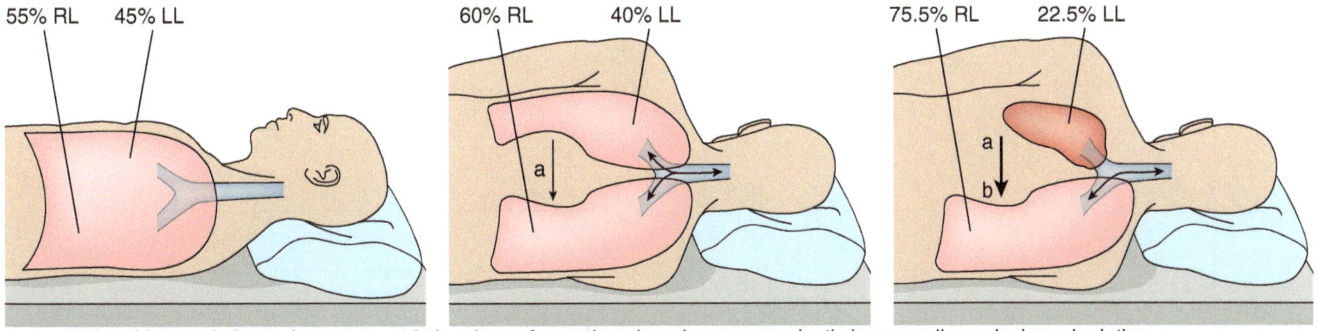

a, gravitational forces; b, hypoxic vasoconstriction, loss of negative pleural pressure, elastic lung recoil, surgical manipulation

A

Supine position, closed chest		
Two-LV	Shunt	No-shunt
	% blood flow	
Left lung	2.5	42.5
Right lung	2.5	55.5

B

Right lateral, closed chest		
Two-LV	Shunt	No-shunt
	% blood flow	
Left lung	1	39
Right lung	4	56

C

Right lateral, open chest		
Two-LV	Shunt	No-shunt
	% blood flow	
Left lung	20	0
Right lung	<5	75

• **Fig. 15.9** Changes in shunted and nonshunted pulmonary blood flow, in supine position (**A**), right lateral decubitus (**B**), and one-lung ventilation (**C**). *a*, Gravitational forces; *b*, hypoxic vasoconstriction, loss of negative pleural pressure, elastic lung recoil, surgical manipulation. *LL*, left lung; *RL*, right lung; *Two-LV*, two lung ventilation.

reduced surface area available for gas diffusion and a variable degree of intrapulmonary shunting mainly through the nondependent lung.[2] Because of the sigmoid shape of the O_2-Hb dissociation curve, significant oxygen desaturation (<90%) only occurs in a minority of patients if the PaO_2 decreases below 7.5 to 8.5 kPa.

Patient position, surgical manipulations, and the HPV response all contribute to improve blood oxygenation as a result of better V/Q matching and reduced shunting through the operated lung (Fig. 15.9).[1,64] As a reminder, the most common cause of intraoperative hypoxemia is related to incorrect placement of the double-lumen tube (DLT) or bronchial blockers (BB).

Body Position

In supine position, CO is distributed through the lungs in proportion to their respective sizes, the left receiving approximately 45% and the right 55% of the total CO. When moving the patient from supine to lateral position, the distribution of blood flow, as well as venous and capillary blood volumes, are partially shifted from the nondependent to the dependent lung.[65] The dependent lung receives a larger proportion of CO (+5%) because the gravitational forces generate a vertical pressure gradient through the pulmonary circulation, PAP (and venous pressure) decreasing by 10 to 20 mm Hg from the bottom of the dependent lung to the top of the nondependent lung. Similar to perfusion, gravitational forces also affect the distribution of ventilation: the pleural pressure decreases by 0.25 cm H_2O per cm from the lower to upper pulmonary areas, the largest part of the V_T being delivered to the middle areas of the lung. This physiologic concept supports the clinical practice of positioning critically ill patients with unilateral hypoxemic pulmonary diseases with the "good lung down" to promote V/Q matching.

Chest Opening, Lung Exclusion, and One-Lung Ventilation

At the start of surgery, the operated (nondependent) lung is "excluded" from the ventilatory circuit, and the inspiratory pressure (P_{Insp}) is only delivered to the dependent lung. The weight of the mediastinal and abdominal organs on the dependent hemithorax causes a higher pleural pressure and in turn a further reduction in FRC; therefore, a higher P_{Insp} is required to deliver the V_T (compared with the supine position), the driving pressure remaining unchanged ($\Delta P = P_{Insp} - P_{Pleural}$).

Within 10 to 20 minutes after chest opening, the nonventilated lung spontaneously tends to collapse as a result of the elastic lung recoil forces and the loss of negative pleural pressure. Additional measures may accelerate lung deflation, namely: (1) mechanical ventilation with 100% O_2 before lung exclusion to enhance resorption atelectasis; (2) transient ventilator disconnection (1–2 minutes) with balloon deflation to facilitate alveolar gas clearance; and (3) external lung compression by the surgeon.

After lung exclusion in lateral position, perfusion of the dependent lung is increased by activation of the HPV response in the nonventilated "hypoxic" lung, whereas mechanical vascular closure that parallels the collapse of bronchoalveolar tissues plays a minor role.[66] These mechanisms minimize shunting (Q_S/Q_T) and venous admixture in the operated lung (from 40%–50% to 20%–25%) and contribute to redirect pulmonary blood flow to the ventilated dependent lung.[67] The distensibility and recruitability of pulmonary vessels in the dependent lung attenuate the

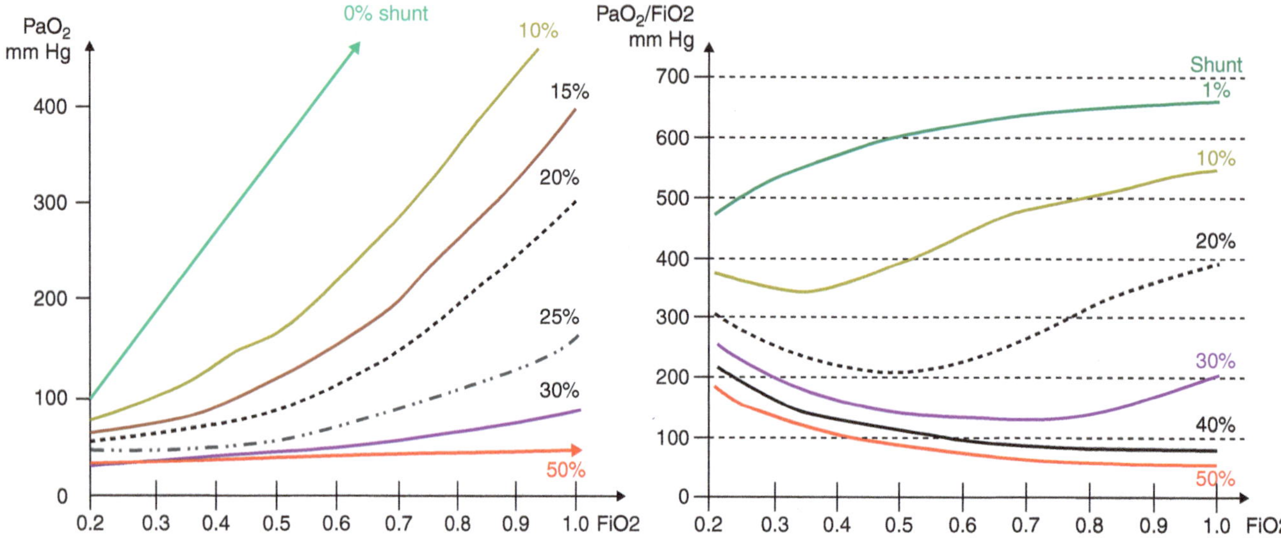

• **Fig. 15.10** Isoshunt diagram describing the relationship between arterial oxygen pressure (*PaO2*) or PaO2/fraction of inspired oxygen (*FiO2*) ratio and FiO2 in the presence of variable pulmonary shunt fraction. (Modified from Feiner JR, Weiskopf RB. Evaluating pulmonary function: an assessment of PaO2/FIO2. *Crit Care Med*. 2017;45(1):e40–e48; and Benatar SR, Hewlett AM, Nunn JF. The use of iso-shunt lines for control of oxygen therapy. *Br J Anaesth*. 1973;45(7):711–718.)

increase in PAP and right ventricular afterload, while providing a larger capillary surface area for gas exchange to mitigate the fall in diffusion capacity. As the increased capillary blood flow tends to match the alveolar ventilation through the dependent lung with increasing V/Q ratios along a vertical bottom-up distance, adequate gas exchange can be ensured during OLV in most cases.

Actually, as long as the intrapulmonary shunt fraction is less than 15% to 20% of the total CO, hypoxemia can be easily corrected by increasing FiO_2, whereas lesser gains in PaO_2 are achieved in the presence of shunt exceeding 20%, as the slope of the PaO_2-FiO_2 curve decreases and flattens when the shunt is over 30% (Fig. 15.10).[68,69] Application of recruitment maneuvers and PEEP titration on the dependent lung are helpful to reopen atelectatic areas, to maintain FRC, to reduce venous admixture, and minimize shear stress and strain by reducing cyclic opening/closing of alveolar tissue.[70] Compared with two-lung ventilation in supine patients, higher external PEEP levels are required to maintain FRC during OLV in lateral position, owing to the compressive extravascular forces and in turn the higher $P_{Pleural}$.[71] These higher PEEP levels have not been associated with increasing shunt (Q_S/Q_T) because of blood flow diversion from the dependent to nondependent lung. Indeed, Spadaro et al. reported that application of PEEP at 10 cm H_2O during OLV with small V_T resulted in lower shunt fraction and driving pressure while improving oxygenation, compared with PEEP at 5 or 0 cm H_2O.[72]

Application of continuous positive airway pressure (CPAP) to the nondependent lung is an effective way to reverse hypoxemia by apneic oxygenation that increase the surface area available for blood gas exchange with a reduction of the HPV response.[73]

Impact of General Anesthetics, Analgesics, and Cardiovascular Drugs (Table 15.1)

In vitro studies[74] using denervated pulmonary arteries and in vivo experiments using isolated perfused lungs strongly support a dose-response inhibition of HPV by volatile anesthetics and few effects of intravenous anesthetics.[74] In studies using intact animal models, the efficacy of HPV varies inversely with CO and is determined by the combined cardio-depressive and vasodilatory effects of volatile anesthetics. The direct inhibition of HPV can partially be offset by the decreased CO causing flow diversion and enhanced vascular responsiveness because of low $P_{mv}O_2$.

In a model of isolated perfused rat lung, the administration of intravenous drugs, such as **ketamine, droperidol, and barbiturates,** failed to alter the HPV response.[75] In chronically instrumented dogs, ketamine was shown to preserve HPV, and propofol was associated with mild potentiation of HPV by inhibition of the pulmonary vasodilatation mediated by K_{ATP} channels.[76]

In thoracic surgery with OLV, **inhalational anesthetics** cause mild-to-moderate inhibition of HPV, whereas intravenous anesthetic drugs result in preserved or even enhanced HPV. A metaanalysis of 23 randomized controlled trials demonstrated that volatile anesthetics compared with intravenous anesthesia was associated with higher intrapulmonary shunt (Q_S/Q_T 33% vs. 27%, mean difference of −5.4%), higher cardiac index (3.2 vs. 2.9 L/min, mean difference of 0.19 L/min), and lower oxygenation index during OLV (PaO_2 with mean difference of −27 mm Hg). These data confirm that volatile anesthetics within the clinical dose range (from 0.5 to 1.5 MAC) slightly impair lung

TABLE 15.1 Impact of Perioperative Drug and Anesthetic Management on Cardiovascular Control and Hypoxic Pulmonary Vasoconstriction

	HR	MAP	SVR	PVR	CO	HPV	Raw
Intravenous anesthetics							
Ketamine	+	+	+	+/0	+	0	-
Etomidate	0	0	0	0	0	0	0
Propofol	0/-	–	–	0	-	0	0
Midazolam	0	0/-	0/-	0	0/-	0	0
Analgesics							
Opiates	0	0	0	0	0	0	0(+)
Dexmedetomidine	-	-	-	0	-	0	0
Nonsteroidal antiinflammatory drugs	0	0	0	0	0	(-/0/+)	0
Volatile anesthetics							
Isoflurane	0/-	–	–	–	–	–	-
Sevoflurane	0/-	-	-	-	-	-	-
Desflurane	0/-	-	-	-	-	-	-
Inotropes, vasopressors, bronchodilators							
Dobutamine, Dopamine	+	+/0/-	0/-	0/-	+	-	0
Phenylephrine	0/-	+	+	+	0/-	0	0
Milrinone							0(-)
Salbutamol	+	+/0/-	+	0/-	+	-	-
Antihypertensive drugs	0/-	–	–	-	0/+	-	
CCB	0/-	–	–	-	0/+	-	0
NTG, NPS	0/+	–	–	-	+	-	0
ACEi, ATA	0	-	-	0/-	+	0/-	0(+)
Beta-blockers	-	-	0/+	0/+	-	0	0/+

0, No change; +, increased; ++, more increased; +++, most increased; -, decreased; *ACEi*, angiotensin-converting enzyme inhibitor; *ATA*, angiotensin II antagonist; *CCB*, calcium-channel blocker; *CO*, cardiac output; *HPV*, hypoxic pulmonary vasoconstriction; *HR*, heart rate; *MAP*, mean arterial pressure; *NPS*, nitroprussiate; *NTG*, nitroglycerine; *PVR*, pulmonary vascular resistance; *Raw*, airway resistance; *SVR*, systemic vascular resistance.

oxygen uptake as a result of an attenuation of the HPV response and consequent increase in intrapulmonary shunt/venous admixture. Besides this mild impairment in blood oxygenation, volatile anesthetics offer the advantage to induce bronchodilatation, which is particularly valuable in patients with COPD and during upper airways instrumentation with a DLT or BB.[77] Moreover, a larger attenuation of the release of alveolar inflammatory mediators coupled with reduced adhesion of platelets and leucocytes in endothelial pulmonary capillaries has been reported when patients were exposed to volatile anesthetics compared with intravenous anesthetics during OLV.[78,79] Therefore better protection of the alveolar-capillary membrane appears to be afforded with inhalational anesthesia, resulting in lesser ischemia-reperfusion injury, attenuated oxidative stress, and reduced capillary leak and edema formation. However, although sevoflurane has been shown to protect the endothelial glycocalix in various organs, damage of the endothelial glycocalyx as expressed by the systemic release of heparin sulfate and syndecan-1 was not attenuated in patients anesthetized with sevoflurane compared with propofol during thoracic surgery.[80–82]

Animal studies have shown that the administration of **opiates** (e.g., morphine, fentanyl, sufentanil, buprenorphine) does not impair the capacity of the pulmonary circulation to respond to hypoxia.[83,84] Clinical data also confirm the lack of interference of opiates with the HPV response and blood oxygenation during OLV.

Dexmedetomidine, an alpha-2 adrenergic agonist, has been shown to preserve (or enhance) HPV response, while facilitating fast-tracking by reducing intraoperative opiate and anesthetic requirements.[85,86] Improvement in oxygenation and the favorable clinical outcome in patients receiving dexmedetomidine could be attributed to blunting of the sympathetic stress response to surgery, higher dynamic lung compliance, reduced need for volatile anesthetics, and lower oxidative stress and antiinflammatory effects by lowering the release of interleukin (IL)-6 and inhibiting the toll-like receptor 4/NF-κB pathway.[87–89]

With **nonsteroidal antiinflammatory drugs**, the HPV response is minimally altered because the balance between vasoconstrictive (TXA_2) and vasodilatory mediators (PGI_2) remains stable with nonselective cyclooxygenase (COX) inhibitors.[90] The production of PGI_2 is predominantly related to COX-1 activity in acute hypoxia and to COX-2 in chronic hypoxia. Therefore celexocib, a COX-2 inhibitor, was reported to attenuate the HPV in subjects exposed to hypoxic environments, as the vasodilatory effects of PGI_2 are unopposed by the lower concentrations of TXA2. In contrast, in patients with chronic hypoxemic pulmonary diseases, the HPV response can be reinforced owing to reduced PGI_2 activity when COX-2 inhibitors are given.[91,92]

Effects of Cardiovascular Drugs

Inotropes, such as dobutamine, dopamine, and epinephrine, stimulate cardiac BAR-1 and vascular BAR-2 with increased ventricular contractility and reduced ventricular afterload. The consequent increase in O_2 transport and O_2 availability may result in improved kidney, splanchnic, or cerebral function in patients with heart failure. However, the BAR-2-mediated dilatation of pulmonary vessels attenuates the HPV response, and a larger part of the increased pulmonary blood flow is distributed to poorly ventilated lung areas indicating a larger intrapulmonary shunt as expressed by greater PA-aO_2 gradient and impaired blood oxygenation.[93]

Phenylephrine, an agonist acting on AAR-1, exerts both pulmonary and systemic vasoconstrictor effects. **Ephedrine**, an alkaloid derived from ephedra herb, exerts mixed effects by releasing NE from the sympathetic nerve endings and also acting directly on AARs and BARs. During OLV, Tanaka et al. have shown that treatment of hypotension with either phenylephrine or ephedrine was effective in restoring normotension without increasing Q_S/Q_T, while preserving (or improving) blood oxygenation.[94] Likewise, Doering et al. reported that, in some patients with ARDS, a continuous infusion of phenylephrine resulted in improved oxygenation (mean gain of 15 mm Hg in PaO_2), suggesting the ability of AAR-1 agonists to enhance HPV along with a minor increase in PAP and unchanged CO.[95]

With inhaled BAR-2 agonists, such as **salbutamol or terbutaline**, the common occurrence of O_2 desaturation in patients with bronchospastic disease is attributed to greater heterogeneity in V/Q ratios, owing to increased blood flow and alveolar ventilation that do not match together in the same lung areas.[96]

Most **antihypertensive drugs**, such as NO donors (nitroglycerin, nitroprussiate), phosphodiesterase inhibitors, AAR-1, CCBs, ACE inhibitors (ACEis), and angiotensin receptor antagonists (ATAs), all attenuate HPV by acting on EC-derived modulators, signal transduction pathways in pulmonary VSMCs to limit Ca^{2+} mobilization, and gene transcription. The vasodilatory effects of these drugs are particularly helpful to unload the right ventricular in patients with "fixed" PH. Interestingly, treatment with ACEis or ATAs has been shown to attenuate the acute pulmonary hypertensive response in volunteers breathing a hypoxic mixture.[23,97] However, after long-term therapy with ACEis in patients with heart failure, improvement in oxygenation has been observed that suggests a limited role in drug-induced V/Q mismatch and prominent effects of better O_2 delivery to respiratory muscles.[98]

Nonselective beta-blockers, such as **propranolol**, have been shown to augment O_2 content in hypoxemic critically ill patients by blocking the pulmonary vasodilatation depending on BAR-2 and by reducing ventricular contractility depending on BAR-1.[99] The diminished CO and in turn the reduced $P_{mv}O_2$ could enhance the HPV response in low V/Q lung areas.[100]

Almitrine besylate, a diphenylmethylpiperazine derivative, was initially used in COPD patients to improve gas exchange by a chemoreflex-mediated increase in minute ventilation and by optimizing V/Q matching along with enhanced HPV.[101] In patients with acute respiratory failure, the intravenous form of almitrine has demonstrated short-term improvement in blood oxygenation, particularly when it was combined with selective vasorelaxant drugs (e.g., inhaled NO and PGI2), but it has been abandoned given the occurrence of lactic acidosis, worsening PH, and liver dysfunction.[102] In thoracic surgery, almitritine has been shown to attenuate or even reverse the fall in PaO_2 during OLV under total intravenous anesthesia (TIVA) but not under sevoflurane anesthesia, where the intrapulmonary remained unchanged, suggesting that volatile anesthetics counteract the vasoconstrictive effects of almitrine.[103–105]

Thoracic epidural anesthesia

Noradrenergic sympathetic nerve endings are mainly located around medium size pulmonary arteries in contrast with their higher densities around small arteries in the systemic circulation.

In unstressed individuals in supine position, the sympatho-adrenergic system is barely activated. Therefore, blocking the sympathetic efferent nerves with thoracic epidural anesthesia produces minor hemodynamic changes, except a mild reduction in mean arterial pressure because of vasodilatory effects in the visceral and cutaneous compartments.[106]

During stressful events (e.g., exercise, hemorrhage, pain), activation of the sympatho-adrenal pathways results in systemic vasoconstriction (AAR-1), cardiac hyperactivity (BAR-1), as well as vasodilatation in the pulmonary circulation and in actively contracting skeletal muscles (BAR-2). Importantly, blunting of cardiac and vascular sympathetic drive induced by thoracic epidural anesthesia (TEA) with even a low dose of local anesthetic (LA) results in vagal predominance along with attenuation of the baroreflex response, rendering patients less tolerant to cope appropriately with sudden blood losses.[107]

Blood oxygenation has been reported to be unaffected, impaired, or enhanced by TEA, depending on the dose of LA, the general anesthetic regimen, and the prevailing hemodynamic conditions.[108–111] A dose-response has been observed between the concentrations of ropivacaine (0.75%, 0.5%, and 0.25%) and the development of intrapulmonary shunting with hypoxemia.[112] At the highest concentrations of ropivacaine (0.75%–0.5%), the potent sympathetic blockade produces prominent cardiac depression and inhibition of alpha-1 adrenergic vasoconstriction in large pulmonary arteries. Attenuation of HPV is mitigated by the TEA-induced reduction in CO, the consequent lower $P_{mv}O_2$, as well as by the lower anesthetic requirement if volatile anesthetics are used. At the lowest concentrations of LA routinely used in thoracic anesthesia, cardiac depression is less pronounced and the HPV response is barely affected or preserved, particularly under TIVA.

Choice of General Anesthetics

Worldwide, the majority of thoracic procedures are performed under inhalational anesthesia.[113] Thoracic anesthesiologists justify this choice by several arguments: (1) ability to control in a simple and reliable way the depth of anesthesia; (2) relaxation of bronchial muscle tone in instrumented airways; (3) potentiation of muscular relaxation; and (4) organ protection against ischemia-reperfusion and septic-induced injuries.

In cardiac surgery, anesthetic preconditioning with volatile agents (e.g., isoflurane, desflurane, or sevoflurane) has failed to provide better survival despite the evidence for lesser myocardial injury and shorter intensive care unit stays.[114,115] In thoracic surgery, a metaanalysis of 23 randomized control trials (RCTs) with trial sequential analysis has revealed a 50% reduction in postoperative pulmonary complications (PPCs) among patients receiving volatile anesthetics compared with those receiving TIVA, the total number of enrolled participants being sufficient to support the protective pulmonary effects.[116] In agreement with these findings, an analysis of a multicentric cohort of patients undergoing noncardiac surgery (n =124,497), including 4880 thoracic interventions, has demonstrated a dose-dependent protective effect of volatile anesthetics against PPCs, along with a reduced 30-day mortality rate and decreased hospital costs among those patients exposed to higher doses of inhalational anesthetics.[117] Although the use of inhalation anesthesia has been associated with improved early postoperative clinical outcome, such anesthetic-organ preconditioning does not translate into better long-term outcome. A higher rate in cancer recurrence and a reduction in long-term survival has been observed among patients anesthetized with volatile agents compared with TIVA, regardless of the comorbidity burden, surgical severity, and presence of metastasis.[118,119] Experimental data have demonstrated that volatile anesthetics exert inhibitory effects on cell-based immunity (e.g., natural killer cell activity) and upregulate the transcription of HIF, insulin growth factor, and vascular endothelial growth factor, which are important for intraoperative "seeding" of tumor cells, remodeling of lymphatic vessels, and angiogenesis-induced tumor growth, all factors that may promote later cancer recurrence and metastasis.[120] In contrast, propofol inhibits the host immunity to a lower extent, as the natural killer cell activity is better preserved. Moreover, propofol has demonstrated antitumor effects in non-small cell lung carcinoma resulting from disrupted regulation of HIF.[121] Co-administration of low doses of ketamine may represent a valuable way to attenuate surgery-induced immunosuppression through its analgesic and antiinflammatory effects, reducing leucocyte reactivity, ROS generation, and cytokines overproduction, while preserving IL-2 activity, a key regulator of both cellular and humoral immune response.[122]

So far, clinical studies comparing TIVA and inhalational anesthesia have reported mixed results regarding long-term clinical outcome. A systematic review including 7800 patients undergoing lung, esophageal, or breast cancer resection found that TIVA was associated with improved recurrence-free survival compared with inhalation anesthesia (hazard ratio of 0.78, 95% CI, 0.65–0.94).[123] Given the heterogeneity of the patient populations, the various surgical procedures, and the retrospective nature of the studies (one RCT, five cohorts), large randomized trials should be designed to confirm or refute the immunomodulatory effects of anesthetic agents.

The initiation of OLV is always associated with a fall in PaO_2, but the incidence of severe hypoxemia is low, and numerous interventions have demonstrated their effectiveness to improve blood oxygenation and prevent hypoxia-induced organ dysfunction.[124]

The HPV response is a local reflex that minimizes intrapulmonary shunt during OLV and tends to optimize V/Q ratios in the dependent ventilated lung. Attention should be paid for correct placement of DLT/BB, the effects of anesthetics, analgesics, and cardiovascular drugs, as well as ventilatory modes, patient positioning, and surgical manipulation that may all influence HPV and pulmonary blood flow distribution (Fig. 15.11).

High-risk patients could potentially benefit from inhalational anesthesia given its preconditioning and protective organ effect. Conversely, switching from inhalational to TIVA could be indicated when the patient becomes hypoxemic and/or if she/he experiences intraoperative complications that will require postoperative ventilatory support. Currently, the scientific evidence is too weak to recommend the utilization of one specific anesthetic regimen instead of another. Further well-designed clinical studies are needed to demonstrate that anesthetic preconditioning may translate into better quality of life and increased survival.

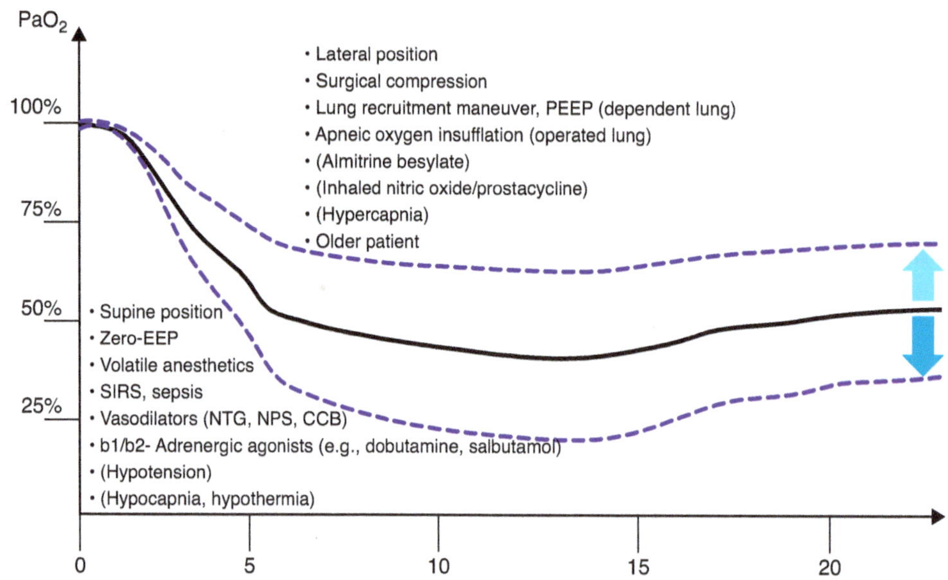

• **Fig. 15.11** Time course of arterial PO2 after initiation of one-lung ventilation and impact of specific factors. *CCB,* Calcium-channel blocker; *EEP*, end-expiratory pressure; *NPS,* nitroprussiate; *NTG*, nitroglycerin; *PAO_2,* partial pressure of oxygen; *PEEP*, positive end-expiratory pressure; *SIRS*, systemic inflammatory response syndrome; *NTG*, Nitroglycerin; *NPS*, nitroprusside; *CCB*, calcium channel blockers.

References

1. Ashok V, Francis J. A practical approach to adult one-lung ventilation. *BJA Educ.* 2018;18(3):69–74.
2. Campos JH, Feider A. Hypoxia during one-lung ventilation-a review and update. *J Cardiothorac Vasc Anesth.* 2018;32(5):2330–2338.
3. Liljestrand G. Regulation of pulmonary arterial blood pressure. *Arch Intern Med (Chic).* 1948;81(2):162–172.
4. Dunham-Snary KJ, Wu D, Syles EA, et al. Hypoxic pulmonary vasoconstriction: from molecular mechanisms to medicine. *Chest.* 2017;151(1):181–192.
5. Morrell NW, Nijran KS, Biggs T, Seed WA. Changes in regional pulmonary blood flow during lobar bronchial occlusion in man. *Clin Sci* (Lond). 1994;86(5):639–644.
6. Hughes JM. Hypoxic pulmonary vasoconstriction: clinical implications. *Eur Respir J.* 2016;47(1):31–34.
7. Shimoda LA, Laurie SS. HIF and pulmonary vascular responses to hypoxia. *J Appl Physiol.* 1985–2014;116(7):867–874.
8. Hirota K. Basic biology of hypoxic responses mediated by the transcription factor HIFs and its implication for medicine. *Biomedicines.* 2020;8(2):32.
9. Kapanci Y, Assimacopoulos A, Irle C, Zwahlen A, Gabbiani G. "Contractile interstitial cells" in pulmonary alveolar septa: a possible regulator of ventilation-perfusion ratio? Ultrastructural, immunofluorescence, and in vitro studies. *J Cell Biol.* 1974;60(2):375–392.
10. al-Tinawi A, Krenz GS, Rickaby A, Linehan JH, Dawson CA. Influence of hypoxia and serotonin on small pulmonary vessels. *J Appl Physiol.* 1985–1994;76(1):56–64.
11. Gao Y, Raj JU. Role of veins in regulation of pulmonary circulation. *Am J Physiol Lung Cell Mol Physiol.* 2005;288(2):L213–L226.
12. Benumof JL, Pirlo JF, Johanson I, Trousdale FR. Interaction of PVO2 with PAO2 on hypoxic pulmonary vasoconstriction. *J Appl Physiol Respir Environ Exerc Physiol.* 1981;51(4):871–874.
13. Marshall BE, Clarke WR, Costarino AT, Chen L, Miller F, Marshall C. The dose-response relationship for hypoxic pulmonary vasoconstriction. *Respir Physiol.* 1994;96(2-3):231–247.
14. Sylvester JT, Shimonda LA, Aaronson PI, Ward JPT. Hypoxic pulmonary vasoconstriction. *Physiol Rev.* 2012;92(1):367–520.
15. Jameson AG. Diffusion of gases from alveolus to precapillary arteries. *Science.* 1963;139(3557):826–828.
16. Sommer N, Strielkov I, Pak O, Weissmann N. Oxygen sensing and signal transduction in hypoxic pulmonary vasoconstriction. *Eur Respir J.* 2016;47(1):288–303.
17. Smith KA, Schumacker PT. Sensors and signals: the role of reactive oxygen species in hypoxic pulmonary vasoconstriction. *J Physiol.* 2019;597(4):1033–1043.
18. Firth AL, Gordienko DV, Yuill KH, Smirnov SV. Cellular localization of mitochondria contributes to Kv channel-mediated regulation of cellular excitability in pulmonary but not mesenteric circulation. *Am J Physiol Lung Cell Mol Physiol.* 2009;296(3):L347–L360.
19. Vaillancourt M, Chia P, Sarji S, et al. Autonomic nervous system involvement in pulmonary arterial hypertension. *Respir Res.* 2017;18(1):201.
20. Shirai M, Tsuchimochi H, Nagai H, et al. Pulmonary vascular tone is dependent on the central modulation of sympathetic nerve activity following chronic intermittent hypoxia. *Basic Res Cardiol.* 2014;109(5):432.
21. Brimioulle S, Vachiéry J-L, Brichant J-F, Delcroix M, Lejeune P, Naeije R. Sympathetic modulation of hypoxic pulmonary vasoconstriction in intact dogs. *Cardiovasc Res.* 1997;34(2):384–392.
22. Gaur P, et al. Regulation, signalling and functions of hormonal peptides in pulmonary vascular remodelling during hypoxia. *Endocrine.* 2018;59(3):466–480.

23. Cargill RI, Lipworth BJ. Lisinopril attenuates acute hypoxic pulmonary vasoconstriction in humans. *Chest.* 1996;109(2):424–429.
24. Hubloue I, Rondelet B, Kerbaul F, et al. Endogenous angiotensin II in the regulation of hypoxic pulmonary vasoconstriction in anaesthetized dogs. *Crit Care.* 2004;8(4):R163–R171.
25. Robin ED, Theodore J, Burke CM, et al. Hypoxic pulmonary vasoconstriction persists in the human transplanted lung. *Clin Sci* (Lond). 1987;72(3):283–287.
26. Grimmer B, Kuebler WM. The endothelium in hypoxic pulmonary vasoconstriction. *J Appl Physiol.* 1985–2017;123(6):1635–1646.
27. Wang L, Yin J, Nickles JT, et al. Hypoxic pulmonary vasoconstriction requires connexin 40-mediated endothelial signal conduction. *J Clin Invest.* 2012;122(11):4218–4230.
28. Pak O, Aldashev A, Welsh D, Peacock A. The effects of hypoxia on the cells of the pulmonary vasculature. *Eur Respir J.* 2007;30(2):364–372.
29. Tawhai MH, Clark AR, Burrowes KS. Computational models of the pulmonary circulation: insights and the move towards clinically directed studies. *Pulm Circ.* 2011;1(2):224–238.
30. Naeije R. Pulmonary circulation in hypoxia. *Int J Sports Med.* 1992;13(suppl 1):S27–S30.
31. Marshall BE, Marshall C, Benumof J, Saidman LJ. Hypoxic pulmonary vasoconstriction in dogs: effects of lung segment size and oxygen tension. *J Appl Physiol Respir Environ Exerc Physiol.* 1981;51(6):1543–1551.
32. Drop LJ, Toal KW, Geffin GA, O'Keefe DD, Haoglin DC, Daggett WM. Pulmonary vascular responses to hypercalcemia and hypocalcemia in the dog. *Anesthesiology.* 1989;70(5):825–836.
33. Galletti PM, Salisbury PF, Rieben A. Influence of blood temperature on the pulmonary circulation. *Circ Res.* 1958;6(3):275–282.
34. Benumof JL, Wahrenbrock EA. Dependency of hypoxic pulmonary vasoconstriction on temperature. *J Appl Physiol Respir Environ Exerc Physiol.* 1977;42(1):56–58.
35. Ketabchi F, Egemnazarov B, Schermuly RT, et al. Effects of hypercapnia with and without acidosis on hypoxic pulmonary vasoconstriction. *Am J Physiol Lung Cell Mol Physiol.* 2009;297(5): L977–L983.
36. Sicard D, Haak AJ, Moo Choi K, Craig AR, Fredenburgh LE, Tschumperlin DJ. Aging and anatomical variations in lung tissue stiffness. *Am J Physiol Lung Cell Mol Physiol.* 2018; 314(6):L946–L955.
37. Balanos GM, Pugh K, Frise MC, Dorrington KL. Exaggerated pulmonary vascular response to acute hypoxia in older men. *Exp Physiol.* 2015;100(10):1187–1198.
38. Luks AM, Swenson ER, Bartsch P. Acute high-altitude sickness. *Eur Respir Rev.* 2017;26(143):160096.
39. Swenson ER. Early hours in the development of high-altitude pulmonary edema: time course and mechanisms. *J Appl Physiol.* 1985–2020;128(6):1539–1546.
40. Sartori C, Rimoldi SF, Rexhaj E, Allemann Y, Scherrer U. Epigenetics in cardiovascular regulation. *Adv Exp Med Biol.* 2016;903:55–62.
41. Petousi N, Croft QPP, Cavalleri GL, et al. Tibetans living at sea level have a hyporesponsive hypoxia-inducible factor system and blunted physiological responses to hypoxia. *J Appl Physiol.* 1985–2014;116(7):893–904.
42. Eichstaedt CA, Antão T, Cardona A, et al. Genetic and phenotypic differentiation of an Andean intermediate altitude population. *Physiol Rep.* 2015;3(5):e12376.
43. Wagner PD. The multiple inert gas elimination technique (MIGET). *Intensive Care Med.* 2008;34(6):994–1001.
44. Riley RL, Cournand A. Ideal alveolar air and the analysis of ventilation-perfusion relationships in the lungs. *J Appl Physiol.* 1949;1(12):825–847.
45. Melot C, Naeije R, Rothschild T, Mertens P, Mols P, Hallemans R. Improvement in ventilation-perfusion matching by almitrine in COPD. *Chest.* 1983;83(3):528–533.
46. Bogaard HJ. Hypoxic pulmonary vasoconstriction in COPD-associated pulmonary hypertension: been there, done that? *Eur Respir J.* 2017;50(1):1701191.
47. Nagaraj C, Tabeling C, Nagy BM, et al. Hypoxic vascular response and ventilation/perfusion matching in end-stage COPD may depend on p22phox. *Eur Respir J.* 2017;50(1):1601651.
48. Kelly VJ, Hibbert KA, Kohli P, et al. Hypoxic pulmonary vasoconstriction does not explain all regional perfusion redistribution in asthma. *Am J Respir Crit Care Med.* 2017;196(7): 834–844.
49. Kholdani C, Fares WH, Mohsenin V. Pulmonary hypertension in obstructive sleep apnea: is it clinically significant? A critical analysis of the association and pathophysiology. *Pulm Circ.* 2015;5(2):220–227.
50. Licker M, Fauconnet P, Villiger Y, Tschopp J-M. Acute lung injury and outcomes after thoracic surgery. *Curr Opin Anaesthesiol.* 2009;22(1):61–67.
51. Licker M, de Perrot M, Spiliopoulos A, et al. Risk factors for acute lung injury after thoracic surgery for lung cancer. *Anesth Analg.* 2003;97(6):1558–1565.
52. Ryan D, Frohlich S, McLoughlin P. Pulmonary vascular dysfunction in ARDS. *Ann Intensive Care.* 2014;4:28.
53. Turzo M, Vaith J, Lasitschka F, Weigand MA, Busch CJ. Role of ATP-sensitive potassium channels on hypoxic pulmonary vasoconstriction in endotoxemia. *Respir Res.* 2018;19(1):29.
54. Benzing A, Mols G, Brieschal T, Geiger K. Hypoxic pulmonary vasoconstriction in nonventilated lung areas contributes to differences in hemodynamic and gas exchange responses to inhalation of nitric oxide. *Anesthesiology.* 1997;86(6):1254–1261.
55. Rossaint R, Falke KJ, López F, Slama K, Pison U, Zapol WM. Inhaled nitric oxide for the adult respiratory distress syndrome. *N Engl J Med.* 1993;328(6):399–405.
56. Robertson HT. Dead space: the physiology of wasted ventilation. *Eur Respir J.* 2015;45(6):1704–1716.
57. Grant BJ. Effect of local pulmonary blood flow control on gas exchange: theory. *J Appl Physiol Respir Environ Exerc Physiol.* 1982;53(5):1100–1109.
58. Nyren S, Radell P, Mure M, et al. Inhalation anesthesia increases V/Q regional heterogeneity during spontaneous breathing in healthy subjects. *Anesthesiology.* 2010;113(6):1370–1375.
59. Tokics L, Hedenstierna G, Svensson L, et al. V/Q distribution and correlation to atelectasis in anesthetized paralyzed humans. *J Appl Physiol.* 1985-1996;81(4):1822–1833.
60. Bates JHT, Smith BJ. Ventilator-induced lung injury and lung mechanics. *Ann Transl Med.* 2018;6(19):378.
61. Duggan M, Kavanagh BP. Pulmonary atelectasis: a pathogenic perioperative entity. *Anesthesiology.* 2005;102(4):838–854.
62. Wolf SJ, Reske AP, Hammermuller S, et al. Correlation of lung collapse and gas exchange—a computer tomographic study in sheep and pigs with atelectasis in otherwise normal lungs. *PLoS One.* 2015;10(8):e0135272.
63. Arai TJ, Henderson AC, Dubowitz DJ, et al. Hypoxic pulmonary vasoconstriction does not contribute to pulmonary blood

flow heterogeneity in normoxia in normal supine humans. *J Appl Physiol.* 1985-2009;106(4):1057–1064.

64. Lumb AB, Slinger P. Hypoxic pulmonary vasoconstriction: physiology and anesthetic implications. *Anesthesiology.* 2015; 122(4):932–946.
65. Wieslander B, Ramos JG, Ax M, Petersson J. Supine, prone, right and left gravitational effects on human pulmonary circulation. *J Cardiovasc Magn Reson.* 2019;21(1):69.
66. Benumof JL. Mechanism of decreased blood flow to atelectatic lung. *J Appl Physiol Respir Environ Exerc Physiol.* 1979;46(6): 1047–1048.
67. Hambraeus-Jonzon K, Bindslev L, Mellgard LJ, Hedenstierna G. Hypoxic pulmonary vasoconstriction in human lungs. A stimulus-response study. *Anesthesiology.* 1997;86(2):308–315.
68. Feiner JR, Weiskopf RB. Evaluating pulmonary function: an assessment of PaO2/FIO2. *Crit Care Med.* 2017;45(1):e40–e48.
69. Benatar SR, Hewlett AM, Nunn JF. The use of iso-shunt lines for control of oxygen therapy. *Br J Anaesth.* 1973;45(7):711–718.
70. Young CC, Harriss EH, Vacchiano C, et al. Lung-protective ventilation for the surgical patient: international expert panel-based consensus recommendations. *Br J Anaesth.* 2019;123(6):898–913.
71. Slinger PD, Hickey DR. The interaction between applied PEEP and auto-PEEP during one-lung ventilation. *J Cardiothorac Vasc Anesth.* 1998;12(2):133–136.
72. Spadaro S, Grasso S, Karbing DS, et al. Physiologic evaluation of ventilation perfusion mismatch and respiratory mechanics at different positive end-expiratory pressure in patients undergoing protective one-lung ventilation. *Anesthesiology.* 2018;128(3): 531–538.
73. Jung DM, Ahn HJ, Jung SH, et al. Apneic oxygen insufflation decreases the incidence of hypoxemia during one-lung ventilation in open and thoracoscopic pulmonary lobectomy: a randomized controlled trial. *J Thorac Cardiovasc Surg.* 2017;154(1): 360–366.
74. Eisenkraft JB. Effects of anaesthetics on the pulmonary circulation. *Br J Anaesth.* 1990;65(1):63–78.
75. Bjertnaes LJ. Hypoxia-induced vasoconstriction in isolated perfused lungs exposed to injectable or inhalation anesthetics. *Acta Anaesthesiol Scand.* 1977;21(2):133–147.
76. Nakayama M, Murray PA. Ketamine preserves and propofol potentiates hypoxic pulmonary vasoconstriction compared with the conscious state in chronically instrumented dogs. *Anesthesiology.* 1999;91(3):760–771.
77. Volta CA, Alvivi V, Petrini S, et al. The effect of volatile anesthetics on respiratory system resistance in patients with chronic obstructive pulmonary disease. *Anesth Analg.* 2005;100(2):348–353.
78. Sun B, Wang J, Bo L, et al. Effects of volatile vs. propofol-based intravenous anesthetics on the alveolar inflammatory responses to one-lung ventilation: a meta-analysis of randomized controlled trials. *J Anesth.* 2015;29(4):570–579.
79. Collins SR, Blank RS, Deatherage LS, Dull RO. Special article: the endothelial glycocalyx: emerging concepts in pulmonary edema and acute lung injury. *Anesth Analg.* 2013;117(3):664–674.
80. Kim HJ, Kim E, Baek SH, et al. Sevoflurane did not show better protective effect on endothelial glycocalyx layer compared to propofol during lung resection surgery with one lung ventilation. *J Thorac Dis.* 2018;10(3):1468–1475.
81. Casanova J, Simon C, Vara E, et al. Sevoflurane anesthetic preconditioning protects the lung endothelial glycocalyx from ischemia reperfusion injury in an experimental lung autotransplant model. *J Anesth.* 2016;30(5):755–762.
82. Chappell D, Heindl B, Jacob M, et al. Sevoflurane reduces leukocyte and platelet adhesion after ischemia-reperfusion by protecting the endothelial glycocalyx. *Anesthesiology.* 2011;115(3): 483–491.
83. Bjertnaes L, Hauge A, Kriz M. Hypoxia-induced pulmonary vasoconstriction: effects of fentanyl following different routes of administration. *Acta Anaesthesiol Scand.* 1980;24(1):53–57.
84. Gibbs JM, Johnson H. Lack of effect of morphine and buprenorphine on hypoxic pulmonary vasoconstriction in the isolated perfused cat lung and the perfused lobe of the dog lung. *Br J Anaesth.* 1978;50(12):1197–1201.
85. Huang SQ, Zhang J, Zhang XX, et al. Can dexmedetomidine improve arterial oxygenation and intrapulmonary shunt during one-lung ventilation in adults undergoing thoracic surgery? A meta-analysis of randomized, placebo-controlled trials. *Chin Med J* (Engl). 2017;130(14):1707–1714.
86. Kernan S, Rehman S, Meyer T, Bourbeua J, Caron N, Tobias JD. Effects of dexmedetomidine on oxygenation during one-lung ventilation for thoracic surgery in adults. *J Minim Access Surg.* 2011;7(4):227–231.
87. Lee SH, Kim N, Lee CY, Ban MG, Oh YJ. Effects of dexmedetomidine on oxygenation and lung mechanics in patients with moderate chronic obstructive pulmonary disease undergoing lung cancer surgery: a randomised double-blinded trial. *Eur J Anaesthesiol.* 2016;33(4):275–282.
88. Wu Y, Liu Y, Huang H, et al. Dexmedetomidine inhibits inflammatory reaction in lung tissues of septic rats by suppressing TLR4/NF-kappaB pathway. *Mediators Inflamm. 2013.* 2013: 562154.
89. Xia R, Xu J, Yin H, et al. Intravenous infusion of dexmedetomidine combined isoflurane inhalation reduces oxidative stress and potentiates hypoxia pulmonary vasoconstriction during one-lung ventilation in patients. *Mediators Inflamm. 2015.* 2015: 238041.
90. Weir EK, McMurtry IF, Tucker A, Reeves JT, Grover RF. Prostaglandin synthetase inhibitors do not decrease hypoxic pulmonary vasoconstriction. *J Appl Physiol.* 1976;41(5 Pt. 1):714–718.
91. Su CL, Yuan DW, Chiang LL, Lee HL, Chen KH, Wang D. Inducible cyclooxygenase expression mediating hypoxia/reoxygenation-induced pulmonary vasoconstriction is attenuated by a cyclooxygenase inhibitor in rats. *Transplant Proc.* 2012; 44(4):929–932.
92. Kylhammar D, Radegran G. The principal pathways involved in the in vivo modulation of hypoxic pulmonary vasoconstriction, pulmonary arterial remodelling and pulmonary hypertension. *Acta Physiol* (Oxf). 2017;219(4):728–756.
93. Bryan TL, van Diepen S, Bhutani M, Shanks M, Welsh RC, Stickland MK. The effects of dobutamine and dopamine on intrapulmonary shunt and gas exchange in healthy humans. *J Appl Physiol* (1985). 2012;113(4):541–548.
94. Tanaka M, Dohi S. Effects of phenylephrine and ephedrine on pulmonary arterial pressure in patients with cervical or lumbar epidural anesthesia, or enflurane anesthesia. *J Anesth.* 1994; 8(2):125–131.
95. Doering EB, Hanson CW, Reily JD, Marshall C, Marshall BE. Improvement in oxygenation by phenylephrine and nitric oxide in patients with adult respiratory distress syndrome. *Anesthesiology.* 1997;87(1):18–25.
96. Tal A, Pasterkamp H, Leahy F. Arterial oxygen desaturation following salbutamol inhalation in acute asthma. *Chest.* 1984;86(6):868–869.

97. Kiely DG, Cargill RI, Lipworth BJ. Angiotensin II receptor blockade and effects on pulmonary hemodynamics and hypoxic pulmonary vasoconstriction in humans. *Chest.* 1996;110(3): 698–703.
98. Stanek EJ, Nara AR, Strohl KP, Nair RN, Decker MJ, Mumger MA. Effect of long-term angiotensin-converting enzyme inhibitor therapy on arterial oxygen saturation in patients with mild to moderate heart failure. *Pharmacotherapy.* 1994;14(3): 321–329.
99. Vincent JL, Lignian H, Gillet JB, Berre J, Contu E. Increase in PaO2 following intravenous administration of propranolol in acutely hypoxemic patients. *Chest.* 1985;88(4):558–562.
100. Pellett AA, Cairo JM, Levitzky MG. Hypoxemia and hypoxic pulmonary vasoconstriction: autonomic nervous system versus mixed venous PO2. *Respir Physiol.* 1997;109(3):249–260.
101. Górecka D, Śliwiński P, Pałasiewicz G, Pachocki R, Zieliński J. Effects of almitrine bismesylate on arterial blood gases in patients with chronic obstructive pulmonary disease and moderate hypoxaemia: a multicentre, randomised, double-blind, placebo-controlled study. *Respiration.* 2003;70(3):275–283.
102. Roch A, Hraiech S, Dizier S, Papazian L. Pharmacological interventions in acute respiratory distress syndrome. *Ann Intensive Care.* 2013;3(1):20.
103. Bermejo S, Gallart L, Silva-Costa-Gomes T, Vallès J, Aguiló R, Puig MM. Almitrine fails to improve oxygenation during one-lung ventilation with sevoflurane anesthesia. *J Cardiothorac Vasc Anesth.* 2014;28(4):919–924.
104. Silva-Costa-Gomes T, Gallart L, Vallès J, Trillo L, Minguella J, Puig MM. Low- vs high-dose almitrine combined with nitric oxide to prevent hypoxia during open-chest one-lung ventilation. *Br J Anaesth.* 2005;95(3):410–416.
105. Dalibon N, Moutafis M, Liu N, et al. Treatment of hypoxemia during one-lung ventilation using intravenous almitrine. *Anesth Analg.* 2004;98(3):590–594, table of contents.
106. Freise H, Van Aken HK. Risks and benefits of thoracic epidural anaesthesia. *Br J Anaesth.* 2011;107(6):859–868.
107. Licker M, Spiliopoulos A, Tschopp JM. Influence of thoracic epidural analgesia on cardiovascular autonomic control after thoracic surgery. *Br J Anaesth.* 2003;91(4):525–531.
108. Garutti I, Quintana P, Olmedilla L, Cruz A, Barranco M, Garcia de Lucas E. Arterial oxygenation during one-lung ventilation: combined versus general anesthesia. *Anesth Analg.* 1999;88(3):494–499.
109. Jung SM, Cho KM, Kim YJ, et al. The effect of thoracic epidural anesthesia on pulmonary shunt fraction and arterial oxygenation during one-lung ventilation. *J Cardiothorac Vasc Anesth.* 2010;24(3):456–462.
110. Ozcan PE, Sentürk M, Sungur Ulke Z, et al. Effects of thoracic epidural anaesthesia on pulmonary venous admixture and oxygenation during one-lung ventilation. *Acta Anaesthesiol Scand.* 2007;51(8):1117–1122.
111. Casati A, Mascotto G, Iemi K, Nzepa-Batonga J, De Luca M. Epidural block does not worsen oxygenation during one-lung ventilation for lung resections under isoflurane/nitrous oxide anaesthesia. *Eur J Anaesthesiol.* 2005;22(5):363–368.
112. Xu Y, Tan Z, Wang S, Shao H, Zhu X. Effect of thoracic epidural anesthesia with different concentrations of ropivacaine on arterial oxygenation during one-lung ventilation. *Anesthesiology.* 2010;112(5):1146–1154.
113. Licker M. Anaesthetic management and unplanned admission to intensive care after thoracic surgery. *Anaesthesia.* 2019; 74(9):1083–1086.
114. Jiao XF, Lin XM, Ni XF, et al. Volatile anesthetics versus total intravenous anesthesia in patients undergoing coronary artery bypass grafting: an updated meta-analysis and trial sequential analysis of randomized controlled trials. *PLoS One.* 2019; 14(10):e0224562.
115. Landoni G, Lomivorotov VV, Neto CN, et al. Volatile anesthetics versus total intravenous anesthesia for cardiac surgery. *N Engl J Med.* 2019;380(13):1214–1225.
116. Pang QY, An R, Liu HL. Effects of inhalation and intravenous anesthesia on intraoperative cardiopulmonary function and postoperative complications in patients undergoing thoracic surgery. *Minerva Anestesiol.* 2018;84(11):1287–1297.
117. Grabitz SD, Farhan HN, Ruscic KJ, et al. Dose-dependent protective effect of inhalational anesthetics against postoperative respiratory complications: a prospective analysis of data on file from three hospitals in New England. *Crit Care Med.* 2017;45(1): e30–e39.
118. Wigmore TJ, Mohammed K, Jhanji S. Long-term survival for patients undergoing volatile versus IV anesthesia for cancer surgery: a retrospective analysis. *Anesthesiology.* 2016;124(1):69–79.
119. Sekandarzad MW, van Zundert AA, Lirk PB, Doornebal CW, Hollmann MW. Perioperative anesthesia care and tumor progression. *Anesth Analg.* 2017;124(5):1697–1708.
120. Longhini F, Bruni A, Garofalo E, et al. Anesthetic strategies in oncological surgery: not only a simple sleep, but also impact on immunosuppression and cancer recurrence. *Cancer Manag Res.* 2020;12:931–940.
121. Xu Y, Pan S, Jiang W, Xue F, Zhu X. Effects of propofol on the development of cancer in humans. *Cell Prolif.* 2020:e12867.
122. Beilin B, Rusabrov Y, Shapira Y, et al. Low-dose ketamine affects immune responses in humans during the early postoperative period. *Br J Anaesth.* 2007;99(4):522–527.
123. Yap A, Lopez-Olivo MA, Dubowitz J, Hiller J, Riedel B, Global Onco-Anesthesia Research Collaboration Group. Anesthetic technique and cancer outcomes: a meta-analysis of total intravenous versus volatile anesthesia. *Can J Anaesth.* 2019;66(5):546–561.
124. Karzai W, Schwarzkopf K. Hypoxemia during one-lung ventilation: prediction, prevention, and treatment. *Anesthesiology.* 2009;110(6):1402–1411.

NON-PRINT ITEMS

Abstract

The inhalational anesthetic (InhA) technique offers a simple and reliable way to control the depth of anesthesia, to protect the organs against ischemia-reperfusion injuries, to potentiate the effects of neuromuscular blocking agents, and to decrease the airway resistance. In experimental models of sepsis, the exposure to halogen-containing hydrocarbons has been shown to improve survival, whereas propofol anesthesia is associated with increased mortality along with larger systemic release of endotoxins. Likewise, in thoracic surgery with one-lung ventilation, the early pulmonary protective effect of InhA is accompanied by a lower level of alveolar inflammatory mediators, as compared with intravenous anesthetic (IVA). In contrast, regarding the long-term effects, the impairment in cell-based immunity induced by InhA may promote "seeding" of tumor cells at the time of cancer resection and could explain a higher rate of cancer recurrence and a reduction in long-term survival, when compared with IVA.

Because hypoxic pulmonary vasoconstriction is inhibited by volatile anesthetics, some anesthesiologists preferentially select IVA to avoid (or to treat) hypoxemia because of intrapulmonary blood shunting. Another reason to select an intravenous agent is the need to continue mechanical ventilation in the intensive care unit, a place where InhAs are usually not used.

Patients with a higher preoperative risk profile caused by advanced respiratory, cardiac, or renal diseases would be the best candidates to receive volatile anesthetics given their preconditioning and protective organ effects. Conversely, switching from InhA to IVA could be indicated if patients present oxygen desaturation because of intrapulmonary shunting and/or if they experience intraoperative complications that justify the continuation of mechanical ventilation after surgery.

Keywords

pulmonary flow, hypoxemia, pulmonary hypertension, intrapulmonary shunt, ventilation-perfusion mismatch, intravenous anesthesia, volatile anesthetics

16

Separation of the Lung: Double-Lumen Endotracheal Tubes and Endobronchial Blockers

JAVIER H. CAMPOS

Introduction

Lung separation techniques are designed to facilitate surgical exposure and provide one-lung ventilation (OLV) in patients undergoing thoracic, mediastinal, cardiac, vascular, esophageal, or selective spine surgery.[1–3] Lung separation can be achieved with two different techniques. **The first** involves the double-lumen endotracheal tube (DLT) technique. This device is made of disposable polyvinyl, chloride material, or silicone material.[4,5] The DLT is a bifurcated tube with both an endotracheal and an endobronchial lumen and can be used to selectively achieve separation of either the right or left lung.[6,7] Over time, several modifications have been made to the DLT to improve quality of placement and patient safety. A newly designed VivaSight® DLT has an integrated camera, allowing continuous visualization of tube position within the trachea.[8] In addition, there is the ECOM (Endotracheal Cardiac output Monitor)-DLT® that has multiple flexible surface sensors attached to the endotracheal cuff of the DLT that, when connected to a monitor measure the aortic blood flow by the bioimpedance method. Based upon an algorithm, it can record cardiac output, stroke volume, and systemic vascular resistances.[9] **The second** technique involves using an endotracheal blocker to block the mainstem bronchus to allow lung collapse distal to the occlusion.[10,11] Currently, there are several bronchial blockers clinically available to facilitate lung separation and provide OLV. Initially, a single-lumen endotracheal tube with an incorporated bronchial blocker, such as the torque control blocker Univent was used.[12] Presently, endobronchial blockers are used independently through a single-lumen endotracheal tube. Several are available: the wire-guided endobronchial blocker (Arndt blocker)[13] (Cook Critical Care, Bloomington, IN), the Cohen tip-deflecting endobronchial blocker[14] (Cook Critical Care, Bloomington, IN), the Fuji Uniblocker[15] (Fuji Corp, Tokyo Japan), or the EZ-Blocker[16,17] (Teleflex Medical, Morrisville, NC).

The most common indications for lung separation and OLV are for providing a still operative field and surgical exposure or for lung isolation, for prevention of contamination to the contralateral lung from bleeding or pus material, and during the application of differential lung ventilation or for continuing of the airway gas exchange, such as bronchopleural fistula, and during a lung lavage.[18]

Double-Lumen Endotracheal Tubes

There are two versions of DLTs; a left-sided and a right-sided, which are designed to accommodate the unique anatomy of each mainstem bronchus. DLTs are available from different manufactures: Mallinckrodt Broncho-Cath (St. Louis, MO), Sheridan Sheri-I Bronch (Argyle, NY), Rüsch (Duluth, GA), Portex (Keene, NH), VivaSight DLT from Ambu (St. Louis, MO), the Silbroncho from Fuji (Japan), and the ECOM-DLT (San Juan Capistrano, CA). The sizes of the DLTs vary among manufactures. The smallest available is 26 French (Fr) followed by 28, 32, 33, 35, 37, 39, and 41 Fr. Table 16.1 displays the external and internal diameters of the different-sized DLTs and the size of the flexible fiberoptic bronchoscope recommended.

Size Selection of the Double-Lumen Endotracheal Tubes

A properly sized DLT is one in which the main body of the tube passes without resistance through the glottis and advances easily within the trachea, and in which the bronchial component passes into the selected bronchus without difficulty or resistance. A DLT that is too small in size requires a larger endobronchial cuff volume (i.e., >3.0 mL) for effective blockade, which might increase the incidence of malposition, or can result in a DLT that is too short to be properly positioned in the target bronchus, resulting in

TABLE 16.1 Displays the External and Internal Diameters of the Different Size of Double-Lumen Tubes and the Size of the Flexible Fiberoptic Bronchoscope Recommended

Double-Lumen Tube French Size (Fr)				
F Size	OD (mm)	Bronchial ID (mm)	Trachea ID (mm)	FOB Size OD (mm)
26	8.7	3.5	3.5	2.2
28	9.3	3.2	3.1	2.2
32	10.7	3.4	3.5	2.2
35	11.7	4.3	4.5	3.5 or 4.2
37	12.3	4.5	4.7	3.5 or 4.2
39	13.0	4.9	4.9	3.5 or 4.2
41	13.7	5.4	5.4	3.5 or 4.2

DLT, Double-lumen endotracheal tube; *ID*, internal diameter; *FOB*, fiberoptic bronchoscope; *OD*, outer diameter.

From Campos J. Lung isolation. In: Slinger P, ed. *Principles and Practice of Anesthesia for Thoracic Surgery*. Switzerland: Springer Nature; 2019:283–309. With permission.

failure to achieve lung separation. A DLT that is too small may migrate deeply into a bronchus, resulting in airway trauma or development of a pneumothorax if both the tracheal and the endobronchial lumen are inserted into one bronchus, resulting in an overinflated large tidal volume into a single lobe.[19,20] Fig. 16.1 displays an undersized left-sided DLT that migrated distally into the left-main stem bronchus producing a pneumothorax and lack of ventilation in the right lung and left lower lobe.

In addition, an undersized DLT might present a higher resistance to gas flow and increase intrinsic autopositive end-expiratory pressure as compared with the wider lumen of larger DLTs.[21] In a study performed in adult cadavers, it was shown

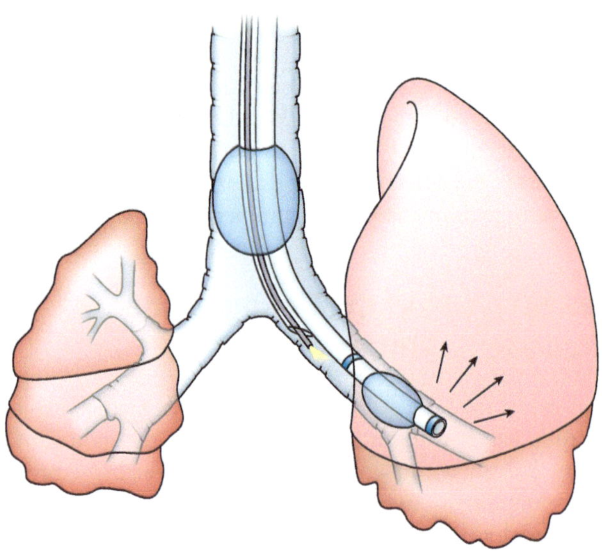

• **Fig. 16.1** Display of a left-sided double-lumen endotracheal tube (undersized) that migrated too distal into the left-main stem bronchus, producing a pneumothorax and lack of ventilation in the right lung and left lower lobe.

that the cricoid ring diameter never exceeds the diameter of the glottis. If a DLT encounters resistance when passing the glottis, it is likely that the DLT would encounter resistance while passing the cricoid ring.[22] An oversized DLT can potentially produce trauma to the airway,[23] therefore it is important to select the appropriate size for the patient to prevent complications.

A common challenge with the appropriate size selection of a DLT is the lack of objective guidelines to demonstrate the optimal method to determine the best size for the patient. There is no universal consensus on the best method of selecting the size of the DLT. Some studies have selected the left-sided DLT based on height and sex of the patient. Using this method, unfortunately, the appropriated size of the left-sided DLT could not be predicted in the Asian patient population.[24] Others have reported that the measurement of the tracheal diameter at the level of the clavicle on the preoperative posterior anterior chest radiograph can be used to determine proper left-sided DLT size. These methods lead to a 90% increase in the use of larger left-sided lumen tubes (i.e., 41 Fr DLT in men and 39 Fr in women).[25] However, a study involving Asian patients by Chow et al.[26] using the same methodology of Brodsky et al.[25] found this approach less reliable. In the Chow et al. study,[26] the overall positive predictive value for the proper left size of a left-sided DLT was 77% for men and 45% for women. This method and the patient's sex and height seem to have limited use in patients with smaller statures.

An interesting study by Amar et al.[27] involving thoracic anesthesiologists, has shown that the use of a smaller DLT (35 Fr left-sided DLT) rather than a conventionally large-sized DLT (i.e., 39 or 41 Fr) was not associated with any difference in clinical intraoperative outcomes, regardless of the patient size or gender in 300 patients undergoing thoracic surgery requiring lung separation. However, in their study, only 51 (35%) of the patients who received a 35 Fr DLT were males and 92 (65%) were females. In practice, women usually receive a 35 Fr DLT; therefore the question of whether or not a 35 Fr is favorable for all patients remains unclear.

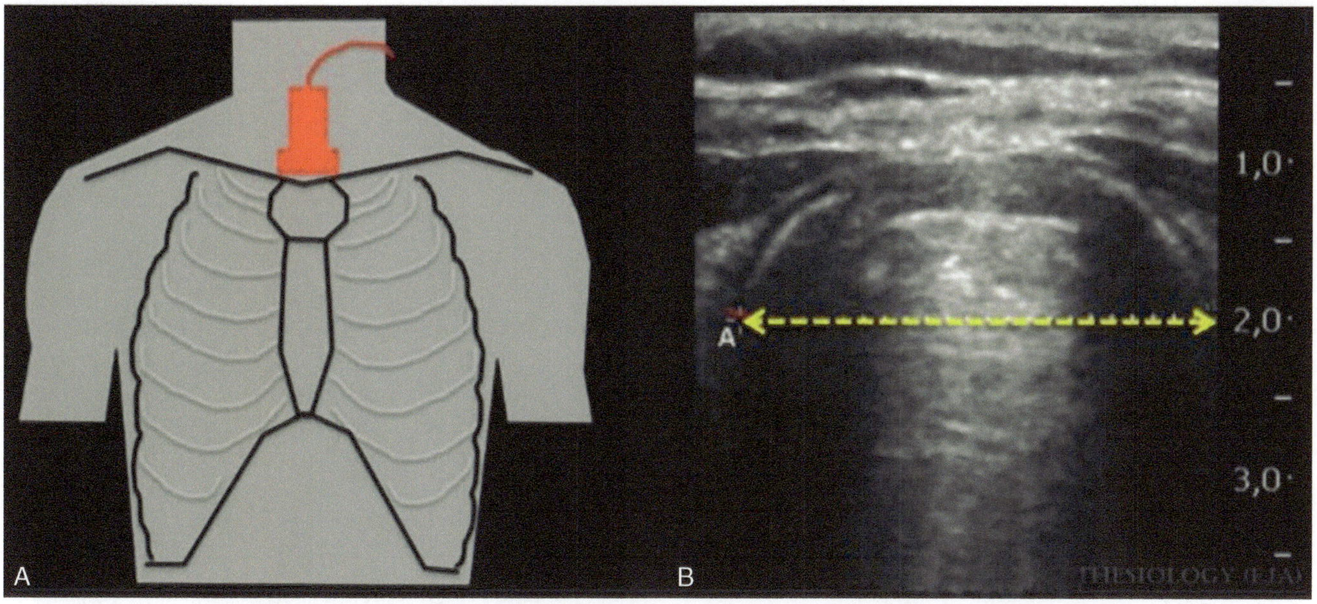

• **Fig. 16.2** Display of the tracheal ultrasound examination with the linear probe placed perpendicular to the neck (A), the outer tracheal diameter is measured on this transverse view (mm) (B). (From Roldi E, Inghileri P, Dransart-Raye O, et al. Use of tracheal ultrasound combined with clinical parameters to select left double-lumen tube size: a prospective observational study. *Eur J Anaesthesiol.* 2019;36:215–220. With permission.)

A different method to predict the proper size of a right-sided or left-sided DLT is a three-dimensional image reconstruction of tracheobronchial anatomy generated from spiral computed tomography (CT) scans combined with superimposed transparencies of DLTs.[28]

Another interesting alternative is the use of tracheal ultrasonography measurements combined with clinical parameters to select the appropriate size of a left-sided DLT. Roldi et al.[29] has combined the ultrasound measurement of the tracheal diameter with the patient lying in supine position, and the probe placed just above the sternoclavicular junction to the neck in transverse view. They were able to estimate the tracheal diameter and measure it in mm. Fig. 16.2 displays the tracheal ultrasound examination with the linear probe placed perpendicular to the neck (panel A), the outer tracheal diameter is measured on this transverse view (mm) (panel B). Their study showed that patients' height and sex, plus the use of tracheal ultrasonography to measure the tracheal diameter, optimized the proper selection of a left-sided DLT, reducing significantly the use of oversized and underside DLTs. One of the limitations with this method is that it requires expertise in tracheal ultrasonography.

The information derived from these studies suggests that chest radiographs, CT scans, and ultrasonography of the trachea are valuable tools when selecting a proper DLT size, in addition to their proven value in assessment of any abnormal tracheobronchial anatomy. These images and measurements should be reviewed before placement of a DLT. Particular emphasis should be made in viewing a posterior-anterior chest radiograph to assess the shadow of tracheobronchial anatomy along with bronchial bifurcation. It is estimated that in 75% of the films, the left mainstem bronchus shadow is seen. Fig. 16.3 shows the anatomic changes that occur in a 60-year-old man with severe chronic obstructive pulmonary disease (COPD) in which the deviated trachea and narrow bronchus can be appreciated. It is crucial to recognize any distorted anatomy identified in the film before placement of DLTs.[30]

Methods of Insertion of Double-Lumen Endotracheal Tubes

Fig. 16.4 shows the most common indications for the use of a DLT for lung separation. Two techniques are most commonly used by anesthesiologists when inserting and placing a DLT. The first is a blind technique, when the DLT is passed with direct laryngoscopy, then it is turned to the left (for a left-sided DLT) or right (for a right-sided DLT) after the endobronchial cuff has passed beyond the vocal cords. The DLT is then advanced until it reaches the depth of insertion at the teeth, which is approximately 29 cm for both men and women if the patient's height is at least 170 cm.[31] The second technique involves the use of the flexible fiberoptic bronchoscope as a guide to the selected main bronchus, where the tip of the endobronchial lumen is guided after the DLT is passed the vocal cords. A study by Boucek et al.[32] comparing the blind technique versus the fiberoptic bronchoscopy–guided technique, showed that of the 32 patients who underwent the blind technique approach, primary success occurred in 30 patients. In contrast, in the 27 patients receiving the brochoscopy-guided technique, primary success was initially achieved only in 21 patients, and eventually successfully placed in 25 patients. In addition, two

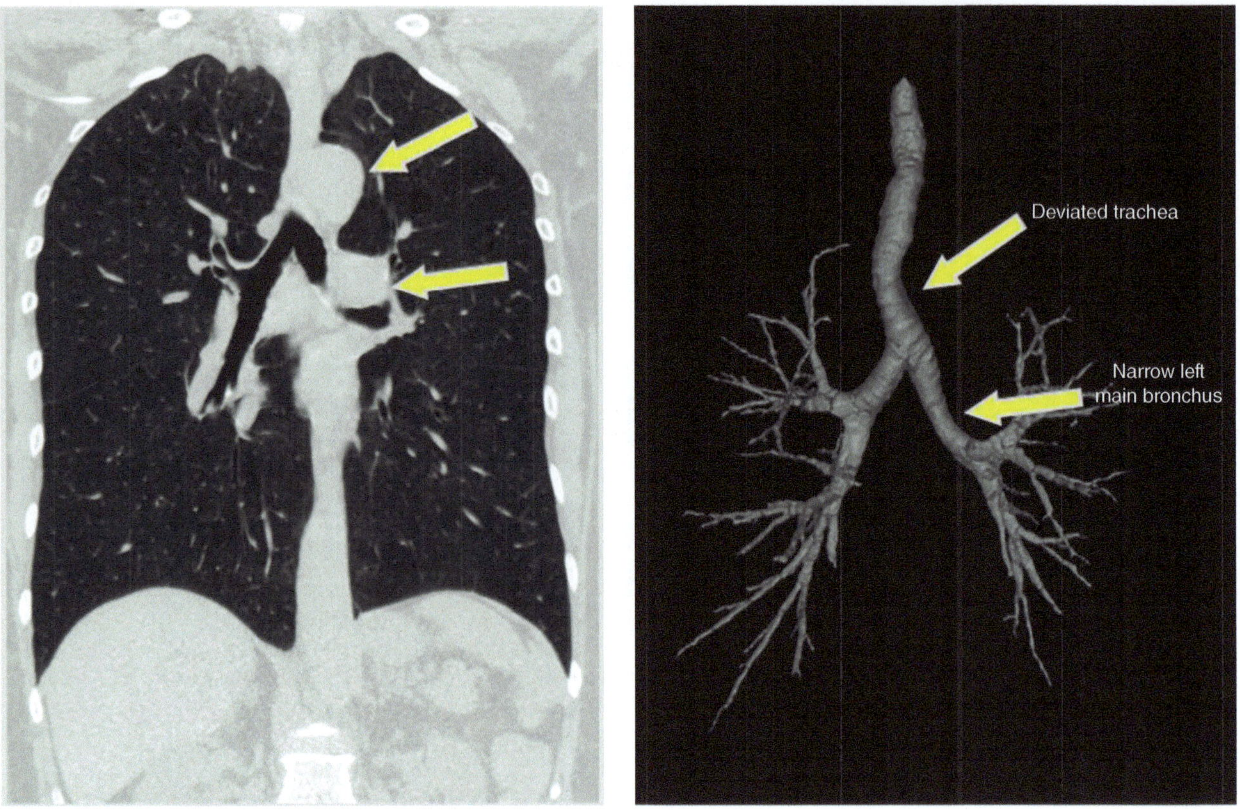

• **Fig. 16.3** Anatomic changes that occur in a 60-year-old man with severe chronic obstructive pulmonary disease, which shows a deviated trachea and narrow bronchus. (From Campos JH. Update on tracheobronchial anatomy and flexible fiberoptic bronchoscopy in thoracic anesthesia. *Curr Opin Anaesthesiol.* 2009;22:4–10. With permission.)

patients in each group required an alternative method for tube placement. Fig. 16.5A shows the blind method technique and Fig. 16.5B shows a flexible fiberoptic bronchoscopy guidance technique for placement of a left-sided DLT.

In recent years, video laryngoscopy has been introduced as an important tool in the management of patients with expected or unexpected difficult airways. Clinical studies have shown that video laryngoscopies improve visualization of laryngeal structures and facilitate insertion of DLTs at first pass.[33] In a study by Purugganan et al.,[34] the use of the C-MAC video laryngoscope has been compared with the standard Macintosh blade and with the Miller blade during DLT intubation in patients with normal airways. The authors showed that video laryngoscopy was similar to the views obtained with a Miller blade while passing a DLT. In contrast, the Macintosh blade group has reported higher

• **Fig. 16.4** The most common indications for the use of a double-lumen endotracheal tubes (*DLTs*) for lung separation. (Courtesy of Edmond Cohen M.D.)

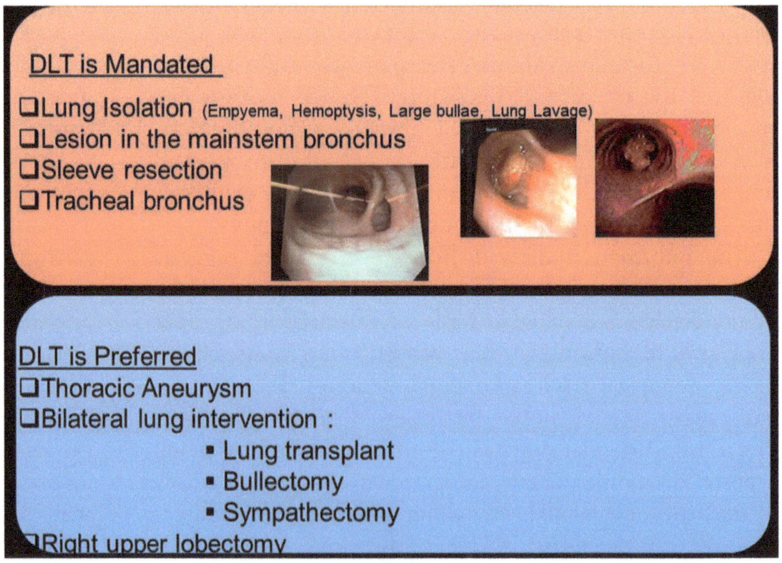

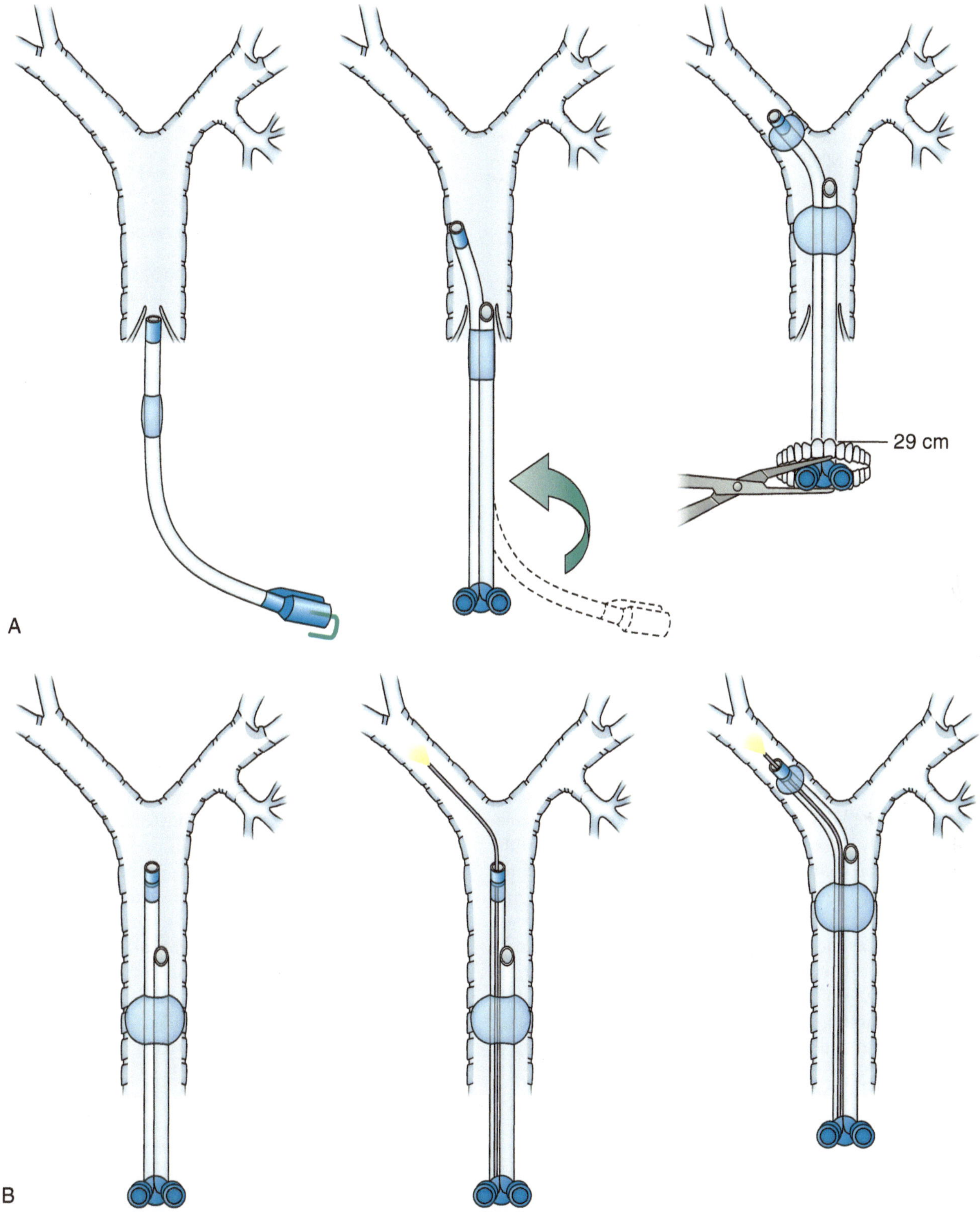

A

B

• **Fig. 16.5** (**A**) A blind technique for placing a left-sided double-lumen tube (DLT). (*Left*) The DLT is passed with direct laryngoscopy passed the vocal cords. (*Center*) The DLT is rotated 90 degrees to the left. (*Right*) The DLT is advanced into the left mainstem bronchus, with a depth at the level of the teeth approximately to the 29 cm mark of the DLT. (**B**) A fiberoptic bronchoscopy–guidance technique for placing a left-sided DLT. (*Left*) The DLT is passed with direct laryngoscopy passed the vocal cords. (*Center*) The fiberoptic bronchoscope is advanced through the endobronchial lumen. The tracheal carina and the left main stem bronchus are visualized. (*Right*) The DLT is rotated 90 degrees to the left and, with the aid of the fiberoptic bronchoscope; the tube is advanced to the optimal position into the left main stem bronchus. (From Campos JH. How to achieve successful lung separation. *SAJAA*. 2008;14:22–26. With permission.)

difficult intubations with the DLTs. Another study by Russell et al.,[35] comparing a GlideScope® with the Macintosh laryngoscope for a DLT intubation, showed that the overall rate of successful endobronchial intubation was easier with the Macintosh blade compared with the GlideScope®. In addition, the incidence of postoperative voice changes was less common in the Macintosh group, therefore the authors do not recommend the routine use of the GlideScope® for DLT insertion in patients with normal airways. In contrast, a recent study by Chastel et al.,[36] using the Airtraq DL® video laryngoscope during placement of a DLT, showed an improved exposure of the supraglottis during insertion of the DLT in patients with normal airways. In the views using the Airtraq DL® video laryngoscopy, patients were graded Cormack and Lehane I (on the Cormack-Lehane grading system), as compared with the Macintosh laryngoscopy. A recent study by El-Tahan et al.,[37] comparing the Macintosh laryngoscope blade with video laryngoscopes (GlideScope®, Airtraq®, and King Vision® video laryngoscope), showed that first pass success while passing a DLT was similar with all the four laryngoscopes studied. However, rupture of the tracheal cuff of the DLT occurred in the Macintosh, the GlideScope®, and the King® video laryngoscopes, whereas none were reported within in the Airtraq®. The incidence of sore throat was not different among the groups studied.

An interesting report was published by Liu et al.,[38] who performed a systematic review and metaanalysis of 12 studies comparing the use of video laryngoscopes versus the Macintosh laryngoscope during intubation with DLTs. They concluded that video laryngoscopy use for DLT intubation was superior to the Macintosh groups. Of interest, the authors showed an increased incidence of malposition rates at first pass of the DLT in the groups intubated with video laryngoscopy. It is possible that diverting the attention to the monitor screen contributed to the loss of orientation of the rotation of the DLT by the anesthesiologist. There is no designated stylet for a DLT. When anon channeled video laryngoscopy devices such as the GlideScope, the DLT should be curved to mimic the shape of the blade prior to intubation. Overall, the use of a video laryngoscope while inserting a DLT has a learning curve and will depend on the experience of the operator and the clinical necessity at laryngoscopy.

Left-Sided Double-Lumen Endotracheal Tubes

Left-sided DLT is the most commonly used device to achieve lung separation because it has a greater margin of safety than right-sided DLT.[39–42] The indications for a left-sided DLT include lung separation: that is, any operation that requires surgical exposure of the chest cavity with a lung collapse. Left-sided DLT is mandatory in cases of lung isolation to protect the dependent lung from a contralateral contamination, such as a lung abscess, lung cyst, pulmonary hemorrhage, or bronchopulmonary lavage. In addition, a left-sided DLT is used in cases for control and continuity of the airway gas exchange when bronchopleural fistula or giant bullae are present. Contraindication for placement, such as difficult airway or obstruction, to the entrance of the left main stem bronchus precludes the use of the left-sided DLT. Box 16.1 displays the indications and contraindications for left-sided DLT.

• BOX 16.1 Displays the Indications and Contraindications for Left-Sided Double-Lumen Tubes

Indications of Left-Sided Double-Lumen Tubes

Any operation that requires surgical exposure through the chest cavity with lung collapse:

- Prevention of and protection from contamination of contralateral lung (lung abscess or cyst, pulmonary hemorrhage or bronchoalveolar lavage)
- Control and continuity of the airway gas exchange (i.e., bronchopleural fistula)
- Application of differential lung ventilation (i.e., positive-end expiratory pressure [PEEP] to the dependent lung and continuous positive airway pressure [CPAP] or apneic oxygen insufflation to the nondependent lung)[41]

Contraindications of Left-Sided Double-Lumen Tubes

- Any double-lumen tube size that cannot be passed through the glottis
- Any obstruction, compression, or absence of left mainstem bronchus
- Any patient that has a fresh tracheostomy in place

Placement Technique for a Left-Sided Double-Lumen Endotracheal Tube

Placement and positioning of a left-sided DLT can be accomplished with either of the following techniques: the blind technique in which the left-sided DLT is passed beyond the vocal cords (endobronchial cuff) and the tube is rotated 90 degrees counterclockwise and advanced until the tip of the tube enters the left mainstem bronchus, or the bronchoscopy guidance technique, in which the endobronchial tip is passed beyond the vocal cords and guided with the aid of the fiberoptic bronchoscope into the entrance of the left mainstem bronchus. The optimal position for a left-sided DLT is confirmed with the fiberoptic bronchoscopy through the tracheal lumen to observe a fully inflated endobronchial cuff with no more than 3 mL of air located at least 5 to 10 mm below the tracheal carina inside the left mainstem bronchus. The second important view is the endobronchial bronchoscopy view, where the fiberoptic bronchoscope is advanced inside the endobronchial lumen and the patency of the lumen is observed before advancing the bronchoscope through the blue portion of the tube; the next view is at the distal end of the endobronchial tip of the tube, where a clear and unobstructed view of bronchial carina with the left upper and left lower lobe bronchus entrance orifices visualized distally. It is important to recognize tracheobronchial anatomy with the fiberoptic bronchoscope to ensure a successful placement of the left-sided DLT.

To identify which is the right mainstem bronchus while placing a left-sided DLT, the fiberoptic bronchoscope is advanced through the tracheal lumen below the main tracheal

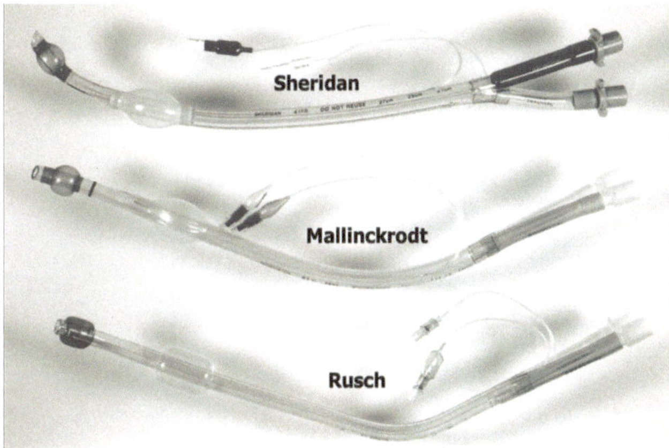

• **Fig. 16.6** The most commonly used double-lumen tubes.

carina to the right side approximately 1 to 2 cm, at which point the orifice of the right upper lobe (RUL) bronchus is seen at 3 to 4 o'clock on the lateral wall. By advancing the fiberoptic bronchoscope inside the right upper bronchus, it should display a clear view of three orifices (apical, anterior, and posterior segments). This is the only structure of the tracheobronchial tree that has three orifices.[42] Identifying the RUL orifice should be part of the routine bronchoscopy in thoracic anesthesia because, with secretion and in the lateral position, it not always easy to recognize the proper cranial orientation. Fig. 16.6 shows the most commonly used DLT. Fig. 16.7 shows the optimal position of the left-sided DLT as seen with a fiberoptic bronchoscope. Fig. 16.8 shows the correct position where the semilunar blue cuff is in view at the carina and the incorrect position in which that cuff edge is not seen by the fiberoptic bronchoscope.

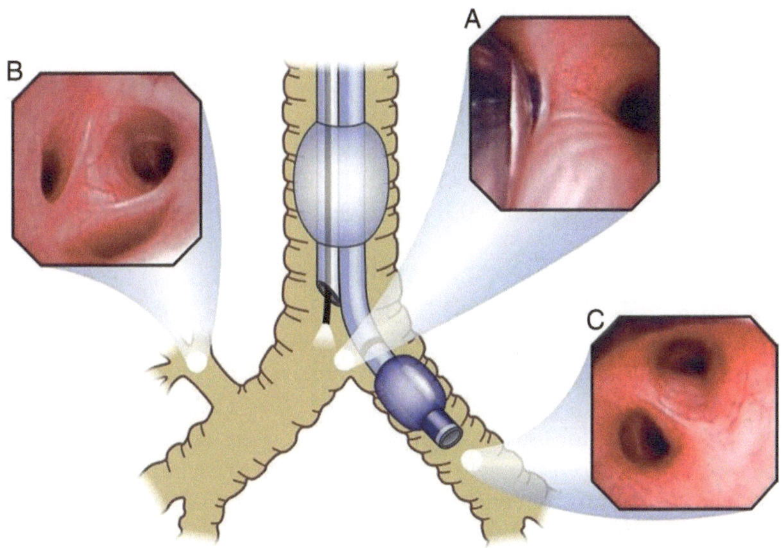

• **Fig. 16.7** The optimal position of the left-sided double-lumen tube (DLT), as seen with a fiberoptic bronchoscope. (**A**) View from the tracheal lumen of the unobstructed entrance of the right b mainstem bronchus. (**B**) View from the tracheal lumen of the right upper bronchus. (**C**) View from the bronchial lumen of the left upper (above) and left lower (below) lobe bronchi. (From Campos JH. Current techniques for perioperative lung isolation in adults. *Anesthesiology*. 2002;97:1295–1301. With permission.)

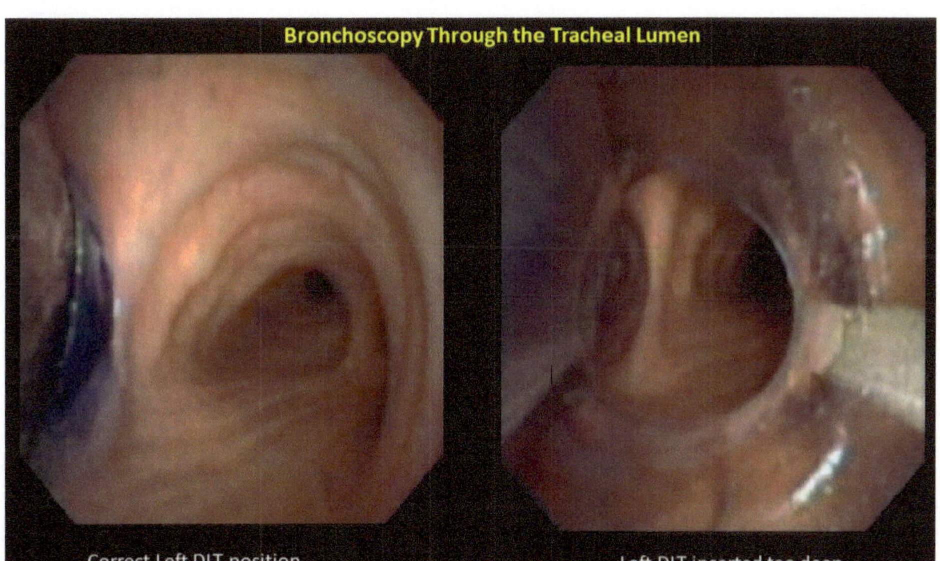

• **Fig. 16.8** The correct position where the semilunar blue cuff is in view at the carina and the incorrect position in which that cuff edge is not seen by the fiberoptic bronchoscope. *DLT,* Double-lumen tube.

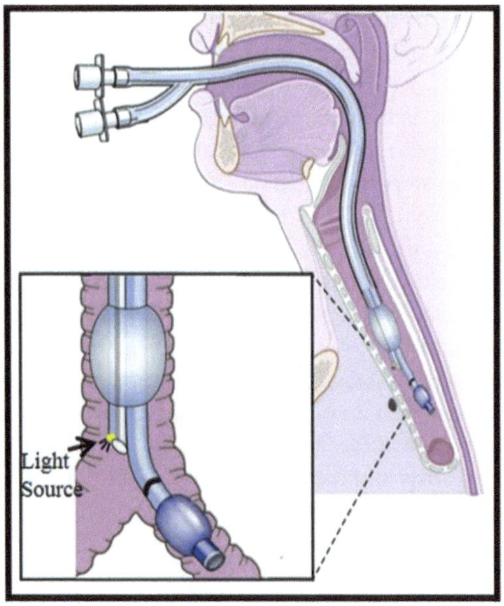

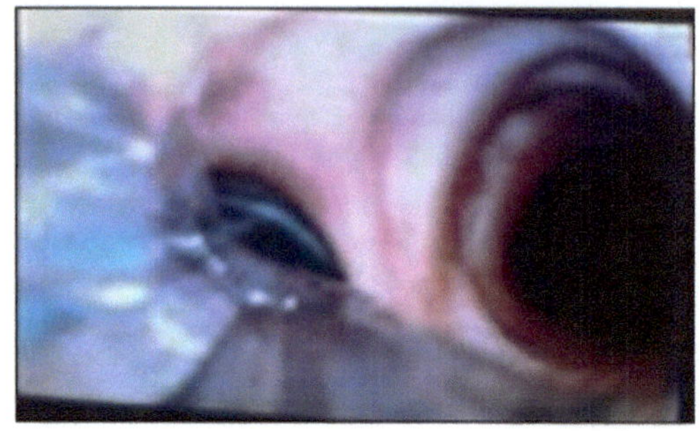

• **Fig. 16.9** A left-sided VivaSight DLT® along with an image of the optimal position when connected to a monitor camera. *DLT,* Double-lumen tube. (From Campos JH, Hanada S. DLT with incorporated fiberoptic bronchoscopy. In: Rosenblatt WH, et al. *Master Techniques in Upper and Lower Airway Management.* Lippincott Williams and Wilkins; 2015:250–251. With permission.)

VivaSight Double-Lumen Tube

ETView Medical (Ambu) has designed a new device, the VivaSight DLT, with an integrated high-resolution camera. This camera is embedded at the end of the endotracheal lumen that is connected to a monitor screen, which allows a continuous view of the tracheal carina. In addition, this DLT device has an integrated flushing system that allows for in situ camera lens cleaning.[43] The main advantage of the VivaSight DLT is that it allows a continuous view of the DLT position and immediately corrects any DLT malpositions at the level of the tracheal carina.[44] To maintain a good visualization with the VivaSight camera, it is recommended that a defogging solution be used before insertion.[45] Fig. 16.9 shows the VivaSight DLT system and a monitor view. In a prospective single-center study by Massot et al.,[46] of the 76 patients included in the study, 99% had correct position of the VivaSight DLT after intubation; however, malposition was present in 40 patients (53%) intraoperatively. These malpositions were easily corrected by the embedded camera of the VivaSight DLT view without the need of a flexible fiberoptic bronchoscope.

Levy-Faber et al.,[47] in a prospective study of 71 adult patients, compared intubation times using either the VivaSight DL or a conventional double-lumen tube. Median duration of intubation with visual confirmation of tube position was significantly reduced using the VivaSight DL compared with the conventional double-lumen tube 51 (42–60 [35–118]) seconds versus 264 (233–325 [160–490]) seconds, respectively ($P < .0001$). None of the patients allocated to the VivaSight DL required fiberoptic bronchoscopy during intubation or surgery. They concluded that the VivaSight DL enables significantly more rapid intubation compared with the conventional double-lumen tube.

One of the limitations of the VivaSight is the presence of secretions on the tip of the camera; using a suction channel and flushing it with normal saline will in part alleviate the problems. Unfortunately, all previous studies have shown more hoarseness and discomfort with the use of the VivaSight DLT. The practitioner should be aware that connecting the camera for prolonged periods of time in vitro may lead to melting the portion of the tube near the light source.[47] The VivaSight DLT is only available for a left-sided DLT version and is placed similar to a conventional DLT.

Right-Sided Double-Lumen Endotracheal Tubes

There are specific clinical situations in which the use of a right-sided DLT is indicated. Box 16.2 lists the indication for use of a right-sided DLT. The anatomic differences between the right and left mainstem bronchus are reflected in fundamentally different designs of the right-sided and left-sided DLTs. Because the right mainstem bronchus is shorter than the left bronchus, and because the RUL bronchus originates at a distance of 1.5 to 2.0 cm from the carina, techniques using right endobronchial intubation must take into account the location and potential obstruction of the orifice of the RUL bronchus. The right-sided DLT incorporates

• BOX 16.2 Right-Sided Double-Lumen Tube

Indications of Right-Sided Double-Lumen Tubes

- Any contraindication to placement of a left-sided double-lumen tube
- Distorted anatomy of the entrance of left mainstem bronchus by an intrabronchial or external compression
- Compression of the entrance of the left mainstem bronchus because of a descending thoracic aortic aneurysm
- Left lung transplantation
- Left-sided sleeve resection
- Left-sided pneumonectomy

Contraindications of Right-Sided Double-Lumen Tubes

- Any anomalous take of the right upper lobe bronchus emerging above the tracheal carina

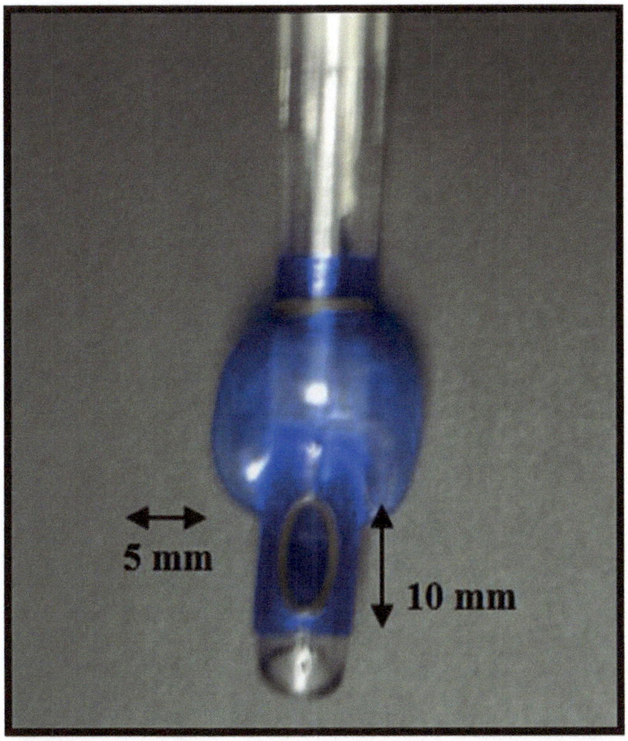

• **Fig. 16.10** A Mallinckrodt right-sided double-lumen tube. An orifice designated to facilitate ventilation of the right upper lobe bronchus.

a modified cuff with a ventilating opening orifice that rides off the orifice of the RUL that allows ventilation of the RUL. Fig. 16.10 displays the Mallinckrodt right-side DLT.

Ehrenfeld et al.[48] retrospectively reviewed thoracic surgical anesthetics automated anesthesia information management systems, comparing the frequency of right- and left-sided Mallinckrodt tube use by thoracic anesthesiologists. They examined the incidence, duration, and severity of hypoxemia (oxygen saturation [SpO_2] < 90%), hypercapnia (end-tidal carbon dioxide [EtCO2] > 45 mm Hg), and high airway pressures (peak inspiratory pressure > 35 cm H_2O) for lung and chest wall surgery patients. Right- (n = 241) and left- (n = 450) sided tubes were almost exclusively used on the side contralateral to surgery. There were no differences in the incidence or duration of hypoxemia, hypercarbia, or high airway pressures.

Because of the additional orifice on the right-sided DLT to allow ventilation through the RUL bronchus, the right-sided DLT requires a precise optimal placement. To increase the margin of safety of the right-sided Broncho-Cath DLT, the opening slot of the ventilating orifice for the right upper bronchus lobe has been widened and consists of an enlarged area of the lateral orifice, this modification has increased the alignment between the opening slot and the RUL bronchus.[49]

Placement Technique for a Right-Sided Double-Lumen Endotracheal Tube

The preferred technique for placement of a right-sided DLT is with the fiberoptic bronchoscopy-guidance technique. After the right-sided DLT is passed beyond the vocal cords under direct laryngoscopy, the fiberoptic bronchoscope is advanced through the endobronchial lumen. Before advancing the DLT, the tracheal carina, the entrance of the right mainstem bronchus, and the entrance of the RUL bronchus are identified, then the DLT is rotated 90 degrees to the right and advanced with the aid of the fiberoptic bronchoscope. The optimal position of a right-sided DLT is one that provides good alignment between the endobronchial lumen opening slot and visualizes the three segments of the RUL bronchus. A clear view of the bronchus intermedius and the right lower lobe bronchus should be seen from the endobronchial lumen. From the tracheal view, the optimal position for a right-sided DLT provides a view of the edge of the blue cuff of the endobronchial balloon when inflated just below tracheal carina and a full view of the entrance of the left mainstem bronchus. Fig. 16.11 shows the optimal position of a right-sided DLT seen from the endobronchial or endotracheal view with a fiberoptic bronchoscope.

Auscultation, Flexible Fiberoptic Bronchoscopy, and Ultrasonography When Placing Double-Lumen Endotracheal Tubes

Evidence strongly suggests that auscultation alone may be unreliable for confirmation of proper DLT placement. However, the basic principle of auscultation and clamping maneuvers while testing the proper placement of a DLT must be routinely applied before the use of fiberoptic bronchoscopy. For a left-sided DLT, the endobronchial lumen should be placed below the tracheal carina into the left mainstem bronchus, the depth of tube in a 170 cm tall subject should be approximately 29 cm at the level of the teeth. With both DLT cuffs inflated clamping the limb connector of the tracheal lumen should reveal the absence of breath sounds in the right side of the chest (right hemothorax). If both lungs are being ventilated, the bronchial lumen is too shallow above the carina. After this maneuver is completed, the next step is to ventilate both lungs. Then clamping the limb connector of the endobronchial lumen should reveal the absence of breath sounds on the left side of the chest (left hemothorax). If these maneuvers are unsuccessful, or confusion ensues with breath sounds and the location of the DLT, a fiberoptic bronchoscopy examinations takes precedent. In a study by Klein et al.,[50] 200 patients were intubated by the blind technique and confirmation of placement of the DLTs was initially done by auscultation, following clamping of one of the ports of the connector of the DLT. A second anesthesiologist with expertise in flexible fiberoptic bronchoscopy reconfirming the placement of the DLT, showed that 35% of the tubes placed were mispositioned with auscultation alone. All detected malpositions were eventually corrected with the use of fiberoptic bronchoscopy.

A study by Campos et al.[51] involving nonthoracic anesthesiologists with very limited experience in lung separation techniques, showed that when placing lung isolation

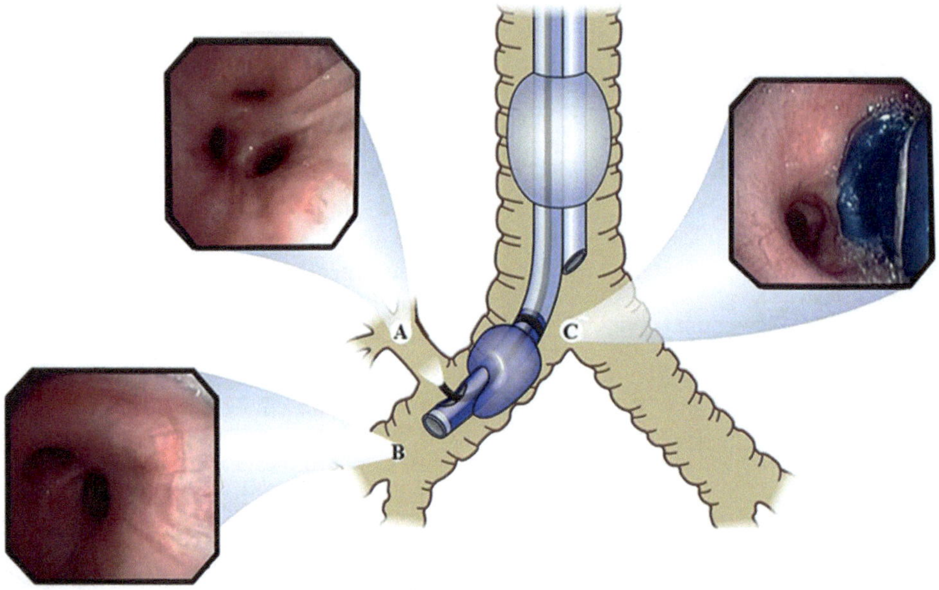

• **Fig. 16.11** The optimal position of a right-sided double-lumen endotracheal tube. (**A**) Shows the take-off of the right-upper bronchus with three segments (apical, anterior, and posterior) when the fiberoptic bronchoscope emerges from the opening slot located in the endobronchial lumen. (**B**) Shows an unobstructed view of the entrance of the right middle and right lower lobe bronchus when the fiberscope is passed through the endobronchial lumen. (**C**) Shows a view of tracheal carina to the right edge of the blue balloon fully inflated, to the left, an unobstructed view of the entrance of the left-mainstem bronchus when the fiberscope is advanced through the tracheal lumen. (From Campos J. Lung isolation. In: Slinger P, ed. *Principles and Practice of Anesthesia for Thoracic Surgery*. Switzerland: Springer Nature; 2019:283–309. With permission.)

devices (DLTs or bronchial blockers), there was a 38% incidence in unrecognized malpositions even when these devices were placed with the fiberoptic bronchoscope. The possible cause was lack of skills with fiberoptic bronchoscopy and lack of recognition of tracheobronchial anatomy.

Fiberoptic bronchoscopy is essential and mandatory to achieve 100% success in placement and positioning of DLTs, as long as the anesthesiologist is able to recognize proper tracheobronchial anatomy and possesses skills with flexible fiberoptic bronchoscopy. In another study by de Bellis et al.[52] involving thoracic anesthesiologists, 104 patients were intubated with a left-sided DLT, and they confirmed the optimal position of the DLT initially by using auscultation only. An endoscopist with experience in flexible fiberoptic bronchoscopy was asked to confirm the optimal and proper position after auscultation, and this showed that in 37% of the patients, there were unrecognized malpositions while placing the DLT. All the malpositions were easily corrected with the use of flexible fiberoptic bronchoscopy. This study clearly demonstrates that even experienced thoracic anesthesiologists cannot rely on the optimal position of the DLT with just auscultation; therefore flexible fiberoptic bronchoscopy must be used to obtain optimal position.[53] Table 16.2 displays the role of flexible fiberoptic bronchoscopy and DLTs.

TABLE 16.2 Displays the Role of Flexible Fiberoptic Bronchoscopy and Double-Lumen Tubes

Author	*n*	End Points	Outcome
Klein et al.[50] *Anesthesiology.* 1998;88:346–350	• 200 L-R DLTs (prospective)	Auscultation/clamping (2nd anesthesiologist) FOB	• 35% malposition • FOB all malpositions corrected
Bellis et al.[52] *Eur J Cardiothorac Surg.* 2011;40:912–916	• *n* = 104 pts, L-DLTs (prospective)	Auscultation/clamping (endoscopist) FOB	• 37% unrecognized malpositions • FOB all corrected
Campos et al.[115] *Euro J Anaesthesiol.* 2011;28:169–174	• *n* = 60 pts, DLTs • *n* = 27 nonthoracic anesth (prospective)	Anesthesia Simulator or Computer DVD training	• 23% unrecognized malpositions • Failed placements with FOB

DLT, double-lumen endotracheal tube; *FOB*, fiberoptic bronchoscopy; *L*, left; *R*, right.

Use of Ultrasonography in the Assessment of Double-Lumen Endotracheal Tube Position and Function

Ultrasonography has been widely used in various aspects of airway management. Previous studies have applied lung ultrasound signs like lung sliding and lung pulse in assessment of regional distribution of ventilation and have reported that lung ultrasonography is a noninvasive technique and effective to confirm lung separation following a DLT placement.[54]

In a study by Álvarez-Díaz et al.,[55] the authors compared the ability of lung ultrasound and a clinical method in the confirmation of a selective bronchial intubation by left double-lumen tube in elective thoracic surgery. Some 105 consecutive patients were included. After blind intubation, the position of the tube was confirmed by clinical and ultrasound assessment. Ultrasound confirmation was obtained by visualizing lung sliding, diaphragmatic movements, and the appearance of lung pulse sign. Finally, the authors' bronchoscopy confirmation as a reference standard was used to confirm the position of the tube. The sensitivity of the clinical method was 84.5%, with a specificity of 41.1%. The sensitivity of the ultrasound method was 98.6%, specificity was 52.9%, They concluded that lung ultrasound was superior to the clinical method in confirming the adequate position of the left double-lumen tube. On the other hand, in confirming the misplacement of the tube, differences between both methods could not be ensured.

A prospective, randomized controlled study by Parab et al.[56] involving 100 patients, comparing auscultation and lung ultrasonography in the assessment of DLT position in thoracic patients requiring OLV, showed that the lung ultrasonography group ($n = 44$) compared with the auscultation group ($n = 47$) had a significantly higher sensitivity (94.1% vs. 73.3%) and improved accuracy in the assessment of the DLT position for confirmation of lung separation, and that ultrasonography is a better complimentary technique for fiberoptic bronchoscopy when compared with auscultation alone.

Hu et al.[57] evaluated 103 patients requiring the use of a DLT, and compared the point-of-care via ultrasonography versus auscultation to determine the optimal position of the DLT in a supine and lateral decubitus position. The sequence of this study included auscultation, followed by ultrasonography of the lung (by a different researcher), and finally examination by flexible fiberoptic bronchoscopy. The results of the study showed that the accuracy of ultrasonography compared with auscultation was 84% versus 59% for a left-sided DLT. When a right-sided DLT was used, the accuracy of ultrasonography was 89% in comparison to auscultation at 67.4% in supine position. The authors concluded that the assessment via point-of-care ultrasonography of the lung is superior to auscultation in determining the position of DLTs.

When using ultrasonography in the lung to assess ventilation, the lung sliding sign can be recognized, as the visceral and parietal pleura slide over each other during ventilation, indicating ventilation of the lung. When the **sliding sign** is abolished, it indicates absence of ventilation on the hemithorax. In addition, the pulsatile movement is apparent at the pleural interface. This pulsatile movement is a sign of lung collapse. In addition, when the ultrasound probe is switched to M-mode, two observations can be made. One is the **seashore sign** along with pleura gliding that indicates ventilation in the lung. In contrast, a **barcode sign** along with a sign of no pleural gliding indicates no ventilation to the lung. This ultrasonography examination of the chest can be done with the use of a linear probe at different reference points in the chest between the second and fourth intercostal space in the midclavicular line and between the fifth and sixth intercostal space in the anterior axillary line. The limitations in the use of ultrasonography include that it requires an expertise on lung ultrasonography, In addition, patients with severe COPD, pleural adhesions, or morbid obesity, present difficulties to accurately perform a lung scan. These two studies previously recommend that the use of ultrasonography of the lung should be used as a complementary method and not a replacement of fiberoptic bronchoscopy examination to enhance the optimal position of DLTs. Fig. 16.12A shows an ultrasound examination of the lung. The pleura sling sign evaluated from the motion of the pleura and the sliding sign show the movement between the parietal pleural and visceral pleura. In Fig. 16.12B, the M-mode ultrasound shows a seashore sign indicating ventilation of a the lung. Fig. 16.12C shows absence of a sliding sign in the pleura, and Fig. 16.12D shows an M-mode bar code image indicating no ventilation.

Newer Technology With Double-Lumen Endotracheal Tubes

Fuji Systems in Tokyo, Japan has introduced the Silbroncho DLT, which is made of silicone material. The unique characteristic of this device relies on the wire-reinforced endobronchial tip to prevent collapse or kinking and collapse of the left mainstem bronchus because of external compression. The short endobronchial cuff tip can provide a greater margin of safety to avoid obstruction of the left upper lobe bronchus. Because of its short endobronchial tip, this tube needs to be inserted 20 mm below the tracheal carina into the left mainstem bronchus, so the outer balloon of the endobronchial lumen is seen below the tracheal carina, to prevent dislodgement of the tube. One advantage of the tube is the ability to prevent kinking and obstruction of the bronchial lumen when the takeoff of the left main bronchus (LMB) is at a 90-degree angle. That type of orientation can be seen in patients who have had a left upper lobectomy previously and are present for a redo procedure. The lower left lobe will expand upward to occupy the empty space, resulting in upward rotation of the LMB. A right- and left-sided Silbroncho® are currently available.[5,58]

A recent study by Kwon et al.[5] involving 108 patients requiring OLV, comparing a displacement of the polyvinyl chloride ($n = 54$) and silicone Silbroncho left-sided DLT ($n = 54$) during lateral positioning, showed that both DLTs produced

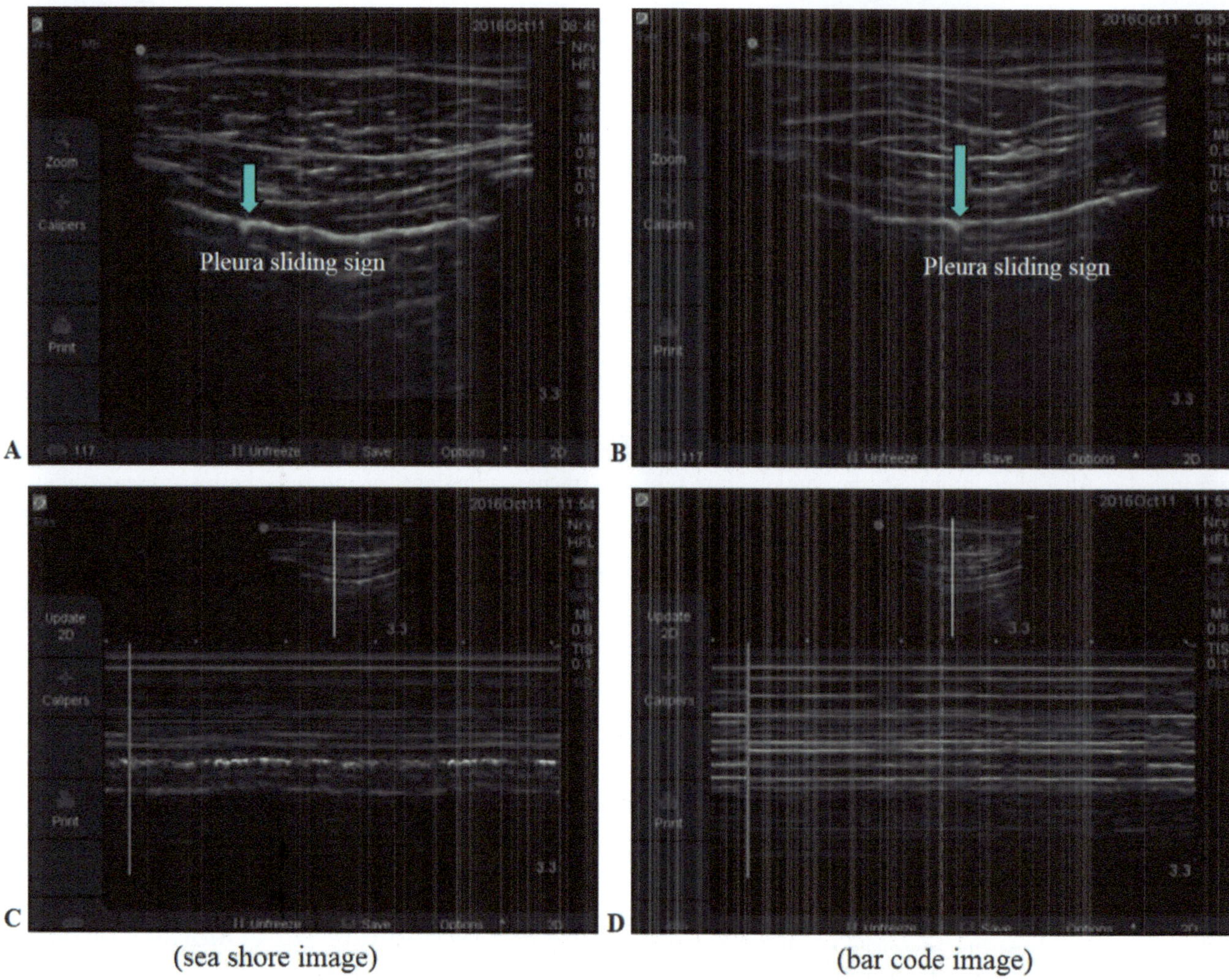

• **Fig. 16.12** (A) An ultrasound examination of the lung. The pleura sling sign evaluated from the motion of the pleura. The sliding sign shows the movement between the parietal pleural and visceral pleura. (B) The M-mode ultrasound shows a seashore sign, indicating ventilation of the lung. (C) Absence of sliding sign in the pleura. (D) M-mode bar code image, indicating no ventilation. (From Hu WC, Xu L, Zhang Q, et al. Point-of-care ultrasound versus auscultation in determining the position of double-lumen tube. *Medicine*. 2018;97:e9311. With permission.)

comparable incidence of clinically significant displacement (DLT group 35.4% vs. Silbroncho group 34.6%) and both devices required similar rates of reposition for successful lung separation after lateral position. Therefore there is no advantage to using conventional left-sided DLT versus left-sided Silbroncho DLT® during OLV. The sizes of the Silbroncho DLT include 33 Fr, 35 Fr, 37 Fr, and 39 Fr. Fig. 16.13A shows a left-sided Silbroncho DLT®; this is a wire-reinforced DLT. Fig. 16.13B shows a right-sided Silbroncho DLT®.

A relatively new DLT called the VivaSight DLT® has an integrated high-resolution camera. The camera is embedded at the end of the endotracheal lumen, which is connected to an external video monitor that allows continuous visualization of the tracheal carina and the blue cuff of the endobronchial lumen, of the DLT.[43] The advantage of this VivaSight DLT® is that the image is displayed in real time allowing the continuous monitoring of the position of the DLT and which can be advantageous on robotic thoracic surgical cases, spine surgery requiring OLV, or prone position patients where access to the airway can be limited. This device can provide improvement in patient safety because of continuous monitor DLT positions. Limitation of the use of the VivaSight DLT® includes that the light source can be obscured by secretions. However, this device has an extra channel that allows saline or air to clean the lens.[45]

The ECOM-DLT: Endotracheal Cardiac Output Monitor (ECOM Medical, Inc., San Juan Capistrano, CA) is another new generation of DLT. It contains multiple flexible sensible electrodes on the cuff and the tube that continuously measure the bioimpedance signal from the ascending aorta, in close proximity to the trachea. This device when connected to the ECOM monitor, in conjunction with an arterial catheter, provides continues cardiac output measurements (Fig. 16.14). This new ECOM-DLT has not been compared with other technology; however, based on the original ECOM ETT, using a single lumen ECOM tube appears to be promising to derive hemodynamic parameters if used in thoracic surgical patients.[59]

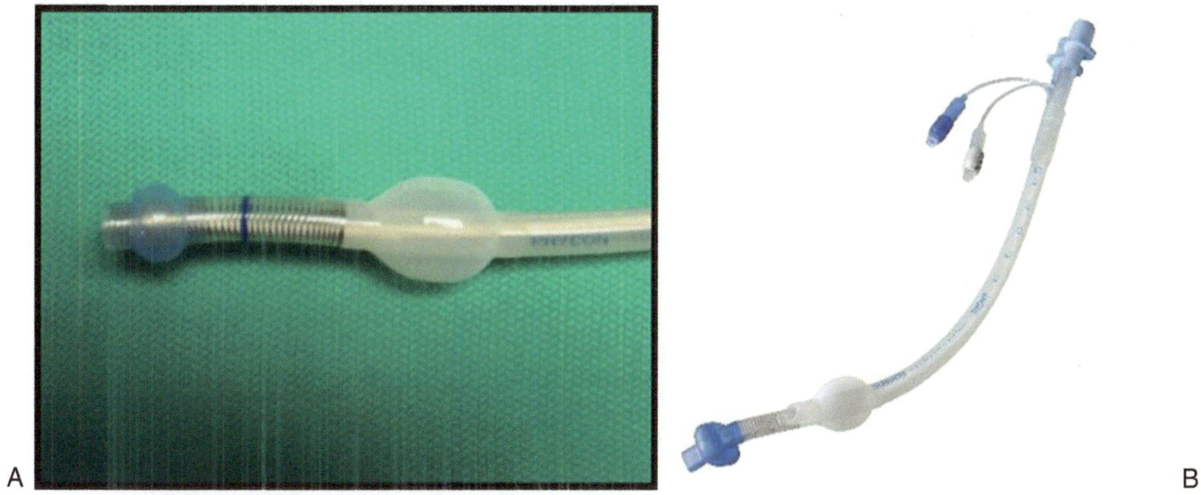

• **Fig. 16.13** (**A**) A left-sided Silbroncho DLT®. This is a wire-reinforced double-lumen tube (DLT). (**B**) A right-sided Silbroncho DLT®.

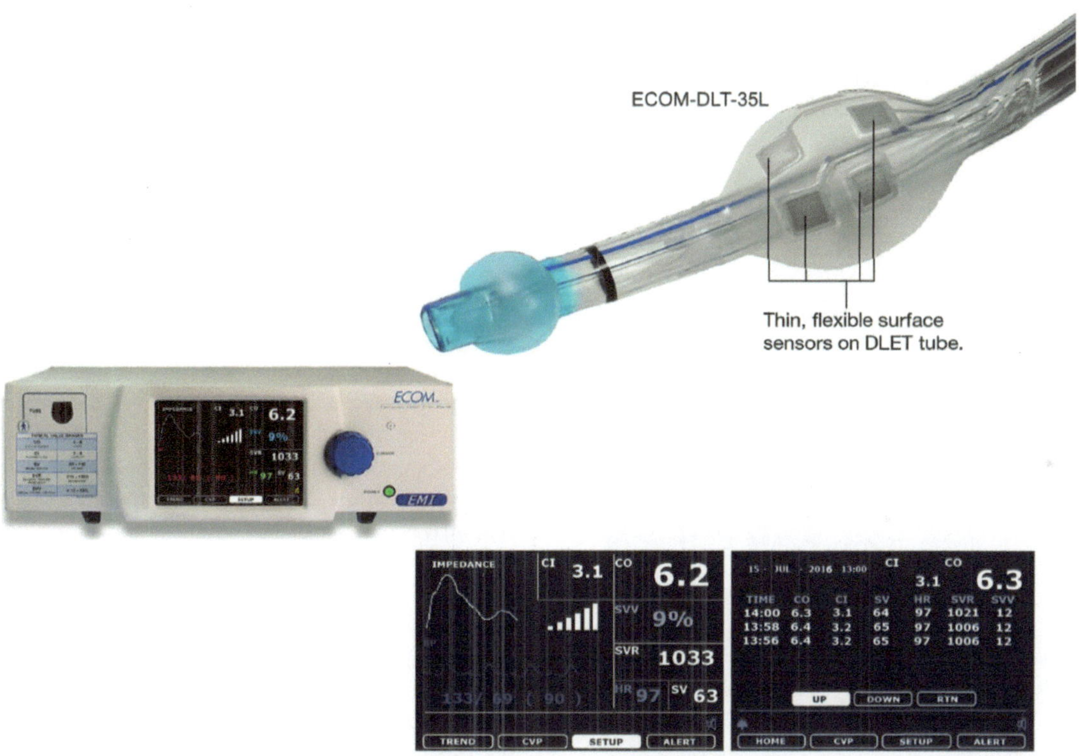

• **Fig. 16.14** The ECOM-DLT has multiple electrodes on the cuff and the tube that continuously measure the bioimpedance signal from the ascending aorta with measurements of cardiac output. *DLT*, Double-lumen tube. (From Slinger PD, Campos JH. Anesthesia for thoracic surgery. In: Miller MD, et al., eds. *Miller's Anesthesia*. ed 9. Saunders; 2020:1648–1716. With permission.)

The Cliny Right-Sided Double-Lumen Endotracheal Tube

There is a newly designed right-sided DLT, the Cliny® (Create Medic Co., Ltd. Yokohmam, Japan). This DLT has a long oblique bronchial cuff and two ventilation slots to facilitate ventilation of the RUL bronchus. The proximal part of the bronchial cuff is located immediately opposite the tracheal orifice. The Cliny® DLT can be useful in patients with a very short right mainstem bronchus.[60] Fig. 16.15 displays the Cliny® right-sided DLT.

The Papworth BiVent tube (P3 Medical, Bristol, UK) is essentially a divided single-lumen tube that rides on the carina and contains a premeasured blocker intended to be inserted into the operative side (not yet approved for use in the United States). Fig. 16.16 displays the Papworth BiVent tube[61], a disposable red rubber Robertshaw design DLT that mimics the old red rubber nondisposable DLT, which were less likely to

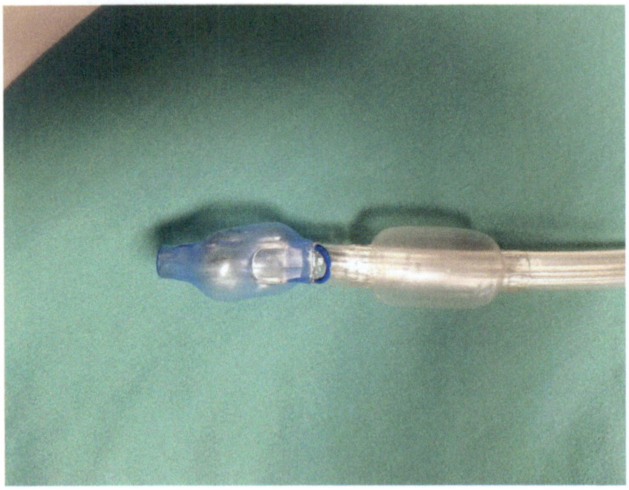

• **Fig. 16.15** The Cliny® right-sided double-lumen tube.

move intraoperatively (P3 Medical, Bristol, UK). Fig. 16.17 displays a disposable red rubber Robertshaw design DLT.

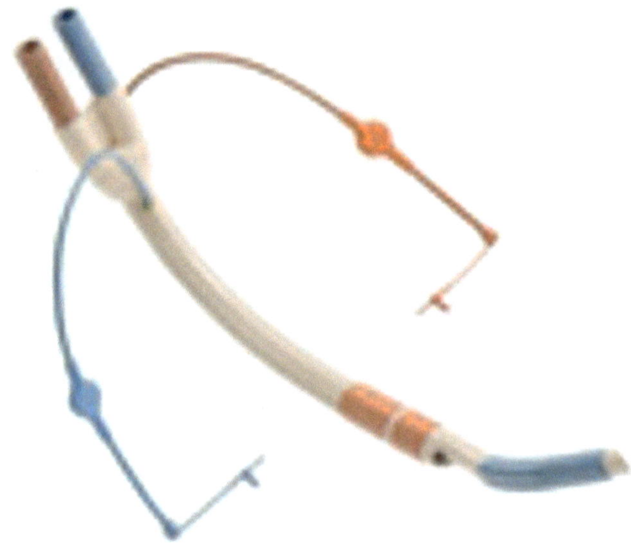

• **Fig. 16.17** A disposable red rubber Robertshaw design double-lumen tube.

Complications Associated With Double-Lumen Endotracheal Tube Placement

The most common problems and complications from the use of DLTs are malpositions and airway trauma. A mispositioned DLT will fail to provide collapse of the lung, causing gas trapping during positive pressure ventilation, or it may partially collapse the ventilated or dependent lung, producing hypoxemia. A common cause of malposition is dislodgement of the endobronchial cuff because of overinflation, surgical manipulation of the bronchus, or extension of the head and neck during or after patient positioning.[62]

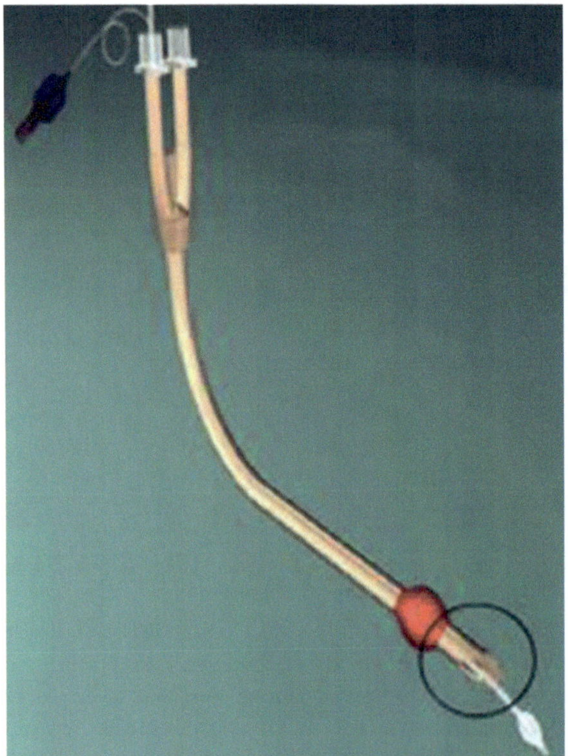

• **Fig. 16.16** The Papworth BiVvent tube. (From Ghosh S, Falter F, Klein AA, Arrowsmith JE. The Papworth BiVent tube: initial clinical experience. *J Cardiothorac Vasc Anesth*. 2011;25:505–508.)

Airway trauma and rupture of the membranous part of the trachea or the bronchus continue to be infrequent problems with the insertion of the DLTs or during reposition of patient in lateral decubitus position.[63,64] These complications can occur, for the most part, during insertion and placement while the case is in progress, or during extubation.[65–67] Another problem that has been reported is the development of bilateral pneumothoraces or a tension pneumothorax in the dependent, ventilated lung.[68,69] A 25-year review of the literature by Fitzmaurice and Brodsky[70] found that most airway injuries were associated with undersized DLTs, particularly in women who received a 35 Fr disposable DLT. It is likely that airway damage occurs when an undersized DLT migrates distally into the bronchus, advancing the large tracheal DLT body into the bronchus, producing lacerations or rupture of the airway. Airway damage during the use of DLTs can present as unexpected air leaks, subcutaneous emphysema, massive bleeding into the lumen of the DLT, or protrusion of the endotracheal or endobronchial cuff into the surgical field, with direct visualization by the surgeon. If any of the aforementioned problems occur, a bronchoscopic examination should be performed and surgical repair performed.

Benign complications with the use of the DLT have been reported by Knoll et al.[71] In their comparative study between the DLT and the endobronchial blocker, the development of postoperative hoarseness occurred significantly more commonly in the DLT group compared with the endobronchial blocker group; however, the incidence of bronchial injuries was comparable between groups. A systemic review and metaanalysis of randomized controlled trials of 10 years by Clayton-Smith et al.[39] compared the efficacy and adverse effects of DLTs and bronchial blockers in thoracic surgery. They showed that it took slightly longer to position the endobronchial blockers and how the time it took to achieve lung collapse, and the quality of the lung collapse, were similar to that of a DLT. DLTs were associated with more patients having a

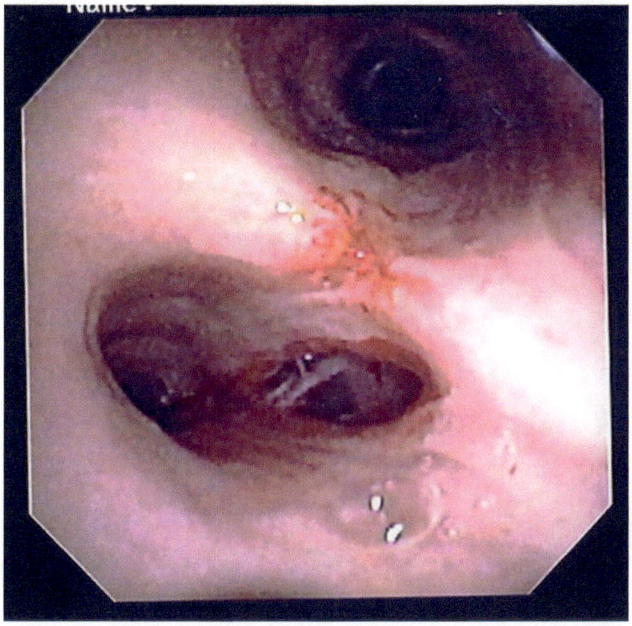

• **Fig. 16.18** An injury of the proximal section of the left main bronchus from left double-lumen tube insertion. (Courtesy of Edmond Cohen MD.)

sore throat and hoarseness and more minor airway injuries. Fig. 16.18 displays an injury of the proximal section of the left main bronchus from left DLT insertion.

In addition, a study on lung isolation for thoracic surgery comparing DLTs with bronchial blockers (Coopdech®, Arndt®, Univent®) in an Asian patient population, reported that the incidence of sore throat or hoarseness was less in the blocker group.[72] A prospective randomized study has shown that the use of dexamethasone 0.1 or 0.2 mg·kg is beneficial before the use of the DLT to reduce the incidence of sore throat and hoarseness up to 24 hours.[73]

Bronchial Blockers

An alternative method to achieve lung separation involves blockage of a mainstem bronchus to allow lung collapse distal to the occlusion.[10] Bronchial blockers can also be used selectively to achieve lobar collapse if needed.[74–78] Currently, there are several bronchial blockers clinically available to facilitate lung separation collapse; these devices are used independently mainly through or alongside a conventional single-lumen endotracheal tube.

Indications of the bronchial blocker include: to facilitate surgical exposure,[10] to prevent contamination of the contralateral lung in case of pulmonary hemorrhage, or to apply differential lung ventilation.[74] Box 16.3 shows specific indications of bronchial blocker.

Independent Bronchial Blockers During Lung Separation

Lung separation can be achieved by using an independent blocker passed through an in situ single-lumen endotracheal tube. Commonly used endobronchial blockers are the wire-guided endobronchial blocker Arndt® blocker,[12] the Cohen® tip-deflecting endobronchial blocker,[14] the Fuji Uniblocker®,[15] or the EZ-Blocker® (Teleflex Medical, Morrisville, NC),[16,17] or a different version of a bronchial blocker where the enclosed blocker is attached already to a single-lumen endotracheal tube (torque control blocker Univent).[12] Fig. 16.19 displays the Arndt blocker, the Cohen blocker, the Uniblocker, and the EZ-Blocker.

• **BOX 16.3 Specific Indications for Bronchial Blockers**

- Difficult airways
- Limited mouth opening
- Nasotracheal intubation
- Awake orotracheal intubation
- Already intubated patient requiring lung isolation
- Tracheostomy patient requiring lung isolation
- Selective lobar blockade
- Potential for mechanical ventilation in the postoperative period

The Arndt blocker

The Arndt® blocker[12] is an independent blocker attached to a 5.0 Fr, 7.0 Fr, or 9.0 Fr catheter that is available in 65- and 78-cm lengths, with an inner lumen measuring 1.4 mm in diameter. The 9.0 Fr Arndt® blockers have, at the distal end of the catheter, side holes incorporated to facilitate lung deflation. The Arndt® blocker has a high-volume, low-pressure cuff with either an elliptical or spherical shape. A unique feature of the Arndt® blocker compared with other blockers is that the inner lumen contains a flexible nylon wire passing through the proximal end of the catheter and extending to the distal end, which exits as a small flexible wire loop. This blocker comes with a multiport connector to accommodate the blocker and the fiberoptic bronchoscope. The wire loop of the Arndt® blocker is coupled with the fiberoptic bronchoscope and serves as a guide wire to introduce the blocker into the bronchus.[10] For the Arndt® blocker to function properly and allow manipulation with the adult fiberoptic bronchoscope, the proper size endotracheal tube must be used. For a 7 Fr blocker, which can be used for a 40-kg patient, a 7.5-mm internal diameter (ID) single-lumen endotracheal tube is used, and the larger 9 Fr Arndt® blocker is best used with an 8.0-mm internal diameter (ID) single-lumen endotracheal tube. Fig. 16.20A displays the placement of an Arndt® blocker through a single-lumen endotracheal tube with the fiberoptic bronchoscope advanced through the guide-wire loop. Fig. 16.20B displays the optimal position of the Arndt® blocker.

The advantages of the Arndt® blocker, as with other blockers, include its use in patients who are already tracheally intubated,[79] or those who present a difficult airway and require an awake orotracheal or nasotracheal intubation,[80] or when OLV is required during acute trauma to the chest.[81,82] In addition, an Arndt® blocker can be used as a selective lobar blocker in patients with previous pneumonectomy who require selective one-lobe ventilation[83] or as a selective blockade during severe pulmonary bleeding.[84] Fig. 16.21A displays the use of a bronchial blocker for selective lobar blockade. Fig. 16.21B displays the use of the Arndt® blocker

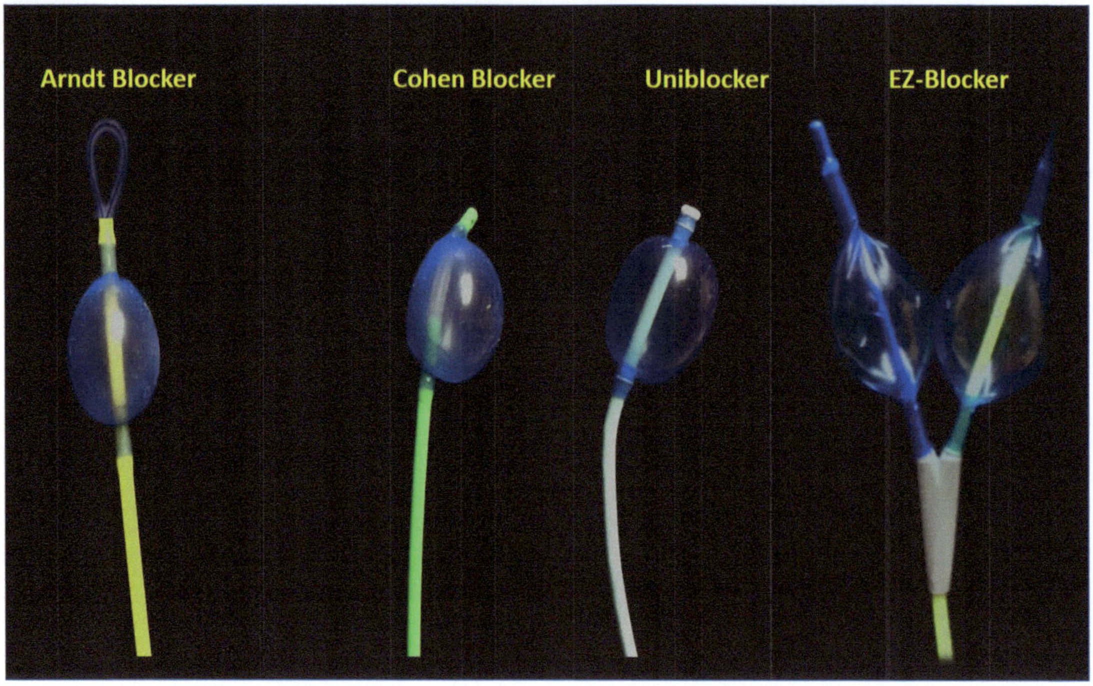

• **Fig. 16.19** The Arndt blocker, the Cohen blocker, the Uniblocker, and the EZ-Blocker.

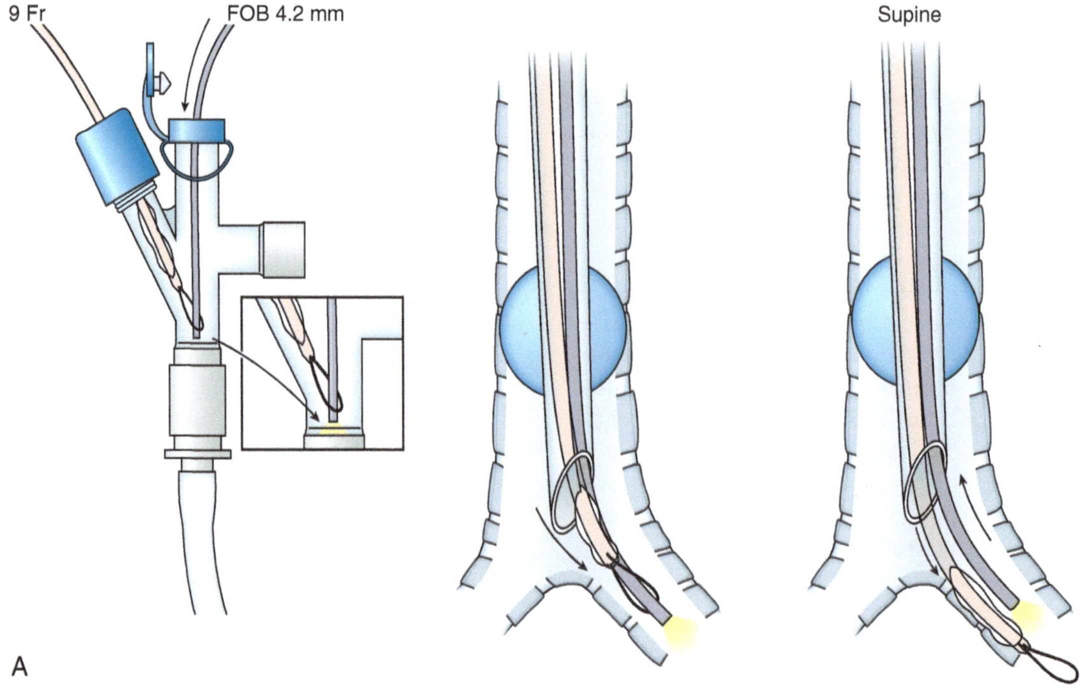

• **Fig. 16.20** (A) The placement of an Arndt® blocker through a single-lumen endotracheal tube, with the fiberoptic bronchoscope (*FOB*) advanced through the guidewire loop into the left mainstem bronchus.

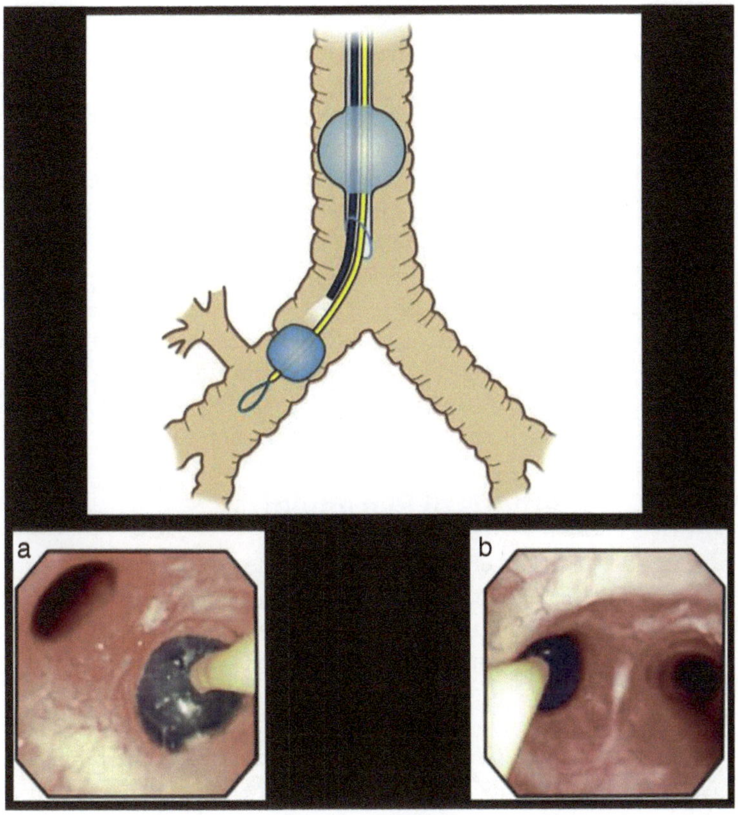

B

• **Fig. 16.20** (*Continued*) (**B**) The optimal position of a bronchial blocker in the right and left mainstem bronchus. The proximal edge of the fully inflated cuff is approximately 5 to 10 mm below the trachea carina. (a) A bronchial blocker in the right mainstem bronchus, and (b) A bronchial blocker in the left mainstem bronchus. (From Campos J. Lung isolation. In: Slinger P, ed. *Principles and Practice of Anesthesia for Thoracic Surgery*. Switzerland: Springer Nature; 2019:283–309. With permission.)

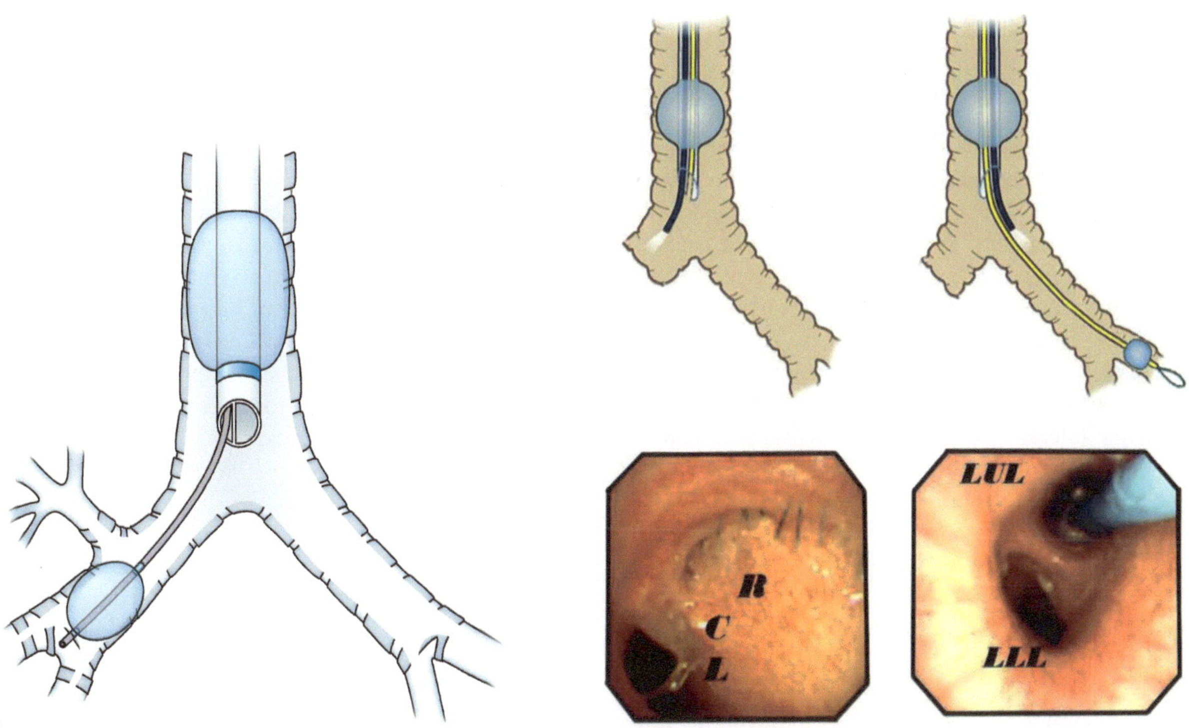

A B

• **Fig. 16.21** (**A**) A selective lobar blockade with a Univent® tube where the blocker is occluding the bronchus intermedius 18. (**B**) A patient with previous pneumonectomy where a selective lobar blockade is occluding the left-upper lobe bronchus. *C*, Carina; *L*, left bronchus; *LLL*, left lower lobe bronchus; *LUL*, left-upper lobe bronchus; *R*, right bronchus.

in a patient with previous contralateral pneumonectomy and segmental lobar blockade.

Methods of Placement

The Arndt® blocker is an independent endobronchial blocker that is passed through an existing single-lumen endotracheal tube. To facilitate insertion through the endotracheal tube, the blocker and the fiberoptic bronchoscope are lubricated. For a right-sided mainstem bronchus intubation, the spherically shaped blocker is recommended; for the left mainstem bronchus intubation, the elliptical or the spherical blocker is used.

The placement of the Arndt® blocker involves placing the endobronchial blocker through the endotracheal tube and using the fiberoptic bronchoscope and wire-guided loop to direct the blocker into a mainstem bronchus. The fiberoptic bronchoscope has to be advanced distally enough so that the Arndt® blocker enters the bronchus while it is being advanced. When the deflated cuff is beyond the entrance of the bronchus, the fiberoptic bronchoscope is withdrawn, and the cuff is fully inflated with fiberoptic visualization with 4 to 8 mL of air to obtain total bronchial blockade.

For right mainstem bronchus blockade, the Arndt® blocker can be advanced independently of the wire loop by observing its entrance into the right mainstem bronchus under fiberoptic visualization. Before turning the patient into a lateral decubitus position, the cuff of the blocker should be deflated, and then advanced 1 cm deeper to avoid proximal dislodgement while changing the patient's position; the placement again is confirmed in the lateral decubitus position. It is not recommended to turn the patient while the bronchial blocker cuff is inflated, unless in cases of lung isolation to prevent contamination of the dependent lung. The wire loop can be withdrawn to convert the 1.4-mm channel into a suction port to expedite lung collapse. The newest version of the Arndt® blocker has a cone-shaped device that is attached to the center channel to connect and facilitate suction.[85,86] It is important to make certain that the wire loop is removed to avoid inclusion in the stapling line of the bronchus.[87] The optimal position of the Arndt® blocker in the left or in the right bronchus is achieved when the blocker balloon's outer surface is seen with the fiberoptic bronchoscope at least 5 mm below the tracheal carina on the targeted bronchus, and the proper seal is obtained, although during a left blockade the cuff can be slightly deeper.

Cohen® Flexitip Endobronchial Blocker

The Cohen® blocker is an independent, endobronchial blocker that is available only in size 9.0 Fr and 65-cm length, with an inner lumen measuring 1.4 mm in diameter. This device comes with a spherically shaped high-volume low-pressure balloon. Near the distal end of the catheter, there are two side holes incorporated to facilitate lung deflation. The Cohen® blocker relies on a wheel-turning device located in the most proximal part of the unit allowing deflection of the flexible tip of the distal part of the blocker into the desired bronchus.[11–14] This device has been purposely preangled at the distal tip to facilitate insertion into a target bronchus. Also, there is a torque grip located at the 55-cm mark to allow rotation of the blocker. The torque grip can be moved and positioned at the level of the multiport adapter to achieve a tight seal and avoid movement of the blocker or air leak. In the distal tip above the balloon, there is a black arrow that, when visualized with the fiberoptic bronchoscope, indicates in which direction the tip deflects. This Cohen® blocker also comes with a multiport adaptor to facilitate an airtight seal when in place. The indications for use of the Cohen® blocker are the same as for the Arndt® blocker. Fig. 16.22A displays the Cohen® Flexitip blocker. Fig. 16.22B displays the Cohen® Flexitip blocker passed through a single-lumen endotracheal tube.

Methods of Placement

The Cohen® blocker is advanced through an 8.0-mm ID single-lumen endotracheal tube; before insertion, the blocker balloon is tested, and then fully deflated. This blocker, as all blockers, needs to be lubricated to facilitate insertion and passage through the single-lumen endotracheal tube.

The placement of the Cohen® blocker involves placing the endobronchial blocker through the endotracheal tube and using the fiberoptic bronchoscope to observe the direction of the blocker into a mainstem bronchus. For blocking the right mainstem bronchus, the optimal position is the one that provides a view of the outer surface of the fully inflated balloon (4–8 mL of air), with the fiberoptic bronchoscope at least 5 mm below the tracheal carina on the right mainstem bronchus.

Directing the blocker into the left mainstem bronchus can be facilitated by allowing the tip of the single-lumen endotracheal tube to be near the entrance of the left bronchus, and then twisting the Cohen® blocker to the left side. After the blocker is seen inside the left bronchus, the single-lumen endotracheal tube is withdrawn a few centimeters. An alternative approach is to turn the head toward the right, allowing the left main bronchus to displace to the midline. This maneuver will facilitate the placement of a Cohen® blocker into the left mainstem bronchus. The optimal position in the left mainstem bronchus is achieved when the blocker balloon's outer surface is seen with the fiberoptic bronchoscope at least 5 mm below the trachea carina inside the left mainstem bronchus.

Fuji Uniblocker®

The Fuji Uniblocker® is a hockey stick shaped tip independent bronchial blocker that is available in 5.0 and 9.0 Fr size, is 65 cm in length, and has a high-volume balloon made of silicone with a gas barrier property to reduce diffusion of gas into or out of the cuff. With its maximal cuff inflation of 6 mL of air, this new bronchial blocker's transmitted pressure tested in vitro was less than 30 mm Hg, which does not exceed the recommended safety limit in relationship to bronchial mucosa.[88] In addition, the Fuji Uniblocker® is equipped with a swivel connector. The swivel connector allows easy insertion of the fiberoptic bronchoscope and continuous ventilation during the blocker positioning. The Fuji Uniblocker® has a torque control

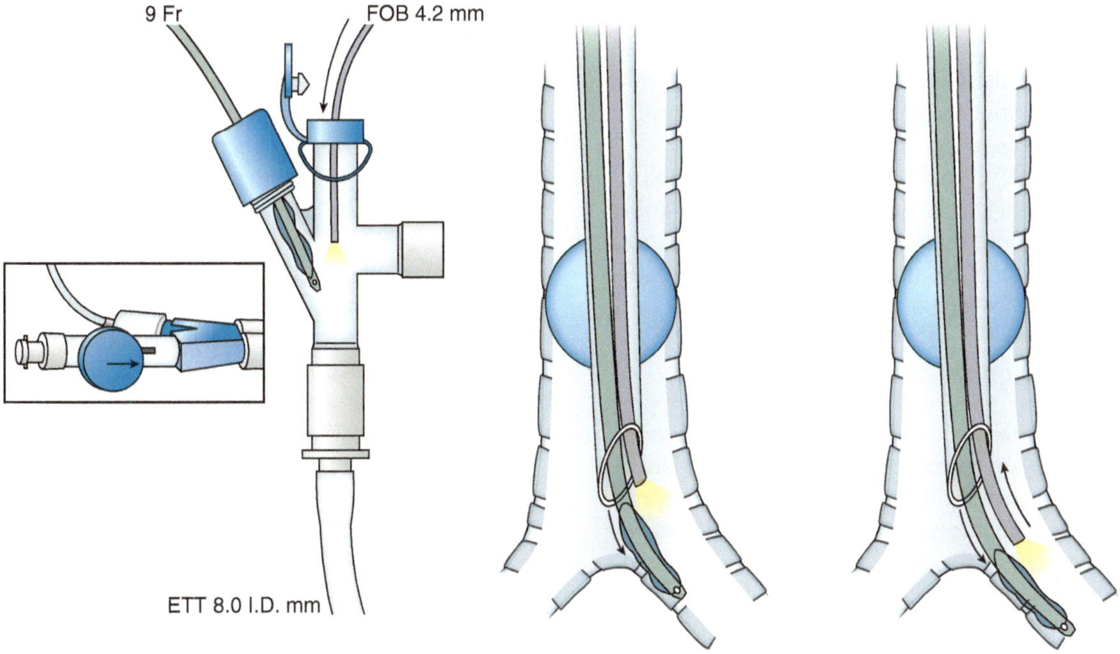

A

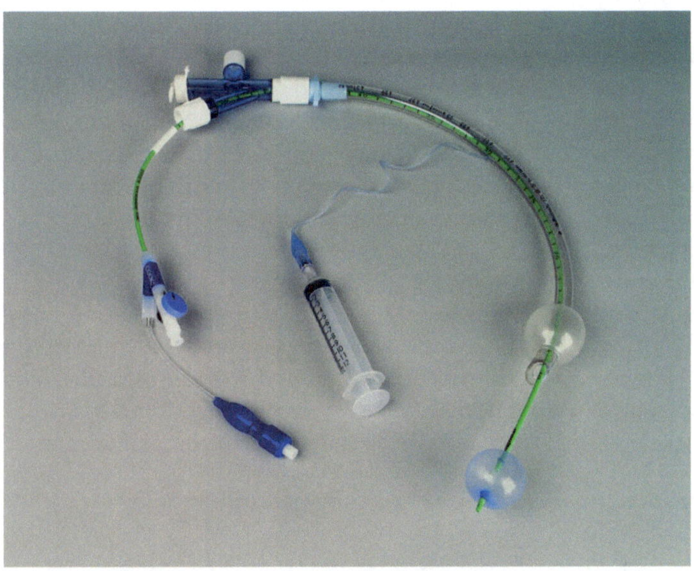

B

• **Fig. 16.22** (**A**) An independent bronchial blocker: Cohen Flexitip blocker going into left mainstem bronchus. (**B**) The Cohen Flexitip blocker through a single-lumen endotracheal tube. *FOB*, Fiberoptic bronchoscope. (A, From Campos J. Lung isolation. In: Slinger P, ed. *Principles and Practice of Anesthesia for Thoracic Surgery*. Switzerland: Springer Nature; 2019:283–309. With permission.)

blocker with an incorporated shaft that allows the guidance through the desired bronchus. A study by Narayanaswamy et al.[15] involved the use of the Fuji Uniblocker® compared with the Arndt® and Cohen® blockers, where the surgeons were blinded to which device was used to provide lung separation. The study showed that surgical exposure, as graded by the surgeons, was clinically equivalent to left-sided DLTs for thoracoscopic or open thoracotomies; however, the bronchial blockers, including the Fuji Uniblocker® took a longer time to position and required more intraoperative repositioning when compared with left-sided DLTs. Another report by Lizuka et al.[89] examining the use of the Fuji Uniblocker® in patients undergoing thoracoscopic surgery, not surprisingly showed a better quality of lung collapse with left-sided procedures than right-sided procedures because a right-sided blockade using a blocker has the potential difficulty in providing a complete seal of the RUL bronchus. The indications for use of the Fuji Uniblocker® are the same as for the Arndt® blocker. The Cohen® and Fuji® blockers can be easily placed through the glottis or tracheostomy external to an endotracheal tube, if required in small patients, and the blocker position confirmed with a fiberoptic bronchoscope passed through the endotracheal tube. As mentioned previously, it also available in 5.0 Fr size for the pediatric population.

The EZ-Blocker

The EZ-Blocker is an independent bronchial blocker that is available in a 7.0 Fr size and made of polyurethane material. The EZ-Blocker is manufactured with a Y-shaped distal end. Both limbs of the distal end are fitted with an inflatable balloon and a central channel to allow suction. Also, each limb is color-coded (yellow or blue) for easy identification with the matching pilot balloon. The EZ-Blocker is inserted through a port on the enclosed multiport adapter that is attached to a single-lumen endotracheal tube. The optimal size of the single-lumen endotracheal tube should be 7.5- or 8.0-mm internal diameter so it allows the blocker and the fiberoptic bronchoscope to navigate together.

The multiport adaptor of the EZ-Blocker is designed to join to a connector of the single-lumen endotracheal tube, and it contains two additional ports, one to allow advancement of the blocker, and the other port for passing the flexible fiberoptic bronchoscope.

Methods of Placement

The EZ-Blocker is tested and lubricated before passing into the lumen of the single-lumen endotracheal tube and the multiport connector. After advancing the blocker, the Y-shaped end should be seated in the tracheal carina, and each independent tip should be located in the entrance of right and left bronchus. Only the balloon where lung isolation is desired should be inflated under direct fiberoptic bronchoscopy. After the tip of the deflated balloon is in the bronchus, inflation of the balloon should be performed under direct vision with flexible fiberoptic bronchoscopy. Unfortunately, the balloon of the EZ-Blocker sometimes requires between 10 and 14 cc of air to block the left or right bronchus.[17] The proper and optimal position is when the outer surface of the balloon is seen 5 to 10 mm below the entrance of the bronchus. A common problem with the EZ-Blocker is that both limbs initially enter the right mainstem bronchus. This requires withdrawing the blocker above the carina and readvancement under direct vision with the bronchoscope. For this reason, the distal end of the single-lumen ETT should be at least 4 cm above the carina to minimize this problem. The distal Y-junction of the two limbs of the blocker must be firmly seated on the carina to minimize displacement of the blocker during surgery. Fig. 16.23 displays the optimal position of the EZ-Blocker.

VivaSight® Single-Lumen Tube With Guided Bronchial Blocker

The VivaSight® single-lumen endotracheal tube (ETView LTD., Ambu) is the new generation of endotracheal tubes incorporating a high-resolution imaging camera and a light source in its tip. The advantage of the light source is that, when connected to a monitor, it displays in real time the placement and positioning of a bronchial blocker without the aid of a fiberoptic bronchoscope.[90] Fig. 16.24A shows a VivaSight® single-lumen endotracheal tube with a cable connected to a video monitor. Fig. 16.24B shows a bronchial blocker used as an independent bronchial blocker within the VivaSight® single-lumen endotracheal tube.

A case report by Qiu et al.[90] involving a patient with a tracheal tumor in the mid-trachea section managed with a VivaSight® single-lumen endotracheal tube, showed that after the patient was intubated and under continuous visualization of the trachea, the endotracheal tube was properly placed above the tumor. Then using the high-resolution camera and light source, a bronchial blocker was placed on the right mainstem bronchus. This is a novel approach to managing patients under tracheal resection and reconstruction. The VivaSight® single-lumen endotracheal tube provides real time and continuous monitoring on the portion of the bronchial blocker.[90] Some limitations with this novel technology include the presence of secretions in the tip of the light source, which can obscure the view of the tracheal carina on the video monitor.

Torque Control Blocker Univent

The Univent® tube consists of a single-lumen endotracheal tube with an enclosed and movable bronchial blocker made of flexible, nonlatex material, and it includes a flexible shaft that is easier to guide into a bronchus.[12] The angled-tip

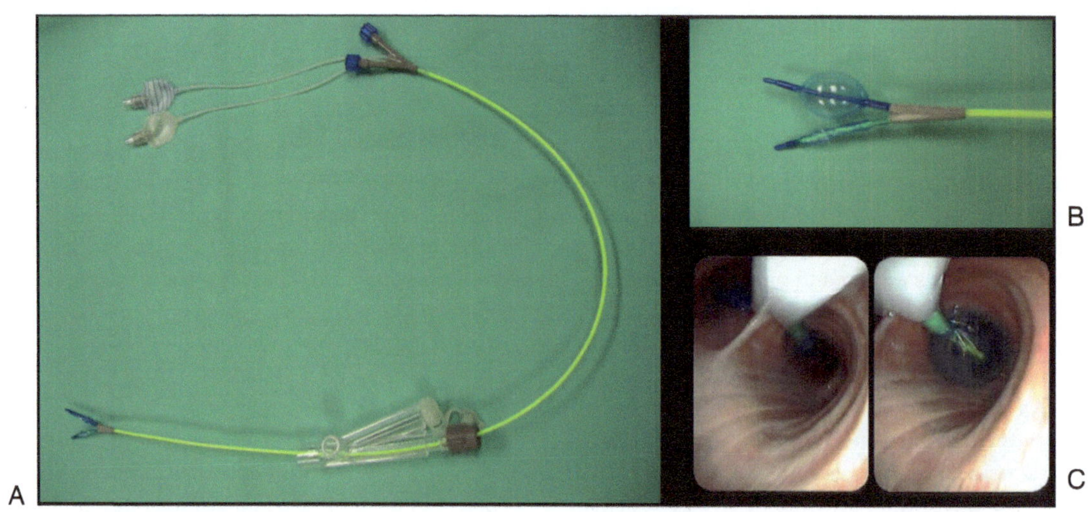

• **Fig. 16.23** The optimal position of the EZ-Blocker. (**A**) The EZ-Blocker and multiport adapter, (**B**) displays the Y-shaped distal end with one balloon fully inflated and the other deflated, (**C**) shows Y-shaped distal end sitting on tracheal carina and to the right the balloon fully inflated. (From Campos J. Lung isolation. In: Slinger P, ed. *Principles and Practice of Anesthesia for Thoracic Surgery*. Switzerland: Springer Nature; 2019:283–309. With permission.)

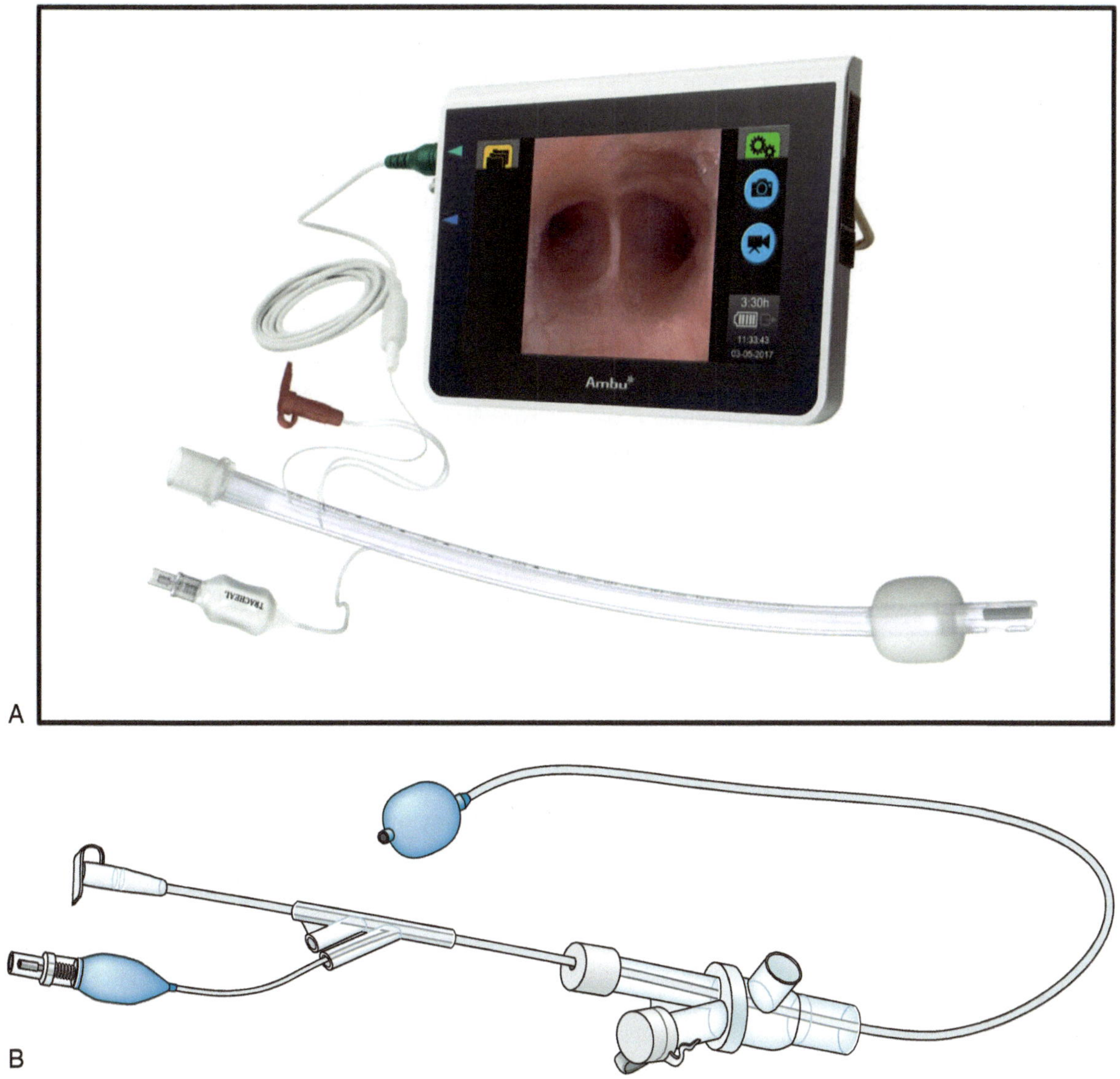

• **Fig. 16.24** (**A**) A VivaSight® single-lumen endotracheal tube with a cable connected to a video monitor, (**B**) a bronchial blocker to be used as an independent bronchial blocker within the VivaSight® single-lumen endotracheal tube.

blocker is host in an anterior separate channel and cannot be detached form the tube. The bronchial balloon has a high-pressure, low-volume cuff that requires approximately 2 mL of air to produce an airtight seal if selective lobar blockade is used, or 4 to 8 mL of air if the total blockade of the bronchus is desired. The bronchial blocker has a 2-mm-diameter lumen that can be used for suctioning or for oxygen administration, and it should be closed before insertion. One of the advantages of the Univent® blocker is its utility in patients in whom the airway is considered difficult for direct laryngoscopy and during unanticipated difficult endotracheal intubation.[91–94] The Univent tube can be left in place if the patient requires postoperative ventilatory support. However, the external diameter of the tube is relatively high (an 8.0-mm tube has an external diameter > 13 mm), which can be undesirable for an extended ventilation period.

Placement of the Univent® blocker is straightforward like any single-lumen endotracheal tube. First the bronchial blocker is lubricated to facilitate passage. Next, the enclosed bronchial blocker is fully retracted into the lumen of the tube. Conventional endotracheal tube placement is performed via direct laryngoscopy, and then a fiberoptic bronchoscope is passed through a Portex swivel adaptor into the endotracheal tube. Under direct vision, the enclosed bronchial blocker is advanced into the targeted bronchus.

Complications With the Use of Bronchial Blockers

Although serious complications have been reported with the use of current bronchial blockers, these complications appear to be more benign than those involving DLTs. A structural complication has been reported in the torque control Univent blocker in which a fracture of the blocker cap connector occurred in 2 of the first 50 tubes used.[95] Failure to achieve lung separation because of abnormal anatomy, in which the entrance of the RUL bronchus was located above the tracheal carina, or lack of seal within the bronchus also has been reported.[96,97] Inclusion of the enclosed bronchial blocker into the stapling line has been reported during a right upper lobectomy.[98] Communication with the surgical team regarding the presence of a bronchial blocker in the surgical side is crucial. Because the blocker cannot be detached from the main tube, a potential and dangerous complication with the bronchial cuff of the Univent has been reported; the cuff of the bronchial blocker was inflated mistakenly near the tracheal lumen, precluding all airflow, and producing respiratory arrest.[99]

Complications with the Arndt® blocker include a report of a sheared balloon that occurred when the blocker was removed through the multiport blocker side.[100] It is advised that when an independent bronchial blocker is not in use, it needs to be removed with the multiport connector in place rather than through the connector to prevent shredded material into the single-lumen endotracheal tube. Another near-fatal complication reported with the use of the Arndt® blocker occurred when the fully inflated balloon of the blocker dislodged into the patient's trachea, leading to a complete airway obstruction. Severe air trapping led to pulseless activity in the patient, who was undergoing a rupture descending thoracic aortic aneurysm. A prompt deflation of the bronchial blocker cuff resolved the problem.[101]

Another complication reported with the Arndt® blocker involved inadvertent resection of the guide wire and part of the tip of the bronchial blocker during stapler resection of the left lower lobe because the surgeon cannot see the thin guide wire. This complication required surgical reexploration after unsuccessful removal of the bronchial blocker during extubation.[87]

In a retrospective review, Ueda et al.[102] evaluated the safety and efficacy of bronchial blocker use in thoracic anesthesia in 302 patients to achieve OLV. Variables recorded from the anesthetic record included type of device used, type and side of surgery, specific indications for OLV, Mallampati score, route of intubation, and complications related to the use of bronchial blockers. The bronchial blockers used include the Arndt wire-guided, Univent, Cohen Flexitip, Fogarty catheter, and Fuji. Of the 251 patients, 216 (86%) had a Mallampati score of I/II and 35 (14%) had a score of III/IV. There were no identified complications related to bronchial blockers. They concluded that endobronchial blockers can be safely used to achieve OLV and offer advantages for OLV in specific situations.

A recent report by Honikman et al.[103] discussed three cases where the balloon of the Fuji blocker failed to deflate at the conclusion of the surgery. In two of the cases, the already inflated bronchial blocker had to be removed along with the single-lumen endotracheal tube during extubation. It is recommended to test the pilot and the balloon before use to ensure that the air that is injected is aspirated and the balloon completely deflates. When the accumulated data on complications during lung separation were compared, complications with the DLTs outnumbered the reported complications with the bronchial blockers.

A recent complication involving a perforation of the bronchus with the use of the EZ-Blocker has been reported[104] in a patient that had received radiation therapy. In this case, the EZ-Blocker was advanced blindly into the single-lumen endotracheal tube, where both distal ends were located below the tracheal carina inside the right mainstem bronchus. One of the blocker tips perforated the bronchial wall and was visualized outside the bronchus during an open thoracotomy. It is very important to advance the blocker with the guidance of the fiberoptic bronchoscope to prevent this complication.

Lung Collapse During Lung Isolation

A challenge for every anesthesiologist is to properly position a lung isolation device and make it work by providing a well collapsed lung and a still surgical field. In a study[12] comparing the Broncho-Cath left-sided DLT with the Univent® torque control blocker and the Arndt® wire-guided blocker, it was shown that the average time for lung collapse is 17 minutes for a DLT (spontaneous lung collapse without suction) versus 19 to 26 minutes for the Univent® or Arndt® bronchial blocker (assisted with suction). A study by Narayanaswamy et al.,[15] involving left-sided DLTs and comparing them with the Arndt®, the Cohen®, or the Fuji® blocker, showed that the surgical exposure was equivalent among the devices studied. The quality of the lung collapse was done by the surgeons grading, who were blinded to the device that was used to achieve lung separation. The bronchial blockers required longer time to position (2 minutes longer) and were more prone to intraoperative reposition. It is important to emphasize that these two studies involved at least one senior thoracic anesthesiologist with broad experience with lung isolation devices.

A study[105] has shown that denitrogenation of the collapsed lung with a fraction of inspired oxygen (FiO2) 1.0 is a useful strategy to improve surgical conditions during OLV; in contrast, the use of air in the inspired gas mixture during two-lung ventilation and before OLV delays lung collapse.

A recent study involving the use of a bronchial blocker showed that the use of nitrous oxide in a mixture of N_2O/O_2 (FiO2 = 0.5) facilitated lung collapse after opening the chest, compared with a comparative group using 100% oxygen. Both groups in this study had a suction assistant in place during OLV.[106] Another study involving morbidly obese patients undergoing OLV, where a left-sided DLT was compared with the Arndt wire-guided blocker, reported that there was no overall advantage of one device over the other during intubation or the success of lung collapse, both devices were very comparable.[107]

A recent study by Bussières et al.[108] compared the Fuji blocker with a left-sided DLT in video-assisted thoracoscopic surgery in 40 patients. The grading of the quality of the lung collapse was performed intraoperatively by the

TABLE 16.3 **Advantages and Disadvantages of Double-Lumen Tubes and Bronchial Blockers**

Double-Lumen Endotracheal Tubes	Bronchial Blockers (Arndt®, Cohen®, Fuji®, EZ-Blocker®)
Advantages	
• Large lumen facilitates suctioning	• Easy recognition of anatomy if the tip of a single tube is above carina
• Best device for absolute indications for lung separation, to protect the lung from soiling	• Best device for patients with difficult airways
• Conversion from 2- to 1-lung ventilation and back easy and reliable	• Cuff damage during intubation rare • No need to replace a tube if mechanical ventilation is needed
Disadvantages	
• Difficulties in selecting proper size	• Small channel for suctioning
• More difficult to place during laryngoscopy	• Conversion from 1- to 2-, then to 1-lung ventilation problematic, more complicated
• Potential damage to tracheal cuff during intubation	• High maintenance device (frequent dislodgement or loss of seal during surgery)
• Rare major tracheobronchial injuries	

surgeons who were blinded to the type of the device used to collapse the lung and by postoperative review of scrambled images of the collapsed lung during various stages of the surgery. The authors reported that the bronchial blocker had a faster time to obtain lung collapse and overall superior quality of lung deflation when compared with a left-sided DLT. The surgeon incorrectly guessed the type of device used in 78% of the bronchial blocker group and 50% of the DLT group.

Combining all studies and recommendation, all anesthesiologists, in addition to the use of DLT, should be familiar with the use of bronchial blockers[109,110] and DLTs[1,2] during lung isolation techniques. It should be part of the "toolbox" of every practitioner. That will allow them to be versatile when the need to use an alternative to DLT will arise. Editorial reports, scientific evidence, and topic of debates support this recommendation.[11,12,17] Table 16.3 displays the advantages and disadvantages of DLTs and bronchial blockers.

Future Trends in Lung Isolation

The advances in thoracic, cardiac, and esophageal surgery, and minimally invasive surgery, led to an increased need for lung isolation techniques among anesthesiologists. A previous study[51] has shown that anesthesiologists with limited thoracic experience often fail to correctly place lung isolation devices. Increased clinical experience would reduce this failure rate. However, a great deal of experience may be limited for anesthesiologists working in centers that perform relatively few thoracic cases. Therefore improved nonclinical training methods are essential.

Two important tools to improve the clinical skills are available worldwide. The first is to attend one of many thoracic workshops and an entire day of thoracic symposiums that are offered during the anesthesia meeting of most anesthesia societies. During these workshops the attendees can familiarize themselves with the various devices used to provide lung separation, aviaries of endobronchial blocker, and DLTs. The one-on-one "hands on" approach will allow the practical use of these devices and allow interaction with the expert faculties.

The second tool is the Anesthesia Simulators, which are available in most institutions, and have been used to enhance learning and improve performance,[111,112] usually under the personal direction of an experienced clinician. These educational approaches to lung isolation techniques might involve training on an airway simulator mentored by an experienced thoracic anesthesiologist. Another alternative is to train in a fiberoptic bronchoscopy simulator[113,114] on lung isolation techniques, particularly for the anesthesiologist who does not perform thoracic cases on a regular basis. A study involving anesthesiologists with limited thoracic experience, comparing the simulator intubation model versus computer didactic–based material in how to place a left-sided DLT, showed that both teaching methods had similar outcomes when this group of anesthesiologists placed the DLTs after their training.[115]

Another study involving high-fidelity simulation of lung isolation with DLTs and bronchial blockers among anesthesiology residents showed that their performance in placing lung isolation devices was very successful.[116] A similar model/study was performed involving senior medical students to teach basic lung isolation skills on a showed that video-didactic and simulation-based methods were very comparable and successful in training novices for lung isolation techniques.[117] This study also reported that the acquired skills particularly decreased without practice. Regardless of the method used to teach lung isolation techniques, it should be used periodically by anesthesiologists with limited thoracic experience to retain their level of skills.

A free online bronchoscopy simulator is available on the website www.thoracicanesthesia.com to learn tracheobronchial anatomy (Fig. 16.25).

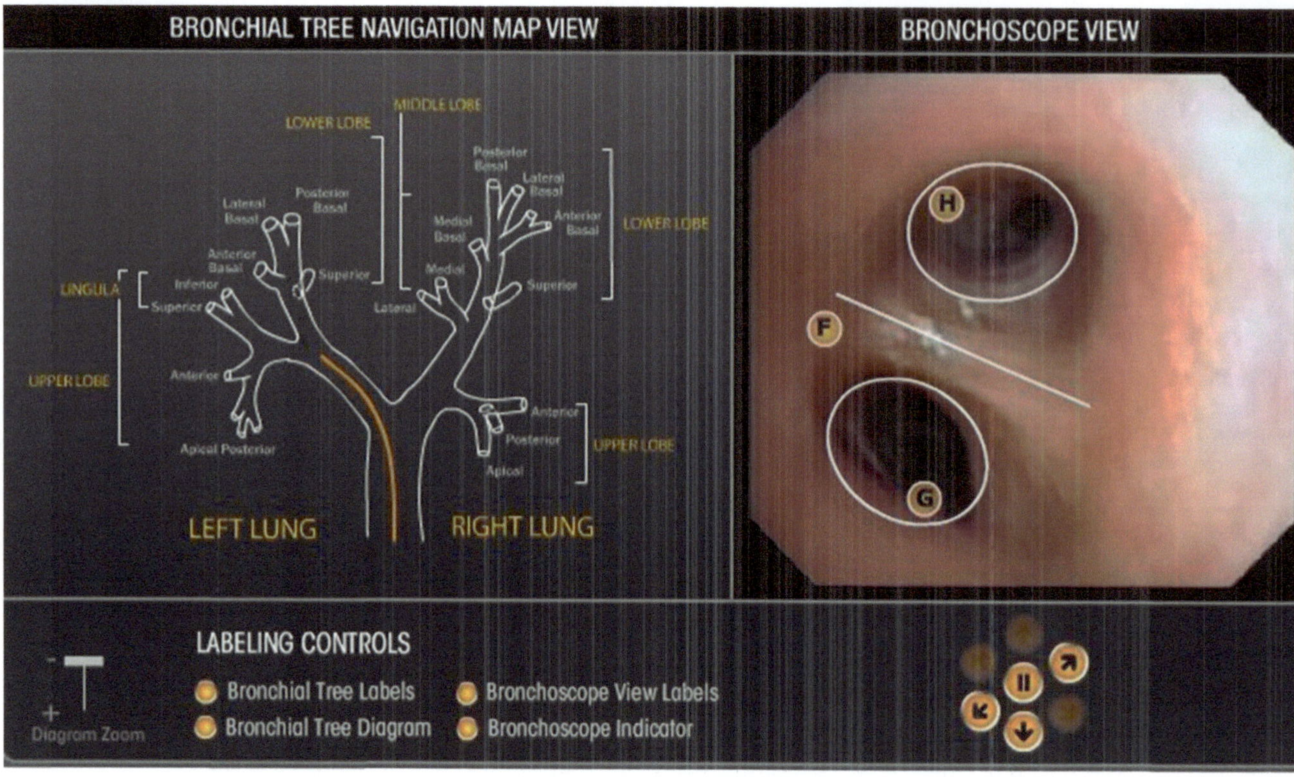

• **Fig. 16.25** The free online bronchoscopy simulator at www.thoracicanesthesia.com. The user can navigate the tracheobronchial tree using real-time video by clicking on the lighted directional arrows under the "Bronchoscopic View" (right). Clicking on the labels on the "Bronchoscopic View" gives details of the anatomy seen. The process is aided by the "Bronchial Tree Navigational Map" (left), which shows the simultaneous location of the bronchoscope as the orange line in the airway. (Source: www.thoracicanesthesia.com.)

Conclusion

The basic principle of successful lung separation requires: (1) recognition of tracheobronchial anatomy with a posteroanterior chest radiograph in the preoperative evaluation and with flexible fiberoptic bronchoscopy in the perioperative period; (2) familiarity and skills with flexible fiberoptic bronchoscopy; and (3) familiarity and expertise with DLTs and bronchial blockers.

Because of its greater margin of safety, a left-sided DLT is the more common and easiest device used during lung separation. A right-sided DLT is recommended for a left-sided pneumonectomy or any contraindication to placement of a left-sided DLT, such as a tumor occupying the LMB. For patients with a difficult abnormal airway or a tracheostomy in place, the use of a bronchial blocker is the preferred choice. Bronchial blockers require more time for placement and are more prone to intraoperative dislodgement. Lung collapse is facilitated with a denitrogenation technique using FiO2 1.0 during two-lung ventilation before lung collapse. Every lung isolation device placement requires auscultation and clamping maneuvers, followed by a fiberoptic bronchoscopy confirmation to obtain 100% success during lung separation techniques. The optimal position of these devices, DLTs or bronchial blockers, is best achieved with the use of fiberoptic bronchoscopy techniques, first in the supine, and then in the lateral decubitus position or whenever repositioning of the device is needed. There are many new devices currently available for clinical use. It would be best to have several of them as part of the practitioner "toolbox" and use them as indicated clinically.

References

1. Campos J. Lung isolation. In: Slinger P, ed. *Principles and Practice of Anesthesia for Thoracic Surgery*. Switzerland: Springer Nature; 2019:283–309.
2. Campos JH. Current techniques for perioperative lung isolation in adults. *Anesthesiology*. 2002;97:1295–1301.
3. Campos JH. Progress in lung separation. *Thorac Surg Clin*. 2005; 15:71–83.
4. Campos J. Lung isolation. In: Slinger P, ed. *Principles and Practice of Anesthesia for Thoracic Surgery*. Switzerland: Springer Nature; 2011:227–246.
5. Kwon NK, Jung SM, Park SJ, et al. Comparison of displacement of polyvinyl chloride and silicone left-sided double-lumen tubes during lateral positioning. *Korean J Anesthesiol*. 2019;72:32–38.

6. Falzon D, Alston RP, Coley E, et al. Lung isolation for thoracic surgery: from inception to evidence-based. *J Cardiothorac Vasc Anesth*. 2017;31:678–693.
7. Campos JH, Massa CF, Kernstine KH. The incidence of right upper lobe collapse when comparing a right-sided double lumen tube versus modified left double lumen tube for left-sided thoracic surgery. *Anesth Analg*. 2000;90:535–540.
8. Heir JS, Guo SL, Purugganan R, et al. A randomized controlled study of the use of video double-lumen endobronchial tubes versus double-lumen endobronchial tubes in thoracic surgery. *J Cardiothorac Vasc Anesth*. 2018;32:267–274.
9. Slinger PD, Campos JH, et al. Anesthesia for thoracic surgery. In: Miller MD, et al., eds. *Miller's Anesthesia*. ed 9. Saunders; 2020:1648–1716.
10. Campos JH. An update on bronchial blockers during lung separation techniques in adults. *Anesth Analg*. 2003;97:1266–1274.
11. Kreft T, Zardo P, Busk H, et al. Modern bronchial blockers in thoracic surgery. *Curr Anesthesiol Rep*. 2016;6:103–110.
12. Campos JH, Kernstine KH. A comparison of a left-sided Broncho-Cath with the torque control blocker Univent and the wire-guided blocker. *Anesth Analg*. 2003;96:283–289.
13. Neustein SM. The use of bronchial blockers for providing one-lung ventilation. *J Cardiothorac Vasc Anesth*. 2009;23:860–868.
14. Cohen E. The Cohen flexitip endobronchial blocker: an alternative to a double lumen tube. *Anesth Analg*. 2005;101:1877–1879.
15. Narayanaswamy M, McRae K, Slinger P, et al. Choosing a lung isolation device for thoracic surgery: a randomized trial of three bronchial blockers versus double-lumen tubes. *Anesth Analg*. 2009;108:1097–1101.
16. Ruetzler K, Grubhofer G, Schmid W, et al. Randomized clinical trial comparing double-lumen tube and EZ-Blocker for single-lung ventilation. *Br J Anaesth*. 2011;106:896–902.
17. Mourisse J, Liesveld J, Verhagen A, et al. Efficiency, efficacy, and safety of EZ-blocker compared with left-sided double-lumen tube for one-lung ventilation. *Anesthesiology*. 2013;118:550–561.
18. Campos JH. How to achieve successful lung separation. *SAJAA*. 2008;14:22–26.
19. Sivalingam P, Tio R. Tension pneumothorax, pneumomediastinum, pneumoperitoneum, and subcutaneous emphysema in a 15-year-old Chinese girl after a double-lumen tube intubation and one-lung ventilation. *J Cardiothorac Vasc Anesth*. 1999;13: 312–315.
20. Sakuragi T, Kumano K, Yasumoto M, et al. Rupture of the left main-stem bronchus by the tracheal portion of a double-lumen endobronchial tube. *Acta Anaesthesiol Scand*. 1997;41:1218–1220.
21. Bardoczky G, d'Hollander A, Yernault JC, et al. On-line expiratory flow-volume curves during thoracic surgery: occurrence of auto-PEEP. *Br J Anaesth*. 1994;72:25–28.
22. Seymour AH, Prakash N. A cadaver study to measure the adult glottis and subglottis: defining a problem associated with the use of double-lumen tubes. *J Cardiothorac Vasc Anesth*. 2002; 16:196–198.
23. Liu H, Jahr JS, Sullivan E, et al. Tracheobronchial rupture after double-lumen endotracheal intubation. *J Cardiothorac Vasc Anesth*. 2004;18:228–233.
24. Ideris SS, Che Hassan MR, Abdul Rahman MR, et al. Selection of an appropriate left-sided double-lumen tube size for one-lung ventilation among Asians. *Ann Card Anaesth*. 2017;20:28–32.
25. Brodsky JB, Macario A, Mark JB. Tracheal diameter predicts double-lumen tube size: a method for selecting left double-lumen tubes. *Anesth Analg*. 1996;82:861–864.
26. Chow MY, Liam BL, Lew TW, et al. Predicting the size of a double-lumen endobronchial tube based on tracheal diameter. *Anesth Analg*. 1998;87:158–160.
27. Amar D, Desiderio DP, Heerdt PM, et al. Practice patterns in choice of left double-lumen tube size for thoracic surgery. *Anesth Analg*. 2008;106:379–383.
28. Eberle B, Weiler N, Vogel N, et al. Computed tomography-based tracheobronchial image reconstruction allows selection of the individually appropriate double-lumen tube size. *J Cardiothorac Vasc Anesth*. 1999;13:532–537.
29. Roldi E, Inghileri P, Dransart-Raye O, et al. Use of tracheal ultrasound combined with clinical parameters to select left double-lumen tube size: a prospective observational study. *Eur J Anaesthesiol*. 2019;36:215–220.
30. Campos JH. Update on tracheobronchial anatomy and flexible fiberoptic bronchoscopy in thoracic anesthesia. *Curr Opin Anaesthesiol*. 2009;22:4–10.
31. Brodsky JB, Benumof JL, Ehrenwerth J, et al. Depth of placement of left double-lumen endobronchial tubes. *Anesth Analg*. 1991;73:570–572.
32. Boucek CD, Landreneau R, Freeman JA, et al. A comparison of techniques for placement of double-lumen endobronchial tubes. *J Clin Anesth*. 1998;10:557–560.
33. Bakshi SG, Gawri A, Divatia JV. McGrath MAC video laryngoscope versus direct laryngoscopy for the placement of double-lumen tubes: a randomised control trial. *Indian J Anaesth*. 2019;63:456–461.
34. Purugganan RV, Jackson TA, Heir JS, et al. Video laryngoscopy versus direct laryngoscopy for double-lumen endotracheal tube intubation: a retrospective analysis. *J Cardiothorac Vasc Anesth*. 2012;26:845–848.
35. Russell T, Slinger P, Roscoe A, et al. A randomised controlled trial comparing the GlideScope(®) and the Macintosh laryngoscope for double-lumen endobronchial intubation. *Anaesthesia*. 2013;68:1253–1258.
36. Chastel B, Perrier V, Germain A, et al. Usefulness of the Airtraq DL™ videolaryngoscope for placing a double-lumen tube. *Anaesth Crit Care Pain Med*. 2015;34:89–93.
37. El-Tahan MR, Khidr AM, Gaarour IS, et al. A comparison of 3 video laryngoscopes for double-lumen tube intubation in humans by users with mixed experience: a randomized controlled study. *J Cardiothorac Vasc Anesth*. 2018;32:277–286.
38. Liu TT, LI L, Wan L, et al. Video laryngoscopy vs. Macintosh laryngoscopy for double-lumen tube intubation in thoracic surgery: a systematic review and meta-analysis. *Anaesthesia*. 2018;73: 997–1007.
39. Clayton-Smith A, Bennett K, Alston RP, et al. A comparison of the efficacy and adverse effects of double-lumen endobronchial tubes and bronchial blockers in thoracic surgery: a systematic review and meta-analysis of randomized controlled trials. *J Cardiothorac Vasc Anesth*. 2015;29:955–966.
40. Benumof JL, Partridge BL, Salvatierra C, Keating J. Margin of safety in positioning modern double-lumen endotracheal tubes. *Anesthesiology*. 1987;67:729–738.
41. Jung DM, Ahn HJ, Jung SH, et al. Apneic oxygen insufflation decreases the incidence of hypoxemia during one-lung ventilation in open and thoracoscopic pulmonary lobectomy: a randomized controlled trial. *J Thorac Cardiovasc Surg*. 2017;154:360–366.
42. Campos J. Fiberoptic bronchoscopy for positioning double-lumen tubes and bronchial blockers. In: Slinger P, ed. *Principles and Practice of Anesthesia for Thoracic Surgery*. Switzerland: Springer Nature; 2019:311–322.

43. Campos JH, Hanada S, et al. DLT with incorporated fiberoptic bronchoscopy. In: Rosenblatt WH, et al., eds. *Master Techniques in Upper and Lower Airway Management*: Lippincott Williams and Wilkins; 2015:250–251.
44. Saracoglu A, Saracoglu KT. VivaSight: a new era in the evolution of tracheal tubes. *J Clin Anesth*. 2016;33:442–449.
45. Heir JS, Purugganan R, Jackson TA, et al. A retrospective evaluation of the use of video-capable double-lumen endotracheal tubes in thoracic surgery. *J Cardiothorac Vasc Anesth*. 2014;28: 870–872.
46. Massot J, Dumand-Nizard V, Fischler M, et al. Evaluation of the double-lumen tube Vivasight-DL (DLT-ETView): a prospective single-center study. *J Cardiothorac Vasc Anesth*. 2015;29: 1544–1549.
47. Levy-Faber D, Malyanker Y, Nir RR, et al. Comparison of VivaSight double-lumen tube with a conventional double-lumen tube in adult patients undergoing video-assisted thoracoscopic surgery. *Anaesthesia*. 2015;70:1259–1263.
48. Ehrenfeld JM, Walsh JL, Sandberg WS. Right- and left-sided Mallinckrodt double-lumen tubes have identical clinical performance. *Anesth Analg*. 2008;106:1847–1852.
49. Bussières JS, Lacasse Y, Côté D, et al. Modified right-sided Broncho-Cath double lumen tube improves endobronchial positioning: a randomized study. *Can J Anaesth*. 2007;54:276–282.
50. Klein U, Karzai W, Bloos F, et al. Role of fiberoptic bronchoscopy in conjunction with the use of double-lumen tubes for thoracic anesthesia: a prospective study. *Anesthesiology*. 1998;88: 346–350.
51. Campos JH, Hallam EA, Van Natta T, Kernstine KH. Devices for lung isolation used by anesthesiologists with limited thoracic experience: comparison of double-lumen endotracheal tube, Univent torque control blocker, and Arndt wire-guided endobronchial blocker. *Anesthesiology*. 2006;104:261–266.
52. de Bellis M, Accardo R, Di Maio M, et al. Is flexible bronchoscopy necessary to confirm the position of double-lumen tubes before thoracic surgery? *Eur J Cardiothorac Surg*. 2011;40:912–916.
53. Slinger P. A view of and through double-lumen tubes. *J Cardiothorac Vasc Anesth*. 2003;17:287–288.
54. Sustić A, Protić A, Cicvarić T, et al. The addition of a brief ultrasound examination to clinical assessment increases the ability to confirm placement of double-lumen endotracheal tubes. *J Clin Anesth*. 2010;22:246–249.
55. Álvarez-Díaz N, Amador-García I, Fuentes-Hernández M, et al. Comparison between transthoracic lung ultrasound and a clinical method in confirming the position of double-lumen tube in thoracic anaesthesia. A pilot study. *Rev Esp Anestesiol Reanim*. 2015;62:305–312.
56. Parab SY, Kumar P, Divatia JV, et al. A prospective randomized controlled double-blind study comparing auscultation and lung ultrasonography in the assessment of double lumen tube position in elective thoracic surgeries involving one lung ventilation at a tertiary care cancer institute. *Korean J Anesthesiol*. 2019;72:24–31.
57. Hu WC, Xu L, Zhang Q, et al. Point-of-care ultrasound versus auscultation in determining the position of double-lumen tube. *Medicine*. 2018;97:e9311.
58. Lohser J, Brodsky JB. Silbronco double-lumen tube. *J Cardiothorac Vasc Anesth*. 2006;20:129–131.
59. Leclercq T, Lilot M, Schulz T, et al. Endotracheal bioimpedance cardiography improves immediate postoperative outcome: a case control study in off-pump coronary surgery. *J Clin Monit Comput*. 2018;32:81.
60. Hagihira S, Takashina M, Mashimo T. Application of a newly designed right-sided, double-lumen endobronchial tube in patients with a very short right mainstem bronchus. *Anesthesiology*. 2008;109:565–568.
61. Ghosh S, Falter F, Klein AA, Arrowsmith JE. The Papworth BiVent Tube: initial clinical experience. *J Cardiothorac Vasc Anesth*. 2011;25:505–508.
62. Saito S, Dohi S, Naito H. Alteration of double-lumen endobronchial tube position by flexion and extension of the neck. *Anesthesiology*. 1985;62:696–697.
63. Hannallah M, Gomes M. Bronchial rupture associated with the use of a double-lumen tube in a small adult. *Anesthesiology*. 1989;71:457–478.
64. Lemay J, Conti M, Somma J, et al. Avoidable tracheal injury using a double-lumen endotracheal tube: a case report. *Can J Anaesth*. 2018;65:735–736.
65. Yüceyar L, Kaynak K, Cantürk E, Aykaç B. Bronchial rupture with a left-sided polyvinylchloride double-lumen tube. *Acta Anaesthesiol Scand*. 2003;47:622–625.
66. Hartman WR, Brown M, Hannon J. Iatrogenic left main bronchus injury following atraumatic double lumen endotracheal tube placement. *Case Rep Anesthesiol*. 2013;2013:524348.
67. Benumof JL, Wu D. Tracheal tear caused by extubation of a double-lumen tube. *Anesthesiology*. 2002;97:1007–1008.
68. Sucato DJ, Girgis M. Bilateral pneumothoraces, pneumomediastinum, pneumoperitoneum, pneumoretroperitoneum, and subcutaneous emphysema following intubation with a double-lumen endotracheal tube for thoracoscopic anterior spinal release and fusion in a patient with idiopathic scoliosis. *J Spinal Disord Tech*. 2002;15:133–138.
69. Weng W, DeCrosta DJ, Zhang H. Tension pneumothorax during one-lung ventilation: a case report. *J Clin Anesth*. 2002;14: 529–531.
70. Fitzmaurice BG, Brodsky JB. Airway rupture from double-lumen tubes. *J Cardiothorac Vasc Anesth*. 1999;13:322–329.
71. Knoll H, Ziegeler S, Schreiber JU, et al. Airway injuries after one-lung ventilation: a comparison between double-lumen tube and endobronchial blocker: a randomized, prospective, controlled trial. *Anesthesiology*. 2006;105:471–477.
72. Zhong T, Wang W, Chen J, et al. Sore throat or hoarse voice with bronchial blockers or double-lumen tubes for lung isolation: a randomised, prospective trial. *Anaesth Intensive Care*. 2009; 37:441–446.
73. Park SH, Han SH, Do SH, et al. Prophylactic dexamethasone decreases the incidence of sore throat and hoarseness after tracheal extubation with a double-lumen endobronchial tube. *Anesth Analg*. 2008;107:1814–1818.
74. Campos JH. Effects of oxygenation during selective lobar versus total lung collapse with or without continuous positive airway pressure. *Anesth Analg*. 1997;85:583–586.
75. Campos JH, Ledet C, Moyers JR. Improvement of arterial oxygen saturation with selective lobar bronchial block during hemorrhage in a patient with previous contralateral lobectomy. *Anesth Analg*. 1995;81:1095–1096.
76. Amar D, Desiderio DP, Bains MS, Wilson RS. A novel method of one-lung isolation using a double endobronchial blocker technique. *Anesthesiology*. 2001;95:1528–1530.
77. Campos JH. Update on selective lobar blockade during pulmonary resections. *Curr Opin Anaesthesiol*. 2009;22:18–22.
78. Campos JH. Which device should be considered the best for lung isolation: double-lumen endotracheal tube versus bronchial blockers. *Curr Opin Anaesthesiol*. 2007;20:27–31.

79. Arndt GA, DeLessio ST, Kranner PW, et al. One-lung ventilation when intubation is difficult-presentation of a new endobronchial blocker. *Acta Anaesthesiol Scand.* 1999;43:356–358.
80. Arndt GA, Buchika S, Kranner PW, DeLessio ST. Wire-guided endobronchial blockade in a patient with a limited mouth opening. *Can J Anaesth.* 1999;46:87–89.
81. Grocott HP, Scales G, Schinderle D, King K. A new technique for lung isolation in acute thoracic trauma. *J Trauma.* 2000;49:940–942.
82. Byhahn C, Habler OP, Bingold TM, et al. The wire-guided endobronchial blocker: applications in trauma patients beyond mere single-lung ventilation. *J Trauma.* 2006;61:755–759.
83. Campos JH, Kernstine KH. Use of the wire-guided endobronchial blocker for one-lung anesthesia in patients with airway abnormalities. *J Cardiothorac Vasc Anesth.* 2003;17:352–354.
84. Kabon B, Waltl B, Leitgeb J, Kapral S, Zimpfer M. First experience with fiberoptically directed wire-guided endobronchial blockade in severe pulmonary bleeding in an emergency setting. *Chest.* 2001;120:1399–1402.
85. Kazari W. Alternative method to deflate the operated lung when using wire-guided endobronchial blockade. *Anesthesiology.* 2003;99:239–240.
86. Campos JH. In response: an alternative method to deflate the operated lung when using wire guided endobronchial blockade. *Anesthesiology.* 2003;99:241.
87. Soto RG, Oleszak SP. Resection of the Arndt bronchial blocker during stapler resection of the left lower lobe. *J Cardiothorac Vasc Anesth.* 2006;20:131–132.
88. Roscoe A, Kanellakos GW, McRae K, Slinger P. Pressures exerted by endobronchial devices. *Anesth Analg.* 2007;104:655–658.
89. Lizuka T, Tanno M, Hamada Y, Shga T, Ohe Y. Uniblocker® bronchial blocker tube to facilitate one-lung ventilation during thoracoscopic surgery. *Anesthesiology.* 2007;108:A1815.
90. Qiu J, Feng M, Zhang C, et al. VivaSight™ single-lumen tube guided bronchial blocker placement for one-lung ventilation in a patient with a tracheal tumor under video-assisted transthoracic surgery: a case report. *BMC Anesthesiol.* 2019;19:2.
91. Shaw AD, Grichnik K, Barbeito, et al. Lung separation techniques. In: Barbelto A, et al., eds. *Thoracic Anesthesia.* The McGraw-Hill Companies; 2012:82–101.
92. Baraka A. The univent tube can facilitate difficult intubation in a patient undergoing thoracoscopy. *J Cardiothorac Vasc Anesth.* 1996;10:693–694.
93. Ransom ES, Carter SL, Mund GD. Univent tube: a useful device in patients with difficult airways. *J Cardiothorac Vasc Anesth.* 1995;9:725–727.
94. Takenaka I, Aoyama K, Kadoya T. Use of the univent bronchial-blocker tube for unanticipated difficult endotracheal intubation. *Anesthesiology.* 2000;93:590–591.
95. Campos JH, Kernstine KH. A structural complication in the torque control blocker Univent: fracture of the blocker cap connector. *Anesth Analg.* 2003;96:630–631.
96. Peragallo RA, Swenson JD. Congenital tracheal bronchus: the inability to isolate the right lung with a univent bronchial blocker tube. *Anesth Analg.* 2000;91:300–301.
97. Asai T. Failure of the Univent bronchial blocker in sealing the bronchus. *Anaesthesia.* 1999;54:97.
98. Thielmeier KA, Anwar M. Complication of the Univent tube. *Anesthesiology.* 1996;84:491.
99. Dougherty P, Hannallah M. A potentially serious complication that resulted from improper use of the Univent tube. *Anesthesiology.* 1992;77:835.
100. Prabhu MR, Smith JH. Use of the Arndt wire-guided endobronchial blocker. *Anesthesiology.* 2002;97:1325.
101. Sandberg WS. Endobronchial blocker dislodgement leading to pulseless electrical activity. *Anesth Analg.* 2005;100:1728–1730.
102. Ueda K, Goetzinger C, Gauger EH, et al. Use of bronchial blockers: a retrospective review of 302 cases. *J Anesth.* 2012;26:115–117.
103. Honikman R, Rodriguez-Diaz CA, Cohen E. A ballooning crisis: three cases of bronchial blocker malfunction and a review. *J Cardiothorac Vasc Anesth.* 2017;31:1799–1804.
104. van de Pas JM, van der Woude MC, Belgers HJ, et al. Bronchus perforation by EZ-Blocker™ endobronchial blocker during esophageal resection after neoadjuvant chemoradiation -a case report. *Korean J Anesthesiol.* 2019;72:184–187.
105. Ko R, McRae K, Darling G, et al. The use of air in the inspired gas mixture during two-lung ventilation delays lung collapse during one-lung ventilation. *Anesth Analg.* 2009;108:1092–1096.
106. Yoshimura T, Ueda K, Kakinuma A, et al. Bronchial blocker lung collapse technique: nitrous oxide for facilitating lung collapse during one-lung ventilation with a bronchial blocker. *Anesth Analg.* 2014;118:666–670.
107. Campos JH, Ueda K, Hallam EA. Lung isolation in the morbidly obese patient: a comparison of a left-sided double-lumen endotracheal tube with the Arndt® Wire-Guided Blocker. *Br J Anaesth.* 2012;109:630–635.
108. Bussières JS, Somma J, Del Castillo JL, et al. Bronchial blocker versus left double-lumen endotracheal tube in video-assisted thoracoscopic surgery: a randomized-controlled trial examining time and quality of lung deflation. *Can J Anaesth.* 2016;63:818–827.
109. Neustein SM. Pro: bronchial blockers should be used routinely for providing one-lung ventilation. *J Cardiothorac Vasc Anesth.* 2015;29:234–236.
110. Cohen E. Strategies for lung isolation: to block or not to block? *Can J Anaesth.* 2016;63:797–801.
111. Hesselfeldt R, Kristensen MS, Rasmussen LS, et al. Evaluation of the airway of the SimMan® full-scale patient simulator. *Acta Anaesthesiol Scand.* 2005;49:1339–1345.
112. Wong AK. Full scale computer simulators in anesthesia training and evaluation. *Can J Anaesth.* 2004;51:455–464.
113. Nyssen AS, Larbuisson R, Janssens M, et al. A comparison of the training value of two types of anesthesia simulators: computer screen-based and mannequin-based simulators. *Anesth Analg.* 2002;94:1560–1565.
114. Duffy CH, Myles PS. Review: thoracic-anesthesia.com. *J Cardiothorac Vasc Anesth.* 2008;22:644.
115. Campos JH, Hallam EA, Ueda K. Training in placement of the left-sided double lumen tube among non-thoracic anesthesiologists: intubation model simulator versus computer-based DVD, a randomized control trial. *Eur J Anaesthesiol.* 2011;28:169–174.
116. Failor E, Bowdle A, Jelacic S, et al. High-fidelity simulation of lung isolation with double-lumen endotracheal tubes and bronchial blockers in anesthesiology resident training. *J Cardiothorac Vasc Anesth.* 2014;28:865–869.
117. Latif RK, VanHorne EM, Kandadai SK, et al. Teaching basic lung isolation skills on human anatomy simulator: attainment and retention of lung isolation skills. *BMC Anesthesiol.* 2016; 20(16):1–7.

NON-PRINT ITEMS

Abstract

Lung separation techniques are designed to facilitate surgical exposure and provide one-lung ventilation (OLV) in patients undergoing thoracic, mediastinal, cardiac, vascular, esophageal, or selective spine surgery. Lung separation can be achieved with two different techniques. The first involves the double-lumen endotracheal tube (DLT) technique. This device is made of disposable polyvinyl, chloride or silicone material. The DLT is a bifurcated tube with both an endotracheal and an endobronchial lumen and can be used to achieve separation of either the right or left lung. Modifications have been made to the DLT to improve quality of placement and patient safety. A newly designed VivaSight® DLT has an integrated camera, allowing continuous visualization of its position within the trachea. In addition, there is the ECOM-DLT®. This device has multiple flexible surface sensors attached to the endotracheal cuff of the DLT that, when connected to a monitor measure the aortic blood flow by the bioimpedance method, and based upon an algorithm, it can record cardiac output, stroke volume, and systemic vascular resistances. The second technique involves blockade of a mainstem bronchus to allow lung collapse distal to the occlusion. Currently, there are different bronchial blockers to facilitate lung separation and provide OLV. These devices are either attached to a single-lumen endotracheal tube with an enclosed bronchial blocker, such as the torque control blocker Univent or can be used independently while advanced over a single-lumen endotracheal tube, such as the wire-guided endobronchial blocker (Arndt blocker), the Cohen tip-deflecting endobronchial blocker, the Fuji Uniblocker, or the EZ-Blocker.

Keywords

double-lumen endotracheal tubes, bronchial blockers, airway management, flexible fiberoptic bronchoscopy, ultrasonography

17

Lung Isolation in Patients With a Difficult Airway in Thoracic Anesthesia

JAVIER H. CAMPOS

Introduction

One-lung ventilation (OLV) in the thoracic surgical patient who presents with a difficult airway can be achieved with the use of a single-lumen endotracheal tube with a bronchial blocker or with the use of a double-lumen endotracheal tube (DLT).[1–4] It is estimated that between 5% and 8% of the patients who presented for thoracic surgery for primary lung carcinoma also have carcinoma of the pharynx, usually in the epiglottic area. Many of these patients have undergone extensive surgery of the airway or neck.[3] In addition, some of these patients had previous radiation to the neck or previous airway surgery, such as hemi-mandibulectomy or hemi-glossectomy, making intubation difficult in general, and particularly for achievement of OLV because of distorted upper airway anatomy. The distorted anatomy can be located at or beyond the tracheal carina, such as descending thoracic aortic aneurysm compressing the left mainstem bronchus or an intrabronchial or extrabronchial tumor near the tracheobronchial bifurcation that make the insertion of a left-sided DLT difficult or impossible.[5]

Preoperative Assessment of the Difficult Airway

An airway is termed difficult when conventional laryngoscopy reveals a class III view (just the epiglottis is seen) or class IV view (just part of the soft palate is seen). Fig. 17.1 displays the airway anatomy and class III and IV according to the modified Mallampati classification. Once the airway is recognized as being potentially difficult, a careful examination of the patient should follow. Previous anesthesia records, if available, should be examined for a history of airway management of the patient. Patients should be asked to open their mouths as wide as possible and extend their tongues. The length of the submental space should also be noted. Patients should be evaluated from side to side to assess any degree of maxillary overbite and their ability to assume the sniffing position. Also the patency of the nostrils must be assessed in patients who cannot open their mouths because a nasotracheal approach might be considered.[6] For patients who have a tracheostomy in place, the inlet of the stoma and the circumferential diameter must be assessed when considering replacing the tracheostomy cannula with the device selected to achieve OLV.[7] Furthermore, depending on the type and the length of surgery, the degree of fluid shift during surgery, an airway that initially was not classified as difficult may become difficult secondary to airway edema, the presence of secretion, and laryngeal trauma from the initial intubation. In addition, 10% of the patients who can be intubated with a single lumen tube can be difficult to insert a DLT into depending on the degree of the mouth opening, the size of the tongue and the composition of the teeth.

Another group of patients considered to have a difficult airway during OLV are those who have distorted anatomy from compression or intraluminal tumor at the orifice of the mainstem bronchus.[5] Such anomalies can be recognized by reviewing chest radiographs and multidetector computed tomography scans to determine the main stem bronchus diameter and anatomy to exclude the presence of distortion or compression.[8] In some cases, the use of flexible fiberoptic bronchoscopy will be necessary to evaluate the degree of distorted anatomy of the airway before the selection of a specific device to achieve OLV. Box 17.1 displays the patients at risk of potentially having difficult intubation during OLV.[3]

Difficult Airways and Lung Isolation: Primary Objective to Secure the Airway

In patients who require OLV and present with a difficult airway, the primary initial goal is to establish an airway with a single-lumen endotracheal tube. Any concern regarding the possibility of losing control of the patient's airway during the induction of anesthesia mandates an awake fiberoptic intubation, following an adequate topicalization of the

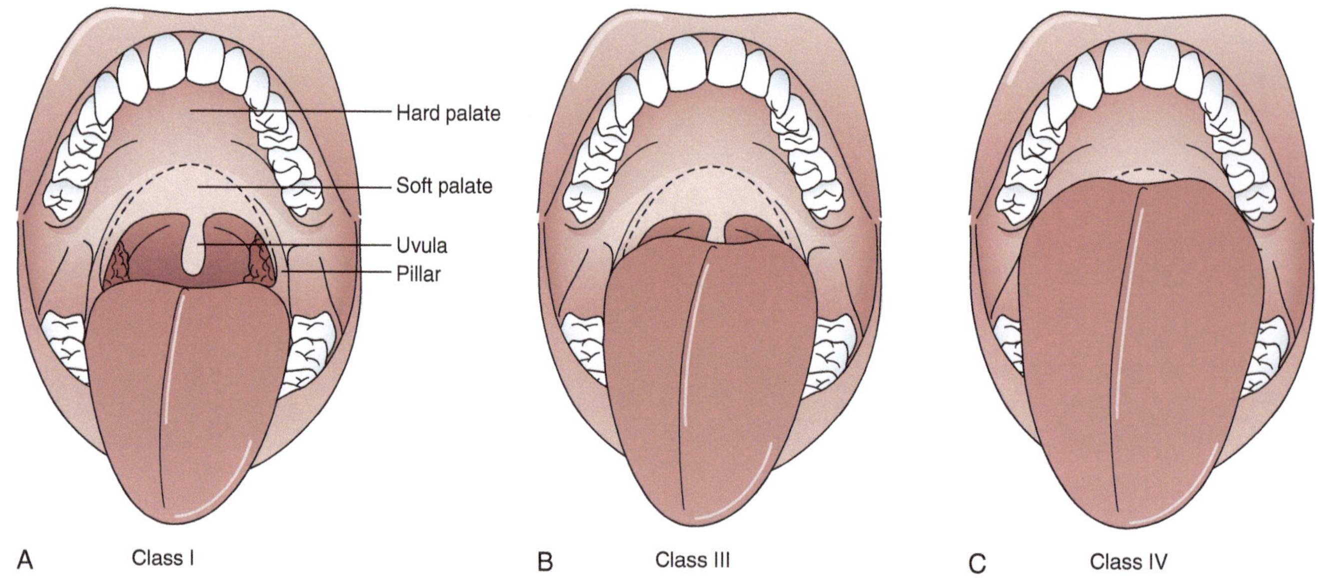

• **Fig. 17.1** Modified Mallampati classification for difficult laryngoscopy and intubation. (**A**) Normal airway anatomy, (**B**) class III, just the epiglottis is seen, and (**C**) class IV, where just part of the soft palate is seen.

airway. In selected patients who seem easy to ventilate, this may be performed after induction of anesthesia with the use of a bronchoscope or with one of several clinically available video laryngoscopes such as the C-MAC blade, GlideScope, King Video laryngoscope, or the Airtraq. All these devices have been shown to facilitate the view of epiglottis and vocal cords.[9–11]

Upper Airway Abnormalities and Lung Isolation

Patients requiring OLV can be identified during the preoperative evaluation to have a potentially difficult airway from distorted airway anatomy caused by previous surgery, radiation therapy with stiff tissues or both. Various methods are available to provide OLV under these circumstances. As mentioned previously, the first step is to establish an airway with a single-lumen endotracheal tube placed orally when the patient is awake, using a flexible fiberoptic bronchoscopy.

• BOX 17.1 Patients With Potential Risk of Having a Difficult Airway During One-Lung Ventilation

Upper Airway

- Short neck and increased neck circumference >42 cm
- Prominent upper incisors with a receding mandible
- Limited cervical mobility and compression of spinal cord
- Limited jaw opening, that is, chronic trismus
- Radiation therapy to the neck region
- Hemi-glossectomy/hemi-mandibulectomy
- Large tumor of the tongue, mouth, and epiglottis

Lower Airway

- Existing tracheostomy in place
- Distorted anatomy within trachea or bronchus
- Compression at the entrance of right or left mainstem bronchus

During the preparation for an awake fiberoptic intubation, the patients should receive oxygen via a nasal cannula and be fully monitored with electrocardiogram, blood pressure, and pulse oximetry. All local anesthetics used via spray or aerosolizer should be quantified to avoid complications from overdose of local anesthetic, such as seizures. Also, these patients should receive an antisialagogue medication, such as glycopyrrolate.

A simple approach to anesthetize the posterior part of the tongue is to apply lidocaine 5% ointment to a tongue blade depressor, and let the patient hold this in the mouth for 5 minutes. After the tongue blade depressor is removed, a mucosal atomization device to spray a local anesthetic with lidocaine 4% directly to pharynx, larynx, and vocal cords should be used. When the patient experiences a cough reflex, it is very likely that the anesthetic has entered the vocal cords.

The next step is to suction all residual secretions that were accumulated in the airway. To test that the gagging reflex is abolished, a Berman intubating pharyngeal airway impregnated with lidocaine 5% ointment at the posterior tip end of the cannula is advanced in the middle of the tongue until it is completely inserted in the oral cavity. The advantage of using the Berman cannula is that it facilitates a view of the epiglottis and allows the direct passage of the fiberscope followed by a single-lumen endotracheal tube. Also, the rigid cannula protects the fiberscope against potential damage from the patient's teeth. The fiberscope must be positioned in the midline such that the single-lumen endotracheal tube faces posteriorly during the attempt for intubation. In some cases, retracting the single-lumen endotracheal tube in a 90-degree counterclockwise rotation will disengage the tip of the tube from the vocal cord and facilitate passage of the tube into the trachea.

Following placement of the fiberoptic bronchoscope and the single-lumen endotracheal tube within the patient's trachea is the direct visualization of the tracheal rings and the tracheal carina with the fiberscope, along with the view of the tip of the single-lumen endotracheal tube inside the trachea.[12] After the patient is intubated with a single-lumen endotracheal tube, then an independent bronchial blocker should be used to achieve OLV.

Common independent bronchial blockers used through, or extraluminal to, the single-lumen endotracheal tube include: a wire-guided endobronchial Arndt blocker sizes 5.0, 7.0, and 9.0 Fr, the Cohen Flexitip blocker size 9.0 Fr, the Fuji Uniblocker sizes 4.5 and 9.0 Fr, or the EZ-Blocker size 7.0 Fr.[13] An alternative for securing the airway if a patient cannot open the mouth because of previous surgery and cannot be intubated orally, is an awake nasotracheal intubation, which can be performed taking all precautions of a nasal intubation, including the application of a vasoconstrictor, followed by a local anesthetic, and the passage of a single-lumen endotracheal tube. Once the airway is established, then an independent bronchial blocker can be advanced under direct fiberoptic view to the selected main bronchus.[14]

When an independent bronchial blocker is used, specifically, size 9.0 Fr, (the smallest acceptable single-lumen endotracheal tube size recommended is 8.0 internal diameter (ID) mm), it is important to have enough space between the bronchial blocker and the flexible fiberoptic bronchoscope so that navigation can be achieved with the single-lumen endotracheal tube. If only a 7.0- or a 7.5-mm single lumen tube was able to be placed, the 9.0 Fr blockers can still be positioned. Following an extensive lubrification of the blocker, it should be passed first blindly to have the blocker cuff beyond the tip of the single lumen tube. Then, the insertion of the fiberoptic bronchoscope will follow for proper positioning. That will avoid having the blocker cuff, which is the limiting factor, and the bronchoscope together in the narrow single lumen tube. An advantage of the Cohen Flexitip, Fuji Uniblocker, or the EZ-Blocker over the Arndt wire-guided endobronchial blocker is that while advancing it to a desired bronchus, the distal tip of the blocker can be seen by the bronchoscope while being directed to the selected bronchus. With the Arndt blocker, the distal tip is looped into the fiberscope and cannot be visualized until disengagement occurs. Because this blocker is advanced blindly, it can be caught in the Murphy eye of the endotracheal tube or at the carina. One of the advantages of the use of a blocker in a patient with a difficult airway, in addition to providing OLV with insertion of a single-lumen endotracheal tube, is that the independent bronchial blocker is simply removed at the end of the procedure if postoperative ventilatory support is needed.[15] The blocker balloon should be inflated only once the patient is turned to the lateral decubitus position. The amount of air needed to achieve a complete seal within the bronchus in an adult varies between 5 and 8 mL. The EZ-Blocker requires higher amounts of air to achieve a seal.[16] It is best to inflate the blocker cuff under direct vision with the bronchoscope.

The optimal position of a bronchial blocker in the left or right bronchus is when the blocker balloon's outer surface is seen at least 10 mm below the tracheal carina inside the blocked bronchus and a proper seal is achieved. Fig. 17.2 shows the optimal position of the Fuji Uniblocker through a single-lumen endotracheal tube. Fig. 23 in Chapter 16 shows the optimal position of an EZ-blocker. Following the inflation of the blocker cuff, the blocker lumen can be attached to a suction while observing the ventilator bellows. If the bellows fail to fill up, it is an indication that the inflated bronchial cuff is not adequately sealing the main bronchus lumen and the tidal volume is being lost.

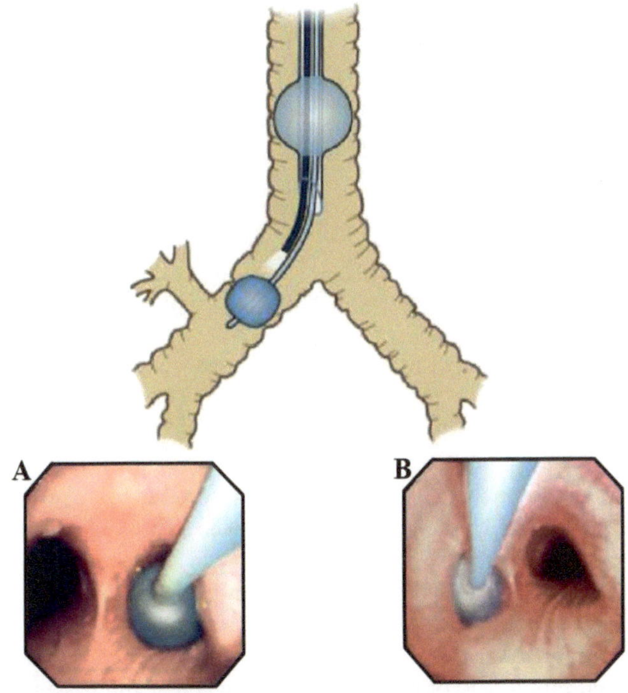

• **Fig. 17.2** The optimal position of the Fuji Uniblocker through a single-lumen endotracheal tube. (**A**) Fully inflated balloon of the Fuji Uniblocker in the right mainstem bronchus. (**B**) Fully inflated balloon of the Fuji Uniblocker in the left mainstem bronchus.

Use of Laryngeal Mask Airway and a Bronchial Blocker During Difficult Airways

An alternative to achieve OLV in a patient with a difficult airway is with the use of a laryngeal mask airway in conjunction with the use of an independent bronchial blocker. The ProSeal laryngeal mask airway has been used with a bronchial blocker in patients in whom the airway was deemed difficult and who required OLV during thoracoscopic surgery.[17,18]

Use of a Double-Lumen Endotracheal Tube in Patients With Difficult Airways

Intubation with a DLT can be more difficult than intubation with a single-lumen endotracheal tube. The larger size, the rigidity, and the shape of the DLT without a bevel at the tip of the tube can obscure the view of the glottis. In practice, there are different ways to place a DLT in a patient with a difficult airway. The first involves the use of airway topical anesthesia, an awake fiberoptic bronchoscopy with passage of the flexible fiberoptic bronchoscope through

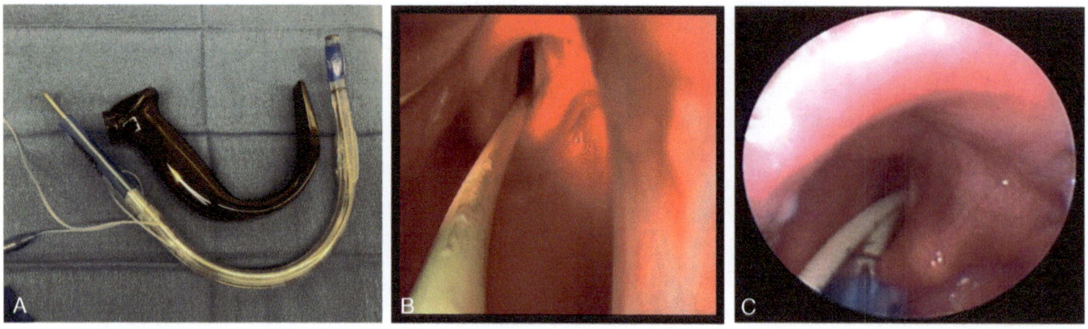

• **Fig. 17.3** The double airway exchange catheter technique. (**A**) The video laryngoscope, with a curve shaped DLT. (**B**) A view of the airway exchange catheter through the vocal cords. (**C**) A DLT advanced with two airway exchange catheters 11 Fr, one through the tracheal lumen, and one through the endobronchial lumen. *DLT,* Double-lumen endotracheal tube.

the endobronchial lumen of the DLT, where the tube is advanced under bronchoscopy guidance.[19] This technique can be limited by the short length of the fiberoptic bronchoscope available for manipulations when placed through the long DLT. The second technique involves the use of ancillary-lighted devices or video laryngoscopes that increase the visualization field of the epiglottis, vocal cords, and passage of the tube. The use of a malleable-lighted stylet has been reported. It was used within the endobronchial lumen of the DLT, where the tip of the bulb was positioned distally at the tip of the DLT in patients with difficult airways.[20]

In the past the use of a prototype fiberoptic laryngoscope, the WuScope, (no longer commercially available) during placement of a DLT in patients with abnormal airway anatomy was described.[21] One of the advantages of the channeled fiberoptic laryngoscope is that it protects against rupture of the endotracheal cuff during laryngoscopy because the DLT is enclosed with the laryngoscope blade. One of the limitations of this device is the need for smaller size DLTs, such as 35 to 37 Fr.[22]

Tube Exchanger Technique for a Double-Lumen Endotracheal Tube

Another alternative to establish lung separation following placement of a single-lumen endotracheal tube during an awake fiberoptic bronchoscopy or after induction of anesthesia, is to use a tube exchanger to replace the existing tube for a DLT.

For an airway exchange catheter to work, it must have a hollow center channel and universal adapter to insufflate oxygen. The exchange catheter must have a flexible tip distally to avoid airway lacerations, be long in length, and have outer markings to control the depth of insertion while in use. For a DLT, the exchange catheter should be at least 83 cm long. The airway Aintree tube exchanger has a large ID that allows fiberoptic bronchoscopy guidance. Also, a 14-Fr airway exchange catheter can be used to facilitate insertion of 39 and 41 Fr DLTs. For a 35 or 37 Fr DLT, an 11 Fr airway exchange catheter can be used.

The airway exchange catheter, single-lumen endotracheal tube, and the DLT combination should be tested in vitro before the exchange.[23] A sniffing position will facilitate tube exchange. After the airway exchange catheter is lubricated, it is advanced through a single-lumen endotracheal tube. The airway catheter should not be inserted deeper than 24 cm from the lips to avoid accidental rupture or laceration of the trachea, bronchi, or lung.[24,25] After cuff deflation, the single-lumen endotracheal tube is withdrawn, then the endobronchial lumen of the DLT is advanced over the exchange catheter. It is optimal to use a video laryngoscope during the tube exchange to guide the DLT through the glottis under direct vision.[26] Fig. 17.3 displays the double airway exchange catheter technique. Fig. 17.3A displays the video laryngoscope; Fig. 17.3B displays a view of the airway exchange catheter through the vocal cords; and Fig. 17.3C displays a DLT advanced with two airway exchange catheters 11 Fr, one through the tracheal lumen, and one through the endobronchial lumen.

If a video laryngoscope is not available, then having an assistant perform a standard laryngoscopy during tube exchange partially straightens out the alignment of the oropharynx and glottis and facilitates the exchange. Proper final position of the DLT is then achieved with auscultation, presence of end-tidal carbon dioxide ($ETCO_2$) waveform, and a fiberoptic bronchoscopy examination. An alternative to facilitating the placement of a DLT in a patient with a difficult airway is with the use of a bougie. Unfortunately, some of these bougies have resulted in shearing material through the lumen of the DLT,[27–29] and the manufacturer clearly indicates in the instructions that the bougie intubating introducer is not intended to use with DLTs.

A recent study[30] investigated three different brands of DLTs (Mallinckrodt BronchoCath, Silbroncho, and the P3 DLTs) and compared the performance of four brands of bougies in a simulation in vitro model. The authors reported that the brand of bougie, brand of the DLT, and size of the DLT all contributed to a degree of shearing of the bougie device when it was passed through and removed from the lumen of the DLTs. The bougies sheared least when used with the Silbroncho DLT. The authors also reported when the Frova bougie was used with the Mallinckrodt DLT, it showed more shearing then the other brands of DLTs. Although bougies are helpful during insertion of a single-lumen endotracheal tube, be aware that misuse, particularly with placement of DLTs of these sheared bougie

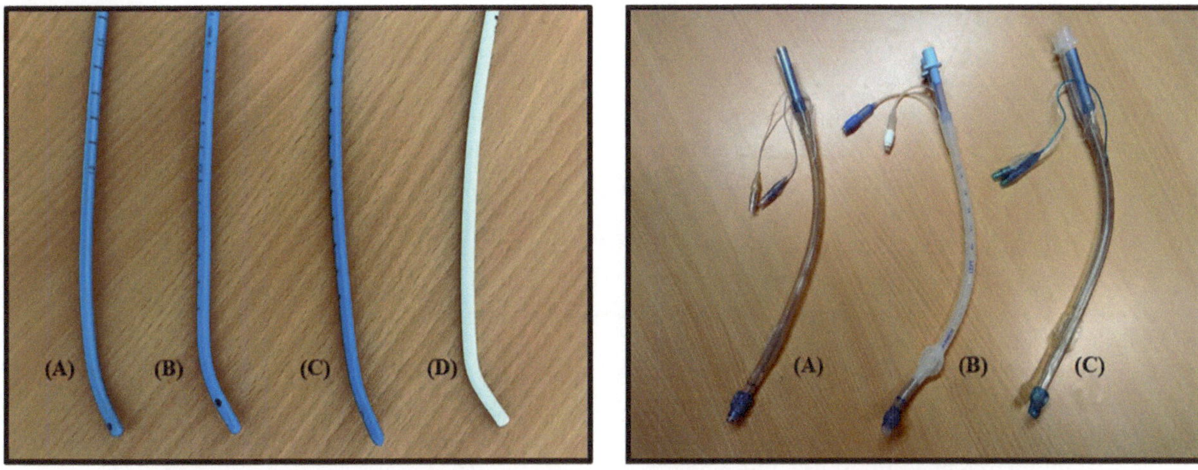

• **Fig. 17.4** **Left:** Bougies (A) Frova, (B) P3, (C) PROACT and (D) Portex. **Right:** Double lumen tubes (A) Mallinckrodt Broncho-Cath, (B) Silbronco and (C) P3. (From Luther DGP, Robertson HF, Suchett-Kaye I, et al. Double-lumen tracheal tubes and bougies: a bench study to investigate factors that influence the risk of shearing. *Anaesthesia*. 2019;74:891–895.)

fragments, can cause short-term airway obstruction and may potentially cause long-term morbidity. The extent to which a bougie shears is not only a function of its physical properties but also depends on the DLT used. The Frova bougie with Mallinckrodt DLT is particularly high risk. In addition, bougies shear less with Silbronco DLTs. Fig. 17.4 displays double-lumen tracheal tubes and bougies.

Exchange of a Double-Lumen Endotracheal Tube for a Single-Lumen Endotracheal Tube

Replacement of a DLT for a single-lumen endotracheal tube can be done at the conclusion of surgery with the use of a double airway exchange catheter. One study using two airway exchange catheters to exchange a DLT for a single-lumen endotracheal tube showed that there was a reduction in the incidence of glottis impingement of the tracheal tube, and that there was a higher success rate of passage of the single-lumen endotracheal tube when compared with the use of a single airway exchange catheter.

The use of a double airway exchange catheter involves various techniques. The most common is using a double-diameter coaxial airway exchange catheter. This consists of a 4.0-mm outer diameter exchanger inside a 7.0-mm outer diameter exchanger. This device allows for a more rigid guide wire for replacing a DLT with a single-lumen endotracheal tube. During tube exchanging techniques, it is recommended to use a video laryngoscope to visualize the proper exchange and move the tongue away from the tube. A second technique is using two 11.0 Fr, 83-cm long airway exchange catheters from Cook Critical Care. One catheter is passed through the endobronchial lumen of the DLT, making sure that the tip of the airway exchanger does not protrude distally in the tip of the DLT. A second exchange catheter is passed through the tracheal lumen; both wires provide easy placement of the new single-lumen endotracheal tube because of the increased rigidity with the two tube exchangers. For this technique to work, an 8.0 ID mm single-lumen endotracheal tube must be used. Fig. 17.5 displays the Aintree airway catheter from Cook Critical Care.

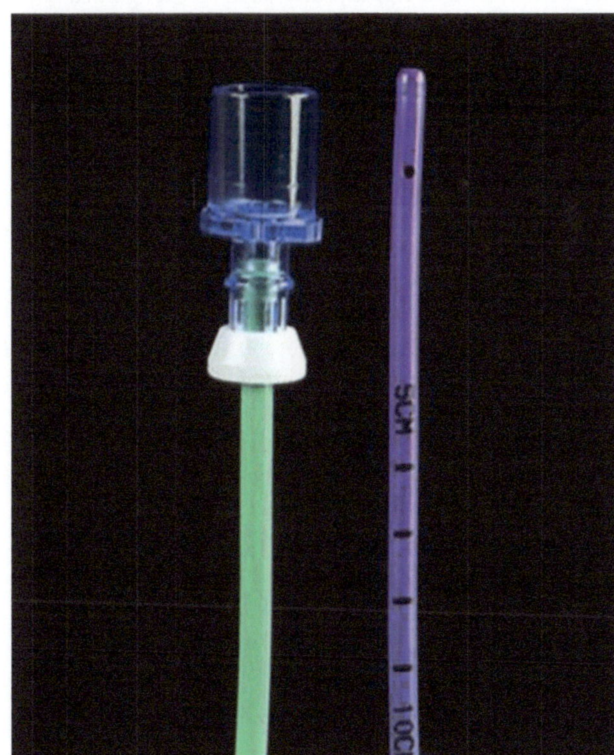

• **Fig. 17.5** The Cook airway catheter Aintree (Cook Critical Care) for exchange between double-lumen endotracheal tubes and a single-lumen endotracheal tube. This recent modification has a soft distal (purple) tip to attempt to decrease the risk of distal airway injury during tube exchange (right). The proximal stiffer green end (left) has detachable connectors for emergency ventilation. Shown is the standard 15-mm outside diameter breathing circuit connector.

Lung Isolation Techniques in Patients With Tracheostomies

The patient with a tracheostomy in situ needs special airway management because the airway has been shortened or because a total laryngectomy will limit oral-tracheal intubation. Opportunities for using a conventional DLT in a patient with a tracheostomy in situ are limited because the DLT is too long or has a large outside diameter and is too rigid, or the tracheostomy stoma may be too small to accommodate the DLT, which can damage the airway easily. Factors to consider when managing lung isolation devices in a tracheostomized patient include early-stage stoma within 7 days of insertion,[31] and that the airway can be lost immediately while attempting to remove the Shiley tube, unlike a long-term well-established tracheostomy with a well-formed stoma.[32] All of these factors are important when selecting the appropriate lung isolation device to be placed through a tracheostomy stoma.[7]

In a patient with a tracheostomy in situ who had an early-stage tracheostomy, the Shiley tube with a bronchial blocker can be used.[7] In contrast for patients with a long-term tracheostomy stoma, a single-lumen endotracheal tube can be used and guided to a selective bronchus where lung isolation takes place. An alternative is the use of a single-lumen endotracheal tube, followed by intraluminal or extraluminal placement of an independent bronchial blocker guided with the use of flexible fiberoptic bronchoscopy to achieve optimal position of the bronchial blocker. One-lung ventilation in tracheostomized patients has been reported with the use of the Arndt wire-guided endobronchial blocker, Cohen Flexitip blocker, Fuji Uniblocker, and EZ-Blocker with good results.[7,33] DLT has been used through a tracheotomy, however,[34] it is recommended as a first choice using a bronchial blocker unless there is an absolute indication for the use of a DLT. For all these cases, a small-size fiberoptic bronchoscope (i.e., 3.5-mm outer diameter) is recommended. In Europe, a short-curved DLT (Portex) that fits through the stoma can be positioned to achieve lung separation (Note that this tube is not presently marked in the United States). Figs. 17.6 and 17.7 display a patient with an existing tracheostomy, where a Cohen blocker has been used to achieve OLV. Table 17.1 displays the recommendations for patients with tracheostomy in situ based upon 70 cases, with permission from Campos et al.[7]

Lung Isolation in Patients With Lower Airway Abnormalities

Another important group of patients to consider when managing the difficult airway and OLV is those who present with lower airway abnormalities, specifically, distal trachea or bronchial lesions. The common problems that will preclude or contraindicate the use of a left-sided DLT include an intraluminal tumor of the left mainstem bronchus or a descending thoracic aortic aneurysm that compressed the entrance of the left main bronchus (Fig. 17.8). In this case, a right-sided DLT guided with flexible fiberoptic bronchoscopy should be used.

Another group of patients that has lower airway abnormalities and requires OLV are those with previous lobectomies. These patients may have a distorted anatomy, which may contribute to difficulties in recognizing the right and left bronchus because of the loss of anatomic landmarks.[35] In these patients, a complete fiberoptic bronchoscopy examination of the trachea and bronchi before placement of lung isolation device is required to properly identify the anatomy of the tracheobronchial tree. Fig. 17.9 displays a patient with a previous lobectomy indicating the missing (stapled) segmental bronchus for a right upper lobectomy.

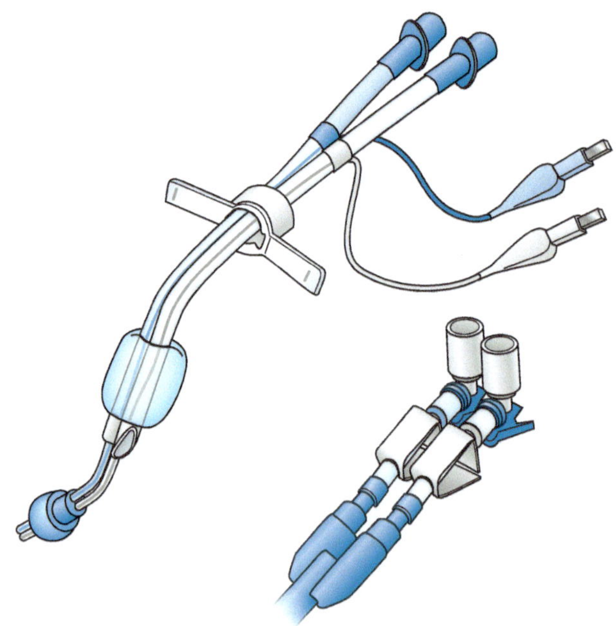

• **Fig. 17.6** A tracheostomy double-lumen endotracheal tube (available in Europe).

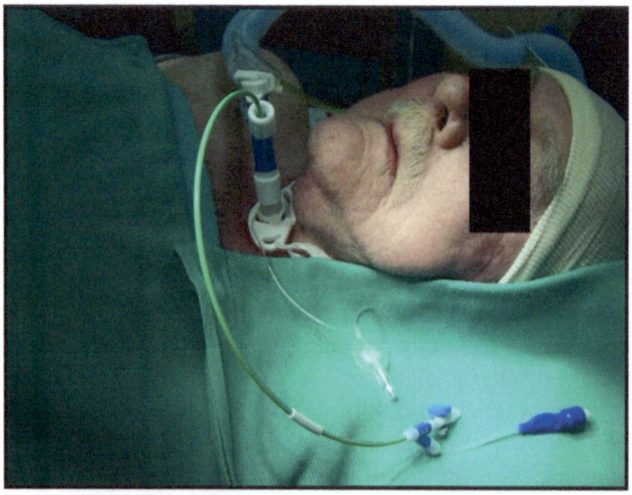

• **Fig. 17.7** A patient with an existing tracheostomy where a Cohen blocker has been used to achieve one-lung ventilation.

TABLE 17.1 Display of the Recommendations to Manage Lung Isolation in a Patient With an Existing Tracheostomy

Recommendations for Patients With Tracheostomy and One-Lung Ventilation	
Early-Stage Tracheostomy <7 days	**Long-Term Tracheostomy >7 days**
Shiley-cuffed low pressure tracheostomy tube in situ	Assess the tracheostomy stoma
	Shiley tracheostomy tube 6 or 8 mm ID or SLT 7.5 or 8.0 mm ID
• Consider a bronchial blocker	• Consider a bronchial blocker intra- or extraluminal placement
• Arndt, Cohen, EZ-Blocker (based upon expertise)	• Arndt, Cohen, EZ-Blocker, Fuji Uniblocker (based upon expertise)
• Flexible fiberoptic bronchoscope—size 3.5 mm OD or size 4.2 mm OD	• Flexible fiberoptic bronchoscope—size 3.5 mm OD or size 4.2 mm OD
	Advance an SLT through the tracheostomy stoma to block a main bronchus or pass a left-sided DLT

DLT, Double-lumen endotracheal tube; *ID*, internal diameter; *OD*, outer diameter; *OLV*, one-lung ventilation; *SLT*, single-lumen endotracheal tube.

(From Campos JH, et al. Lung isolation techniques in patients with early stage or long-term tracheostomy: a case series report of 70 cases and recommendations. *J Cardiothorac Vasc Anesth*. 2019;33:433–439. With permission.)

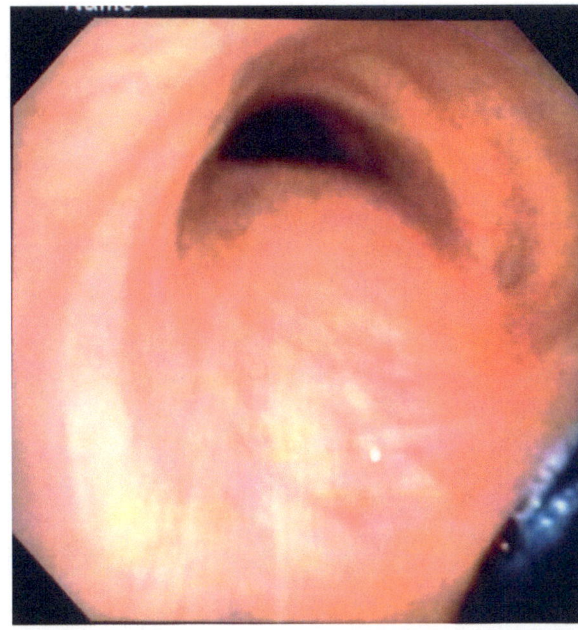

• **Fig. 17.8** A tracheal carina view with the fiberoptic bronchoscope. Toward the left, there is a compression of the entrance of the left mainstem bronchus because of an aortic thoracic aneurysm. Toward the right, shows the blue edge of the balloon of the endobronchial lumen of a right-sided double-lumen endotracheal tube. (Courtesy of Edmond Cohen M.D).

Extubation or Mechanical Ventilation After Surgery

Extubation at the completion of surgery in a patient who has a difficult airway represents a challenge. Fig. 17.10 displays the approach to extubation or tube exchange at the end of the procedure. Factors to consider before extubation include any mucosal edema, bleeding, secretion, or lacerations to the pharynx during intubation, the length of surgery, and the amount of fluid administered during the intraoperative period. Continuous access to the airway should be maintained in case reintubation is needed. The single-lumen endotracheal tube or the DLT can be removed with an airway catheter exchanger in place before extubation (stage extubation).[36] Another alternative technique is to exchange a DLT for a single-lumen endotracheal tube using an airway catheter exchanger under direct vision with a laryngoscope or video laryngoscope.[37–39] In some circumstances, a patient with a difficult airway and a DLT may require mechanical ventilation in the postoperative period. One option for extubation of these patients is to deflate both cuffs of the DLT, withdraw the tube above the carina, then reinflate the tracheal cuff, and convert the DLT to two-lung ventilation, particularly if the conversion to exchange a DLT for a single-lumen endotracheal tube is considered too risky. This is only recommended as the last option because the intensive care unit staff is not always familiar with the DLT management, and it opens the gate to potential complications.

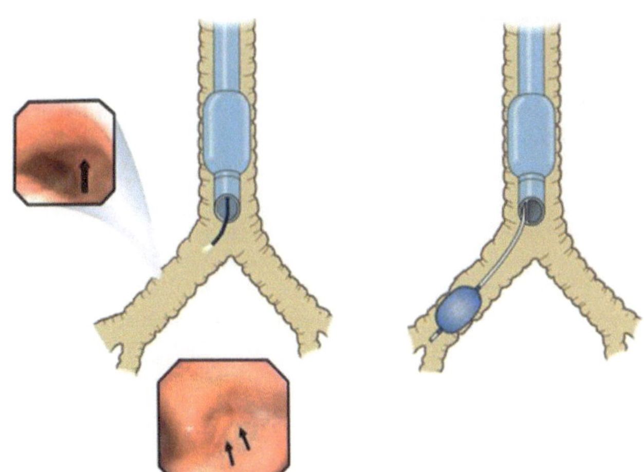

• **Fig. 17.9** A patient with a previous lobectomy, indicating the missing (stapled) segmental bronchus for a right upper lobectomy. Arrows indicate the staple line. (From Campos JH. Update on selective lobar blockade during pulmonary resections. *Curr Opin Anaesthesiol*. 2009;22:18–22. With permission.)

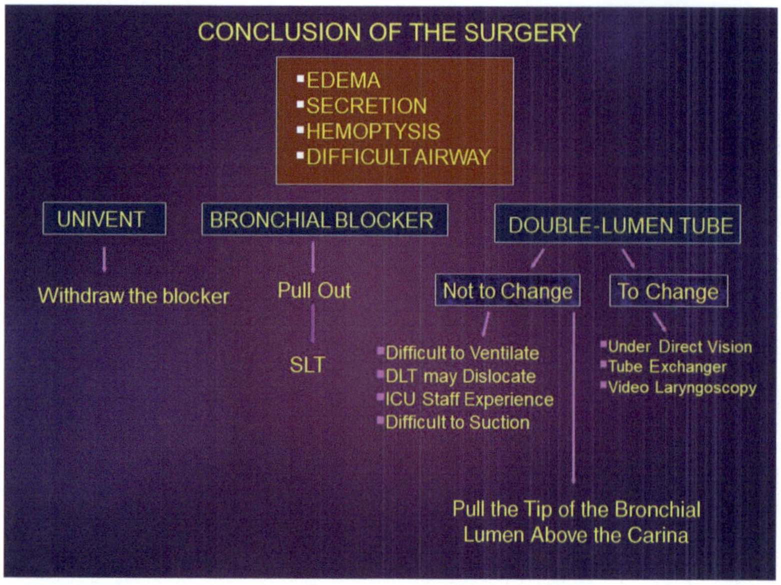

• **Fig. 17.10** The approach to extubation or tube exchange at the end of the procedure. *DLT,* Double-lumen endotracheal tube; *ICU*, intensive care unit; *SLT* single-lumen endotracheal tube.

Conclusion

In patients who require OLV, a key element during the preoperative assessment is the recognition and identification of the potentially difficult airway.[40] The safest way to establish an airway is by securing the airway with a single-lumen endotracheal tube placed orally or nasotracheally with the aid of flexible fiberoptic bronchoscopy. Lung isolation in these patients is achieved best with the use of an independent bronchial blocker.[41] An alternative can be the use of a DLT with an airway exchange technique. For the patient who has a tracheostomy in place, the use of an independent bronchial blocker through a single-lumen endotracheal tube or through a Shiley tracheostomy cannula in place is recommended. For all these devices, a flexible fiberoptic bronchoscopy examination is recommended prior, during placement, and at the conclusion of the use of lung isolation device.[7,42]

References

1. Campos J. Lung isolation in patients with difficult airways. In: Slinger P, ed. *Principles and Practice of Anesthesia for Thoracic Surgery*: Springer Publisher; 2011:247–258.
2. Campos J, Granell M. Difficult airway management in thoracic surgery. In: Granell Gil M, Sentürk M, eds. *Anesthesia in Thoracic Surgery*. Switzerland AG: Springer Nature; 2020.
3. Campos JH. Lung isolation techniques for patients with difficult airway. *Curr Opin Anaesthesiol.* 2010;23:12–17.
4. Collins SR, Titus BJ, Campos JH, Blank RS. Lung isolation in the patient with a difficult airway. *Anesth Analg*. 2018;126:1968–1978.
5. Campos JH, Ajax TJ, Knutson R, et al. Case Conference a 76-year-old needs an emergency surgery for a descending thoracic aortic aneurysm repair, has multiple intraoperative and postoperative complications. *J Cardiothorac Anesth*. 1990;5:631–645.
6. Campos JH, Kernstine KH. Use of the wire-guided endobronchial blocker for one-lung anesthesia in patients with airway abnormalities. *J Cardiothorac Vasc Anesth*. 2003;17:352–354.
7. Campos JH, Musselman ED, Hanada S, Ueda K. Lung isolation techniques in patients with early stage or long-term tracheostomy: a case series report of 70 cases and recommendations. *J Cardiothorac Vasc Anesth*. 2019;33:433–439.
8. Campos JH. Update on tracheobronchial anatomy and flexible fiberoptic bronchoscopy in thoracic anesthesia. *Curr Opin Anaesthesiol.* 2009;22:4–10.
9. Poon KH, Eh Liu. The Airway Scope for difficult double-lumen tube intubation. *J Clin Anesth*. 2008;20:319.
10. El-Tahan MR, Khidr AM, Gaarour IS, et al. A comparison of 3 videolaryngoscopes for double-lumen tube intubation in humans by users with mixed experience: a randomized controlled study. *J Cardiothorac Vasc Anesth*. 2018;32:277–286.
11. Liu TT, Li L, Wan L, et al. Video laryngoscopy vs. Macintosh laryngoscopy for double-lumen tube intubation in thoracic surgery: a systematic review and meta-analysis. *Anaesthesia*. 2018;73:997–1007.
12. Campos JH. Fiberoptic bronchoscopy in anesthesia. *Curr Rev Clin Anesth*. 2008;29:61–72.
13. Campos J. Lung isolation. In: Slinger P, ed. *Principles and Practice of Anesthesia for Thoracic Surgery*. Switzerland: Springer Publisher; 2019:283–309.
14. Angie Ho CY, Chen CY, Yang MW, et al. Use of the Arndt wire-guided endobronchial blocker via nasal for one-lung ventilation in patient with anticipated restricted mouth opening for esophagectomy. *Eur J Cardiothorac Surg*. 2005;28:174–575.
15. Cohen E. Pro: the new bronchial blockers are preferable to double-lumen tubes for lung isolation. *J Cardiothorac Vasc Anesth*. 2008; 22:920–924.
16. Mourisse J, Liesveld J, Verhagen A, et al. Efficiency, efficacy, and safety of EZ-Blocker compared with left-sided double-lumen tube for one-lung ventilation. *Anesthesiology*. 2013;118:550–561.
17. Ozaki M, Murashima K, Fukutome T. One-lung ventilation using the ProSeal laryngeal mask airway. *Anaesthesia*. 2004;59:726.
18. Tsuchihashi T, Ide S, Nakagawa H, et al. Differential lung ventilation using laryngeal mask airway and a bronchial blocker tube for a patient with unanticipated difficult intubation. *Masui*. 2007; 56:1075–1077.

19. Patane PS, Sell BA, Mahla ME. Awake fiberoptic endobronchial intubation. *J Cardiothorac Anesth*. 1990;4:229–231.
20. O'Connor CJ, O'Connor TA. Use of lighted stylets to facilitate insertion of double-lumen endobronchial tubes in patients with difficult airway anatomy. *J Clin Anesth*. 2006;18:616–619.
21. Smith CE, Kareti M. Fiberoptic laryngoscopy (WuScope) for double-lumen endobronchial tube placement in two difficult-intubation patients. *Anesthesiology*. 2000;93:906–907.
22. Hernandez AA, Wong DH. Using a GlideScope for intubation with a double lumen endotracheal tube. *Can J Anaesth*. 2005;52: 658–659.
23. Benumof JL. Difficult tubes and difficult airways. *J Cardiothorac Vasc Anesth*. 1998;12:131–132.
24. Thomas V, Neustein SW. Tracheal laceration after the use of an airway exchange catheter for double-lumen tube placement. *J Cardiothorac Vasc Anesth*. 2007;21:718–719.
25. deLima LG, Bishop MJ. Lung laceration after tracheal extubation over a plastic tube changer. *Anesth Analg*. 1991;73:350--351.
26. Chen A, Lai HY, Lin PC, et al. GlideScope-assisted double-lumen endobronchial tube placement in a patient with an unanticipated difficult airway. *J Cardiothorac Vasc Anesth*. 2008;22:170–172.
27. Vlachtsis H, Veltman M. Shearing of a Frova Intubating Introducer by a BronchoCath double lumen tube. *Anaesthesia*. 2006; 61:197–198.
28. Huitink JM, Bisschops M. A complication with an intubating introducer and a double-lumen tube: tip of the iceberg? *Anaesthesia*. 2012;67:926–927.
29. Graham JM, Von Heldreich C, Howard WV, et al. Frova Intubating Introducers and double-lumen tubes. *Anaesth Intensive Care*. 2013;41:127–128.
30. Luther DGP, Robertson HF, Suchett-Kaye I, et al. Double-lumen tracheal tubes and bougies: a bench study to investigate factors that influence the risk of shearing. *Anaesthesia*. 2019;74:891--895.
31. Mitchell RB, Hussey HM, Setzen G, et al. Clinical consensus statement: tracheostomy care. *Otolaryngol Head Neck Surg*. 2013; 148:6–20.
32. De Leyn P, Bedert L, Delcroix M, et al. Tracheotomy: clinical review and guidelines. *Eur J Cardiothorac Surg*. 2007;32:412–421.
33. Rispoli M, Nespoli MR, Salvi R, et al. One-lung ventilation in tracheostomized patients: our experience with EZ-Blocker. *J Clin Anesth*. 2016;31:288–290.
34. Yaney LL. Double-lumen endotracheal tube for one-lung ventilation through a fresh tracheostomy stoma: a case report. *AANA J*. 2007;75:411–415.
35. Campos JH. Update on selective lobar blockade during pulmonary resections. *Curr Opin Anaesthesiol*. 2009;22:18–22.
36. Mort TC. Continuous airway access for the difficult extubation: the efficacy of the airway exchange catheter. *Anesth Analg*. 2007;105: 1357–1362.
37. Merli G, Guarino A, Della Rocca G, et al. Recommendations for airway control and difficult airway management in thoracic anesthesia and lung separation procedures. *Minerva Anestesiol*. 2009; 75:59–78.
38. Campos JH. Guidelines, algorithms, and recommendations during the management of the difficult airways in the thoracic surgical patient: are they supported by evidence based. *Rev Esp Anestesiol Reanim*. 2018;65:1–4.
39. Thong SY, Lim Y. Video and optic laryngoscopy assisted tracheal intubation—the new era. *Anaesth Intensive Care*. 2009;37:219–233.
40. Campos JH. Progress in lung separation. *Thorac Surg Clin*. 2005; 15:71–83.
41. Ueda K, Goetzinger C, Gauger EH, et al. Use of bronchial blockers: a retrospective review of 302 cases. *J Anesth*. 2012;26:115–117.
42. Clayton-Smith A, Bennett K, Alston RP, et al. A comparison of the efficacy and adverse effects of double-lumen endobronchial tubes and bronchial blockers in thoracic surgery: a systematic review and meta-analysis of randomized controlled trials. *J Cardiothorac Vasc Anesth*. 2015;29:955–966.

18

Pathophysiology of Perioperative Lung Injury

ALEXANDER WHITE, ANDREW C. STEEL

Introduction

Postoperative pulmonary complications remain a significant cause of morbidity and mortality after surgery.[1] Approximately 230 million major surgical procedures are conducted annually worldwide. Perioperative pulmonary complications are common, occurring in up to 59% of patients. Approximately 2.7% of surgical patients will develop severe acute lung injury (ALI) causing postoperative respiratory failure.[2] The risk is not uniform, and is significantly higher in surgery on the esophagus (23.8%) than most orthopedic procedures. Should the patient recover from the episode and is discharged, the long-term prognosis for survivors of ALI is still significantly worse than those without ALI. A 2-year follow-up study reported that survivors of perioperative ALI required an average of two episodes of readmission and 6 days of hospital stay per year.[2] Another study reported 30-day mortality to be 27% following thoracic surgery,[3] and 90-day mortality to be 55%.[4]

The term "perioperative lung injury" has been known by a number of different terms in the past, including "permeability pulmonary edema" and "postoperative lung injury."[5] The current definition of perioperative lung injury is the development of acute respiratory distress syndrome (ARDS) immediately after surgery, using the Berlin definition of 2012[6] (Table 18.1). Although this definition is not without controversy, it is currently the most widely used and accepted definition.

Epidemiology

ARDS was initially described by Laennec in 1821, as a new syndrome characterized by pulmonary edema without heart failure.[7] Subsequently, terms such as "double pneumonia" and "shock lung" were used to describe this syndrome, before the term "acute respiratory distress syndrome" was coined by Ashbaugh and colleagues in 1967.[8] ARDS may result from intrapulmonary or extrapulmonary mechanisms, and indeed the cause is often multifactorial. It develops most commonly in the context of severe bacterial and viral pneumonia, nonpulmonary sepsis, aspiration, and trauma. Some of the less common causes of ARDS are included in Table 18.2. Perioperative lung injury results from a complex interaction between the patient's physiologic state, the underlying surgical diagnosis and technique, and interaction with the mechanical ventilator. Although ARDS is a common entity, it is important to understand that there are many clinical pathologies that mimic ARDS and should be considered, especially in the absence of an inciting factor (Table 18.3).[9]

Several comorbidities and exposures have been implicated in elevating the risk for developing ALI, and or worse outcomes, including excessive alcohol consumption,[10] cigarette smoking,[11] and environmental pollutants.[12] Data from the United States and the United Kingdom suggest there is also an association between mortality, ethnicity, and gender. Black, Asian, and minority ethnicity patients and male patients have a higher than average mortality from ALI than White and female patients.[13] The biologic cause for such disparities, beyond social inequality, is not clear. Erickson and colleagues concluded that it appeared to be mediated by increased severity of illness at presentation for Black patients but could not explain the increase seen among Hispanics in the United States.[13]

Imaging

The plain chest radiograph appearance that is consistent with ARDS is that of bilateral diffuse alveolar opacification, although it has been demonstrated that there is significant interobserver variability, and the findings may be subtle.[14] As the severity worsens, the consolidation becomes more apparent.[14] Computed tomography (CT) scanning of patients with ARDS reveals a more detailed picture of the heterogeneous nature of the lung injury than chest x-ray. The information gained from the CT scan can help quantify the extent of the abnormalities and localize them.[15]

The classic findings of early ARDS on CT scan are: (1) normal (or near-normally) aerated lung regions with minimal pathologic findings, most commonly in the least dependent

TABLE 18.1 Berlin Definition of Acute Respiratory Distress Syndrome

Oxygenation	Mild	Moderate	Severe
Timing	Onset within 1 week of a known clinical insult		
Chest imaging	Bilateral opacifications not fully explained by pleural effusions or lobar collapse		
Origin	Not fully explained by cardiogenic pulmonary edema		
P_aO_2/F_iO_2 ratio	200–300 with PEEP or CPAP ≥ 5 cm H_2O	100–200 with PEEP ≥5 cm H_2O	PaO_2/FiO_2 < 100 with PEEP ≥5 cm H_2O

Chest imaging may refer to a conventional chest x-ray or computed tomography thorax.

F_iO_2, Fraction of inspired oxygen; *P_aO_2*, partial pressure of oxygen taken from an arterial blood gas; *PEEP*, positive end expiratory pressure.

zones of the lung. These tend to be ventral when the patient is supine; (2) a hazy increase in lung attenuation, with preservation of bronchial and vascular margins, known as ground glass opacification in the middle lung; and (3) consolidative changes in the most dependent (dorsal) zones of the lung, appear as a homogeneous increase in lung attenuation that obscures bronchovascular margins in which air-bronchograms may be present.[15,16]

Lung ultrasound (LUS) is being used with increasing frequency to aid in the diagnosis of ARDS, and to help differentiate it from other lung pathologies (see Ch. 54). It has been demonstrated that LUS can identify the principal pathologic findings in ARDS with reasonable sensitivity and specificity.[17] International evidence-based recommendations for the use of LUS were established in 2012.[18] LUS is recommended as a tool to help evaluate and differentiate between fibrotic lung disease, pulmonary edema, and ARDS.[18]

The four main patterns that are seen on LUS are summarized from these guidelines as follows:

1. Normally aerated lung, represented by **lung sliding** and artifactual horizontal repetitions of the pleural line, known as **A-lines**.
2. Alveolar-interstitial syndrome, represented by the presence of three or more discrete laser-like vertical hyperechoic reverberation artifacts arising from the pleural line, extending to the bottom of the screen without fading, and moving synchronously with lung sliding, known as **B-lines**.
3. Consolidation, represented as a subpleural area consisting of tissue-like echodensities interlaced with echo-poor areas which are indicative of **dynamic air bronchograms**.
4. **Pleural effusions**, represented by an anechoic space between the parietal and visceral pleura, with respiratory movement of the lung within the effusion.[18,19]

TABLE 18.2 Different Causes of Acute Respiratory Distress Syndrome

Intrapulmonary	Extrapulmonary
Pneumonia	Sepsis
Aspiration	Trauma
Pulmonary contusion	Acute pancreatitis
Fat embolism	Cardiopulmonary bypass
Drowning	TRALI
Inhalational injury	Intracranial hemorrhage
Reperfusion syndrome	

TRALI, Transfusion associated acute lung injury.

When compared with CT scanning, LUS has shown reasonable sensitivity and specificity (82.7%–92.3% and 90.2%–98.6%, respectively) in the diagnosis of ARDS.[19] Its portability, lack of radiation, and steep learning curve make it an ideal tool in many situations to assist in diagnosis ARDS.

The Normal Lung

The alveolocapillary barrier separates alveolar gas from pulmonary blood. It is by necessity extremely thin and has a large surface area to allow sufficient and rapid diffusion of gases. The alveolar epithelial cells form the external layer and the endothelial cells the internal layer. Both cell layers are supported by their respective basement membranes and separated by the pulmonary interstitial space—a "potential space" in the gas exchange regions. **Type I alveolar epithelial cells** are large, extremely flattened cells that cover approximately 95% of the lung's surface area. These cells form a thin lining over the external interface (alveolar surface) and bind to adjacent cells via tight intercellular junctions. The cuboidal **type II alveolar epithelial cell** is the more complex and metabolically active alveolar cell; whose functions include: surfactant production, proliferation, and differentiation into type I cells following injury, and sodium and chloride ion transport.[20] The pulmonary endothelial cells line the capillaries within the lung parenchyma (Fig. 18.1).

Pathophysiology of the Injured Lung

The pathology of the injured lung in ARDS was first described in 1977 by Marianne Bachofen and Ewald Weibel in their seminal publication on respiratory insufficiency

TABLE 18.3 Diseases That May Be Mistaken for Acute Respiratory Distress Syndrome

Disease	Characteristic Findings That May Help Differentiate From Acute Respiratory Distress Syndrome
Congestive heart failure	Usually central symmetric interstitial and alveolar opacifications; pleural effusions, pulmonary venous congestion
Idiopathic pulmonary fibrosis	Traction bronchiectasis, honeycombing, predominantly in bases, scattered ground glass opacification
Cryptogenic organizing pneumonia	Bilateral, peripheral opacifications; diffuse or patchy ground glass opacifications, patchy air-space opacification, and small nodules
Nonspecific interstitial pneumonitis	Interstitial opacifications, symmetric, peripheral, subpleural
Granulomatosis with polyangiitis	Hemoptysis; alveolar and interstitial opacifications; multiple nodules 2–8 cm diameter, frequently with cavitation, may present with glomerulonephritis
Diffuse alveolar hemorrhage	Hemoptysis; diffuse alveolar infiltrates, usually bilateral, increasingly bloody lavage return
Goodpasture syndrome	Hemoptysis; may present with acute kidney failure, increasingly bloody lavage return
Acute hypersensitivity pneumonitis	Presents within several hours of offending antigen
Acute eosinophilic pneumonia	Eosinophilia
Drug-induced lung disease	Known exposure to amiodarone, bleomycin, or other pneumotoxic drug

Modified from Guérin C, Thompson T, Brower R. The ten diseases that look like ARDS. *Intensive Care Med.* 2015;41:1099–1102.

in septicaemia.[21] Since their early clinical and pathologic descriptions, considerable basic and clinical research has been devoted to understanding the pathogenesis and determinants of clinical outcomes in ALI.

Genotype

There has been significant investment in research to identify genetic factors that: increase susceptibility to ALI or delineate genetic subtypes. The advantages of identifying the "gene for ALI" would be to determine those at risk and to appropriately match intervention(s) with subtype.

Although no specific gene has been identified for ARDS, there has been some success identifying candidates that are associated with the pathologic mechanisms that in turn confer higher mortality, for example, lung vascular permeability and the *angiopoietin 2* gene (*ANGPT2*).[22]

Pathologic Phenotype

The pathologic phenotype of ALI is "diffuse alveolar damage," (Fig. 18.2). The degree of alveolar epithelial injury and increased vascular permeability, leading to the formation of pulmonary edema, is a valuable predictor of outcome. Biopsies taken from the lungs of patients, within the first 7 days of ALI, display the histologic features of cell death, epithelial hyperplasia, inflammation, disordered coagulation, and fibrinolysis. In addition, there is an alveolar cellular

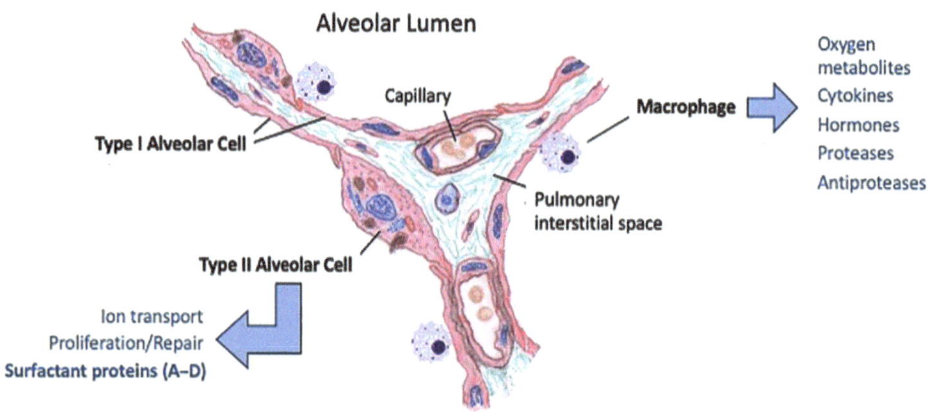

• **Fig. 18.1** The normal alveolus. Schematic representing the continuous monolayer of thin type I alveolar cells (allowing gas exchange), and the type II alveolar cells (which produce surfactant). (Modified from Adeniji K, Steel AC. Effects of intraoperative fluid management on postoperative outcomes after lobectomy. *Anesthesiol Clin* 2012;30:573–590.)

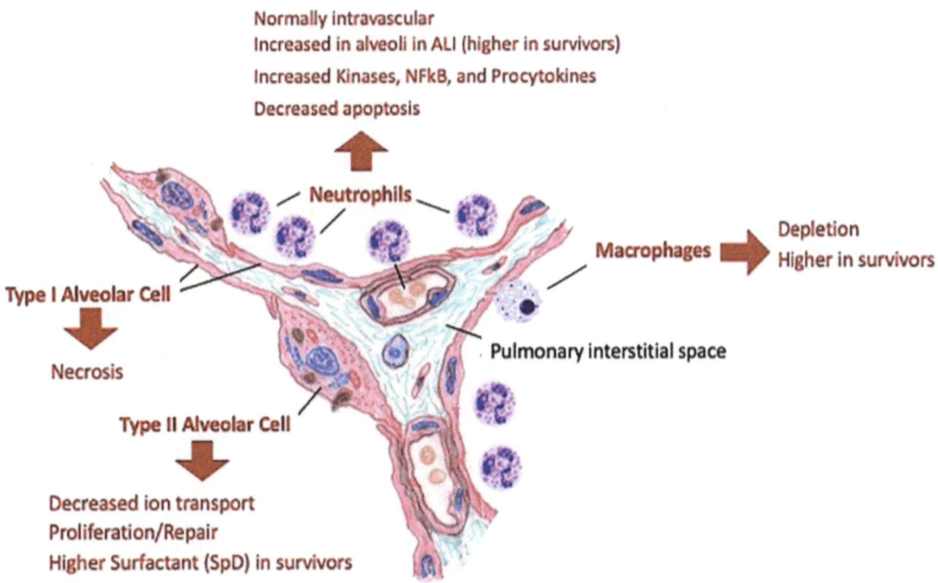

• **Fig. 18.2** The injured alveolus. Schematic representing the effects (*red arrows*) of the inflammatory cascade on cellular components of the alveolar capillary barrier that influence prognosis. *ALI*, Acute lung injury; *NFkB*, nuclear factor κB; *SpD*, surfactant protein D. (From Adeniji K, Steel AC. Effects of intraoperative fluid management on postoperative outcomes after lobectomy. *Anesthesiol Clin* 2012;30:573–590. With permission.)

infiltrate, rich with neutrophils, macrophages, and erythrocytes. The normal alveolar epithelium of type I and type II alveolar cells is anatomically and functionally disrupted. The tight barrier that selectively restricts the movement of solutes is denuded and becomes lined by fibrin-rich hyaline exudates.[23]

Edema Formation

The reabsorption of fluid in the alveolus depends on the integrity and health of the barrier of type I and type II alveolar cells. This monolayer of cells is linked by tight junctions and adherens junctions, and both are key to the transport of ions and fluid from the airspace. Loss of epithelial integrity and injury to type II cells will disrupt normal fluid and cellular transport; leading to impaired fluid removal from the alveolar space,[24] septic shock in patients with pneumonia,[25] and impaired surfactant production.[26]

Surfactant Production

The type II alveolar epithelial cell is the more complex alveolar epithelial cell. It is a highly metabolically active cell, most appreciated for the synthesis and secretion of pulmonary surfactant proteins. There are four such proteins, A to D, responsible for reducing alveolar surface tension, enabling them to remain open. Dysfunction contributes to inhomogeneous airspace collapse, and low levels of protein D are associated with increased mortality.

Surfactant release is initially enhanced by high-volume ventilation. However, the increased surface area of the alveoli increases the rate at which surfactant is released, eventually exceeding the rate of production.[27] Higher tidal volumes also increase the conversion of the large aggregate surfactant on epithelial cells. Eventually, the basement membrane gives way, leading to alveolar hemorrhage.[28] Finally, the increasing alveolar pulmonary edema fluid contains serum proteins and proteases that disable surfactant proteins.[29]

The clinical significance of flooding of the alveolar airspaces is that it rapidly impairs adequate ventilation, resulting in hypoxemia from ventilation-perfusion mismatch and intrapulmonary shunt. Additional right-to-left shunt from reabsorption atelectasis, secondary to alveolar denitrogenation, may also contribute when high levels of oxygen are administered.[30] In the presence of protein-rich pulmonary edema fluid, cellular infiltrate, and a reduction in functionally active surfactant, will results in a dramatic reduction in thoracic compliance.

Humoral Factors

A complex network of cytokines and other proinflammatory compounds initiate and amplify the inflammatory response in ALI/ARDS. Shear-stress and stretch of the injured lung will induce and amplify an inflammatory response in patients with ALI. Proinflammatory cytokines are released from endothelial, epithelial, and macrophage cells. Specifically, there is upregulation of nuclear factor κB (interleukin 8 [IL-8] and 1b [IL-1β] and tumor necrosis factor [TNF-α]). IL-8 complexes with anti-IL-8 and this complex are potent chemotactic agents for cell migration. TNF-α is responsible for membrane permeability and the increased production of IL-1β—an important proinflammatory cytokine. Damage to cell membranes also causes an increase in intracellular calcium ions, which results in membrane deformation. This in turn activates genes involved in paracrine signaling and the production of factors, such as transforming growth factor 1 and basic fibroblast growth factor. Genes responsible for the synthesis of collagen, fibronectin, and matrix metalloproteinase are also activated and or upregulated.[31,32] It is not only the production of proinflammatory cytokines that is important, but also the balance between proinflammatory and antiinflammatory mediators (e.g., IL-1–receptor antagonist, soluble TNF receptor, and autoantibodies against IL-8, IL-10, and IL-11). It also appears that the biologic activity of cytokines, rather than static levels that may not reflect tissue pathophysiology, may be the key to effective immunomodulatory therapy.

Whether this humoral response is directly responsible for the activation of proinflammatory genes, or if its initiation is secondary to cell necrosis and cell membrane exposure, is not clear.[33] It does appear that it is the mechanism of injury-induced cell death that determines the pulmonary response to an injury. Stress modifies the important balance between apoptosis and necrosis. Low mechanical stress causes primarily pulmonary apoptosis. High stress, (such as hyperoxia) leads to more necrosis (secondary to toxic oxygen metabolites).[34] Apoptosis (programmed cell death) plays a role in protecting the lung against mechanical stress and is vital in maintaining alveolar-epithelial integrity. It is suppressed by the key mitogen-activated protein kinase cell membrane–nucleus transduction pathway. Overexpression of mitogen-activated protein kinases, as seen in high-stretch ventilation strategies, therefore results in the inhibition of less-damaging proapoptotic mechanisms.[35]

This is important because apoptosis occurs without the release of cell contents. Whereas necrosis causes disruption of the cell membrane, thus resulting in release of nuclear debris and inflammation. The inflammatory reaction, as described previously, is chemotactic; priming and activating polymorphonuclear leukocytes. These neutrophils migrate to the lung parenchyma, and macrophages migrate to the alveolar air spaces. Ordinarily there are few (<5%) neutrophils in the bronchoalveolar lavage (BAL) of mechanically ventilated patients, as they should be intravascular. Whereas in patients with ALI, this rises rapidly to more than 60%. Higher concentrations are found in survivors on day 7 and 14, although not in the trauma population. Macrophages are also decreased in those who die, compared with survivors, and so must be essential for normal resolution of inflammation.

Microthrombosis

Lung biopsy specimens of ALI patients contain microthrombi within pulmonary capillaries in addition to capillary endothelial injury. It is therefore hypothesized that aberrant activation of the coagulation system is implicated in the pathogenesis of ALI. The humoral response in ALI activates thrombotic and antifibrinolytic pathways that favor fibrin deposition with microthrombosis. BAL specimens from patients contain increased tissue factor and factor VIIIa—which are potent stimulators of the extrinsic coagulation cascade. Tissue factor (TF) activity increases (a procoagulant) and plasminogen activator inhibitor-1 (PAI-1) increases. TF itself is a procoagulant, and PAI-1 is an inhibitor of urokinase plasminogen activator (i.e., a fibrinolytic defect). Additional markers of this altered prothrombotic and antifibrinolytic state include: decreasing circulating protein C levels and increased thrombomodulin.[36] The role played by endothelial cell injury activation within the pulmonary microvasculature is reflected in elevated plasma levels of von Willebrand factor and plasma endothelin-1 observed in ALI patients.

The clinical significance of this direct injury of microthrombi is that it leads to compromised blood flow of the alveoli, and the subsequent damage to the pulmonary microvascular bed. This in turn results in an increased physiologic pulmonary dead space fraction,[37] and worsening gas exchange. Therefore these markers are all associated with increased mortality and fewer ventilation-free days.[30]

Fibroproliferative Recovery Phase

Following a severe ALI, survivors may follow an uncomplicated course and experience rapid resolution of their disease. In others, the alveolar space becomes filled with mesenchymal cells, their products, and neovascularization (interstitial granulation tissue). These patients progress to fibrotic lung injury, which can be observed histologically as early as day 5 following initiation of mechanical ventilation.[38] This process of fibrosing alveolitis may begin even earlier in the course of the disorder promoted by early profibroinflammatory mediators, such as IL-1, and it correlates with worse clinical outcomes, including mortality.[39]

Translation Into the Operating Room

Mechanical ventilation is an unavoidable and integral component of many major operations. Furthermore, it is a supportive therapy in many patients who develop ALI. However, most patients undergoing surgery do not present with preexisting ARDS, and so the predominant intraoperative strategy against perioperative lung injury will be prevention rather than treatment.

Ventilator-Induced Lung Injury

Mechanical ventilation itself can have injurious effects on lung tissue, and this process is known as ventilator-induced lung injury (VILI). VILI can lead to inflammation, pulmonary edema, and hypoxemia (Fig. 18.3). The first description of VILI was reported in 1744 when John Fothergill proposed that "the lungs of one man may bear, without injury, as great a force as those of another man can exert; which by the bellows cannot always be determined."[40] During the polio epidemic, it was noted that patients receiving mechanical ventilation could develop structural damage,[41] and the term "respirator lung" was coined in 1967 after postmortem analyses of patients having undergone mechanical

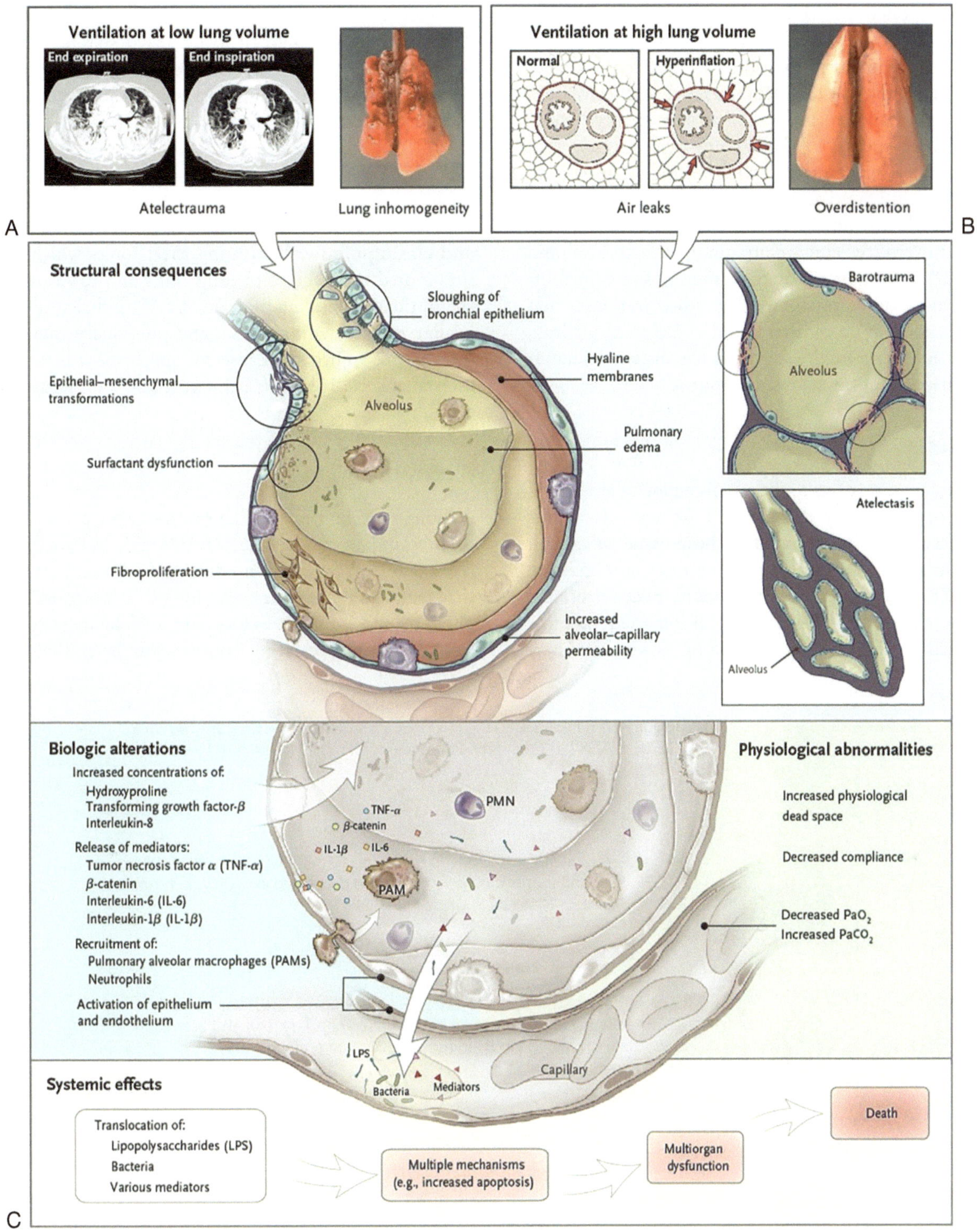

• **Fig. 18.3** Pathogenesis of acute lung injury by forces generated by ventilation at low and high tidal volumes. At low lung volume ventilation, lung injury may be induced by the opening and closing of lung units (atelectrauma), as well as by other mechanisms. This injury is magnified when there is increased lung inhomogeneity, as shown on computed tomography (**A**), and especially in patients with established acute respiratory distress syndrome (ARDS). In addition, ventilation may be very inhomogeneous, a status that may be partially or fully reversed by the use of positive end-expiratory pressure, as shown in a ventilated ex vivo rat lung. At high lung volumes, overdistention can lead to gross barotrauma (air leaks) (**B**). Overdistention can also lead to increased alveolar-capillary permeability and gross pulmonary edema. Ventilation at both high and low lung volumes has structural, physiologic, biologic, and systemic effects (**C**). *$PaCO_2$*, partial pressure of arterial carbon dioxide; *PaO_2*, partial pressure of arterial oxygen; *PMN*, polymorphonuclear leukocytes. (From Slutsky AS, Ranieri VM. Ventilator-induced lung injury. *N Engl J Med*. 2013;369:2126–2136. With permission.)

ventilation revealed diffuse alveolar infiltrates and hyaline membranes.

The clinical importance of VILI was first demonstrated in 2000, when investigators demonstrated that ventilation strategies aimed at reducing VILI had a mortality benefit among ARDS patients.[42] A 2004 study demonstrated that VILI can occur even in patients with healthy lungs who received mechanical ventilation.[43] The principal mechanisms that are thought to contribute to the development of VILI are alveolar overdistension (volutrauma), atelectrauma, and biotrauma.[44] Barotrauma is often referred to as a contributing factor to the development of VILI; however, this mechanism refers to rupture of alveoli and consequent air leak, and this is actually a result of alveolar overdistension rather than the presence of high airway pressures.[44]

Volutrauma

The term volutrauma refers to the overdistension of alveoli and the incipient lung injury that results.[45] Animal experiments revealed that it is the **stretching of the lung tissue** rather than the pressure present within the alveolus that contributed to lung injury.[46] Although high tidal volumes have been associated with the development of volutrauma, it is important to know that "protective" tidal volumes delivered by the ventilator may still result in volutrauma from regional overdistension of alveoli. The heterogeneous nature of ARDS may result in certain lung regions receiving a disproportionate amount of the delivered tidal volumes and thus being overdistended, with other regions of consolidated lung receiving much less.[47]

Atelectrauma

Mechanical ventilation can result in the **repetitive opening and closing of alveoli**, creating shear forces which disrupt the normal architecture of lung units and can cause damage to the surrounding lung units.[47–50] Epithelial sloughing, hyaline membrane formation, and pulmonary edema characterize this injury.[44] Because the mechanism is a result of cyclical atelectasis and reopening, it has been termed "atelectrauma."[44]

Biotrauma

Although mechanical ventilation has direct physical effects on lung units that can result in injury, it can also trigger a **release of inflammatory mediators** from within these cells that results in more widespread lung inflammation.[51,52] This phenomenon is known as biotrauma.[53] The increased capillary permeability resulting from tears in the epithelial cells[44]

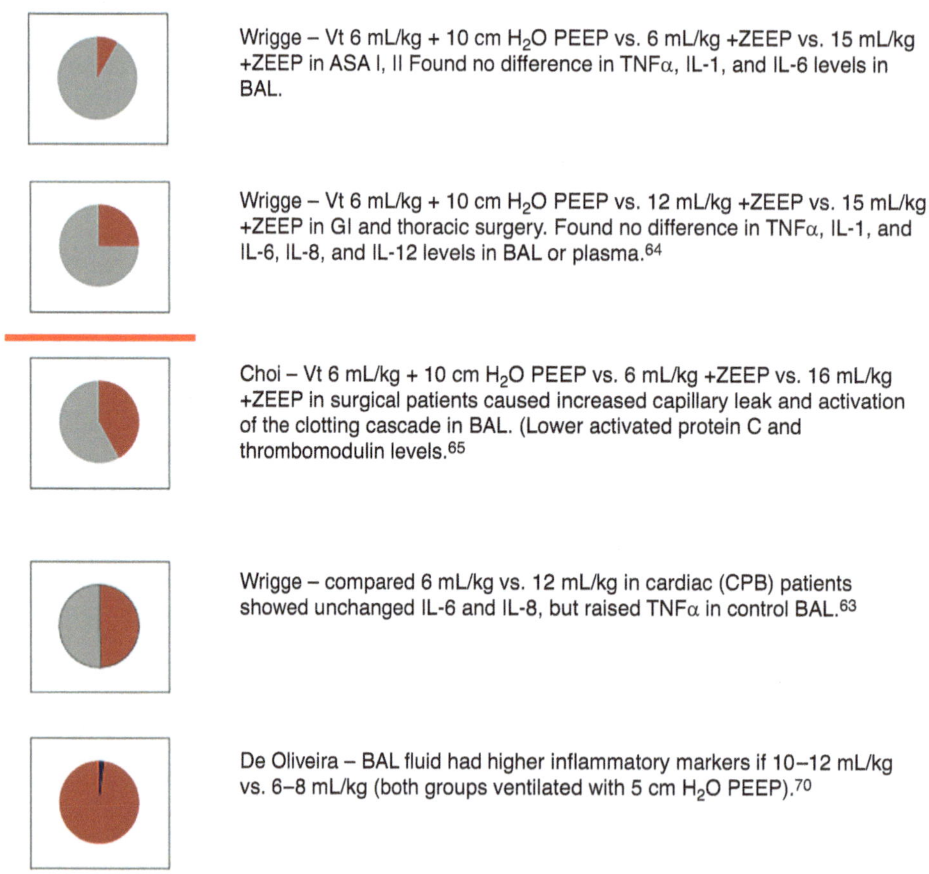

• **Fig. 18.4** Pathogenesis of acute lung injury by ventilation technique over time (1 h, 3 h, 5 h, 6 h, and 12 h). The *red bar* denotes period after which ventilation strategy impacts on inflammatory response. *BAL*, Bronchoalveolar lavage; *CPB*, cardiopulmnary bypass; *GI*, gastrointestinal; *IL*, interleukin; *PEEP*, positive end expiratory pressure; *TNF*, tumor necrosis factor; *Vt*, tidal volume; *ZEEP*, zero end expiratory pressure.

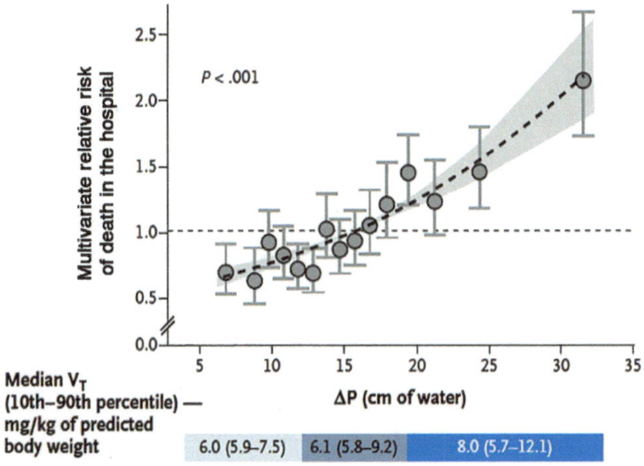

• **Fig. 18.5** Relative risk of death in the hospital versus driving pressure in the combined cohort after multivariate adjustment. *Vt*, Tidal volume. (From Amato MB, Meade MO, Slutsky AS, et al. Driving pressure and survival in the acute respiratory distress syndrome. *N Engl J Med*. 2015;372:747–755. With permission).

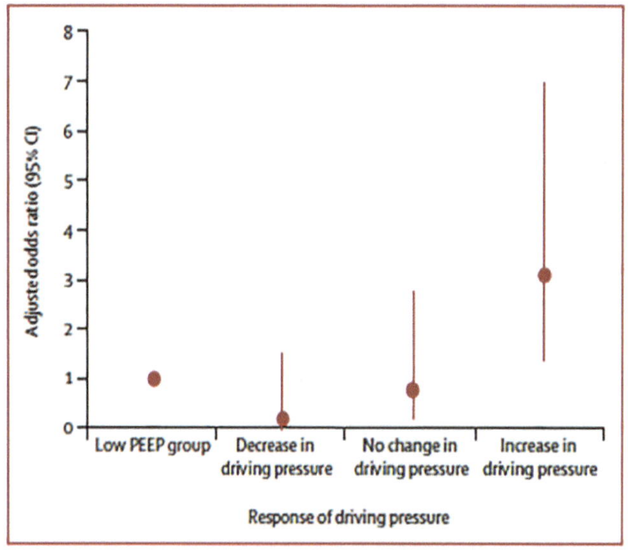

• **Fig. 18.6** Odds of postoperative pulmonary complications according to response of driving pressure after increase of positive end expiratory pressure (*PEEP*). *CI*, Confidence interval. (From Neto AS, Hemmes SN, Barbas CS, et al., PROVE Network Investigators. Association between driving pressure and development of postoperative pulmonary complications in patients undergoing mechanical ventilation for general anaesthesia: a meta-analysis of individual patient data. *Lancet Respir Med*. 2016;4:272–280. With permission.)

results in systemic distribution of inflammatory mediators, bacteria, and toxins (see Fig. 18.3, panel C).[54–56]

Protective Ventilation (See Chapters 19, 20)

As in the intensive care unit, low tidal volumes should be used as a preventative strategy in the operating room. A 2013 study demonstrated that VILI may occur in elective surgical patients after only a few hours of mechanical ventilation in the operating theater, and prophylactic intraoperative ventilation strategy (6–8 mL/kg of predicted body weight, using the formula defined in the ARDSnet trial)[42] was demonstrated to reduce major intrapulmonary and extrapulmonary complications.[57] A 2020 systematic review of intraoperative ventilation strategies found that low tidal volume (4–8 mL/kg predicted body weight) reduced the risk of postoperative pulmonary complications.[58]

The optimal positive end-expiratory pressure (PEEP) strategy and the use of recruitment maneuvers intraoperatively is not clear, and likely varies considerably based on patient characteristics. Several studies comparing the use of high versus low PEEP strategies intraoperatively have failed to show a benefit of a high PEEP strategy,[59,60] even in obese patients.[61] A 2018 trial examining individualized PEEP titration has shown that it may reduce atelectasis and improve intraoperative oxygenation,[62] but its effect on perioperative lung injury has yet to be elucidated.

Fig. 18.4 summarizes the pathogenesis of the humoral response to different ventilation strategies over time. If the patient's procedure, and period of mechanical ventilation, is less than 4 hours, Wrigge and colleagues found that there was no detectable difference in the concentrations of inflammatory markers in lavage specimens.[63] However, where there is protracted use of high tidal volumes and zero PEEP, a progressive increase in inflammatory mediators in the lavage, and later in the serum is found, indicating early perioperative lung injury.[64–66]

Data over the past decade have revealed that a key ventilator variable in preventing lung injury is the driving pressure (DP), defined as the difference between plateau pressure and PEEP.[67] Using a statistical tool known as multilevel mediation analysis, Amato and colleagues analyzed individual data from 3562 patients with ARDS enrolled in nine previously reported randomized trials. They found that ventilator changes that resulted in decreases in DP were strongly associated with survival. One-standard deviation increment in DP (approximately 7 cm H_2O) was associated with increased mortality (relative risk, 1.41; 95% confidence interval [CI], 1.31–1.51; $P < .001$), even in patients receiving "protective" plateau pressures and tidal volumes (relative risk, 1.36; 95% CI, 1.17–1.58; $P < .001$) (Fig. 18.5).

In perioperative patients, the PROtective VEnetilation Network investigators conducted a metaanalysis of 17 randomized controlled trials and the data of 2250 patients undergoing a variety of surgical procedures.[68] Like Amato and colleagues, and further to the work by Wrigge and Choi, they were able to demonstrate that DP was independently associated with the risk of a worse composite outcome (Fig. 18.6); the development of a postoperative pulmonary complication ($P = .009$).

Conclusion

Perioperative ALI is a complex condition which involves the activation of inflammatory pathways, increased endovascular permeability, increased oxidative stress, and change in stress hormones. It occurs as a result of the interaction among surgical technique, anesthetic management, and patient's perioperative condition.

Improvements in perioperative care have led to significant improvement in the outcomes following major surgery. However, perioperative pulmonary complications remain common and ALI, when it occurs, portends to significantly worse outcomes.[69] Patients with ALI are twice as likely to be admitted to intensive care, and 5 to 10 times more likely to die than a comparative population without ALI.[2]

Currently, the treatment options are limited to supportive care and conservative respiratory support. Hopefully, with increasing understanding of the pathophysiology of ALI and the biochemical pathways involved, novel treatments will emerge, and help to improve patient outcome.

References

1. Lawrence VA, Cornell JE, Smetana GW. American College of Physicians. Strategies to reduce postoperative pulmonary complications after noncardiothoracic surgery: systematic review for the American College of Physicians. *Ann Intern Med.* 2006;144:596–608.
2. Canet J, Gallart L. Postoperative respiratory failure: pathogenesis, prediction, and prevention. *Curr Opin Crit Care.* 2014;20:56–62.
3. Alam N, Park BJ, Wilton A, et al. Incidence and risk factors for lung injury after lung cancer resection. *Ann Thorac Surg.* 2007;84:1085–1091, discussion 1091.
4. Canet J, Mazo V. Postoperative pulmonary complications. *Minerva Anestesiol.* 2010;76:138–143.
5. Slinger P. Perioperative lung injury. In: Slinger P, ed. *Principles and Practice of Anesthesia for Thoracic Surgery.* Springer International Publishing; New York City, USA. 2019:143–151.
6. ARDS Definition Task Force, Ranieri VM, Rubenfeld GD, Thompson BT, et al. Acute respiratory distress syndrome: the Berlin Definition. *JAMA.* 2012;307:2526–2533.
7. Bernard GR. Acute respiratory distress syndrome: a historical perspective. *Am J Respir Crit Care Med.* 2005;172:798–806.
8. Ashbaugh DG, Bigelow DB, Petty TL, Levine BE. Acute respiratory distress in adults. *The Lancet*, Saturday 12 August 1967. *Crit Care Resusc.* 2005;7:60–61.
9. Guerin C, Thompson T, Brower R. The ten diseases that look like ARDS. *Intensive Care Med.* 2015;41:1099–1102.
10. Moss M, Bucher B, Moore FA, Moore EE, Parsons PE. The role of chronic alcohol abuse in the development of acute respiratory distress syndrome in adults. *JAMA.* 1996;275:50–54.
11. Calfee CS, Matthay MA, Kangelaris KN, et al. Cigarette smoke exposure and the acute respiratory distress syndrome. *Crit Care Med.* 2015;43:1790–1797.
12. Ware LB, Zhao Z, Koyama T, et al. Long-term ozone exposure increases the risk of developing the acute respiratory distress syndrome. *Am J Respir Crit Care Med.* 2016;193:1143–1150.
13. Erickson SE, Shlipak MG, Martin GS, et al. National Institutes of Health National Heart, Lung. Racial and ethnic disparities in mortality from acute lung injury. *Crit Care Med.* 2009;37:1–6.
14. Rubenfeld GD, Caldwell E, Granton J, Hudson LD, Matthay MA. Interobserver variability in applying a radiographic definition for ARDS. *Chest.* 1999;116:1347–1353.
15. Gattinoni L, Caironi P, Pelosi P, Goodman LR. What has computed tomography taught us about the acute respiratory distress syndrome? *Am J Respir Crit Care Med.* 2001;164:1701–1711.
16. Copolla S, Froio S, Chiumello D. *Lung injury in ARDS, Acute Respiratory Distress Syndrome*: Springer International; 2017:155–171.
17. Lichtenstein D, Goldstein I, Mourgeon E, Cluzel P, Grenier P, Rouby JJ. Comparative diagnostic performances of auscultation, chest radiography, and lung ultrasonography in acute respiratory distress syndrome. *Anesthesiology.* 2004;100:9–15.
18. Volpicelli G, Elbarbary M, Blaivas M, et al. International Liaison Committee on Lung Ultrasound (ILC-LUS) for International Consensus Conference on Lung Ultrasound (ICC-LUS). International evidence-based recommendations for point-of-care lung ultrasound. *Intensive Care Med.* 2012;38:577–591.
19. Chiumello D, Umbrello M, Sferrazza Papa GF, et al. Global and regional diagnostic accuracy of lung ultrasound compared to CT in patients with acute respiratory distress syndrome. *Crit Care Med.* 2019;47:1599–1606.
20. Matthay MA, Robriquet L, Fang X. Alveolar epithelium: role in lung fluid balance and acute lung injury. *Proc Am Thorac Soc.* 2005;2:206–213.
21. Bachofen M, Weibel ER. Alterations of the gas exchange apparatus in adult respiratory insufficiency associated with septicemia. *Am Rev Respir Dis.* 1977;116:589–615.
22. Reilly JP, Wang F, Jones TK, et al. Plasma angiopoietin-2 as a potential causal marker in sepsis-associated ARDS development: evidence from Mendelian randomization and mediation analysis. *Intensive Care Med.* 2018;44:1849–1858.
23. Pelosi P, D'Onofrio D, Chiumello D, et al. Pulmonary and extrapulmonary acute respiratory distress syndrome are different. *Eur Respir J Suppl.* 2003;42:48s–56s.
24. Sznajder JI. Strategies to increase alveolar epithelial fluid removal in the injured lung. *Am J Respir Crit Care Med.* 1999;160:1441–1442.
25. Kurahashi K, Kajikawa O, Sawa T, et al. Pathogenesis of septic shock in Pseudomonas aeruginosa pneumonia. *J Clin Invest.* 1999;104:743–750.
26. Walker MG, Tessolini JM, McCaig L, Yao LJ, Lewis JF, Veldhuizen RA. Elevated endogenous surfactant reduces inflammation in an acute lung injury model. *Exp Lung Res.* 2009;35:591–604.
27. Hillman NH, Kallapur SG, Pillow JJ, et al. Inhibitors of inflammation and endogenous surfactant pool size as modulators of lung injury with initiation of ventilation in preterm sheep. *Respir Res.* 2010;11:151.
28. Greene KE, Wright JR, Steinberg KP, et al. Serial changes in surfactant-associated proteins in lung and serum before and after onset of ARDS. *Am J Respir Crit Care Med.* 1999;160:1843–1850.
29. Baker CS, Evans TW, Randle BJ, Haslam PL. Damage to surfactant-specific protein in acute respiratory distress syndrome. *Lancet.* 1999;353:1232–1237.
30. Ware LB, Matthay MA, Parsons PE, Thompson BT, Januzzi JL, Eisner MD. National Heart, Lung, and Blood Institute Acute

Respiratory Distress Syndrome Clinical Trials Network. Pathogenetic and prognostic significance of altered coagulation and fibrinolysis in acute lung injury/acute respiratory distress syndrome. *Crit Care Med.* 2007;35:1821–1828.
31. Wang HM, Bodenstein M, Duenges B, et al. Ventilator-associated lung injury superposed to oleic acid infusion or surfactant depletion: histopathological characteristics of two porcine models of acute lung injury. *Eur Surg Res.* 2010;45:121–133.
32. Kilpatrick B, Slinger P. Lung protective strategies in anaesthesia. *Br J Anaesth.* 2010;105(suppl 1):108.
33. Jaecklin T, Otulakowski G, Kavanagh BP. Do soluble mediators cause ventilator-induced lung injury and multi-organ failure? *Intensive Care Med.* 2010;36:750–757.
34. Mathru M, Rooney MW, Dries DJ, Hirsch LJ, Barnes L, Tobin MJ. Urine hydrogen peroxide during adult respiratory distress syndrome in patients with and without sepsis. *Chest.* 1994; 105:232–236.
35. Muders T, Wrigge H. New insights into experimental evidence on atelectasis and causes of lung injury. *Best Pract Res Clin Anaesthesiol.* 2010;24:171–182.
36. Ware LB, Fang X, Matthay MA. Protein C and thrombomodulin in human acute lung injury. *Am J Physiol Lung Cell Mol Physiol.* 2003;285:514.
37. Gattinoni L, Bombino M, Pelosi P, et al. Lung structure and function in different stages of severe adult respiratory distress syndrome. *JAMA.* 1994;271:1772–1779.
38. Matthay MA, Wiener-Kronish JP. Intact epithelial barrier function is critical for the resolution of alveolar edema in humans. *Am Rev Respir Dis.* 1990;142:1250–1257.
39. Martin C, Papazian L, Payan MJ, Saux P, Gouin F. Pulmonary fibrosis correlates with outcome in adult respiratory distress syndrome. A study in mechanically ventilated patients. *Chest.* 1995;107:196–200.
40. Fothergill J. Observations on a case published in the last volume of the medical essays, c. of recovering a man dead in appearance, by distending the lungs with air. *Philos Trans R Soc Lond.* 1744;43:275–281.
41. Avignon PD, Hedenstrom G, Hedman C. Pulmonary complications in respirator patients. *Acta Med Scand Suppl.* 1956;316:86–90.
42. Acute Respiratory Distress Syndrome Network, Brower RG, Matthay MA, Morris A, et al. Ventilation with lower tidal volumes as compared with traditional tidal volumes for acute lung injury and the acute respiratory distress syndrome. *N Engl J Med.* 2000; 342:1301–1308.
43. Gajic O, Dara SI, Mendez JL, et al. Ventilator-associated lung injury in patients without acute lung injury at the onset of mechanical ventilation. *Crit Care Med.* 2004;32:1817–1824.
44. Slutsky AS, Ranieri VM. Ventilator-induced lung injury. *N Engl J Med.* 2013;369:2126–2136.
45. Caironi P, Cressoni M, Chiumello D, et al. Lung opening and closing during ventilation of acute respiratory distress syndrome. *Am J Respir Crit Care Med.* 2010;181:578–586.
46. Dreyfuss D, Soler P, Basset G, Saumon G. High inflation pressure pulmonary edema. Respective effects of high airway pressure, high tidal volume, and positive end-expiratory pressure. *Am Rev Respir Dis.* 1988;137:1159–1164.
47. Gattinoni L, Pesenti A. The concept of "baby lung." *Intensive Care Med.* 2005;31:776–784.
48. Gattinoni L, Protti A, Caironi P, Carlesso E. Ventilator-induced lung injury: the anatomical and physiological framework. *Crit Care Med.* 2010;38:539.
49. Muscedere JG, Mullen JB, Gan K, Slutsky AS. Tidal ventilation at low airway pressures can augment lung injury. *Am J Respir Crit Care Med.* 1994;149:1327–1334.
50. Bilek AM, Dee KC, Gaver DP. Mechanisms of surface-tension-induced epithelial cell damage in a model of pulmonary airway reopening. *J Appl Physiol (1985).* 2003;94:770–783.
51. Tremblay L, Valenza F, Ribeiro SP, Li J, Slutsky AS. Injurious ventilatory strategies increase cytokines and c-fos m-RNA expression in an isolated rat lung model. *J Clin Invest.* 1997;99:944–952.
52. Tremblay LN, Slutsky AS. Ventilator-induced lung injury: from the bench to the bedside. *Intensive Care Med.* 2006;32: 24–33.
53. Tremblay LN, Slutsky AS. Ventilator-induced injury: from barotrauma to biotrauma. *Proc Assoc Am Physicians.* 1998;110:482–488.
54. Ranieri VM, Suter PM, Tortorella C, et al. Effect of mechanical ventilation on inflammatory mediators in patients with acute respiratory distress syndrome: a randomized controlled trial. *JAMA.* 1999;282:54–61.
55. Nahum A, Hoyt J, Schmitz L, Moody J, Shapiro R, Marini JJ. Effect of mechanical ventilation strategy on dissemination of intratracheally instilled *Escherichia coli* in dogs. *Crit Care Med.* 1997;25:1733–1743.
56. Murphy DB, Cregg N, Tremblay L, et al. Adverse ventilatory strategy causes pulmonary-to-systemic translocation of endotoxin. *Am J Respir Crit Care Med.* 2000;162:27–33.
57. Futier E, Constantin JM, Paugam-Burtz C, et al. IMPROVE Study Group. A trial of intraoperative low-tidal-volume ventilation in abdominal surgery. *N Engl J Med.* 2013;369:428–437.
58. Deng QW, Tan WC, Zhao BC, Wen SH, Shen JT, Xu M. Intraoperative ventilation strategies to prevent postoperative pulmonary complications: a network meta-analysis of randomised controlled trials. *Br J Anaesth.* 2020;124:324–335.
59. PROVE Network Investigators for the Clinical Trial Network of the European Society of Anaesthesiology, Hemmes SN, Gama de Abreu M, Pelosi P, Schultz MJ. High versus low positive end-expiratory pressure during general anaesthesia for open abdominal surgery (PROVHILO trial): a multicentre randomised controlled trial. *Lancet.* 2014;384:495–503.
60. Barbosa FT, Castro AA, de Sousa-Rodrigues CF. Positive end-expiratory pressure (PEEP) during anaesthesia for prevention of mortality and postoperative pulmonary complications. *Cochrane Database Syst Rev.* 2014(6):CD007922.
61. Writing Committee for the PROBESE Collaborative Group of the PROtective VEntilation Network (PROVEnet) for the Clinical Trial Network of the European Society of Anaesthesiology-PROBESE Collaborative Group, Bluth T, Serpa Neto A, Schultz MJ, Pelosi P, Gama de Abreu M, et al. Effect of intraoperative high positive end-expiratory pressure (PEEP) with recruitment maneuvers vs low PEEP on postoperative pulmonary complications in obese patients: a randomized clinical trial. *JAMA.* 2019;321:2292–2305.
62. Pereira SM, Tucci MR, Morais CCA, et al. Individual positive end-expiratory pressure settings optimize intraoperative mechanical ventilation and reduce postoperative atelectasis. *Anesthesiology.* 2018;129:1070–1081.
63. Wrigge H, Uhlig U, Baumgarten G, et al. Mechanical ventilation strategies and inflammatory responses to cardiac surgery: a prospective randomized clinical trial. *Intensive Care Med.* 2005;31: 1379–1387.

64. Wrigge H, Zinserling J, Stuber F, et al. Effects of mechanical ventilation on release of cytokines into systemic circulation in patients with normal pulmonary function. *Anesthesiology*. 2000;93:1413–1417.
65. Choi G, Wolthuis EK, Bresser P, et al. Mechanical ventilation with lower tidal volumes and positive end-expiratory pressure prevents alveolar coagulation in patients without lung injury. *Anesthesiology*. 2006;105:689–695.
66. Gajic O, Dara SI, Mendez JL, et al. Ventilator-associated lung injury in patients without acute lung injury at the onset of mechanical ventilation. *Crit Care Med*. 2004;32:1817–1824.
67. Amato MB, Meade MO, Slutsky AS, et al. Driving pressure and survival in the acute respiratory distress syndrome. *N Engl J Med*. 2015;372:747–755.
68. Neto AS, Hemmes SN, Barbas CS, et al. PROVE Network Investigators. Association between driving pressure and development of postoperative pulmonary complications in patients undergoing mechanical ventilation for general anaesthesia: a meta-analysis of individual patient data. *Lancet Respir Med*. 2016;4:272–280.
69. Canet J, Gallart L. Predicting postoperative pulmonary complications in the general population. *Curr Opin Anaesthesiol*. 2013; 26:107–115.
70. de Oliveira R, Hetzel MP, Silva MA, et al. Mechanical ventilation with high tidal volume induces inflammation in patients without lung disease. *Critical Care*. 2010;14:R39.

19

Intraoperative Lung Injury During One-Lung Ventilation: Causes and Prevention

WAHEEDULLAH KARZAI

Introduction

The intraoperative period is critical for the patient undergoing thoracic surgery, frequently performed for resection of lung cancer. Both surgery and anesthesia are required to help the patient to overcome and survive a disease amenable to surgical treatment, however, both come at a cost to the patient. The cost of surgery is tissue destruction, bleeding, and ischemia-reperfusion injury which may lead to a varying degree of local and systemic inflammatory response in the perioperative period. The cost of undergoing anesthesia is among other problems, cardiovascular instability, and pulmonary injury. The cardiovascular consequences may include hypotension, sometimes aggravated by bleeding, which usually requires treatment with vasoactive substances and volume repletion, which when inappropriate, may lead to volume overload and its sequelae. Pulmonary injuries from positive pressure ventilation, even if protective lung ventilation strategy is applied, may lead to postoperative pulmonary complications (PPCs). Patients' comorbidities, especially cardiovascular and pulmonary diseases or preoperative chemotherapy, may aggravate these problems.

This chapter will mainly review the ventilation strategies during thoracic surgery which when inappropriately applied may contribute to intraoperative lung injury. Although the inflammatory reaction of the lungs in response to ventilation or thoracic surgery may emerge and can be measured during one-lung ventilation, these do not predictably lead or correspond to the incidence of PPCs.[1,2] Therefore the relevant clinical hallmark of any intraoperative-inflicted lung injury is the increased incidence of PPC. Once present, PPCs contribute to an increased length of stay in high dependency units and may increase mortality and cost.[3,4]

Characterizing Postoperative Pulmonary Complication

Because PPCs are used as a measure of intraoperative lung injury, we need to better define them before reviewing the literature. Postoperative morbidities which are defined in clinical trials as PPCs, consist of atelectasis, pneumonia, lung edema, poor oxygenation, need for supplemental oxygen, postoperative invasive or noninvasive ventilation, reintubation, pleural effusion, pneumothorax, acute lung injury, acute respiratory distress syndrome (ARDS), pulmonary aspiration, postoperative fever over 38°C, bronchospasm, pulmonary embolism, radiologic consolidation, and more.[5] Usually, a composite subset of these signs has been used to increase the chances of identifying complications and help evaluate the severity of respiratory complications.[6,7] In one major study in a general population of surgical patients, Canet et al.[6] used a carefully chosen set of such signs with appropriate definitions (Table 19.1), which was subsequently used in some studies to evaluate the incidence of postoperative lung injury after lung surgery.[8,9] There are some inherent problems in using the items of PPCs. Some of the items may have some degrees of overlap, that is, "pneumonia," "consolidation," and "atelectasis" or "respiratory failure" and "need for intubation." Some of the complications, such as "need for oxygen" are considered a "minor" complication, whereas others such as acute lung injury or ARDS are "major" complications. Furthermore, the endpoints may or may not be appropriate depending on the clinical circumstances. For example, when evaluating the postoperative impact of intraoperative ventilation, endpoints such as atelectasis, pneumonia, need for oxygen, and pneumothorax may seem pathophysiologically linked to mechanical ventilation. Although aspiration pneumonitis or pulmonary embolism may contribute to PPCs as such,

TABLE 19.1 Definitions of Postoperative Pulmonary Complications

Complication	Definition
Respiratory infection	When a patient received antibiotics for a suspected respiratory infection and meet at least one of the following criteria: new or changed sputum, new or changed lung opacities, fever, leukocyte count > 12,000/μL
Respiratory failure	When postoperative PaO_2 < 60 mm Hg on room air, a ratio of PaO_2 to inspired oxygen fraction < 300 mm Hg or arterial oxyhemoglobin saturation measured with pulse oximetry < 90% and requiring oxygen therapy
Pleural effusion	Chest x-ray demonstrating blunting of the costophrenic angle, loss of the sharp silhouette of the ipsilateral hemidiaphragm in upright position, evidence of displacement of adjacent anatomical structures, or (in supine position) a hazy opacity in one hemithorax with preserved vascular shadows
Atelectasis	Lung opacification with a shift of the mediastinum, hilum, or hemidiaphragm toward the affected area, and compensatory overinflation in the adjacent nonatelectatic lung
Pneumothorax	Air in the pleural space with no vascular bed surrounding the visceral pleura
Bronchospasm	Newly detected expiratory wheezing treated with bronchodilators
Aspiration pneumonitis	Acute lung injury after the inhalation of regurgitated gastric contents

PaO_2, Partial pressure of oxygen in arterial blood.

From Canet J, et al. Prediction of postoperative pulmonary complications in a population-based surgical cohort. *Anesthesiology*. 2010;113:1338–1350. With permission.

they may not necessarily be related to intraoperative ventilation. In general, linking specific intraoperative injurious interventions, such as mechanical ventilation, to PPCs may be difficult if they are not adequately controlled for unrelated intraoperative events (major bleeding, extent of tissue injury) or related to postoperative events (wound infections, anastomoses leakage, peritonitis), which may independently lead to PPCs. Thus consensual definitions of outcome measures in view of their pathophysiologic relevance have been attempted to standardize outcome measures for clinical studies.

At least two consensus papers on the issue of PPC and its use in perioperative studies have been published with quite different results. In 2015, a European Society of Anaesthesiology and European Society of Intensive Care Medicine (ESA/ESICM) task force published outcome measures for postoperative outcomes which included PPCs.[7] The ESA/ESAICM closely followed Canets' items and definitions of PPC issued in 2010,[6] with minor changes (see Table 19.1). A more recent consensus statement by Abbott et al.[10] used a systematic review and a three-stage Delphi process to choose appropriate items. Briefly, items were first procured from relevant available literature. Then, in three consecutive steps, investigators assessed and scored the items in terms of quality and validity, excluded items with low scores, and ultimately defined only four items: **atelectasis**, as detected with chest x-ray or chest computer tomography; **pneumonia**, using U.S. Centers for Disease Control and Prevention criteria; **acute respiratory distress syndrome** (ARDS) using the Berlin definition;[11] and **pulmonary aspiration** using "clear clinical history and radiologic evidence." Unfortunately, none of the two consensual agreements are used consistently among investigators studying PPCs. Despite the controversies on items included in endpoint of PPCs among studies, it would seem prudent to at least relate some of the intraoperative issues under assessment, that is, intraoperative lung ventilation to pathophysiologically related and well-defined postoperative complications.

The Incidence of Postoperative Morbidity and Mortality in Thoracic Surgery

The incidence of PPC following lung resection or thoracic surgery varies in accordance with the data surveyed and items used to define the entity of the pulmonary complication. Licker et al.,[12] as well as Serpa Neto et al.[13] used the definitions of acute lung injury and ARDS as a measure of PPCs and found an incidence of 4.2% and 4.3%, respectively in thoracic surgical patients. Significantly, once a patient suffered from these complications, the mortality rate rose to 26%. In a study using a relevant clinical database, Blank and colleagues[14] used postoperative events such as tracheostomy, empyema requiring treatment, pneumonia, reintubation, initial ventilator support greater than 48 hours, ARDS, bronchopleural fistula, pulmonary embolism, air leak greater than 5 days, atelectasis requiring bronchoscopy, and respiratory failure to define their primary outcome of "respiratory complications" and found an incidence of 18% among patients undergoing pneumonectomy. Adjusting for patient characteristics, such as age, gender, body mass index, and American Society of Anesthesiologists status, the length of hospital stay in patients who developed respiratory failure

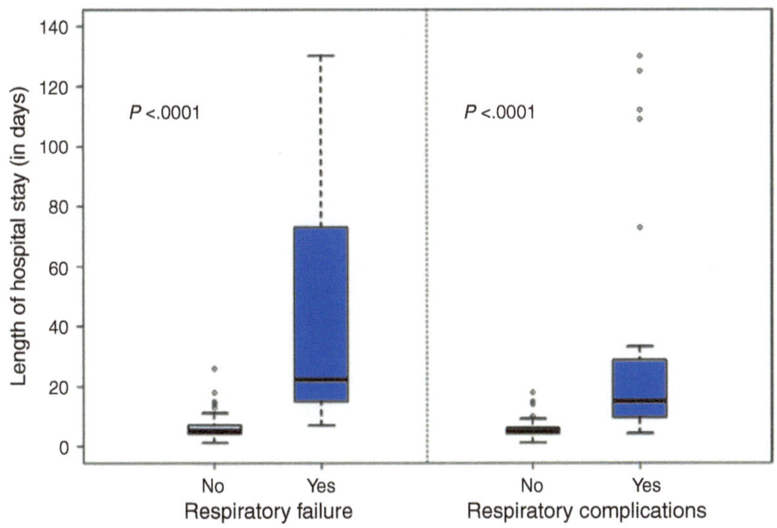

• **Fig. 19.1** Box plot of relationships between incidence of postoperative respiratory failure or respiratory complications and length of hospital stay in days in patients undergoing pneumonectomy. Boxes indicate the interquartile range. The bold horizontal line corresponds to the 50th quartile (median value). The *P* values were estimated using nonparametric Wilcoxon rank sum tests. (From Blank RS, Hucklenbruch C, Gurka KK, et al. Intraoperative factors and the risk of respiratory complications after pneumonectomy. *Ann Thorac Surg.* 2011;92(4):1188–1194. With permission.)

and respiratory complications was increased by a factor of 4.7 and 3.5 respectively (Fig. 19.1). Alam et al.[4] found an incidence of lung injury consisting of pneumonitis, acute lung injury, and ARDS of 5.3% after thoracic surgery; they report a 25% mortality rate in patients with PPC compared with 2.6% in those without. These studies show that postoperative pulmonary complications are highly relevant and, once developed, caused considerable increased in mortality.

Predisposing Condition for Postoperative Pulmonary Complication

Preoperative factors, such as age, preoperative peripheral oxygen saturation (SpO_2), respiratory infection before surgery, and preoperative anemia have been identified as risk factors contributing significantly to the development of PPCs.[6] Some of these factors (smoking, preoperative lung function, preoperative infections) are potentially amenable to preoperative improvement with proper preoperative rehabilitation, which, if pragmatically practicable, would be mandatory before surgery (see Chapter 9).[5]

Intraoperative Lung Injury and Postoperative Pulmonary Complications

Intraoperative events which may injure or initiate injury in the lungs during the surgical procedure can be related to the surgery itself and/or to the anesthesiologic management. In the individual patient, both disciplines may contribute in a varying degree to PPCs. Some studies consistently show that both short- and long-term survival of lung cancer patients after surgery depend on the volume or number of operations performed at hospitals.[15] Pezzi et al.[16] evaluated this issue in the National Cancer Database for major lung resections from 2007 to 2011. There were 124,418 major pulmonary resections identified in 1233 facilities. The 30-day and 90-day mortality rates were, respectively, 2.8% and 5.4%. Hospital volume of cases was significantly associated with 30-day mortality, with a mortality rate of 3.7% for an annual volume of cases less than 10, and 1.7% for a volume of 90 or more cases. The lowest volume centers had a 1.5- to 2-fold increase in 30-day and 90-day mortality in comparison to highest volume centers. This finding is significant considering that other improvements in care usually do not translate to a large difference in outcome.

Surgical Causes of Lung Injury

Surgery leads to a systemic inflammatory response, which involves the activation and interaction among cytokines and inflammatory cells, which contribute considerably to alveolar dysfunction.[17,18] The extent of surgery has been consistently shown to be closely associated with an increased inflammatory response[19,20] and increased perioperative morbidity.[21] Salati M et al.[22] report from the European Society of Thoracic Surgeons Database 2017 on patterns of care and perioperative outcomes of surgery for malignant lung neoplasm in 62,774 patients submitted to lung resections. They show that cardiopulmonary complications and mortality increase with the extent of the lung resection, respectively, 11.5% and 1.6% in segmentectomy, 17.6% and 2% in lobectomy, and 26.4% and 6.7% in pneumonectomy. The overall mortality in lung resection surgery is about 3%. Surgical approach is important, and although no large scale multicenter, randomized controlled clinical trials comparing minimally invasive video-assisted lobectomy (VATS) to open thoracotomy has so far been conducted, most retrospective studies using propensity matching show lower PPCs in the VATS group.[23] Lower systemic inflammatory response, lower pain scores, and shorter duration of chest tubes in the VATS group may be the cause of the positive short-term effects and a decrease in length of hospital stay. Blank et al.[14] show that increased blood transfusion is an independent predictor of increase in PPC in patients undergoing pneumonectomy. In summary, the extent of surgery and surgical stress is a major contributary cause of PPCs after lung surgery. When there is a choice, decreasing the extent of surgery and surgical stress might lead to decrease in postoperative complications.

Anesthesiologic Causes of Lung Injury

In recent years, mechanical ventilation has been the focus of utmost attention in preventing intraoperative lung injury, which may then be manifested in PPCs. Mechanical ventilation as a possible cause of intraoperative lung injury will therefore be the focus of this chapter. Anesthetic regime, which may modify intraoperative lung inflammatory response and possibly postoperative morbidity. Other factors, especially intraoperative fluid administration (see Chapter 21) and postoperative sequelae of muscle relaxation are contributing factors.[24]

Pathogenesis of Intraoperative Lung Injury Through Mechanical Ventilation

During mechanical ventilation, kinetic energy is necessarily expended on lung tissue to inflate the lung. However, kinetic energy may also overstretch and/or deform lung structures to potentially damage the lung. Stress and strain are concepts used to measure these changes.[25–27] Briefly, **stress** is defined as force per unit of area as induced by an external force applied onto a specific material. In terms of pulmonary physiology, the transpulmonary pressure (difference between alveolar and pleural pressure) would best represent stress. **Strain** is defined as the consequent change in dimension over the initial or resting value of that specific material. Strain during mechanical ventilation may be defined as the change in tidal volume relative to functional residual capacity (FRC). Stress and strain are conceptually related and are linked mathematically (stress = constant × strain).

How much strain (tidal volume in relation to FRC) is needed to injure a healthy lung? Because strain is related to tidal volume, Protti et al.[25] studied the effects of increasing levels of tidal volume corresponding to strain levels of 0.45 to 3.3 on lung injury in a large-animal study. They found that healthy pigs whose lungs were ventilated for over 50 hours with tidal volumes equivalent to strain values less than 1.5 (i.e., tidal volumes < 1.5 times the volume of the FRC in healthy pig lungs) showed neither physiologic nor histologic signs of lung injury. This is an interesting and intriguing finding because most recent studies on protective ventilation during surgery consider low tidal volumes in the approximate range of 0.20 to 0.25 of FRC (assuming a FRC of 2000–2200 mL) protective, and those in the range of 0.35 to 0.40 of FRC potentially injurious. Both ranges are far below the levels this study deems noninjurious in subjects with healthy lungs. However, atelectasis, which is prevalent during anesthesia, and anesthesia as such, will decrease the FRC, which might then make a low tidal volume a realistic option within a comprehensive protective ventilation strategy.

When is stress injurious? Stress is especially injurious when it is not evenly distributed throughout the healthy lung but concentrated in small areas.[28] Atelectasis, that is not recruited, leads to a cyclic concentration of stress in the interface between the aerated and nonaerated lung areas during inspiration and expiration, and is thus an important stress potentiator during mechanical ventilation.[28]

Clinically, the injurious aspects of mechanical ventilation are also characterized by the terms barotrauma, volutrauma, and atelectrauma. **Barotrauma** is the injurious effects of high airway pressure leading to excess stress deforming and disrupting lungs tissue. Although barotrauma was previously used for any lung injury attributable to mechanical ventilation,[29] today it is reserved for direct effects of pressure on lung parenchyma leading to airway rupture, pneumothorax or pneumomediastinum. In pioneering studies,[30,31] Dreyfuss et al. showed that ventilating the lungs of rats with high airway pressure led to overt lung injury when the high airway pressure translated into high tidal volumes. The same level of high airway pressure alone did not lead to lung injury when it was deterred from leading to high tidal volumes by straps around the chest of the animals. The authors concluded that tidal volume and not airway pressure per se was the injurious factor and coined the term "**volutrauma**" for this entity.[32] Further studies by other groups showed that low tidal volumes applied without positive end-expiratory pressure (PEEP) may promote atelectasis and allow repetitive recruitment and derecruitment of lungs, and thus lead to or potentiate lung injury.[33,34] Repetitive cyclic recruitment and derecruitment of atelectatic alveoli generates shear forces (in terms of stress), which lead to lung injury. This injurious mechanism of lung injury, theoretically prevalent during anesthesia, is called **atelectrauma.** Recently, the various damaging aspects of mechanical ventilation have been subsumed under one, all encompassing, "**mechanical power.**"[35,36] The higher the mechanical power expended on the lung, the higher the chance that the lung will be injured. The components of mechanical power are not only pressure (stress) and volume (strain) but also respiratory rate (stress and strain increase with rate) and the rate of inspiratory pressure change. This model attempts to provide a comprehensive explanation of the mechanical causes of lung injury and may in the future help us in better understanding of the potential risk when applying mechanical ventilation.[37]

The damaging mechanical effects of ventilation lead to mechanical disruptions or breaks in alveolar endothelial and epithelial cell membranes[38,39] (Fig. 19.2). Any damage to these cells activates a local inflammatory response, which although ultimately needed in the repair process of these injuries, may first lead to release of cytokines, activation and recruitment of inflammatory cells, and release of enzymes and active oxygen species, which intensify the injury.[40] This inflammatory reaction in the lung is the primary substrate of intraoperative lung injury which may ultimately lead to PPC (see Chapter 18 for a more detailed account of this topic). It is therefore imperative to define and to implement

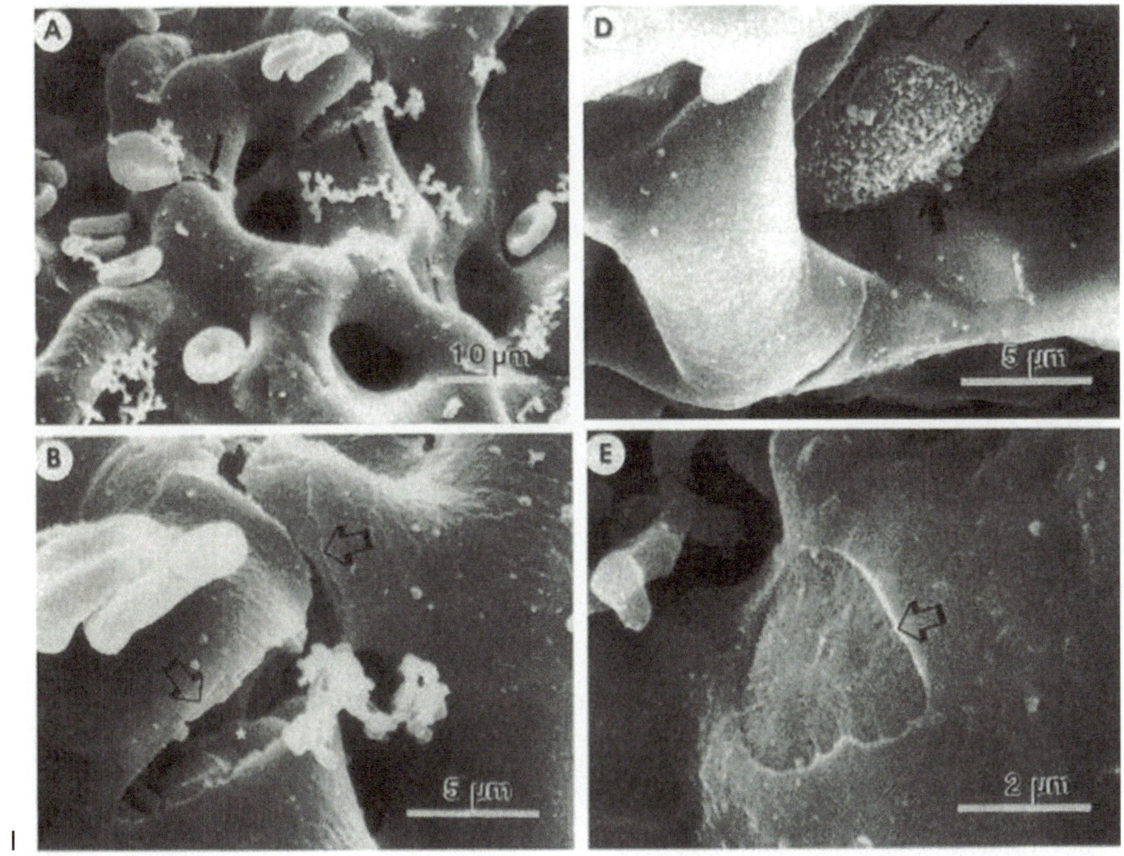

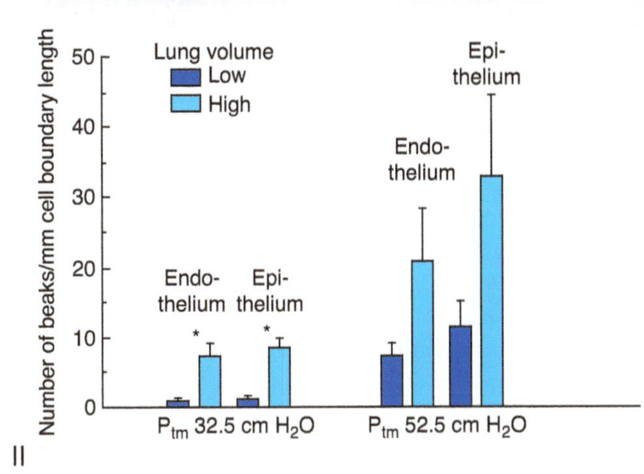

• **Fig. 19.2 Upper panels:** (I) Scanning electron micrographs showing examples of disruptions of blood-gas barrier in rabbit lungs perfused at 20 cm H_2O transpulmonary pressure and 52.5 cm H_2O Ptm. (**A**) Adjacent capillaries with complete ruptures of blood-gas barrier (*solid arrows*) at various angles relative to capillary axis (higher magnifications are shown in **B**). (**B**) higher magnification of A showing retraction of epithelial layer on edge of break (*open arrows*). (**D**) Slits of blood-gas barrier (*solid arrows*). (**E**) Round rupture involving only epithelial layer (*open arrow*). **Left panel:** (II) Epithelium at 20 (high lung volume) and 5 cm H_2O transpulmonary pressure. $^*P < .05$. (Modified from Fu Z, Costello ML, Tsukimoto K, et al. High lung volume increases stress failure in pulmonary capillaries. *J Appl Physiol* (1985). 1992;73(1):123–133. With permission.)

a ventilation strategy which would avoid mechanical and inflammatory injury to the lung.

Mechanical Ventilation During Anesthesia and Lung Injury

Two pathophysiologic aspects of lung injury have been given substantial attention in defining new protective ventilation strategies during anesthesia and surgery.

The first is lung injury through atelectrauma, which develops when atelectasis has developed in the ventilated lung. Atelectasis, as supported by clinical and experimental evidence, has been long recognized as a very frequent and serious perioperative problem.[41,42] In the conscious subject, thoracic and diaphragm muscle tone and body posture are major determinants of the FRC, which is the lung volume at which the balance between the natural tendency of the lung to retract and that of the rib cage to expand occurs.[43] In the conscious subject during spontaneous ventilation, physiologic variability in tidal volume, variability in respiratory cycles,[44] and frequent sighs[45,46] superimposed on a lung kept inflated by chest wall and diaphragm muscle tone prevent atelectasis. During anesthesia, with or without paralysis, the chest and diaphragm muscle tone is decreased leading to lung compression and decreased FRC.[47] Compression of the lung leads to small airway closure and subsequent resorption of air and especially oxygen within the nonventilated alveoli, which will cause alveolar collapse and atelectasis. Lung compression and airway closure is a main determinant for the development of atelectasis and is highlighted by the fact that any further increase in lung compression increases atelectasis. Examples of increase in lung compression may occur in obese patients,[48,49] owing to the increased weight and pressure of thoracic and abdominal fat, and during laparoscopic abdominal operations[50] from increased lung compression through increased intraabdominal pressure. Beyond the more common atelectasis caused by compression of airways during anesthesia, atelectasis may also occur when an airway is blocked by tumor, pus, or mucus plug. Ventilation with high fraction of inspired oxygen (FiO_2) increases the incidence and prevalence of atelectasis because in alveoli distal to airway closure, oxygen more readily passes across a concentration gradient from the alveoli to the capillaries, whereas nitrogen, once it reaches a concentration equilibrium does not and will keep the alveoli open.[41,51]

Atelectasis during intraoperative ventilation may cause lung injury by allowing repetitive cyclic opening and closing alveoli and thus generating shear trauma.[28,33,34] In addition, with parts of the lung now atelectatic, the remaining lung would overstretch with large tidal volumes.[52] Finally, atelectasis formed during the intraoperative period may, in vulnerable surgical patients, persist beyond the intraoperative period with an increased incidence of PPC.[5,53]

The second mechanism of intraoperative lung injury is high tidal volumes leading to alveolar overstretch and thus volutrauma. A significant event in the history and practice of mechanical ventilation was the publication of the ARDS Network study.[54] In that study, it was shown that low tidal ventilation (6 mL/kg predicted body weight [PBW]) as compared with 12 mL/kg PBW decreased mortality and increased ventilator-free days. In fact, the study was terminated prematurely, because considering the preliminary results, it was felt that it was unethical to ventilate the lungs of the patients at 12 mL/kg PBW. Anesthesiologists reasoned that because low tidal volumes are evidently beneficial for critically ill patients with severe lung injury, they may likewise be beneficial and should be applied in patients with healthy lungs undergoing surgery. However, the ARDS lung is not comparable with a healthy lung of a surgical patient. First, extensive consolidation of lung tissue in ARDS patients leaves only a small amount of lung able to accommodate the tidal volume. Because the amount of lung open to ventilation is as small as the size of a lung of a baby, the concept of a "baby lung" was introduced over 15 years ago by Gattinoni.[55] Using large or even moderate tidal volumes would excessively overinflate the baby lung (Fig. 19.3). Second, systemic and local lung inflammation present during ARDS would amplify any lung injury occurring in these open units.[56] Clearly, these pathophysiologic principles can not be translate to the mechanical ventilation in surgical patients with healthy lungs. Because most of the data addressing the effect of protective lung ventilation strategy are derived from studies conducted on critically ill, intensive care patients, there is no evidence to confirm that the same ventilation strategy is applicable to patients undergoing a general surgical or thoracic surgical procedure. Patients presenting for thoracic surgery, unlike patients suffering from ARDS, do not have areas of the lung that cannot be recruited and have no systemic inflammation. In fact, many thoracic surgery patients have a lung lesion that was discovered during a routine screening evaluation in an otherwise healthy individual.

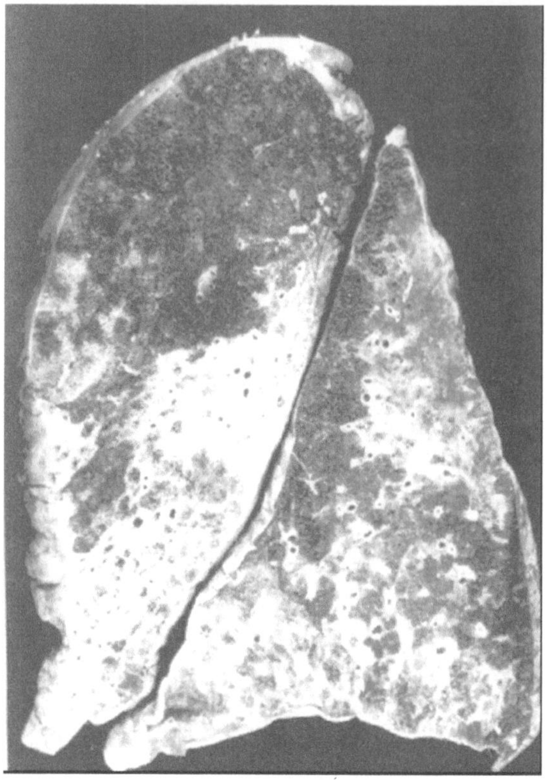

• **Fig. 19.3** This figure shows why the concept of the "baby lung" holds in patients suffering from acute respiratory distress syndrome. As can be seen, only the very small area of upper part of the upper lobe (baby lung equivalent) is open for ventilation. (From Wright JL. The pathology of ARDS. In: Russel JA, Walley WR, eds. *Acute Respiratory Distress Syndrome*. Cambridge University Press; 1999:49. With permission.)

The previously cited animal study by Protti et al.[25] on strain and tidal volume, as well as the reassessment of the ARDs trial by Amato et al.[57] on driving pressure (see later), clearly demonstrates the shortcoming of pinpointing tidal volume and the accompanying strain as the only culprit. High tidal volumes may lead to lung injury in a healthy lung as well when other conditions such as significant atelectasis, are present, and high tidal volumes may then potentiate atelectrauma.[28,58] The many studies applying low tidal volumes during anesthesia in patients with mostly healthy lungs, although not always conclusive, have over the past decade nevertheless led to a net decrease in tidal volume, but fortunately also in an overall change of ventilation practice,[59] which is a welcome improvement in quality of care.

Protective Ventilation and Postoperative Pulmonary Complications

In light of volutrauma and atelectrauma, many studies on protective ventilation during anesthesia and surgery used different combinations of at least three protective measures to decrease intraoperative lung injury and PPCs: (1) low tidal volume in the range of 6 to 8 mL/kg PBW to avoid overinflation; (2) PEEP of at least 5 or higher or adjusted to patients lung capacity to avoid the development of atelectasis; and (3) alveolar recruitment using inflating pressure up to 35 to 40 cm H_2O to open existing atelectasis.[60,61] In one randomized controlled study, Futier et al.[62] randomized 400 patients at risk of PPCs undergoing abdominal surgery, either to protective ventilation (tidal volume 6–8 mL/kg PBW, PEEP 6–8 cm H_2O and recruitment every 30 min) or conventional ventilation, (tidal volume 10–12 mL/kg PBW, no PEEP, no recruitment). The primary endpoint was pulmonary (pneumonia or need for invasive or noninvasive ventilation) and extrapulmonary complications (sepsis, severe sepsis, septic shock, or death). Of the protective group, 10.5% developed the primary outcome, of the conventional group 27.5% (P = .001), with no difference in mortality at 30 days. One limitation of the report is that the incidence of anastomoses leakage and sepsis was significantly higher in the conventional group. These complications are most probably unrelated to the ventilation strategy and may have also contributed to worst outcome in the control group. In another large study[63] (PROVHILO trial), Prove Network Investigators randomized 900 patients, all ventilated with low tidal volume (8 mL/kg PBW), in two groups: a higher PEEP group of 12 cm H_2O with recruitment maneuvers or a lower PEEP group of 2 cm H_2O without recruitment maneuvers. PPC developed in 40% versus 39% of the patients in the two groups. However, patients in the high PEEP group developed more hypotension and needed more vasoactive drugs. This trial shows that indiscriminately applying high PEEP is not protective and leads to other complications. In a recent large randomized controlled protective ventilation trial (PROBESE trial),[64] 2013 obese patients (of whom 1976 completed the trial) who underwent noncardiac surgery and all ventilated with low tidal volumes, were randomized in two groups; either a low PEEP group of 2 cm H_2O with no alveolar recruitment or a high PEEP group of 12 cm H_2O with alveolar recruitment. The two groups did not differ in terms of PPCs; however, hypoxemia was less likely in the high PEEP group and hypotension and bradycardia less likely in the low PEEP group. Finally, Ferrando et al.[65] randomized 1012 patients undergoing abdominal surgery in four groups with either individualized PEEP (mean 10 cm H_2O) or standard PEEP (mean 5 cm H_2O) and either individualized postoperative continuous positive airway pressure (CPAP) or standard CPAP. Low tidal volume was used in all groups. The incidence of PPCs did not differ among groups. A Cochrane Review published in 2018[66] studying the effects of low tidal volume on outcomes showed that low tidal volume ventilation had no impact on mortality, may have possibly led to moderate reductions in postoperative pneumonia (moderate quality of evidence), but had no meaningful decrease in intensive care unit (ICU) stay (low quality of evidence). However, many small sample size studies with inherent problems were included in this review and contributed to the results. On the other hand, a retrospective analysis by Levin et al., who reviewed records of over 29,000 patients who had undergone elective nonthoracic, noncardiac general surgery and found that the 30-day mortality rate was lower when a tidal volume of 8 to 10 mL/kg PBW as compared with a lower tidal volume of 6 to 8 mL/kg PBW was used intraoperatively[67] (Fig. 19.4).

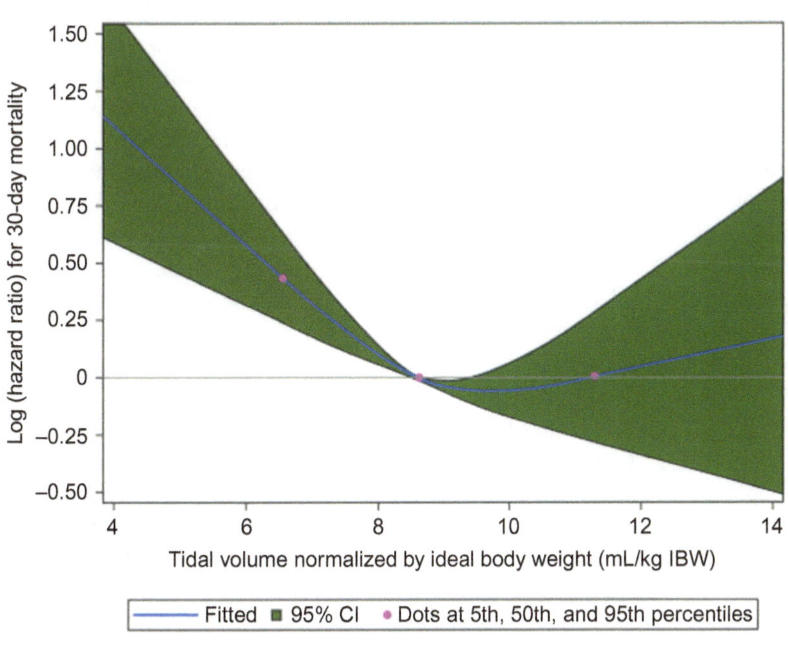

• **Fig. 19.4** The effect of intraoperative tidal volume V_T on 30-day mortality. RCS curve showing the dose–response relationship between median V_T per kg ideal body weight (IBW) and 30-day mortality. Dots show the 5th, 50th, and 95th percentiles of V_T per kg IBW. The shaded area shows the 95% confidence interval (*CI*). The CI > 0.00 indicates a significant association between V_T per kg IBW < 9.7 mL per kg IBW and 30-day mortality. *RCS*, regional curve standardization. (From Levin MA, McCormick PJ, Lin HM, et al. Low intraoperative tidal volume ventilation with minimal PEEP is associated with increased mortality. *Br J Anaesth*. 2014; 113:97–108. With permission).

Despite these controversial outcomes, there is some consensus[61] that the triad of a protective lung ventilation "bundle" of low tidal volume, low to moderate PEEP, and recruitment may best avoid PPCs. However, because of inconclusive evidence, the authors do not go much beyond these broad recommendations.

Lately, low driving pressure (plateau pressure – PEEP) has been shown to be a good measure of applying and managing protective ventilation.[26,57,68] Driving pressure is a means of adjusting tidal volume to lung compliance. Using low driving pressure as a measure of protective ventilation strategy shows more pathophysiologic rationale because it adjusts the tidal volume to actual lung compliance. In comparison, a low tidal volume strategy alone adjusts tidal volume to the predicted body weight, irrespective of possible lung pathology, such as consolidation or fibrosis. Neither low tidal volume nor high PEEP reduces driving pressure predictably and may be the reason for many failed protective ventilation trials. Amato et al.[57] reassessed previous ARDS study trials and convincingly showed that neither low tidal volume nor the applied PEEP, but only low driving pressure, was associated with outcome. The authors conducted a multilevel mediation analysis of individual data from 3562 patients with ARDS. They found that among the ventilation variables, driving pressure was most strongly associated with survival. An increment in driving pressure of approximately 7 cm H_2O was associated with increased mortality even in patients receiving "protective" lung ventilation. Individual changes in tidal volume or PEEP after randomization were not independently associated with survival; they were associated with survival only if they were among the changes that led to reductions in driving pressure. Further observational studies in 778 ARDS patients have shown that variations in tidal volume or PEEP have no impact on mortality. As depicted in Fig. 19.5, rather, driving pressures above 19 cm H_2O and plateau pressures above 20 cm H_2O were associated with risk of death.[69]

We thus see that even within the context of ARDS, low tidal volume is not the magic bullet, and more is needed to adjust ventilation strategy to individual patient's pathophysiology and improve outcome.

Driving pressure has also been evaluated in ventilation studies during surgery. A recent reanalysis of previous protective ventilation studies during anesthesia[70] shows that high driving pressure was independently associated with PPCs, and that increases in PEEP, which increased driving pressure increased the rate of PPCs. Driving pressure is a valuable instrument to adapt ventilation to lung pathophysiology during intraoperative mechanical ventilation. However, large prospective studies are needed to substantiate the strong pathophysiologic rationale and its momentary appeal.

Protective Ventilation During One-Lung Ventilation

Like the general discussion on ventilation strategy during anesthesia outlined earlier, ventilation strategies during OLV have also undergone changes. Previously, oxygenation and avoidance of hypoxemia was the main issue defining a good ventilation practice. Now, avoiding intraoperative lung injury through protective ventilation is the main issue in recent ventilation literature on OLV.[71]

There are, however, similarities but also major differences in having two or one lung to ventilate.

First, maintaining oxygenation is a cardinal factor during OLV. Because ventilation of the dependent lung and its perfusion are interconnected to the perfusion of the nonventilated lung, a ventilation strategy which impedes the distribution of the perfusion of the dependent, ventilated lung will lead to an increase in the perfusion of the nonventilated lung resulting in hypoxemia. Low tidal volumes in the dependent lung without adequate PEEP will promote atelectasis in the dependent lung and likewise promote hypoxemia and hence be counterproductive. Hypoxemia during OLV may endanger the patient and necessitate interrupting surgery. Any ventilation strategy must therefore provide sufficient oxygenation during OLV.

Second, there is an increased likelihood of atelectasis generation in the dependent lung during OLV in the lateral decubitus position. An increase in the compressive forces on the dependent lung leads to reduced compliance and atelectasis during OLV. They include not only the pressure of the abdominal contents, particularly in the paralyzed patient causing cephalad displacement, especially of the dependent diaphragm, but also from the weight of the mediastinum and the upper, collapsed lung and the pressure of the thoracic wall. Clinical studies show that changing the position of the anesthetized patient from supine to the lateral decubitus reduces the compliance of the dependent lung.[72,73] In addition, because FiO_2 during OLV is usually kept high, absorption of alveolar oxygen may accelerate atelectasis behind compressed airways.[41,51] Finally, atelectasis may also occur as a result of dislocation of a double-lumen tube or a bronchial blocker. Therefore, atelectasis is a frequent problem during OLV in the lateral decubitus body position. The "clinical proof" of atelectasis occurrence during OLV is revealed when a recruitment maneuver is performed: if lung compliance increases (driving pressure and plateau pressure decrease during volume controlled ventilation or tidal volume increases during pressure-controlled ventilation) and oxygenation improves after the maneuver, it is most probable that atelectatic areas of the lung were reexpanded by the recruitment maneuvers.[74] Because of the occurrence of atelectasis during OLV, cyclic recruitment of atelectatic or poorly aerated lung regions may occur readily and could, in susceptible patients and during long and critical operations, lead to intraoperative lung injury.

This has been recently shown in an elegant study using a large animal model during two-lung ventilation (TLV) and OLV by Kozian et al.[58] To ventilate the lungs of the anesthetized pig, the authors used either low (5 mL/kg) or high (10 mL/kg) tidal volumes in combination with a PEEP of 5 cm H_2O. Using computer tomography to assess lung tissue density and hence atelectasis, they found that atelectasis

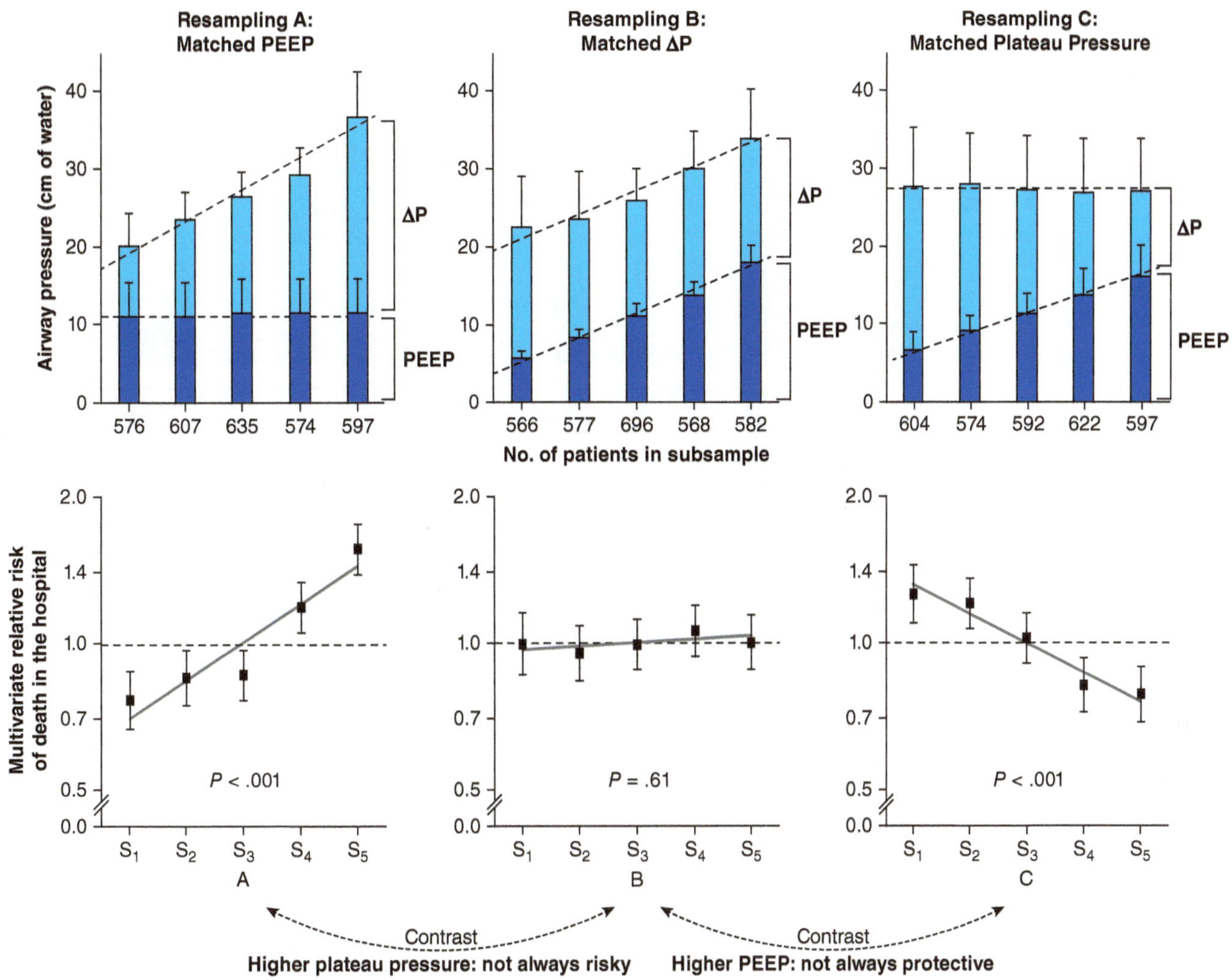

• **Fig. 19.5** Relative risk of death in the hospital by ventilation pressure quintile. Acute respiratory distress syndrome (ARDS) patients from nine previously reported randomized controlled trials were grouped into quintiles (of approximately 600 patients) based on mean ventilation pressure variable (matched positive end-expiratory pressure [*PEEP*] with variable driving pressure [*ΔP*], matched ΔP with variable PEEP, and matched plateau pressure [P_{plat}] with variable ΔP and PEEP) and relative risk of in-hospital mortality was calculated, adjusted for five covariates (trial, age, APACHE score or SAPS, arterial pH, PaO_2:FiO_2). Independent of PEEP and P_{plat}, higher ΔP was associated with a higher relative risk of in-hospital death, and lower ΔP was associated with a lower risk of in-hospital death. *SAPS*, simplified acute physiologic score. (From Amato MB, Meade MO, Slutsky AS, et al. Driving pressure and survival in the acute respiratory distress syndrome. *N Engl J Med*. 2015;372(8):747–755.)

developed in the dependent lung, and that it led to a significant tidal recruitment and derecruitment during OLV. Cyclic recruitment of frankly atelectatic lung areas occurred both at low and high tidal volumes. However, of the poorly aerated lung areas, 53% were recruited at every inspiration in the low tidal volume compared with 82% in the high tidal volume (Fig. 19.6). After the 60-minute OLV period, the lungs of the pigs, which were ventilated with 10 mL/kg, showed a significantly higher proportion of poorly ventilated lung areas, suggesting lung injury occurred through the cyclic recruitment (see Fig. 19.6). Unfortunately, these significant pathophysiologic findings were not substantiated by any measurement of lung injury indices. Nevertheless, this study shows that cyclic recruitment, which is a known mechanism of lung injury, may occur especially when using a high tidal volume and may lead to functional changes in regional lung physiology. In a recent discussion on volutrauma and atectrauma, Gattinoni notes that the deleterious effects of high tidal volumes during ventilation may be more caused by atelectrauma and less caused by hyperinflating the lung.[28] Indeed, as discussed previously, very high tidal volumes will be required (>20 mL/kg) to produce the needed injurious strain (1.5–2) to injure a healthy lung, and even then, it would need a long time to develop, which is more than the usual length of most surgeries.[25]

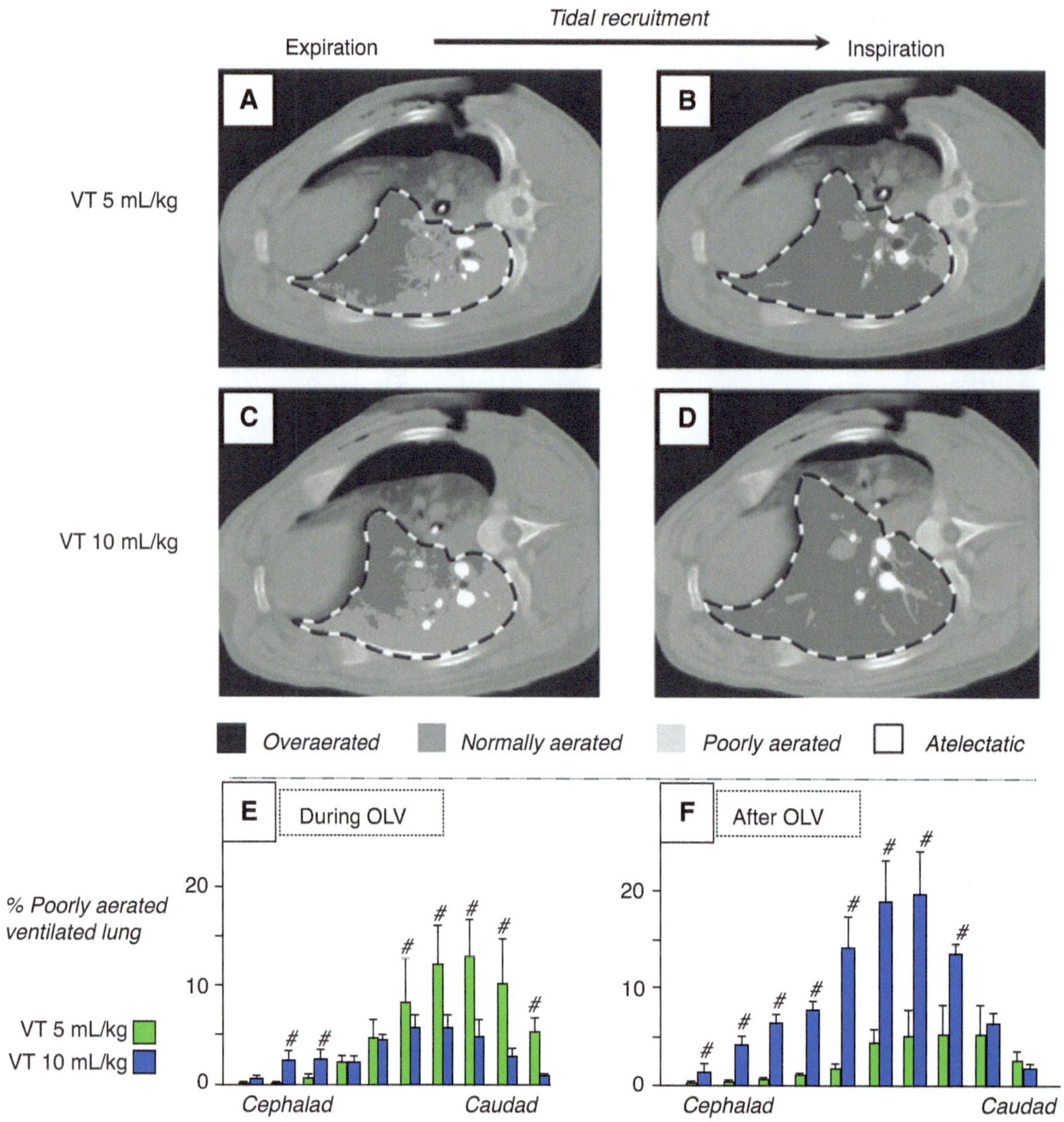

• **Fig. 19.6** Tidal recruitment and lung overdistension during one-lung ventilation (*OLV*) in a pig model. Lung aeration was determined at end-expiration and end-inspiration based on radiologic densities (Hounsfield units [HU]) on computed tomography (CT) scans in a pig OLV model: overaerated (from −1000 to −900 HU), normally aerated (from −900 to −500 HU), poorly aerated (from −500 to −100 HU), and atelectatic (from −100 to 100 HU) lung areas. (**A–D**), CT images during OLV with tidal volumes (V_T) of 5 or 10 mL/kg (fraction of inspired oxygen 0.4 and positive end-expiratory pressure 5 cm H_2O). Lung regions are coded by *gray scale* for the degree of lung aeration. End-expiratory images demonstrate marked alveolar collapse with either V_T (**A** and **C**). End-inspiratory images demonstrate increased tidal recruitment with V_T 10 mL/kg, with near-complete elimination of poorly aerated lung areas (**D**). End-inspiratory panels further demonstrate ventilated lung overdistension with mediastinal shift, which is markedly increased at V_T 10 mL/kg (**D**). (**E** and **F**), Schematic representation of lung aeration at end-inspiration in craniocaudal direction (CT slices 1–100) during OLV and during two-lung ventilation thereafter. Data are summarized in blocks of 10 slices of the dependent lung and presented as means. Lungs exposed to high V_T OLV exhibited more tidal recruitment during OLV, resulting in increased amounts of poorly aerated lung tissue on resumption of two-lung ventilation ($^{\#}P < .05$; V_T 5 vs. 10 mL/kg). (Modified from Lohser J, Slinger P. Lung injury after one-lung ventilation: a review of the pathophysiologic mechanisms affecting the ventilated and the collapsed lung. *Anesth Analg*. 2015;121(2):302–318. With permission. This is an adaptation from reference 58 with permission.)

Protective Ventilation Strategy and Postoperative Pulmonary Complication During One-Lung Ventilation

In an early study on the immune effects of low (5 mL/kg actual body weight [abw]) vs. high tidal volume (10 mL/kg abw) without PEEP during OLV, Schilling et al.[1] showed modest increases in some mediators of the inflammatory immune response in the lung lavage fluid of the patients in the high tidal volume group. However, a lavage performed 2 hours after reestablishing TLV showed no significant differences. Clinical outcome measures were not assessed. In another similar study in patients undergoing esophagectomy, Michelet et al.[2] showed significant increases in blood cytokine levels of patients in the conventional ventilation strategy group (9 mL/kg PBW without PEEP) as compared with the protective ventilation strategy group (5 mL/kg PBW with PEEP = 5 cm H_2O) during OLV. However, although oxygenation was better preserved in the protective ventilation group, no differences in postoperative morbidity or mortality were found between the groups. Shen et al.[75] randomized 101 patients undergoing minimally invasive esophagectomy in a protective group (5 mL/kg abw with PEEP = 5 cm H_2O) and a conventional group (8 mL/kg abw without PEEP) with the incidence of PPCs as endpoints of the study. PPC was defined as the need for bronchoscopy/tracheostomy for bronchial secretions, pneumonia, acute lung injury, and ARDS requiring reintubation, pleural effusion requiring drainage, and pulmonary embolism. Although the authors reported significantly more pulmonary complications in the conventional group, they failed to distinguish the side on which the pathology was found. This makes the study difficult to assess because the operated lung was not ventilated during OLV, and the surgical procedure causes radiologic changes on the operated side, which makes defining "ARDS" difficult. Furthermore, overall morbidity and mortality were not affected. Another randomized study by Yang et al.[76] likewise reported reduced PPCs in patients undergoing lobectomy with low tidal volumes (pressure-controlled ventilation, tidal volume 5 mL/kg PBW and PEEP = 5 cm H_2O) versus high tidal volume (volume-controlled ventilation, tidal volume 10 mL/kg PBW with PEEP). However, they too used the sum of ipsilateral (side of surgery) and contralateral "infiltrates" and "atelectasis" to achieve a significant result. A small randomized study by Ahn et al.[77] in 50 patients undergoing VATS using either a tidal volume of 10 mL/kg abw without PEEP versus 6 mL/kg abw with PEEP = 5 cm H_2O did not find postoperative differences between groups in terms of oxygenation, atelectasis, hospital stay, or postoperative inflammatory response. The largest prospective study to date is that by Marret et al.[78] who randomized 346 patients undergoing lobectomy or pneumectomy in a lung protective ventilation group (tidal volume 5 mL/kg PBW and PEEP = 5–8 cm H_2O) versus a conventional group (tidal volume 10 mL/kg PBW without PEEP). The primary outcome was major pulmonary complications (pneumonia, acute respiratory failure requiring ventilation, pulmonary embolism) and nonpulmonary complications (acute myocardial infarction and hemodynamic shock). The authors showed a significant increase in pulmonary complications, as defined by the primary outcome in the conventional group, but failed to show any increase in ICU stay or mortality. Finally, Park et al.[79] randomized 292 patients scheduled for thoracic surgery into two groups, one conventional ventilation group (tidal volume 6 mL/kg PBW, PEEP = 5 cm H_2O and recruitment maneuver) and a driving pressure group (tidal volume 6 mL/kg PBW with recruitment maneuver and PEEP adjusted stepwise to achieve "lowest" driving pressure for each individual patient). The authors reported lower rates of PPCs and lower rates of pneumonia and ARDS in the driving pressure group. This study, however, has major shortcomings, such as including esophagectomy patients and also using radiologic data from the operated lung to define PPCs. Furthermore, the low driving pressure was achieved by decreasing PEEP, which seems counterintuitive (see Table 19.2 for a summary of randomized trials). All these studies stress the urgent need to conduct meticulous clinical research on the effects of lung injury during OLV and must define sound pathophysiologically relevant endpoints to be used in clinical studies.

Because randomized studies are neither conclusive nor consistent to allow recommendations, we may need to focus our attention on observational studies. Two studies are remarkable. In 2014, Serpa Neto et al.[13] conducted a systematic review and metaanalysis including both observational *and* randomized controlled protective ventilation trials in abdominal and thoracic surgery patients. The overall 30-day incidence of PPC was 3.9%, with rates similar between abdominal and thoracic patients. Lung protective ventilation during both thoracic and abdominal surgery was associated with a significantly lower rate of PPC as compared with conventional ventilation, although the mortality rate was similar. Of note, in the thoracic arm, the observation study by Licker and coworkers[12] with over 1100 patients far outnumbered the total sum of patients in all the small randomized trials. Even then, not all trials could provide postoperative data which makes definitive conclusions difficult. In a large database study, Blank et al.[80] scrutinized data collected by the Society of Thoracic Surgery between 2012 and 2014. The data of 1019 patients available for analysis were included in the study. Mean tidal volume during OLV was 4.9 mL/kg PBW, mean PEEP 4.2 cm H_2O, and mean driving pressure 17.5 cm H_2O. They found that tidal volume was inversely related to the incidence of respiratory complications (odds ratio 0.837; CI, 0.729–0.958) (Fig. 19.7). They reported that an increase in tidal volume of 1 mL/kg PBW was associated with approximately a 16% reduction in the risk of respiratory complications. Low tidal volume with insufficient PEEP was inversely related to the incidence of complication, whereas increases in driving pressure were predictive of increases in PPCs.

TABLE 19.2 Summary of Randomized Studies on Protective One-Ventilation

Study	Nos.*	Study Setting	One-Lung-Ventilation in Study Group	One-Lung Ventilation in Control Group	Outcome	Comment
Michelet 2006[2]	52	Patients undergoing minimally invasive esophagectomy	VCV, V_T = 5 mL/kg PBW, PEEP = 5 cm H_2O, FiO_2 = 1.0, no recruitment	VCV, V_T = 9 mL/kg PBW, PEEP = 5 cm H_2O, FiO_2 = 1.0, no recruitment	Control group had marginal increases in alveolar cytokines and oxygenation No difference in overall morbidity, mortality, or hospital stay	Extra vascular lung water was increased in the control group However, the measurement does not differentiate between lungs
Ahn 2012[77]	50	Patients without pulmonary functional abnormalities undergoing VATS lobectomy	V_T = 6 mL/kg abw, PEEP = 5 cm H_2O, FiO_2 0.5, no recruitment	V_T = 10 mL/kg abw, No PEEP, FiO_2 0.5, no recruitment	No difference in rate of atelectasis, oxygenation or hospital stay	
Yang 2011[76]	100	Patients undergoing open or VATS lobectomy	VCV, V_T = 5 mL/kg PBW, PEEP = 5 cm H_2O, FiO_2 = 1.0, no recruitment	PCV, V_T = 10 mL/kg PBW, No PEEP, FiO_2 = 0.5, no recruitment	Higher incidence of PaO_2/FiO_2 <300 (8 vs. 1) and of atelectasis and acute lung injury in the control group No difference in ICU or hospital stay	Assessment of atelectasis and/or infiltrations were made on both operated and nonoperated lung sides
Shen 2012[75]	101	Patients undergoing minimally invasive esophagectomy	V_T = 5 mL/kg abw, PEEP = 5 cm H_2O, no recruitment	V_T = 8 mL/kg abw, No PEEP, no recruitment	Marginally worse oxygenation and higher incidence of PPC in the control group No difference in mortality or morbidity otherwise	Assessment of atelectasis and/or infiltrations were made on both operated and nonoperated lung sides
Marret 2018[78]	346	Patients undergoing lobectomy or pneumonectomy	V_T 5 mL//kg PBW and PEEP = 5–8 cm H_2O	V_T 10 mL/kg PBW without PEEP	Major postoperative (pulmonary and cardiac) complications occurred in 13.4% in the study group vs. 22.2% in the control group (*P* = .03). No increase in mortality or ICU stay	
Park 2019[79]	292	Patient undergoing lung resection and esophagectomy	V_T 6 mL/kg PBW and respiratory rate of 12 PEEP was adjusted before staring the study to get the lowest driving pressure	V_T 6 mL/kg PBW, PEEP = 5 cm H_2O and recruitment No optimizing of driving pressure	There was a mean difference of 1 cm H_2O in driving pressure between the groups. The authors report lower rates of PPC and lower rates of pneumonia and ARDS in the optimized driving pressure group	Assessment of chest x-ray for pneumonia and ARDS diagnosis were made on both the operated and nonoperated lung sides Discarding these data, no significant effect is seen

abw, Actual body weight; *ARDS*, acute respiratory distress syndrome; *ICU*, intensive care unit; *nos.*, number of patients included in the analysis; *PBW*, predicted body weight; *PEEP*, positive end-expiratory pressure; *PPC*, postoperative pulmonary complications; *VCV* and *PCV*, volume-controlled and pressure-controlled ventilation; V_T, tidal volume.

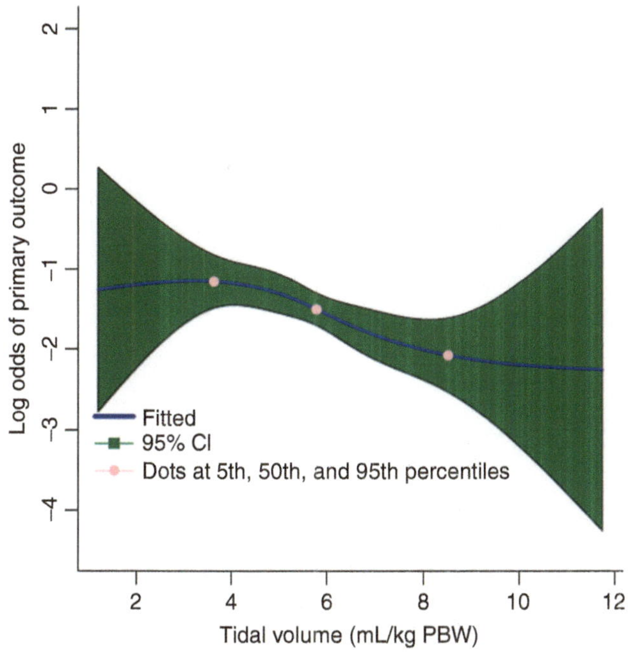

• **Fig. 19.7** Log odds of primary outcome versus tidal volume and driving pressure. The logarithm of the odds of developing the primary outcome (respiratory complications) is plotted against the tidal volume during one-lung ventilation. *PBW*, Predicted body weight. See text for discussion. (From Blank RS, Colquhoun DA, Durieux ME, et al. Management of one-lung ventilation: impact of tidal volume on complications after thoracic surgery. *Anesthesiology*. 2016;124(6):1286–1295. With permission.)

The existing literature relating intraoperative protective ventilatory regimes during OLV to postoperative PPC is contradictory at best and calls for better prospective studies, which include a larger number of patients and better defined outcome parameters to pinpoint the pathophysiologic variable causally related to the injury afflicted. The physiologic rationale of using a protective ventilation to reduce volutrauma, but especially atelectrauma during surgery, seems rather convincing, but the clinical data reviewed does not offer a clear strategy for protective ventilation during OLV. On the other hand, the results reported thus far may reflect the possibility that the rather small differences between ventilation strategies in the study and control groups do not suffice to produce measurable clinical differences. Despite these reservations, progress has been made, and the present data suggests that merely using a low tidal volume strategy alone is not the sole answer. Rather, we need a more comprehensive approach, which allows adapting components of a protective ventilation strategy to fit the individual patient. The approach, which at this time would most probably be least injurious with the least likelihood associated with hypoxemia, and easily adaptable to the individual patient during OLV, would be an open lung approach. While ventilating a presumably healthy dependent single lung (as can be readily substantiated by referring to lung function and radiologic studies), the following open lung approach can be suggested using either volume controlled or pressure controlled ventilation (Table 19.3).

TABLE 19.3 Summary of Recommendations

Item	Recommendation	Comment
Ventilation mode	Volume-controlled ventilation	Allows control of tidal volume, that is, tidal volume does not change when adjustments in respiratory rate or inspiration-to-expiration ratio are made This is not the case with pressure-controlled ventilation.
Tidal volume	5–6 mL/kg PBW	Start with 6 mL/kg PBW. A lower tidal volume should be used if plateau pressure exceeds 30 cm H_2O and is not treatable by tube correction nor recruitment.
Positive end-expiratory pressure (PEEP)	5–8 cm H_2O	Starting with 8 cm H_2O will provide better oxygenation and less hypoxemia especially in the obese patient
Respiratory rate	15–18 breaths/min	Set to achieve a $PaCO_2$ in the upper normal range (45 mm Hg)
Recruitment	Only when oxygenation deteriorates or driving pressure increases beyond 15 cm H_2O	In lean patients, increasing PEEP to 15 cm H_2O for 30–60 s will suffice to open the lung. In obese patients, inflating the lung with a manual inspiratory hold 35–40 cm H_2O for 10 s may be necessary.
Driving pressure	<15 cm H_2O	If driving pressure exceeds 15 cm H_2O, consider recruitment and a subsequent increase in PEEP

The recommendations are based on the literature discussed in the chapter and personal, practical preference of the author. Optimal double-lumen tube or bronchial blocker management is a prerequisite for any ventilation strategy.

PBW, Predicted body weight; *$PaCO_2$*, partial pressure of carbon dioxide in arterial blood; *PEEP*, positive end-expiratory pressure.

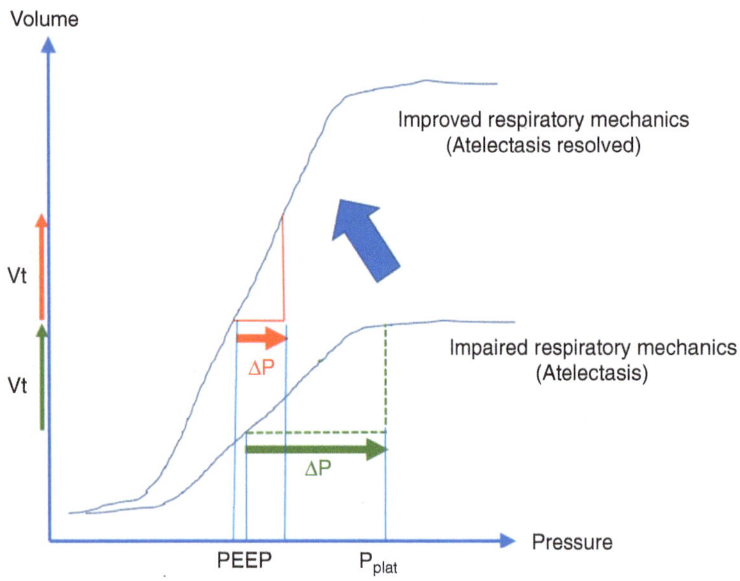

• **Fig. 19.8 Pressure-volume curves and respiratory mechanics.** When driving pressure (*ΔP*) increases beyond 15 cm H_2O (*green*), respiratory mechanics are impaired (lower curve). During anesthesia and one-lung ventilation, this increase in driving pressure is mostly because of atelectasis. Recruitment (*blue arrow*) can resolve atelectasis, increase lung compliance, and thereby decrease driving pressure (*red*). Note that tidal volume (*Vt*) remains the same in both curves. *PEEP*, Positive end expiratory pressure; P_{plat}, plateau pressure. (Modified from PulmCCM.org with permission.)

Tidal volume in the range of 5 to 6 mL/kg PBW, (because this corresponds to 10 to 12 mL/kg PBW for two-lung ventilation), may be seen as too high. This is not so because the FRC of the single healthy lung is still in the range of 1000 to 1200 mL, which means the strain we are applying is far below 1.0, which would not overstretch the lung.[25,81] When using volume controlled ventilation, the tidal volume would not change when adjustments in respiratory rate or inspiration-to-expiration ratio are made (this is not the case with pressure control ventilation). When considering PEEP in the range of 5 to 8 cm H_2O, the author prefers PEEP = 8 cm H_2O because it usually achieves the best oxygenation. These levels of PEEP are suggested because the dependent lung is prone to developing atelectasis, and using lower PEEP levels may frequently lead to atelectasis and hypoxemia and possibly to lung injury.[80] Respiratory rates are set to achieve a partial pressure of carbon dioxide in arterial blood in the upper normal range (45–50 mm Hg). In a healthy lung, using the strategy described should lead to driving pressure below 15 cm H_2O. If driving pressure is greater than 15 cm H_2O, and especially when oxygenation is also impaired, one should suspect atelectasis formation and consider recruiting the lung through appropriate recruitment maneuvers thus improving ventilation (Fig. 19.8). It might be necessary to increase PEEP to a higher level after recruitment because atelectasis occurred despite the PEEP level before recruitment. In lean patients, recruitment maneuvers by increasing PEEP to 15 cm H_2O for 30 to 60 seconds will suffice to open the lung. In obese patients, inflating the lung with a manual inspiratory hold 35 to 40 cm H_2O for 10 seconds may be necessary. Note that driving pressure might also be high and not responsive to recruitment when the ventilated lungs have other pathologic problems, such as frank consolidations or fibroses, which would need alternative strategies of ventilation to provide adequate oxygenation.

Modulating the Inflammatory Response During Ventilation With Anesthetics

Lung injury in experimental and clinical settings is accompanied by increases in the pulmonary and systemic immune responses.[82,83] Attenuating the effects of these immune responses (such as tumor necrosis factor-alpha [TNF-alpha]) in animal studies reduces the development of ventilator-induced lung injury.[84] This shows that these cytokines are not innocent bystanders and may, when released in sufficiently high quantities, contribute causally to lung injury. Surgery and mechanical ventilation lead to increases both in pulmonary and systemic immune response during thoracic surgery.[1,85] The question arises whether modulation of the immune response can ameliorate ventilation-induced lung inflammation and possibly ventilator-induced lung injury (VILI) during OLV.

Volatile anesthetics have been shown to differentially decrease lung immune inflammatory response. In experimental lipopolysaccharide-induced lung injury in rats, sevoflurane was found to reduce cytokine release and reduce neutrophil influx into the lung, but also to reduce lung damage and improve oxygenation.[86] In a mouse model of VILI, sevoflurane posttreatment was found to decrease lung injury.[87] In clinical studies, anesthesia with volatile anesthetic was associated with lower increases or lower levels of inflammatory cytokines in lung lavage of patients than with anesthesia with propofol. Schilling and coworkers[88] showed that lung inflammatory mediator release (TNF-alpha, interleukin [IL]-1β, IL-8) was significantly less pronounced in lungs of patients under volatile anesthetics desflurane and sevoflurane as compared with the propofol group (Fig. 19.9). In a clinical study, De la Gala et al.[9] randomized 180 patients to either propofol or sevoflurane anesthesia and assessed intraoperative pulmonary inflammatory response and PPCs. They report, increases in cytokines concentration in the dependent and nondependent lung, which were more pronounced in the propofol group as compared with sevoflurane. They also reported a 2-fold higher incidence of PPCs in the propofol as compared with the sevoflurane group. However, PPC was not a primary endpoint of the study, and the patients in the propofol group seemed older and sicker. In a much larger prospective study, Beck-Schimmer and coworkers[89] randomized 460 patients to propofol or desflurane anesthesia during lung surgery and assessed the incidence of major complications for up to 6 months using the Clavien-Dindo classification. ICU and hospital stay did not differ between the groups, and the authors found no significant differences in the incidence or severity of complications during the first 30 days or in the 6 months after surgery (Table 19.4). In conclusion, although anesthetics may differentially modulate the inflammatory response in the lung, the available evidence at this point does not justify any clinical preference on this basis.

Injury in the Nondependent Lung

The nondependent lung has not been the object of many studies. However, there is some experimental and clinical evidence which suggests that applying CPAP on the nonventilated lung during OLV would not only improve oxygenation by apneic oxygenation, but also ameliorate the inflammatory response (mediator release) to both lungs.[90,91] The published evidence so far does not provide definite proof nor

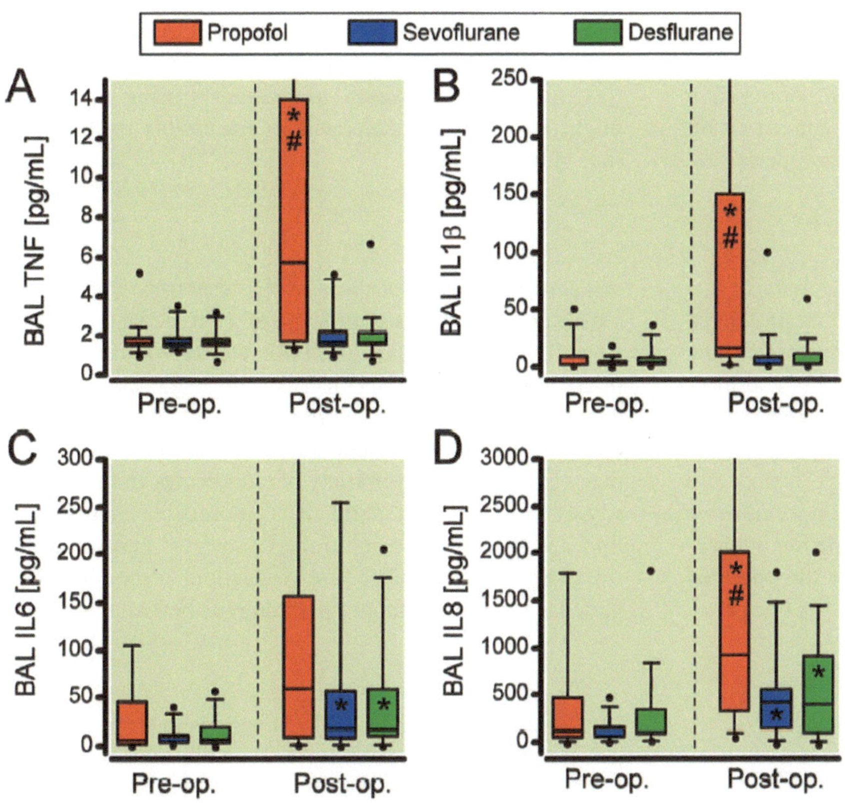

• **Fig. 19.9** The time-dependent changes of the intraalveolar concentrations of tumor necrosis factor (*TNF*)-alpha **A,** interleukin (IL)-1 **B,** IL-6 **C,** and IL-8 **D,** in patients undergoing one-lung ventilation and open thoracic surgery. Data are given as medians, ranges, and interquartile ranges (25–75 percentile). The *black dots* indicate the outliers in each group. The symbol * indicates differences within a single study group, and # marks differences between the propofol and both volatile anesthesia patient groups. *BAL*, Bronchoalveolar lavage; *Post-op*, postoperatively; *Pre-op*, preoperatively. (From Schilling T, Kozian A, Senturk M, et al. Effects of volatile and intravenous anesthesia on the alveolar and systemic inflammatory response in thoracic surgical patients. *Anesthesiology*. 2011;115(1):65–74. With permission.)

TABLE 19.4 Comparison of Overall Incidence of Related Major Complications During Hospitalization and up to 6-Months Follow-Up in Patients Undergoing Lung Surgery Anesthetized With Either Propofol or Desflurane

	Propofol (n = 230)	Desflurane (n = 230)	Unadjusted Incidence Rate Ratio	Adjusted Incidence Rate Ratio*
Incidence of complications during hospitalization (%)	22 (9.6)	20 (8.7)	0.94 (95% CI, 0.52–1.73; *P* = .85)	0.94 (95% CI, 0.51–1.74; *P* = .85)
Incidence complications up to 6 months follow-up.	33 (14.3)	36 (15.7)	1.10 (95% CI, 0.68–1.76; *P* = .70)	1.09 (95% CI, 0.68–1.76; *P* = .71)

*Adjusted for prestratification variables (study cite, major disease, and pneumonectomy) and age.

Table reproduced with permission from Beck-Schimmer B, Bonvini JM, Braun J, et al. Which anesthesia regimen is best to reduce morbidity and mortality in lung surgery? A multicenter randomized controlled trial. *Anesthesiology*. 2016;125(2):313–321.

recommendations to use CPAP routinely as a lung protective measure. It is mainly because of the poor visibility associated with the application of CPAP that presents serious problems for the surgical procedure, specifically during minimally invasive video-assisted or robotics procedures. However, using the low levels of CPAP or oxygen insufflation to the nonventilated lung to treat hypoxemia is standard practice.

Oxygen Toxicity

During OLV, although one lung is ventilated, both lungs are perfused. Because perfusion of the nonventilated lung causes varying degrees of shunt, high FiO_2 is frequently used in the ventilated lung to avoid hypoxemia. High FiO_2, which is associated with generation of reactive oxygen species, can theoretically cause lung injury. Although there is ample experimental evidence that reactive oxygen species do injure cells and tissues, this does not readily translate into clinical evidence.[92] In a large randomized trial,[93] 1400 patients undergoing abdominal surgery were randomized to ventilation with either 30% or 80% oxygen concentration during surgery and extended for 2 hours postoperatively. The incidence of PPC did not differ among the two groups. In a large data-based study by Staehr-Rye AK et al.,[94] intraoperative FiO_2 and PPC data were available for more than 5000 patients. The authors produced some evidence that high FiO_2 as compared with low FiO_2 is associated with an increased rate of PPCs. However, a high FiO_2 may generate PPCs through an increase in the incidence of atelectasis, and this study can at best generate hypothesis and can make no judgement on causation. Cohen et al.[95] used data from an alternating cohort quality improvement project in the Cleveland Clinic, in which the target FiO_2 was altered every 2 weeks between 30% and 80% for a total of 39 months from 2013 to 2016. This resulted in a large cohort of more than 8000 patients assigned to intraoperative administration of either 30% or 80% oxygen. The authors found that intraoperative hyperoxia did not change the postoperative SpO_2/FiO_2 ratio or the risk for pulmonary complications. As can be discerned, the data to date does not support the claim that high FiO_2 during surgery necessarily poses a significant hazard. However, unnecessarily using high FiO_2 might lead to more atelectasis in susceptible patients and should be avoided.[51]

Conclusion

In conclusion, lung injury does occur during thoracic surgery and can, in predisposed patients undergoing prolonged and major thoracic surgery, induce intraoperative lung injury, lead to overt PPCs and increase morbidity and mortality. Patient factors such as age, pulmonary comorbidity and lung function, preoperative care, extent of surgery, the experience of the surgical and anesthesiologic teams, and the quality of postoperative care, all play an important role in the occurrence and severity of PPCs. Among the intraoperative factors, ventilation strategy does have the potential for lung injury although clinical data are neither consistent nor conclusive on a specific strategy to prevent them. Consensus opinion at this stage suggests a protective open lung strategy consisting of the triad of low tidal volumes, appropriate levels of PEEP, and recruitment maneuvers to avoid or treat atelectasis. Driving pressure is a valuable tool to help diagnose problems and help adapt ventilation to lung compliance. Because of the variety of pathologies and the diversity of the clinical scenario, it is improbable that we will find a one-size-fits-all solution. Rather, we need to adapt the components of protective ventilation to the individual patients' lung function and pathology as best as possible.

References

1. Schilling T, Kozian A, Huth C, et al. The pulmonary immune effects of mechanical ventilation in patients undergoing thoracic surgery. *Anesth Analg*. 2005;101:957–965, table of contents.
2. Michelet P, D'Journo XB, Roch A, et al. Protective ventilation influences systemic inflammation after esophagectomy: a randomized controlled study. *Anesthesiology*. 2006;105:911–919.
3. Agostini P, Cieslik H, Rathinam S, et al. Postoperative pulmonary complications following thoracic surgery: are there any modifiable risk factors? *Thorax*. 2010;65(9):815–818.
4. Alam N, Park BJ, Wilton A, et al. Incidence and risk factors for lung injury after lung cancer resection. *Ann Thorac Surg*. 2007; 84(4):1085–1091; discussion 1091.
5. Miskovic A, Lumb AB. Postoperative pulmonary complications. *Br J Anaesth*. 2017;118(3):317–334.
6. Canet J, Gallart L, Gomar C, et al. Prediction of postoperative pulmonary complications in a population-based surgical cohort. *Anesthesiology*. 2010;113:1338–1350.
7. Jammer I, Wickboldt N, Sander M, et al. Standards for definitions and use of outcome measures for clinical effectiveness research in perioperative medicine: European Perioperative Clinical Outcome (EPCO) definitions: a statement from the ESA-ESICM joint taskforce on perioperative outcome measures. *Eur J Anaesthesiol*. 2015;32(2):88–105.
8. iPROVE Network investigators, Belda J, Ferrando C, et al. The effects of an open-lung approach during one-lung ventilation on postoperative pulmonary complications and driving pressure: a descriptive, multicenter national study. *J Cardiothorac Vasc Anesth*. 2018;32(6):2665–2672.
9. de la Gala F, Pineiro P, Reyes A, et al. Postoperative pulmonary complications, pulmonary and systemic inflammatory responses after lung resection surgery with prolonged one-lung ventilation. Randomized controlled trial comparing intravenous and inhalational anaesthesia. *Br J Anaesth*. 2017;119(4):655–663.
10. Abbott TEF, Fowler AJ, Pelosi P, et al. A systematic review and consensus definitions for standardised end-points in perioperative medicine: pulmonary complications. *Br J Anaesth*. 2018;120(5): 1066–1079.

11. Force ADT, Ranieri VM, Rubenfeld GD, et al. Acute respiratory distress syndrome: the Berlin Definition. *JAMA*. 2012; 307(23):2526–2533.
12. Licker M, de Perrot M, Spiliopoulos A, et al. Risk factors for acute lung injury after thoracic surgery for lung cancer. *Anesth Analg*. 2003;97:1558–1565.
13. Serpa Neto A, Hemmes SN, Barbas CS, et al. Incidence of mortality and morbidity related to postoperative lung injury in patients who have undergone abdominal or thoracic surgery: a systematic review and meta-analysis. *Lancet Respir Med*. 2014;2:1007–1015.
14. Blank RS, Hucklenbruch C, Gurka KK, et al. Intraoperative factors and the risk of respiratory complications after pneumonectomy. *Ann Thorac Surg*. 2011;92(4):1188–1194.
15. Bach PB, Cramer LD, Schrag D, et al. The influence of hospital volume on survival after resection for lung cancer. *N Engl J Med*. 2001;345(3):181–188.
16. Pezzi CM, Mallin K, Mendez AS, et al. Ninety-day mortality after resection for lung cancer is nearly double 30-day mortality. *J Thorac Cardiovasc Surg*. 2014;148(5):2269–2277.
17. Desborough JP. The stress response to trauma and surgery. *Br J Anaesth*. 2000;85(1):109–117.
18. Manou-Stathopoulou V, Korbonits M, Ackland GL. Redefining the perioperative stress response: a narrative review. *Br J Anaesth*. 2019;123(5):570–583.
19. Craig SR, Leaver HA, Yap PL, et al. Acute phase responses following minimal access and conventional thoracic surgery. *Eur J Cardiothorac Surg*. 2001;20(3):455–463.
20. Nagahiro I, Andou A, Aoe M, et al. Pulmonary function, postoperative pain, and serum cytokine level after lobectomy: a comparison of VATS and conventional procedure. *Ann Thorac Surg*. 2001;72(2):362–365.
21. Paul S, Altorki NK, Sheng S, et al. Thoracoscopic lobectomy is associated with lower morbidity than open lobectomy: a propensity-matched analysis from the STS database. *J Thorac Cardiovasc Surg*. 2010;139(2):366–378.
22. Salati M, Brunelli A, Decaluwe H, et al. Report from the European Society of Thoracic Surgeons Database 2017: patterns of care and perioperative outcomes of surgery for malignant lung neoplasm. *Eur J Cardiothorac Surg*. 2017;52(6):1041–1048.
23. Berfield KS, Farjah F, Mulligan MS. Video-assisted thoracoscopic lobectomy for lung cancer. *Ann Thorac Surg*. 2019;107(2):603–609.
24. Kirmeier E, Eriksson LI, Lewald H, et al. Post-anaesthesia pulmonary complications after use of muscle relaxants (POPULAR): a multicentre, prospective observational study. *Lancet Respir Med*. 2019;7(2):129–140.
25. Protti A, Cressoni M, Santini A, et al. Lung stress and strain during mechanical ventilation: any safe threshold? *Am J Respir Crit Care Med*. 2011;183:1354–1362.
26. Williams EC, Motta-Ribeiro GC, Vidal Melo MF. Driving pressure and transpulmonary pressure: how do we guide safe mechanical ventilation? *Anesthesiology*. 2019;131(1):155–163.
27. Cipulli F, Vasques F, Duscio E, et al. Atelectrauma or volutrauma: the dilemma. *J Thorac Dis*. 2018;10(3):1258–1264.
28. Gattinoni L, Quintel M, Marini JJ. Volutrauma and atelectrauma: which is worse? *Crit Care*. 2018;22(1):264.
29. Dreyfuss D, Saumon G. Ventilator-induced lung injury: lessons from experimental studies. *Am J Respir Crit Care Med*. 1998; 157(1):294–323.
30. Dreyfuss D, Basset G, Soler P, et al. Intermittent positive-pressure hyperventilation with high inflation pressures produces pulmonary microvascular injury in rats. *Am Rev Respir Dis*. 1985;132(4): 880–884.
31. Dreyfuss D, Soler P, Basset G, et al. High inflation pressure pulmonary edema. Respective effects of high airway pressure, high tidal volume, and positive end-expiratory pressure. *Am Rev Respir Dis*. 1988;137(5):1159–1164.
32. Dreyfuss D, Saumon G. Barotrauma is volutrauma, but which volume is the one responsible? *Intensive Care Med*. 1992;18(3): 139–141.
33. Muscedere JG, Mullen JB, Gan K, et al. Tidal ventilation at low airway pressures can augment lung injury. *Am J Respir Crit Care Med*. 1994;149:1327–1334.
34. Chu EK, Whitehead T, Slutsky AS. Effects of cyclic opening and closing at low- and high-volume ventilation on bronchoalveolar lavage cytokines. *Crit Care Med*. 2004;32:168–174.
35. Gattinoni L, Tonetti T, Cressoni M, et al. Ventilator-related causes of lung injury: the mechanical power. *Intensive Care Med*. 2016;42(10):1567–1575.
36. Cressoni M, Gotti M, Chiurazzi C, et al. Mechanical power and development of ventilator-induced lung injury. *Anesthesiology*. 2016;124(5):1100–1108.
37. Huhle R, Serpa Neto A, Schultz MJ, et al. Is mechanical power the final word on ventilator-induced lung injury?-no. *Ann Transl Med*. 2018;6(19):394.
38. Fu Z, Costello ML, Tsukimoto K, et al. High lung volume increases stress failure in pulmonary capillaries. *J Appl Physiol (1985)*. 1992;73(1):123–133.
39. West JB. Invited review: pulmonary capillary stress failure. *J Appl Physiol* (1985). 2000;89(6):2483–2489; discussion 2497.
40. Slutsky AS. Ventilator-induced lung injury: from barotrauma to biotrauma. *Respir Care*. 2005;50:646–659.
41. Hedenstierna G, Edmark L. Mechanisms of atelectasis in the perioperative period. *Best Pract Res Clin Anaesthesiol*. 2010;24:157–169.
42. Duggan M, Kavanagh BP. Pulmonary atelectasis: a pathogenic perioperative entity. *Anesthesiology*. 2005;102:838–854.
43. Wahba RW. Perioperative functional residual capacity. *Can J Anaesth*. 1991;38:384–400.
44. Fadel PJ, Barman SM, Phillips SW, et al. Fractal fluctuations in human respiration. *J Appl Physiol*. 2004;97:2056–2064.
45. Bendixen HH, Smith GM, Mead J. Patterns of ventilation in young adults. *J Appl Physiol*. 1964;19:195–198.
46. Grim PS, Freund PR, Cheney FW Jr. Effect of spontaneous sighs on arterial oxygenation during isoflurane anesthesia in humans. *Anesth Analg*. 1987;66:839–842.
47. Hedenstierna G, Strandberg A, Brismar B, et al. Functional residual capacity, thoracoabdominal dimensions, and central blood volume during general anesthesia with muscle paralysis and mechanical ventilation. *Anesthesiology*. 1985;62:247–254.
48. Eichenberger A, Proietti S, Wicky S, et al. Morbid obesity and postoperative pulmonary atelectasis: an underestimated problem. *Anesth Analg*. 2002;95:1788–1792, table of contents.
49. Pelosi P, Gregoretti C. Perioperative management of obese patients. *Best Pract Res Clin Anaesthesiol*. 2010;24:211–225.
50. Andersson LE, Bååth M, Thörne A, et al. Effect of carbon dioxide pneumoperitoneum on development of atelectasis during anesthesia, examined by spiral computed tomography. *Anesthesiology*. 2005;102:293–299.
51. Rothen HU, Sporre B, Engberg G, et al. Influence of gas composition on recurrence of atelectasis after a reexpansion maneuver during general anesthesia. *Anesthesiology*. 1995;82:832–842.
52. Tsuchida S, Engelberts D, Peltekova V, et al. Atelectasis causes alveolar injury in nonatelectatic lung regions. *Am J Respir Crit Care Med*. 2006;174:279–289.

53. Strandberg A, Tokics L, Brismar B, et al. Atelectasis during anaesthesia and in the postoperative period. *Acta Anaesthesiol Scand.* 1986;30:154–158.
54. Ventilation with lower tidal volumes as compared with traditional tidal volumes for acute lung injury and the acute respiratory distress syndrome. The Acute Respiratory Distress Syndrome Network. *N Engl J Med.* 2000;342:1301–1308.
55. Gattinoni L, Pesenti A. The concept of "baby lung." *Intensive Care Med.* 2005;31(6):776–784.
56. Schreiber T, Hueter L, Schwarzkopf K, et al. Increased susceptibility to ventilator-associated lung injury persists after clinical recovery from experimental endotoxemia. *Anesthesiology.* 2006;104:133–141.
57. Amato MB, Meade MO, Slutsky AS, et al. Driving pressure and survival in the acute respiratory distress syndrome. *N Engl J Med.* 2015;372(8):747–755.
58. Kozian A, Schilling T, Schutze H, et al. Ventilatory protective strategies during thoracic surgery: effects of alveolar recruitment maneuver and low-tidal volume ventilation on lung density distribution. *Anesthesiology.* 2011;114(5):1025–1035.
59. Bender SP, Paganelli WC, Gerety LP, et al. Intraoperative lung-protective ventilation trends and practice patterns: a report from the Multicenter Perioperative Outcomes Group. *Anesth Analg.* 2015;121(5):1231–1239.
60. Serpa Neto A, Schultz MJ, Slutsky AS. Current concepts of protective ventilation during general anaesthesia. *Swiss Med Wkly.* 2015;145:w14211.
61. Young CC, Harris EM, Vacchiano C, et al. Lung-protective ventilation for the surgical patient: international expert panel-based consensus recommendations. *Br J Anaesth.* 2019;123(6):898–913.
62. Futier E, Constantin JM, Paugam-Burtz C, et al. A trial of intraoperative low-tidal-volume ventilation in abdominal surgery. *N Engl J Med.* 2013;369:428–437.
63. The PROVE Network investigators. High versus low positive end-expiratory pressure during general anaesthesia for open abdominal surgery (PROVHILO trial): a multicentre randomised controlled trial. *Lancet.* 2014;384(9942):495–503.
64. Writing Committee for the PROBESE Collaborative Group Effect of intraoperative high positive end-expiratory pressure (PEEP) with recruitment maneuvers vs low PEEP on postoperative pulmonary complications in obese patients: a randomized clinical trial. *JAMA.* 2019;321(23):2292–2305.
65. Ferrando C, Soro M, Unzueta C, et al. Individualised perioperative open-lung approach versus standard protective ventilation in abdominal surgery (iPROVE): a randomised controlled trial. *Lancet Respir Med.* 2018;6(3):193–203.
66. Guay J, Ochroch EA, Kopp S. Intraoperative use of low volume ventilation to decrease postoperative mortality, mechanical ventilation, lengths of stay and lung injury in adults without acute lung injury. *Cochrane Database Syst Rev.* 2018;7:CD011151.
67. Levin MA, McCormick PJ, Lin HM, et al. Low intraoperative tidal volume ventilation with minimal PEEP is associated with increased mortality. *Br J Anaesth.* 2014;113:97–108.
68. Bugedo G, Retamal J, Bruhn A. Driving pressure: a marker of severity, a safety limit, or a goal for mechanical ventilation. *Crit Care.* 2017;21(1):199.
69. Villar J, Martín-Rodríguez C, Domínguez-Berrot AM, et al. A quantile analysis of plateau and driving pressures: effects on mortality in patients with acute respiratory distress syndrome receiving lung-protective ventilation. *Crit Care Med.* 2017;45(5):843–850.
70. Neto AS, Hemmes SN, Barbas CS, et al. Association between driving pressure and development of postoperative pulmonary complications in patients undergoing mechanical ventilation for general anaesthesia: a meta-analysis of individual patient data. *Lancet Respir Med.* 2016;4(4):272–280.
71. Lohser J, Slinger P. Lung injury after one-lung ventilation: a review of the pathophysiologic mechanisms affecting the ventilated and the collapsed lung. *Anesth Analg.* 2015;121(2):302–318.
72. Larsson A, Malmkvist G, Werner O. Variations in lung volume and compliance during pulmonary surgery. *Br J Anaesth.* 1987;59:585–591.
73. Rehder K, Hatch DJ, Sessler AD, et al. The function of each lung of anesthetized and paralyzed man during mechanical ventilation. *Anesthesiology.* 1972;37:16–26.
74. Tusman G, Bohm SH, Sipmann FS, et al. Lung recruitment improves the efficiency of ventilation and gas exchange during one-lung ventilation anesthesia. *Anesth Analg.* 2004;98:1604–1609 table of contents.
75. Shen Y, Zhong M, Wu W, et al. The impact of tidal volume on pulmonary complications following minimally invasive esophagectomy: a randomized and controlled study. *J Thorac Cardiovasc Surg.* 2013;146(5):1267–1273; discussion 1273–1264.
76. Yang M, Ahn HJ, Kim K, et al. Does a protective ventilation strategy reduce the risk of pulmonary complications following lung cancer surgery? A randomized controlled trial. *Chest.* 2011;139(3):530–537.
77. Ahn HJ, Kim JA, Yang M, et al. Comparison between conventional and protective one-lung ventilation for ventilator-assisted thoracic surgery. *Anaesth Intensive Care.* 2012;40(5):780–788.
78. Marret E, Cinotti R, Berard L, et al. Protective ventilation during anaesthesia reduces major postoperative complications after lung cancer surgery: A double-blind randomised controlled trial. *Eur J Anaesthesiol.* 2018;35(10):727–735.
79. Park M, Ahn HJ, Kim JA, et al. Driving pressure during thoracic surgery: a randomized clinical trial. *Anesthesiology.* 2019;130(3):385–393.
80. Blank RS, Colquhoun DA, Durieux ME, et al. Management of one-lung ventilation: impact of tidal volume on complications after thoracic surgery. *Anesthesiology.* 2016;124(6):1286–1295.
81. Hedenstierna G, Edmark L. Protective ventilation during anesthesia: is it meaningful? *Anesthesiology.* 2016;125(6):1079–1082.
82. dos Santos CC, Slutsky AS. The contribution of biophysical lung injury to the development of biotrauma. *Annu Rev Physiol.* 2006;68:585–618.
83. Dos Santos CC, Slutsky AS. Invited review: mechanisms of ventilator-induced lung injury: a perspective. *J Appl Physiol* (1985). 2000;89(4):1645–1655.
84. Imai Y, Kawano T, Iwamoto S, et al. Intratracheal anti-tumor necrosis factor-alpha antibody attenuates ventilator-induced lung injury in rabbits. *J Appl Physiol* (1985). 1999;87(2):510–515.
85. Wrigge H, Uhlig U, Zinserling J, et al. The effects of different ventilatory settings on pulmonary and systemic inflammatory responses during major surgery. *Anesth Analg.* 2004;98:775–781, table of contents.
86. Voigtsberger S, Lachmann RA, Leutert AC, et al. Sevoflurane ameliorates gas exchange and attenuates lung damage in experimental lipopolysaccharide-induced lung injury. *Anesthesiology.* 2009;111(6):1238–1248.
87. Wagner J, Strosing KM, Spassov SG, et al. Sevoflurane posttreatment prevents oxidative and inflammatory injury in ventilator-induced lung injury. *PLoS One.* 2018;13(2):e0192896.
88. Schilling T, Kozian A, Senturk M, et al. Effects of volatile and intravenous anesthesia on the alveolar and systemic inflam-

matory response in thoracic surgical patients. *Anesthesiology*. 2011;115(1):65–74.
89. Beck-Schimmer B, Bonvini JM, Braun J, et al. Which anesthesia regimen is best to reduce morbidity and mortality in lung surgery? A multicenter randomized controlled trial. *Anesthesiology*. 2016; 125(2):313–321.
90. Verhage RJ, Boone J, Rijkers GT, et al. Reduced local immune response with continuous positive airway pressure during one-lung ventilation for oesophagectomy. *Br J Anaesth*. 2014;112(5): 920–928.
91. Verhage RJ, Croese AC, van Hillegersberg R. Reduced local immune response with continuous positive airway pressure during one-lung ventilation for oesophagectomy. *Br J Anaesth*. 2015; 114(6):1009–1010.
92. Martin DS, Grocott MP. Oxygen therapy and anaesthesia: too much of a good thing. *Anaesthesia*. 2015;70(5):522–527.
93. Meyhoff CS, Wetterslev J, Jorgensen LN, et al. Effect of high perioperative oxygen fraction on surgical site infection and pulmonary complications after abdominal surgery: the PROXI randomized clinical trial. *JAMA*. 2009;302(14):1543–1550.
94. Staehr-Rye AK, Meyhoff CS, Scheffenbichler FT, et al. High intraoperative inspiratory oxygen fraction and risk of major respiratory complications. *Br J Anaesth*. 2017;119(1):140–149.
95. Cohen B, Ruetzler K, Kurz A, et al. Intra-operative high inspired oxygen fraction does not increase the risk of postoperative respiratory complications:alternating intervention clinical trial. *Eur J Anaesthesiol*. 2019;36(5):320–326.

NON-PRINT ITEMS

Abstract

Lung injury may occur during thoracic surgery and can, in predisposed patients undergoing prolonged and major thoracic surgery, induce intraoperative lung injury and lead to overt postoperative pulmonary complications (PPCs). PPC is a serious problem for thoracic anesthesia because it increases morbidity and mortality. Patient factors such as age, pulmonary comorbidity and lung function, preoperative care, extent of surgery, experience of the surgical and anesthesiologic teams, and quality of postoperative care may all play a role in the occurrence and severity of PPCs. Among intraoperative factors, ventilation strategy does have the potential of causing harm although clinical data are neither consistent nor conclusive on a specific strategy to prevent them. Consensus opinion at this stage suggests a protective open lung strategy with low tidal volumes, appropriate levels of positive end-expiratory pressure, and recruitment maneuvers to avoid or treat atelectasis. Driving pressure is a valuable tool to help diagnose problems, and help adapt ventilation to lung compliance. It is improbable that we will find a one-size-fits-all solution. Rather, we need to adapt the components of protective ventilation to the individual patients' lung function.

Keywords

intraoperative lung injury, postoperative pulmonary complications, protective ventilation, one-lung ventilation, atelectasis

20

Management of One-Lung Ventilation: Protective Lung Ventilation

MARCELO GAMA DE ABREU, JAKOB WITTENSTEIN

Introduction

One-lung ventilation (OLV) was first described in 1931, and the first pneumonectomy for cancer was performed in 1933. Although technology has evolved since then, OLV still poses a challenge for the anesthesiologist. For several decades, the impairment of gas exchange during OLV represented the focus of the attention. Accordingly, intraoperative mechanical ventilation settings were aimed at avoiding or reversing hypoxemia, as well as hypercapnia, without much concern about the potentially harmful effects of the mechanical stress on the lung parenchyma. Those settings included tidal volume (V_T) of 10–12 mL/kg of the actual body weight (for a single lung), and zero positive end-expiratory pressure (PEEP). Since then, however, the concept of ventilator-induced lung injury (VILI) emerged and became the cornerstone of mechanical ventilation. The so-called "lung-protective ventilation" strategy, which is based on the use of low V_T with low distending pressures, gained much attention when a multicenter randomized trial showed that V_T of 6 mL/kg of the predicted body weight (pbw) led to lower mortality in patients with the acute respiratory distress syndrome (ARDS) when compared with V_T of 12 mL/kg pbw.[1] It is worth noting that the lung-protective strategy was associated with lower oxygenation than the nonprotective strategy in that study. Furthermore, a meta-analysis showed that use of low V_T is associated with favorable outcomes also in patients without injured lungs.[2]

The use of protective ventilation strategies is not limited to the intensive care unit setting and became widespread also among anesthesiologists to be applied in the operating room. A recent compilation of recommendations for intraoperative mechanical ventilation emphasized the role of low V_T and distending pressures, as well as of adequate PEEP levels, during general anesthesia, as a means to reduce the risk of postoperative pulmonary complications (PPCs).[3] However, those recommendations did not address OLV because protective ventilation during OLV has not been investigated yet with adequately powered trials.[4,5] Clearly, it must be taken into account that mediastinal displacement, surgical manipulation and chest immobilization, external pressure on the dependent lung,[6] and atelectasis formation increased during thoracic surgery as compared with the other types of surgeries. To date there is no convincing evidence that the data derived from patients with ARDS in the ICU can be translated to the thoracic surgical patients.[7]

In this chapter, we will review the mechanisms of VILI, and explore the basic concepts of protective mechanical ventilation during OLV for thoracic surgery, with emphasis on the maintenance of adequate gas exchange, while avoiding injury that might increase the risk of PPCs.

Ventilator-Induced Lung Injury

During mechanical ventilation, atelectatic and overdistended lung regions may coexist, increasing vulnerability of lungs to the potentially detrimental effects of mechanical ventilation.[8,9] Accordingly, the regional stress of the lungs is not well reproduced by gross measurements of lung mechanics.[10,11]

Different mechanisms have been proposed for VILI, most of which are interrelated (Fig. 20.1). Increased airway pressure (**barotrauma**) or the application of relatively high V_T (**volutrauma**) may generate excessively high stretch (strain) and transpulmonary pressures (stress), exceeding the elastic properties of the lung parenchyma above its resting volume and causing direct physical damage of the alveolar-capillary barrier and the cells attached.[12,13] Also, tidal close-and-reopening of lung units, so-called **atelectrauma,**[14] can occur in regions close to atelectasis. Importantly, barotrauma, volutrauma, and atelectrauma can have effects on both epithelial and endothelial cells,[15,16] and cause fragmentation of the fragile extracellular matrix.[17,18] The mechanical damage of the extracellular matrix favors the formation of interstitial edema and activation of metalloproteinases, may not necessarily cause inflammation, however, these fragments of the extracellular matrix have the potential to activate inflammatory mediators.[19,20] Furthermore, the damage of the extracellular matrix induced by mechanical ventilation might be exacerbated by fluid load,[21] which is not uncommon to be underestimated during general anesthesia.

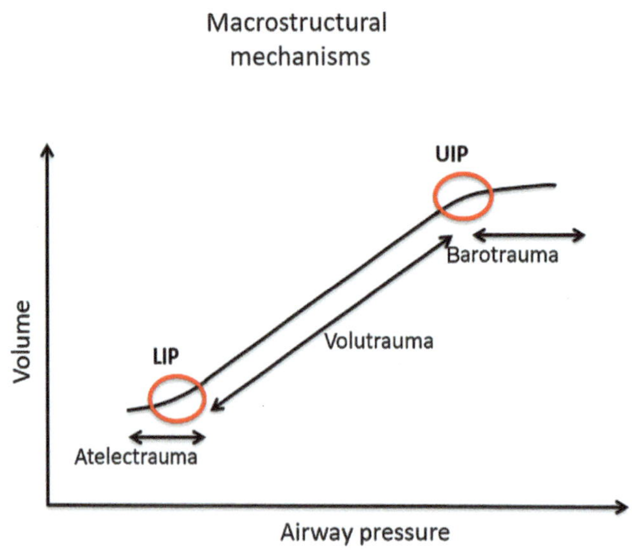

• **Fig. 20.1 Panel 1:** Macrostructural mechanisms of ventilator-induced lung injury (VILI). Volume versus pressure curve of the respiratory system. **Atelectrauma,** repetitive closing, and reopening of lung units—more common in the region of the lower inflection point (*LIP*); **volutrauma,** overdistension of lung parenchyma—more common at higher lung volumes; **barotrauma**—more likely when the curve flattens and the airway pressure increases disproportionally to the volume, with breaks in the lung structure. *UIP,* Upper inflection point.

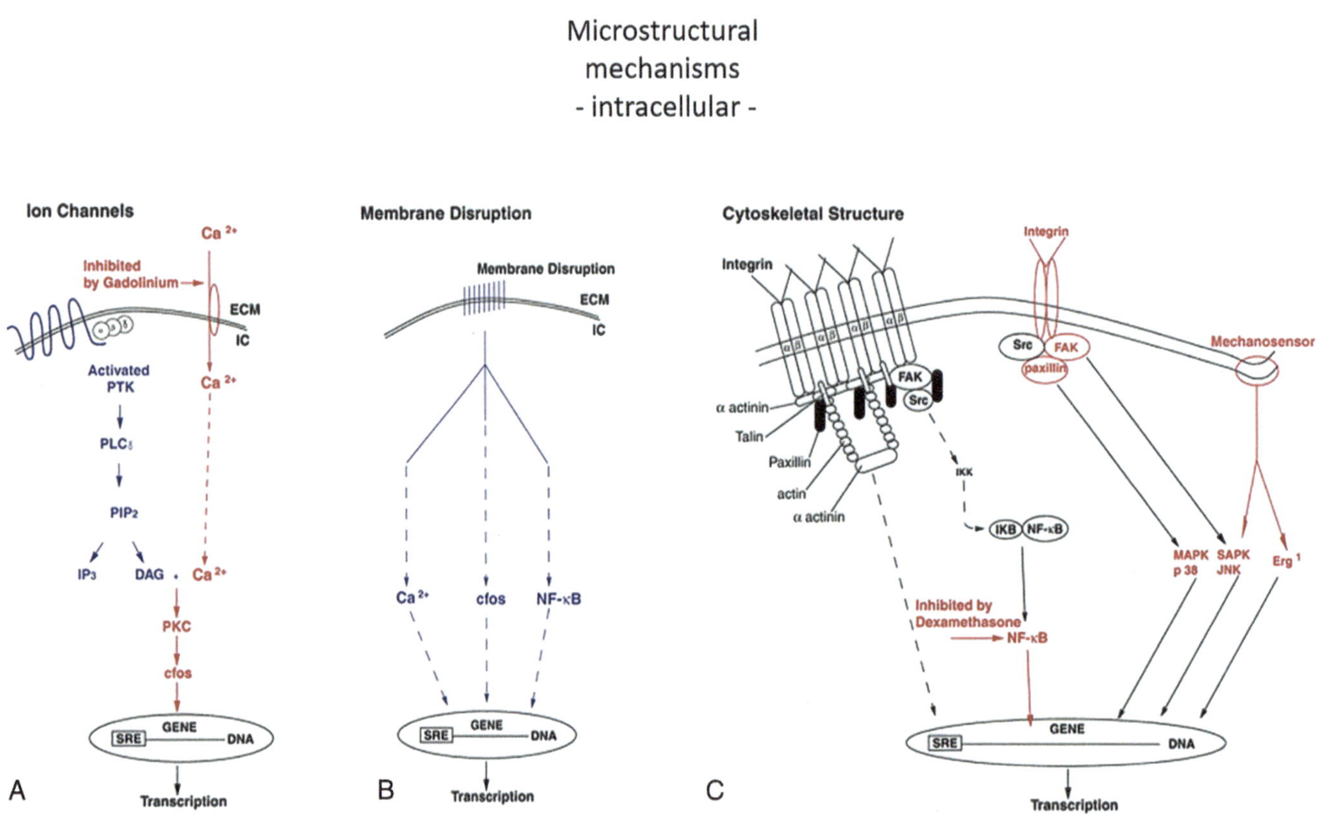

Panel 2: Microstructural mechanisms of VILI. (**A**) Activation of calcium channels. (**B**) Partial disruption of the cell membrane. (**C**) Deformation of the cytoskeletal structure. All mechanisms lead to the transduction of mechanical stress into an inflammatory response. (From Dos Santos CC, Slutsky AS. Invited review: mechanisms of ventilator-induced lung injury: a perspective. *J Appl Physiol* (1985). 2000 Oct;89(4):1645-55. With permission.)

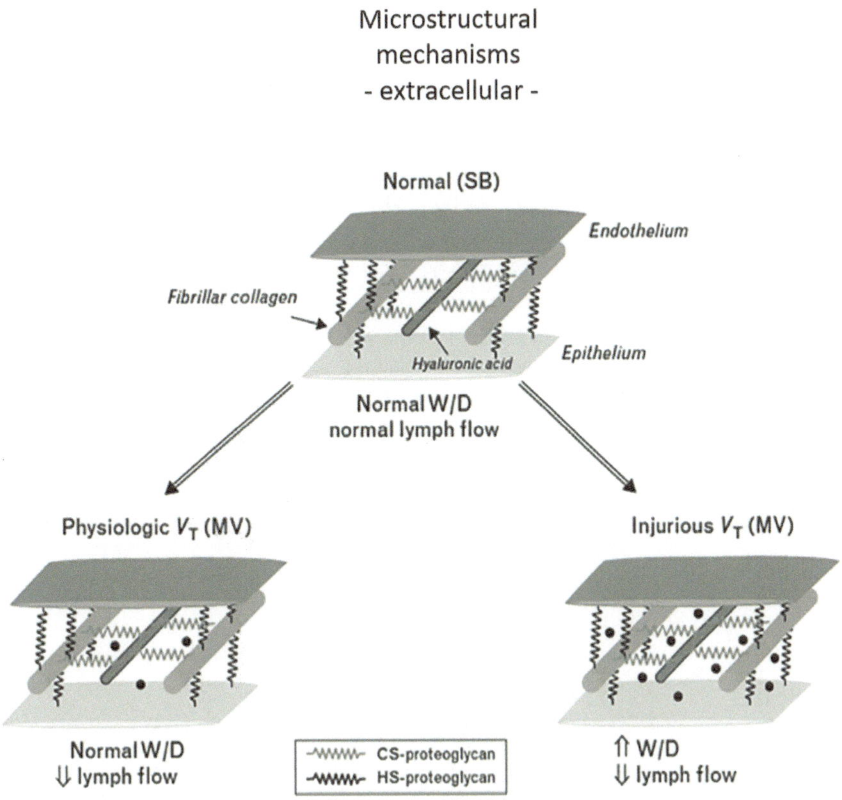

Panel 3 Microstructural mechanisms of VILI. Extracellular matrix (ECM), during spontaneous breathing (SB), and mechanical ventilation (MV) with physiologic (low) or high injurious tidal volume (V_T). In mechanical ventilation at physiologic tidal volume, an initial fragmentation of both heparan sulphate (HS) and chondroitin sulphate (CS) proteoglycans is triggered by activation of a few metalloproteases (•). Deeper degradation of both heparin sulphate and chondroitin sulphate proteoglycans and loss of the entire ECM structure and function is observed in mechanical ventilation at high tidal volume. In healthy lungs, matrix breakdown is associated with enhanced metalloproteases degradative digestion and is not associated with release of inflammatory mediators. *W/D*, Wet-to-dry weight ratio. (From Pelosi P, Negrini D. Extracellular matrix and mechanical ventilation in healthy lungs: back to baro/volotrauma? *Curr Opin Crit Care*. 2008 Feb;14(1):16-21. With permission.)

In cells, especially those from the alveolar epithelium, mechanical stress can be transducted into chemical signals through different pathways, which elicit proinflammatory and profibrotic responses. This process is known as "**mechanotransduction**".[22] Mechanotransduction can lead to cell apoptosis, and release of homing molecules that promote homing and remote activation of neutrophils and macrophages in lungs and peripheral organs.[23] These effects are termed "**biotrauma**".[24]

In the alveolar-epithelial barrier, mechanical stress can disrupt endothelial cells and lead to capillary stress failure.[25,26] Also in the presence of structurally intact cells, disruption of adherence junctions ("tight junction") can occur.[27] Together, those mechanisms increase the epithelial permeability of inflammatory factors and the formation of edema. On the alveolar side of the barrier, the permeability of the alveolar epithelium can also increase with mechanical stress.[28] Those phenomena are more likely during overstretching, but have been described also during atelectrauma.[29,30] Besides the increased permeability during ventilation with high V_T, there is also a risk that excessive stretch impairs the Na, K-adenosine triphosphatase activity,[31] further contributing to edema formation. Ventilation with low V_T reduces this risk of excessive stretch, but on the other hand, it favors hypoxia, and may impair fluid clearance.[32] Independently of the mechanism, alveolar edema interferes with surfactant function.[33] In addition to those phenomena, translocation of pathogens and proinflammatory mediators is more likely to occur when the alveolar-capillary barrier loses integrity, which may result in damage of distal organs.[34]

During OLV, presence of atelectasis favors the inhomogeneity of ventilation, which in turn can increase the forces applied to the lung parenchyma.[9] Those forces increase the likelihood that one or more of the mechanisms mentioned earlier takes place, and VILI can result even in previously noninjured lungs.

Mechanical ventilation settings may affect the risk of VILI and subsequent development of PPCs, which increase morbidity and result in a longer duration of in-hospital stay and even increased risk of death.[35–37] Therefore protective mechanical ventilation settings should be known in detail by anesthesiologists performing OLV (Table 20.1).

Protective One-Lung Ventilation

As shown in Fig. 20.2, there are at least two possible mechanical ventilation strategies to reduce the risk of VILI, namely, the so-called open-lung approach and the lung rest strategy

TABLE 20.1 Settings of Protective One-Lung Ventilation

Mechanical ventilation mode	Pressure- or volume-controlled mode – Volume-controlled ventilation preferred to keep tidal volume constant independently of surgical manipulation; can result in higher peak pressures – Pressure-controlled ventilation preferred to keep peak pressure within safety margins, and during bronchoscopy; can result in derecruitment
Tidal volume (V_T)	≤6 mL/kg predicted body weight (pbw) - Consider 6–8 mL/kg pbw when severe hypercapnia is present and in patients with COPD
Respiratory rate	≤20/min and titrated to arterial pH ≥ 7.25, provided there are no contraindications for permissive hypercapnia - Obstructive lung diseases: lower respiratory rates preferred
Positive end-expiratory pressure (PEEP)	5–10 cm H_2O in most patients, 3–12 cm H_2O range possible depending on the other ventilator settings - Consider PEEP titration according to compliance of the respiratory system or driving pressure if hypoxemia occurs - Be aware of auto-PEEP, and its potential consequences
Driving pressure	≤14 cm H_2O
Plateau pressure	≤30 cm H_2O - Consider values ≤ 25 cm H_2O
Inspiratory to expiratory ratio (I:E)	1:1 to 1:2 - consider I:E 1:2 to 1:3 in case of auto-PEEP
Fraction of inspired oxygen (F_iO2)	When switching from TLV to OLV = 1.0 - During OLV, titration to SpO2 ≥ 92%, as individually appropriate
Recruitment maneuvers of the ventilated lung	Not indicated routinely - Potentially useful for reversal of intraoperative hypoxemia, especially if followed by titration of PEEP - Stepwise increase of V_T or PEEP during tidal ventilation preferred over manual bag squeezing

COPD, Chronic obstructive pulmonary disease; *OLV*, one-lung ventilation; *SpO2*, peripheral oxygen saturation; *TLV*, two-lung ventilation.

(permissive atelectasis). **The open-lung approach** is based on alveolar recruitment maneuvers (RM) (open the lungs), high levels of PEEP (keep the lungs open),[38] and the use of low V_T. The **lung rest strategy** is based on the concept that atelectatic-collapsed lung regions, when not subjected to repetitive opening and closing, are protected from inflammation,[39] and aims at a minimal PEEP level to assure adequate gas exchange (oxygen saturation ≥ 88%–90%), low V_T and low respiratory rate.[40]

In a porcine model of experimental pneumonia, both exogenous surfactant administration and ventilation according to the open-lung approach attenuated bacterial growth and systemic translocation by minimizing alveolar collapse and atelectasis formation.[41] In a similar model of experimental pneumonia in mechanically ventilated pigs, bacterial translocation was lowest with individually tailored PEEP levels, whereas low and high PEEP promoted bacterial translocation.[42]

In isolated nonperfused mouse lungs, both an open-lung approach (V_T of 6 mL/kg, RM and PEEP of 14–16 cmH_2O) as well as a lung rest strategy (V_T of 6 mL/kg, PEEP of 8–10 cmH_2O, no RM) were associated with reduced pulmonary inflammatory response and improved respiratory mechanics compared with injurious mechanical ventilation (V_T of 20 mL/kg, PEEP of 0 cmH_2O).[43] Interestingly, the lung rest strategy was associated with less apoptosis but more ultrastructural cell damage, most likely because of increased activation of mitogen-activated protein kinase pathways as compared with the open-lung strategy.[43]

In healthy mice, mechanical ventilation with a V_T of 8 mL/kg and PEEP of 4 cmH_2O induced a reversible increase in plasma and lung tissue cytokines, as well as increased leukocyte infiltration, but the integrity of the lung tissue was preserved.[44] In another investigation, even least-injurious ventilator settings were able to induce VILI in the absence of a previous pulmonary insult in mice.[45] Of note, the deleterious effects of mechanical ventilation in noninjured lungs are only partly dependent on its duration.[46] However, an experimental study demonstrated that large V_T had only minor (if any) deleterious effects on the lungs, despite prolonged mechanical ventilation.[13] Possibly, this finding is explained by the lack of a previous inflammatory insult, as surgery, for example. In fact, it is the systemic inflammation that may prime the lungs to injury by mechanical ventilation.[47]

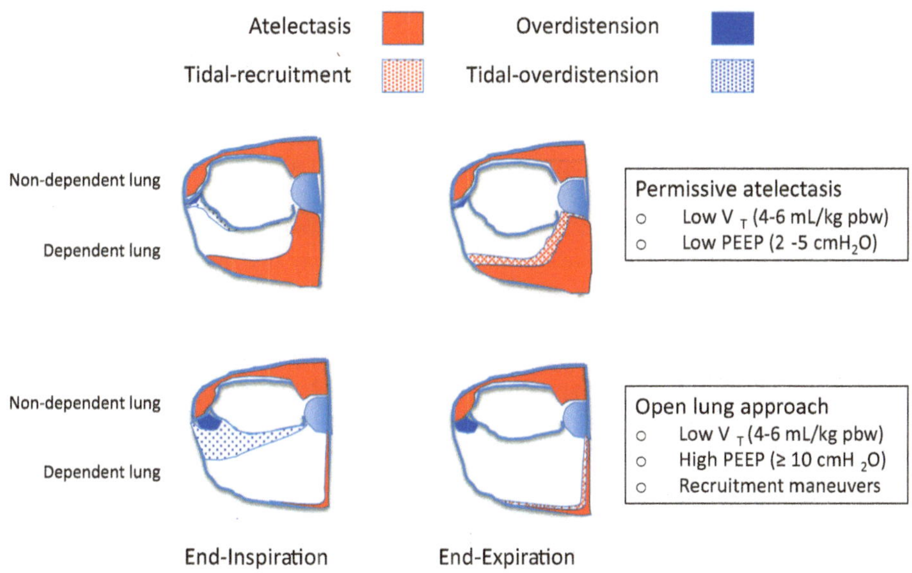

• **Fig. 20.2** Possible strategies for protective one-lung ventilation (OLV). During permissive atelectasis, a low PEEP (2–5 cmH_2O) is used, and recruitment maneuvers only for rescue because of hypoxemia; during the Open-lung approach, high PEEP (≥10 cmH_2O) is used to keep the lungs open after periodic recruitment maneuvers. PBW, Predicted body weight; *PEEP*, positive end-expiratory pressure; V_T, tidal volume.

Tidal Volume

OLV with high V_T has been shown to induce lung overdistension (volutrauma), promoting VILI.[48,49] In patients undergoing abdominal surgery, an intraoperative ventilation strategy with low V_T and PEEP improved postoperative lung function[50] and even outcome.[51] OLV with a V_T of 10 mL/kg pbw compared with 5 mL/kg pbw resulted in a higher inflammatory response in a small randomized control trial (RCT).[52] In another RCT, OLV with a V_T of 6 mL/kg pbw as compared with 10 mL/kg pbw resulted in a lower incidence of postoperative lung dysfunction.[5] A meta-analysis of randomized trials on low versus high V_T during OLV in patients undergoing thoracic surgery showed a lower incidence of pulmonary infiltrations and ARDS, but the incidence of PPCs did not differ between both strategies.[53] A retrospective analysis suggested that the use of low protective V_T during OLV may be not sufficient to improve clinical outcomes if not accompanied by appropriate levels of PEEP. In the thoracic surgical patients, Blank et al. analyzed the data (medical records and the Society of Thoracic Surgery database) for postthoracic procedure complications of 1019 patients. Associations between ventilator parameters and clinical outcomes were examined by multivariate linear regression. They found that a V_T of 8 to 9 mL/kg pbw was associated with fewer PPCs. In the large proportion of the patients, the large V_T during OLV was inversely propositional to the incidence of respiratory complications.[54]

The estimation of pbw is crucial when setting the mechanical ventilator for OLV. The use of pbw is based on the assumption that volutrauma might be minimized by delivering a volume appropriate to the patient's lung capacity.[1] Lung capacity and respiratory system compliance are more closely related to height than weight.[55–57] pbw for male and female patients can be calculated by the following formulas:

Male: pbw = 50 + 0.91 (centimeters of height − 152.4)
Female: pbw = 45.5 + 0.91 (centimeters of height − 152.4)

It has been suggested that the forced vital capacity (FVC) is a more reliable predictor of appropriate V_T for thoracic surgery than pbw,[58] and that FVC values below 3.5 L are associated with reduced compliance of the respiratory system. Accordingly, V_T equal to functional residual capacity (FRC)/8, as measured preoperatively, could be used to guide the selection of V_T during OLV.[58]

Although adequately powered trials are still missing for a strong recommendation of low protective V_T during OLV, values should not exceed 6 mL/kg pbw in most cases.[59,60]

Respiratory Rate

Low respiratory rates combined with low V_T during OLV likely result in hypercapnia. When deliberately conducted, this approach is usually termed permissive hypercapnia, and aims at minimizing VILI.[61] Mild hypercapnia can also improve hypercapnic pulmonary vasoconstriction,[62] shift the oxyhemoglobin dissociation curve rightward, improve oxygenation,[63] thus enhancing oxygen delivery to tissue and, potentially improving wound healing and reducing infectious complications. Besides that, moderate respiratory acidosis resulting in arterial pH of approximately 7.25 can decrease the proinflammatory response during OLV.[64] Recently, a comprehensive appraisal of the mechanisms of VILI suggested that the mechanical power transferred from the ventilator to the lung is associated with lung damage.[65] Mechanical power represents the energy per unit of time that is delivered to the lungs, and depends directly on the respiratory rate.[66] In each breath delivered by the mechanical ventilator, a certain amount of energy is transferred to the patient's respiratory system, which is mainly used to overcome resistance of the airways and to expand the thorax wall. It has been hypothesized that the extent of lung injury depends on the total amount of "mechanical power" delivered by the ventilator per unit of time. Mechanical power is a single variable which combines volume, pressures, flow, and respiratory rate. Accordingly, lower respiratory rates might contribute to reduce the mechanical power and minimize VILI during OLV. Especially in patients with obstructive lung diseases who show expiratory flow limitation, low respiratory rates should be preferred, to avoid formation of auto-PEEP.[67]

Because respiratory acidosis may have also undesirable side effects, including increased intracranial pressure, pulmonary hypertension, myocardial depression, and decreased renal perfusion,[68–70] its use must be considered judiciously.

Positive End-Expiratory Pressure and Recruitment Maneuvers

During OLV, especially in the lateral decubitus position, the dependent lung can by compressed by the mediastinal and intraabdominal structures, as well as surgical manipulation, resulting in further reduction of FRC. PEEP has the potential to keep lung units open at the end of expiration preventing the formation of atelectasis and thereby increasing FRC above the closing capacity of the lungs. Also, appropriate levels of PEEP may result in ventilation within a linear part of the pressure-volume curve of the respiratory system, minimizing atelectrauma.[40] However, PEEP can lead also to hyperinflation, increasing the alveolar dead space, and compressing lung capillaries. This might result in an increased afterload of the right ventricle with cardiovascular depression, need for fluid loading, and inotropic support. Furthermore, PEEP in the ventilated lung can shift perfusion to the nonventilated lung, resulting in an increased intrapulmonary shunt. Special caution is needed when setting PEEP in patients with severe obstructive disease, because inspiratory flow limitation may result in dynamic hyperinflation because of auto-PEEP.

The appropriate level of PEEP has been a matter of intensive debate in the last decade, and higher levels of PEEP are frequently used. However, recent clinical trials failed to show that high PEEP could improve outcome. In nonobese patients, as well in obese patients submitted to abdominal surgery, a PEEP of 12 cmH_2O did not reduce the incidence of PPCs.[71,72] Besides using a fixed value, PEEP can be individualized according to different characteristics: (1) the best compliance by a decremental PEEP titration to reach the best compliance;[73] (2) the lowest driving pressure;[74] and (3) according to electrical impedance tomography (EIT).[75] The titrated PEEP may vary depending on the titration method used. PEEP titrated according to the compliance of the respiratory system in patients submitted to abdominal surgery did not reduce the occurrence of PPCs when compared with low PEEP.[76] In a small RCT, PEEP level titrated to the lowest driving pressure during OLV, as compared with a fixed level of PEEP of 5 cmH_2O, resulted in improved lung protection.[74] PEEP values determined with EIT effectively improved oxygenation and lung mechanics during OLV in elderly patients undergoing thoracoscopic surgery.[75] However, adequately powered studies on the effects of different PEEP levels on lung protection are missing.

The effects of a particular level of PEEP may vary when PEEP is used isolated or in combination with an RM.[77] Currently, high-quality evidence is lacking to recommend a routine RM for all patients and further research is required.[3] An RM is a maneuver aimed at increasing the transpulmonary pressure in an attempt to revert alveolar collapse.[78] Different RMs have been described to achieve this aim in the ventilated, and also the nonventilated, lung. All RMs lead to a temporary increase of the airway pressure, usually with values of 40 cmH_2O or more, during 20 to 40 seconds. Most frequently, this is achieved by switching the mechanical ventilator to manual ventilation and using bag squeezing along with appropriate fresh gas flow and setting of the adjustable pressure-limiting valve, as shown schematically in Fig. 20.3. Albeit popular, this procedure is not standardized and may be less effective because loss of airway pressure may occur when resuming mechanical ventilation. The preferred approach is to conduct an RM under pressure-controlled ventilation (PCV), as shown illustratively in Fig. 20.3. If PEEP titration is necessary, changing for volume-controlled ventilation (VCV), followed by decremental PEEP steps of 2 to 3 cmH_2O to identify the value leading to maximal compliance of the respiratory system is likely adequate. Alternatively, the RM can be conducted under VCV by increasing V_T in increments of 4 mL/kg pbw under a constant high PEEP level of 12 cmH_2O. RMs that are conducted under tidal ventilation are usually known as "stepwise RM." Importantly, during the stepwise RMs, the respiratory rate is reduced to 10/min at an inspiratory to expiratory ratio (I:E) of 1:1, and 1 minute is spent at each V_T or PEEP step to allow enough time for lung recruitment during inspiration (3 seconds).

During OLV in lateral decubitus position, an RM of the dependent lung can result in increased compliance and improved arterial oxygenation.[79,80] To keep the recruited alveoli open after the RM, PEEP can be set to optimize respiratory mechanics, while minimizing alveolar overdistension.[77] Nevertheless, the potential of high PEEP and RM during OLV to protect the lungs from injury and improve clinical outcome variables has not been investigated in adequately powered trials. Currently, an international multicenter RCT is being conducted to fill this information gap.[7]

In patients with severe obstructive disease, auto-PEEP may develop. Accordingly, the resulting total PEEP in these patients is unpredictable. In fact, application of external PEEP might result in increase, decrease, or no change of total PEEP.[81] Therefore PEEP should be used cautiously in these patients, and total PEEP measured whenever possible to avoid overdistension and hemodynamic impairment. If auto-PEEP measurement is not available, it can be estimated using inline spirometry. Thereby, an interruption of the end-expiratory flow curve indicates existence of auto-PEEP.[82]

Driving, Plateau, and Peak Pressures

At constant inspiratory flow, the peak inspiratory pressure depends mainly on the resistance, which is determined by the diameter of the endotracheal tube. Therefore peak

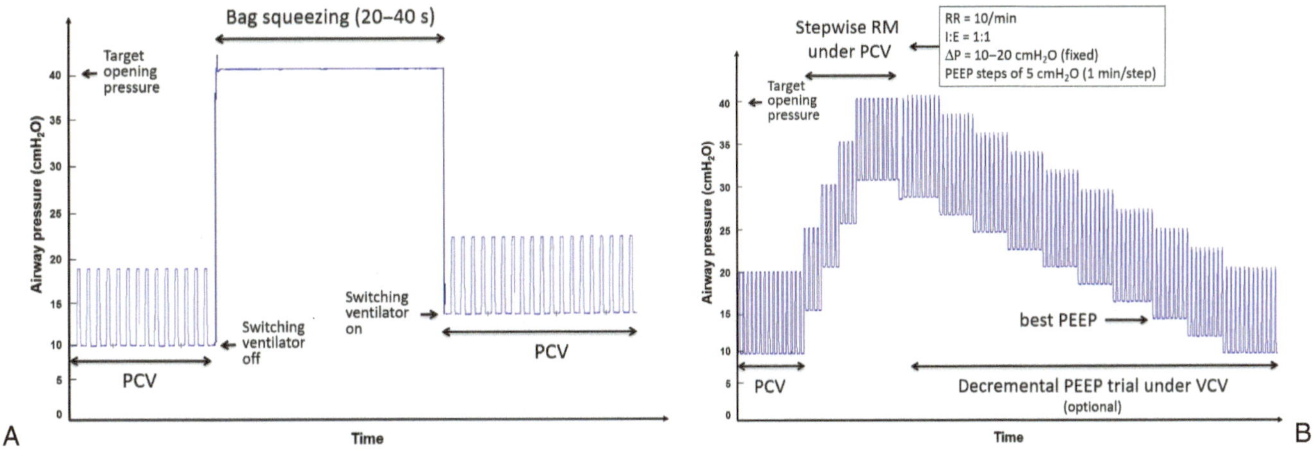

• **Fig. 20.3** Diagrammatic representation of airway pressure versus time recordings during common lung recruitment maneuvers for one-lung ventilation. (A) Bag squeezing; (B) stepwise recruitment maneuver. *ΔP*, Driving pressure; *I:E*; inspiratory to expiratory time ratio; *PCV*, pressure-controlled ventilation; *PEEP*, positive end-expiratory pressure; *RM*, recruitment maneuvers; *RR*, respiratory rate; *VCV*, volume-controlled ventilation.

inspiratory pressure during constant inspiratory flow likely plays a minor role regarding VILI. However, the inspiratory plateau airway pressure, which is a surrogate of the alveolar pressure, is key in determining the potential for injury. Whereas in VCV, the plateau pressure can be measured using an appropriate inspiratory pause, in PCV, inspiratory pressure equals the plateau pressure when flow decreases to zero at the end of inspiration. Thus in both modes, zero-flow is necessary to determine the plateau pressure. To protect the lungs from high distending pressures and to avoid barotrauma, the plateau pressure should ideally be kept at values of 30 cmH_2O or less, but values of 25 cmH_2O or less are likely more protective.[83]

In ARDS patients, it was proposed that driving pressure resamples another parameter which should be limited because it normalizes the V_T to functional lung size ($\Delta P = V_T/\text{Compliance}$). In a retrospective study, a driving pressure of 15 cmH_2O or more was associated with a higher mortality in patients with ARDS.[84] In a meta-analysis in patients who underwent surgery, intraoperative high driving pressure and changes in the level of PEEP that increased driving pressure were associated with more PPCs,[85] but a cutoff value was not proposed. In a clinical study, titration of PEEP during OLV to minimize the driving pressure at a V_T of 5 mL/kg pbw reduced the severity of PPCs. Park et al. confirmed the significance of ΔP during OLV. In a double-blind randomized controlled study of 292 patients undergoing thoracic surgery, they compared ΔP–guided ventilation with conventional protective ventilation. The protective ventilation group ($n = 147$) received conventional protective ventilation during OLV: V_T 6 mL/kg pbw, PEEP 5 cm H_2O, and RM. The ΔP group ($n = 145$) received the same V_T and recruitment, but with titrated individualized PEEP to produce the lowest ΔP during OLV. The number of patients who developed pneumonia or ARDS was smaller in the ΔP group than in the protective ventilation group.[74] Nevertheless, compelling evidence from adequately powered trials is missing to recommend this approach. Furthermore, one must keep in mind that the transpulmonary driving pressure is the real lung-distending pressure, which effectively results in lung strain, which can be estimated using the esophageal pressure. Transpulmonary driving pressure may be useful to understand how much of the driving pressure is caused by elastance of the lungs and how much to chest wall elastance.[86] Accordingly, ΔP 15 cmH_2O or more resulting from increased chest-wall elastance might be, at least theoretically, acceptable if other ventilatory settings, especially V_T, is situated in the protective range (≤6 mL/kg pbw), and PEEP is low to moderate (5–10 cmH_2O).

Inspiratory-to-Expiratory Ratio

A prolonged inspiratory time with a I:E of 1:1 during OLV can result in a modest improvement in oxygenation and decreased shunt fraction.[87] However, in patients with obstructive lung disease, expiratory time must be long enough, to allow complete expiration and avoid air trapping and consecutive auto-PEEP. Expiratory flow limitation has been implicated in the deterioration of hemodynamics because of dynamic hyperinflation.[88] Theoretically, auto-PEEP can contribute to a shift of pulmonary perfusion from the ventilated to the nonventilated lung. Furthermore, the distribution of auto-PEEP across the lungs may be heterogeneous depending on regional time constants.[89] Therefore high I:E during OLV should be ideally either avoided or applied under judicious evaluation of its effects on hemodynamic and gas exchange.

Mechanical Power

The role of V_T in lung protection has been well established in both experimental[90] and clinical studies.[91] Also the importance of choosing adequate levels of PEEP has been well documented in patients with ARDS.[92] More recently, the importance of limiting the driving pressure has been emphasized even when combinations of low V_T and adequate PEEP are used.[84] Furthermore, experimental studies have shown that respiratory rate,[93] the inspiratory[94] and

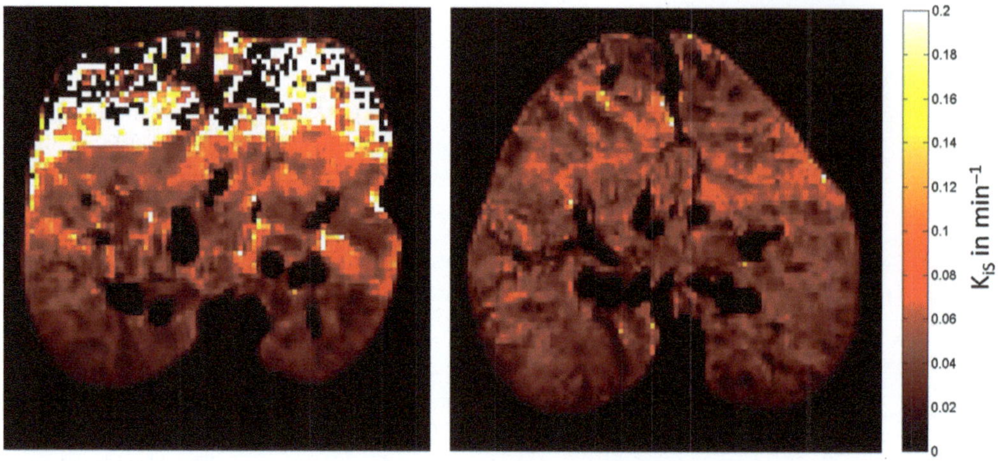

• **Fig. 20.4** Regional distribution of inflammation as measured by intake of 18F Fluorodeoxyglucose (KiS) using positron emission tomography in mechanically ventilated pigs. Left panel: low tidal volume (V_T) with positive end-expiratory pressure (PEEP) below the lower inflection point (LIP) of the pressure versus volume curve of the respiratory system; right panel: low V_T with PEEP above the LIP. Note the difference in magnitude and distribution of inflammation despite similar settings of V_T and respiratory rate.

expiratory[95] airflow, as well as the airway pressure versus time product[96] modulate the severity of lung injury. Combined, these variables determine the mechanical energy across time, or power, that is transferred from the mechanical ventilator to the lungs, which was estimated[65,97] as shown in Equation 20.1:

$$MP = RR \cdot \left\{ V_T^2 \cdot \left[\frac{1}{2} \cdot E + RR \cdot \frac{(1 + I{:}E)}{(60 \cdot I{:}E)} \cdot R \right] + V_T \cdot PEEP \right\} \quad (20.1)$$

where MP is the mechanical power, E is the elastance of the respiratory system, I:E is the inspiratory-to-expiratory ratio, and R is the airway resistance.

Increased mechanical power as described in Eq. 20.1, which should correspond to mechanical energy over time, led to the deterioration of lung function and formation of lung edema in pigs without previous lung injury,[65] as well as in rats.[98] Recently, it was shown that high mechanical power of ventilation is associated with increased mortality in critically ill patients. In a 2018 trial, Serpa Neto et al., in analysis of 8207 patients from 59 hospitals of critically ill patients, found an association between higher mechanical power and worse outcomes in mechanically ventilated, critically ill patients.[99]

However, the equation of mechanical power as originally proposed (Eq. 20.1) by Gattinoni et al.[97] contains inconsistencies, and was validated only using the extent of edematous lung tissue as a surrogate of VILI. The most important inconsistency in that equation is the computation of the contribution of PEEP, which is multiplied by the variation of lung volume and respiratory rate as RR·ΔV·PEEP. Certainly, PEEP increases the static stress and, thereby, the energy stored in mechanically ventilated lungs, but this contribution is independent of V_T. Also Eq. 20.1 predicts that VILI would be minimal at zero PEEP, which is not supported by the literature.[92] Recently, an attempt to estimate the contribution of PEEP to VILI within the concept of mechanical power was conducted.[100] Authors suggested the presence of a "U-shaped" relationship between injury and PEEP, that is, reduced VILI in a PEEP range of 4 to 7 cmH_2O, as compared with lower and higher PEEP.

Certainly, PEEP and plateau pressure have effects on the mechanical energy stored in the lungs, but their contribution is poorly defined. Recently, our group showed that VILI is associated essentially with the dynamic components of MP (MPdyn),[66] as represented in Equation 20.2:

$$MPdyn = \left(R \cdot \frac{I{:}E + 1}{I{:}E \cdot 60} \cdot RR + \frac{1}{2} E \right) \cdot V_T^2 \cdot RR \quad (20.2)$$

According to that equation, MPdyn during OLV can be minimized mainly through limitation of V_T 6 mL/kg pbw or less, provided the elastance of the respiratory system is within the normal range, that is, the driving pressure is 14 cmH_2O or less. Importantly, as expected, limitation of respiratory rate, for example, 20 or less per minute with permissive hypercapnia, also reduces MPdyn. Theoretically, MPdyn (according to Eq. 20.2) of ≤ 8 J/min might be protective, but there is no sound evidence to support such a recommendation during OLV. Also the mechanical energy may dissipate differently across the lungs depending on the set PEEP value, a concept that is known as mechanical energy intensity. Fig. 20.4 illustrates how the distribution of inflammation can differ at similar values of V_T and respiratory rate, when PEEP is set below the lower inflection point of the volume versus pressure curve of the respiratory system, or above it.

Inspiratory Oxygen Concentration

Provided there is no contraindication, the fraction of inspired oxygen (FiO_2) should be set at 100% when switching from two-lung ventilation (TLV) to OLV to avoid hypoxemia, and to allow faster collapse of the nonventilated lung. In a denitrogenated and nonventilated lung, oxygen

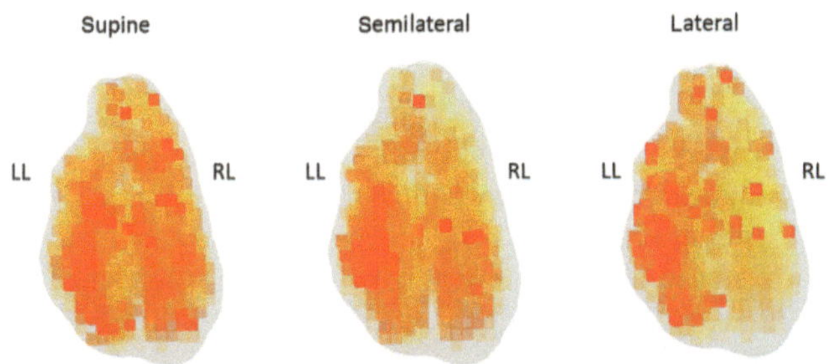

• **Fig. 20.5** Distribution of relative perfusion during one-lung ventilation (OLV) in a pig in supine, semilateral, and lateral decubitus position (*yellow*—low perfusion, *red*—high perfusion). The left lung (*LL*) was ventilated, while the right lung (*RL*) was allowed to collapse. Note that the relative lung perfusion of RL is reduced as compared with the RL (shift of perfusion because of hypoxic pulmonary vasoconstriction), and lowest in the lateral decubitus position. Failure in perfusion shifting is a frequent cause of severe hypoxemia during OLV.

will be absorbed, contributing to achieve an adequate surgical field. The oxygenation nadir is usually reached 15 to 20 minutes after the onset of OLV. Thereafter, F_iO_2 can be titrated according to the desired level of peripheral oxygen saturation (SpO_2). In most patients, SpO_2 of 90% to 92% might contribute to avoid negative side effects of high F_iO_2, namely, toxicity with histopathologic changes similar to VILI, ischemia-reperfusion injury, and oxidative stress.[101] However, if clinically relevant hypoxemia develops, F_iO_2 should be kept, or increased, to 100% until a treatable cause can be identified and reverted.

Mechanical Ventilation Mode

During OLV, VCV guarantees that the desired V_T is achieved irrespective of external pressures on the ventilated lung. In turn, PCV guarantees that the driving pressure is constant, and peak pressure is lower than during VCV. When switching from TLV to OLV, the pressure-control modus might be useful to avoid overdistension because of inadvertently high V_T. However, if the respiratory system compliance is reduced, hypoventilation can occur. In a relatively small clinical trial, the ventilation mode termed "pressure-control with volume guaranty" (PC-VC) reduced airway pressures in patients undergoing thoracotomy, kept V_T approximately constant, and decreased the inflammatory response and lung injury compared with volume-controlled ventilation.[102]

Evidence from large trials is missing to allow recommendations regarding a particular mechanical ventilation mode for OLV. In our experience, PCV can be particularly useful when leakage in the respiratory system is present, for example, when fiberscopes are used because the inspiratory flow is increased and partially compensates the escape of gas. Also PCV might be valuable when the pressure in the airways cannot exceed a given value. PCV is valuable during the use of endobronchial blockers in which the peak pressure should ideally maintain under 30 mm H_2O, or during procedures with carbon dioxide insufflation to avoid excessive peak airway pressure. However, PCV, and even PC-VC, may allow reduction of V_T over multiple cycles, which can result in atelectasis of the ventilated lung. VCV is less prone to such fluctuations but can lead to higher peak airway pressures if the compliance of the respiratory system is reduced.

Rescue Maneuvers in Case of Hypoxemia

The incidence of hypoxemia during OLV decreased in recent years, but it can be as high as 10%.[103] Usually, hypoxic pulmonary vasoconstriction shifts perfusion from the nonventilated to the ventilated lung, as illustrated in Fig. 20.5, reducing the transpulmonary shunt and preventing severe hypoxemia during OLV (see Chapter 15). Possible predictors are the side of operation with a higher risk for hypoxemia when the left lung is the dependent lung because the right lung is larger than the left lung. In addition, OLV in

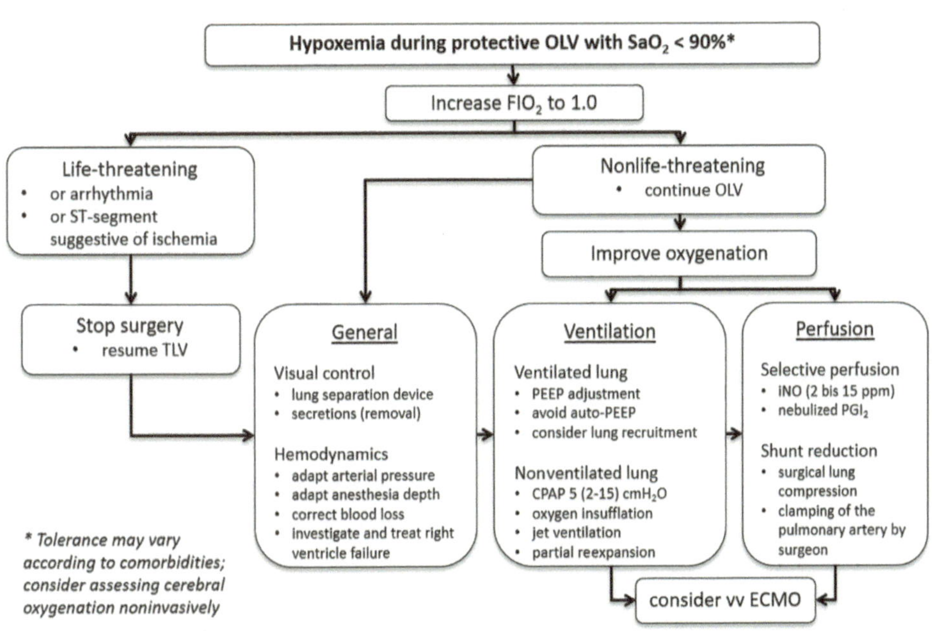

• **Fig. 20.6** Schematic diagram of an algorithm to treat arterial hypoxemia during one-lung ventilation (*OLV*) without abandoning protective ventilation settings. *CPAP*, Continuous positive airway pressure; *DLT*, double lumen tube; *F_iO2*, inspiratory oxygen fraction; *iNO*, inhaled NO; *PEEP*, positive end-expiratory pressure; *PGI_2*, prostacyclin; *SaO2*, arterial partial pressure of oxygen; *TLV*, two-lung ventilation; *vv ECMO*, venous-venous extracorporeal membrane oxygenation. (Modified from Rozé H, Lafargue M, Ouattara A. Case scenario: Management of intraoperative hypoxemia during one-lung ventilation. *Anesthesiology*. 2011 Jan;114(1):167-74.)

the supine position as compared with lateral position will increase the incidence of hypoxemia because of lack of gravity increase in blood flow to the dependent lung. Furthermore, a low arterial partial pressure of oxygen during spontaneous breathing and TLV are predictive of increased risk of hypoxemia during OLV.[104] When severe hypoxemia occurs, protective OLV should not be abandoned, but, instead, the following steps undertaken:

- Increase F_iO_2 to 100%.
- Use visual control (fiberoptic bronchoscopy, endotracheal tube with embedded cameras) to check if the lung isolation device is appropriately placed. Displacement of lung separation devices is not uncommon following changes in patient position and surgical manipulation of the airways.[105]
- Check for occlusion of major bronchi by secretions, mucus plugs, or blood cloth.
- Optimize ventilation (adjust the respiratory rate, PEEP, and consider RM).
- Continuous positive airway pressure if possible, high frequency jet ventilation, O_2 insufflation to the nonventilated lung.
- Optimize perfusion (hypovolemia, increased pulmonary vascular resistance, and auto-PEEP), consider inhaled nitric oxide or extracorporeal membrane oxygenation.

TABLE 20.2 ARISCAT-Score

Parameter	Score
Age (Year)	
≤50	0
51–80	3
>80	16
Preoperative peripheral oxygen saturation (SpO2) %	
≥96	0
91–95	8
≤90	24
Respiratory infection in the last month	
No	0
Yes	17
Preoperative anemia (Hb ≤ 10 g/dL)	
No	0
Yes	11
Surgical incision	
Peripheral	0
Upper abdominal	15
Intrathoracic	24
Duration of surgery (hours)	
>2	0
2–3	16
>3	23
Emergency procedure	
No	8
Yes	0

Hb, Hemoglobin.

Low risk < 24, moderate risk 24–44, high-risk ≥ 45

Modified from Mazo V, Sabate S, Canet J, et al. Prospective external validation of a predictive score for postoperative pulmonary complications. *Anesthesiology.* 2014;121:219–231.

- In some rare cases, if the surgeon has access to the nondependent lung main pulmonary artery, he can temporarily occlude it with a noncrashing clamp.

If the gas exchange despite protective OLV is still inadequate, it might be justifiable resuming TLV at least temporarily. In selected cases, extracorporeal gas exchange could be considered. Fig. 20.6 depicts a possible detailed algorithm for rescue caused by hypoxemia while keeping protective OLV settings, as used in our own department.

The Nonventilated Lung

At the end of surgery, reexpansion of the nonventilated lung is usually necessary. To protect the lung from high pressures, this can be accomplished with gentle sustained inflation at low levels of positive airway pressure of up to 20 cmH_2O for 15 to 30 seconds. This procedure must be carefully conducted to avoid rupture of airways and lung tissue.

Equipment (See Chapter 16)

For lung separation and OLV, either a double-lumen tube or endobronchial blocker can be used. In a metaanalysis, endobronchial blockers were associated with a lower incidence of airway injury and lower severity of airway injury, while double-lumen tubes could be placed quicker and more reliably.[106] Furthermore, when performing OLV, a fiberoptic bronchoscope must be available. A detailed discussion of the methods of lung separation can be found in Chapter 16.

Risks Assessment

The ARISCAT score provides a simple and safe way of preoperative risk stratification of PPCs[37,107] (Table 20.2). Four patient risk factors (low preoperative peripheral oxygen saturation, recent respiratory tract infection, age, and low hemoglobin concentration) and three procedural risk factors (intrathoracic and upper abdominal surgery, duration of surgery, and emergency surgery) are evaluated. According to the calculated score, classification into a low, medium, and high PPC risk can be made. Although the result of large randomized studies[7] remains to be seen, measures to minimize risk should be taken, especially in the high-risk group. These include nicotine withdrawal from 8 weeks before surgery, cough and breathing training, and preoperative therapy optimization in patients with chronic obstructive pulmonary disease (COPD).

Conclusion

OLV is associated with an increased risk for VILI and PPC. Therefore so-called protective OLV settings consisting of low V_T, limited plateau, and driving pressure, as well as appropriate PEEP and low respiratory rate adjusted to the concept of permissive hypercapnia, should be considered. Use of routine RMs is not recommended, but they may be valuable as part of the strategy to revert hypoxemia. In such case, a decremental PEEP trial should follow to preserve the effects. In patients with expiratory flow limitation, most notably those with COPD, V_T may be higher and PEEP lower, while RMs are better avoided. Because of the lack of sound evidence, protective settings must be always critically appraised and adapted to the patient's needs.

References

1. Acute Respiratory Distress Syndrome Network, Brower RG, Matthay MA, et al. Ventilation with lower tidal volumes as compared with traditional tidal volumes for acute lung injury and the acute respiratory distress syndrome. *N Engl J Med.* 2000;342:1301–1308.
2. Serpa Neto A, Cardoso SO, Manetta JA, et al. Association between use of lung-protective ventilation with lower tidal volumes and clinical outcomes among patients without acute respiratory distress syndrome: a meta-analysis. *JAMA.* 2012;308:1651–1659.
3. Young CC, Harris EM, Vacchiano C, et al. Lung-protective ventilation for the surgical patient: international expert panel-based consensus recommendations. *Br J Anaesth.* 2019;123:898–913.
4. Shen Y, Zhong M, Wu W, et al. The impact of tidal volume on pulmonary complications following minimally invasive esophagectomy: a randomized and controlled study. *J Thorac Cardiovasc Surg.* 2013;146:1267–1273; discussion 1273–1264.
5. Yang M, Ahn HJ, Kim K, et al. Does a protective ventilation strategy reduce the risk of pulmonary complications after lung cancer surgery? A randomized controlled trial. *Chest.* 2011;139:530–537.
6. Tusman G, Bohm SH, Sipmann FS, et al. Lung recruitment improves the efficiency of ventilation and gas exchange during one-lung ventilation anesthesia. *Anesth Analg.* 2004;98:1604–1609, table of contents.
7. Kiss T, Wittenstein J, Becker C, et al. Protective ventilation with high versus low positive end-expiratory pressure during one-lung ventilation for thoracic surgery (PROTHOR): study protocol for a randomized controlled trial. *Trials.* 2019; 20:213.
8. Higuita-Castro N, Mihai C, Hansford DJ, et al. Influence of airway wall compliance on epithelial cell injury and adhesion during interfacial flows. *J Appl Physiol.* 2014;117:1231–1242.
9. Mead J, Takishima T, Leith D. Stress distribution in lungs: a model of pulmonary elasticity. *J Appl Physiol.* 1970;28:596–608.
10. Needham DM, Colantuoni E, Mendez-Tellez PA, et al. Lung protective mechanical ventilation and two year survival in patients with acute lung injury: prospective cohort study. *BMJ.* 2012;344:e2124.
11. Hager DN, Krishnan JA, Hayden DL, et al. Tidal volume reduction in patients with acute lung injury when plateau pressures are not high. *Am J Respir Crit Care Med.* 2005;172:1241–1245.

12. Chiumello D, Carlesso E, Cadringher P, et al. Lung stress and strain during mechanical ventilation for acute respiratory distress syndrome. *Am J Respir Crit Care Med.* 2008;178: 346–355.
13. Protti A, Cressoni M, Santini A, et al. Lung stress and strain during mechanical ventilation: any safe threshold? *Am J Respir Crit Care Med.* 2011;183:1354–1362.
14. Davidovich N, Dipaolo BC, Lawrence GG, et al. Cyclic stretch-induced oxidative stress increases pulmonary alveolar epithelial permeability. *Am J Respir Cell Mol Biol.* 2013;49:156–164.
15. Hussein O, Walters B, Stroetz R, et al. Biophysical determinants of alveolar epithelial plasma membrane wounding associated with mechanical ventilation. *Am J Physiol Lung Cell Mol Physiol.* 2013;305:L478–L484.
16. Suki B, Hubmayr R. Epithelial and endothelial damage induced by mechanical ventilation modes. *Curr Opin Crit Care.* 2014;20:17–24.
17. Moriondo A, Pelosi P, Passi A, et al. Proteoglycan fragmentation and respiratory mechanics in mechanically ventilated healthy rats. *J Appl Physiol.* 2007;103:747–756.
18. Moriondo A, Marcozzi C, Bianchin F, et al. Impact of respiratory pattern on lung mechanics and interstitial proteoglycans in spontaneously breathing anaesthetized healthy rats. *Acta Physiol* (Oxf). 2011;203:331–341.
19. Pelosi P, Rocco PR. Effects of mechanical ventilation on the extracellular matrix. *Intensive Care Med.* 2008;34:631–639.
20. Negrini D, Passi A, Moriondo A. The role of proteoglycans in pulmonary edema development. *Intensive Care Med.* 2008;34: 610–618.
21. Moriondo A, Marcozzi C, Bianchin F, et al. Impact of mechanical ventilation and fluid load on pulmonary glycosaminoglycans. *Respir Physiol Neurobiol.* 2012;181:308–320.
22. Spieth PM, Bluth T, Gama De Abreu M, et al. Mechanotransduction in the lungs. *Minerva Anestesiol.* 2014;80:933–941.
23. Rocco PR, Dos Santos C, Pelosi P. Pathophysiology of ventilator-associated lung injury. *Curr Opin Anaesthesiol.* 2012;25:123–130.
24. Uhlig S. Ventilation-induced lung injury and mechanotransduction: stretching it too far? *Am J Physiol Lung Cell Mol Physiol.* 2002;282:L892–L896.
25. Parker JC, Hernandez LA, Longenecker GL, et al. Lung edema caused by high peak inspiratory pressures in dogs. Role of increased microvascular filtration pressure and permeability. *Am Rev Respir Dis.* 1990;142:321–328 1990.
26. West JB, Tsukimoto K, Mathieu-Costello O, et al. Stress failure in pulmonary capillaries. *J Appl Physiol.* 1991;70:1731–1742.
27. Del Maschio A, Zanetti A, Corada M, et al. Polymorphonuclear leukocyte adhesion triggers the disorganization of endothelial cell-to-cell adherens junctions. *J Cell Biol.* 1996; 135:497–510.
28. Cavanaugh KJ Jr, Oswari J, Margulies SS. Role of stretch on tight junction structure in alveolar epithelial cells. *Am J Respir Cell Mol Biol.* 2001;25:584–591.
29. Pecchiari M, Monaco A, Koutsoukou A, et al. Plasma membrane disruptions with different modes of injurious mechanical ventilation in normal rat lungs*. *Crit Care Med.* 2012;40:869–875.
30. D'angelo E, Koutsoukou A, Della Valle P, et al. Cytokine release, small airway injury, and parenchymal damage during mechanical ventilation in normal open-chest rats. *J Appl Physiol.* 2008;104:41–49.
31. Lecuona E, Saldias F, Comellas A, et al. Ventilator-associated lung injury decreases lung ability to clear edema in rats. *Am J Respir Crit Care Med.* 1999;159:603–609.
32. Planes C, Escoubet B, Blot-Chabaud M, et al. Hypoxia down-regulates expression and activity of epithelial sodium channels in rat alveolar epithelial cells. *Am J Respir Cell Mol Biol.* 1997;17:508–518.
33. Bhattacharya J, Matthay MA. Regulation and repair of the alveolar-capillary barrier in acute lung injury. *Annu Rev Physiol.* 2013;75:593–615.
34. Imai Y, Parodo J, Kajikawa O, et al. Injurious mechanical ventilation and end-organ epithelial cell apoptosis and organ dysfunction in an experimental model of acute respiratory distress syndrome. *JAMA.* 2003;289:2104–2112.
35. Canet J, Sabate S, Mazo V, et al. Development and validation of a score to predict postoperative respiratory failure in a multicentre European cohort: a prospective, observational study. *Eur J Anaesth.* 2015;32:458–470.
36. Bluth T, Teichmann R, Kiss T, et al. Protective intraoperative ventilation with higher versus lower levels of positive end-expiratory pressure in obese patients (PROBESE): study protocol for a randomized controlled trial. *Trials.* 2017;18:202.
37. Mazo V, Sabate S, Canet J, et al. Prospective external validation of a predictive score for postoperative pulmonary complications. *Anesthesiology.* 2014;121:219–231.
38. Lachmann B. Open up the lung and keep the lung open. *Intensive Care Med.* 1992;18:319–321.
39. Chu EK, Whitehead T, Slutsky AS. Effects of cyclic opening and closing at low- and high-volume ventilation on bronchoalveolar lavage cytokines. *Crit Care Med.* 2004;32:168–174.
40. Pelosi P, Rocco PRM, Gama De Abreu M. Close down the lungs and keep them resting to minimize ventilator-induced lung injury. *Crit Care.* 2018;22:72.
41. Van Kaam AH, Lachmann RA, Herting E, et al. Reducing atelectasis attenuates bacterial growth and translocation in experimental pneumonia. *Am J Respir Crit Care Med.* 2004;169:1046–1053.
42. Lachmann RA, Van Kaam AH, Haitsma JJ, et al. High positive end-expiratory pressure levels promote bacterial translocation in experimental pneumonia. *Intensive Care Med.* 2007;33:1800–1804.
43. Fanelli V, Mascia L, Puntorieri V, et al. Pulmonary atelectasis during low stretch ventilation: "open lung" versus "lung rest" strategy. *Crit Care Med.* 2009;37:1046–1053.
44. Vaneker M, Halbertsma FJ, Van Egmond J, et al. Mechanical ventilation in healthy mice induces reversible pulmonary and systemic cytokine elevation with preserved alveolar integrity: an in vivo model using clinical relevant ventilation settings. *Anesthesiology.* 2007;107:419–426.
45. Wolthuis EK, Vlaar AP, Choi G, et al. Mechanical ventilation using non-injurious ventilation settings causes lung injury in the absence of pre-existing lung injury in healthy mice. *Crit Care.* 2009;13:R1.
46. Hegeman MA, Hemmes SN, Kuipers MT, et al. The extent of ventilator-induced lung injury in mice partly depends on duration of mechanical ventilation. *Crit Care Res Pract.* 2013;2013:435236.
47. Wellman TJ, Winkler T, Costa EL, et al. Effect of local tidal lung strain on inflammation in normal and lipopolysaccharide-exposed sheep. *Crit Care Med.* 2014;42:e491–e500.
48. Slutsky AS, Ranieri VM. Ventilator-induced lung injury. *N Engl J Med.* 2013;369:2126–2136.

49. Marret E, Cinotti R, Berard L, et al. Protective ventilation during anaesthesia reduces major postoperative complications after lung cancer surgery: a double-blind randomised controlled trial. *Eur J Anaesth*. 2018;35:727–735.
50. Severgnini P, Selmo G, Lanza C, et al. Protective mechanical ventilation during general anesthesia for open abdominal surgery improves postoperative pulmonary function. *Anesthesiology*. 2013;118:1307–1321.
51. Hemmes SN, De Abreu MG, Pelosi P, et al. ESA Clinical Trials Network 2012: LAS VEGAS–Local Assessment of Ventilatory Management During General Anaesthesia for Surgery and Its Effects on Postoperative Pulmonary Complications: a prospective, observational, international, multicentre cohort study. *Eur J Anaesth*. 2013;30:205–207.
52. Schilling T, Kozian A, Huth C, et al. The pulmonary immune effects of mechanical ventilation in patients undergoing thoracic surgery. *Anesth Analg*. 2005;101:957–965, table of contents.
53. El Tahan MR, Pasin L, Marczin N, et al. Impact of low tidal volumes during one-lung ventilation. A meta-analysis of randomized controlled trials. *J Cardiothorac Vasc Anesth*. 2017;31:1767–1773.
54. Blank RS, Colquhoun DA, Durieux ME, et al. Management of one-lung ventilation: impact of tidal volume on complications after thoracic surgery. *Anesthesiology*. 2016;124:1286–1295.
55. Ball L, Robba C, Gama De Abreu M, et al. Lung protection during one-lung ventilation: another piece in the puzzle. *Eur J Anaesth*. 2018;35:724–726.
56. Cressoni M, Gallazzi E, Chiurazzi C, et al. Limits of normality of quantitative thoracic CT analysis. *Crit Care*. 2013;17:R93.
57. Martin DC, Richards GN. Predicted body weight relationships for protective ventilation—unisex proposals from pre-term through to adult. *BMC Pulm Med*. 2017;17:85.
58. Hoftman N, Canales C, Leduc M, et al. Positive end expiratory pressure during one-lung ventilation: selecting ideal patients and ventilator settings with the aim of improving arterial oxygenation. *Ann Card Anaesth*. 2011;14:183–187.
59. Sundar S, Novack V, Jervis K, et al. Influence of low tidal volume ventilation on time to extubation in cardiac surgical patients. *Anesthesiology*. 2011;114:1102–1110.
60. Slinger PD. Optimizing one-lung ventilation: moving beyond tidal volume. *J Cardiothorac Vasc Anesth*. 2018;32:2673–2675.
61. Della Rocca G, Coccia C. Acute lung injury in thoracic surgery. *Curr Opin Anaesthesiol*. 2013;26:40–46.
62. Balanos GM, Talbot NP, Dorrington KL, et al. Human pulmonary vascular response to 4 h of hypercapnia and hypocapnia measured using Doppler echocardiography. *J Appl Physiol*. 2003;94:1543–1551.
63. Lee J, Kim Y, Mun J, et al. Effects of hypercarbia on arterial oxygenation during one-lung ventilation: prospective randomized crossover study. *Korean J Anesthesiol*. 2020;73(6):534–541.
64. Gao W, Liu DD, Li D, et al. Effect of therapeutic hypercapnia on inflammatory responses to one-lung ventilation in lobectomy patients. *Anesthesiology*. 2015;122:1235–1252.
65. Cressoni M, Gotti M, Chiurazzi C, et al. Mechanical power and development of ventilator-induced lung injury. *Anesthesiology*. 2016;124:1100–1108.
66. Huhle R, Serpa Neto A, Schultz MJ, et al. Is mechanical power the final word on ventilator-induced lung injury?—No. *Ann Translat Med*. 2018;6:394.
67. Szegedi LL, Barvais L, Sokolow Y, et al. Intrinsic positive end-expiratory pressure during one-lung ventilation of patients with pulmonary hyperinflation. Influence of low respiratory rate with unchanged minute volume. *Br J Anaesth*. 2002;88:56–60.
68. Viitanen A, Salmenpera M, Heinonen J. Right ventricular response to hypercarbia after cardiac surgery. *Anesthesiology*. 1990;73:393–400.
69. Kontos HA, Raper AJ, Patterson JL. Analysis of vasoactivity of local pH, PCO2 and bicarbonate on pial vessels. *Stroke*. 1977;8:358–360.
70. Anderson RJ, Pluss RG, Pluss WT, et al. Effect of hypoxia and hypercapnic acidosis on renal autoregulation in the dog: role of renal nerves. *Clin Sci* (Lond). 1983;65:533–538.
71. Writing Committee for The PROBESE Collaborative Group of the PROtective VEntilation Network (PROVEnet) for the Clinical Trial Network of the European Society of Anaesthesiology. Effect of intraoperative high positive end-expiratory pressure (PEEP) with recruitment maneuvers vs low PEEP on postoperative pulmonary complications in obese patients: a randomized clinical trial. *JAMA*. 2019;321:2292–2305.
72. The PROVE Network investigators. High versus low positive end-expiratory pressure during general anaesthesia for open abdominal surgery (PROVHILO trial): a multicentre randomised controlled trial. *Lancet*. 2014;384:495–503.
73. PNI I, Belda J, Ferrando C, et al. The effects of an open-lung approach during one-lung ventilation on postoperative pulmonary complications and driving pressure: a descriptive, multicenter national study. *J Cardiothorac Vasc Anesth*. 2018;32:2665–2672.
74. Park M, Ahn HJ, Kim JA, et al. Driving pressure during thoracic surgery: a randomized clinical trial. *Anesthesiology*. 2019;130:385–393.
75. Liu J, Meng Z, Lv R, et al. Effect of intraoperative lung-protective mechanical ventilation on pulmonary oxygenation function and postoperative pulmonary complications after laparoscopic radical gastrectomy. *BLMBR*. 2019;52:e8523.
76. Ferrando C, Soro M, Unzueta C, et al. Individualised perioperative open-lung approach versus standard protective ventilation in abdominal surgery (iPROVE): a randomised controlled trial. *Lancet Respir Med*. 2018;6:193–203.
77. Ferrando C, Mugarra A, Gutierrez A, et al. Setting individualized positive end-expiratory pressure level with a positive end-expiratory pressure decrement trial after a recruitment maneuver improves oxygenation and lung mechanics during one-lung ventilation. *Anesth Analg*. 2014;118:657–665.
78. Choi YS, Bae MK, Kim SH, et al. Effects of alveolar recruitment and positive end-expiratory pressure on oxygenation during one-lung ventilation in the supine position. *Yonsei Med J*. 2015;56:1421–1427.
79. Cinnella G, Grasso S, Natale C, et al. Physiological effects of a lung-recruiting strategy applied during one-lung ventilation. *Acta Anaesthesiol Scand*. 2008;52:766–775.
80. Madke GR, Forgiarini LA Jr, Grun G, et al. Effect of positive end-expiratory pressure after porcine unilateral left lung transplant. *Exp Clin Transplant*. 2013;11:50–55.
81. Slinger PD, Hickey DR. The interaction between applied peep and auto-peep during one-lung ventilation. *J Cardiothorac Vasc Anesth*. 1998;12:133–136.
82. Bardoczky GI, D'hollander AA, Cappello M, et al. Interrupted expiratory flow on automatically constructed flow-volume curves may determine the presence of intrinsic positive end-expiratory pressure during one-lung ventilation. *Anesth Analg*. 1998;86:880–884.

83. Hess DR. Respiratory mechanics in mechanically ventilated patients. *Respir Care.* 2014;59:1773–1794.
84. Amato MB, Meade MO, Slutsky AS, et al. Driving pressure and survival in the acute respiratory distress syndrome. *N Engl J Med.* 2015;372:747–755.
85. Neto AS, Hemmes SN, Barbas CS, et al. Association between driving pressure and development of postoperative pulmonary complications in patients undergoing mechanical ventilation for general anaesthesia: a meta-analysis of individual patient data. *Lancet Respir Med.* 2016;4:272–280.
86. Rauseo M, Mirabella L, Grasso S, et al. Peep titration based on the open lung approach during one lung ventilation in thoracic surgery: a physiological study. *BMC Anesthesiol.* 2018;18:156 2018.
87. Lee SM, Kim WH, Ahn HJ, et al. The effects of prolonged inspiratory time during one-lung ventilation: a randomised controlled trial. *Anaesthesia.* 2013;68:908–916.
88. Georgopoulos D, Giannouli E, Patakas D. Effects of extrinsic positive end-expiratory pressure on mechanically ventilated patients with chronic obstructive pulmonary disease and dynamic hyperinflation. *Intensive Care Med.* 1993;19:197–203.
89. Kurahashi K, Ohtsuka M, Usuda Y. Central airway occlusion underestimates intrinsic positive end-expiratory pressure: a numerical and physical simulation. *Exp Lung Res.* 2009;35:756–769.
90. Samary CS, Silva PL, Gama De Abreu M, et al. Ventilator-induced lung injury: power to the mechanical power. *Anesthesiology.* 2016;125:1070–1071.
91. Putensen C, Theuerkauf N, Zinserling J, et al. Meta-analysis: ventilation strategies and outcomes of the acute respiratory distress syndrome and acute lung injury. *Ann Intern Med.* 2009;151:566–576.
92. Briel M, Meade M, Mercat A, et al. Higher vs lower positive end-expiratory pressure in patients with acute lung injury and acute respiratory distress syndrome: systematic review and meta-analysis. *JAMA.* 2010;303:865–873.
93. Rich PB, Douillet CD, Hurd H, et al. Effect of ventilatory rate on airway cytokine levels and lung injury. *J Surg Res.* 2003;113:139–145.
94. Maeda Y, Fujino Y, Uchiyama A, et al. Effects of peak inspiratory flow on development of ventilator-induced lung injury in rabbits. *Anesthesiology.* 2004;101:722–728.
95. Schumann S, Goebel U, Haberstroh J, et al. Determination of respiratory system mechanics during inspiration and expiration by FLow-controlled EXpiration (FLEX): a pilot study in anesthetized pigs. *Minerva Anestesiol.* 2014;80:19–28.
96. Spieth PM, Silva PL, Garcia CS, et al. Modulation of stress versus time product during mechanical ventilation influences inflammation as well as alveolar epithelial and endothelial response in rats. *Anesthesiology.* 2015;122:106–116.
97. Gattinoni L, Tonetti T, Cressoni M, et al. Ventilator-related causes of lung injury: the mechanical power. *Intensive Care Med.* 2016;42:1567–1575.
98. Santos RS, Maia LA, Oliveira MV, et al. Biologic impact of mechanical power at high and low tidal volumes in experimental mild acute respiratory distress syndrome. *Anesthesiology.* 2018;128:1193–1206.
99. Serpa Neto A, Deliberato RO, Johnson AEW, et al. Mechanical power of ventilation is associated with mortality in critically ill patients: an analysis of patients in two observational cohorts. *Intensive Care Med.* 2018;44:1914–1922.
100. Collino F, Rapetti F, Vasques F, et al. Positive end-expiratory pressure and mechanical power. *Anesthesiology.* 2019;130:119–130.
101. Jordan S, Mitchell JA, Quinlan GJ, et al. The pathogenesis of lung injury following pulmonary resection. *Eur Respir J.* 2000;15:790–799.
102. Yao W, Yang M, Cheng Q, et al. Effect of pressure-controlled ventilation-volume guaranteed on one-lung ventilation in elderly patients undergoing thoracotomy. *Med Sci Monitor.* 2020;26:e921417.
103. Liu TJ, Shih MS, Lee WL, et al. Hypoxemia during one-lung ventilation for robot-assisted coronary artery bypass graft surgery. *Annals Thorac Surg.* 2013;96:127–132.
104. Karzai W, Schwarzkopf K. Hypoxemia during one-lung ventilation: prediction, prevention, and treatment. *Anesthesiology.* 2009;110:1402–1411.
105. Brodsky JB, Lemmens HJ. Left double-lumen tubes: clinical experience with 1,170 patients. *J Cardiothorac Vasc Anesth.* 2003;17:289–298.
106. Clayton-Smith A, Bennett K, Alston RP, et al. A comparison of the efficacy and adverse effects of double-lumen endobronchial tubes and bronchial blockers in thoracic surgery: a systematic review and meta-analysis of randomized controlled trials. *J Cardiothorac Vasc Anesth.* 2015;29:955–966.
107. Canet J, Gallart L, Gomar C, et al. Prediction of postoperative pulmonary complications in a population-based surgical cohort. *Anesthesiology.* 2010;113:1338–1350.

21

Fluid Management During Lung Resection

FELICE EUGENIO AGRÒ, CHIARA PILIEGO

Introduction

Managing fluid administration during lung resection by the anesthesiologist is very similar to a tightrope walker trying to balance the risk of acute lung injury (ALI) and that of acute kidney injury (AKI); there is a narrow margin of safety between fluid overload and hypovolemia, two conditions that may impair lung and renal function, respectively.

Maintaining fluid and electrolyte homeostasis represents a crucial challenge because of the profound impact on perioperative morbidity and mortality. The evolution in surgical techniques lead to reduction of in-hospital mortality rates to less than 2% for lobectomies and less than 6% for pneumonectomies.[1,2] The length of hospital stay is also shorter, and with cumulative experience, procedural complications are less frequent. The main causes of mortality are not from surgical or cardiac complications, but rather being replaced by pulmonary pathology, such as pneumonia, empyema, and ALI.[3]

Pulmonary complications are caused by a combination of multiple factors acting together and among them, the volume of intravenous fluids administered intraoperatively plays an important role.[4]

The aim of this chapter is to provide a guide for fluid management during lung resection, answering some question, yet raising some others.

From Postpneumonectomy Pulmonary Edema to Acute Lung Injury

Postpneumonectomy pulmonary edema (PPPE) was first reported by Zeldin, who described the correlation between the amount of perioperative fluid, over 37 mL/kg intraoperatively and for the first 24 hours after surgery, and pulmonary complications.[5]

This article laid the foundations for establishing an association between fluid overload and development of lung injury but has some issues to consider. First, the edema affected only 10 patients, which makes the sample size low for current standards. Most of the PPPE occurred in patients who had right pneumonectomies, which has a larger parenchymal tissue. These pulmonary complications can be present not only in pneumonectomies, but also after less extensive resections or even after thoracotomies without resections.[6]

However, after Zeldin, several investigators attempted to explore the correlation between fluid administration and lung outcome.[7–10]

Licker et al.[11] in a multivariate analysis, described two independent risk factors for ALI: the extent of lung resection (pneumonectomy was associated to the highest risk) and fluid overload (meaning 9.1 mL/kg/h intraoperatively and 1 mL/kg/h for the first 24 hours). This study however, did not provide for protective lung ventilation (PLV): a latter comparison with a group of patients with adoption of PLV showed a pronounced decrease in the incidence of ALI/acute respiratory distress syndrome (ARDS), despite no change in fluid administration. This finding suggests the importance of ventilation strategy in lung outcomes. However, some studies report the presence of lung injury even when applying a "very restrictive ventilatory strategy."[12]

Postoperative lung injury usually occurs 1 to 4 days after surgery, and presents with a low pulmonary capillary wedge pressure, which raises questions if the fluid overload is the sole accountable factor. Certainly, this measure confirms that this type of edema has not its origin from heart failure, but—au contraire—it challenges the hypothesis of hypervolemia. In addition, the edema fluid has high concentrations of proteins.[13] This type of pulmonary edema seems to be the result of an increase in pulmonary capillary permeability, associated with a rise in plasma protein content; it suggests that this lung injury could occur despite normovolemia, and most likely is being just exacerbated by fluid overload.

The clinical pattern formerly known as PPPE shares many clinical and histologic features with ARDS. It is unclear which studies are referring to ALI or postoperative lung injury rather than PPPE.

TABLE 21.1 Risk, Injury, Failure, Loss, End-Stage Renal Disease Criteria of Acute Kidney Injury

Stage	Glomerular Filtration Rate	Urinary Output
Risk	↑SCr × 1.5 or ↓GFR >25%	<0.5 mL/kg/h for 6 hours
Injury	↑SCr × 2 or ↓GFR >50%	<0.5 mL/kg/h for 12 hours
Failure	↑SCr × 3 or ↓GFR >75% or SCr 4 mg/dL with acute rise of 0.5	<0.3 mL/kg/h for 24 hours or anuria >12 hours
Loss	Complete loss of kidney function for > 4 weeks	
End-stage	End-stage kidney disease >3 months	

GFR, Glomerular filtration rate; *SCr*, serum creatinine.

Definitions and Epidemiology

Postthoracotomy Acute Lung Injury

The definition of ALI and ARDS, according to the American-European Consensus Conference on ARDS,[14] consists of a syndrome of inflammation and increased permeability with:

- **Acute onset**
- **Bilateral infiltrates on chest radiograph**
- **Hypoxemia (partial pressure of arterial oxygen [PaO2] ≤300 mm Hg for ALI and PaO2 ≤200 for ARDS), despite positive end-expiratory pressure**
- **No evidence of left atrial hypertension or pulmonary capillary occlusion pressure below 18 mm Hg**

This definition can be applied to postthoracotomy ALI, even if there is a broad spectrum of clinical pictures described in patients with postthoracotomy lung injury.[15]

Lung injury following lung resection occurs in 2.5% of all lung resections, with increased incidence of 7.9% after pneumonectomy.[16]

Acute Kidney Insufficiency

Historically, the incidence of kidney damage in thoracic surgery was reported to be quite low. The Society of Thoracic Surgeons database cited an overall incidence of 1.4%.[2] These data pertained only to patients who required renal suppurative replacement therapy, and a subsequent assessment using standardized criteria reported a much higher incidence.

In 2002, the Acute Dialysis Quality Initiative Group presented a classification system for AKI named **RIFLE** (risk, injury, failure, loss, and end-stage renal disease), based on increased serum creatinine (SCr) associated with a decrease in glomerular filtration rate (GFR) and urinary output.[17] A more recent system was reported, called **AKIN** (Acute Kidney Injury Network) criteria:[18] this system is considering an absolute increase in SCr of 0.3 mg/dL as a diagnostic criteria in identifying stage 1 disease. These criteria attracted much criticism by clinicians, questioning the clinical relevance of a minimal increase in SCr. However, Basile et al.[19] showed worse outcomes in patients with postoperative AKI, even with slight increases of SCr and with complete restoration of kidney function; postthoracotomy AKI, specifically, was associated with a hazard ratio of 1.6 in terms of long-term survival.

Studies using the AKIN criteria report a higher incidence of kidney injury. Ishikawa et al. reported an incidence of renal impairment in 5.9% of thoracic surgical patients,[20] and Hobson reached 33% of incidence in a high-risk group.[21]

The classification systems are summarized in Tables 21.1 and 21.2.

Ventilator-Induced Lung Injury

Ventilation can cause a broad spectrum of local and systemic pathophysiologic changes, in particular in patients requiring lung surgery and one-lung ventilation (OLV), defined as ventilator-induced lung injury (VILI). The causes of these adverse effects are barotrauma (direct consequence of high pressure on the lung), volutrauma (effect of excessive distension of the lung), atelectotrauma (cyclic opening and closing of alveoli) and biotrauma (inflammatory cascades triggered by cytokines release).[22,23]

TABLE 21.2 Acute Kidney Injury Network Criteria of Acute Kidney Injury

Stage	Creatinine	Urinary Output
I	↑SCr × 1.5–2 or ↑SCr 0.3 mg/dL	<0.5 mL/kg/h for 6 hours
II	↑SCr × 2–3	<0.5 mL/kg/h for 12 hours
III	↑SCr × 3 or ↓GFR >75% or SCr 4 mg/dL with acute rise of 0.5 or any dialysis	<0.3 mL/kg/h for 24 hours or anuria >12 hours

GFR, Glomerular filtration rate; *SCr*, serum creatinine.

Transfusion-Related to Acute Lung Injury

Transfusion-related to acute lung injury (TRALI) diagnosis was classically based upon development of a new ALI within 6 hours of transfusion, not ascribable to another ALI risk factor.[24]

Recently, an updated TRALI definition/classification scheme has been published with several modifications. Among them is the distinction between two types of TRALI that should be noted TRALI type I applies to patients without an ARDS risk factor, TRALI type II to cases with an ARDS risk factor or even with mild preexisting ARDS. At first glance, one should immediately notice that this second type is in contrast with the old definition.

This new diagnostic criteria for TRALI is listed in Box 21.1.[25]

Physiopathology

Acute Lung Injury

Understanding the two main mechanisms that play a crucial role in the development of pulmonary edema following thoracic surgery, which are an increase in pulmonary capillary hydrostatic pressure and/or an increase in capillary permeability, is essential to improve patient outcomes.

Starling Forces

In 1896, Ernest Starling working on an animal model, stated that the mechanism of fluid exchange (a combination of filtration and reabsorption between capillaries and interstitial space) was found in differences between hydrostatic and osmotic pressures, as well as in the capillary wall structure.[26]

This observation led to the formulation of Starling equation as follows:

$$J_v/A = L_p\,[(P_c - P_i) - \sigma\,(\pi_c - \pi_i)]$$

Likewise J_v / A is the rate of fluid exchange per unit area of the vessel, Lp is the permeability of the vessel wall, $(P_c - P_i)$ and $(\pi_c - \pi_i)$ with a difference between capillary and interstitial fluid in terms of hydrostatic and osmotic pressure, and σ is the reflection coefficient of the vessel wall to plasma proteins.

This equation depicts fluid exchange as a balance between opposing forces with capillary hydrostatic pressure representing the filtration force and the capillary osmotic pressure representing the reabsorption force; the larger is the difference, the greater is the exchange (Fig. 21.1).

Hydrostatic Edema

Pulmonary circulation is endowed with the ability to respond to significant variations in cardiac output without raising its capillary pressure, thanks to capillary recruitment mechanisms.[27] This system maintains stable pulmonary pressure even if the left atrial pressure is doubled and pulmonary capillary filtration remains unvaried.[28] Only when adaptive mechanisms are overcome, fluids start to collect in the interstitium. Because of the low compliance of this compartment and owing to the role of lymphatic drainage, there is an initial limitation to the accumulation of interstitial fluid. This protection cannot last long, because of fragmentation of the proteoglycan network of the interstitial matrix.[29] The last protective mechanism is represented by the alveolar epithelium clearance of alveolar fluid is carried on through the epithelial sodium channels, stimulated by beta-adrenergic agonists[30] (which are gaining attention as therapeutic agents in this field) and inhibited by endothelin-1.[31]

Revised Starling and Role of Endothelial Glycocalyx Layer

The Starling equation has some limitations different studies described deviations from it, both in vitro and in vivo[32] (Fig. 21.2).

• BOX 21.1 New Consensus Transfusion-Related to Acute Lung Injury Definition

TRALI type I: Patients who have no risk factors for ARDS and meet the following criteria

- Clinical features:
  - Acute onset
  - Hypoxemia (PaO2/FiO2 <300 or SpO2 <90% on room air)
  - Clear evidence of bilateral pulmonary edema on imaging
  - No evidence of LAH or, if LAH is present, it is not main contributor to hypoxemia
- Onset during or within 6 hours of transfusion
- No temporal relationship to an alternative risk factor for ARDS

TRALI type II: Patients who have risk factors for ARDS (but who have not been diagnosed with ARDS) or who have preexisting mild ARDS (PaO2/FiO2 of 200–300), but whose respiratory status deteriorates and is judged to be caused by transfusion based.

- Findings as described in categories a and b of TRALI type I, and
- Stable respiratory status in the 12 h before transfusion

ARDS, Acute respiratory distress syndrome; *FiO2*, fraction of inspired oxygen; *LAH*, left atrial hypertension; *PaO2*, partial pressure of arterial oxygen; *TRALI*, transfusion related acute lung injury.

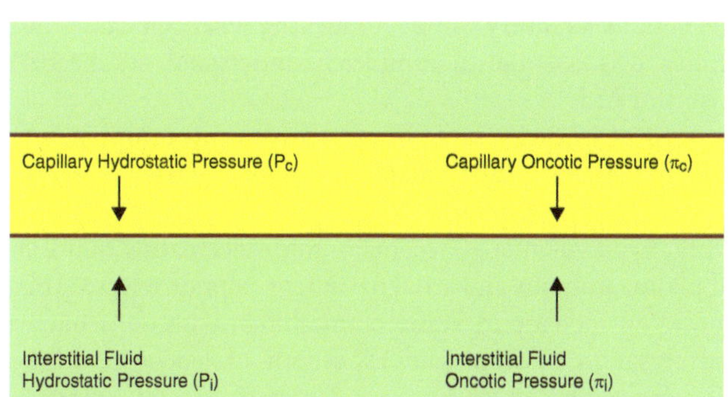

• Fig. 21.1 Starling forces across the capillary wall.

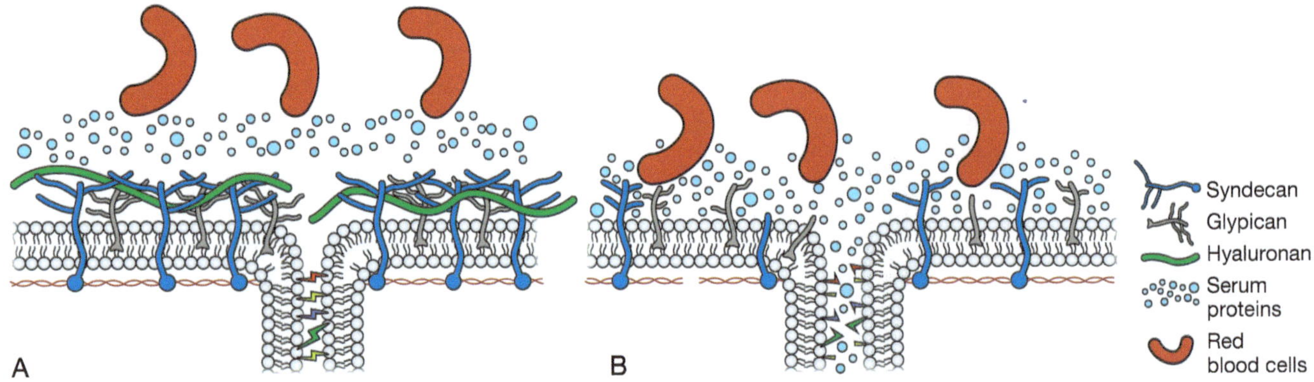

• **Fig. 21.2** Transcapillary fluid flux: classic Starling relationship versus active mechanotransduction. (**A**) Classic Starling principle (*black line*) predicts a linear relationship between capillary pressure (cm H_2O) and transcapillary fluid flux (µm/s). (**B**) Active endothelial mechanotransduction (*maroon line*), capillary hydrostatic pressure activates signaling pathways that increase endothelial permeability resulting in nonlinear dynamics and a higher water flux than would be predicted by the summation of net Starling forces. (From Collins SR, Blank RS, Deatherage LS, Dull RO. The endothelial glycocalyx. *Anesth Analg*. 2013;117:664–674.)

These studies focused on the role of non-Starling mechanisms of barrier regulation, which involve the endothelium and more specifically, the endothelial glycocalyx layer (EGL).[33]

Fluids cross capillary endothelium through breaks in tight junctions, vesicles and leaky junctions, allowing the transport of molecules of various dimensions.

EGL is a layer of proteoglycans and glycoprotein bound to the membrane, covering the luminal surface of vascular endothelium, with function of molecular barrier. It is a complex mesh of glycosaminoglycans and proteins, which filters circulating cells and macromolecules, so that they cannot enter the interstitium. The composition and dimensions of the glycocalyx fluctuate as it continuously replaces material sheared by flowing plasma.[34]

This brings us to the so-called revised Starling equation, which takes the EGL role in capillary fluid dynamics in considerations; the role it plays is carried out in two different functions. First, it represents a strainer for plasmatic proteins, altering the balance in oncotic pressure between plasma and interstitium as predicted by the traditional Starling's equation.[35] Secondly, it responds to fluid shear stress as a mechanosensory, eliciting an increase in capillary permeability in response to a raised capillary blood flow.[36]

It is easy to understand how important this structure is in maintaining fluid homeostasis, and, consequently, how deleterious its injury can be; to identify what can cause this injury, it is essential to completely understand the mechanisms of ALI.

Loss of integrity in EGL can derive from multiple factors, for instance, inflammatory cytokines release,[37] surgical trauma, and ischemia-reperfusion injury.[38] In this framework, hypervolemia plays a major role exacerbating dilution of plasma proteins and atrial natriuretic peptide release. This causes an increase in vessel permeability, with consequent extravasation of fluid and exposition of leucocyte adhesion molecules (which fosters inflammation), and triggers a vicious cycle, inevitably leading to ALI.[39]

Some colloids do appear to be markedly superior as resuscitation fluids expansion because they preserve the glycocalyx. In hemorrhagic shock, for example, resuscitation with higher ratios of plasma seems to result in lower mortality than crystalloid, despite there being seemingly little advantage in terms of preservation of coagulation factors. The explanation may lie not with the Starling equation but rather that certain colloids act to preserve the endothelial glycocalyx.

Risk Factors for Acute Lung Injury and Multiple-Hit Hypothesis

Multiple risk factors seem to be involved in this clinical pattern development and are summarized in Box 21.2.

Rather than a single risk factor being responsible for ALI, it is likely that a combination of multiple-hit series of damages harms the alveolar epithelial and capillary endothelium, as well as extracellular matrix.[40]

In ARDS, the multiple-hit hypothesis presents several pathophysiologic injuries, which may not cause lung damage when presented separately, but, when collected, result in the clinical syndrome of ALI or ARDS. In postthoracotomy ALI, the "first hit" is represented by an activation

• BOX 21.2 Risk Factors for Postthoracotomy Acute Lung Injury

Preoperative severe pulmonary disfunction
Neoadjuvant chemotherapy
Chronic alcohol consumption
Pneumonectomy or extended lung resection
Suboptimal lymphatic drainage
Ventilatory trauma
Fluid overload transfusion
Aspiration
Infection
Oxidative stress
Ischemia-reperfusion damage because of one-lung ventilation

of the systemic inflammatory response (because of surgical trauma, manipulation, or atelectasis).[41] Among the possible "second hits" we can find all the risk factors described before, which aggravates the injury and results in increasing lung insult.

The Role of Fluid Overload

Alam et al. conducted a retrospective case-control study of consecutive patients undergoing resection for lung cancer. The severity of lung injury was defined using the American European Consensus Conference on ARDS. Patients with lung injury were compared with matched control patients, based on age, sex, and extent of resection, for examination of a priori defined risk factors. Some 1428 patients underwent lung cancer resection. Postoperative lung injury occurred in 76 (5.3%) cases, 44 (3.1%) of which met criteria for ARDS. After univariate and multivariate analysis, increasing perioperative fluid administration and decreasing postoperative predicted lung function were significant risk factors for the development of lung injury. The overall mortality for patients with lung injury was 25%, compared with 2.6% for the control group. They concluded that the odds ratio of developing ALI after lung resection of 1.17 for every 500 mL increase in perioperative fluid administration.[42]

Several studies and meta analyses demonstrated that fluid overload is constantly related to postoperative lung injury; this led to the adoption of restrictive fluid management. On the other hand, recent literature encourage an optimal strategy for fluid management, rather than towards a restrictive one.

Excessive fluid administrations are not only responsible for postthoracotomy ALI, they is important anesthetic- and surgery-related risk factors. With fluids "we can make the lung injury worse, but we do not cause it."[43]

Acute Kidney Injury

As is the case for lung, the kidney is insulted by a multifactorial process in this clinical setting.

It is well known that anesthetic drugs generally impair renal function, decreasing GFR, urinary output, and sodium excretion,[44] and that surgery may sometimes unmask latent kidney disease often underlying, hypertension-, diabetes- or atherosclerosis-related.

Thoracic surgery triggers a systemic inflammatory response that may result in kidney injury.

Hypervolemia as well as hypovolemia may be related to the appearance of AKI. Hypervolemia increases the kidney workload to maintain fluid clearance. Hobson et al. investigated the incidence of AKI after thoracic surgery, and described its association with larger amounts of crystalloid administration.[21] However, patients who received higher volumes had longer operative times, and it is unclear which factor caused the worsening of kidney function.

On the other hand, hypotension because of hypovolemia causes decreased renal perfusion, which when associated with the surgery-related inflammatory state, may promote the development of AKI.[45,46]

Ventilator-Induced Lung Injury

The role of mechanical ventilation worsening capillary and (subsequently) lung damage has to be briefly presented.

Gattinoni et al.[47] demonstrated the role of high tidal volumes used during mechanical ventilation of healthy lungs. High tidal volumes, indeed, cause barotraumas, stress ruptures because of the excessive stretching of the alveolar maximal physiologic strain is overtaken, beyond total lung capacity.

The tidal volume ventilation of a patient with ARDS can causes stress rupture and should be reduced to protect the lung. This consideration represents the foundation for the concept of "baby lung", which exposes lungs to a greater risk for VILI.

This concept originates from the analysis of computed tomography lung scans of adult patients with severe ARDS: the images showed an amount of aerated lung of only 200 to 500 g, that corresponds to the lung tissue of a 6-year-old child.[48]

Thus OLV has even more adverse effects.[49] It has been demonstrated that by applying two-lung ventilation tidal volume to a single lung ventilation, the peak inspiratory pressure will rise to about 55% and plateau pressure increases to 42%. Peak inspiratory pressure is dependent on tidal volume, inspiratory time, endotracheal size, and presence or absence of bronchospasm. It does not represent the distending pressure transmitted to the alveoli, meaning it is not necessarily the actual cause of alveolar trauma. Plateau pressure elevation, on the other hand, is the real culprit of the lung damage, reflecting the actual distention pressure of the alveoli. No threshold has been identified to be actually safe. Plateau pressure is inherently related to lung volume; analyzing the physiopathology of VILI, this is an important consideration because it helps to understand that barotrauma and volutrauma proceed at the same pace (or, better that increase of the plateau pressure proceeds at the same pace to create lung distension).

Stress strain inducing deformation causes rapid lipid transport to the plasma membrane, to increase the surface area, prevent membrane disruption and repair the damaged cells.[50] When these protective mechanisms are overtaken, though, cells are detached from the basement membrane, cell junctions in epithelium and endothelium are smashed losing the tight junction between the cells, and the formation of intracapillary blebs, alveolar, will initiate the formation of interstitial edema.[51]

Protective ventilation strategies are applied in an attempt to protect the lung from barotrauma, limiting plateau pressures, as well as from volutrauma, avoiding overdistension.

In ARDS, both increased weight of the edematous lung and surfactant dysfunction are involved in regional atelectasis; atelectatic lung units are still recruitable, so that during ventilation, cyclic opening and collapse of these units occur.[52] Recruitment at the interface air-collapsed airway

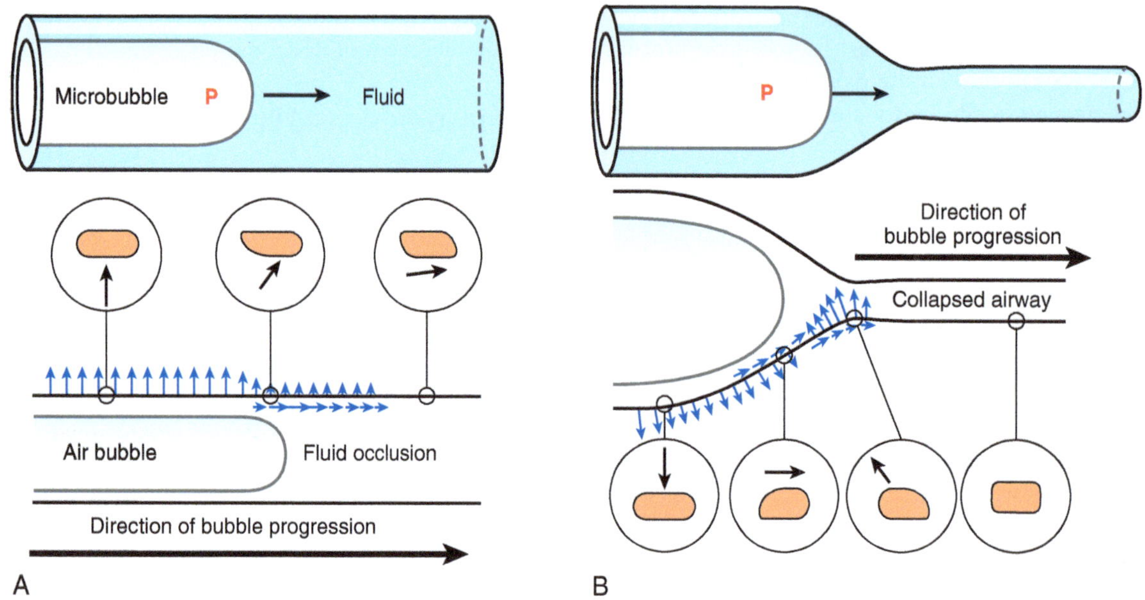

• **Fig. 21.3** (A) Airway reopening in a noncollapsed fluid-filled airway. (B) Collapsed airway.

causes mechanical injuries to the atelectasis alveoli. The flooded alveoli that are responsible for interfacial stress, disrupting the plasma membrane-cytoskeleton adhesion, results in formation and destruction of foam bubbles at the gas-liquid interface. Although the exact nature of airway/alveolar "closure" might include both compliant collapse and/or the flooding of noncollapsed airways, in either case, airway "reopening" involves the movement of an air-liquid interface or a microbubble of air that displaces the surrounding fluid. As shown schematically (in Fig. 21.3) these "microbubble" flows will result in the application of a complex, nonuniform, and transient hydrodynamic stress field on the epithelial cell lining the airway/alveolar walls.[53,54]

Microbubble flows exert complex fluid mechanical forces on the airway wall. The schematic diagrams of airway reopening in a noncollapsed fluid-filled airway forces, shown schematically as arrows, include normal pressure and tangential shear stresses, as well as temporal and spatial gradients in these stresses. Hypothetical cell deformations because of these stresses at different locations are shown schematically in the circular inserts.[53]

Repetitive inflation/deflation cycles of lung units are therefore involved in the multifactorial genesis of perioperative ALI.

Lastly, in response to mechanical lung injury, a systemic biologic cascade is triggered, releasing proinflammatory and proinjurious cytokines. This response may promote damage in lung regions even when not initially influenced by mechanical insult, and also spread extrapulmonary organ injury, predisposing to multiorgan failure.[55]

This pathway, named biotrauma, may not seem so significant. It should be remembered, though, that the epithelial surface area of one single adult lung is about 60 to 80 square meters, so that the release of proinjurious mediators is amplified.[56] In addition, the blood flow through the pulmonary circulation is substantial, so that any mediator produced by the lung is rapidly transported with the blood stream throughout the whole body.

In conclusion, referring to the multiple hit hypothesis, VILI (promoted by the combination of barotrauma, volutrauma, atelectotrauma, and biotrauma) represents a first hit. In thoracic surgery in particular, OLV and surgical manipulation should be considered as the second hit, and the third hit may result from reexpansion/reperfusion lung injury.[57]

Transfusion-Related to Acute Lung Injury

During the initial stages of TRALI, neutrophils and endothelial cells of the pulmonary capillary come into contact and bond, establishing a firm cell adhesion; this causes the retention of neutrophils, which induces endothelial damage and capillary leakage. This first insult allows the flux of proteinaceous fluid from the vessels to the air spaces.[58]

Immune Transfusion-Related to Acute Lung Injury

The antibodies involved in TRALI are mostly directed against human leukocyte antigen (HLA) and human neutrophilic alloantigen (HNA).

Multiple mechanisms of neutrophil activation have been proposed: antibodies against HLA and HNA could bind to neutrophil receptors and trigger their activation, or antibodies from donors could bind HLA class II antigens in monocytes, causing the release of cytokines, which could activate primed neutrophils.[59]

Transfusion-Related to Acute Lung Injury Not Immune or of Two Events

In this other situation, the first event is an injury that activates the pulmonary endothelium. This activation triggers the recruitment and adherence of neutrophils to endothelial

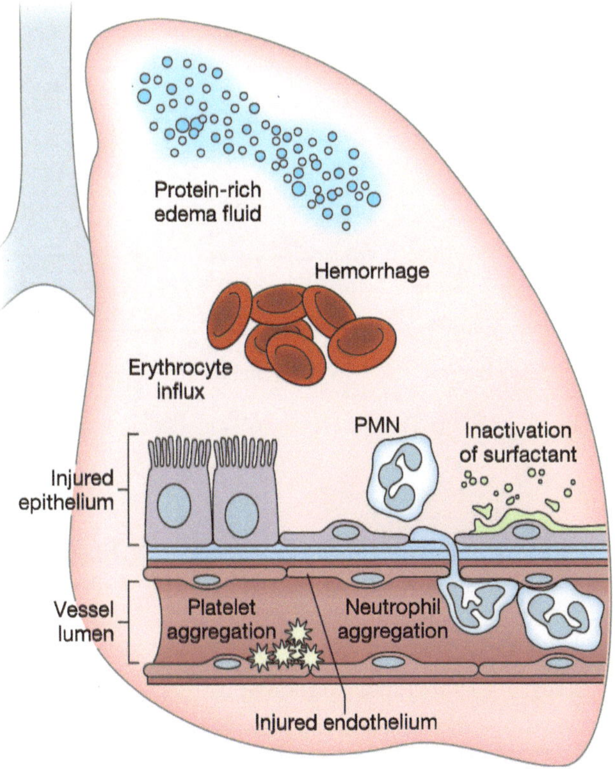

• **Fig. 21.4** Pathogenesis of transfusion-related to acute lung injury. *PMN*, Polymorphonuclear leukocytes. (From IMMUCOR 2015. www.immucor.com)

cells. The **first event** may be represented by sepsis, trauma, surgery, massive transfusion, or general anesthesia.

The **second event** is caused by some trigger that activates the neutrophils, causing the release of cytotoxic factors and endothelial damage. Capillary damage will then occur, because of the exposure of biologically active agents.[58]

Before TRALI, one could witness an increase in levels of interleukin (IL)-8, IL-6, and alpha1-antitrypsin elastase complex: IL-8, released by endothelial cells, promotes neutrophil attraction to the lung compartment. Adherence to endothelial cells, mediated by beta2-integrins, L-selectin, E-selectin, P-selectin, and intracellular adhesion molecules, is the first event in this genetic pathway. Factors responsible for host neutrophil activation, for the second event, can be antibodies, or biologic response modifiers, such as bioactive lipids, lysophosphatidylcholines, ceramides, and soluble CD40 ligand (Fig. 21.4).

Fluid Administration Strategies

As mentioned previously, good clinical practice does not require simple restriction in fluid administration, but rather an "optimal" fluid balance management. This definition may seem reasonable, but is vague and not quite helpful in clinical practice.

Liberal Versus Restrictive

Several studies compared liberal and restrictive strategies, with many limitations.[60]

The majority of them were retrospective, so that, in the absence of a standardized protocol, causal relationship is impossible to be defined. Moreover, there is a significant causality dilemma: the more critical the patient is, the more fluids are needed.[61]

Furthermore, there is not a definition for "liberal" or "restrictive", so similar strategies are depicted in one study restrictive, in another one liberal. Sometimes, in addition, a "restrictive" case rapidly became a "liberal" one because of intraoperative rescue strategies, which made the fluid total amount larger than predicted. Finally, none of these studies adopted PLV, which represents an unacceptable bias when analyzing postoperative lung injury. A randomized control trial (RCT) comparing liberal and restrictive strategy in thoracic anesthesia can have significant approval obstacles from the hospital ethical committee.

Normovolemia as a Target

Two studies by Assaad et al.[62,63] attempted to apply a standardized fluid protocol targeting normovolemia, in association with PLV. The authors reported an absence of increase in the extravascular lung water (EVLW), compared with basal levels, and an improvement in cardiac index and serum creatinine levels.

The fluid strategy they applied established the administration of maintenance fluids at 1.5 mL/kg/h, in addition to replacement of blood losses and deficit; fluids were continued until oral intake was resumed in the postoperative period.

This approach, which was able to protect the kidney and limit the increase in EVLW, however, was not goal directed. It is well accepted that goal-directed approaches, as shown by recent metaanalysis involving nonthoracic surgery,[64–67] were associated with a slight reduction in postoperative morbidity, when compared with standard protocols.

Goal-Directed Strategies

The Goal-Directed Therapy Role

The goal the anesthesiologist pursues is the optimal balance between hypervolemia and hypovolemia, namely, between edema and hypoperfusion.[68]

Certainly, the definition of "optimal" remains elusive, and nowadays the approaches are basically oriented to limit fluid intraoperative administration and in the postoperative period. In general, besides thoracic anesthesia, the trend is toward more restrictive, avoiding weight gain and related postoperative complications. As mentioned previously, however, impaired tissue perfusion may protect from postoperative edema while restrictive strategies may lead to organ dysfunction, in particular the kidney.

Several studies investigated the relationship between kidney function and fluid administration. Many of them however, found no correlation between AKI and the amount of fluid administration[21,69]; this could suggest that fluid restriction does not cause renal impairment. In fact, in comparing groups of patients with and without postoperative AKI, no significant differences in fluid administration was pointed out. Different strategies did not seem to affect the intraoperative urinary outcome,[70] and perioperative oliguria (<0.5 mL/kg/h) is not a marker of postoperative renal failure.[71]

This clarifies why goal-directed approaches (targeting urinary output, weight gain, or other variables) may not be completely reliable.

The goal-directed therapy (GDT) approach has been applied in numerous types of surgery, and meta analyses showed better outcomes in patients receiving it. On the other hand, two recent RCTs, which included patients undergoing abdominal aortic surgery and colorectal surgery, found no benefits of GDT strategy over conventional clinical choice, as far as intensive care stay and length of hospital stay. Egal et al.[71] performed a systematic review and meta analysis to which they compared "conventional fluid management" (CFM) with GDT using cardiac output, urine output, or oxygen delivery parameters, and reported the occurrence of AKI in critically ill or surgical patients. They divided the studies into groups with and without oliguria reversal as a target for hemodynamic optimization. Based on analyses of 28 studies, GDT resulted in less AKI than CFM when compared with CFM were oliguria reversal was the target therapy. However, other studies comparing GDT with CFM in which the reversal of oliguria was targeted in both or in neither group did not provide enough evidence to conclude a superiority of GDT.[72,73]

Despite this controversial result in nonthoracic surgery, GDT has probably played a role in thoracic surgery, in which fluid administration needs a careful guide[74] (Fig. 21.5).

GDT aimed at optimizing tissue perfusion and oxygenation can have different targets, but classically considered the most important is oxygen delivery by optimizing cardiac output. Optimization does not mean maximization[75] maximization is crucial in patients with shock who require resuscitation. In these patients, it is often necessary to administer cardiovascular drugs (vasopressors, inotropes, beta blockers, vasodilators, alpha-2 agonists) to influence preload afterload, heart rate, cardiac contractility, and relaxation, to control the cardiac output and to match flow/oxygen delivery (DO2) to the different metabolic needs and consumption of oxygen.

Fluid Responsiveness and Its Prediction

The rational approach to fluid administration in GDT is based on the prediction of fluid responsiveness. A central role is played by identification of patients who, according to Starling's law, will benefit from fluid loading, in terms of hemodynamic stability and DO2, avoiding the administration of unnecessary fluid loads; these patients are defined as fluid responders.

The response to a fluid challenge is sometime difficult to predict because of cardiovascular physiology; the Frank-Starling curve can assume many different shapes depending

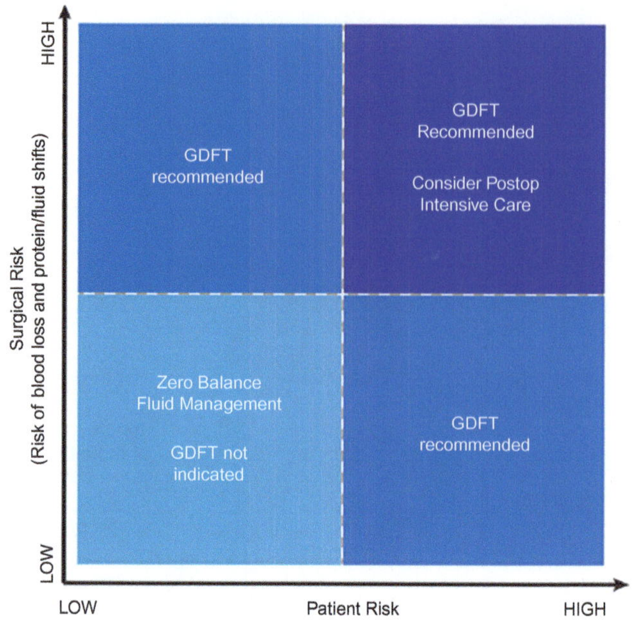

• **Fig. 21.5** Fluid management and goal-directed therapy (GDT) as an adjunct to enhanced recovery after surgery (ERAS). Goal-directed fluid therapy (GDFT) is unlikely either to cause harm or to add benefit in healthy patients undergoing uneventful surgery within an ERAS pathway. (From Miller TE, Pearse RM. Perioperative fluid management: moving toward more answers than questions-a commentary on the RELIEF study. *Perioper Med (Lond)*. 2019;8:2.)

on the ventricular systolic function.[76] Depending on which kind of curve we are dealing with, a fluid challenge can lead to a significant increase in stroke volume and cardiac output, or have no effect at all. When a fluid bolus is administered to a patient without attempts to predict fluid responsiveness, a significant hemodynamic improvement takes place in only half the patients.[77] In the other half, the clinician has to deal with hemodilution, increased cardiac filling pressure, and fluid overload. For that reason a careful evaluation of the effects of fluid before its administration is mandatory.

Established hemodynamic variables are used to test fluid responsiveness and can be divided into static and dynamic ones. **Static variables** indicate hemodynamic status at a specific time, providing a preload value at that defined time. One example may be the value of the cardiac index obtained in a single thermodilution through a Swan-Ganz catheter. **Dynamic variables** identify hemodynamic changes in response to a periodic variation in preload; they are more reliable in evaluating fluid responsiveness, compared to static ones.[78]

Static Variables

For decades, cardiac filling pressures (central venous pressure [CVP] and pulmonary artery occlusion pressure [PAOP]) were used to guide intravascular volume therapy. Several studies and meta analyses established that CVP is not a reliable predictor of fluid responsiveness.[79,80] This inadequacy derives from the fact that a static value of CVP can have completely different meanings depending on the shape of the Frank-Starling curve (different from one patient to another and, in the same patient, from one time to another).

Despite this evidence, surveys report that clinicians still continue to use it; for instance, the FENICE study (involving intensive care units [ICUs] around the world) showed that static variables are still used to test fluid responsiveness in one-third of cases.[81]

This unreliability is not limited to CVP; all static indicators of cardiac preload, such as PAOP, the global end-diastolic volume measured with transpulmonary thermodilution and the flow time of aortic flow by esophageal Doppler, can be as inadequate.

Dynamic Variables

The stroke volume variations (SVVs), induced by mechanical ventilation, allow a dynamic evaluation of preload responsiveness. During positive pressure ventilation, insufflation will lower right ventricle preload, which results in a decreased left ventricle preload. If stroke volume of left ventricle changes in response to ventilation, which means that both ventricles are preload dependent: that is how mechanical ventilation, used to measure SVV, can be useful to define the slope of the Frank-Starling curve.

To obtain a reliable evaluation of stroke volume, the amplitude of arterial pulse pressure (in particular the gap between systolic and diastolic pressures) during mechanical ventilation was proposed and used: large amounts of evidence from several studies confirmed it as a marker.[82–84] Several meta analysis have confirmed its reliability,[85,86] even though a study underlined a grey zone (between 9% and 13%) where its sensitivity or specificity is below 90%, and within which 24% of pulse pressure variation (PPV) values measured in clinical practice fall.[87] The clinical meaning of the grey zone is that, the farther PPV values diagnostic threshold, the more reliable its evaluation as a predictor of fluid responsiveness (see Fig. 21.4).

Other less-invasive surrogates of stroke volume have been explored in recent years, with greater feasibility in the operating room.[88–96] These include the volume-clamp photoplethysmography (to evaluate the ventilation-related variations in arterial pulse pressure), pulse contour analysis, the echocardiography-obtained velocity time integral of the flow in left ventricular outflow track (even if a recent study questioned its validity in mechanically ventilated patients), the aortic blood flow by esophageal Doppler and the amplitude of plethysmography.

There are some conditions, however, in which PPV and SVV are unreliable:

- Spontaneous breathing, even in intubated patients (leading to false positive results)
- Cardiac arrhythmias (leading to false positive results)
- Low tidal volume/low lung compliance, as in ARDS (leading to false negative results)
- Open chest (leading to false negative results)
- Increased intraabdominal pressure (leading to false positive results)
- Very high respiratory rate, HR/RR ratio under 3.6 (leading to false negative results)
- Right heart failure (leading to false positive results)

In patients with ARDS, low tidal volume is commonly used to follow the concept of a "baby lung", leading to lower changes in intrathoracic pressure. A transient increase in tidal volume to 8 mL/kg was proposed, called "tidal volume challenge." The interpretation of the response to the tidal volume challenge seems to be useful to predict fluid responsiveness.[97,98] It is however, less valid in patients with ARDS who have a low lung compliance, which reduces the transmission of alveolar pressures to intravascular and cardiac compartment.[99]

A limitation to keep in mind when interpreting SVV and PPV values to guide fluid therapy, was raised by a study published in 2017, which suggested that dynamic preload indicators are not useful for predicting fluid responsiveness in video-assisted thoracoscopic surgery (VATS) or open thoracic surgery. Jeong et al.[100] evaluated SVV and PPV used as indicators of fluid responsiveness during thoracic surgery. They enrolled 80 patients scheduled for an elective lobectomy requiring OLV including: n = 40, VATS; n = 40, open thoracotomy. Some 20 minutes after opening the thoracic cavity, 7 mL/kg hydroxyethyl starch was administered for 30 minutes and various hemodynamic parameters were measured before and after fluid challenge. Among the 80 patients enrolled in this study, 37% were fluid responders (increase in stroke volume index ≥10%). SVV before fluid challenge was not different between nonresponders and responders (mean ± standard deviation [SD]: 7.1 ± 2.7% vs. 7.4 ± 2.6%,) regardless of whether the surgery involved open thoracotomy or VATS. PPV before fluid challenge showed no difference between no responders and responders (mean ± SD: 6.9 ± 3.0% vs. 8.4 ± 3.2%). In general, open thorax has been seen as a limitation, but not as a contraindication of these measurements.[101] Two other recent studies have investigated this subject, one suggesting that SVV may be used to guide fluid treatment in thoracic surgery but without a significant reduction in the complications rate,[102] the other indicating that OLV requires different thresholds to predict fluid responsiveness and that the interpretation of PPV during OLV should be done with caution. Lema et al.[103] in a prospective study evaluated 112 patients undergoing lung resection surgery with OLV. Intravenous fluid therapy with crystalloids was set at 2 mL/kg/h and OLV was managed with a tidal volume of 6 mL/kg/h. They found that SVV values were influenced by lung collapse (before lung collapse 14.6 [DS] vs. OLV 9.9% [DS], $P < .0001$), or after restoring two-lung ventilation (11.01 [DS], $P < .0001$). During two-lung ventilation there was a significant correlation between airway pressures and SVV; however, this correlation was lacking during OLV.

Respiratory variation in inferior vena cava diameter has been proposed as a predictor, but in addition to the difficulty in investigating it, a recent systematic review underlined how its reliability is limited to definite ventilatory settings.[104] It may be more accurate, but it also more complex because it requires transesophageal echocardiography. The collapsibility of the superior vena cava seems to be a useful marker.[105]

Passive Leg Raising

Passive leg raising (PLR) represents an "internal" preload challenge. It is equivalent to a preload challenge of around 300 mL of blood, which can be repeated as many times as needed, without actually administering any fluid.[106] Fluid responders, in addition to an increase in mean systemic pressure, present an increase in pressure gradient of venous return and in cardiac output.[107]

The great reliability of this test, as confirmed by many studies,[108–110] and its feasibility caused its popularity and diffusion. In contrast to ICU conditions, however, it is not practical during anesthesia.

End-Expiratory Occlusion Test

During mechanical ventilation, as mentioned before, insufflation lowers cardiac preload, impeding venous return as well. A brief interruption (at least 15 seconds) of the mechanical ventilation removes this obstacle, causing a transient increase in cardiac preload. If cardiac output (measured through pulse contour analysis or echocardiography)[111,112] rises as well, the patient can be considered a fluid responder.

Even though very easy to perform and valid in patients with ARDS,[113] it is useless during tubeless procedures (which, with the recent implementation of tubeless anesthetic techniques for thoracic surgery, may represent a significant limitation[114,115]). The sedated patient is not able to tolerate a 15-seconds respiratory hold.

Fluid Challenge

Administering fluid is inevitably the most direct way to test fluid responsiveness. The "traditional" fluid challenge consist of administration of an intravenous bolus of crystalloids or colloids over a short time, followed by a precise assessment of the cardiovascular response.[116,117]

The risk of fluid overload and hemodilution, in particular in critical patients needing multiple assessment, should not be ignored.

For this reason, an initial mini-fluid challenge has been proposed.[118] Several studies reported that changes in velocity-time integral measured by transthoracic ecochardiography,[119] cardiac output analysis through pulse contour,[118] as well as changes in SVV[120] induced by the infusion of 100 mL of saline was reliable to assess fluid responsiveness.

The main issue associated with this mini-fluid strategy is that such a small volume of fluid inducing slight variations in cardiac preload results in only a minimal change in cardiac output in patients who are fluid responders. For this reason the test requires a very precise monitor of cardiac output with very precise techniques.

Clinical Practice

Whatever monitor or maneuver is chosen to guide the fluid administration, once it is determined whether the patient is a fluid responder, the need for additional fluids must be questioned. Volume responsiveness, in fact, is not equal to volume deficiency[121]; "giving volume to fluid responders as long as they respond, should not become the iatrogenic syndrome of the decade."[122]

Careful, continuous and dynamic monitoring should be used to assess the volume status and to guide a correct fluid strategy.

The anesthesiologist should keep the pathophysiology in mind during thoracic surgery. Although sudden volume loss is rare but not unusual (because of injuries of central vessels), when facing a hypotension during thoracic anesthesia, this is rarely to ascribe to absolute hypovolemia. It is frequently because of the manipulation of pulmonary vessels, vasodilation related to thoracic epidural, or anesthetic drugs. Low doses of catecholamine are more appropriate than the risk of fluid overloads.

Choice of Fluids: Crystalloids Versus Colloid Solutions

Analysis on perioperative fluid management during thoracic anesthesia must include a brief comparison between different types of fluids used both for maintenance and for resuscitation. Finding the balance between renal and lung injury becomes even more difficult when facing this choice.

Large amounts of crystalloids, indeed, may precipitate pulmonary edema; colloid solutions, on the other hand, may be associated with kidney dysfunction and coagulopathy as well.

Colloids are divided into hyperoncotic and hypooncotic. Hyperoncotic colloids, increasing the intravascular oncotic pressure, promote the extravascular fluid shift into the bloodstream; this property makes them rapid plasma expanders. Hydroxyethyl starch (HES) is one of them (Fig. 21.6).

Considering ALI pathophysiology, they may have beneficial effects in patients suffering from lung injury, potentially removing water from the lungs to deposit it into the vascular compartment.[123] Verheij et al. in a prospective trial of 67 mechanically ventilated patients who were randomly assigned to receive saline, gelatin 4%, HES 6% or albumin 5%, according to a 90 minute fluid loading protocol with target central venous pressure of 13 mm Hg and pulmonary

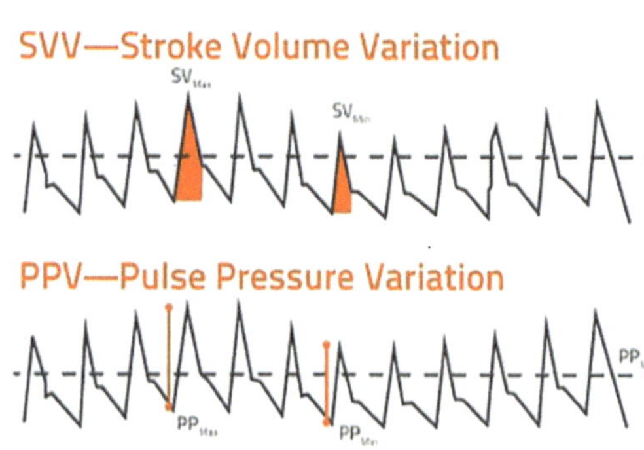

• **Fig. 21.6** Hydroxyethyl starch are obtained by the substitution of hydroxyl groups of natural starches with hydroxyethyl groups (yellow circles) at carbon position C2, C3, and C6 of the anhydroglucose residues.

capillary wedge pressure of 15 mm Hg, within 3 hours after cardiac or major vascular surgery. They found that more saline was infused than colloid solutions ($P < .005$). The plasma colloid osmotic pressure increased in the colloid groups and decreased in patients receiving saline. Cardiac output increased more in the colloid groups. The oxygenation ratio improved in all groups. In the colloid groups, the lung injury score increased because of a decrease in total respiratory compliance, probably associated with an increase in intrathoracic plasma volume. Provided that fluid overloading is prevented, the type of fluid used for volume loading does not affect pulmonary permeability and edema. Huang et al. reported a rapid improvement of hemodynamics without lung impairment in patients with early ARDS.[124]

Other studies have not observed any pulmonary beneficial effects from the use of colloids and, above all, a Cochrane systematic review (even when including patients with sepsis or following nonthoracic surgeries) could not prove any outcome improvement when administering colloids instead of crystalloids.[125]

In addition, the impact of colloids on kidney function must be mentioned; a hyperoncotic renal damage following colloid administration has been reported.[126] This clinical picture can be the result of a high plasma oncotic pressure overtaking the hydraulic pressure of glomerular filtration, blocking urinary output, or from osmotic nephrosis.

Different studies were conducted on this subject, which concluded that HES increases kidney impairment, and sometimes mortality rate.[127–130] In most of these studies, however, large amounts of colloids were used, often exceeding the maximal manufacturer recommended doses and, thus, failing to provide enough free water at glomerular level, precipitating the development of hyperoncotic syndrome. The previously mentioned study of Ahn[69] suggests an increased risk of postoperative AKI because of colloid administration, in particular in high-risk patients.

On the other hand, there are studies demonstrating no impact on renal function or renal replacement therapy,[131] even in patients with baseline injury.[132] One published work showed that volume expansion with a combination of 6% HES and crystalloids can even improve renal function, compared with 4% gelatin administration.[133]

It is crucial to underline that all these studies established the use of 6% HES always in combination with crystalloids, and never exceeding the maximal manufacturer recommended daily dose of 20 mL/kg.

Another work by Vives et al.[134] attempted to determine the renal safety of 6% HES use in cardiac surgery, and found no association between its administration and increased risk of AKI or renal replacement therapy.

In conclusion, few studies address this issue in patients undergoing lung resection, and most of the data is extrapolated from studies performed on different populations or retrospective databases.

The admonition of crystalloid should be balanced, and it appears that HES is best used in combination with crystalloids, as part of a multimodal fluid resuscitation, or even limiting its use for a replacement of rapid losses.

References

1. Licker MJ, Widikker I, Robert J, et al. Operative mortality and respiratory complications after lung resection for cancer: impact of chronic obstructive pulmonary disease and time trends. *Ann Thorac Surg.* 2006;81:1830–1837.
2. Boffa DJ, Allen MS, Grab JD, et al. Data from The Society of Thoracic Surgeons General Thoracic Surgery database: the surgical management of primary lung tumors. *J Thorac Cardiovasc Surg.* 2008;135:247–254.
3. Licker M, Fauconnet P, Villiger Y, Tschopp JM. Acute lung injury and outcomes after thoracic surgery. *Curr Opin Anaesthesiol.* 2009;22:61–67.
4. Marret E, Miled F, Bazelly B, et al. Risk and protective factors for major complications after pneumonectomy for lung cancer. *Inter Cardiovasc Thorac Sur.* 2010;10:936–939.
5. Zeldin RA, Normandin D, Landtwing D, Peters RM. Postpneumonectomy pulmonary edema. *J Thorac Cardiovasc Surg.* 1984;87:359–365.
6. Gothard J. Lung injury after thoracic surgery and one-lung ventilation. *Curr Opin Anaesthesiol.* 2006;19:5–10.
7. Parquin F, Marchal M, Mehiri S, et al. Postpneumonectomy pulmonary edema: analysis and risk factors. *Eur J Cardiothorac Surg.* 1996;10:929–932.
8. Blank RS, Hucklenbruch C, Gurka KK, et al. Intraoperative factors and the risk of respiratory complications after pneumonectomy. *Ann Thorac Surg.* 2011;92:1188–1194.
9. Licker M, de Perrot M, Spiliopoulos A, Robert J, Diaper J, Chevalley C, et al. Risk factors for acute lung injury after thoracic surgery for lung cancer. *Anesth Analg.* 2003;97:1558–1565.
10. Arslantas MK, Kara HV, Tuncer BB, et al. Effect of the amount of intraoperative fluid administration on postoperative pulmonary complications following anatomic lung resections. *J Thorac Cardiovasc Surg.* 2015;149:314–320.
11. Licker M, Diaper J, Villiger Y, et al. Impact of intraoperative lung-protective interventions in patients undergoing lung cancer surgery. *Crit Care.* 2009;13:R41.
12. Slinger P. Fluid management during pulmonary resection surgery. *Ann Card Anaesth.* 2002;5:220–224.
13. Ware LB, Fremont RD, Bastarache JA, et al. Determining the aetiology of pulmonary edema by the edema fluid-to-plasma protein ratio. *Eur Respir J.* 2010;35:331–337.
14. Bernard GR, Artigas A, Brigham KL, et al. The American-European Consensus Conference on ARDS. Definitions, mechanisms, relevant outcomes, and clinical trial coordination. *Am J Respir Crit Care Med.* 1994;149:818–824.
15. Villar J, Perez-Mendez L, Lopez J, et al. An early PEEP/FiO2 trial identifies different degrees of lung injury in patients with acute respiratory distress syndrome. *Am J Respir Crit Care Med.* 2007;176:795–804.
16. Dulu A, Pastores SM, Park B, et al. Prevalence and mortality of acute lung injury and ARDS after lung resection. *Chest.* 2006;130:73–78.
17. Shaw A. Update on acute kidney injury after cardiac surgery. *J Thorac Cardiovasc Surg.* 2012;143:676–681.

18. Mehta RL, Kellum JA, Shah SV, et al. Acute Kidney Injury Network: report of an initiative to improve outcomes in acute kidney injury. *Crit Care.* 2007;11:R31.
19. Basile DP. Rarefaction of peritubular capillaries following ischemic acute renal failure: a potential factor predisposing to progressive nephropathy. *Curr Opin Nephrol Hypertens.* 2004;13:1–7.
20. Ishikawa S, Griesdale DE, Lohser J. Acute kidney injury after lung resection surgery: incidence and perioperative risk factors. *Anesth Analg.* 2012;114:1256–1262.
21. Hobson CE, Yavas S, Segal MS, et al. Acute kidney injury is associated with increased long-term mortality after cardiothoracic surgery. *Circulation.* 2009;119:2444–2453.
22. Grichnik KP, Shaw A. Update on one-lung ventilation: the use of continuous positive airway pressure ventilation and positive end-expiratory pressure ventilation - clinical application. *Curr Opin Anaesth.* 2009;22:23–30.
23. Lipes J, Bojmehrani A, Lellouche F. Low tidal volume ventilation in patients without acute respiratory distress syndrome: a paradigm shift in mechanical ventilation. *Crit Care Res Pract.* 2012;2012:416862.
24. Toy P, Popovsky MA, Abraham E, et al. Transfusion-related acute lung injury: definition and review. *Crit Care Med.* 2005;33:721–726.
25. Vlaar APJ, Toy P, Fung M, et al. A consensus redefinition of transfusion-related acute lung injury. *Transfusion.* 2019;59(7):2465–2476.
26. Starling EH. On the absorption of fluids from the connective tissue spaces. *J Physiol.* 1896;19:312–326.
27. West JB. *Respiratory Physiology: The Essentials.* Philadelphia: Wolters Kluwer/Lippincott Williams & Wilkins; 2008.
28. Dull RO, Cluff M, Kingston J, et al. Lung heparan sulfates modulate K(fc) during increased vascular pressure: evidence for glycocalyx-mediated mechanotransduction. *Am J Physiol Lung Cell Mol Physiol.* 2012;302:L816–L828.
29. Miserocchi G, Negrini D, Passi A, De Luca G. Development of lung edema: interstitial fluid dynamics and molecular structure. *News Physiol Sci.* 2001;16:66–71.
30. Downs CA, Kriener LH, Yu L, et al. Beta-adrenergic agonists differentially regulate highly selective and nonselective epithelial sodium channels to promote alveolar fluid clearance in vivo. *Am J Physiol Lung Cell Mol Physiol.* 2012;302:L1167–L1178.
31. Berger MM, Rozendal CS, Schieber C, et al. The effect of endothelin-1 on alveolar fluid clearance and pulmonary edema formation in the rat. *Anesth Analg.* 2009;108:225–231.
32. Levick JR, Michel CC. Microvascular fluid exchange and the revised Starling principle. *Cardiovasc Res.* 2010;87:198–210.
33. Collins SR, Blank RS, Deatherage LS, Dull RO. The endothelial glycocalyx. *Anesth Analg.* 2013;117:664–674.
34. Alphonsus CS, Rodseth RN. The endothelial glycocalyx: a review of the vascular barrier. *Anaesthesia.* 2014;69:777–784.
35. Tarbell JM. Shear stress and the endothelial transport barrier. *Cardiovasc Res.* 2010;87:320–330.
36. Weinbaum S, Tarbell JM, Damiano ER. The structure and function of the endothelial glycocalyx layer. *Annu Rev Biomed Eng.* 2007;9:121–167.
37. Chappell D, Hofmann-Kiefer K, Jacob M, et al. TNF-alpha induced shedding of the endothelial glycocalyx is prevented by hydrocortisone and antithrombin. *Basic Res Cardiol.* 2009;104:78–89.
38. Bruegger D, Jacob M, Rehm M, et al. Atrial natriuretic peptide induces shedding of endothelial glycocalyx in coronary vascular bed of guinea pig hearts. *Am J Physiol Heart Circ Physiol.* 2005;289:H1993–H1999.
39. Ait-Oufella H, Maury E, Lehoux S, Guidet B, Offenstadt G. The endothelium: physiological functions and role in microcirculatory failure during severe sepsis. *Intensive Care Med.* 2010;36:1286–1298.
40. Ware LB. Pathophysiology of acute lung injury and the acute respiratory distress syndrome. *Semin Respir Crit Care Med.* 2006;27:337–349.
41. Guarracino F. Perioperative acute lung injury: reviewing the role of anesthetic management. *J Anesth Clin Res.* 2012;4:312.
42. Alam N, Park BJ, Wilton A, Seshan VE, Bains MS, Downey RJ, et al. Incidence and risk factors for lung injury after lung cancer resection. *Ann Thorac Surg.* 2007;84:1085–1091.
43. Slinger PD. Postpneumonectomy pulmonary edema: good news, bad news. *Anesthesiology.* 2006;105:2–5.
44. Cousins MJ, Skowronski G, Plummer JL. Anaesthesia and the kidney. *Anaesth Intensive Care.* 1983;11:292–320.
45. Sanders G, Mercer SJ, Saeb-Parsey K, et al. Randomized clinical trial of intravenous fluid replacement during bowel preparation for surgery. *Br J Surg.* 2001;88:1363–1365.
46. Grocott MP, Mythen MG, Gan TJ. Perioperative fluid management and clinical outcomes in adults. *Anesth Analg.* 2005;100:1093–1106.
47. Gattinoni L, Protti A, Caironi P, Carlesso E. Ventilator-induced lung injury: the anatomical and physiological framework. *Crit Care Med.* 2010;38:S539–S548.
48. Gattinoni L, Pesenti A. The concept of baby lung. *Intensive Care Med.* 2005;31:776–784.
49. Szegedi LL, Bardoczky GI, Engelman EE, et al. Airway pressure changes during one-lung ventilation. *Anesth Analg.* 1997;84:1034–1037.
50. Vlahakis NE, Hubmayr RD. Cellular stress failure in ventilator-injured lungs. *Am J Respir Crit Care Med.* 2005;171(12):1328–1342.
51. Beitler JR, Malhotra A, Taylor Thompson B. Ventilator-induced lung injury. *Clin Chest Med.* 2016;37:633–646.
52. Albert RK. The role of ventilation-induced surfactant dysfunction and atelectasis in causing acute respiratory distress syndrome. *Am J Respir Crit Care Med.* 2012;185(7):702–708.
53. Ghadiali SN, Gaver DP. Biomechanics of liquid-epithelium interactions in pulmonary airways. *Respir Physiol Neurobiol.* 2008;163(1–3):232–243.
54. Oeckler RA, Lee W-Y, Park M-G, et al. Determinants of plasma membrane wounding by deforming stress. *Am J Physiol Lung Cell Mol Physiol.* 2010;299(6):L826–L833.
55. Dolinay T, Kim YS, Howrylak J, et al. Inflammasome-regulated cytokines are critical mediators of acute lung injury. *Am J Respir Crit Care Med.* 2012;185(11):1225–1234.
56. Slutsky AS. Ventilator-induced lung injury: from barotrauma to biotrauma. *Respir Care.* 2005;50(5):646–659.
57. Kozian A, Schilling T, Rocken C, et al. Increased alveolar damage after mechanical ventilation in a porcine model of thoracic surgery. *J Cardiothorac Vasc Anesth.* 2010;24:617–623.
58. Benjamin RJ. Tracking TRALI in target populations. *Blood.* 2011;117(16):4163–4164.
59. Bux Jürgen, Sachs UJ. The pathogenesis of transfusion-related acute lung injury (TRALI). *Br J Hematol.* 2007;136(6):788–799.
60. Şentürk M, Sungur Orhan M, Sungur Zerrin. Fluid management in thoracic anesthesia. *Minerva Anestesiol.* 2017;83(6):652–659.

61. Licker M, Triponez F, Ellenberger C, Wolfram W. Fluid therapy in thoracic surgery: a zero-balance target is always best! *Turk J Anaesthesiol Reanim.* 2016;44:227–229.
62. Assaad S, Perkal M, Kyriakides T, et al. Does liberalized fluid protocol increase lung water post lung resection surgery? *Anesth Analg.* 2012;114(Supp l):01–493 SCA.
63. Assaad S, Perkal M, Kyriakides T, et al. Liberalized fluid protocol and tissue perfusion biomarkers in lung resection surgery. *Anesth Analg.* 2012;114(Suppl):01–493 SCA.
64. Ripollés J, Espinosa A, Martínez-Hurtado E, et al. EAR Group (Evidence Anestesia Review Group). Intra-operative goal directed hemodynamic therapy in noncardiac surgery: a systematic review and meta-analysis. *Braz J Anesthesiol.* 2016;66:513–528.
65. Pearse RM, Harrison DA, MacDonald N, et al. OPTIMISE Study Group. Effect of a perioperative, cardiac output-guided hemodynamic therapy algorithm on outcomes following major gastrointestinal surgery: a randomized clinical trial and systematic review. *JAMA.* 2014;311:2181–2190.
66. Rollins KE, Lobo DN. Intraoperative goal-directed fluid therapy in elective major abdominal surgery: a meta-analysis of randomized controlled trials. *Ann Surg.* 2016;263:465–476.
67. Benes J, Giglio M, Brienza N, Michard F. The effects of goal-directed fluid therapy based on dynamic parameters on post-surgical outcome: a meta-analysis of randomized controlled trials. *Crit Care.* 2014;18:584.
68. Doherty M, Buggy DJ. Intraoperative fluids: how much is too much? *Br J Anaesth.* 2012;109:69–79.
69. Ahn HJ, Kim JA, Lee AR, Yang M, Jung HJ, Heo B. The risk of acute kidney injury from fluid restriction and hydroxyethyl starch in thoracic surgery. *Anesth Analg.* 2016;122: 186–193.
70. Matot I, Dery E, Bulgov Y, Cohen B, Paz J, Nesher N. Fluid management during video-assisted thoracoscopic surgery for lung resection: a randomized, controlled trial of effects on urinary output and postoperative renal function. *J Thorac Cardiovasc Surg.* 2013;146:461–466.
71. Egal M, Erler NS, de Geus HRH, van Bommel J, Groeneveld ABJ. Targeting oliguria reversal in goal-directed hemodynamic management does not reduce renal dysfunction in perioperative and critically ill patients: a systematic review and meta-analysis. *Anesth Analg.* 2016;122:173–185.
72. Challand C, Struthers R, Sneyd JR, et al. Randomized controlled trial of intraoperative goal-directed fluid therapy in aerobically fit and unfit patients having major colorectal surgery. *Br J Anaesth.* 2012;108:53–62.
73. Bisgaard J, Gilsaa T, Ronholm E, Toft P. Optimizing stroke volume and oxygen delivery in abdominal aortic surgery: a randomized controlled trial. *Acta Anaesthesiol Scand.* 2013;57(2): 178–188.
74. Assaad S, Popescu W, Perrino A. Fluid management in thoracic surgery. *Curr Opin Anesthesiol.* 2013;26(1):31–39.
75. Licker M, Triponez F, Ellenberger C, Karenovics W. Less fluids and a more physiological approach. *Turk J Anaesthesiol Reanim.* 2016;44:230–232.
76. Monnet X, Pinsky MR. Predicting the determinants of volume responsiveness. *Intensive Care Med.* 2015;41:354–356.
77. Michard F, Teboul JL. Predicting fluid responsiveness in ICU patients: a critical analysis of the evidence. *Chest.* 2002;121: 2000–2008.
78. Lees N, Hamilton M, Rhodes A. Clinical review: Goal-directed therapy in high risk surgical patients. *Crit Care.* 2009;13:231.
79. Bentzer P, Griesdale DE, Boyd J, MacLean K, Sirounis D, Ayas NT. Will this hemodynamically unstable patient respond to a bolus of intravenous fluids? *JAMA.* 2016;316:1298–1309.
80. Marik PE, Cavallazzi R. Does the central venous pressure predict fluid responsiveness? An updated meta-analysis and a plea for some common sense. *Crit Care Med.* 2013;41:1774–1781.
81. Cecconi M, Hofer C, Teboul JL, et al. Fluid challenges in intensive care: the FENICE study: a global inception cohort study. *Intensive Care Med.* 2015;41:1529–1537.
82. Michard F, Boussat S, Chemla D, et al. Relation between respiratory changes in arterial pulse pressure and fluid responsiveness in septic patients with acute circulatory failure. *Am J Respir Crit Care Med.* 2000;162:134–138.
83. Yang X, Du B. Does pulse pressure variation predict fluid responsiveness in critically ill patients? A systematic review and meta-analysis. *Crit Care.* 2014;18:650.
84. Marik PE, Cavallazzi R, Vasu T, Hirani A. Dynamic changes in arterial waveform derived variables and fluid responsiveness in mechanically ventilated patients: a systematic review of the literature. *Crit Care Med.* 2009;37:2642–2647.
85. Piccioni F, Bernasconi F, Tramontano GTA, Langer M. A systematic review of pulse pressure variation and stroke volume variation to predict fluid responsiveness during cardiac and thoracic surgery. *J Clin Monitor Comput.* 2017;31(4):677–684.
86. Myatra SN, Prabu NR, Divatia J, Monnet X. The changes in pulse pressure variation or stroke volume variation after a "tidal volume challenge" reliably predict fluid responsiveness during low tidal volume ventilation. *Crit Care Med.* 2017;45(3):415–421.
87. Cannesson M, Le Manach Y, Hofer CK, et al. Assessing the diagnostic accuracy of pulse pressure variations for the prediction of fluid responsiveness: a "gray zone" approach. *Anesthesiology.* 2011;115(2):231–241.
88. Monnet X, Dres M, Ferre A, et al. Prediction of fluid responsiveness by a continuous non-invasive assessment of arterial pressure in critically ill patients: comparison with four other dynamic indices. *Br J Anaesth.* 2012;109:330–338.
89. Wagner JY, Negulescu I, Schöfthaler M, et al. Continuous non-invasive arterial pressure measurement using the volume clamp method: an evaluation of the CNAP device in intensive care unit patients. *J Clin Monitor Comput.* 2015;29(6):807–813.
90. Bartels K, Thiele RH. Advances in photoplethysmography: beyond arterial oxygen saturation. *Can J Anaesth.* 2015;62(12): 1313–1328.
91. Grensemann J. Cardiac output monitoring by pulse contour analysis, the technical basics of less-invasive techniques. *Front Med.* 2018;5:64.
92. Saugel B, Reuter DA. Perioperative goal-directed therapy using invasive uncalibrated pulse contour analysis. *Front Med.* 2018;5:12.
93. Michard F, Giglio MT, Brienza N. Perioperative goal-directed therapy with uncalibrated pulse contour methods: impact on fluid management and postoperative outcome. *Br J Anaesth.* 2017;119(1):22–30.
94. Blancas R, Martínez-González Ó, Ballesteros D, et al. Lack of correlation between left ventricular outflow tract velocity time integral and stroke volume index in mechanically ventilated patients. *Med Intensiva* (English Edition). 2019;43(2): 73–78.
95. Monnet X, Rienzo M, Osman D, et al. Esophageal Doppler monitoring predicts fluid responsiveness in critically ill ventilated patients. *Intensive Care Med.* 2005;31:1195–1201.

96. Tusman G, Bohm SH, Suarez-Sipmann F. Advanced uses of pulse oximetry for monitoring mechanically ventilated patients. *Anesth Analg.* 2017;124(1):62–71.
97. Myatra SN, Monnet X, Teboul J-L. Use of tidal volume challenge to improve the reliability of pulse pressure variation. *Crit. Care.* 2017;21(1):60.
98. Messina A, Montagnini C, Cammarota G, et al. Tidal volume challenge to predict fluid responsiveness in the operating room: an observational study. *Eur J Anaesthesiol.* 2019;36(8):583–591.
99. Liu Y, Wei LQ, Li GQ, Yu X, Li GF, Li YM. Pulse pressure variation adjusted by respiratory changes in pleural pressure, rather than by tidal volume, reliably predicts fluid responsiveness in patients with acute respiratory distress syndrome. *Crit Care Med.* 2016;44:342–351.
100. Jeong DM, Ahn YJ, Park HW, Yang M, Kim JA, Park J. Stroke volume variation and pulse pressure variation are not useful for predicting fluid responsiveness in thoracic surgery. *Anesth Analg.* 2017;125(4):1158–1165.
101. Michard F, Chemla D, Teboul JL. Applicability of pulse pressure variation: how many shades of grey? *Crit Care.* 2015;19:144.
102. Sahutoglu C, Turksal E, Kocabas S, Askar FZ. Influence of stroke volume variation on fluid treatment and postoperative complications in thoracic surgery. *Ther Clin Risk Manag.* 2018;14:575.
103. Lema Tome M, De la Gala FA, Piñeiro P, Olmedilla L, Garutti I. Behavior of stroke volume variation in hemodynamic stable patients during thoracic surgery with one-lung ventilation periods. *Rev Bras Anestesiol.* 2018;68(3):225–230.
104. Si X, Xu H, Liu Z, et al. Does respiratory variation in inferior vena cava diameter predict fluid responsiveness in mechanically ventilated patients? A systematic review and meta-analysis. *Anesth Analg.* 2018;127(5):1157–1164.
105. Cheng Z, Yang Q-Q, Zhu P, Feng J-I, Zhang X-B, Zhao Z-B. Transesophageal echocardiographic measurements of the superior vena cava for predicting fluid responsiveness in patients undergoing invasive positive pressure ventilation. *J Ultrasound Med.* 2019;38(6):1519–1525.
106. Jabot J, Teboul JL, Richard C, Monnet X. Passive leg raising for predicting fluid responsiveness: importance of the postural change. *Intensive Care Med.* 2009;35:85–90.
107. Guerin L, Teboul JL, Persichini R, Dres M, Richard C, Monnet X. Effects of passive leg raising and volume expansion on mean systemic pressure and venous return in shock in humans. *Crit Care.* 2015;19:411.
108. Cooke K, Sharvill R, Sondergaard S, Aneman A. Volume responsiveness assessed by passive leg raising and a fluid challenge: a critical review focused on mean systemic filling pressure. *Anaesthesia.* 2018;73(3):313–322.
109. Pickett JD, Bridges E, Kritek PA, Whitney JD. Noninvasive blood pressure monitoring and prediction of fluid responsiveness to passive leg raising. *Am J Crit Care.* 2018;27:228–237.
110. Monnet X, Marik P, Teboul JL. Passive leg raising for predicting fluid responsiveness: a systematic review and meta-analysis. *Intensive Care Med.* 2016;42(12):1935–1947.
111. Jozwiak M, Depret F, Teboul J-L, et al. Predicting fluid responsiveness in critically ill patients by using combined end-expiratory and end-inspiratory occlusions with echocardiography. *Crit Care Med.* 2017;45(11):e1131–e1138.
112. Monnet X, Bleibtreu A, Ferré A, et al. Passive leg raising and end-expiratory occlusion tests perform better than pulse pressure variation in patients with low respiratory system compliance. *Crit Care Med.* 2012;40:152–157.
113. Silva S, Jozwiak M, Teboul JL, Persichini R, Richard C, Monnet X. End expiratory occlusion test predicts preload responsiveness independently of positive end-expiratory pressure during acute respiratory distress syndrome. *Crit Care Med.* 2013;41:1692–1701.
114. Gonzalez-Rivas D, Bonome C, Fieira E, et al. Non-intubated video-assisted thoracoscopic lung resections: the future of thoracic surgery? *Eur J Cardiothorac Surg.* 2015;49(3):721–731.
115. Armenta-Flores R, Sanchez-Quiroz J, Castillo-Delgado S, Camarena-Arredondo V. Non-intubated video-assisted thoracic surgery: breaking down paradigms. *Eur J Cardiothorac Surg.* 2016;51(1):197.
116. Weil MH, Henning RJ. New concepts in the diagnosis and fluid treatment of circulatory shock. Thirteenth annual Becton, Dickinson and Company Oscar Schwidetsky Memorial Lecture. *Anesth Analg.* 1979;58:124–132.
117. Vincent JL, Weil MH. Fluid challenge revisited. *Crit Care Med.* 2006;34:1333–1337.
118. Biais M, de Courson H, Lanchon R, et al. Mini-fluid challenge of 100 ml of crystalloid predicts fluid responsiveness in the operating room. *Anesthesiology.* 2017;127:450–456.
119. Muller L, Toumi M, Bousquet PJ, et al. An increase in aortic blood flow after an infusion of 100 ml colloid over 1 minute can predict fluid responsiveness: the mini-fluid challenge study. *Anesthesiology.* 2011;115:541–547.
120. Mallat J, Meddour M, Durville E, et al. Decrease in pulse pressure and stroke volume variations after mini-fluid challenge accurately predicts fluid responsiveness. *Br J Anaesth.* 2015;115(3):449–456.
121. Della Rocca G, Vetrugno L. Fluid therapy today: where are we? *Turk J Anaesth Reanim.* 2016;44:233–235.
122. Takala J. Volume responsive, but does the patient need volume? *Intensive Care Med.* 2016;42:1461–1463.
123. Verheij J, van Lingen A, Raijmakers PG, et al. Effect of fluid loading with saline or colloids on pulmonary permeability, edema and lung injury score after cardiac and major vascular surgery. *Br J Anaesth.* 2006;96:21–30.
124. Huang CC, Kao KC, Hsu KH, et al. Effects of hydroxyethyl starch resuscitation on extravascular lung water and pulmonary permeability in sepsis-related acute respiratory distress syndrome. *Crit Care Med.* 2009;37:1948–1955.
125. Perel P, Roberts I. Colloids versus crystalloids for fluid resuscitation in critically ill patients. *Cochrane Database Syst Rev.* 2012:CD000567.
126. Honore PM, Joannes-Boyau O, Boer W. Hyperoncotic colloids in shock and risk of renal injury: enough evidence for a banning order? *Intensive Care Med.* 2008;34:2127–2129.
127. Schortgen F, Girou E, Deye N, Brochard L. The risk associated with hyper oncotic colloids in patients with shock. *Intensive Care Med.* 2008;34:2157–2168.
128. Brunkhorst FM, Engel C, Bloos F, et al. Intensive insulin therapy and pentastarch resuscitation in severe sepsis. *N Engl J Med.* 2008;358:125–139.
129. Perner A, Haase N, Guttormsen AB, et al. Hydroxyethyl starch 130/0.42 versus Ringer's lactate in severe sepsis. *N Engl J Med.* 2012;367:124–134.

130. Myburgh JA, Finfer S, Bellomo R, et al. Hydroxyethyl starch or saline for fluid resuscitation in intensive care. *N Engl J Med.* 2012;367:1901–1911.
131. Sakr Y, Payen D, Reinhart K, et al. Effects of hydroxyethyl starch administration on renal function in critically ill patients. *Br J Anaesth.* 2007;98:216–224.
132. Godet G, Lehot JJ, Janvier G, et al. Safety of HES 130/0.4 (Voluven(R)) in patients with preoperative renal dysfunction undergoing abdominal aortic surgery: a prospective, randomized, controlled, parallel-group multicenter trial. *Eur J Anaesthesiol.* 2008;25:986–994.
133. Mahmood A, Gosling P, Vohra RK. Randomized clinical trial comparing the effects on renal function of hydroxyethyl starch or gelatin during aortic aneurysm surgery. *Br J Surg.* 2007;94:427–433.
134. Vives M, Callejas R, et al. Modern hydroxyethyl starch and acute kidney injury after cardiac surgery: a prospective multicenter cohort. *Br J Anaesth.* 2016;117(4):458–463.

22

Perioperative Arrhythmias During Thoracic Surgery

SPENCER P. WALSH, DAVID AMAR

Introduction

Cardiac arrythmias are the most frequent postoperative complication affecting up to 20% of patients undergoing thoracic surgery. The most common arrhythmia is postoperative atrial fibrillation (POAF), which typically presents on postoperative day 1 to 5, peaks on postoperative day 2, and resolves within 4 to 6 weeks in more than 90% of patients.[1] Despite its transient nature, POAF is associated with increased length of stay, costs, incidence of stroke, morbidity, and mortality.[2] In addition, it presents several vexing clinical problems in the acute perioperative period. Most significantly, POAF can cause hemodynamic instability, and if persistent can put the patient at an increased risk of thromboembolic events. This scenario presents the conundrum of whether and when to initiate anticoagulation in a postoperative patient potentially at increased risk of bleeding. Therefore attempts to prevent POAF may be warranted.

Key Points

- Most common complication after thoracic surgery, up to 20% of patients
- Recently published risk factors are increased age, body mass index (BMI), preoperative brain natriuretic peptide (BNP), extent of surgery, and prior history of atrial fibrillation (AF)
- Prevention is most effective with amiodarone or calcium channel blockers; beta blockers were recently shown to also be effective
- Treat unstable patients with synchronized cardioversion
- Stable patients should first be treated with rate control and then with rhythm control drugs
- An early rhythm control strategy (including cardioversion) may be warranted to avoid anticoagulation in patients at high risk of bleeding
- Anticoagulation in the first 48 hours is based on CHA_2DS_2-VASc (congestive heart failure, hypertension, age ≥ 75 years, diabetes mellitus, stroke or transient ischemic attack [TIA], vascular disease, age 65 to 74 years, sex category) score, and should be considered if ≥2
- Most POAF will resolve within 48 hours, and nearly all within 4 to 6 weeks without severe sequelae. However, those in AF for more than 48 hours require anticoagulation for stroke prevention

Core Chapter

Predictive Factors

For atrial fibrillation (AF), including POAF, to develop and be sustained requires the combination of atrial pathology to promote a vulnerable substrate and a trigger to initiate the arrhythmia. Using heart rate variability, the authors have demonstrated the presence of competing autonomic mechanism in the 2 hours before POAF onset.[3] In that study, the patients were postoperatively monitored with Holter technology which showed an increased vagal tone in the setting of heightened adrenergic tone occurred before POAF onset, which suggests that a vagal surge could be an important trigger.[3] Although the exact mechanisms underlying this are complex and only partially understood, several risk factors associated with AF are highly predictive including: increased age, atrial dilation, pulmonary hypertension, myocardial ischemia, volume overload, and a history of heart failure.[1] Other risk factors, such as postoperative pericarditis, electrolyte imbalance, and hypoxemia, have all been proposed to trigger POAF but have not been proven. In addition, the extent of surgery is highly predictive and is directly related to the risk of POAF. Table 22.1 shows that wedge resections have a low risk of less than 5%, which is similar to patients undergoing nonthoracic surgery. However, anatomic lung resections have a greater than 10% risk of POAF.[1] These large anatomic resections of lung or esophageal structures are associated with higher rates of POAF because of the degree of unavoidable trauma to sympathovagal fibers located within the deep and superficial cardiac plexi.

Studies have shown that whether an operation is performed by open thoracotomy or minimally invasive surgery

TABLE 22.1 **RISK of Postoperative Atrial Fibrillation by Surgical Procedure**

Type of Procedures	Risk of POAF by Surgical Procedures		
	Low Risk Procedures (<5% Incidence)	Intermediate Risk Procedures (5%–15% Incidence)	High Risk Procedures (>15% Incidence)
Intrathoracic/ airway procedures Minor procedures	Flexible bronchoscopy with and without biopsy Photodynamic therapy Tracheal stenting Placement of thoracostomy tube or PleurX catheter (CareFusion Corporation, San Diego, Calif) Pleuroscopy, pleurodesis, decortication		
Procedures with moderate stress	Tracheostomy Rigid bronchoscopy Mediastinoscopy Thoracoscopic wedge resection Bronchoscopic laser surgery	Thoracoscopic sympathectomy	
Major procedures		Segmentectomy	Resection of anterior mediastinal mass Thoracoscopic lobectomy Open thoracotomy for lobectomy Tracheal resection and reconstruction/carinal resection Pneumonectomy Pleurectomy Volume reduction/bullectomy Bronchopleural fistula repair Clagett window Lung transplantation Esophagectomy
Esophageal procedures	Esophagoscopy/PEG/ esophageal dilation and/or stenting	Laparoscopic Nissen fundoplication/ myotomy Zenker diverticulectomy	
Other procedures			Pericardial window

PEG, Percutaneous endoscopic gastrostomy; *POAF*, postoperative atrial fibrillation.

(Modified from Frendl G, Sodickson AC, Chung MK, et al. 2014 AATS guidelines for the prevention and management of perioperative atrial fibrillation and flutter for thoracic surgical procedures. *J Thorac Surg*. 2014;148.)

the rates of POAF are similar. Park et al.[4] analyzed 122 patients undergoing video-assisted thoracic surgery and 122 patients undergoing an open thoracotomy. AF occurred in 12% of patients (15/122) undergoing video-assisted thoracic surgery and 16% of patients (20/122) undergoing thoracotomy (P = .36). Length of stay for patients that developed AF was greater in both video-assisted thoracic surgery (6.0 ± 1.5 days vs. 4.7 ± 2.5 days) and thoracotomy groups (9.2 ± 4.3 days vs. 6.8 ± 3.6 days). The authors concluded that regardless of surgical approach, AF after lobectomy occurred with equal frequency. This supports the theory that autonomic denervation and stress-mediated neurohumoral mechanisms are responsible for the pathogenesis of postoperative AF. Prophylaxis regimens against AF should be the same for either operative approach.

Although use of transthoracic echocardiography before surgery and presence of indices of atrial dysfunction are more sensitive than preoperative brain natriuretic peptide, the latter blood test is easier to perform and does not require expertise to acquire and analyze complex echocardiography.[5,6] Amar et al.[7] most recently created an online prediction model that incorporates age, BMI, history of AF, extent of surgery, and preoperative BNP for quick bedside calculation. This model is also displayed graphically in Fig. 22.1 for visual estimation. Finally, POAF is also correlated strongly with other complications that are sources of sympathetic stress, such

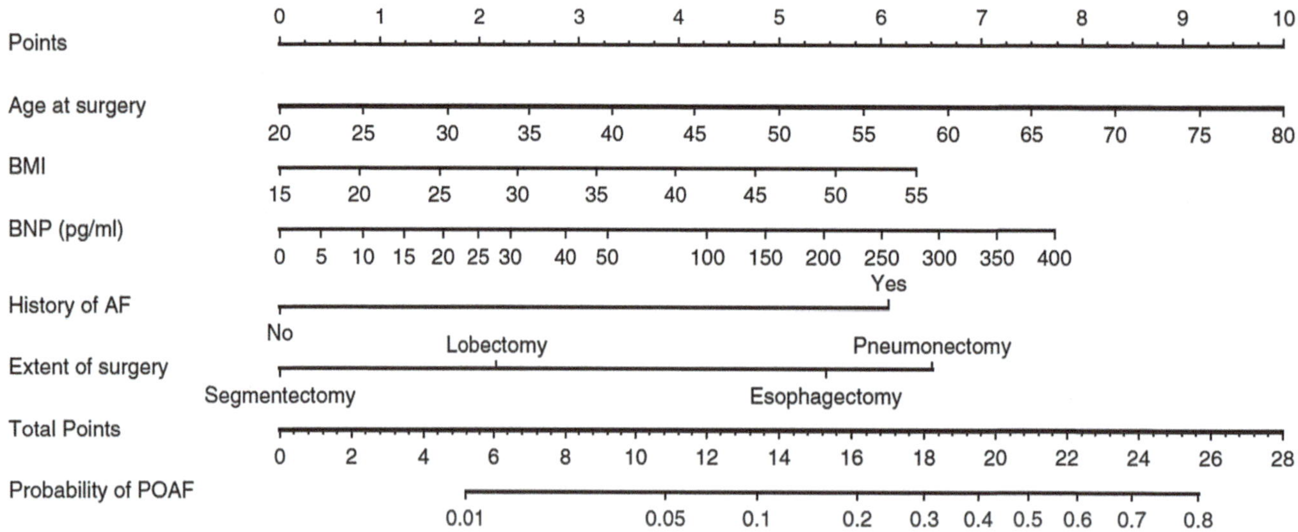

• **Fig. 22.1** The nomogram presents a visual method to calculate the probability of postoperative atrial fibrillation (*POAF*) based on a patient's combination of characteristics. To calculate the probability of POAF, sum up the point identified on the scale for each of the five variables (age, body mass index [*BMI*], brain natriuretic peptide [*BNP*] level, history of atrial fibrillation [*AF*], and extent of surgery) to obtain the total points. Draw a vertical line down from the total points scale to the last axis to obtain the corresponding probability of POAF. (Modified from Amar D, Zhang H, Tan KS, Piening D, Rusch VW, Jones DR. A brain natriuretic peptide-based prediction model for atrial fibrillation after thoracic surgery: development and internal validation. *J Thorac Surg*. 2019;157.)

as pneumonia, sepsis, and systemic inflammation.[8] In these latter settings, POAF usually occurs beyond the initial postoperative period (first 7 days) after the index surgery.

Monitoring

A common clinical question is how to determine who should be monitored with telemetry postoperatively, which has the practical implication of what inpatient units constitute a safe disposition for the patient. The 2014 American Association of Thoracic Surgeons (AATS) guidelines recommend continuous electrocardiogram monitoring for 48 to 72 hours for all patients with more than intermediate risk (>5%), that is, all patients undergoing a segmentectomy or larger resection, if their CHA_2DS_2-VASc score is 2 or more for stroke (Fig. 22.2), or if they have a history of AF.[1]

Prevention

Given the common incidence of POAF complicating the postoperative course, it stands to reason that an effective prevention program would assist in the management of these patients. In pursuit of a prevention strategy, several approaches have been tried but the ideal solution remains elusive. There is a lack of data confirming that prophylaxis leads to improved outcomes in thoracic surgery, and many of the recommendations are extrapolated from the cardiac surgery literature. The strongest recommendation with a class I indication is to continue beta blockers, if patients are taking them preoperatively for other indications (Fig. 22.3). Furthermore, restarting beta blockers on postoperative day 1 is associated with a lower POAF rate; however no difference was seen if they were restarted on the day of surgery. Khanna et al.[9] evaluated 1924

Components of CHA_2DS_2-VASc

Risk Factor	Score
Cardiac failure	1
HTN	1
Age ≥75 y	2
Diabetes	1
Stroke	2
Vascular disease (MI, PAD, aortic atherosclerosis)	1
Age 65-74 y	1
Sex category (female)	1

CHA_2DS_2-VASc Score	Annual Risk of Stroke (%)
0	0
1	1.3
2	2.2
3	3.2
4	4.0
5	6.7
6	9.8
7	9.6
8	6.7
9	15.2

• **Fig. 22.2** Stroke risk stratification in atrial fibrillation. (Modified from Frendl G, Sodickson AC, Chung MK, et al. 2014 AATS guidelines for the prevention and management of perioperative atrial fibrillation and flutter for thoracic surgical procedures. *J Thorac Surg*. 2014;148.)

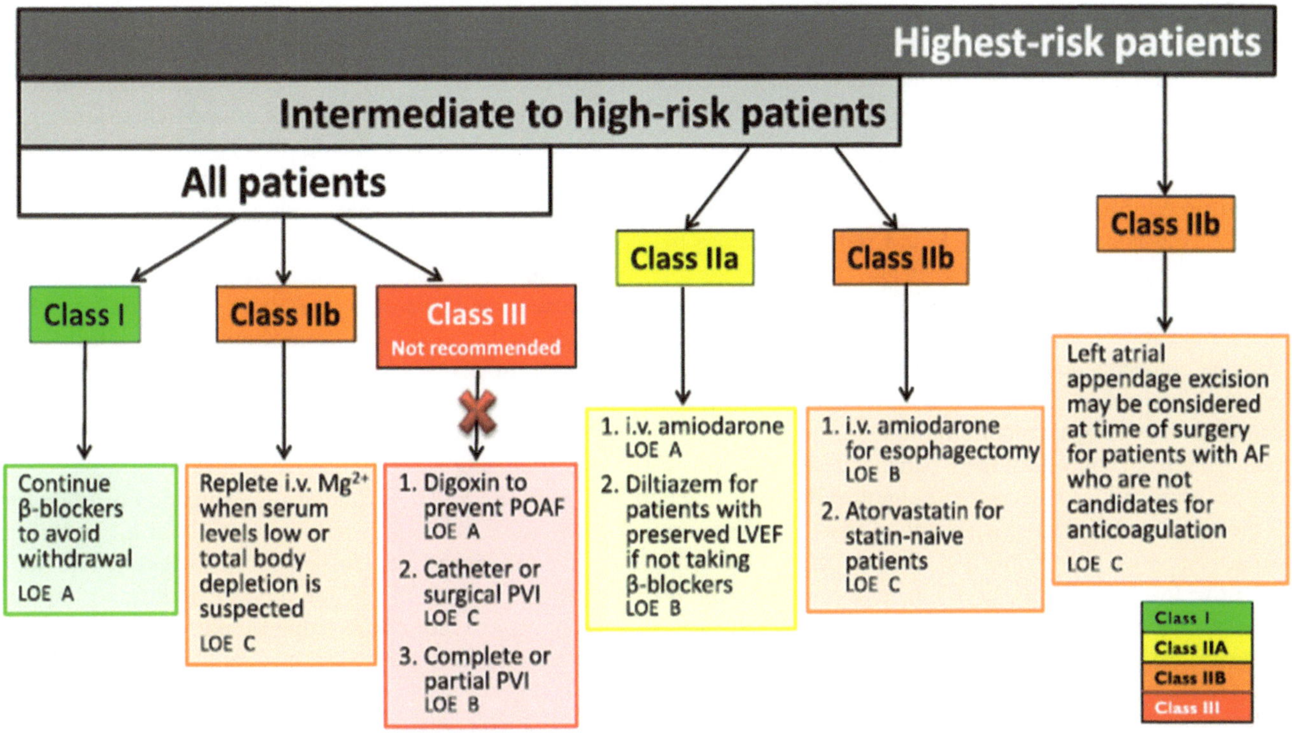

• **Fig. 22.3** Prevention strategies and their efficacy for postoperative atrial fibrillation (*POAF*). *AF*, Atrial fibrillation; *i.v.*, intravenous; *LOE*, level of evidence; *LVEF*, left ventricular ejection fraction; *PVI*, pulmonary vein isolation. (Modified from Frendl G, Sodickson AC, Chung MK, et al. 2014 AATS guidelines for the prevention and management of perioperative atrial fibrillation and flutter for thoracic surgical procedures. *J Thorac Surg*. 2014;148.)

patients who did resume beta blockers by the end of postoperative day 1 with 973 patients who had not resumed beta blockers by that time. A secondary matched analysis compared 3198 patients who resumed beta blockers on the day of surgery with 3198 who resumed thereafter. Of propensity score-matched patients who resumed beta blockers by end of postoperative day 1, 4.9% (94 of 1924) developed AF, compared with 7.0% (68 of 973) of those who resumed thereafter. Patients who resumed beta blockers on the day of surgery had an AF incidence of 4.9% versus 5.8% for those who started thereafter. The authors concluded that resuming beta blockers in chronic users by the end of the first postoperative day may be associated with lower odds of in-hospital AF.

The initiation of beta blockers or other medications for prevention is limited by their side effect profile, which varies, but nearly all can lead to hypotension and bradycardia. In the large PeriOperative ISchemic Evaluation (POISE)-I trial of de novo initiation of beta blockade on the day of surgery, in clinically effective doses, there was a significant reduction of myocardial ischemia and nonfatal myocardial infarction but at the expense of a greater incidence of perioperative stroke because of hypotension and related mortality.[10] The most commonly used medications are amiodarone, beta blockers, and calcium channel blockers. Zhao et al. found that beta blockers may be the most effective with a number needed to treat (NNT) of 5, whereas the other medications were in the 6 to 8 range.[11] The NNT offers a measurement of the impact of a medicine or therapy by estimating the number of patients that need to be treated to have an impact on one person. However, these results were derived from a meta-analysis and require additional confirmation from properly powered prospective trials. One such trial was the PRESAGE (Prevention of Atrial Fibrillation in High-risk Patients Undergoing Lung Cancer Surgery) trial that looked at a prophylactic strategy of either metoprolol or losartan in patients with elevated N-terminal pro-BNP (NT-proBNP) levels. The authors had previously studied NT-proBNP as a predictor of POAF and found a greater incidence in those with elevated levels (64% vs. 5%; $P < .001$). Cardinale et al.[12] performed a prospective, randomized study to assess whether prophylactic treatment with metoprolol or losartan, initiated soon after lung cancer surgery in patients with elevated NT-proBNP levels, reduces the incidence of postoperative AF. Some 328 patients showed a high NT-proBNP value and were enrolled: 108 were assigned to the metoprolol group, 102 to the losartan group, and 110 to the control group. Overall, the incidence of POAF was 20% ($n = 64$); it was significantly lower in the metoprolol and losartan groups compared with the control group (6%, 12%, and 40%, respectively). The authors concluded that a prophylactic treatment with metoprolol or losartan, initiated soon after lung cancer surgery in patients with high NT-proBNP levels, significantly reduced the occurrence of POAF.

As mentioned earlier, the use of beta blockers is limited by their potential side effects of bradycardia, hypotension, and bronchospasm. A promising small study showed fewer of these adverse effects with landiolol, which is a short acting β-1 selective beta blocker which can be given as an infusion.[13] Landiolol is not yet commercially available in the United States. Magnesium could be useful in patients who are depleted, and statins have also shown some efficacy but larger trials in cardiac surgery did not support their global use in prevention. Digoxin has been shown to potentially increase the incidence of POAF and should therefore be avoided as part of a prevention strategy.[1]

Studies by Tisdale et al.[14] and Riber et al.[15] have shown that amiodarone is effective in prevention of POAF, with an absolute risk reduction around 20%. Neither reported any serious adverse effects except occasional bradycardia which is expected. However, acceptance of amiodarone as a prevention strategy in thoracic surgery patients is complicated by the perceived risk of rare cases of pulmonary toxicity, which is thought to result from an idiopathic allergic reaction to the drug.[16] Although this is only a concern in patients on long-term therapy, and there is no risk in short-term exposure of less than 1 month, which can be reasonable in the immediate postoperative period. Additional concerns were raised following a small, randomized trial that was stopped because of development of acute respiratory distress syndrome in three of 11 patients undergoing right-sided pneumonectomy. However, this complication is a known risk of pneumonectomy, and the results have not been replicated or supported in subsequent observational and prospective studies. Furthermore, the cumulative dose of amiodarone in this study was more than 2 g over 24 hours, and prevention strategies targeting cumulative doses under 2 g have not shown this adverse effect. In addition, in the lung transplantation literature, although there is some retrospective evidence that amiodarone use for AF may be associated with increased mortality, the preponderance of evidence suggests that there is no increase in adverse effects.[17–19]

Finally, in terms of surgical approaches, prophylactic catheter or surgical pulmonary vein isolation and ablation is not recommended as a means of preventing POAF associated with major general thoracic surgery in contrast to that of cardiac surgery. In rare circumstances, for patients with preexisting AF who are considered too high risk for anticoagulation in the perioperative period, the insertion of a Watchman device (Boston Scientific, Marlborough, MA) for closure of the left atrial appendage may be considered before extensive lung surgery.[1] Because there are no studies to support this recommendation in this clinical setting, risk/benefit discussions between the patient, cardiac electrophysiologist, and surgeon should be undertaken to inform individualized decisions of care.

Treatment of Postoperative Atrial Fibrillation

Once a patient has developed POAF, there are several issues that need to be addressed before establishing proper treatment. The first and most important is to determine if that patient is hemodynamically stable. If the patient is unstable with symptomatic severe hypotension, acute myocardial ischemia, or pulmonary edema, then treatment should proceed promptly with a synchronized direct current cardioversion. If unsuccessful, repeat cardioversion attempts with concurrent intravenous pharmacologic treatment with either beta blockers, such as metoprolol or esmolol, L-type calcium channel blockers, such as diltiazem or verapamil, or rhythm control drugs, such as amiodarone or ibutilide. Digoxin may be added in patients with heart failure. In addition, if feasible, catecholaminergic agents should be stopped, fluid balance be optimized, and electrolytes should be normalized. The care team should evaluate for potential triggers of POAF: bleeding, pneumothorax, pericardial processes, airway issues with possible hypoxemia, infection, or the presence of sepsis. Often, none of these are present, as the triggering factor is the inflammation provoked by the surgery itself. Unless there is high suspicion or evidence of myocardial ischemia or pulmonary embolism, the 2014 and 2019 American Heart Association (AHA) guidelines for the management of AF do not support performing expensive laboratory or radiologic testing to rule out these conditions, because the likelihood of positive results is extremely small.[20]

Rate Control

In the hemodynamically stable patient, the goal becomes to establish lenient rate control of less than 110 beats per minute. The rationale is that up to 80% of patients with POAF will return to sinus rhythm in under 24 hours, and nearly all within 4 to 6 weeks. In addition, the Atrial Fibrillation Follow-Up Investigation of Rhythm Management (AFFIRM) trial in patients with chronic AF unrelated to surgery showed no difference in outcomes between patients managed with a rate versus rhythm control strategy. Wyse et al.,[21] evaluated the impact of individual antiarrhythmic drugs on mortality and hospital stay in AF. Cardiovascular outcomes in AF patients receiving pharmacologic rhythm control therapy have not been compared with rate control therapy on the basis of antiarrhythmic drug selection. The authors included 729 amiodarone patients, 606 sotalol patients, and 268 class 1C patients were matched. The composite outcome of mortality or cardiovascular hospital stays showed better outcomes with rate control therapy compared with amiodarone. There was a nonsignificant increase in mortality with amiodarone; however, the risk of noncardiovascular death was significantly higher with amiodarone versus rate control.

The medications used for rate control are similar to those used for prevention and as such, they are limited by their side effect profile. Notably, the major adverse effect of **beta blockers** is bronchospasm in patients with asthma and exacerbation of heart failure symptoms in patients with decompensated heart failure. **Diltiazem** is another option, however in combination with beta blockers can lead to profound hypotension. **Digoxin** has a very narrow therapeutic window and should be avoided in patients with hypertrophic cardiomyopathy; however, it may be useful in patients with decreased ejection fraction or history of heart failure.

Amiodarone is an acceptable option for rate control and is preferred in patients with hypotension or decreased ejection fraction. It also has the advantage of being an antiarrhythmic medication and can restore sinus rhythm. In patients with Wolff-Parkinson-White syndrome, atrioventricular nodal blocking agents should be avoided as they can potentiate rapid conduction through the accessory pathway; an antiarrhythmic medication should be chosen for these conditions. Cardiology consultation should be considered if the patient develops recurrent/refractory POAF, has a high risk for stroke, requires a second-line antiarrhythmic medication, or develops acute kidney injury. In a landmark trial comparing a rate control strategy to rhythm control strategy for the management of acute POAF associated with cardiac surgery, Gillinov et al.[22] showed that there were no differences in any measured outcome at 30 or 60 days between the groups. **Both AHA and AATS guidelines recommend a rate control strategy first for the acute management of AF or POAF.**[1,21]

Rhythm Control

Despite the high rate of spontaneous conversion to sinus rhythm in the first 24 hours, some patients will remain in AF. The risk for stroke increases significantly enough after 48 hours in AF to mandate anticoagulation therapy. Some postoperative patients are at a high risk for significant bleeding if anticoagulated. In these patients, it is reasonable to pursue a rhythm control strategy in the first 24- to 48-hour window after POAF onset to restore sinus rhythm, thus potentially avoiding the need for anticoagulation and bleeding risk. A rhythm control strategy is also indicated for patients that fail rate control therapy or who remain symptomatic and difficult to achieve adequate rate control. Of the antiarrhythmic medications, amiodarone is the most common followed by sotalol, flecainide, propafenone, and dofetilide. Of interest, despite the wide use of amiodarone for the management of patients with AF in the general population its use for this indication is still off label. Notably, flecainide and propafenone are very effective medications to restore sinus rhythm; unfortunately, they should be avoided in patients with structural heart disease, such as those with ischemia, valvular heart disease, or significant left ventricular hypertrophy.[1] The treatment of the hemodynamically stable patient with new onset POAF is summarized in Fig. 22.4.

Anticoagulation

For all patients with POAF lasting longer than 48 hours, anticoagulation is indicated. Anticoagulation is recommended for 3 to 4 weeks before and 4 weeks after cardioversion. Alternatively, in patients in whom anticoagulation is relatively contraindicated, one can perform a transesophageal echocardiogram and if no thrombus is identified can proceed with immediate cardioversion and consider anticoagulation for 4 weeks after the procedure. Alternatively, as mentioned previously, in very rare circumstances an insertion of a Watchman device (Boston Scientific, Marlborough, MA) for closure of the left atrial appendage can be considered. This approach has been referred to as the "fast-track" pathway and has been shown to be safe when compared with the conventional approach.[1]

Anticoagulation can be accomplished with warfarin for a target international normalized ratio 2.0 to 3.0 or with the more recent nonvitamin K oral anticoagulants (NOACs). The NOACs have been shown to be noninferior to warfarin for prevention of AF-related thromboembolism and offer several advantages including: lower risk of fatal bleeding and intracranial hemorrhage, fixed dosing schedule that does not require coagulation monitoring, fewer drug-drug interactions, and shorter half-lives. Conversely, disadvantages include an increased risk of gastrointestinal bleeding. Notably, patients with valvular AF (AF secondary to prosthetic heart valve, rheumatic mitral stenosis, or mitral valve repair) were left out of safety studies and therefore the NOACs are not approved in these patients. Other contraindications include: mechanical prosthetic heart valve, severe renal dysfunction with creatinine clearance less than 15 mL/min, severe liver dysfunction, pregnancy, and need to take concomitant potent inhibitors of p-glycoprotein. An additional difference between the NOACs and warfarin is that prothrombin time and partial thromboplastin time coagulation studies do not accurately reflect the medication's effect nor adequate cessation of effect. The level of NOACs effects can be monitored by specialized tests that may not be readily available in all settings.[23] The NOACs and their sites of action are summarized in Fig. 22.5.

The particularly difficult question in postoperative thoracic surgery patients who develop POAF is the need to anticoagulate within the first 48 hours. This is determined by their CHA_2DS_2-VASc score (see Fig. 22.2). Reviewing the scoring system shows an overlap with many typical comorbidities in thoracic surgery patients. In patients with 0 points anticoagulation is not recommended. A score of 1 is equivocal and it is recommended to consider anticoagulation if the benefits outweigh the bleeding risks. For patients with a score of 2 or more, anticoagulation is highly recommended if its benefits outweigh the risk of bleeding. These patients are often at high risk of bleeding and therefore a joint discussion between the surgeon and cardiologist must take place to assess this risk. The frequency of POAF and the balancing of potentially catastrophic risks of bleeding versus stroke in this subset of patients reinforces the needed for an effective and safe prevention strategy. Although not developed for postoperative patients, calculation of the HAS-BLED (Hypertension, Abnormal renal/liver function, Stroke, Bleeding history or predisposition, Labile international normalized ration, Elderly [>65 years], Drugs/alcohol concomitantly) score can help the treating physicians involved to assess the risk of bleeding.[24] (HAS-BLED is a scoring system developed to assess 1-year risk of bleeding in patients taking anticoagulant with AF.) A HAS-BLED score greater than 3 indicates a higher risk of bleeding (Fig. 22.6).

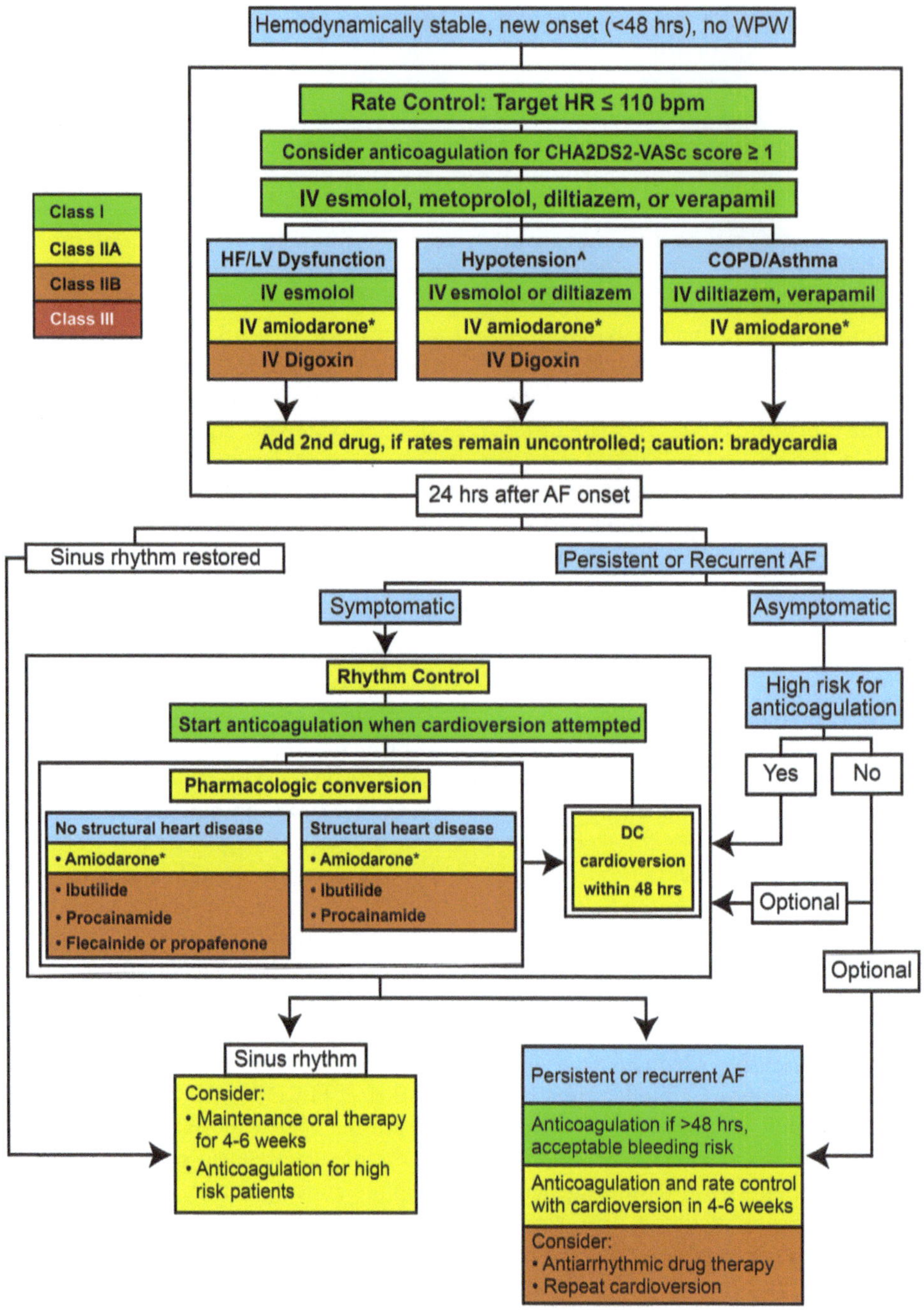

*Caution should be exercised and a TEE considered if amiodarone is used after 48 hours after the onset of AF, as there is a possibility that the rhythm could convert with risk of thromboembolism.
^Esmolol or diltiazem first line depending on degree of hypotension

• **Fig. 22.4** Management of the hemodynamically stable patient with new onset postoperative atrial fibrillation (POAF) of less than 48 hours duration. *AF*, Atrial fibrillation; *COPD*, chronic obstructive pulmonary disease; *DC*, direct current; *HF*, heart failure, *HR*, heart rate; *IV*, intravenous; *TEE*, transesophageal echocardiography; *WPW*, Wolff-Parkinson-White syndrome. (Modified from Frendl G, Sodickson AC, Chung MK, et al. 2014 AATS guidelines for the prevention and management of perioperative atrial fibrillation and flutter for thoracic surgical procedures. *J Thorac Surg*. 2014;148.)

Other Arrhythmias

Although POAF is the most common postoperative arrhythmia in thoracic surgery patients, it is not the only arrhythmia. Similar to POAF, any unstable rhythm is an indication for synchronized cardioversion or defibrillation. For stable supraventricular tachycardia that is not caused by AF or atrial flutter, it is recommended to treat the patient in the following stepwise fashion until sinus rhythm is returned: vagal maneuvers followed by medical therapy with either adenosine, beta blockers, diltiazem, or verapamil, and, if still ineffective, synchronized cardioversion.[25] Notably, for

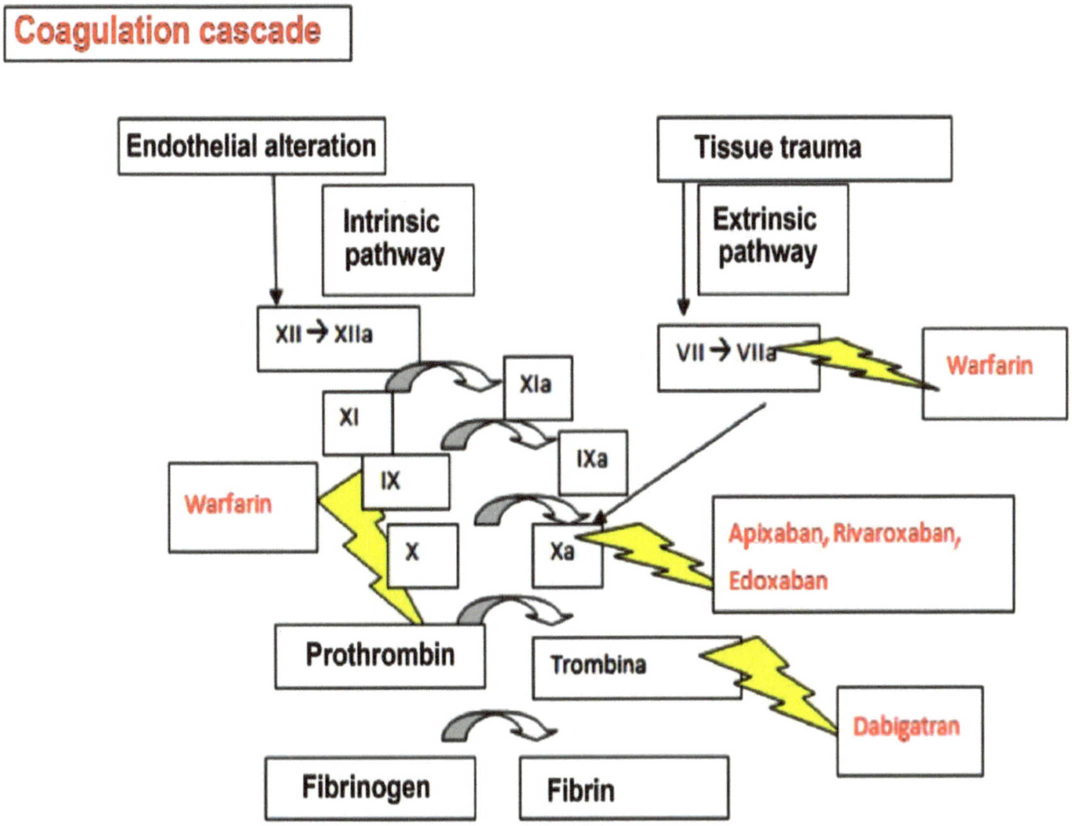

	Dabigatran	Apixaban	Edoxaban	Rivaroxaban
Standard dosing*	150 mg or 110 mg twice daily	5 mg twice daily	60 mg once daily	20 mg once daily
Dose adjustment in patients with chronic kidney disease and for age, weight, co-medication*	No (creatinine clearance <30 mL/min contraindicated)	2.5 mg twice daily in patients with atrial fibrillation and severe chronic kidney disease (creatinine clearance 15–29 mL/min) or at least 2 of the following criteria: age ≥ 80 years; body weight ≤ 60 kg or serum creatinine ≥ 1.5 mg/dL	30 mg once daily, in the presence of the following factors: Creatinine clearance 15–49 mL/min, body weight ≤ 60 kg, co-medication with cyclosporine, dronedarone, erythromycin or ketoconazole	15 mg once daily in patients with atrial fibrillation, if creatinine clearance 15–49 mL/min
Bioavailability	3–7%	50%	62%	66% without food, almost 100% with food
Prodrug	Yes	No	No	No
Non-renal/renal clearance of the absorbed dose (with normal renal function)	20% / 80%	73% / 27%	50% / 50%	65% / 35%
Hepatic drug metabolism: CYP450 involved	No	Yes (elimination; low CYP3A4 involvement)	minimal (<10% of elimination)	Yes (elimination)
Absorption with concomitant food intake	No effect	No effect	No effect	+39% more
Recommended to take with food?	No	No	No	Compulsory
Absorption with H2 blocker/ proton pump inhibitor treatment	–12–30%	No effect	No effect	No effect
Asian patients	+25%	No effect	No effect	No effect
Gastrointestinal tolerability	Dyspepsia 5–10%	No problems	No problems	No problems
Elimination half-life	12–17 hrs	12 hrs	9–11 hrs	5–9 hrs (younger) 11–13 hrs (older)
Specific antidote available	Yes	No	No	No

• **Fig. 22.5** Non-Vitamin K oral anticoagulants and their sites of action.

Letter	Clinical Characteristic[a]	Points Awarded
H	Hypertension	1
A	Abnormal renal and liver function (1 point each)	1 or 2
S	Stroke	1
B	Bleeding	1
L	Labile INRs	1
E	Elderly	1
D	Drugs or alcohol (1 point each)	1 or 2

• **Fig. 22.6** ***HAS-BLED***, Hypertension, Abnormal renal/liver function, Stroke, Bleeding history or predisposition, Labile international normalized ration, Elderly (>65 years), Drugs/alcohol concomitantly; *INR*, international normalized ratio. (Modified from Pisters R, Lane DA, Nieuwlaat R, Vos CBD, Crijns HJ, Lip GY. A novel user-friendly score (HAS-BLED) to assess 1-year risk of major bleeding in patients with atrial fibrillation. *Chest*. 2010; 138:1093–1100.)

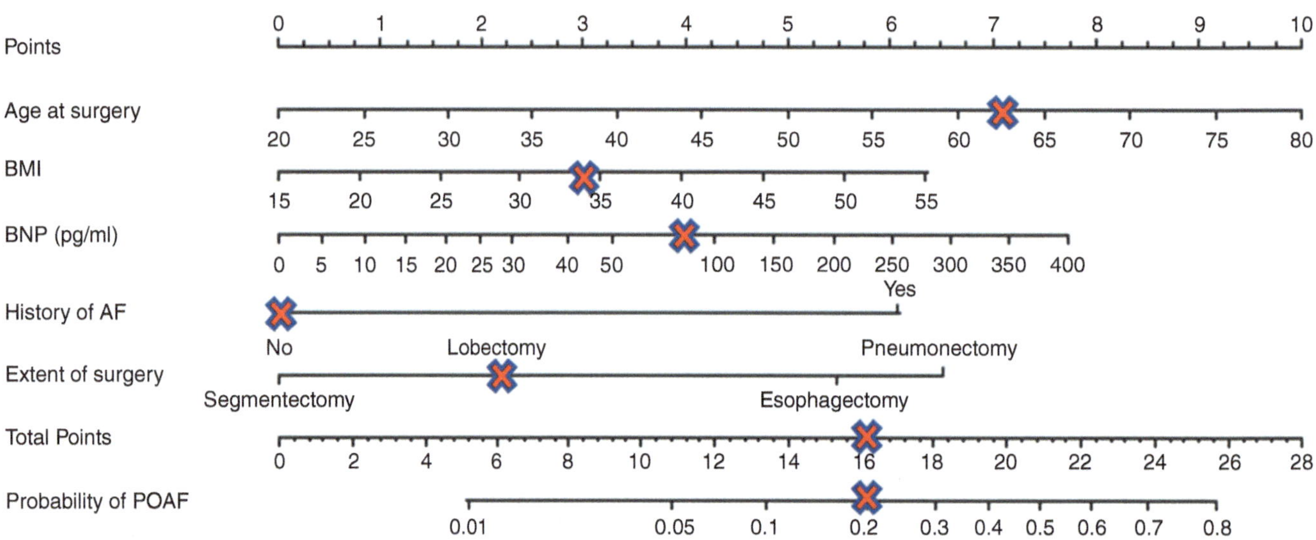

• **Fig. 22.7** Using the nomogram from Fig. 22.1, the patient has approximately a 20% chance of developing postoperative atrial fibrillation (*Red X's* indicate where this patient falls on scale). *AF,* Atrial fibrillation; *BNP,* brain natriuretic peptide; *BMI,* body mass index; *POAF,* postoperative atrial fibrillation.

patients in atrial flutter, anticoagulation is indicated following the same guidelines as AF. In general, atrial flutter can be converted to sinus rhythm with electrical cardioversion more successfully than AF. Clinically significant bradyarrhythmias are rare, with complete heart block reported in 0.1% of patients who had noncardiac surgery.[1] Patients with complete heart block can be managed with either medications and/or temporary noninvasive cardiac pacing until more definitive therapy is done. Lastly, transient nonsustained ventricular tachycardia (VT) occurs frequently (15%) in the postoperative period and is usually benign and associated with a favorable outcome. More malignant sustained VT and/or ventricular fibrillation are rare events. Amar et al.[26] evaluated the incidence and significance of ventricular arrhythmias early after thoracic surgery. The database from 412 patients who had lobectomy ($n = 243$) or pneumonectomy ($n = 169$) and were continuously monitored with Holter recorders for 72 to 96 hours postoperatively was analyzed. The primary end point of the study was the occurrence of VT defined as three or more consecutive wide complexes. Some 61 of 412 patients (15%) developed one or more episodes of VT. There were no episodes of sustained (>30 seconds) VT and no patient required treatment for hemodynamic compromise associated with any VT episode.

Case Discussion

A 62-year-old male, former 20 pack year smoker, with hypertension, hyperlipidemia, and chronic obstructive pulmonary disease presents for right upper lobectomy for adenocarcinoma. He has no allergies and takes amlodipine, atorvastatin, losartan, and metoprolol daily. His BMI is 34 kg/m^2, hemoglobin 14, Cr 1.1, BNP 84.

Question 1: What is his risk of developing POAF?

Question 2: What would you suggest to your surgical colleagues for prevention?

Question 3: On postoperative day 3, he develops POAF. What is his CHA_2DS_2-VASc score and does he require anticoagulation?

Answers 1: Following the subsequent nomogram (Fig. 22.7), you can see that his probability of developing POAF is approximately 20%.

Answer 2: The most effective strategy is to make sure his beta blocker therapy is continued throughout the perioperative period. The AATS Task Force recommends using amiodarone or diltiazem for prevention in patients at intermediate or high risk for POAF.

Answer 3: His CHA_2DS_2-VASc score is 1 for hypertension. This is fairly low risk and means anticoagulation should be considered but is not necessarily indicated in the first 48 hours. If he should remain in AF for more than 48 hours, then he will require anticoagulation.

Conclusion

POAF is the most common complication after thoracic surgery and increases in frequency with older age and more extensive surgical resection. It is associated with an increase in length of stay, costs, and long-term stroke risk. Prevention strategies are effective and reasonable but can be limited by their side effects. Prompt rate control should be initiated once POAF develops and anticoagulation considered based on a patient's CHA_2DS_2-VASc score. Those patients at significant risk for bleeding can be considered for rhythm control to avoid needing anticoagulation. AF persisting beyond 48 hours requires anticoagulation given the increased risk of thromboembolic complications.

References

1. Frendl G, Sodickson AC, Chung MK, et al. 2014 AATS guidelines for the prevention and management of perioperative atrial fibrillation and flutter for thoracic surgical procedures. *J Thorac Surg.* 2014;148:e153–e193.
2. Bhave PD, Goldman LE, Vittinghoff E, Maselli J, Auerbach A. Incidence, predictors, and outcomes associated with postoperative atrial fibrillation after major noncardiac surgery. *Am Heart J.* 2012;164:918–924.
3. Amar D, Zhang H, Miodownik S, Kadish AH. Competing autonomic mechanisms precede the onset of postoperative atrial fibrillation. *J Am Coll Cardiol.* 2003;42:1262–1268.
4. Park BJ, Zhang H, Rusch VW, Amar D. Video-assisted thoracic surgery does not reduce the incidence of postoperative atrial fibrillation after pulmonary lobectomy. *J Thorac Surg.* 2007;133: 775–779.
5. Brecher O, Gulati H, Roistacher N, et al. Preoperative echocardiographic indices of diastolic dysfunction and brain natriuretic peptide in predicting postoperative atrial fibrillation after noncardiac surgery. *Anesth Analg.* 2017;124:1099–1104.
6. Raman T, Roistacher N, Liu J, et al. Preoperative left atrial dysfunction and risk of postoperative atrial fibrillation complicating thoracic surgery. *J Thorac Surg.* 2012;143:482–487.
7. Amar D, Zhang H, Tan KS, Piening D, Rusch VW, Jones DR. A brain natriuretic peptide-based prediction model for atrial fibrillation after thoracic surgery: development and internal validation. *J Thorac Surg.* 2019;157:2493–2499.
8. McCormack O, Zaborowski A, King S, et al. New-onset atrial fibrillation post-surgery for esophageal and junctional cancer. *Ann Surg.* 2014;260:772–778.
9. Khanna AK, Naylor DF, Naylor AJ, et al. Early resumption of β blockers is associated with decreased atrial fibrillation after noncardiothoracic and nonvascular surgery. *Anesthesiology.* 2018;129: 1101–1110.
10. Devereaux PJ, Yang H, Yusuf S, et al. Effects of extended-release metoprolol succinate in patients undergoing non-cardiac surgery (POISE trial): a randomised controlled trial. *Lancet.* 2008; 371:1839–1847.
11. Zhao B-C, Huang T-Y, Deng Q-W, et al. Prophylaxis against atrial fibrillation after general thoracic surgery. *Chest.* 2017;151:149–159.
12. Cardinale D, Sandri M, Colombo A, et al. Prevention of atrial fibrillation in high-risk patients undergoing lung cancer surgery: the PRESAGE trial. *Ann Surg.* 2016:264.
13. Balik M, Sander M, Trimmel H, Heinz G. Landiolol for managing postoperative atrial fibrillation. *Eur Heart J Suppl.* 2018:20.
14. Tisdale J, Jaynes H, Watson M, Corya A, Kesler K. Intravenous amiodarone for prevention of atrial fibrillation following esophagectomy: a propensity score-matched analysis. *J Am Coll Cardiol.* 2017;69:545.
15. Riber LP, Larsen TB, Christensen TD. Postoperative atrial fibrillation prophylaxis after lung surgery: systematic review and meta-analysis. *Ann Thorac Surg.* 2014;98:1989–1997.
16. Schwaiblmair M, Berghaus T, Haeckel T, Wagner T, Scheidt WV. Amiodarone-induced pulmonary toxicity: an under-recognized and severe adverse effect? *Clin Res Cardiol.* 2010;99:693–700.
17. Henri C, Giraldeau G, Dorais M, et al. Atrial fibrillation after pulmonary transplantation. *Circ Arrhythm Electrophysiol.* 2012;5: 61–67.
18. Isiadinso I, Meshkov AB, Gaughan J. Atrial arrhythmias after lung and heart–lung transplant: effects on short-term mortality and the influence of amiodarone. *J Heart Lung Transplant.* 2011;30:37–44.
19. Berry MF, D'Amico TA, Onaitis MW. Use of amiodarone after major lung resection. *Ann Thorac Surg.* 2014;98:1199–1206.
20. January CT, Wann LS, Calkins H, et al. 2019 AHA/ACC/HRS focused update of the 2014 AHA/ACC/HRS guideline for the management of patients with atrial fibrillation. *Circulation.* 2019;140(2).
21. Wyse DG, Waldo AL, DiMarco JP, et al., Atrial Fibrillation Follow-up Investigation of Rhythm Management (AFFIRM) Investigators. A comparison of rate control and rhythm control in patients with atrial fibrillation. *N Engl J Med.* 2002;347:1825–1833.
22. Gillinov AM, Bagiella E, Moskowitz AJ, et al. Rate control versus rhythm control for atrial fibrillation after cardiac surgery. *N Engl J Med.* 2016;374(20):1911–1921.
23. Verma A, Ha A, Rutka J, Verma S. What surgeons should know about non–vitamin K oral anticoagulants. *JAMA Surg.* 2018;153(6):577–585.
24. Pisters R, Lane DA, Nieuwlaat R, Vos CBD, Crijns HJ, Lip GY. A novel user-friendly score (HAS-BLED) to assess 1-year risk of major bleeding in patients with atrial fibrillation. *Chest.* 2010;138:1093–1100.
25. Al-Khatib SM, Page RL. Acute treatment of patients with supraventricular tachycardia. *JAMA Cardiol.* 2016;1:483.
26. Amar D, Zhang H, Roistacher N. The incidence and outcome of ventricular arrhythmias after noncardiac thoracic surgery. *Anesth Analg.* 2002;95:537–543.

23

Anesthesia for Pediatric Thoracic Surgery

CESAR RODRIGUEZ-DIAZ

Introduction

Pediatric patients undergoing thoracic surgery can be particularly challenging because of the differences in anatomy, physiology, and behavior in comparison to adult patients. The anesthesiologists must be cognizant of these to successfully manage these patients. The availability of proper pediatric size equipment, such as bronchoscopes and bronchial blockers (BBs), allows the anesthesiologist to achieve optimal operating conditions particularly during minimally invasive procedures. However, oftentimes, because of the small size of some patients, the anesthesiologist is required to modify the standard adult techniques to achieve one-lung ventilation (OLV). In this chapter, we will review the specific anatomic and physiologic characteristics that make pediatric thoracic patients different from adult patients. In addition, we will review techniques that have been proven successful even in the smallest patients.

Pediatric Anatomy and Physiology

Anatomy

Pediatric patients have several key differences in anatomy as compared with the adult, of which anesthesiologists must be aware to successfully take care of these patients during thoracic surgery. The most prominent airway characteristics are listed here[1]:

- Large head, short neck, and a prominent occiput.
- Tongue is relatively large.
- Larynx is high and anterior, at the level of C3–C4.
- Epiglottis is long, stiff, and U-shaped.
- Preferential nasal breathing.
- Airway is funnel shaped and narrowest at the level of the cricoid cartilage.
- Airway is small and prone to develop edema resulting in airway obstruction.

Physiology

Pediatric patients have a baseline limited respiratory reserve during normal two-lung ventilation compared with adults because of several reasons listed here[2]:

- Horizontal ribs prevent the "bucket handle" action seen in adult breathing and limit an increase in tidal volume. Ventilation is primarily diaphragmatic.
- The chest wall is significantly more compliant than that of an adult. Subsequently, the functional residual capacity (FRC) is relatively low. FRC decreases with apnea and anesthesia causing lung collapse.
- Minute ventilation is rate dependent because there few ways to increase tidal volume.
- The closing volume is larger than the FRC until 6 to 8 years of age. This causes an increased tendency for airway closure at end expiration. Thus neonates and infants generally need intermittent positive pressure ventilation during anesthesia and would benefit from a higher respiratory rate and the use of positive expiratory end-pressure (PEEP).
- Muscles of ventilation are easily subject to fatigue because of low percentage of type I muscle fibers in the diaphragm. This number increases to the adult level over the first year of life.
- The alveoli are thick walled at birth. There is only 10% of the total number of alveoli found in adults. The alveoli clusters develop over the first 8 years of life.
- Apneas are common postoperatively in premature infants.
- High oxygen (O_2) consumption compared with adult.

In addition to the baseline limited respiratory reserve in two-lung ventilation, the respiratory physiology of pediatric patients is also different from adults in the lateral decubitus OLV. Unlike adults, oxygenation is higher in the nondependent lung rather than the dependent one (healthy lung), especially in neonates and infants. The reason for this is that children have an easily compressible chest wall and FRC becomes equal to the residual volume in the dependent lung, and small airways begin to close even in tidal volume values. Hydrostatic pressure between dependent and nondependent lungs is minimal because of the small size of children. Therefore the advantage of better oxygenation in the nondependent lung is not present in children. As a result, compared with adults, children are at greater risk for developing hypoxemia or airway complications during thoracoscopic surgery or thoracotomy.

Preoperative Evaluation

A standard preoperative evaluation assessing for allergies, comorbidities, and current medication use, is necessary to reduce perioperative complications children undergoing thoracic surgery. Fasting time should be reviewed. Two hours nil per os (NPO) for clear fluids, 4 hours for breast milk, and at least 6 hours for formula milk or a light meal, is recommended per the American Society of Anesthesiology guidelines.[3] It is imperative for the anesthesiologist to evaluate for the presence of acute and chronic pulmonary and cardiac pathology. Dyspnea and decreased tolerance to exercise are signs indicating decreased pulmonary reserve.

The presence of a current or recent upper respiratory tract infection must be ascertained because the risk of perioperative complications increases for the following 2 to 4 weeks from the initial illness. Sometimes it might be prudent to delay the surgery for such time to pass. However, on occasions it might be advisable to proceed with surgery if it is deemed that the outcome would supersede the increased risk. The decision to proceed or delay the surgery should be made after a thoughtful discussion between the surgeon, the anesthesiologist, and the parents.

Lung auscultation must be performed to evaluate for the presence of pathologic breath sounds, such as rhonchi or wheezing. Ancillary tests, such as arterial blood gas analysis, radiographies, echocardiograms, or respiratory function tests should be reviewed if present, but not necessarily ordered routinely. Blood gas analysis is not mandatory in children. It is usually sufficient to evaluate peripheral oxygen saturation and venous bicarbonate concentrations, which is always elevated in children with chronic carbon dioxide (CO_2) retention.[4,5] Radiographic studies may help the anesthesiologist to anticipate for possible problems, such as difficult intubation, potential blood loss if a lesion is adherent to a great vessel, or even cardiovascular collapse from anterior mediastinal mass following induction of anesthesia. Although respiratory function tests are not routinely recommended in asymptomatic patients, they may be useful to determine the progression of disease. Since they require patient's cooperation it is only feasible from a certain age. It is also necessary for the anesthesiologists to investigate whether the indication for surgery is related to a congenital disease. In adults, the indication is usually limited to infections, and commonly for tumors and lobe resections, whereas in younger children, congenital diseases, such as pulmonary sequestration, congenital diaphragmatic hernia, tracheoesophageal fistulas, congenital lobar emphysema, vascular rings, and tracheal stenosis are most common. In these cases, it is necessary to rule out the presence of a cardiac disease that is often associated with many congenital pathologies.

Anesthetic Techniques

Bronchoscopy

Flexible bronchoscopy is helpful in the diagnosis of chronic respiratory ailments. It allows the evaluation of the airway for fixed or dynamic changes occurring with ventilation, such as in vascular rings or tracheomalacia, respectively. Maintaining spontaneous ventilation is necessary to diagnose dynamic changes in airway patency. Intravenous sedation along with topicalization is often the preferred choice of anesthetic for older children. Younger children will often require general anesthesia, which can be facilitated with an airway device such as a laryngeal mask airway, but as mentioned previously, spontaneous ventilation must be insured. If the flexible bronchoscopy is being done for other purposes, such as for biopsy samples or performing an alveolar lavage, general endotracheal anesthesia with or without paralysis is often preferred. It is not uncommon to have to upsize the endotracheal tube (ETT) size to accommodate a flexible fiberoptic scope with a working channel.

Rigid bronchoscopy (RB) is another diagnostic and therapeutic modality. It is most commonly used in pediatric patients for the treatment of aspirated foreign bodies to be removed through the rigid bronchoscope lumen. Because of the highly stimulating effects from the rigid bronchoscope, it is performed under general anesthesia. The plan for maintaining either spontaneous ventilation or providing controlled ventilation should be discussed and coordinated with the surgeon. The techniques can vary but can be summarized as: (1) insufflating sevoflurane on the airway of a spontaneously breathing patient; (2) intermittent controlled ventilation via the bronchoscope; or (3) intermittent jet ventilation. Each technique has its benefits and downsides. **Insufflating sevoflurane** on a spontaneously breathing patient, in theory, should minimize dislodgement of a foreign body but can risk hypoventilation if deeply anesthetized, or unwanted motion, cough, retching, laryngospasm and even bronchospasm if the anesthetic depth is not sufficient.[6–8] Another concern is operating room pollution with volatile anesthetic and aerosol particles spread. **Intermittent controlled ventilation via the bronchoscope** can work for a deeply anesthetized and perhaps paralyzed patient, but has the downside of air leak through the outer part of the rigid bronchoscope leading to suboptimal tidal volumes. In addition, the positive pressure can dislodge a foreign body distally. During positive pressure ventilation, the viewing port must be occluded, interfering with the procedure, to deliver an effective breath through the ventilation port of the rigid bronchoscope.[9] **Jet ventilation** offers the advantages of allowing bronchoscopic interventions to be performed without cessations. Complications include barotrauma, inability to predict fraction of inspired oxygen (FiO_2) and monitor end-tidal CO_2, foreign body dislocation, and blowing of blood and debris materials to distal airways resulting in inadequate gas exchange. Low-frequency jet ventilation should not be used in patients with tracheobronchial mucosa injury or low respiratory compliance.[10] A total intravenous anesthetic should be considered in cases where controlled ventilation is planned, to minimize operating room air pollution with inhaled anesthetic. It is advised to use spontaneous ventilation for the removal of proximally located foreign bodies and positive pressure ventilation for the removal of distally located foreign bodies.[11] Regardless of the technique used, adequate depth of anesthesia and airway patency need to be ensured. The key to an uncomplicated procedure is the cooperation of the surgeon and the anesthesiologist.

It should be considered that aspirated foreign body retrieval is usually performed emergently. Foreign bodies can swell, progressively occluding the airway, can cause an inflammatory reaction on the airway, or can cause airway perforation leading to pneumomediastinum or subcutaneous emphysema. Fortunately, most patient do not present with many comorbidities because there is minimal time for optimization. Premedication targeting a decrease in the production of saliva and anxiety is beneficial. Albuterol sulfate and budesonide inhalations are reported to be advantageous in reducing perioperative pulmonary complications.[6] The knowledge of the type, place, and aspiration time of the foreign body is important. If it is above the carina, there is a total obstruction risk, which could be precipitated with positive pressure ventilation. Inhalational or intravenous agents or both may be administered. During maintenance, short-acting agents, such as propofol, dexmedetomidine, remifentanil and short-acting muscle relaxants are administered as the procedure is generally quite short. Nitrous oxide is not recommended because many patients undergoing RB have air trapping to some extent.

Severe complications can occur during RB,[12] which are closely related to the patient's condition, the severity of the pathology, the experience of the surgeon and the anesthesiologist. Failure to retrieve the foreign body might necessitate an emergent thoracotomy or tracheostomy.

Sternotomy

In children, sternotomy is generally performed for the biopsy or removal of the mediastinal tumors. A detailed history and physical examination are extremely important. Anesthesiologists should focus on the respiratory system symptoms, such as difficulty in breathing, cyanosis, or stridor aggravated by motion, cough, or straining. Wheezing unresponsive to the bronchodilators, recurrent pneumonia, persistent atelectasis, pericardial invasion, arrhythmias, pulsus paradoxus, or signs of the superior vena cava syndrome are the warning pathologies for a complicated perioperative period. Echocardiographic examination is mandatory in children with mediastinal tumors to determine a possible mass effect from compression of the surrounding structures. The riskiest period is the induction of anesthesia especially in previously symptomatic children. Decrease in the sympathetic tonus, loss of the spontaneous ventilation and physiologic changes related to patient position diminish compensatory mechanisms. Children with mediastinal mass are at increased risk of severe airway obstruction and hemodynamic instability on induction. The pediatric surgeon must be ready to perform emergent RB during the anesthesia induction of children with a mediastinal mass in cases of total obstruction as a result of a mass effect. During induction of anesthesia, preservation of the spontaneous ventilation to secure the airway continuity (and to never burn your bridges), is recommended. If airway obstruction occurred during induction of anesthesia, turning the child to the lateral position will move the obstructing mass away from the trachea and help to open the airways. In cases of superior vena cava obstruction symptoms, induction must be performed in the sitting position and intravenous lines must be inserted into the lower limb veins. If possible, biopsy must be taken under local anesthesia. Chemotherapy or radiotherapy must be done to shrink tumors before surgery. A cardiopulmonary bypass circuit on standby should be considered for extremely high-risk cases.

Two-Lung Ventilation With Manual Retraction

Several thoracic procedures, for example, patent ductus arteriosus ligation, vascular ring resection, and tracheoesophageal fistula repair, can be performed with a single lumen tube positioned in the trachea providing ventilation to both lungs, with the surgeon gently retracting the lungs as necessary. This is typically done for short procedures in small infants where the surgeon is operating in the chest cavity but not directly on the lungs. This technique is especially helpful in the management of emergencies, such as acute hemorrhagic conditions or tension pneumothorax. Lung injury is a concern, and thus retraction should be kept to the minimum necessary. It is also possible for the surgeon to insufflate CO_2 into the pleural space to displace the lung if a thoracoscopy is being performed. That may influence the delivered tidal volume, displace the lung isolation device, and cause hypercarbia and hypotension.

Lung Isolation and One-Lung Ventilation

OLV is a ventilation strategy that facilitates surgical exposure and provides still lung in thoracoscopy or thoracotomy.[13] Unlike adult patients, OLV presents a challenge in children, especially in neonates and infants because of equipment limitations. Nevertheless, technology is advancing daily and equipment available to help anesthesiologists in performing OLV has been developed. OLV has other advantages other than surgical exposure, they include:

- Decreasing the over distention of the pathologic lobe, in congenital lobar emphysema.

- Differentiating the normal lung tissue from the pathologic one.
- Decreasing the potential trauma to the lung tissue, caused by the retractors.
- Decreasing the risk of contamination of the healthy lung by secretions, blood, or infected materials originating from the diseased lung.

Providing Lung Separation in the Pediatric Patients (Table 23.1)

Selective Bronchial Intubation

Selective bronchial intubation with a regular single lumen tube can be achieved readily and is the simplest method to achieve OLV. The ETT is advanced while auscultating breath sounds until the sound is lost on the desired side. Confirmation can be obtained by noting an acute drop in end-tidal CO_2 or by auscultation as the tube enters a mainstem bronchus. Being that the left bronchus has a more acute angle of separation from the trachea than the right bronchus (45 vs. 25 degrees) it is much more common for the tube to be advanced into the right mainstem bronchus. Rotating the patient's head to the right side helps to decrease the angle of the left bronchus improving the chance of a left mainstem bronchus intubation. Also rotating the ETT 180 degrees so the bevel is pointing to the left helps direct the tube to the left bronchus. Alternatively, and with a higher first pass success rate, the tube can be vision guided with a fiberoptic bronchoscope (FOB). It should be noted that the bronchi have a smaller diameter than the trachea and thus a tube that is too big could cause trauma to the bronchus or may not advance into the selected bronchus. If an uncuffed tube is being used, there is chance of a leak, which might not allow for full lung collapse. Cuffed tubes should not be placed too far into the bronchus because the cuff can occlude the upper lobe of the selected bronchus, especially when intubating the right mainstem bronchus.[14] It is recommended that the cuff partially remains in the trachea. A major downside to selective bronchial intubation is that if it is not possible to ventilate in the presence of hypoxemia, apply suction to the nondependent lung, or continuous positive airway pressure (CPAP) to the nondependent lung. Several variations of this technique have been described. Marraro described an endobronchial bi-lumen tube consisting of two uncuffed tubes joined together with the bronchial tube being longer than the tracheal one. It was developed for children under 3 years old.[15] Tsujimoto et al. described a microlaryngeal ETT that can be advanced into the desired bronchus, through the intubating laryngeal mask airway with the aid of flexible fiberoptic bronchoscopy.[16] High-frequency jet ventilation and high-frequency oscillatory ventilation is another option and can be indicated in short procedures. They provide optimal surgical field while allowing blood gas exchange. There is an inability to monitor end-tidal CO_2 that might be overcome by transcutaneous CO_2($PtcCO_2$) monitoring.

Bronchial Blocker (Fig. 23.1)

Another option for lung separation is the placement of a BB in the operative side. A major advantage of this technique is that the BB balloon can be deflated allowing quick ventilation to the operative lung if necessary. The smallest BBs in the market are the 5.0 Fr Arndt blocker (Cook Medical, Indiana, USA) and the Uniblocker (Fuji System Corporation, Tokyo, Japan). They are both smaller versions of the 9.0 Fr blockers from the same manufacture and are intended to be used in the same way, inside (also called coaxial) the ETT (Fig. 23.2). The 5.0 Fr Uniblocker, however, does not have a suction port. It should be noted that the 5.0 Fr BB has a higher-pressure balloon than the 9.0 Fr BB balloon used in adults and caution is warranted when inflating it.[17] Being that a FOB is necessary for the placement of all BBs, placing them becomes a challenge when the ETT inner diameter is small. The most common pediatric FOB size available is 2.2 mm in outer diameter. Because both the FOB (2.2 mm) and the 5 Fr BB (1.67 mm) must fit inside the ETT plus some room for maneuvering them, the minimum recommended ETT inner diameter is 4.5 mm. There are many different models and sizes of FOBs in the market, therefore it is best if the anesthesiologist checks both the FOB being used and the BB fitting inside the intended tube ex vivo. In small patients where the BB and the FOB do not fit inside the tube, that is, ETT 4 mm or smaller, lung separation can still be achieved with a BB; however, it must be placed outside (also referred as parallel) the ETT (Fig. 23.3). Our routine practice is, after

TABLE 23.1 Approach to One-Lung Ventilation by Age

Age	Endotracheal Tube	Feasible One-Lung Ventilation Technique	Fiberoptic Size
Newborn to 2 years	3.0–4.5 mm	Endobronchial intubation/5 Fr parallel bronchial blocker (BB)	<2.2 mm
2–8 years	4.5–6.0 mm	5 Fr BB coaxial/endobronchial intubation	2.2–2.8 mm
8–10 years	6.0–7.0 mm	5 Fr BB coaxial/4.0 Univent tube	2.8–4.0 mm
>10 years	7.0 mm plus	7 Fr BB coaxial/≥26 double lumen tube/≥4.0 Univent tube	2.8–4.0 mm

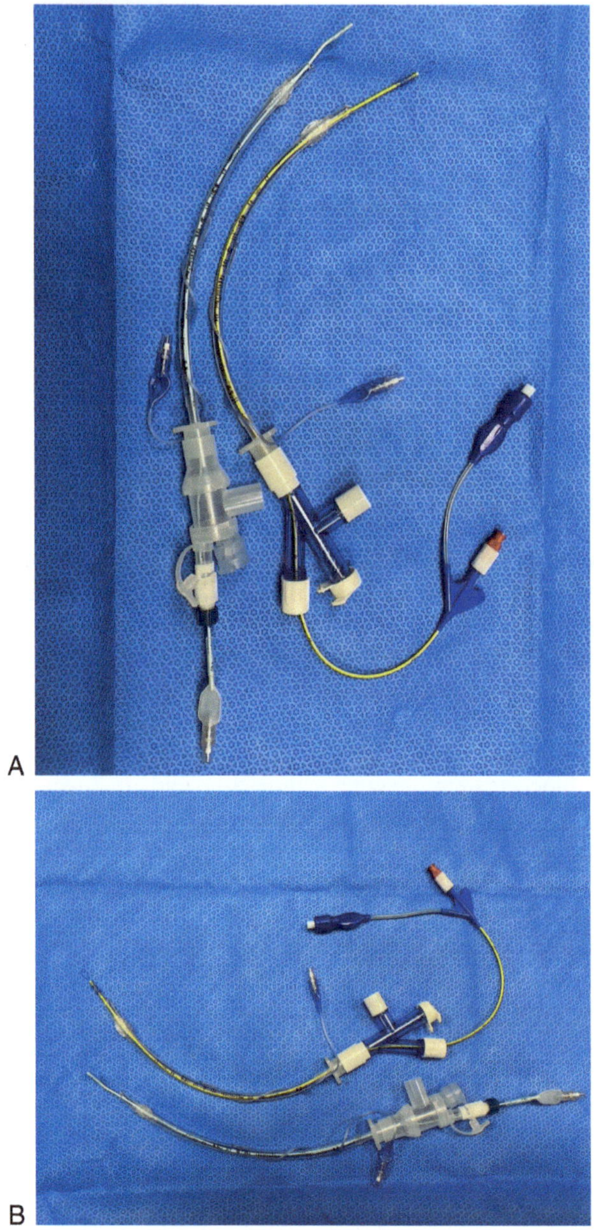

• **Fig. 23.1** A 5 French (Fr) Arndt blocker (**A**) and 5 Fr Uniblocker (**B**) with its own ventilator adapter when used inside the tube (coaxially).

assuring the patent is fully anesthetized and paralyzed, to perform a laryngoscopy with the adequate size blade, passing the 5 Fr blocker through the glottis and advancing it gently until soft resistance is met, followed by intubation of the trachea with the desired ETT tube. Typically, we use a cuffed ETT to minimize having to reintubate for leaks. After verifying that the trachea has been properly intubated and end-tidal CO_2 is confirmed, an FOB is placed inside the tube to visualize the carina and position the BB into the proper bronchus (Fig. 23.4). The adapter included with the BB can be used to ventilate while the FOB is being used. Most of the time, the BB will enter the right mainstem bronchus and needs to be pulled back and redirected. If collapse of the right lung is desired, the balloon of the BB is placed very shallow in the right mainstem bronchus to avoid blocking the right

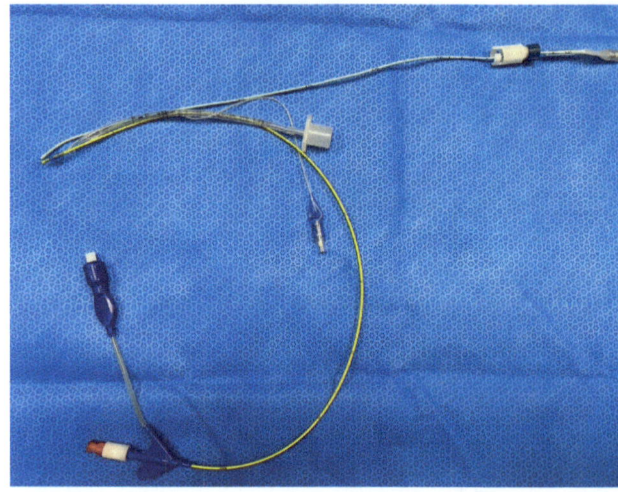

• **Fig. 23.2** A 5 French (Fr) Uniblocker and 5 Fr Arndt blocker when used outside the tube (parallel), adapter removed.

upper lobe. Visualization of the cuff as it is being inflated is mandatory to avoid injuring the bronchus or herniation of the cuff into the trachea. If it is desired to block the left mainstem bronchus then the BB must be pulled above the carina and, taking advantage of the hockey stick design of the Uniblocker (or alternatively manually shaping the distal end of the Arndt blocker into a hockey stick because we do not use the lasso with this technique), rotating it so that the hockey stick shape directs the BB into the left bronchus. As mentioned previously, rotating the head of the patient to the right side can help bring the left bronchus into a more direct angle. It must be recognized that when placing a BB outside the tube, it can be much more difficult to manipulate the BB into the left bronchus compared with placing it inside the ETT, especially if it migrates out of the bronchus mid-procedure. Care must be taken to ensure the ETT and BB are properly secured in place and not to allow any motion, such as neck flexion or any undue pulling on the circuit that can displace the BB. Our preference is to advance the BB deep into the desired bronchus while the patient is supine

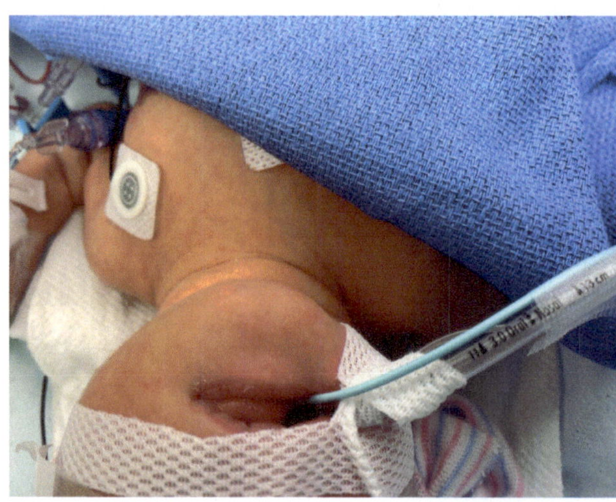

• **Fig. 23.3** Uniblocker placed outside a 3.0-mm endotracheal tube in a very small infant.

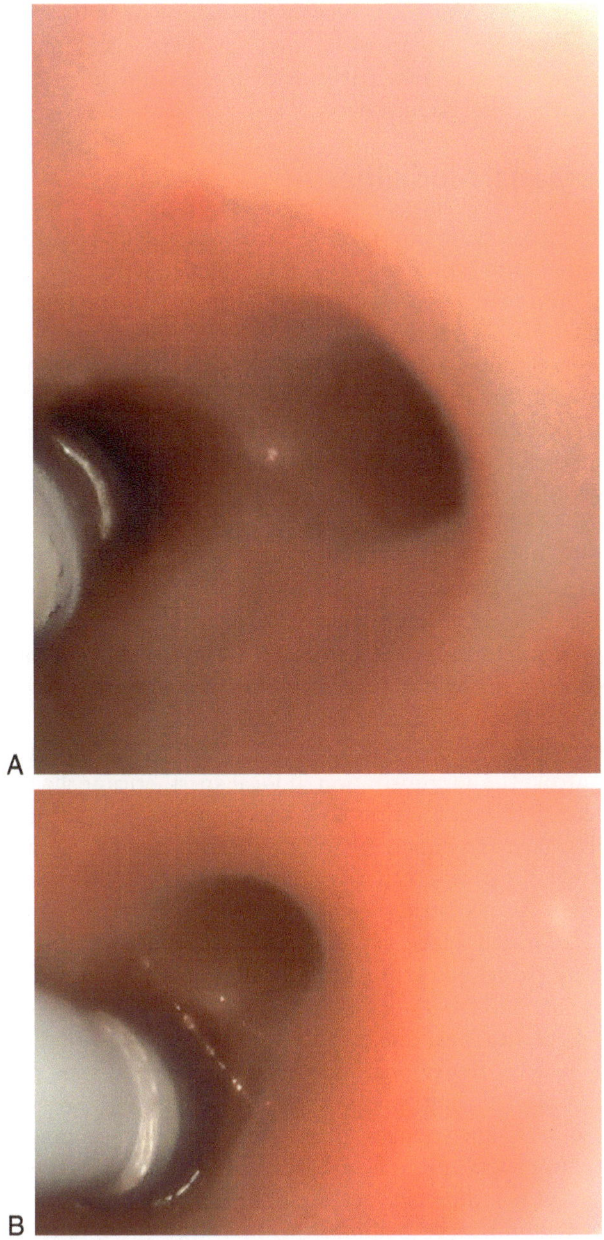

• **Fig. 23.4** (A and B). A 5.0 French Uniblocker, balloon down and balloon inflated placed in left mainstem bronchus outside a 3.0-mm endotracheal tube visualized through a 2.2 fiberoptic scope.

and, after the patient has been fully positioned, to pull the BB out the correct distance into the bronchus after we are certain the patient will remain immobile. Alternatively, Fogarty catheters or Miller atrial septostomy balloons have been described when small BBs have not been available, but considering that they have a high-pressure, low-volume balloon means that caution is recommended to avoid injuring the bronchus.

Univent Tube

The Univent tube (Fuji System Corporation, Tokyo, Japan) is a single lumen tube with a BB balloon already integrated in the wall of the tube through a designated channel. The blocker has a hockey stick shape tip and is advanced and rotated into position. Albeit narrow, the lumen of the second tube may be served to deliver oxygen, inhalational agents, or to suction the operated lung; this property is only present in Univent tubes with an inner diameter of 6 mm or greater. The Univent tube's blocker balloon has low-volume, high-pressure properties, so overdistention or long-term use may cause damage of the tracheal mucosa.[18] Dislodgement of the balloon during surgery is quite difficult because it is strictly connected to the main ETT. Owing to the simplicity of its design, it would seem ideal for lung isolation in small pediatric patients. However, the limiting factor is the outer tube diameter which is much larger than a regular single lumen tube with the same inner diameter. For example, the smallest Univent tube in the market has a 3.5-mm inner diameter but an outer diameter of at least 7.5 to 8 mm according to the manufacturer, which would compare to a regular 5.5-mm tube. Thus it is useful for children older than 6 years of age, in which case it is preferable to use a regular single lumen tube with a BB inside, which provides a larger area to ventilate and less resistance to flow. In the scenario of a patient needing to remain intubated postprocedure, the BB can be simply pulled out instead of requiring the Univent tube to be replaced by a regular single lumen tube owing to its large external diameter.

Double-Lumen Tube

Double-lumen tubes (DLT) are the preferred method for lung separation in older children and it allows for suction and application of CPAP. The smallest DLT available is 26 Fr Rusch (Teleflex, North Carolina, USA) and is available in both right- and left-sided tubes. Its outer diameter is 8.67 mm, which is close to the outer diameter of a 6.5-mm regular single tube (8.9 mm). Other pediatric sizes available in the market are 28 and 32 Fr, both made by Rusch and Mallinckrodt (United Kingdom). Thus they are recommended for children older than 8 years of age.[19] A small pediatric FOB (2.2 mm) is required to be able to enter each lumen. In adults, the correct length of the tube is directly proportionate to the height of the patient, but there is no clear proportion in children. The use of right DLTs is not preferred in small children because of the high risk of occluding the right upper lobe. This is an anatomic disadvantage of children, and tube manipulation does not overcome it. A similar disadvantage is present in left-sided DLTs, such as occluding the left upper lobe bronchus by the advanced bronchial tip. The technique for placement is the same as in adults described elsewhere in this book (see Chapter 16).

Hypoxemia Management During One-Lung Ventilation

Hypoxemia during OLV is almost inevitable, especially in small children. As in adults, CPAP use or intermittent ventilation of the nondependent lung, PEEP application to the dependent lung may improve oxygenation.

Monitoring

Standard monitoring including electrocardiogram, pulse oximeter, blood pressure measurement, end-tidal CO_2 monitoring, and temperature are the minimum requirement for any thoracic procedure involving general anesthesia. Invasive arterial blood pressure monitoring is encouraged and is required if there is expectation of a long or complicated procedure, poor cardiopulmonary status, or possibility of large blood loss. If in doubt, it is probably best to err on the side of caution and obtain arterial access. In terms of venous access, most cases can be done with two large bores, for age, peripheral intravenous catheter. Central venous access is rarely required, but if there is poor peripheral venous access or any comorbidity that might require the patient to need any vasoactive infusions, it is reasonable to obtain. $PtcCO_2$ is recommended, if available, when the operative procedure does not allow for end-tidal CO_2 monitoring.

Postoperative Period

The choice of the ventilation technique after the procedure depends on the severity of the pathology, the patient's medical condition, the effectiveness of the ventilation, and the degree of edema in airways. In uncomplicated cases, spontaneous ventilation is assisted via a face mask; however, endotracheal intubation should be preferred in patients having severe pathologies together with impotent airways and ineffective ventilation. After the recovery, hospital stay is strictly recommended.[20] If the patient has no previous respiratory failure and has completed the procedure without complication, he/she may be referred to the ward or to a monitored unit. Otherwise, follow-up in intensive care unit is recommended.

Pain Management (see Chapters 25, 26)

Pain management following thoracic surgery in pediatric patients presents unique challenges. Young patients may not be able to communicate properly and the identification and assessment of pain presents a challenge in itself. Even when pain has been properly identified and assessed, providing adequate analgesia without risking oversedation and respiratory depression can be difficult. Pain is a very complex experience involving a multitude of factors, the most obvious being the tissue trauma, but also just as important, the anxiety and coping mechanisms of the child along with the parents.[21] Left untreated, pain can have physical consequences, such as hyperglycemia, protein catabolism, increased oxygen consumption, increased blood pressure, diaphragmatic splinting, decreased cough, decreased tidal volume, decreased FRC, and decreased bowel motility.[22]

Chronic pain after thoracotomy, also referred to as post-thoracotomy pain syndrome, is defined by the International Association for the Study of Pain as pain along the thoracotomy incision that persist after 2 months following the surgical procedure.[23] Its incidence is estimated around 50% in adults but appears to be lower in 20% of children.[24,25] Preemptive analgesia, particularly regional anesthesia, may help to reduce its incidence.[26,27]

Regional Modalities

The most basic form of regional anesthesia is surgical wound infiltration with local anesthetic. It has low risk and can be easily performed by the surgeon. Care must be taken not the exceed the toxic amount of local anesthetic. Doses of bupivacaine of up to 3 mg/kg, and lidocaine up to 5 mg/kg have been found to be below the toxic range.[28,29] It should be noted that clearance and protein binding for local anesthetic agents are reduced in infants under 6 months of age, thus the dose is recommended to be halved in these patients. In a study by Cerfolio et al., preemptive local anesthetic infiltration before incision for thoracotomy did not reduce postoperative pain during the hospital stay or at 3, 6, and 12 months after surgery.[30]

Thoracic epidural catheters are the most common modality for pain management in adult thoracic anesthesia.[31] It seems obvious that local anesthetic delivered at the corresponding thoracic level will provide superior pain control. The administration of local anesthetics at the thoracic level is easily titratable and provides the additional advantage of sympathetic blockade and superior blunting of stress response otherwise not achieved by other techniques. In pediatric patients, epidural catheter placement is performed in the same manner and following the same safety guidelines as for adults. One major difference being that both the American Society of Regional Anesthesia and the European Society of Regional Anesthesia recommend that all regional anesthesia in children should be performed during general anesthesia or deep sedation.[32,33] Also in infants younger than 1 year, it is common practice to thread the epidural catheter from the caudal space to the desired thoracic location.[34] Ultrasound imaging has been found to be helpful in guiding the catheter to the proper location.[35] Maximum infusion rates for lidocaine of 1 mg/kg/h, and for bupivacaine of 0.2 to 0.3 mg/kg/h have been recommended for young infants.[36,37] Again, the dose should be halved for infants younger than 6 months. The concomitant use of opioids allows the use of lower concentrations of local anesthetics and decreases the risk of local anesthetic toxicity.

Paravertebral catheters have emerged as an alternative to the epidural catheter route for management of postthoracotomy pain. When performed unilaterally, they have been found to provide comparable pain control with fewer side effects, such as nausea, vomiting, and hypotension, when compared with an epidural catheter technique.[38]

Single-shot epidural techniques are typically administered in younger children at the caudal epidural space. Because administering a local anesthetic at the caudal or even lumbar epidural level will not reach adequate thoracic levels, single-shot caudal techniques are mostly limited to the use of hydrophilic opioids and in particular preservative free morphine. Morphine, easily administered via the caudal space in younger children (typically but not limited to children <5 years of age), will provide a long-lasting analgesic effect. Its peak analgesic effect is 4 to 7 hours,[39] and its duration of action has been reported up to 24 hours.[40] Dose can range from 30mcg/kg to as high as 100mcg/kg. Dose should be halved for neonates. Even though neuraxial opioids do not offer the potential advantages of a sympathetic thoracic epidural block achieved with local anesthetic agents, epidurally administered opioids have been shown to provide excellent analgesia, pulmonary function, and early ambulation.[41] Side effects related to neuraxial opioids include nausea and vomiting, pruritus, somnolence, respiratory depression, and urinary retention. Close postoperative monitoring for 24 hours is mandatory when neuraxial opioids are used, importantly to identify any potential respiratory depression. Alternative drugs, such as the alpha 2 receptor agonist clonidine, ketamine, and magnesium have been used in the epidural space to minimize undesirable side effects of opioids, such as respiratory depression, and to prolong analgesic effects.[42–44]

Insertion of an epidural catheter can lead to several complications such as misplacement, knotting, and migration, (especially if advanced too far), rupture, infection, leakage, epidural hematoma, and neurologic injury. The true incidence of neuraxial anesthesia complications is not known. Severe complications of epidural catheters, defined as infection (epidural abscess), include local anesthetic toxicity, cardiac arrest, drug error causing harm, or neurologic injury. In pediatric patients, complications have been estimated around one in 2000 patients in one study, with permanent neurologic injury at one in 10,000 patients[45] whereas another reported no neurologic complication in 150,000 single-shot caudal anesthetics.[46] At the moment, it does not appear that children are at higher risk from neuraxial techniques than adults.[47]

Intravenous Modalities

Intravenous opioids although highly effective for pain management, have the downside of having periods of heavy sedation, respiratory depression, early after being administered, transitioning into periods of low analgesic effect when wearing off. In addition, nausea, pruritus, urinary retention, and constipation are common side effects. Long-acting opioids, such as morphine, hydromorphone, and even methadone provide a steadier pain control than short acting opioids, such as fentanyl.

Acetaminophen is a nonopioid, centrally acting analgesic. Acetaminophen used in combination with opioids leads to improved analgesia and a decrease in opioid dosing and their side effects.[48] Nonsteroidal antiinflammatory drugs, particularly ketorolac, have been shown to reduce postoperative opioid requirements in pediatric surgical patients, including neonates and premature babies.[49]

Dexmedetomidine is a sedative agent that confers sedation by selectively binding to central alpha 2 adrenoceptors. Although at this point it is only approved by the U.S. Food and drug Administration for use in adults for up to 24 hours, it has been widely used, off label, in children even for prolonged periods of time.[50] It has become popular in pediatric anesthesia because it is associated with a lower incidence of emergence delirium after inhalational anesthesia in children.[51,52] Preemptive use of intravenous dexmedetomidine was reported to reduce the incidence of postthoracotomy pain syndrome in adults undergoing coronary artery bypass grafting.[53] However, in another study, when administered via a paravertebral catheter, even though it was associated with lower postoperative pain and opioid consumption, it had no effect in the incidence of postthoracotomy pain syndrome. It must be noted that preoperative teaching also plays a role in anxiety reduction.[54]

Ketamine, an N-methyl D-aspartic acid (NMDA) receptor antagonist, is a dissociative hypnotic with analgesic properties when used in low doses. It has been shown to reduce lower pain scores in the postoperative period in adults.[55]

In summary, a complete multimodal approach to pain management covers different factors involved in the experience of pain. Suggestions include anesthetic to block the transition of the nociceptive signal, and antiinflammatory to reduce tissue trauma, an NMDA receptor antagonist to prevent central sensitization to pain, opioids to enhance inhibitory pathways, and a preoperative teaching and/or a sedative for anxiolysis.

Conclusion

Anesthesia for pediatric thoracic surgery is challenging. It is essential to perform a detailed preoperative evaluation, know the characteristics of different age groups and applicable two-lung ventilation or OLV strategies, and also have a full anesthetic plan that includes pain management strategies. Furthermore, it must be stressed that communication between the surgeon and the anesthesiologist, such as sharing the surgical plan, any acute changes in ventilation parameters, heart rate or blood pressure, and the postoperative plan, is extremely important to reduce complications.

References

1. Sunder RA, Haile DT, Farrell PT, Sharma A. Pediatric airway management: current practices and future directions. *Pediatr Anesth.* 2012;22(10):1008–1015.
2. Madden K, Khemani RG, Newth CJ. Paediatric applied respiratory physiology–the essentials. *Paediatr Child Health.* 2009; 19(6):249–256.
3. American Society of Anesthesiologists Committee. Practice guidelines for preoperative fasting and the use of pharmacologic agents

to reduce the risk of pulmonary aspiration: application to healthy patients undergoing elective procedures: an updated report by the American Society of Anesthesiologists Committee on Standards and Practice Parameters. *Anesthesiology.* 2011;114(3): 495.
4. Yuan N, Skaggs DL, Davidson Ward SL, Platzker AC, Keens TG. Preoperative polysomnograms and infant pulmonary function tests do not predict prolonged post-operative mechanical ventilation in children following scoliosis repair. *Pediatr Pulmonol.* 2004;38:256–260.
5. Stocks J. Infant respiratory function testing: is it worth all the effort? *Paediatr Anaesth.* 2004;13:537–540.
6. Cai Y, Li W, Chen K. Efficacy and safety of spontaneous ventilation technique using dexmedetomidine for rigid bronchoscopic airway foreign body removal in children. *Paediatr Anaesth.* 2013;23:1048–1053.
7. Chai J, Wu XY, Han N, Wang LY, Chen WM. A retrospective study of anesthesia during rigid bronchoscopy for airway foreign body removal in children: propofol and sevoflurane with spontaneous ventilation. *Paediatr Anaesth.* 2014;24:1031–1036.
8. Chen KZ, Ye M, Hu CB, Shen X. Dexmedetomidine vs remifentanil intravenous anaesthesia and spontaneous ventilation for airway foreign body removal in children. *Br J Anaesth.* 2014;112: 892–897.
9. Annigeri RV, Patil RS. A retrospective analysis on anesthetic management during rigid bronchoscopy in children with foreign body aspiration: propofol and sevoflurane with controlled ventilation. *Anesth Essays Res.* 2017;11(4):871.
10. Evans E, Biro P, Bedforth N. Jet ventilation. *Contin Educ Anaesth Crit Care Pain.* 2007;1:2–5.
11. Liu Y, Chen L, Li S. Controlled ventilation or spontaneous respiration in anesthesia for tracheobronchial foreign body removal: a meta-analysis. *Pediatr Anesth.* 2014;24(10):1023–1030.
12. Roberts S, Thornington RE. Paediatric bronchoscopy. *Contin Educ Anaesth Crit Care Pain.* 2005;5(2):41–44.
13. Fabila TS, Menghraj SJ. One lung ventilation strategies for infants and children undergoing video assisted thoracoscopic surgery. *Indian J Anaesth.* 2013;57:339–344.
14. Lammers CR, Hammer GB, Brodsky JB, Cannon WB. Failure to isolate the lungs with an endotracheal tube positioned in the bronchus. *Anesth Analg.* 1997;85:944.
15. Pawar DK, Marraro GA. One lung ventilation in infants and children: experience with Marraro double lumen tube. *Paediatr Anaesth.* 2005;15:204–208.
16. Tsujimoto S, Fujiwara S, Tashiro C. How to perform differential lung ventilation in pediatric cases? *Anesthesiology.* 1999;91:327.
17. Golianu B, Hammer GB. Pediatric thoracic anesthesia. *Curr Opin Anesthesiol.* 2005;18(1):5–11.
18. Hammer GB, Brodsky JB, Redpath JH, Cannon WB. The Univent tube for single-lung ventilation in paediatric patients. *Paediatr Anaesth.* 1998;8:55–57.
19. Semmelmann A, Kaltofen H, Loop T. Anesthesia of thoracic surgery in children. *Paediatr Anaesth.* 2018;28(4):326–331.
20. Andreoli SM, Kofmehl E, Sobol SE. Is inpatient admission necessary following removal of airway foreign bodies? *Int J Pediatr Otorhinolaryngol.* 2015;79(9):1436–1438.
21. Rabbitts JA, Groenewald CB, Tai GG, Palermo TM. Presurgical psychosocial predictors of acute postsurgical pain and quality of life in children undergoing major surgery. *J Pain.* 2015;16(3): 226–234.
22. Kehlet H. Manipulation of the metabolic response in clinical practice. *World J Surg.* 2000;24(6):690–695.
23. Gerner P. Postthoracotomy pain management problems. *Anesthesiol Clin.* 2008;26(2):355–367.
24. Karmakar MK, Ho AM. Postthoracotomy pain syndrome. *Thorac Surg Clin.* 2004;14:345–352.
25. Kristensen AD, Pedersen TA, Hjortdal VE, Jensen TS, Nikolajsen L. Chronic pain in adults after thoracotomy in childhood or youth. *Br J Anaesth.* 2009;104(1):75–79.
26. Gottschalk A, Cohen SP, Yang S, Ochroch EA. Preventing and treating pain after thoracic surgery. *Anesthesiology.* 2006; 104(3):594–600.
27. Andreae MH, Andreae DA. Regional anaesthesia to prevent chronic pain after surgery: a Cochrane systematic review and meta-analysis. *Br J Anaesth.* 2013;111(5):711–720.
28. Berde CB. Toxicity of local anesthetics in infants and children. *J Pediatr.* 1993;122(5):S14–S20.
29. Morton NS. Local and regional anaesthesia in infants. *Contin Educ Anaesth Crit Care Pain.* 2004;4(5):148–151.
30. Cerfolio RJ, Bryant AS, Bass CS, Bartolucci AA. A prospective, double-blinded, randomized trial evaluating the use of preemptive analgesia of the skin before thoracotomy. *Ann Thorac Surg.* 2003; 76:1055–1058.
31. Goto T. What is the best pain control after thoracic surgery? *J Thorac Dis.* 2018;10(3):1335.
32. Ivani G, Suresh S, Ecoffey C, et al. The European Society of Regional Anaesthesia and Pain Therapy and the American Society of Regional Anesthesia and Pain Medicine joint committee practice advisory on controversial topics in pediatric regional anesthesia. *Reg Anesth Pain Med.* 2015;40(5):526–532.
33. Horlocker TT, Vandermeulen E, Kopp SL, Gogarten W, Leffert LR, Benzon HT. Regional anesthesia in the patient receiving antithrombotic or thrombolytic therapy: American Society of Regional Anesthesia and Pain Medicine evidence-based guidelines. *Reg Anesth Pain Med.* 2018;43(3):263–309.
34. Gunter JB, Eng C. Thoracic epidural anesthesia via the caudal approach in children. *Anesthesiology.* 1992;76:935–938.
35. Ponde VC, Bedekar VV, Desai AP, Puranik KA. Does ultrasound guidance add accuracy to continuous caudal-epidural catheter placements in neonates and infants? *Pediatr Anesth.* 2017;27(10): 1010–1014.
36. Biebuyck JF, Yaster M, Maxwell LG. Pediatric regional anesthesia. *Anesthesiology.* 1989;70(2):324–338.
37. Morton NS. Local and regional anaesthesia in infants. *Contin Educ Anaesth Crit Care Pain.* 2004;4(5):148–151.
38. Davies R, Myles P, Graham J. A comparison of the analgesic efficacy and side-effects of paravertebral vs epidural blockade for thoracotomy—a systematic review and meta-analysis of randomized trials. *Br J Anaesthesia.* 2006;96:418–426.
39. Bailey BL, Rhondeau S, Schafer PG, et al. Dose-response pharmacology of intrathecal morphine in human volunteers. *Anesthesiology.* 1993;79:49–59.
40. Stoelting RK. Intrathecal morphine—an under used combination for postoperative pain management. *Anaesth Analg.* 1989;68: 707–709.
41. Glenski JA, Warner MA, Dawson B, Kaufman B. Postoperative use of epidurally administered morphine in children and adolescents. *Mayo Clin Proc.* 1984;59(8):530–533.
42. De Negri P, Ivani G, Visconti C, et al. The dose-response relationship for clonidine added to a postoperative continuous epidural infusion of ropivacaine in children. *Anesth Analg.* 2001;93: 71–76.
43. Cook B, Grubb DJ, Aldridge LA, Doyle E. Comparison of the effects of adrenaline, clonidine and ketamine on the duration

of caudal analgesia produced by bupivacaine in children. *Br J Anaesth.* 1995;75:698–701.

44. Bilir A, Gulec S, Erkan A, Ozcelik A. Epidural magnesium reduces postoperative analgesic requirement. *Br J Anaesth.* 2007; 98:519–523.
45. Llewellyn N, Moriarty A. The national pediatric epidural audit. *Pediatr Anesth.* 2007;17(6):520–533.
46. Giaufre E, Dalens B, Gombert A. Epidemiology and morbidity of regional anesthesia in children: a one-year prospective survey of the French-Language Society of Pediatric Anesthesiologists. *Anesth Analg.* 1996;83(5):904–912.
47. De Tommaso O, Caporuscio A, Tagariello V. Neurological complications following central neuraxial blocks: are there predictive factors? *Eur J Anaesthesiol.* 2002;19(10):705–716.
48. Walker SM. Pain after surgery in children: clinical recommendations. *Curr Opin Anaesthesiol.* 2015;28(5):570.
49. Papacci P, De Francisci G, Iacobucci T, et al. Use of intravenous ketorolac in the neonate and premature babies. *Paediatr Anaesth.* 2004;14:487–492.
50. Hammer GB, Philip BM, Schroeder AR, et al. Prolonged infusion of dexmedetomidine for sedation following tracheal resection. *Pediatr Anesth.* 2005;15:616–620.
51. Isik B, Arslan M, Tunga AD, Kurtipek O. Dexmedetomidine decreases emergence agitation in pediatric patients after sevoflurane anesthesia without surgery. *Paediatr Anaesth.* 2006;16:748–753.
52. Ibacache ME, Munoz HR, Brandes V, Morales AL. Single-dose dexmedetomidine reduces agitation after sevoflurane anesthesia in children. *Anesth Analg.* 2004;98:60–63.
53. Moghaddam MJ, Barkhori A, Mirkheshti A, Hashemian M, Mohajerani SA. The effect of pre-emptive dexmedetomidine on the incidence of post-thoracotomy pain syndrome in patients undergoing coronary artery bypass grafting. *Anesthesiol Pain Med.* 2016;6(3).
54. Guo P. Preoperative education interventions to reduce anxiety and improve recovery among cardiac surgery patients: a review of randomised controlled trials. *J Clin Nursing.* 2015;24(1-2):34–46.
55. Gorlin AW, Rosenfeld DM, Ramakrishna H. Intravenous subanesthetic ketamine for perioperative analgesia. *J Anaesthesiol Clin Pharmacol.* 2016;32(2):160.

24

Postoperative Management of Acute Pain

JEFFREY J. MOJICA, ERIC S. SCHWENK, UZUNG YOON, MARK S. KIM, OMAR BEN AMER, EUGENE R. VISCUSI

Introduction

In 2021, noncardiac thoracic surgery can range from minimally invasive, robot-assisted procedures, such as lung biopsies or resections, to more invasive procedures requiring thoracotomy such as pneumonectomy, esophagectomy, tracheal resection, or lung transplantation.

The noxious stimulus associated with thoracic surgery is among the most severe sources of postoperative pain and carries one of the highest incidences of persistent postsurgical pain (PPSP).[1,2] These procedures can be associated with intense pain throughout the perioperative encounter. In addition, inadequately controlled pain can compromise respiratory function, inhibiting coughing and deep breathing in the postoperative period and leading to atelectasis and pneumonia. The consequences of these acute conditions can negatively impact long-term outcomes, leading to increased patient morbidity and mortality.[3,4]

The incidence of severe postoperative pain after thoracic surgery was already documented in the anesthesia literature of the 1960s.[5] Subsequent investigations have shown that postoperative respiratory compromise was associated with surgical incision site.[6,7] By the 1980s, the benefits of adequate intraoperative and postoperative analgesia on respiratory function were being elucidated.[8,9] Today, pain after thoracic surgery is viewed as multifactorial. Patients experience acute pain in the days after surgery and some develop PPSP.[10] A detailed understanding of the mechanisms of pain after thoracic surgery will allow for optimal management.

The evidence suggests that effective perioperative pain control can improve postoperative pain and recovery, reduce time to extubation, improve pulmonary function and gas exchange, and increase patient satisfaction.[9,11,12] Aggressive pain management strategies have also been identified as a method to reduce the incidence of chronic postthoracotomy pain.[1,10,13,14] In this chapter, we will discuss the pathophysiology of pain after thoracic surgery and how multimodal analgesia (MMA) with systemic and regional anesthesia techniques are used for pain management.

Description of Pain in Thoracic Surgery

Acute pain from thoracic surgery can arise from multiple pathways. Nociceptive, inflammatory, neuropathic, and referred pathways can each produce and modulate pain that becomes a total subjective experience for the patient undergoing thoracic surgery (Table 24.1).

Nociceptive stimuli can be transmitted via somatic afferent fibers or visceral afferent fibers. Nociceptive pain is the pain that results from activation of high-threshold peripheral (nociceptor) neurons by intense mechanical, chemical, or thermal noxious stimuli. It signals the presence, location, intensity, and duration of a noxious stimulus and fades once the peripheral driving force is removed.[15]

Nociceptive somatic stimuli are initially gathered by the anterior cutaneous branch (anterior midline to midclavicular line) and the lateral cutaneous branch (midclavicular line to side wall to back) of the intercoastal nerve for afferent transmission to the ipsilateral dorsal horn of the spinal cord. At the spinal cord, somatic afferent fibers ascend via the contralateral anterolateral system in the spinal cord to reach the limbic system of the thalamus and finally terminating at the somatosensory cortex. Skin incision, separation of muscle fibers, retraction of ribs, and the interruption of the parietal pleura all provide nociceptive somatic stimuli that can be perceived by the patient as nociceptive somatic pain.[16]

Nociceptive visceral stimuli are transmitted by the phrenic and vagus nerves following injury to the internal organs of the thorax, such as the thymus gland, heart, lungs and its tracheobronchial tree, and visceral pleura. These stimuli can be perceived by the patient as a dull, poorly localized pain.[16]

The tissue injury of thoracic surgery activates an inflammatory response. This response can be observed peripherally at nociceptors and centrally at the spinal cord and brain. The peripheral inflammatory response consists of the release of sensitizing inflammatory mediators that decrease the activation threshold of nociceptors that innervate the injured tissue.[16] Examples of inflammatory mediators include prostaglandins, histamine, bradykinin, and potassium. Together, these mediators heighten pain sensitivity and describe the peripheral inflammatory pathway of pain

TABLE 24.1 Sources of Pain in Thoracic Surgery

Classification of Pain in Thoracic Surgery	Example
Nociceptive Somatic	Skin incision, retraction of ribs, surgical dissection of muscle fibers and the parietal pleura, insertion of thoracostomy tube
Nociceptive Visceral	Dissection, retraction, excision or resection of the thymus gland, heart, lungs, tracheobronchial tree and/or visceral pleura
Inflammatory	Tissue injury from surgical dissection and cautery
Neuropathic	Intercostal nerve and phrenic nerve injuries, postthoracotomy pain
Referred pain	Ipsilateral shoulder pain from phrenic nerve injury
Chronic pain	Persistent postsurgical pain (postthoracotomy pain syndrome)

as a component of the pain experience related to thoracic surgery. As a consequence of continued nociception and peripheral sensitization of pain, the central nervous system can undergo sensitization at the spinal cord through activation of N-methyl-D-aspartate (NMDA) receptors in response to central mediators, such as substance P, calcitonin gene-related peptide, and glutamate.[15] Inflammatory pain can present soon after tissue injury and persist for days if inflammation is present. Patients are likely to report a tense, throbbing pain and hyperalgesia to heat with sensory and motor function remaining intact. Inflammatory pain and the related sensitization can be reversed and is the focus of acute pain management after thoracic surgery.

Neuropathic pain can also be produced from nerve injury during thoracic surgery to the intercostal nerves located within the neurovascular bundle at the inferior aspect of each rib (Fig. 24.1). Neuropathic pain has the unique characteristic of combining simultaneous sensory deficit to touch, pressure, and temperature with pain hypersensitivity, such as allodynia, hyperalgesia, or dysesthesia.[15] This new sensory experience can contribute to pain and results from abnormal neuronal function. This hypersensitivity of neuropathic pain, which can spread beyond the distribution of the damaged intercostal nerve, can mask sensory loss. Neuropathic pain can be difficult to discriminate from inflammatory pain because both can arise spontaneously after tissue damage. Patients are likely to report neuropathic pain as a burning pain, spasmodic in onset with sensory loss along the nerve distribution in the affected intercostal space.

Referred pain to the ipsilateral shoulder following thoracic surgery can add to the burden of a patient's pain experience. Prevalence of ipsilateral shoulder pain was observed to be 97% following thoracotomy.[17] Studies concerning the etiology of this ipsilateral shoulder pain have identified the phrenic nerve as being the most likely source.[18] There is direct evidence that blockade of the periphrenic fat pad at the diaphragm relieves postthoracotomy ipsilateral shoulder pain.[19,20] There is also supporting evidence that interscalene and stellate ganglion blockade have relieved ipsilateral shoulder pain, likely from concomitant blockade of the phrenic nerve that is commonly associated with these blocks.[21,22] Irritation or injury of the visceral pleura, the mainstem bronchi, diaphragm, or pericardium will produce sensory input carried by the phrenic nerve. Thoracostomy tubes can also irritate the phrenic nerve and produce ipsilateral shoulder pain.[16] Because the phrenic nerve originates from C3 to C5, pain to the shoulder is thought to be referred most likely from phrenic nerve input at the site of thoracic surgery.

In summary, acute pain in thoracic surgery involves multiple nerve fibers and pathways (nociceptive, inflammatory, neuropathic, and referred) that produce and modulate the pain experienced by a patient. The pain experienced in the perioperative period has the potential to progress to PPSP, defined as discomfort that lasts for more than 3 to 6 months after surgery and wound healing. Furthermore, PPSP can progress to chronic pain with an incidence of 30% to 40% among those undergoing thoracotomy (see Chapter 25).[15] Therefore it is imperative for the perioperative physician to understand and implement strategies to treat pain related to thoracic surgery, both to decrease acute postoperative pain and decrease the incidence of PPSP.

Multimodal Analgesia and Perioperative Analgesic Strategies

MMA incorporates two or more analgesic agents of different pharmacologic classes to provide superior analgesia and reduce individual class side effects. MMA targets various receptors along the pain pathway to block the transmission of nociceptive stimuli. Because the pain following thoracic surgery involves multiple nociceptive fibers and pathways, a multimodal analgesic strategy is recommended.[23] Combination therapy with different nonopioid analgesics can produce additive or synergistic effects, thereby minimizing opioid use and their associated adverse effects.[24,25]

MMA has been shown to be superior to traditional opioid-based therapies for a variety of surgical procedures and is an integral component of enhanced recovery after surgery (ERAS) and anesthesia protocols.[23,25–27] An MMA regimen that incorporates regional and systemic anesthesia is strongly recommended by the ERAS Society and European Society of

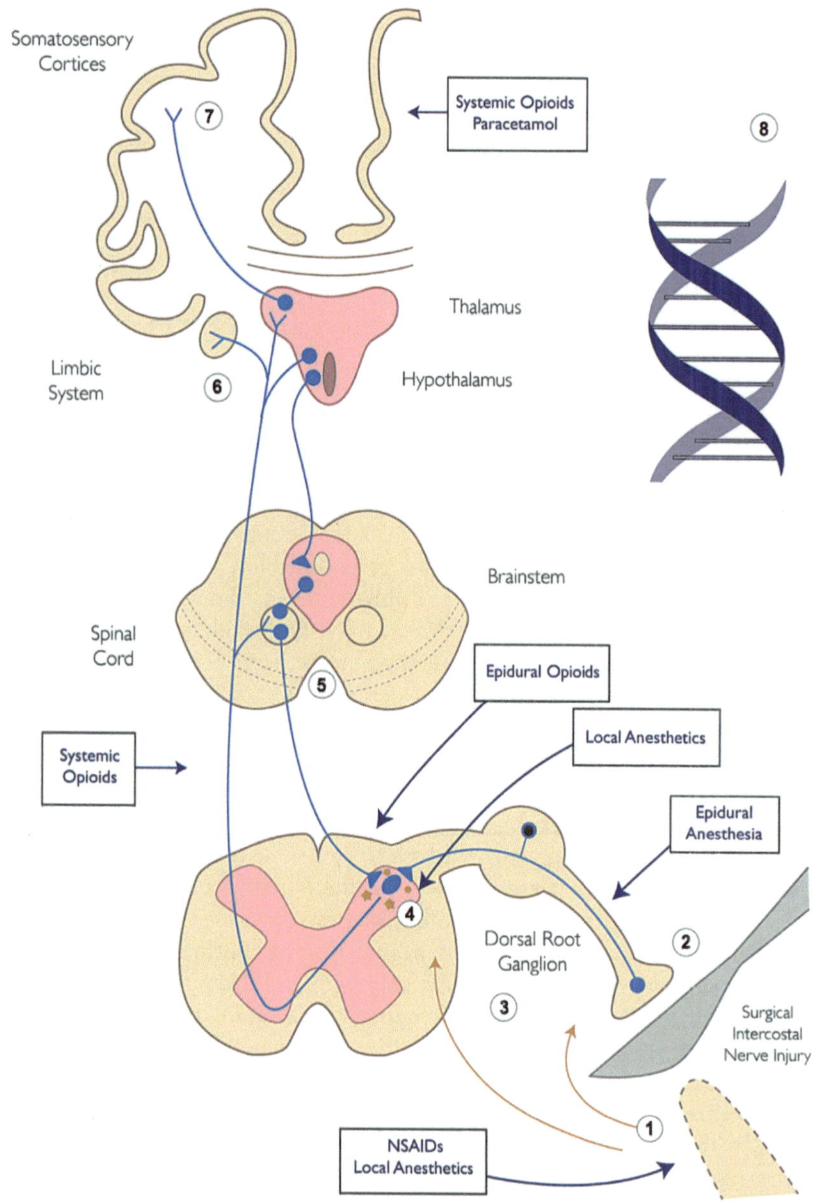

• **Fig. 24.1** Mechanism of persistent postsurgical neuropathic pain. **(1)** Denervated Schwann cells and infiltrating macrophages distal to nerve injury produce local and systemic chemicals that drive pain signaling. **(2)** Neuroma at site of injury is source of ectopic spontaneous excitability in sensory fibers. **(3)** Changes in gene expression in dorsal root ganglion alter excitability, responsiveness, transmission, and survival of sensory neurons. **(4)** Dorsal horn is site of altered activity and gene expression, producing central sensitization, loss of inhibitory interneurons, and microglial activation, which together amplify sensory flow. **(5)** Brainstem descending controls modulate transmission in spinal cord. **(6)** Limbic system and hypothalamus contribute to altered mood, behavior, and autonomic reflexes. **(7)** Sensation of pain generated in cortex (past experiences, cultural inputs, and expectations converge to determine what patient feels). **(8)** Genomic deoxyribonucleic acid (DNA) predispose (or not) patient to chronic pain and affect their reaction to treatment. (From Kehlet H, Jensen TS, Woolf CJ. Persistent postsurgical pain: risk factors and prevention. *Lancet.* 2006;367(9522):1618–1625. With permission.)

Thoracic Surgeons.[23] Thoracic surgery impairs pulmonary function and the respiratory depressant effects of opioid medications can lead to postoperative complications in this at-risk population. Opioids are also associated with an increase in postoperative nausea/vomiting (PONV), ileus, and can impair ambulation and possibly delay a patient's recovery from thoracic surgery.[28] Nonopioids should be administered on a scheduled basis, reserving opioids for severe pain that is not relieved by other modalities. The advantages and disadvantages of various systemic analgesics are summarized in Table 24.2.

Opioids

Postthoracotomy pain was traditionally managed with opioid-based therapies.[1] Various routes of opioid administration have been investigated, including intramuscular (IM),[29] subcutaneous (SC),[30] continuous intravenous (IV) infusions,[31] and epidural administration.[32] IV opioids administered via patient-controlled analgesia (PCA) has been shown to be more effective than IM and SC injections and is also associated with higher patient satisfaction and recovery after surgery.[33–36] As discussed later in this chapter, epidural opioids can be administered in combination with local anesthetics or as a single solution. Regardless of the route or mode of administration, opioid-related adverse effects, such as PONV, constipation, sedation, cough suppression, and respiratory depression, have been shown to impede postoperative recovery.[24] MMA techniques that focus on opioid minimization have replaced opioid-based therapies as the preferred perioperative pain management strategy.

Acetaminophen

Acetaminophen has been incorporated into many enhanced recovery pathways and has been shown to reduce morphine consumption after major surgery.[37] In postthoracotomy

TABLE 24.2 Systemic Analgesics

Systemic Therapies	Advantages	Disadvantages
Opioids	• Simple to administer • Familiar dosing	• Impair respiratory mechanics • Respiratory depression • Ileus
Acetaminophen	• Established safety record	• Mostly effective for mild to moderate pain
NSAIDs	• Lower NNT than opioids	• Increased CV risks, especially for those with CV disease • Causes platelet dysfunction • Can result in slight increase in postop creatinine
Ketamine	• Preserves respiratory drive	• Psychomimetic effects • May not be permitted outside of intraoperative setting at some locations
Glucocorticoids	• Analgesic and antiemetic properties	• Can impair wound healing • Hyperglycemia
Gabapentinoids	• Reduces pain in the immediate postoperative period	• Sedation, especially in the elderly
Intravenous lidocaine	• Possibly helpful for inflammatory pain	• May not be permitted outside of intraoperative setting at some locations

CV, Cardiovascular; *NNT*, number needed to treat; *NSAIDs*, nonsteroidal antiinflammatory drugs.

patients, acetaminophen has been successful in reducing ipsilateral shoulder pain in patients with a thoracic epidural.[17] It is available in oral, rectal, and IV formulations. IV formulations have greater drug bioavailability, but do not appear to enhance the quality of analgesia when compared with oral formulations.[38] IV formulations may be an alternative to patients not tolerating oral intake.[38]

Acetaminophen is a well-tolerated medication that does not have the cardiovascular, gastrointestinal, and renal adverse effects associated with nonsteroidal antiinflammatory drugs (NSAIDs). High doses of acetaminophen can be hepatotoxic, and the total daily dose should be limited to less than 4000 mg per day. It is considered safe for patients at risk for renal failure.

Nonsteroidal Antiinflammatory Drugs

NSAIDs are a diverse class of analgesics that inhibit prostaglandin production via cyclooxygenase (COX) enzymes. NSAIDs can reduce opioid consumption and when combined with opioids can result in improved analgesia and a reduction in PONV and sedation compared with opioids alone.[39] In addition, the combination of NSAIDs and acetaminophen has been shown to be more efficacious than either class of medication alone.[40] High-quality evidence supports the combination of acetaminophen and NSAIDs for thoracic surgery and is strongly recommended by guidelines published by the ERAS Society.[23,41–43]

Several small studies suggested that the antiinflammatory effects of NSAIDs may reduce the efficacy of surgical pleurodesis.[44] However, a recent randomized trial demonstrated that NSAIDs were noninferior to opioids when assessing pleurodesis efficacy.[45] NSAIDs may worsen renal function in patients who are elderly, hypovolemic, or have preexisting renal dysfunction. Many patients who undergo thoracic surgery are at risk for these conditions and an examination of their comorbidities should be accessed before administration.[23]

Nonselective NSAIDs are associated with an increased risk of major cardiovascular events.[46] However, these adverse effects are more likely to be of concern with the long-term use of NSAIDs.[46] Multiple randomized controlled trials (RCTs) have demonstrated that the short-term use of perioperative NSAIDs does not increase the risk of mortality, cardiovascular events, surgical bleeding, or renal dysfunction.[47] Nevertheless, the U.S. Food and Drug Administration recently expanded its warning about NSAIDs increasing the risk of stroke and heart attack to include all classes of NSAIDs.[48]

N-Methyl-D-Aspartate-Receptor Antagonists

Ketamine is a potent analgesic that mediates its effects through the antagonism of the NMDA receptor. In a large metaanalysis of 70 RCTs, ketamine was shown to reduce postoperative opioid consumption.[49] The greatest reduction in opioid consumption was seen in upper abdominal and thoracic surgeries. The opioid-sparing effects of ketamine were independent on the dose or timing of ketamine administration or the type of intraoperative opioid used.[49] In a prospective, randomized double-blinded study after thoracic surgery, the addition of ketamine to a morphine PCA reduced morphine consumption and decreased the number of nocturnal desaturations.[50]

The use of ketamine in thoracic surgery is supported by both the ERAS Society and the 2018 American Society of Regional Anesthesia and Pain Medicine (ASRA) guidelines for IV ketamine for acute pain.[23,51] In the acute pain setting, subanesthetic doses of ketamine are used. Current recommendations state that bolus dosing should not exceed 0.35 mg/kg and infusions should not exceed 1 mg/kg/h in settings without intensive monitoring.[51]

Gabapentinoids

Gabapentinoids (gabapentin and pregabalin) are antiepileptic agents commonly used to treat neuropathic pain. Gabapentinoids have analgesic properties mediated by the alpha 2-delta subunits of presynaptic voltage-gated calcium channels and decreased excitatory neurotransmitter release.[52]

In an RCT that studied its efficacy in postthoracotomy patients, perioperative gabapentin was ineffective in treating acute postthoracotomy pain or for the prevention of persistent postthoracotomy pain.[53] In a separate RCT, pregabalin was also ineffective in reducing the incidence of persistent postthoracotomy pain.[54] Perioperative gabapentinoids are currently not recommended for perioperative pain management in patients undergoing thoracic surgery.[23]

Glucocorticoids

Glucocorticoids, including dexamethasone and methylprednisolone, are commonly administered during surgery because of their analgesic, antiemetic, antipyretic, and antiinflammatory properties.[55] The analgesic effect of dexamethasone is dose-dependent and at intermediate doses (0.11–0.20 mg/kg), a reduction in postoperative pain, opioid consumption, and PONV can be achieved.[56,57] The effect of a single administration of high-dose methylprednisolone (125 mg) in patients undergoing a video-assisted thoracoscopic surgery (VATS) lobectomy was a significant reduction in pain ratings, nausea, and fatigue without an increase in complications.[58]

Glucocorticoids can be considered as part of a multimodal approach to treating PONV, postoperative pain, and airway edema. Compared with the evidence in PONV, the strength of evidence as part of a multimodal analgesic strategy for thoracic surgery is comparatively weak. Nevertheless, dexamethasone has a variety of systemic benefits that are useful in thoracic surgery and is strongly recommended.[23]

Intravenous Lidocaine

High-quality evidence supports the use of perioperative intravenous lidocaine infusions for abdominal surgery.[59] Its utility in thoracic surgery is less clear. In a single, randomized trial of 40 patients, systemic infusions of lidocaine reduced acute postoperative pain and morphine consumption after thoracotomy.[60] In a separate study, systemic lidocaine failed to demonstrate benefit after VATS.[61] More evidence is needed to determine the utility of perioperative lidocaine infusions for thoracic surgery.

Regional Anesthesia

Several regional anesthetic techniques are available for treating pain after thoracic surgery (Table 24.3). Techniques, such as the thoracic epidural anesthesia (TEA), thoracic

TABLE 24.3 Regional Anesthesia Techniques

Regional Anesthesia Techniques	Advantages	Disadvantages
Thoracic epidural analgesia	• Gold standard • Attenuates stress response • Reduces opioid requirements • Improves respiratory mechanics • Improves GI motility	• Invasive and technically challenging • Incompatibility with anticoagulation
Thoracic paravertebral block	• Analgesia comparable to TEA with more favorable side effect profile • Reduces risk of PONV, pruritus, hypotension, and urinary retention	• Invasive and technically challenging • Pneumothorax • Incompatibility with anticoagulation
Intercostal nerve block	• Less technically challenging to perform	• Inferior analgesia compared with TEA and PVB • Pneumothorax • Highest systemic absorption of local anesthetics
Erector spinae plane block	• Less technically challenging to perform • Favorable side effect profile	• Clinical evidence is limited • Little guidance on best dosing strategy
Serratus anterior plane block	• Easy to perform • Reduced risk of pneumothorax	• Clinical evidence is limited • Little guidance on best dosing strategy

GI, Gastrointestinal; *PONV*, postoperative nausea/vomiting; *PVB*, paravertebral block; *TEA*, thoracic epidural.

paravertebral block (TPVB), and intercostal nerve block (ICNB) have been used for many decades in thoracic surgery and their benefits are well established in the literature.[62–64] In recent years, newer techniques, such as the erector spinae plane (ESP) block and the serratus anterior plane block (SAPB), have been developed. Early studies indicate that these blocks provide good analgesia, but additional evidence into their mechanism of action and safety is needed.[65]

The choice of regional anesthetic technique should be dependent on the surgical approach, clinical circumstances, and the presence or absence of contraindications. For example, coagulopathy is a contraindication for a TEA, TPVB, and ICNB, but the risk-benefit ratio might be more favorable when considering ESP or SAPB. However, current guidelines from the ASRA for patients taking anticoagulants do not address the risks associated with newer blocks, such as ESP or SAPB, and caution should still be exercised because few data are available to guide clinicians.[66]

In the era of enhanced recovery, TEA has for the most part been limited to patients undergoing an open thoracotomy. Patients undergoing minimally invasive procedures (robotic-assisted and thoracoscopic surgery) are more likely to receive either a TPVB, ICNB, ESPB, or SAPB. Each of these techniques can be performed as either a single injection, repeat injections, or via continuous infusions.

Thoracic Epidural Analgesia

It could be argued that the "gold standard" for analgesia after open thoracotomy is the thoracic epidural. TEA has been shown in multiple studies to provide effective analgesia and an epidural may be used intraoperatively as an infusion or intermittent bolus dosing. Large-scale meta-analyses have concluded that TEA is superior to systemic analgesia for postoperative pain relief.[62,67] TEA also reduces overall opioid consumption, which is often a goal of surgeons, anesthesiologists, and patients alike.[62] Additional TEA benefits include decreased pulmonary complications, decreased bowel dysfunction, and improved patient satisfaction.[68]

Typically, TEA serves as an adjunct to general anesthesia. Initiation of the epidural infusion intraoperatively is useful in establishing an adequate dermatomal band of analgesia and can reduce the intraoperative opioid requirements, as well as anesthetic requirements.[10,13] TEA infusions may consist of local anesthetic alone, opioid alone, or a combination. The optimal solution is debatable, although some evidence suggests that combining TEA local anesthetics and opioids produces superior analgesia compared with using epidural opioids or local anesthetics alone.[62] Local anesthetic infusions alone in a multimodal platform with supplemental IV or oral opioids likely produces the most opioid reduction and least opioid-related adverse events. There are many local anesthetic-opioid mixtures using TEA with the common characteristics of long duration of action of the local anesthetic (ropivacaine or bupivacaine) and lipophilicity of the opioid (fentanyl or to a lesser degree hydromorphone). In a systematic review comparing various regional anesthetic techniques with systemic opioids, TEA with local anesthetic plus opioid, local anesthetic alone, or lipophilic opioid alone was superior to systemic routes of opioid administration.[32] The studies yielded mixed results when comparing TEA with hydrophilic opioids alone and systemic opioid administration.[32] Continuous delivery of an opioid by any route of administration, including the epidural route, is associated with a higher rate of respiratory depression than intermittent on-demand opioids. All current acute pain guidelines recommend a multimodal analgesic approach with intermittent delivery of opioids at the lowest possible dose. Thoracic epidural analgesia is best used within the context of MMA minimizing opioids and preferentially using opioids only intermittently as needed. Because patients recovering from thoracic surgery are at an increased risk for respiratory impairment, special consideration should be given to reducing overall opioid doses, and it is particularly crucial in patient with myasthenia gravis. Maintenance of analgesia throughout the postoperative period may be administered as a bolus or continuous infusion with the possibility of patient-controlled delivery. TEA is generally continued until chest tubes are removed a few days after surgery.

Technique

Placement of a thoracic epidural is typically guided by anatomic landmarks between the T4 and T6 levels (Fig. 24.2). Compared with the lumbar spine, the thoracic spinous processes are longer and have a steeper angulation that makes the midline approach potentially more difficult. A paramedian approach to the thoracic epidural space may facilitate epidural placement.

In addition to producing segmental analgesia, blockade of the cardiac sympathetic fibers can occur if infusions spread cephalad to anesthetize the T1–T5 sympathetic nerves.[69] This can result in decreases in preload, suppression of the baroreceptor reflex, and activation of the reverse Bainbridge reflex, leading to hypotension and bradycardia.[69]

Complications and Safety Considerations

Compared with lumbar epidurals, TEA is technically more challenging and carries a higher risk of neurologic complications. Fortunately, the overall incidence of neurologic complications is rare and reported to be around 3.1%.[70] The development of an epidural hematoma is another devastating, but fortunately very rare, complication of epidural placement.[66,71] Because coagulopathy is a relative contraindication to TEA, patient history should be obtained with focus on easy bleeding and bruising. Although routine coagulation studies are not needed, such studies should be reviewed if already obtained to ensure unexpected coagulopathy is not present. We recommend that anticoagulant medications should be managed in accordance with the anticoagulation guidelines published by the ASRA.[66]

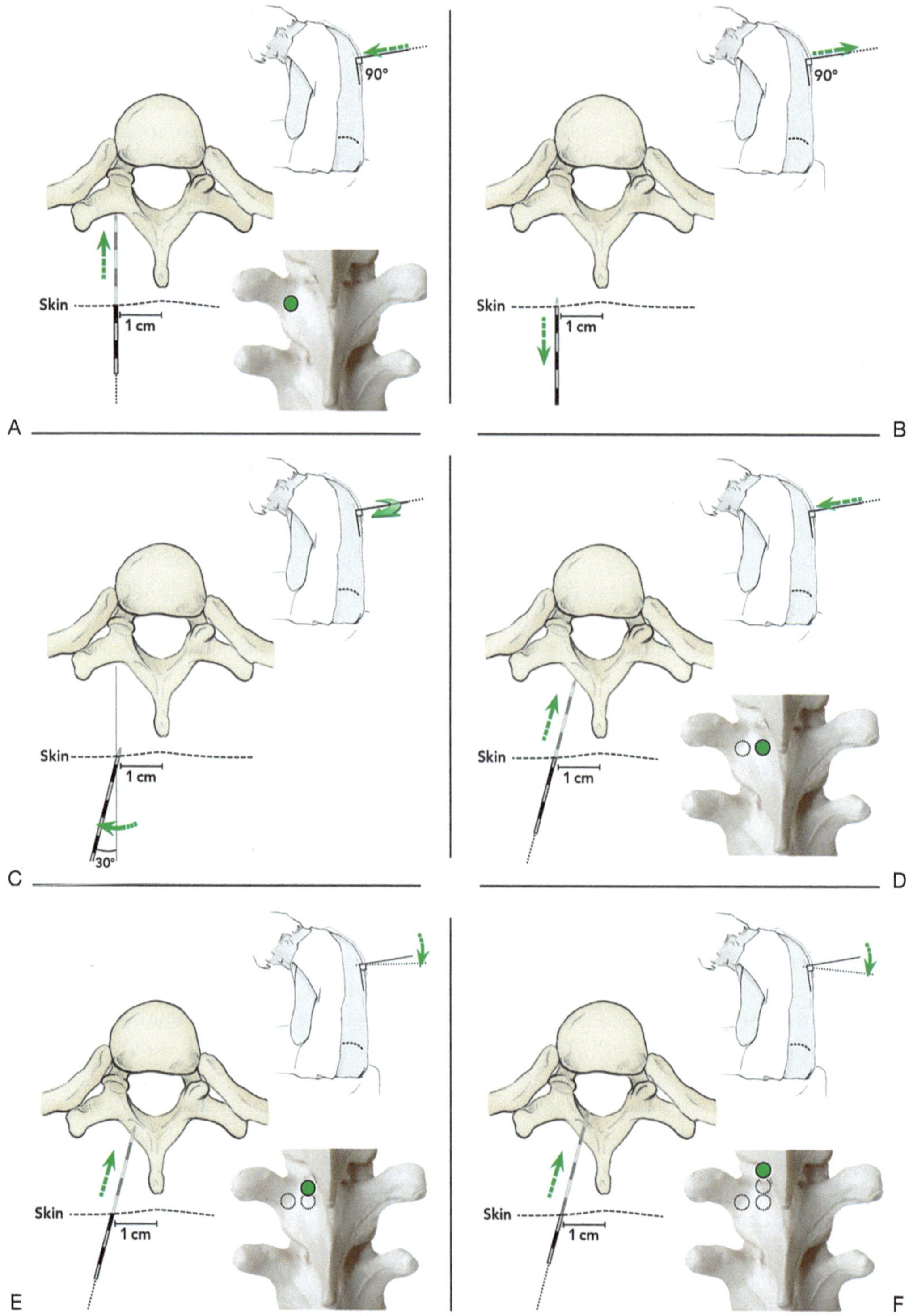

• **Fig. 24.2** Thoracic epidural catheter placement. Schematic of thoracic epidural catheter placement using transverse and posterior views of drawings of the thoracic spine. Hustead (or Tuohy) needle with the bevel directed cephalad is introduced perpendicular to the anesthetized skin approximately 1 cm lateral to the spinous process of the targeted segment and advanced until the ipsilateral lamina or medial transverse process is contacted. If lamina is not contacted, avoid advancing the needle laterally, which will place the needle in the paravertebral space. Note the needle depth to the lamina (**A**). Withdraw the needle back to skin (**B**). Readvance the needle slightly medially without a change in cephalocaudal direction (**C**). With advancement, lamina again should be contacted (**D**). Slight medial revisions of the needle are performed until the needle contacts bone at a slightly more superficial (about 2–5 mm) depth than the original depth (A) of the lateral lamina. This suggests the epidural needle tip is midline at the junction of the lamina and spinous process. If the needle contacts bone much shallower than the original depth of the lateral lamina (≥1 cm), it is likely the needle has contacted the posterior part of the spinous process and the angle is too medial. If this is the case, the needle should be withdrawn and repositioned slightly more lateral. After the correct medial angle is determined, the needle is withdrawn and advanced with the same medial angle but in small increments cephalad to the same depth as in D (**E**). If bone is contacted, direct the needle slightly more cephalad and advance. If bone is no longer contacted and the depth exceeds the depth previously noted, the epidural needle stilette is removed and loss-of-resistance technique is begun (**F**). (From Manion SC, Brennan TJ. Thoracic epidural analgesia and acute pain management. *Anesthesiology*. 2011;115(1):181–188. With permission.)

Clinical Advantages

Following thoracic surgery, TEA reduces overall opioid consumption while improving analgesia.[32,62] Reduced opioid consumption may allow for patients to ambulate earlier and could help in reducing sedation and postoperative cognitive dysfunction, especially in the elderly.

Inadequate analgesia and oversedation in the postoperative period may compromise pulmonary function and increase pulmonary complications. TEA has been shown to improve pulmonary function when compared with systemic analgesia. TEA decreases the degree of postoperative diaphragmatic dysfunction after thoracic surgery by minimizing the impact of surgical injury on phrenic motor nerve activity.[72] A metaanalysis of the protective effects of TEA showed that from 1971 to 2006 the incidence of pneumonia with TEA remained about 8% but decreased from 34% to 12% with systemic analgesia.[73] This difference reached statistical significance and suggests that the relative benefit of TEA has lessened over time. Finally, a metaanalysis of 65 RCTs comparing TEA using opioids and local anesthetics versus systemic opioids demonstrated a significant decrease in the incidence of atelectasis, pulmonary infections, hypoxemia, and overall pulmonary complications.[74]

Postoperative ileus is a common concern related to systemic opioids. TEA with local anesthetics results in faster return of bowel function compared with systemic opioids.[75] In fact, TEA infusions of local anesthetic, with or without opioids, have been shown to enhance gastrointestinal recovery from surgery.[76] The prevailing understanding is that TEA can selectively block nociceptive afferent fibers and the sympathetic nervous system but spares the parasympathetic nervous system. Specifically, the preservation of vagal tone may increase gastrointestinal motility postoperatively and limit the duration of ileus after thoracic surgery.

The partial blockade of the sympathetic nervous system with TEA may reduce some specific cardiac complications. Injury to cardiac parasympathetic nerves during thoracic surgery may be the source of tachyarrhythmias in the postoperative period because of the relatively unopposed innervation of the sympathetic nervous system. Investigators have found that postoperative thoracic sympathetic blockade with continuous thoracic epidural bupivacaine infusion after pulmonary resection reduced supraventricular tachyarrhythmias compared with epidural morphine infusion.[77]

Another clinical advantage of TEA is decreased postoperative catabolism and decreased muscle protein synthesis. TEA has been observed to reduce amino acid oxidation and nitrogen excretion to preserve lean body mass in the postoperative period.[78,79]

Controversies

Although many studies suggest that TEA provides excellent analgesia for thoracic surgery, there is evidence that epidural analgesia with opioids alone does not necessarily improve **pulmonary function**. A comparison of epidural fentanyl and IV morphine concluded that epidural fentanyl provided superior analgesia, but there was no difference in postoperative forced vital capacity between the two groups following thoracic surgery.[80] Another study comparing IV fentanyl with lumbar epidural fentanyl demonstrated no difference in analgesia following thoracic surgery but a difference in the amount of fentanyl consumed. However, a secondary finding was the lack of difference in respiratory rates, arterial carbon dioxide partial pressure, or changes in pulmonary function as measured by forced vital capacity and forced expiratory volume in 1 second.[81]

TEA has been reported to reduce the duration of **postoperative ileus** but the suggestion that utilization of epidural analgesia in the postoperative period can reduce the patient's length of hospitalization is questionable. This is primarily because of typically insufficient subject numbers to detect differences in currently low incidences of postoperative complications.[75,76]

Finally, **thoracic versus lumbar epidural catheters** can both be used for analgesia following thoracic surgery. TEA with local anesthetics is thought to target the dermatomes corresponding to surgery, thereby improving analgesia and limiting the total amount of opioids required when compared with a lumbar epidural placement. However, several studies have indicated that the quality of analgesia is comparable in patients receiving either a thoracic or lumbar epidural for postthoracotomy pain.[82–85] Furthermore, a reduction in opioid consumption was not consistently observed in the thoracic epidural group.[82,85] The literature has also been inconsistent in demonstrating an advantage of thoracic epidural placement over lumbar epidural placement in terms of postoperative pulmonary function.[74,83] Arguments have been made that not every patient undergoing a thoracotomy requires a thoracic epidural for pain management because of the lack of strong evidence.[86] Nevertheless, the role of a lumbar epidurals has not been as extensively studied, and there is a greater abundance of evidence that supports the use of TEA for thoracic surgery. Dynamic pain control is important to maintain pulmonary function, and in general, local anesthetics are superior opioids in relieving dynamic pain. A thorough risk-benefit discussion should take place before TEA is initiated and, in some cases, an alternative technique may be more appropriate. Some of these techniques will be discussed in the following sections.

Thoracic Paravertebral Block

The TPVB is an alternative to TEA and is useful for ipsilateral pain of the thorax and abdomen. Local anesthetic is injected into the paravertebral space to anesthetize the somatic and sympathetic nerves of contiguous dermatomes. This technique has been used for surgical anesthesia, postoperative analgesia, and other acute and chronic pain conditions.

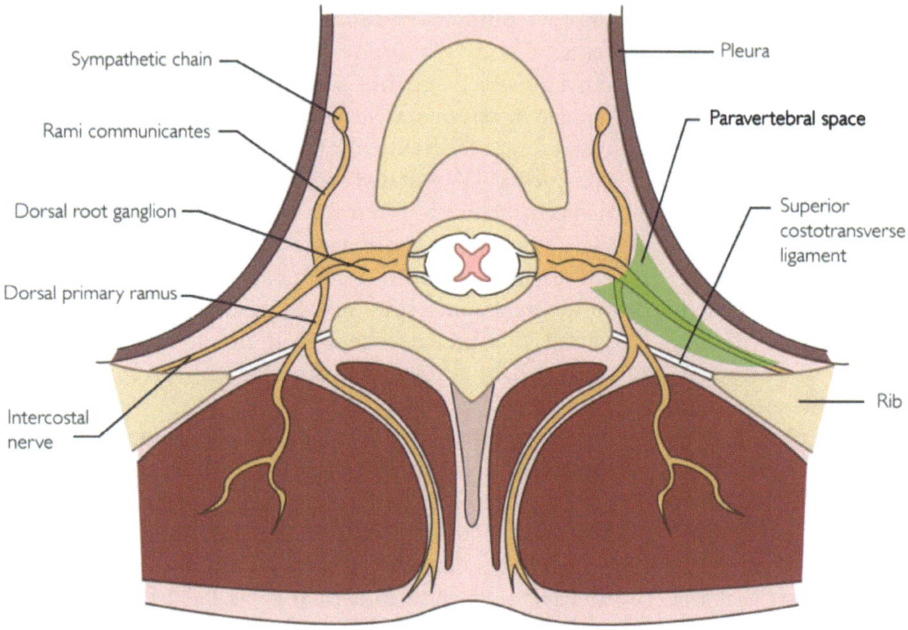

• **Fig. 24.3** Anatomy of the thoracic paravertebral space where the local anesthetic should be deposit. (From Mesbah A, Yeung J, Gao F. Pain after thoracotomy. *BJA Educ*. 2016;16(1):1–7. With permission.)

Anatomy of the Paravertebral Space

The thoracic paravertebral space (TPVS) is a wedge-shaped space located on either side of the vertebral column (Fig. 24.3).[87] The parietal pleura forms the anterolateral boundary, while the superior costotransverse ligament forms the posterior wall of the TPVS. The medial border of the TPVS is formed by the posterolateral aspect of the vertebral body, the intervertebral disc, the intervertebral foramen, and its contents.[87,88] The endothoracic fascia divides the TPVS into two fascial compartments: the anterior (extrapleural) paravertebral compartment and the posterior (subendothoracic) paravertebral compartments.[89,90] The anterior compartment contains the sympathetic trunk.[87,88] The posterior compartment contains the intercostal (spinal nerve), the dorsal ramus, intercostal vessels, and the rami communicantes.[87,88]

Mechanism of Blockade and Distribution of Spread

Injections into the thoracic paravertebral space can spread in a cephalad-caudad direction to anesthetize somatic and sympathetic nerve fibers of contiguous dermatomes.[91,92] Injections can also spread in a medial and lateral direction to involve the epidural space and intercostal space, respectively.[92] The distribution of blockade usually results in unilateral analgesia, however, instances of bilateral anesthesia have been described.[93,94] The contribution of epidural spread after TPVB is unclear, but ipsilateral epidural spread likely occurs in the majority of patients, resulting in a greater distribution of anesthesia than occurs with paravertebral spread alone.[95] Injections into the lower TPVS can anesthetize lumbar spinal nerves within the retroperitoneal space via connections between the endothoracic fascia and transversalis fascia of the abdomen.[96]

The distribution of blockade after a single paravertebral injectate is unpredictable and may be related to spread within the endothoracic fascia.[97] A study by Cheema et al. demonstrated that 15 mL of 0.5% bupivacaine produced a mean unilateral somatic block over five dermatomes and a sympathetic block over eight dermatomes.[91] If dense anesthesia spanning several dermatomes is desired, multiple small-volume injections at consecutive levels can be considered, and may be preferable over a single, large-volume injection.[95]

Technique

The classical approach for thoracic paravertebral blockade is a blind, loss-of-resistance technique that uses surface landmarks to access the TPVS (Fig. 24.4).[88] Ultrasound-guided approaches have gained in popularity and may improve

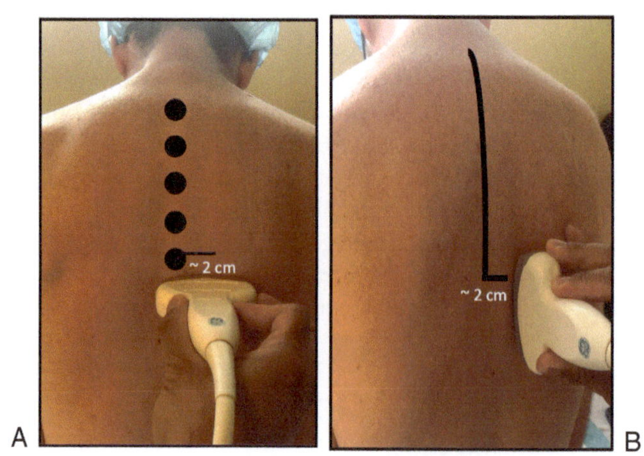

• **Fig. 24.4** Patient positioning for thoracic paravertebral block. (**A**) Transverse probe orientation. (**B**) Parasagittal probe placement for a thoracic paravertebral block. The thoracic paravertebral space is located approximately 1.5 to 3 cm lateral to the spinous processes.

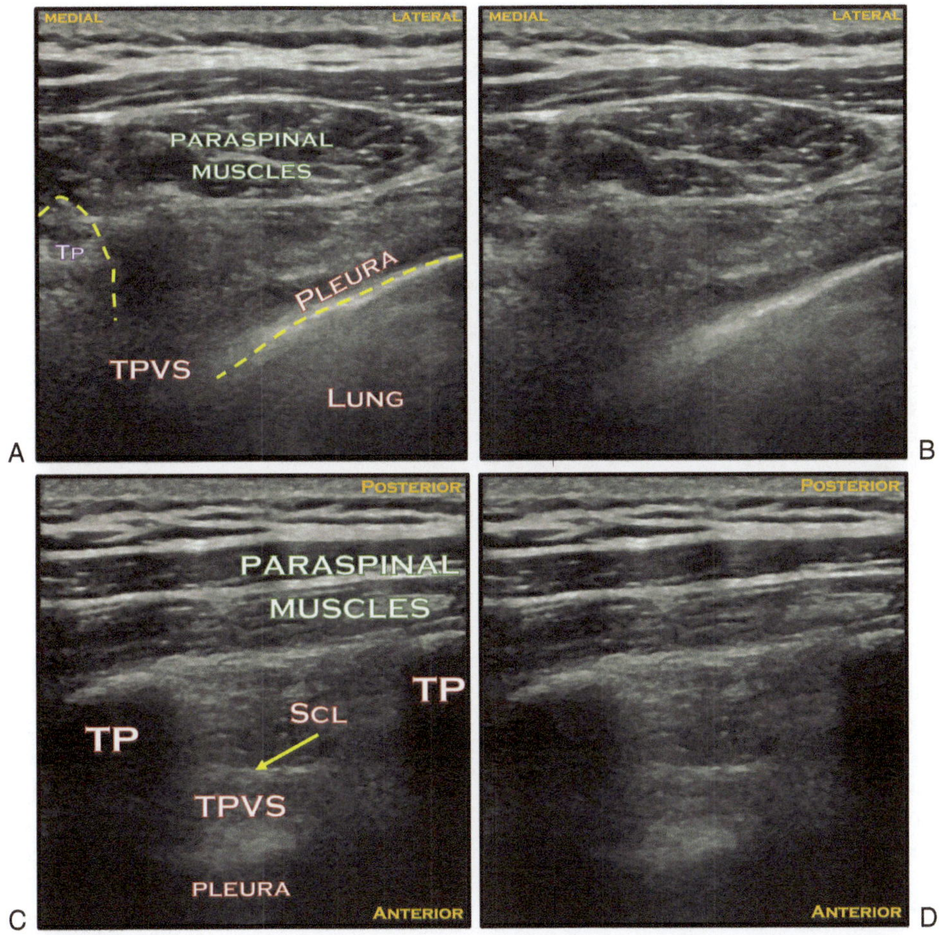

• **Fig. 24.5** Ultrasound anatomy of the thoracic paravertebral space (*TPVS*). (**A** and **B**) Transverse sonogram. The TPVS is lateral to the transverse process (TP) and medial to the pleura. (**C** and **D**) Parasagittal sonogram. The TPVS lies anterior to the superior costotransverse ligament (*SCL*).

block success, minimize block-related complications, and reduce the number of needle redirections (Fig. 24.5).[98] Downward displacement of the parietal pleural can be seen on ultrasound in some patients and may represent objective, sonographic evidence of a properly performed TPVB.[99]

Paravertebral catheters may be used to extend the duration of analgesia but should not be advanced beyond 2 to 3 to avoid inadvertent placement in the pleural, epidural, intercostal, or prevertebral space.[100] An injection of 5 to 10 mL of saline can be used to expand the TPVS and facilitate catheter insertion.

Complications and Safety Considerations

Complications associated with TPVB are rare, occurring in about 2.6% to 5% of cases.[101,102] Complications include vascular puncture (3.8%), hypotension (4.6%), pleural puncture (1.1%), and pneumothorax 0.5%).[103] Compared with TEA, euvolemic patients are less likely to experience hypotension because the sympathectomy is unilateral.[91,104] Pulmonary hemorrhage after a single-shot TPVB has been reported in a patient undergoing a repeat thoracotomy.[105]

Choosing Between Thoracic Epidural Analgesia and Paravertebral Block

TEA is still considered the "gold standard" analgesic technique for thoracic surgery.[106] However, side effects, such as potential respiratory depression, hypotension, urinary retention, incomplete (or failed) block, and spinal cord injury may limit its use. TPVB is an alternative to TEA and produces comparable analgesia[107] with a more favorable side effect profile.[108] In a metaanalysis comparing TEA and TPVB after thoracotomy, TPVB was associated with fewer pulmonary complications, less urinary retention, less nausea and vomiting, less hypotension, and a lower rate of failed blocks.[108]

Intercostal Nerve Block

Anatomy and Mechanism of Blockade

An ICNB anesthetizes the intercostal nerve along the inferior border of the corresponding rib, producing ipsilateral numbness and motor blockade of the adjacent intercostal muscles. The intercostal nerves arise from the anterior divisions of the T1 to T11 spinal nerves. The intercostal

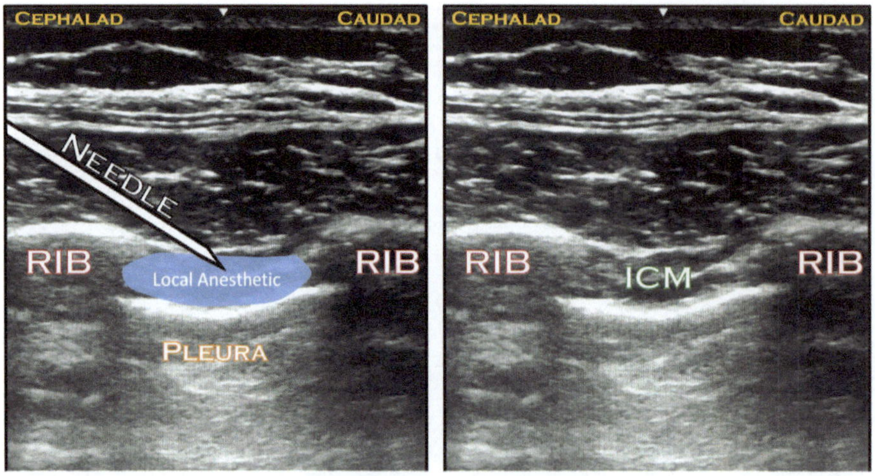

• **Fig. 24.6** Ultrasound guided intercostal nerve block with in-plane needle advancement. The needle is advanced towards the intercostal muscles (*ICM*) and local anesthetic is deposited superficial to the pleura.

nerves travel in the fascial plane between the innermost intercostal muscle and the internal intercostal muscle. At the midaxillary line, a lateral cutaneous branch arises from each of the intercostal muscles (ICN). The continuation of the ICN terminates as an anterior cutaneous branch. The ICN and its branches provide sensory and motor innervation to skin and musculature of the chest and abdominal wall.

Technique and Technical Considerations

ICNBs can be performed anywhere along the inferior border of the rib. However, injections beyond the midaxillary line may fail to anesthetize the lateral cutaneous branch, sparing the muscular, and cutaneous fibers of the lateral thorax. For this reason, injections proximal to the midaxillary line and along the angle of the rib are recommended (Fig. 24.6). Blocks performed at this location are believed to confer a larger margin of safety because the rib is superficial, easily palpated, and the subcostal groove is the widest.

Compared with TEA, patients receiving ICNBs report higher pain scores and consume more opioids.[32] Only one study comparing the efficacy of an ICNB to TPVBs has been performed and it demonstrated no significant difference between the two techniques.[109] Nevertheless, ICNBs can still be useful in the treatment of postthoracotomy pain. For example, in the setting of a failed TEA or TPVB, a single injection ICNB can offer temporary relief, until the TEA or TPVB can be replaced. Furthermore, in the presence of neuraxial contraindications, repeat injections or continuous ICNBs can be considered as a primary analgesic or as an adjunct to systemic analgesia. Each of these techniques has been shown to reduce postoperative pain when compared with systemic analgesia alone.[110–112] Continuous intercostal catheters have the advantage of extending the duration of analgesia and minimize the discomfort associated with repeat injections.

Complications and Safety Considerations

Pneumothorax is a well-recognized, but fortunately very rare, complication of an ICNB. If a pneumothorax is suspected, the patient should be monitored closely for tension physiology. Additional complications include injury to the abdominal viscera, hypotension, inadequate dermatomal spread, and spinal anesthesia.[113,114] ICNB can be considered a "deep" peripheral nerve block according to ASRA and the same anticoagulation guidelines for neuraxial techniques may be followed.[66]

The plasma levels of local anesthetics after an ICNB are the highest among all regional anesthetic techniques, making local anesthetic systemic toxicity a significant concern.[63,115] The addition of epinephrine to local anesthetics may slow systemic absorption of local anesthetic, and increase the maximal allowable dose.[116] Dilute concentrations of local anesthetics should be considered for continuous intercostal catheters.[1] It is advisable to leave a wide safety margin between the doses given and the maximum recommended dosages, especially in young children, the elderly, debilitated patients, and those with underlying cardiac, hepatic, or renal impairment. The maximum single injection dose of plain bupivacaine is 2 and 3 mg/kg with epinephrine.[117,118] The maximum single dose of plain ropivacaine is 2.5 and 4 mg/kg with epinephrine.[117,118]

Erector Spinae Plane Block

The erector spinae plane block (ESPB) was first described in 2016 by Forero et al. for the treatment of chronic thoracic neuropathic pain and postoperative pain in thoracic surgery.[119] The main advantages offered by an ESPB are the ease of performance and possibility of fewer complications, although the latter has not yet been proven.

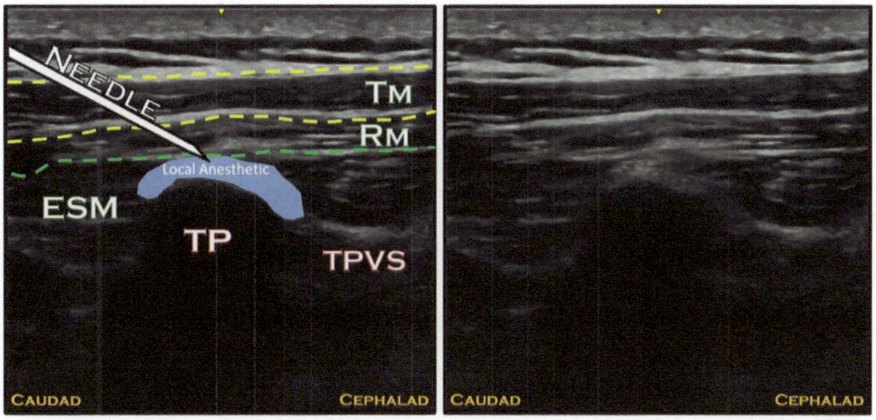

• **Fig. 24.7** Ultrasound guided erector spinae plane block with in-plane needle advancement. The needle is directed towards the transverse process (*TP*) and local anesthetic is deposited in the fascial plane between the TP and the erector spinae muscle (*ESM*). *TM*, trapezius muscle; *RM*, rhomboid muscle; *TPVS*, thoracic paravertebral space.

Mechanism of Blockade and Distribution of Spread

The erector spinae are a group of muscles that include the longissimus, iliocostalis, and spinalis muscles. These muscles span the length of the axial spine and primarily function to stabilize and extend the spine. Injectates are deposited in the fascial plane deep to the erector spinae muscles and spread in a craniocaudal direction of contiguous vertebral levels (Fig. 24.7).[119] Although the exact mechanism is unknown, the ESPB is believed to produce somatic and visceral analgesia via blockade of the intercostal nerves, the dorsal and ventral rami, and the sympathetic fibers. Anterior diffusion into the thoracic paravertebral space was observed in some cadaver studies but not others.[119–121]

Technique and Technical Considerations

The goal of the block is to deposit local anesthetic in the fascial plane between the erector spinae muscle and transverse process of the vertebra. A properly performed block is confirmed by observation on ultrasound of the injectate "lifting" the erector spinae muscles off the tip of the transverse process and the fascial plane filling with hypoechoic local anesthetic. On average, 3.4 mL of injected local anesthetic results in the cephalad or caudad spread of one dermatome fascial plane.[122]

Single-Shot Erector Spinae Plane Versus Continuous Erector Spinae Plane

The ESPB is a fascial plane block, and large volume injectates are recommended to maximize the spread of local anesthetics. Single-shot ESPB with long-acting local anesthetics or continuous infusions through catheters can be used to provide adequate analgesia.[123] Existing evidence does not support the superiority of single-shot versus continuous techniques. Analgesia with the single-shot ESPB will be limited to postoperative day 0.

Eng et al.[124] reported that pain relief occurred immediately after performance of an ESPB, but pain recurred within 2 to 3 hours of the block, despite the use of long-acting local anesthetics. The authors suggested that systemic absorption of local anesthetic may have been a contributing factor to the short duration. ESPBs have not been well studied in thoracic surgery but one prospective study[125] in patients undergoing a thoracotomy and one case series[65] in patients undergoing VATS have shown promising results.

Complications and Safety Considerations

Although theoretically the ESPB should carry a lower risk of pneumothorax and minimal risk of spinal hematoma, given the distance from the spinal cord, safety has still not been demonstrated. A case series of five patients, all of whom received an ESPB and had altered coagulation, reported that no patients developed a hematoma after block placement.[126] One of the larger RCTs included 100 patients undergoing mastectomy, 50 of whom received an ESPB, and reported no vascular punctures or pneumothoraces, but the study was not powered for complications, which may be rare.[127] Local anesthetic systemic toxicity risk has not been evaluated with ESPBs. Early reports have been encouraging but more data are clearly needed before safety can be established.

Serratus Anterior Plane Block

The SAPB was first described by Blanco et al. in 2013.[128] This block anesthetizes the lateral cutaneous branch of the intercostal nerves and provides analgesia to the anterolateral

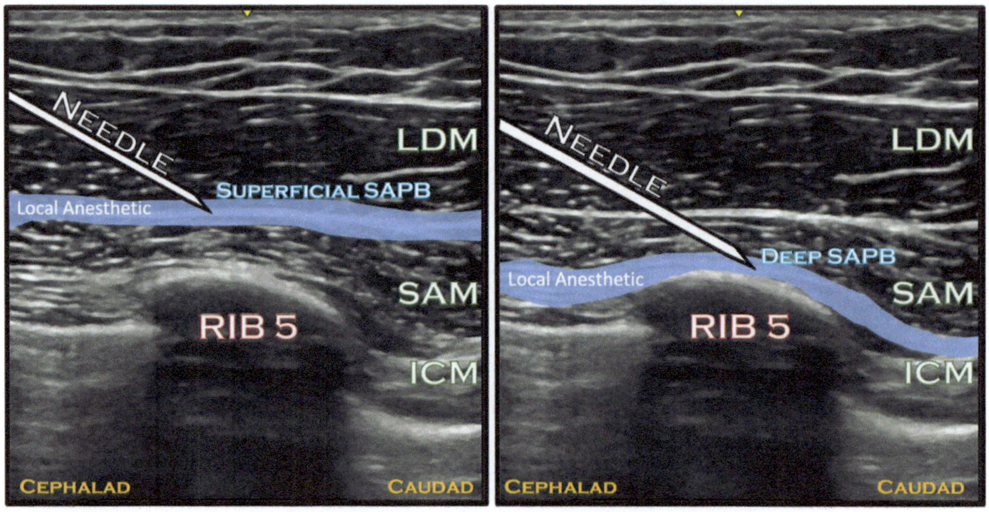

• **Fig. 24.8** Ultrasound guided serratus anterior plane block (*SAPB*) with in-plane needle advancement. Local anesthetic can be deposited in the fascial plane between the latissimus dorsi muscle (*LDM*) and the serratus anterior muscle (*SAM*) or in the fascial plane between the SAM and the intercostal muscle (*ICM*).

thoracic wall. Early reports indicate that this block may be a safe and effective technique for thoracic surgery and other surgical procedures involving the chest wall.[129,130]

Technique and Technical Considerations

The SAPB is performed by depositing local anesthetic in either the superficial or deep fascial layers of the serratus anterior muscle (Fig. 24.8). The superficial SAPB targets the fascial plane between the latissimus dorsi muscle and the serratus anterior muscle. The deep SAPB targets the fascial plane between the serratus anterior muscle and the intercostal muscles. The optimal plane of injection is not clear, but blockade of the lateral cutaneous branch of the intercostal nerve is the purported mechanism of analgesia for both techniques.[128] Similar to the ESPB, the volume of local anesthetic influences the spread of the injectate.

There are only a handful of studies that have evaluated the utility of the SAPB in thoracic surgery, and the available evidence indicates that this block may be an effective alternative for both open and thoracoscopic surgeries.[129,131–134] When compared with TEA and TPVB, the SAPB produced comparable levels of postoperative analgesia in patients undergoing open thoracotomies.[129,132] Unlike TEA, reductions in mean arterial pressure do not occur in patients receiving SAPB.[129,132] Investigations in thoracoscopic surgery have shown an opioid sparing effect, reduction in pain, and PONV when SAPB was added to systemic analgesic therapy.[131,133,134]

Complications and Safety Considerations

The SAPB was designed to be a safer alternative to TEA, TPVB, and ICNB; however, more studies are necessary to support this assertion. The block is performed in the fascial planes along the posterior axillary line, thereby eliminating, or at least substantially reducing, the risks of spinal cord injury and pneumothorax.[128] The block produces ipsilateral blockade of somatic nerve fibers and spares sympathetic nerve fibers, making hypotension less likely.[128] Complication risks are not yet defined.

Conclusion

Thoracic surgery is considered to be one of the most painful surgical procedures. Inadequately controlled postoperative pain can impair functional recovery, limit participation in rehabilitation, and is associated with a substantial risk of PPSP. The pain can also impair respiratory mechanics, leading to atelectasis and other postoperative pulmonary complications.[1,2,13] Traditional opioid-based strategies are often inadequate and opioid escalation risks respiratory depression in a patient population with already impaired respiratory mechanics. As a result, the reliance on opioids for acute postoperative pain has waned, and most modern-day analgesic strategies incorporate MMA with regional anesthesia. Regional anesthetic techniques such as TEA, TPVC, and the more novel fascial plane blocks have proven to be safe and effective in managing postoperative pain after thoracic surgery, although more research is warranted for the newer techniques. Like any modality these techniques also have drawbacks that must be factored into the risk-benefit discussion. When combined with MMA, the quality of analgesia with regional anesthesia techniques is enhanced and facilitates postoperative recovery. The influence of pain management on patient outcomes has made it an integral consideration when caring for patients undergoing thoracic surgery.

References

1. Kavanagh BP, Katz J, Sandler AN. Pain control after thoracic surgery. A review of current techniques. *Anesthesiology.* 1994;81(3):737–759.
2. Richebe P, Capdevila X, Rivat C. Persistent postsurgical pain: pathophysiology and preventative pharmacologic considerations. *Anesthesiology.* 2018;129(3):590–607.
3. Muehling BM, Halter GL, Schelzig H, et al. Reduction of postoperative pulmonary complications after lung surgery using a fast track clinical pathway. *Eur J Cardiothorac Surg.* 2008;34(1):174–180.
4. Wijeysundera DN, Beattie WS, Austin PC, Hux JE, Laupacis A. Epidural anaesthesia and survival after intermediate-to-high risk non-cardiac surgery: a population-based cohort study. *Lancet.* 2008;372(9638):562–569.
5. Loan WB, Morrison JD. The incidence and severity of postoperative pain. *Br J Anaesth.* 1967;39(9):695–698.
6. Ali J, Weisel RD, Layug AB, Kripke BJ, Hechtman HB. Consequences of postoperative alterations in respiratory mechanics. *Am J Surg.* 1974;128(3):376–382.
7. Johnson WC. Postoperative ventilatory performance: dependence upon surgical incision. *Am Surg.* 1975;41(10):615–619.
8. Bromage PR, Camporesi E, Chestnut D. Epidural narcotics for postoperative analgesia. *Anesth Analg.* 1980;59(7):473–480.
9. Shulman M, Sandler AN, Bradley JW, Young PS, Brebner J. Post-thoracotomy pain and pulmonary function following epidural and systemic morphine. *Anesthesiology.* 1984;61(5):569–575.
10. Ochroch EA, Gottschalk A, Augostides J, et al. Long-term pain and activity during recovery from major thoracotomy using thoracic epidural analgesia. *Anesthesiology.* 2002;97(5):1234–1244.
11. Sabanathan S. Has postoperative pain been eradicated? *Ann R Coll Surg Engl.* 1995;77(3):202–209.
12. Sabanathan S, Eng J, Mearns AJ. Alterations in respiratory mechanics following thoracotomy. *J R Coll Surg Edinb.* 1990;35(3):144–150.
13. Gottschalk A, Cohen SP, Yang S, Ochroch EA. Preventing and treating pain after thoracic surgery. *Anesthesiology.* 2006;104(3):594–600.
14. Obata H, Saito S, Fujita N, Fuse Y, Ishizaki K, Goto F. Epidural block with mepivacaine before surgery reduces long-term post-thoracotomy pain. *Can J Anaesth.* 1999;46(12):1127–1132.
15. Kehlet H, Jensen TS, Woolf CJ. Persistent postsurgical pain: risk factors and prevention. *Lancet.* 2006;367(9522):1618–1625.
16. Mesbah A, Yeung J, Gao F. Pain after thoracotomy. *BJA Education.* 2016;16(1):1–7.
17. Mac TB, Girard F, Chouinard P, et al. Acetaminophen decreases early post-thoracotomy ipsilateral shoulder pain in patients with thoracic epidural analgesia: a double-blind placebo-controlled study. *J Cardiothorac Vasc Anesth.* 2005;19(4):475–478.
18. MacDougall P. Postthoracotomy shoulder pain: diagnosis and management. *Curr Opin Anaesthesiol.* 2008;21(1):12–15.
19. Danelli G, Berti M, Casati A, et al. Ipsilateral shoulder pain after thoracotomy surgery: a prospective, randomized, double-blind, placebo-controlled evaluation of the efficacy of infiltrating the phrenic nerve with 0.2%wt/vol ropivacaine. *Eur J Anaesthesiol.* 2007;24(7):596–601.
20. Scawn ND, Pennefather SH, Soorae A, Wang JY, Russell GN. Ipsilateral shoulder pain after thoracotomy with epidural analgesia: the influence of phrenic nerve infiltration with lidocaine. *Anesth Analg.* 2001;93(2):260–264, 261st contents page.
21. Burgess FW, Anderson DM, Colonna D, Sborov MJ, Cavanaugh DG. Ipsilateral shoulder pain following thoracic surgery. *Anesthesiology.* 1993;78(2):365–368.
22. Garner L, Coats RR. Ipsilateral stellate ganglion block effective for treating shoulder pain after thoracotomy. *Anesth Analg.* 1994;78(6):1195–1196.
23. Batchelor TJP, Rasburn NJ, Abdelnour-Berchtold E, et al. Guidelines for enhanced recovery after lung surgery: recommendations of the Enhanced Recovery After Surgery (ERAS(R)) Society and the European Society of Thoracic Surgeons (ESTS). *Eur J Cardiothorac Surg.* 2019;55(1):91–115.
24. Wick EC, Grant MC, Wu CL. Postoperative multimodal analgesia pain management with nonopioid analgesics and techniques: a review. *JAMA Surg.* 2017;152(7):691–697.
25. American Society of Anesthesiologists Task Force on Acute Pain M. Practice guidelines for acute pain management in the perioperative setting: an updated report by the American Society of Anesthesiologists Task Force on Acute Pain Management. *Anesthesiology.* 2012;116(2):248–273.
26. Practice guidelines for acute pain management in the perioperative setting: an updated report by the American Society of Anesthesiologists Task Force on Acute Pain Management. *Anesthesiology.* 2012;116(2):248–273.
27. Rafiq S, Steinbruchel DA, Wanscher MJ, et al. Multimodal analgesia versus traditional opiate based analgesia after cardiac surgery, a randomized controlled trial. *J Cardiothorac Surg.* 2014;9:52.
28. Kaban JM, Kurtz J, Parsikia A, et al. Adherence to non-opioid multimodal analgesia (NOMA) protocol is associated with a shorter length of stay after thoracic surgery. *J Clin Anesth.* 2020;60:113–114.
29. Jenkins AV, Das B. The use of phenoperidine in thoracic surgery. A preliminary report. *Anaesthesia.* 1966;21(1):51–56.
30. Larsen VH, Christensen P, Brinklov MM, Axelsen F. Postoperative pain relief and respiratory performance after thoracotomy: a controlled trial comparing the effect of epidural morphine and subcutaneous nicomorphine. *Dan Med Bull.* 1986;33(3):161–164.
31. Salomaki TE, Laitinen JO, Nuutinen LS. A randomized double-blind comparison of epidural versus intravenous fentanyl infusion for analgesia after thoracotomy. *Anesthesiology.* 1991;75(5):790–795.
32. Joshi GP, Bonnet F, Shah R, et al. A systematic review of randomized trials evaluating regional techniques for postthoracotomy analgesia. *Anesth Analg.* 2008;107(3):1026–1040.
33. Boldt J, Thaler E, Lehmann A, Papsdorf M, Isgro F. Pain management in cardiac surgery patients: comparison between standard therapy and patient-controlled analgesia regimen. *J Cardiothorac Vasc Anesth.* 1998;12(6):654–658.
34. Dolin SJ, Cashman JN, Bland JM. Effectiveness of acute postoperative pain management: I. Evidence from published data. *Br J Anaesth.* 2002;89(3):409–423.
35. Hudcova J, McNicol E, Quah C, Lau J, Carr DB. Patient controlled opioid analgesia versus conventional opioid analgesia for postoperative pain. *Cochrane Database Syst Rev.* 2006(4):CD003348.
36. Patak LS, Tait AR, Mirafzali L, Morris M, Dasgupta S, Brummett CM. Patient perspectives of patient-controlled analgesia (PCA) and methods for improving pain control and patient satisfaction. *Reg Anesth Pain Med.* 2013;38(4):326–333.
37. Remy C, Marret E, Bonnet F. Effects of acetaminophen on morphine side-effects and consumption after major surgery:

meta-analysis of randomized controlled trials. *Br J Anaesth.* 2005;94(4):505–513.
38. Jibril F, Sharaby S, Mohamed A, Wilby KJ. Intravenous versus oral acetaminophen for pain: systematic review of current evidence to support clinical decision-making. *Can J Hosp Pharm.* 2015;68(3):238–247.
39. Elia N, Lysakowski C, Tramer MR. Does multimodal analgesia with acetaminophen, nonsteroidal antiinflammatory drugs, or selective cyclooxygenase-2 inhibitors and patient-controlled analgesia morphine offer advantages over morphine alone? Meta-analyses of randomized trials. *Anesthesiology.* 2005;103(6):1296–1304.
40. Ong CK, Seymour RA, Lirk P, Merry AF. Combining paracetamol (acetaminophen) with nonsteroidal antiinflammatory drugs: a qualitative systematic review of analgesic efficacy for acute postoperative pain. *Anesth Analg.* 2010;110(4):1170–1179.
41. Keenan DJ, Cave K, Langdon L, Lea RE. Comparative trial of rectal indomethacin and cryoanalgesia for control of early postthoracotomy pain. *Br Med J (Clin Res Ed).* 1983;287(6402):1335–1337.
42. Pavy T, Medley C, Murphy DF. Effect of indomethacin on pain relief after thoracotomy. *Br J Anaesth.* 1990;65(5):624–627.
43. Rhodes M, Conacher I, Morritt G, Hilton C. Nonsteroidal antiinflammatory drugs for postthoracotomy pain. A prospective controlled trial after lateral thoracotomy. *J Thorac Cardiovasc Surg.* 1992;103(1):17–20.
44. Hunt I, Teh E, Southon R, Treasure T. Using non-steroidal anti-inflammatory drugs (NSAIDs) following pleurodesis. *Interact Cardiovasc Thorac Surg.* 2007;6(1):102–104.
45. Rahman NM, Pepperell J, Rehal S, et al. Effect of opioids vs NSAIDs and larger vs smaller chest tube size on pain control and pleurodesis efficacy among patients with malignant pleural effusion: the TIME1 randomized clinical trial. *JAMA.* 2015;314(24):2641–2653.
46. Mathiesen O, Wetterslev J, Kontinen VK, et al. Adverse effects of perioperative paracetamol, NSAIDs, glucocorticoids, gabapentinoids and their combinations: a topical review. *Acta Anaesthesiol Scand.* 2014;58(10):1182–1198.
47. Moore RA, Derry S, Aldington D, Wiffen PJ. Adverse events associated with single dose oral analgesics for acute postoperative pain in adults - an overview of Cochrane reviews. *Cochrane Database Syst Rev.* 2015(10):CD011407.
48. Pirlamarla P, Bond RM. FDA labeling of NSAIDs: Review of nonsteroidal anti-inflammatory drugs in cardiovascular disease. *Trends Cardiovasc Med.* 2016;26(8):675–680.
49. Laskowski K, Stirling A, McKay WP, Lim HJ. A systematic review of intravenous ketamine for postoperative analgesia. *Can J Anaesth.* 2011;58(10):911–923.
50. Michelet P, Guervilly C, Helaine A, et al. Adding ketamine to morphine for patient-controlled analgesia after thoracic surgery: influence on morphine consumption, respiratory function, and nocturnal desaturation. *Br J Anaesth.* 2007;99(3):396–403.
51. Schwenk ES, Viscusi ER, Buvanendran A, et al. Consensus guidelines on the use of intravenous ketamine infusions for acute pain management from the American Society of Regional Anesthesia and Pain Medicine, the American Academy of Pain Medicine, and the American Society of Anesthesiologists. *Reg Anesth Pain Med.* 2018;43(5):456–466.
52. Dunkman WJ, Manning MW. Enhanced recovery after surgery and multimodal strategies for analgesia. *Surg Clin North Am.* 2018;98(6):1171–1184.
53. Grosen K, Drewes AM, Hojsgaard A, Pfeiffer-Jensen M, Hjortdal VE, Pilegaard HK. Perioperative gabapentin for the prevention of persistent pain after thoracotomy: a randomized controlled trial. *Eur J Cardiothorac Surg.* 2014;46(1):76–85.
54. Brulotte V, Ruel MM, Lafontaine E, Chouinard P, Girard F. Impact of pregabalin on the occurrence of postthoracotomy pain syndrome: a randomized trial. *Reg Anesth Pain Med.* 2015;40(3):262–269.
55. Gan TJ, Diemunsch P, Habib AS, et al. Consensus guidelines for the management of postoperative nausea and vomiting. *Anesth Analg.* 2014;118(1):85–113.
56. De Oliveira GS, Jr., Almeida MD, Benzon HT, McCarthy RJ. Perioperative single dose systemic dexamethasone for postoperative pain: a meta-analysis of randomized controlled trials. *Anesthesiology.* 2011;115(3):575–588.
57. Weren M, Demeere JL. Methylprednisolone vs. dexamethasone in the prevention of postoperative nausea and vomiting: a prospective, randomised, double-blind, placebo-controlled trial. *Acta Anaesthesiol Belg.* 2008;59(1):1–5.
58. Bjerregaard LS, Jensen PF, Bigler DR, et al. High-dose methylprednisolone in video-assisted thoracoscopic surgery lobectomy: a randomized controlled trial. *Eur J Cardiothorac Surg.* 2018;53(1):209–215.
59. Beaussier M, Delbos A, Maurice-Szamburski A, Ecoffey C, Mercadal L. Perioperative use of intravenous lidocaine. *Drugs.* 2018;78(12):1229–1246.
60. Cui W, Li Y, Li S, Wang R, Li J. Systemic administration of lidocaine reduces morphine requirements and postoperative pain of patients undergoing thoracic surgery after propofol-remifentanil-based anaesthesia. *Eur J Anaesthesiol.* 2010;27(1):41–46.
61. Slovack M, Taylor B, Bryce R, Ong D. Does intravenous lidocaine infusion during video-assisted thoracoscopic surgery reduce postoperative analgesia? A randomized controlled study. *Can J Anaesth.* 2015;62(6):676–677.
62. Block BM, Liu SS, Rowlingson AJ, Cowan AR, Cowan JA, Jr., Wu CL. Efficacy of postoperative epidural analgesia: a meta-analysis. *JAMA.* 2003;290(18):2455–2463.
63. Baxter CS, Fitzgerald BM. *Intercostal Nerve Block.* StatPearls. Treasure Island (FL): StatPearls Publishing LLC; 2019.
64. Hughes R, Gao F. Pain control for thoracotomy. *Contin Educ Anaesth Crit Care Pain.* 2005;5(2):56–60.
65. Luis-Navarro JC, Seda-Guzman M, Luis-Moreno C, Lopez-Romero JL. The erector spinae plane block in 4 cases of video-assisted thoracic surgery. *Rev Esp Anestesiol Reanim.* 2018;65(4):204–208.
66. Horlocker TT, Vandermeuelen E, Kopp SL, Gogarten W, Leffert LR, Benzon HT. Regional anesthesia in the patient receiving antithrombotic or thrombolytic therapy: American Society of Regional Anesthesia and Pain Medicine Evidence-Based Guidelines (Fourth Edition). *Reg Anesth Pain Med.* 2018;43(3):263–309.
67. Wu CL, Cohen SR, Richman JM, et al. Efficacy of postoperative patient-controlled and continuous infusion epidural analgesia versus intravenous patient-controlled analgesia with opioids: a meta-analysis. *Anesthesiology.* 2005;103(5):1079–1088; quiz 1109–1010.
68. Manion SC, Brennan TJ. Thoracic epidural analgesia and acute pain management. *Anesthesiology.* 2011;115(1):181–188.
69. Wink J, Veering BT, Aarts L, Wouters PF. Effects of thoracic epidural anesthesia on neuronal cardiac regulation and cardiac function. *Anesthesiology.* 2019;130(3):472–491.

70. Giebler RM, Scherer RU, Peters J. Incidence of neurologic complications related to thoracic epidural catheterization. *Anesthesiology.* 1997;86(1):55–63.
71. Horlocker TT, Wedel DJ. Anticoagulation and neuraxial block: historical perspective, anesthetic implications, and risk management. *Reg Anesth Pain Med.* 1998;23(6 Suppl 2):129–134.
72. Manikian B, Cantineau JP, Bertrand M, Kieffer E, Sartene R, Viars P. Improvement of diaphragmatic function by a thoracic extradural block after upper abdominal surgery. *Anesthesiology.* 1988;68(3):379–386.
73. Popping DM, Elia N, Marret E, Remy C, Tramer MR. Protective effects of epidural analgesia on pulmonary complications after abdominal and thoracic surgery: a meta-analysis. *Arch Surg.* 2008;143(10):990–999, discussion 1000.
74. Ballantyne JC, Carr DB, deFerranti S, et al. The comparative effects of postoperative analgesic therapies on pulmonary outcome: cumulative meta-analyses of randomized, controlled trials. *Anesth Analg.* 1998;86(3):598–612.
75. Liu SS, Wu CL. Effect of postoperative analgesia on major postoperative complications: a systematic update of the evidence. *Anesth Analg.* 2007;104(3):689–702.
76. Guay J, Nishimori M, Kopp SL. Epidural local anesthetics versus opioid-based analgesic regimens for postoperative gastrointestinal paralysis, vomiting, and pain after abdominal surgery: a Cochrane review. *Anesth Analg.* 2016;123(6):1591–1602.
77. Oka T, Ozawa Y, Ohkubo Y. Thoracic epidural bupivacaine attenuates supraventricular tachyarrhythmias after pulmonary resection. *Anesth Analg.* 2001;93(2):253–259, 251st contents page.
78. Lattermann R, Wykes L, Eberhart L, Carli F, Meterissian S, Schricker T. A randomized controlled trial of the anticatabolic effect of epidural analgesia and hypocaloric glucose. *Reg Anesth Pain Med.* 2007;32(3):227–232.
79. Schricker T, Meterissian S, Wykes L, Eberhart L, Lattermann R, Carli F. Postoperative protein sparing with epidural analgesia and hypocaloric dextrose. *Ann Surg.* 2004;240(5):916–921.
80. Benzon HT, Wong HY, Belavic AM, Jr., et al. A randomized double-blind comparison of epidural fentanyl infusion versus patient-controlled analgesia with morphine for postthoracotomy pain. *Anesth Analg.* 1993;76(2):316–322.
81. Grant RP, Dolman JF, Harper JA, et al. Patient-controlled lumbar epidural fentanyl compared with patient-controlled intravenous fentanyl for post-thoracotomy pain. *Can J Anaesth.* 1992;39(3):214–219.
82. Grant GJ, Zakowski M, Ramanathan S, Boyd A, Turndorf H. Thoracic versus lumbar administration of epidural morphine for postoperative analgesia after thoracotomy. *Reg Anesth.* 1993;18(6):351–355.
83. Hurford WE, Dutton RP, Alfille PH, Clement D, Wilson RS. Comparison of thoracic and lumbar epidural infusions of bupivacaine and fentanyl for post-thoracotomy analgesia. *J Cardiothorac Vasc Anesth.* 1993;7(5):521–525.
84. Guinard JP, Mavrocordatos P, Chiolero R, Carpenter RL. A randomized comparison of intravenous versus lumbar and thoracic epidural fentanyl for analgesia after thoracotomy. *Anesthesiology.* 1992;77(6):1108–1115.
85. Coe A, Sarginson R, Smith MW, Donnelly RJ, Russell GN. Pain following thoracotomy. A randomised, double-blind comparison of lumbar versus thoracic epidural fentanyl. *Anaesthesia.* 1991;46(11):918–921.
86. Grant RP. Con: every postthoracotomy patient does not deserve thoracic epidural analgesia. *J Cardiothorac Vasc Anesth.* 1999;13(3):355–357.
87. Macintosh RR, Bryce-Smith R. *Local Analgesia: Abdominal Surgery.* 2nd ed. Edinburgh, London: E&S Livingstone; 1962.
88. Eason MJ, Wyatt R. Paravertebral thoracic block-a reappraisal. *Anaesthesia.* 1979;34(7):638–642.
89. Karmakar MK, Chung DC. Variability of a thoracic paravertebral block. Are we ignoring the endothoracic fascia? *Reg Anesth Pain Med.* 2000;25(3):325–327.
90. Karmakar MK, Kwok WH, Kew J. Thoracic paravertebral block: radiological evidence of contralateral spread anterior to the vertebral bodies. *Br J Anaesth.* 2000;84(2):263–265.
91. Cheema SP, Ilsley D, Richardson J, Sabanathan S. A thermographic study of paravertebral analgesia. *Anaesthesia.* 1995; 50(2):118–121.
92. Conacher ID, Kokri M. Postoperative paravertebral blocks for thoracic surgery. A radiological appraisal. *Br J Anaesth.* 1987;59(2):155–161.
93. Evans PJ, Lloyd JW, Wood GJ. Accidental intrathecal injection of bupivacaine and dextran. *Anaesthesia.* 1981;36(7):685–687.
94. Purcell-Jones G, Pither CE, Justins DM. Paravertebral somatic nerve block: a clinical, radiographic, and computed tomographic study in chronic pain patients. *Anesth Analg.* 1989;68(1): 32–39.
95. Karmakar MK. Thoracic paravertebral block. *Anesthesiology.* 2001;95(3):771–780.
96. Saito T, Gallagher ET, Yamada K, Tanuma K, Ogawa R. Broad unilateral analgesia. *Reg Anesth.* 1994;19(5):360–361.
97. Dugan DJ, Samson PC. Surgical significance of the endothoracic fascia. The anatomic basis for empyemectomy and other extrapleural technics. *Am J Surg.* 1975;130(2):151–158.
98. Riain SCO, Donnell BO, Cuffe T, Harmon DC, Fraher JP, Shorten G. Thoracic paravertebral block using real-time ultrasound guidance. *Anesth Analg.* 2010;110(1):248–251.
99. Hara K, Sakura S, Nomura T, Saito Y. Ultrasound guided thoracic paravertebral block in breast surgery. *Anaesthesia.* 2009;64(2):223–225.
100. Luyet C, Eichenberger U, Greif R, Vogt A, Szucs Farkas Z, Moriggl B. Ultrasound-guided paravertebral puncture and placement of catheters in human cadavers: an imaging study. *Br J Anaesth.* 2009;102(4):534–539.
101. Coveney E, Weltz CR, Greengrass R, et al. Use of paravertebral block anesthesia in the surgical management of breast cancer: experience in 156 cases. *Ann Surg.* 1998;227(4):496–501.
102. Richardson J, Sabanathan S. Thoracic paravertebral analgesia. *Acta Anaesthesiol Scand.* 1995;39(8):1005–1015.
103. Lonnqvist PA, MacKenzie J, Soni AK, Conacher ID. Paravertebral blockade. Failure rate and complications. *Anaesthesia.* 1995;50(9):813–815.
104. Tenicela R, Pollan SB. Paravertebral-peridural block technique: a unilateral thoracic block. *Clin J Pain.* 1990;6(3):227–234.
105. Thomas PW, Sanders DJ, Berrisford RG. Pulmonary haemorrhage after percutaneous paravertebral block. *Br J Anaesth.* 1999;83(4):668–669.
106. Wildsmith JA. Developments in local anaesthetic drugs and techniques for pain relief. *Br J Anaesth.* 1989;63(2):159–164.
107. Casati A, Alessandrini P, Nuzzi M, et al. A prospective, randomized, blinded comparison between continuous thoracic paravertebral and epidural infusion of 0.2% ropivacaine after lung resection surgery. *Eur J Anaesthesiol.* 2006;23(12):999–1004.
108. Davies RG, Myles PS, Graham JM. A comparison of the analgesic efficacy and side-effects of paravertebral vs epidural blockade for thoracotomy–a systematic review and meta-analysis of randomized trials. *Br J Anaesth.* 2006;96(4):418–426.

109. Perttunen K, Nilsson E, Heinonen J, Hirvisalo EL, Salo JA, Kalso E. Extradural, paravertebral and intercostal nerve blocks for post-thoracotomy pain. *Br J Anaesth.* 1995;75(5):541–547.
110. Liu M, Rock P, Grass JA, et al. Double-blind randomized evaluation of intercostal nerve blocks as an adjuvant to subarachnoid administered morphine for post-thoracotomy analgesia. *Reg Anesth.* 1995;20(5):418–425.
111. Sabanathan S, Richardson J, Mearns AJ. Efficacy of continuous intercostal bupivacaine for pain relief after thoracotomy. *Br J Anaesth.* 1993;71(3):463–464.
112. Chan VW, Chung F, Cheng DC, Seyone C, Chung A, Kirby TJ. Analgesic and pulmonary effects of continuous intercostal nerve block following thoracotomy. *Can J Anaesth.* 1991;38(6):733–739.
113. Karmakar MK, Ho AM. Acute pain management of patients with multiple fractured ribs. *J Trauma.* 2003;54(3):615–625.
114. Moore DC. Anatomy of the intercostal nerve: its importance during thoracic surgery. *Am J Surg.* 1982;144(3):371–373.
115. Hadzic A. *Hadzic's Textbook of Regional Anesthesia and Acute Pain Management.* 2nd ed. New York: McGraw-Hill Education; 2017.
116. Neal JM. Effects of epinephrine in local anesthetics on the central and peripheral nervous systems: Neurotoxicity and neural blood flow. *Reg Anesth Pain Med.* 2003;28(2):124–134.
117. McLure HA, Rubin AP. Review of local anaesthetic agents. *Minerva Anestesiol.* 2005;71(3):59–74.
118. Rosenberg PH, Veering BT, Urmey WF. Maximum recommended doses of local anesthetics: a multifactorial concept. *Reg Anesth Pain Med.* 2004;29(6):564–575, discussion 524.
119. Forero M, Adhikary SD, Lopez H, Tsui C, Chin KJ. The erector spinae plane block: a novel analgesic technique in thoracic neuropathic pain. *Reg Anesth Pain Med.* 2016;41(5):621–627.
120. Chin KJ, Malhas L, Perlas A. The erector spinae plane block provides visceral abdominal analgesia in bariatric surgery: a report of 3 cases. *Reg Anesth Pain Med.* 2017;42(3):372–376.
121. Kot P, Rodriguez P, Granell M, et al. The erector spinae plane block: a narrative review. *Korean J Anesthesiol.* 2019;72(3):209–220.
122. De Cassai A, Tonetti T. Local anesthetic spread during erector spinae plane block. *J Clin Anesth.* 2018;48:60–61.
123. Jain K, Jaiswal V, Puri A. Erector spinae plane block: relatively new block on horizon with a wide spectrum of application - A case series. *Indian J Anaesth.* 2018;62(10):809–813.
124. Eng HC, Chin KJ, Adhikary S. How I do it: erector spinae block for rib fractures: the Penn State Health Experience. In. ASRA News. *Am Soc Reg Anesth Pain Med.* 2018:16–20.
125. Wang Q, Zhang G, Wei S, He Z, Sun L, Zheng H. Comparison of the effects of ultrasound-guided erector spinae plane block and wound infiltration on perioperative opioid consumption and postoperative pain in thoracotomy. *J Coll Physicians Surg Pak.* 2019;29(12):1138–1143.
126. Galacho J, Veiga M, Ormonde L. Erector spinae plane block and altered hemostasis: is it a safe option? a case series. *Korean J Anesthesiol.* 2020.
127. Seelam S, Nair AS, Christopher A, Upputuri O, Naik V, Rayani BK. Efficacy of single-shot ultrasound-guided erector spinae plane block for postoperative analgesia after mastectomy: A randomized controlled study. *Saudi J Anaesth.* 2020;14(1):22–27.
128. Blanco R, Parras T, McDonnell JG, Prats-Galino A. Serratus plane block: a novel ultrasound-guided thoracic wall nerve block. *Anaesthesia.* 2013;68(11):1107–1113.
129. Khalil AE, Abdallah NM, Bashandy GM, Kaddah TA. Ultrasound-guided serratus anterior plane block versus thoracic epidural analgesia for thoracotomy pain. *J Cardiothorac Vasc Anesth.* 2017;31(1):152–158.
130. Okmen K, Okmen BM, Uysal S. Serratus anterior plane (SAP) block used for thoracotomy analgesia: a case report. *Korean J Pain.* 2016;29(3):189–192.
131. Kim DH, Oh YJ, Lee JG, Ha D, Chang YJ, Kwak HJ. Efficacy of ultrasound-guided serratus plane block on postoperative quality of recovery and analgesia after video-assisted thoracic surgery: a randomized, triple-blind, placebo-controlled study. *Anesth Analg.* 2018;126(4):1353–1361.
132. Saad FS, El Baradie SY, Abdel Aliem MAW, Ali MM, Kotb TAM. Ultrasound-guided serratus anterior plane block versus thoracic paravertebral block for perioperative analgesia in thoracotomy. *Saudi J Anaesth.* 2018;12(4):565–570.
133. Lee J, Kim S. The effects of ultrasound-guided serratus plane block, in combination with general anesthesia, on intraoperative opioid consumption, emergence time, and hemodynamic stability during video-assisted thoracoscopic lobectomy: A randomized prospective study. *Medicine (Baltimore).* 2019; 98(18):e15385.
134. Semyonov M, Fedorina E, Grinshpun J, et al. Ultrasound-guided serratus anterior plane block for analgesia after thoracic surgery. *J Pain Res.* 2019;12:953–960.

25

Postthoracotomy Chronic Pain

PAUL RYAN HAFFEY, NEAL RAKESH, GRANT H. CHEN, AMITABH GULATI

Introduction

According to the International Association for the Study of Pain, chronic postthoracotomy pain is defined as "pain that recurs or persists along a thoracotomy incision at least 2 months following the surgical procedure".[1] The condition may also be referred to as postthoracotomy pain syndrome (PTPS) or postthoracotomy neuralgia. The first cases were described in soldiers after World War II. Patients often describe pain along the thoracotomy scar and a burning, aching sensation that resides along the back or the chest. It may be accompanied by painful dysesthesia or allodynia.[2,3] The prevalence of chronic postthoracotomy pain is highly variable, with reports ranging from 33% to 91% in the literature.[4,5]

One of the most significant predictors of PTPS is inadequate analgesia in the acute postoperative period.[2] For this reason effective pain control during this time is critical. Other contributors to the development of PTPS include preexisting pain conditions, age, sex, psychosocial factors, and genetic predisposition. It has been hypothesized that minimally invasive techniques may reduce postoperative pain after any procedure; however, this remains unclear in the case of PTPS.[4]

Pathophysiology

The exact mechanisms that lead to PTPS are unclear, and additional investigation is warranted. In addition to surgical approach and genetic contributions, some evidence suggests that intercostal neuroma formation, healing rib fracture, costochondral dislocation, and suprasensitization may all play a role in the development of PTPS.[2]

Genetic contributions may be important in the development of any type of persistent pain. The exact role that genes play, however, has not been made clear. Some potential genetic influences may arise from the following: genetic polymorphisms of catechol-O-methyltransferase, genetic variants to determine voltage-gated sodium channels, and guanosine triphosphate (GTP) cyclohydrolase.[6,7] Additional research into the genetics contributing to the development of many types of persistent painful conditions is needed.

Postsurgical nerve injury is a well-described phenomenon in the literature, and it is the most commonly implicated culprit behind the development of PTPS. This is likely because many patients present with distinctly neuropathic symptoms. The patients describe a sensation of burning and numbness along the surgical site, which is typical for neuropathic pain. Some studies have found electrodiagnostic evidence that nerve injury has a causal role in the development of long-lasting postoperative pain after thoracotomy.[8]

Nerve injury and other factors may also lead to central or peripheral sensitization. Immediately following local injury, a series of inflammatory mediators (i.e., substance P, prostaglandins, adenosine triphosphate, histamine) are released with the aim of attracting immune cells that release cytokines, such as tumor necrosis factor and interleukin-1.[9] This inflammatory milieu causes increases in sodium and calcium at the nociceptor nerve terminal thereby generating action potentials leading to the perception of pain. Peripheral sensitization can be characterized by a decreased threshold for activation of this chain of events and may lead to activation of inflammatory mediators without an inciting event such as nerve injury.[10] If these pain signals persist, it may lead to a lasting change in the central nervous system that can result in the development of central sensitization. This is a condition in which a patient may experience chronic hypersensitivity and a heightened sensation of pain because of a persistent decreased threshold for activation in the central nervous system.[11] The prevention of this unfortunate cascade is just one reason why it is imperative to control pain in the immediate postoperative procedure, particularly in the case of chronic PTPS.

Clinical Presentation

Patients often present with pain at or along the incision site, chest tube, or drain site. Some patients also report painful symptoms in the shoulder and, in some cases, diffusely along the T5–T6 dermatomes.[12] It is typically characterized as burning, aching, tender, and sensitive in the area surrounding the scar. Patients also report numbness and additional features characteristic of neuropathic pain including tingling, decreased sensation, and allodynia.[13] Between 80% and 90% of patients report pain directly at the surgical site.[14] In addition, myofascial pain in adjacent areas (i.e., scapula, neck, shoulder, pectoral musculature) is not uncommon and is likely caused by disruption of the fascial planes during surgery. Some patients also report experiencing sudomotor derangements similar to those experienced in chronic regional pain syndrome.

Prevention

There are some reports that 70% of patients who undergo thoracic surgery may develop PTPS.[15] It has been postulated that open thoracic procedures may result in greater incidence of PTPS, but the prevalence of PTPS is roughly equal in both open and video-assisted procedures.[13] Based on this information, it is reasonable to conclude that modifications in surgical approach will not have an effect on preventing PTPS.

Effective postoperative pain management, however, is essential for the prevention of the development of PTPS. Greater consumption of analgesics during the immediate postoperative period has been associated with a greater incidence of PTPS.[16] Therefore using a multimodal protocol to address immediate postoperative pain is essential. This may include a variety of pharmacologic medications including nonsteroidal antiinflammatory drugs (NSAIDs), opioids, neuromodulating medications, and acetaminophen. Preemptive multimodal analgesia may, in fact, prevent hypersensitization of the central nervous system that leads to the development of chronic pain.[2,17,18] Incorporating regional anesthesia techniques should also be considered. One highly favored approach includes preoperative NSAIDs, opioid medications, preoperative regional block, and either epidural anesthesia or continuous paravertebral block; this combination was found to result in a lower than average incidence of PTPS.[2,17–19] The goal of this technique is to use analgesic therapies with different mechanisms of action to block or modulate different pain pathways, while decreasing the incidence of related adverse effects.[20] With this in mind, it is imperative that the clinician take into consideration the patient's psychosocial history and surgical approach when establishing a pain management regimen with the aim of controlling postoperative pain and taking measures to prevent the development of chronic pain.

The utility of preoperative or intraoperative administration of steroids to prevent postoperative pain remains controversial. Studies on the analgesic effects of glucocorticoids have focused primarily on dexamethasone. There have been numerous studies demonstrating the efficacy of a single intraoperative dose, 4 to 8 mg intravenously, in reducing postoperative pain scores and increasing the period to first analgesic request.[21] Concerns with its use include raised blood glucose levels and possibly an increased incidence of surgical site infections. However, the latter has been shown to be false by numerous studies.[22–24] Nonetheless, in diabetics with poor glycemic control, the intraoperative use of dexamethasone may warrant frequent blood glucose monitoring.

Treatment

Gabapentin and Pregabalin

Gabapentin and pregabalin are two of the most commonly prescribed neuromodulating medications largely because of their ability to titrate and their reasonably favorable side-effect profile. Similar to many other neuromodulating medications, the mechanism by which these drugs confer pain relief is not completely understood. It is theorized that they work through modulation of voltage-gated calcium channels in the dorsal horn.[25] Because many patients suffering from PTPS experience symptoms corresponding with neuropathy, these agents have been especially beneficial.[26] Their role in prevention of PTPS, however, has not been fully evaluated. Several studies have looked at the effectiveness of both gabapentin and pregabalin on acute postoperative pain with mixed results. In two studies, the authors found that both gabapentin and pregabalin use reduced opioid consumption and improved pain scores postoperatively.[27] In these same studies, pregabalin was also shown to reduce opioid-related side-effects following surgery.[28] The optimal dosage was not elucidated in either of these studies and side effects were seen at the doses needed for clinical effect including sedation, dizziness, drowsiness, and visual disturbances.

Acetaminophen

Acetaminophen offers benefits as part of a multimodal analgesic regimen owing to its relative ease of administration, favorable side-effect profile and dependable pharmacokinetics.[15] Although the mechanism of action of this medication remains unclear, it appears to exert its effects through the central nervous system providing both analgesic and antipyretic properties, as well as being a weak inhibitor of the cyclooxygenase (COX) enzymes.[29] Acetaminophen exhibits a more favorable side-effect profile than NSAIDs, particularly in the postoperative and cancer populations for whom bleeding may be a concern. However, hepatotoxicity is a concern when doses exceed 4000 mg/day in adults or in patients with preexisting liver pathology. As such, caution is advised when used in patients with severe alcoholic liver disease, cirrhosis, or hepatitis. Formulations have been available for both oral and rectal routes of administration for many years and have frequently been used in the perioperative period owing to its low cost. More recently, with the U.S. Food and Drug Administration approval of the intravenous formulation in 2010, the use of acetaminophen for thoracic surgery has increased despite the cost as compared with the other formulations as several studies have demonstrated a benefit in this population of patients. Specifically, studies have shown intravenous acetaminophen to reduce postoperative pain scores and opioid consumption when used as a part of a multimodal analgesic regimen.[30] Therefore it is a commonly used perioperative adjunct to a multimodal pain management protocol and may have use in the prevention of PTPS. The utility of acetaminophen in treating PTPS, however, remains unclear; particularly because, much like NSAIDs and COX-2 specific inhibitors, acetaminophen will reach a "ceiling effect" at which point no further benefit will be seen despite increasing concentration of the drug.[31]

Nonsteroidal Antiinflammatory Drugs

NSAIDs have become more popular for the management of postoperative pain following the advent of parenteral formulations for this class of drugs (i.e., ketorolac). Considerable research has already been devoted to examining their utility in the perioperative period and much of it has shown them to decrease opioid requirements, improve pain scores, and decrease opioid-related side-effects in patients following surgery.[32] Much of these same results have also been seen in patients following thoracic surgery. One study was able to show that use of NSAIDs as part of multimodal pain management regimen decreased opioid consumption by about 30% and reduced pain scores by about 60% following thoracotomy.[33] Like acetaminophen, however, the utility of NSAIDs in the treatment of PTPS is unclear and most of the research focuses on adequate pain control immediately following surgical intervention. In this capacity, they are likely to be used as a preventative agent. Potential side effects include bleeding, kidney injury, and gastrointestinal mucosal damage. These are of particular concern in the perioperative and cancer populations in whom bleeding risk is increased.

Ketamine

Ketamine acts on central N-methyl-D-aspartate receptors with antagonistic effects to produce analgesia and dissociative anesthesia. Despite the usefulness of ketamine in the treatment of acute postoperative pain, no benefit, to date, has been seen in the prevention of chronic postthoracotomy pain syndrome.[33]

Opioid Analgesic Medications

Opioid analgesics have long been the mainstay for treatment in postoperative pain, but their utility in chronic pain is limited by their extensive side-effect profile, limited benefit for neuropathic pain, dependency, and risk of abuse. Although it is available in a variety of formulations, the versatility of opioid medications does not outweigh their risks. Their large side-effect profile includes constipation, nausea, vomiting, pruritis, sedation, and importantly respiratory depression, which can have negative effects on recovery from thoracic surgery.[34] Specifically, respiratory depression can have deleterious consequences in patients who are status postlung resection, especially those with poor preexisting pulmonary function. In light of this information, opioid medications should be used sparingly and as a last resort option after all other potential pharmacologic and nonpharmacologic options have been exhausted.

Cryoablation

Cryoablation following thoracic surgery involves exposing one or more intercostal nerves in the vicinity of the surgical incision to hypothermic conditions (between −20°C and −100°C) to induce temporary nerve damage and subsequently hinder action potential transmission.[35] This will produce a temporary area and period of sensory loss (~1–4 days) including the sensation of pain. The goal of this procedure is to reduce postoperative opioid use through a temporary loss of neural function.[36] However, the effects of cryoablation are not instantaneous, and it is prudent therefore that patients are continued on a multimodal analgesic regimen postoperatively to ensure adequate pain control.[37] Controlled trials, on the other hand, have called the utility of this technique into question with one study showing that patients who received cryoablation following surgery had a higher incidence of moderate and severe pain that effectively interfered with daily function.[38] Another study concluded that, when compared with epidural analgesia alone, patients in the cryoanalgesia group reported a higher incidence of a neuropathic component to their pain following a thoracotomy.[39]

Transcutaneous Electrical Nerve Stimulation

Transcutaneous electrical nerve stimulation (TENS) is an attractive option for pain control because it is both noninvasive and nonpharmacologic. Patients can easily apply the device for pain control, but pain may return upon removal of the device. Research evaluating the utility of TENS is extremely limited, but there have been few studies examining the effectiveness of TENS as an adjunct to other analgesic therapies following both cardiac and thoracic surgery. In one study, the results showed that the benefits of TENS were seen on the fourth postoperative day and continued for at least 2 months following surgery, which is especially relevant for the PTPS population.[40]

Intercostal Nerve Approach

Intercostal nerve blockage is commonly performed before closure during thoracotomy; however, there is likely significant utility to performing this procedure in managing PTPS. If successful, some practitioners elect to perform cryoneurolysis or ablation of the intercostal nerve. Caution must be taken to prevent pneumothorax.[41] Although literature is scarce, this is practiced clinically with relative frequency. Relevant ultrasound anatomy can be seen in Fig. 25.1.

Serratus Anterior Plane Approach

Another approach to PTPS is through targeting the serratus anterior plane. The intervention is performed in the midaxillary region in the fascial plane between the serratus anterior and latissimus dorsi muscles. Within the compartment,

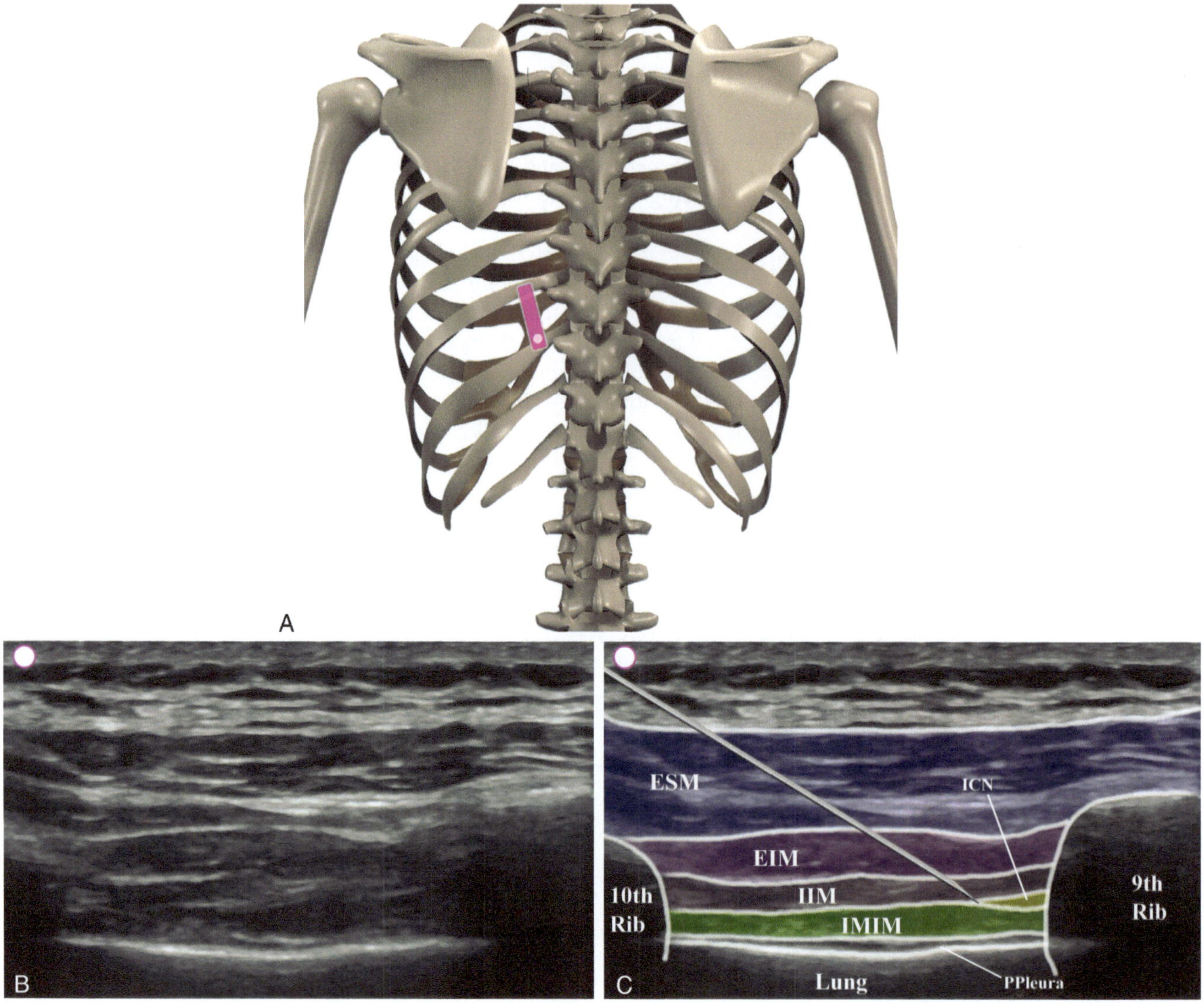

• **Fig. 25.1** (**A**) Probe placement in a sagittal oblique plane on the posterior aspect between the ninth and tenth ribs. (**B**) Ultrasound image of the posterior thoracic spine between T9 and T10. (**C**) Labeled ultrasound image of an in-plane needle approach of the T9 intercostal nerve in short-axis. *ESM*, Erector spinae muscle; *EIM*, external intercostal muscle; *IIM*, internal intercostal muscle; *IMIM*, innermost intercostal muscle; *ICN*, intercostal neurovascular bundle; *PPleura,* parietal pleura.

medication can spread to affect the lateral cutaneous branches of the T3–T9 intercostal nerves, long thoracic nerve, thoracodorsal nerve and, dependent on injectate volume, the intercostobrachial nerve.[42] Thus the approach would target the innervation to the anterior and lateral chest wall, which would help to alleviate PTPS. Madabushi et al. described a patient with severe refractory PTPS to intravenous pain medications but significantly improved pain on the visual analog scale and respiratory status with the placement of a serratus anterior plane block and continuous catheter infusion. Relevant ultrasound anatomy can be seen in Fig. 25.2.[43]

Paravertebral Analgesia

Paravertebral blocks (PVBs) can be achieved using either a posterior loss of resistance, ultrasound-guided technique, or alternatively under direct visualization by the surgeon at the end of surgery and postoperatively in the treatment of PTPS. The goal of this procedure is to inject local anesthetic into the paravertebral space while avoiding the potential complications associated with thoracic epidural analgesia (TEA).

Studies comparing TEA and PVB have often been heterogeneous and inadequately powered. A prospective trial in patients undergoing pneumonectomy comparing TEA with PVB showed that the PVB group experienced a lower incidence of hypotension requiring inotropes, arrhythmias, respiratory complications, and need for surgical reexploration.[44] However, multiple reviews and metaanalysis, including a Cochrane review of 14 studies with about 700 thoracotomy patients, have shown no difference in pain scores, postoperative pulmonary function, and major complications in patients undergoing thoracic procedures between PVB and TEA.[45] Nonetheless, the Cochrane review did report that paravertebral blockade reduced the risks of developing minor

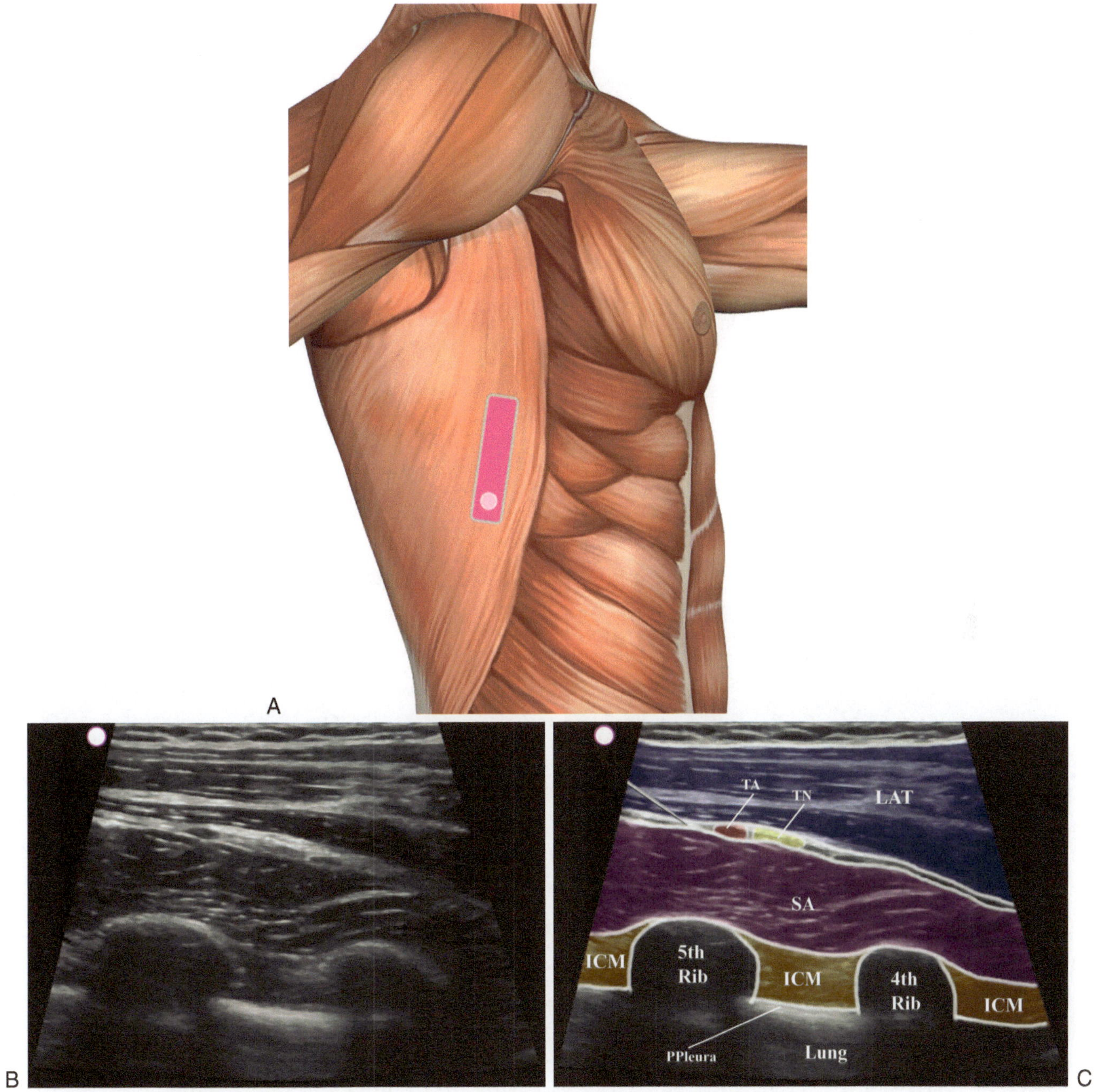

• **Fig. 25.2** (**A**) Probe placement in a coronal oblique plane in the midaxillary region between the fourth and fourth ribs. (**B**) Ultrasound image of the midaxillary region between the fourth and fifth ribs. (**C**) Labeled ultrasound image of an in-plane needle approach of the serratus anterior plane in short-axis. *ICM*, Intercostal muscles; *LAT*, latissimus dorsi; *PPleura,* parietal pleura; *SA*, serratus anterior; *TA*, thoracodorsal artery; *TN*, thoracodorsal nerve.

complications, such as hypotension, nausea/vomiting, pruritis, and urinary retention as compared with thoracic epidural blockade. Despite these benefits, this was confounded by a lack of evidence in other outcomes, including no difference in reported 30-day mortality and major complications. When comparing the two for certain surgeries requiring bilateral analgesia, that is, bilateral lung transplant or heart-lung transplant requiring bilateral thoracotomy incisions with sternal transection, TEA might make more intuitive sense, but bilateral PVBs is a viable alternative.[46]

One of the concerns with paravertebral blockade has been epidural spread of local anesthetic. This has been reported to occur in up to 70% of patients receiving PVBs. The use of ultrasound and single large volume injection techniques seem to increase the risk of this spread.[47] Despite this possible occurrence, the resultant side effects tend to be relatively mild and limited to transient hypotension and lower limb weakness. Other potential complications of PVBs include vascular and pleural injury. However, the likelihood of hematoma formation resulting in significant

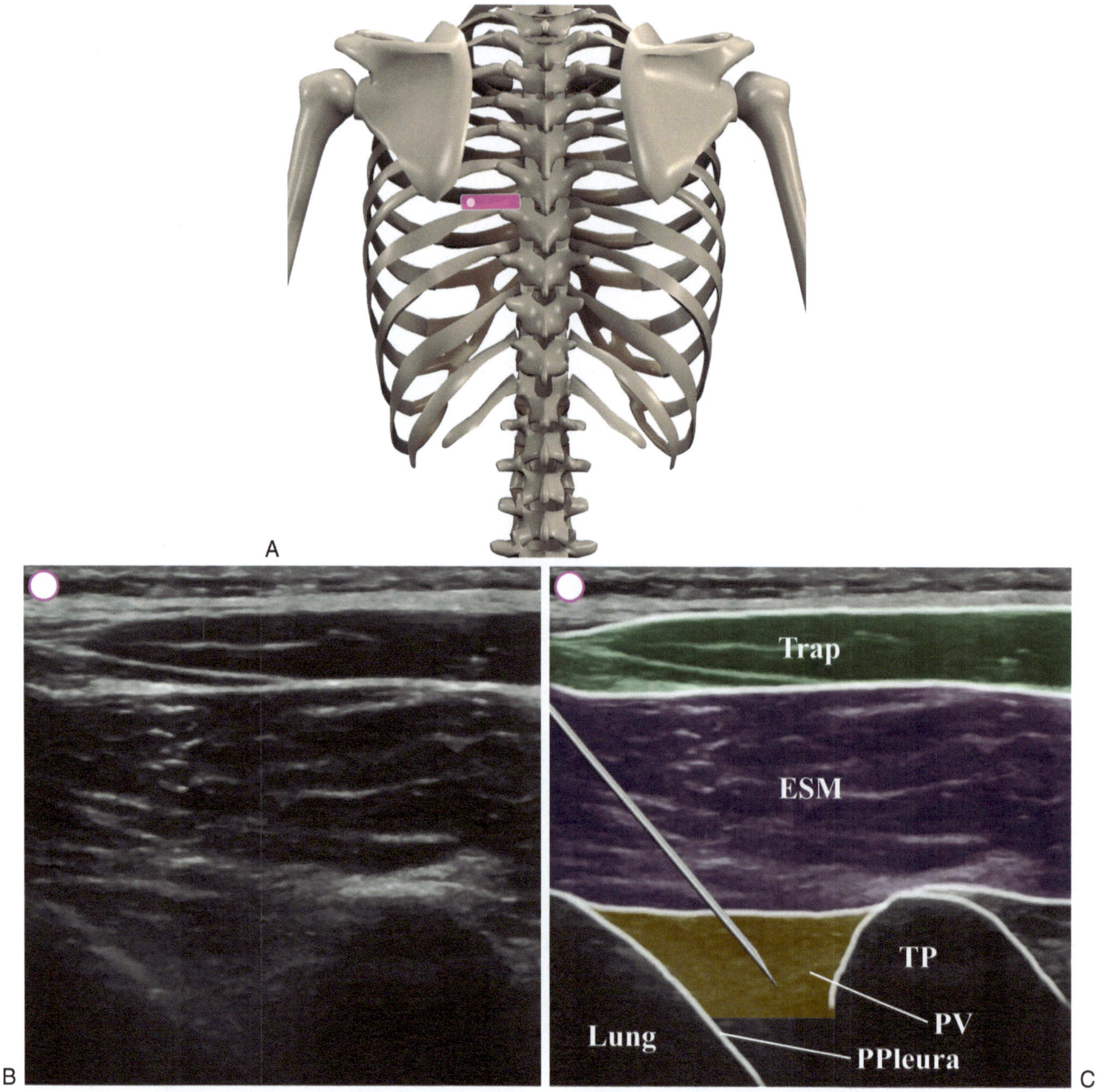

• **Fig. 25.3** (**A**) Probe placement in an axial plane on the posterior aspect the T8 level slightly cephalad to the rib. (**B**) Labeled ultrasound image of in-plane needle approach to the paravertebral space in long-axis. (**C**) Labeled ultrasound image of in-plane needle approach to the paravertebral space in long-axis. *ESM*, Erector spinae muscle; *PPleura*, parietal pleura; *PV*, paravertebral space; *TP*, transverse process; *Trap*, trapezius.

morbidity is very rare because of the large volume of the paravertebral space. Pleural injury and pneumothorax can be minimized by performing the procedure under direct visualization and with the use of ultrasound in the hands of an experienced anesthesiologist.[48] In addition, the block failure rate with thoracic PVBs is reported to be lower than that with TEA at about 6%.[49]

Although limited by practitioner expertise, given its favorable side-effect profile and similar efficacy, paravertebral analgesia has seen a steady resurgence in clinical practice. Relevant ultrasound anatomy can be seen in Fig. 25.3.

Thoracic Epidural Analgesia

TEA has long been considered the gold standard for thoracic surgical pain relief. There have been some studies evaluating the effectiveness of various analgesia techniques on long-term postthoracotomy pain. Based on these studies, it appears important not only whether the patient received epidural analgesia, but also how the epidural was managed.[41] This is particularly relevant in the prevention of PTPS. However, thoracic epidural injections are also commonly performed for the treatment of PTPS.

There are two practiced approaches to performing a thoracic epidural with the most important determinant between the use of either one being practitioner level of expertise and comfort. However, it is of the opinion that a paramedian approach permits a markedly less angled trajectory with thoracic vertebral segments, enabling an approach to the epidural space at a predictable depth in most patients, especially above T11 vertebral level.[50]

On the other hand, besides the risks and complications, some studies have shown a rate of TEA failure owing to various causes between 10% and 15% to as high as 32%.[51,52] Over the decades, the relative benefits of TEA in reducing postoperative pulmonary complications have decreased in studies, likely because of improved surgical techniques, prophylactic antibiotics, improved postoperative care (i.e., the avoidance of nasogastric tubes), improved pulmonary physiotherapy, and early mobilization.

Neuromodulation

Little evidence has been published regarding the utility of neuromodulation in treating PTPS, but it is practiced clinically. One case report describes a patient who experienced full resolution of symptoms 4 months after implantation of spinal cord stimulator (SCS) device.[53] SCS leads were placed at the T3 level in this case, which appears to be common in clinical practice to ensure adequate coverage of painful areas. There are many potential hypotheses speculating the mechanism by which SCS works. The most prominent of these is the "gate control theory" by which vibratory sensations made by the SCS device may interfere with pain signals.[54] A variety of other theories exist including central desensitization, and inhibition of phenotypic switching in A-beta fibers.[54] As occurred in the case study listed earlier, it is likely that the pain will return once the SCS device is turned off. Similarly, clinicians have been using peripheral nerve stimulation (PNS) to achieve the same effects of SCS. Even less evidence exists demonstrating the effectiveness of PNS and peripheral nerve field stimulation. However, there has been some case reports showing potential benefit of stimulation around the scar and paravertebral regions,[55–57] but further exploration into the area would be necessary before it becomes common practice.

Conclusion

PTPS is a complex condition that is often a diagnosis of exclusion. Incidence is highly variable, with many sources reporting a greater than 70% incidence in patient's status postthoracotomy.[15] Patients complain of burning, hypersensitivity, aching, and numbness most commonly along the incision site. Some will experience sudomotor and myofascial symptoms associated with PTPS. Adequate postoperative analgesia is essential in preventing the development of PTPS. An aggressive, multimodal approach is the most appropriate, particularly when more invasive surgical methods are used. Like prevention, treatment requires a multimodal approach that may include regional anesthesia techniques, pharmacologic management, and neuromodulation. Additional research into the pathophysiology and treatment of this often difficult to treat condition is warranted.

References

1. Merskey H, Bogduk N, et al. *Classification of Chronic Pain: Descriptions of Chronic Pain Syndroms and Definitions of Pain Terms.* 2nd ed. IASP Press; 1994:143–144.
2. Dzjczman E, Gordon A, Kreisman H, et al. Long-term postthoracotomy pain. *Chest.* 1991;99(2):270–274.
3. Rogers ML, Duffy JP. Surgical aspects of chronic post-thoracotomy pain. *Eur J Cardiothorac Surg.* 2000;18(6):711–716.
4. Arends S, Böhmer AB, Poels M, et al. Post-thoracotomy pain syndrome: seldom severe, often neuropathic, treated unspecific, and insufficient. *Pain Rep.* 2020;5(2):e810.
5. Wildgaard K, Ravn J, Kehlet H. Chronic post-thoracotomy pain: a critical review of pathogenic mechanisms and strategies for prevention. *Eur J Cardiothorac Surg.* 2009;36(1):170–180.
6. Hetmann F, Kongsgaard UE, Sandvik L. Schou-Bredal I. Post-thoracotomy pain syndrome and sensory disturbances following thoracotomy at 6- and 12-month follow-ups. *J Pain Res.* 2017;10:663–668.
7. d'Amours RH, Riegler FX, Little AG. Pathogenesis and management of persistent postthoracotomy pain. *Chest Surg Clin North Am.* 1998;8(3):703–722.
8. Benedetti F, Vighetti S, Ricco C, et al. Neurophysiologic assessment of nerve impairment in posterolateral and muscle-sparing thoracotomy. *J Thorac Cardiovasc Surg.* 1998;115:841–847.
9. Pergolizzi J, Ahlbeck K, Aldington D, et al. The development of chronic pain: physiological CHANGE necessitates a multidisciplinary approach to treatment. *Curr Med Res Opin.* 2013;29(9):1127–1135.
10. Costigan M, Scholz J, Woolf CJ. Neuropathic pain: a maladaptive response of the nervous system to damage. *Annu Rev Neurosci.* 2009;32:1–32.
11. Sandkuhler J. Models and mechanisms of hyperalgesia and allodynia. *Physiol Rev.* 2009;89:707–758.
12. Hopkins KG, Hoffman LA, Dabbs Ade V, et al. Postthoracotomy pain syndrome following surgery for lung cancer: symptoms and impact on quality of life. *J Adv Pract Oncol.* 2015;6(2):121–132.
13. Landreneau RJ, Mack MJ, Hazelrigg SR. Prevalence of chronic pain after pulmonary resection by thoracotomy or videoassisted thoracic surgery. *J Thorac Cardiovasc Surg.* 1994;107:1079–1086.
14. Maguire MF, Ravenscroft A, Beggs D, Duffy JP. A questionnaire study investigating the prevalence of the neuropathic component of chronic pain after thoracic surgery. *Eur J Cardiothorac Surg.* 2006;29(5):800–805.

15. Kinney MA, Hooten WM, Cassivi SD, et al. Chronic postthoracotomy pain and health-related quality of life. *Ann Thorac Surg.* 2012;93:1242–1247.
16. Pertunnen K, Tasmuth T, Kalso E. Chronic pain after thoracic surgery: a follow-up study. *Acta Anaesthesiol Scand.* 1999;43:563–567.
17. Sabanathan S. Has postoperative pain been eradicated? *Ann R Coll Surg Engl.* 1995;77:202–209.
18. Eng J, Sabanathan S. Post-thoracotomy analgesia. *J R Coll Surg Edinb.* 1993;38:62–68.
19. Richardson J, Sabanathan S, Mearns AJ, Sides C, Goulden CP. Postthoracotomy neuralgia. *Pain Clin.* 1994;7:87–97.
20. Joshi GP. Multimodal; analgesia techniques and postoperative rehabilitation. *Anesthesiol Clin N Am.* 2005;23:185–202.
21. De Oliveira GS, Almeida MD, Benzon HT, et al. Perioperative single dose systemic dexamethasone for postoperative pain: a meta-analysis of randomized controlled trials. *Anesthesiology.* 2011;115:575–588.
22. Thangaswamy CR, Rewari V, Trikha A, et al. Dexamethasone before total laparoscopic hysterectomy: a randomized controlled dose-response study. *J Anesth.* 2010;24:24–30.
23. Coloma M, Duffy LL, White PF, et al. Dexamethasone facilitates discharge after outpatient anorectal surgery. *Anesth Analg.* 2001;92:85–88.
24. Worni M, Schudel HH, Seifert E, et al. Randomized controlled trial on single dose steroid before thyroidectomy for benign disease to improve postoperative nausea, pain, and vocal function. *Ann Surg.* 2008;248:1060–1066.
25. Gee NS, Brown JP, Dissanayake VU, et al. The novel anticonvulsant drug gabapentin (Neurontin) binds to the alpha2delta subunit of a calcium channel. *J Biol Chem.* 1996;10:5768–5776.
26. Solak O, Metin M, Esme H, et al. Effectiveness of gabapentin in the treatment of chronic post-thoracotomy pain. *Eur J Cardiothorac Surg.* 2007;32:9–12.
27. Ho KY, Gan TJ, Habib AS. Gabapentin and postoperative pain – a systematic review of randomized controlled trials. *Pain.* 2006;126:91–101.
28. Zhang J, Ho KY, Wang Y. Efficacy of pregabalin in acute postoperative pain: a meta-analysis. *Br J Anaesth.* 2011;106:454–462.
29. Chaim E, Weinberg L, Bellomo R. Paracetamol: a review with specific focus on the haemodynamic effects of intravenous administration. *Heart Lung Vessel.* 2015;7(2):121–132.
30. Hahn TW, Morgensen T, Lund LS, et al. Analgesic effect of I.V. Paracetamol: possible ceiling effect of paracetamol in postoperative pain. *Acta Anesthesiol Scand.* 2003;47:138–145.
31. Maund E, McDaid C, Rice S, et al. Paracetamol and selective and non-selective nonsteroidal anti-inflammatory drugs for the reduction in morphine-related side-effects after major surgery: a systematic review. *Br J Anaesth.* 2011;106:292–297.
32. Pavy T, Medley C, Murphy DF. Effect of indomethacin on pain relief after thoracotomy. *Br J Anaesth.* 1990;65:624–627.
33. Duale C, Sibaud F, Guastella V, et al. Perioperative ketamine does not prevent chronic pain after thoracotomy. *Eur J Pain.* 2009;13: 497–505.
34. Joshi GP, Bonnet F, Shah R, et al. A systemic review of randomized trials evaluating regional techniques for postthoracotomy analgesia. *Anesth Analg.* 2008;107:1026–1040.
35. Keller BA, Kabagambe SK, Becker JC, et al. Intercostal nerve cryoablation versus thoracic epidural catheters for postoperative analgesia following pectus excavatum repair: preliminary outcomes in twenty-six cryoablation patients. *J Ped Surg.* 2016;51: 2033–2038.
36. Oates HB. Non-pharmacological pain control for the CABG patient. *Dimens Crit Care Nurs.* 1993;12:296–304.
37. Whittaker DK. Degeneration and regeneration of nerves following cryosurgery. *Br J Exp Pathol.* 1974;55:595–600.
38. Ju H, Feng Y, Yang BX, Wang J. Comparison of epidural analgesia and intercostal nerve cryoanalgesia for postthoracotomy pain control. *Eur J Pain.* 2008;12:378–384.
39. Mustola ST, Lempinen J, Saimanen E, Vilkko P. Efficacy of thoracic epidural analgesia with or without intercostal nerve cryoanalgesia for postthoracotomy pain. *Ann Thorac Surg.* 2011;91: 869–873.
40. Solak O, Turna A, Pekcolaklar A, et al. Transcutaneous electric nerve stimulation for the treatment of postthoracotomy pain: a randomized prospective study. *Thorac Cardiovasc Surg.* 2007;55: 182–185.
41. Gerner P. Postthoracotomy pain management problems. *Anesthesiol Clin.* 2008;26(2):355 vii.
42. https://www.nysora.com/regional-anesthesia-for-specific-surgical-procedures/thorax/pectoralis-serratus-plane-blocks/.
43. Madabushi R, Tewari S, Gautam SK, Agarwal A, Agarwal A. Serratus anterior plane block: a new analgesic technique for postthoracotomy pain. *Pain Physician.* 2015;18(3):E421–E424.
44. Powell ES, Cook D, Pearce AC, et al. A Prospective, multicentre, observational cohort study of analgesia and outcome after pneumonectomy. *Br J Anaesth.* 2011;106:364–370.
45. Yeung JH, Gates S, Naidu BV, et al. Paravertebral block versus thoracic epidural for patients undergoing thoracotomy. *Cochrane Database Syst Rev.* 2016;2:CD009121.
46. Richardson J, Lönnqvist PA, Naja Z. Bilateral thoracic paravertebral block: potential and practice. *Br J Anaesth.* 2011;106:164–171.
47. Chelly JE. Paravertebral blocks. *Anesthesiol Clin.* 2012;30:75–90.
48. Kus A, Gurkan Y, Gul Akgul A, et al. Pleural puncture and intrathoracic catheter placement during ultrasound guided paravertebral block. *J Cardiothorac Vasc Anesth.* 2013;27:11–12.
49. Naja Z, Lönnqvist PA. Somatic paravertebral nerve blockade: incidence of failed block and complications. *Anaesthesia.* 2001; 56:1184–1188.
50. Manion SC, Brennan TJ. Thoracic epidural analgesia and acute pain management. *Anesthesiology.* 2011;115:181–188.
51. Hermanides J, Hollmann MW, Stevens MF, et al. Failed epidural: causes and management. *Br J Anaesth.* 2012;109:144–154.
52. Ready LB. Acute pain: lessons learned from 25,000 patients. *Reg Anesth Pain Med.* 1999;24:499–505.
53. Graybill J, Conermann T, Kabazie AJ, Chandy S. Spinal cord stimulation for treatment of pain in a patient with post thoracotomy pain syndrome. *Pain Physician.* 2011;14(5):441–445. PMID: 21927048.
54. Linderoth B, Foreman R. Mechanisms of spinal cord stimulation in painful syndromes: Role of animal models. *Pain Med.* 2006;7:14–26.
55. McJunkin TL, Berardoni N, Lynch PJ, Amrani J. An innovative case report detailing the successful treatment of post-thoracotomy syndrome with peripheral nerve field stimulation. *Neuromodulation.* 2010;13(4):311–314.
56. Goyal GN, Gupta D, Jain R, Kumar S, Mishra S, Bhatnagar S. Peripheral nerve field stimulation for intractable post-thoracotomy scar pain not relieved by conventional treatment. *Pain Pract.* 2010;10(4):366–369.
57. Hegarty D, Goroszeniuk T. Peripheral nerve stimulation of the thoracic paravertebral plexus for chronic neuropathic pain. *Pain Physician.* 2011;14(3):295–300.

26

Postoperative Care of the Thoracic Patient

EVREN ŞENTÜRK, FUNDA GÖK, MERT ŞENTÜRK

Introduction

Anesthesiologists are responsible for the management of the surgical cases not only during the intraoperative stage, but rather through the entire perioperative period. In the multidisciplinary context of perioperative medicine, anesthesiology is an important component in addressing the challenges from all practical, financial, and scientific points of view. Providing anesthesia to thoracic procedures is probably the prime example within the field of anesthesiology to have a crucial responsibility as a perioperative medicine physician. In general, the postoperative care of thoracic surgical patients is controlled by the intensive care unit (ICU) anesthesiologists either exclusively or as part of a multidisciplinary team with thoracic surgeons and pulmonologists. This chapter aims to review the postoperative care of the thoracic surgical patient. Postoperative complications, postoperative analgesia, as well as the postoperative part of the enhanced recovery after surgery (ERAS) protocol are discussed in Chapter 53 of the book.

In recent years, there have been significant advances in surgery, anesthesia, and intensive care techniques; however, thoracic surgery is still associated with a high incidence of postoperative complications recently reported, as being 27%.[1] That high complication rate can be attributed to the fact that patients who were not surgical candidate decades ago are now offered major resections.

To decrease the high incidence of complications, enhanced recovery after thoracic surgery (ERATS) has been reported as a possible approach[2]: these recommendations should be considered as a very promising pioneer step with a beneficial philosophy, but it should be underlined that they are based rather on strong recommendations than scientific evidence; therefore it is not surprising that the ERAS pathway is available in different protocols, with similar, but not the same recommendations, from different centers in different countries.[3–5]

As a matter of fact, there are still very few obvious evidences to support any suggestion for possible challenges of the postoperative care after thoracic surgery.

However, the philosophy of ERAS is very appropriate in that all the stages of the perioperative period, namely preoperative evaluation and preparation, intraoperative management, and postoperative care should focus on enhanced recovery with decreased complications. We want to underline as an important note that enhanced does not mean necessarily fast.

Location and Structure of Postoperative Care: Intensive Care Unit, High-Dependency Unit or Postanesthetic Care Unit?

There are still no clear cut criteria for deciding whether to send the patient to the ICU or the postanesthetic care unit (PACU). In the past, patients post thoracotomy were almost routinely sent to the ICU. However in recent years, it is progressively difficult to find available ICU beds which are more expensive but not necessarily more beneficial. In fact, it has been shown that although elective transfer to the ICU has reduced the total morbidity and frequency of complications it has not changed the mortality rate (7.3% vs. 7.3%); moreover, elective transfer to the ICU has caused a longer hospital stay.[6] The increasing quality of the PACUs has ensured a cost-effective and reliable alternative for postoperative admission.

The current trend is to move away from ICU admission and toward PACU or high dependency units (HDUs). In most institutions patients who undergo pneumonectomy, esophagectomy, or tracheal resection, are admitted to the ICU. In a recent retrospective study with 451 patients who underwent video-assisted thoracoscopic surgery (VATS) lobectomy, it has been shown that in selected patients (except: chronic obstructive pulmonary disease [COPD], nonstage I cancer, multiple port VATS, and age ≥60 years), selective intensive monitoring in the general ward—with the motto routine intensive monitoring but not routine intensive care—was safe and feasible without a poor outcome.[7] Well-equipped units with appropriate monitoring would be a reasonable consideration when choosing the postoperative care location.

Preoperative criteria for transferring a patient to the ICU will depend on the patient's medical condition, the type and the extent of the surgical procedure, and the hospital organization. We propose that a standardized preoperative prediction of whether the patient will be sent to the ICU or the PACU will help to establish a more appropriate organization of patient care. An interesting recent study has shown that patients who had an unplanned admission to ICU had higher mortality (29% vs. 0.03%).[8]

How Helpful Are the Scoring Systems to Predict the Postoperative Status Preoperatively?

In general, three factors affect the decision of the location of the postoperative care: patient-related risks (whereby modifiable and nonmodifiable factors should be evaluated), surgical risks, and intraoperative events which are usually unexpected.

Some patient-related factors, such as age over 70 years, American Society of Anesthesiologists—score of 3 or more, fibrotic lung disease, or preoperative neoadjuvant chemotherapy are generally considered as potential indications for ICU admission.[9,10] Surgical procedures, such as pneumonectomy, tracheal and bronchial resection, esophagectomies, lung volume reduction, and transplantation are considered (not exclusively) as high-risk operations.

The difference between modifiable (e.g., smoking) and nonmodifiable factors (e.g., age) is the most clinically relevant measure; preoperative interventions on modifiable factors may decrease the need for ICU treatment.[11] Some factors (e.g., preexisting lung disease, obesity, comorbidities, such as cardiovascular diseases, hypertension, diabetes mellitus) are partly modifiable. To achieve improvements in modifiable and partly modifiable factors, preoperative habilitation/prehabilitation programs have been shown to have a positive impact on the occurrence and severity of postoperative complications after thoracic operations by minimally invasive surgery.[12] From this point of view it can be argued that the postoperative care of the thoracic patients starts in the preoperative period (see Chapter 9).

Scoring systems[13] and risk factor definitions have been reported in several studies and reviews, can be helpful in defining the composite of patient-related surgical risks and provide some objective criteria regarding the location of postoperative care. Although it can differ among different centers, the overall recommendations of different scoring systems regarding the decision for sending the patient to ICU are:[14]

- >5 points in the Surgical Mortality Probability Model (S-MPM)
- ≥3 points in the Revised Cardiac Risk Index
- >2.5 points in the Thoracic Revised Cardiac Risk Index (ThRCRI)
- ≤5 points in the Surgical Apgar Score.
- >45 points in the ARISCAT Score.

The ARISCAT study has reported a risk score for the development of postoperative pulmonary complications (PPCs) includes seven independent risk factors,[15] both patient-related and surgical risk factors, that contributed equally to global risk and has been shown to have a predictive power.[16] This scoring system is being used for several studies and clinical practice today.

Yet, there is still a big grey zone regarding the decision of the location of postoperative care of thoracic patients, because:

1. First, the scoring systems were not originally defined for this purpose.
2. Even in high-volume centers, a high number of patients unexpectedly become candidate for ICU admission because of intraoperative (e.g., longer duration of operation, longer duration of one-lung ventilation [OLV], excessive blood loss, and air leak) or postoperative (e.g., respiratory insufficiency, air leak, and atelectasis) factors.
3. By calculating the balance between ICU versus PACU, incidence, and cost of readmission to ICU, and also failure to rescue of PPCs should also be taken in account. An important advantage of high-volume centers compared with the ones with less thoracic operations is that they have the resources and experience to address these problems.
4. Local conditions play a very important role: the postoperative admission criteria for various institutions differ based on their individual preferences and organization schemes. Numerous reasons, such as the number and experience of nurses and health personnel, the ratio of postoperative patients/ICU beds, the conditions of PACU influence different hospitals' decision to transfer patients, with the same preoperative conditions and similar surgical procedures, to the ICU or the PACU.

Management of Chest Tubes

Chest tubes are considered mandatory in all intrathoracic operations. Therefore the physician should be familiar with proper management of the thorax drainage, diagnosis, and treatment of its complications. Chest tubes remove air (ventral or cranial placement) and/or fluid (dorsal or caudal placement). Thus the physician's goal is to monitor, prevent, or treat air leaks and excessive pleural drainage.[17]

Although digital chest drainage systems are being used increasingly since approximately 10 years, the principle of the classical 3-bottle chest tube drainage system (Fig. 26.1) should still be mastered by the clinician dealing with a post-thoracotomy patient.

The introduction of ERATS protocols has again shown the controversies in the management of chest tubes. There are several issues regarding the chest tube management:

1. Suction Versus No Suction?

   The air from the pleura can be sucked passively (with a water seal) or actively (with a wall suction). ERATS protocol[2] sufficiently summarizes the pros and cons of

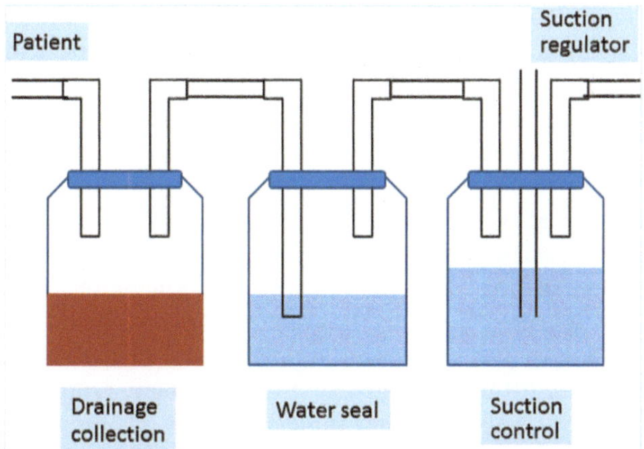

• **Fig. 26.1** Three-bottle system: using the **first (drainage collection) bottle** only would cause an increased resistance to drainage as a result of rising fluid/blood level and/or the foamy mixture of blood and air in the bottle. Adding a **second bottle** (water seal) allows fluid to drain into the first bottle only and the air into the second, preventing also the foam forming. However, the added length of the tubing can increase the dead space and add further resistance, causing a reversal of flow back up into the tube and back into the pleural space. Therefore a **third bottle** (suction control) allows for active suction to be exerted on the system, preventing the chest tube effluent from going back toward the patient.

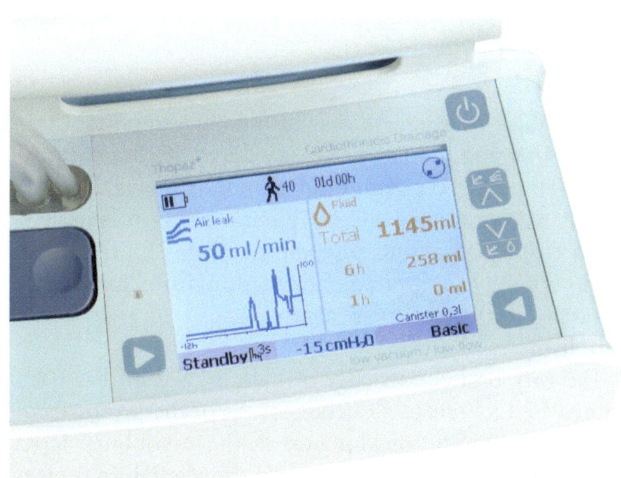

• **Fig. 26.2** The screen of a digital chest tube system: continuous monitoring of both air leak and the drainage facilitates the removal of the chest tube.

both suction and the so-called water seal. The relationship between the suction approach and clinical outcome is relatively weak that it can be easily biased by other components of the protocol of chest tube management.[18] Yet, there are some common approaches:

a. As a general rule, routine use of negative suction is to be avoided, and should be limited to persisting air leakages and nonexpandable lungs
b. The negative pressure should not exceed 15 to 20 cm H_2O.
c. After pneumonectomy, no negative pressure should be applied because of the risk of mediastinal shift.

2. Drainage and Removal

After a thoracic procedure, blood drainage should be carefully monitored especially in the early phase, and excessive drainage should signal an emergency alarm to immediately contact the surgical team. There have been empirically determined thresholds (e.g., 200 or 250 mL/day) for chest tube removal, however these dogmas have been refuted with stronger studies showing that the chest tubes can be removed if the drainage is <450 mL/day as long as there is no air leak or cerebrospinal fluid, chyle, or blood in the fluid.[19] Even a high drainage of 500 mL/day following VATS lobectomy resulted in an incidence of clinically relevant recurrent effusions, that needing drainage or aspiration, in only 2.8% of patients.[20]

3. Other Relevant Issues

- Any discrepancy between chest x-rays (or lung ultrasonography) and chest tubes output, may indicate failing thorax drainage because of tube blockage with a kink, blood clot, or suction failure.
- Chest tubes should never be clamped during patient transport because of the risk of pneumothorax.
- During removal of the chest tube, a Valsalva maneuver should be applied (preferably after full expiration instead of full inspiration)[21] to ensure positive intrathoracic pressure—combined with rapid removal—to prevent pneumothorax.
- Digital chest tube systems, commercially available since approximately 10 years, have been shown to reduce the risk of prolonged air leak, shorten the duration of both chest drainage and hospital stay compared with the traditional chest drainage system[18,22] (Fig. 26.2).

Specific Monitoring Tools

Routine monitoring after thoracic surgery outside the ICU consists of continuous pulsated oximetry (SpO2) and chest x-ray (CXR) in predetermined certain times. However, this paradigm of routine CXR is subject to change: studies examining the advantages of routine daily CXR versus selective clinical evaluation were not able to report any change in mortality rate, hospital length of stay, or adverse events on the basis of schedule CXR,[18] with the only exception in hypoxic patients. On the other hand, selective CXR only caused by clinical suspicion of a potential problem carries the risk of missing the initial phase of pulmonary complications. Low-radiation dose computer tomography (CT) allows reliable evaluation of pulmonary edema, but does not appear to be a widespread alternative because of the high cost, the risk of transport, and radiation exposure. Lung ultrasound (LUS) appears to solve the dilemma, in addition to its other advantages.

Another challenge is the decision about optimal fluid management, as the fluid therapy has been a classical problem especially in the intra- and postoperative period of thoracic surgery. New techniques not only help to determine whether to give more fluids, they can also help to monitor right ventricle function.

Lung Ultrasound as a New Tool (See Chapter 54)

LUS is a quick, inexpensive, easy-to-use and—importantly—reliable imaging modality.[23] It can diagnose cases of possible or undetected pneumothorax in CXR[24] (Fig. 26.3A); as well as pulmonary edema, pleural effusion, subcutaneous emphysema, and pneumonia (Fig. 26.3B–D). In conjunction with limited information from cardiac or vascular ultrasound, LUS aids diagnosis of pulmonary embolism.[25]

The very basic knowledge of LUS evaluation has been defined by Lichtenstein.[26] The pioneer of the protocols of this approach: in normal lung tissue, the interlobular septa are not detected by ultrasound and the pleural lines yield horizontal repetition artifacts, which have been termed the A-lines (Fig 26.3E). When the subpleural alveoli become edematous in the setting of increased extravascular lung water (EVLW), the resulting mixture of air and fluid yields the pathologic B-lines by ultrasound. These B-lines represent reverberation artifacts arising from the air-fluid interface between the fluid-filled and aerated alveoli[26] (see Fig. 26.3B). There is a linear correlation of the numbers of B-lines and increasing EVLW that reaches from interstitial edema showing four to eight B-lines to severe states of the alveolar-interstitial syndrome (AIS) with the confluence of multiple B-lines to the appearance of white lung[27] (see Fig. 26.3B and F). Sonographic appearance of AIS can also help to differentiate its possible causes, whereby a uniform distribution pattern of B-lines, with normal lung sliding and a high incidence of homogeneous appearing pleural effusions indicates left atrial hypertension and increased hydrostatic pressure. While in acute respiratory distress syndrome (ARDS) there are increased amounts of B-lines, seen in combination with pleural line abnormalities, lack of lung sliding, uneven tissue patterns like spared areas, consolidations, such as lung pulse and air bronchograms.[28]

Using transthoracic echocardiography (TTE), ventricular function can be evaluated. Especially right ventricular functions during and after thoracic surgery has been considered to be very difficult, and also often underestimated.[29]

Furthermore, the evaluation of the diaphragm with ultrasonography (DUS) may provide additional benefits to the clinician. A diaphragmatic dysfunction has been documented after thoracic surgery, as a condition that contribute to an increase in postoperative pulmonary complications.[30,31] The diaphragmatic ultrasonography is a noninvasive method which can be performed at the bedside. For this purpose, the diaphragm is evaluated in two different ways. These include the functional evaluation of the diaphragmatic excursion (DE) and the diaphragmatic thickening (DT) fraction (Fig. 26.3G and H). In a study where DE was used for the functional evaluation of the diaphragm, it has been shown that the diaphragmatic dysfunction detected within the first 24 hours was associated with the PPC occurring within the first 7-day period. Spadaro et al.

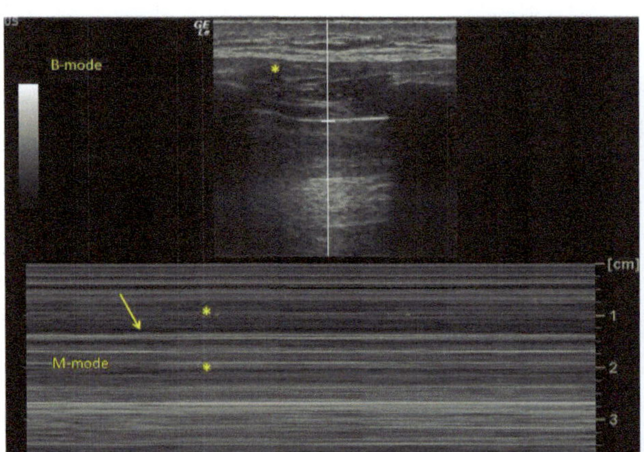

A

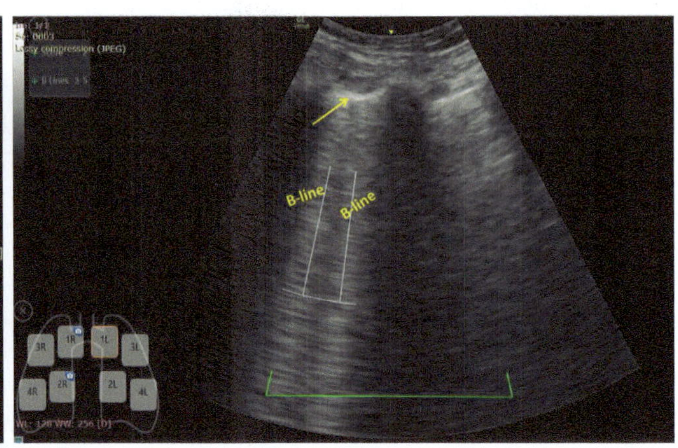

B

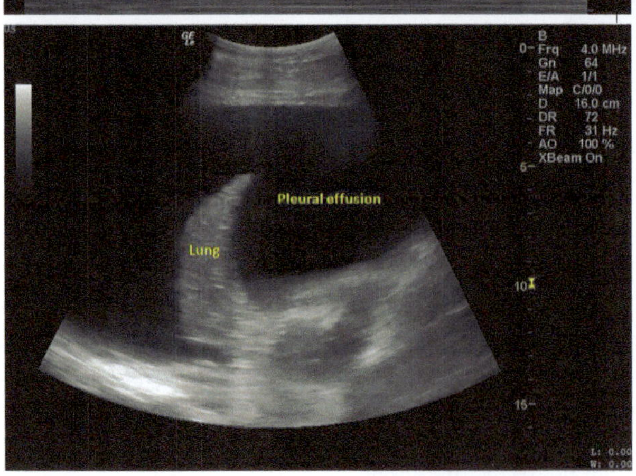

C

• **Fig. 26.3 Lung ultrasound screenings.**
(A) Barcode (stratosphere) sign. This pattern is the typical of the patients with pneumothorax. On M-mode image, the static thoracic wall consisting of subcutaneous and muscular tissues above the parietal pleura (*yellow arrow*), the parietal pleura and the reflections of the static thoracic wall structures located under the pleura are seen. The image obtained on M-mode is called the sign of barcode or stratosphere. * Static thoracic wall.
(B) **Sonographic image of B-lines.** It is the artifact of a hyperechoic, vertical reverberation originating from the pleura and extending to the end of the screen due to the lung ventilation. The number of B-lines is associated with the amount of extravascular lung water. The pleura looks thickened (*yellow arrow*).
(C) **Pleural effusion.** The pleural effusion is usually visualized as an anechoic space between the visceral and parietal layers of the pleura. The evaluation is performed at the point of PLAPS (posterolateral alveolar or pleural syndromes). On this image, too many effusions are noteworthy. Note that the lower lobe becomes atelectatic because of the effusion. (*continued*)

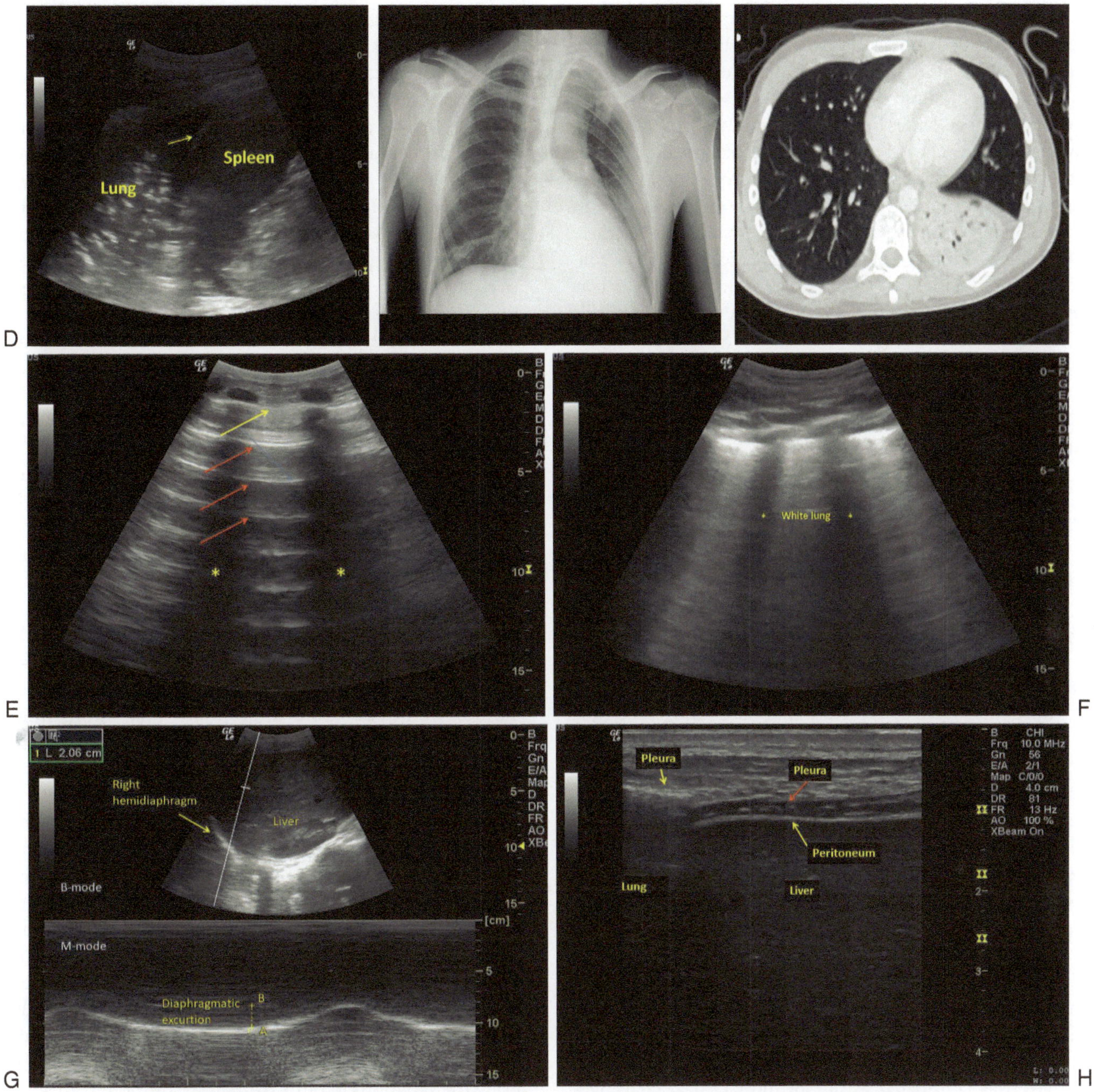

• **Fig. 26.3** *(Continued)* **(D) Sonographic, chest x-ray and computerized tomography (CT) images** of the same patient with lobar pneumonia. On the sonographic image, there is the consolidated area seen in the form of hyperechoic punctuation. In addition, a minimal pleural effusion is observed around the diaphragm (*yellow arrow*). Although the sonographic images and CT (consolidation and air bronchogram) show a marked pathology, the images are not pathognomonic on the chest x-ray.

(E) Sonographic image of the normally ventilated lung. A-lines (*red arrow*) are the artifact of horizontal reverberation extending at even intervals below the pleura (*yellow arrow*). These intervals are equal to the distance between the pleura and the transducer. A-lines can be seen in some cases of pneumothorax. * Shadow of costa.

(F) Image of white lung developing because of the confluence of multiple B-lines. Thickened pleura. * Shadow of costa. The image was taken from a patient with acute respiratory distress syndrome in the prone position.

(G) Sonographic view of the right hemidiaphragm upon examining through a convex probe. The upper image was obtained when the diaphragm was examined through B mode. The diaphragm appears as a hyperechoic line around the liver. The subsequent image was obtained when the diaphragm was examined with M-mode. The end points of expiration (A) and inspiration (B) are marked by a caliper. Diaphragmatic excursion is the difference between these two points. The excursion was measured as 2.06 cm in the figure.

(H) The image obtained by assessing the diaphragm with a linear probe. The diaphragm is the hypoechoic striated muscle layer located between the peritoneum and the pleura.

in a prospective study enrolled 75 patients undergoing VATS versus those undergoing thoracotomy. Diaphragmatic dysfunction was defined as a diaphragmatic excursion less than 10 mm. The ultrasound evaluations were carried out before (preoperative) and after (i.e., 2 hours and 24 hours postoperatively). The incidence of postoperative diaphragmatic dysfunction at 24 hours was higher in the thoracotomy group as compared with VATS group (83% vs. 55%, respectively). Patients with diaphragmatic dysfunction on the first day after surgery had higher percentage of PPCs (odds ratio = 5.5; 95% confidence interval [CI], 1.9–16.3; $P = .001$).[32] Although there are few studies addressing the issue, the value of the available evidence indicates the significance of DUS and the need for further studies.

Consequently, LUS should be considered as a beneficial diagnostic tool in the practice of postoperative thoracic surgery:

1. Compared with CXR, it is more specific and sensitive in diagnosing pathologic entities.
2. It can monitor EVLW, which can be challenging especially in the perioperative period of thoracic surgery; and differentiate in some cases between the possible causes of EVLW increase.
3. By switching to TTE, it can monitor the functions of right ventricle.
4. Finally, ultrasound can be used as a guide in procedures like vascular catheterization and nasogastric tube replacement.

It should be taken in account that for the patient undergoing thoracic surgery, abnormal anatomy because of preexisting diseases or changes because of surgery can limit the diagnostic value of LUS; preoperative LUS evaluation can be a rational approach to eliminate this limitation.[23]

Fluid Management and its Monitoring

Since Zeldin's first definition of postpneumonectomy pulmonary edema (PPE), a series of studies have shown the direct relation of fluid overload in the perioperative period and the incidence of postoperative respiratory failure. Fluid therapy was considered as one of most critical challenges of perioperative care of thoracic surgery. It has been shown that fluid challenges often fail to increase the intravascular volume but instead results in fluid leakage into the interstitial space.[33] Even the definitions of liberal and restrictive regimens differ essentially among different studies. The debate about different regimens like goal-directed therapy or zero-balance is true for all types of surgeries[34,35] and the challenge is even more dramatic in thoracic surgery because of several additive factors.

On the other hand, the thought of the less, the better is also not appropriate: the evidence of fluid restriction is weaker than its reputation: in fact, inadequate fluid administration can be associated with tissue hypoperfusion as seen in acute kidney injury and other end-organ failure.[36] The assertion that lungs do not have a third space is accurate, yet one must be reminded that any other organ does not have a third space either, so that this elusive third space should be considered as an urban myth.[37] Moreover, it has to be kept in mind that earlier studies that showed the relationship between high fluids administration and lung injury are often biased because many other factors, such as lung injury from mechanical ventilation with high tidal volumes, were applied. A very important pathophysiologic pathway of leakage of fluids into the interstitial space is the damage of endothelial glycocalyx,[38] a fragile network structure lining the endothelium. Many factors (such as nonprotective mechanical ventilation, surgical trauma) have been reported to cause or at least associated with a damage of glycocalyx. Similar to ARDS and ventilator-associated lung injury, administering fluids is not the only cause; but may be a contributing factor to worsening symptoms of PPE. With intravenous fluids, we can make it worse, but we do not cause it.[39]

Fluid overload should be avoided both during and after thoracotomies. Slinger has suggested a limit for the intraoperative period (<2 L), and limit the fluid to (<3 L) for the entire day of surgery.[40] Newer guidelines suggest not to exceed the perioperative positive fluid balance of 1500 mL (or 20 mL/kg/24 hours).[2] Hypotension during and after thoracotomy is only rarely caused by hypovolemia; it is more often caused by vasodilation (e.g., caused by thoracic epidural anesthesia.). Low doses of catecholamines would be more appropriate than more fluids considering that hypotension is likely caused by relative hypovolemia.[41]

Monitoring the fluid balance is mandatory, especially in patients at risk of acute lung injury (ALI). Pulmonary artery catheters have been almost entirely replaced by newer, noninvasive, such as LUS, or semi-invasive devices.[23] Among them, the single-indicator transpulmonary thermodilution (TPTD) method can assess quantitatively the EVLW index (EVLWI)[42] and can monitor cardiac output using pulse contour analysis of the arterial pressure.[43] Pulse-pressure variation analysis can predict the fluid responsiveness also intraoperatively.[44] Another method, called the pleth variability index, provides information about the volume status using the variations in pulse oximetry;[45] the noninvasiveness of this method is advantageous and existing studies seem promising.

There is a concern about usefulness of these techniques during OLV in both VATS and open thoracotomy. In spite of controversies, the majority of the studies report that stroke volume variation and pulse pressure variation are not useful for predicting fluid responsiveness in thoracic surgery.[46] However, the postoperative period differs from the conditions of OLV, where the concern about the accuracy of single thermodilution measurement to estimate EVLW after lung resection was validated against double dye technique and found to be well correlated for up to 12 hours.[47] Yet, TPTD also has some limitations: measurement takes place only in areas of perfused lungs, assuming there is a homogeneous distribution of pulmonary perfusion. That homogeneous distribution can be impaired by several perioperative factors, such as lung resection, hypoxic pulmonary vasoconstriction, and others.[23]

The ability to measure the EVLW has obtained a more rational fluid management. Indeed, EVLW was shown to be an independent predictor of survival in critically ill patients,[48] so that the clinicians can change their historical approach of restrictive fluid management to achieving normovolemia with a goal-directed treatment.[49] For patients with sepsis or ARDS, the threshold of EVLW appears to be between 8 and 9 mL/kg.[42] Although the inhomogeneity in patients following thoracic surgery can make the decision more complicated, this threshold can still be helpful. Using the results of TPTD measurements in combination with LUS (changes between preoperative and postoperative LUS findings) can obtain more reliable decisions.[23] The decision regarding the fluid treatment or vasoactive drugs should be based on several parameters as depicted in Box 26.1.[42,49]

The type of fluids is also a subject of discussion. As the indication of colloids, mainly hydroxy-ethyl starch (HES), is currently limited only to acute blood loss, their use in the postoperative period in PACU or in ICU appears to be the exception. Yet, it has to be kept in mind that most of the available data are not from thoracic patients, but extrapolated from studies performed on septic, critically ill patients in ICUs, or from patients undergoing cardiovascular surgery. In a retrospective study, the incidence of acute kidney injury (AKI) after thoracic surgery was found to be 5.1% (74 in 1442 patients). There was no correlation between crystalloid restriction and AKI; interestingly, AKI occurred more often when HES were administered to the patients with decreased renal function or having more than two risk factors with normal renal function. The authors concluded that HES should be administered with caution in high-risk patients undergoing thoracic surgery.[36] Besides the drawback in patients with renal risks, this study limits the concern about HES only to these patients. Thoracic anesthesiologists tend to use HES in combination with balanced crystalloids (rather than saline), as part of a multimodal fluid resuscitation.[2,49]

• BOX 26.1 Fluid Management

1. The classical target of fluid management is: Cardiac index >3 L/min/m² (in some clinical conditions normotension would be also a simpler—and maybe more appropriate—target)
2. Maintain normovolemia (restrictive approach only in extreme cases)
3. Extravascular lung water index should be monitored
   a. by transpulmonary thermodilution (threshold: 10 mL/kg; in sepsis and ARDS 8–9 mL/kg)
   b. by lung ultrasound:
      i. compare preoperative and postoperative LUS views
      ii. compare operated and nonoperated lungs
4. Evaluate tissue oxygenation
5. Decide: fluid/diuretics, vasoconstrictors, inotropes

ARDS, Acute respiratory distress syndrome; *LUS*, lung ultrasound.

Monitoring of Right Ventricular Function

It is well-known that there is a reduction of up to 25% in right ventricular ejection fraction (RVEF) following lung resection[50] that can result in postoperative right ventricular (RV) dysfunction. The evaluation of RV and pulmonary vascular function has remained limited until recently because of the lack of a simple inexpensive technology to obtain reliable diagnostic criteria.[51] Perioperative factors, such as preexisting pulmonary disease, ventilation strategies, including OLV and analgesia methods like thoracic epidural anesthesia, can all adversely affect RV function.[52] Recently, the relationship between lung resection and RV dysfunction has been shown using cardiac magnetic resonance. McCall et al. evaluated 27 patients using cardiovascular magnetic resonance imaging to assess the RV response to lung resection. Cardiovascular magnetic resonance imaging with volume and flow analysis, preoperatively, on postoperative day 2 and at 2 months. They found that RVEF deteriorated from 50.5% ± 6.9% preoperatively to 45.6% ± 4.5% on postoperative day 2 and remained decreased at 44.9% ± 7.7% by 2 months ($P = .003$). They concluded that RV dysfunction occurs following lung resection and persists 2 months after surgery.[53] In another study, the utility of TTE was examined to aid in the diagnosis of RV dysfunction following pulmonary resection.[29] The studies show that RV dysfunction persists for up to 2 months postoperatively, and is more severe in patients undergoing pneumonectomy, whereas thoracoscopy may be protective.

Using a relatively simple and noninvasive method like TTE can be helpful to put a new target in pre- and postoperative care of thoracic surgery. The prevention of RV dysfunction can change our current practice of mechanical ventilation, fluid management, and even postoperative analgesia.

Ventilatory Support for Patients After Thoracic Surgery

This section will focus on and limit itself to the specific features of ventilatory support in the postthoracotomy period. Postoperative ventilatory support is indicated when there are:

- Severe comorbidities of the patient (preoperatively planned) (preventive)
- Intraoperative complications (e.g., bleeding) (preventive or grey zone)
- Postoperative complications (importantly postoperative lung injury) (curative), whereas almost all of the potential complications after thoracic surgery result in acute respiratory failure (ARF) (Fig. 26.4).

There are two serious complications associated with postoperative mechanical ventilation:

1. Damage to the lung parenchyma and tracheobronchial tree: the risk of lung injury is a general challenge of mechanical ventilation. In thoracic surgery patients,

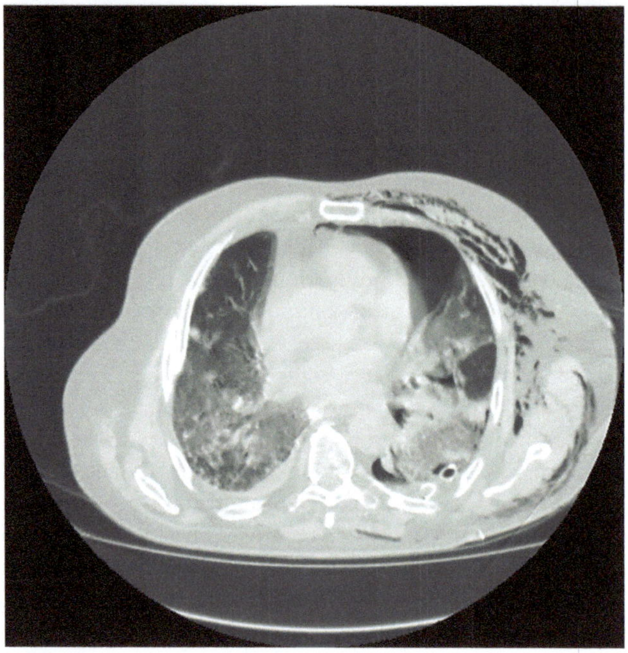

• **Fig. 26.4** Computerized tomography scan of a postthoracotomy (left upper lobectomy) patient with acute respiratory distress syndrome: space at the operation area of the resected tissue; atelectatic areas at the rest lung; infiltrations in both (also right) lungs (without any clinical sign of infection); subcutaneous emphysema.

the trauma to the suture line may disrupt the bronchial stump as a result of positive airway pressure and constitutes an additional risk.

2. Ventilator-associated pneumonia (VAP)

Mechanical ventilation as a method of treatment/prevention of respiratory failure can per se cause ALI (i.e., ventilatory-associated or -related lung injury).[54] As relative newer methods like noninvasive ventilation (NIV) or high-flow oxygen (HFO) therapy have been introduced in practice, conventional mechanical ventilation is currently indicated in a limited group of patients, in whom—paradoxically—it can be even more hazardous: devil or the deep blue sea.

The specific group of patients after thoracic surgery might have already undergone a multi-hit of ventilatory traumas by both thoracic surgeons and the anesthetists: surgeons remove larger parts of the lungs; in addition, they manipulate the remaining lung tissue in a traumatic way, and cause damage to the respiratory muscles. A thoracotomy is one of the most painful operations, which can cause further impaired ventilation. OLV can cause lung injury, especially if the OLV-management is inappropriate and nonprotective[55]; in addition, excessive fluid infusion and blood transfusion can further directly harm the lungs. Interestingly, the possibility of a postoperative lung injury in the nonsurgical dependent lung is higher than the surgical collapsed lung, indicating that the intraoperative ventilation affect the postoperative lung functions.[56]

Therefore in PACU or ICU, mechanical ventilation should be continued or restarted only if absolutely necessary; less invasive methods of respiratory support should be considered before indicating the invasive mechanical ventilation.

The pathway of ventilatory support can be considered as a stairway, where in every step the risks increase (Fig. 26.5).

There are some practical generalized rules for deciding to continue mechanical ventilation in the postoperative period:

1. If possible, the decision should be made pre- or intraoperatively, and preoperative predictive decisions should be reevaluated at the end of the operation.
2. In patients in which postoperative mechanical ventilation is predicted, using bronchial blockers for the operation may be safer, as no tube exchange would be necessary.
3. If a double-lumen tube (DLT) has been used, it should be replaced with a normal ETT at the end of the operation. In some institutions, in patients who expected to be extubated shortly within 2 hours of the conclusion of the surgery, assuming the ICU staff is familiar with the use of a DLT, the DLT may remain (caveat: the cuff of the bronchial lumen should be deflated). If a Univent® tube was used for OLV, the tube can remain, and the blocker should be pulled back into the main lumen.
4. Spontaneous breathing is better than mechanical ventilation, and assisted ventilation is better than controlled ventilation; however, obligatory reintubation can be the worst scenario. NIV and/or HFO therapy should be preferred.
5. Weaning is a process that starts with the admission of an intubated patient.

Protective Ventilation After Thoracic Surgery

Protective lung ventilation (PLV) is currently the method of choice of mechanical ventilation; and is crucial when it is applied to the vulnerable lungs of the patients after thoracic surgery. PLV is a bundle of several components:

- applying a low V_T (<7 mL/kg),
- limiting the ventilation pressure (<30 cm H_2O),
- having an appropriate positive end-expiratory pressure (PEEP), and
- applying recruitment maneuvers (RM).

PLV has been shown to be effective and protective both in ARDS in the ICU[57] and in OLV.[58] Although these common rules can generally be extrapolated to PLV in patients after thoracic surgery, there are also some specific limitations and conditions regarding this patient group:

- **An intraoperative V_T of 6 to 8 mL/kg** (ideal body weight) is associated with a decreased frequency of postoperative pulmonary failure. Moreover, there is already a reduction of functional lung tissue (similar to the baby lung of the ARDS).[55] In this manner, it can even be questioned whether a V_T of 6 mL/kg is protective enough. In some patients, high ventilatory pressures can be necessary even for these low V_Ts, so that an extracorporeal ventilatory support can be indicated.
- In patients after thoracic surgery, **monitoring the difference between inspiratory and expiratory V_Ts** is extremely important, as it is a very easy, reliable and objective measure of air leakage.

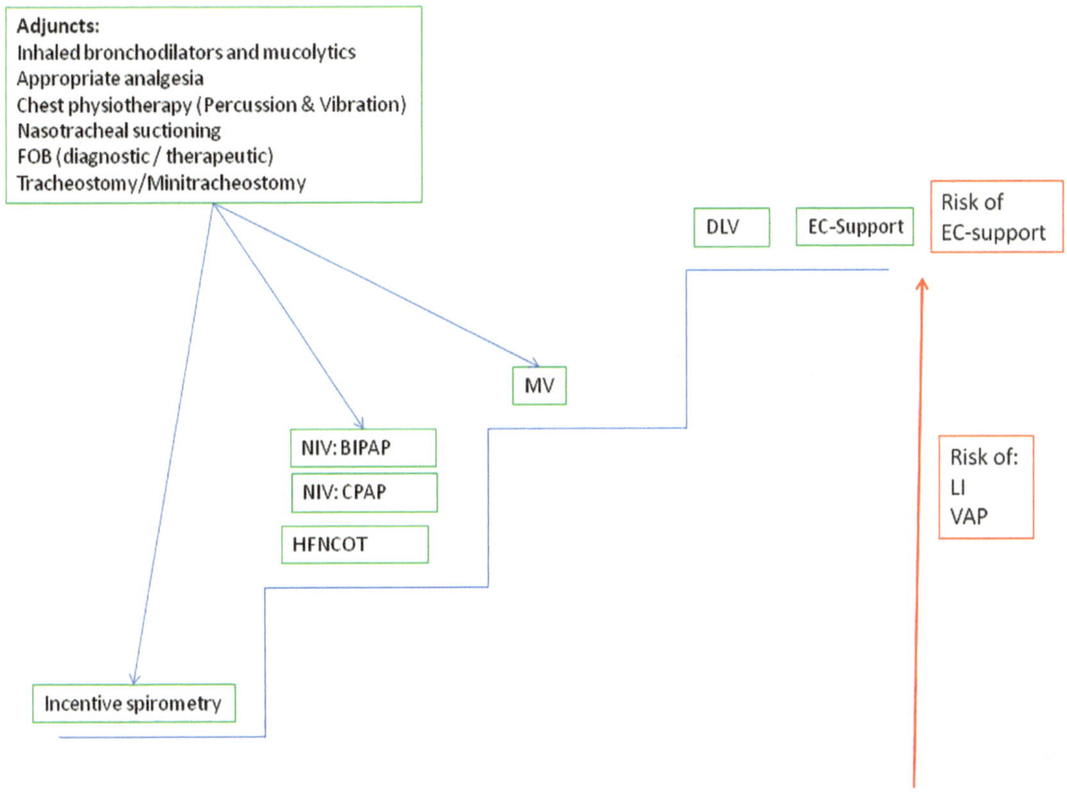

• **Fig. 26.5 Stairs of ventilatory support in patients after thoracic surgery.** Note that the higher the stairs, the higher the risks. Climbing the stairs should be avoided and descending (weaning) should be targeted, as possible. Adjuncts would be helpful to descend. *DLV*, Differential lung ventilation; *EC-Support*, extracorporeal lung support; *FOB*, fiberoptic bronchoscopy; *HFNOT*, high-flow nasal oxygen treatment; *LI*, lung injury; *MV*, mechanical ventilation; *NIV-BIPAP*, noninvasive ventilation-biphasic positive airway pressure; *NIV-CPAP*, noninvasive ventilation-continuous positive airway pressure; *VAP*, ventilator-associated pneumonia.

- Even if the decrease in V_T can be compensated by an increase in frequency, this approach has some drawbacks: shorter inspiration can generate high ventilation pressures and shorter expiration can lead to air-trapping and auto-PEEP. More importantly, mild hypercapnia is permitted in many cases[59] and can even be therapeutic for several hours.[60] However, hypercapnia enhances hypoxic pulmonary vasoconstriction; thus **permissive hypercapnia** is contraindicated in the presence of pulmonary hypertension (which is more frequent in post-thoracotomy patients). In the remaining population, permissive hypercapnia can be considered as a rational part of PLV.
- **The inspiratory fraction of O_2 (F_iO_2)** also plays an important role for both mechanically ventilated and spontaneously breathing patients: the fact that O2 consumption is increased in postoperative patients has led to a routine administration of supplemental O2 in all postoperative patients. Moreover, the World Health Organization has recently recommended to use high F_iO2 (0.80) also during the postoperative period to prevent surgical site infections.[61] This recommendation is based on some studies,[62,63] which are not confirmed in later larger studies;[64] and is recently an important issue of discussion of our discipline.[65] Disadvantages of high F_iO2 appear to be more prominent than its advantages: high F_iO2 is known to cause absorption atelectasis; and second, hyperoxia causes both coronary and systemic vasoconstriction and results in the deterioration of hemodynamic parameters, such as decreased stroke volume and increased systemic vascular resistance.[66] Effects on the glycocalyx is unclear and is being examined in ongoing studies.
- Whether to use **volume or pressure-controlled ventilation** (VCV or PCV) is another controversy: previous studies have shown the benefits of PCV in OLV,[67] but more recent studies have not confirmed these findings,[68] so most likely there is probably no difference between these modes with regard to injury to the lung. One study has shown that PCV was associated with an improvement of RV functions compared with VCV, because of reduced airway pressures.[69]
- The more appropriate approach is to **avoid high ventilatory pressures**. High maximum airway pressures (Pmax: defined as P-max in pressure-controlled assist modes and plateau pressure in volume-controlled assist modes) were found to be a potentially modifiable variable associated with in-hospital mortality.[70] In this study, a Pmax of 18 cm H_2O was defined as a cut-off value for all patients (both at risk and not at risk of ARDS). Although in several studies, high plateau pressure levels (which includes

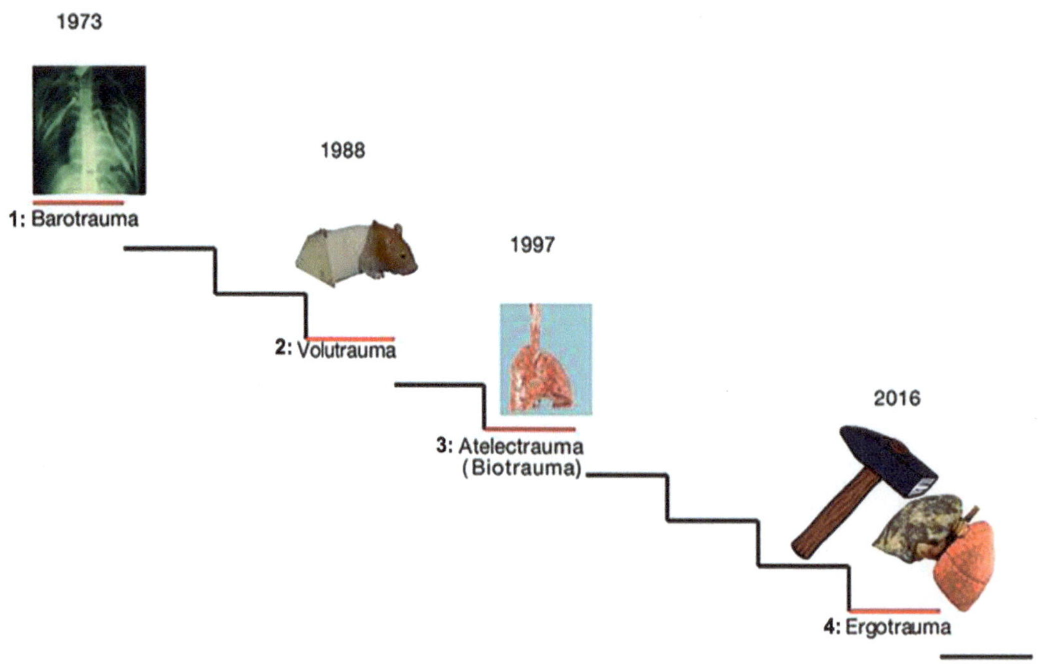

• **Fig. 26.6** Evolution of the concept of VILI. From left to right: barotrauma (**1**), volutrauma (**2**), atelectrauma/biotrauma (**3**), ergotrauma (**4**). *VILI*, Ventilator-induced lung injury. (From Tonetti T, Vasques F, Rapetti F, et al. Driving pressure and mechanical power: new targets for VILI prevention. *Ann Transl Med*. 2017;5:286.)

PEEP), and high PEEP per se have been shown as risk factors, a pioneer study of Amato et al. has reported that the main parameter to monitor is the **driving pressure** (driving pressure = plateau pressure—PEEP).[71] Following these data regarding ARDS patients, newer studies have also confirmed the relationship between the driving pressure and lung injury, and concluded that even in patients ventilated with protective V_T, higher driving pressure is associated with worse long-term pulmonary function and structure.[72] Regarding the effects of intraoperative mechanical ventilation, driving pressure was found again to be the only significant parameter associated with the development of pulmonary complications and mortality.[73] Also in thoracic surgery, application of driving pressure-guided ventilation during OLV has been found to be associated with a lower incidence of PPCs.[74] Again, it should be underlined that this is a study about the intraoperative ventilation strategy. We assume that a similar approach should also be valid for the postoperative mechanical ventilation. It is worth mentioning that there is a discrepancy between the ICU data and the thoracic surgical populations that can be explained by the fact that to date, there is no evidence to confirm that the data derived from ICU patients are applicable to patients undergoing a thoracic surgical procedure. Importantly, the majority of thoracic patients who presented for lung resection, unlike the ICU patients, have no ARDS or areas of the lung that cannot be recruited.

- A relative new entity, **mechanical power**, takes several parameters like PEEP, peak pressure, and also frequency into account: this philosophy imposes that driving pressure is one of the components of the mechanical power, which also includes respiratory rate, flow, and PEEP. Mechanical power is the energy delivered from the ventilator to the respiratory system per unit of time. This approach introduces ergotrauma, among the classical baro-, volu-, and atelectotrauma (Fig. 26.6).[75]

$$\text{Simplified Power formula: } 0.098 \times RR \times V_T \times [P_{peak} - \tfrac{1}{2} \times (P_{plat} - PEEP)]$$

In ICU setting, a high mechanical power is associated with a higher risk. Serpa Neto et al. analyzed the data from Medical Information Mart for Intensive Care (MIMIC)-III, and the eICU Collaborative Research Database (eICU) of 59 hospitals of critically ill patients receiving invasive ventilation for at least 48 hours with the primary outcome was in-hospital mortality. Data from 8207 patients were analyzed. Median mechanical power (MP) during the second 24 hours was 21.4 (16.2–28.1) J/min in MIMIC-III and 16.0 (11.7–22.1) J/min in eICU. MP was independently associated with in-hospital mortality. High MP was also associated with ICU mortality, 30-day mortality, and with ventilator-free days, ICU and hospital length of stay. Even at low V_T, high MP was associated with in-hospital mortality. They concluded MP unifies variables known to be related to development of ventilator-induced lung injury. MP is independently associated with worse outcomes in patients receiving invasive ventilation. Of additional interest, even at low V_T and low driving pressure, high MP is associated with worse patient-centered outcomes.[76] Whether and how this new tool can affect the strategy of mechanical ventilation in patients after thoracic surgery, has to be studied.

This new approach inspires two new discussions:

1. **The respiratory rate,** which was not included in former suggestions for the prevention of lung injury, has now become an important part.
2. **PEEP** plays an important role in PPC (which is—probably—contrary to the driving pressure only approach).
   - The advantages and disadvantages of PEEP constitute a continuous ongoing discussion. Several studies have showed that PEEP improves the oxygenation[77] and—more importantly—prevents cyclic closing-reopening of the alveoli during ventilation;[78,79] it also allows the decrease of F_iO2 without compromising the oxygenation: PEEP is considered as an important part of PLV. However, preventing atelectasis with PEEP can also lead to overinflation, which can be even more harmful to lungs. The debate between open lung and resting lung is an ongoing discussion.[80,81] An individualized PEEP-titration to evaluate the best PEEP in each patient appears to be a smart approach.[82] This approach consists of an alveolar RM followed by a descending PEEP titration adjusted to best respiratory system compliance; and has been found to be associated with a decreased incidence of PPCs compared with similar patients.[82]

     Another method to determine the optimal PEEP is again an individualized approach, with the help of electrical impedance tomography (EIT).[83] EIT can be considered as a reliable monitor of mechanical ventilation, even more in the ICU than in the operating room, as it can inform about both atelectasis and overinflation continuously.

     Starting from the classical F_iO2-PEEP table in the ARDS-Net study, there are several ways defined to measure the best or optimal PEEP value (Table 26.1). Explanation of different methods of PEEP titration can be found in Chapter 31. Whatever method is chosen, keep in mind that individualization should be preferred. To define the best PEEP in patients after thoracic surgery, effects on anastomoses and sutures should also be taken into account.
   - RM: PEEP can keep the lung open but is not capable of opening the lung. To open collapsed regions, a physical opening with RM is necessary.[84] After opening the lung with RM, PEEP will prevent a recollapse. PEEP and RM are therefore obligatory components of the PLV; however, there are no studies examining the effects of RM in patients after thoracic surgery: RM is absolutely contraindicated in patients with a risk of air leakage. Moreover, the high pressure of RM and PEEP may have unwarranted effects of overpressured stress on bronchial stumps and anastomoses. Therefore indication of RM in patients after thoracic surgery appears to be limited in exceptional cases.

TABLE 26.1 Different Methods of Positive End-Expiratory Pressure Titration

Different Methods	Short Explanation	Comments
F_iO2-PEEP chart	The higher F_iO2 requirement; the higher PEEP. Classical from ARDS-Net study	Still used, but not very appropriate
Stress index	A straight incline (not convex, not concave) in pressure-time curve during inspiration with constant flow	Reliable, but requires technology
Best static compliance	Lowest pressure changes after a constant tidal volume application (rather than decremental)	Should be performed in a decremental way after a recruitment maneuver[82]
EIT	Visual differentiation of areas with optimal ventilation	Continuous, noninvasive ventilation. Requires experience with belts[83]
CT	Visual differentiation of areas of atelectasis, overinflation and ventilation	Sophisticated and reliable; but obviously not a bedside test
Mechanical power	Measurement via the equation	Very new approach; probably lower measurements than other methods[75]
Highest PaO2	Blood gas measurement at each level At least 10 minutes at each level	Price of an (unnecessary high) PaO2 can be high; too high measurement; hemodynamic compromises
Highest DO2	DO2 measurement necessary at each level At least 10–15 minutes at each level	Too long (and sometimes too invasive) process
None of them	None of the possible methods above can obtain perfect results	Titration by feel

ARDS, Acute respiratory distress syndrome; *CT*, computerized tomography; *DO2*, oxygen delivery; *EIT*, electrical impedance tomography; *F_iO2*, inspiratory oxygen fraction; *PaO2*, arterial oxygen partial pressure; *PEEP*, positive end-expiratory pressure.

• **BOX 26.2 Mechanical Ventilation in a Patient After Thoracic Surgery**

1. Do not apply if the problem can be solved with less invasive methods (noninvasive or high-flow oxygen treatment)
2. Plan and try to wean: always
3. Oxygenation goal: PaO2 >55 mm Hg or SpO2 >88%
4. Low ventilatory pressures (low pressures are more important than low tidal volume)
   a. Plateau pressure: as low as possible (<30 cm H_2O)
   b. Driving pressure ($P_{Plateau}$ – PEEP) (<15 cm H_2O) or (<18 cm H_2O)
5. Low tidal volume: 5–7 mL/kg ideal body weight (the less the better)
6. Low mechanical power
7. Permit a hypercapnia until pH ≤7.3 (do not increase the respiratory rate to keep normocapnia)
8. Individual PEEP titration
9. Recruitment maneuver (only if absolutely necessary): should be avoided, if possible
10. If specific cases: consider differential lung ventilation or extracorporeal support

PaO2, Arterial oxygen partial pressure; *PEEP*, positive end-expiratory pressure; *SpO2*, pulsated oximetry.

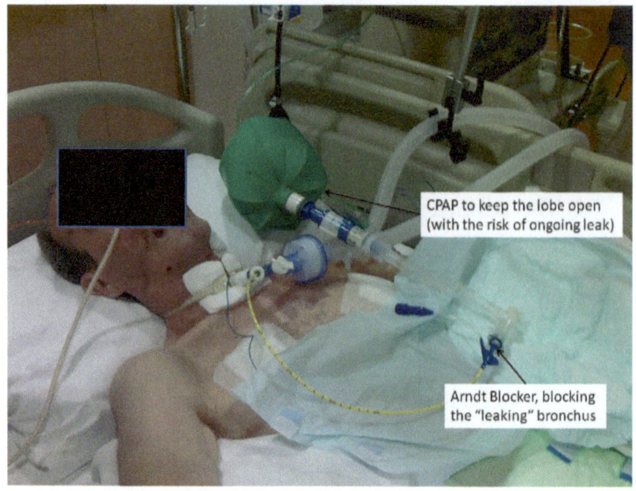

• **Fig. 26.7** In a patient with persistent bronchopleural fistula and requirement of mechanical ventilation, the lung (or the lobe) with the fistula can be blocked with a bronchial blocker (in this case an Arndt Blocker). The remaining lung can be ventilated in the necessary way, whereby in the blocked part, a low level of continuous positive airway pressure (*CPAP*) can be applied to prevent a full collapse without forcing the fistula.

As a short conclusion for PLV in patients after thoracic surgery, clinicians should be aware that the lungs after thoracic surgery are at risk of injury. PLV should be a part of mechanical ventilation, mandatory during the intraoperative period; but also, during the postoperative period. Indeed, several studies have shown the effects of an intraoperative ventilation strategy on pulmonary complications in postoperative period,[85] and new multicentric studies are currently being performed.[86] Similarly, several studies concerning protective ventilation in non-ARDS patients in the ICU setting have shown its beneficial effects. Therefore a protective approach would be also rational for the ventilation of patients after thoracic surgery, even if there are fewer studies in this patient group (Box 26.2).

Differential Lung Ventilation

Differential lung ventilation (DLV) can be considered as the ICU variation of OLV. The objective is to ventilate both lungs—synchronized or not—with different V_Ts and/or PEEPs. This method has been shown to be beneficial in bilateral ARDS in the lateral decubitus position.[87] Two essential indications of DLV are related to thoracic surgery: unilateral lung processes and air leaks.[88]

Two coupled ventilators (master and slave) with synchronized inspiration and expiration can be used. Two ventilators can also be used in an asynchronized manner but there is a risk causing a mediastinal shift from differential pressure ventilation. Another solution is to ventilate one lung (the healthy one) with the conventional setting, whereas continuous positive airway pressure (CPAP) or high frequency ventilation can be applied to the sick lung (Fig. 26.7).

DLV can:

- Protect the healthy lung against the spillage of the pathologic processes of the diseased other lung (massive unilateral hemoptysis, bronchiectasis, and lung abscesses).
- Help to maintain adequate ventilation for oxygenation and gas exchanges in intractable air leaks, such as with a bronchopleural fistula, making a conventional ventilation impossible.
- In cases with an inhomogeneous distribution of infiltrations—until the process in the sick lung can be treated DLV will, in the meanwhile, permit less trauma to the healthy lung.
- DLV can be applied with all possible methods of OLV; however, the long-term use of these techniques is limited because of the obligatory muscle relaxation and the potential risks from displacement of the DLT.

High-Frequency Ventilation

To avoid high ventilatory pressures that can cause overinflation during mechanical ventilation, high-frequency ventilation (HFV) can be an alternative solution. There are different ways to achieve HFV: in many of them, the V_T is less than the dead space, but gas exchange is possible by combining different factors, such as convection, diffusion, and others. The types of HFV differ in setting (such as in frequency or driving pressure and inspiratory/expiratory [I:E] ratio) and can be applied alone or in combination with other methods, such as DLV. In one study, high-frequency percussive ventilation, a variant of HFV has been shown to effectively improve oxygenation, help to remove produced secretions, and decrease the frequency of pneumonia and the length of the hospital stay.[89] However, there are no randomized control trials that examine the effects of HFV in postthoracotomy patients.

Noninvasive Ventilation

NIV is defined as a partial or complete support of the breathing without an endotracheal tube or tracheostomy cannula. As with mechanical ventilation, ventilatory support with positive pressure in patients after thoracic surgery is not without risks (if not contraindicated) and should therefore be always limited to selected cases where it is absolutely necessary. As in mechanical ventilation, NIV is also classified for curative and prophylactic treatment, and for a group between them (grey zone).[90] Both noninvasive positive pressure ventilation (NIPPV: referring to two positive airway pressures) and CPAP (referring to one positive airway pressure) can be used in all clinical situations.

The beneficial clinical results with NIV have been reported mostly in patients with COPD.[91] Several studies have shown the prophylactic and therapeutic beneficial effects of NIV after thoracic surgery:[92] NIV is associated with an increase in oxygenation, gas exchange, a decrease in the work of breathing (which can be of great importance in postthoracotomy patients) and better management of air leaks.[93] Lefebvre et al. prospectively evaluated early NIV use for ARF after lung resection in the medical and a surgical ICU of 690 patients at risk of severe complications following lung resection. They reported 113 (16.3%) experienced ARF, which was initially supported by NIV in 89 (78.7%), including 59 with hypoxemic ARF (66.3%) and 30 with hypercapnic ARF (33.7%). The overall success rate of NIV was 85.3% (76/89). In-ICU mortality was 6.7% (6/89). In conclusion, their survey confirms the feasibility and efficacy of NIV in ARF following lung resection.[94]

The simple method involves applying CPAP with a tight mask in a spontaneously breathing patient. In a hypoxemic patient during the immediate postoperative period, CPAP application would address the etiology of the hypoxia more than the more frequently used basic O2 application. NIPPV can also be used for both curative and prophylactic strategies, in spite of the fear of physicians that in postthoracotomy patients, positive pressure could stress the bronchial sutures and anastomoses. With a careful titration of NIPPV, the transanastomotic pressure gradient (corresponding to transpulmonary pressure) can be adjusted within safe limits.[95] Hereby, a temporary suspension of negative suction of the chest tube would help to keep the pressure gradient as a precautionary measure.[96] Moreover, adjusting the ventilatory setting to provide the lowest pressures (starting with a pressure support ventilation [PSV] of 3–5 cm H_2O) would also improve patient comfort and adjustment to the NIV[97] (Fig. 26.8).

In general, NIV aims to achieve the advantages of mechanical ventilation to provide adequate oxygenation and gas exchange, without carrying its risks. Compared with mechanical ventilation, NIV has the advantages of avoiding the risks related to intubation and extubation maneuvers, and loss of airway defense mechanisms because the upper airways are preserved. The incidence of respiratory infections is reduced, expectoration of the secretions is allowed; and speaking, sometimes drinking and eating is possible. One important logistic advantage is that some types of NIV can be applied also in the ward; but only with a very dedicated and experienced team, and adequate monitoring.

NIV is also considered as a weaning tool: the recent European Respiratory Society (ERS)/American Thoracic Society guidelines suggest that NIV:[98]

- Should be used to facilitate weaning from MV in patients with hypercapnic acute respiratory failure (ARF) only in centers with adequate experience.
- Should not be used in the treatment of patients with established postextubation ARF (should be reconsidered, especially in patients after thoracic surgery).
- Should be used to prevent postextubation ARF in high-risk patients but not used to prevent postextubation ARF in nonhigh-risk patients.

NIV has also some limitations: as a prerequisite the patient should be cooperable able to protect the airway and has a pH greater than 7.1 and arterial carbon dioxide partial pressure (PaCO2) less than 90 mm Hg. The contraindications are shown in Table 26.2.[99] Adaptation problems are always a challenge (increased in older patients). Beside several unwarranted effects (like claustrophobia), a relatively new unwarranted finding with NIV is that it can worsen lung injury leading to so-called patient self-inflicted lung injury (P-SILI).[100] As a general rule, if no improvement in oxygenation is observed after 15 to 30 minutes after NIV initiation, invasive mechanical ventilation should be considered.

Several interfaces for the application of NIV are available, such as nose masks, oronasal masks, full-face masks, and helmets (Fig. 26.9). Inappropriate usage can cause skin lesions. Moreover, in all these devices, a leak of the inspired volume is almost inevitable, even if the device fits well. However, many ventilators can compensate for this leakage by increasing the inspiratory flow.

High-Flow Nasal Cannula Oxygen Therapy

High-flow nasal cannula oxygen therapy (HFNCOT) is a new promising technique to improve lung function and possibly also patient outcome, not only in the post-, but also in pre- and intraoperative period,[101] whereby a humidified and heated mixture of air and oxygen with a F_iO2 between 0.21 and 1.0 is delivered at a flow of up to 80 L/min.[102]

HFNCOT is a relative new technique; the majority of the studies have shown its advantages and benefits compared with NIV; that means: NIV has been implemented as an alternative to mechanical ventilation (same benefits, lower risks); now HFNCOT appears to be an alternative to NIV and also to mechanical ventilation.

HFNCOT offers similar benefits as NIV: improved oxygenation, reduction of dyspnea, work of breathing, and

1. Appropriately monitored location; oximetry, vital signs as clinically indicated
2. Patient in bed sitting at > 30 degree angle
3. Select and fit interface
4. Check initial settings in the ventilator before connecting to the mask of the patient:
- *Ventilatory mode: PSV*
- *Inspiratory trigger: -1 to -2 L/min or -1 to -2 cm H_2O (i.e, lowest level without induced auto-triggering)*
- *Slope delivered pressure: moderate to maximal*
- *Initial PSV level: 3 to 5 cm H_2O*
- *Expiratory trigger (expiratory cycling setting if available): flow: 40 to 60% or time cycled: fixed inspiratory time between 0.8 to 1.2 second.*
- *Initial PEEP level: 3 to 5 cm H_2O*
- *Initial Fi_{O2}: 50-60%*

5. After briefly explaining the NIV method to the patient, apply headgear; avoid excessive strap tension (one or two fingers under strap); encourage patient to hold mask. Propose to the patient to breathe through the mask for few seconds without connect to ventilator
6. Connect interface to ventilator tubing and turn on ventilator
7. Start with low pressures (as set previously) and gradually increase PSV (usually 5 to 15 cm H_2O) and PEEP (5 to 10 cm H_2O) as tolerated without major leaks to achieve alleviation of dyspnea, decreased respiratory rate, increased **expiratory** tidal volume (to achieve 6- to 10 ml/kg) and good patient-ventilator synchrony. Never exceed total inspiratory pressure (PSV+PEEP) more than 25 cm H_2O (ideally < 20 cm H_2O)
8. Set Fi_{O2} to keep $Sp_{O2} \geq 95\%$ (for COPD patients keep $SpO2 \geq 90\%$)
9. Check for air leaks, readjust straps as needed or decreased pressure levels if major leaks
10. Add humidifier as indicated (heated humidifier or heated and moisture exchanger with low internal volume to avoid excess dead space)
11. Encouragement, reassurance, and frequent checks and adjustments as needed
12. Monitor blood gases (within 1 to 2 h and then as needed)
13. Duration: initial period for 60 to 90 min at 2-to 3-h intervals (range, 6 to12 hours per day)

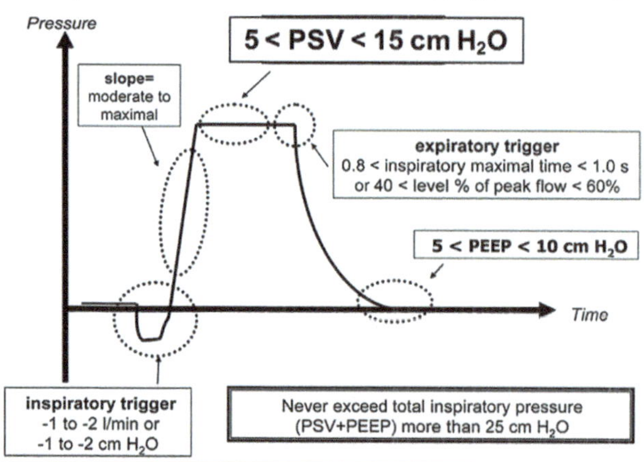

• **Fig. 26.8** A possible protocol for postoperative noninvasive ventilation (NIV). *COPD*, Chronic obstructive pulmonary disease; *F_iO2*, fraction of inspired oxygen; *PEEP*, positive end-expiratory pressure; *PSV*, pressure support ventilation; *SpO2*, pulsated oximetry. (With kind permission of Prof S Jaber; Jaber S, De Jong A, Castagnoli A, Futier E, Chanques G. Noninvasive ventilation after surgery. *Ann Fr Anesth Reanim*. 2014;33:487–491.)

TABLE 26.2 The Contraindications of Noninvasive Ventilation

Central Nervous System
- Decreased level of consciousness
- Severe agitation or encephalopathy
- Inability to cooperate
- Inability to protect airway

Cardiorespiratory
- Cardiac or respiratory arrest
- Hemodynamic instability or unstable cardiac arrhythmia
- Severe respiratory failure
- Copious secretions or hemoptysis

Gastrointestinal (GI)
- Vomiting/gastric distension: high risk of aspiration
- Upper GI bleeding

Other
- Facial trauma or other condition preventing facemask application
- Multiple organ failure

(Modified from Jaber S, Chanques G, Jung B. Postoperative noninvasive ventilation. *Anesthesiology* 2010;112:453–461.)

respiratory rate[103] (Fig. 26.10). Moreover, there are some further advantages, mostly as a result of high flow:[101]

- High flow creates a PEEP up to 5 cm H_2O—especially when the mouth is kept closed.[104]
- The flush decreases anatomic dead space and so leads to washout of CO2.[105] The CO2 clearance seems to be flow-dependent.
- The method offers a heated and humidified gas, and so helps to maintain mucociliary function.
- The device is well-tolerated by the patients compared with NIV, helping to overcome the limitations of eating, drinking, and communicating. Fortunately, the higher flow, the better the tolerance to the device, and therefore the more successful the therapy.
- Contrary to NIV, there is no risk of so-called P-SILI,[100] an advantage that is especially important in patients after thoracic surgery in whom avoiding high transpulmonary pressures have an important role to reduce ARF.

As a relatively new method, there is for now almost no evidence-based suggestion regarding the setting (i.e., F_iO2,

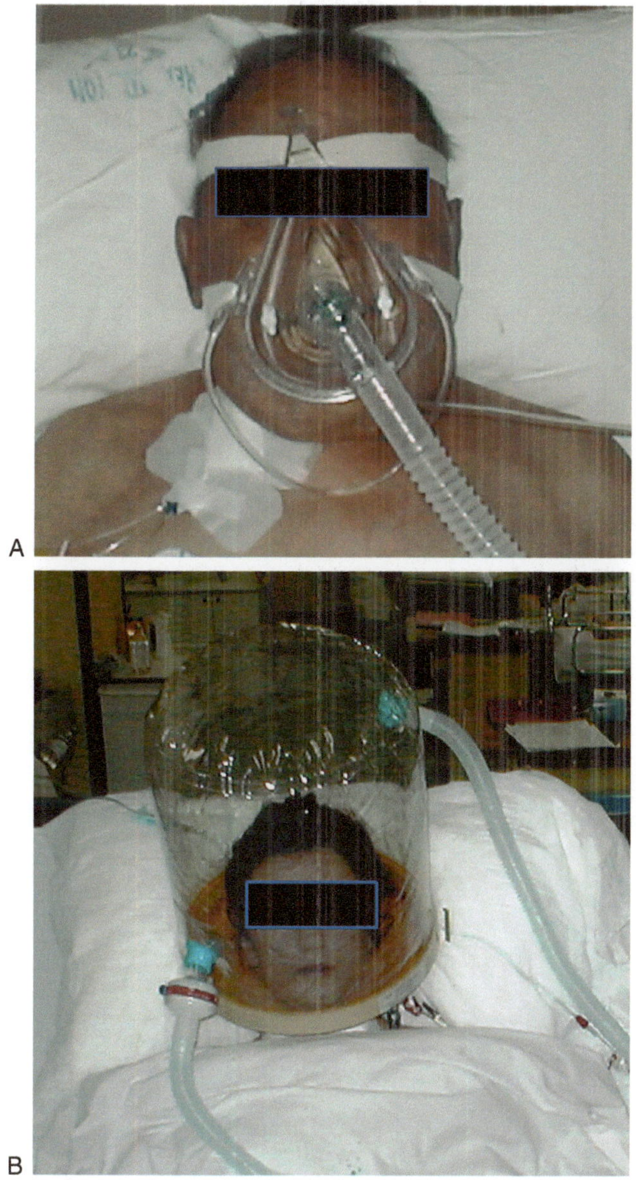

• **Fig. 26.9** Interfaces for the application of noninvasive ventilation: (**A**) Oronasal mask; (**B**) Helmet.

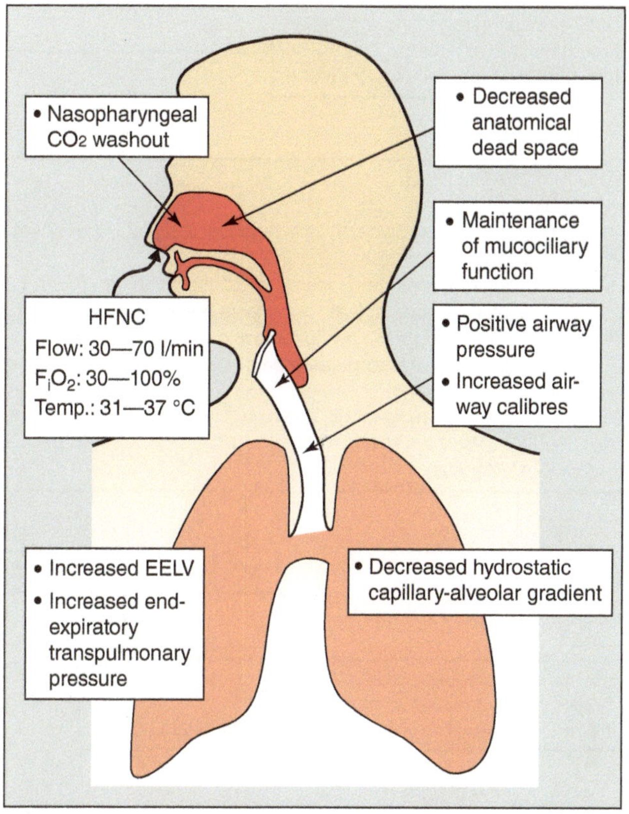

• **Fig. 26.10** Application information and benefits of high-flow nasal cannula (*HFNC*) oxygen therapy. *EELV*, End-expiratory lung volume; *F_iO2*, inspiratory oxygen fraction; *Temp.*; temperature. (With kind permission of the authors Wittenstein J, Ball L, Pelosi P, Gama De Abreu M. High-flow nasal cannula oxygen therapy in patients undergoing thoracic surgery: current evidence and practice. *Curr Opin Anesthesiol.* 2019;32:44–49.)

flow, temperature) and duration of the treatment. A general approach is to start with the highest flow tolerated by the patient, and the F_iO2 to maintain a rational SpO2; and then decrease both of them, as the status of the patient, until weaning the patient from the therapy.

Similar to NIV, if there is no improvement of oxygenation, and decrease in the respiratory rate within 20 to 60 minutes after start of HFNCOT, the risk of failure is high.

Weaning

Weaning from mechanical ventilation is one of the most important challenges: the longer the mechanical ventilation, the worse the prognosis. In the specific group of patients after thoracic surgery, the challenge is even more significant. An unsuccessful weaning can be also caused by the extension of the resection of the pulmonary tissue itself. Weaning should begin at the start of the mechanical ventilation, and it should be performed as fast as possible with careful monitoring of the patient respiratory parameters.

Different guidelines and consensus reports have been published by different groups, importantly by the National Association for Medical Direction of Respiratory Care[106] and by the ERS Task Force;[107] a more recent definition (Weaning according to New Definition)[108] has suggested a new approach. The fact that a new definitions are required even after 10 to 12 years of the former guidelines, shows that the problem of weaning has not been solved adequately. Moreover, it should be underlined that in the years when the former guidelines[106,107] were published, NIV was just a promising newcomer, and HFNCOT did even not exist.

One of the key points of successful weaning is to follow a certain protocol.[109] There should be protocols defining (Fig. 26.11):

- Patients in whom weaning can be tried
- Methods and strategies of weaning
- The success of weaning

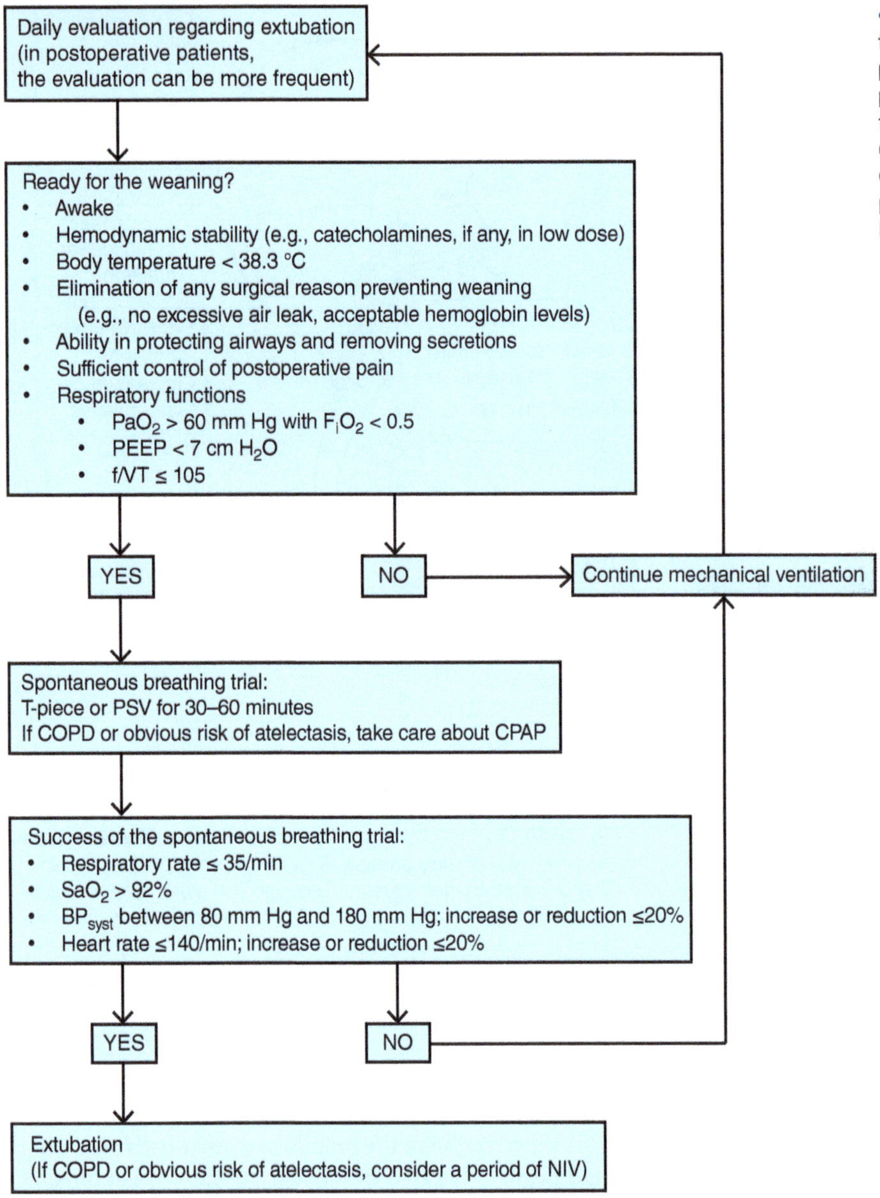

• **Fig. 26.11** A weaning-protocol for delayed extubation of postoperative (incl. postthoracotomy) patients of Istanbul Medical Faculty. Note that protocols can differ between centers, but a certain basic protocol should exist and be followed. *COPD,* Chronic obstructive pulmonary disease; *CPAP,* continuous positive airway pressure; *PEEP,* positive end-expiratory pressure. (Source: The Istanbul Medical Faculty.)

There are some important general practical recommendations:

- In every ventilated patient (>24 hours), daily spontaneous breathing trials (SBTs) should be performed. First, this trial would identify patients who are ready for weaning (without such daily trials, more than half of the patients would not be recognized).[106] Second, if a patient could not pass the trial, physicians would be motivated to find the underlying reason(s) for the failure, which leads back to the protocol of consideration for weaning. The very first attempt of weaning should be considered as the milestone of the process.[110]
- Weaning modalities can differ among centers and patients. Obviously, the weaning of a COPD patient is harder and different than weaning a postoperative patient (failure rate up to 80% vs. approximately 5%). There must be a protocol to rationalize and standardize the applications during the weaning process. A stepdown from controlled to supported ventilation or from invasive to NIV are considered components of weaning. Similarly, T-piece trials can also be performed. There is no ideal SBT.[109] Applying all of these possible methods in a documented algorithm can prevent unpredicted drawbacks (e.g., oversedation) during a trial.[111]
- In every patient, the success of the weaning should also be evaluated following a protocol. An example is shown in Table 26.3.

Electronic data recording systems are being used more frequently in the ICUs. These systems can be helpful to apply the center-specific weaning protocols in a more appropriate way. Algorithms consisting all the parameters in the weaning process—possibly with different factors for each parameter—can automatically calculate a weaning factor, that informs the clinician whether the patient is above the threshold for weaning or SBT; or whether there is a decline

TABLE 26.3 Criteria of a Successful Weaning

- Oxygenation
  ($PaO2 \geq 60$ mm Hg or $SaO2 \geq 90\%$ with $F_iO2 \leq 0.40$ or $PaO2/F_iO2 > 200$ with PEEP ≤ 5 cm H_2O)
- Ventilation
  (increase in PaCO2 ≥ 10 mm Hg or reduction of pH ≥ 0.10)
- Arterial pressure
  (systolic arterial pressure ≥ 90 mm Hg or ≤ 180 mm Hg; increase or reduction $\leq 20\%$)
- Cardiac frequency
  (≥ 50 or ≤ 140 beats per minute; increase or reduction $\leq 20\%$)
- Respiratory rate
  (≥ 35 breaths/min)
- No signs of excessive work of breathing
  (no paradoxical breathing and/or exaggerated use of accessory muscles)
- No agitation, exaggerated depression or manifest distress

F_iO2, Inspiratory oxygen fraction; *PaCO2*, arterial carbon dioxide partial pressure; *PaO2*, arterial oxygen partial pressure; *PEEP*, positive end-expiratory pressure; *SaO2*, oxygen saturation.

in the score compared with the previous calculation. An example is shown in Fig. 26.12A and B.

Current strategies used to achieve successful weaning are:[111]

- Pressure support ventilation (PSV) with decreasing (<8 cm H_2O) support.
- Progressive longer periods of SBT through the tube (the authors prefer a fixed period of 30 minutes)
- Synchronized intermittent mandatory ventilation
- Neurally adjusted ventilatory assist
- Noninvasive ventilation (NIV)
- HFO (for NIV and HFO, see also earlier)

Weaning should be considered as a process both covering the whole period of mechanical ventilation, and other associated tools:

- **Tracheostomy:** prolonged mechanical ventilation (>7 days) with unsuccessful weaning trials is associated with additional problems. In these cases, a tracheostomy should be considered. Even in cases in which prolonged mechanical ventilation is predicted during the early period of mechanical ventilation, an earlier tracheostomy can be rational, which can reduce the need for sedation and ease the mobilization of the patient and facilitate removal of the secretions, which is even more important in the subgroup of patients after thoracic surgery. Prophylactic application of a mini tracheostomy can facilitate sputum clearance, however as an invasive approach, its use should be—probably—limited to high-risk patients.[2]
- **Early mobilization and physiotherapy:** there is a strong evidence (but there are still also controversial studies) of benefits of early mobilization and physiotherapy;[112] helping to decrease the risks of PPCs and venous thromboembolism. It is recommended that following thoracic operations (even after less invasive VATS)[113] all patients should receive routine postoperative physiotherapy assessment, to be started as soon as possible. Physiotherapeutic approaches should include active and passive muscle training as well as cough augmentation techniques, such as percussive ventilation.
- **Sedation:** a titrated (or tailored) sedation is crucial, not only during the weaning process. Usually, sedation is considered as a component of sedo-analgesia. Drugs that can lead to respiratory depression and other complications, such as opioids, should be avoided. Being opioid-free can be an appropriate target, but the price may not be an agitated and painful patient. Dexmedetomidine or small doses of propofol, appear to be good choices for sedation in this group of patients, helping also for analgesia without adhering the ventilatory drive.[114]

Ventilator-Associated Pneumonia (VAP) and Its Prevention

VAP is one of the most common and most serious complications in patients after thoracic surgery during prolonged mechanical ventilation. In this chapter, we will focus rather on definition (to assure the awareness of VAP), and the prevention of VAP than its treatment.

Unfortunately, there are different definitions, different suggestions for diagnosis, prevention, and treatment for VAP. In general, it is defined as pneumonia developing more than 48 hours after initiating mechanical ventilation with absence before intubation,[115] whereby we have to differentiate between ventilator-associated tracheobronchitis (VAT), infection-related ventilator-associated complications (IVAC), ventilator-associated events (VAE) and possible others.

There are host-related and intervention-related risk factors of VAP: First thoracic surgery is per se one of the host-related risk factors; moreover medical history and underlying illness, male gender, extreme age, immunocompromised patient, and ARDS are some of the host-related factors which are also seen in thoracic surgery patients. In addition, almost all intervention-related risk factors can be found also in thoracic surgery (such as perioperative transfusion of blood products, enteral nutrition, inappropriate antibiotic therapy, etc.).[116] Because only the intervention-related risk factors are accessible to prevention,

1. clinicians have to be aware of these interventions to prevent VAP
2. prevention of VAP is harder to prevent than other nosocomial infections.

Different bundles have been recommended to prevent VAP. Although there is a lack of evidence to support some of them, many can be considered as appropriate

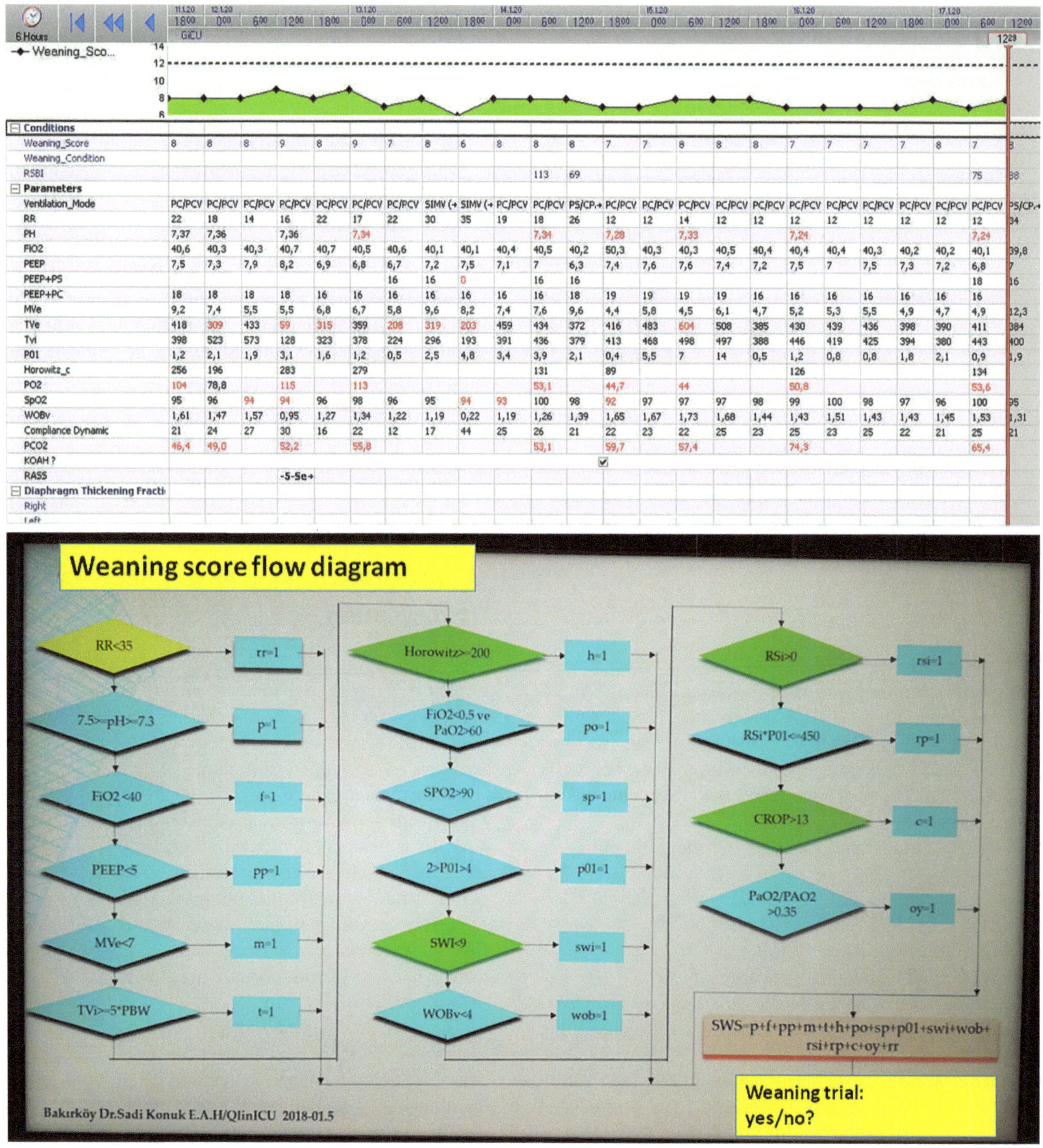

• **Fig. 26.12** Electronic data recording systems can be helpful to alert on weaning process. Additional data on the recorded variables show the weaning score (**A**); the weaning score can be determined with different factors of the parameters (**B**). (With kind permission from Prof Zafer Çukurova.)

recommendations; using the initials of VAP can be helpful to memorize (Fig. 26.13).[117] It should be noted that avoidance of intubation is a general rule with a strong evidence level that is also valid to prevent ventilation-induced/associated lung injury. However, some suggestions can be associated with some compromises, even contradictions:

- Oral rinse 0.2% chlorhexidine is a general suggestion that reduces the occurrence of VAP,[118] but selective oral or digestive decontamination is not preferred in some centers as they can cause/exacerbate antibiotic resistance;
- Early enteral nutrition is generally associated with decreased mortality and also a part of ERAS protocols;[2] but considered as a risk factor for VAP.[119]

Regarding the diagnostic procedure in suspicion of VAP, there are differences in European and U.S. guidelines, different definitions (VAC, VAT, IVAC, etc.) make it even

V | **Ventilation: risk reduction**
Avoid intubation if possible (NIV, etc.)
Minimize sedation (sedation breaks, etc.)
Physical conditioning (exercise and mobilization)

A | **Accompanying measures**
Education
Measuring performance,
Improvement in "overall safety culture"
Public reporting

P | **Preventive measures**
Do not change the ventilator circuit unless soiled or malfunctioning
SOD: selective oral/digestive decontamination
Endotracheal tube with subglottic drainage of secretions
Chlorhexidine
Prophylactic probiotics
Head elevation

• **Fig. 26.13** Preventive measures of ventilator-associated pneumonia. (Modified from Timsit JF, Esaied W, Neuville M, Bouadma L, Morvillier B. Update on ventilator-associated pneumonia [version 1; peer review: 2 approved]. *F1000Research* 2017; 6(F1000 Faculty Rev):2061.)

more complicated. Obviously, the presence of clinical signs and symptoms, such as leukocytosis/leucopenia, fever/hypothermia, changes in color or amount of secretion, new infiltration in CXR, and impairment in oxygenation requiring an increase in F_iO2 and/or PEEP in mechanically ventilated patients more than 48 hours should make the clinician suspicious of VAP. Invasive techniques, such as bronchoalveolar lavage or protected specimen brush with quantitative culture, require qualified clinicians. U.S. guidelines recommend noninvasive sampling with semi-quantitative culture,[120] whereas the European guidelines suggest obtaining distal samples with quantitative cultures to improve the accuracy of results.[121] No matter which approach is followed, both guidelines agreed that a bacteriologic sample should be performed before any antibiotic treatment to reduce antibiotic exposure.

Initial empiric antibiotic treatment, which may be an inappropriate initial choice, is associated with increased mortality. Even if it is based on empirical choices, an inappropriate antibiotic treatment can lead to multi-drug resistant bacteria, which is clearly associated with an increased risk of inappropriate therapy of VAP. In accordance with recent North American guidelines, authors prefer to start an empiric treatment with piperacillin-tazobactam 4.5 g IV/6 hours or levofloxacin 750 mg IV daily. If there is an increased likelihood of Gram-negative and/or Gram-positive bacteria, meropenem 1 g IV/8 hours and/or linezolid 600 mg IV/12 hours, respectively, are added.

Extracorporeal Ventilatory Support

Does extracorporeal ventilatory support have a place in postoperative care after thoracic surgery? Yes, for few patients, such as:

A

B

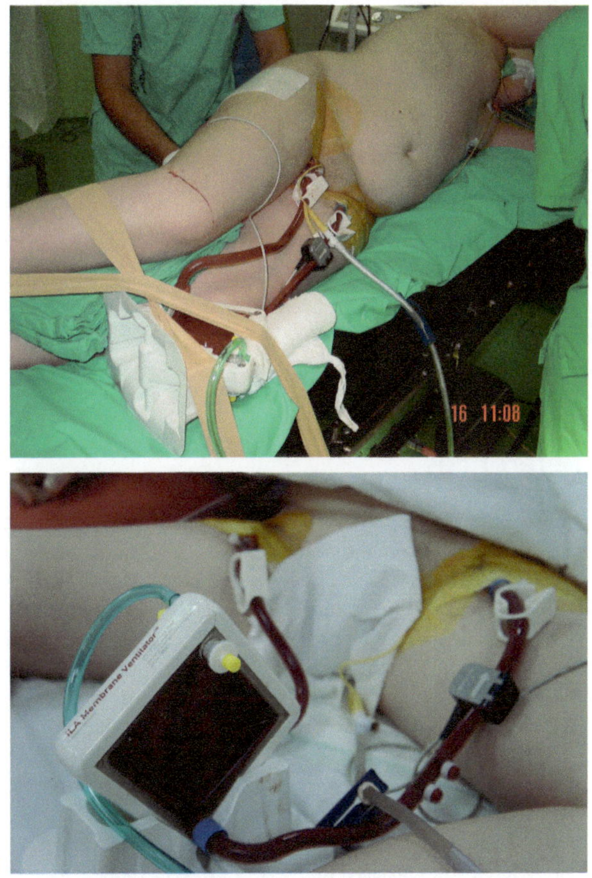

• **Fig. 26.14** Use of Novalung ® ('Interventional Lung Assist') in the intraoperative (**A**) and postoperative (**B**) period.

1. Even if the protective ventilation is the main approach, in some very seriously ill patients (e.g., with a very limited compliance), the ventilatory settings cannot be protective enough: high ventilatory pressures can be necessary even for a low V_T.
2. Following an unusually large parenchymal resection of the lung, the remaining tissue could temporarily be insufficient for an adequate oxygenation during the acute period after surgery. Allowing the lung to rest until it heals is a rational approach.

To create a safe zone between the hazardous effects of high positive pressure of the mechanical ventilation and insufficient oxygenation and gas exchange, extracorporeal lung support can be applied. As the newer technologies are less complicated and provide less invasive devices that require less or no anticoagulant, experienced teams more likely prefer to use this form of support.

It can serve as a bridge to recovery' or also a bridge to transplantation.[122] The author's experience is with a child who has a previous right pneumonectomy, and had to be reoperated because of the metastases in the left mediastinum. The interventional lung assist was initiated before the operation and continued for 24 hours after the operation, and the device was removed 18 hours after the extubation (Fig. 26.14A and B).

Conclusion

Challenges for the postoperative care following thoracic surgery change their guidelines based on scientific and technologic developments. Invasive mechanical ventilation should be avoided when possible to prevent both ventilation induced/associated lung injury and VAP. Methods like NIV, HFO treatment, and even extracorporeal support are expected to decrease the requirement for classical invasive mechanical ventilation. New monitoring devices can help to follow-up on important parameters via a less invasive way; monitoring of RV function, which was previously complicated to monitor and was underestimated, is now clinically more feasible. Among the future aspects, are:

- A shorter mechanical ventilation period
- More reliable, but less invasive monitoring
- A protocol of optimal (for all organs) fluid management
- Easier and less complicated weaning protocols

ERATS protocols are in place and their philosophy outlines the way to the pragmatic target: enhanced outcome; more scientific evidence will help us to achieve more reliable suggestions to reach this target.

References

1. Fernandez FG, Kosinski AS, Furnary AP, et al. Differential effects of operative complications on survival after surgery for primary lung cancer. *J Thorac Cardiovasc Surg.* 2018;155:1254–1264.
2. Batchelor TJP, Rasburn NJ, Abdelnour-Berchtold E, et al. Guidelines for enhanced recovery after lung surgery: recommendations of the Enhanced Recovery After Surgery (ERAS (R)) Society and the European Society of Thoracic Surgeons (ESTS). *Eur J Cardiothorac Surg.* 2019;55:91–115.
3. Giménez-Milà M, Klein AA, Martinez G. Design and Implementation of an Enhanced Recovery Program in Thoracic Surgery. *J Thorac Dis.* 2016;8(Suppl 1):S37–S45.
4. Hubert J, Bourdages-Pageau E, Paradis Garneau CA, Labbé C, Ugalde PA. Enhanced Recovery Pathways in Thoracic Surgery: The Quebec Experience. *J Thorac Dis.* 2018;10(Suppl 4):S583–S590.
5. Eustache J, Ferri LE, Feldman LS, Lee L, Spicer JD. Enhanced recovery after pulmonary surgery. *J Thorac Dis.* 2018;10(Suppl 32): S3755–S3760.
6. Brunelli A, Pieretti P, Al Refai M, et al. Elective intensive care after lung resection: a multicentric propensity-matched comparison of outcome. *Interact Cardiovasc Thorac Surg.* 2005;4:609–613.
7. Lee SE, Cho WH, Lee SK, et al. Routine intensive monitoring but not routine intensive care unit-based management is necessary in video-assisted thoracoscopic surgery lobectomy for lung cancer. *Ann Transl Med.* 2019;7(7):129.
8. Shelley BG, McCall PJ, Glass A, Orzechowska I, Klein AA. Association of Cardiothoracic Anaesthesia and collaborators. Association between anaesthetic technique and unplanned admission to intensive care after thoracic lung resection surgery: The Second Association of Cardiothoracic Anaesthesia and Critical Care (ACTACC) National Audit. *Anaesthesia.* 2019;74: 1121–1129.
9. Damhuis RA, Schütte PR. Resection rates and postoperative mortality in 7,899 patients with lung cancer. *Eur Respir J.* 1996;9:7–10.
10. Jordan S, Evans TW. Predicting the need for intensive care following lung resection. *Thorac Surg Clin.* 2008;18:61–69.
11. Bryant AS, Cerfolio RJ. The influence of preoperative risk stratification on fast tracking patients after pulmonary resection. *Thorac Surg Clin.* 2009;18:113–118.
12. Sanchez-Lorente D, Navarro-Ripoll R, Guzman R, et al. Prehabilitation in thoracic surgery. *J Thorac Dis.* 2018;10(Suppl 22): S2593–S2600.
13. Brunelli A, Varela G, Refai M, et al. A scoring system to predict the risk of prolonged air leak after lobectomy. *Ann Thorac Surg.* 2010;90:204–209.
14. Kreienbühler L, Cassina T, Licker M. Where should I send my patient after the operation? In: Şentürk M, Sungur MO, eds. *Postoperative Care in Thoracic Surgery.* 1st ed.: Springer International Publishing: Switzerland; 2017:13–28.
15. ARISCAT GroupCanet J, Gallart L, Gomar C, et al. Prediction of postoperative pulmonary complications in a population-based surgical cohort. *Anesthesiology.* 2010;113:1338–1350.
16. PERISCOPE Group; Canet J, Sabate S, Mazo V, et al. Development and validation of a score to predict postoperative respiratory failure in a multicentre European cohort: a prospective, observational study. *Eur J Anaesthesiol.* 2015;32:458–470.
17. Cerfolio RJ, Bryant AS. The management of chest tubes after pulmonary resection. *Thorac Surg Clin.* 2010;20:399–405.
18. French DG, Dilena M, LaPlante S, et al. Optimizing postoperative care protocols in thoracic surgery: best evidence and new technology. *J Thorac Dis.* 2016;8(Suppl 1):S3–S11.
19. Cerfolio RJ, Bryant AS. Results of a prospective algorithm to remove chest tubes after pulmonary resection with high output. *J Thorac Cardiovasc Surg.* 2008;135:269–273.
20. Bjerregaard LS, Jensen K, Petersen RH, Hansen HJ. Early chest tube removal after video-assisted thoracic surgery lobectomy with serous fluid production up to 500 mL/day. *Eur J Cardiothorac Surg.* 2014;45:241–246.
21. Cerfolio RJ, Bryant AS, Skylizard L, Minnich DJ. Optimal technique for the removal of chest tubes after pulmonary resection. *J Thorac Cardiovasc Surg.* 2013;145:1535–1539.
22. Wang H, Hu W, Ma L, Zhang Y. Digital chest drainage system versus traditional chest drainage system after pulmonary resection: a systematic review and meta-analysis. *J Cardiothorac Surg.* 2019;14:13.
23. Assaad S, Kratzert WB, Perrino AC. Extravascular lung water monitoring for thoracic and lung transplant surgeries. *Curr Opin Anesthesiol.* 2019;32:29–38.
24. Chiappetta M, Meacci E, Cesario A, et al. Postoperative chest ultrasound findings and effectiveness after thoracic surgery: a pilot study. *Ultrasound Med Biol.* 2018;44:1960–1967.
25. Lichtenstein DA. BLUE-protocol and FALLS-protocol: two applications of lung ultrasound in the critically ill. *Chest.* 2015; 147:1659–1670.
26. Lichtenstein DA. Lung ultrasound in the critically ill. *Ann Intensive Care.* 2014;4:1.
27. Picano E, Pellikka PA. Ultrasound of extravascular lung water: a new standard for pulmonary congestion. *Eur Heart J.* 2016; 37:2097–2104.
28. Assaad S, Kratzert WB, Shelley B, et al. Assessment of pulmonary edema: principles and practice. *J Cardiothorac Vasc Anesth.* 2018;32:901–914.

29. McCall P, Soosay A, Kinsella J, et al. The utility of transthoracic echocardiographic measures of right ventricular systolic function in a lung resection cohort. *Echo Res Pract.* 2019;6:7–15.
30. Fratacci MD, Kimball WR, Wain JC, Kacmarek RM, Polaner DM, Zapol WM. Diaphragmatic shortening after thoracic surgery in humans. Effects of mechanical ventilation and thoracic epidural anesthesia. *Anesthesiology.* 1993;79:654–665.
31. Sasaki N, Meyer MJ, Eikermann M. Postoperative respiratory muscle dysfunction: pathophysiology and preventive strategies. *Anesthesiology.* 2013;118:961–978.
32. Spadaro S, Grasso S, Dres M, et al. Point of care ultrasound to identify diaphragmatic dysfunction after thoracic surgery. *Anesthesiology.* 2019;131:266–278.
33. Nishimura A, Tabuchi Y, Kikuchi M, Masudo R, Goto K, Iijima T. The amount of fluid given during surgery that leaks into the interstitium correlates with infused fluid volume and varies widely between patients. *Anesth Analg.* 2016;123:925–932.
34. Della Rocca G, Vertrugno L. what is the goal of fluid management "optimization"? *Turk J Anaesthesiol Reanim.* 2016;44:224–226.
35. Licker M, Triponez F, Ellenberger C, Karenovics W. Fluid therapy in thoracic surgery: a zero-balance target is always best! *Turk J Anaesthesiol Reanim.* 2016;44:227–229.
36. Ahn HJ, Kim JA, Lee AR, Yang M, Jung HJ, Heo B. The risk of acute kidney injury from fluid restriction and hydroxyethyl starch in thoracic surgery. *Anesth Analg.* 2016;122:186–193.
37. Sentürk M, Sungur MO, Sungur Z. Fluid management in thoracic anesthesia. *Minerva Anestesiol.* 2017;83:652–659.
38. Lohser J, Slinger P. Lung injury after one-lung ventilation: a review of the pathophysiologic mechanisms affecting the ventilated and the collapsed lung. *Anesth Analg.* 2015;121:302–318.
39. Slinger PD. Postpneumonectomy pulmonary edema: good news, bad news. *Anesthesiology.* 2006;105:2–5.
40. Slinger PD. Perioperative fluid management for thoracic surgery: the puzzle of postpneumonectomy pulmonary edema. *J Cardiothorac Vasc Anesth.* 1995;9:442–451.
41. Chappell D, Jacob M, Hofmann-Kiefer K, Conzen P, Rehm M. A rational approach to perioperative fluid management. *Anesthesiology.* 2008;109:723–740.
42. Assaad S, Shelley B, Perrino A. Transpulmonary thermodilution: its role in assessment of lung water and pulmonary edema. *J Cardiothorac Vasc Anesth.* 2017;31:1471–1480.
43. Monnet X, Anguel N, Osman D, Hamzaoui O, Richard C, Teboul JL. Assessing pulmonary permeability by transpulmonary thermodilution allows differentiation of hydrostatic pulmonary edema from ALI/ARDS. *Intensive Care Med.* 2007;33:448–453.
44. Lee JH, Jeon Y, Bahk JH, et al. Pulse pressure variation as a predictor of fluid responsiveness during one-lung ventilation for lung surgery using thoracotomy: randomised controlled study. *Eur J Anaesthesiol.* 2011;28(1):39–44.
45. Loupec T, Nanadoumgar H, Frasca D, et al. Pleth variability index predicts fluid responsiveness in critically ill patients. *Crit Care Med.* 2011;39:294–299.
46. Jeong DM, Ahn HJ, Park HW, Yang M, Kim JA, Park J. Stroke volume variation and pulse pressure variation are not useful for predicting fluid responsiveness in thoracic surgery. *Anesth Analg.* 2017;125:1158–1165.
47. Naidu BV, Dronavalli VB, Rajesh PB. Measuring lung water following major lung resection. *Interact Cardiovasc Thorac Surg.* 2009;8:503–506.
48. Sakka SG, Klein M, Reinhart K, Meier-Hellmann A. Prognostic value of extravascular lung water in critically ill patients. *Chest.* 2002;122:2080–2086.
49. Assaad S, Popescu W, Perrino A. Fluid management in thoracic surgery. *Curr Opin Anaesthesiol.* 2013;26:31–39.
50. Lewis J, Bastanfar M, Gabriel F, Mascha E. Right heart function and prediction of respiratory morbidity in patients undergoing pneumonectomy with moderately severe cardiopulmonary dysfunction. *J Thorac Cardiovasc Surg.* 1994;108:169–175.
51. Gelzinis T, Assaad S, Perrino Jr AC. Right ventricular function during and after thoracic surgery. *Curr Opin Anesthesiol.* 2020;33:27–36.
52. Elrakhawy H, Alassal M, Shaalan A, et al. Impact of major pulmonary resections on right ventricular function: early postoperative changes. *Heart Surg Forum.* 2018;21:E009–E017.
53. McCall P, Arthur A, Glass A, et al. The right ventricular response to lung resection. *J Thorac Cardiovasc Surg.* 2019;158:556–565, e5.
54. Licker M, Fauconnet P, Villigr Y, Tschopp JM. Acute lung injury and outcomes after thoracic surgery. *Curr Opin Anaesthesiol.* 2009;22:61–67.
55. Sentürk M. New concepts of the management of one-lung ventilation. *Curr Opin Anaesthesiol.* 2006;19:1–4.
56. Padley SPG, Jordan SJ, Goldstraw P, Wells AU, Hansell DM. Asymmetric ARDS following pulmonary resection: CT findings initial observations. *Radiology.* 2002;223:468–473.
57. Verbrugge SJ, Lachmann B, Kesecioglu J. Lung protective ventilatory strategies in acute lung injury and acute respiratory distress syndrome: from experimental findings to clinical application. *Clin Physiol Funct Imaging.* 2007;27:67–90.
58. Kozian A, Schilling T, Schütze H, Senturk M, Hachenberg T, Hedenstierna G. Ventilatory protective strategies during thoracic surgery: effects of alveolar recruitment maneuver and low-tidal volume ventilation on lung density distribution. *Anesthesiology.* 2011;114:1025–1035.
59. Eichenbaum KD, Neustein SM. Acute lung injury after thoracic surgery. *J Cardiothorac Vasc Anesth.* 2010;24:681–690.
60. Kavanagh BP, Laffey JG. Hypercapnia: permissive and therapeutic. *Minerva Anestesiol.* 2006;72:567–576.
61. Allegranzi B, Zayed B, Bischoff P, et al. The WHO Guidelines Development Group. New WHO recommendations on intraoperative and postoperative measures for surgical site infection prevention: an evidence-based global perspective. *Lancet Infect Dis.* 2016;16:e288–e303.
62. Belda FJ, Aguilera L, García de la Asunción J, et al. Spanish Reduccion de la Tasa de Infeccion Quirurgica Group. Supplemental perioperative oxygen and the risk of surgical wound infection: a randomized controlled trial. *JAMA.* 2005;294:2035–2042.
63. Outcomes Research GroupGreif R, Akça O, Horn EP, Kurz A, Sessler DI. Supplemental perioperative oxygen to reduce the incidence of surgical-wound infection. *N Engl J Med.* 2000;342:161–167.
64. Meyhoff CS, Wetterslev J, Jorgensen LN, et al. Effect of high perioperative oxygen fraction on surgical site infection and pulmonary complications after abdominal surgery: the PROXI randomized clinical trial. *JAMA.* 2009;302:1543–1550.
65. Akca A, Ball L, Belda FJ, et al. Who needs high FIO2? *Turk J Anaesthesiol Reanim.* 2017;45:181–192.
66. Cornet AD, Kooter AJ, Peters MJL, Smulders YM. Supplemental oxygen therapy in medical emergencies: more harm than benefit? *Arch Intern Med.* 2012;172:289–290.
67. Tuğrul M, Camci E, Karadeniz H, Sentürk M, Pembeci K, Akpir K. Comparison of volume controlled with pressure controlled ventilation during one-lung anaesthesia. *Br J Anaesth.* 1997;79:306–310.

68. Unzueta MC, Casas JI, Moral MV. Pressure-controlled versus volume-controlled ventilation during one-lung ventilation for thoracic surgery. *Anesth Analg.* 2007;104(5):1029–1033.
69. Al Shehri A, El-Tahan M, et al. Right ventricular function during one-lung ventilation: effects of pressure-controlled and volume-controlled ventilation. *J Cardiothorac Vasc Anesth.* 2014;28: 880–884.
70. Simonis FD, Barbas CSV, Artigas-Raventos A, Canet J, et al. PRoVENT investigators, PROVE Network investigators. Potentially modifiable respiratory variables contributing to outcome in ICU patients without ARDS: a secondary analysis of PRoVENT. *Ann Intensive Care.* 2018;8:39.
71. Amato MB, Meade MO, Slutsky AS, et al. Driving pressure and survival in the acute respiratory distress syndrome. *N Engl J Med.* 2015;372:747–755.
72. Toufen Junior C, De Santis Santiago RR, Hirota AS, et al. Driving pressure and long-term outcomes in moderate/severe acute respiratory distress syndrome. *Ann Intensive Care.* 2018;8:119.
73. Neto AS, Hemmes SN, Barbas CS, et al. PROVE Network Investigators: Association between driving pressure and development of postoperative pulmonary complications in patients undergoing mechanical ventilation for general anaesthesia: a meta-analysis of individual patient data. *Lancet Respir Med.* 2016;4: 272–280.
74. Park M, Ahn HJ, Kim JA, et al. Driving pressure during thoracic surgery: a randomized clinical trial. *Anesthesioloogy.* 2019; 130:385–393.
75. Tonetti T, Vasques F, Rapetti F, et al. Driving pressure and mechanical power: new targets for VILI prevention. *Ann Transl Med.* 2017;5:286.
76. Serpa Neto A, Deliberato RO, Johnson AE, et al. PROVE Network Investigators. Normalization of mechanical power to anthropometric indices: impact on its association with mortality in critically ill patients. *Intensive Care Med.* 2019;45:1835–1837.
77. Sentürk NM, Dilek A, Camci E, et al. Effects of positive end-expiratory pressure on ventilatory and oxygenation parameters during pressure-controlled one-lung ventilation. *J Cardiothorac Vasc Anesth.* 2005;19(1):71–75.
78. Grichnik KP, Shaw A. Update on one-lung ventilation: the use of continuous positive airway pressure ventilation and positive end-expiratory pressure ventilation–clinical application. *Curr Opin Anaesthesiol.* 2009;22:23–30.
79. Farias LL, Faffe DS, Xisto DG, et al. Positive end-expiratory pressure prevents lung mechanical stress caused by recruitment/ derecruitment. *J Appl Physiol.* 2005;98:53–61.
80. Pelosi P, Ball L, Gama De Abreu M, Rocco PRM. General anesthesia closes the lungs: keep them resting. *Turk J Anaesthesiol Reanim.* 2016;44:163–164.
81. Hedenstierna G. Optimum PEEP during anesthesia and in intensive care is a compromise but is better than nothing. *Turk J Anaesthesiol Reanim.* 2016;44:161–162.
82. iPROVE Network investigators. Belda J, Ferrando C, Garutti I. The Effects of an open-lung approach during one-lung ventilation on postoperative pulmonary complications and driving pressure: a descriptive, multicenter national study. *Cardiothorac Vasc Anesth.* 2018;32:2665–2672.
83. Pereira SM, Tucci MR, Morais CCA, et al. Individual positive end-expiratory pressure settings optimize intraoperative mechanical ventilation and reduce postoperative atelectasis. *Anesthesiology.* 2018;129:1070–1081.
84. Dyhr T, Nygård E, Laursen N, Larsson A. Both lung recruitment maneuver and PEEP are needed to increase oxygenation and lung volume after cardiac surgery. *Acta Anaesthesiol Scand.* 2004;48:187–197.
85. Blank RS, Colquhoun DA, Durieux ME, et al. Management of one-lung ventilation: impact of tidal volume on complications after thoracic surgery. *Anesthesiology.* 2016;124:1286–1295.
86. Kiss T, Wittenstein J, Becker C, et al. PROTHOR investigators and the Research Workgroup PROtective VEntilation Network (PROVEnet) of the European Society of Anaesthesiology (ESA): Protective ventilation with high versus low positive end-expiratory pressure during one-lung ventilation for thoracic surgery (PROTHOR): study protocol for a randomized controlled trial. *Trials.* 2019;20:213.
87. Borges JB, Senturk M, Ahlgren O, Hedenstierna G, Larsson A. Open lung in lateral decubitus with differential selective positive end-expiratory pressure in an experimental model of early acute respiratory distress syndrome. *Crit Care Med.* 2015;43:e404–e411.
88. Anantham D, Jagadesan R, Tiew PE. Clinical review: independent lung ventilation in critical care. *Crit Care.* 2005;9:594–600.
89. Lucangelo U, Antonaglia V, Zin WA. High-frequency percussive ventilation improves perioperatively clinical evolution in pulmonary resection. *Crit Care Med.* 2009;37:1663–1669.
90. Jaber S, Antonelli M. Preventive or curative postoperative noninvasive ventilation after thoracic surgery: still a grey zone? *Intensive Care Med.* 2014;40:280–283.
91. Burns KE, Adhikari NK, Keenan SP, Meade M. Use of non-invasive ventilation to wean critically ill adults off invasive ventilation: meta-analysis and systematic review. *BMJ.* 2009;338: b1574.
92. Chiumello D, Chevallard G, Gregoretti C. Non-invasive ventilation in postoperative patients: a systematic review. *Intensive Care Med.* 2011;37:918–929.
93. Auriant I, Jallot A, Hervé P, et al. Noninvasive ventilation reduces mortality in acute respiratory failure following lung resection. *Am J Respir Crit Care Med.* 2001;164:1231–1235.
94. Lefebvre A, Lorut C, Alifano M, et al. Noninvasive ventilation for acute respiratory failure after lung resection: an observational study. *Intensive Care Med.* 2009;35:663–670.
95. Ball L, Dameri M, Pelosi P. Pros and cons of non-invasive ventilation. In: Şentürk M, Sungur MO, eds. *Postoperative Care in Thoracic Surgery.* 1st Edition: Springer International Publishing: Switzerland; 2017:183–197.
96. Barbagallo M1, Ortu A, Spadini E, et al. Prophylactic use of helmet CPAP after pulmonary lobectomy: a prospective randomized controlled study. *Respir Care.* 2012;57(9):1418–1424.
97. Jaber S, De Jong A, Castagnoli A, Futier E, Chanques G. Non-invasive ventilation after surgery. *Ann Fr Anesth Reanim.* 2014; 33:487–491.
98. Burns KEA, Meade MO, Premji A, Adhikari NKJ. Noninvasive positive pressure ventilation as a weaning strategy for intubated adults with respiratory failure: a Cochrane systematic review. *CMAJ.* 2014;186:E112–E122.
99. Jaber S, Chanques G, Jung B. Postoperative noninvasive ventilation. *Anesthesiology.* 2010;112:453–461.
100. Brochard L, Slutsky A, Pesenti A. Mechanical ventilation to minimize progression of lung injury in acute respiratory failure. *Am J Respir Crit Care Med.* 2017;195:438–442.
101. Wittenstein J, Ball L, Pelosi P, Gama De Abreu M. High-flow nasal cannula oxygen therapy in patients undergoing thoracic surgery: current evidence and practice. *Curr Opin Anesthesiol.* 2019; 32:44–49.

102. Roca O, Riera J, Torres F, et al. High-flow oxygen therapy in acute respiratory failure. *Respir Care.* 2010;55:408–413.
103. Papazian L, Corley A, Hess D, et al. Use of high-flow nasal cannula oxygenation in ICU adults: a narrative review. *Intensive Care Med.* 2016;42:1336–1349.
104. Parke RL, McGuinness SP. Pressures delivered by nasal high flow oxygen during all phases of the respiratory cycle. *Respir Care.* 2013;58:1621–1624.
105. Hernandez G, Roca O, Colinas L. High-flow nasal cannula support therapy: new insights and improving performance. *Crit Care.* 2017;21:62.
106. MacIntyre NR, Epstein SK, Carson S, Scheinhorn D, Christopher K, Muldoon S. Management of patients requiring prolonged mechanical ventilation: report of a NAMDRC consensus conference. *Chest.* 2005;128:3937–3954.
107. Boles JM, Bion J, Connors A, et al. Weaning from mechanical ventilation. *Eur Respir J.* 2007;29:1033–1056.
108. Béduneau G, Pham T, Schortgen F, et al. Epidemiology of weaning outcome according to a new definition. The WIND study. *Am J Respir Crit Care Med.* 2017;195:772–783.
109. Ambrosino N, Vitacca M. The patient needing prolonged mechanical ventilation: a narrative review. *Multidisciplinary Respir Med.* 2018;13:6.
110. Lago AF, Gastaldi AC, Mazzoni AAS, et al. Comparison of International Consensus Conference guidelines and WIND classification for weaning from mechanical ventilation in Brazilian critically ill patients: a retrospective cohort study. *Medicine.* 2019;98:42.
111. Ouellette DR, Patel S, Girard TD, et al. Liberation from mechanical ventilation in critically ill adults: an official American College of Chest Physicians/American Thoracic Society clinical practice guideline. Inspiratory pressure augmentation during spontaneous breathing trials, protocols minimizing sedation, and noninvasive ventilation immediately after extubation. *Chest.* 2017;151:166–180.
112. Connolly B, O'Neill B, Salisbury L, Blackwood B. Physical rehabilitation interventions for adult patients during critical illness: an overview of systematic reviews. *Thorax.* 2016;71:881–890.
113. Agostini P, Lugg ST, Adams K, et al. Video-assisted thoracoscopic lobectomy: which patients require postoperative physiotherapy? *Physiotherapy.* 2020;106:87–93.
114. Białka S, Copik M, Karpe J, et al. Effect of dexmedetomidine or propofol sedation on haemodynamic stability of patients after thoracic surgery. *Anaesthesiol Intensive Ther.* 2018;50:359–366.
115. Spalding MC, Cripps MW, Minshall CT. Ventilator-associated pneumonia: new definitions. *Crit Care Clin.* 2017;33:277–292.
116. Fitch ZW, Whitman GJ. Incidence, risk, and prevention of ventilator-associated pneumonia in adult cardiac surgical patients: a systematic review. *J Card Surg.* 2014;29:196–203.
117. Timsit JF, Esaied W, Neuville M, Bouadma L, Morvillier B. Update on ventilator-associated pneumonia [version 1; peer review: 2 approved]. *F1000Research.* 2017;6(F1000 Faculty Rev):2061.
118. Lin YJ, Xu L, Huang XZ, et al. Reduced occurrence of ventilator-associated pneumonia after cardiac surgery using preoperative 0.2% chlorhexidine oral rinse: results from a single-centre single-blinded randomized trial. *J Hosp Infect.* 2015;91:362–366.
119. Reignier J, Darmon M, Sonneville R, et al. Impact of early nutrition and feeding route on outcomes of mechanically ventilated patients with shock: a post hoc marginal structural model study. *Intensive Care Med.* 2015;4:875–886.
120. Kalil AC, Metersky ML, Klompas M, et al. Management of adults with hospital-acquired and ventilator-associated pneumonia: 2016 Clinical Practice Guidelines by the Infectious Diseases Society of America and the American Thoracic Society. *Clin Infect Dis.* 2016;63:e61–e111.
121. Torres A, Niederman MS, Chastre J, et al. International ERS/ESICM/ESCMID/ALAT guidelines for the management of hospital-acquired pneumonia and ventilator-associated pneumonia: Guidelines for the management of hospital-acquired pneumonia (HAP)/ventilator-associated pneumonia (VAP) of the European Respiratory Society (ERS), European Society of Intensive Care Medicine (ESICM), European Society of Clinical Microbiology and Infectious Diseases (ESCMID) and Asociación Latinoamericana del Tórax (ALAT). *Eur Respir J.* 2017:50.
122. Meyer A, Strüber M, Fischer S. Advances in extracorporeal ventilation. *Anesthesiol Clin.* 2008;26(2):381–391.

27

Postthoracotomy Complications

THOMAS HACHENBERG, TORSTEN LOOP

Introduction

Thoracotomy is required to get surgical access to the thoracic cavity through the chest wall to the pleural space and the thoracic organs, such as heart, lung, thymus, and esophagus. The principles and techniques of thoracotomy are differentiated in the anterolateral (= muscle sparing) and posterolateral (= nonmuscle sparing) approach, which requires a lateral position of the patient. In addition, sternotomy, anterior or axillary thoracotomy, clamshell, or hybrid techniques are further techniques that are performed in supine positioning.

Despite extensive and aggressive perioperative management, postoperative respiratory failure or cardiac complications may still occur. Postoperative complications because of thoracotomy encompasses serious risks in general, such as bleeding or hemorrhage or mainly because of the procedure per se, such as bronchopleural fistula, atelectasis, infection, or persistent organ damage.

Postoperative cardiopulmonary complications occur in 10% to 40% of patients undergoing lung resection surgery, resulting in prolonged hospital stay and increased healthcare costs.[1–4] The most common factors contributing to this high rate are postoperative respiratory complications with respiratory insufficiency. The various causes are shown in Table 27.1.

Cao et al. evaluated 1264 patients who underwent robotic anatomic pulmonary resections, and 64 major complications occurred in 54 patients (4.3%) (Fig. 27.1).[5] Male sex, decreased forced expiratory volume in 1 second (FEV_1), reduced diffusion capacity of the lung for carbon monoxide, neoadjuvant therapy, and extent of resection are associated with increased likelihood of a major postoperative complication.

Morbidity and mortality further depend on the type, invasiveness, and extent of the thoracic surgical procedure. The planned admission to the intensive care unit (ICU), high dependency unit (HDU), or postanesthetic care unit depends on the clinician's pre- and intraoperative prediction of potentially preventable major complications. In addition, adverse events may demand unplanned admission to the HDU or ICU for further diagnosis and treatment of complications. The overall risk profile for thoracic surgical patients is shown in Fig. 27.2.

The definition of postoperative pulmonary complications (PPCs) is heterogeneous. Typically, PPCs are categorized as a composite outcome measure.[6] The PPCs after thoracotomy are defined as need for noninvasive ventilation because of hypercapnia or hypoxia, need for tracheal intubation because of hypercapnia or hypoxia, prolonged air leak for 5 or more days after surgery, new thoracic drainage from an increased pleural effusion with respiratory compromise, and the presence of pleural empyema. Pneumonia was diagnosed according to the European Perioperative Clinical Outcome definition. This included new pulmonary infiltrate with associated leukocytosis, fever, new purulent sputum, need for antibiotic therapy, and increased oxygen demand via face mask. PPCs are ranked as the leading causes of early mortality after lung surgery, whereas sepsis and cardiac events are ranked second and third, respectively.[7] Thoracotomy by itself was defined as a risk factor for PPCs.[8] There is more compelling evidence that the thoracoscopic approach reduces the incidence of PPCs. Chen et al. performed a metaanalysis of 20 studies with 3457 patients comparing video-assisted thoracoscopic surgery (VATS) lobectomy with open lobectomy.[9] There was no difference in operation time between the two groups ($P = .14$), but distinct advantages in terms of intraoperative blood loss, chest drainage time, hospital stay, and complication incidence were found in the VATS group ($P < .01$). Moreover, the 5-year survival rate of VATS group was significantly higher than the thoracotomy group.

Prediction of Postoperative Pulmonary Complications

The preoperative identification of risk factors and the prediction of PPCs has the potential to optimize the perioperative care of patients and could help to reduce PPC. Canet et al. assessed the incidence and characteristics of PPCs in a large sample of 2464 patients and built a scoring system with a reduced number of significant variables that would identify PPC risk in most clinical settings (Assess Respiratory Risk in Surgical Patients in Catalonia [ARISCAT]) (Tables 27.2 and 27.3).[10,11]

TABLE 27.1 Causes and Frequencies of Respiratory Insufficiency

Atelectasis/secret retention	Nearly all patients
With the need for bronchoscopy	3.6%
Pneumonia	Up to 25%
Therapeutic atrial arrhythmia	10.7%
Bronchopleural fistula >5 d	8%
Reintubation	3.4%
ARDS	1.1%
Phrenic/recurrent nerve paresis	0.5%
Pulmonary embolism	0.4%
Empyema	0.3%

ARDS, Acute respiratory distress syndrome.

Modified from Cao C, Louie BE, Melfi F, et al. Outcomes of major complications after robotic anatomic pulmonary resection. *J Thorac Cardiovasc Surg*. 2019;159(2):681–686.

Postthoracotomy Complications in General and/or Specific to the Thoracic Procedure

Postthoracotomy complications may be categorized in general and/or specific to the thoracic procedure and may be related to patient- and procedure-specific risk factors.

Risk Factors

Patient-specific risk factors for the occurrence of PPCs include continued nicotine abuse, the male sex, the presence of chronic obstructive pulmonary disease (COPD), increased comorbidity (American Society of Anesthesiologists [ASA] ≥3), cachexia, increased age, obesity, preoperative impaired lung function, and preexisting hypoxia.[1,2,4,8]

With regard to surgical risk factors, the extent of parenchymal resection, thoracotomy compared with thoracoscopy, as well as an extended duration of surgery, contribute to an increase in risk factors for the occurrence of PPCs.[8,12,13] As previously mentioned, thoracoscopy as an alternative procedure to thoracotomy is the most important surgical factor in reducing PPCs.[13–15] During the intraoperative management, a liberal intraoperative volume therapy, a high tidal volumes >8 mL/kg body weight) to the dependent lung were identified as the main risk factors for the occurrence of PPCs.[4,13,16] Serpa Neto et al. evaluated 15 randomized controlled trials (2127 patients).[17] There were 97 cases of PPC in 1118 patients (8.7%) assigned to protective ventilation and 148 cases in 1009 patients (14.7%) assigned to conventional ventilation. Patients who developed postthoracotomy complications were older, presented higher ASA scores, had a higher prevalence of sepsis or pneumonia, received more frequent blood transfusions, and were ventilated with higher tidal volumes, lower positive end-expiratory pressure (PEEP) levels, or both.[18,19] These factors increase postoperative respiratory failure after thoracic procedures. Additional patient-specific risk factors are expiratory peak flow limitations during COPD, which result in increased work of breathing and muscle fatigue and ultimately respiratory failure. The frequent presence of postoperative atelectasis formed intraoperatively often persists postoperatively and may increase intrapulmonary shunt and predisposes acute lung injury. The incidence of postoperative lung injury after thoracotomy and thoracic surgery may be as high as 4.3%.[18]

Postthoracotomy Complications

Despite the developments and improvements in surgical technique, examples of general complications after thoracic surgical procedures are extra- or intrathoracic

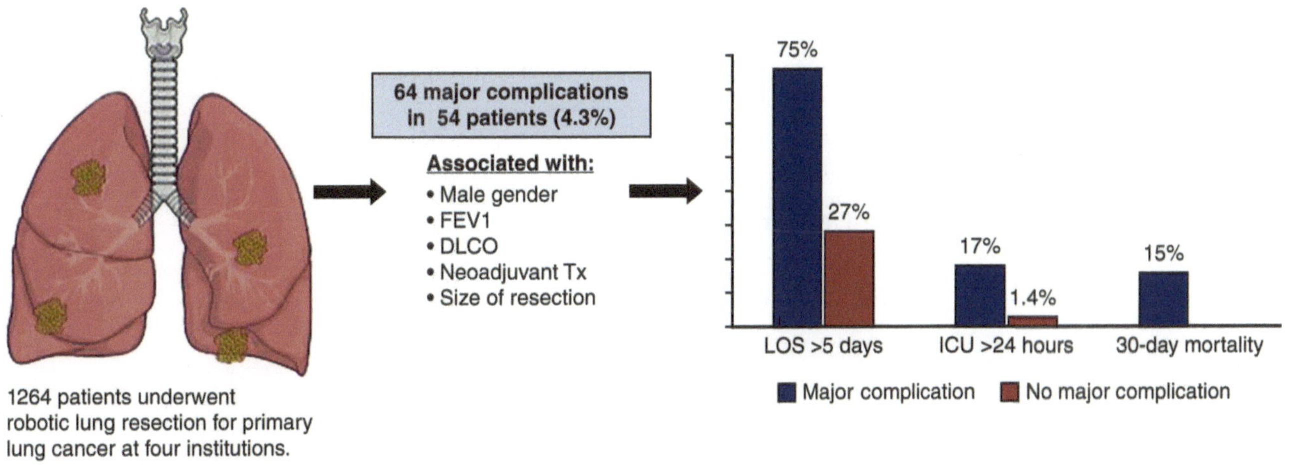

• **Fig. 27.1** Outcomes of major complications after robotic anatomic pulmonary resection. *DLCO*, Diffusing capacity for the lung for carbon monoxide; *FEV1*, forced expiratory volume in 1 second; *ICU*, intensive care unit; *LOS*, length of stay; *Tx*, Treatment. (From Meert AP, Grigoriu B, Licker M, Van Schil PE, Berghmans T. Intensive care in thoracic oncology. *Eur Respir J*. 2017;49(5):1602189.)

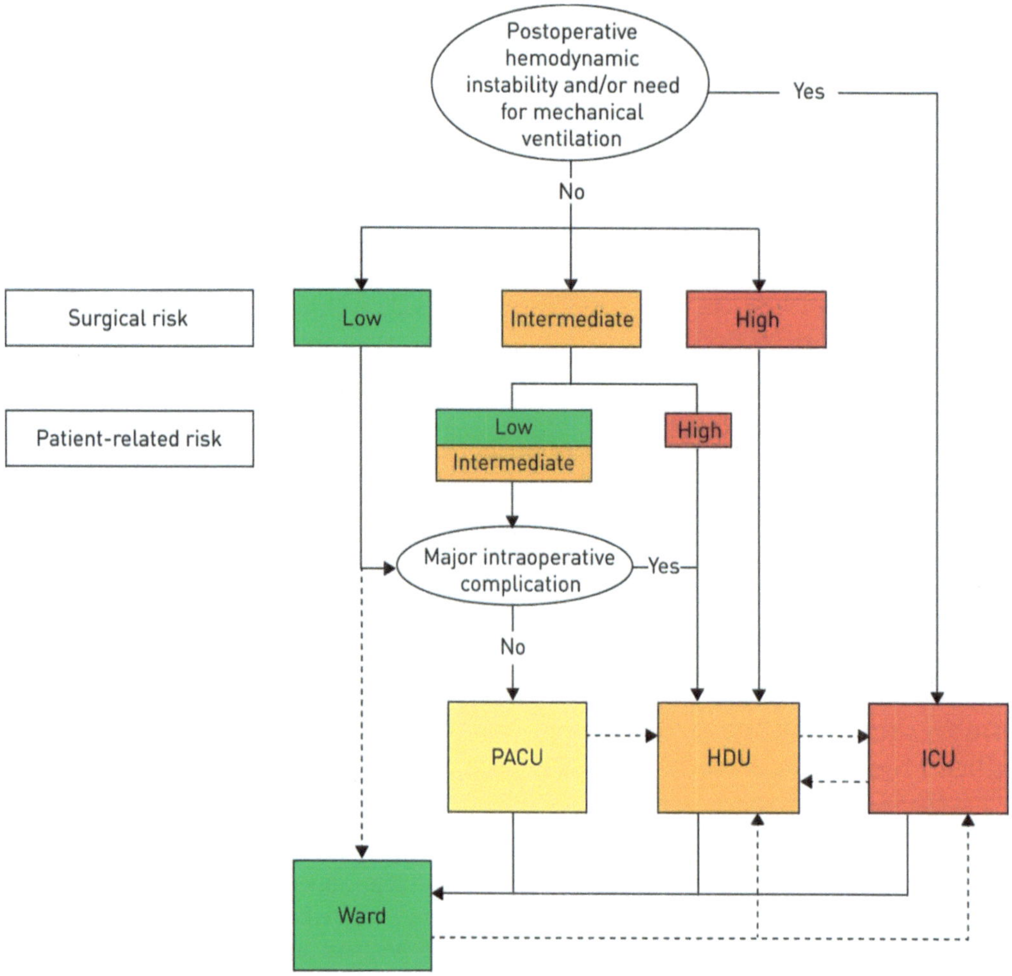

• **Fig. 27.2** Overall risk profile for thoracic surgical patients. *HDU,* High dependency unit; *ICU,* intensive care unit; *PACU,* postanesthesia care unit. (Modified from Jammer I, Wickboldt N, Sander M, et al. Standards for definitions and use of outcome measures for clinical effectiveness research in perioperative medicine: European Perioperative Clinical Outcome (EPCO) definitions: a statement from the ESA-ESICM joint taskforce on perioperative outcome measures. *Eur J Anaesthesiol.* 2015;32(2):88–105.)

bleeding after hemorrhage, hemothorax, pleural effusion, nerve injuries, chylothorax, acute, and postthoracotomy pain, pneumonia without/with septic condition. More specific complications particularly during thoracic procedures are: air leakage and/or bronchopleural fistula, pneumothorax, subcutaneous emphysema, lung torsion, lung infarction after pulmonary resection, anastomotic insufficiency after esophagectomy, and airway complications: aspiration of gastric contents and retained secretions.

TABLE 27.2 ARISCAT Score for Postoperative Pulmonary Complications[10]

Age, years	≤50 (0)	51 – 80 (+3)	>80 (+16)
Preoperative SpO_2	≥96% (0)	91 – 95% (+8)	≤90% (+24)
Respiratory infection in the last month	No (0)		Yes (+17)
Preoperative anemia (Hb <10 g*dL^{-1}) (6.2 mmol*L^{-1})	No (0)		Yes (+11)
Surgical incision	Peripheral (0)	Upper abdominal (+15)	Intrathoracic (+24)
Duration of surgery	<2 hours (0)	2 – 3 hours (+16)	> 3 hours (+23)
Emergency procedure	No (0)		Yes (+8)

TABLE 27.3 Postoperative Pulmonary Complications Risk Score

	Risk Score Intervals		
	Low Risk <26 Points	Intermediate Risk 26–44 Points	High Risk >45 Points
Postoperative pulmonary complication rate in %	1.6	13.3	42.1

From Chen FF, Zhang D, Wang YL, Xiong B. Video-assisted thoracoscopic surgery lobectomy versus open lobectomy in patients with clinical stage non-small cell lung cancer: a meta-analysis. *Eur J Surg Oncol*. 2013;39(9):957–963.

Postoperative Thoracic Complications

Bleeding

Postoperative bleeding after thoracic surgery is a rare but life-threatening complication. A national database with over 33,000 patients found an incidence of intraoperative bleeding of 1.9% for open, 1.3% for VATS, and 1.7% for robotic-assisted lobectomy resections.[19] Not all postoperative bleedings are subject to immediate exploration in the operating room (OR). A chest tube drainage of 1000 mL of bloody secretion within the first hour after lung resection must be considered for immediate exploration in the OR. Furthermore, a serial drainage rate of more than 200 mL/h over 2 to 4 hours postoperatively indicates an intrathoracic hemorrhage and requires surgical revision as well.

Lobe Torsion

The torsion of a pulmonary lobe after previous lung resection leads to a circulatory disorder and bronchial stenosis because of rotation around the supplying vessels and bronchial structures. The incidence is stated to be about 0.1% to 0.3%.[20] Lobar torsion was frequently reported after upper lobectomy (74.4%) and the middle lobe was the most vulnerable to torsion (29.4%). The main clinical presentations were dyspnea (38.4%), fever (23.3%), and chest pain (17.4%). Radiologic findings (computed tomography [CT] scan) included worsening consolidation and abrupt truncation/tapering of the pulmonary artery. The overall mortality was 8.3%.[21] Lobe torsion is a life-threatening situation; if a pulmonary lobe torsion was detected after clinical and CT diagnostics, an immediate surgical revision must be performed (Figs. 27.3 and 27.4).

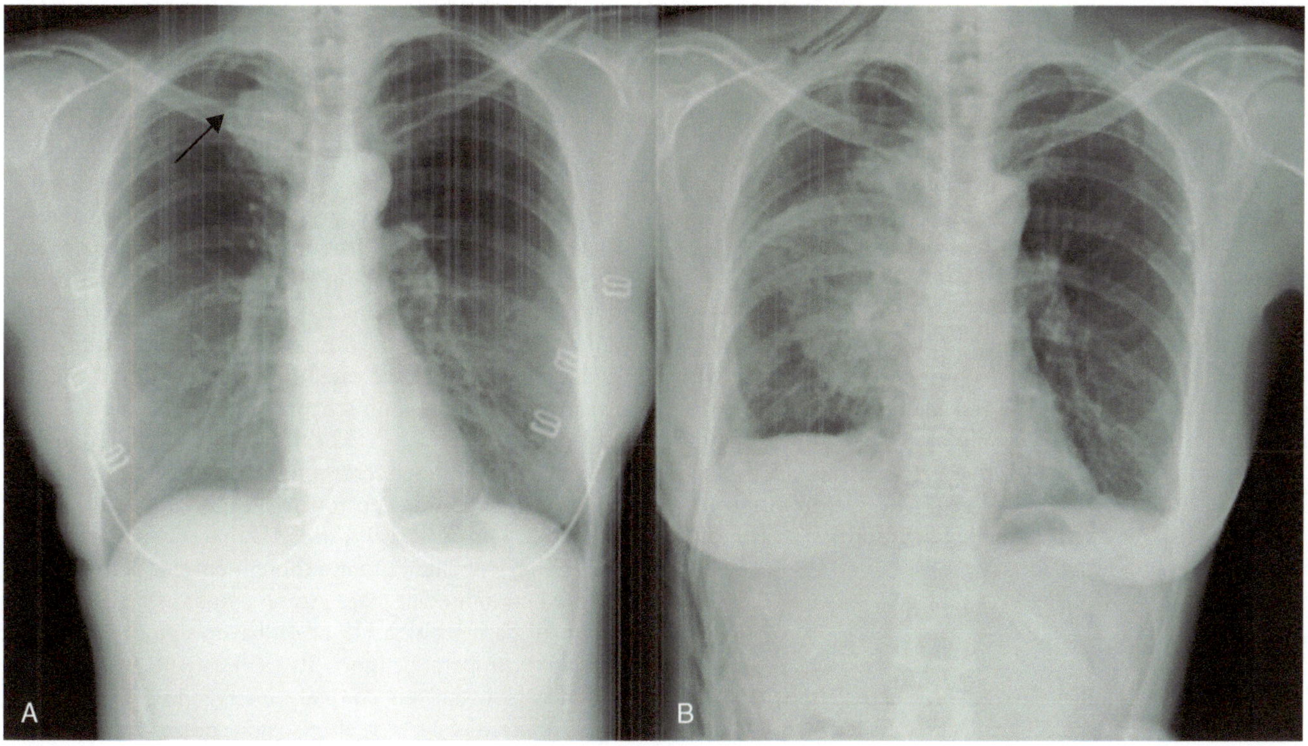

• **Fig. 27.3** (**A**) Mass (*arrow*) measuring around 3.5 cm in greatest diameter in right upper lung field. (**B**) Follow-up chest radiograph showed a wedge-shaped opacity of large area in the middle lung field.

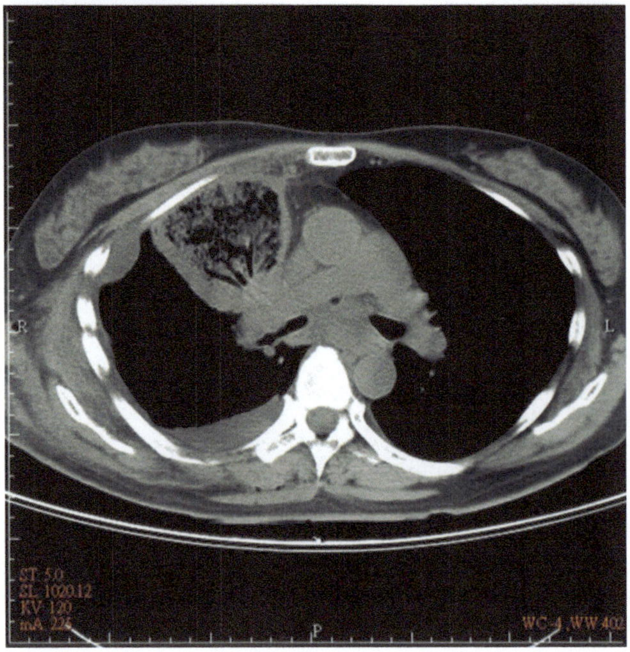

• **Fig. 27.4** Computed tomography scan show collapsed (see Fig. 27.3) and hemorrhagic consolidation of the right middle lobe. (From Froehlich JB, Fleisher LA. Noncardiac surgery in the patient with heart disease. *Med Clin North Am*. 2009;93(5):995–1016.)

A chest x-ray and a CT scan were taken of a 50-year-old woman who presented with a 2-month cough and mild symptoms of hemoptysis. On routine examination, the patient was found to have a mass measuring around 3.5 cm in right upper lung field. The patient underwent right upper lobectomy through a standard right posterolateral thoracotomy. The chest radiographs on postoperative day 1 and 2 showed adequate lung expansion with no obvious abnormality. Five days postoperatively, the patient presented fever and mild dyspnea. Follow-up chest radiograph showed a wedge-shaped opacity of large area in the middle lung field. Bedside bronchoscopy showed tight orifice of right middle lobe. CT scan showed collapse and hemorrhagic consolidation from right middle lobe torsion (see Fig. 27.4).

Postthoracotomy Cardiac Complications

Major adverse cardiac events (MACE) and myocardial infarction (MI) significantly contribute to postoperative morbidity and mortality. The vast majority of the patients admitted for lung resection are current smokers or ex-smokers at the time of surgery and have at least one risk factor for coronary artery disease (CAD). The identification of patients at risk may help to guide the utilization of clinical resources and preventive interventions.

Myocardial Ischemia

Perioperative myocardial ischemia is a strong predictor of adverse cardiac events in different surgical specialties, including thoracic surgery.[22] The diagnosis of perioperative MI is associated with a 30% to 50% risk of death after vascular surgery.[23,24] Age over 70 years and FEV_1 of 70% or less combined with coronary heart disease are independent prognostic factors for postoperative major complications.[25] Myocardial ischemia results from an imbalance between oxygen supply and demand, which may result from multiple factors before, during, and after thoracic surgery. Major determinants include intravascular fluid shifts, blood loss, alterations of coagulation, increased production and release of inflammatory substances, and pain, which increases production of catecholamines. A combination of tachycardia, decreased mean diastolic aortic pressure, and hypoxemia, which may occur during one-lung ventilation (OLV), are particularly detrimental for the development of perioperative myocardial ischemia. Thus the intraoperative prevention and/or control of these determinants is crucial in thoracic surgical patients.

The incidence of a MACE, death, or MI perioperatively is mainly related to the baseline risk. The revised cardiac risk index was developed for prediction of major cardiac complications after elective noncardiac surgery (Table 27.4).

Prolonged anticoagulation has to be considered before, during, and after thoracic surgery in patients with cardiac stents. The duration of anticoagulation depends on the type of the stent. Bare-metal stents are subjected to dual antiplatelet therapy for 4 to 6 weeks, whereas drug eluting stents are treated with acetylsalicylate and clopidogrel for 6 to 12 months.[23] Low-molecular-weight heparin is initiated preoperatively once antiplatelet therapy is temporarily paused. Patients who have not had previous coronary stenting, but are daily taking acetylsalicylate, should continue acetylsalicylate therapy throughout the perioperative period (class IIb recommendation). Continuation of acetylsalicylate perioperatively is certainly reasonable in patients with high-risk CAD or cerebrovascular disease, unless there is concern for an increased bleeding risk in certain thoracic procedures. However, some practitioners have concerns regarding giving a full dose acetylsalicylate (325 mg) when thoracic epidural is planned. Current guidelines provide a class III recommendation against initiating acetylsalicylate therapy preoperatively because of a higher risk of bleeding.[26]

Prophylactic coronary artery revascularization before thoracic surgery offers no further benefits over optimal medical treatment.[27,28] Van Diepen et al. evaluated the postoperative risks for patients with CAD undergoing noncardiac surgery, patients with heart failure (HF), and atrial fibrillation (AF). They created four cohorts of consecutive patients with either nonischemic HF (NIHF; $n = 7700$), ischemic HF (IHF; $n = 12{,}249$), CAD ($n = 13{,}786$), or AF ($n = 4312$) who underwent noncardiac surgery (Fig. 27.5). The unadjusted 30-day postoperative mortality was 9.3% in NIHF, 9.2% in IHF, 2.9% in CAD, and 6.4% in AF (Fig. 27.6). They concluded that although current perioperative risk prediction models place greater emphasis on CAD than HF or AF, patients with HF or AF have a significantly higher risk of postoperative mortality than patients with CAD.[27]

When percutaneous coronary intervention is performed before noncardiac surgery, elective noncardiac surgery should be delayed 14 days after balloon angioplasty, 30 days after bare-metal stent implantation, and 365 days after drug-eluting

TABLE 27.4 Summary of Risk Scores

ASA		Revised Cardiac Risk Index		Thoracic Revised Cardiac Risk Index	
Risk Factors	**Points**	**Risk Factors**	**Points**	**Risk Factors**	**Points**
ASA I	0	History of coronary artery disease	1	History of coronary artery disease	1.5
ASA II	2				
ASA III	4	History of heart failure	1	History of cerebrovascular disease	1.5
ASA IV	5	History of cerebrovascular disease	1		
ASA V	6			Pneumonectomy	1.5
Surgical risk: low/ intermediate/ high/ emergency intervention	0/1/2/1	High-risk surgery (vascular, intraperitoneal, or intrathoracic)	1	Serum creatinine >2 mg/dL >177 μmol/L	1
		Preoperative insulin therapy	1		
		Serum creatinine >2 mg/dL >177 μmol/L	1		

ASA, American Society of Anesthesiologists.

(From Jammer I, Wickboldt N, Sander M, et al. Standards for definitions and use of outcome measures for clinical effectiveness research in perioperative medicine: European Perioperative Clinical Outcome (EPCO) definitions: a statement from the ESA-ESICM joint taskforce on perioperative outcome measures. *Eur J Anaesthesiol*. 2015;32(2):88–105.)

stent (DES) implantation. The recent European Society of Cardiology (ESC) guidelines suggest that with newer-generation DES implantation, a 6-month duration of dual-antiplatelet therapy may be considered if there is increased need for noncardiac surgery. The American College of Cardiology (ACC)/American Heart Association (AHA) 2014 Guideline for the Management of Patients with Non–ST-Elevation Acute Coronary Syndromes recommends that if the risk of morbidity from bleeding outweighs the anticipated benefit of a recommended duration of antiplatelet drug—P2Y12 inhibitor therapy after stent implantation, earlier discontinuation (e.g., <12 months) of P2Y12 inhibitor therapy is reasonable.[29]

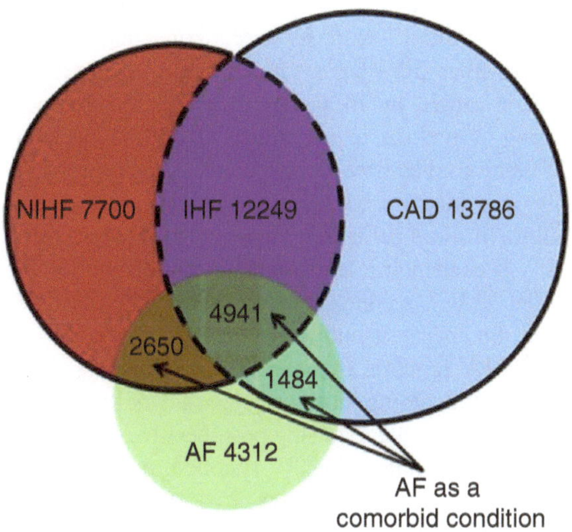

• **Fig. 27.5** Overlap between nonischemic heart failure (*NIHF*), ischemic heart failure (*IHF*), coronary artery disease (*CAD*), and atrial fibrillation/flutter (*AF*) cohorts. (From van Diepen S, Bakal JA, McAlister FA, Ezekowitz JA. Mortality and readmission of patients with heart failure, atrial fibrillation, or coronary artery disease undergoing noncardiac surgery: an analysis of 38 047 patients. *Circulation*. 2011;124(3):289–296.)

Valvular Heart Disease

Valvular heart disease (VHD) is frequently diagnosed in the United States and in the European population and may present as symptomatic or asymptomatic patient.[30] Mitral regurgitation (MR), often caused by leaflet prolapse, is the most frequent form of VHD in the United States, and its prevalence increases with age. ACC/AHA guidelines recommend surgical intervention in adult patients with significant MR and preserved left ventricular function. However, current estimates indicate that only one in 40 patients with moderate or severe MR undergoes surgical treatment. Approximately 45% of native VHD involves the aortic valve, and 2% to 7% of people above 65 years and about 13% of those aged above 75 years, have a clinical diagnosis of symptomatic aortic stenosis (AS). Current data suggest that approximately 500,000 people in the United States suffer from severe AS, and 250,000 patients with severe AS are symptomatic. Without a new valve placement, approximately half of these patients will die within 2 to 3 years.

The risk of postoperative cardiovascular complications is increased in patients with VHD. Agarwal et al., matching 634 patients with AS to 2536 controls patients, found that death or MI within 30 days after noncardiac surgery was significantly more frequent in patients with moderate AS

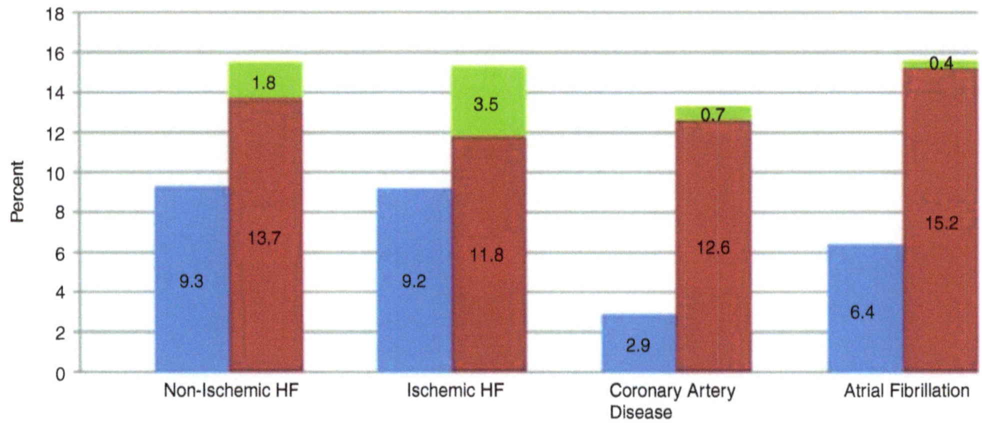

• **Fig. 27.6** Unadjusted 30-day perioperative mortality (*blue*), rehospitalization (*red*), and cardiac rehospitalization (*green*); *HF*, Heart failure. (From van Diepen S, Bakal JA, McAlister FA, Ezekowitz JA. Mortality and readmission of patients with heart failure, atrial fibrillation, or coronary artery disease undergoing noncardiac surgery: an analysis of 38 047 patients. *Circulation*. 2011;124(3):289–296.)

(4.4% vs. 1.7%) and severe AS (5.7% vs. 2.7%).[31] However, the difference between the control group and the study groups was significant only in symptomatic patients. Lai et al. compared 167 patients with chronic moderate-severe aortic regurgitation (AR) with other 167 case-matched control peers.[32] Patients with advanced AR risked potential hazards of serious hemodynamic instability (0.6%) and circulatory collapse (1.2%) during surgery. A 5-fold increase of in-hospital mortality rate (9.0% vs.1.8%) has been reported in patients with moderate-to-severe and severe AR compared with case-matched controls without AR. Main determinants of in-hospital death were decreased left ventricular ejection fraction (LVEF) under 55%, high surgical risk, and lack of cardiac medication, and creatinine greater than 2 mg/dL (>177 µmol/L).

In patients with severe MR, 30-day composite outcomes (death and postoperative MI, HF, and stroke) were worse than in patients without MR (22.2% vs. 16.4%).[33] Key predictors of adverse postoperative outcomes after noncardiac surgery included LVEF under 35%, ischemic mitral disease, and diabetes mellitus. There are no data available on perioperative care for patients with symptomatic VHD undergoing thoracic surgery. The ACC/AHA and the European Society of Cardiologists (ESC) guidelines emphasize the importance of general measures in the management of patients with untreated VHD undergoing noncardiac surgery.[34]

Careful selection of the mode of anesthesia, use of invasive hemodynamic monitoring (arterial line, transesophageal echocardiography, etc.), avoidance of rapid changes in volume status, aggressive treatment of arrhythmia, and high-intensity postoperative ward care are strongly recommended.

Heart Failure

Actively decompensated HF significantly increases the risk for perioperative MACE. As previously mentioned, from the work of van Diepen et al., 30-day postoperative mortality rates are higher in patients with NIHF (9.3%), ischemic HF (9.2%), and AF (6.4%) than in those with stable CAD (2.9%).[27] Diastolic dysfunction with and without systolic dysfunction is associated with a significantly higher rate of MACE, prolonged length of hospital stays, and higher rates of postoperative HF. However, few data are available on the prevalence and impact of diastolic dysfunction in patients undergoing thoracic surgery. Flu et al. performed echocardiography preoperatively in 1005 consecutive vascular surgery patients. Left ventricular dysfunction was diagnosed in 506 (50%) patients of which 80% were asymptomatic. In open vascular surgery ($n = 649$), both asymptomatic systolic and isolated diastolic LV dysfunctions were associated with 30-day cardiovascular events.[35] The 30-day cardiovascular event rate of 49% was observed in patients with symptomatic HF, in 23% of patients with asymptomatic systolic LV dysfunction, in 18% of patients with asymptomatic diastolic LV dysfunction, and in 10% of patients with normal LV function. Preoperative evaluation of LV function is strongly recommended in patients with decompensated HF to decrease the risk of perioperative MACE. In addition, acute LV dysfunction may result from right ventricular (RV) failure, for example, an interventricular shifting caused by an acutely increased RV afterload, by decreasing LV preload, or a combination of both mechanisms.

Different studies have demonstrated a decrease of RVEF of 25% after lung resection surgery which may lead to acute RV failure in some patients.[36] However, the evaluation of RV function is challenging and there are few diagnostic criteria to predict MACE secondary to RV failure.[37] A clinical study analyzed the effects of pulmonary resection on perioperative changes in RV function by transthoracic echocardiography in 86 patients undergoing lobectomy ($n = 47$) or pneumonectomy ($n = 39$).[38] On the following postoperative days, pneumonectomy patients had higher RV systolic pressure than lobectomy patients (31 ± 15 mm Hg vs. 25 ± 10 mm Hg, $P < .05$). Postoperative pulmonary hypertension was not associated with RV systolic dysfunction. In contrast, a recent study analyzed tricuspid annular plane systolic excursion, tricuspid annular systolic velocity, RV fractional area change, two-dimensional speckle tracking, and tissue Doppler imaging of the RV and RV freewall in patients undergoing thoracic noncardiac surgery

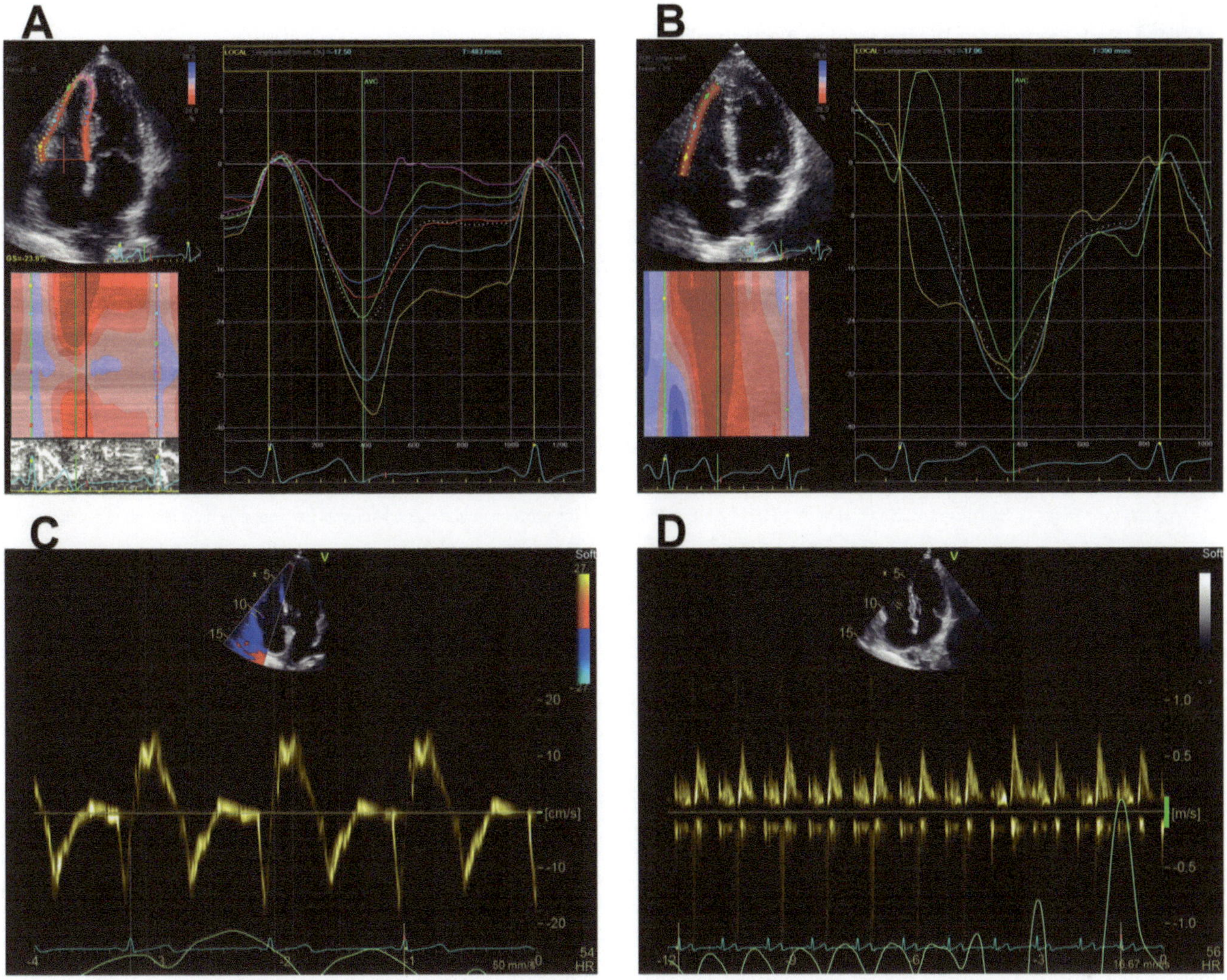

• **Fig. 27.7** Selected right ventricular (RV) measurements. (**A**) Global longitudinal strain of RV measured in four chamber (4CH) view. (**B**) Global longitudinal strain of RV freewall measured in 4CH. (**C**) Tricuspid annular systolic velocity estimated from tissue Doppler imaging. (**D**) Pulsed Doppler of the tricuspid valve inflow. (From Steffen HJ, Kalverkamp S, Zayat R, et al. Is systolic right ventricular function reduced after thoracic non-cardiac surgery? A propensity matched echocardiographic analysis. *Ann Thorac Cardiovasc Surg*. 2018;24(5):238–246.)

and coronary artery bypass grafting (CABG) surgery. Lung resection surgery had no early postoperative effect on RV function, whereas CABG surgery with pericardiotomy significantly impaired global RV function[39] (Fig. 27.7).

The risk of RV dysfunction may be increased by mechanical ventilation, particularly in patients with COPD, which is common in thoracic surgical patients, and in pulmonary hypertension.[40] During OLV the dependent lung is subjected to increased strain caused by nonphysiologic tidal volumes and the loss of functional residual capacity.[41] Oxidative stress, the production and release of proinflammatory substances, increased capillary shear stress from capillary hyperperfusion, and ischemia-reperfusion injury may increase PVR and induce RV-pulmonary artery uncoupling. Current practice of ventilation during OLV uses the protective lung ventilation strategy to decrease the risk of lung injury.[42] Because intraoperative effects on mechanical ventilation persist in the postoperative period, efforts should be taken to avoid additional lung injury with extubation in the OR if possible.

Older clinical studies suggest that intravenous fluid therapy may significantly contribute to postoperative complications, such as acute lung edema. However, a restrictive approach may put the patient at risk for hypovolemia, RV and LV dysfunction, and organ hypoperfusion, such as renal injury. Thus adequate fluid administration, that is, normovolemia, in most patients is recommended to maintain cardiac performance while avoiding acute lung injury particularly if the lung tissue resection is extended.

Cardiac Arrhythmias (See Chapter 22)

Cardiac arrhythmias are associated with prolonged HDU or ICU stay and increased morbidity and mortality after thoracic surgery. Risk factors can be classified into patient and surgery related (Tables 27.4 and 27.5).

TABLE 27.5 Risk Factors for Perioperative Arrhythmias

Patient-Related Risk Factors	Surgery-Related Risk Factors
• Increased age >60 years	• Surgical trauma (type of procedure/operation, magnitude of lung resection, dissection around the atria, mechanical factors, such as instrumentation)
• Male sex	• Hemodynamic stress (volume overload or depletion, hypertension, endogenous catecholamines)
• Structural heart disease (coronary artery disease, valve disease, left ventricular hypertrophy, systolic and diastolic left ventricular dysfunction)	• Metabolic changes (hypoxemia, hypercarbia, acid-base imbalances)
• Extracardiac risk factors (obesity, previous stroke, concomitant lung disease)	• Electrolyte disturbances (particularly hypokalemia)
• History of arrhythmias	• Drug effects (beta blocker withdrawal, digoxin, exogenous catecholamines, phosphodiesterase inhibitors [milrinone], levosimendan)

Modified from Frendl G, Sodickson AC, Chung MK, et al. 2014 AATS guidelines for the prevention and management of perioperative atrial fibrillation and flutter for thoracic surgical procedures. *J Thorac Cardiovasc Surg*. 2014;148(3):e153–e193.

Patient-Related Risk Factors

Various patient-related clinical and nonclinical risk factors for postoperative arrhythmias have been identified. Age-related structural and/or electrophysiologic changes may lower the threshold for atrial and ventricular arrhythmias. Patients undergoing noncardiac thoracic surgery often have the substrate of atrial enlargement or elevation in atrial pressures, which predispose to atrial tachyarrhythmias. Reported extracardiac risk factors for postoperative atrial tachyarrhythmias include obesity, previous stroke, and history of COPD. These risk factors are identical to those known to increase the propensity to the development of AF in the nonsurgical setting.

Surgery-Related Risk Factors

The surgical trauma predisposes patients to supraventricular and ventricular arrhythmias. Inflammatory mechanisms have been proposed in the development of postoperative arrhythmias because their incidence peaks during the first week after surgery. Hemodynamic stress favoring arrhythmias may result from surgical trauma, hypervolemia or hypovolemia, hypertension, and increased levels of endogenous catecholamines. Hypoxemia, hypercarbia, acid-base imbalances as well as mechanical factors such as instrumentation, often predispose to electrophysiologic changes favoring the occurrence of arrhythmias. In particular, hypokalemia may provoke postoperative atrial and ventricular arrhythmias. Beta blocker withdrawal in the perioperative period has been associated with an increased rate of postoperative supraventricular tachyarrhythmias. A state of heightened catecholamine effect occurs because chronic beta blocker use leads to a higher density of beta-adrenergic receptors. Intravenous administration of catecholamines, digoxin, phosphodiesterase inhibitors, such as milrinone or enoximone and levosimendan have been reported to cause ventricular premature beats, short runs of ventricular tachycardia, and AF.

Atrial Fibrillation and Other Supraventricular Arrhythmias

AF after thoracic surgery is associated with prolonged ICU and hospital stays, higher costs, and an increased morbidity and mortality (Table 27.6). However, because many patients with postoperative AF often have complex comorbidities, the impact of arrhythmia on mortality is not clear.[43] The incidence of postoperative AF was 12.3% in an analysis of 2588 patients undergoing noncardiac thoracic surgery. Retrospective analysis was carried out by Elrakhawy et al. on 987 patients after noncardiac thoracic surgery to define the prevalence, associated risk factors, and clinical course of postoperative arrhythmias.[43] The patients were divided into two groups depending on the occurrence or absence of supraventricular arrhythmia. Group I consisted of 876 patients who were free from rhythm disturbances. The remaining 111 patients exhibited episodes of supraventricular arrhythmia (29 supraventricular tachycardia; 82 AF). Significant risk factors for the occurrence of AF were male sex, advanced age (relative risk [RR] in patients with age >70 years 5.3), a history of congestive HF (RR, 2.51), a history of arrhythmias (RR, 1.92), a history of peripheral vascular disease (RR, 1.65), resection of mediastinal tumor or thymectomy (RR, 2.36), lobectomy (RR 8.91), bilobectomy (RR, 7.16), pneumonectomy (RR, 8.91), esophagectomy (RR, 2.95), and intraoperative transfusions (RR, 1.39).

Treatment of Atrial Fibrillation

Atrial premature beats are usually benign and do not need specific treatment. Paroxysmal supraventricular tachycardia which may occur from time to time often respond

TABLE 27.6 Risk of Postoperative Atrial Fibrillation Stratified by Thoracic Surgery Procedures

Low Risk (<5% Incidence)	Intermediate Risk (5%–15% Incidence)	High Risk (>15% Incidence)
• Bronchoscopy with/without biopsy	• Thoracoscopic sympathectomy	• Resection of anterior mediastinal mass
• Photodynamic therapy	• Segmentectomy	• Thoracoscopic lobectomy
• Tracheal stenting	• Laparoscopic Nissen fundoplication	• Open thoracotomy for lobectomy
• Placement of thoracostomy tube or catheter	• Myotomy	• Tracheal resection and reconstruction/ carinal resection
• Pleuroscopy, pleurodesis, decortication	• Zenker diverticulectomy	• Pneumonectomy
• Tracheostomy		• Pleurectomy
• Mediastinoscopy		• Volume reduction/bullectomy
• Thoracoscopic wedge resection		• Bronchopleural fistula repair
• Bronchoscopic laser surgery		• Clagett window
• Esophagoscopy/PEG		• Lung transplantation
• Dilation and/or stenting		• Esophagectomy
		• Pericardial window

PEG, percutaneous endoscopic gastrostomy.

Modified from Frendl G, Sodickson AC, Chung MK, et al. 2014 AATS guidelines for the prevention and management of perioperative atrial fibrillation and flutter for thoracic surgical procedures. *J Thorac Cardiovasc Surg*. 2014;148(3):e153–e193.

to treatment. If vagal maneuvers are not successful, adenosine can be used in increasing doses (Table 27.4). Success rates exceed 95% and electrical cardioversion is rarely needed unless the patient is hemodynamically unstable. The management of AF is much more complex. Given the often-transient nature of new-onset postoperative AF (the arrhythmia frequently resolves within 4–6 weeks), control of the ventricular response rate is usually the initial therapy. Conventionally, nondihydropyridine calcium-channel antagonists (verapamil and diltiazem) and digitalis have been used for treating postoperative AF (Table 27.7).[44,45] However, because calcium antagonists may be associated with hypotension and are contraindicated in patients with HF, they may not be the ideal drugs in patients with compromised heart function. Digitalis acts primarily by increasing vagal tone and its effects are attenuated when sympathetic tome is markedly increased. Beta blockers have been shown to be effective particularly when AF occurs after surgery. Patients taking beta blockers before surgery should have beta blockade continued; abrupt withdrawal is associated with an increased risk of complications and should be avoided. Amiodarone intravenously should be preferred in patients with known severe systolic dysfunction. The drug also exerts antiarrhythmic effects, which may lead to termination of the arrhythmias. Preliminary studies indicate that amiodarone may have a beneficial effect on mortality and survival in certain groups of patients with ventricular arrhythmias, an action probably related to both its antiarrhythmic and anti fibrillatory effects.[46]

Acute pulmonary toxicity has been reported with amiodarone in patients undergoing lung resection. Amiodarone or at least high amiodarone doses (>1000 mg/day) should be avoided in these patients. Preexisting pulmonary disease is associated with an increased risk of amiodarone pulmonary toxicity.[47]

Class I antiarrhythmic drugs may be used in patients without structural heart disease. However, even in those patients these agents may exert proarrhythmic effects (e.g., convert to a well-tolerated AF compromising atrial flutter). Immediate electrical cardioversion is indicated in patients who demonstrate severe hemodynamic deterioration in response to new-onset AF. It is highly effective with a greater than 90% conversion rate. However, early recurrences are frequent. Cardioversion from well-tolerated postoperative AF is usually not necessary because of a frequent self-limited course. New AF after thoracic surgery often resolves within 4 to 6 weeks, regardless of treatment.

Patients who develop AF after surgery are at risk of thromboembolic events, including stroke. In the individual postsurgical patient with an embolic event, the cause may be unclear because underlying comorbidities may be responsible for these strokes, rather than the arrhythmia itself. Anticoagulant therapy prevents episodes of systemic embolization in the broad population of patients with AF; therefore anticoagulation is reasonable therapy for patients with postoperative AF who have stroke risk factors (age >65 years, female gender, prior stroke, hypertension, congestive HF, diabetes mellitus).

TABLE 27.7 **Drugs Used for Postoperative Arrhythmias**

Drug	Dosing	Indication	Side Effects
Adenosine	6 or 12 mg, 18 mg intravenous (IV)	Paroxysmal SVT	Transient heart block, flushing, chest pain, induction of AF
Atropine	0.4–1 mg IV	Bradycardia or AV-block	Excessive tachycardia
Verapamil	5–10 mg IV	Rate control of AF, paroxysmal SVT	Hypotension, exacerbation of CHF, AV block
Diltiazem	10–20 mg IV, then infusion at 5–15 mg/h	Rate control of AF, I paroxysmal SVT	Hypotension, exacerbation of CHF, AV block
Esmolol	0.5 mg/kg IV, then infusion at 0.05 mg/kg/h; increase by 0.05 mg/kg/h every 5 min	Rate control of AF	Hypotension, bronchospasm, exacerbation of CHF
Metoprolol	5 mg IV every 5 min × 3	Rate control of AF	Hypotension
Digoxin	0.25 mg IV every 4–6 h up to 1 mg	Rate control of persisting AF	Delayed onset, nausea, vomiting
Amiodarone	Prophylaxis: 300 mg IV then 600 mg orally for 3–5 days; treatment: 150 mg IV over 10 min, then 1 mg/min × 6 hours, then 0.5 mg/min	Rate control and conversion of AF, frequent nonsustained/sustained VT, VF	Hypotension, bradycardia abnormal QTc prolongation with torsade de pointes (rare), acute respiratory distress syndrome (rare, after supra-therapeutic doses)

AF, Atrial fibrillation; *CHF*, congestive heart failure; *SVT*, supraventricular tachycardia; *VF*, ventricular fibrillation; *VT*, ventricular tachycardia.

Modified from Frendl G, Sodickson AC, Chung MK, et al. 2014 AATS guidelines for the prevention and management of perioperative atrial fibrillation and flutter for thoracic surgical procedures. *J Thorac Cardiovasc Surg*. 2014;148(3):e153–e193.

Ventricular Arrhythmia

Isolated ventricular premature beats postoperatively are not associated with an increased risk for malignant ventricular tachyarrhythmias, and generally there is no need for treatment. Nonsustained and sustained ventricular tachyarrhythmias are observed in 0.5% to 1.0% of noncardiac surgical patients, who often suffer from severe heart disease with depressed left ventricular function or severe acute postoperative complications (e.g., hemodynamic instability, myocardial ischemia, septic shock, major surgical complications).[45] In the case of frequent and complex premature beats and nonsustained ventricular tachycardia the correction of any reversible cause of arrhythmias (see earlier) should be pursued. Antiarrhythmic drugs may be indicated when longer repeated episodes of nonsustained or sustained ventricular tachycardia develop. The preferred antiarrhythmic drug is amiodarone administered intravenously. Class I antiarrhythmic drugs, such as lidocaine, have also been used successfully; however, they are also associated with an increased risk for ventricular arrhythmias. Currently, with hemodynamic deterioration because of sustained ventricular tachyarrhythmias, either R-wave triggered DC cardioversion or immediate defibrillation and cardiopulmonary resuscitation may become necessary. Most patients with known, previously documented, ventricular tachyarrhythmias have an implanted cardioverter/defibrillator, which effectively shocks the patient to terminate spontaneous arrhythmias. All devices should be thoroughly evaluated before and after surgery to make sure that their function has not been damaged or changed and may need to be reprogrammed if the patient is also pacemaker dependent.

Bradyarrhythmias

Bradyarrhythmias are relatively rare after noncardiac thoracic surgery. In most cases, they consist of transitory episodes of low ventricular heart rate resulting from (usually preexisting) sick sinus syndrome or various degrees of atrioventricular blocks. Bradyarrhythmias may be hemodynamically relevant because of a decrease in cardiac output. Atropine can reverse symptomatic bradycardia. It is prudent to stop all unnecessary medications that can cause increased AV block like beta blockers or calcium channel blockers. Temporary electrical pacing may be required in symptomatic bradycardias not responding to atropine. In some cases, when the conduction defect does not revert, permanent pacing may be necessary.

Postthoracotomy Pulmonary Complications

Respiratory Insufficiency

Resection of functionally borderline parenchyma in patients with preexisting lung diseases, hypoxia or hypercapnia may occur postoperatively because of insufficient gas exchange after thoracic surgery. This can be treated early with continuous positive airway pressure or high-flow oxygen therapy via nasal cannula.[48–50] The goal in the treatment of respiratory insufficiency after thoracic surgery should be to provide inspiratory muscle assistance and appreciation of the pathophysiologic underlying causes. Causes of hypoxemic respiratory failure are hypoventilation, V/P-mismatch through consolidation (i.e., atelectasis or infection), and edematous lung. Causes of hypercapnic respiratory failure are decreased muscle function, structural and/or mechanical problems (pneumothorax, pain), and decreased central respiratory drive.

Pneumonia

Normally the lower respiratory tract is sterile. Pneumonia often results from a transfer of bacteria into the lower respiratory tract (Fig. 27.8). The risk factors, causes, and pathophysiology for postoperative pneumonia are the result of a combination of several causative factors. These include preoperative bacterial colonization of the airways, a restricted cough with reduced mucociliary clearance, altered immunocompetence of pulmonary neutrophil leukocytes, aspiration from the upper airways, and direct and indirect trauma to the lungs by surgery and anesthesia. Patients scheduled for lung parenchyma resection procedures carry a high rate of bronchial colonization with potentially pathogenic microorganisms (up to 50%).[51,52] The most common strains of bacteria isolated are *Haemophilus influenzae* (35%), *Streptococcus pneumoniae* (13%), *Pseudomonas aeruginosa* (9%), *Escherichia coli*, *Proteus mirabilis*, and fungi-like *Candida albicans* and *Aspergillus fumigatus*. Colonization with bacteria represents a mortality factor. Laroumagne et al. aimed to prospectively define the prevalence and nature of bronchial colonization in patients at the time of diagnosing lung cancer.[52] Some 210 consecutive patients with lung cancer underwent a flexible bronchoscopy. In their patient population, pathogens were found in 48.1% of samples: mainly the gram-negative bacilli *Escherichia coli* (8.1%), *Haemophilus influenzae* (4.3%), and *Enterobacter* spp. (2.4%); gram-positive *cocci*, *Staphylococcus* spp. (12.9%) and *Streptococcus pneumoniae* (3.3%); atypical mycobacteria (2.9%); *Candida albicans* (42.9%); and *Aspergillus fumigatus* (6.2%). Older patients with COPD were significantly more frequently colonized. Postoperative survival analyses postulate that 50% of patients with colonization have mortality after 10.7 months, whereas 50% of patients without colonization die only after 14.3 months.

Pneumonia is a significant morbidity and mortality factor of thoracic surgery. In addition to general hygiene measures, specific interventions should place great emphasis on avoidance of aspiration and bacterial colonization of the deeper airways. Optimization of anesthetic techniques, such as lung protective ventilation, or the use of regional analgesia procedures, such as epidural or paravertebral anesthesia, can reduce the perioperative pneumonia risk.

Atelectasis

Atelectasis is a common complication following thoracic surgical procedures and is aggravated by ineffective analgesic therapy, inadequate coughing, and retention of secretion. The loss of lung volume results in a lower FRC, an increased transpulmonary pressure to achieve an adequate tidal volume, possibly from residual muscle relaxants, leading to increased work of breathing.

Atelectasis therefore significantly affects systemic oxygenation by the loss of adequate ventilation to perfused lung units.[53,54] Patients present with symptoms such as hypoxia, tachypnea, tachycardia, and clinical and radiologic signs of lung consolidation. Chest physiotherapy with incentive deep breathing spirometry, bronchial toilet with fiberoptic bronchoscopy, or positive pressure breathing may recruit the collapsed lung units (Fig. 27.8).

The penetration of air into the soft tissues around the thoracotomy is normal to a small extent. A soft tissue emphysema increasing over days after lung resection is an expression of a larger parenchyma leakage or bronchial

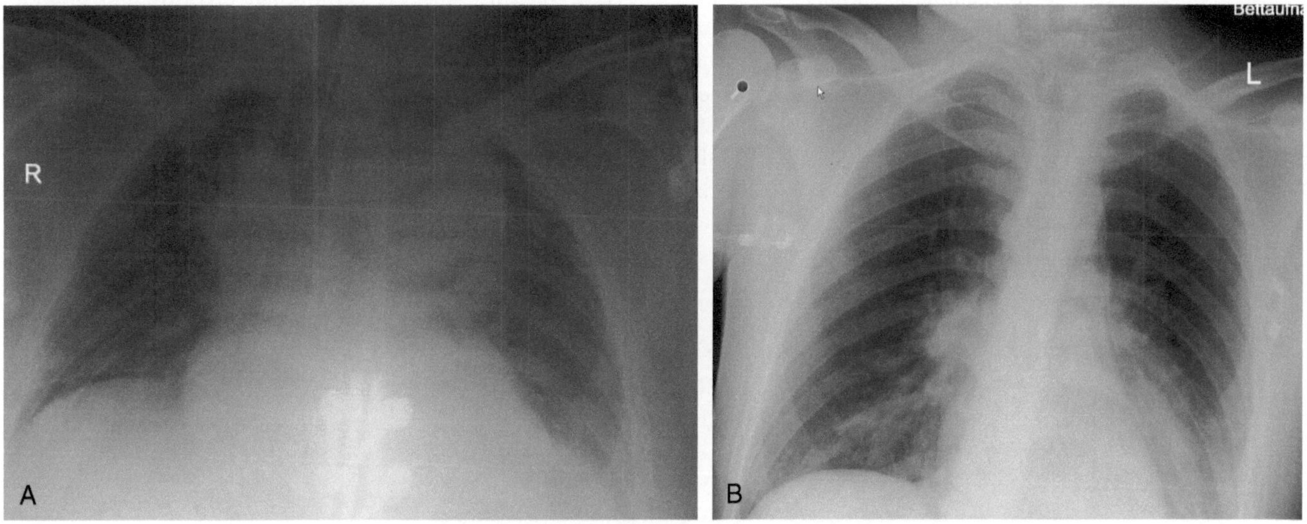

• **Fig. 27.8** X-ray thorax image with atelectasis (*left*) and pneumonic infiltrate (*right*). Air leakage and mediastinal and subcutaneous soft tissue emphysema and pneumothorax.

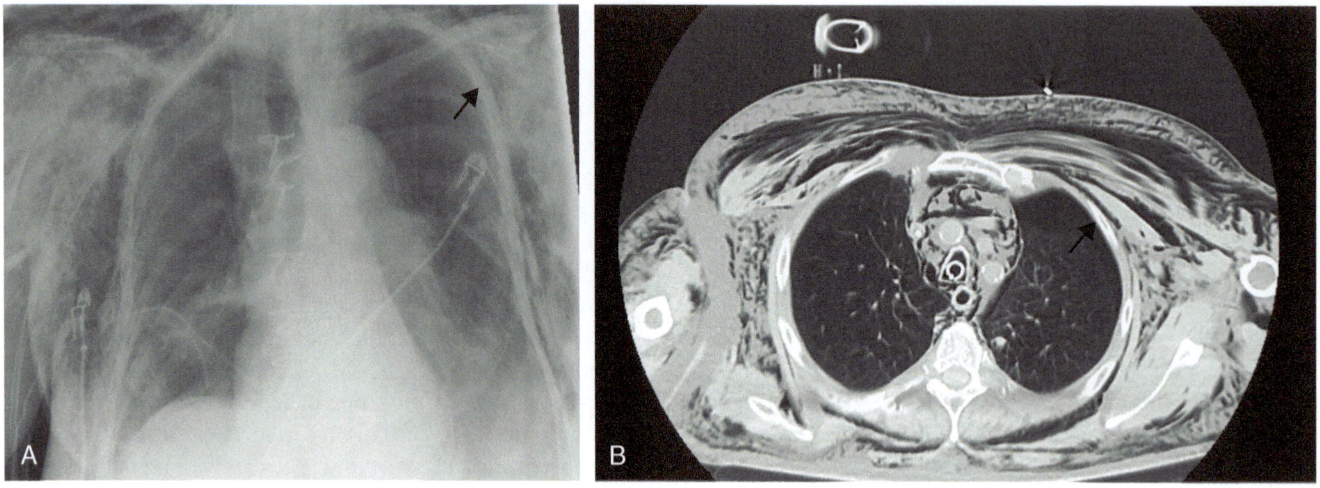

• **Fig. 27.9** X-ray (*left*) and computed tomography scan (*right*) thorax image with pneumothorax (*arrows*) and soft tissue emphysema in a patient with chronic obstructive pulmonary disease.

fistula.[55] The function and position of the drains should be first checked; if necessary, a further drain can be inserted or the suction increased. If this does not lead to any improvement, the only remaining option is revision by means of VATS or re-thoracotomy. Postsurgical air leaks continue to be the most common complication following surgical resection and a leading cause of increased hospitalization, morbidity, and cost, with a reported incidence ranging from 8% up to 26%.[56] Risk factors for postoperative air leak are impaired pulmonary function (FEV_1 <50%), steroid medication, and the presence of pleural adhesions.[56] Most patients with an air leak require nonoperative management by means of intercostal drains connected to an underwater seal or suction[56,57] (Fig. 27.9). Inconsistencies in the interpretation of air leaks and in chest tube management are likely contributors to the conflicting results found in the literature.[58] Besides personal preferences and experience, chest tube removal appears to be safe in absence of air leak (leakage <50 mL/min in 12 hours or <20 mL/min in 8 hours).[59]

In an effort to use alternatives to lung volume reduction for the treatment of end-stage COPD, several methods are offered including the placement of unidirectional valves. These bronchoscopic therapies aimed at reducing lung volumes have evaluated the use of various one-way valves, which cause distal atelectasis, lung volume reduction coils that mechanically reduce lung volume, and thermal ablation (see Chapter 32). Unidirectional valves are commercially available for the treatment of emphysema in many countries worldwide outside the United States. The Spiration Valve (Olympus Respiration System, Center Valley, PA), which was developed for this purpose, is a small, umbrella-shaped, one-way valve that is placed inside the airways using a delivery system via a fiberoptic bronchoscopy of the diseased lung (Fig. 27.10). The Spiration Valve redirects air away from areas most affected by emphysema and toward healthier lung areas allowing the patient to breathe more easily. However, in the United States, this valve is approved for the treatment of persisting air leak during postsurgical period. The Spiration Valve System procedure is minimally invasive and provides

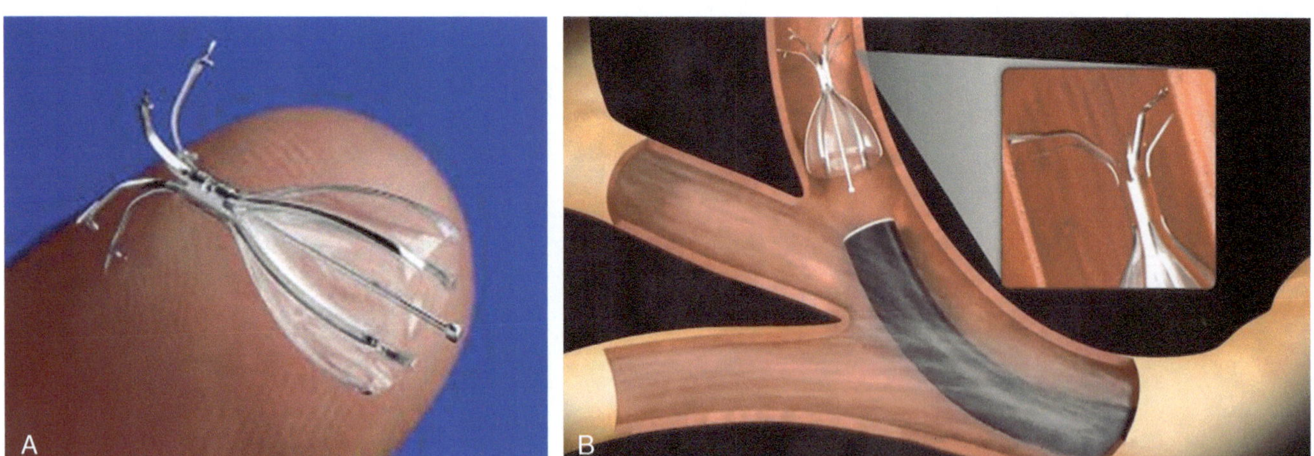

• **Fig. 27.10** Spiration Valve System. (**A**) The Spiration valve. (**B**) Deployment of the Spiration valve through a flexible bronchoscope.

surgeons and pulmonologists a novel method for limiting distal airflow to the damaged lung while allowing trapped air and secretions to escape naturally along the airway wall. It is a proactive option in the management of prolonged air leaks. A reduction in airflow to the damaged lung has been shown to accelerate resolution of a persisting air leak. In most patients, following a tissue healing of approximately 6 weeks, the valve is removed using flexible bronchoscopy forceps.[60]

Pulmonary Hypertension

Surgical resection of lung parenchyma decreases the cross-sectional area of the pulmonary vasculature with an elevated pulmonary vascular resistance (PVR), which impacts RV function in the early postoperative phase.[61] Comparing the two cohorts, Elrakhawy et al. reported that the patients undergoing pneumonectomy had higher mean pulmonary arterial pressure (MPAP), PVR, and pulmonary capillary wedge pressure (PCWP) than patients with lobectomy, and some had mild pulmonary hypertension, with MPAP more than 30 mm Hg. The patients with pneumonectomy had a larger RV end-diastolic volume index (RVEDVI), signifying greater RV dilation, a higher incidence of postoperative arrhythmias, and a greater reduction in RV ejection fraction (RVEF) than the patients with lobectomy.[61] This may be tolerated and/or compensated by most patients, but in COPD patients, the reduced ability to compensate will lead to acute RV dysfunction, which may be present intraoperatively and postoperatively, persisting for up to 2 months after surgery.[36] The treatment should focus on reversible causes of pulmonary vasoconstriction, such as hypoxia, hypercapnia, acidosis, and pain. Optimizing the volume status with echocardiographic, as well as right heart catheter assessment of right- and left-ventricular filling pressures and/or pulmonary vasodilation as earlier described, may reduce pulmonary hypertension.

Pulmonary Edema and Acute Respiratory Distress Syndrome

ARDS is one of the major causes of mortality after lung resection surgery. Currently, the reported mortality rates following lung resection range from 4% to 9% after pneumonectomy and from 1% to 3% after lobectomy.[1,62,63] The mortality rate has been reported as 40% to 64.6%.[63–66] Diagnosis is dependent on the presentation of acute, refractory hypoxemia and diffuse, uni- or bilateral infiltrates on chest radiograph consistent with alveolar edema. In most cases, symptoms begin between 1 and 3 postoperative days. The management of ARDS postlung resection is supportive with protective lung mechanical ventilation using higher PEEP, nitric oxide with a short-lived effect on arterial oxygenation, and ultimately extracorporeal membrane oxygenation (ECMO).

Conclusion

Postthoracotomy complication after procedures of the lung, mediastinum, or thoracic wall are frequent and are caused by the generally high cardiopulmonary comorbidity of thoracic surgery patients. In individual cases, borderline indications for surgery, inadequacies in the course of the operation and anesthesia, deficits in postoperative care, are often fateful events. This underlines the importance of close and continuous postoperative monitoring, whereas the detection of complications is mostly based on characteristic clinical signs and typical "time periods."

References

1. LaPar DJ, Bhamidipati CM, Lau CL, Jones DR, Kozower BD. The Society of Thoracic Surgeons General Thoracic Surgery Database: establishing generalizability to national lung cancer resection outcomes. *Ann Thorac Surg.* 2012;94(1):216–221; discussion 21.
2. Ellenberger C, Garofano N, Reynaud T, et al. Patient and procedural features predicting early and mid-term outcome after radical surgery for non-small cell lung cancer. *J Thorac Dis.* 2018; 10(11):6020–6029.
3. Im Y, Park HY, Shin S, et al. Prevalence of and risk factors for pulmonary complications after curative resection in otherwise healthy elderly patients with early stage lung cancer. *Respir Res.* 2019;20(1):136.
4. Kaufmann KB, Loop T, Heinrich S, Working Group of the German Thorax Registry. Risk factors for post-operative pulmonary complications in lung cancer patients after video-assisted thoracoscopic lung resection: results of the German Thorax Registry. *Acta Anaesthesiol Scand.* 2019;63(8):1009–1018.
5. Cao C, Louie BE, Melfi F, et al. Outcomes of major complications after robotic anatomic pulmonary resection. *J Thorac Cardiovasc Surg.* 2019;159(2):681–686.
6. Meert AP, Grigoriu B, Licker M, Van Schil PE, Berghmans T. Intensive care in thoracic oncology. *Eur Respir J.* 2017;49(5):1602189.
7. Jammer I, Wickboldt N, Sander M, et al. Standards for definitions and use of outcome measures for clinical effectiveness research in perioperative medicine: European Perioperative Clinical Outcome (EPCO) definitions: a statement from the ESA-ESICM joint taskforce on perioperative outcome measures. *Eur J Anaesthesiol.* 2015;32(2):88–105.
8. McMillan RR, Berger A, Sima CS, et al. Thirty-day mortality underestimates the risk of early death after major resections for thoracic malignancies. *Ann Thorac Surg.* 2014;98(5):1769–1774; discussion 74–75.
9. Traibi A, Grigoroiu M, Boulitrop C, et al. Predictive factors for complications of anatomical pulmonary segmentectomies. *Interact Cardiovasc Thorac Surg.* 2013;17(5):838–844.
10. Chen FF, Zhang D, Wang YL, Xiong B. Video-assisted thoracoscopic surgery lobectomy versus open lobectomy in patients with

clinical stage non-small cell lung cancer: a meta-analysis. *Eur J Surg Oncol.* 2013;39(9):957–963.

11. Canet J, Gallart L, Gomar C, et al. Prediction of postoperative pulmonary complications in a population-based surgical cohort. *Anesthesiology.* 2010;113(6):1338–1350.
12. Mazo V, Sabate S, Canet J, et al. Prospective external validation of a predictive score for postoperative pulmonary complications. *Anesthesiology.* 2014;121(2):219–231.
13. Yang J, Xia Y, Yang Y, et al. Risk factors for major adverse events of video-assisted thoracic surgery lobectomy for lung cancer. *Int J Med Sci.* 2014;11(9):863–869.
14. Licker M, de Perrot M, Spiliopoulos A, et al. Risk factors for acute lung injury after thoracic surgery for lung cancer. *Anesth Analg.* 2003;97(6):1558–1565.
15. Ceppa DP, Kosinski AS, Berry MF, et al. Thoracoscopic lobectomy has increasing benefit in patients with poor pulmonary function: a Society of Thoracic Surgeons Database analysis. *Ann Surg.* 2012;256(3):487–493.
16. Mehta H, Osasona A, Shan Y, Goodwin JS, Okereke IC. Trends and outcomes of thoracoscopic lobectomy or segmentectomy: a national surgical quality improvement project analysis. *Semin Thorac Cardiovasc Surg.* 2018;30(3):350–359.
17. Fernandez-Perez ER, Keegan MT, Brown DR, Hubmayr RD, Gajic O. Intraoperative tidal volume as a risk factor for respiratory failure after pneumonectomy. *Anesthesiology.* 2006;105(1):141–148.
18. Serpa Neto A, Hemmes SN, Barbas CS, et al. Protective versus conventional ventilation for surgery: a systematic review and individual patient data meta-analysis. *Anesthesiology.* 2015;123(1):66–78.
19. Serpa Neto A, Hemmes SN, Barbas CS, et al. Incidence of mortality and morbidity related to postoperative lung injury in patients who have undergone abdominal or thoracic surgery: a systematic review and meta-analysis. *Lancet Respir Med.* 2014;2(12):1007–1015.
20. Kent M, Wang T, Whyte R, Curran T, Flores R, Gangadharan S. Open, video-assisted thoracic surgery, and robotic lobectomy: review of a national database. *Ann Thorac Surg.* 2014;97(1):236–242; discussion 42–44.
21. Cable DG, Deschamps C, Allen MS, et al. Lobar torsion after pulmonary resection: presentation and outcome. *J Thorac Cardiovasc Surg.* 2001;122(6):1091–1093.
22. Dai J, Xie D, Wang H, et al. Predictors of survival in lung torsion: a systematic review and pooled analysis. *J Thorac Cardiovasc Surg.* 2016;152(3):737–745 e3.
23. Senbaklavaci O, Taspinar H, Hartert M, Ergun S, Keranen S, Vahl CF. Lobar lung resection in elderly patients with non-small cell lung carcinoma: impact of cardiac comorbidity on surgical outcome. *Swiss Med Wkly.* 2012;142:w13742.
24. Froehlich JB, Fleisher LA. Noncardiac surgery in the patient with heart disease. *Med Clin North Am.* 2009;93(5):995–1016.
25. Patel AY, Eagle KA, Vaishnava P. Cardiac risk of noncardiac surgery. *J Am Coll Cardiol.* 2015;66(19):2140–2148.
26. Wang Z, Zhang J, Cheng Z, et al. Factors affecting major morbidity after video-assisted thoracic surgery for lung cancer. *J Surg Res.* 2014;192(2):628–634.
27. van Diepen S, Bakal JA, McAlister FA, Ezekowitz JA. Mortality and readmission of patients with heart failure, atrial fibrillation, or coronary artery disease undergoing noncardiac surgery: an analysis of 38 047 patients. *Circulation.* 2011;124(3):289–296.
28. Marcucci C, Chassot PG, Gardaz JP, et al. Fatal myocardial infarction after lung resection in a patient with prophylactic preoperative coronary stenting. *Br J Anaesth.* 2004;92(5):743–747.
29. Levine GN, Bates ER, Bittl JA, et al. 2016 ACC/AHA guideline focused update on duration of dual antiplatelet therapy in patients with coronary artery disease: a report of the American College of Cardiology/American Heart Association Task Force on Clinical Practice Guidelines: an update of the 2011 ACCF/AHA/SCAI guideline for percutaneous coronary intervention, 2011 ACCF/AHA guideline for coronary artery bypass graft surgery, 2012 ACC/AHA/ACP/AATS/PCNA/SCAI/STS guideline for the diagnosis and management of patients with stable ischemic heart disease, 2013 ACCF/AHA guideline for the management of ST-elevation myocardial infarction, 2014 AHA/ACC guideline for the management of patients with non-ST-elevation acute coronary syndromes, and 2014 ACC/AHA guideline on perioperative cardiovascular evaluation and management of patients undergoing noncardiac surgery. *Circulation.* 2016;134(10):e123–e155.
30. Nkomo VT, Gardin JM, Skelton TN, Gottdiener JS, Scott CG, Enriquez-Sarano M. Burden of valvular heart diseases: a population-based study. *Lancet.* 2006;368(9540):1005–1011.
31. Agarwal S, Rajamanickam A, Bajaj NS, et al. Impact of aortic stenosis on postoperative outcomes after noncardiac surgeries. *Circ Cardiovasc Qual Outcomes.* 2013;6(2):193–200.
32. Lai HC, Lai HC, Lee WL, et al. Impact of chronic advanced aortic regurgitation on the perioperative outcome of noncardiac surgery. *Acta Anaesthesiol Scand.* 2010;54(5):580–588.
33. Bajaj NS, Agarwal S, Rajamanickam A, et al. Impact of severe mitral regurgitation on postoperative outcomes after noncardiac surgery. *Am J Med.* 2013;126(6):529–535.
34. Nishimura RA, Otto CM, Bonow RO, et al. 2017 AHA/ACC focused update of the 2014 AHA/ACC guideline for the management of patients with valvular heart disease: a report of the American College of Cardiology/American Heart Association Task Force on Clinical Practice Guidelines. *Circulation.* 2017;135(25):e1159–e1195.
35. Flu WJ, van Kuijk JP, Hoeks SE, et al. Prognostic implications of asymptomatic left ventricular dysfunction in patients undergoing vascular surgery. *Anesthesiology.* 2010;112(6):1316–1324.
36. Gelzinis T, Assaad S, Perrino Jr AC. Right ventricular function during and after thoracic surgery. *Curr Opin Anaesthesiol.* 2020;33(1):27–36.
37. Venuta F, Sciomer S, Andreetti C, et al. Long-term Doppler echocardiographic evaluation of the right heart after major lung resections. *Eur J Cardiothorac Surg.* 2007;32(5):787–790.
38. Amar D, Burt ME, Roistacher N, Reinsel RA, Ginsberg RJ, Wilson RS. Value of perioperative Doppler echocardiography in patients undergoing major lung resection. *Ann Thorac Surg.* 1996;61(2):516–520.
39. Steffen HJ, Kalverkamp S, Zayat R, et al. Is systolic right ventricular function reduced after thoracic non-cardiac surgery? A propensity matched echocardiographic analysis. *Ann Thorac Cardiovasc Surg.* 2018;24(5):238–246.
40. Alviar CL, Miller PE, McAreavey D, et al. Positive pressure ventilation in the cardiac intensive care unit. *J Am Coll Cardiol.* 2018;72(13):1532–1553.
41. Kozian A, Schilling T, Schutze H, Senturk M, Hachenberg T, Hedenstierna G. Ventilatory protective strategies during thoracic surgery: effects of alveolar recruitment maneuver and low-tidal volume ventilation on lung density distribution. *Anesthesiology.* 2011;114(5):1025–1035.
42. Lohser J, Slinger P. Lung injury after one-lung ventilation: a review of the pathophysiologic mechanisms affecting the ventilated and the collapsed lung. *Anesth Analg.* 2015;121(2):302–318.

43. Haverkamp W, Hachenberg T. Post-thoracotomy dysrhythmia. *Curr Opin Anaesthesiol.* 2016;29(1):26–33.
44. Elrakhawy HM, Alassal MA, Elsadeck N, Shaalan A, Ezeldin TH, Shalabi A. Predictive factors of supraventricular arrhythmias after noncardiac thoracic surgery: a multicenter study. *Heart Surg Forum.* 2014;17(6):E308–E312.
45. Frendl G, Sodickson AC, Chung MK, et al. 2014 AATS guidelines for the prevention and management of perioperative atrial fibrillation and flutter for thoracic surgical procedures. *J Thorac Cardiovasc Surg.* 2014;148(3):e153–e193.
46. Frendl G, Sodickson AC, Chung MK, et al. 2014 AATS guidelines for the prevention and management of perioperative atrial fibrillation and flutter for thoracic surgical procedures. Executive summary. *J Thorac Cardiovasc Surg.* 2014;148(3):772–791.
47. Riber LP, Christensen TD, Jensen HK, Hoejsgaard A, Pilegaard HK. Amiodarone significantly decreases atrial fibrillation in patients undergoing surgery for lung cancer. *Ann Thorac Surg.* 2012; 94(2):339–344; discussion 45–46.
48. Gill J, Heel RC, Fitton A. Amiodarone. An overview of its pharmacological properties, and review of its therapeutic use in cardiac arrhythmias. *Drugs.* 1992;43(1):69–110.
49. Del Sorbo L, Vendramin A, Mehta S. High flow oxygen therapy in adult critically ill patients. *Minerva Anestesiol.* 2017;83(4):402–411.
50. Stephan F, Barrucand B, Petit P, et al. High-flow nasal oxygen vs noninvasive positive airway pressure in hypoxemic patients after cardiothoracic surgery: a randomized clinical trial. *JAMA.* 2015;313(23):2331–2339.
51. Ansari BM, Hogan MP, Collier TJ, et al. A randomized controlled trial of high-flow nasal oxygen (optiflow) as part of an enhanced recovery program after lung resection surgery. *Ann Thorac Surg.* 2016;101(2):459–464.
52. Schussler O, Alifano M, Dermine H, et al. Postoperative pneumonia after major lung resection. *Am J Respir Crit Care Med.* 2006;173(10):1161–1169.
53. Laroumagne S, Lepage B, Hermant C, et al. Bronchial colonisation in patients with lung cancer: a prospective study. *Eur Respir J.* 2013;42(1):220–229.
54. Hedenstierna G, Rothen HU. Respiratory function during anesthesia: effects on gas exchange. *Compr Physiol.* 2012;2(1):69–96.
55. Hedenstierna G. Oxygen and anesthesia: what lung do we deliver to the post-operative ward? *Acta Anaesthesiol Scand.* 2012;56(6): 675–685.
56. Cerfolio RJ, Bryant AS. The benefits of continuous and digital air leak assessment after elective pulmonary resection: a prospective study. *Ann Thorac Surg.* 2008;86(2):396–401.
57. Singhal S, Ferraris VA, Bridges CR, et al. Management of alveolar air leaks after pulmonary resection. *Ann Thorac Surg.* 2010; 89(4):1327–1335.
58. Brunelli A, Sabbatini A, Xiume F, Refai MA, Salati M, Marasco R. Alternate suction reduces prolonged air leak after pulmonary lobectomy: a randomized comparison versus water seal. *Ann Thorac Surg.* 2005;80(3):1052–1055.
59. Leo F, Duranti L, Girelli L, et al. Does external pleural suction reduce prolonged air leak after lung resection? Results from the AirINTrial after 500 randomized cases. *Ann Thorac Surg.* 2013;96(4): 1234–1239.
60. Zardo P, Busk H, Kutschka I. Chest tube management: state of the art. *Curr Opin Anaesthesiol.* 2015;28(1):45–49.
61. Abu-Hijleh M, Styrvoky K, Anand V, et al. Intrabronchial valves for air leaks after lobectomy, segmentectomy, and lung volume reduction surgery. *Lung.* 2019;197(5):627–633.
62. Elrakhawy HM, Alassal MA, Shaalan AM, Awad AA, Sayed S, Saffan MM. Impact of major pulmonary resections on right ventricular function: early postoperative changes. *Heart Surg Forum.* 2018;21(1):E009–E017.
63. Licker MJ, Widikker I, Robert J, et al. Operative mortality and respiratory complications after lung resection for cancer: impact of chronic obstructive pulmonary disease and time trends. *Ann Thorac Surg.* 2006;81(5):1830–1837.
64. Kutlu CA, Williams EA, Evans TW, Pastorino U, Goldstraw P. Acute lung injury and acute respiratory distress syndrome after pulmonary resection. *Ann Thorac Surg.* 2000;69(2):376–380.
65. Dulu A, Pastores SM, Park B, Riedel E, Rusch V, Halpern NA. Prevalence and mortality of acute lung injury and ARDS after lung resection. *Chest.* 2006;130(1):73–78.
66. Kozower BD, Sheng S, O'Brien SM, et al. STS database risk models: predictors of mortality and major morbidity for lung cancer resection. *Ann Thorac Surg.* 2010;90(3):875–881; discussion 81–83.

28 Extracorporeal Ventilatory Therapies

STEVEN P. KELLER

Introduction

Clinical use of extracorporeal ventilatory support technologies is increasing exponentially with an expanding range of indications for patients with cardiopulmonary disease.[1–3] Rapid adoption is occurring despite limited basic and translational research on extracorporeal support and only a handful of large-scale multicenter trials to inform clinical practice.[4–6] At present, clinicians must rely on pathophysiologic reasoning and understanding of device technology to guide the initiation, titration, and weaning of support.

Expanding deployment of extracorporeal devices has also led to an evolution in the methods used to initiate support. From its early role as an extension of the cardiopulmonary bypass circuit, in which support was initiated in the operating room for patients unable to wean from bypass following cardiotomy, extracorporeal support is increasingly a component of advanced critical care and is available for bedside deployment in intensive care units at tertiary medical centers.[7,8] As support expands to new indications and different patient populations, cannulation of peripheral vessels has also expanded to include not only surgical vascular cutdowns but also percutaneous methods more common to the intensivist. The use of extracorporeal ventilatory therapies to provide circulatory support, including in cases of active cardiopulmonary arrest, further fuels demand for clinicians to become familiar with the management and physiologic effects of these new devices.[9]

This chapter will review the development of extracorporeal ventilatory therapies and discuss their implementation and management in supporting patients with respiratory and circulatory failure and issues specific to perioperative management. The chapter concludes with a brief discussion of future trends in development of novel means of providing extracorporeal support and will emphasize avenues for ongoing investigation.

Development of Extracorporeal Ventilatory Therapies

Historical Overview

The development of extracorporeal support technologies is intrinsically linked to the work of 19th century physiologists investigating methods to support isolated limbs and ex vivo organs.[10,11] Experimental physiologists sought to replicate the perfusion and respiratory functions of the heart and lungs. Efforts to achieve extracorporeal ventilation through direct exposure of blood to air led to the bubble oxygenator, in which small bubbles of oxygen were passed through reservoirs of blood, and the film oxygenator, in which blood was conveyed as a thin film over which oxygen was passed to achieve gas exchange.[12] The subsequent discovery of heparin enabled controlled anticoagulation and clinical use of oxygenator methods that relied on direct contact of blood and gas. Concurrent with exploration of extracorporeal ventilation methods was the development of perfusion systems to maintain blood flow to ex vivo organs.[13] These efforts led to the first clinically used cardiopulmonary bypass circuit consisting of a peristaltic roller pump coupled to a film oxygenator to maintain perfusion and provide gas exchange.[14]

Hollow Fiber Membrane Devices and Modern Oxygenators

Early oxygenators relying on direct air and blood contact were plagued by complications, such as gas embolization and the propensity to form clots. These difficulties motivated efforts to develop gas exchange devices modeled on the lung, in which blood is separated from inspired air by the alveolar epithelial and capillary endothelial membranes.[15] The first membrane oxygenator consisted of polyethylene tubing wrapped around a central longitudinal axis. This design was adapted from early efforts to produce an artificial kidney and was inspired by the observation that aerated dialysates led to oxygenation of blood pumped through the device.[16] This work prompted the search for the ideal oxygenator biomaterial capable of providing gas transfer, while limiting plasma diffusion across the membrane to maintain device function and operational life. The ability to make silicone into a thin film, coupled with its excellent gas diffusion properties, led to its use in the first membrane oxygenator widely deployed in clinical practice.[17] Improvements in fabrication techniques and device construction led to the widespread adoption of silicone membrane oxygenators in the 1980s.

The advent of poly-4-methyl-1-pentene (PMP) as a biomaterial, with its highly efficient gas transfer properties and

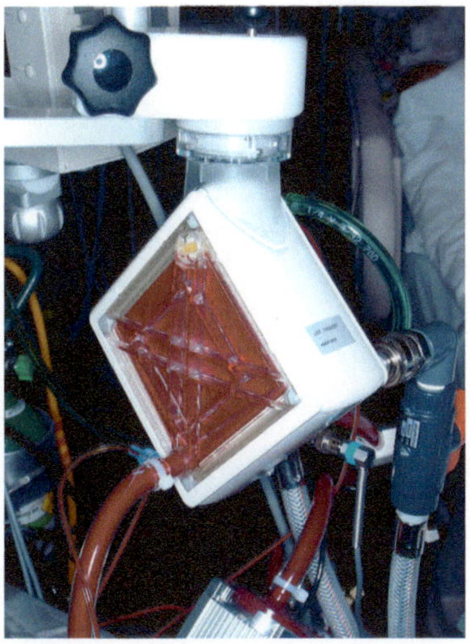

• **Fig. 28.1** Modern hollow fiber membrane oxygenator. Blood passes around the fibers which carry a sweep gas. Diffusion across fiber membranes achieves gas exchange. Heated water is passed through the housing of the oxygenator to maintain blood temperature. (From Gutsche JT, Harish R. *Extracorporeal Membrane Oxygenation, Kaplan's Cardiac Anesthesia*. 2017:1214–1228. © 2017. Polymethylpentene membrane oxygenator. With permission.)

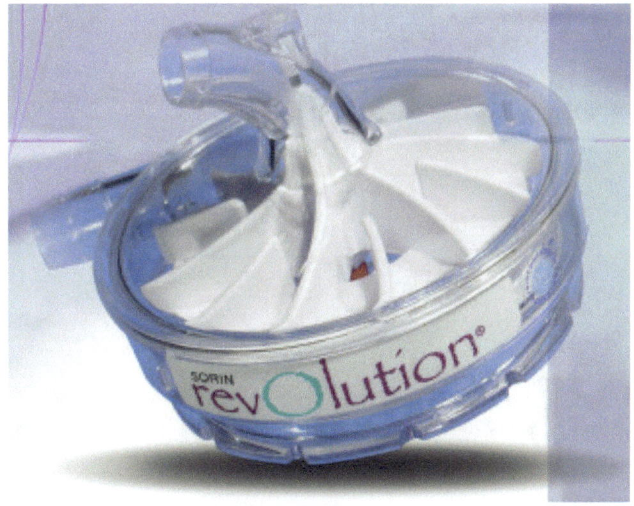

• **Fig. 28.2** Example of a centrifugal pump representative of pumps used in modern extracorporeal membrane oxygenation circuits. (From Groom RC, Fitzgerald, D. *Extracorporeal Devices and Related Technologies, Kaplan's Cardiac Anesthesia*. 2017:1162–1213. © 2017. (Courtesy Sorin Group, Arvada, CO. With permission.)

limited plasma leakage, led to the development of the modern oxygenator.[18] Newer devices based on PMP are capable of providing prolonged support, often several weeks or longer, before the need for replacement because of reduced performance. An example of a commercially available PMP-based hollow fiber oxygenator is shown in Fig. 28.1. In modern oxygenators, blood is pumped through the device where it comes into contact with sheets of hollow fibers carrying a sweep gas. As carbon dioxide diffuses more rapidly into blood than oxygen because of its higher solubility, oxygenators are designed for blood transiting through the device to have multiple interactions with fiber bundles to achieve adequate oxygenation. Carbon dioxide removal by the device, in turn, is determined by: (1) blood flow rate through the device; (2) sweep gas flow rate; and (3) sweep gas composition.[19]

Pump Technology

Early extracorporeal devices relied on peristaltic pumps, widely used in a variety of clinical applications, such as dialysis machines, infusion pumps, and cardiopulmonary bypass machines, to withdraw blood and pass it through the circuit.[13] Ease of implementation, minimal priming volume, and a set relationship between revolutions per minute (RPMs) and the flow delivered motivated their adoption in early devices. However, these pumps generate flow through physical compression of the tubing, causing trauma to the blood and activation of platelets and leukocytes, while friction of the pump rollers on the tubing creates wear over time, and may lead to tubing rupture and embolization of small pieces of the tubing.[20]

Centrifugal pumps produce less heating and markedly reduced platelet and leukocyte activation compared with peristaltic pumps, resulting in their rapid integration into modern extracorporeal circuits.[21] Centrifugal pumps can still induce hemolysis, but this is partially dependent on pump speed, with increased levels of red blood cell destruction observed at extremes of device function.[22] Priming of centrifugal pumps is more challenging, and entrained air can be difficult to extract. The high operational speed of centrifugal pumps, typically 2500 to 5000 RPMs, is also a hurdle to the integration of autoregulatory feedback into device operation. An example of a commonly used and commercially available centrifugal pump is shown in Fig. 28.2.

The Modern Extracorporeal Membrane Oxygenation Circuit

Extracorporeal ventilatory support therapies in current clinical practice largely consist of implementations of extracorporeal membrane oxygenation (ECMO) circuits such that the terms can be used interchangeably. However, with the advance of newer, more specialized extracorporeal ventilatory therapies, the terminology of ECMO will likely become associated with a specific device configuration. ECMO itself is a confusing term because it is simultaneously used to refer both to circulatory and ventilatory support implementations of the same device. The specific therapeutic function is dependent on the cannulation strategy used.

The core components of the ECMO circuit consist of: (1) membrane oxygenator; (2) centrifugal pump and pump controller; (3) heater; and (4) vascular cannula and circuit tubing.[23,24] A schematic of the core components of an ECMO circuit is shown in Fig. 28.3. Additional circuit components, such as flow meters and air bubble detectors, can be integrated to provide expanded monitoring capabilities and safeguards to reduce complications. Modern oxygenators also maintain blood at a desired temperature by the passage of heated water through the device housing.

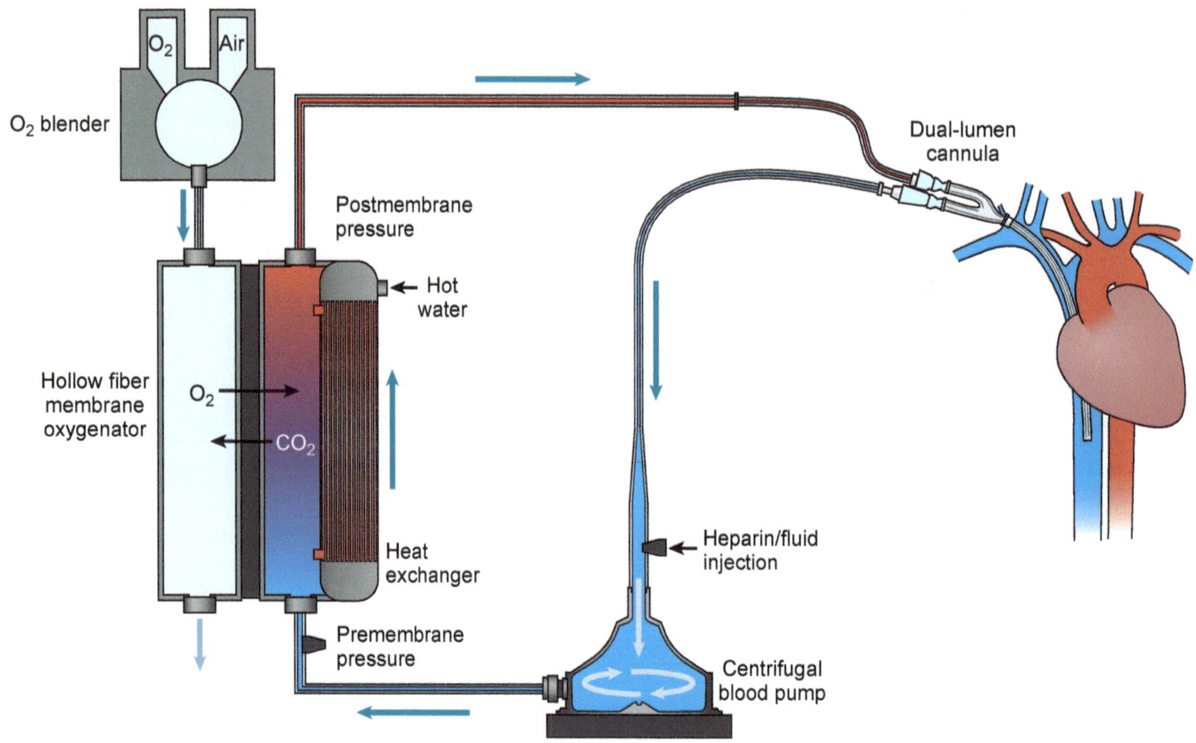

• **Fig. 28.3** Schematic of components of a typical extracorporeal membrane oxygenation circuit. Core components include: (1) vascular cannula and tubing to provide blood flow to and from the device; (2) centrifugal pump to maintain perfusion through the device; (3) oxygenator to provide gas exchange with a blender and flow meter to vary fraction of oxygen and flow rate for sweep gas; and (4) heater to maintain body temperature. (Modified with permission from a figure created by Dr. Brian Y. Chang.)

An example of a modern ECMO using an integrated pump and oxygenator unit mounted on the controller is shown in Fig. 28.4.

Clinical Adoption of Extracorporeal Membrane Oxygenation Support

The first widely reported successful clinical use of ECMO took place at the California Pacific Medical Center in San Francisco in 1971, in which a 24-year-old man with trauma-related acute respiratory distress syndrome (ARDS) was supported for 75 hours with a modified form of extracorporeal bypass, followed by gradual recovery and hospital discharge.[25] Further anecdotal case experience motivated a National Institutes of Health sponsored prospective, randomized, multicenter controlled trial in the early 1970s to compare outcomes for patients with acute respiratory failure supported by conventional medical therapy versus ECMO.[26] In the setting of mortality rates of 90% for both groups, the trial was halted prematurely following enrollment of only 90 patients in total. The lack of success of this and subsequent trials dampened enthusiasm for the use of extracorporeal support for adult patients and hampered research and development efforts.

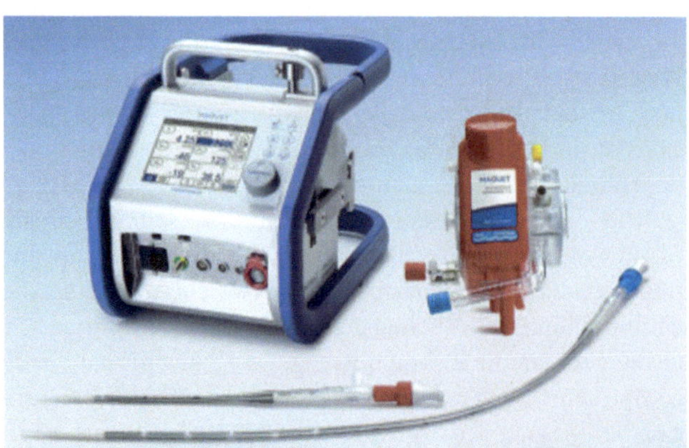

• **Fig. 28.4** Modern extracorporeal membrane oxygenation circuit consisting of vascular cannula, integrated oxygenator and centrifugal pump, and circuit controller. (Reprinted with permission from Getinge AB.)

Despite negative trials in adult patients, case experience with ECMO support in neonatal respiratory failure demonstrated marked improvement in mortality compared with predicated outcomes with traditional therapy.[8] Multiple factors likely contributed to the different outcomes observed in neonates compared with adults, which included prompt initiation of support; different etiology of lung disease in neonates with the primary cause being airway immaturity; and plasticity of the newborn lung. Subsequent clinical trials and accumulating evidence of efficacy led to ECMO becoming the preferred support modality for some forms of neonatal respiratory failure.

Although ECMO gained an increasing presence in pediatric hospitals, it was used on a limited basis as a means of supporting postcardiotomy adult patients unable to wean from cardiopulmonary bypass. By the time of the H1N1 influenza pandemic in 2009, expanding ECMO capability in adult cardiac surgical intensive care units made extracorporeal support an accessible salvage therapy for adult ARDS patients. The pandemic caused a surge in previously healthy patients now critically ill with severe ARDS generating renewed interest in ECMO as a support modality. A large-scale multicenter trial comparing ECMO with traditional ARDS therapy, although flawed by variations in practices and experience level between clinical sites, favored treatment of patients with ARDS at centers capable of providing ECMO support.[5]

Following the H1N1 pandemic, the global number of ECMO centers doubled within seven years.[2] The increase in ECMO centers coincided with concomitant growth in use of ECMO as support modality. Clinical indications in adult patients are expanding beyond postcardiotomy circulatory failure and salvage therapy in ARDS to providing support for patients as a bridge to transplant and for patients with medical cardiogenic shock.[27–29] Potential indications continue to expand as extracorporeal approaches are being trialed as an alternative to conventional therapies for procedural and operative support.

Extracorporeal Membrane Oxygenation Circuit Operational Parameters

Cannulation Approaches and Support Modality

ECMO can be categorized as providing two primary forms of support: ventilatory and circulatory. A third possibility consists of a combination of both forms for the patient in circulatory shock with profound concomitant lung failure. The cannulation strategy deployed determines the form of support provided by the ECMO circuit. For this chapter, the following terminology will be used:

- Venovenous (VV) ECMO: ventilatory support
- Venoarterial (VA) ECMO: circulatory support
- Venoarteriovenous (VAV) ECMO: ventilatory and circulatory support

These terms are used to describe the source of blood entering the circuit (venous) followed by the anatomic site of the blood returned to the patient from the circuit (venous or arterial or a combination of both). VA ECMO can be further described depending on whether the site of cannulation is central VA ECMO, consisting of direct bicaval or right atrial drainage of venous blood and return of oxygenated blood to the aortic arch, or peripheral VA ECMO, in which cannula are inserted into the peripheral vasculature, most commonly the femoral vessels, for drainage and return.[30–32] The differences in anatomic site of cannulation in central and peripheral VA ECMO are shown in Fig. 28.5. In the case of central VA ECMO, the return cannula supplies oxygenated blood to the proximal aortic arch and provides physiologic support for both ventilatory and circulatory failure. As clinical use of ECMO has expanded and initiation of support has extended from the surgical theater to the intensive care unit and emergency department, peripheral cannulation methods relying on the Seldinger technique and serial dilation have become more common to establish vascular access and initiate support.[33–36]

For this chapter, the cannula used to remove blood from the patient and direct it to the ECMO circuit is termed the **withdrawal cannula**, whereas the cannula carrying oxygenated blood from the ECMO circuit to the patient will be referred to as the **return cannula**. To accommodate high blood flow rates (≥4 L/min), withdrawal cannula typically are large bore (21 or 25 Fr). The withdrawal cannula can be single stage, with a single inlet at the end of the cannula, or multistage, in which small holes are placed at intervals along the length of the cannula to achieve improved drainage.[37] Percutaneously placed withdrawal cannula are typically advanced in the inferior vena cava to the level right atrium, with the cannula ranging in length from 50 to 60 cm. Return cannula are frequently shorter, 18 cm is a common length to accommodate placement in the internal jugular vein or femoral artery, depending on the modality of support, and vary in diameter from 15 to 21 Fr. Double lumen cannula, designed for placement in the internal jugular vein with the distal tip residing in the inferior vena cava (IVC) and with holes in the superior vena cava (SVC) to provide for drainage of both upper body and lower body venous blood and an outlet for return of oxygenated blood to the right atrium, are used in VV ECMO to facilitate ambulation.[38] The different approaches to cannulation for providing VV ECMO support are shown in Fig. 28.6.

This terminology applies to the most commonly used configurations utilized in clinical practice. Because VV ECMO provides for gas exchange to support lung failure, use of this configuration requires adequate heart function to maintain end-organ perfusion. VA ECMO achieves circulatory support through shunting blood from the systemic venous to the systemic arterial circulation. This configuration profoundly alters systemic hemodynamics with specific effects depending on support titration and the physiologic state of the patient. VAV ECMO is less commonly used and is primarily attempted in patients with combined respiratory and circulatory failure.[35]

Circuit Operational Parameters

The basic components of the ECMO circuit have few functional parameters for titration of support. ECMO circuit flow is a function of: (1) pump speed; (2) afterload to the pump including circuit resistance and patient vascular resistance; (3) patient volume status and the negative pressure threshold for vascular collapse around the withdrawal cannula; and (4) cardiac function.[27] Oxygenator gas exchange is a function of the sweep gas flow rate and composition of the sweep gas. Increasing the sweep gas flow rate increases removal of carbon dioxide whereas increasing the oxygen fraction increases the diffusion gradient to increase

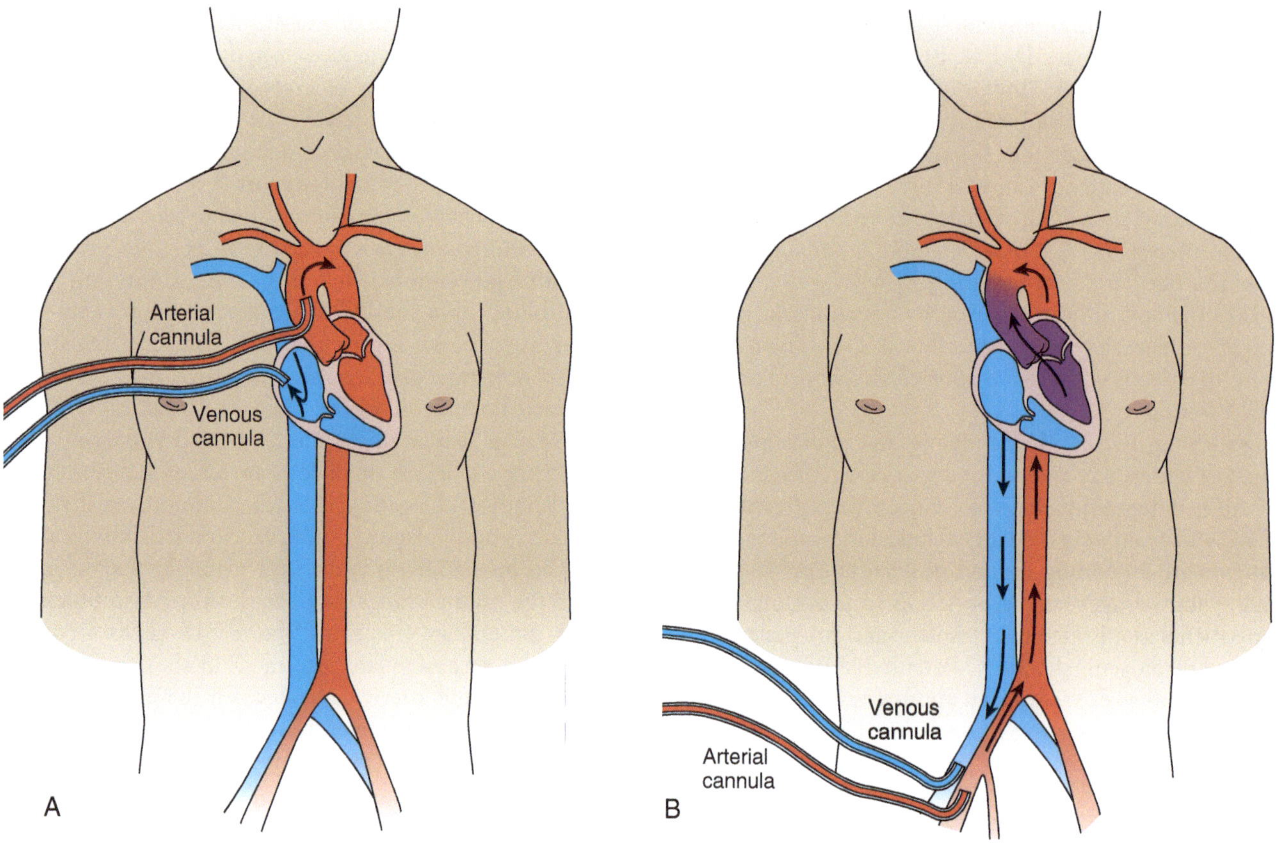

• **Fig. 28.5** Schematic of the cannulation approach in venoarterial extracorporeal membrane oxygenation (VA ECMO). (**A**) Central VA ECMO with placement of withdrawal cannula in the right atrium and return cannula carrying oxygenated blood in the aortic arch. (**B**) Peripheral VA ECMO with placement of withdrawal cannula in the femoral vein and advanced to the right atrium inferior vena cava junction. Return cannula is placed in the femoral artery.

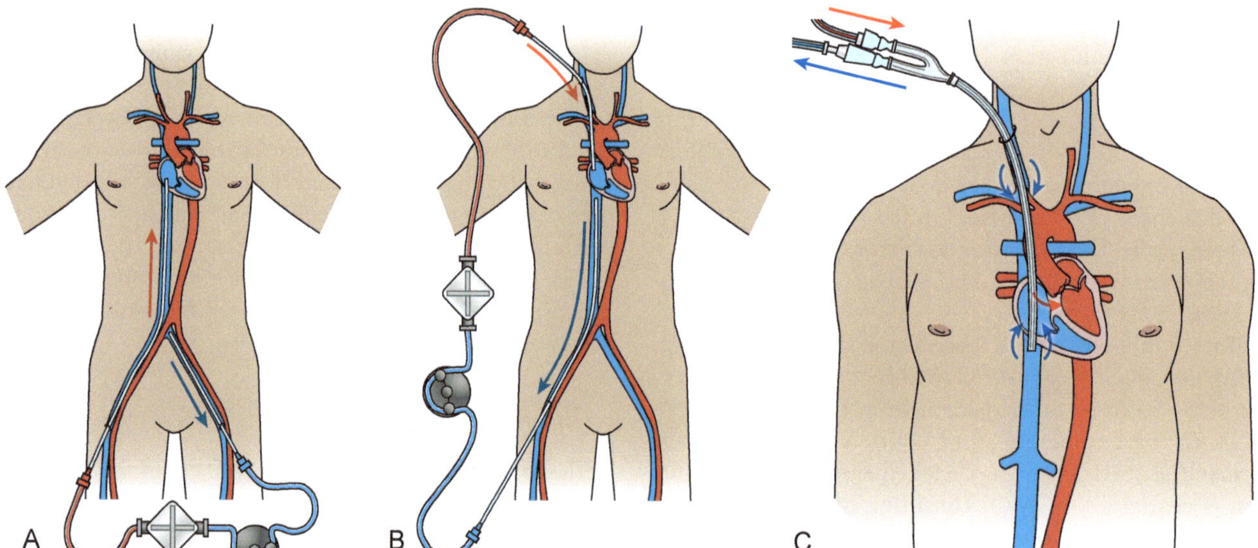

• **Fig. 28.6** Representation of venovenous extracorporeal membrane oxygenation cannulation strategies. (**A**) Femoral-femoral vein cannulation approach. Withdrawal cannula is placed within the inferior vena cava (IVC) inferior to the return cannula which terminates in the right atrium. (**B**) Femoral-internal jugular (IJ) vein cannulation approach with blood withdrawal via the femoral cannula and return via the IJ cannula. (**C**) Single dual lumen bicaval cannula advanced via the IJ into the IVC with the return outlet directed towards the tricuspid valve. (Modified from Marasco SF, Lukas G, et al. Review of ECMO (extra corporeal membrane oxygenation) support in critically ill adult patients. *Heart Lung Circulation*. 2008;17(4):S41–S47. © 2008. Figures 1 (Central ECMO cannulation.) and 2 (Peripheral ECMO cannulation.).)

delivery to the blood. Support provided by ECMO is a complex integration of device operation and patient physiologic state and anatomy.

Pump speed is the major parameter available to readily adjust circuit flow. The RPM range that constitutes safe operation is specific to a given pump with speeds at either extreme associated with increased risk of hemolysis. High RPMs damage cells from accelerated velocities and increased shear stress, whereas low RPMs result in inefficient propulsion of flow with blood circulating multiple times through a pump before being expelled causing accumulated stress.[39,40] Circuit blood flow is also partially determined by **pump afterload**. Factors that increase afterload include clot formation within the oxygenator or at connection points in the circuit, kinking or obstruction of the return cannula, and high pressure within the return circulation of the patient. For VV ECMO, in which the return cannula is placed in the venous system, this is less of an issue than for VA ECMO where the pump must work against the pressure of the arterial system. As vascular pressure increases, the amount of flow provided by the ECMO circuit decreases resulting in a reduction in support. Flow is also limited by drain pressure generated by the pump at the withdrawal cannula. As pump RPMs are increased, negative pressure is generated at the drain site within the venous system risking venous collapse around the cannula resulting in a suction event and temporary cessation of flow.

Blood contact with cannulas, tubing, pump, and oxygenator promotes clotting cascade activation increasing the risk of thromboemboli to the patient and circuit failure from thrombosis.[41] Whereas novel antithrombotic coatings and new biomaterials hold promise in reducing clot formation, anticoagulation remains an important consideration.[42–44] This is particularly relevant in circulatory support, in which blood is returned to the systemic arterial circulation where a thromboembolism may cause a stroke or end-organ damage. Anticoagulation is also used in an effort to reduce clot formation within the oxygenator and to extend the operational life of the circuit. Heparin is most commonly used because of its availability, familiarity, and reversibility in the setting of active bleeding. The site of administration, whether delivered systemically or into the circuit, the therapeutic target range, and the laboratory test used to titrate therapy vary between centers all lack definitive evidence to guide a specific approach.

Common ECMO circuit measurements include withdrawal and return pressures and pressures measured across the oxygenator. An increasing pressure drop across the oxygenator can signify clot formation leading to increased flow resistance. Some devices include continuous oxygen saturation measurements of the venous blood, which is a useful marker of recirculation of blood from the return to the withdrawal cannula during VV ECMO support. Additional features include bubble detectors to identify the presence of entrained air in the circuit and flow alarms.

Physiologic Basis of Extracorporeal Lung Support

The development of extracorporeal ventilatory therapies enables new approaches to care for the patient with respiratory failure while requiring determination of how to deploy these therapies to optimize clinical outcomes. Improved understanding of ventilator-associated lung injury motivates interest in ECMO for salvage support for patients with severe ARDS unable to be safely maintained with mechanical ventilation alone. For patients with end-stage lung disease, ECMO is a means of maintaining vitality while being listed or undergoing evaluation for lung transplantation.[29,45–47] The specific role, optimal timing of initiation, and how to titrate ECMO support are areas of active investigation without clear guidelines to aid the clinician in determining the approach to maximize clinical outcomes. This section details the physiologic basis of ECMO and discusses considerations in management of ECMO to provide ventilatory support.

Motivation of Extracorporeal Membrane Oxygenation Use as Bridge to Recovery in Lung Failure

Mechanical ventilation is the mainstay of support for the patient with respiratory failure, but it carries the risk of ventilator-induced lung injury (VILI).[48,49] Animal models of ARDS demonstrate that excessive distending pressures exacerbate underlying injury whereas hyperoxia leads to progressive lung inflammation and eventual death.[50,51] Multicenter clinical studies evaluating ventilation strategies in ARDS demonstrate improved mortality with low tidal volume ventilation (LTVV) approaches while subsequent analysis demonstrating that low lung compliance and high driving pressures are associated with worse patient outcomes.[52]

In the setting of severe disease, patients may either: (1) not be able to maintain homeostasis with LTVV or (2) may experience ongoing VILI and progressive lung disease despite ventilator optimization. The emergence of ECMO provides an alternative approach to supporting patients unable to be safely maintained with mechanical ventilation alone.[53] The motivation for use of ECMO is to maintain physiologic homeostasis while optimizing mechanical ventilation to limit lung injury and facilitate recovery from the underlying disease process. Similar reasoning applies to the use of ECMO for patients with bronchopleural fistulas in which extracorporeal support enables reduced need for positive pressure ventilation to promote lung healing.

The ability of ECMO to achieve its intended therapeutic purpose is dependent on multiple factors: (1) the severity of lung injury and residual gas exchange capacity of the lungs; (2) the specific physiologic impairment; and (3) the fraction of the cardiac output entrained into the ECMO circuit. Increasing severity of lung injury necessitates an increased load on the ECMO circuit to provide physiologic gas exchange. The specific nature of the impairment,

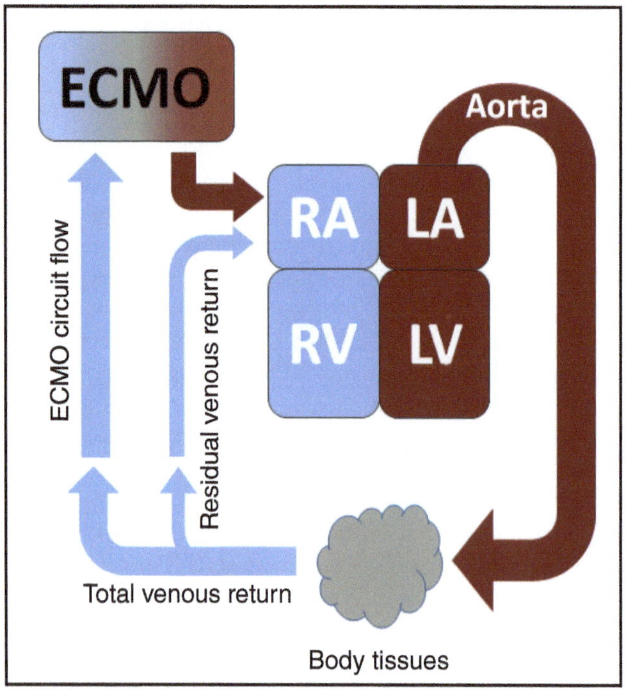

• **Fig. 28.7** Schematic of venovenous extracorporeal membrane oxygenation (*ECMO*) circulation. Venous blood is withdrawn from the inferior vena cava via a multistage withdrawal cannula and into the ECMO circuit. Nonoxygenated venous blood not entrained into the ECMO circuit enters the right atrium to mix with oxygenated blood returned from the ECMO circuit. Total oxygen delivery is a function of oxygenation provided by the ECMO circuits and lungs.

whether predominantly hypoxic or hypercapnic, determines the amount of blood flow required to be entrained into the device to achieve its physiologic support goal. The function of the ECMO circuit as a support modality in respiratory failure is intrinsically linked to gas transport in the body. A schematic of the integration of VV ECMO with the systemic venous circulation is shown in Fig. 28.7.

Physiology of Hypoxic and Hypercapnic Respiratory Failure

Approximately 97% of the oxygen content in the arterial circulation is bound to hemoglobin within red blood cells with the residual 3% of oxygen present as dissolved gas.[54] For ECMO to provide meaningful support to patients with predominantly hypoxic respiratory failure, a large fraction of the total circulating hemoglobin must be entrained into the ECMO circuit to provide adequate oxygen delivery. This reality determines the cannulation strategy and choice of cannula to achieve adequate circuit blood flow.

Unlike oxygen transport, carbon dioxide (CO_2) has an additional carrier in the form of bicarbonate ion which acts as a CO_2 reservoir in the blood. In arterial blood, approximately 90% of the total CO_2 is carried as bicarbonate ion with the remainder present equally as either dissolved gas or bound to hemoglobin.[55] The enzyme carbonic anhydrase, ubiquitous in red blood cells, reversibly interconverts bicarbonate and CO_2 via carbonic acid. The presence of the large reservoir provides additional CO_2 that can be ventilated as blood passes through the circuit.

Physiologic differences in oxygen and CO_2 transport in the body translate into differing efficacies in extracorporeal support. ECMO is more readily able to support a patient primarily suffering from hypercapnic respiratory failure at a lower blood flow rate in comparison to a patient with predominantly hypoxic failure. The function of the membrane oxygenator also provides for additional titration of gas exchange for CO_2 removal not readily available for oxygenation. Increasing the sweep gas rate allows for increased CO_2 clearance in comparison with oxygenation in which increasing the fraction of inspired oxygen (FiO_2) achieves only modestly increased total levels of oxygen delivery once hemoglobin is fully saturated.[19,56]

Cannulation Approaches to Provide Extracorporeal Lung Support

There are three primary VV cannulation approaches for providing ECMO lung support: (1) femoral vein and right internal jugular (RIJ) vein cannulation; (2) dual lumen bicaval cannulation via the RIJ vein; and (3) femoral vein-femoral vein cannulation. **The femoral-RIJ approach** generally provides for high blood flow levels (>4 liters per minute [LPM]) and is straightforward to manage. **Dual lumen bicaval cannula** offer upper and lower body venous drainage but typically achieve lower flow rates because of a smaller comparable lumen size in comparison to what can be achieved with a multistage withdrawal cannula. The return outlet of the dual lumen bicaval cannula is also prone to malpositioning and may induce turbulent flow to the right ventricle or cause recirculation within the cannula. An example of the positioning of a dual lumen bicaval cannula as seen on a chest radiograph is shown in Fig. 28.8 with a Doppler ultrasound demonstrating the flow from the return outlet shown in Fig. 28.9. **The femoral-femoral vein approach** is limited in achievable total flow because the withdrawal cannula must be positioned inferior to the return cannula, which reduces the amount of lower body venous return captured into the circuit. Each cannulation strategy offers specific benefits and drawbacks with a combination of patient anatomic factors, cannulating physician expertise, and physiologic demands of extracorporeal support determining the strategy used.

Clinical Management of Extracorporeal Membrane Oxygenation in Acute Respiratory Distress Syndrome

Despite the growing use of ECMO to support patient with ARDS, there is limited evidence from animal models or clinical studies to guide the clinician on the optimal use of this support modality. Key questions on the role of ECMO in ARDS which include: (1) when to initiate therapy; (2)

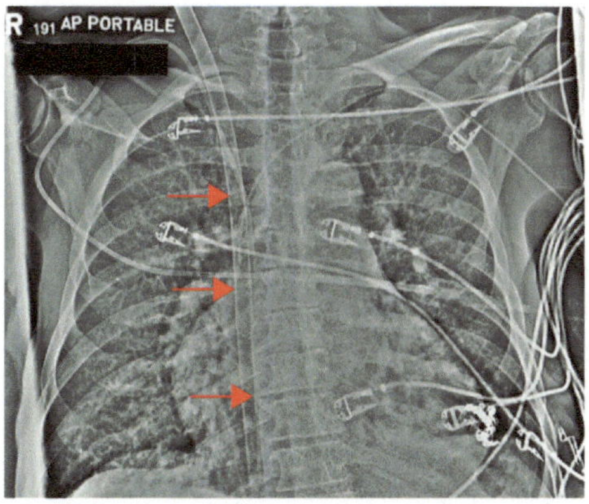

• **Fig. 28.8** Patient chest x-ray with dual lumen bicaval cannula placed via the right internal jugular and terminating in the inferior vena cava *(red arrows)*.

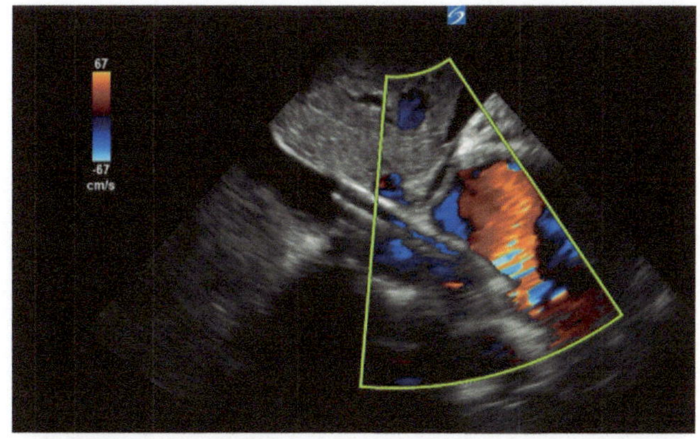

• **Fig. 28.9** Surface ultrasound with Doppler demonstrating return flow from the dual lumen bicaval cannula directed toward the tricuspid valve.

how to titrate mechanical ventilation; (3) how to manage persistent hypoxia; and (4) what is the optimal cannulation strategy.[53] This section discusses these questions and provides a framework for clinical management pending the availability of evidence-based guidelines.

Criteria to Initiate Extracorporeal Membrane Oxygenation Support

At present, ECMO is an advanced therapy for patients with ARDS unable to be safely maintained on mechanical ventilation. Clinicians must determine when in a patient's clinical course, the potential benefit from initiation of ECMO support outweighs the associated risks of this intensive resource. Factors such as circuit and personnel availability, cost, and patient selection criteria, must be weighed before cannulation, in addition to determining if ECMO support is capable of achieving the physiologic goals of support, which primarily consists of reducing VILI to provide for lung recovery.

Patient trajectory is a major challenge in determining the optimal time to initiate ECMO support. The argument for earlier initiation is that by preemptively limiting VILI, a patient's course will be shortened and survival improved. The counter argument is that earlier initiation deploys limited resources and exposes patients to the risk of cannulation and extracorporeal support unnecessarily. Increased availability of ECMO with advancing expertise will allow this argument to be determined by physiologic benefit as clinical practice evolves and evidence accumulates.

There are currently no evidence-based criteria to determine the threshold at which initiation of ECMO is recommended. Whereas prior clinical studies relied on patient mortality predictors such as the Lung Injury Score (also called the Murray Score) to determine if ECMO is indicated, there are no definitive metrics to guide the exact point at which cannulation will lead to improved outcomes.[4] An alternative approach to clinical scores is to deploy ECMO when mechanical ventilation parameters required to maintain patient homeostasis are at thresholds associated with VILI. Clinical judgement is required in managing an evolving patient requiring ventilatory support above the threshold for initiating ECMO, but who may experience improvement (such as in the case of a patient requiring high levels of oxygen in the setting of pulmonary edema that subsequently improves with diuresis, or a patient undergoing a trial of prone ventilation) and then no longer meet the criteria for ECMO.

Multiple factors are taken into consideration before the initiation of support which, include patient age, comorbidities and presence of any existing diagnoses with an anticipated survival of months to a year, preexisting lung disease, and severity of current illness.[57] Additional factors include duration of mechanical ventilation before initiation of ECMO, bleeding risks or contraindication to anticoagulation, and anatomic factors that may preclude safe cannulation. A proposed list of key physiologic criteria to use to guide the threshold for initiating ECMO support in ARDS is presented in Table 28.1. Determining which patients are most likely to benefit from ECMO respiratory support is an area of active investigation and definitive guidance is lacking. Table 28.2 provides suggested absolute and relative contraindications for use of ECMO in ARDS.

Initial Management of Extracorporeal Support

Following cannulation, circuit flow is gradually increased over a period of a few minutes. Contact of patient blood with the circuit, as well as rapid instillation of room temperature saline typically used to prime the circuit, can induce vasodilation and require fluid resuscitation or administration of vasopressors. Circuit RPMs are increased while monitoring flow rate and pressure at the circuit withdrawal and return sites. RPMs are increased until either: (1) the goal flow rate is achieved, (2) the RPM safe upper limit is reached, or (3) suction events occur at the withdrawal cannula limiting titration further up. Sweep gas flow rate is typically set to match the blood flow rate after which it is adjusted based on blood gas analysis and titration of ventilatory support. An important exception to this approach

TABLE 28.1 Criteria to Initiate Extracorporeal Membrane Oxygenation Support in Acute Respiratory Distress Syndrome Patients

Indications to Initiate Extracorporeal Membrane Oxygenation Lung Support

• PaO2:FiO2 ratio <80 mm Hg for >6 h in setting of ventilator optimization as listed subsequently:
  • FiO2 titrated to maintain goal PaO2 >60 mm Hg with goal FiO2 <75%
  • PEEP optimization
  • Prone position ventilation
  • Neuromuscular blockade

• P_{pl} >30 cm H_2O or DP >15 cm H_2O
• pH <7.15
• No trend toward improvement or presence of rapidly reversible process

ARDS, Acute respiratory distress syndrome; *DP*, driving pressure (calculated as DP = P_{pl} − PEEP); *ECMO*, extracorporeal membrane oxygenation; *FiO2*, fraction of inspired oxygen; *PaO2*, arterial partial pressure of oxygen; *PEEP*, positive end expiratory pressure; P_{pl}, plateau pressure.

is the case of severe hypercapnic failure.[58] For patients with hypercapnic failure of more than 48 hours duration, the rapid decrease in serum CO_2 levels enabled by ECMO is associated with worse neurologic outcomes, which motivates a strategy of gradual normalization of CO_2 levels over a period of 48 to 72 hours. To achieve this starting at a low sweep, often 0.5 LPM, and then titrating up slowly as guided by serial blood gas measurement is preferred to avoid overly rapid correction.

Management of Mechanical Ventilation

A key consideration following the initiation of ECMO support is how to optimally titrate mechanical ventilatory support to reduce VILI and promote lung recovery. General practice is to target "lung rest" ventilation settings, but what exactly constitutes these settings is undefined.[6,59] Conceptually, lung rest consists of reducing driving pressure, limiting plateau pressure, and maintaining nontoxic levels of oxygen support. In practice, these settings vary widely between centers with titration of ventilatory support also depending on the physiology of a specific patient.

Coupled with the uncertainty of specific parameters is whether mechanical ventilatory support itself is beneficial when patients are adequately supported on ECMO. Multiple centers have reported variable success in isolated case series of ARDS patients extubated and maintained on ECMO.[60–62] The benefit of this approach is the ability to limit sedation and engage in physical therapy. The uncertainty is whether removal of positive pressure promotes lung collapse and induces further injury from cyclic alveolar collapse and expansion during passive breathing.

Although definitive evidence is lacking to guide the optimal ventilation strategy, an approach that integrates insight

TABLE 28.2 Contraindications for Extracorporeal Membrane Oxygenation Support in Acute Respiratory Distress Syndrome Patients

Criteria	Consideration
Absolute contraindications:	
• Age >75 years	Specific age threshold is controversial
• Active solid or liquid malignancy	Limited or treatable disease may not be an absolute contraindication
• High-grade shock	Unstable septic shock or severe cardiogenic shock associated with poor outcomes; however, RV failure because of ARDS and/or high PEEP is an indication for ECMO support
• Multiorgan failure	Associated with poor outcomes
• Inability to tolerate anticoagulation	Anticoagulation required for initiation of support
• Irreversible neurologic injury	May be unable to access neurologic status in some patients before decision on whether to proceed with ECMO support
• Life expectancy <6 months	Underlying poor health with limited life expectancy before current illness is a contraindication to ECMO support
• Anatomic limitations on cannulation	
Relative contraindications:	
• Neutropenia or immune deficiency	ANC <500
• Thrombocytopenia	Platelets <50,000
• Unable to perform ADLs at baseline	Patients with a poor functional baseline unable to participate in rehabilitation
• Chronic respiratory insufficiency	FEV_1 <1 L or need for chronic oxygen therapy
• Morbid obesity or high body mass	ECMO may be unable to sustain patients requiring very high flows

ADL, Activities of daily living; *ANC*, absolute neutrophil count; *ARDS*, acute respiratory distress syndrome; *ECMO*, extracorporeal membrane oxygenation; FEV_1, forced expiratory volume in 1 second; *PEEP*, positive end expiratory pressure; *RV*, right ventricular.

from the mechanisms of VILI and understanding from animal models defines a clinical pathway. Maintaining positive pressure to promote an open lung following initiation of ECMO is a reasonable first approach. Static high pressures are well tolerated by the lung compared with dynamic pressure changes.[63,64] Using ventilator pressure-volume tools, esophageal balloon measures of intrathoracic pressure, or empiric best positive end-expiratory pressure (PEEP) measurements to titrate initial PEEP maintains an open lung on initiation of ECMO.

Selection of a ventilation mode is another area lacking definitive evidence. Regardless of the specific mode, limiting the driving pressure and tidal volume are the major emphasis, while achieving patient-ventilator synchrony are the primary parameters. Use of a pressure control mode, titrated to a low driving pressure (<10 cm H_2O), allows for both low tidal volumes and reduced transpulmonary pressure while also providing for a means of tracking patient recovery through the increase in tidal volumes as a marker of improving lung compliance.

Persistent Hypoxia in the Extracorporeal Membrane Oxygenation Supported Patient

In the setting of persistent hypoxia requiring potentially injurious ventilatory support in addition to ECMO, interventions must be pursued to reduce lung injury and increase the likelihood of survival.[65,66] Key interventions can be grouped into the following categories: (1) increase extracorporeal oxygen delivery; (2) decrease oxygen consumption; and (3) advanced ventilator management to decrease VILI. The most straightforward means to augment extracorporeal oxygen delivery is to **increase venous drainage** through the placement of larger or additional cannula to provide for more flow to the ECMO circuit. Practically, this may be challenging to achieve in a critically ill patient, and other interventions may be easier to perform. For patients with venous drainage achieved via a multistage cannula inserted into the femoral vein and advanced to the IVC-right atrial (RA) junction, drainage of venous blood from the upper body achieved via a drainage cannula inserted into the subclavian vein, may provide adequate additional circuit flow to maintain adequate oxygenation and permit lung rest ventilation.

Increasing hemoglobin concentration via transfusion is another means of increasing oxygen delivery while also increasing oxygen saturation. Physiologically, transfusion increases the oxygen carrying capacity of blood entrained into the ECMO circuit such that more oxygen is delivered to the body and the saturation of venous blood is higher. By increasing oxygen delivery with each heartbeat, transfusion acts to decrease cardiac output thereby increasing the fraction of total cardiac output entrained into the ECMO circuit. Use of beta blockers to reduce cardiac output and increase the fraction of total flow entrained into the circuit is an approach used to increase oxygen saturation but at the expense of likely decreasing total oxygen delivery. This approach may have a role in the patient with active coronary disease and evidence of cardiac ischemia in the setting of low oxygen saturation but otherwise may not provide substantive therapeutic benefit.

Decreasing oxygen consumption by the body is an alternative approach and can be accomplished by inducing mild hypothermia. The challenge of this approach is that patients may require paralysis to eliminate the effects of shivering to successfully achieve lower body temperatures. Optimizing ventilator strategies, such as using prone ventilation while on ECMO support, is another means of attempting to maintain patient homeostasis while limiting VILI.

Approach to Right Ventricular Dysfunction

Right ventricular (RV) dysfunction in ARDS is a common finding and is associated with poor prognosis.[67] Many factors contribute to RV dysfunction in the setting of severe lung injury and include the effects of hypoxia on pulmonary vasoconstriction and resultant increased RV afterload and the effects of high PEEP often used in patients with severe ARDS. Initiation of ECMO support, permitting the use of lung rest ventilation settings with lower PEEP and the introduction of oxygenated blood into the venous circulation, reduces the main drives of increased RV afterload in ARDS. Patients with persistent RV failure not responsive to inotropic therapy and volume optimization may require isolated RV mechanical support or the use of alternative ECMO cannulation strategies, such as VAV cannulation.

Weaning of Extracorporeal Membrane Oxygenation Support

Patients with improving lung function, typically demonstrated by increasing lung compliance and better gas exchange, are candidates for weaning of ECMO support.[68] The optimal timing of weaning and decannulation is unknown but a reasonable approach is to ensure that the patients can be stably supported by mechanical ventilation alone with settings considered to be noninjurious and well tolerated. Weaning of support requires that patients are able to both maintain oxygenation and ventilation safely.

For patients with predominantly hypoxic respiratory failure, the amount of extracorporeal oxygen delivery provided is largely a function of blood flow through the ECMO circuit. Because it is not possible to provide less than room air levels of oxygen through the ECMO oxygenator in typical circuit configurations, the lower bound of oxygen titration in the gas supply is limited and is sufficient to fully oxygenate the blood. To wean oxygen delivery, blood flow through the ECMO circuit is gradually reduced. The lower bound here is also limited by the functional capabilities of the ECMO pump. Decreasing flows too much prolongs the contact time for blood within the device and increases the risk of clotting and thrombus formation. In addition, low flows also result in recirculation within the pump with the risk of hemolysis. Functionally, this acts to limit how low the flows through the circuit can be reduced meaning that weaning of oxygenation requires a significant step down before decannulation. This is easy to test as gas flow through the oxygenator can be capped so that no gas exchange is occurring with the circuit. Because hypoxia develops relatively quickly, within minutes, in the setting of insufficient oxygen delivery, the ability to assess if a patient can be safely decannulated within acceptable ventilation support is relatively straightforward.

Weaning of ECMO support for patients with predominantly hypercapnic failure is more involved. Because ECMO provides ventilatory support for all patients, the approach to weaning for hypercapnic failure is the predominant weaning strategy. As patient lung function improves, the ventilatory burden shifts from the ECMO circuit to the patient. Reduction in ECMO ventilatory support is achieved through the gradual reduction in sweep gas flow rate. Sweep gas is decreased in 0.5 to 1 LPM increments every 2 to 8 hours, depending on patient response, while targeting a normal systemic pH and maintaining ventilatory support within goal parameters. As sweep gas decreases to less than 2 LPM, continued weaning by 0.5 LPM increments is performed while monitoring any patient response to the decreased support. Serial blood gas analysis is used to measure systemic pH and CO_2 levels to ensure that the patient is tolerating the weaning of support.

Because hypercapnic failure can progress more slowly than hypoxic failure, weaning of support requires a prolonged gradual reduction in support and longer periods of observation. Once sweep gas is decreased to 0.5 LPM of flow, decreasing flow to 2.5 to 3 L through the circuit is the final reduction in support before a capping trial. This allows for the maintenance of a base level of flow through the device to limit clotting risks while functionally transferring the work of ventilation from the ECMO circuit to the patient's lungs. Patients able to tolerate a capping trial for a period of 12 to 24 hours without any change in their respiratory status or ventilator requirements are likely able to be safely decannulated. VV ECMO can be safely decannulated at the bedside and is increasingly being performed by intensivists. Percutaneous venous cannula can be removed with the cannulation sites closed by purse string sutures and application of pressure in the setting of anticoagulation being held for 2 or more hours before removal.

Failure of Support and Goals of Care

Not all patients are able to be successfully maintained by ECMO support. Whereas ECMO is able to achieve total support for the CO_2 elimination for the majority of patients at a basal metabolic state, ECMO may only provide partial oxygenation support. It may not be possible to adequately support a patient to achieve lung rest mechanical ventilation. In such scenarios, clarifying goals of care and determining if further support is warranted is imperative as the ECMO may permit prolonged survival but unfortunately without the possibility of recovery.

The occasional remarkable case of recovery inspires caution in premature cessation of extracorporeal support but likely leads to prolonged support for otherwise terminal disease. Various scoring systems have been developed in an effort to prognosticate and guide clinical decision making for patients initiated on extracorporeal support. Although helpful in estimating survival, the systems can be summarized by the observation that **the sicker patients are at the time of cannulation, the lower the expected survival**.

Given the evolving nature of the ongoing development of extracorporeal support, one approach to determine timing of withdrawal of support is whether lung safe ventilation can be achieved. As the major goal of ECMO for ARDS is to maintain homeostasis while reducing VILI, if lung safe ventilation cannot be achieved, then ongoing lung injury is anticipated and meaningful recovery is unlikely. Using this as a metric is one approach to avoid prolonged support in a patient with minimal hope for recovery.

Use of Extracorporeal Membrane Oxygenation as Bridge to Lung Transplantation

Before the adoption of the lung allocation score (LAS) in 2005, donor organs were awarded based on recipient time on the waiting list.[69] This system prioritized early evaluation for lung transplantation and listing of healthier patients able to survive the wait of months to several years until matched donor lungs became available. In an effort to reduce waiting list mortality rates, the LAS prioritized potential transplant recipients based on estimated life expectancy.[70] In the new regime, as patients became sicker and their lung disease advanced, they gained priority on the waiting list to reflect their decreasing expected transplant-free survival. Transplant centers adapted to this new environment by developing strategies to maintain the vitality of patients with advancing disease, so they were better equipped to withstand the rigors of surgery and postoperative recovery while also bridging high priority critically ill patients to transplantation.[29]

As transplant centers grappled with the changing requirements, physicians turned to ECMO as a means of providing lung support for patients either listed or undergoing evaluation for lung transplantation. Unlike its use during ARDS, where ECMO serves as a bridge to lung recovery, its use in transplant is targeted toward maintaining patient vitality with less focus on preserving existing lung function. And, unlike typical care of the ECMO-supported ARDS patient, the patient undergoing consideration for lung transplantation while supported on ECMO is awake, active, and commonly maintained without mechanical ventilation.

Candidate Selection for Extracorporeal Membrane Oxygenation Bridge to Transplant

Identification of the appropriate patient to initiate on ECMO support as a bridge to lung transplantation is challenging because treatment failure leads to prolonged support of a patient with otherwise terminal disease. Even more challenging is the growing use of ECMO as a bridge to decision for patients with end-stage lung disease not listed prior to undergoing any formal evaluation for lung transplantation. A significant ethical consideration is that a patient with end-stage disease may be initiated on ECMO support before listing and then determined not to be a candidate for transplantation. This creates the possibility of caring for an awake, well-supported patient maintained via a support device that is only available within the hospital in a critical care environment. Although the transplant community works to determine processes and guidelines for addressing such situations, careful patient selection is the most important first step before ECMO cannulation.

Key considerations before initiation of ECMO support include ensuring the patient meets the following: (1) adequate social support to ensure medical adherence and ability to maintain posttransplant care; (2) lack of any comorbidities or preexisting conditions that would preclude transplantation; and, (3) lack of concerns regarding patient compliance or behaviors that would jeopardize the health of the transplant organ.[28] Some of these criteria, such as behavioral assessments or cancer screening, may be difficult to ascertain in the critically ill patient before initiation of ECMO support, thereby creating the potential for ethical challenges. At present, patient selection is evolving rapidly and is determined independently by each transplant center.

Clinical Criteria to Initiate Extracorporeal Membrane Oxygenation Support

Determining the optimal timing for initiation of ECMO support in a patient with end-stage lung disease requires balancing risk of cannulation and initiation of support against the effects of further deterioration of the patient's functional status. Initiation too soon exposes the patient to unnecessary risks when support with conventional means, such as supplemental oxygen via high flow nasal cannula, may be sufficient. Alternatively, initiation after a patient has clinically deteriorated, risks providing insufficient support to enable activity and rehabilitation while waiting for lung transplantation. Because ECMO provides only partial lung support, maintenance of some residual lung function is needed for the patient to be able to maintain homeostasis and participate in physical activity.

Factors to consider when initiating ECMO support for this patient population include: (1) physiologic goal of support; (2) specific cannulation strategy to meet provide desired support; (3) availability of required personnel and needed resources; and (4) patient stability and urgency of needed support. For most patients, progressive end-stage lung disease evolves over days to weeks and provides the opportunity to determine the optimal cannulation strategy and prepare for nonurgent cannulation in a controlled environment. Exceptions to this, such as in cases of rapidly progressive idiopathic pulmonary fibrosis or severe exacerbations of cystic fibrosis (CF), may require emergent cannulation for initiation of extracorporeal support. Table 28.3 provides a list of criteria for use in determining the appropriate threshold for initiating ECMO support for the pretransplant patient.

TABLE 28.3 Threshold to Initiate Extracorporeal Membrane Oxygenation Support in Pretransplant Patient

Criterial to Initiate Extracorporeal Membrane Oxygenation Lung Support for Lung Transplant Candidates
• Oxygen saturation via pulse oximetry <90% while on high-flow nasal cannula at rest
• Inability to participate in physical therapy despite noninvasive ventilation or oxygen support
• Hemodynamic or cardiac instability attributed to impaired gas exchange

Cannulation of the Pretransplant Patient

Unlike cannulation of the intubated patient with ARDS or other causes of profound respiratory failure, initiation of ECMO support in pretransplant patients often necessitates cannulation of an awake and nonintubated patient. This scenario requires specific considerations as obtaining large bore vascular access in the spontaneously breathing patient, often in varying degrees of respiratory distress, presents challenges to the cannulating physician and risks to the patient. Cannulation in a controlled environment, such as an operating room where access to required supplies may be easier and space for personnel less limited, is preferred although bedside cannulation is feasible and safe for experienced providers.

Both femoral-IJ and bicaval double lumen cannulation approaches are commonly used by transplant centers to support pretransplant patients. The higher flows typically achieved with the femoral-IJ approach may provide improved support of patients with profound hypoxic failure whereas the bicaval double lumen cannula may facilitate ambulation and more stable flows during patient movement, while simultaneously being more susceptible to cannula malpositioning. A major consideration in the approach selected is the comfort level and familiarity of a given center with the chosen cannulation strategy. A comparison of VV ECMO cannulation strategies is provided in Table 28.4.

Placement of a cannula in the RIJ, whether a return cannula in the femoral-IJ configuration or a bicaval double lumen cannula, is technically challenging in an awake and spontaneously breathing patient. Percutaneous cannulation consists of obtaining vascular access and then performing serial dilation

TABLE 28.4 **Comparison of Venovenous Extracorporeal Membrane Oxygenation Cannulation Strategies**

Cannulation Strategy	Typical Flow Rates	Considerations
Femoral-internal jugular (IJ) vein	3.5–5 liters per minute (LPM)	• Provides most reliable high flow rates and highest range of support
Dual lumen bicaval	2.8–4.5 LPM	• Single insertion point; can facilitate ambulation; susceptible to decreased flow with cannula rotation or movement
Femoral-Femoral	2.5–4 LPM	• Lowest flow support strategy best used for hypercapnic respiratory failure when IJ not accessible

over a guidewire. Adequate topical anesthetic is vital to limit patient discomfort during the procedure. Use of anxiolytics, such as dexmedetomidine, are commonly used to reduce patient distress while reserving patient respiratory drive. Physician control of the skin tract into the vessel is vital to both limit bleeding and, importantly, to reduce the risk of entrainment of air into the IJ and the right heart during spontaneous breathing. An additional consideration is that patients undergoing cannulation are often hypovolemic in the setting of aggressive diuresis to optimize lung function before cannulation, which may complicate efforts to safely obtain vascular access. Use of surface ultrasound or fluoroscopy is needed to guide advancement of guidewires and cannula, especially with use of a bicaval double lumen cannula, to avoid risk of cardiac injury and malpositioning of the cannula.

Clinical Management of the Prelung Transplant Patient on Extracorporeal Membrane Oxygenation Support

Unlike in bridge to recovery support of ARDS patients, where the primary motivation for use of ECMO is to reduce VILI, the goal of ECMO support for pretransplant patients is to maintain viability and facilitate ongoing activity. This difference presents unique challenges in clinical management of the pretransplant patient on ECMO. Patients who are awake, mobile, and engaged in physical activity, experience rapid changes in intrathoracic pressure affecting venous return and blood flow entrainment into the ECMO circuit. Patients with advanced lung disease, particularly those with CF and interstitial lung disease, experience frequent coughing which itself causes extreme changes in intrathoracic pressure and resultant changes in ECMO flow. Excessive negative pressure at the withdrawal cannula can result in temporary cessation of flow as the IVC collapses around the cannula. The resulting visible recoil in the circuit tubing produced by the cessation of flow is termed **"circuit chugging"** and is typically self-limited in the stable and awake patient.

Typical management of circuit chugging resulting in flow limitation on ECMO support is to perform volume expansion through the administration of crystalloid or colloid fluid infusions or via transfusions of blood products. In the case of the prelung transplant patient, volume administration can precipitate pulmonary edema and impair residual lung function. For patients who are comfortable and well supported by ECMO, tolerating circuit chugging during coughing episodes or with activity is preferable to fluid resuscitation, which should be used primarily in the treatment of hypotension in this patient cohort.

Approaches to the Prelung Transplant Patient With Right Ventricular Failure

RV dysfunction in patients with end-stage lung disease is a particularly complex challenge with no definitive optimal extracorporeal support strategy.[38,71] In some patients, initiation of VV ECMO and the infusion of highly oxygenated blood into the cardiopulmonary circulation reduces hypoxic vasoconstriction thereby lowering pulmonary vascular resistance and improving RV function. For other patients, and particularly for patients with group I pulmonary hypertension, alternative cannulation strategies are required to provide adequate support to bridge successfully to transplantation. Centers report multiple different approaches, but an optimal strategy is yet to be identified. Each method presents technical and management challenges that require substantial expertise to master and complicate efforts to compare approaches.

Strategies for extracorporeal lung support in the setting of RV failure include: (1) VV ECMO with atrial septostomy; (2) upper body VA ECMO; and (3) RV bypass ECMO. An atrial septostomy provides a means of offloading the RV when right-sided filling pressures exceed those of the left atrium. Coupling the septostomy to VV ECMO allows for shunting of oxygenated blood to the systemic circulation while retaining systemic VAV coupling to allow for pretransplant assessment of left ventricular function. Upper body VA ECMO consists of shunting a fraction of total cardiac output, typically 2 to 3 LPM, from the venous circulation to the systemic arterial circulation via a return cannula sutured to an axillary artery. This approach achieves titratable offloading of the RV but provides limited support in the setting of hypoxic respiratory failure because of uncertain distribution within the aorta of oxygenated blood from the ECMO circuit. For patients with profound hypoxic respiratory failure complicated by RV failure, an alternative approach is to surgically place a withdrawal cannula in the right atrium with a return cannula placed in the pulmonary vein (either accessed directly or inserted via the right upper pulmonary vein with the cannula advanced to the left atrium). This approach allows for bypass of the cardiopulmonary circulation and achieves high flow support but risks an invasive surgery in a patient with advanced lung disease and may complicate subsequent transplant surgery.

Extracorporeal Circulatory Support

A detailed discussion of the use and management of ECMO as a circulatory support device in the setting of heart failure is beyond the scope of this chapter. However, use of ECMO to provide circulatory support provides gas exchange for the tissues perfused by the circuit markedly affects cardiopulmonary circulation with specific considerations important for the management of ventilatory support.[27] Briefly, VA ECMO shunts blood from the venous to the systemic arterial circulation bypassing the cardiopulmonary circulation. Central VA ECMO, in which the blood is withdrawn via the right atrium or a bicaval cannulation approach and returned via a cannula placed in the aortic arch, shunts blood across the cardiopulmonary circulation and provides both circulatory and ventilatory support to the entire body. As use of ECMO to provide circulatory support has grown, it is increasingly common to place a return cannula in the femoral artery, either percutaneously or via arterial cutdown, which is then advanced to the iliac artery or distal aorta to provide retrograde perfusion of the aortic vascular tree. This cannulation approach is referred to as peripheral VA ECMO. Cannulation of other arterial branches, such as the axillary artery via a vascular graft as in the previously described upper body VA ECMO, can also be considered as forms of peripheral VA ECMO while recognizing that each cannulation site induces its own unique effects on perfusion and specific interactions with the failing heart that have yet to be fully described.

Central Venoarterial Extracorporeal Membrane Oxygenation

In the case of central VA ECMO, the entire cardiopulmonary circulation is bypassed with only residual blood not entrained into the circuit then passing through the lungs. In this cannulation strategy, ECMO is providing both circulatory and ventilatory support. Because these patients commonly have an open chest postcardiotomy, they are typically deeply sedated, intubated, and maintained on mechanical ventilation. In this setting, maintenance of lung rest ventilation is a common strategy to avoid lung injury. The specific settings are variable, but example parameters are a volume control mode of ventilation with a tidal volume of 4 to 8 mL/kg of ideal body weight, PEEP of 5 to 10 to maintain lung inflation, and an FiO2 less than or equal to 60% to avoid hyperoxic injury. Minimal mechanical ventilatory support is typically needed in these cases because of the support provided by the ECMO circuit. As the return cannula is inserted in the proximal aorta, there are limited means of determining how to titrate mechanical ventilation to optimize gas exchange on the blood perfusing the lungs.

An uncommon but important special consideration is central ECMO cannulation of the postlung transplant or postheart/lung transplant patient. These patients typically lack a bronchial circulation and their lungs are dependent on the blood supply from the pulmonary artery for perfusion. In these cases, high blood flow rates through the ECMO circuit produces markedly decreased lung perfusion and risks ischemia and subsequent failure of the allograft. Because of the need to maintain perfusion through the cardiopulmonary circulation, cases of postlung transplant initiated on central VA ECMO support need to limit the total flow through the ECMO circuit. The minimum flow through the cardiopulmonary circulation required to maintain lung viability is unknown. However, extrapolating from ex vivo lung perfusion experimental work, a flow of 20% to 40% of normal basal cardiac output through the cardiopulmonary circulation is likely sufficient to meet lung metabolic demands.

Peripheral Venoarterial Extracorporeal Membrane Oxygenation

The ECMO-failing heart circulation created from the initiation of peripheral VA ECMO is profoundly nonphysiologic. Continuous retrograde perfusion from the ECMO circuit collides with pulsatile antegrade perfusion from the failing heart to form a dynamic watershed region within the aorta. A schematic of the ECMO-failing heart circulation in peripheral VA ECMO support is shown in Fig. 28.10. In the setting of concomitant lung failure, regional differential hypoxia can develop, in which tissues perfused by the heart may receive inadequate oxygen delivery compared with the oxygenated blood provided distally in the aorta by the ECMO circuit. This scenario is also termed **North-South syndrome** to

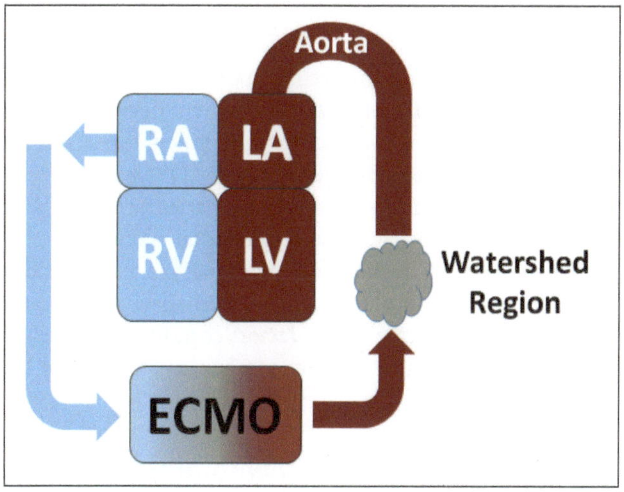

• **Fig. 28.10** Schematic of peripheral venoarterial extracorporeal membrane oxygenation (*ECMO*) with return cannula directing retrograde perfusion in the aorta where it collides with antegrade perfusion from the heart to form a dynamic watershed region whose position varies over the cardiac cycle.

describe the difference in oxygen delivery experienced by superior and inferior tissue beds. The location of the watershed region defines the boundary between these two regions and is dependent on the relative contributions to perfusion from the failing heart and the ECMO circuit.

Except in cases of profound heart failure, in which 90% or more of total perfusion is supplied by the ECMO circuit, perfusion to the aortic arch during peripheral VA ECMO support is supplied by the heart. Peripheral VA ECMO primarily is a form of circulatory support and does not provide gas exchange support to the head or upper extremities, which are dependent on the lungs for adequate oxygenation. Management of mechanical ventilatory support for intubated patients, or supplemental oxygen for nonintubated patients, is vital to ensure appropriate delivery of oxygen. Monitoring of oxygenation of the aortic arch, typically via blood gas monitoring from samples drawn from the radial artery or pulse oximetry performed on the right arm or right ear, is a means of guiding oxygenation support to ensure adequate oxygen delivery.

Titration of mechanical ventilation in the setting of VA ECMO is itself challenging given the nonphysiologic blood flow through the cardiopulmonary circulation. Decreased blood flow through the pulmonary artery may decrease pulmonary capillary pressure and the distribution of lung perfusion zones. In addition, titration of PEEP will also alter the lung zones with an increase in PEEP coupled with low blood flow conceivably creating type I lung zones in which alveolar pressure exceeds pulmonary arterial pressure. Optimal titration of mechanical ventilation during peripheral VA ECMO support is unknown. Given the uncertainties, being mindful of the effects of altered perfusion patterns is important in determining the appropriate titration for a given patient.

Perioperative Management of the Extracorporeal Membrane Oxygenation Patient

The introduction of the extracorporeal circuit generates multiple additional considerations when determining an appropriate sedation or anesthetic regimen for a specific patient.[72] Factors to consider include: (1) specific cannulation strategy, such as whether the patient is on VV or VA ECMO support; (2) fraction of total blood flow that is being delivered to the cardiopulmonary circuit; (3) distribution and origin of perfusion within the aorta; and (4) severity of lung disease. These factors combine to guide the appropriate agent and delivery mechanism to achieve the therapeutic goal.

Effect of Extracorporeal Membrane Oxygenation Circuit on Pharmacokinetics

The impact of the ECMO circuit on drug distribution and metabolism is poorly elucidated for the majority of commonly used drugs.[73] The contact surface of the oxygenator and circuit tubing tends to bind drugs that are lipophilic or highly protein-bound resulting in significant sequestration of such drugs within the circuit. The sequestration phenomenon can be unpredictable as drugs may be initially bound to the circuit and then continue to be released over time.[74] The circuit also acts to change the volume of distribution of drugs in ways that are difficult to predict. Drugs with a small volume of distribution are most likely affected as the ECMO circuit functionally expand the circulating volume, whereas drugs with a very large volume of distribution are less likely to be as affected. The sum of these effects leads to profoundly altered drug kinetics for patients on ECMO support, which require close monitoring and regular titration of drugs to desired concentration levels or physiologic effect.

Sedation Management

For patients requiring prolonged sedation while being maintained on ECMO support, a scenario common in severe ARDS in which sedation is used to reduce respiratory effort and maintain synchrony with mechanical ventilation to limit VILI, sedation management can be complicated by both the interactions of drugs with the circuit and the effects of patient tolerance because of prolonged exposure. Infusions of narcotics are the mainstay of most sedation regimens for ARDS patients on ECMO. Fentanyl is commonly used but is a lipophilic drug that is highly sequestered within the ECMO circuit and frequently requires very high infusion rates to achieve sedation targets.[75] Hydromorphone is an alternative agent frequently used in ECMO support but is also highly lipophilic. Benzodiazepines are commonly used as adjuvant sedatives but with similar caveats to narcotics. Midazolam, a frequently used benzodiazepine in the intensive care unit, is highly lipophilic and binds to proteins leading to sequestration within the ECMO circuit. Use of propofol is controversial because it is also highly lipophilic and tightly protein-bound, while reports that it may separate from blood within the oxygenator lead to concerns for degrading device performance with prolonged use.

In the setting of prolonged ECMO support, common for patients with severe ARDS who may require a lengthy period before recovery, a transition to oral sedation and use of atypical antipsychotics and mood stabilizers may provide an alternative approach. This is particularly important as patients become tolerant to the effects of sedating agents and require escalating doses to achieve sedation targets. As support progresses, this can lead to significant amounts of intravenous fluid, which may have harmful effects on lung function and recovery. Use of oral sedation regimens is a means to limit fluid intake while also providing for slowly tapering agents as lung function improves.

Lung Disease and Altered Perfusion

Patients with advanced lung disease supported by ECMO have variable and uncertain absorption of inhaled anesthetic. This is particularly challenging in the setting of patients being bridged to lung transplant who require anesthetic induction before surgery. Given uncertain uptake of inhaled anesthetic in the setting of profound end-stage lung disease, use of intravenous anesthetic in such cases is preferred.

A similar consideration is required in patients maintained on VA ECMO support. In the case of central VA ECMO, limited perfusion of the lungs translates into unclear efficacy of inhaled anesthetic. Peripheral VA ECMO represents an even more complex case in which perfusion of the aortic arch, and hence the brain, may come from the heart, but also partially from the ECMO circuit. In addition, intravenous administration of anesthetic may be at least partially taken up by the ECMO circuit and then returned to the inferior tissue beds and not to the brain. Careful planning of anesthesia delivery and a thorough understanding of a patient's perfusion is required before initiation of any anesthesia for this patient population.

Approach to the Use of Extracorporeal Membrane Oxygenation for Procedural Support

A rapidly evolving area of extracorporeal ventilatory support is the use of ECMO to facilitate procedures and surgery in patients in whom traditional mechanical ventilation is either difficult or impossible. Less invasive than cardiopulmonary bypass, ECMO provides an alternative means of supporting patients requiring tracheal or mediastinal surgery in whom mechanical ventilation is not easily achieved. Expanding capacity and increasing comfort with ECMO will lead to its further use to facilitate procedures that would otherwise require more invasive heart and lung support.

Experimental Therapies and Future Directions

The physiologic principles of extracorporeal ventilatory support are actively being leveraged to create a new generation of extracorporeal support modalities targeting specific respiratory failure indications. This is most advanced in the development of extracorporeal CO_2 removal (ECCO2R) devices, which aim to remove physiologically significant amounts of CO_2 at low (<800 mL/min) and ultra-low (<300 mL/min) blood flow rates.[76] The lower blood flow rates of these devices enable use of smaller cannulas more widely familiar to critical care and emergency medicine physicians. Such technology will likely alter the care of patients with exacerbations of obstructive lung disease by providing alternatives to positive pressure ventilation. ARDS care may change as ECCO2R devices will more widely permit use of ultraprotective lung ventilation (tidal volumes of 4 mL/kg of predicted body weight) currently limited by the associated development of hypercapnia. Multiple ECCO2R devices are currently in clinical trials with many already available in Europe and other healthcare markets.

Longer-term research is focused on the development of ambulatory extracorporeal ventilatory support devices capable of providing expanded support. Such devices will offer an alternative to lung transplantation for patients with end-stage lung disease and will be a life-extending option for patients who are not transplant candidates.

REFERENCES

1. Pasrija C, Kronfli A, George P, et al. Utilization of veno-arterial extracorporeal membrane oxygenation for massive pulmonary embolism. *Ann Thorac Surg.* 2018;105(2):498–504.
2. Lorusso R, Alexander P, Rycus P, Barbaro R. The Extracorporeal Life Support Organization Registry: update and perspectives. *Ann Cardiothorac Surg.* 2019;8(1):93–98.
3. Paden ML, Conrad SA, Rycus PT, Thiagarajan RR, Registry ELSO. Extracorporeal Life Support Organization Registry Report 2012. *ASAIO J.* 2013;59(3):202–210.
4. Sidebotham D, Allen SJ, McGeorge A, Ibbott N, Willcox T. Venovenous extracorporeal membrane oxygenation in adults: Practical aspects of circuits, cannulae, and procedures. *J Cardiothorac Vasc Anesth.* 2012;26(5):893–909.
5. Peek GJ, et al. Efficacy and economic assessment of conventional ventilatory support versus extracorporeal membrane oxygenation for severe adult respiratory failure (CESAR): a multicentre randomised controlled trial. *Lancet.* 2009;374(9698):1351–1363.
6. Combes A, et al. Extracorporeal membrane oxygenation for severe acute respiratory distress syndrome. *N Engl J Med.* 2018; 378(21):1965–1975.
7. Le Gall A, Follin A, Cholley B, Mantz J, Aissaoui N, Pirracchio R. Veno-arterial-ECMO in the intensive care unit: from technical aspects to clinical practice. *Anaesth Crit Care Pain Med.* 2018;37(3):259–268.
8. Bartlett RH. Historical perspectives: extracorporeal membrane oxygenation (ECMO). *Neoreviews.* 2005;6:e251–e254.
9. de Chambrun MP, et al. Venoarterial extracorporeal membrane oxygenation for refractory cardiogenic shock post-cardiac arrest. *Intensive Care Med.* 2016;42(12):1999–2007.
10. Jing L, Yao L, Zhao M, Peng L-P, Liu M. Organ preservation: from the past to the future. *Acta Pharmacol Sin.* 2018;39(5):845–857.
11. Boettcher W, Merkle F, Weitkemper HH. History of extracorporeal circulation: the conceptional and developmental period. *J Extra Corpo Technol.* 2003;35(3):172–183.
12. Iwahashi H, Yuri K, Nos Y. Development of the oxygenator: past, present, and future. *J Artif Organs.* 2004;7(3):111–120.
13. Boettcher W, Merkle F, Weitkemper H-H. History of extracorporeal circulation: the invention and modification of blood pumps. *J Extra Corpor Technol.* 2003;35(3):184–191.
14. Hessel EA. A brief history of cardiopulmonary bypass. *Semin Cardiothorac Vasc Anesth.* 2014;18(2):87–100.
15. Palanzo D, Qui F, Baer L, Clark JB, Myers JL, Ündar A. Evolution of the ECLS circuitry. *Artif Organs.* 2011;34(11):869–873.
16. Melchior R, Sutton S, Harris W, Dalton H. Evolution of membrane oxygenator technology for utilization during pediatric cardiopulmonary bypass. *Pediatr Heal Med Ther.* 2016;7:45–56.
17. Federspiel W, Lung Henchir K. artificial: basic principles and current applications. *Encyclopedia of Biomaterials and Biomedical Engineering.* 2004:910–920.
18. Drummond M, Braile DM, Lima-Oliveira APM, Camim AS, Oyama RSK, Sandoval GH. Technological evolution of

membrane oxygenators. *Brazilian J Cardiovasc Surg.* 2005; 20(4):432–437.
19. Epis F, Belliato M. Oxygenator performance and artificial-native lung interaction. *J Thorac Dis.* 2018;10(S5):S596–S605.
20. Rubens FD, Mesana T. The inflammatory response to cardiopulmonary bypass: a therapeutic overview. *Perfusion.* 2004;19(1): S5–S12.
21. Palanzo D, Qui F, Baer L, Clark JB, Myers JL, Ündar A. Evolution of the ECLS circuitry. *Artif Organs.* 2011;34(11):869–873.
22. Toomasian JM, Bartlett RH. Hemolysis and ECMO pumps in the 21st Century. *Perfusion.* 2011;26(1):5–6.
23. Lequier L, Horton S, McMullan D, Bartlett RH. Extracorporeal membrane oxygenation circuitry. *Pediatr Crit care.* 2013;14:1–10.
24. Bartlett RH, Gattinoni L. Current status of extracorporeal life support (ECMO) for cardiopulmonary failure. *Minerva Anestesiol.* 2010;76(7):534–540.
25. Hill JD, et al. Prolonged extracorporeal oxygenation for acute post-traumatic respiratory failure (shock-lung syndrome). *N Engl J Med.* 1972;286(12):629–634.
26. Zapol WM, Snider MT, Hill JD, et al. Extracorporeal membrane oxygenation in severe acute respiratory failure: a randomized prospective study. *JAMA.* 1979;242(20):2193–2196.
27. Keller SP. Management of peripheral venoarterial extracorporeal membrane oxygenation in cardiogenic shock. *Crit Care Med.* 2019;47(9):1235–1242.
28. Keller SP. Contemporary approaches in the use of extracorporeal membrane oxygenation to support patients waiting for lung transplantation. *Ann Cardiothorac Surg.* 2020;9(1):29–41.
29. Biscotti M, et al. Awake extracorporeal membrane oxygenation as bridge to lung transplantation: a 9-year experience. *Ann Thorac Surg.* 2017;104(2):412–419.
30. Truby LK, et al. Incidence and implications of left ventricular distention during venoarterial extracorporeal membrane oxygenation support. *ASAIO J.* 2017;63(3):257–265.
31. Rao P, Khalpey Z, Smith R, Burkhoff D, Kociol RD. Venoarterial extracorporeal membrane oxygenation for cardiogenic shock and cardiac arrest. *Circulation Heart Fail.* 2018;11(9):e004905.
32. Guglin M, et al. Venoarterial ECMO for adults. *J Am Coll Cardiol.* 2019;73(6):698–716.
33. Napp LC, et al. Cannulation strategies for percutaneous extracorporeal membrane oxygenation in adults. *Clin Res Cardiol.* 2016;105(4).
34. Jayaraman A, Cormican D, Shah P, Ramakrishna H. Cannulation strategies in adult veno-arterial and veno-venous extracorporeal membrane oxygenation: techniques, limitations, and special considerations. *Ann Card Anaesth.* 2017;20(5):11.
35. Pavlushkov E, Berman M, Valchanov K. Cannulation techniques for extracorporeal life support. *Ann Transl Med.* 2017;5(4): 70 -70.
36. Rupprecht L, Lunz D, Philipp A, Lubnow M, Schmid C. Pitfalls in percutaneous ECMO cannulation. *Heart Lung Vessel.* 2015;7(4):320–326.
37. Kohler H, Valchanov K, Voylsteke A. Review ECMO cannula review. *Perfusion.* 2012;28(2):114–124.
38. Fuehner T, et al. Extracorporeal membrane oxygenation in awake patients as bridge to lung transplantation. *Am J Respir Crit Care Med.* 2012;185(7):763–768.
39. Wang S, Moroi MK, Kunselman AR, Myers JL, Ündar A. Evaluation of centrifugal blood pumps in term of hemodynamic performance using simulated neonatal and pediatric ECMO circuits. *Artif Organs.* 2020;44(1):16–27.
40. Gross-Hardt S, et al. Low-flow assessment of current ECMO/ECCO2R rotary blood pumps and the potential effect on hemocompatibility. *Crit Care.* 2019;23(1).
41. Millar JE, Fanning JP, McDonald CI, McAuley DF, Fraser JF. The inflammatory response to extracorporeal membrane oxygenation (ECMO): a review of the pathophysiology. *Crit Care.* 2016;20(1):387.
42. Murphy DA, et al. Extracorporeal membrane oxygenation—hemostatic complications. *Transfus Med Rev.* 2015;29(2):90–101.
43. Martucci G, et al. Anticoagulation and transfusions management in veno-venous extracorporeal membrane oxygenation for acute respiratory distress syndrome: assessment of factors associated with transfusion requirements and mortality. *J Intensive Care Med.* 2019;34(8):630–639.
44. Maul TM, Massicotte MP, Wearden PD. ECMO biocompatibility: surface coatings, anticoagulation, and coagulation monitoring*Extracorporeal Membrane Oxygenation: Advances in Therapy*: InTech; 2016.
45. Abrams D, Brodie D. Extracorporeal membrane oxygenation for adult respiratory failure. *Chest.* 2017;152(3):639–649.
46. Abrams D, Brodie D. Novel uses of extracorporeal membrane oxygenation in adults. *Clin Chest Med.* 2015;36(3):373–384.
47. Garcia JP, et al. Ambulatory veno-venous extracorporeal membrane oxygenation: innovation and pitfalls. *J Thorac Cardiovasc Surg.* 2011;142(4):755–761.
48. Pham T, Brochard LJ, Slutsky AS. Mechanical ventilation: state of the art. *Mayo Clin Proc.* 2017;92(9):1382–1400.
49. Curley GF, J. Laffey JG, Zhang H, Slutsky AS. Biotrauma and ventilator-induced lung injury: clinical implications. *Chest.* 2016;150(5):1109–1117.
50. Kallet RH, Matthay MA. Hyperoxic acute lung injury. *Respir Care.* 2013;58(1):123–141.
51. Bautista AF, Akca O. Hypercapnia: is it protective in lung injury?. *Med Gas Res.* 2013;3(1):23.
52. Acute Respiratory Distress Syndrome Network, et al. Ventilation with lower tidal volumes as compared with traditional tidal volumes for acute lung injury and the acute respiratory distress syndrome. *N Engl J Med.* 2000;342(18):1301–1308.
53. Shekar K, Davies AR, Mullany DV, Tiruvoipati R, Fraser JF. To ventilate, oscillate, or cannulate?. *J Crit Care.* 2013;28(5): 655–662.
54. Gas Transport & pH. Ganong's Review of Medical Physiology, 26e. AccessMedicine. McGraw-Hill Medical. [Online]. Available: https://accessmedicine.mhmedical.com/content.aspx?bookid=2525&sectionid=204297654. [Accessed: 03-Aug-2020].
55. Sheldon M, Ali E. Practical approach to physical-chemical acid-base management: Stewart at the bedside. *Ann Am Thorac Soc.* 2015;12(1):111–117.
56. Schmidt M, et al. Blood oxygenation and decarboxylation determinants during venovenous ECMO for respiratory failure in adults. *Intensive Care Med.* 2013;39(5):838–846.
57. Zampieri FG, et al. Extracorporeal membrane oxygenation for severe respiratory failure in adult patients: A systematic review and meta-analysis of current evidence. *J Crit Care.* 2013;28(6): 998–1005.
58. Cavayas YA, Munshi L, Del Sorbo L, Fan E. The early change in PaCO2 after extracorporeal membrane oxygenation initiation is associated with neurological complications. *Am J Respir Crit Care Med.* 2020;201(12):1525–1535.
59. Abrams D, et al. Mechanical ventilation for acute respiratory distress syndrome during extracorporeal life support research and practice. *Am J Respir Crit Care Med.* 2020;201(5):514–525.

60. Xia J, et al. Spontaneous breathing in patients with severe acute respiratory distress syndrome receiving prolonged extracorporeal membrane oxygenation. *BMC Pulm Med.* 2019;19(1).
61. Abrams D, Garan AR, Brodie D. Awake and fully mobile patients on cardiac extracorporeal life support. *Ann Cardiothorac Surg.* 2019;8(1):44–53.
62. Langer T, et al. Awake' extracorporeal membrane oxygenation (ECMO): pathophysiology, technical considerations, and clinical pioneering. *Crit Care.* 2016;20(1).
63. Nieman GF, et al. Physiology in Medicine: Understanding dynamic alveolar physiology to minimize ventilator-induced lung injury. *J Appl Physiol.* 2017;122(6):1516–1522.
64. Marini JJ, Rocco PRM, Gattinoni L. Static and dynamic contributors to ventilator-induced lung injury in clinical practice pressure, energy, and power. *Am J Respir Crit Care Med.* 2020;201(7):767–774.
65. Montisci A, Maj G, Zangrillo A, Winterton D, Pappalardo F. Management of refractory hypoxemia during venovenous extracorporeal membrane oxygenation for ARDS. *ASAIO J.* 2015;61(3):227–236.
66. Messai E, Bouguerra A, Guarracino F, Bonacchi M. Low blood arterial oxygenation during venovenous extracorporeal membrane oxygenation: proposal for a rational algorithm-based management. *J Intensive Care Med.* 2016;31(8):553–560.
67. Zochios V, Parhar K, Tunnicliffe W, Roscoe A, Gao F. The right ventricle in ARDS. *Chest.* 2017;152(1):181–193.
68. Broman LM, Malfertheiner MV, Montisci A, Pappalardo F. Weaning from veno-venous extracorporeal membrane oxygenation: how I do it. *J Thorac Dis.* 2018;10(5):S692–S697.
69. Maxwell BG, et al. Increased resource use in lung transplant admissions in the lung allocation score era. *Am J Respir Crit Care Med.* 2015;191(3):302–308.
70. Russo MJ.Who is the high-risk recipient? Predicting mortality after lung transplantation using pretransplant risk factors. *J Thorac Cardiovasc Surg.* 2009;138(5):1234–1238 e1.
71. Camboni D, et al. Use of venovenous extracorporeal membrane oxygenation and an atrial septostomy for pulmonary and right ventricular failure. *Ann Thorac Surg.* 2011;91(1):144–149.
72. Shah AG, Peahota M, Thoma BN, Kraft WK. Medication Complications in Extracorporeal Membrane Oxygenation. *Crit Care Clin.* 2017;33(4):897–920.
73. Cheng V, Abdul-Aziz M-H, Roberts JA, Shekar K. Optimising drug dosing in patients receiving extracorporeal membrane oxygenation. *J Thorac Dis.* 2018;10(5):S629–S641.
74. Raffaeli G, et al. Drug disposition and pharmacotherapy in neonatal ECMO: from fragmented data to integrated knowledge. *Front Pediatr.* 2019;7.
75. Ha MA, Sieg AC. Evaluation of altered drug pharmacokinetics in critically ill adults receiving extracorporeal membrane oxygenation. *Pharmacotherapy.* 2017;37(2):221–235.
76. Cove ME, MacLaren G, Federspiel WJ, Kellum JA. Bench to bedside review: extracorporeal carbon dioxide removal, past present and future. *Crit Care.* 2012;16(5):232.

29 Lung Volume Reduction Surgery

EDMOND COHEN

Introduction

Chronic obstructive pulmonary disease (COPD) is the third leading cause of death in the United States.[1–3] Emphysema is one component of COPD, and it is estimated that 3.1 million adults in the United States are currently diagnosed with emphysema. Emphysema is associated with permanent enlargement and destruction of the lung alveoli. The destruction of the alveolar walls of the distal terminal bronchioles results in loss of gas exchange surface area, air-trapping, and hyperinflation of the alveoli.[4] Emphysema often manifests with large air-containing bullae that do not contribute to gas exchange. These bullae are overventilated and underperfused, creating ventilation-perfusion (V/Q) mismatch from increased dead-space ventilation. They can physically compress neighboring normal tissue, thus worsening gas exchange. The progression of the disease ultimately results in compromised lung mechanics, hyperinflation, hypercapnia, dyspnea through airflow limitation, and hypoxia that often require oxygen therapy.

Emphysema

Emphysema changes are widespread in the general population and in the smoking population in particular. In smokers, there appears to be an augmented response to tobacco byproducts resulting in an excessively inflammatory destructive cycle. It is a progressive, debilitating disease, which in its final stages, greatly impacts the patient's quality of life (QOL), his/her family, as well as the cost of medical care.

Other components of COPD, such as chronic bronchitis and bronchospasm usually coexist with emphysema and contribute to obstructive dysfunction and expiratory airflow obstruction.

The hyperinflation leads to flattening of the diaphragm and widening of the chest cavity and intercostals spaces, putting the mechanics of these respiratory muscles at a tension-length disadvantage. Smoking-related emphysema most commonly manifests heterogeneously distributed throughout the lung, which predominantly affects the upper lobes of the lung. Destruction of lung tissue may lead to increased compliance of the remaining lung, with change in compliance directly related to the amount and severity of emphysema present.[5] In normal lungs, the diameter of airways during exhalation progressively decreases in conjunction with the decrease in lung volume. This leads to progressively decreasing flow rates throughout expiration, as exemplified by the characteristic downward slope of the expiratory limb of the flow-volume loop measured by spirometry. The airways are tethered open during exhalation by the integrity of the lung parenchyma. The degree to which the diameter of the airways decreases during exhalation is directly related to this tethering effect, measured as the elastic recoil of the lung. The obstruction to expiratory airflow may become severe enough to prevent complete exhalation of inspired air. Progressive "air trapping" may eventually lead to chronic hyperinflation of the lungs and increased total lung capacity (TLC). Hyperinflation in turn disrupts the mechanical advantage in the ventilatory design of the thorax, pushing the diaphragm downward toward the abdomen and pushing the ribcage outward. Hyperinflation is a significant contributor to dyspnea and decreased exercise tolerance in such patients, with a commensurate negative impact on QOL.

The increase in TLC in a patient with COPD is mostly caused by an increase in residual volume (RV) in patients with very severe emphysema and hyperinflation; the RV may be as high as 150% to 200% of its predicted value.

Thus patients with emphysema have been categorized as "pink puffers": cachectic with increased anterior-posterior (AP) dimensions of the chest and demonstrable increased work of breathing. They do not generally exhibit the abundant sputum production of chronic bronchitis or the periodic exacerbations of asthma.[6]

As depicted in Fig. 29.1 several attempts were made in the past to treat emphysema. Some of them were directed in an effort to reduce the size of the hyperinflated chest cavity to improve the lung mechanics. These techniques were not clinically effective.

There is no cure for the reduction of the gas exchange surface in emphysema, and the treatment only focuses on

Surgical treatment of end-stage emphysema

Unproven Efficacy	Proven Efficacy
■ Costochondrectomy	■ Transtracheal Oxygen Catheter
■ Transverse Sternotomy	■ Tracheostomy
■ Thoracoplasty	■ Needle Aspiration of Bullae
■ Phrenic Nerve resection	■ Tube Thoracostomy
■ Pneumoperitoneum	■ Bullectomy
■ Abdominal Belting	■ Lung Volume Reduction
■ Talc Pleurodesis	■ Lung Transplant
■ Sympathectomy	
■ Vagotomy	

• **Fig. 29.1** Past and current treatment for emphysema.

attempting to slow the progression of the disease by offering symptomatic therapy. These may includes steroids, bronchodilators, expectorant nebulizers, treatment of infection, and oxygen therapy or ventilatory support at the end-stage phase. When advanced, emphysema causes severe dyspnea that markedly diminishes QOL. Despite medical therapy, the course of advanced disease is slowly and relentlessly progressive. Lung transplantation is the only definitive treatment, but this has its own associated morbidity and mortality. However, donor availability and patient suitability do not make this an option for many patients with emphysema. Surgical techniques, such as lung volume reduction surgery (LVRS) and newer endoscopic lung reduction surgery (see Chapter 32), are the only effective procedures that have been developed to alleviate the dyspnea and can temporarily improve the patient QOL.

As mentioned earlier, no procedure can cure the disease except bilateral lung transplant, an option available to extremely select few patients because of assorted available organs. It became clear that these sick, debilitated patients would need innovative, alternative, nonsurgical procedures to potentially alleviate their symptoms. In recent years, a variety of noninvasive endoscopic lung volume reduction procedures were developed with the hope of improving the respiratory status of these patients. The common principle behind bronchoscopic lung volume reduction (BLVR) is the goal of reducing the extent of the hyperinflation because of emphysema via a flexible bronchoscope, which would result in a similar beneficial effect to surgical resection.[7–9]

Lung Volume Reduction Surgery

LVRS was initially introduced in 1957 by Otto C. Brantigan who published a series of 16 patients who underwent surgical treatment for nonbullous emphysema.[10] The procedure attempted to reduce overall lung volume as a means to restoring the outward traction on the smaller airways, thereby reducing airway resistance and air trapping. The Brantigan procedure, consisting of multiple wedge excisions, would restore the elastic "pull" on the small airways and thereby improve pulmonary mechanics. Because surgical staplers were not yet introduced, surgery was performed with a hand-sutured line of resection. Surgery resulted in a high incidence of persistent air leaks and a significant mortality rate of 16%. Because no surgeon would associate with such a high mortality, the procedure did not gain wide acceptance.

Interest in the Brantigan proposal was renewed by Cooper et al., following their experience with lung transplantation.[11] Initially, concern was that the smaller donor lung would not fit inside the overexpanded thorax, which will result in continuous air leak; instead they noticed that the lung recipient's distended chest reconfigured to the smaller volume of the donor lung. The idea behind LVRS is that by reducing the large RV, the diaphragm will reverse its flattened shape to resume its normally curved shape configuration. This will reduce the mismatching between the hyperinflated lungs and the chest cavity and improve the lung function, thereby restoring the outward circumferential pull and improving expiratory airflow. The first report by Dr. Cooper's group was of 20 patients who underwent this revived "pneumectomy" procedure.[12] As described in this landmark report: "We undertook surgical bilateral lung volume reduction in 20 patients with severe COPD to relieve thoracic distention and improve respiratory mechanics. The operation, done through median sternotomy, involves excision of 20% to 30% of the volume of each lung. The most affected portions are excised with the use of a linear stapling device fitted with strips of bovine pericardium attached to both the anvil and the cartridge to buttress the staple lines and eliminate air leakage through the staple holes (see Fig. 29.2 A and B). Preoperative and postoperative assessment of results has included grading of dyspnea and QOL, exercise performance, and objective measurements of lung function by spirometry and plethysmography. There has been no early or late mortality and no requirement for immediate postoperative ventilatory assistance. Follow-up ranges from 1 to 15 months (mean 6.4 months). The mean forced expiratory volume in 1 second (FEV_1) has improved by 82% and the reduction in TLC, RV, and trapped gas has been highly significant. These changes have been associated with marked relief of dyspnea and improvement in exercise tolerance and QOL. Although the follow-up period is short, these preliminary results suggest that bilateral surgical volume reduction may be of significant value for selected patients with severe COPD."

LVRS gained in popularity despite evidence of limited short-term beneficial effects.[13–15] These favorable results and a patient population eager to improve their QOL, led to a dramatic increase in the number of centers offering LVRS for COPD patients via thoracoscopic LVRS and laser pneumoplasty.[16]

In a subsequent prospective cohort study of 200 stringently selected patients undergoing LVRS from 1993 to 1998, at Washington University in St Louis, there were substantial beneficial effects far more beneficial than those achieved with optimized medical therapy. They enrolled 200 patients who underwent LVRS with a follow-up of 6 months, 3 years, and 5 years after surgery; dyspnea scores were improved in 81%, 52%, and 40% of patients, respectively. Good-to-excellent

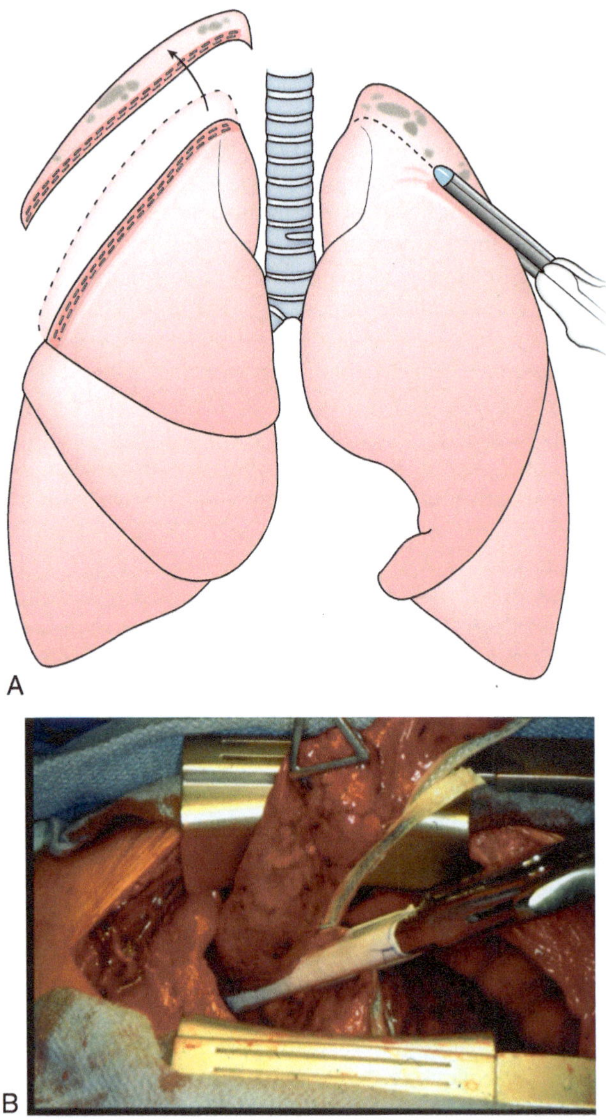

• **Fig. 29.2** (**A**) Schematic illustration of lung volume reduction surgery. (**B**) Lung resection with bovine pericardium attached to both the anvil and the stapler cartridge to buttress the staple lines.

satisfaction with the outcomes was reported by 96% (6 months), 89% (3 years), and 77% (5 years) of patients. The FEV_1 was improved in 92% (6 months), 72% (3 years), and 58% (5 years) of patients. During follow-up, 15 of these patients underwent subsequent lung transplantation.[17]

In a later study from the same group, LVRS produced significant functional improvement for selected patients with emphysema, and the benefits appeared to last at least 5 years. The authors enrolled a total of 250 consecutive patients who underwent bilateral LVRS through median sternotomy. All patients had end-stage COPD with disabling dyspnea, thoracic hyperinflation, and a heterogeneous pattern of emphysema that is a suitable target area for resection. Preoperative pulmonary rehabilitation was required and postrehabilitation data were used as the baseline for data analysis. Follow-up ranged from 1.8 to 9.1 years (Figs. 29.3–29.5). The authors reported that prolonged air leaks of at least 7 days were the most common complication

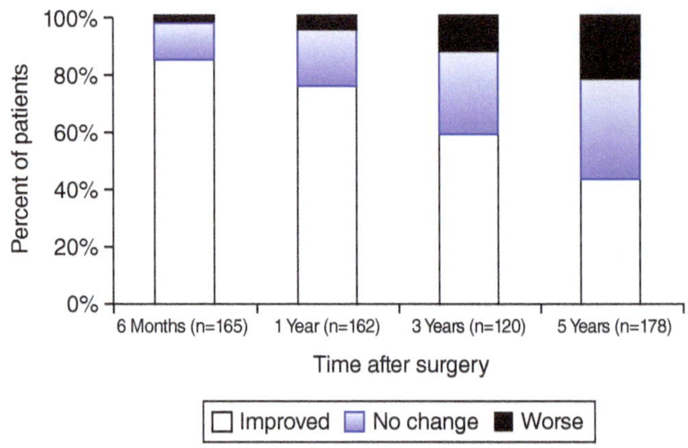

• **Fig. 29.3** Score changes in Modified Medical Research Council Dyspnea Scale after lung volume reduction surgery. (From Ciccone AM, Meyers BF, Guthrie TJ, et al. Long-term outcome of bilateral lung volume reduction in 250 consecutive patients with emphysema. *J Thorac Cardiovasc Surg*. 2003;125:513–525) (Courtesy of Joel Cooper M.D.)

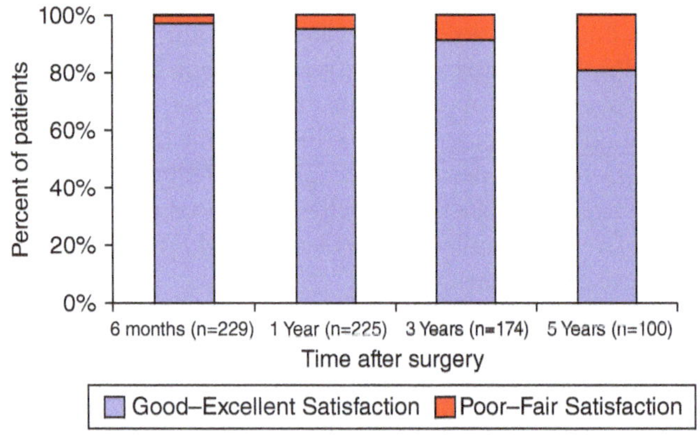

• **Fig. 29.4** Postoperative patient overall satisfaction over 5 years follow-up lung volume reduction surgery. (From Ciccone AM, Meyers BF, Guthrie TJ, et al. Long-term outcome of bilateral lung volume reduction in 250 consecutive patients with emphysema. *J Thorac Cardiovasc Surg*. 2003;125:513–525.)

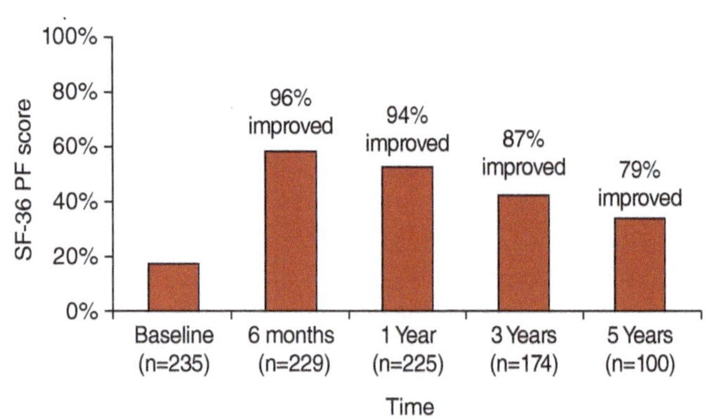

• **Fig. 29.5** SF-36 PF scale scores from before lung volume reduction surgery (baseline) and after surgery over 5 years follow-up. *PF*, Physical functioning; *SF-36*, short form health survey. (From Ciccone AM, Meyers BF, Guthrie TJ, et al. Long-term outcome of bilateral lung volume reduction in 250 consecutive patients with emphysema. *J Thorac Cardiovasc Surg*. 2003;125:513–525.)

(45.2%). Reexploration rates for air leak and bleeding were 3.2% and 1.2%, respectively. Eighteen patients (7.2%) required reintubation and support by mechanical ventilation. The in-hospital mortality in this series was 4.8%. Survivals after LVRS were 93.6%, 84.4%, and 67.7% at 1, 3, and 5 years, respectively. Spirometry values, lung volumes, and gas exchange parameters improved after surgery. The FEV_1 and the RV and health-related QOL showed significant improvements between preoperative values and each time.[18]

It must be emphasized that LVRS is a palliative procedure. It does not remove the pathology, or restore the destructed alveoli. It is however allowing for some restoration in the elastic recoil so that smaller airways have a reduced tendency to prematurely collapse and therefore have a lower resistance to airflow to the intact alveoli and improve the gas exchange.

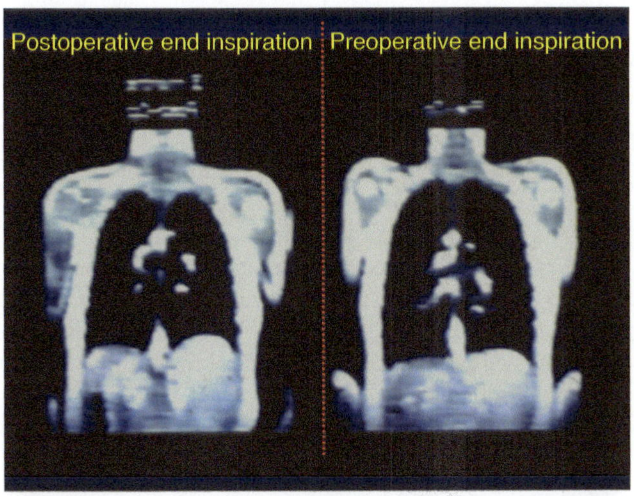

• **Fig. 29.6**

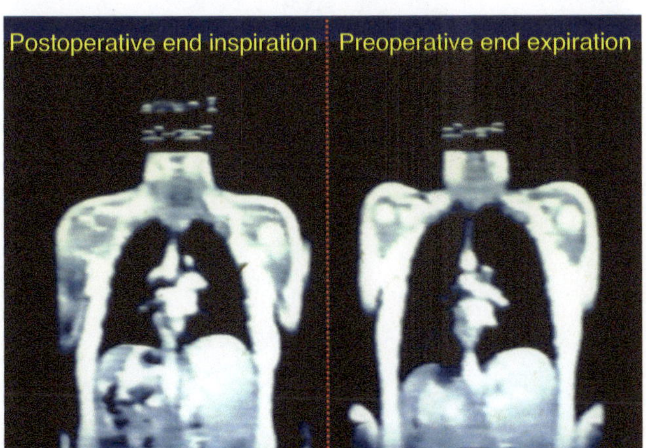

• **Fig. 29.7**

• **Figs. 29.6 and 29.7** Consequence of lung volume reduction surgery as depicted in the dynamic magnetic resonance imaging: reduction of the hyperinflation and air which restores the diaphragm to a more curved position and the chest wall to a less expanded diameter thereby improving the tension-length relationship and the respiratory mechanical advantage. The comparison between preoperative and postoperative during end-expiration (Fig. 29.6) and end-inspiration (Fig. 29.7) is illustrated. In the preoperative image, the diaphragm is flat from hyperinflation. (Courtesy of Joel Cooper M.D.)

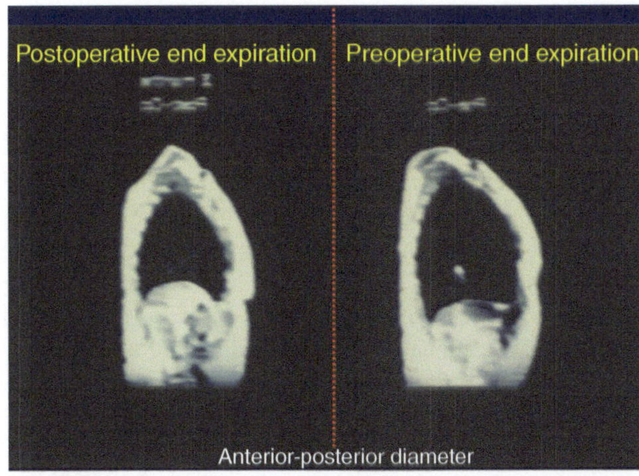

• **Fig. 29.8** The anterior-posterior diameter is larger and the patient is using his accessory muscles during inspiration. In the postoperative image the size of the chest decreased, the diaphragm has assumed its dome-shape and the shoulders of the patient are more relaxed because the accessory muscles to help with inspiration are not engaged. (Courtesy of Joel Cooper M.D.)

Another positive consequence of LVRS as depicted in the dynamic magnetic resonance imaging (Figs. 29.6–29.8) is the reduction of the hyperinflation and air which restores the diaphragm to a more curved position and the chest wall to a less expanded diameter, thereby improving the tension-length relationship and the respiratory mechanical advantage. The comparison between preoperative and postoperative is illustrated. In the preoperative images, the diaphragm is flat from hyperinflation, the AP diameter is large, and the patient sits using his accessory muscles to help in inspiration. In the postoperative images, the size of the chest decreased, the diaphragm has assumed its dome-shape, and shoulders of the patient are more relaxed because the accessory muscles are not engaged to help with inspiration.

Facing a nationwide increase in LVRS, the enthusiasm was tempered by the purported lack of convincing evidence of this new surgical intervention's safety, efficacy, and appropriate patient selection. The large number of potential procedures, specifically targeting the older population, could increase cost in the Medicare patient population. In the absence of sufficient evidence of beneficial outcome, the National Institutes of Health and the Health Care Financing Administration concluded in 1995 that "although initial results were promising, LVRS was often being performed with sufficient evaluation and a randomized study should be undertaken to evaluate the procedure critically." In an attempt to determine the potential beneficial outcome of the procedure, a nationwide "National Emphysema Treatment Trial" (NETT) was proposed.[19] This was a randomized multicenter prospective clinical trial of medical versus surgical treatments of patients with severe bilateral emphysema. Initially, the NETT would enroll 4700 patients with the primary outcomes of survival and maximum exercise capacity. Secondary outcomes studied would include QOL, cost effectiveness, oxygen requirements, cardiovascular measures, and surgical approach (thoracoscopy versus median sternotomy).

In 2001 the NETT Research Group published a preliminary report (n = 1033 patients) entitled "Patients at High Risk of Death After Lung Volume–Reduction Surgery." This report recommended not performing surgery on the highest-risk patients with emphysema. These high-risk patients were defined as having an FEV_1 under 20% predicted and either homogeneous distribution of emphysema on computed tomography (CT) scan or a carbon monoxide diffusing capacity (DLCO) under 20% predicted. When compared with the medically treated group, the surgical patients had a higher 30-day mortality rate after surgery (16% vs. 0%; 95% confidence interval [CI], 8.2–26.7%, $P < .001$) and overall mortality rate was higher in surgical patients than medical patients (0.43 deaths per person-year vs. 0.11 deaths per person-year; relative risk, 3.9; 95% CI, 1.9–9.0). The investigators concluded that the operation harmed some patients and did not benefit those who survived.[20] In an accompanying editorial, Dr. Jeffrey Drazen, the Editor-in-Chief of the New England Journal of Medicine, agreed: "At this time, it does not make sense to use lung-volume–reduction surgery in patients whose emphysema is so severe that they meet these exclusion criteria."[21] These preliminary results decreased dramatically the number of LVRS performed nationwide because of the lack of beneficial evidence for the procedure.

The final NETT study results were reported in 2003 and were somewhat disappointing. There were 1228, randomized patients were divided into four subgroups, depending on the extent of the emphysema and their exercise capacity[22]:

- Patients with **upper lobe predominant emphysema and a low exercise capacity**. Surgery was significantly more likely to lead to short-term and long-term improvement of exercise capacity and health-related QOL (Fig. 29.9).
- Patients with **upper lobe predominant emphysema and high exercise capacity**. Surgery did not impact the 90-day, short-term, or long-term mortality of this group (Fig. 29.10).
- Patients with **diffuse emphysema and low exercise capacity**. LVRS slightly increased 90-day mortality, but did not affect mortality at 24 months (Fig. 29.11).
- Patients with **diffuse emphysema and high exercise capacity**. LVRS increased 90-day mortality (Fig. 29.12).

Because of that initial impression that the mortality risk was higher with surgery, LVRS was met with significant skepticism by the pulmonary community. Concerns were raised relating to safety, patient selection, effectiveness, choice of surgical technique, and cost. The concern was based on the risk of performing a major thoracic surgery on patients with very poor lung function, which inherently imparts significant risk to individual patients while providing benefit to only a limited subgroup of patients with emphysema. The cost-effectiveness ratio in this subgroup was $98,000 per quality-adjusted life-year gained at 3 years and $21,000 at 10 years. The authors concluded that LVRS is costly relative to medical therapy, but that it may be cost effective if benefits can be maintained over time.[23,24] Because of these concerns, general acceptance by the medical community rapidly declined, from the peak of 1990s when more than 4000

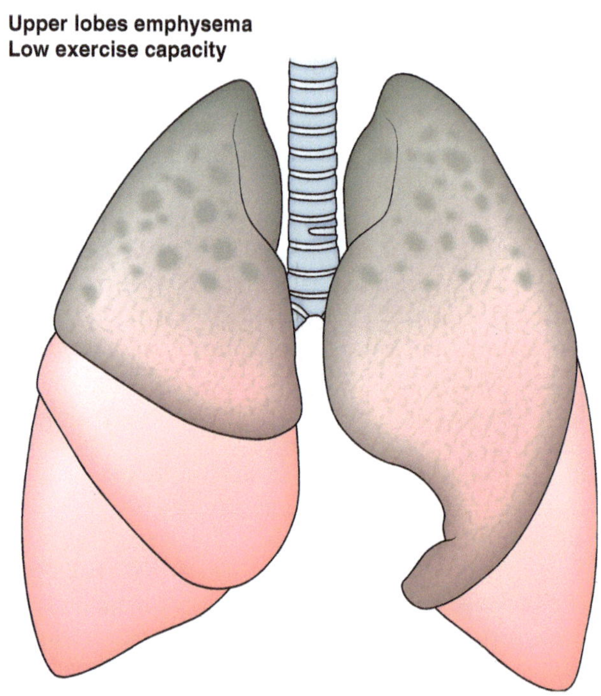

• **Fig. 29.9** Some 290 patients with upper lobe predominant emphysema and low exercise capacity. This surgical group had lower risk of death (risk ratio 0.47), and were significantly more likely to have an improvement of exercise capacity and health-related quality of life. (From NETT Research Group.)[22]

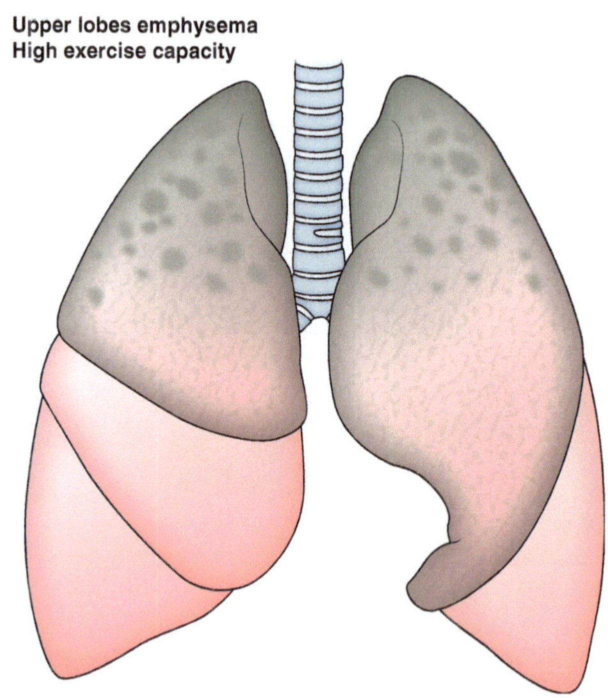

• **Fig. 29.10** Some 419 patients with upper lobe predominant emphysema and high exercise capacity. This surgical group had similar risk of death (risk ratio 0.98), but greater improvement in maximum workload. (From NETT Research Group.)[22]

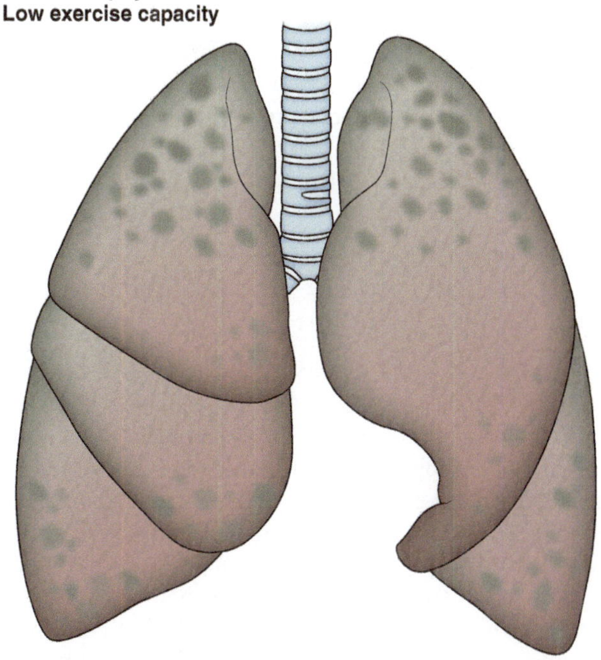

• **Fig. 29.11** 149 patients with nonupper lobe predominant emphysema and low exercise capacity. This surgical group had similar risk of mortality at 24 months (risk ratio 0.81) and similar improvement in maximum workload. (From NETT Research Group.)[22]

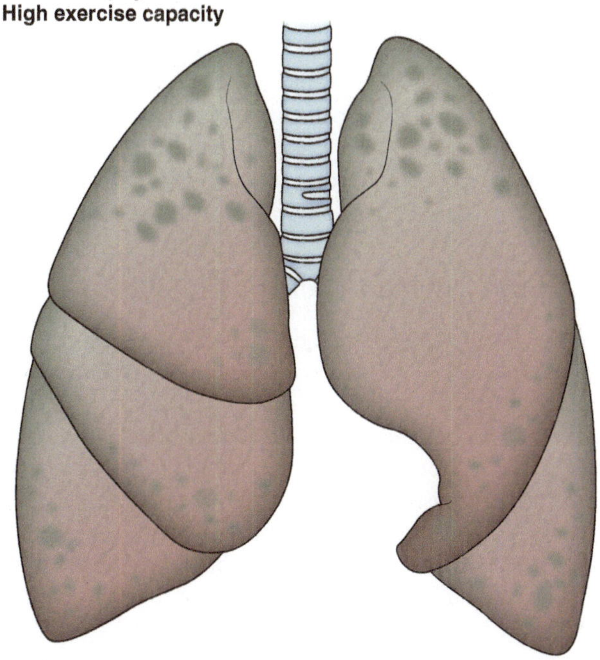

• **Fig. 29.12** 220 patients with predominantly nonupper lobe emphysema and high exercise capacity. This surgical group had higher risk of 90-day mortality (risk ratio 2.06), low improvement in maximum workload. (From NETT Research Group.)[22]

LVRS were done annually in the United States.[25] Several other studies reported the potential benefit of LVRS,[26–28] including some that compared medical therapy with surgical therapy.[29–31] Rather than acceptance of LVRS by the medical community, effort was focused on improving the less invasive endoscopic techniques, broadly described as BLVR (as described in Chapter 32).

Patient Selection and Rehabilitation

To be considered for LVRS, the patients should have end-stage emphysema, and that despite maximal medical therapy and rehabilitation may be a potential candidate to benefit from the procedure. Appropriate patients selection is crucial to ensure best outcomes with the least perioperative mortality. Most patients will have severe dyspnea despite optimal medical therapy and maximal pulmonary rehabilitation. Before considering a patient for LVRS, smoking cessation for longer than 6 months is an absolute requirement.[32,33] Testing typically includes pulmonary function tests, a six-minute walk test, arterial blood gas (ABG), electrocardiogram, echocardiogram with measurement of pulmonary artery pressures, a cardiopulmonary exercise test, and high-resolution computed tomography (HRCT).

The best-suited patients for LVRS are those who have distended chest walls and flattened diaphragms and who have a disease distribution that has a clear-cut distinction between normal and diseased lung tissue on CT scan rather than a homogeneous distribution throughout the lung.[34,35]

HRCT will confirm the heterogeneously distributed emphysema, quantitate the amount of lung affected, and assess the anatomic distribution. Diffuse and homogeneous distribution of emphysema on HRCT are less likely to benefit from LVRS than patients with a heterogeneous distribution of emphysema, particularly those with upper lobe predominant disease.[36]

Other criteria include age less than 75 years, severe airflow obstruction on spirometry with FEV_1 of less than 45% predicted, and a DLCO of at least 20% predicted. Other criteria include RV greater than 150% predicted, TLC greater than 100% predicted, and an increased RV/TLC ratio, which are all indicative of air trapping. As mentioned earlier, the patient must complete a course of postrehabilitation with postrehabilitation six-minute walk distance greater than 140 meters, but a low maximal achieved cycle ergometry.[37,38]

Exclusion Criteria (Fig. 29.13)

1. Patients who have an increased risk of surgical mortality from coronary heart disease, heart failure with a left ventricular ejection fraction less than 30%, or significant right heart dysfunction or pulmonary hypertension, pulmonary artery systolic pressure greater than 45 mm Hg, mean pulmonary artery pressure greater than 35 mm Hg would be excluded as a candidate for LVRS.[23,32]

Lung volume reduction

Patients' selection

- Progressive emphysema
- Severe, symptomatic dyspnea
- Radiographic evidence of diffuse emphysema
- Identifiable distention and hyperinflated lung tissue
- FEV_1 < 40%, RV > 150%, TLC > 120% predicted
- No previous chest surgery
- Smoking cessation
- Acceptable cardiac function

Contraindication

- Age > 75 years
- Uniformly destroyed lungs
  - FEV_1 < 15%
  - PaCO2 > 55 mm Hg
  - O2 > 6 L/min
- Pulmonary hypertension
- Severe kyphoscoliosis
- Predominance of chronic bronchitis, asthma
- Active infection
- Inability to complete preoperative rehabilitation program

• **Fig. 29.13** Criteria for patients' selection and contraindications. *FEV_1*, Forced expiratory volume in 1 second; *PaCO2*, arterial partial pressure of carbon dioxide; *RV*, residual volume; *TLC*, total lung capacity.

2. If severe hypercapnia is present which, is usually indicative of extensive emphysema, or hypoxemia with arterial partial pressure of carbon dioxide (PaCO2) greater than 60 mm Hg, or an arterial partial pressure of oxygen (PaO2) greater than 60 mm Hg.
3. Patients with prior thoracotomy or pleurodesis or chest deformity. The NETT data showed a significantly greater mortality in the sickest subgroups (16% at 30 days vs. 0 without surgery) and adjusted their exclusion criteria as a result to eliminate those with DLCO or FEV_1 less than 20% predicted or homogeneous distribution of disease.
4. Patients with continuous cigarette smoking within the prior six months[23]
5. Patients with severe cachexia or obesity: body mass index (BMI) over 31.1 kg/m^2
6. Patients unable to complete a 6-week to 10-week program of pulmonary rehabilitation
7. Patients who have lower lobe emphysema from severe alpha-1 antitrypsin deficiency, appear less likely to benefit from LVRS and should be considered with caution.

Preoperative Rehabilitation

Preoperative assessment typically includes ensuring that medical therapy for COPD is optimized and that comorbid illnesses (e.g., coronary heart disease, heart failure) have been evaluated and treated, as necessary. Optimizing patients preoperatively includes not only medical therapy, but exercise and nutritional rehabilitation as well. Patients who are below normal BMI, need to demonstrate improved nutritional status and weight gain in the weeks before surgery.[39] Most centers enroll patients in a supervised exercise rehabilitation program for 6 to 10 weeks preoperatively with specific goals, such as walking for 30 minutes on a treadmill at 1 mile/hour without stopping. Exercise rehabilitation also involves upper extremity strengthening and improved flexibility. Lastly, psychosocial counseling support needs to be available to patients and their families.[19]

Anesthetic Considerations

Preoperative Evaluation

Preoperative evaluation of these patients includes initial chest x-ray, which defines the degree of the hyperinflated thorax and CT scan, possibly HRCT, that shows heterogeneous areas of clear-cut distinction between normal and emphysematous lung. As mentioned previously, diffused and homogeneous distribution of emphysema on HRCT are less likely to benefit from LVRS than patients with a heterogeneous distribution of emphysema. Therefore, the radiologic findings will determine if the patient can be a candidate for LVRS. Pulmonary function tests should confirm that DLCO or FEV_1 are more than 20%, markedly abnormal alveolar gas exchange with a DLCO less than 20% of predicted mm Hg ABG, often present with hypercarbia a PaCO2 greater than 60 mm Hg, and hypoxemia or a PaO2 less than 45 mm Hg.[40,41] The electrocardiogram may present with electrical axis as normal (rightward axis P pulmonale which may be a sign of significant pulmonary hypertension). Echocardiography in these patients is performed via transesophageal echocardiography (TEE) because the transthoracic echocardiography (TTE) would most likely provide poor images in these patients, secondary to the intervening hyperinflated lungs.[42] Patients with signs of pulmonary hypertension or right heart failure or significant coronary artery disease most likely would not tolerate the procedure or recovery period. These patients should have a more invasive cardiac evolution, such as cardiac catherization, to clearly define the extent of the cardiac function and the pulmonary pressures.

Intraoperative Management (Fig. 29.14)

The anesthetic plan must be designed for the goal of early extubation in these patients with medically challenged pulmonary disease. For these patients in particular, there is no benefit to placing them on a positive-pressure ventilation (PPV), which should be kept to a minimal period as possible. PPV increases the risk of pulmonary complications in these patients including breath-stacking, barotrauma, and, most importantly for LVRS, increasing the risk of postoperative air leaks, which is a frequent complication in these patient population.[43,44] Therefore anesthetics of short duration with minimal postoperative respiratory depression should be used, which will allow early extubation and should be used with full reversal of any short action neuromuscular blockade.

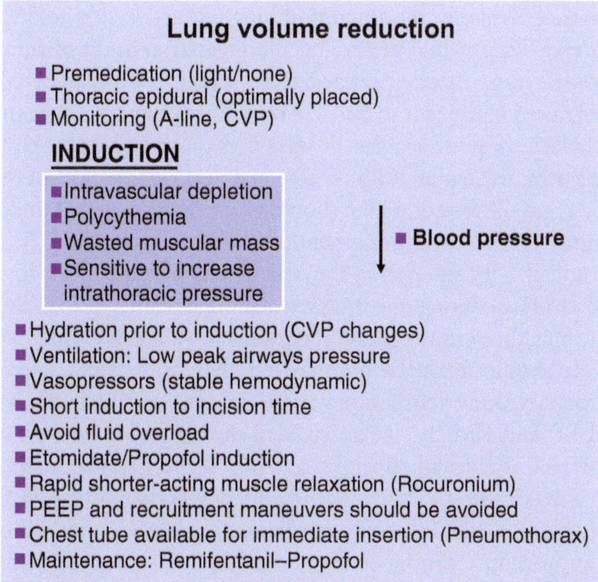

• **Fig. 29.14** Anesthetic management of lung volume reduction surgery. *CVP*, Central venous pressure; *PEEP*, positive end-expiratory pressure.

Thoracic epidural anesthesia and excellent postoperative pain management is the best approach for achieving this goal. A thoracic epidural is placed with the catheter tip at the T4 level preinduction and should be tested for proper function. Initially, in some institutions, given the importance of postoperative pain control, and in some institutions the correct placement of the epidural catheter is confirmed by fluoroscopic guidance. Because these patients are typically hypovolemic, only a small volume (4–5 cc) of a more dilute solution (1.5% lidocaine or 0.25% bupivacaine) should be enough to detect a sensory block without inducing significant hypotension. Correcting their volume status with a large fluid bolus before induction should also be avoided because of the concern over postoperative pulmonary edema, as most of these patients have a compromised right ventricular function of a variable degree owing to the presence of pulmonary hypertension.[45]

In the operating room, in addition to standard monitoring during the procedure, including blood pressure, pulse oximetry, capnography, core temperature, and continuous electrocardiogram, an arterial line is placed for blood pressure monitoring and serial assessment of ABGs. Central venous pressure monitoring is indicated in patients with significant cardiovascular disease. Pulmonary artery catheter placement is used in patients with significant pulmonary hypertension, otherwise they have not been found to provide additional benefit. Before induction of anesthesia, bronchodilator inhalers and stress-dose steroids can be given because that is part of the medical regime of most of these patients. An antisialagogue agent may be beneficial as well and is helpful to reduce the secretion to optimize the view for fiberoptic placement of the double lumen endotracheal tube (DLT).

LVRS is typically performed under general anesthesia. After induction, intravenous agents are preferable because the severe bullous disease may make the uptake and distribution of inhalational agents unpredictable. Propofol (2–3 mg/kg) is the preferred induction agent because of its inherent smooth muscle relaxant properties and minimal residual sedative effects. Owing to the risk of auto-positive end-expiratory pressure (auto-PEEP), hypovolemia and subsequent hypotension, one may consider administering a small dose of phenylephrine (0.5–1.0 mcg/kg) with the induction agent. A small amount of fentanyl, 1 to 2 mcg/kg, may be given with induction, but larger doses or continued administration are avoided as it could result in respiratory depression during emergence. Alternatively, remifentanil infusion, with its rapid clearance, can be safely used intraoperatively.[46,47] However, narcotics also increase the risk of postoperative nausea and vomiting, which is particularly undesirable in these patients shorter-acting neuromuscular blocking agents, such as rocuronium, are chosen for neuromuscular blockade to reduce risk of residual weakness complicating recovery and can be promptly reversed with sugammadex administration.

After induction of anesthesia, appropriate positioning, and sterile draping, a DLT is placed using propofol, low-dose fentanyl, or remifentanil infusion and rocuronium. Correct placement of the endotracheal tube is confirmed with fiberoptic bronchoscopy. Deflation of the operative lung may be slow because of the underlying obstructive airways disease and may require gentle suctioning and external pressure. Endobronchial blockers are less desirable for LVRS unless the patient has a difficult airway and a DLT is not an option. DLTs are preferred for bilateral procedure because deflation of the operative lung may be slow owing to the underlying obstructive airways disease and may require gentle suctioning and external pressure.

During single lung ventilation, patients with advanced COPD may develop air trapping and hyperinflation, causing hemodynamic instability. Modified protective lung ventilatory techniques, using low tidal volumes (5–6 mL/kg), lower respiratory rates, and longer expiratory times (I:E 1:3 or 1:4), can help prevent this complication. Lowering minute ventilation in this way may lead to alveolar hypoventilation and elevation in the PaCO2. Accepting deliberate alveolar hypoventilation to mitigate auto-PEEP is an acceptable permissive hypercapnic.[48,49]

If the strategies of permissive hypercapnia cause the pH to drop below 7.2, strategies such as a cautious increase in ventilatory rate, suctioning of airway secretions, optimizing muscle relaxation, and administering inhaled bronchodilator therapy, should help to improve alveolar ventilation. If hyperinflation and hemodynamic instability develop despite measures to minimize air trapping and auto-PEEP, transient disconnection of the endotracheal tube from the ventilator usually leads to resolution over several seconds.

Recruitment maneuvers (RM) should be avoided in patients with significant lung disease because these patients are at an increased risk of bullae rupture under positive pressure breaths that could cause tension pneumothorax. More commonly, intrinsic PEEP can complicate the expiratory phase, and, if not careful, stacked breaths with incomplete exhalation can result in overexpanded lungs.[6] This creates essentially a tamponade effect on the heart that decreases its preload and cardiac output. PPV with excessive tidal volumes or PEEP can increase pulmonary vascular resistance (PVR) and place an afterload strain on the right ventricle, further decreasing cardiac output. This "pulmonary tamponade" must be in the differential diagnosis of significant and refractory hypotension, and as mentioned before, the effect can often be relieved by disconnecting the breathing circuit from the ventilator and letting the lungs passively exhale.[50]

Maintenance and the Surgical Procedure

If inhaled anesthetic is used, less-soluble volatile anesthetics, either sevoflurane or desflurane, are ideal. For the longer procedures, the lower fat solubility of desflurane may confer a wakeup benefit and can relax smooth airway muscles. Nitrous oxide should be avoided owing to the risk of bullae rupture, and possible increase in PVR. Maintenance of anesthesia is best achieved with techniques including propofol infusion combined with remifentanil infusions. The depth of anesthesia should be monitored with bispectrality index (BIS) to facilitate emergence from anesthesia.[51,52] Lower concentrations of volatile anesthetics together with minimal doses of narcotics can be used in addition to boluses through an epidural catheter with local anesthetic. Intraoperatively this combination would have a MAC-sparing effect in addition to creating a sensory blockade from the surgical stimuli. If the epidural is activated during the surgery, sympathectomy may occur from higher concentrations of local anesthetics. Bupivacaine can have more profound sensory effect but the, motor blockade may induce hypotension that can be offset with the infusion of phenylephrine.

Given that these patients are often hypovolemic, hypotension is expected and treatment primarily involves vasopressor drugs rather than volume because postoperative pulmonary edema increases mortality. Capillary leak is probably the biggest culprit in this phenomenon. Typical fluid replacement is usually in the range of 1 to 2 L of crystalloid by arrival into the postanesthesia care unit (PACU). Ringer's lactate is usually chosen as the fluid of choice because the hyperchloremic metabolic acidosis induced by normal saline may aggravate the postoperative acidosis. Bilateral LVRS may be performed through a median sternotomy, staged anterolateral thoracotomies, or video-assisted thoracoscopy. When bilateral LVRS is planned, the more severely affected side is operated first. Unilateral LVRS is typically performed through a lateral thoracotomy or a video-assisted thoracoscopic approach.[53,54]

The operation is done through a standard median sternotomy incision or thoracoscopically. Oxygen at 100% is recommended before institution of one-lung ventilation. After a few minutes, absorption atelectasis promotes collapse of the perfused alveoli, leaving the most damaged areas that have no functional gas exchange, distended. That will provide some delineation of the emphysematous diseased area to be resected. Once identified, these areas are resected using a linear stapling device. Volume reduction is generally achieved by making a series of wedge excisions in areas where the emphysematous changes are most marked. Typically, the amount of lung resected is 20% to 35% of each lung, while preserving the greatest amount of functioning lung. Bovine pericardial strips and/or other materials were used in the past to buttress the suture line and reduce the incidence of postoperative air leaks.[55] Because the highest postoperative risk comes from persistent air leaks, the surface of the lung and the resection lines should be carefully inspected under saline for air leaks during gentle reinflation of the lung. It is prudent to try and restrict the peak airway pressure to less than 25 cm H_2O during one-lung ventilation and after reexpanding the lung. The entire operation typically takes 2 to 3 hours.

It should again be emphasized that the current use of protective lung ventilation which includes low tidal volume, PEEP, and RM should be avoided during LVRS because of the risk of alveolar ruptures. Owing to the strict adherence to a maximum peak airway pressure of less than 25 cm H_2O once one side is resected, ventilation for the second half of the procedure can be challenging. Tidal volumes are therefore often smaller than desired, especially given the need for a prolonged I:E ratio. Permissive hypercapnia is the end result and PCO_2s in the 60s mm Hg or higher are not unusual during the second phase of the operation. This permissive hypercapnia is well tolerated by these patients without significant cardiovascular issues.[56] Continuous positive airway pressure (CPAP) to the operative lung interferes with the identification of diseased versus normal lung tissue, and therefore is not recommended routinely.

The decision about whether to perform LVRS via thoracotomy or thoracoscopy depends in large part on the surgical and institutional expertise.[57] In a nonrandomized analysis of NETT data, morbidity and mortality were similar when LVRS was performed via thoracotomy or thoracoscopy. Thoracoscopic LVRS was associated with lower costs and shorter hospitalizations (9 vs. 10 days) than median sternotomy.

Emergence (Fig. 29.15)

After the second side is complete, a propofol infusion is added to the maintenance of our anesthetic to facilitate emergence. Adding dexmethomidine infusion would help to achieve a smooth emergence for anesthesia. Before extubation, an aggressive pulmonary suctioning through a bronchoscope at the end of surgery requires transient deepening of the anesthetic, making propofol an ideal choice. Most importantly, adequate epidural analgesia must be present before emergence.

Once the chest is closed and the chest tubes are connected to water seal or suction, the DLT may be changed to an 8.0 or 9.0 single lumen endotracheal tube to facilitate pulmonary toilet through the bronchoscope. However, if the secretions are not excessive, this step may be unnecessary and, once the airways are well-suctioned, the patient's neuromuscular blockade is reversed best with sugammadex if rocuronium was used, and the patient is placed in a semi-sitting position and allowed to spontaneously ventilate. Severe coughing and bucking on the endotracheal tube should be avoided. Mask ventilation with gentle CPAP assists the patient's spontaneous efforts after extubation until tidal volumes are adequate.[58]

Lung volume reduction

Intubation

DLT not Univent Blocker

- Easy to switch ventilation between the two lungs
- Frequent manipulation may cause desaturation
- Easy to deflate the operative lung
- Fiberoptic bronchoscopy is not absolutely necessary with a DLT
  - DLT or Univent MUST be optimally positioned

Postoperative

- Postoperative mechanical ventilation is undesirable
- Patients should be extubated at the end of the surgery
- Emergence should be smooth
- Fluid overload or hypovolemia may affect outcome
- Long-lasting narcotics/anesthetics may affect outcome
- Pain management should start in the OR.
  (Bupivacaine 0.5% intraoperatively)
  (Bupivacaine 0.25% postoperatively)

• **Fig. 29.15** Method of lung separation for lung volume reduction surgery and postoperative care. *DLT*, Double lumen endotracheal tube; *OR*, operating room.

Before extubation, the patient should be assessed for anemia because of excessive intraoperative blood loss, cardiac ischemia, electrolyte abnormalities, hypercapnia, hypoxemia, and inadequate lung reexpansion caused by air leak or suboptimal function of chest tubes. Every effort should be done to extubate the patient in the operating room to minimize the duration of PPV.

The patient should be monitored for at least 30 minutes before transfer to the PACU. Postintubation respiratory insufficiency can result from bronchoconstriction from the underlying COPD, atelectasis, pneumothorax, hypoventilation caused by postoperative pain. In these patients, even a small amount of anesthetic (0.1 MAC) can cause decreased respiratory drive to hypoxia or hypercarbia.[6] During emergence and the first few hours postoperatively, the patient is often hypercapnic and acidotic, but this is usually well tolerated. ABGs are frequently monitored during this period.

Early Recovery in the Postanesthesia Care Unit

The anticipated improvement in pulmonary function does not occur for a few weeks. In fact, pulmonary function undoubtedly may worsen in the immediate postoperative period. A decrease in FRC and VC are seen immediately postoperatively in upper abdominal and thoracic surgery, an effect that may last up to 2 weeks and that occurs despite adequate pain control.[6,53,54] Epidural anesthesia has been shown to be safe and effective even in patients with severe COPD with minimal effect on respiratory function.[59,60] In these high-risk patients, epidural local anesthetics can improve arterial oxygen tension, as well as decrease pulmonary infections and overall complications.

Nebulized albuterol and ipratropium bromide are administered immediately upon arrival to the PACU, followed by humidified 100% oxygen by face mask. The fraction of inspired oxygen (FiO2) is titrated down as tolerated to maintain an oxygen saturation between 92% and 95%. It is not necessary to keep inspired oxygen concentrations low in these patients to improve their hypoxic drive in the immediate postoperative period because oxygen therapy helps them tolerate their respiratory acidosis. Hypercarbia is seen in most patients in the PACU. One study stated that 25% patients had PCO2 over 80 mm Hg and 50% with PCO2 greater than 70 mm Hg in their first postoperative ABG,[33] whereas another reported a mean pH 7.26 (standard deviation [SD] 0.07) and PCO2 of 64.4 (SD 15). The patient remains in the PACU and chest x-ray and serial ABGs are drawn until the PCO2 is less than 60 mm Hg and the pH over 7.30.

Care must be taken to reduce risk of air leaks, and chest tubes should be placed to −10 cm water seal and not to excessive suction. Intravenous fluid maintenance is about 60 to 80 cc/h crystalloid while boluses should be given judiciously. Hypotension should not be treated with volume alone, and the liberal use of phenylephrine is common in the early postoperative period.

Postoperative pain control is achieved primarily with the epidural catheter. Good analgesia is a crucial element in the reduction of morbidity in these patients. Epidural local anesthetic allows the patients to avoid splinting and hypoventilation and helps them participate in chest physiotherapy and early ambulation. Inadequate pain control can lead to respiratory failure and reintubation, which should be avoided. Combining local anesthetic and narcotic, such as bupivacaine 0.1%, plus fentanyl 2 to 4 mcg/mL can provide excellent analgesia with fewer side effects; lower concentrations of each can be used because of synergistic effect. Triantafillou et al. reported that infusions containing bupivacaine 0.2% resulted in 40% to 50% patients requiring phenylephrine drips after discharge from PACU. In summary, fluids should be given judiciously, but should not be restricted to the point where high doses of vasopressors are required leading to a decreased end organ perfusion.[61,62]

Epidural narcotics carry the risk of respiratory depression, but those with high-lipid solubility have a lower risk when compared with hydrophilic opioids or intravenous supplementation. Therefore in a high thoracic epidural catheter, fentanyl or sufentanil is preferred to morphine.[63,64] Small doses are sufficient when added to a local anesthetic infusion. Indeed, higher concentrations of epidural narcotic can cause unwanted side effects, such as nausea and pruritis.[30] Multimodal analgesic regimen should also include a nonsteroidal antiinflammatory drug (NSAID), such as ketorolac. NSAIDs can help patients tolerate the chest tube irritation that is not adequately covered by the epidural. Similarly, selective cyclooxygenase (COX)-2 inhibitors can be considered, with their reduced effect on platelets being a potential advantage.[65] However, both NSAIDs and COX-2 inhibitors should be administered with caution because the incidence of renal failure is increased when they are given in the presence of relative hypovolemia, a situation common to LVRS patients.[65–69]

Persistent air leak, lasting more than 1 week, is the most common complication with an incidence as high as 46%. Pneumonia, phrenic nerve palsy, respiratory failure with need for reintubation, empyema, wound infection, intrathoracic bleeding, and myocardial ischemia or infarction are also reported. Patients with prolonged air leak can be discharged home with a chest tube with a Heimlich one-way valve.[70–72]

The Value of BODE Index

A multidimensional index called BODE (BMI, degree of airflow obstruction assessed by spirometry, grade of dyspnea, and exercise capacity), quantified by 6-minute walk distance (6MWD), has excellent predictive power with respect to outcome in COPD.[73,74] Whether the BODE index is able to predict survival after LVRS was investigated. The authors retrospectively evaluated 186 patients with severe emphysema who underwent bilateral thoracoscopic LVRS. BMI, pulmonary function, 6MWD, and the modified Medical Research Council dyspnea score were assessed before and 3 months after LVRS, and the BODE index was calculated. The patients were followed up with respect to survival for a median time of 40 months after surgery. The mean BODE index decreased from 7.2 ± 1.6 preoperatively to 4.0 ± 2.0 at 3 months after LVRS (P <. 001). The postoperative but not the preoperative BODE correlated with survival, although preoperative patient characteristics were comparable between short-term (<5 years) and long-term (>5 years) survivors. A decrease to a lower BODE score class was associated with a reduced mortality. The C statistic for the ability of the BODE index to predict the risk of death was larger (0.74) than that for the FEV_1 (0.63), the degree of dyspnea (0.64), or the 6MWD (0.62). The authors concluded that the postoperative BODE index is a powerful predictor of survival in COPD patients after LVRS.[75]

Martinez et al.[76] evaluated a cohort of 610 patients treated medically and 608 treated surgically with LVRS, all had severe airflow obstruction, moderate breathlessness, and increased modified BODE (mBODE) at baseline. A wide distribution of change in mBODE was seen at follow-up. An increase in mBODE of more than 1 point was associated with increased mortality in surgically and medically treated patients. Surgically treated patients were less likely to experience death or an increase greater than 1 in mBODE. Indices of concordance showed that mBODE change predicted survival better than its separate components.

The issue of LVRS as a bridge to lung transplantation and as it compared with lung transplanting is well described in a recent publication by Martinez.[77]

"LVRS and lung transplantation When emphysema is advanced, both LVRS and lung transplantation are often considered.

Comparison: A retrospective series compared functional outcomes (pulmonary function tests, ABG analysis, 6 MWD) in 33 patients who underwent LVRS versus 39 patients who had single lung transplantation and 27 patients who had bilateral sequential lung transplantation. The patients were evaluated before the operation and at 3, 6, and 12 months after surgery. The following results were noted:

- The mean FEV_1 improved by 79% at 6 months and 82% at 12 months in the LVRS group, 231% and 212% in the single lung transplant group, and 498% and 518% in the bilateral lung transplant group.
- The 6 MWD at 6 months after surgery improved by 28% in the LVRS group, 47% in the single lung transplant recipients, and 79% in the bilateral lung transplant recipients.
- All lung transplant recipients required supplemental oxygen before surgery, whereas none needed oxygen at rest or during exercise after the transplant. Eighty-eight percent of the patients who underwent LVRS required oxygen before surgery, and only 5.5% were oxygen-dependent during exercise and none at rest after LVRS.

Thus although LVRS results in substantial improvements, single and bilateral lung transplantation result in superior lung function. Interpretation of these results must be cautious given the retrospective nature of the study and the baseline differences in age and pulmonary physiology between the groups.

Bridging procedure: Patients who undergo LVRS are not automatically excluded from undergoing lung transplantation. Limited experience with patients who initially undergo LVRS suggests that subsequent successful transplantation is possible. In one prospective study, LVRS before lung transplantation improved symptoms and lung function enough to delay lung transplantation for a median of 33 months in eight of 58 potential lung transplant candidates, while not impairing recovery or survival after transplantation. Outcomes of lung transplantation following LVRS are discussed separately."

Conclusion

LVRS is not a widespread procedure. Although the NETT study identified a subgroup of patients who may benefit from the procedure, as described earlier in this chapter, concerns were raised relating to safety, patient selection, effectiveness, choice of surgical technique, and cost. The concern was based on the risk of performing a major thoracic surgery on patients with very poor lung function, which inherently imparts significant risk to individual patients while providing benefit to only a limited subgroup of patients with emphysema. Endoscopic lung volume reduction with endobronchial valves is expanding in the treatment of end-stage emphysema patients. These valves, made of silicon and nitinol, prevent air from entering the diseased segments but allow mucus and air out. They can be placed and removed by a bronchoscopic approach. Other means, such as fibrin glue, metal coils, and thermal application are all under investigation and presently are not approved by the U.S. Food and Drug Administration (see Chapter 32). These investigations are encouraging that further studies and technologic development may improve the quality and length of life in patients with end-stage COPD without the need for surgery.

References

1. May SM, Li JT. Burden of chronic obstructive pulmonary disease: healthcare costs and beyond. *Allergy Asthma Proc.* 2015;36(1):4–10.
2. Global Initiative for Chronic Obstructive Lung Disease. *Chronic Obstructive Pulmonary Disease: A Definition and Implications of Structural Determinants of Airflow Obstruction for Epidemiology*; 2020 Report.
3. Guarascio AJ, Ray SM, Finch CK, Self TH. The clinical and economic burden of chronic obstructive pulmonary disease in the USA. *Clinicoecon Outcomes Res.* 2013;5:235–245.
4. Snider GL. Chronic obstructive pulmonary disease: a definition and implications of structural determinants of airflow obstruction for epidemiology. *Am Rev Respir Dis.* 1989;140:(3) Pt 2 S3–S8.
5. Hogg JC, Senior RM. Chronic obstructive pulmonary disease c2: pathology and biochemistry of emphysema. *Thorax.* 2002;57:830–834.
6. Seigne PW, Hartigan PM, Body SC. Anesthetic considerations for patients with severe emphysematous lung disease. *Int Anesthesiol Clin.* 2000;38:1–23.
7. Wan IY, Toma TP, Geddes DM, et al. Bronchoscopic lung volume reduction for end-stage emphysema: report on the first 98 patients. *Chest.* 2006;129(3):518–526.
8. Sterman DH, Mehta AC, Wood DE, et al. A multicenter pilot study of a bronchial valve for the treatment of severe emphysema. *Respiration.* 2010;79(3):222–233.
9. Sciurba FC, Ernst A, Herth FJ, et al. A randomized study of endobronchial valves for advanced emphysema. *N Engl J Med.* 2010;363(13):1233–1244.
10. Brantigan OC, Mueller E. Surgical treatment of pulmonary emphysema. *Am Surg.* 1957;23:789–804.
11. Cooper JD, Trulock EP, Triantafillou AN, et al. Bilateral pneumectomy (volume reduction) for chronic obstructive pulmonary disease. *J Thorac Cardiovasc Surg.* 1995;109:106–116.
12. Cooper JD, Patterson GA. Lung volume reduction surgery for severe emphysema. *Semin Thorac Cardiovasc Surg.* 1996;8:52–60.
13. Cooper JD, Lefrak SS. Lung-reduction surgery: 5 years on. *Lancet.* 1999;353:SI26–SI127.
14. Attaway AH, Hatipoğlu U, Murthy S, Zein J. Lung volume reduction surgery in the United States From 2007 to 2013: increasing volumes and reason for caution. *Chest.* 2019;155:1080.
15. Meyers BF, Yusen RD, Lefrak SS, et al. Outcome of Medicare patients with emphysema selected for, but denied, a lung volume reduction operation. *Ann Thorac Surg.* 1998;66:331–336.
16. Brenner M, McKenna RJ Jr, Chen JC, et al. Survival following bilateral staple lung volume reduction surgery for emphysema. *Chest.* 1999;115:390–396.
17. Yusen RD, Lefrak SS, Gierda DS, et al. A prospective evaluation of lung volume reduction surgery in 200 consecutive patients. *Chest.* 2003;123:1026–1037.
18. Ciccone AM, Meyers BF, Guthrie TJ, et al. Long-term outcome of bilateral lung volume reduction in 250 consecutive patients with emphysema. *J Thorac Cardiovasc Surg.* 2003;125:513–525.
19. National Emphysema Therapy Trial Research Group. Rationale and design of the national emphysema treatment trial. A prospective randomized trial of lung volume reduction surgery. *J Cardiopulm Rehabil.* 2000;20:24–36.
20. NETT Research Group. Patients at high risk of death after lung-volume-reduction surgery. *N Engl J Med.* 2001;345:1075–1083.
21. Drazen JM, Epstein AM. Guidance concerning surgery for emphysema. *N Engl J Med.* 2003;348:2134.
22. NETT Research Group. A randomized trial comparing lung-volume-reduction surgery with medical therapy for severe emphysema. *N Engl J Med.* 2003;348:2059–2073.
23. Ault A. US government to pay for lung volume reduction surgery. *Lancet.* 2003;362:712.
24. Ramsey SD, Berry K, Etzioni R, et al. Cost effectiveness of lung-volume-reduction surgery for patients with severe emphysema. *N Engl J Med.* 2003;348:2092–2102.
25. Decker MR, Leverson GE, Jaoude WA, Maloney JD. Lung volume reduction surgery since the National Emphysema Treatment Trial: study of Society of Thoracic Surgeons Database. *J Thorac Cardiovasc Surg.* 2014;148:2651.
26. Martinez FJ, de Oca MM, Whyte RI, et al. Lung-volume reduction improves dyspnea, dynamic hyperinflation, and respiratory muscle function. *Am J Respir Crit Care Med.* 1997;155:1984.
27. Keller CA, Ruppel G, Hibbett A, et al. Thoracoscopic lung volume reduction surgery reduces dyspnea and improves exercise capacity in patients with emphysema. *Am J Respir Crit Care Med.* 1997;156:60.
28. van Agteren JE, Carson KV, Tiong LU, Smith BJ. Lung volume reduction surgery for diffuse emphysema. *Cochrane Database Syst Rev.* 2016;10. CD001001.
29. Miller JD, Berger RL, Malthaner RA, et al. Lung volume reduction surgery vs medical treatment: for patients with advanced emphysema. *Chest.* 2005;127:1166.
30. Miller JD, Malthaner RA, Goldsmith CH, et al. A randomized clinical trial of lung volume reduction surgery versus best medical care for patients with advanced emphysema: a two-year study from Canada. *Ann Thorac Surg.* 2006;81:314.
31. Fishman A, Martinez F, Naunheim K, et al. A randomized trial comparing lung-volume-reduction surgery with medical therapy for severe emphysema. *N Engl J Med.* 2003;348:2059.
32. McKenna RJ Jr, Brenner M, Fischel RJ, et al. Patient selection criteria for lung volume reduction surgery. *J Thorac Cardiovasc Surg.* 1997;114:957–964.
33. Markos J, Mullan BP, Hillman DR, et al. Preoperative assessment as a predictor of mortality and morbidity after lung resection. *Am Rev Respir Dis.* 1989;139:902–910.
34. Hunsaker A, Ingenito E, Topal U, et al. Preoperative screening for lung volume reduction surgery: usefulness of combining thin-section CT with physiologic assessment. *AJR Am J Roentgenol.* 1998;170:309.
35. Cederlund K, Tylén U, Jorfeldt L, Aspelin P. Classification of emphysema in candidates for lung volume reduction surgery: a new objective and surgically oriented model for describing CT severity and heterogeneity. *Chest.* 2002;122:590.
36. Slone RM, Pilgram TK, Gierada DS, et al. Lung volume reduction surgery: comparison of preoperative radiologic features and clinical outcome. *Radiology.* 1997;204:685–693.
37. National Emphysema Therapy Trial Research Group. Rationale and design of the national emphysema treatment trial. A prospective randomized trial of lung volume reduction surgery. *J Cardiopulm Rehabil.* 2000;20:24–36.
38. DeCamp MM Jr, Lipson D, Krasna M, et al. The evaluation and preparation of the patient for lung volume reduction surgery. *Proc Am Thorac Soc.* 2008;5:427.
39. Tschernko EM, Kritzinger M, Gruber EM, et al. Lung volume reduction surgery: preoperative functional predictors for postoperative outcome. *Anesth Analg.* 1999;88:28–33.
40. American Thoracic Society, European Respiratory Society. Standards for the diagnosis and management of patients with COPD.

http://www.thoracic.org/clinical/copd-guidelines/index.php. Accessed March 29, 2010.
41. Shrager JB, Kaiser LR, Edelman JD. Lung volume reduction surgery. *Curr Prob Surg.* 2000;37:257–317.
42. Bach DS, Curtis JL, Christensen PJ, et al. Preoperative echocardiographic evaluation of patients referred for lung volume reduction surgery. *Chest.* 1998;114:972–980.
43. Triantafillou AN. Anesthetic management for bilateral volume reduction surgery. *Semin Thorac Cardiovasc Surg.* 1996;8:94–98.
44. Cohen E. Surgical treatment of end-stage emphysema: current status? *Curr Opin Anesthesiol.* 2003;16:53.
45. Buettner AU, McRae R, Myles PS, et al. Anaesthesia and postoperative pain management for bilateral lung volume reduction surgery. *Anaesth Intensive Care.* 1999;27:503.
46. Zollinger A, Pasch T. Anaesthesia for lung volume reduction surgery. *Curr Opin Anaesthesiol.* 1998;11:45–49.
47. Conacher ID. Anasthesia for the surgery of emphysema. *Br J Anaesth.* 1997;79:530–538.
48. Hillier J, Gillbe C. Anaesthesia for lung volume reduction surgery. *Anaesthesia.* 2003;58:1210.
49. Brister NW, Barnette RE, Kim V, Keresztury M. Anesthetic considerations in candidates for lung volume reduction surgery. *Proc Am Thorac Soc.* 2008;5:432.
50. Liu EH, Gillbe CE, Watson AC. Anaesthetic management of patients undergoing lung volume reduction surgery for treatment of severe emphysema. *Anaesth Intensive Care.* 1999; 27:459–463.
51. Drover DR, Lemmens HJ, Pierce ET, et al. Patient State Index: titration of delivery and recovery from propofol, alfentanil, and nitrous oxide anesthesia. *Anesthesiology.* 2002;97:82–89.
52. Gan TJ, Glass PS, Windsor A, et al. Bispectral index monitoring allows faster emergence and improved recovery from propofol, alfentanil, and nitrous oxide anesthesia. *Anesthesiology.* 1997;87:808–815.
53. Alvarez JM, Bairstow BM, Tang C, Newman MA. Post-lung resection pulmonary edema: a case for aggressive management. *J Cardiothorac Vasc Anesth.* 1998;12:199–205.
54. Mathru M, Blakeman BP. Don't drown the "down lung." *Chest.* 1993;103:1644–1645.
55. Fischel RJ, McKenna RJ Jr. Bovine pericardium versus bovine collagen to buttress staples for lung reduction operations. *Ann Thorac Surg.* 1998;65:217.
56. Morisaki H, Serita R, Innami Y, Kotake Y, Takeda J. Permissive hypercapnia during thoracic anaesthesia. *Acta Anaesthesiol Scand.* 1999;43:845–849.
57. McKenna RJ Jr, Benditt JO, DeCamp M, et al. Safety and efficacy of median sternotomy versus video-assisted thoracic surgery for lung volume reduction surgery. *J Thorac Cardiovasc Surg.* 2004;127:1350.
58. Krucylak PE, Naunheim KS, Keller CA, Baudendistel LJ. Anesthetic management of patients undergoing unilateral video-assisted lung reduction for treatment of end-stage emphysema. *J Cardiothorac Vasc Anesth.* 1996;10:850–853.
59. Gruber EM, Tschernko EM, Kritzinger M, et al. The effects of thoracic epidural analgesia with bupivacaine 0.25% on ventilatory mechanics in patients with severe chronic obstructive pulmonary disease. *Anesth Analg.* 2001;92:1015–1019.
60. Groeben H, Schafer B, Pavlakovic G, Silvanus MT, Peters J. Lung function under high thoracic segmental epidural anesthesia with ropivacaine or bupivacaine in patients with severe obstructive pulmonary disease undergoing breast surgery. *Anesthesiology.* 2002;96:536–541.
61. Gruber EM, Tschernko EM, Kritzinger M, et al. The effects of thoracic epidural analgesia with bupivacaine 0.25% on ventilatory mechanics in patients with severe chronic obstructive pulmonary disease. *Anesth Analg.* 2001;92:1015–1019.
62. Ballantyne JC, Carr DB, deFerrant S, et al. The comparative effects of postoperative analgesic therapies on pulmonary outcome: cumulative meta-analyses of randomized, controlled trials. *Anesth Analg.* 1998;86:598–612.
63. Mahon SV, Berry PD, Jackson M, Russell GN, Pennefather SH. Thoracic epidural infusions for post-thoracotomy pain: a comparison of fentanyl-bupivacaine mixtures vs. fentanyl alone. *Anaesthesia.* 1999;54:641–646.
64. Kahn L, Baxter FJ, Dauphin A, et al. A comparison of thoracic and lumbar epidural techniques for post-thoracoabdominal esophagectomy analgesia. *Can J Anesth.* 1999;46:415–422.
65. Liu SS, Allen HW, Olsson GL. Patient-controlled epidural analgesia with bupivacaine and fentanyl on hospital wards: prospective experience with 1,030 surgical patients. *Anesthesiology.* 1998;88:688–695.
66. Burgess FW, Anderson DM, Colonna D, Cavanaugh DG. Thoracic epidural analgesia with bupivacaine and fentanyl for postoperative thoracotomy pain. *J Cardiothorac Vasc Anesth.* 1994;8:420–424.
67. de Leon-Casasola OA, Lema MJ. Postoperative epidural opioid analgesia: what are the choices? *Anesth Analg.* 1996;83:867–875.
68. Bernards CM. Rostral spread of epidural morphine: the expected and the unexpected. *Anesthesiology.* 2000;92:299–301.
69. Schnitzer TJ. Cyclooxygenase-2-specific inhibitors: are they safe? *Am J Med.* 2001;110:46S–49S.
70. Vaughn CC, Wolner E, Dahan M, et al. Prevention of air leaks after pulmonary wedge resection. *Ann Thorac Surg.* 1997;63:864.
71. Moser C, Opitz I, Zhai W, et al. Autologous fibrin sealant reduces the incidence of prolonged air leak and duration of chest tube drainage after lung volume reduction surgery: a prospective randomized blinded study. *J Thorac Cardiovasc Surg.* 2008;136:843.
72. DeCamp MM, Blackstone EH, Naunheim KS, et al. Patient and surgical factors influencing air leak after lung volume reduction surgery: lessons learned from the National Emphysema Treatment Trial. *Ann Thorac Surg.* 2006;82:197.
73. Lederer DJ, Thomashow BM, Ginsburg ME, et al. Lung-volume reduction surgery for pulmonary emphysema: improvement in body mass index, airflow obstruction, dyspnea, and exercise capacity index after 1 year. *J Thorac Cardiovasc Surg.* 2007; 133:1434.
74. Pompeo E, Mineo TC. Two-year improvement in multidimensional body mass index, airflow obstruction, dyspnea, and exercise capacity index after nonresectional lung volume reduction surgery in awake patients. *Ann Thorac Surg.* 2007;84:1862.
75. Imfeld S, Bloch KE, Weder W, Russi EW. The BODE index after lung volume reduction surgery correlates with survival. *Chest.* 2006;129(4):873–878.
76. Martinez FJ, MeiLan KH, Andrei A-C, et al. and for the National Emphysema Treatment Trial Research Group. Longitudinal change in the BODE index predicts mortality in severe emphysema. *Am J Respir Crit Care Med.* 2008;178(5):491–499.
77. Martinez FJ. *Lung volume reduction surgery in COPD*; 2019 *UpToDate.* June.

30

The Patient With Cardiovascular Disease for Lung Resection Surgery

ANAHITA DABO-TRUBELJA, GREGORY W. FISCHER

Introduction

The patient with cardiovascular disease (CVD) presenting for lung resection surgery has special concern. Identifying significant cardiac risk factors provides information to better quantify the risks of a possible cardiac event in the perioperative period. Cardiac complications in the perioperative period may prolong recovery in the immediate postoperative period and may also affect outcome following the surgery. Over the past decades, research initially focused on identifying cardiac risk factors in patients with CVD presenting for noncardiac surgery (NCS). Recent research focused on randomized controlled trials identifying strategies to reduce perioperative cardiac complications. Cardiac risk is specific to each patient and to the extent of the surgery. Guidelines from the American College of Cardiology (ACC) and the American Heart Association (AHA) provide information and guidelines for the evaluation and management of the cardiac risk and best practices to reduce morbidity and mortality for patients with CVD presenting for NCS.[1] This chapter will outline risk assessment, identify appropriate noninvasive testing in patients with suspected or known coronary artery disease (CAD), and outline management of perioperative medical therapies to reduce the risk of cardiac complications during and after lung resection surgery including anticoagulation therapies.

Incidence

A national database review of over 10 million hospitalized patients from 2003 to 2014 presenting for NCS revealed a perioperative incidence of cardiovascular events of 3%.[2] Over 5% of major cardiac events (in-hospital, all cause death, acute myocardial infarction [MI], or acute ischemic stroke) occurred in thoracic, vascular, and transplant surgery. In addition, those with an estimated decrease in systolic function of less than 40% had a higher incidence of perioperative cardiac morbidity. The perioperative period is characterized by a catecholamine surge, prothrombotic milieu, altered platelet function, increased oxygen demand from fluctuating heart rate and blood pressure, as well as volume shifts and blood loss. This predisposes and contributes to a higher incidence of myocardial ischemia in patients with CVD. Patients with CVD, because of their underlying disease, have an increased risk of perioperative cardiac complications compared with those patients without CVD.[2]

Assessment of Risk

Every patient scheduled for lung surgery should have an assessment of risk of a cardiac event in the perioperative period. Many risk models have been developed over the past decades based on preoperative evaluation of patient history, physical examination, electrocardiogram (ECG), and type of surgery. The original cardiac risk index (CRI) was developed in 1977 by Goldman et al.[3] and was known as the Goldman Index. It included nine variables associated with an increased risk of a cardiovascular event in the perioperative period. The Goldman index has been validated since its inception and was revised in 1999 by Lee et al.[4] to include six independent variables and revised again by Davis et al.[5] in 2013 to five variables. This simplified index of five independent variables was validated in 9519 patients over the age of 50 years undergoing major NCS with an expected length of stay longer than 2 days at two major tertiary teaching hospitals. Five independent variables were identified that predicted an increased risk for perioperative cardiac complications. The risk increased with the number of variables that were present in the patient (Table 30.1). Patients with less than 1% are in the low risk group and no further testing is required. In the higher risk group, further testing determines whether there will be a change in management and improved outcome, especially in the long term. Another model has been developed by the American College of Surgeons National Surgical Quality Improvement Program (ACS NSQIP) called the Gupta myocardial infarction or cardiac arrest (MICA) NSQIP database risk model.[6] The NSQIP MICA is an online risk calculator that is comprehensive and procedure specific. It is based on a national database evaluation of risk factors in over 200,000 patients who underwent surgery in 2007. This

TABLE 30.1 Revised Cardiac Risk Index

Independent Predictors of Major Cardiac Complications		
High-Risk Surgery		Thoracic, Vascular, Open Abdominal
Ischemic heart disease		History of MI
		Positive stress test
		Current chest pain
		Nitrate therapy
		Pathologic Q waves on ECG
History of congestive heart failure		
History of cerebrovascular disease		
Preoperative glomerular filtration rate (GFR) <30 mL/min		
Risk of Cardiac Death, Nonfatal MI, Noncardiac Death		
Risk Factors	**Percentage (%)**	**95% CI**
0	0.4	0.1–0.8
1	1.0	0.5–1.4
2	2.4	1.3–3.5
3 or >	5.4	2.8–7.9
Risk of MI, Pulmonary Edema, VF, Primary Cardiac Arrest, Complete Heart Block		
Risk Factors	**Percentage (%)**	**95% CI**
0	0.5	0.2–1.1
1	1.3	0.7–2.1
2	3.6	2.1–5.6
3 or >	9.1	5.5–13.8

CI, Confidence interval; *ECG*, electrocardiography; *MI*, myocardial infarction; *VF*, ventricular fibrillation.

study showed a 0.65% rate of perioperative MI or cardiac arrest. Five factors were associated with an increased risk of a perioperative MI or cardiac arrest:

- Type of surgery
- Functional status
- Preoperative creatinine level
- American Society of Anesthesiology (ASA) physical status classification
- Increased age

The newer NSQIP MICA calculator is more comprehensive and cumbersome and includes over 20 patient risk factors, as well as surgical procedures. Also developed by the ACS, is the ACS NSQIP surgical risk calculator. This has not been externally validated because confounding factors, such as institution, surgeon experience, and different definitions of risk, complications, and outcomes may increase or lower the overall risk in the perioperative period. A comparison of Revised CRI, NSQIP MICA, and the NSQIP surgical risk calculator is shown in Table 30.2.

The Revised CRI remains the standard for assessing perioperative cardiac risk in the preoperative evaluation of the patient presenting for NCS. It also guides the decision for further testing and management protocols in preparing the patient for NCS.

Ischemic Heart Disease

The patient with coronary ischemic heart disease (CAD) may be evaluated by a primary caregiver or by a cardiologist. However, many patients are evaluated by the surgeon or anesthesiologist immediately before surgery. According to the Society of Thoracic Surgeons national database, the incidence of CAD in patients undergoing lung resection is greater than 20%.[7] The preoperative evaluation should focus on identifying the presence of stable or unstable CAD because these patients have a higher risk of cardiac decompensation leading to a cardiac event in the perioperative period. In addition, the stress of undergoing a thoracic procedure may elevate the heart rate and further contribute to myocardial ischemia from an increase in oxygen demand in the symptomatic or asymptomatic patient. Identification of risk factors would determine the extent of preoperative

TABLE 30.2 Comparison of the Revised Cardiac Risk Index, the American College of Surgeons NSQIP Myocardial Infarction or Cardiac Arrest, and the American College of Surgeons National Surgical Quality Improvement Program Surgical Risk Calculator

Revised Cardiac Risk Index	American College of Surgeons NSQIP Myocardial Infarction or Cardiac Arrest	American College of Surgeons NSQIP Surgical Risk Calculator
Criteria	**Increasing age**	**Age**
Ischemic heart disease	—	Previous cardiac event
GFR <30 mL/min	Creatinine >1.5 mg/dL	Acute renal failure
Heart failure	—	Heart failure
IDDM	—	DM
History of CVA	—	—
Intrathoracic surgery	Based on surgery type: Neurosurgery Head and neck Cardiac and thoracic Abdominal Vascular Orthopedic	Based on current procedural terminology (CPT)
		Single point for the following ASA class, wound class, ascites, sepsis, emergency surgery, ventilator dependent, widespread cancer, steroid use, hypertension, sex, dyspnea, smoker, COPD, dialysis, acute kidney injury, BMI
Calculation method		
One point per risk factor	www.surgicalriskcalculator.com/miorcardiacarrest	www.riskcalculator.facs.org

ASA, American Society of Anesthesiologists; *BMI*, body mass index; *COPD*, chronic obstructive pulmonary disease; *CVA*, cerebrovascular accident; *DM*, diabetes mellitus; *IDDM*, insulin-dependent diabetes mellitus; *GFR*, glomerular filtration rate; *MICA*, myocardial infarction or cardiac arrest; *NSQIP*, National Surgical Quality Improvement Program.

testing that should be performed and if their results will affect perioperative management. Changes in management may include delay of surgery for prohibitive risks, delay of surgery for further medical management and optimization before surgery, coronary interventions such as stents placement, or if indicated, preoperative admission to the hospital for medical optimization, and monitoring.

Angina or dyspnea, which manifests with mild exertion may be a sign of significant CAD. Additional testing and monitoring should be considered as these patients are at high risk of perioperative cardiovascular events such as ventricular dysfunction, congestive heart failure, myocardial ischemia, or infarction. The patient with angina who is on strenuous exertion or stress test and does not manifest signs of left ventricular dysfunction can be medically managed with aspirin, beta blockers, nitrates, and statins. These patients can be considered optimized and no further cardiac testing is required.

In the event a patient has a history of prior MI, the timing between MI and surgery is crucial. Within 30 days of an MI, plaque and myocardial healing occurs. After this period, risk stratification is based on the presenting symptoms. Some patients will continue to have myocardium at risk; most patients however, were likely to have been reevaluated and their coronary stenosis revascularized if indicated or be on maximal medical therapy. The current practice of improved perioperative management, thrombolytics, and revascularization procedures have decreased the risk of reinfarction rate following NCS even if the prior MI was within 6 months.[8–10]

Hypertension

Several large prospective studies have failed to establish mild to moderate hypertension as an independent predictor of postoperative cardiac complications, including arrhythmias, MI, heart failure, and cardiac death. Chronic hypertension may lead to increased risk of perioperative MI because these patients have a higher occurrence of CAD. However, in the Perioperative Ischemic Evaluation (POISE) trial of beta blocker therapy, the incidence of hypertension was 62% among 8351 patients and did not show hypertension as an independent predictor of postoperative stroke or death. Poorly controlled hypertension is often associated with hemodynamic fluctuations during anesthesia. The approach to the hypertensive patient relies on management strategies from nonsurgical literature where the recommendation being to continue antihypertensive agents in the perioperative period for optimal control of blood pressure. Blood pressure should be maintained at or near preoperative levels to reduce the risk of myocardial ischemia. In patients with severe hypertension, such as diastolic blood pressure higher than 110 mm Hg, the decision to delay surgery for optimization of blood pressure control should be weighed against the benefit or the urgency of surgery. A study by Hartle et al.[11] of 989 patients, compared the preoperative use of rapid-acting intravenous agents to lower blood pressure with a control group admitted for blood pressure control with 10-mg nifedipine intranasally. Control of blood pressure was rapidly achieved within a few hours and there was no statistical difference observed in postoperative complications between the two groups, suggesting that this subset of patients without significant cardiovascular comorbidities can proceed with surgery despite elevated blood pressure on the day of surgery.

Heart Failure

The clinical approach to the preoperative evaluation of the patient with heart failure should focus on risk assessment to determine whether to proceed with surgery, how to manage the patient intraoperatively, and postoperative care. This should be in agreement with the 2013 and 2014 ACC/AHA perioperative guidelines.[12] The initial step should take into consideration the following:

- The assessment of functional status
- Determining if patients are medically stable and optimized
- Signs and symptoms of heart failure
- Risk factors for developing heart failure
- Comorbidities that may exacerbate heart failure in the perioperative period: underlying myocardial disease, CAD, valvular disease

Patients with heart failure have a higher risk of perioperative morbidity and mortality. Improvement in medical care has led patients to live longer with chronic diseases. Elderly patients who often lead a sedentary lifestyle because of chronic comorbidities and deconditioning, and have a higher incidence of heart failure. Symptoms of heart failure, such as fatigue and dyspnea, are not specific and may be confused with other chronic conditions, such as obesity and lung disease, which contribute to the delay in diagnosis and treatment. Careful preoperative evaluation is often required to differentiate heart failure from other debilitating comorbidities. For this reason, the elderly patient may present with an advanced stage of heart failure for preoperative evaluation. Elderly patients with heart failure have an increased risk of readmission compared with those with CAD admitted for the same diagnosis. A population-based analysis of 38,047 patients revealed a higher 30-day postoperative rate mortality for patients with nonischemic heart failure compared with other cardiac comorbidities, as shown in Table 30.3.

Although emphasis has been made on predicting cardiac perioperative risk in patients with CAD, patients with heart failure have a significantly higher risk of perioperative death than those with CAD. Certain risk factors and triggers should be identified as these contribute to the increased risk for major adverse events in the perioperative period. Identifying the severity of morbidities, such as CAD, hypertension, arrythmias, kidney disease, and diabetes in the patient with heart failure would influence the patient management in the perioperative period. These optimization measures may include early postoperative dialysis, preoperative beta blockers or antiarrhythmic medications, and optimal pain control to prevent hypertension.[13] It is important to differentiate the etiology of the cardiomyopathy: dilated, obstructive, or ischemic. They have different perioperative management, which can affect influence postoperative morbidity. Dilated cardiomyopathy may require inotropic support; ischemic cardiomyopathy may develop further ischemia in the perioperative period. Obstructive cardiomyopathy has long been viewed as high risk for perioperative complications because of its high preload dependence with consequences of further dynamic obstruction, decreased cardiac output, and potential untoward results. Studies related to perioperative outcomes in patients with hypertrophic cardiomyopathy had small sample sizes, reflected different perioperative management, and have had mixed results.[14] Most postoperative events were related to heart failure. Important independent risk factors for increased morbidity were major surgery and increased duration of surgery. Several studies show the 30-day cardiovascular event rate at 14% among heart failure patients with normal left ventricular function, 31% with left ventricular diastolic dysfunction, and up to 54% among patients with symptomatic heart failure. Risk classification remains a challenge because there is no model that can reliably predict who will experience a perioperative event opposed to those who will not across all levels of risk. Therefore the goals in the perioperative period, in addition to identifying the etiology and precipitating factors, should be to maintain stability, including symptomatic relief, maintain normal oxygenation, optimize volume status, and maintain organ perfusion.

The routine measurement of brain natriuretic peptide (BNP) is recommended in patients when the diagnosis is uncertain. BNP levels may also be helpful to identify disease severity, and in patients at increased risk for adverse outcome. Karthikeyan et al.[15] evaluated nine studies, which included a total of 3281 patients, among whom 314 experienced

TABLE 30.3 The 30-Day Postoperative Mortality in Patients With Nonischemic Heart Failure Compared With Other Cardiac Morbidities

Cardiac Comorbidity	30-Day Postoperative Mortality
Nonischemic heart failure	9.3%
Ischemic heart failure	9.2%
Atrial fibrillation	6.4%
Coronary artery disease	2.9%

one or more perioperative cardiovascular complications. The average proportion of patients with elevated BNP was 24.8%. All studies showed a statistically significant association between an elevated preoperative BNP level and various cardiovascular outcomes, such as a composite of cardiac death and nonfatal myocardial infarction or atrial fibrillation. The preoperative BNP measurement was an independent predictor of perioperative cardiovascular events in the first 30 days after NCS.

Valvular Heart Disease

The patient with valvular heart disease has significant risks for perioperative complications in the perioperative period. Suspected patients with valvular heart disease should undergo echocardiography evaluation for quantification of severity of stenosis or regurgitation, systolic function, and heart pressures if there has been no prior echocardiography performed within the past year or there is a change in clinical status since last evaluation. Patients should also undergo appropriate evaluation for the extent of the CAD. Over the past decades, improvements in anesthetic and surgical techniques have seen a significant decrease in 30-day perioperative morbidity and mortality from 13% to 2.1%. The mechanism of an acute perioperative event is likely associated with anesthetic agents and surgical stress leading to hemodynamic instability, decreased coronary perfusion with myocardial ischemia, arrythmias, heart failure, and possible death. Agarwal et al.[16] evaluated the risk for perioperative complication in patients undergoing NCS with moderate aortic stenosis (AS) (valve area: 1.0–1.5 cm^2) or severe AS (valve area: <1.0 cm^2) from an echocardiographic database. Using propensity score analysis, they obtained four matched control patients without AS for each patient with AS undergoing NCS, matching 634 patients with AS undergoing NCS to 2536 controls. There were 244 patients with severe AS and 390 patients with moderate AS. The 30-day mortality was 2.1% for AS patients compared with 1.0% in non-AS controls (P = .036). Postoperative myocardial infarction was more frequent in patients with AS compared with controls (3.0% vs. 1.1%; P = .001). High-risk surgery, symptomatic severe AS, coexisting mitral regurgitation (MR), and preexisting coronary disease were significant predictors of primary outcome in patients with AS. Predictors of 30-day mortality in patients with moderate or severe AS are shown in Table 30.4.[16]

Patients who are candidates for aortic valve replacement (AVR) before lung resection surgery have several options available depending on their risk criteria. Options include AVR, transcatheter aortic valve replacement (TAVR), or percutaneous balloon dilation, as a bridge to definitive treatment after lung resection surgery. If they are considered high risk or ineligible, these patients may proceed with lung resection surgery with invasive monitoring for optimal hemodynamic monitoring. Simultaneously performed AVR and lung resection surgery on bypass have been carried out with success.

Patients with moderate to severe MR undergoing NCS had a higher perioperative mortality rate (1.7%) than those without MR (<1%). The 30-day primary outcomes, including postoperative death, MI, heart failure, and stroke, were 22.2% in those with MR compared with 16.4% without MR. Important predictors of morbidity in these patients were left ventricular ejection fraction less than 35%, ischemic etiology of MR, a history of diabetes mellitus, and a history of carotid endarterectomy. Perioperative management should include invasive hemodynamic monitoring and echocardiography and admission to the intensive care unit for postoperative management and care.[17]

TABLE 30.4 Predictors of 30-Day Postoperative Mortality and Myocardial Infarction in Patients With Moderate or Severe Aortic Stenosis

Associated Cardiac Comorbidity	Odds Ratio	95% Confidence Interval
High-risk surgery	7.3	2.6–20.6
Symptomatic severe AS	2.7	1.1–7.5
Moderate or severe MR	9.8	3.1–20.4
Preexisting CAD	2.7	1.1–6.2

AS, Aortic stenosis; *CAD*, coronary artery disease; *MR*, mitral regurgitation.

Prosthetic Valves

An estimated 13% of patients with prosthetic heart valves will require noncardiac surgical procedure. These patients are at an increased risk of bleeding because of their anticoagulation therapy or for a thrombotic event from holding anticoagulation therapy in the perioperative period. The risk of a thrombotic event is higher in the immediate postoperative period and diminishes over time. In patients with an international normalizing ration (INR) maintained at 2.5 to 3.5, it is recommended to stop oral anticoagulation 5 days before surgery to let the INR decrease to a normal level. The INR should be tested on the day of surgery as individual responses are unpredictable and may vary. If the INR level is greater than 1.5 on the day of the procedure, oral administration of vitamin K, 1 to 2 mg, is an acceptable practice to lower the INR below 1.5 and proceed with surgery. Oral anticoagulation therapy may be resumed 12 to 24 hours after surgery. In cases of high risk for bleeding, the patient should be bridged with low-molecular-weight heparin (LMWH). Oral anticoagulation should be stopped 4 to 5 days before surgery and LMWH initiated. The last dose should be given 24 hours before surgery and may be resumed 48 to 72 hours after surgery when adequate hemostasis is secured. Different options for bridging therapies are available for outpatients and inpatients, depending on the clinical scenarios. The decision on how to bridge anticoagulation therapy with LMWH or unfractionated heparin should be decided with the clinical care management team following current guidelines. If the patient is at high risk for a perioperative thrombotic event, aspirin should be continued during the perioperative period. The decision should be based on the risk of bleeding versus the risk of a thrombotic event.[18] Aspirin should be discontinued before spine, intracranial, or intraocular procedures.

Pulmonary Hypertension

Progressive dyspnea, unexplained dyspnea, fatigue, or syncope are clinical symptoms susceptive of pulmonary hypertension (PH). Once PH is suspected, transthoracic echocardiography is the initial test of choice. Echocardiography evidence includes: pulmonary artery systolic pressure (PASP) over 40 mm Hg, tricuspid regurgitant jet velocity exceeding 2.8 m/s, and signs of right ventricular (RV) dysfunction (size, thickness, and/or function). Other parameters of RV pressure overload, including RV failure, right atrial enlargement, decreased pulmonary acceleration time, and increase in inferior vena cava diameter can be found. The left-sided heart disease contribution to PH includes left ventricular systolic dysfunction, left ventricular diastolic dysfunction, and mitral valvular disease. Right heart catheterization remains the gold standard for PH diagnosis. It is important to distinguish left heart disease from right heart disease in the etiology of PH because the approach to therapies is different. The presence of shunting in congenital heart disease and its relation to PH must be also evaluated for the presence of possible Eisenmenger syndrome. PH is further discussed in Chapter 36.

Arrhythmias

Cardiac arrhythmias and conduction disorders are common findings in the perioperative period, particularly in thoracic surgery. The presence of arrhythmia in the perioperative period, such as the presence of atrial fibrillation, should prompt investigation into the underlying etiology of the arrhythmia. This subject is discussed in detail in Chapter 22 on perioperative arrythmia.

Congenital Heart Disease in Adults

The patient with congenital heart disease should be evaluated in a center that specializes in preoperative evaluation of patients with congenital heart disease. These patients have an increased risk of perioperative events related to the nature of their congenital cardiac disease and the surgery performed, especially if there is a residual cyanotic lesion. These patients may also have developmental and psychologic concerns that must be addressed in the perioperative period. Maxwell et al.[19] compared patients with adult congenital heart disease (ACHD) who underwent NCS with a non-ACHD comparison cohort matched on age, sex, race, year, elective, or urgent or emergency procedure. They evaluated 10,004 ACHD patients who were compared with a matched comparison cohort of 37,581 patients. Inpatient mortality was greater in the ACHD cohort (407 of 10,004 [**4.1%**] vs. 1355 of 37,581 [**3.6%**]; $P < .001$). The authors concluded that, compared with a matched control cohort, ACHD patients undergoing NCS experienced increased perioperative morbidity and mortality. Within the limitations of a retrospective analysis of a large administrative dataset, this finding demonstrates that this is a vulnerable population and suggests that better efforts are needed to understand and improve the perioperative care they receive.

Diagnostic Test

The patient presenting for thoracic surgery should have a stepwise approach to perioperative cardiac assessment. Functional status is good predictor of perioperative cardiac events.[20] It also is reliable in predicting long-term cardiac outcome. Functional capacity status can be estimated from the activities of daily living in terms of **metabolic equivalent (METs)** as shown in Table 30.5.

One MET is the equivalent of resting or basal oxygen consumption of a 40-year-old 70-kg male. Functional capacity is described as excellent if greater than 10 METs, good 7 to 10 METs, moderate 4 to 7 METs, poor less than 4 METs or unknown. In a highly functional patient, it is often acceptable to proceed to surgery without any additional preoperative testing. In a patient with reduced or unknown functional status, preoperative testing can be used as assessment of risk of a likely perioperative cardiac event. Functional status can also be assessed using the more formal DUKE activity scale as shown in Table 30.6. The **DUKE Activity Status Index** is an assessment tool used to evaluate the functional capacity of patients with CVD, such as CAD, myocardial infarction, and heart failure. In clinical practice, it can be used to assess the effects of medical treatments and cardiac rehabilitation as well.[2] Positive responses are summed up to get a total score, which ranges from 0 to 58.2. Higher scores would indicate a higher functional capacity.[21] Using this activity scale, it was shown that patients with poor preoperative functional status were at higher risk of a perioperative cardiac event even when adjusted for other factors. Poor functional status was defined as the inability to walk four blocks or climb two flight of stairs.

TABLE 30.5 Metabolic Equivalents (METS) of Various Activities

METS	Activity Level
1	Light: reading, getting dressed, eating, watching TV
2–3	Light: housework, walking 3–4 km/h
4	Moderate: golf, walking 6 km/h, climbing few stairs, heavy housework
>10	Strenuous: tennis, swimming, running, skiing

TABLE 30.6 DUKE Activity Functional Status Questionnaire

Activity Question: Are You Able To?	Weighted Score
Perform daily personal needs (dress, bath)	2.75
Walk around the house	1.75
Walk two blocks	2.75
Climb a flight of stairs	5.50
Run a short distance	8.00
Light housework	2.70
Moderate housework—vacuum	3.50
Move furniture	8.00
Yardwork	4.50
Have sexual relations	5.25
Moderate physical activities—tennis	6.00
Strenuous physical activities	7.50

The **ACS National Surgical Quality Improvement Program (ACS NSQIP®)** is a nationally validated, risk-adjusted, outcomes-based program to measure and improve the quality of surgical care. It provides participating hospitals with tools, analyses, and reports to make informed decisions about improving quality of care. Further, peer-reviewed studies have shown that ACS NSQIP is effective in improving the quality of surgical care while also reducing complications and costs. The ACS NSQIP relied on formal activities of daily living questionnaire rather than METs. National dataset analysis has shown that the need for assistance in daily activities was associated with significant risk of perioperative morbidity and mortality.[22,23]

Cardiac Risk Stratification for Thoracic Procedures

To quantify cardiac risk for patients undergoing pulmonary resection, Brunelli et al.[24] in 2010 proposed a new risk score, the **Thoracic Revised Cardiac Risk Index** (ThRCRI). This assessment of risk calculator was derived from patients undergoing lung resection surgery. There were 1426 patients undergoing pulmonary lobectomies and 270 patients with pneumonectomies. Four different factors were taken into account to calculate the ThRCRI score and each was assigned 1.5 points for a maximum of 5.5 points. This identified four different classes, A, B, C, and D, and the incidence of a major perioperative cardiac event in each class was assessed. A major cardiac event was defined as occurring within 30 days of pulmonary resection and included acute myocardial infarction-diagnosed by ECG changes and increased serum troponin level, pulmonary edema as confirmed by consistent findings on chest x-ray, ventricular fibrillation or primary cardiac arrest, complete heart block, and any cardiac-related death. The ThRCRI was validated in outside studies and was revised in 2011 after a large series of pulmonary resections in two different external populations of more than 3000 patients (Table 30.7). A comparison of RCRI and ThRCRI is shown in Table 30.8.

TABLE 30.7 Recalibrated Thoracic Revised Cardiac Index

Risk Factor	Points	
Ischemic heart disease	1.5	
History of cerebrovascular accident	1.5	
Serum creatinine >2 mg/dL	1.0	
Planned pneumonectomy	1.5	
Class	**Points**	**Risk of Cardiac Complication**
A	0	1.5%
B	1–1.5	5.8%
C	2–2.5	19%
D	>2.5	23%

These studies revealed that a patient with a score greater than C2 should be referred for a formal cardiology evaluation because of increased perioperative cardiac risk. The recalibrated ThRCRI may be used as a first-line screening tool in risk stratification to identify the patients who present for lung resection surgery who may require a cardiac evaluation, from those who may proceed to surgery without further cardiac testing. Brunelli et al.[24] analyzed 2431 patients undergoing lobectomy and 190 patients undergoing pneumonectomy. Patients were grouped into four classes of risk (A, B, C, and D) according to the recalibrated ThRCRI. The outcome variable measured was the occurrence of major cardiac complications as defined by the ThRCRI. (Incidence of major cardiac events was assessed in the four risk class groupings to assess the discriminative ability of the index score. The incidence of major cardiac morbidity was 2.2%

TABLE 30.8 Comparison Revised Cardiac Risk Index and Thoracic Revised Cardiac Risk Index

Risk Classes	Revised Cardiac Risk Index (%)	Thoracic Revised Cardiac Risk Index (%)
A	1	1.5
B	2.3	5.8
C	6	19
D	7.3	23

[59 cases].) Patients were grouped into four risk classes according to their recalibrated ThRCRI. Incidence of major cardiac morbidity in risk classes A, B, C, and D were 0.9%, 4.2%, 8%, and 18%, respectively ($P < .0001$). The authors concluded that the recalibrated ThRCRI is a reliable instrument that can be used during preoperative workup to differentiate patients needing further cardiologic testing from those who can proceed without any further cardiac testing.

Inclusion of Biomarkers

As previously discussed, preoperative BNP and C-reactive protein have been studied as risk indices to identify patients with increased risk of a perioperative cardiac event. Meta-analysis has suggested that these biomarkers may prove useful as a predictive value. However, the time frame in obtaining levels of biomarkers varied and studies did not include a control arm nor were biomarkers followed serially in the postoperative period. Studies also failed to prove that targeting these biomarkers for treatment in the perioperative period reduced perioperative cardiac complications.[25,26]

Electrocardiogram

In a patient with a history of CAD, a resting 12-lead ECG contained information relating to perioperative morbidity and mortality. Prognostic significance of numerous abnormalities appreciated, such as pathologic Q-waves, left ventricular hypertrophy, ST depressions, QTc prolongation, and bundle branch blocks, have been well established in prospective observational studies. A baseline standard ECG to which changes can be measured in the postoperative period is important information to obtain in all patients scheduled for thoracic surgery. Abnormalities increase with patient age and with risk factors for CAD. However, a standard risk factor cutoff or age has not been determined for the use of ECG in the preoperative evaluation, or knowing the optimal time to obtain an ECG for elective surgery. Expert consensus is between 1 and 3 months before surgery if the patient is stable, and as part of the preoperative evaluation if there has been a change in clinical status.[27,28]

Recommendation for Coronary Revascularization

The decision to perform coronary bypass surgery (CABG) or percutaneous coronary intervention (PCI) depends on current risk stratification guidelines. Patients with significant CAD whose risk stratification recommends CABG surgery should undergo coronary revascularization before lung resection surgery. In patients who are not candidates for coronary revascularization, PCI should be performed. In patients whose surgery is time sensitive, balloon angioplasty or bare-metal stent (BMS) implantation can be considered. However, prospective randomized control trials (RCTs) do not support coronary revascularization with either CABG or PCI to reduce the risk of perioperative cardiac event. In the Coronary Artery Revascularization Prophylaxis (CARP) RCT trial, there was no difference appreciated in perioperative cardiac events and long-term cardiac outcomes in patients with CAD who underwent preoperative coronary revascularization by CABG or PCI. In a prospective study, McFalls et al.[29] included 510 patient who were randomly assigned to either coronary-artery revascularization before surgery or no revascularization before surgery. The indications for a vascular operation were an expanding abdominal aortic aneurysm (33%) or arterial occlusive disease of the legs (67%). Among the patients assigned to preoperative coronary-artery revascularization, PCI was performed in 59%, and bypass surgery was performed in 41%. The median time from randomization to vascular surgery was 54 days in the revascularization group and 18 days in the group not undergoing revascularization ($P < .001$). At 2.7 years after randomization, mortality in the revascularization group was 22% and, in the no revascularization group, 23%. Within 30 days after the vascular operation, a postoperative myocardial infarction, defined by elevated troponin levels, occurred in 12% of the revascularization group and 14% of the no revascularization group. The exceptions were patients with left main disease, reduced left ventricular function less than 20%, and severe AS. Recommendations for coronary revascularization and timing of surgery in patients with previous PCI are shown in Table 30.9.[29]

TABLE 30.9 Recommendations of Coronary Revascularization and Timing of Elective Surgery

Recommendation	Level of Recommendation
Coronary Revascularization Before Noncardiac Surgery	**Class**
Indicated by existing cardiac procedural guidelines	I
To reduce perioperative cardiac events	III—no benefit
Timing of Elective Noncardiac Surgery in Patients With Previous Percutaneous Coronary Intervention	
Delay surgery—14 days after balloon angioplasty	I
Delay surgery—30 days after bare metal stent implantation	I
Delay surgery—90 days after drug eluding stent placement	I

Cardiac Implantable Devices and Left Ventricular Assist Devices

Patients with cardiac implantable electric devices (CIEDs) presenting for lung resection surgery should have their devices reprogrammed before surgery. The patient should be on cardiac monitoring continuously and external defibrillator equipment at the patient's bedside while the device is inactive. The proximity of the device and the surgical field has the potential for interaction between the CIED and the electrocautery used by the surgeon. This is especially important if the patient is pacemaker dependent because electrocautery may cause inhibition of pacing. Depending on the underlying cardiac condition necessitating placement of pacemaker or internal cardiac defibrillator (ICD), the clinical care team should be familiar with the type of device, patient program, whether the patient is dependent on the pacemaker, programmability of the device, if there is a concurrent ICD, and last recording events. Advances in pacemaker/ICD technology is rapidly evolving, necessitating communication between the cardiologist and clinical care team in the perioperative period concerning best management of the CIED in the perioperative period.[30]

Left ventricular assist devices (LVADs) are becoming more common in the patient population presenting for NCS. The LVAD has prolonged patients' lives, and patients are able to live a relatively normal life with an LVAD in place. Although the patients with LVADs require a different approach, lung resection surgery is feasible in a patient with an implantable LVAD. Evidence on best practice is limited to expert opinion and case series. The effects of one-lung ventilation (OLV) on the right heart and pulmonary vascular resistance and device function must be considered. Preoperative risk assessments are not valid in this patient population as significant perioperative hemodynamic changes involving LVAD flow occurs. A balanced LVAD flow that is preload dependent and afterload sensitive must be considered. The anesthesiologist must be aware of LVAD-related complications, balancing protective mechanical ventilation and right ventricular hemodynamics, and be familiar with invasive monitoring, including transesophageal echocardiography. It is recommended that patients with LVADs should have their surgery performed at an institution provided by clinical care teams that are familiar with both thoracic and LVAD surgery.[31]

Recommendation for Perioperative Therapy

The use of beta blockers in the perioperative period in improving long-term outcomes has been validated in many studies over the past decades. It is unclear, however, whether starting beta blocker therapy in the perioperative period has any effect on immediate or long-term outcome. Initiating beta blocker therapy less than 1 day before surgery may be ineffective and even harmful because tight control of heart rate may contribute to an adverse event in the perioperative period. The POISE trial in 2008 has demonstrated that perioperative blockade was effective in reducing cardiac events but at a cost of increased mortality and stroke.[32–34]

There are limited RCTs and observational studies on the use of statins in the perioperative period. Evidence suggests the use of statins in the perioperative period has a protective effect on perioperative cardiac complications. Observational studies showed that even if started in the immediate preoperative period compared with patients with no statin therapy, there was an overall 5-times reduction in 30-day perioperative myocardial injury and a reduction in mortality at 2-year follow-up in the statin patients. The mechanism in which statin benefits in cardiac protection remains unclear, but this may be an opportunity to contribute to long-term health in patients presenting preoperatively for NCS.[35,36]

Angiotensin converting enzyme (ACE) inhibitors are the most prescribed drug in the United States; however, only observational studies have data on its effects in the perioperative period on patients undergoing NCS. Metaanalysis of available trials reveals that patients continuing ACE inhibitors or angiotensin receptor blockers (ARB), such as losartan, even on the day of surgery had more hypotension throughout the perioperative period but there was no difference in cardiovascular outcomes of death, stroke, MI, and kidney failure.[37]

Patients with a BMS or a drug eluding stent (DES) are at higher risk of stent thrombosis 4 to 6 weeks after implantation. Should the patient with a BMS or DES require surgery, the decision to continue dual antiplatelet therapy (DAPT) should be on an individualized basis, made between the patient and the physician care teams, with the risk of bleeding weighed against the risk of thrombosis. After 6 weeks of stent implantation, the risk of thrombosis is lower and varies from study to study. The decision whether to continue DAPT or to proceed with aspirin alone should be decided based on risk–benefit ratio as there is no definitive data but is based on expert consensus. Continuing aspirin throughout the perioperative period may seem reasonable if the risk of a thrombotic event outweighs the risk of bleeding.[38–44] Recommendations for perioperative therapy are outlined in Table 30.10.

Supplemental recommendations for preoperative evaluation of the patient with CVD for NCS and the level of recommendation are outlined in Tables 30.11 and 30.12. The stepwise approach to the cardiac patient presenting for NCS based on the 2014 ACC/AHA guidelines is outlined in Fig. 30.1.

Hypoxemia and Coronary Artery Disease

A major concern in the anesthetic management of patients with CAD undergoing lung resection surgery is the occurrence of hypoxemia during OLV. There is no absolute value that is universally acceptable as the lowest oxygen saturation during OLV. An oxygen saturation of 90% equals a partial arterial oxygen pressure (PaO2) of 60 mm Hg which is usually accepted as the lowest limit. The balance between oxygen supply and demand is regulated by a variety of factors, including the autonomic nervous system, arterial pressure, arterial oxygen tension, and myocardial metabolism, collectively contributing to coronary vasculature resistance. Decreases in PaO2 result in coronary vasodilation and the oxygen supply–demand balance is well maintained to the level of 40 mm Hg PaO2. Below this value, activation of the sympathetic nervous system occurs with an increase in aortic pressure, heart rate, and myocardial oxygen consumption.

TABLE 30.10 Recommendations for Perioperative Therapy

Recommendations	Level of Recommendation
Perioperative Beta Blocker	**Class**
Continue in patients who are on beta blockers	I
Postoperative beta blocker by clinical circumstances	IIa
High-risk preoperative testing begin beta blocker	IIb
>3 Revised Cardiac Risk Index factors, begin beta blocker	IIb
To reduce perioperative risk with no Revised Cardiac Risk Index	IIb
Begin >1 day preoperatively to assess tolerability	IIb
Do not start beta blocker on day of surgery	III—harm
Perioperative Statin Therapy	
Continue statins if currently on statins	I
Initiate if clinical risk factor and high-risk surgery	IIb
Alpha-2 Agonist	
Not recommended to prevent cardiac event	III—no benefit
Angiotensin-Converting Enzyme Inhibitors	
Continue angiotensin-converting enzyme inhibitor or angiotensin receptor blocker	IIa
If discontinued, resume postoperatively as soon clinically feasible	IIa
Antiplatelet Agents in Patients With Coronary Stents	
Continue dual antiplatelet therapy during 4–6 weeks after bare-metal stent or drug-eluting stent, unless risk of bleeding outweighs risk of rethrombosis	I
Discontinuing P2Y12 should be bridged with American Society of Anesthesiologists, and P2Y12 restarted as soon as possible	I
Management should be consensus between patient and treating physicians	I
American Society of Anesthesiologists in Patients Without Coronary Stents	
Continue if risk of perioperative cardiac event is greater than risk of bleeding	IIb

The partial pressure of oxygen in myocardial tissue is reduced yielding local metabolic vasodilator activation and increased myocardial oxygen consumption. The coronary vascular response depends on metabolic and endothelial vasodilatory factors that are produced in direct proportion to the degree of hypoxemia. Effects of hypoxic coronary vasodilation are appreciated as ischemic ST segment changes on ECG, lactate production, and decreased cardiac contractile function.[45–47]

Anesthetic Goals in Patients With Coronary Artery Disease

The goals in the perioperative period of a patient with CAD is to prevent, detect, and treat to avert myocardial injury after NCS (MINS).[48] Negative oxygen balance ischemia rather than acute thrombosis is in most cases the etiology by which an acute ischemic event occurs.[49] Therefore it is important to optimize hemodynamics and maximize oxygen supply and minimize oxygen demand with the following objectives in the perioperative period:

1. **Maintain normal to low heart rate.** Tachycardia increases oxygen demand and is associated with an increased risk of MINS. This relationship is nonlinear but more exponential. Doubling the heart rate more than doubles the risk of MINS in the perioperative period. Tachycardia that last longer than 30-min duration had a higher risk of MINS, with an odds ratio (OR) of 2.22; 95% confidence interval (CI), 1.71–2.88. Intraoperative tachycardia greater than 100 beats per minute was associated with increased:
   - MINS OR, 1.27; 95% CI, 1.07 to 1.5
   - MI OR, 1.34; 95% CI, 1.05 to 1.07
   - Mortality OR, 2.65; 95% CI, 2.06 to 3.41

   Bradycardia less than 55 beats per minute was associated with a decreased risk of MINS.[48]
2. **Blood pressure should be maintained within 20% of baseline** for optimal oxygen supply–demand. Hypotension reduces myocardial oxygen supply, whereas hypertension

TABLE 30.11 Supplemental Preoperative Cardiac Evaluation for Noncardiac Surgery and Level of Recommendation

Preoperative Testing	Recommendation	Level of Recommendation
ECG	Patients with known CAD, structural heart disease except low-risk surgery	Class IIa
	Consider for asymptomatic patients as baseline except for low-risk surgery	Class IIb
	Routine asymptomatic patients for low-risk surgery	Class III—no benefit
Assessment of LV function	Dyspnea of unknown origin	Class IIa
	Heart failure patients with change in clinical status	Class IIa
	Reassessment in clinically stable patients	Class IIb
	Routine preoperative evaluation	Class III—no benefit
Exercise stress testing for functional capacity and myocardial ischemia	Excellent functional capacity and elevated risk—no further testing, proceed to surgery	Class IIa
	Unknown functional capacity and elevated risk—if will change management proceed with preoperative exercise stress testing	Class IIb
	Moderate to good functional capacity and elevated risk—no further testing, proceed to surgery	Class IIb
	Poor or unknown functional capacity and elevated risk—proceed with preoperative exercise stress testing	Class IIb
	Routine screening for low-risk surgery	Class III—no benefit
Cardiopulmonary exercise testing	Consider for elevated risk procedures	Class IIb
Noninvasive pharmacologic stress testing	Poor functional capacity and elevated risk—DSI or MPI if will change management	Class IIa
	Routine for low-risk surgery—not recommended	Class III—no benefit
Coronary angiogram	Routine preoperative coronary for noncardiac surgery—not recommended	Class III—no benefit

CAD, Coronary artery disease; *DSI*, dobutamine stress imaging; *ECG*, electrocardiography; *LV*, left ventricular; *MPI*, myocardial perfusion imaging.

TABLE 30.12 Classification of Recommendations Based on Level of Evidence

Classification	Recommendation—Level of Evidence
Class I	Useful and effective
Class IIa	In favor of usefulness/effectiveness
Class IIb	Less well-established usefulness/effectiveness
Class III	No proven benefit
Grading	**Recommendation—Quality of Evidence**
A	Sufficient evidence
B	Limited evidence
C	Based on expert opinion, case studies, standard of care

increases demand. In a study of 955 patients undergoing NCS, hypotension was defined as systolic blood pressure less than 90 mm Hg for more than 10 minutes. The incidence of hypotension was associated with MI or death within 30 days of surgery in 16.4% patients with CAD compared with 6.7% patients with CAD but no hypotension and only in 2.7% of patients without CAD or hypotension. Hypertension increases systolic wall stress and left ventricular end-diastolic pressure leading to a demand-mediated ischemia. In patients with systolic blood pressure greater than 160 mm Hg, increased risk of MINS and MI: which suggests that both hypotension and hypertension extremes should be avoided in the perioperative period.[48,50]

3. **Maintain normal left ventricular end diastolic volume (LVEDV)** by avoiding left ventricular distension caused by fluid overload. This causes an increase in left ventricular wall stress and oxygen demand. Estimates of LVEDV using central venous pressure (CVP) or pulmonary catheter (PAC) have been used; however these modalities have limitations.[51–53]

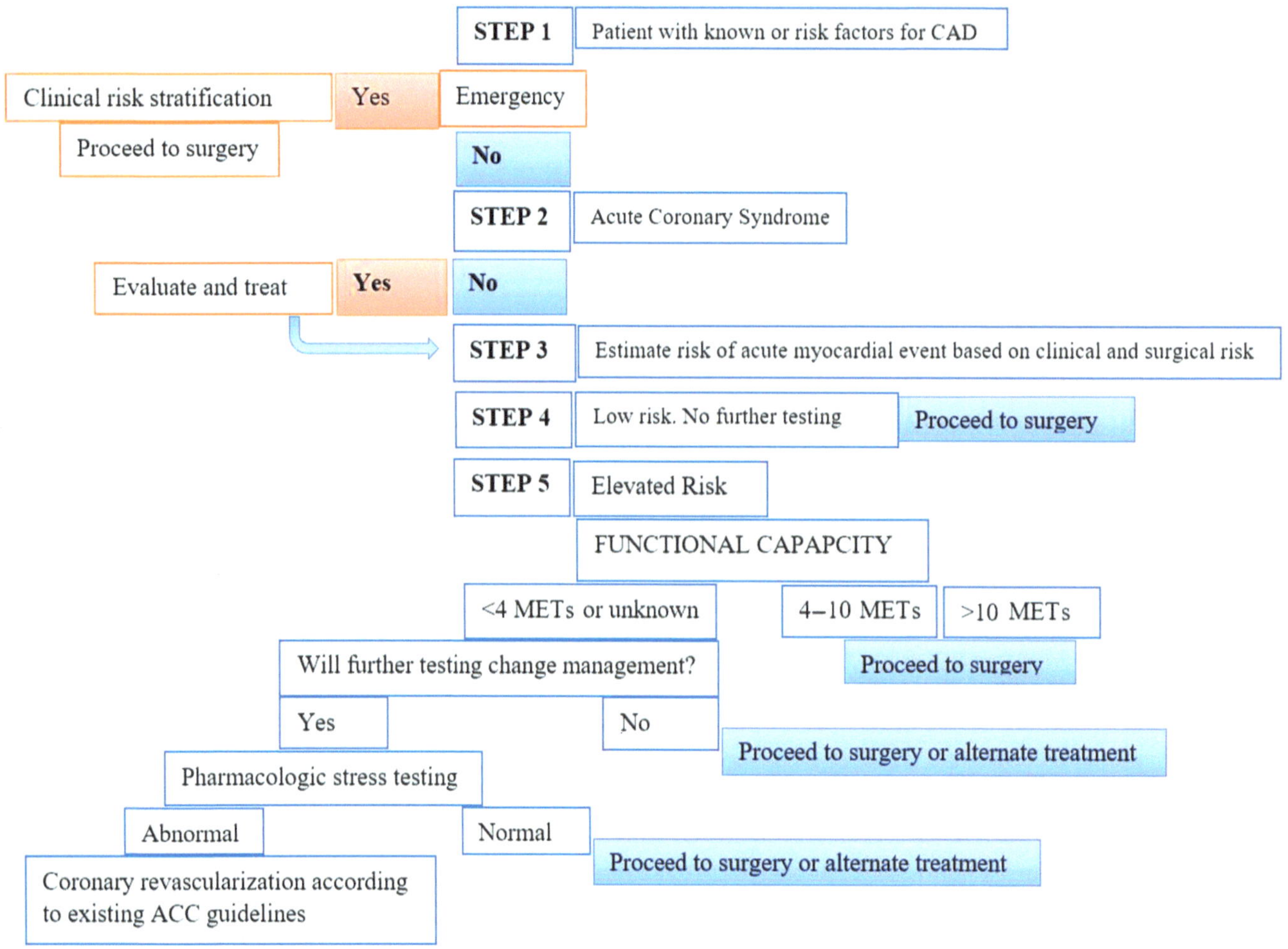

• **Fig. 30.1** Stepwise algorithm based on ACC/AHA 2014 Guidelines on Preoperative Cardiac Evaluation of Patient Presenting for Noncardiac Surgery. *ACC*, American College of Cardiology; *AHA*, American Heart Association; *CAD*, coronary artery disease; *METs*, metabolic equivalents.

4. **Maximize oxygen content in coronary arterial blood** with packed red blood cell transfusions as necessary, to maintain hemoglobin level between 7 and 8 g/dL. Liberal versus restrictive transfusion practices in patients with CAD with ongoing signs of bleeding or ischemia have shown that an optimal hemoglobin of 9 g/dL is recommended. Supplemental oxygen is given in the perioperative period to maintain oxygen saturation greater than 95% and monitored with pulse oximetry.[54,55]
5. **Maintaining normothermia** in the perioperative period is important for optimal tissue oxygenation. Hypothermia induces shivering, which in turn increases oxygen demand and may lead to myocardial ischemia.

Cardiovascular Monitoring in Patients With Coronary Artery Disease

All patients should have continuous ECG monitoring for arrhythmias and cardiac ischemia in the perioperative period. Even though ECG has shown to be poorly sensitive for cardiac ischemia, leads II and V5 detect over 80% of ischemic episodes in a 12-lead ECG. Lead V5 alone is more sensitive, and ST segment changes are associated with a high risk of cardiac morbidity and mortality in patients with CAD.[56,57]

Intraarterial line placement is warranted when continuous blood pressure measurement is required. Instances where hemodynamic instability is anticipated, major blood loss is likely to occur, large fluid shifts expected, and detection of hypotension is vital, an intraarterial catheter is best placed before induction of anesthesia. In addition, an intraarterial line is placed for most of the thoracic procedures useful to guide continuous management of blood pressure where vasoactive substances are required. In these circumstances, patients may also require frequent sampling of blood gases and other laboratory values, which are facilitated with an intraarterial catheter line in place.[58] A CVP is placed when major fluid shifts are anticipated during surgery, major blood loss is expected, and the transfusion of blood products and infusion of vasoactive drugs is contemplated. The applicability of CVP in providing data for fluid status has been studied for many decades and has shown to be a poor predictor of fluid responsiveness.[59,60] The use of a PAC by monitoring a change in pulmonary capillary wedge pressure has shown to be a poor predictor of cardiac ischemia in comparison to ECG and transesophageal echocardiography. In patients where severe cardiac conditions affect hemodynamics, placement of a PAC is warranted to follow trends in pulmonary artery pressures and cardiac output. The decision whether to place a PAC is based on a risk–benefit ratio in the context of the surgical procedure performed.[61–64] In recent years, the use of the PAC has lost momentum in favor of transesophageal echocardiography for NCS. Continuous transesophageal echocardiography monitoring is sensitive for detection of new wall motion abnormalities, especially in high-risk cardiac patients undergoing major surgery and for evaluating volume responsiveness. Transesophageal echocardiography is more sensitive than ECG or PAC in the detection of a cardiac ischemic event. Transesophageal echocardiography is also indicated in identifying life-threatening hemodynamic compromise and differentiating causes of hypotension. The use of transesophageal echocardiography is limited by equipment availability and the level of expertise required for interpretation of echocardiographic findings.[65,66]

Conclusion

Identifying significant cardiac risk factors provides information to better quantify risks of a possible cardiac event in the perioperative period. Cardiac risk is specific to patient and surgery-specific characteristics. Guidelines from the ACC and AHA provide information for the evaluation and management of cardiac risk and best practices to reduce morbidity and mortality for the patient with CVD presenting for NCS.

References

1. Wijeysundera DN. 2014 ACC/AHA guideline on perioperative cardiovascular evaluation and management of patients undergoing noncardiac surgery: a report of the American College of Cardiology/American Heart Association Task Force on Practice Guidelines. *Circulation.* 2014;130:e278–e333.
2. Smilowitz NR, Gupta N, Ramakrishna H, et al. Perioperative major adverse cardiovascular and cerebrovascular events associated with noncardiac surgery. *JAMA Cardiol.* 2017;2:181.
3. Goldman L, Caldera DL, Nussbaum SR. Multifactorial index of cardiac risk in noncardiac surgical procedures. *N Engl J Med.* 1977;297:845–885.
4. Lee TH, Marcantonio ER, Mangione CM, et al. Derivation and prospective validation of a simple index for prediction of cardiac risk of major noncardiac surgery. *Circulation.* 1999;100(10): 1043–1049.
5. Davis C, Tait G, Carroll J, et al. The Revised Cardiac Risk Index in the new millennium: a single-center prospective cohort re-evaluation of the original variables in 9,519 consecutive elective surgical patients. *Can J Anaesth.* 2013;124:855–863.
6. Gupta PK, Gupta H, Sundaram A, et al. Development and validation of a risk calculator for prediction of cardiac risk after surgery. *Circulation.* 2011;124:381.
7. Kitamura Y, Suzuki K, Teramukai S, et al., Japanese Association for Chest Surgery. Feasibility of pulmonary resection for lung cancer in patients with coronary artery disease or atrial fibrillation. *Ann Thorac Surg.* 2017;103(2):432–440.
8. Devereaux PJ, Chan MT, Alonso-Coello P, et al. Association between postoperative troponin levels and 30-day mortality among patients undergoing noncardiac surgery. *JAMA.* 2012;307: 2295–2304.
9. Shah KB, Kleinman BS, Rao TL, et al. Angina and other risk factors in patients with cardiac diseases undergoing noncardiac operations. *Anesth Analg.* 1990;70:240–247.
10. Livhits M, Ko CY, Leonardi MJ, et al. Risk of surgery following recent myocardial infarction. *Ann Surg.* 2011;253:857–864.
11. Hartle A, McCormack T, Carlisle J, et al. The measurement of adult blood pressure and management of hypertension before elective surgery. Joint Guidelines from the Association of Anaesthetists of Great Britain and Ireland and the British Hypertension Society. *Anaesthesia.* 2016;71(3):326–337.
12. Yancy CW. 2013 ACC/AHA guideline on perioperative cardiovascular evaluation and management of patients with heart failure: a report of the American College of Cardiology/American Heart Association Task Force on Practice Guidelines. *Circulation.* 2013; 128:e240.
13. van Diepen S, Bakal JA, McAlister FA, Ezekowitz JA. Mortality and readmission of patients with heart failure, atrial fibrillation, or coronary artery disease undergoing noncardiac surgery: an analysis of 38 047 patients. *Circulation.* 2011;124(3):289–296.
14. Xuan T, Zeng Y, Zhu W. Risk of patients with hypertrophic cardiomyopathy undergoing noncardiac surgery. *Chin Med Sci J.* 2007;22:211–215.
15. Karthikeyan G, Moncur RA, Levine O, et al. Is a preoperative brain natriuretic peptide or N-terminal pro-B-type natriuretic peptide measurement an independent predictor of adverse cardiovascular outcomes within 30 days of noncardiac surgery? A systematic review and meta-analysis of observational studies. *J Am Coll Cardiol.* 2009;54:1599–1606.
16. Agarwal S, Rajamanickam A, Bajaj NS, et al. Impact of aortic stenosis on postoperative outcomes after noncardiac surgeries. *Circ Cardiovasc Qual Outcomes.* 2013;6:193–200.
17. Bajaj NS, Agarwal S, Rajamanickam A, et al. Impact of severe mitral regurgitation on postoperative outcomes after noncardiac surgery. *Am J Med.* 2013;126:529–535.
18. Tan CW, Wall M, Rosengart TK, RK Ghanta. How to bridge? Management of anticoagulation in patients with mechanical heart valves undergoing noncardiac surgical procedures. *C J Thorac Cardiovasc Surg.* 2019;158:200–203.
19. Maxwell BG, Wong JK, Kin C, et al. Perioperative outcomes of major noncardiac surgery in adults with congenital heart disease. *Anesthesiology.* 2013;119:762–769.
20. Ford MK, Beattie WS, Wijeysundera DN. Systematic review: prediction of perioperative cardiac complications and mortality by the Revised Cardiac Risk Index. *Ann Intern Med.* 2010;152:26–35.
21. Hlatky MA, Boineau RE, Higginbotham MB, et al. A brief self-administered questionnaire to determine functional capacity (the Duke Activity Status Index). *Am J Cardiol.* 1989;64:651–654.
22. Goswami S, Brady JE, Jordan DA, et al. Intraoperative cardiac arrests in adults undergoing noncardiac surgery: incidence, risk factors, and survival outcome. *Anesthesiology.* 2012;117:1018–1026.
23. Tsiouris A, Horst HM, Paone G, et al. Preoperative risk stratification for thoracic surgery using the American College of Surgeons National

Surgical Quality Improvement Program data set: functional status predicts morbidity and mortality. *J Surg Res*. 2012;177: 1–6.

24. Brunelli A, Cassivi SD, Fibla J, Halgren LA, Wigle DA, Allen M. External validation of the recalibrated thoracic revised cardiac risk index for predicting the risk of major cardiac complications after lung resection. *Ann Thorac Surg*. 2011;92:445–448.
25. Choi J-H, Cho DK, Song Y-B, et al. Preoperative NT-proBNP and CRP predict perioperative major cardiovascular events in non-cardiac surgery. *Heart*. 2010;96:56–62.
26. Farzi S, Stojakovic T, Marko T, et al. Role of N terminal pro B-type natriuretic peptide in identifying patients at high risk for adverse outcome after emergent non-cardiac surgery. *Br J Anaesth*. 2013;110:554–560.
27. Noordzij PG, Boersma E, Bax JJ, et al. Prognostic value of routine preoperative electrocardiography in patients undergoing noncardiac surgery. *Am J Cardiol*. 2006;97:1103–1106.
28. Biteker M, Duman D, Tekkesin AI. Predictive value of preoperative electrocardiography for perioperative cardiovascular outcomes in patients undergoing noncardiac, nonvascular surgery. *Clin Cardiol*. 2012;35:494–499.
29. McFalls EO, Ward HB, Moritz TE, et al. Coronary artery revascularization before elective major vascular surgery. *N Engl J Med*. 2004;351:2795–2804.
30. Tracy CM, Epstein AE, Darbar D, et al. 2012 ACCF/ AHA/HRS focused update of the 2008 guidelines for device-based therapy of cardiac rhythm abnormalities: a report of the American College of Cardiology Foundation/American Heart Association Task Force on Practice Guidelines. *J Am Coll Cardiol*. 2012;60:1297–1313.
31. Hayes T, Charlesworth M, Garcia M. Patients with left ventricle assist devices presenting for thoracic surgery and lung resection: tips, tricks and evidence. *Curr Opin Anesthesiol*. 2020;33:17–26.
32. Devereaux PJ, Yang H, Guyat GH, et al. Rationale, design, and organization of the PeriOperative ISchemic Evaluation (POISE) trial: a randomised controlled trial of metoprolol versus placebo in patients undergoing noncardiac surgery. *Am Heart J*. 2006;152: 223–230.
33. Andersson C, Mérie C, Jørgensen M, et al. Association of beta-blocker therapy with risks of adverse cardiovascular events and deaths in patients with ischemic heart disease undergoing noncardiac surgery: a Danish nationwide cohort study. *JAMA Intern Med*. 2014;174:336–344.
34. Dai N, Xu D, Zhang J, et al. Different betablockers and initiation time in patients undergoing noncardiac surgery: a meta-analysis. *Am J Med Sci*. 2014;347:235–244.
35. Raju MG, Pachika A, Punnam SR, et al. Statin therapy in the reduction of cardiovascular events in patients undergoing intermediate-risk noncardiac, nonvascular surgery. *Clin Cardiol*. 2013; 36:456–461.
36. Desai H, Aronow WS, Ahn C, et al. Incidence of perioperative myocardial infarction and of 2-year mortality in 577 elderly patients undergoing noncardiac vascular surgery treated with and without statins. *Arch Gerontol Geriatr*. 2010;51:149–151.
37. Rosenman DJ, McDonald FS, Ebbert JO, et al. Clinical consequences of withholding versus administering renin-angiotensin-aldosterone system antagonists in the preoperative period. *J Hosp Med*. 2008;3:319–325.
38. Tokushige A, Shiomi H, Morimoto T, et al. Incidence and outcome of surgical procedures after coronary bare-metal and drug-eluting stent implantation: a report from the CREDO-Kyoto PCI/CABG registry cohort-2. *Circ Cardiovasc Interv*. 2012;5: 237–246.
39. Sharma AK, Ajani AE, Hamwi SM, et al. Major noncardiac surgery following coronary stenting: when is it safe to operate? *Catheter Cardiovasc Interv*. 2004;63:141–145.
40. Reddy PR, Vaitkus PT. Risks of noncardiac surgery after coronary stenting. *Am J Cardiol*. 2005;95:755–757.
41. Van Werkum JW, Heestermans AA, Zomer AC, et al. Predictors of coronary stent thrombosis: the Dutch Stent Thrombosis Registry. *J Am Coll Cardiol*. 2009;53:1399–1409.
42. Iakovou I, Schmidt T, Bonizzoni E, et al. Incidence, predictors, and outcome of thrombosis after successful implantation of drug-eluting stents. *JAMA*. 2005;293:2126–2130.
43. Gandhi NK, Abdel-Karim A-RR, Banerjee S, et al. Frequency and risk of noncardiac surgery after drug eluting stent implantation. *Catheter Cardiovasc Interv*. 2011;77:972.
44. Brichon P-Y, Boitet P, Dujon A, et al. Perioperative in-stent thrombosis after lung resection performed within 3 months of coronary stenting. *Eur J CardioThorac Surg*. 2006;30:793–796.
45. Roach R, Wagner P. *Hypoxia and the Circulation. Experimental Medicine and Biology*. Springer Science; 2007:618.
46. Hajime A, Hiroaki S, Norihiko T. The roles of hypoxia signaling in the pathogenesis of cardiovascular diseases. *J Atheroscler Thromb*. 2017;24:884–894.
47. Spoelstra-de Man AME, Smit B, Oudemans-van Straaten HM, Smulder YM. Cardiovascular effects of hyperoxia during and after cardiac surgery. *Anaesthesia*. 2015;70:1307–1319.
48. Abbott TEF, Pearse RM, Archbold RA, et al. A prospective international multicentre cohort study of intraoperative heart rate and systolic blood pressure and myocardial injury after noncardiac surgery: results of the VISION study. *Anesth Analg*. 2018;126: 1936.
49. Helwani MA, Amin A, Lavigne P, et al. Etiology of acute coronary syndrome after noncardiac surgery. *Anesthesiology*. 2018; 128(6):1084.
50. Roshanov PS, Sheth T, Duceppe E, et al. Relationship between perioperative hypotension and perioperative cardiovascular events in patients with coronary artery disease undergoing major noncardiac surgery. *Anesthesiology*. 2019;130:756.
51. Marik PE, Baram M, Vahid B. Does central venous pressure predict fluid responsiveness? A systematic review of the literature and the tale of seven mares. *Chest*. 2008;134:172.
52. Mark JB. Central venous pressure monitoring: clinical insights beyond the numbers. *J Cardiothorac Vasc Anesth*. 1991;5: 163.
53. Barone JE, Tucker JB, Rassias D, Corvo PR. Routine perioperative pulmonary artery catheterization has no effect on rate of complications in vascular surgery: a meta-analysis. *Am Surg*. 2001;67:674.
54. American Society of Anesthesiologists Task Force on Perioperative Blood Management. Practice guidelines for perioperative blood management: an updated report by the American Society of Anesthesiologists Task Force on Perioperative Blood Management. *Anesthesiology*. 2015;122:241.
55. Carson JL, Brooks MM, Abbott JD, et al. Liberal versus restrictive transfusion thresholds for patients with symptomatic coronary artery disease. *Am Heart J*. 2013;165:964.
56. Maile MD, Engoren MC, Tremper KK, Tremper TT, Jewell ES, Kheterpal S. Variability of automated intraoperative ST segment values predicts postoperative troponin elevation. *Anesth Analg*. 2016;122(3):608–701.

57. Landesberg G, Mosseri M, Wolf Y, Vesselov Y, Weissman C. Perioperative myocardial ischemia and infarction: identification by continuous 12-lead electrocardiogram with online ST-segment monitoring. *Anesthesiology*. 2002;96(2):264–270.
58. Cockings JG, Webb RK, Klepper ID, Currie M, Morgan C. The Australian Incident Monitoring Study. Blood pressure monitoring–applications and limitations: an analysis of 2000 incident reports. *Anaesth Intensive Care*. 1993;21(5):565–569.
59. Marik PE, Cavallazzi R. Does the central venous pressure predict fluid responsiveness? An updated meta-analysis and a plea for some common sense. *Crit Care Med*. 2013;41:1774.
60. Bentzer P, Griesdale DE, Boyd J, et al. Will this hemodynamically unstable patient respond to a bolus of intravenous fluids? *JAMA*. 2016;316:1298.
61. van Daele ME, Sutherland GR, Mitchell MM, et al. Do changes in pulmonary capillary wedge pressure adequately reflect myocardial ischemia during anesthesia? A correlative preoperative hemodynamic, electrocardiographic, and transesophageal echocardiographic study. *Circulation*. 1990;81:865.
62. Sandham JD, Hull RD, Brant RF, et al. A randomized, controlled trial of the use of pulmonary artery catheters in high-risk surgical patients. *N Engl J Med*. 2003;348:5.
63. Polanczyk CA, Rohde LE, Goldman L, et al. Right heart catheterization and cardiac complications in patients undergoing noncardiac surgery: an observational study. *JAMA*. 2001;286:309.
64. Rajaram SS, Desai NK, Kalra A, et al. Pulmonary artery catheters for adult patients in intensive care. *Cochrane Database Syst Rev*. 2013:CD003408.
65. Poldermans D, Bax JJ, Boersma E, et al., Task force for preoperative cardiac risk assessment and perioperative cardiac management in non-cardiac surgery, European Society of Cardiology (ESC). Guidelines for pre-operative cardiac risk assessment and perioperative cardiac management in non-cardiac surgery. *Eur Heart J*. 2009;30:2769.
66. American Society of Anesthesiologists Task Force on Perioperative Transesophageal Echocardiography. Practice guidelines for perioperative transesophageal echocardiography. *Anesthesiology*. 2010;112(5):1084–1096.

31

Video-Assisted Thoracoscopy: Multiportal Uniportal

ZERRIN SUNGUR, MERT ŞENTÜRK

Introduction

Video-assisted thoracoscopic surgery (VATS) is one of the major innovations in surgery. Within less than 30 years after its modern introduction, almost all of the operations, with only few exceptions, can be performed via VATS. It provides several benefits for the patients, as well as several challenges for the anesthetist. It is an "intentionally created" pneumothorax followed by the introduction of instruments into the cavity to perform the operation.

History

Though thoracoscopic surgery has prospered in the 1990s in terms of surgical spectrum and variability of patients, its history dates back to 19th century. Bozzini was the first to describe a primitive endoscope with a thin cannula and mirrors illuminated by candle in 1806 and named it "Lichleiter," which is still exhibited in Josephinum of Vienna. However, this device was not largely adopted by the medical community because of low image quality and cumbersome access. Later, modifications, such as introduction of a lens to focus with a direct light source improved visualization,[1] and endoscopes were developed to remove foreign bodies from the esophagus (esophagoscope) or diagnose and treat diseases of the bladder and urethra (cystoscope).

The ontogenesis of thoracoscopic procedures overlaps with the history of discovery and treatment of tuberculosis disease. Artificial pneumothorax was suggested and later published about in an Italian journal[2] for phthisis by Forlany within the same year of the discovery of tuberculosis bacillus. The technique was based on insertion of a needle via and the anterior axillary line and insufflation of air or nitrogen, but the presence of adhesions in the chest wall seemed to limit the expected benefit of the technique. An internist in Sweden, Hans Christian Jacobaeus, who performed the initial step in thoracoscopic history by dividing these adhesions using the two cannula technique via fluoroscopy guidance: the first cannula was the thoracoscope and the second was galvanocautery to be heated at red glow. Ironically, the aforementioned first phases of thoracoscopy were established by pulmonologists and not by surgeons. However, thoracoscopic procedures soon lost their popularity, and thoracoscopy became mostly limited to diagnostic practices with the introduction of antituberculosis chemotherapy in the 1940s. Its rediscovery in trauma surgery was heralded by Branco from Brazil in the 1940s.[1] During the transition period, Bloomberg from the United States continued to perform thoracoscopic procedures and shared his experience at the end of the 1970s. Meanwhile, in Europe, thoracoscopy was not totally abandoned and was applied in the treatment of empyema. During this time, scopes and staple devices further evolved yielding a breakthroughs in minimally invasive surgery, and the once-forgotten technique was revived. The thoracoscopic lobectomy was eventually performed in the 1990s, redefined as VATS, by Roviaro from Milan.[3] Indications have extended beyond the diagnostic issues to achieve a surgical spectrum of thoracoscopic procedures of extended lung resections, including mediastinal mass, thoracic trauma, thoracic wall abnormalities, and esophageal operations. Today, VATS has evolved to subxyphoid, uniportal, or robotic procedures with the goal to minimize surgical injury.

Thoracoscopic surgery today is implemented worldwide. In the 1930s, Dr. Nissen, one of the Jewish academicians who left Germany for Istanbul University before the Second World War, has contributed to the advancement of thoracic surgery in Turkey. Historical progress was similar, starting with surgical treatment of tuberculosis in the 1940s to VATS in the late 1990s,[4] and robotic and uniportal VATS in the 2010s.[5] Today, in the institution of the authors, and in most other institutions worldwide, the majority of the thoracic surgical procedures are performed with VATS.

Techniques of Video-Assisted Thoracoscopic Surgery and Its Advantages

The classical (almost historical) approach of VATS is performed with the standard three-port (up to five ports) technique (camera port, utility port, and posterior/grasping port), in different degrees of lateral position. A video camera is introduced to allow for direct visualization of the entrance of trocars into the thorax.

Unlike laparoscopic procedures, insufflation of carbon dioxide (CO2) into the hemithorax to enhance the view of the working-space (better collapse of the lung; less adhesion etc.) is an uncommon approach in thoracoscopic operations; drawbacks exceeding the evidence of benefit. Insufflation of CO2 into the closed cage of the hemithorax can be associated with hemodynamic instability, hypercarbia, and hypotension. Although non routinely done, more spread during robotic thoracic procedures, the intrathoracic insufflation pressure should be kept below 10 cm H_2O.

Following its introduction to clinical practice, VATS has been shown to be a reliable method to safely replace—almost—every possible open procedure: "medical thoracoscopies" are performed almost exclusively by pulmonologists for diagnostic purposes; "surgical thoracoscopies" can be diagnostic, where the traditional "diagnostic mini-thoracotomy" has become almost historical, or therapeutic. Because thoracoscopy is a less invasive approach, it has permitted that patients who were not considered to be operated because of their severe comorbidities, are now offered major resections.

Video-Assisted Thoracoscopic Surgery Versus Open Thoracotomy

Contrary to conventional incisions—such as posterolateral thoracotomy—port holes require smaller incisions which would be associated with reduced inflammatory response, better respiratory mechanics, improved respiratory muscle recovery, and certainly lesser pain. Thoracoscopic procedures have become more frequently comprising a wide range of procedures and represent a reliable minimal invasive alternative for high-risk patients.

Initial reports highlighted benefits of VATS in reducing overall complications and decreasing hospital stay.[6] Furthermore, the thoracoscopic approach was found to be more favorable in terms of intensive care unit (ICU) stay time and postoperative pneumonia despite preoperative comorbidities.[7] In several studies, it was shown that VATS minimized complications and enhanced the quality of life in the postoperative period,[8] with less postoperative pain,[9] better pulmonary function outcomes,[10] shorter overall hospital length of stay, and faster return to normal activities.[11,12] In 2010, the American College of Surgeons Oncology Group published data of approximately 1000 patients and found that thoracoscopic lobectomy was associated with lower pulmonary complications (atelectasis, chest tube drainage) and shorter length of stay.[13] In 2016, the European Society of Thoracic Surgeons reported results from 235 centers which included 5500 patients (selected among 26,000 according to propensity score).[14] Major cardiopulmonary complications were significantly lower in the VATS group compared with the thoracotomy group (15.9% vs. 16.9%; $P = .0094$). Length of stay was shorter among the thoracoscopic group as expected ($P = .003$). Mortality at discharge was also lower in the VATS group, which, however, needs to be cautiously commented according to authors because of some missing data. A more recent trial by Nwogu et al. has compared VATS with open thoracotomies as length of stay (LOS) for primary outcome. The VATS group had significantly lower LOS (5.4 vs. 8 days; $P < .001$). Moreover, incidence of complications was consistent with the primary outcome favoring the VATS group (6% vs. 16%; $p = .0001$). Thoracoscopic surgery is associated with reduced injury, stress response, and may enhance recovery of patients in thoracic surgery. The short-term outcome appeared favorable for thoracoscopic surgery.[15]

In the recently published: "Guidelines for enhanced recovery after thoracic surgery (ERATS)," VATS was recommended for lung resection for early-stage lung cancer with a "high" evidence level and "strong" recommendation grade, stating that "the benefits are even more marked in patients with poor respiratory reserve."[16]

Long-term results are controversial; studies show either similar results of both approaches, or better results for VATS in terms of survival. Sugi et al. reported a similar oncologic outcome in VATS compared with conventional lobectomy for the following 5 years.[17] Similarly, Whitson et al. did not find any difference in survival between thoracoscopy and thoracotomy.[7] Recently, one center study by Oda et al. in patients with early lung cancer, reported better 5-year survival in patients undergoing thoracoscopic resection.[18] Short-term variables (blood loss, hospital stay, C-reactive protein [CRP] levels) were also significantly advantageous in the thoracoscopy group. The authors speculated that it could be related to lesser tissue damage and inflammatory response screened by CRP values. Other studies confirm that the long-term (5 years) survival was better with VATS when compared with open surgery for early-stage lung cancer[19,20] (Fig. 31.1). Another recent study comparing VATS to open thoracotomy for cT1–T2 N1 M0 nonsmall cell lung cancer (NSCLC) showed that VATS had no significant difference in long-term survival, with shorter LOS and similar nodal upstaging rates, considering it suitable for the treatment of NSCLC.[21]

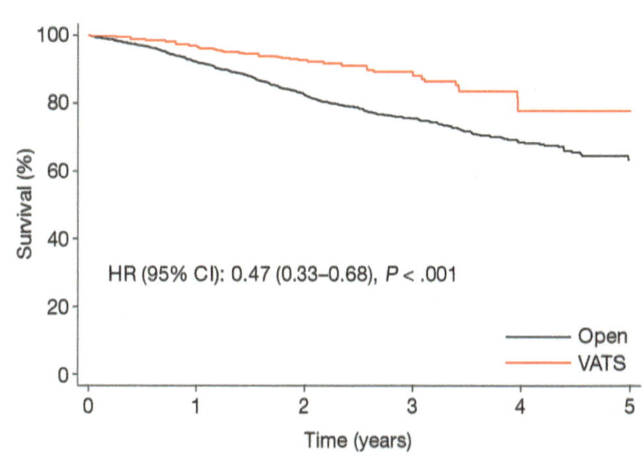

• **Fig. 31.1 Kaplan-Meier curve of the survival after open thoracotomy or VATS.** *CI*, Confidence interval; *HR*, hazard ratio; *VATS*, video-assisted thoracoscopic surgery. (From Al-Ameri M, Bergman P, Franco-Cereceda A, et al. Video-assisted thoracoscopic versus open thoracotomy lobectomy: a Swedish nationwide cohort study. *J Thorac Dis*. 2018;10:3499–3506.)

Today, VATS is recognized by international guidelines as preferred over thoracotomy for treatment of early-stage NSCLC.[22]

An interesting retrospective study revealed similar costs for thoracoscopic or traditional lobectomies.[23] Operative cost was significantly higher with VATS, whereas total hospital cost was similar with traditional lobectomy, but a shorter stay in the thoracoscopic group and increased patients' turnover abolished the temporary economic issue of conventional approach.

Uniportal Video-Assisted Thoracoscopic Surgery

In a period of less than 20 years, there has been a rapid evolution in the surgical technique of VATS: the classical three-port approach was initially changed to a two-port strategy, and soon afterwards, there was a trend toward a one-port technique, where the camera was moved to the utility port, the camera's port was abandoned, and the entire procedure was completed using just one incision. Uniportal VATS was first described in 2001, and then reported for simple procedures, such as lung biopsies and spontaneous pneumothorax in 2005.[24]

The expansion of the technique was achieved following the developments by Gonzalez-Rivas et al. in the next 10 years, where the technique was used for more complex procedures, such as pulmonary anatomic and complex resections for the treatment of lung cancer.[25] This strategy achieves a direct vision of the targeted tissue and of the pulmonary hilum. This fact, together with the accession of parallel instrumentation, achieves an approach similar to the open surgery view and maneuvers, making the surgeons feel more comfortable while operating, compared with other VATS strategies. Today, the technique has been adopted, reproduced, and reinforced by the surgical community; however, it is limited by the significant learning curve.[26,27]

Compared with conventional VATS, UniVATS has been shown to be beneficial with shorter LOS in the hospital, duration of drainage, and reduced overall morbidity.[28] One—instead of three—incision is associated with less inflammation and less pain, leading to reduced postoperative complications, with an overall better outcome. It has been used not only in operations like lobectomy or wedge resection but also in more complicated procedures like pneumonectomy, sleeve resection or tracheal and carinal resections.[27]

It should be noted that some trials report no difference between uniportal and multiport VATS lobectomy. Perna et al. have compared uniportal video-assisted lobectomy (group A; $n = 51$) and other video-assisted thoracoscopic lobectomy techniques (group B; $n = 55$). The median visual analog pain score in the first 3 days did not show statistically significant differences. Likewise, the median morphine use in the first 3 days did not show statistically significant differences. There was no difference in timing to remove the paravertebral catheter and the chest drain and the duration of the postoperative hospital stay. There was no difference in postoperative complications.[29] In ERATS protocols, it has been stated that "The number of ports used does not appear to affect outcomes, and so, one VATS approach cannot be recommended over another."[16] As a matter of fact, more and more high quality studies are still necessary to evaluate the potential benefits of this technique. The anesthetic management, including ventilation, for uniportal VATS does not differ from that performed for classical VATS.[30]

Subxiphoid Uniportal Video-Assisted Thoracoscopic Surgery

The subxiphoid approach began its evolution in 1999.[31] First implemented for mediastinal pathologies, in 2014, a subxiphoid UniVATS left upper lobectomy was reported.[32] Following that, many procedures, such as wedge resections, segmentectomies, lobectomies, and even pneumonectomies have been performed by this approach. There are two major advantages of this technique: (1) intercostal nerve injury related to the incision and instrumentation is avoided, and (2) it will allow approaching bilateral lesions from a single incision without changing the patient's position. Avoidance of intercostal nerve injury has been shown to be associated with significantly lower postoperative pain compared with intercostal UniVATS.[33]

Robotic-Assisted Thoracic Surgery

Robotic-assisted thoracic surgery (RATS) is covered in Chapter 52 in this book in detail. It should be considered as an important step of the rapid changes in the practice of thoracic surgery and anesthesia. A subcostal VATS approach (with or without robotic help) is also one of these promising steps.[34]

Preoperative Evaluation and Prehabilitation

Preoperative Risk Stratification

Preoperative evaluation with risk stratification and scoring systems are extensively explained in Chapter 8 of this book. Regarding VATS, it should be noted that some systems take also "operation-related" risk factors into consideration (e.g., considering pneumonectomy as "high-risk"); however, to our knowledge, none of these risk stratifications and scoring systems differentiated between open thoracotomy and VATS as different risk factors. The risk of a patient undergoing open thoracotomy with similar comorbidities and extent of resection is higher than the patient undergoing VATS. This part will therefore focus on "common" criteria.

Improvements of surgical techniques and advances in anesthesia have resulted in an overall improved outcome. But at the same time, those improvements allowed patients who previously were not considered surgical candidates to now be offered major resections. These patients are older, with multiple comorbidities which in many cases are uncontrolled or

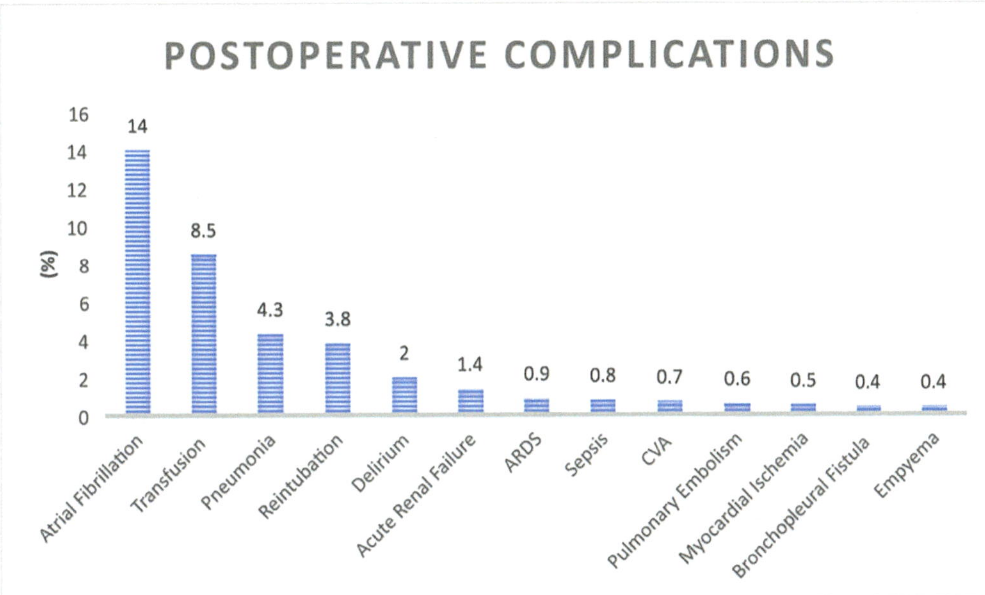

• **Fig. 31.2** Incidence of postoperative complications after lung resection. Complications affect survival at different times in the postoperative period. *ARDS*, Acute respiratory distress syndrome; *CVA*, cerebrovascular accident. (From Pedoto A, Perrino AC Jr. Delayed recovery following thoracic surgery: persistent issues and potential interventions. *Curr Opin Anesthesiol*. 2019;32:3–9.)

not treatable, making the perioperative period challenging, and probably leading to an increase in postoperative complications and decrease survival.[35] Therefore preoperative evaluation and preparation of patients who will undergo a VATS procedure should be revised separately.

Perioperative mortality represents a serious worldwide public health problem. Thoracic surgery deserves special interest because postoperative complications are significantly high (up to 27% in a recent review) (Fig. 31.2).[36] Preoperative assessment and screening of high-risk patients must identify the patient that would benefit from optimizing measures. Increase in patient comorbidities and an increase in awareness during the perioperative period is a relatively new topic which is part of the ERAS (enhance recovery after thoracic surgery) guidelines.[16] A team approach makes sense for this population while assessing cardiac risk, planning optimizing measures, organizing oncologic follow-up, and judging operability. Thus an experienced team should be composed of a pulmonologist, oncologist, thoracic surgeon, and anesthesiologist as well as the patient and the relatives.

The first step of preparation can be initiated with cardiac evaluation to determine preexisting risk factors and to treat before surgery. The revised cardiac risk index has been adapted for thoracic surgery (Table 31.1).[37] Three to four subgroups are defined in this scoring system as A (0 point), B (1–1.5 points), C (2–2.5 points), or D (>2.5 points); the latter two described as high risk. The incidence of cardiac event varies in groups for A less than 1.5%, for B 5.8%, for C 19%, and for D 23%. The thoracic revised cardiac risk index (ThRCRI) can discriminate high-risk patients—groups C and D[38]—and may allow for identification of patients who would benefit from additional cardiac evaluation.

A subsequent cardiac issue—generally neglected—is right ventricular (RV) function, which remains affected from the second postoperative day to the second month.[39] Postthoracotomy impaired RV ejection fraction is a recognized phenomenon usually related to elevated pulmonary vascular pressures but also to reduced compliance. Thoracoscopic surgery compared with thoracotomy offers advantages in terms of RV function in the early postoperative course for elderly patients.[40] Not surprisingly, the extent of lung resection directly affects RV changes. Pneumonectomy is found to be associated with more pronounced RV dysfunction compared with lobectomy.[41] Further studies are needed to determine the best predictor for preoperative assessment of RV. Natriuretic peptides seem promising in thoracic patients to detect some CV complications, especially for prediction of postoperative atrial fibrillation.[42,43]

Pulmonary evaluation for lung surgery includes spirometry, diffusion capacity, and exercise tests if needed, as summarized in Fig. 31.3.[37] Although patients with low risk can be cleared for surgery, in high-risk patients, cardiopulmonary exercise testing should be considered. In a newly introduced algorithm, a slope of minute ventilation to CO2 output ratio seems promising.[44] A slope of more than 34 was associated with increased mortality. In fact, an increased ratio could be explained by respiratory inefficiency and appeared to be associated with increased mortality.[45]

TABLE 31.1 Thoracic Revised Cardiac Risk Index

	Point
History of coronary artery disease	1.5
Cerebrovascular disease	1.5
Creatinine >2 mg/dL	1
Pneumonectomy	1.5

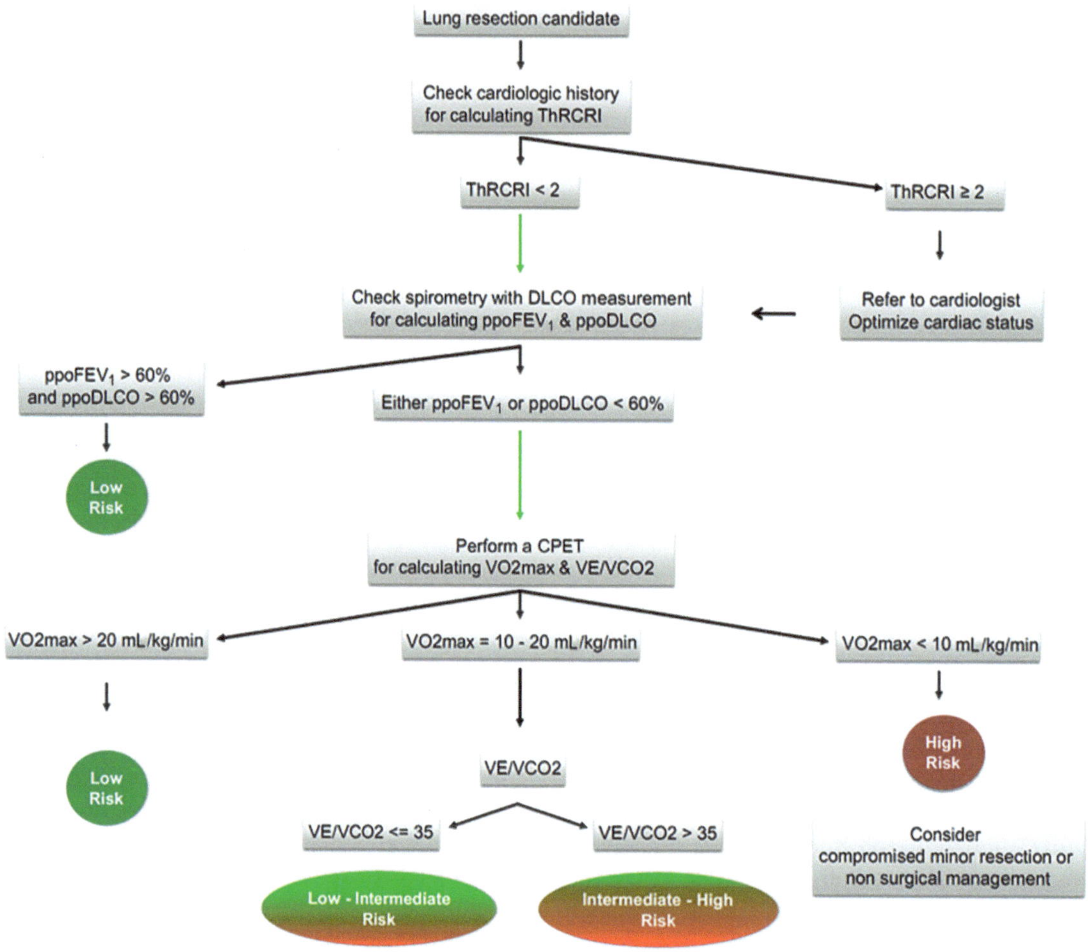

• **Fig. 31.3** Risk stratification for thoracic surgery. Note that this algorithm is defined for all thoracic operations, including both open thoracotomies and video-assisted thoracoscopic surgery (VATS). It could be considered that for a patient with similar risk factors, undergoing VATS would be less risky than an open thoracotomy. *CPET*, Cardiopulmonary exercise testing; *DLCO*, diffusing capacity for the lung for carbon monoxide; *FEV_1*, forced expiratory volume in one second; *ThRCRI*, thoracic revised cardiac risk index; *PPO*, predictive post operative; *VO_2 max*, maximum rate of oxygen consumption; *VCO2*, carbon dioxide output; *VE*, minute ventilation; *VE/VCO_2 slope*, minute ventilation/CO_2 production.

Preoperative Optimization and "Prehabilitation" (See Chapter 9)

Besides risk stratification, the aim of a preoperative evaluation is optimization and rehabilitation. The anesthesiologist as perioperative physician has to manage treatable conditions to reduce complications. The initial measure should be **smoking cessation**, as it is a considerable risk factor in lung cancer for both short- and long-term outcomes.[46,47] Smoking impairs mucociliary ability to remove pathogens or foreign bodies from the airway and alveolar macrophage activity. In a retrospective study performed with more than 20,000 subjects, smoking cessation was found to be associated with reduced in-hospital morbidity and mortality independent of time interval and amount of smoking.[48] A prospective study affirmed similar results among thoracoscopic lung surgery patients; with incidence of postoperative pulmonary complications (PPCs) 10 times greater in active smokers compared with never smokers and 2 times compared with ex-smokers.[49] Cessation of more than 6 weeks resulted in reduced LOS. However, optimal timing for cessation before surgery has yet to be determined.

Iron deficiency anemia is very common worldwide and affects surgical populations. Screening and treatment of anemia is recommended for expected blood loss greater than 500 mL before surgery. The target value of hemoglobin commonly accepted for preoperative iron therapy is 13 g/dL and replacement is achieved by intravenous (IV) iron if there is a window of less than 6 weeks to surgery.[50] In case of chronic inflammation, diagnosis requires additional findings; serum ferritin levels less than 100 mcg/L or transferrin saturation less than 20% can be considered as inadequate iron stores. Anemia has been associated with worse survival in lung cancers.[51] On the other hand, transfusion itself was related with early recurrence and shorter survival in a meta-analysis of 23 studies.[52] The authors conclude with recommendation of stricter transfusion policy, especially for early stages. Supporting recent results from 15 years' data of a single center with worse outcome and increased recurrence of blood transfusion.[53] The difference seemed to appear with more than one unit of blood transfusion. Patient blood management, a concept that aims to rationalize blood transfusion, should be applied as possible also in VATS operations.

A relatively new issue of optimization is preoperative habilitation "**prehabilitation,**" which consists of training patients with respiratory or cardiopulmonary exercises before surgery. The expectation is to improve physical performance, to increase exercise tolerance, and to improve health-related quality of life for a well-conditioned patient. Types of exercise are endurance or high-intensity interval trainings (HIIT). The first one consists of moderate intensity efforts and 60 to 120 minutes in daily practice over 6 to 12 weeks. On the other hand, the second one is performed at a high intensity in relatively brief training periods. Licker et al. investigated effects of HIIT and conventional preoperative optimization (nutritional measures, smoking, and alcohol cessation) in patients undergoing lobectomy.[54] The training group attained significantly better peak O2 consumption and 6-minute walking values. Pulmonary complications were significantly lower in the prehabilitation group because of decreased incidence of atelectasis. However, composite outcome, death, and in-hospital complications which was the primary outcome, were similar between groups. Moreover, beneficial effects of a rehabilitation program can be more prominent in patients with respiratory impairment during induction chemotherapy.[55] Initial reports are encouraging with improved aerobic performance and respiratory volumes. Is this progress sufficient to prevent postoperative complications? An adequately powered randomized controlled trial (RCT) that is presently ongoing multicentric study (INSPIRE) hopefully will provide more concrete information.

Lung Isolation (See Chapters 16,17)

Airway management is a crucial topic of thoracic anesthesia and is covered in different chapters in this book. Here, we aim to inform about specific conditions in VATS operations within a range of general aspects.

History

Historically, lung isolation essays were started with physiologic animal studies by C. Bernard and E. Pflüger in the 19th century. The setup was adapted to volunteers by Loewe and von Schrotter at the beginning of the 1900s, again, for cardiopulmonary physiologic studies.[56] Introduction of the endotracheal tube (ETT), by Gale and Waters, followed by the introduction of the double-lumen tubes (DLTs). The 1950s presented the first double-cuffed double-lumen tube described by Carlens. DLTs designed by Robertshaw were introduced first in red rubber in the 1960s; 20 years later, they are marketed as disposable polyvinyl chloride, and are used worldwide. A rubber bronchial blocker (BB) was first used (positioned by radiography) in the 1930s by Archibald.[57] The use of the fiberoptic bronchoscope was considerably later in the 1980s and constituted a huge advancement in thoracic anesthesia.

Indications

The historical classification of indications for one-lung ventilation (OLV; namely, absolute vs. relative) is not target-oriented and sometimes confusing. From that historical point of view, every VATS operation should be considered as an "absolute" indication of OLV. Currently, thoracic anesthetists agree on the classification of **lung isolation versus lung separation:** the isolation of the lungs means a completed "anatomic" sealing (conditions like massive pulmonary bleeding, air leak as a result of bronchopleural fistulae, pneumonia with pus, etc.); whereas the separation of the lung means a "functional" sealing.[58] Because most VATS operations require just lung separation and not isolation, both DLTs and BBs can be used. DLT is the most common device used in OLV, but it should be known that in some conditions, BBs can be a more rational alternative (Table 31.2).

Challenges During Video-Assisted Thoracoscopic Surgery

The primary objective of lung isolation is to protect the healthy lung to ensure gas exchange in the presence of pulmonary hemorrhage, bronchopleural fistula, etc. On the other hand, lung separation (and sometimes also isolation) is necessary to improve surgical exposure especially in thoracic and also cardiac, mediastinal, orthopedic, or esophageal surgeries.

- Anesthesiologists must be aware of the necessity of lung collapse for thoracoscopic surgeries to ensure adequate exposure. In fact, it can be considered that the smaller the incision, the better collapsed the lung should be. If the lung is not adequately collapsed, it would not be possible to achieve an optimal still surgical exposure. In some open thoracotomies, this compromise can be compensated by the large incision; however, it can lead easily to a failure during VATS.
- A total collapse is necessary not only for an optimal surgical exposure: in VATS, stapling devices are used for resection. If the lung is not well collapsed, the risk of air leak from the staple lines increases.
- Continuous positive airway pressure (CPAP) to the nondependent lung is considered as a method of choice to treat—and prevent—hypoxemia during OLV. In VATS, the application of this technique is not practical since the inflate lung reduce the surgeon view.

Double-Lumen Tubes Versus Bronchial Blockers (See Table 31.2)

Using the DLTs is the most common method for lung isolation; referred to as the "gold standard" by Cohen[59]: many anesthesiologists consider it as the easiest method, mainly

TABLE 31.2 Comparison of Tools for Lung Isolation

	Indications	Advantages	Disadvantages
Double-lumen tube	Lung separation (unilateral abscess or cyst; unilateral hemorrhage; bronchoalveolar fistula; unilateral giant bullae, lung transplantation; bronchoalveolar lavage lung isolation (all other indications of OLV, including all kinds of lung resections, and other operations, such as esophagectomy, orthopedic surgery etc.)	Familiarity Easy insertion Malposition uncommon Faster, effective lung collapse Bronchoscopy possible for each lung (operative or other) Feasible in absence of bronchoscope Differential ventilation available if needed	Problematic in difficult airway Not available for each size Not suitable for postoperative ventilation Risk of airway (tracheal or bronchial) trauma
Bronchial blocker (BB)	Lung isolation (i.e., the majority of cases undergoing VATS)	Patient with tracheotomy Selective lobar placement Difficult airway Pediatric patients Nasal intubation Postoperative ventilation	Experience required Malposition more common Bronchoscope mandatory Difficult to alternate OLV for each lung (except EZ-Blocker)

OLV, One-lung ventilation; *VATS*, video-assisted thoracoscopic surgery.

because they are familiar with it. A left DLT is preferable for the vast majority of thoracic procedures because a right DLT is more difficult to place and it is more complicated to maintain the optimal position to ventilate the right upper lobe. There are some limited indications for use of a right DLT, such as left main bronchial lesions with associated surgery (e.g., left pneumonectomy or sleeve resection) or an external cause of obstruction of the left main bronchus by an aneurysm of the descending aorta.

Available sizes of DLTs for adults vary between 26 Fr and 41 Fr and smallest sizes can be selected in children over 8 to 10 years old. One of the major challenges of a DLT is the lack of an accurate method to select the proper size and also the optimal insertion depth.

*Proper size: For a left-sided DLT, it is recommended to measure the width of the left main bronchus and to choose the largest tube that can fit safely that bronchus[60] (Table 31.3). For a right-sided DLT, this issue remains unsolved.

*Optimal insertion depth: The depth of the DLT can be most accurately determined with fiberoptic bronchoscopy (FOB). A blind technique could easily be associated with 50% incidence of malposition.[61] Formulas based on height have been proposed to estimate optimal DLT depth.[62]

A major concern regarding DLTs is airway trauma because of tube and stiffness and the larger diameter. Other risk factors are lack of flexibility (especially compared with BB), malposition (and multiple attempts to place), or rotation angle in one study (safer with 180 degrees instead of 90 degrees).[63] A new meta-analysis comparing a DLT with BB affirmed that a DLT was more commonly associated with an increase in airway trauma presenting as sore throat.[64] However, a DLT had significantly less malposition and was more rapidly inserted with a difference of 1 minute, which may be statistically significant but is obviously clinically irrelevant.

A relative new innovation of DLTs has an embedded camera at the tip of the tracheal lumen. This camera enables a continuous view of the carina and ensures the optimal position of the tube. The authors suggest that these types of DLTs can be a good choice especially for (but not excluded to) robotic VATS procedures, where the approach of the anesthetist to the patient can sometime be limited.

Bronchial Blockers

There are several types of BBs:

- Cohen BB contains a small wheel in the proximal tip that enables the movement of the distal tip.
- Arndt BB has a wired loop at the distal end, where the FOB is passed through to direct the BB.
- Several BBs (Fuji Uniblocker, Tappa, VivaSight) have a "hockey-stick" distal tip enabling a torque movement to

TABLE 31.3 Double-Lumen Tubes With Size and Diameters

French Size	Double-Lumen External Diameter (Fr)	Bronchial Lumen Internal Diameter (mm)
26	8.7	3.2
28	9.3	3.4
32	10.7	3.5
35	11.7	4.3
37	12.3	4.5
39	13	4.9
41	13.7	5.4

rotate and direct into the main bronchus. Univent tube has the same principle.
- EZ-Blocker has a biforked distal extremity in a Y shape to be inserted into both main bronchi.

Details of these devices are covered in other chapters in this book.

It should be noted that in cases where a lung isolation is indicated, unless absolutely necessary, there is no place for BBs. In clinical practice, in most VATS cases, only lung separation is required; therefore if preferred, BBs can be used. Moreover, there are numerous clinical challenges where BBs have to be preferred to DLTs:

1. Patients with tracheotomy: in the largest tracheotomy series Arndt, Cohen, and EZ-Blockers were safe and effective.[65]
2. Patients with previous lung resections, where a lobar blockade is required.[66]
3. Difficult airway: a difficult intubation is even more difficult when using a DLT.
4. OLV in children: although small sizes of DLT can be used in children, their use is difficult; and only suitable for above 8 to 10 years of age. Uniblocker, and Arndt blockers have pediatric sizes of 5.0 mm.
5. Use in nasal intubation.
6. Patients arrived intubated to the operating room and/or planned for prolonged mechanical ventilation after the operation: Specific tube exchangers can also be used to switch from ETT to DLT or from DLT to ETT, but this can be complicated because of edema formation.
7. Intraoperative new indication of OLV: changing to a DLT may present a challenge.

There is a perception of slower or poor lung deflation with the BB. However, Buissière et al. obtained excellent lung collapse with BB and faster than the DLT group.[67] Metaanalysis comparing DLT with BB did not find any difference for both tools in terms of lung collapse, most likely because of diverse evaluation of collapse.[64] One possible complication of BBs (rarely also of DLTs) is that the malposition may push the tip of BBs into the stapling line.[68] The position of the BB (and of DLT) should be controlled before bronchial stapling, and communication with the surgical team is crucial.

Among these alternatives, the choice would be based on a patient characteristics (airway anatomy, underlying disease, need to protect one lung, etc.), type of surgery (site of lesion, possibility of sleeve resection, need for sequential lung separation), and possible adverse effects of devices. The thoracic anesthesiologists should be skilled in different techniques and should have both in their "tool box": courses and workshops are organized for these purposes.

Fiberoptic Bronchoscopy

Use of FOB in thoracic anesthesia, and especially during VATS, is crucial:

- One of the most common reasons of hypoxemia during OLV is dislocation of OLV devices, which is much more common (e.g., 38%) for less experienced anesthesiologists in low-volume centers.[69] In another study, more than one-third of the DLTs, which were thought to be correctly positioned according to auscultation, required repositioning after use of FOB.[70]
- For the intubation with a DLT, there are two possible methods:
  - After passing a DLT with direct laryngoscopy, confirmation with FOB is essential to ensure that the bronchial tube is in the correct bronchus, and its depth is optimal (cuff 3–5 mm below the carina).
  - FOB can be used from the beginning as a guide: the intubation is performed with the FOB in the bronchial lumen of the DLT to guide under direct vision into the correct bronchus. Afterwards, the depth should be confirmed with via bronchoscopy through the tracheal lumen.
- Cohen, Arndt, and Uniblocker BBs have to be positioned with FOB.
- Position of the DLT or BB should be checked again with FOB:
  - After lateral decubitus position.
  - In changes in oxygenation, gas exchange, ventilation pressures.
- Specific for VATS: contrary to open thoracotomies, reinflation of the remaining lobe(s) during the stapling process can impair the surgical visualization. At this stage, visual control via FOB can ensure the patency of the bronchi of not resected lobe(s).

Although it is strongly suggested to use FOB, it may not be available, especially in hospitals with a low volume of thoracic operations. There can be some hints to avoid the drawbacks, as possible:

1. DLTs have to be preferred to Arndt, Cohen, and Uniblocker.
2. EZ-Blocker can be used because the resistance of the Y at the distal tip on carina can be positioned without FOB. In this case, careful auscultation would avoid the possibility that both ends of the blocker have been introduced to the same bronchus.
3. Position control of DLT should be performed with auscultation: first in two-lung ventilation, followed by the sequential blockade of both lumens.
4. New, but extensively introduced in anesthesia practice, ultrasound (US) was found to be useful in confirming adequate position of left DLT.[71] It is feasible in the intercostal view to distinguish the ventilating lung from the collapsed one. To and from movement of ventilated lung is associated with pleura seen as "lung sliding," whereas collapsed lung appears with "lung-pulse sign" because of pleural movement with heartbeat.
5. Electric impedance tomography (EIT) can be used to confirm the correct placement of a DLT.[72]
6. Finally, DLT and ETT with an embedded camera (VivaSight®). The DLT has the camera at the tip of the tracheal lumen to monitor the position of the bronchial lumen continuously. The ETT has the camera

at the distal tip so that BBs (including the one of the same companies) can be positioned under continuous view.[73,74]

Total Collapse of the Nonventilated Lung (Fig. 31.4)

In open thoracotomies, some degree of "partial" collapse can be tolerated by the surgeons. On the contrary, in VATS, a total collapse of the lung is inevitable. Even apneic periods can be necessary to create an immobile surgical area for manipulation in the hilum or mediastinum.

Some maneuvers can help to create a total collapse:

1. Immediately after starting the OLV, open to air or suction to the lumen of DLT or BB to the nonventilated lung should be applied. A relatively low level of negative pressure (–20 cm H_2O) is usually enough to improve the speed and quality of lung collapse. The negative pressure and the suction catheter itself achieve both the suction of air from the lung and the prevention of passive entrainment of air into the lung.
2. Although it is a general rule to keep the time of OLV as short as possible, it can make sense to start the OLV immediately after the positioning of the patient to the lateral position. This would not require a significantly long time, but can help to achieve a collapsed lung when the trocar enters the thorax. Moreover, this time can also be used for a positive end-expiratory pressure (PEEP)-titration in the patients (see the next part of this chapter). Remember that in "OLV with closed chest," if the lumen of the DLT to the nonventilated lung is open to atmosphere, so-called "passive paradoxical ventilation" can occur, and a tidal volume (V_T) of approximately 130 mL can be inhaled to the nonventilated lung (during expiration).[75] This means, starting OLV earlier may lead to a delayed collapse, which can be avoided by applying the suction immediately after OLV.

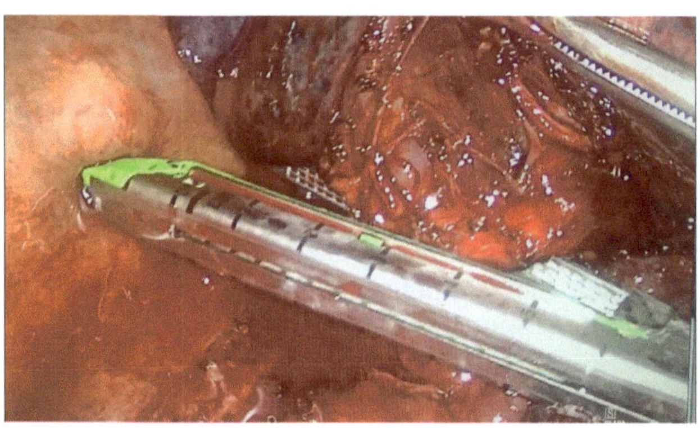

• **Fig. 31.4** A stapling device about to resect left upper lobe. Total collapse of the lung is necessary to avoid several problems including air leaks, limitations of exposure, removal of the resected tissue through a little hole, etc.

3. During two-lung ventilation before OLV, lungs can be ventilated with a fraction of inspired oxygen (F_iO2) of 1.0 for a period of some minutes. Nitrogen is the "natural CPAP" of the alveoli preventing/delaying the collapse. Wash-out of the pure oxygen from the denitrogenated lung would obtain a faster and better collapse of the lung. After the initiation of OLV, a recruitment maneuver (RM) to "open" the dependent lung would be necessary; adding some air (if the oxygen saturation [SpO2] >90%) would also prevent further atelectasis of the dependent lung.
4. To repeat one suggestion in this chapter that the use of CPAP during VATS is limited, however oxygen insufflation without expanding the lung may provide some improvement in oxygenation through apneic oxygenation.

One-Lung Ventilation During Video-Assisted Thoracoscopic Surgery

Challenges of One-Lung Ventilation

Although VATS is associated with better outcomes for the patient, it is by no means an "easier" or "simpler" procedure for the anesthetist, nor less invasive than thoracotomy. In some cases, the challenges of OLV can be even more complicated.

During OLV, one lung is excluded from ventilation, but the perfusion to the nonventilated lung continues, leading to a significant increase in intrapulmonary shunt (Qs/Qt) and consequently a higher risk of hypoxemia. In the 1970s, the incidence of hypoxemia during OLV was assumed to be between 20% and 25%. Therefore the historical (classical) recommendations for OLV have mainly focused on preventing and treating the hypoxemia (Table 31.4).[76]

Several mechanisms (above all, hypoxic pulmonary vasoconstriction [HPV]) cause a decrease of blood flow to the nonventilated lung, resulting in a decreased Qs/Qt. For anesthesia and intensive care practitioners, the knowledge of the basic (patho) physiology of HPV is essential.[77] This is also the reason why the historical guidelines suggest the use of IV anesthetics, as inhalational agents are known to inhibit HPV, leading to a further increase in pulmonary shunt.

Today, the incidence of hypoxemia has declined to less than 10%, but it should still be considered as an important challenge of OLV.

In the last decades, a growing number of studies have shifted the attention to lung injury (acute lung injury [ALI]) associated with/induced by the OLV.[78] One can assume that the postoperative lung injury would be more likely because of the surgical trauma; however, it has been shown that the degree of radiologic density increase was significantly greater in the nonoperative lung compared with operative lung after lobectomy.[79] This finding implicates that the intraoperative ventilation strategy is one of the factors that can lead to postoperative lung injury.

TABLE 31.4 Historical and Current Recommendations for One-Lung Ventilation

4A: Historical Recommendation for One-Lung Ventilation (OLV) (to Avoid Hypoxemia)
- F_iO2: 1.0
- High tidal volume (e.g., 10 mL/kg)
- Normocapnia (if necessary, increase respiratory rate)
- CPAP, if necessary
- PEEP, only if necessary, should be < CPAP
- TIVA instead of inhalational anesthetics

4B: Current Recommendation for OLV (to Avoid Hypoxemia and Lung Injury)
- F_iO2: <1.0
- Low tidal volume (max. 6 mL/kg)
- Low driving pressure of ventilation
- Permissive hypercapnia
- Inhalational anesthetics
- Routine use of CPAP (if not contraindicated [VATS])
- One-lung RM
- Routine use of PEEP

CPAP, Continuous positive airway pressure; *F_iO2*, fraction of inspired oxygen; *PEEP*, positive end-expiratory pressure; *RM*, recruitment maneuvers; *TIVA*, total intravenous anesthesia; *VATS*, video-assisted thoracoscopic surgery.

The mechanism of ALI and/or increased inflammation induced by the OLV has been explained recently.[78,80] In fact, there are similarities between OLV and acute respiratory distress syndrome (ARDS): OLV can be assumed as a variation of ventilation in ARDS because they both deal with smaller ventilated volumes of lung (baby lung in ARDS, and the one-lung in OLV).[81]

Consequently, the ventilation strategy during OLV should deal not only with the maintenance of the adequate gas exchange, but also with the protection of the lung: "protect both the lung and its functions." It should be noted that some methods of "prevention of hypoxemia" can be associated with postoperative ALI; and some methods of "protective ventilation" can increase the possibility of hypoxemia.

Mechanisms of Hypoxemia During One-Lung Ventilation

- **Dislocation of OLV device:** One of the most common causes of hypoxemia (e.g., 38%) during OLV is dislocation of OLV devices, as mentioned previously[70]: the decline in the incidence of hypoxemia from 20% to 25% in the 1970s to less than 10% today is probably because of the wide usage and increased familiarity of FOB to prevent the change of the optimal position of the airway device together with the application of protective lung ventilation.
- **Shunt:** During OLV, the ventilation of one lung is interrupted, while the perfusion persists: Qs/QT increases. Because of the effect of HPV, a shunt ratio of less than 30% could be expected.
- **Atelectasis:** Hypoventilation in the dependent lung as a result of derecruitment of the alveoli (increased risk of atelectasis).
- **Inhibition of HPV:** The older inhalational agents are claimed to have a relevant inhibitory effect on HPV. In addition, there is a list of possible inhibitors of HPV during the intraoperative period.
- Any application causing **a diversion of blood flow** to the nonventilated lung (e.g., high airway pressures in ventilated lung) can lead, even without any impact of HPV, to hypoxemia.[82]

Mechanisms of Lung Injury During One-Lung Ventilation (Fig. 31.5)

- **High V_T:** Application of the whole V_T into the ventilated lung (as suggested in classical guidelines) can lead to baro- and/or volutrauma, similar to experience in ARDS ventilation.
- **Inappropriate PEEP:** No or very low PEEP to the ventilated lung can lead to atelectasis, as this lung is already under external pressure; opening of this collapse during inhalation can result in "cyclic recruitment" and, consequently, in atelectotrauma. On the other side, unnecessarily high PEEP can lead to overinflation, another possible cause of ALI.
- **High F_iO2:** Atelectasis and the possible atelectotrauma can worsened by application of high F_iO2 (i.e., 1.0).[83]
- **Biotrauma** (immune response and oxidative stress): OLV is also associated with an increased pulmonary immune response[84] ("biotrauma"), and furthermore, the alveolar damage during OLV can be even more exaggerated than during two-lung ventilation.[85] Recent findings have shown that the atelectasis and the reexpansion at the end of OLV lead to "oxidative stress" with formation of reactive oxygen and reactive nitrogen species.[80]
- **Duration of OLV:** The magnitude of oxidative stress correlates with the duration of OLV.[80]

Protective Ventilation

The protective ventilation was defined and determined in ARDS patients with a "bundle" of some parameters:

1. Low V_T
2. Low ventilation pressures
3. RM
4. PEEP

This approach is also appropriate in healthy lungs undergoing mechanical ventilation for nonthoracic surgery.[86] In this study by Severgnini et al., intraoperative protective ventilation (a combination of RM, low V_T, and PEEP)—to both lungs—was associated with an improvement in oxygenation (higher SpO2), fewer alterations on chest x-ray, and a lower "modified Clinical Pulmonary Infection Score" during 5 postoperative days. However, note that during OLV, the classical guidelines controvert to all of the components of protective ventilation in some degree (RM and PEEP diverting the blood flow away from the dependent lung to nondependent; and low V_T decreasing the ventilation). Therefore precise changes in the "classical" guidelines have been necessary (see Table 31.4B).

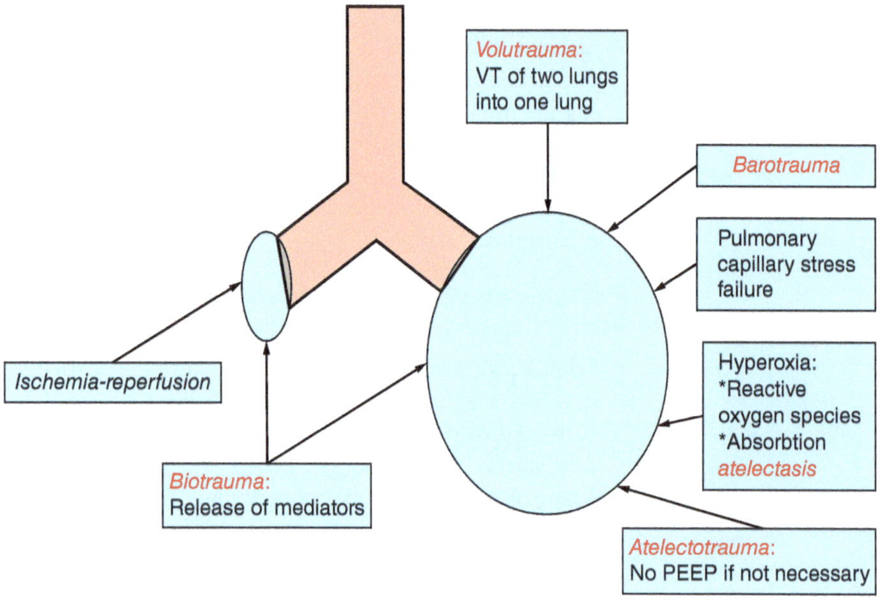

• **Fig. 31.5** Mechanisms of lung injury during one-lung ventilation: application of older recommendations (such as "tidal volume of two lungs into one lung") can be harmful to the ventilated lung. Note that inflammatory processes also occur in nonventilated lung. *PEEP,* Positive end-expiratory pressure; *VT* tidal volume.

We can assume that the application of the combination of all components of protective ventilation can be beneficial for both oxygenation and lung protection during OLV.[87] In healthy lungs, applying PEEP and recruitment maneuver does not improve the postoperative outcome and is even associated with intraoperative hemodynamic instability, as shown in the PROVHILO study.[88] The debate about this so-called "permissive atelectasis" approach continues.[89] New studies entitled PROTHOR and iPROVE are currently testing the effects of PEEP and recruitment maneuvers during OLV.[90]

Tidal Volume

The detrimental effects of high V_T during OLV are well documented. High V_T during OLV produces end-inspiratory lung overdistension, a recognized risk factor of lung injury from parenchymal stretching.[78,91,92] Several clinical studies showed that low V_T is associated with a lower incidence of postoperative ALI.[92,93] Low V_T compared with high V_T decreases the proinflammatory systemic response.[94,95] On the contrary, high V_T during OLV induces diffuse alveolar damage.[85]

Low V_T ventilation based on predicted body weight (pbw) should be routinely applied to avoid the use of excess V_T. The pbw is calculated by a formula based on gender and height. V_T should be restricted to 4 to 5 mL/kg pbw. The use of a V_T of 4mL/kg during OLV was associated with less lung water content than with larger V_Ts of 6 to 8 mL/kg.[96]

A meta-analysis has reported that low V_T was associated with the reduced incidence of PPCs.[97] Another recent meta-analysis has shown that the use of low V_T can worsen gas exchange but reduces airway pressure. Preservation of postoperative oxygenation and reduction in infiltrates suggest a lung-protective modality with low V_T.[98] It is understandable that lower V_T would lead to a decrease in ventilation (Fig. 31.6, left panel), but this problem can be addressed by adding an appropriate PEEP rather than increasing V_T. In fact, it has been shown that low V_T without adequate PEEP does not prevent postoperative respiratory complications. In the thoracic surgical patients, Blank et al. analyzed the data (medical records and the Society of Thoracic Surgery database) for postthoracic procedure complications. They found that a V_T of 8 to 9 mL/kg was associated with fewer PPCs. In the large proportion of the patients, the large V_T during OLV was inversely propositional to the incidence of respiratory complications.[99] Thus use of physiologic V_T may represent a necessary, but not independently sufficient, component of lung protective ventilation (LPV).[99] This finding leads again to the recent question of how the different components of LPV should be combined to achieve the best results.

Lung Recruitment Maneuvers (Fig. 31.7)

RMs are part of the ventilatory strategies with the goal of improving lung aeration by applying a brief and controlled increment in airways pressures. RMs were originally defined for ARDS patients in the ICU. Today, RMS are applied in the operating rooms either routinely, or in suspected atelectasis.

There are two types of RM described in the literature: one is the **sustained inflation** (SI) maneuver, which consists of the application of 40 cm H_2O of continuous airways pressure during 10 to 30 seconds.[100] The other type, the **cycling RM,** is characterized by a stepwise increment in PEEP keeping a constant driving pressure in pressure-controlled ventilation (PCV) mode. Each step of PEEP is increased every 5 cm H_2O and maintained for five breaths, until reaching a final PEEP of 20 cm H_2O and a plateau pressure of 40 cm H_2O.[101] As the first method was easier to perform, most anesthesiologists have preferred to use it. But it may be related to unacceptable hemodynamic repercussion and high stress on the lung tissue[102,103]; moreover, many new anesthesia machines and ventilators are equipped with

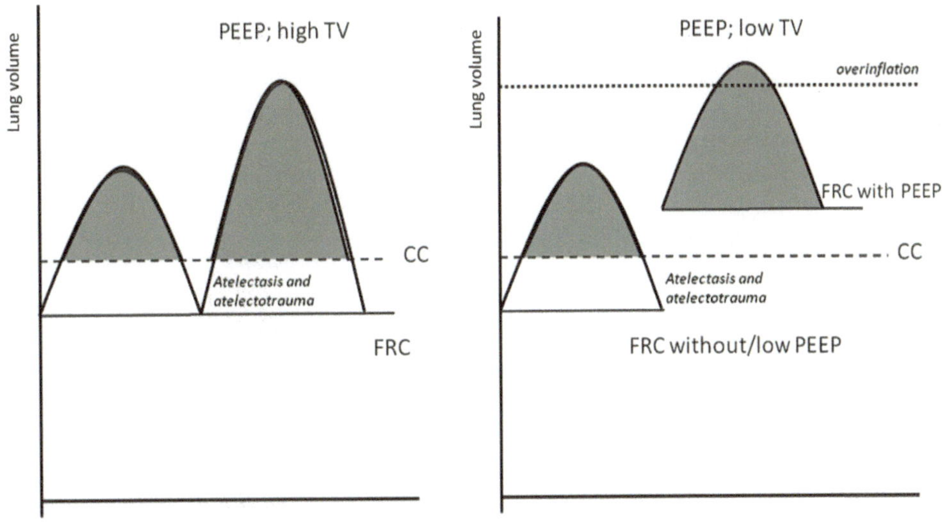

• **Fig. 31.6** Effects of different tidal volumes and positive end-expiratory pressure (*PEEP*) on ventilation and lung injury: mechanical ventilation is associated with a decrease of functional residual capacity (*FRC*) so that the closing capacity (*CC*) can exceed the FRC. This would lead to a decrease in ventilation (only the grey area above the CC [*dashed line*] can contribute to ventilation) and to so-called cyclic opening-closing of alveoli. Increasing the tidal volume **(left panel)** can just improve the ventilation but cannot prevent the cyclic opening-closing of the alveoli (which in turn can lead to "atelectotrauma"). Instead, **(right panel)** application of an appropriate PEEP can both improve the ventilation (*enlarged grey area*) and prevent the atelectasis and atelectotrauma. However, this approach can also lead to exceed the limit of overinflation (*dotted line*), especially in upper zones of the ventilated lung: overinflation is another cause of lung injury. *TV*, tidal volume.

the stepwise RM technique, so that this approach is easy to apply now and should be preferred.

Pros of RM: The increase in pulmonary shunt during OLV is not solely caused by the continuing perfusion of the nonventilated lung. An experimental animal model using computed tomography–scan images showed atelectasis in the most dependent zones of the ventilated lung and hypoventilated areas in the rest of the lung parenchyma.[104] Atelectasis was successfully treated and most of the ventilated lungs became well aerated after lung recruitment, the positive effect of RM applied to ventilated lung aims to "open" the atelectasis in this lung[105] (see Fig. 31.7C). Beneficial effects of RM during OLV have been confirmed as an improvement in gas exchange, functional residual capacity (FRC), and lung

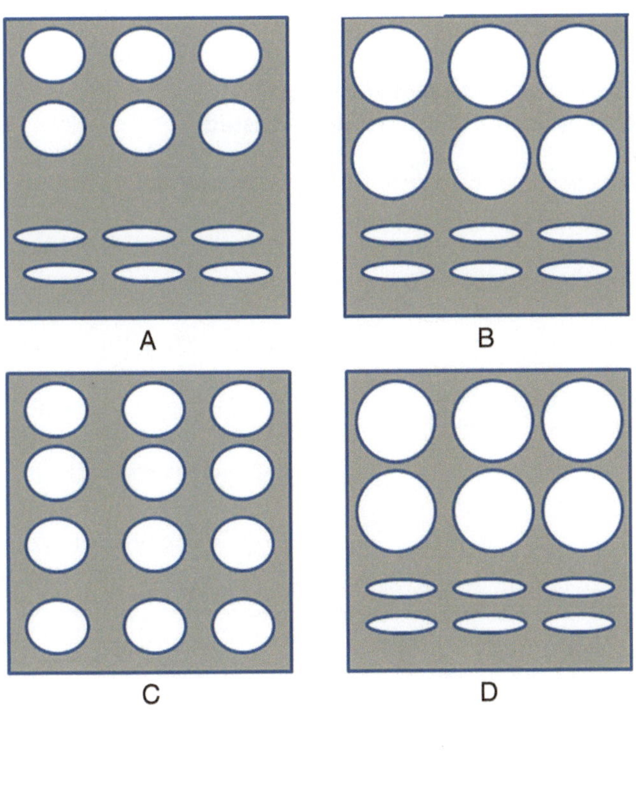

• **Fig. 31.7** Schematic presentation of the distribution of ventilation of the lung. (**A**) Because of several reasons (e.g., decrease in functional residual capacity), the lower parts tend to atelectasis, which is undesired for both ventilation (as this area receives the majority of perfusion) and occurrence of atelectasis. (**B**) Application of positive end-expiratory pressure (PEEP; without a recruitment maneuver) cannot solve this problem, as it would affect only the already "open" alveoli. This is even more undesired, for it can additionally lead to an overinflation. (**C**) A homogeneous distribution of the alveoli can be possible only by application of a supranormal pressure to open the collapsed alveoli. Note that this achievement can sustain only with application of appropriate PEEP. (**D**) Unfortunately, these positive effects of recruitment maneuver can be only possible if the atelectatic area is "recruitable." If not, the maneuver can cause an even worse distribution ventilation.

mechanics.[106,107] The decrease in dead space enables a higher elimination of CO2 per breath during OLV.[108]

Lung mechanics improved after RM because normalizing FRC decreases airways resistance and increases compliance. The final result is a decrease in driving pressure, which is a key factor that can cause ALI[109]:

$$\text{Driving pressure}\,(\text{DP}) = \text{PPlateau} - \text{PEEP}$$

$$\text{Cstat} = \text{V}_\text{T} / (\text{PPlateau} - \text{PEEP}) = \text{V}_\text{T}/\text{DP}\,.$$

PPlateau (plateau pressure) is the airway pressure at the end of inspiration with zero flow in both directions and so shows solely the pressure needed to inflate the alveoli. Combining the RM with an individually titrated PEEP can increase its benefits compared with RM with a fixed PEEP.[106] A recent study of the same group has shown that this combination was also associated with a decrease in PPCs compared with the incidence of previous studies.[110]

Controversies about RM: Obviously, RM is a nonphysiologic maneuver because of the application of supranormal pressures even for a short period. Therefore it can lead to hemodynamic compromise and lung tissue stress.[88] RM can be effective only when:

1. There should be an atelectatic area in the ventilated lung;
2. This atelectatic area should be "recruitable," that is, can be "opened" with RM (see Fig. 31.7D)

If these conditions do not exist in the case, an RM can only lead to hemodynamic instability: a short-term desaturation can also be seen, as the overpressure in the ventilated parts of the ventilated lung can divert the blood flow to the nondependent lung.

Most of the hypotension episodes that are caused by the positive pressure of the RM are rather transient and are resolved at the conclusion of the applied pressure and they have no negative clinical consequences unless the patient is extremely debilitated. Clinical and hemodynamic stabilization of the patient before RM can be helpful to avoid these complications. Moreover, some of the general contraindications of RM can be seen more commonly in patients undergoing VATS (Table 31.5).[111]

Positive End-Expiratory Pressure

PEEP during OLV is a historical controversy: Even when historically, the only challenge of OLV was hypoxemia, there were studies showing that PEEP increased,[112] decreased,[113] or did not change[114] arterial oxygen partial pressure (PaO2). Regarding the classical guidelines, PEEP should be applied only if the patient is hypoxemic and CPAP to the nondependent lung fails to improve the oxygenation during OLV,[76,112] and even in these cases, the PEEP level should not exceed the CPAP to prevent the diversion of blood flow to the nondependent lung.[113] Current practice suggest that an "appropriate" PEEP is good for both oxygenation and lung protection. (Caveat: in some cases the appropriate level of PEEP can be zero.)

An appropriate PEEP is beneficial for lung protection: Although the RM opens the collapsed alveoli, their effects are usually transitory or insufficient when they are not accompanied by an appropriate (this word can be replaced with: "best," "optimal," "titrated," "individualized," etc.) PEEP to "open the lung and keep the lung open" (see Figs. 31.7 and 31.8). The physiologic and clinical effects of a particular level of PEEP are different when only PEEP is used in isolation or in combination with an RM. A recent study has also shown that during low VT, OLV, high PEEP levels improve pulmonary

TABLE 31.5 Contraindications of Recruitment Maneuver and Cases With Least Benefits of a Recruitment Maneuver Application During Video-Assisted Thoracoscopic Surgery Operations

Contraindications of RM (during VATS):

- Patients with severe uncontrolled hypotension
- Head trauma/intercranial hypertension
- (Undrained) pneumothorax/any risk of pneumothorax in the dependent lung
- Bronchospasm
- Pulmonary emphysema
- Lung bullae

Cases with less expectation to have a benefit of RM during VATS:

- Lung fibrosis
- Focal changes in image studies
- Requirement of high PEEP levels
- Poor chest wall elastance
- Asthma-COPD

COPD, Chronic obstructive pulmonary disease; *PEEP*, positive end-expiratory pressure; *RM*, recruitment maneuver; *VATS*, video-assisted thoracoscopic surgery. Modified from García-Fernández J, Romero A, Blanco A, Gonzalez P, Abad-Gurumeta A, Bergese SD. Recruitment manoeuvres in anaesthesia: how many more excuses are there not to use them? *Rev Esp Anestesiol Reanim*. 2018;65(4):209–217.

function without increasing the V/Q and reduce driving pressure. Spadaro et al. studied 41 patients during general anesthesia for thoracic surgery. Shunt fraction, high V/Q, and respiratory mechanics were measured at PEEP 0 cm H_2O during bilateral lung ventilation and OLV and, subsequently, during OLV at 5 or 10 cm H_2O of PEEP. During OLV, increasing PEEP from 0 cm H_2O to 5 cm H_2O and 10 cm H_2O resulted in a shunt fraction decrease of 5% (0–11) and 11% (5–16), respectively ($P < .001$). The PaO2/F_iO2 ratio increased significantly only at a PEEP of 10 cm H_2O ($P < .001$). Driving pressure decreased from 16 ± 3 cm H_2O at a PEEP of 0 cm H_2O to 12 ± 3 cm H_2O at a PEEP of 10 cm H_2O ($P < .001$).[115]

An appropriate PEEP is good for the oxygenation: Earlier studies showing the negative effects of PEEP on oxygenation were probably associated with an unnecessary high level of PEEP (which most likely was associated with a higher VT)[116] (referring to point C in Fig. 31.8). PEEP per se does not restore FRC and an unnecessary higher PEEP not only can increase the shunt by diverting pulmonary blood flow to nonaerated areas, but also can lead to an overinflation in a dependent lung, causing undesirable hemodynamic side effects, especially in heterogeneous lungs. That is not the case when an appropriate PEEP level is applied.

How to determine the appropriate PEEP? For decades, numerous methods have been described to find the "best" PEEP. The lungs of the patients undergoing OLV are heterogeneous, that is, there are patients with obstructive, restrictive pulmonary diseases or patients with healthy lungs. Therefore a fixed, empiric PEEP value probably would have different effects on lung mechanics, oxygenation, and also on lung protection. A tailored or individualized PEEP titration should be applied. Some previously reported methods are not applicable or not appropriate for thoracic surgery: for example, there is no linear relationship between PEEP and oxygenation because of the possibility of diversion of the blood flow to a nonventilated lung, therefore the F_iO2-PEEP table from the ARDS-Net study is not appropriate during OLV. Similarly, PEEP for best oxygen delivery (DO2) is also not applicable because of the difficulties of DO2 measurement and time reasons.

1. The most appropriate method appears to be decremental PEEP **titration to find the PEEP for best static compliance.** Following an RM with a stepwise incline, the static compliance is measured with different PEEP levels, starting usually with 20 cm H_2O and declining in steps of 2 or 3 cm H_2O (Fig. 31.9A). The benefits of this method have been shown both in intraoperative oxygenation and lung mechanics,[106] and also in PPCs.[110] Patients undergoing thoracic surgery benefit most from this combination of RM + PEEP titration.[111] Many modern anesthesia machines are equipped with software to facilitate this type of PEEP titration. In one study by Park et al., the application of lowest driving pressure-guided ventilation during OLV has been found to be associated with a lower incidence of PPCs compared with conventional protective lung ventilation.[117] As a limitation of this study, the PEEP titration was made in an incremental manner (from lower levels to higher ones), but still, the philosophy is similar to other studies searching for the least pressure for the same V_T.
2. An alternative method uses **airway pressure and flow waveforms** obtained at the tracheal tube to derive nonlinear respiratory system mechanical parameters. In particular, the volume-dependent elastance index ("%E2") can quantify the nonlinearity of the lung pressure-volume curve during inspiration. Software helps to draw the elastance (pressure-volume) curves: to make it simple: if the shape of the curve is concave or convex, this would imply that the current PEEP is associated with an overinflation or tidal recruitment; the PEEP level obtaining a straight line is considered as the best PEEP[118] (Fig. 31.9B).
3. **Electrical dependence tomography (EIT)** can also be used to determine the best PEEP. EIT can be

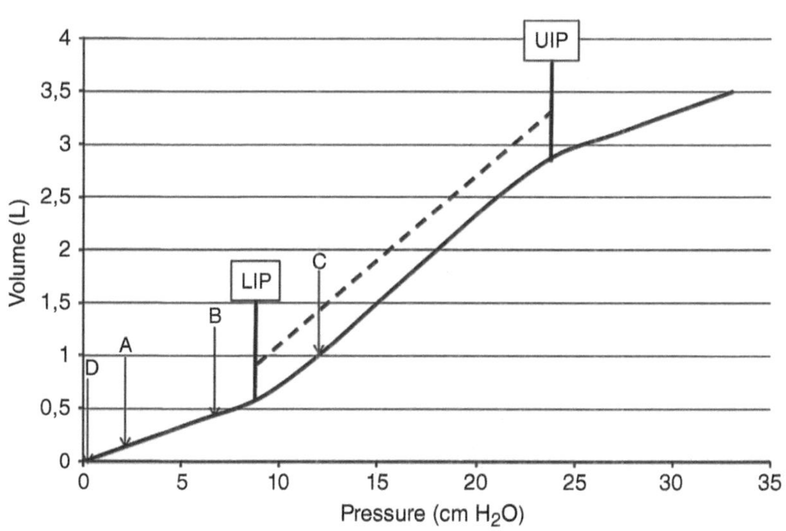

• **Fig. 31.8 Relationship of positive end-expiratory pressure (PEEP) to static compliance curve:** like every "balloon," lungs have also a sigmoid-shaped compliance curve with a lower inflection point (*LIP*) and upper (*UIP*) inflection point. The optimal ventilation should be within the area of these two points (*dashed line*). External PEEP can help to approach the total PEEP (extrinsic + intrinsic) to LIP. (**B**) Too low PEEP (**like A**) can lead to cyclic opening-closing of the alveoli; too high PEEP (**like C**) can lead to exceed the ventilation above the UIP, and, consequently, to overinflation; during one-lung ventilation, this condition can lead to a diversion of perfusion to a nonventilated lung and so worsen the oxygenation. Both A and C are associated with a decreased compliance (more pressure for the same tidal volume; or less volume achieved with the same pressure). Note that in some patients, LIP can be zero (**Point D**). (From Slinger PD, Kruger M, McRae K, Winton T. Relation of the static compliance curve and positive end-expiratory pressure to oxygenation during one-lung ventilation. *Anesthesiology*. 2001;95(5):1096–1102.)

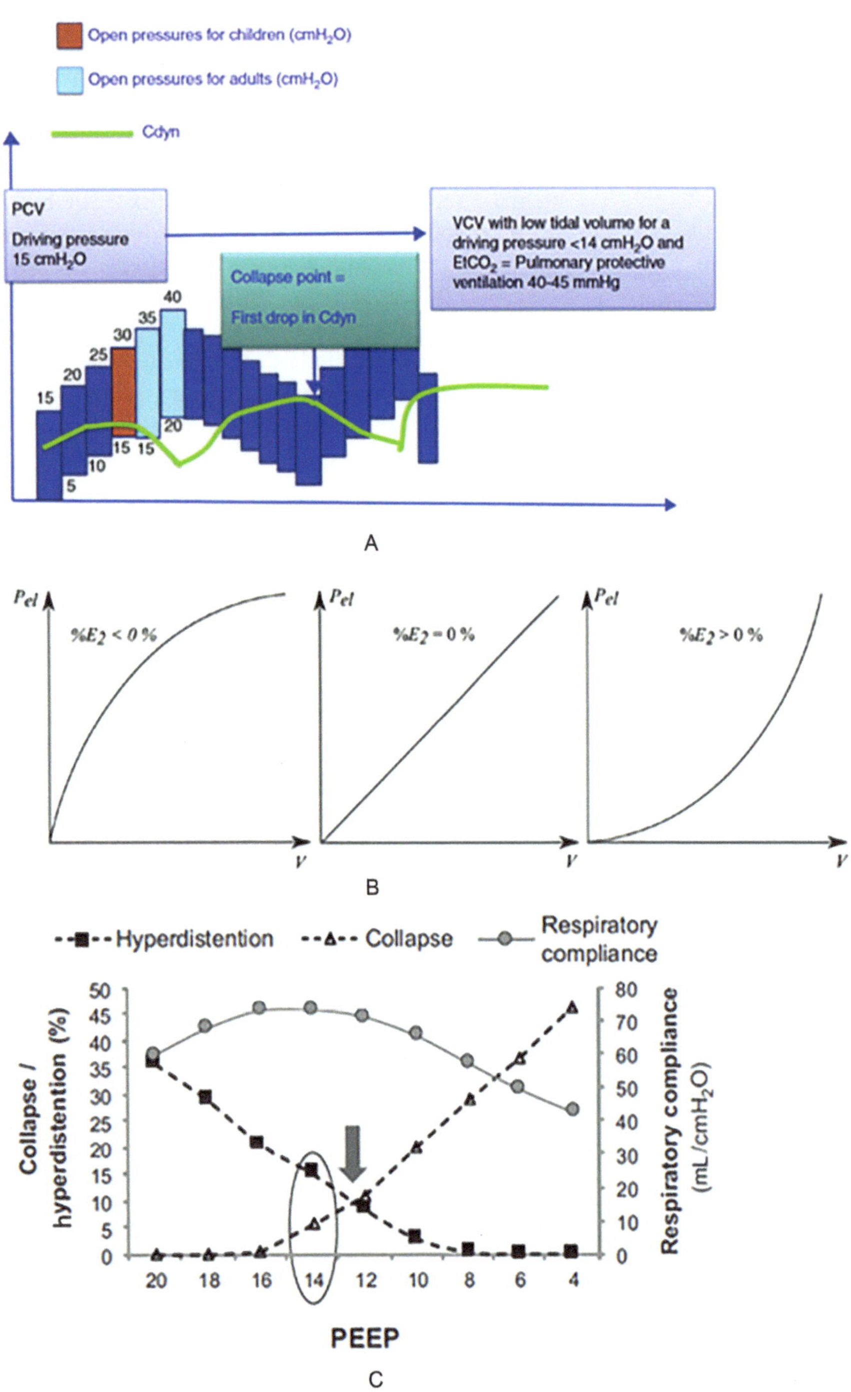

• **Fig. 31.9** Some methods of positive end-expiratory pressure (*PEEP*) titration. (**A**) Following a recruitment maneuver (RM) to open the whole lung, a decremental PEEP titration is performed to find the best compliance (*green line*), a second RM is necessary to open the alveoli again. (**B**) The relationship of airway pressure and flow can help to find the appropriate PEEP. The curve should be "straight" (in the middle); convex and concave curves in regard to tendencies to cyclic opening-closing and overinflation. (**C**) Electric impedance tomography shows the areas of collapse and hyperdistention: these areas change regarding PEEP. The balance between these two variables approximates to the PEEP level achieving the best compliance. *PCV,* Pressure control ventilation; *VCV,* volume control ventilation. **A**, from García-Fernández J, Romero A, Blanco A, Gonzalez P, Abad-Gurumeta A, Bergese SD. Recruitment manoeuvres in anaesthesia: how many more excuses are there not to use them? *Rev Esp Anestesiol Reanim*. 2018;65(4):209–217; Ferrando C, Mugarra A, Gutierrez A, et al. Setting individualized positive end-expiratory pressure level with a positive end-expiratory pressure decrement trial after a recruitment maneuver improves oxygenation and lung mechanics during one-lung ventilation. *Anesth Analg*. 2014;118:657–665.)

considered as a reliable monitor of mechanical ventilation, as it can provide information on both atelectasis and overinflation continuously in real time. Application of the optimal PEEP guided by this method in patients with healthy lungs undergoing general anesthesia intraoperatively has been shown to reduce driving pressure and improve respiratory compliance and oxygenation, and reduce the incidence and severity of postoperative atelectasis[119] (Fig. 31.9C).

4. While using the incremental PEEP titration, some authors suggest evaluating not only the static compliance, but also other **bedside parameters like dead space.**[120]
5. A relative new entity, **mechanical power**, takes several parameters like PEEP, peak pressure, and also respiratory frequency into account. Mechanical power is the energy delivered from the ventilator to the respiratory system per unit of time:

$$\text{Power: } 0.098 \times RR \times V_T \times \left[\text{Ppeak} - \tfrac{1}{2} \times (\text{PPlat} - \text{PEEP})\right]$$

A high mechanical power is associated with a higher risk of ALI.[121] Changes during the intraoperative period in thoracic surgery have also been examined.[122] Obviously, the "best" PEEP calculated with this method would be lower the others.

Does every patient need a PEEP? In some patients, best end-expiratory pressure can be zero (see Fig. 31.8D). Even in patients with a "ideal" PEEP, it is not obvious whether the patient will benefit from this ventilation in the postoperative period.

The debate between "open lung" and "resting lung" is also ongoing.[123,124] Some reports argue that preventing atelectasis (with the possible price of overinflation) is not absolutely necessary. Some multicentric studies have shown that the combination of RM + high PEEP does not improve postoperative outcome, and can even cause some intraoperative instabilities.[88] The protective role of PEEP and its potential beneficial effects have not been clearly established, either in patients during anesthesia (two-lung ventilation or OLV)[89] or in ARDS patients.[125,126]

PEEP level has been always controversial because of the negative effects in oxygenation described in several clinical studies.[113] This may be because just an arbitrarily set higher level of PEEP rather than individualized PEEP can contribute to parenchymal overdistension.

Inspiratory Oxygen Fraction

The recommendation regarding F_iO2 during OLV has also showed a fluctuation in recent decades.

The "classical" recommendation had been to use an F_iO2 of 1.0 during OLV. This approach should serve not only a higher margin of safety, but also vasodilatation of the vessels in the ventilated lung, which augments the blood flow redistribution because of HPV in the nonventilated lung.

On the other hand, it has been shown that even the short period of preoxygenation with an F_iO2 of 1.0 can cause atelectasis[127] and RMs helps less if the F_iO2 is high. Displacement of nitrogen ("the natural CPAP") would lead to a collapse of the alveoli, meaning that an approach that aims to improve the oxygenation can ultimately worsen it, and it is more pronounced in patients undergoing thoracic surgery.

Recently, the World Health Organization has recommended to use high F_iO2 (0.80) during the intraoperative (and postoperative) period to prevent surgical site infections.[128] This recommendation is based on some studies,[129,130] which are not confirmed in later, larger studies[131]; and is recently an important subject of debate in our discipline.[132]

Overall, the disadvantages of high F_iO2 appear to overcome its advantages: high F_iO2 has been shown to be one of the few factors within the intraoperative ventilatory setting to be associated with PPCs.[83]

It is appropriate to keep the F_iO2 at the lowest possible level that maintain adequate oxygenation; it makes sense to start with an empiric level of, for example, 0.7 and increase if necessary, rather than start with 1.0 and decrease. Other maneuvers to prevent and treat hypoxemia would help to prevent unnecessary increases of F_iO2.

Ventilatory Modes

There has been controversy both in ICU patients and also in patients undergoing OLV, whether PCV or volume-controlled ventilation (VCV) can be preferred as the mode of ventilation, considering their effects on both oxygenation and lung protection.

In VCV, the V_T is preset and constant, delivered with a constant flow with a square waveform. In PCV, the inspiratory pressure is set, and the pattern in flow is decelerating. From a physiologic point, the decelerating flow pattern could allow a more homogeneous gas distribution than a square flow pattern. Initial studies had suggested a possible advantage in terms of gas exchange.[133] However, several other studies have not observed the alleged benefits of PCV.[134–136] Thus the beneficial effect on gas exchange of PCV compared with VCV remains inconclusive.

The main advantage of PCV versus VCV appears to be lower peak airway pressure that might decrease the risk for barotrauma during mechanical ventilation. However, peak airway pressure does not reflect peak alveolar pressure: peak airway pressure is much greater and depends on ETT resistance, inspiratory flow, and the respiratory mechanics of the lung. The correlation between plateau airway pressure and the incidence of barotrauma is much stronger than the peak airway pressure. A plateau pressure (Pplat) of more than 35 mm Hg has been shown to induce (or be associated with) a ventilation-induced barotrauma.[137] There is almost no difference in Pplat between VCV and PCV, and, consequently, in lung protection. On the other hand, another study has shown that the use of PCV improved RV function than the use of VCV during OLV.[138] When carbon dioxide is insufflated into the operated hemithorax, the V_Ts that are actually delivered can vary in proportion to the changes in insufflating pressure.

To date, there is no clear evidence to support the advantage of any one of these ventilation modes over the others. It is rather more important to keep the "driving pressure" (plateau pressure—PEEP) as low as possible.[109,139]

Continuous Positive Airway Pressure to the Nondependent Lung

In contrast to open thoracotomies, there is no place for CPAP application to the nondependent lung in VATS. CPAP can:

- Impair the vision, and decrease the surgical exposure and quality.
- Increase the risk of air leaks from the staple lines.

A total collapse of the lung is mandatory in VATS.

Inhalational Versus Intravenous Anesthetics

Historically, the only factor that guided the decision of whether to apply inhalational or IV anesthetics during OLV was their effects on HPV and oxygenation. There are three topics in this debate: effects on oxygenation, on inflammatory response, and on cancer recurrence.

Effects on Oxygenation

Historical guidelines discourage using inhalational anesthetics, as they inhibit HPV, and recommends total IV anesthesia (TIVA) during OLV, which was found to be associated with an increased PaO2 and a decreased Qs/Qt.[140,141] Today, it accepted that in equianesthetic doses, inhalational agents do not aggravate hypoxemia when compared with IV propofol; at least the difference in PaO2 is not clinically relevant, probably because of the interaction of other hemodynamic effects of both, inhalational and IV, anesthetics.[142] Whether this difference in oxygenation was solely caused by the inhibition of HPV is not clearly defined. An RCT has shown that sevoflurane and propofol at equivalent doses, as measured by the bispectral index, were not associated with a significant difference in oxygenation between the two types of anesthetic.[143]

Effects on Inflammatory Response

Most of the studies comparing the effects of inhalational versus IV anesthesia on inflammatory response, direct or indirect organ protection, and immunomodulation, have favored inhalation anesthesia for pre- and postconditioning after biologic insults, such as ischemia reperfusion injury.

Studies performed in OLV have shown similar results: IV anesthesia is associated with an increased inflammatory response during OLV; this has been shown in the increase of the release of different mediators in bronchoalveolar lavage fluid of dependent[144] and nondependent lung;[145] and in some studies was also associated with lower postoperative complications. A more recent study by de la Gala et al. investigated the effects of sevoflurane compared with propofol on the incidence of pulmonary complications and pulmonary and systemic inflammatory response in 180 patients undergoing thoracic surgery. PPCs were higher in the propofol group together with increased systemic and pulmonary cytokine levels and higher first-year mortality.[146]

On the contrary, a multicenter RCT comparing the effects of desflurane versus propofol in 460 patients undergoing thoracic surgery has found no difference in major complications during hospitalization and within the first 6 months after surgery between these interventions.[147]

A recent meta-analysis by Pang et al., which included 23 RCTs with a total of 1349 patients concluded: "Inhalation anesthesia can preserve intraoperative cardiac function and reduce PPCs in patients undergoing thoracic surgery with OLV; although it decreases intraoperative pulmonary function, inhalation anesthesia may be superior to IV anesthesia in thoracic surgery."[148]

Effects on Cancer Recurrence

In vitro and preclinical studies have supported the hypothesis that the cytoprotective effects of inhalational anesthetics when applied to cancer cells together with their effects on immunosuppression may facilitate the development of a promalignant environment that supports the growth of residual cancer cells.[149]

Inhalation agents have been reported to suppress natural killer cell activity and promote tumor metastasis. A retrospective study involving more than 7000 patients reported that the long-term survival after curative resection in a propofol-based TIVA group outpaced that of the inhalation agent group.[150] Another retrospective study conducted in patients who received propofol-based TIVA after surgery for esophageal cancer also showed better overall survival (OS) and recurrence-free survival (RFS), compared with an inhalation-based anesthetic group.[151]

Although this topic is mainly pursued in the general cancer field, its relevance to lung cancer resection and thoracic anesthesia is still questionable. A recent study aimed to compare the favorable effects of TIVA versus inhalation agents on RFS and OS after curative resection of NSCLC in 943 patients has showed that there was no difference between the two strategies.[152]

There are no sufficient data to recommend which technique is preferable at the present time. The decision regarding the choice of the agent for the maintenance of anesthesia is still a topic of discussion. New studies should focus mainly on the balance of possible benefits and drawbacks on different (possibly PPC and cancer recurrence) parameters.

Monitoring: Hemodynamic Status, Tissue Oxygenation, and Fluid Management

Questions About Functional Hemodynamic Monitors

Surgical approaches have become less invasive owing to technologic improvements; similar progress was fortunately observed in monitoring devices. Invasive pulmonary arterial catheters are now substituted by new generation of cardiac output (CO) measurement modalities. In the perioperative period, the aim is to prevent CO decreases and thereby to avoid tissue hypoperfusion. On the other hand, lung resection usually requires restrictive fluid management, which creates a substantial challenge for the anesthesiologist to maintain adequate perfusion and to titrate fluid management attentively.

Perioperative goal directed therapy (GDT) has recently been shown to reduce mortality in nontrauma and nonpregnant patients.[153] Meanwhile, in the newest ERAS guideline, the use of noninvasive CO monitors is not routinely suggested, as they do not offer additional benefits.[16] Optimization of oxygen delivery is often commented through CO or dynamic parameters via new generation noninvasive monitors.

Usefulness of stroke volume variation (SVV) or pulse pressure variation (PPV) or similar new methods is a newer and complex topic for thoracic surgery. There is a 2-fold drawback for these innovative so-called functional hemodynamic monitors:

1. Because they use the cardiopulmonary interaction for accurate measurement, a closed chest is necessary: in this regard, VATS is also an entity where the chest is not anymore, a "closed chamber of pressure." However, there may be differences in measurements between open thoracotomies and VATS.
2. They need controlled ventilation with a "high" V_T to generate pressure changes, as a result of volume changes, that can be evaluated. During OLV, low V_Ts are applied, and the distribution of this volume within the lung is heterogenic since only one lung is ventilated.

Recently, Jeong et al. investigated if SVV and PPV could predict fluid responsiveness in OLV and also if a threshold could be established. Both SVV and PPV were not found to be useful for that purpose.[154] However, the authors identified a threshold value for PPV (7%) with lower specificity and sensitivity (62% and 58%, respectively). This result is consistent with a previous study demonstrating the prediction of fluid responsiveness of PPV during protective OLV.[155] Piccioni et al. examined dynamic measurement in cardiothoracic procedures in a meta-analysis and found that with an open chest setting, both parameters seemed inaccurate in predicting fluid responsiveness.[156] The principle of PPV and SVV is based on heart-lung interaction under mechanical ventilation with conventional settings (not the protective ones). Open thorax, lateral decubitus position for most lung resections, hypoxic pulmonary vasoconstriction of nondependent lung, and increased pulmonary arteriovenous shunt affect heart-lung interaction; and thus cyclic changes under positive pressure ventilation. In a reciprocal way, extravascular lung water was investigated during OLV for different V_T (4, 6, and 8 mL/kg) in a small study. Lowest V_T was associated with least lung water.[96] This study indicates that low V_T should be preferred and extravascular lung water measurements can be performed during OLV.

Monitoring of Tissue Oxygenation

CO monitoring seems a reliable tool to ensure tissue oxygenation in the perioperative setting but could be supplemented with venous saturation and lactate levels, as recommended in a recent review.[157] New technologies offered near-infrared spectroscopy to screen noninvasively cerebral oximetry, which has been largely used/experienced in cardiac surgery. Tissue oxygen saturation—cerebral in this case—can be measured by the difference in the intensity between transmitted and received light wavelengths specially chosen for oxyhemoglobin and deoxyhemoglobin.[158] Cerebral desaturation is widely accepted as a decrease of more than 20% compared with baseline or an absolute value of less than 50%. OLV represents a critical period of impaired tissue oxygenation. In a small study with OLV, authors found that 28% of patients had cerebral desaturation more than 20% and underlined a lack of correlation between peripheral oxygen saturation and cerebral desaturation.[159] In patients undergoing pneumonectomy, 56% had at least a 20% decrease compared with baseline.[160] A remarkable result of this study was the correlation between decreased cerebral saturation values and postoperative complications. Moreover, two studies revealed that cerebral desaturations during OLV might be correlated with cognitive dysfunction, as a sign of neurologic injury. The aforementioned data about cerebral oximetry look promising, and this tool can be used in selected patients.

Adequacy of tissue oxygenation is an attractive myth in the perioperative period. Despite scientific and technologic progress, gold standards are still lacking, and it seems rational and wise to follow multiparametric management strategies.

Fluid Management (See Chapter 21)

Fluid strategy in lung resection should be tailored neither to cause lung edema nor to kidney hypoperfusion, nor acute kidney injury (AKI). Guidelines advocate in favor of euvolemia, considering the negative side effects of very restrictive or liberal strategies.[16] However, until now, concrete definitions of euvolemia, restrictive and liberal, were unsuccessful. Whether the optimal fluid for the lung would be optimal for other organs, such as the kidneys is not clear.[161]

In a dose-based study, Matot et al. compared 8 and 2 mL/kg/h of fluid administration during thoracoscopic surgery. Total fluid volume infused was significantly different between groups (2130 mL vs. 1035 mL; p= .001). However, overall complications were similar, without any increase in kidney injury in the low volume group.[162] A slight increased amount of fluid (6.6 mL/kg/h) was found to be associated with pulmonary complications when intraoperative volume exceeded 2500 mL.[163]

On the other hand, long-term mortality has been shown to be in close correlation with any degree of kidney dysfunction, even in cases of complete recovery. Late incidence of AKI was found as high as 6% to 10% in two studies following thoracic surgery[164,165]; the new approaches like risk, injury, failure loss, end-stage (RIFLE) or Acute Kidney Injury Network (AKIN) would result in higher incidences.

These data explain the dilemma of fluid management in thoracic surgery, and specifically in VATS: there is a narrow safety margin between overload (leading to edema and lung injury) and restrictive (leading to kidney injury) fluid administration; and unfortunately, the existing monitors that should help to justify the amount of fluid do not work reliably in thoracic operations.

Fortunately, VATS appears to have a broader safety margin compared with open thoracotomies. The incidence and severity of AKI has been shown to correspond with a magnitude of surgery.[165] The attenuation of inflammatory response can lead to a decrease in risk of AKI.[164] Open thoracotomy has been defined as a risk factor for AKI.[161]

GDT seems to be associated with reduced mortality.[153,166] CO is commonly selected for GDT to optimize O2 delivery. Monitoring dynamic parameters combined with other optimization goals, such as cardiac output or cardiac index (CI) could improve clinical outcome.[167]

Although several guidelines have excluded the use of central venous pressure as a reliable monitor, anesthesiologists continue to use it as a follow-up parameter in conjunction with other monitoring evaluations: The combination of arterial blood pressure, central venous pressure, plus cerebral oximetry, and/or venous oxygen saturation would provide sufficient reliable information in the majority of cases. Moreover, in thoracic anesthesia, hypotension is rare because of acute hypovolemia and is caused usually by vasodilation or surgical manipulations. Low doses of catecholamines would be more appropriate than more fluids, administration if hypotension is likely caused by relatively minor hypovolemia.[168] Newer guidelines suggest not exceeding a perioperative positive fluid balance of 1500 mL (or 20 mL/kg/24 h).[16] The type of fluid is the most agreed point of the topic: balanced crystalloids are the first-line therapy.[16,169] ERAS protocols allow clear fluid until 2 hours before induction would ameliorate volume state.[16]

As mentioned earlier, an acute hypovolemia caused by massive hemorrhage is not common during thoracic anesthesia. But when it occurs, mainly from pulmonary veins of artery laceration it can be life-threatening. Controlling large vessels during VATS is more difficult than open thoracotomies and more time-consuming. Until the surgical team can control the source of bleeding, which often requires a conversion to open thoracotomy, preservation of the stability of hemodynamics can be challenging:

- Large bore IV catheters at least 16 G or larger, are even more necessary than open thoracotomies
- Central catheter for possible infusions (e.g., catecholamines)
- In specific cases (such as cases with a possible vascular involvement or mediastinal masses), venous access from lower extremities can be necessary.

Mediastinal Surgery, Anesthesia in Thymectomy in Patients With Myasthenia Gravis (See Chapter 47)

Evolution of thoracoscopic procedures affected mediastinal surgery concurrently with lung resection. Diagnostic or operative approaches for mediastinal masses, such as thymomas, teratomas, or cysts have been developed. Moreover, larger masses surrounded by major vascular structures are now successfully removed under thoracoscopic surgery. The minimally invasive feature of the thoracoscopic approach improves patients' outcome, especially in myasthenia gravis (MG). The less invasive thoracoscopic approach replaced most of transsternal thymectomy because of reduced pain, blood loss, length of hospital stay, and number of complications.[170,171] MG is the most common neuromuscular junction disease with autoimmune characteristics, with formation of autoantibodies most frequently to acetylcholine receptors (Ach-R). It affects particularly women and appears mainly in their 30s.

Muscle weakness is the main feature which improves at rest and worsens with activity. Ocular signs are very common in half of the affected subjects, presenting with diplopia or ptosis. Proximal muscle weakness is more frequent in the limbs, whereas dysphagia or dysarthria is associated with bulbar impairment and with a more severe clinical course. The clinical classification of the Myasthenia Gravis Foundation of America is summarized in Table 31.6.

MG presents with antibodies for components of motor end plate; the most encountered type of antibodies is for Ach-R, called seropositive. It is associated with thymic hyperplasia or thymoma, which constitutes an indication for thymectomy. Other antibodies appear against muscle specific kinase or lipoprotein related protein 4. The Ach R antibodies decrease the number of receptors (by increasing degradation and forming a complex, which will bind to complement and damage the postsynaptic membrane), finally resulting in reduction of neuromuscular transmission presented as muscle weakness.[172]

Therapy is based on medical and surgical modalities. Pyridostigmine is the key drug for enhancement of neuromuscular transmission in MG acting against anticholine esterase. Immunosuppressive therapy consists of corticosteroids, azathioprine, methotrexate, and tacrolimus.[173] Thymectomy is the surgical component of immunotherapy since the 1930s, particularly with early onset, Ach-R (+) type of MG.[174] Thymomas are present in 10% to 21% of MG cases; thymectomy is recommended as a part of the treatment of thymomatous and sometimes also in nonthymomatous MG.[175] It is rarely recommended in late onset MG or the seronegative type; and debatable in ocular myasthenia.[176] In some cases, where all other therapeutic measures have failed, plasmapheresis for a period of 2 weeks may be performed in an attempt to wash out the antibodies.

TABLE 31.6 Myasthenia Gravis Foundation of America Clinical Classification

Stage	Clinical Status
I	Only ocular involvement
II	Generalized mild muscle weakness
IIa	Predominantly affects limb and axial muscles
IIb	Predominantly bulbar involvement or respiratory weakness
III	Generalized moderate muscle weakness
IIIa	Predominantly affects limb and axial muscles
IIIb	Predominantly bulbar involvement or respiratory weakness
IV	Generalized severe muscle weakness
IVa	Predominantly affects limb and axial muscles
IVb	Predominantly bulbar involvement or respiratory weakness
V	Tracheal intubation or mechanical ventilation

Preoperative evaluation is crucial and mandates a team approach by the neurologist, thoracic surgeon, and anesthesiologist. Elective surgery should be planned for a stable period of MG and with minimal medication to reduce perioperative complications.[176] Neuromuscular optimization is the key issue, and medical therapy needs to be upgraded. Duration of the action of pyridostigmine is about 3 to 4 hours, and continuation of the drug is highly recommended to maintain neuromuscular stability. Intraoperative dosing is suggested for prolonged surgery.[177] Patients with severe MG (MGFA class III or more) could be preoperatively considered for IV immunoglobulin therapy or as mentioned earlier, plasmapheresis for bridge therapy. Other autoimmune diseases often occur with MG like hypothyroidism, worsening symptoms.

Prediction of postoperative myasthenic crisis (POMC) determines the perioperative course and need for postoperative mechanical ventilation because MGFA classification cannot be predictive in this challenge. Leuzzi suggested a scoring system of four parameters to predict POMC (Table 31.7). A score of more than 4 would be associated with POMC about 50%, whereas a score of less than 2.5 would indicate a probability of POMC less than 10%.[178] Previous myasthenic crisis appeared a significant factor in two series.[179,180] Bulbar

TABLE 31.7 Postoperative Myasthenic Crisis Score by Leuzzi

Variables Associated With Postoperative Myasthenic Crisis	Assigned Points
Osserman scale	
I–IIA	0
IIB	1
III–IV	3
Duration of MG (years)	
<1	0
1–2	1
>2	2
BMI (kg/m²)	
<28	0
≥28	1
Lung resection	
No	0
Yes	2.5

BMI, Body mass index; *MG*, myasthenia gravis.

symptoms, duration of the disease, and antibodies level, or presence of thymoma are associated with controversial results. Furthermore, the anesthesiologist should be aware of the presence of thymoma and its localization (with pericardial or vascular involvement) to plan the perioperative course rationally.

Anesthetic management is targeted to preserve neuromuscular function at best in an optimized myasthenic patient. Premedication is reserved for highly anxious patients, but pyridostigmine therapy should be continued.

Besides neuromuscular blockers (NMBs), inhalation and IV anesthetics, and opioids all impair neuromuscular function. Sevoflurane inhibits neuromuscular transmission in a dose-dependent manner in healthy and prominently myasthenic subjects.[181] NMBs should be avoided in myasthenic patients. However, insertion of DLTs and need for a "still" lung during surgery requires NMB use. Succinylcholine is not recommended, as its effect is unpredictable in this population (depending on pyridostigmine therapy). A variety of nondepolarizing blockers have been safely used. A reduced dose of mivacurium achieved adequate muscle relaxation and also safe recovery at the end of surgery.[182] Sugammadex, the selective antagonist of steroidal NMB, has been introduced in 2008 in Europe and later in the United States. The drug encapsulates rocuronium (or vecuronium to a lesser extent) in an irreversible manner and removes it from the nicotinic receptor. Case series affirmed safe neuromuscular recovery under neuromuscular monitoring with a dose of 2 to 4 mg/kg.[183–185] In the largest series from Japan reporting the national database of nearly 800 patients,[186] sugammadex was found to be associated with reduced incidence of POMC and decreased hospital costs as well, compared with neostigmine. In some cases, adequate recovery cannot be established with sugammadex reversal.[187] Neuromuscular monitoring is mandatory for myasthenic patients.

Postoperative analgesia is multimodal to reduce opioid requirement. Epidural analgesia has been associated with improved pulmonary function and faster recovery.[188] Newer thoracic plane blocks could also achieve adequate analgesia, which will be discussed later.

Myasthenic patients constitute a special group which particularly benefits from minimally invasive effects of VATS, with reduced surgical stress and faster recovery. Interruption of anticholinesterase or immunotherapy should be avoided with the purpose of maintaining function of the neuromuscular junction. An optimal perioperative course which aims for a faster and safe recovery with rational use of NMBs, with neuromuscular monitoring and reversal by sugammadex, is a preferable management.

Video-Assisted Thoracoscopic Surgery With Local or Regional Anesthesia: Nonintubated Video-Assisted Thoracoscopic Surgery

In recent years, several case series have been reported about nonintubated, or tubeless VATS (NIVATS). This topic is covered in Chapter 37 in this book; here, we will only give some short information to be comprehensive.

OLV is associated with several challenges and complications, such as hypoxemia and lung injury. A relative novel alternative to general anesthesia with invasive ventilation is the so-called tubeless, nonintubated anesthetic management. NIVATS might be safe in a broad range of operations up to lobectomy.[189–191] The major disadvantage of this method is that the patient has to breathe spontaneously: a collapse of the surgical lung is therefore limited; and only a partial collapse can be achieved with the air within the pleural cavity. This suboptimal surgical exposure can be tolerated for relatively minor operations for a short period of time, but for major operations, the authors suggest—at least for now—classical general anesthesia with OLV.

Although NIVATS is advertised as a more simple anesthetic strategy, the authors would like to underline that it is more complicated and challenging than the usual approach with general anesthesia and OLV, at least until an adequate experience will be collected. There are four targets to be achieved:

1. **Analgesia:**
   - Local-regional anesthesia: the simplest technique is to apply a local anesthetic (LA) infiltration to the lateral thoracic wall and parietal pleura with sedation and supplemental oxygen, most preferably intercostals nerve blocks at the level of incision and at two interspaces around. That is usually supplemented by IV sedation, which in turn can compromise spontaneous breathing.
   - Thoracic epidural anesthesia (TEA) or paravertebral block (PVB) can be used. Even with TEA or PVB, coughing as a result of surgical irritation of the hilum is a problem and should be prevented by an ipsilateral stellate ganglion block or—more appropriately—intrathoracic vagal blockade which can inhibit the cough.

2. **Sedation:**
   Patients who are candidates for a NIVATS should be also evaluated regarding their willingness and cooperation to maintain their control. Even in these patients, sedation, in addition to regional analgesia, is most likely necessary. Dexmedetomidine in appropriate, tailored doses can be a good choice, as it is not associated with respiratory depression. In several case series, sedative doses of propofol infusion with/without remifentanil are also reported.
3. **Oxygenation and gas exchange:**
   The risk of hypoxemia and hypercapnia during NIVATS is an important concern.[192] A recent concept, high-flow nasal catheter oxygen therapy (HFNCOT) offers a chance to reduce the risk of hypoxemia.[192] Under spontaneous breathing during VATS, a paradox respiratory pattern may cause carbon dioxide rebreathing from the nondependent, collapsed lung. Hypotension from a mediastinal shift from a vertical downward movement of the mediastinum and paradoxic breathing causes movement of air from the nondependent lung into the dependent lung in inspiration and the opposite occurs during exhalation. This wasted ventilation that results in hypoxemia and hypercarbia can be treated by applying slight positive pressure with the face mask that will usually immediately stabilize the patient[189]; HFNCOT with an adequate flow can also avoid this complication. However, it should be kept in mind that higher rates of airflow can also recruit the nondependent lung during VATS and worsen the surgical exposure.
4. Possible **airway management** problems:
   There are several causes, such as sedation that can lead to hypoxemia and hypercapnia: the conversion rate to general anesthesia and endotracheal intubation lies between 3% and 10%.[192] An intubable supralaryngeal airway (of recent generations) can be used in these cases, so that a fiberoptic intubation through the device can be performed. HFNCOT can be used in combination with noninvasive ventilation, so that the advantages of both techniques can be merged.[193]

Again, it should be kept in mind that NIVATS is not a simple procedure; it is more difficult for the surgeon who must be comfortable with the technique, more importantly, it is much more challenging for the anesthetist: it should be conducted by experienced anesthesiologists competent in these techniques, and the patients should be carefully selected. The patient must be able to cooperate, have a body mass index under 40 kg/m^2, and should not have a difficult airway in case an emergency intubation is needed.

Postoperative Analgesia After Video-Assisted Thoracoscopic Surgery

Thoracotomy is one of the most painful operations, whereas VATS is associated with lower pain scores. However, anesthesiologists should not underappreciate thoracoscopic surgery as simple three-hole to chest.[194] Postthoracotomy pain ensues from rib retraction (or even fractures), costovertebral joint retraction, pleural lining, muscle damage, or intercostal nerve injury. Although VATS can decrease the extent of surgical trauma, it cannot totally eliminate all of these components. Multimodal, well-established pain therapy is sine qua non of thoracic anesthesia independent of surgical approach.

Thoracic epidural analgesia (TEA) remains essential in open thoracotomies, especially with posterolateral thoracotomy or chest wall procedures. It achieves adequate analgesia in high and midthoracic dermatomes. Universally accepted contraindications are coagulopathy, antiplatelet use, and infection at the puncture site. Hypotension is a common side effect that limits its use, especially for minimally invasive surgery, where the primary objective is early recovery.

Paravertebral block (PVB) which was first described in the beginning of the 20th century, gained widespread use under nerve stimulation or US-guidance for a large variety of operations. Single injection or a catheter placement are described during thoracic surgery. Meta-analyses confirmed its analgesic efficiency in thoracic surgery.[195–197] The apparent advantage of PVB over TEA is a better side effect profile, while achieving adequate analgesia.[198] Similarly, the recent Cochrane analysis affirmed that PVB was associated with a decrease in complications (low blood pressure, nausea, vomiting, itching, urinary retention) compared with TEA with comparable pain control. The authors concluded that "PVB reduced the risks of developing minor complications compared with thoracic epidural blockade. PVB was as effective as thoracic epidural blockade in controlling acute pain. There was a lack of evidence in other outcomes. There was no difference in 30-day mortality, major complications, or length of hospital stay."[197] The decreased side effects profile can be explained by unilateral sympathetic block. PVB is the block of choice in the ERAS guidelines with a high evidence level and is strongly recommended[16] (Figs. 31.10–31.12). Local anesthetics (LA) choices or doses may vary between institutions.[199] In the systematic review, Kotze et al. found that an increased dose of LA and continuous infusion resulted in better pain control.[200] Higher doses were also associated with improved respiratory mechanics, whereas adjuncts did not improve analgesia. Of note, strict contraindication

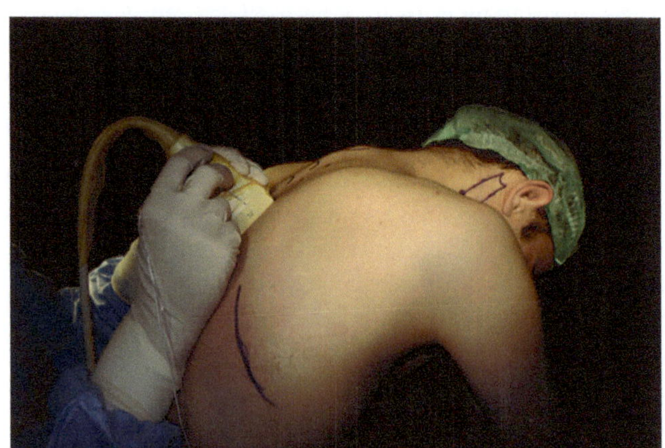

• **Fig. 31.10** Paravertebral block under ultrasonographic guidance with the "out-of-plane" technique.

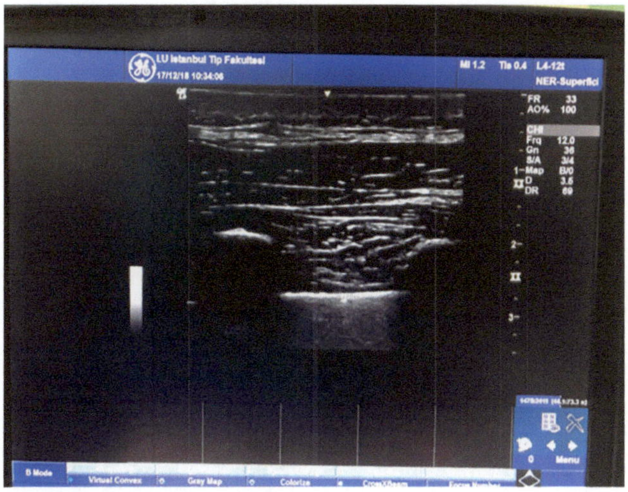

• **Fig. 31.11** Visualization of pleura.

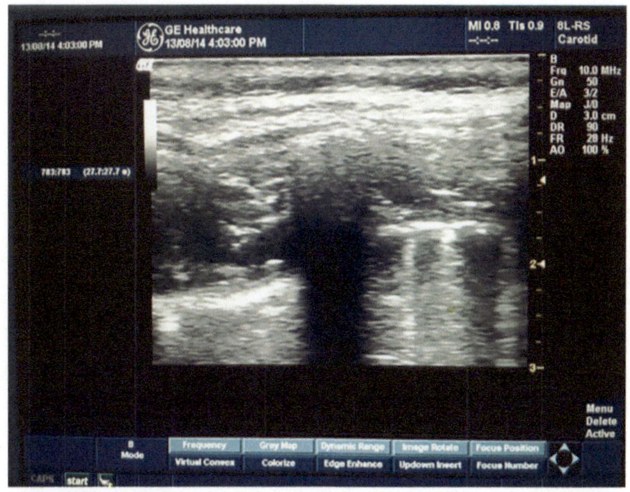

• **Fig. 31.12** Descent of pleura after administration of local anesthetic for paravertebral block.

of TEA in coagulation abnormalities also applies for consideration of PVB. Deep plexus or peripheral blocks should be regarded as neuraxial blocks according to the American Society of Regional Anesthesia guidelines.[201] However, there are some liberal papers describing PVB as a block with minor concern for neuraxial hematoma.[202–204] In patients in whom TEA is contraindicated, the eligibility of PVB should also be questioned in the same manner: Paravertebral space is highly vascular, and incidence of hematoma is 3.8% to 5.4%.[199] Spinal hematoma is a quite rare but a catastrophic complication. Thus we should practice on the conservative site, and it would be wiser to use peripheral plane blocks in patients with compromised coagulation pathway.

Use of US brought an enormous vision to anesthesiologists in pain control, and regional components of multimodal analgesia can be achieved by the recently described blocks. Initially introduced for breast surgery, fascial plane blocks are safe and usually easy to perform under US guidance. In the following part, we will discuss erector spinae plane block (ESPB), serratus anterior block (SAB), and pectoral plane block (PACS).

ESPB has been first described by Forero in 2016.[205] This is a PVB by proxy, affecting dorsal ventral rami of spinal nerves. The usual volume is 15 to 20 mL with a concentration of 0.25% to 0.5% bupivacaine. LA injected at the fifth thoracic vertebra extents epidural and paravertebral spaces via the superior costotransverse ligament in ESPB. Moreover, cutaneous branches of intercostal nerves are also affected. In a modest case series, we have found that ESPB appeared effective after thoracoscopy with slightly higher dynamic scores, and that rescue analgesic was mostly introduced at mobilizing time.[206] Furthermore, ESPB was not inferior to PVB except for the first postoperative hours, where pain scores were in acceptable limits after thoracoscopic surgery.[207] Dermatomal analysis showed a weak analgesic effect on the parasternal region. The LA spread determines both extent and type of block, and there are controversial findings in the literature. Unpredictable spread, small volume reaching paravertebral space, and effective spread to epidural space are all reported.[208–210] In daily practice, multimodal analgesia can help to support in cases if regional techniques are not adequate. On the other hand, Fang et al. have shown that ESPB is associated with a significantly lower rate of complication compared with PVB with effective pain control at rest and at cough.[211]

SAB is a newly introduced block of the anterior chest wall by Blanco.[212] It achieves postoperative analgesia in mastectomy and thoracic surgery. The block was described as superficial and deep planes consistent with LA spread under US guidance (Fig. 31.13). Cutaneous branches of intercostal

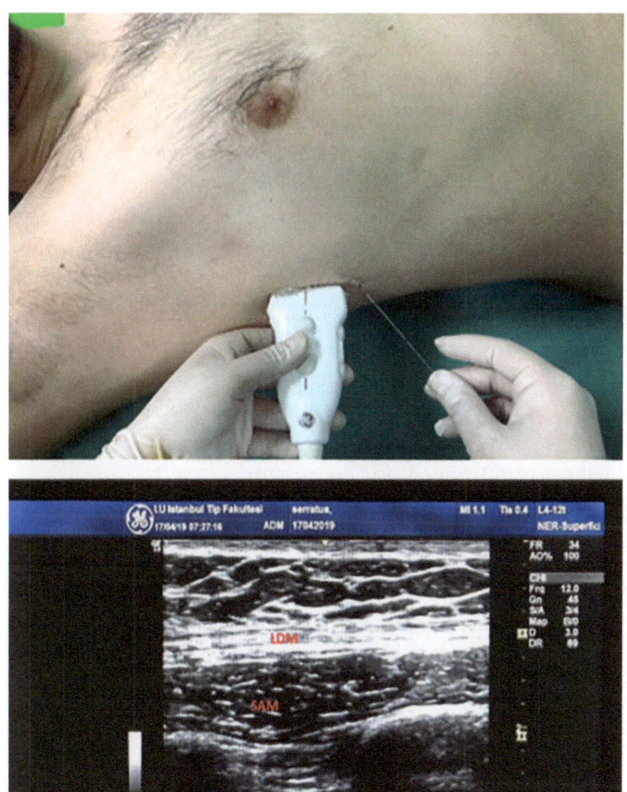

• **Fig. 31.13** Serratus anterior block under ultrasound-guidance. *LDM*, M. latissimus dorsi; *SAM*, m. serratus anterior.

nerves are mainly affected. A superficial plane is situated between serratus anterior muscle, pectoralis major, and minor muscles; the deep plane between serratus anterior muscle, intercostal muscle, and ribs. Cadaver studies investigating LA spread is fairly different within the narrower area from the initial report of Blanco et al.[212] The authors explained the discrepancy by clinical versus anatomic evaluation. Biswas et al. found the extent of dye spread was mostly influenced by the volume of injection rather than the plane of injection (superficial vs. deep to serratus anterior muscle). Increasing the volume from 20 to 40 mL doubled the area of injectate spread and promoted dye spread preferentially to the anterior chest wall, with some impact on cephalad-to-caudad spread, and no impact on posterior spread. Dye spread over anterolateral chest wall—not reaching posterior wall, nor axilla—was consistent with clinical practice. A recently published report on cadaveric work revealed that LA spread was not always predictable, as affected dermatomes vary 2 to 6 hours after injection.[213] Volume and number of injections appeared to determine attitude of LA. Unfortunately, we have limited information about optimal volume for SAB. It is recommended at fourth rib level for single injection or at third and fifth ribs levels for two injections to obtain a dermatomal analgesia between T2 and T6. Although retrospective, an interesting study compared three different analgesic strategies (IV opioid, PVB, or SAB) for uniportal thoracoscopic surgery.[214] Both PVB and SAB were superior to the IV opioid group in postoperative pain scores, as well as in opioid consumption. In clinical practice, Kim et al. investigated the effect of postoperative analgesia on recovery.[215] Patients who were treated by SAB had significantly higher quality of recovery scores compared with the control group of IV opioid patient-controlled analgesia. Pain scores were significantly better in the SAB group for the first 6 hours, but the significance did not persist during the study time. The duration of the single dose correlated with Blanco's results. Thus authors concluded that **SAB could not replace PVB or TEA but could be a part of multimodal analgesia.** When compared with TEA in thoracotomy, SAB with catheter insertion resulted in comparable analgesia with lower hypotensive episode.[216]

There are two pectoral plane blocks (PECs) defined. Pectoral blocks target nerves between pectoralis major and minor muscles for PECs I and adding lateral cutaneous intercostal branches for PECs II. A comparison of bilateral PECs II with infiltration block resulted in lower pain scores in cardiac surgery.[217]

Novel thoracic plane blocks can achieve adequate analgesia in thoracoscopic surgeries with reduced opioid consumption. They are easy to perform using US guidance and have a reduced side effect profile as major advantages. However, a larger RCT to assess their effectiveness and safety, as well as long-term outcome are needed. Currently, PVB is most commonly used with proven efficacy and an acceptable side effect profile. A recent study has found that single-shot PVB (30 mL of 0.5% ropivacaine) compared with both TEA and catheter-PVB can be preferred in VATS, especially in patients who are not ideal candidates for TEA.[218] Actual knowledge indicates that **plane blocks cannot provide reliably comparable analgesia to well-functioning TEA or PVB; rather they can be used where these two are unavailable.**

Conclusion

The future of thoracic surgery (and anesthesia) is in VATS and in its relatives (like robotic and/or subxiphoid VATS). Several devices help the anesthetist to support the patient overcome the perioperative process: FOB, different airway devices, US, near-infrared spectroscopy, functional hemodynamic monitors, etc. Some of these devices are obligatory, some for now are not, but they are obviously supportive. However, to gain the best benefit from these devices, we have to define the problems in a more concrete way.

References

1. Das K, Rothberg M. Thoracoscopic surgery: historical perspectives. *Neurosurg Focus*. 2000;9:e10.
2. Braimbridge MV. The history of thoracic surgery. *Ann Thorac Surg*. 1993;56:610–614.
3. Yan TD, Cao C, D'Amico TA, et al. International VATS Lobectomy Consensus Group. Video-assisted thoracoscopic surgery lobectomy at 20 years: a consensus statement. *Eur J Cardiothorac Surg*. 2014;45:633–639.
4. Toker A, Erus S, Tanju S, Kaya S. Video-assisted thoracoscopic resection of destroyed lung. *Ann Thorac Surg*. 2012;94:632–634.
5. Turna A. Asian perspective in surgery: thoracic surgery in Turkey. *J Thorac Dis*. 2016;8:601–605.
6. Flores RM, Ihekweazu U, Dycoco J, et al. Video-assisted thoracoscopic surgery (VATS) lobectomy: catastrophic intraoperative complications. *J Thorac Cardiovasc Surg*. 2006;138:11.
7. Whitson BA, Andrade RS, Boettcher A, et al. Video-assisted thoracoscopic surgery is more favorable than thoracotomy for resection of clinical stage I non-small cell lung cancer. *Ann Thorac Surg*. 2007;83:1965–1970.
8. Shigemura N, Akashi A, Funaki S, et al. Long-term outcomes after a variety of video-assisted thoracoscopic lobectomy approaches for clinical stage IA lung cancer: a multiinstitutional study. *J Thorac Cardiovasc Surg*. 2006;132:507–512.
9. Yan TD, Black D, Bannon PG, McCaughan BC. Systematic review and meta-analysis of randomized and nonrandomized trials on safety and efficacy of video-assisted thoracic surgery lobectomy for early-stage non-small-cell lung cancer. *J Clin Oncol*. 2009;27:2553–2562.
10. Kaseda S, Aoki T, Hangai N, Shimizu K. Better pulmonary function and prognosis with video-assisted thoracic surgery than with thoracotomy. *Ann Thorac Surg*. 2000;70:1644–1646.
11. Onaitis MW, Petersen RP, Balderson SS, et al. Thoracoscopic lobectomy is a safe and versatile procedure: experience with 500 consecutive patients. *Ann Surg*. 2006;244:420–425.
12. Yang X, Wang S, Qu J. Video-assisted thoracic surgery (VATS) compares favorably with thoracotomy for the treatment of

lung cancer: a five-year outcome comparison. *World J Surg.* 2009;33:1857–1861.
13. Scott WJ, Allen MS, Darling G, et al. Video-assisted thoracic surgery versus open lobectomy for lung cancer: a secondary analysis of data from the American College of Surgeons Oncology Group Z0030 randomized clinical trial. *J Cardiothorac Vasc Surg.* 2010;139:976–981.
14. Falcoz PE, Puyraveau M, Thomas PA, et al. Video-assisted thoracoscopic surgery versus open lobectomy for primary non-small cell lung cancer: a propensity-matched analysis of outcome from the European Society of Thoracic Surgeon database. *Eur J Cardio-Thorac Surg.* 2016;49:602–609.
15. Nwogu CE, D'Cunha J, Pang H, et al. VATS lobectomy has better perioperative outcomes than open lobectomy: CALGB 31001, an ancillary analysis of CALGB 140202 (Alliance). *Ann Thorac Surg.* 2015;99:399–405.
16. Batchelor TJP, Rasburn NJ, Abdelnour-Berchtold E, et al. Guidelines for enhanced recovery after lung surgery: recommendations of the Enhanced Recovery After Surgery (ERAS (R)) Society and the European Society of Thoracic Surgeons (ESTS). *Eur J Cardiothorac Surg.* 2019;55:91–115.
17. Sugi K, Kaneda Y, Esato K. Video-assisted thoracoscopic lobectomy achieves a satisfactory long-term prognosis in patients with clinical stage IA lung cancer. *World J Surg.* 2000;24:27–30.
18. Oda R, Okuda K, Watanabe T, et al. Long-term outcomes of video-assisted thoracoscopic surgery lobectomy vs. thoracotomy lobectomy for stage IA non-small cell lung cancer. *Surg Today.* 2019;49:369–377.
19. Yang CJ, Kumar A, Klapper JA, et al. A national analysis of long-term survival following thoracoscopic versus open lobectomy for stage I non-small-cell lung cancer. *Ann Surg.* 2019;269:163–171.
20. Al-Ameri M, Bergman P, Franco-Cereceda A, et al. Video-assisted thoracoscopic versus open thoracotomy lobectomy: a Swedish nationwide cohort study. *J Thorac Dis.* 2018;10:3499–3506.
21. Yang CJ, Kumar A, Deng JZ, et al. A national analysis of short-term outcomes and long-term survival following thoracoscopic versus open lobectomy for clinical stage II non-small-cell lung cancer. *Ann Surg.* 2019. (Epub ahead of print).
22. Howington JA, Blum MG, Chang AC, Balekian AA, Murthy SC. Treatment of stage I and II non-small cell lung cancer: diagnosis and management of lung cancer, 3rd ed: American College of Chest Physicians evidence-based clinical practice guidelines. *Chest.* 2013;143:e278S–e313S.
23. Lipinska J, Wawrzycki M, Jabłoński S. Comparison of costs of hospitalization of patients with primary lung cancer after lobectomy with access through classic thoracotomy and VATS in the conditions of financing based on diagnosis-related groups. *J Thorac Dis.* 2019;11(8):3490–3495.
24. Jutley RS, Khalil MW, Rocco G. Uniportal vs standard three-port VATS technique for spontaneous pneumothorax: comparison of post-operative pain and residual paraesthesia. *Eur J Cardiothorac Surg.* 2005;28:43–46.
25. Gonzalez D, Paradela M, Garcia J, de la Torre M. Single-port video-assisted thoracoscopic lobectomy. *Interact Cardiovasc Thorac Surg.* 2011;12:514–515.
26. Bertolaccini L, Batirel H, Brunelli A, et al. Uniportal video-assisted thoracic surgery lobectomy: a consensus report from the Uniportal VATS Interest Group (UVIG) of the European Society of Thoracic Surgeons (ESTS). *Eur J Cardiothorac Surg.* 2019;56:224–229.
27. Bulgarelli Maqueda L, García-Pérez A, Minasyan A, Gonzalez-Rivas D. Uniportal VATS for non-small cell lung cancer. *Gen Thorac Cardiovasc Surg.* 2020;68(7):707–715.
28. Harris CG, James RS, Tian DH, et al. Systematic review and meta-analysis of uniportal versus multiportal video-assisted thoracoscopic lobectomy for lung cancer. *Ann Cardiothorac Surg.* 2016;5:76–84.
29. Perna V, Carvajal AF, Torrecilla JA, Gigirey O. Uniportal video-assisted thoracoscopic lobectomy versus other video-assisted thoracoscopic lobectomy techniques: a randomized study. *Eur J Cardiothorac Surg.* 2016;50:411–415.
30. Soultanis KM, Gonzalez-Rivas D. Devising the guidelines: the concept of uniportal video-assisted thoracoscopic surgery-incisions and anesthetic management. *J Thorac Dis.* 2019;11(16):S2053–S2061.
31. Zieliński M. Technique of transcervical-subxiphoid-VATS "maximal" thymectomy in treatment of myasthenia gravis. *Przegl Lek.* 2000;57(5):64–65.
32. Liu CC, Wang BY, Shih CS. Ubxiphoid single-incision thoracoscopic left upper lobectomy. *J Thorac Cardiovasc Surg.* 2014;148:3250–3251.
33. Song N, Zhao DP, Jiang L, et al. Subxiphoid uniportal videoassisted thoracoscopic surgery (VATS) for lobectomy: a report of 105 cases. *J Thorac Dis.* 2016;8(suppl 3):S251–S257.
34. Gonzalez-Rivas D, Ismail M. Subxiphoid or subcostal uniportal robotic-assisted surgery: early experimental experience. *J Thorac Dis.* 2019;11(1):231–239.
35. Nathan H, Yin H, Wong SL. Postoperative complications and long-term survival after complex cancer resection. *Ann Surg Oncol.* 2017;24:638–644.
36. Pedoto A, Perrino AC Jr. Delayed recovery following thoracic surgery: persistent issues and potential interventions. *Curr Opin Anesthesiol.* 2019;32:3–9.
37. Salati M, Brunelli A. Risk stratification in lung resection. *Curr Surg Rep.* 2016;4:37.
38. Thomas DC, Blasberg JD, Arnold BN, et al. Validating the Thoracic Revised Cardiac Risk Index following lung resection. *Ann Thorac Surg.* 2017;104:389–394.
39. Mc Call PJ, Arthur A, Glass A, et al. The right ventricular response to lung resection. *J Thorac Cardiovasc Surg.* 2019;158:556–565.
40. Mikami I, Koizumi K, Tanaka S. Changes in right ventricular performance in elderly patients who underwent lobectomy using video-assisted thoracic surgery for primary lung cancer. *Japan J Thorac Cardiovasc Surg.* 2001;49:153–159.
41. Elrakhawy HM, Alassal MA, Shaalan AM, Awad AA, Sayed S, Saffan MM. Impact of major pulmonary resections on right ventricular function: early postoperative changes. *Heart Surg Forum.* 2018;21(1):E009–E017.
42. Amar D, Zhang H, Tan KS, Piening D, Rusch VW, Jones DR. A brain natriuretic peptide-based prediction model for atrial fibrillation after thoracic surgery: Development and internal validation. *J Thorac Cardiovasc Surg.* 2019;157:2493–2499.
43. Cagini L, Andolfi M, Leli C, et al. B-type natriuretic peptide following thoracic surgery: a predictor of postoperative cardiopulmonary complications. *Eur J Cardiothorac Surg.* 2014;46:74–80.
44. Torchio R, Guglielmo M, Giardino R, et al. Exercise ventilatory inefficiency and mortality in patients with chronic obstructive pulmonary disease undergoing surgery for non-small-cell lung cancer. *Eur J Cardiothorac Surg.* 2010;38:14–20.
45. Shafiek H, Valera JL, Togores B, Torrecilla JA, Sauleda J, Cosío BG. Risk of postoperative complications in chronic

obstructive lung diseases patients considered fit for lung cancer surgery: beyond oxygen consumption. *Eur J Cardiothorac Surg.* 2016;50:772–779.

46. Agostini P, Cieslik H, Rathinam S, et al. Postoperative pulmonary complications following thoracic surgery: are there any modifiable risk factors? *Thorax.* 2010;65:815–818.
47. Maeda R, Yoshida J, Ishii G, Hishida T, Nishimura M, Nagai K. The prognostic impact of cigarette smoking on patients with non-small cell lung cancer. *J Thorac Oncol.* 2011;6:735–742.
48. Turan A, Koyuncu O, Egan C, et al. Effect of various durations of smoking cessation on postoperative outcomes: a retrospective cohort analysis. *Eur J Anaesthesiol.* 2018;35:256–265.
49. Lugg ST, Tikka T, Agostini PJ, et al. Smoking and timing of cessation on postoperative pulmonary complications after curative-intent lung cancer surgery. *J Cardiothorac Surg.* 2017;12:52.
50. Munoz M, Acheson AG, Auerbach M, et al. International consensus statement on the peri-operative management of anaemia and iron deficiency. *Anaesthesia.* 2017;72:233–247.
51. Panagopoulos ND, Karakantza M, Koletsis E, et al. Influence of blood transfusions and preoperative anemia on long-term survival in patients operated for non-small cell lung cancer. *Lung Cancer.* 2008;62:273–280.
52. Wang T, Luo L, Huang H, et al. Perioperative blood transfusion is associated with worse clinical outcomes in resected lung cancer. *Ann Thorac Surg.* 2014;97:1827–1837.
53. Latif MJ, Tan KS, Molena D, et al. Perioperative blood transfusion has a dose-dependent relationship with disease recurrence and survival in patients with non-small cell lung cancer. *J Thorac Cardiovasc Surg.* 2019;157:2469–2477.
54. Licker M, Karenovics W, Diaper J, et al. Short-term preoperative high-intensity interval training in patients awaiting lung cancer surgery: a randomized controlled trial. *J Thorac Oncol.* 2017;12:323–333.
55. Tarumi S, Yokomise H, Gotoh M, et al. Pulmonary rehabilitation during induction chemoradiotherapy for lung cancer improves pulmonary function. *J Thorac Cardiovasc Surg.* 2015;149:569–573.
56. Mc Grath M, Tennuci C, Lee G. The history of one-lung anesthesia and the double-lumen tube. *J Anaesth.* 2017;3:3763–3786.
57. Brodsky JB, Lemmens HJ. The history of anesthesia for thoracic surgery. *Minerva Anesthesiol.* 2007;73:513–524.
58. Cohen E. Pro: the new bronchial blockers are preferable to double-lumen tubes for lung isolation. *J Cardiothorac Vasc.* 2008;22:920–924.
59. Cohen E. Strategies for lung isolation: to block or not to block? *Can J Anesth.* 2016;63:797–801.
60. Brodsky JB, Lemmens HJ. Tracheal width and left double-lumen tube size: a formula to estimate left-bronchial width. *J Clin Anesth.* 2005;17:267–270.
61. Liu Z, Zhao L, Jia Q, Yang X, Liang SJ, He W. Chest computed tomography image for accurately predicting the optimal insertion depth of left-sided double-lumen tube. *J Cardiothorac Vasc Anesth.* 2018;32:855–859.
62. Lin WL, Cherng CH. Predicting optimal insertion depth of a left-sided double-lumen endobronchial tube. *J Cardiothorac Vasc Anesth.* 2016;30:942–946.
63. Seo JH, Kwon TK, Jeon Y, Hong DM, Kim HJ, Bahk JH. Comparison of techniques for double-lumen endobronchial intubation: 90° or 180° rotation during advancement through the glottis. *Br J Anaesth.* 2013;111:812–817.
64. Clayton-Smith A, Bennett K, Alston RP, et al. A comparison of the efficacy and adverse effects of double-lumen endobronchial tubes and bronchial blockers in thoracic surgery: a systematic review and meta-analysis of randomized controlled trials. *J Cardiothorac Vasc Anesth.* 2015;29:955–966.
65. Campos JH, Musselman ED, Hanada S, Ueda K. Lung isolation techniques in patients with early-stage or long-term tracheostomy: a case series report of 70 cases and recommendations. *J Cardiothorac Vasc Anesth.* 2019;33:433–439.
66. Kozian A, Schilling T, Strang C, Hachenberg T. Anesthetic considerations in patients with previous thoracic surgery. *Curr Opin Anaesthesiol.* 2006;19:26–33.
67. Buissière JS, Omma J, Del Castillo JL, et al. Bronchial blocker versus left double-lumen endotracheal tube in video-assisted thoracoscopic surgery: a randomized-controlled trial examining time and quality of lung deflation. *Can J Anaesth.* 2016;63:818–827.
68. Soto RG, Oleszak SP. Resection of the Arndt Bronchial Blocker during stapler resection of the left lower lobe. *J Cardiothorac Vasc Anesth.* 2006;20:131.
69. Campos JH, Hallam EA, Van Natta T, Kernstine KH. Devices for lung isolation used by anesthesiologists with limited thoracic experience: comparison of double-lumen endotracheal tube, Univent torque control blocker, and Arndt wire-guided endobronchial blocker. *Anesthesiology.* 2006;104:261–266.
70. Klein U, Karzai W, Bloos F, et al. Role of fiberoptic bronchoscopy in conjunction with the use of double-lumen tubes for thoracic anesthesia. *Anesthesiology.* 1998;88:346–350.
71. Alvarez-Diaz N, Amador-García I, Fuentes-Hernández M, Dorta-Guerra R. Comparison between transthoracic lung ultrasound and a clinical method in confirming the position of double-lumen tube in thoracic anaesthesia. A pilot study. *Rev Esp Anesthesiol Reanim.* 2015;62:305–312.
72. Steinmann D, Stahl CA, Minner J, et al. Electrical impedance tomography to confirm correct placement of double-lumen tube: a feasibility study. *Br J Anaesth.* 2008;101(3):411–418.
73. Granell Gil M, Solís Albamonte P, Córdova Hernández C, Cobo I, Guijarro R, de Andrés Ibañez JA. Intubation in two patients with difficult airway management and tracheal stenosis after tracheostomy in thoracic surgery. *Rev Esp Anestesiol Reanim.* 2018;65:347–350.
74. Heir JS, Guo SL, Purugganan R, et al. A randomized controlled study of the use of video double-lumen endobronchial tubes versus double-lumen endobronchial tubes in thoracic surgery. *J Cardiothorac Vasc Anesth.* 2018;32:267–274.
75. Pfitzner J, Peacock MJ, McAleer PT. Gas movement in the non-ventilated lung at the onset of single-lung ventilation for video-assisted thoracoscopy. *Anaesthesia.* 1999;54(5):437–443.
76. Benumof JL. Conventional and differential lung management of one-lung ventilation editor. In: Benumof JL, ed. *Anesthesia for Thoracic Surgery*: Philadelphia: WB Saunders; 1995:406–431.
77. Lumb AB, Slinger P. Hypoxic pulmonary vasoconstriction: physiology and anesthetic implications. *Anesthesiology.* 2015; 122:932–946.
78. Lohser J, Slinger P. Lung injury after one-lung ventilation: a review of the pathophysiologic mechanisms affecting the ventilated and the collapsed lung. *Anesth Analg.* 2015;121:302–318.
79. Padley SP, Jordan SJ, Goldstraw P, et al. Asymmetric ARDS following pulmonary resection: CT findings initial observations. *Radiology.* 2002;223:468–473.
80. Heerdt PM, Stowe DF. Single-lung ventilation and oxidative stress: a different perspective on a common practice. *Curr Opin Anaesthesiol.* 2017;30(1):42–49.

81. Sentürk M. New concepts of the management of one-lung ventilation. *Curr Opin Anaesthesiol.* 2006;19:1–4.
82. Conacher ID. 2000–time to apply Occam's razor to failure of hypoxic pulmonary vasoconstriction during one lung ventilation. *Br J Anaesth.* 2000;84:434–436.
83. Okahara S, Shimizu K, Suzuki S, Ishii K, Morimatsu H. Associations between intraoperative ventilator settings during one-lung ventilation and postoperative pulmonary complications: a prospective observational study. *BMC Anesthesiol.* 2018;18(1):13.
84. Schilling T, Kozian A, Huth C, et al. The pulmonary immune effects of mechanical ventilation in patients undergoing thoracic surgery. *Anesth Analg.* 2005;101:957–965.
85. Kozian A, Schilling T, Röcken C, et al. Increased alveolar damage after mechanical ventilation in a porcine model of thoracic surgery. *J Cardiothorac Vasc Anesth.* 2010;24:617–623.
86. Severgnini P, Selmo G, Lanza C, et al. Protective mechanical ventilation during general anesthesia for open abdominal surgery improves postoperative pulmonary function. *Anesthesiology.* 2013;118:1307–1321.
87. Şentürk M, Slinger P, Cohen E. Intraoperative mechanical ventilation strategies for one-lung ventilation. *Best Pract Res Clin Anaesthesiol.* 2015;29:357–369.
88. Hemmes SN, Gama de Abreu M, Pelosi P, Schultz MJ. High versus low positive end-expiratory pressure during general anaesthesia for open abdominal surgery (PROVHILO trial): A multicentre randomised controlled trial. *Lancet.* 2014;384:495–503.
89. Güldner A, Kiss T, Serpa Neto A, Hemmes SN. Intraoperative protective mechanical ventilation for prevention of postoperative pulmonary complications: a comprehensive review of the role of tidal volume, positive end-expiratory pressure, and lung recruitment maneuvers. *Anesthesiology.* 2015;123:692–713.
90. Kiss T, Wittenstein J, Becker C, et al. PROTHOR investigators; Research Workgroup PROtective VEntilation Network (PROVEnet) of the European Society of Anaesthesiology (ESA): Protective ventilation with high versus low positive end-expiratory pressure during one-lung ventilation for thoracic surgery (PROTHOR): study protocol for a randomized controlled trial. *Trials.* 2019;20:213.
91. Jeon K, Yoon JW, Suh GY, et al. Risk factors for post-pneumonectomy acute lung injury/acute respiratory distress syndrome in primary lung cancer patients. *Anaesth Intensive Care.* 2009;37:14–19.
92. Fernández-Pérez ER, Keegan MT, Brown DR, Hubmayr RD, Gajic O. Intraoperative tidal volume as a risk factor for respiratory failure after pneumonectomy. *Anesthesiology.* 2006;105:14–18.
93. Licker M, Diaper J, Villiger Y, et al. Impact of intraoperative lung-protective interventions in patients undergoing lung cancer surgery. *Crit Care.* 2009;13:R41.
94. Shen Y, Zhong M, Wu W, Wang H, Feng M, Wang Tan L. The impact of tidal volume on pulmonary complications following minimally invasive esophagectomy: a randomized and controlled study. *J Thorac Cardiovasc Surg.* 2013;146:1267–1273.
95. Michelet P, D'Journo XB, Roch A, et al. Protective ventilation influences systemic inflammation after esophagectomy: a randomized controlled study. *Anesthesiology.* 2006;105:911–919.
96. H1 Qutub, MR El-Tahan, Mowafi HA, El Ghoneimy YF, Regal MA, Al Saflan AA. Effect of tidal volume on extravascular lung water content during one-lung ventilation for video-assisted thoracoscopic surgery: a randomised, controlled trial. *Eur J Anaesthesiol.* 2014;31(9):466–473.
97. Liu Z, Liu X, Huang Y, Zhao J. Intraoperative mechanical ventilation strategies in patients undergoing one-lung ventilation: a meta-analysis. *Springerplus.* 2016;5(1):1251.
98. El Tahan MR, Pasin L, Marczin N, Landoni G. Impact of low tidal volumes during one-lung ventilation. a meta-analysis of randomized controlled trials. *J Cardiothorac Vasc Anesth.* 2017;31(5):1767–1773.
99. Blank R, Colquhoun D, Durieux M, Kozower B, McMurry T. Management of one-lung ventilation. impact of tidal volume on complications after thoracic surgery. *Anesthesiology* 216;124:1286-1295.
100. Rothen HU, Sporre B, Wegenius G, et al. Reexpansion of atelectasis during general anaesthesia: a computed tomography study. *Br J Anaesth.* 1993;71:788–795.
101. Tusman G, Böhm SH, Vazquez de Anda GF, do Campo JL, Lachmann B. Alveolar recruitment strategy improves arterial oxygenation during general anaesthesia. *Br J Anaesth.* 1999;82:8–13.
102. Marini JJ. Recruitment by sustained inflation: time for a change. *Intensive Care Med.* 2011;37:1572–1574.
103. Tusman G, Bohm SH, Suarez-Sipmann F. Alveolar recruitment during mechanical ventilation – where are we in 2013? *Trends Anesth Crit Care.* 2013;3:238–245.
104. Kozian A, Schilling T, Schütze H, Heres F, Hachenberg T, Hedenstierna G. Lung computed tomography density distribution in a porcine model of one-lung ventilation. *Br J Anaesth.* 2009;102:551–560.
105. Tusman G, Böhm SH, Suarez-Sipmann F, et al. Lung recruitment improves the efficiency of ventilation and gas exchange during one-lung ventilation anesthesia. *Anesth Analg.* 2004;98:1604–1609.
106. Ferrando C, Mugarra A, Gutierrez A, et al. Setting individualized positive end-expiratory pressure level with a positive end-expiratory pressure decrement trial after a recruitment maneuver improves oxygenation and lung mechanics during one-lung ventilation. *Anesth Analg.* 2014;118:657–665.
107. Unzueta C, Tusman G, Suarez-Sipmann F, Bohm SH, Moral V. Alveolar recruitment improves ventilation during thoracic surgery: a randomized controlled trial. *Br J Anaesth.* 2012;108:517–524.
108. Tusman G, Böhm SH, Suarez-Sipmann F. Dead space during one-lung ventilation. *Br J Anaesth.* 2015;28:10–17.
109. Neto AS, Hemmes SN, Barbas CS, et al. PROVE Network Investigators: Association between driving pressure and development of postoperative pulmonary complications in patients undergoing mechanical ventilation for general anaesthesia: a meta-analysis of individual patient data. *Lancet Respir Med.* 2016;4:272–280.
110. iPROVE Network investigators, Belda J, Ferrando C, Garutti I. The Effects of an open-lung approach during one-lung ventilation on postoperative pulmonary complications and driving pressure: a descriptive, multicenter national study. *Cardiothorac Vasc Anesth.* 2018;32(6):2665–2672.
111. García-Fernández J, Romero A, Blanco A, Gonzalez P, Abad-Gurumeta A, Bergese SD. Recruitment manoeuvres in anaesthesia: how many more excuses are there not to use them? *Rev Esp Anestesiol Reanim.* 2018;65(4):209–217.
112. Senturk NM, Dilek A, Camci E, et al. Effects of positive end-expiratory pressure on ventilatory and oxygenation parameters during pressure-controlled one-lung ventilation. *J Cardiothorac Vasc Anesth.* 2005;19:71–75.
113. Capan LM, Turndorf H, Patel C, et al. Optimization of arterial oxygenation during one-lung anesthesia. *Anesth Analg.* 1980;59:847–851.

114. Mascotto G, Bizzarri M, Messina M, et al. Prospective, randomized, controlled evaluation of the preventive effects of positive end-expiratory pressure on patient oxygenation during one-lung ventilation. *Eur J Anaesthesiol.* 2003;20:704–710.
115. Spadaro S, Grasso S, Karbing DS, et al. Physiologic evaluation of ventilation perfusion mismatch and respiratory mechanics at different positive end-expiratory pressure in patients undergoing protective one-lung ventilation. *Anesthesiology.* 2018:531–538.
116. Slinger PD, Kruger M, McRae K, Winton T. Relation of the static compliance curve and positive end-expiratory pressure to oxygenation during one-lung ventilation. *Anesthesiology.* 2001;95(5):1096–1102.
117. Park M, Ahn HJ, Kim JA, et al. Driving pressure during thoracic surgery: a randomized clinical trail. *Anesthesiology.* 2019;130:385–393.
118. D'Antini D, Huhle R, Herrmann J, et al. European Society of Anaesthesiology and the PROtective VEntilation Network. Respiratory system mechanics during low versus high positive end-expiratory pressure in open abdominal surgery: A substudy of PROVHILO randomized controlled trial. *Anesth Analg.* 2018;126:143–149.
119. Pereira SM, Tucci MR, Morais CCA, et al. Individual positive end-expiratory pressure settings optimize intraoperative mechanical ventilation and reduce postoperative atelectasis. *Anesthesiology.* 2018;129:1070–1081.
120. Maisch S, Reissmann H, Fuellekrug B, et al. Compliance and dead space fraction indicate an optimal level of positive end-expiratory pressure after recruitment in anesthetized patients. *Anesth Analg.* 2008;106:175–181.
121. Serpa Neto A, Deliberato RO, Johnson AE, et al. PROVE Network Investigators. Normalization of mechanical power to anthropometric indices: impact on its association with mortality in critically ill patients. *Intensive Care Med.* 2019;45:1835–1837.
122. Chiumello D, Formenti P, Bolgiaghi L, et al. Body position alters mechanical power and respiratory mechanics during thoracic surgery. *Anesth Analg.* 2020;130:391–401.
123. Pelosi P, Ball L, Gama De Abreu M, Rocco PRM. General anesthesia closes the lungs: keep them resting. *Turk J Anaesthesiol Reanim.* 2016;44:163–164.
124. Hedenstierna G. Optimum PEEP during anesthesia and in intensive care is a compromise but is better than nothing. *Turk J Anaesthesiol Reanim.* 2016;44:161–162.
125. Meade MO, Cook DJ, Guyatt GH, et al. Stewart TE for the lung open ventilation study investigators. Ventilation strategy using low tidal volumes, recruitment maneuvers, and high positive end-expiratory pressure for acute lung injury and acute respiratory distress syndrome. A randomized controlled trial. *JAMA.* 2008;299:637–645.
126. Mercat A, Richard JC, Vielle B, et al. Expiratory pressure (Express) study group. Positive end-expiratory pressure setting in adults with acute lung injury and acute respiratory distress syndrome: a randomized controlled trial. *JAMA.* 2008;299: 646–655.
127. Edmark L, Auner U, Enlund M, Ostberg E, Hedenstierna G. Oxygen concentration and characteristics of progressive atelectasis formation during anaesthesia. *Acta Anaesthesiol Scand.* 2011;55(1):75–81.
128. Allegranzi B, Zayed B, Bischoff P, et al. the WHO Guidelines Development Group. New WHO recommendations on intraoperative and postoperative measures for surgical site infection prevention: an evidence-based global perspective. *Lancet Infect Dis.* 2016;16:e288–e303.
129. Belda FJ, Aguilera L, García de la Asunción J, et al. Spanish Reduccion de la Tasa de Infeccion Quirurgica Group: Supplemental perioperative oxygen and the risk of surgical wound infection: a randomized controlled trial. *JAMA.* 2005;294:2035–2042.
130. Greif R, Akça O, Horn EP, Kurz A, Sessler DI, Outcomes Research Group. Supplemental perioperative oxygen to reduce the incidence of surgical-wound infection. *N Engl J Med.* 2000;342:161–167.
131. Meyhoff CS, Wetterslev J, Jorgensen LN, et al. Effect of high perioperative oxygen fraction on surgical site infection and pulmonary complications after abdominal surgery: The PROXI randomized clinical trial. *JAMA.* 2009;302:1543–1550.
132. Akca A, Ball L, Belda FJ, et al. WHO needs high FIO2? *Turk J Anaesthesiol Reanim.* 2017;45:181–192.
133. Tugrul M, Camci E, Karadeniz H, et al. Comparison of volume controlled with pressure-controlled ventilation during one-lung anaesthesia. *Br J Anaesth.* 1997;79:306–310.
134. Unzueta MC, Casas JI, Moral MV. Pressure-controlled versus volume-controlled ventilation during one-lung ventilation for thoracic surgery. *Anesth Analg.* 2007;104:1029–1033.
135. Pardos PC, Garutti I, Piñeiro P, Olmedilla L, de la Gala F. Effects of ventilator mode during one-lung ventilation on intraoperative and postoperative arterial oxygenation in thoracic surgery. *J Cardiothorac Vasc Anesth.* 2009;23:770–774.
136. Choi Y, Shim J, Na S, Hong S, Hong Y, Oh Y. Pressure-controlled versus volume-controlled ventilation during one-lung ventilation in the prone position for robot-assisted esophagectomy. *Surg Endosc.* 2009;23:2286–2291.
137. Boussarsar M, Thierry G, Jaber S, et al. Relationship between ventilatory settings and barotrauma in the acute respiratory distress syndrome. *Intensive Care Med.* 2002;28:406–413.
138. Al Shehri AM, El-Tahan MR, Al Metwally R, et al. Right ventricular function during one-lung ventilation: effects of pressure-controlled and volume-controlled ventilation. *J Cardiothorac Vasc Anesth.* 2014;28:880–884.
139. Amato MB, Meade MO, Slutsky AS, et al. Driving pressure and survival in the acute respiratory distress syndrome. *N Engl J Med.* 2015;372:747–755.
140. Abe K, Shimizu T, Takashina M, et al. The effects of propofol, isoflurane, and sevoflurane on oxygenation and shunt fraction during one-lung ventilation. *Anesth Analg.* 1998;87:1164–1169.
141. Karzai W, Haberstroh J, Priebe HJ. Effects of desflurane and propofol on arterial oxygenation during one-lung ventilation in the pig. *Acta Anaesthesiol Scand.* 1998;42:648–652.
142. Ng A, Swanevelder J. Hypoxaemia associated with one-lung anaesthesia: new discoveries in ventilation and perfusion. *Br J Anaest.* 2011;106:761–763.
143. Pruszkowski O, Dalibon N, Moutafis M, et al. Effects of propofol vs sevoflurane on arterial oxygenation during one-lung ventilation. *Br J Anaesth.* 2007;98:539–544.
144. Schilling T, Kozian A, Senturk M, et al. Effects of volatile and intravenous anesthesia on the alveolar and systemic inflammatory response in thoracic surgical patients. *Anesthesiology.* 2011;115:65–74.
145. De Conno E, Steurer MP, Wittlinger M, et al. Anesthetic-induced improvement of the inflammatory response to one-lung ventilation. *Anesthesiology.* 2009;110:1316–1326.
146. de la Gala F, Piñeiro P, Reyes A, Vara E, Olmedilla L, Cruz P, Garutti I. Postoperative pulmonary complications, pulmonary

and systemic inflammatory responses after lung resection surgery with prolonged one-lung ventilation. Randomized controlled trial comparing intravenous and inhalational anaesthesia. *Br J Anaesth.* 2017;119(4):655–663.

147. Beck-Schimmer B, Bonvini JM, Braun J, et al. Which anesthesia regimen is best to reduce morbidity and mortality in lung surgery? A multicenter randomized controlled trial. *Anesthesiology.* 2016;125(2):313–321.
148. Pang QY, An R, Liu HL. Effects of inhalation and intravenous anesthesia on intraoperative cardiopulmonary function and postoperative complications in patients undergoing thoracic surgery. *Minerva Anestesiol.* 2018;84:1287–1297.
149. Melamed R, Bar-Yosef S, Shakhar G, Shakhar K, Ben-Eliyahu S. Suppression of natural killer cell activity and promotion of tumor metastasis by ketamine, thiopental, and halothane, but not by propofol: mediating mechanisms and prophylactic measures. *Anesth Analg.* 2003;97:1331–1339.
150. Wigmore TJ, Mohammed K, Jhanji S. Long-term survival for patients undergoing volatile versus IV anesthesia for cancer surgery: a retrospective analysis. *Anesthesiology.* 2016;124:69–79.
151. Jun IJ, Jo JY, Kim JI. Impact of anesthetic agents on overall and recurrence-free survival in patients undergoing esophageal cancer surgery: a retrospective observational study. *Sci Rep.* 2017;7:14020.
152. Oh TK, Kim K, Jheon S, Lee J, Do SH, Hwang JW, Song IA. Long-term oncologic outcomes for patients undergoing volatile versus intravenous anesthesia for non-small cell lung cancer surgery: a retrospective propensity matching analysis. *Cancer Control.* 2018;25(1):1073274818775360.
153. Chong MA, Wang Y, Berbenetz NM, McConachie I. Does goal-directed haemodynamic and fluid therapy improve perioperative outcomes? A systematic review and meta-analysis. *Eur J Anaesthesiol.* 2018;35:469–483.
154. Jeong AM, Ahn HJ, Park HW, Yang M, Kim JA, Park J. Stroke volume variation and pulse pressure variation are not useful for predicting fluid responsiveness in thoracic surgery. *Anesth Analg.* 2017;125:1158–1165.
155. Lee J, Jeon Y, Bahk JH, et al. Pulse pressure variation as a predictor of fluid responsiveness during one-lung ventilation for lung surgery using thoracotomy: randomised controlled study. *Eur J Anaesthesiol.* 2011;28:39–44.
156. Piccioni F, Bernasconi F, Tramontano GTA, Langer M. A systematic review of pulse pressure variation and stroke volume variation to predict fluid responsiveness during cardiac and thoracic surgery. *J Clin Monit Comput.* 2017;31:677–684.
157. Hofer CK, Rex S, Ganter MT. Update on minimally invasive hemodynamic monitoring in thoracic anesthesia. *Curr Opin Anesthesiol.* 2014;27:28–35.
158. Murkin JM, Arango M. Near-infrared spectroscopy as an index of brain and tissue oxygenation. *Br J Anaesth.* 2009;103(1): 3–13.
159. Brinkman R, Amadeo RJ, Funk DJ, Girling LG, Grocott HP, Mutch WA. Cerebral oxygen desaturation during one-lung ventilation: correlation with hemodynamic variables. *Can J Anaesth.* 2013;60:660–666.
160. Kazan R, Bracco D, Hemmerling TM. Reduced cerebral oxygen saturation measured by absolute cerebral oximetry during thoracic surgery correlates with postoperative complications. *Br J Anaesth.* 2009;103:811–816.
161. Ahn HJ, Kim JA, Lee AR, Yang M, Jung HJ, Heo B. The risk of acute kidney injury from fluid restriction and hydroxyethyl starch in thoracic surgery. *Anesth Analg.* 2016;122:186–193.
162. Matot I, Dery E, Bulgov Y, Cohen B, Paz J, Nesher N. Fluid management during video-assisted thoracoscopic surgery for lung resection: a randomized, controlled trial of effects on urinary output and postoperative renal function. *J Thorac Cardiovasc Surg.* 2013;146:461–466.
163. Arslantaş MK, Kara HV, Tuncer BB, et al. Effect of the amount of intraoperative fluid administration on postoperative pulmonary complications following anatomic lung resections. *J Thorac Cardiovasc Surg.* 2015;149:314 312.
164. Ishikawa S, Griesdale DE, Lohser J. Acute kidney injury after lung resection surgery: incidence and perioperative risk factors. *Anesth Analg.* 2012;114:1256–1262.
165. Cardinale D, Cosentino N, Moltrasio M, et al. Acute kidney injury after lung cancer surgery: Incidence and clinical relevance, predictors, and role of N-terminal pro B-type natriuretic peptide. *Lung Cancer.* 2018;123:155–159.
166. Ripolles-Melchor J, Espinosa Á, Martínez-Hurtado E, et al. Perioperative goal-directed hemodynamic therapy in noncardiac surgery: a systematic review and meta-analysis. *J Clin Anesth.* 2016;28:105–115.
167. Deng QW, Tan WC, Zhao BC, Wen SH, Shen JT, Xu M. Is goal-directed fluid therapy based on dynamic variables alone sufficient to improve clinical outcomes among patients undergoing surgery? A meta-analysis. *Crit Care.* 2018;22:298.
168. Chappell D, Jacob M, Hofmann-Kiefer K, Conzen P, Rehm M. A rational approach to perioperative fluid management. *Anesthesiology.* 2008;109:723–740.
169. Şentürk M, Orhan Sungur M, Sungur Z. Fluid management in thoracic anesthesia. *Minerva Anesthesiol.* 2017;83:652–659.
170. Siwachat S, Tantraworasin A, Lapisatepun W, Ruengorn C, Taioli E, Saeteng S. Comparative clinical outcomes after thymectomy for myasthenia gravis: thoracoscopic versus trans-sternal approach. *Asian J Surg.* 2018;41:77–85.
171. Raza A, Woo E. Video-assisted thoracoscopic surgery versus sternotomy in thymectomy for thymoma and myasthenia gravis. *Ann Cardiothorac Surg.* 2016;5:33–37.
172. Hirsch NP. Neuromuscular junction in health and disease. *Br J Anaesth.* 2007;99:132–138.
173. Sieb JP. Myasthenia gravis: an update for the clinician. *Clin Exp Immunol.* 2013;175:408–418.
174. Gilhus M, Verschuuren JJ. Myasthenia gravis: subgroup classification and therapeutic strategies. *Lancet Neurol.* 2015;14:1023–1036.
175. Cata JP, Lasala JD, Williams W, Mena GE. Myasthenia gravis and thymoma surgery: a clinical update for cardiothoracic anesthesiologist. *J Cardiothorac Vasc Anesth.* 2019;33:2537–2545.
176. Mi W, Silvestri NJ, Wolfe GI. A neurologist's perspective on thymectomy for myasthenia gravis: current perspective and future trials. *Thorac Surg Clin.* 2019;29:143–150.
177. Sungur Z, Sentürk M. Anaesthesia for thymectomy in adult and juvenile myasthenic patients. *Curr Opin Anaesthesiol.* 2016; 29(1):14–19.
178. Leuzzi G, Meacci E, Cusumano G, et al. Thymectomy in myasthenia gravis: proposal for a predictive score of postoperative myasthenic crisis. *Eur J Cardiothorac Surg.* 2014;45:76–88.
179. Yu S, Lin J, Fu X, et al. Risk factors of myasthenic crisis after thymectomy in 178 generalized myasthenia gravis patients in a five-year follow-up study. *Int J Neurosci.* 2014;124:792–798.
180. Chigurapati K, Gadhinglajkar S, Sreedhar R, Nair M, Unnikrishnan M, Pillai M. Criteria for postoperative mechanical ventilation after thymectomy in patients with myasthenia gravis: a retrospective analysis. *J Cardiothorac Vasc Anesth.* 2018;32:325–330.

181. Nitahara K, Sugi Y, Higa K, Shono S, Hamada T. Neuromuscular effects of sevoflurane in myasthenia gravis patients. *Br J Anaesth*. 2007;98:337 334.
182. Sungur Ulke Z, Senturk M. Mivacurium in patients with myasthenia gravis undergoing video-assisted thoracoscopic thymectomy. *Br J Anaesth*. 2009;103:310–311.
183. Sungur Ulke Z, Yavru A, Camci E, Ozkan B, Toker A, Senturk M. Rocuronium and sugammadex in patients with myasthenia gravis undergoing thymectomy. *Acta Anesthesiol Scand*. 2013;57:745–748.
184. de Boer, Shields MO, Booij LH. Reversal of neuromuscular blockade with sugammadex in patients with myasthenia gravis: a case series of 21 patients and review of the literature. *Eur J Anaesthesiol*. 2014;31:715–721.
185. Vymazal T, Krecmerova M, Bicek V, Lischke R. Feasibility of full and rapid neuromuscular blockade recovery with sugammadex in myasthenia gravis patients undergoing surgery - a series of 117 cases. *Ther Clin Risk Manag*. 2015;11:1593–1596.
186. Mouri H, Jo T, Matsui H, Fushimi K, Yasunaga H. Effect of sugammadex on postoperative myasthenic crisis in myasthenia gravis patients: propensity score analysis of a Japanese nationwide database. *Anesth Analg*. 2020;130:367–373.
187. Fernandes HDS, Ximenes JLS, Nunes DI, Ashmawi HA, Vieira JE. Failure of reversion of neuromuscular block with sugammadex in patient with myasthenia gravis: case report and brief review of literature. *BMC Anesthesiol*. 2019;19:160–163.
188. Liu XZ, Wei CW, Wang HY, et al. Effects of general-epidural anaesthesia on haemodynamics in patients with myasthenia gravis. *West Indian Med J*. 2015;64:99–103.
189. Hung MH, Hsu HH, Cheng YJ, et al. Nonintubated thoracoscopic surgery: state of the art and future directions. *J Thorac Dis*. 2014;6:2–9.
190. Guo Z, Yin W, Pan H, et al. Video-assisted thoracoscopic surgery segmentectomy by nonintubated or intubated anesthesia: a comparative analysis of short-term outcome. *J Thorac Dis*. 2016;8:359–368.
191. Liu J, Cui F, He J. Nonintubated video-assisted thoracoscopic surgery anatomical resections: a new perspective for treatment of lung cancer. *Ann Transl Med*. 2015;3:102.
192. Wang ML, Hung MH, Chen JS, et al. Nasal high-flow oxygen therapy improves arterial oxygenation during one-lung ventilation in nonintubated thoracoscopic surgery. *Eur J Cardiothorac Surg*. 2018;53:1001–1006.
193. Jaber S, Molinari N, De Jong A. New method of preoxygenation for orotracheal intubation in patients with hypoxaemic acute respiratory failure in the intensive care unit, noninvasive ventilation combined with apnoeic oxygenation by high flow nasal oxygen: the randomised OPTINIV study protocol. *BMJ Open*. 2016;6:e011298.
194. Fischer GW, Cohen E. An update on anesthesia for thoracoscopic surgery. *Curr Opin Anaesthesiol*. 2010;23(1):7–11.
195. Davies RG, Myles PS, Graham JM. A comparison of the analgesic efficacy and side-effects of paravertebral vs epidural blockade for thoracotomy—a systematic review and meta-analysis of randomized trials. *Br J Anaesth*. 2006;96:418–426.
196. Harky A, Clarke CG, Kar A, Bashir M. Epidural analgesia versus paravertebral block in video-assisted thoracoscopic surgery. *Interact Thorac Cardiovasc Surg*. 2019;67:404–406.
197. Yeung JHY, Gates S, Naidu BV, Wilson MJ. Gao Smith F. Paravertebral block versus thoracic epidural for patients undergoing thoracotomy. *Cochrane Database Syst Rev*. 2016; 2:CD009121.
198. Scarci M, Joshi A, Attia R. In patients undergoing thoracic surgery is paravertebral block as effective as epidural analgesia for pain management? *Interact Cardiovasc Thorac Surg*. 2010;10:92–96.
199. D'Ercole F, Arora H, Kumar PA. Paravertebral block for thoracic surgery. *J Cardiothorac Vasc Anesth*. 2018;32:915–927.
200. Kotze A, Scally A, Howell S. Efficacy and safety of different techniques of paravertebral block for analgesia after thoracotomy: a systematic review and metaregression. *Br J Anaesth*. 2009;103:626–636.
201. Horlocker TT, Wedel DJ, Rowlingson JC, et al. Regional anesthesia in the patient receiving antithrombotic or thrombolytic therapy: American Society of Regional Anesthesia and Pain Medicine Evidence-Based Guidelines (Third Edition). *Reg Anesth Pain Med*. 2010;35:64–101.
202. Richardson J, Lönnqvist PA, Naja Z. Bilateral thoracic paravertebral block: potential and practice. *Br J Anaesth*. 2011;106:164–171.
203. Katayama T, Hirai S, Kobayashi R, Hamaishi M, Okada T, Mitsui N. Safety of the paravertebral block in patients ineligible for epidural block undergoing pulmonary resection. *Gen Thorac Cardiovasc Surg*. 2012;60:811–814.
204. Okitsu K, Iritakenishi T, Iwasaki M, Imada T, Fujino Y. Risk of hematoma in patients with a bleeding risk undergoing cardiovascular surgery with a paravertebral catheter. *J Cardiothorac Vasc Anesth*. 2017;31:453–457.
205. Forero M, Adhikary SD, Lopez H, Tsui C, Chin KJ. The erector spinae plane block: a novel analgesic technique in thoracic neuropathic pain. *Reg Anesth Pain Med*. 2016;41:621–627.
206. Turhan O, Sungur Z, Sivrikoz N, Şentürk M. Analgesic efficacy of erector spinae plane block in thoracoscopic lung surgery. *J Cardiothorac Vasc Anesth*. 2019;33:s143.
207. Taketa Y, Irisawa Y, Fujitani T. Comparison of ultrasound-guided erector spinae plane block and thoracic paravertebral block for postoperative analgesia after video-assisted thoracic surgery: a randomized controlled non-inferiority clinical trial. *Reg Anesth Pain Med*. 2020;45:10–15.
208. Yang HM, Choi YJ, Kwon HJ, O J, Cho TH, Kim SH. Comparison of injectate spread and nerve involvement between retrolaminar and erector spinae plane blocks in the thoracic region: a cadaveric study. *Anaesthesia*. 2018;73:1244–1250.
209. Dautzenberg KHW, Zegers MJ, Bleeker CP, et al. Unpredictable injectate spread of the erector spinae plane block in human cadavers. *Anesth Analg*. 2019;129:e162–e166.
210. Adhikary SD, Bernard S, Lopez H, Chin KJ. Erector spinae plane block versus retrolaminar block: a magnetic resonance imaging and anatomical study. *Reg Anesth Pain Med*. 2018;43:756–762.
211. Fang B, Wang Z, Huang X. Ultrasound-guided preoperative single-dose erector spinae plane block provides comparable analgesia to thoracic paravertebral block following thoracotomy: a single center randomized controlled double-blind study. *Ann Transl Med*. 2019;7:174.
212. Blanco R, Parras T, McDonnell JG, Prats-Galino A. Serratus plane block: a novel ultrasound-guided thoracic wall nerve block. *Anaesthesia*. 2013;68:1107–1113.
213. Biswas A, Castanov V, Li Z, Perlas A, Kruisselbrink R, Agur A, Chan V. Serratus plane block: a cadaveric study to evaluate optimal injectate spread. *Reg Anesth Pain Med*. 2018;43:854–858.
214. Wang L, Wang Y, Zhang X, Zhu X, Wang G. Serratus anterior plane block or thoracic paravertebral block for postoperative pain treatment after uniportal video-assisted thoracoscopic

surgery: a retrospective propensity-matched study. *J Pain Res.* 2019;12:2231–2237.

215. Kim DH, Oh YJ, Lee JG, Ha D, Chang YJ, Kwak HJ. Efficacy of ultrasound-guided serratus plane block on postoperative quality of recovery and analgesia after video-assisted thoracic surgery: a randomized, triple-blind, placebo-controlled study. *Anesth Analg.* 2018;126:1353–1361.
216. Khalil AE, Abdallah NM, Bashandy GM, Kaddah TA. Ultrasound-guided serratus anterior plane block versus thoracic epidural analgesia for thoracotomy pain. *J Cardiothorac Vasc Anest.* 2017;31:152–158.
217. Kumar KN, Kalyane RN, Singh NG, et al. Efficacy of bilateral pectoralis nerve block for ultrafast tracking and postoperative pain management in cardiac surgery. *Ann Card Anaesth.* 2018;21:333–338.
218. Yeap YL, Wolfe JW, Backfish-White KM, et al. Randomized prospective study evaluating single-injection paravertebral block, paravertebral catheter, and thoracic epidural catheter for postoperative regional analgesia after video-assisted thoracoscopic surgery. *J Cardiothorac Vasc Anesth.* 2020;34(7):1870–1876.

32

Endoscopic Treatment of Chronic Obstructive Pulmonary Disease

TIMOTHY J. HARKIN, JOHN PAWLOWSKI

One Way Valves in the Treatment of Emphysema and Persistent Air Leaks

Emphysema

Emphysema is one component of chronic obstructive pulmonary disease (COPD), the third leading cause of death in the United States.[1–3] Emphysema has been defined as "a condition of the lung characterized by abnormal permanent enlargement of the airspaces distal to the terminal bronchioles accompanied by destruction of their walls and without obvious fibrosis."[4] Emphysema often manifests with large air-containing bullae that do not contribute to gas exchange. Smoking-related emphysema is most commonly heterogeneously distributed throughout the lung, with upper lobe predominance (Fig. 32.1). Destruction of lung tissue may lead to increased compliance of the remaining lung, with change in compliance directly related to the amount and severity of emphysema present. Whereas other components of COPD, such as chronic bronchitis and bronchospasm usually coexist with emphysema to varying degrees in individual patients and contribute to obstructive dysfunction, the presence of severe emphysema alone is sufficient to cause expiratory airflow obstruction. In normal lungs, the diameter of airways during exhalation progressively decreases in conjunction with the decrease in lung volume. This leads to progressively decreasing flow rates throughout expiration, as exemplified by the characteristic downward slope of the expiratory limb of the flow-volume loop measured by spirometry (Fig. 32.2). The airways are tethered open during exhalation by the integrity of the lung parenchyma. The degree to which the diameter of the airways decreases during exhalation is directly related to this tethering effect, measured as the elastic recoil of the lung.

The destruction of lung parenchyma by emphysema decreases elastic recoil (inversely increasing lung compliance), thereby increasing airway obstruction during exhalation by diminishing the tethering effect of the lung on the airways. This effect is exaggerated during forced expiratory maneuvers (Fig. 32.3), causing decreased values for measurements such as the forced expiratory volume in 1 second (FEV_1). The obstruction to expiratory airflow may become severe enough to prevent complete exhalation of inspired air. Progressive "air trapping" may eventually lead to chronic hyperinflation of the lungs and increased total lung capacity (TLC). Hyperinflation in turn disrupts the mechanical advantage in the ventilatory design of the thorax, pushing the diaphragm downward toward the abdomen and pushing the ribcage outward. The degree of hyperinflation may be measured in the pulmonary function lab and expressed by the residual volume (RV), which is the amount of air that cannot be exhaled and remains in the lung at the end of a forced exhalation. Measurements in pulmonary function tests (PFTs) are usually expressed in absolute values and compared with predicted values based on the individual's demographics, including age, sex, race, and height (percent or % predicted). The increase in TLC in a patient with COPD is mostly caused by an increase in RV in patients with very severe emphysema and hyperinflation, the RV may be increased to 150% to 200% of its predicted value or even more (Fig. 32.4). Hyperinflation is a significant contributor to dyspnea and decreased exercise tolerance in such patients, with a commensurate negative impact on quality of life (QOL). Many studies in emphysema treatment measure QOL using the St. George's Respiratory Questionnaire (SGRQ). The *SGRQ* is a disease-specific quality of life assessment tool validated in both COPD and asthma. The questionnaire consists of 76 items divided into 3 parts measuring symptoms, activity limitation, and social impact. Higher scores indicate poorer QOL. A decrease of 4 points in the score is considered a significant improvement in QOL. Functional impairments in patients with COPD are also commonly measured with the 6-minute walk test (6MWT), which measures the distance walked during 6 minutes on a standardized course (6-minute walk distance [6MWD]). Current medical management focuses primarily on optimizing bronchodilation and minimizing airway inflammation with a complement of medications including beta-agonists, antimuscarinics, and inhaled corticosteroids, which do not address the loss of elastic recoil from emphysema.

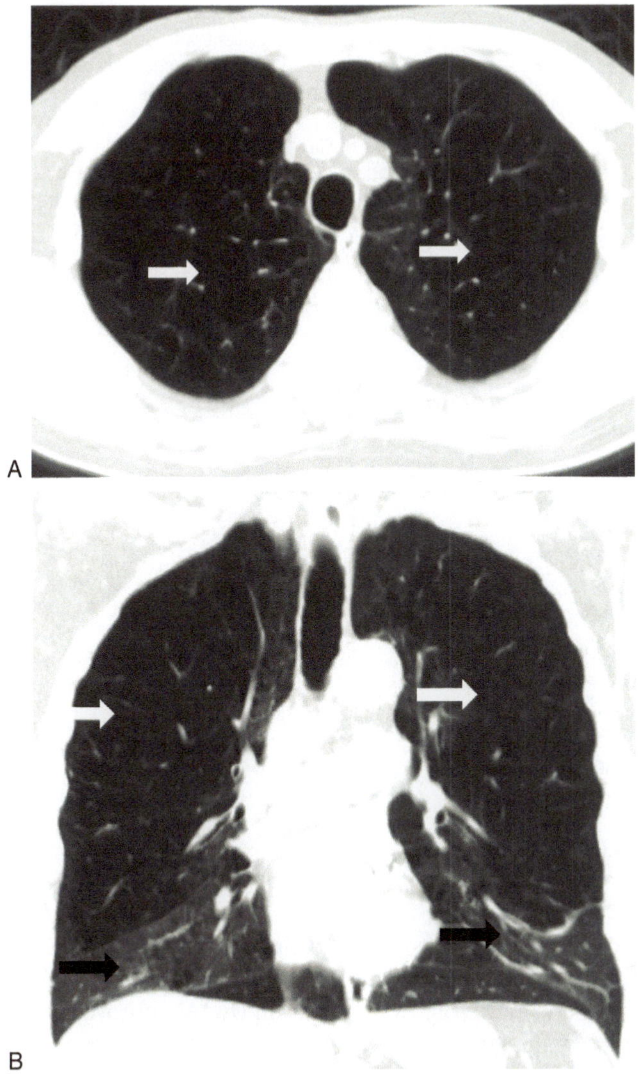

• **Fig. 32.1** Chest computed tomography images demonstrating widespread destruction of lung parenchyma with enlargement of air spaces predominantly in the upper lobes, characteristic of emphysema (*white arrows*). (**A**) Axial view through upper lobes. (**B**) Coronal view showing heterogeneous emphysema with upper lobe predominance (*white arrows*) and compression of remaining lobes (*black arrows*) by upper lobe hyperinflation.

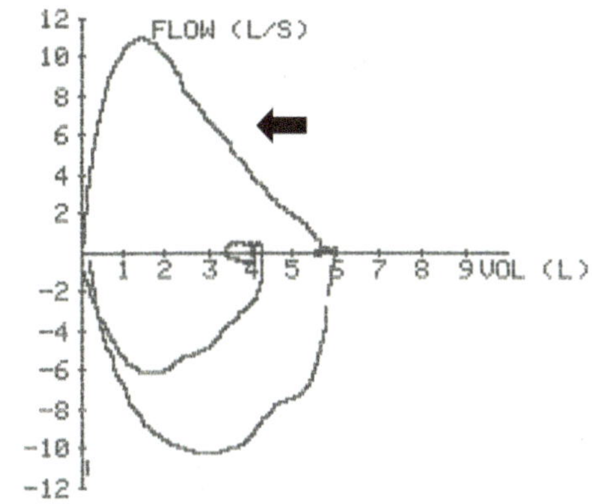

• **Fig. 32.2** Normal flow volume loop measured by spirometry. Note the downward slope of the expiratory limb, demonstrating normal decrease in air flow during expiration (*arrow*).

Recent estimates place the direct cost of COPD treatment in the USA at about $30 billion per year[3]; given that more than 3 million individuals in the United States suffer from emphysema, the need for improved treatment options is compelling.

Surgical Treatment of Emphysema and its Offspring (see Chapter 29)

The goal of specifically decreasing hyperinflation in emphysema has been recognized as a potential means of improving symptoms and QOL if enough of the natural mechanical advantage of the thorax in ventilation can be restored. This led to exploration of surgical methods targeted to removal of portions of the most severely destroyed lung, as the absence of a significant portion of hyperinflated lung would presumably allow the diaphragm and ribcage to return to a more normal position. In the 1990s, Cooper pioneered the modern technique of lung volume reduction surgery (LVRS),[5,6] building upon earlier work by Brantigan in 1959.[7] This work led to the landmark National Emphysema Treatment Trial (NETT), which randomized patients with severe emphysema and dyspnea to standard medical therapy or surgical removal of the most severe regions of emphysema. Although the majority of patients experienced either no benefit or increased mortality from surgery, a subgroup of patients, with both upper-lobe predominant emphysema and low exercise capacity at baseline, derived a significant mortality benefit that extended throughout the 5-year follow-up (30% surgery vs. 50% medical therapy, $P = .005$). Importantly, this subgroup also experienced significant improvements in exercise capacity and health-related QOL, which was related to the decrease in hyperinflation. Unfortunately, the LVRS technique itself was also associated with significant morbidity

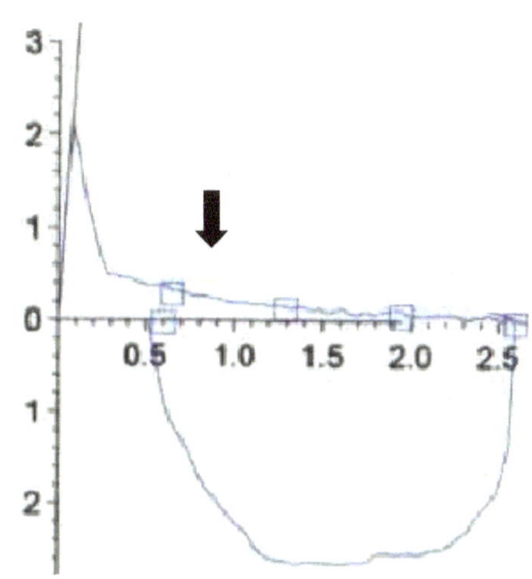

• **Fig. 32.3** Flow volume loop measured by spirometry in a patient with severe emphysema. Severe airflow obstruction is demonstrated by the flattening of the expiratory limb throughout nearly all of expiration (*arrow*).

Spirometry

	Ref	Pre	Pre%ref	LLN	ULN
FVC	2.66	2.61	98	1.95	
FEV 1	2.11	0.60	29	1.53	
FEV1/FVC	80	23		68	91
FEF 25-75%	1.95	0.12	6	0.83	
PIF		2.65			
FET100%		25.62»			
PEF	5.97	2.36	40	4.49	
FIVC	2.66	2.10	79	1.95	
FIF50%		2.61			
PEF50%	1.95	0.13	7	0.83	
PEF/FIF50		0.05			
SPIR_ECODE		000000			

Lung Volumes

		Ref	Pre	Pre%Ref	LLN	ULN
TLC	L	4.90	6.44	131	3.92	5.89
VC	L	2.66	2.61	98	1.95	3.36
FRCpleth	L	2.69	5.27	196	1.87	3.51
RV	L	1.91	3.84	201	1.33	2.48
RV%TLC	%	40	60	150	30	49
ERV	L	1.01	0.82	81	0.78	1.23
VTG	L		5.36			
IC	L	2.02	1.17	58	2.02	2.02

• **Fig. 32.4** Spirometry and lung volume measurements from a patient with severe emphysema (discussed values *outlined in red*). Note the severely reduced FEV_1 (29% of predicted value) and FEV_1/FVC ratio of 23% (predicted value is 80%), demonstrating very severe airflow obstruction. The TLC is 131% predicted, and the RV is 201% predicted, demonstrating very severe hyperinflation and air trapping. *FEV_1*, Forced expiratory volume in 1 second; *FVC*, forced vital capacity; *TLC*, total lung capacity; *RV*, residual volume.

(e.g., prolonged air leaks, prolonged hospitalizations) and mortality (5.2% vs. 1.5% at 90 days).[8]

Although NETT was invaluable in proving that selected patients with severe emphysema and dyspnea may benefit from decreasing hyperinflation via removal of a portion of destroyed lung, LVRS remains an uncommonly used technique.[9] The incidence of postoperative complications were greater than the potential benefits. LVRS simply has not been a very appealing option to patients with severe emphysema and disabling dyspnea nor to the clinicians managing them. At its core, LVRS by definition is major thoracic surgery on patients with very poor lung function, which inherently imparts significant risk to individual patients and a major burden to the healthcare system in terms of costs and hospital days, while, at best, providing benefit to only a subgroup of patients with emphysema. These concerns naturally led to a new question: can a minimally invasive method be devised to specifically treat hyperinflation in chronically ill patients with very poor lung function and frequent comorbidities that is at least as efficacious as LVRS, with fewer complications, and applicable to a greater proportion of patients? Attempts to answer this question have revolved around bronchoscopic techniques, broadly described as **bronchoscopic lung volume reduction (BLVR)**. A variety of BLVR modalities including methods to focally deflate (one-way valves or airway bypass) or minimize ventilation to areas of air trapping (coils), or functionally "remove" emphysematous lobes by focal fibrosis (tissue engineering with lung sealant or steam) have been explored in recent years. In 2018, the U.S. Food and Drug Administration (FDA) approved two different designs of one-way valves for the treatment of emphysema.

A Brief History of Valves in the Treatment of Emphysema

The principle of one-way or unidirectional valves in bronchi leading to emphysematous areas of lung is based on a simple concept: valves that permit air to flow from the lung to the airway and thereby to the atmosphere during exhalation but do not allow air to flow from the atmosphere through the bronchus into the lung. This may reduce overall lung hyperinflation by means of regional deflation of the most emphysematous areas of the lung. Currently, there are two available valves with different designs, both made with a nitinol frame. **Pulmonx** (Redwood City, CA) manufactures the **Zephyr valve** with a silicone "duckbill" design (Fig. 32.5). **Spiration** (Redmond, WA) manufactures the Spiration Valve System (SVS), with an umbrella-like structure covered with a plastic polymer (Fig. 32.6). Both valves came under investigation nearly simultaneously soon after the NETT results were known. (Author's note: Such valves have at times been described as "intrabronchial" or "IBV" usually referring to the Spiration valve, or "endobronchial" or "EBV" often referring to the Pulmonx

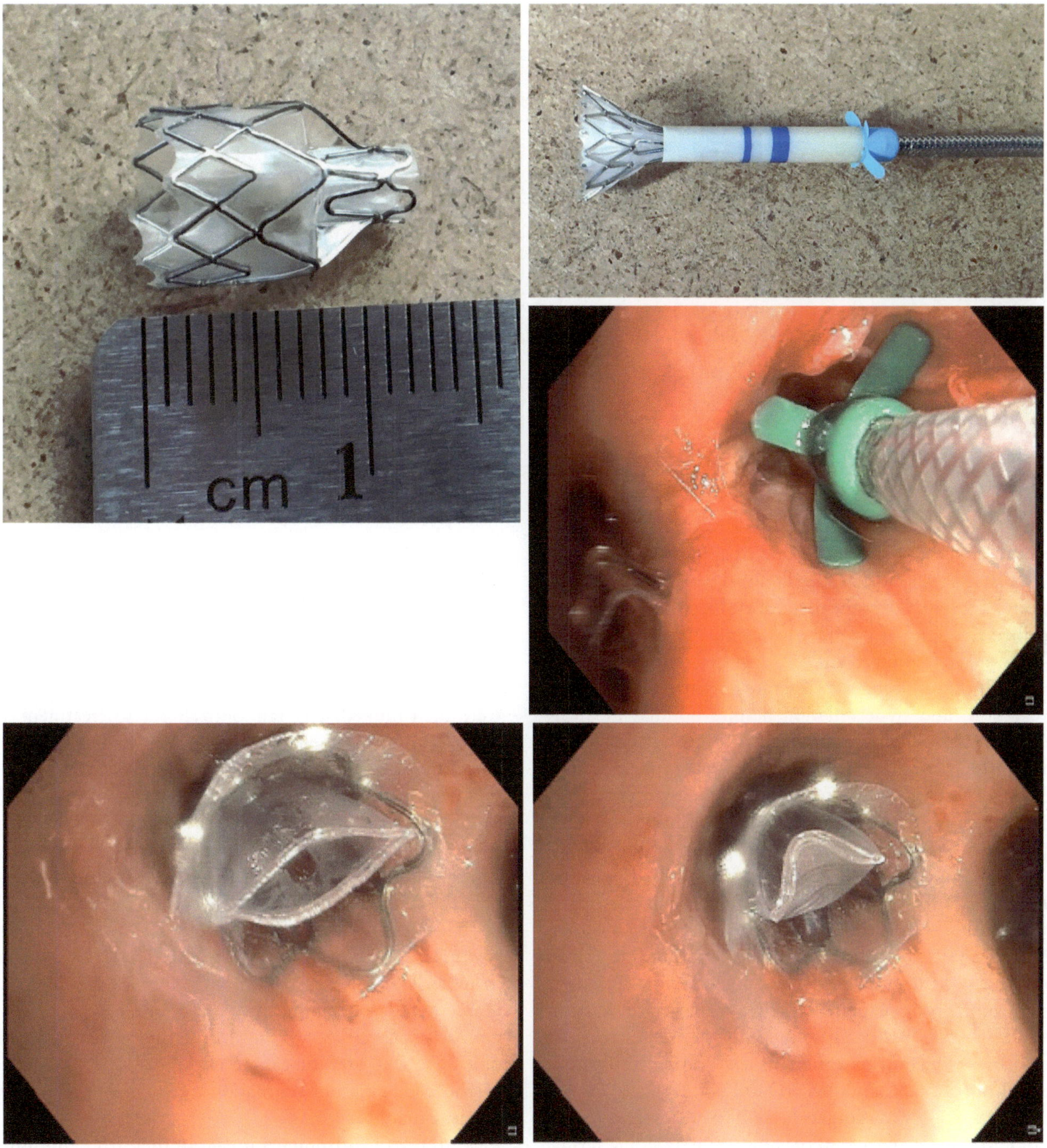

A B C D

• **Fig. 32.5** (**A**) Pulmonx Zephyr valve. (**B**) Zephyr valve partially deployed from catheter. (**C**) Sizing of airway using Pulmonx deployment catheter. A previously placed valve is visible on the left. (**D**) Pulmonx valve appropriately placed in segmental airway. On left, the duckbill component of valve is open during exhalation. On right, the duckbill component is closed during inhalation.

valve; whereas these terms may be considered synonymous, "endobronchial valve" or "EBV" seems to have become the more commonly used term in discussions of these valves, often meant to apply to both currently available valves.) The one-way nature of the valves also permits lung secretions to move from the lungs to the airways, to minimize pooling of secretions in airways distal to the valves, thereby theoretically reducing the risk of postobstructive pneumonia. Both valves have a similar deployment strategy, using a catheter inserted through a flexible bronchoscope to deliver the valve to a segmental or subsegmental airway that ventilates a targeted area of emphysematous lung. Both valves are currently available in four sizes to enhance full occlusion of targeted airways and use different simple sizing techniques during the procedure. In distinction to LVRS, both valves are easily removed by bronchoscopy should clinical circumstances or

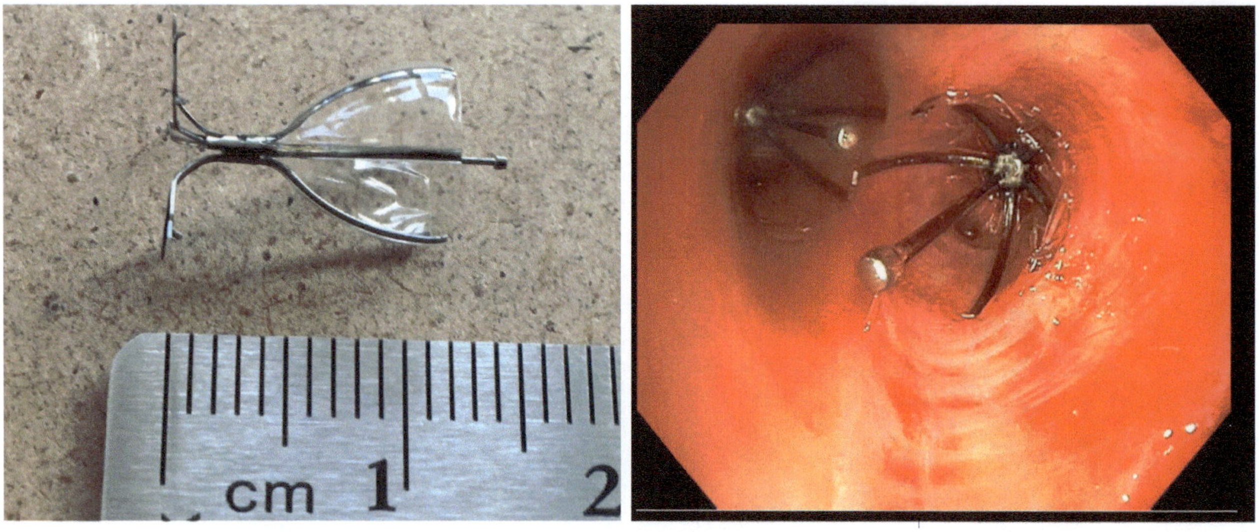

A B

• **Fig. 32.6** (**A**) Spiration intrabronchial valve (IBV), Spiration valve system (SVS). (**B**) Two Spiration valves appropriately seated in segmental airways.

patient preference dictate. Selection of appropriate patients for BLVR, as well as which specific airways and areas of lung to treat, has evolved over the past decade based on key studies described later.

Early, nonrandomized studies suggested that certain patients with the combination of severe emphysema, dyspnea on exertion, and hyperinflation despite optimal medical therapy would benefit from the insertion of EBV. These studies primarily relied on some type of quantitative analysis of high-resolution chest computed tomography (CT) scans to confirm severity and regional distribution of emphysema and to target specific areas, primarily individual or bilateral upper lobes. In a study of the first 98 patients treated with an early version of the Zephyr valve, FEV_1 increased by 11% and 6MWD improved by 23%.[10] Similarly, in the Spiration pilot study, patients with severe upper lobe predominant emphysema and hyperinflation treated in both upper lobes experienced significant improvements in QOL, with an 8.2 decrease in SGRQ. This was accompanied by redirection of airflow to less diseased untreated lobes, although FEV_1 and 6MWD did not change.[11] However, results of early randomized studies were less encouraging or disappointing.

In the Endobronchial Valve for Emphysema Palliation Trial (VENT) study, 321 patients with severe heterogeneous emphysema and hyperinflation (FEV_1 15%–45%, TLC > 100%, RV > 150% predicted values) were randomized to treatment with the Zephyr valve in the most emphysematous lobe by quantitative CT (QCT) or medical therapy. VENT found small but significant improvements from baseline at 6 months for the primary endpoints FEV_1 (increased 4.3%) and 6MWD (increased 2.5%) in the treatment group, whereas both FEV_1 and 6MWD decreased in the control group (2.5% and 3.2%, respectively).[12] The improvements found in the VENT trial were so modest that the FDA did not grant approval for use of the Zephyr valve based on the results.

The IBV Valve Trial was a double-blinded, sham-controlled study of the Spiration valve in upper-lobe predominant severe emphysema with hyperinflation. All patients received bronchoscopy with appropriate anesthesia, during which airways in the upper lobes were measured with a balloon catheter for potential valve insertion. The patients were then immediately randomized 1:1 to treatment and control groups. Patients in the treatment group received valves in both upper lobes, although at least one segment or subsegment in each lobe was intentionally not treated (bilateral-partial lobe occlusion). Patients in the control group had continued bronchoscopy with simulation of valve insertion to provide the sham experience. Similarly to VENT, this study did not show clinically meaningful benefit in the treatment group. Only 5% of patients in the treatment group were considered responders by disease-related QOL measured by the SGRQ. Changes in treated lobe volume was significantly greater than in the control group (–224 mL vs. –17 mL), but the primary endpoint of a 10% or greater increase in nonupper lobe volume (signifying redirection of ventilation to less diseased lung) was not reached.[13]

Thus the improvements found in the early randomized trials were so slight that they were not likely to provide clinically significant benefit across the treatment group. In sum, the results of these studies seemed confusing. Why did some patients with severe emphysema clearly benefit from EBV treatment, while others with the same degree of hyperinflation and similar distribution of emphysema did not? The answer was suggested by subgroup analysis in the VENT study. Individuals whose QCT identified greater heterogeneity of emphysema had greater improvements in FEV_1 and 6MWT (Fig. 32.7), and those whose QCT found complete fissures separating targeted from nontargeted lobes had greater improvements in FEV_1. Specifically, at 6 months postprocedure, patients

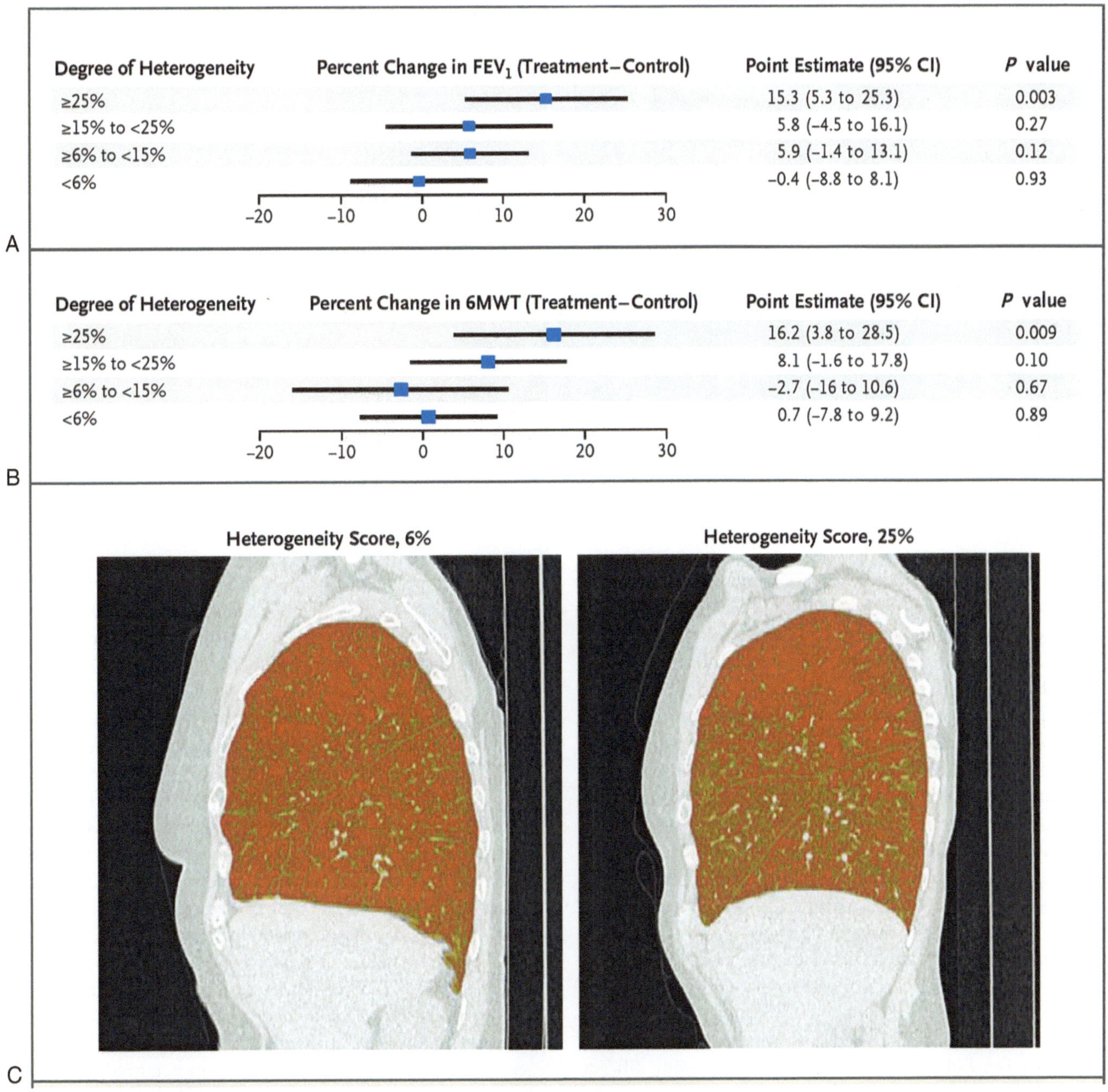

• **Fig. 32.7** Effect of the percentage of heterogeneity on the response to endobronchial valve therapy at 6 months in the Endobronchial Valve for Emphysema Palliation Trial study. Quantitative emphysema score was defined as proportion of pixels less than –910 Hounsfield units, a commonly used cutoff for emphysema. Percentage of heterogeneity was defined as the difference in quantitative emphysema score between the targeted lobe and the ipsilateral nontargeted lobe. (**A**) Effect of heterogeneity on forced expiratory volume in 1 second (*FEV_1*). (**B**) Effect of heterogeneity on 6-minute walk test (*6MWT*). (**C**) Sagittal computed tomography views using density-mask images with color overlay with pixels less than –910 Hounsfield units in red show low heterogeneity (6% on left) and high heterogeneity (25% on right). (From Sciurba FC, Ernst A, Herth FJ, et al. A randomized study of endobronchial valves for advanced emphysema. *N Engl J Med.* 2010;363(13):1233–1244. With permission.)

in the treatment group with complete fissures had improvement in FEV_1 of 16.2% versus 2.0% in patients with incomplete fissures ($P < .001$). The authors noted: **"Greater heterogeneity of emphysema between lobes and intact interlobar fissures appear to identify patients with a greater likelihood of clinically important functional and physiologic responses to endobronchial-valve therapy."**[12]

The significance in this finding is related to the role of intact fissures in preventing air from passing directly from one lobe to another within the lung parenchyma as opposed to ventilation exclusively provided by the bronchi. The knowledge of **collateral ventilation (CV)** between adjacent lobes of the lung in certain people was not new, but the amount of CV across presumed fissural boundaries, its frequency, and

A
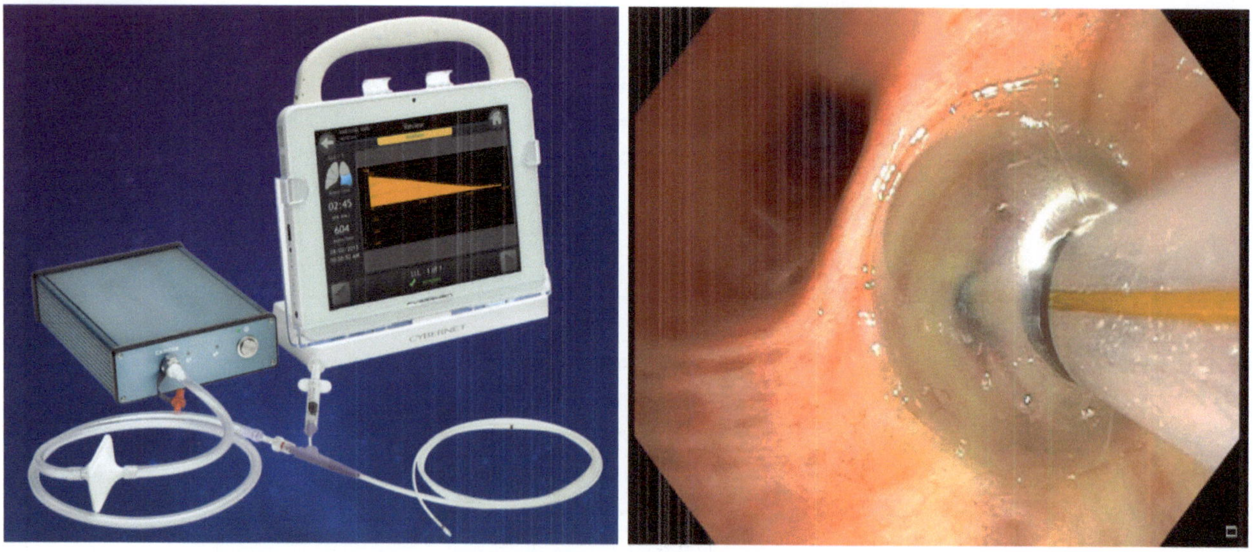
B

• **Fig. 32.8** (A) Chartis System with screen demonstrating decreasing flow (in orange) through balloon catheter consistent with lack of collateral ventilation. (B) Chartis balloon catheter occluding right lower lobe bronchus to assess for collateral ventilation.

clinical significance had not fully been appreciated previously.[14] Based on this finding, the Pulmonx Chartis System was designed to confirm isolation of lobar ventilation and lack of CV between adjacent lobes.[15] This system uses a balloon-tipped catheter passed through a flexible bronchoscope to occlude a lobar bronchus, and measures air flow and airway pressure from the lobe into the catheter. As the lobe cannot be ventilated from proximal airways while occluded by the balloon, air flow will gradually diminish if CV from an adjacent lobe is not present (Fig. 32.8). Using Chartis to identify presence or absence of CV in 80 patients immediately before insertion of Pulmonx EBV, Herth et al. found evidence of CV in 29 patients. The 51 patients without CV had significantly greater improvements in FEV_1 and greater reductions in volume of the treated lobe as measured by QCT than patients with CV.[16] Selection of patients for BLVR with valves who are likely to have little or no CV based on presence of complete fissures on QCT analysis and/or evaluation with Chartis proved critical in subsequent trials showing efficacy of EBV treatment.

For instance, additional support for the importance of assessment of CV in targeted lobes was provided by the Bronchoscopic Lung Volume Reduction for patients with Heterogeneous emphysema and Intact Fissures **(BeLieVeR HIFi) study, (BLVR)** in which entry criteria included FEV_1 under 50%, TLC greater than 100%, and RV over 150% in patients with heterogeneous emphysema and more than 90% intact fissures on chest CT. Davey et al.[16b] reported on this single center double-blind sham-controlled study in which 50 patients had a target lobe identified by CT destruction scores and were randomized 1:1 before bronchoscopy. During bronchoscopy, CV in the target lobe was assessed by Chartis, and then valves were inserted in the target lobe in the treatment group irrespective of Chartis findings, whereas the control group had sham valve placement. Among the treated group in whom absence of CV was confirmed by Chartis, 47% had more than 15% improvement in FEV_1, 58% had greater than 0.35 L improvement in RV, and 58% had significant improvement in QOL measured by SGRQ.

In contrast to most other valve trials, which exclusively included patients with heterogeneous emphysema, patients with homogeneous emphysema and severe hyperinflation (FEV_1 < 45%, TLC > 100%, and RV ≥ 200%) were studied in the **Informing the Pathway of COPD Treatment (IMPACT) trial**. Homogeneous emphysema was defined as less than 15% difference in emphysema destruction score between target and ipsilateral lobes. Lack of CV in primary or secondary target lobes was confirmed by Chartis, after which 93 subjects were randomized 1:1 to immediate treatment with the Zephyr valve (n = 43) or standard of care (n = 50). Improvement in FEV_1 of at least 15% was achieved in 35% of the treated subjects, with significant improvement in QOL measured by SGRQ in 57%. COPD exacerbation requiring hospitalization occurred in 16% of treated patients versus 12% in control group (not significant), and 25.6% of treated patients experienced pneumothorax (vs. none of controls).[17]

The Definitive Valve Trials: LIBERATE and EMPROVE

The Zephyr Endobronchial Valve Treatment in Heterogeneous Emphysema (LIBERATE) study examined use of the Zephyr EBV in patients with severe emphysema and hyperinflation (FEV_1 15%–45%, TLC > 100%, RV ≥ 175% predicted values). Exclusion criteria included severe carbon dioxide retention (partial pressure of carbon dioxide [PCO2] > 50 mm Hg breathing room air) and pulmonary hypertension (systolic pulmonary artery pressure [SPAP] > 45 mm Hg). Subjects were randomized to either EBV or standard of care (SoC) immediately after lack of CV was confirmed by Chartis, whereas subjects found to have CV with Chartis exited the study. The single target lobe treated with EBV was selected based on greater than 50% emphysema destruction score and heterogeneous emphysema defined by degree of difference in destruction between target and ipsilateral lobes as measured by a QCT analysis (Fig. 32.9). A median of four valves were placed per subject. At 12 months, 48% of EBV patients achieved the primary outcome of 15% or more improvement in FEV_1 compared with 17% of SoC patients. All secondary endpoints improved with statistical significance in favor of EBV. The difference of FEV_1 from baseline at 12 months was 0.106 L compared with SoC. 6MWD improved 39 m, and QOL measured by SGRQ also significantly improved, by 7 points. The most important and common adverse event was pneumothorax, which occurred in 27% of EBV subjects, with none in the SoC group. Importantly, 76% of pneumothoraces occurred within 3 days of bronchoscopy.[18]

The Evaluation of the Spiration Valve System for Emphysema to Improve Lung Function (EMPROVE) study examined use of the SVS in subjects with severe emphysema and hyperinflation (FEV_1 < 45%, TLC ≥ 100%, RV ≥ 150% predicted values). Exclusion criteria included severe carbon dioxide retention (PCO2 > 50 mm Hg breathing room air) and severe pulmonary hypertension. At a preprocedural visit, 174 subjects were randomized 2:1 to either treatment with SVS or the control group. The single target lobe treated with SVS was selected based on 40% or more emphysema destruction and 10% or more difference in emphysema severity between target and ipsilateral lobes as measured by a QCT analysis. The primary outcome was the mean change in FEV_1 at 6 months, which found a 0.1 L difference from baseline in the treatment group, with a

SUMMARY

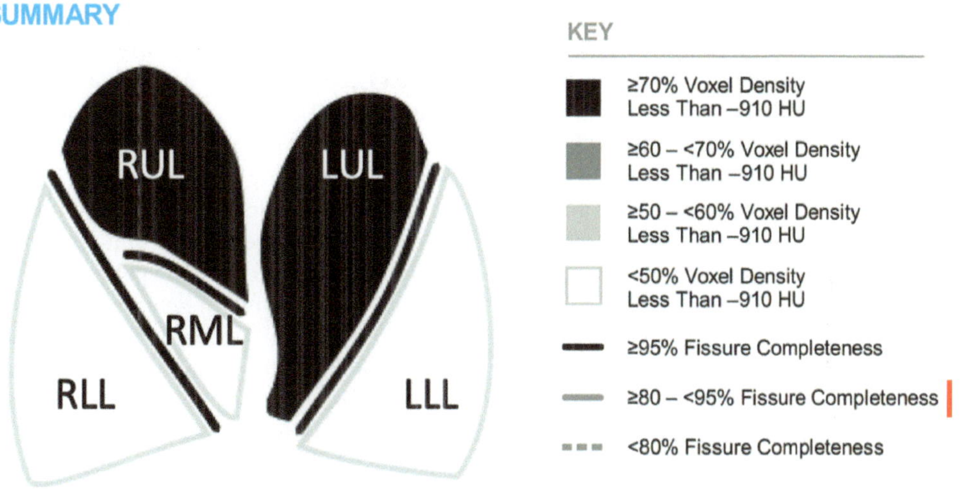

RESULTS

	RIGHT LUNG				LEFT LUNG	
	RUL	RUL+RML	RML	RLL	LUL	LLL
% Fissure Completeness	100	100	100	100	100	100
% Voxel Density Less Than −910 HU	73	65	2	12	70	15
% Voxel Density Less Than −950 HU	54	48	0	3	49	3
Inspiratory Volume (mL)	2919	3275	356	949	2882	852

• **Fig. 32.9** Representative quantitative computed tomography (CT) analysis (Pulmonx *Stratx* Lung Report) demonstrates severe emphysema in both upper lobes (*black areas* labeled right upper lobe [*RUL*] and left upper lobe [*LUL*]) in the schematic diagram, and greater than 95% fissure completeness between each lobe (*thick black line*). This is the analysis of the CT shown in Fig. 32.1. The volume measurements show that each upper lobe is severely hyperinflated, each containing nearly 3 liters of air (*red boxes*). This analysis suggests that either upper lobe would be an excellent target for valve placement.

between-group difference of 0.1 L compared with controls. A mean of about four valves were placed per subject. At 6 months, 37% of SVS patients achieved the secondary outcome of 15% or more improvement in FEV_1 compared with 10% of control patients. All secondary endpoints improved with statistical significance in favor of SVS, including SGRQ, which improved by 9.5 points. Mean reduction in target lobe volume (TLV) was nearly 1 L; 75% of the treatment group experienced a clinically meaningful reduction of TLV of least 350 mL, and 40% experienced complete atelectasis of the treated lobe. The 6MWD improved by only 6.9 m in the treatment group. Serious adverse events occurred in 31% of the treatment group compared with 11.9% in controls. A total of 32 pneumothoraces occurred in 30 treated patients (27%), 66% of which occurred within 3 days of bronchoscopy.[19]

Building on nearly 2 decades of investigation of BLVR, the LIBERATE and EMPROVE studies achieved the goal of finding a minimally invasive means to treat hyperinflation that is safe and effective in a significant number of patients. The recognition of the essential contribution of intact fissures in the selection of patients most likely to benefit from valve treatment was the key factor that led to successful trials of the two valves. Based on the results of LIBERATE and EMPROVE, in 2018, the FDA granted approval to both the Pulmonx Zephyr valve and the Spiration SVS for the treatment of severe emphysema.

Pneumothorax Following Valve Insertion

As previously discussed, pneumothorax is the most common serious complication following EBV treatment and may manifest as either an early (<3 days, up to 76%) or late complication up to 12 months after valve insertion (three pneumothoraces during 6–12-month follow-up in EMPROVE). Serious pneumothoraces may require removal of one or more valves to resolve, and both LIBERATE and EMPROVE followed pneumothorax management protocols that were defined in the respective study design. A recent metaanalysis of five randomized controlled trials (not including LIBERATE or EMPROVE) with 703 patients found a relative risk of 8.16 for pneumothorax after EBV treatment.[20]

In general, the lobe with the most lung destruction should be targeted. This may not be possible if CV is present in that lobe, and if there is good candidate lobe for treatment on the contralateral side that may be considered for treatment. However, if the target lobe is not the most diseased, and the contralateral lung had more than 60% lung destruction, the LIBERATE trial suggests that valve treatment has increased risk of pneumothorax, which may be fatal.[18] Death related to pneumothorax occurred in three patients in LIBERATE (two on day 3 and one on day 13), and one in EMPROVE (on day 95). Given the significant risk of pneumothorax within 3 days of valve insertion, patients must be observed in the hospital for a minimum of 3 days following the procedure. All staff involved in the care of the patient must be alerted to the manifestations of pneumothorax, and all relevant equipment to treat pneumothorax urgently should be kept at the bedside. Patients also must be educated regarding the symptoms of pneumothorax and instructed to seek medical care immediately if these symptoms develop.

Practical Details of Valve Treatment: Procedural Issues, Patient Selection, and Other Complications

Because most studies excluded patients with varying degrees of pulmonary hypertension or hypercapnia, there are virtually no data regarding safety in such patients. Recently, an expert panel issued best practice recommendations acknowledging that pulmonary hypertension is not an absolute contraindication for BLVR, but advised that patients with right ventricular systolic pressure (RVSP) greater than 45 mm Hg should be treated with caution. They also recommended exclusion of patients with severe respiratory failure (room air measurements of PCO2 >60 mm Hg or PO2 <45 mm Hg) and severe heart failure (left ventricular ejection fraction <35%).[21] A recent report of six patients with pulmonary hypertension who underwent right heart catheterization before and 90 days after BLVR, found that mean pulmonary artery pressure (PAP) decreased by 2.5 mm Hg in five of six patients, while PAP worsened in one patient by 3 mm Hg.[22]

Both valves require a deployment catheter that must be passed through a flexible bronchoscope with a minimum instrument channel of 2.8 mm. Current commercially available bronchoscopes that meet this requirement have an outer diameter up to 6.2 mm; accommodation of large bronchoscopes needs to be taken into consideration when planning airway management during the procedure. Mean procedure time was 10 minutes shorter in EMPROVE compared with LIBERATE (24 vs. 34 minutes), which was related in part to the time required for the Chartis evaluation in LIBERATE (mean 19 minutes).[18,19] General anesthesia was used in 65% of patients in LIBERATE; its use was not reported in EMPROVE.

Patients may require repeat procedures to either adjust valves, for example, because of loss of atelectasis, or to remove valves. In LIBERATE, 11 patients (8.6%) required a second procedure for valve adjustment to improve treatment effect and 28 patients (21.9%) required valves removed, either for treatment of pneumothorax (12 patients, 9.4%) or other complications, or at patient request because of lack of improvement (3 patients).

Both valves are readily identifiable on a standard chest radiograph, each with a unique appearance (Fig. 32.10); radiologists interpreting chest x-rays (CXRs) in such patients need to be aware of the characteristic appearance of each valve. In successfully treated patients, atelectasis in the treated lobe may be present, and the ipsilateral hemidiaphragm is returned to its normal domed shape (Fig. 32.11).

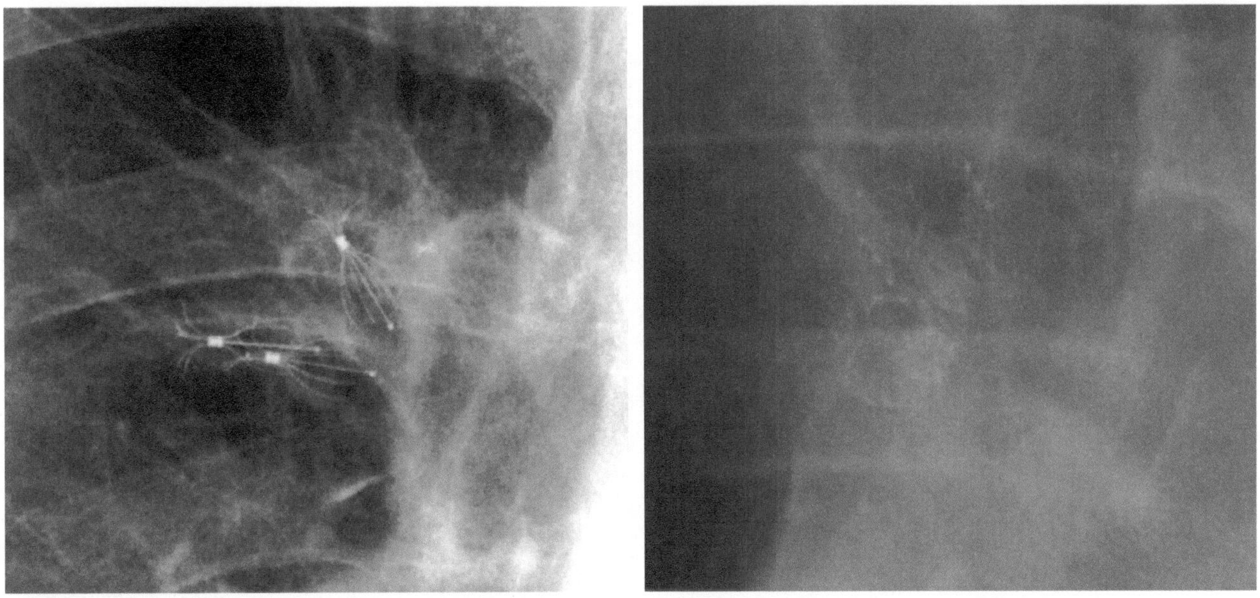

• **Fig. 32.10** Both valves are visible on standard chest radiographs (CXRs) and are readily distinguished from each other. (**A**) Close up view of three Spiration valves on CXR. (**B**) Close up view of two Pulmonx valves on CXR.

Acute exacerbation of COPD (AECOPD) occurred in 8% of treated patients in LIBERATE and 17% in EMPROVE. These may be treated in a standard fashion similar to AECOPD in patients without valves.[2] Pneumonia occurred in 9% of patients in EMPROVE and 5% in LIBERATE. Valve migration is very uncommon, occurring in less than 1% of patients. There was no difference in nonrespiratory adverse events between treatment and control groups in either study.

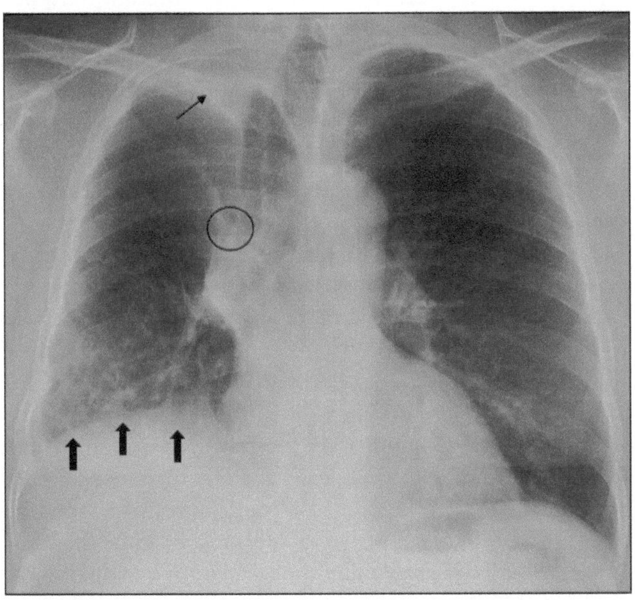

• **Fig. 32.11** Chest radiograph 14 days after treatment with two pulmonx valves visible in the right upper lobe (*black circle*). Note complete atelectasis of right upper lobe (*thin arrow*) and raised, domed contour of right hemidiaphragm (*thick arrows*).

Valve Treatment of Persistent Air Leak

The design of the EBV with its goal of medium size airway occlusion has been recognized for its potential in the treatment of bronchopleural or alveolar-pleural fistula causing persistent air leak (PAL). In acknowledgement of this possibility, the FDA granted the Spiration valve the status of humanitarian use of a device (HUD) in 2008. Using a humanitarian device exemption (HDE), the valve is considered experimental by the FDA but simultaneously approved for use in the treatment of a PAL in selected postoperative settings. According to FDA regulations, experimental devices may be considered for HUD status if clinical evidence suggests that the appropriate clinical setting is reasonably expected to affect no more than 4000 patients per year. Thus the FDA approved use of the Spiration valve for PAL in three postoperative settings, following lobectomy, segmentectomy, or LVRS. PAL in this approval is defined as air leak lasting 5 to 7 days postoperatively depending on severity. Since the HDE was granted in 2008, Spiration valves have been used to treat PAL in hundreds of patients, most commonly off-label, that is, for PAL because of reasons not listed in the HDE, such as secondary spontaneous pneumothorax in patients with chronic lung disease. Use of the SVS has provided a benefit in the majority of patients reported thus far. A multicenter registry reported complete resolution of air leak in 28/32 patients (87.5%) after valves were inserted for PAL, following lobectomy, segmentectomy, or LVRS.[23] In the experience of one author, valve insertion led to complete closure of air leaks, allowing chest tube removal in 74% of 27 patients. Two-thirds of the patients had secondary spontaneous pneumothoraces because

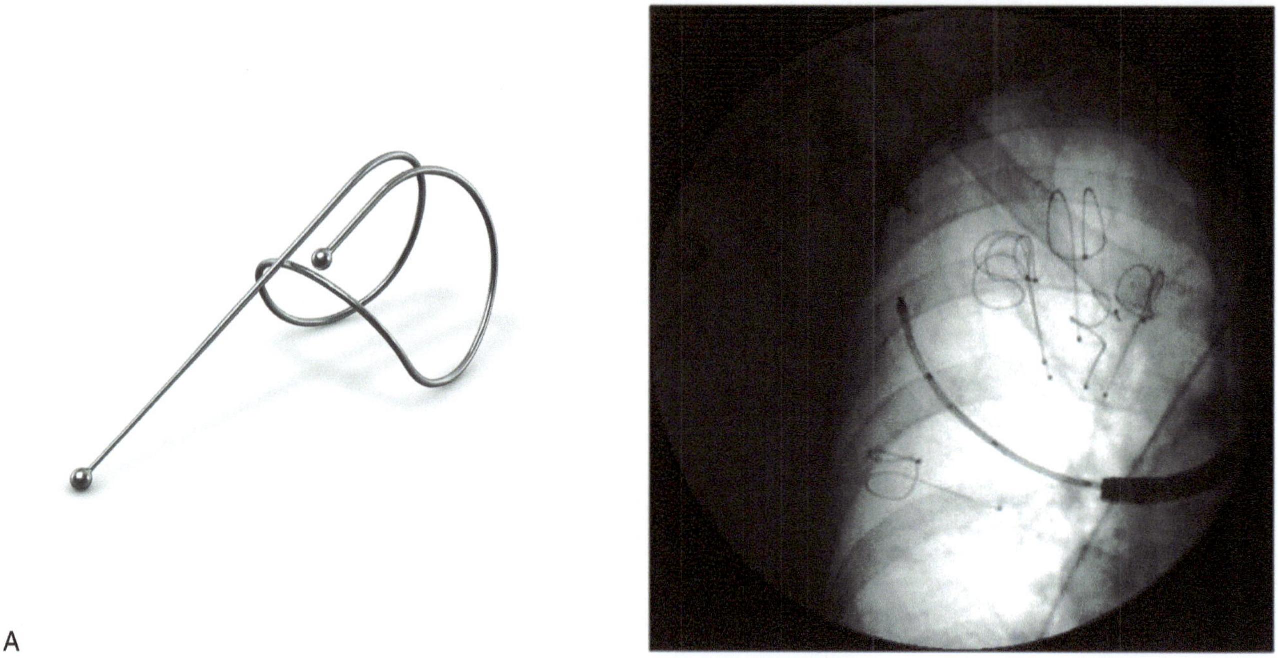

A B

• **Fig. 32.12** (**A**) PneumRx endobronchial coil. (**B**) Fluoroscopic image of coils being deployed in a patient's right upper lobe. The deployment catheter and six previously deployed coils are easily visible. (From Herth FJ, Eberhard R, Gompelmann D, Slebos D-J, Ernst A. Bronchoscopic lung volume reduction with a dedicated coil: a clinical pilot study. *Ther Adv Respir Dis*. 2010;4:225–231. With permission.)

of underlying lung diseases, half from emphysema, and the remainder were postoperative PAL.[24] Despite FDA approval of valve treatment for emphysema, valve treatment of PAL remains an investigational technique under the HDE at this time.

Alternative Bronchoscopic Lung Volume Reduction Procedures: Coils, Lung Sealant, Thermal Ablation, and Airway Bypass

A variety of bronchoscopic treatments of severe hyperinflation in emphysema using techniques other than one-way valves have been explored in recent years. These techniques have shown varying degrees of efficacy in several studies, mostly with modest to no clinical improvement, and some with relatively high serious complication rates. None are currently approved for use by the FDA.

Endobronchial coils (PneumRx, Mountain View, CA) made of nitinol wires that are inserted bronchoscopically, compress emphysematous lung and reduce volume of treated areas by regaining their coiled shape after deployment (Fig. 32.12). The largest study of coils, Lung Volume Reduction Coil Treatment in Patients With Emphysema (RENEW), was a randomized controlled, assessor-blinded trial in 315 patients with severe heterogeneous or homogeneous emphysema. Coils were placed in two targeted contralateral lobes in two sequential single-lobe procedures 4 months apart. The median improvement in 6MWD was 10.2 m in the treatment group versus −7.6 m in controls, whereas the between-group difference in FEV_1 was 7.0%, and SGRQ improved 8.9 points. Major complications occurred in nearly 35% of the treated group.[25]

A lung sealant system using a synthetic polymer (Aeris Therapeutics, Woburn, MA) to cause irreversible atelectasis and scarring was studied in the randomized controlled ASPIRE trial, which was halted prematurely because of financial issues after 95 of planned 300 patients were randomized. Results were published regarding 57 patients in whom results were available 3 months after treatment. Treated patients had significant improvements in FEV_1, SGRQ, and 6MWD. However, 44% of the 37 patients in the treatment group had adverse events requiring hospitalization, with two deaths and four episodes of respiratory failure requiring mechanical ventilation.[26]

Bronchoscopic thermal vapor ablation or BTVA (Uptake Medical Corporation, Seattle, WA) uses water vapor heated to deliver 8.5 calories per gram of lung tissue, causing local inflammation and volume loss. This technique has the advantage of targeting he most severely diseased lung at the segmental rather than lobar level, and efficacy is not affected by presence of CV (Fig. 32.13). The Controlled Sequential Stage Treatment of Emphysema With Upper-Lobe Predominance (STEP-UP) was a randomized, controlled open-label study of BTVA treatment of two or three emphysematous segments in two treatment sessions that found a mean difference of 14.7% in FEV_1 and 9.7 points on SGRQ in the treatment group.[27]

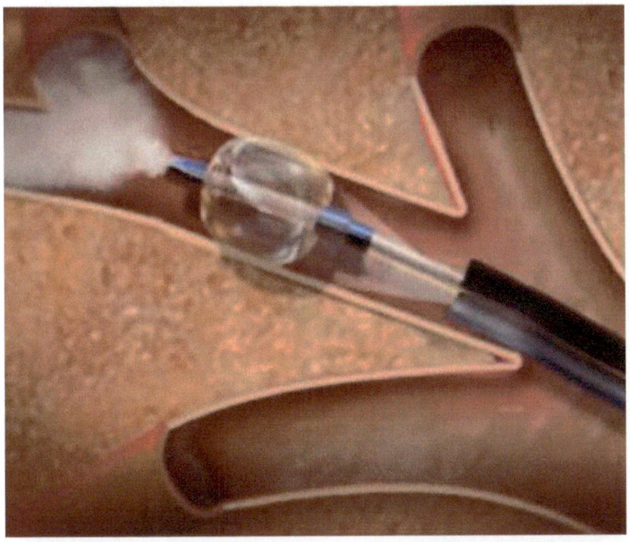

• **Fig. 32.13** Bronchoscopic thermal vapor ablation delivers heated water vapor to targeted segmental airway. The image demonstrates target strategy for selected airway, placement of ablation catheter in target airway, and delivery of vapor to target airway only. (From Trotter MA, Hopkins PM. Advanced therapies for COPD–What's on the horizon? Progress in lung volume reduction and lung transplantation. *J Thorac Dis*. 2014;6:1640–1653. With permission.)

In the **airway bypass technique**, artificial passages are created from airways into emphysematous lung, with patency maintained by insertion of paclitaxel-coated stents, permitting trapped air to decompress directly into central airways (Fig. 32.14). Airway bypass was studied in the Exhale Airway Stents for Emphysema (EASE) trial, a randomized, double-blind, sham-controlled study in patients with homogeneous emphysema. No differences in hyperinflation or QOL scores were found between the two groups.[28]

The Future of Bronchoscopic Lung Volume Reduction

The 2020 report from the Global Initiative for Chronic Obstructive Lung Disease (GOLD) notes that "in select patients with advanced emphysema, bronchoscopic interventions reduce end-expiratory lung volume and improve exercise tolerance, health status and lung function at 6 to 12 months following treatment," with endobronchial valves supported by level A evidence. Both lung coils and vapor ablation were supported by level B evidence.[2] Given the limited treatment options for this group of patients with end-stage lung disease and poor QOL, BLVR with valves is expected to be performed with increasing frequency given safety and efficacy data that compare quite well with LVRS, while avoiding major surgery (Fig. 32.15). With growing experience, improved patient selection and avoidance of major complications may be cautiously anticipated. Further investigation of the alternative forms of BLVR may also lead to new and improved bronchoscopic treatments of emphysema, particularly if effective techniques that are not dependent on the absence of CV are developed.

Anesthetic Management of Endoscopic Treatment of Chronic Obstructive Respiratory Disease

COPD occurs frequently as a comorbidity in patients undergoing surgery and interventional procedures and can lead to increased hospital length of stay and increased morbidity and risk for mortality. For the anesthesiologists, the challenges continue through the intraoperative period and into

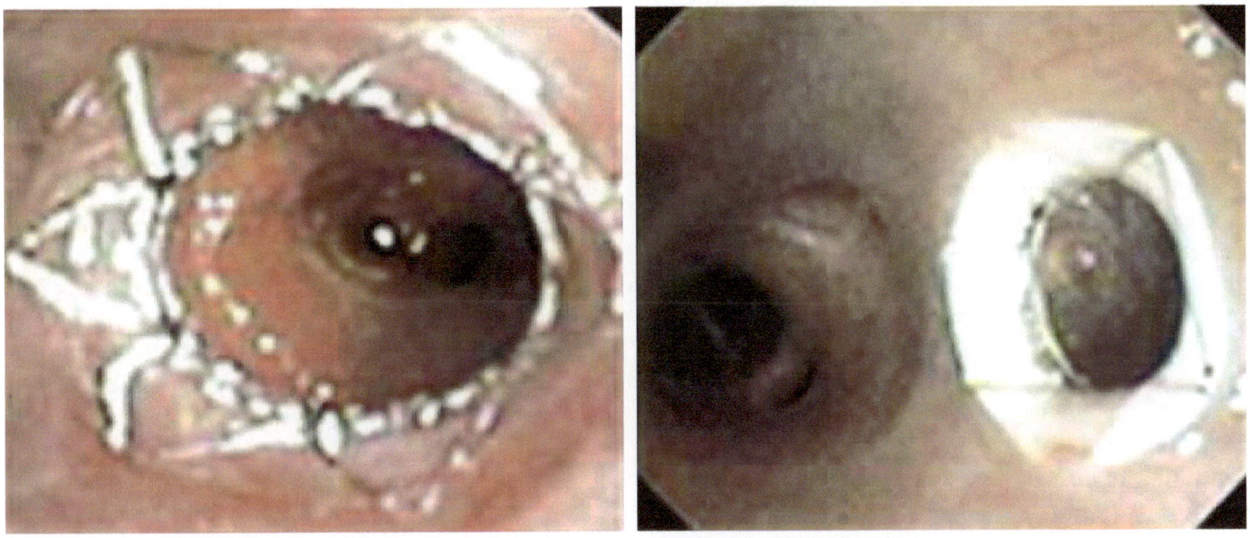

A B

• **Fig. 32.14** (**A**) Airway bypass stent at time of placement in airway, tunneled through into area of emphysematous lung. (**B**) Airway bypass stent at 13 weeks, demonstrating patency maintained by paclitaxel-eluting design of stent. (From Choong CK, Phan L, Massetti P, et al. Prolongation of patency of airway bypass stents with use of drug-eluting stents. *J Thorac Cardiovasc Surg*. 2006;131:60–64. With permission.)

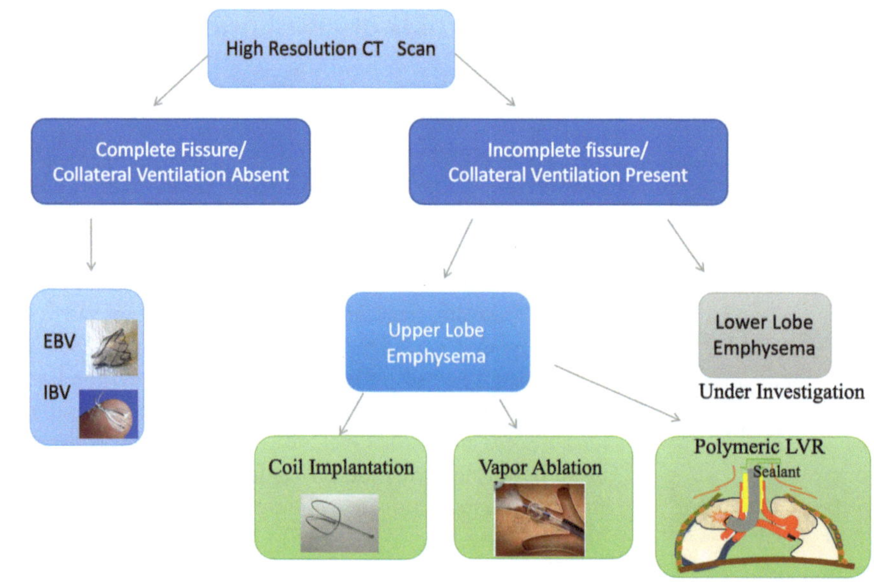

• **Fig. 32.15** Proposed algorithm for bronchoscopic lung volume reduction. *EBV,* Endobronchial valve; *IBV,* intrabronchial valve; *LVR,* lung volume reduction. (Courtesy of Edmond Cohen.)

th postoperative recovery. The remaining sections of this chapter will focus on the current bronchoscopic procedures and the anesthetic management for patients who undergo these therapies.

The Patient With Chronic Obstructive Respiratory Disease

The underlying condition of COPD is a progressive inflammation of both the central and peripheral airways with associated changes in the lung parenchyma, as well as the pulmonary vasculature.[29] There is a remodeling of the airway smooth muscle walls and a proliferation of Goblet cells and mucous glands. The vascular changes result in progressive pulmonary hypertension. Narrowing of the airways causes an expiratory limitation of flow because of both obstructive bronchiolitis and destructive changes of emphysema. With bronchiolitis comes obstruction and air trapping, which can affect ventilation/perfusion (V/Q) matching and, over time, can cause flattening of the diaphragm and impaired respiratory muscle mechanics. With emphysema, the elastin breaks down, and the loss of functional alveoli can lead to impaired gas exchange, a loss of pulmonary capillary architecture, and significant worsening of the V/Q matching.

In advanced emphysema, distended airspaces impinge on normal alveoli, causing compression and dysfunction. The V/Q mismatch worsens. Airway resistance, which is normally very low, such as 2 cm H_2O/L/second, continues to increase with emphysema. The effects of hyperinflation on the chest wall and diaphragm cause an increase in the work of breathing and dyspnea ensues. Resting pleural pressures in emphysema will progressively rise, associated with a decrease in the QOL, decrease in exercise function, and shortness of breath. Left unchecked, respiratory failure can occur. Smoking and genetic factors can influence the progression of COPD. Extrapulmonary effects can also arise, such as weight loss, skeletal muscle atrophy, cardiovascular disease, osteoporosis, and clinical depression.

The patient with COPD has an increased risk of hospitalizations, and the survival during hospitalization and, especially, with admission to an intensive care unit is poor, when compared with those without COPD.[30] In particular, the condition of ventilator-associated pneumonia confers a much greater risk of mortality in patients with underlying COPD. In addition, patients with COPD are more likely to suffer significant episodes of hypoxemia during the hospitalization, which require reintubation and carry a higher mortality at 30 days.[31]

Several diagnostic tests can predict a greater likelihood of postoperative respiratory complications. The FEV_1 can identify significant expiratory obstruction, for example. The body mass index and the presence of dyspnea at rest can also suggest increased risk.[32] Finally, a measure of exercise tolerance, such as the 6MWT can be predictive of both perioperative morbidity and the prospect of a rapid recuperation. Other diagnostic tests can include the carbon monoxide transfer factor. Clinical details, such as the frequency of exacerbations and the response to bronchodilators, can also be useful.

Preoperative Treatment

Stopping smoking before a procedure is critical for improving the perioperative course and for altering the progression of this chronic disease. Cessation of smoking can prolong the time before significant disability and can also extend life. Every effort should be made to encourage active quitting of a smoking habit.

Inhaled therapies can be optimized before a procedure. For example, short-acting bronchodilators are commonly prescribed for mild COPD and can improve shortness of breath and extend exercise limits. In more moderate cases of COPD, where there exist symptoms of dyspnea at rest, more long-acting therapeutic agents can be used such as long-acting muscarinic agonist or a long-acting beta agonist. These bronchodilators may be paired with a corticosteroid, usually also in an inhaled form. More persistent or distressing breathlessness can be treated with nebulizers.

Other chronic therapies for COPD include oral corticosteroids, theophylline, and mucolytics. In general, the chronic use of oral corticosteroids is not recommended because of its significant side effect profile. Steroids can cause hyperglycemia, peptic ulcer disease, osteoporosis, impaired wound healing and immunosuppression, and adrenal insufficiency. The use of selective biologic agents targeting specific inflammatory pathways can also be adjusted before the scheduling of an invasive procedure.[33] Theophylline also has an extensive side effect profile, such as tachyarrhythmias, nausea and vomiting, seizures, and rhabdomyolysis. In addition, there is a narrow therapeutic window for theophylline, often necessitating monitoring of plasma levels; theophylline may be affected by other drugs, which either raise or lower the activity of cytochrome P-450, such as phenytoin, barbiturates or carbamazepine or cimetidine, ciprofloxacin, or erythromycin. Mucolytics, such as carbocysteine, must be used chronically to improve a chronic productive cough and sputum.

Supplemental oxygen therapy can improve mortality, but it must be used for at least 15 hours each day, and it must maintain the oxygen saturation more than 90% for most of that time.[34] In addition, chronic oxygen therapy can lower the PAP and slow the progression of nocturnal hypoxemia, peripheral edema, and polycythemia, as well as pulmonary hypertension.[35]

In the treatment of respiratory failure in patients with COPD, some form of continuous positive airway pressure (continuous positive airway pressure [CPAP] or bilevel positive airway pressure [BiPAP]) has been demonstrated as an effective early intervention. The use of CPAP can decrease treatment failures, avoid endotracheal intubation, and even reduce mortality. Early use of CPAP, along with antibiotics and oral steroids has been shown to reduce the length and seriousness of clinical exacerbations.

In the immediate preoperative period, several additional investigations can help improve the risk stratification and have the potential to improve clinical outcome (see Chapter 8). Routine bloodwork, such as a complete blood count, may be helpful to detail a significant anemia from chronic disease or a polycythemia from chronic hypoxemia. An elevated white blood cell count may indicate an unresolved pneumonia. The polycythemia can also suggest right-sided heart failure, which can be confirmed using cardiac ultrasound. Although a CXR may not be sensitive in diagnosing pneumonia, the presence of bullae on a CXR can demonstrate increased risk for pneumothorax. A low albumen can suggest poor nutritional status and does correlate with poor wound healing and prolonged recovery. Nutritional status can be improved in the preoperative period with nutritional supplements that include vitamins, electrolytes, calories, and protein. An arterial blood gas may provide a basis for comparison during the perioperative period, and low oxygen, high carbon dioxide, and metabolic acidosis are predictive for respiratory problems in the postoperative period, as well as a higher mortality.

The routine use of preoperative PFTs may be useful in categorizing the relative risk for postoperative respiratory complications.[36] Both the National Institute for Health and Clinical Excellence and the GOLD guidelines predict higher severity scores with worsened FEV_1 or when normalized to the forced vital capacity (FEV_1/FVC). The BODE (Body mass index, airflow flow Obstruction, dyspnea and Exercise) score provides a similar assessment of the functional capacity and predicts the relative difficulty of rehabilitation following thoracic procedures. In the BODE score, measurements of body mass index, obstruction (e.g., FEV_1), dyspnea, and exercise tolerance (e.g., 6MWT) are combined together.[37]

Certain preoperative interventions should be attempted before elective thoracic procedures (see Chapter 9).[38] As previously mentioned, smoking cessation should be strongly urged, and programs should be offered and encouraged. Exercise regimens can also improve the course of rehabilitation. The value of nutritional support and counseling has already been mentioned. For patients with wheezing, bronchodilator therapies should be optimized. Patients with pyrexia, productive cough, and dyspnea should be evaluated for treatment of respiratory infections. Targeted physiotherapy to clear secretions can also be of value, along with incentive spirometry.

Types of Anesthesia for Endoscopic Treatment

Monitored Anesthesia Care Versus General

There are obvious advantages to the use of monitored anesthesia care (MAC), in comparison with general anesthesia. In addition to avoiding positive pressure ventilation, a major advantage is the reduction of total anesthetic agent exposure to the patient. For most patients who undergo general anesthesia, there is full unconsciousness, insensibility to pain, full amnesia, and immobility in the face of surgical stimulation. The anesthetic agents can be a combination of inhaled and injected medications but usually involve anesthetic gases, sedatives/amnestic, hypnotics, analgesics, and muscle relaxants.[39] Often, general anesthesia provides such a deep level of sedation that the airway must be protected and ventilation supported during the course of the anesthetic.

The MAC anesthetic may involve the same combination of sedatives and analgesics, but varies as to the depth of anesthesia. For example, the sedative propofol may be combined with the analgesic remifentanil but at a lower dose and with less chance of overdose and accumulation of sedative effects. Usually, MAC cases maintain spontaneous ventilatory efforts and do not require special airways to protect against aspiration or to support airway patency. In practice, very few procedures to improve the condition of patients with COPD can be accomplished using MAC anesthesia. In medical thoracoscopy, for example, blebectomy and pleurodesis can be accomplished under MAC, (known as "tubeless procedures") but only with patients who are cooperative and who have favorable anatomy. The blebs need to be accessible to the pleuroscope and the patients need to be able to tolerate being in the lateral position.

Regional Versus General

Although there may be direct evidence of the superiority of regional anesthesia compared with general anesthesia for thoracic surgery, the usual clinical practice often combines both.[40] When compared directly, epidural anesthesia alone, for example, resulted in one-half the rate of pneumonia than did the general anesthetic alone; however, epidural is not used during endoscopic procedures.[41] In addition, general anesthesia is associated with a higher rate of bronchospasm, laryngospasm, hypoxemia, cardiovascular instability, and ventilation-associated injuries, such as barotrauma and pneumonia. Patients who receive general anesthesia may also have higher rates of postoperative nausea and vomiting than those receiving regional anesthetic techniques alone.

Several problems do exist with the use of regional anesthesia, however. The patient often needs to be cooperative and assume an unconformable or a difficult position, such as sitting up or lying flat. The technique may be blind or may require ultrasound guidance, which requires particular training and benefits from regular practice. Local anesthetic toxicities are possible. Adjacent nerves, such as the phrenic nerve, which innervates the diaphragm, may become paralyzed during brachial plexus block, for example. This complication may be worse in patients with COPD.

In thoracic surgery and some interventional pulmonary procedures, either paravertebral or erector spinae block may be helpful in reducing the amount of postoperative pain and lessening the reliance on postoperative opioid treatments. Both the paravertebral and erector spinae block allow for direct visualization of the emerging spinal nerves in the thoracic region. Both techniques can lessen the postoperative pain scores in thoracic surgery patients who undergo video-assisted thoracic surgery procedures. These patients also enjoyed improved PFTs in the postoperative period, when compared with systemic opioid medication alone.[42]

Consideration of Anesthetic Depth

The indications for bronchoscopy along with the complexity of the procedure, can dictate the required depth of anesthesia.[43] For example, flexible bronchoscopy with dynamic maneuvers requires a cooperative patient who can deliver vital capacity breaths, both inspiratory and expiratory holds, and can phonate on demand.[44] This type of procedure usually involves the topicalization of the vocal cords and airways with minimal sedation (Table 32.1). For simple diagnostic bronchoscopies, the American College of Chest Physicians recommends some degree of sedation unless contraindicated for medical comorbidity reasons. Medical pleuroscopy and thoracoscopy may also proceed with minimal conscious sedation.[45] Most interventional pulmonary procedures, however, require substantially deeper depths of anesthesia to tolerate the larger instruments and more painful manipulations and treatments.[46] In a recent study, a survey from Switzerland reviewed the patterns of nearly 300 pulmonologists, who conducted over 27,000 bronchoscopies.[47] This study revealed that most pulmonologists were using propofol with or without the addition of midazolam or fentanyl. There was a very low complication rate of 0.02%, and these complications were mostly apnea and hypotension.

For more advanced diagnostic and therapeutic bronchoscopic procedures, such as for endoscopic treatment of COPD, total intravenous anesthetic techniques (TIVA) have been described.[48] Most of these infusion techniques pair propofol with some type of analgesic.[49] Usual propofol regimens begin with an initial bolus of 0.5 to 1.0 mg/kg, followed by an infusion rate between 75 to 250 mcg/kg/min, titrated to the desired anesthetic depth.[50,51] Although not currently available in the United States, closed-loop or target-controlled systems can automatically titrate the propofol dose based on pharmacokinetic principles, vital signs, and electroencephalographic data.

The advantages to propofol are its rapid onset, efficacy as a sedative, and favorable antiemetic properties. Propofol use has largely supplanted all other sedative-hypnotics in allowing

TABLE 32.1 Anesthetic Recommendations and Airway Recommendations in the Endoscopic Treatment of Chronic Obstructive Respiratory Disease

Bronchoscopy Type	Anesthesia Type	Airway
With dynamic maneuvers	Top + light sed	Nasal cannulae
Basic diagnostic	Top + MAC	Nasal cannulae
Medical Thoracoscopy/pleuroscopy	Top + MAC	Nasal cannulae
Advanced diagnostic	Top + TIVA	LMA
Advanced therapeutic-flexible	Top + TIVA	LMA
Advanced therapeutic-rigid	Top + TIVA	Rigid, HFJV; LMA

All procedures have complications of desaturation, hypoventilation, hypotension, hemorrhage, laryngospasm, bronchospasm, pneumothorax and postprocedure cough.

HFJV, High-frequency jet ventilation; *LMA*, laryngeal mask airway; *MAC*, monitored anesthesia care (see text); *Rigid*, rigid bronchoscope; *sed*, sedation; *TIVA*, total intravenous anesthesia (see text); *Top*, topical local anesthesia.

for both moderate and deep sedation techniques.[52] Disadvantages include pain at the site of injection because of its lipid emulsion properties, as well as hypotension and respiratory depression. Pretreatment with intravenous lidocaine (50 mg) can ameliorate some of the pain on injection from propofol. Hypotension can be offset with the use of vasoconstricting agents, such as phenylephrine (50–100 mcg).[53] To counteract the respiratory depressant effects of propofol, some mode of pressure-support ventilation can be added to any case that uses a supraglottic airway device, such as a laryngeal mask airway.

The addition of analgesics to the propofol infusion has been found to improve hemodynamic stability and to blunt the coughing and movement associated with bronchoscopic manipulation. Such analgesics as remifentanil, fentanyl, alfentanil, oxycodone, ketamine, and dexmedetomidine have been described, along with others.[54] One of these analgesics, remifentanil, has a unique method of metabolism via esterase activity. The advantage of being metabolized by ubiquitous esterases is that the metabolism is not affected by the presence of other drugs with a similar metabolic pathway, and also is not affected by selective organ dysfunction, such as liver or kidney failure. Remifentanil does not demonstrate a context-sensitive half-time change, as do the other sedatives and analgesics. Therefore the half-time of 9 minutes is preserved, whether the infusion runs for 10 minutes or for 10 hours. In combination with a propofol infusion, remifentanil is usually administered at a rate of 0.1 mcg/kg/min. Boluses of 25 to 50 mcg of remifentanil can be used to quiet coughing or muscle movement.[55] In cases where movement persists despite several boluses of remifentanil, this author will use 10 to 20 mg of rocuronium to further reduce the movement, with careful attention to the adequacy of pressure-support ventilation, as described subsequently.

Volatile anesthetic agents are usually discouraged in bronchoscopic cases because of issues of reliability in the delivery of anesthetic to the patient during open airways procedures and by issues of contamination of the operating room staff. With frequent suctioning and continuous insertion of devices into the bronchoscope, the delivery of potent anesthetic gases is often compromised. The patient could receive a low concentration and experience inadequate depth of anesthesia. This inadequate depth could manifest as increased movement, increased blood pressure and heart rate, or, later, as intraoperative awareness. In addition, the frequent interruption of the breathing circuit during bronchoscopic procedures means that more anesthetic agent is leaked into the operating room. The people closest to the patient, often the pulmonologists and nurses and anesthesiologists, would contact the highest amounts of the airborne gases or infected particles, which is of crucial importance in limiting potential exposure to COVID-19. For these reasons, volatile agents are usually avoided in interventional pulmonary procedures.

Every patient should receive topical lidocaine to the vocal cords, unless contraindicated because of documented allergic reaction. Topical lidocaine is recommended by the American College of Chest Physicians and has been shown to both decrease cough and decrease the need for sedatives in routine bronchoscopy. The gag reflex can be successfully blocked by directly spraying the vocal cords, oropharynx, and aryepiglottic folds. Usually 1% lidocaine is used. In our practice, this topical spray is administered at the beginning and at the end of the procedure, to prevent both coughing and laryngospasm.

To help protect the patient's teeth and to preserve the bronchoscope, a bite block is used on every patient. For most of the advanced diagnostic and therapeutic procedures, a form of supraglottic airway (SGA) that has its own bite block (I-gel SGA, Intersurgical, Wokingham, UK) is used. Sizes 4 and 5 are appropriate for most patients. For example, the size 4 I-gel has a 12.3 mm internal diameter, which can accommodate either a therapeutic (5.9 mm) or an endobronchial ultrasound (EBUS) scope (6.9 mm) without difficulty.

With the constant insertion and withdrawal of the bronchoscope during a procedure, the SGA can become dislodged and can develop an air leak. Audible sounds from the mouth, change in shape of the end-tidal capnography, and auscultation can be used to detect the leak. Direct bronchoscopic inspection of the SGA position relative to the vocal cords can be assessed using the bronchoscope, and this view can be useful in repositioning the SGA. In cases of a difficult SGA placement, persistent leak, severe obesity, or severe gastroesophageal reflux, an endotracheal tube (ETT) can be a reasonable option. Usually, an 8 to 9.0 mm tube is needed to allow for the passage of an EBUS scope, for instance.

Ventilatory Support During Flexible Bronchoscopy

When using an SGA, a maximum peak pressure of 20 to 30 cm H_2O is preferable, to minimize both external air leaks and also to prevent gastric distention. Most often, the patient has some spontaneous ventilatory efforts, and pressure support mode is added at 10 breaths per minute. Reliable end-tidal measurements of CO2 may be episodic in the presence of near-constant suctioning. The circuit and breathing bag may be emptied, as a result of suctioning, and would require higher fresh gas flows. In general, the fraction of inspired oxygen (FiO2) is 1.0, unless some form of cautery is anticipated, such as electrosurgical units, laser, or argon plasma coagulation.[56] In these cases, both low FiO2 (<30%) and apnea are used to mitigate the risk of fire.[57]

In the patient with COPD, ventilator support is about providing oxygenation without causing injury. Intermittent positive pressure ventilation is the most frequently used ventilation mode but has certain hazardous potentials in the COPD patient. The patient's lungs are less compliant and require higher inflation pressures. The narrowed airways provide slower expiratory flow rates and delays in exhalation, which makes air-trapping more likely. Breaths can "stack" on subsequent breaths and develop intrinsic positive end-expiratory pressure (iPEEP). iPEEP can further increase the intrathoracic pressure, causing pulmonary barotrauma and volutrauma, as well as hypercapnia and acidosis.

The cardiovascular effects of increased intrathoracic pressure can lead to elevated PAP, elevated pulmonary vascular resistance, and right heart strain and failure.

Strategies to mitigate the trauma of positive pressure ventilation center around low tidal volumes, the addition of PEEP, and an attendance to bronchospasm and bronchial secretions. Tidal volumes of 5 cc/kg are generally used, with the goal to keep peak airway pressures around 30 cm H_2O. The expiratory time is usually lengthened, to allow for adequate exhalation. To accomplish this level of expiratory time, it may be necessary to allow the end tidal CO2 to rise, a condition known as "permissive hypercapnia." PEEP levels are added until oxygen saturation levels fail to improve or cardiovascular conditions deteriorate significantly. Audible wheezes or changes in the peak pressures, capnography tracings, or ventilator alarms may indicate acute bronchospasm, which can be treated with both beta agonists and glucocorticoids. The exacerbation of bronchospasm needs to be well controlled before extubation.

Before extubation, the patient should be warm, oxygenated, and with nearly normal CO2 values. Neuromuscular blockade should be fully reversed, usually by using sugammadex if rocuronium was used as a muscle relaxant. Accommodations should be made to have available both nebulized treatments for bronchospasm, as well as forms of noninvasive ventilation, such as CPAP or BiPAP. Overall, the total amount of opioids should be restricted, and adjuvant measures and medications should be discussed and available.

Rigid Bronchoscopy

Rigid bronchoscopy is preferred whenever a large working channel is needed or there is significant risk for airway obstruction or significant bleeding.[58] The rigid scope is as long as 43 cm and has an internal diameter as wide as 14 mm.[59] There is also a wider field of vision with the rigid compared with flexible bronchoscopes.[60] In patients with COPD, the rigid bronchoscope can be used to stent airways or place endobronchial valves.[12]

More stimulating than the flexible bronchoscope, the rigid scope requires a deeper level of anesthesia.[61] An infusion rate for both propofol and remifentanil are indicated. Usually propofol infusions have rates of between 150 to 250 mcg/kg/min and remifentanil rates are 0.1 to 0.3 mcg/kg/min. Muscle relaxants are used to prevent the trauma from coughing or bucking with the scope in the airway, and the train of four monitor is kept between 0 and 2 twitches, using bolus doses of rocuronium (0.3 mg/kg).

Ventilatory Support During Rigid Bronchoscopy

To minimize chest movement and to reliably ventilate the patient during rigid bronchoscopy, usually high frequency jet ventilation (HFJV) is used[62] (see Chapter 14). Based on a number of physical principles of diffusion and dispersion,[63] the jet ventilator can deliver adequate oxygen and remove CO2, while causing little chest wall movement and allowing for instruments in the airways. Although a Sanders type of ventilator is often useful for the delivery of recruiting breaths of near vital capacity size, the HFJV delivers smaller tidal volumes (1–3 cc/kg) at high rates (120 breaths/minute).[64] Usual settings of the HFJV are 120 beats per minute, an inspiratory duration of 0.4 of the respiratory cycle and a driving pressure of 20 to 30 pounds per square inch. Certain ventilators have a driving pressure alarm that shuts off the jet and alarms if the drive tubing pressure exceeds the set driving pressure (Monsoon High Frequency Jet Ventilator®; Acutronic Medical Systems AG, Hirzel, Switzerland). In this way, the ventilator attempts to prevent "stacked" breaths as described previously. Ventilation can be adjusted using serial blood gas analysis or, more frequently, using oxygen saturation as the guide. Reverse Trendelenburg positioning, suctioning, and recruiting breaths can also improve oxygen saturation (SaO2).

Bolus doses of propofol (1–2 mg/kg) with muscle relaxants (1–2 mg/kg succinylcholine or 0.5–1 mg/kg rocuronium) are given to facilitate the placement of the rigid bronchoscope. In the rare event that the rigid scope cannot be passed, an ETT can be placed by the anesthesiologist using conventional laryngoscopes. Once the ETT is in place, the rigid scope can be brought along side to the level of the vocal cords, using the ETT as a guide. Any instance of difficult intubation should generate a discussion about extubation or, even, prolonged intubation and ventilation after the procedure. Usually, at the end of the procedure, the rigid bronchoscope is removed, and an SGA inserted for the period of time to wake up the patient.

Common and Specific Complications of Endoscopy

Most of the endoscopic procedures and placement of the pulmonary valves are deployed through a flexible bronchoscope. Flexible bronchoscopy is generally reported to be relatively safe, with a major complication rate of 1% and a mortality of 0.04%.[65] Most common major complications include laryngospasm, bronchospasm, bleeding, arrhythmias, and pneumothorax.[66] Most cases of bleeding with flexible bronchoscopy involve less than 20 cc, and do not cause hemodynamic consequences. Severe bleeding may be an indication to convert to rigid bronchoscopy or to isolate the hemorrhaging lung with a double-lumen tube or a bronchial blocker.[67] Use of color Doppler during EBUS, for example, may help detect major blood vessels during needle aspiration.[68] In addition, attention to the patient's preoperative anticoagulation status is warranted.

In contrast to flexible, bronchoscopy rigid bronchoscopy has a major complication rate of 9% and a mortality of 0.3%. The most common complications are laryngospasm, laryngeal edema, atelectasis, and pneumothorax. In selected groups of patients, such as those with malignant central airway obstruction, the 30-day mortality is as high as 14.8%.[69,70] Specific to jet ventilation are complications of barotrauma, subcutaneous emphysema, and mucociliary desiccation.[71] For jet ventilation cases lasting longer than 2 hours, airway humidification is recommended.[72] Endobronchial valves can become dislodged, resulting in airway obstruction.[73] Ineffective endobronchial valves can also occur in the setting of collateral mixture of gases across an incomplete lobar fissure, which may require a surgical completion of the fissure to accomplish the desired volume reduction.

Conclusion

The most reliable predictor of postoperative respiratory problems is the presence of significant preoperative respiratory problems. Patients with COPD have issues with oxygenation, ventilation, secretions, and work of breathing. Not surprisingly, the postoperative recovery of these patients is often a labor-intensive and medication medley of therapeutic interventions. Although a variety of advanced bronchoscopic procedures extend life and improve symptoms, these gains are not always immediate. Many procedures show temporary worsening before symptoms improve.[74] With bronchothermoplasty, photodynamic therapy, and Goblet cell rheoplasty, for example, the patients usually wake up feeling worse. Managing expectations, and then treating symptoms becomes paramount. Early evaluation and constant communication between patient, anesthesiologist, and pulmonologist are essential for providing the safest and best care for our patients.[75]

References

1. May SM, Li JT. Burden of chronic obstructive pulmonary disease: healthcare costs and beyond. *Allergy Asthma Proc.* 2015;36(1):4–10.
2. Global Initiative for Chronic Obstructive Lung Disease. *Chronic Obstructive Pulmonary Disease: A Definition and Implications of Structural Determinants of Airflow Obstruction for Epidemiology. 2020 Report.* 2020.
3. Guarascio AJ, Ray SM, Finch CK, Self TH. The clinical and economic burden of chronic obstructive pulmonary disease in the USA. *Clinicoecon Outcomes Res.* 2013;5:235–245.
4. Snider GL. Chronic obstructive pulmonary disease: a definition and implications of structural determinants of airflow obstruction for epidemiology. *Am Rev Respir Dis.* 1989;140(3 Pt 2):S3–S8.
5. Cooper JD, Trulock EP, Triantafillou AN, et al. Bilateral pneumectomy (volume reduction) for chronic obstructive pulmonary disease. *J Thorac Cardiovasc Surg.* 1995;109(1):106–116 discussion 116–109.
6. Yusen RD, Lefrak SS, Gierada DS, et al. A prospective evaluation of lung volume reduction surgery in 200 consecutive patients. *Chest.* 2003;123(4):1026–1037.
7. Brantigan OC, Mueller E, Kress MB. A surgical approach to pulmonary emphysema. *Am Rev Respir Dis.* 1959;80(1, Part 2):194–206.
8. Fishman A, Martinez F, Naunheim K, et al. A randomized trial comparing lung-volume-reduction surgery with medical therapy for severe emphysema. *N Engl J Med.* 2003;348(21):2059–2073.
9. Decker MR, Leverson GE, Jaoude WA, Maloney JD. Lung volume reduction surgery since the National Emphysema Treatment Trial: study of Society of Thoracic Surgeons Database. *J Thorac Cardiovasc Surg.* 2014;148(6):2651–2658 e2651.
10. Wan IY, Toma TP, Geddes DM, et al. Bronchoscopic lung volume reduction for end-stage emphysema: report on the first 98 patients. *Chest.* 2006;129(3):518–526.
11. Sterman DH, Mehta AC, Wood DE, et al. A multicenter pilot study of a bronchial valve for the treatment of severe emphysema. *Respiration.* 2010;79(3):222–233.
12. Sciurba FC, Ernst A, Herth FJ, et al. A randomized study of endobronchial valves for advanced emphysema. *N Engl J Med.* 2010;363(13):1233–1244.
13. Wood DE, Nader DA, Springmeyer SC, et al. The IBV Valve trial: a multicenter, randomized, double-blind trial of endobronchial therapy for severe emphysema. *J Bronchology Interv Pulmonol.* 2014;21(4):288–297.
14. Koster TD, Slebos DJ. The fissure: interlobar collateral ventilation and implications for endoscopic therapy in emphysema. *Int J Chron Obstruct Pulmon Dis.* 2016;11:765–773.
15. Gompelmann D, Eberhardt R, Michaud G, Ernst A, Herth FJ. Predicting atelectasis by assessment of collateral ventilation prior to endobronchial lung volume reduction: a feasibility study. *Respiration.* 2010;80(5):419–425.
16. Herth FJ, Eberhardt R, Gompelmann D, et al. Radiological and clinical outcomes of using Chartis to plan endobronchial valve treatment. *Eur Respir J.* 2013;41(2):302–308.

16b. Claire D, Zaid Z, Simon J, et al. Bronchoscopic lung volume reduction with endobronchial valves for patients with heterogeneous emphysema and intact interlobar fissures (the BeLieVeR-HIFi study): a randomised controlled trial. *Lancet.* 2015;386:1066–1073.

17. Valipour A, Slebos DJ, Herth F, et al. Endobronchial valve therapy in patients with homogeneous emphysema. Results from the IMPACT study. *Am J Respir Crit Care Med.* 2016;194(9):1073–1082.
18. Criner GJ, Sue R, Wright S, et al. A multicenter randomized controlled trial of Zephyr Endobronchial Valve Treatment in Heterogeneous Emphysema (LIBERATE). *Am J Respir Crit Care Med.* 2018;198(9):1151–1164.
19. Criner GJ, Delage A, Voelker K, et al. Improving Lung Function in Severe Heterogenous Emphysema with the Spiration Valve System (EMPROVE). A multicenter, open-label randomized controlled clinical trial. *Am J Respir Crit Care Med.* 2019;200(11):1354–1362.
20. Low SW, Lee JZ, Desai H, Hsu CH, Sam AR, Knepler JL. Endobronchial valves therapy for advanced emphysema: a meta-analysis of randomized trials. *J Bronchology Interv Pulmonol.* 2019;26(2):81–89.
21. Slebos DJ, Shah PL, Herth FJ, Valipour A. Endobronchial valves for endoscopic lung volume reduction: best practice recommendations from expert panel on endoscopic lung volume reduction. *Respiration.* 2017;93(2):138–150.
22. Eberhardt R, Gerovasili V, Kontogianni K, et al. Endoscopic lung volume reduction with endobronchial valves in patients

with severe emphysema and established pulmonary hypertension. *Respiration.* 2015;89(1):41–48.
23. Abu-Hijleh M, Styrvoky K, Anand V, et al. Intrabronchial valves for air leaks after lobectomy, segmentectomy, and lung volume reduction surgery. *Lung.* 2019;197(5):627–633.
24. Madisi N Madisi NY, Harkin TJ. Endobronchial Y, Harkin TJ. Endobronchial valves for persistent air leaks of various etiologies. *Am Thorac Soc.* 2019; A1099.
25. Sciurba FC, Criner GJ, Strange C, et al. Effect of endobronchial coils vs usual care on exercise tolerance in patients with severe emphysema: The RENEW randomized clinical trial. *JAMA.* 2016;315(20):2178–2189.
26. Come CE, Kramer MR, Dransfield MT, et al. A randomised trial of lung sealant versus medical therapy for advanced emphysema. *Eur Respir J.* 2015;46(3):651–662.
27. Herth FJ, Valipour A, Shah PL, et al. Segmental volume reduction using thermal vapour ablation in patients with severe emphysema: 6-month results of the multicentre, parallel-group, open-label, randomised controlled STEP-UP trial. *Lancet Respir Med.* 2016;4(3):185–193.
28. Shah P, Slebos D, Cardoso P, et al. Bronchoscopic lung-volume reduction with Exhale airway stents for emphysema (EASE trial): randomised, sham-controlled, multicentre trial. *The Lancet.* 2011;378(9795):997–1005.
29. Licker M, Schweizer A, Ellenberger C, Tschopp J-M, Diaper J, Clergue F. Perioperative medical management of patients with COPD. *Int J Chron Obst Pulm Dis.* 2007;2:493–515.
30. Ramachandran SK, Nafiu OO, Ghaferi A, Tremper KK, Shanks A, Kheterpal S. Independent predictors and outcomes of unanticipated early postoperative tracheal intubation after non-emergent, non-cardiac surgery. *Anesthesiology.* 2011;115:44–53.
31. National Institute for Clinical Excellence. Chronic obstructive pulmonary disease. Guideline 101. June 2010.
32. Global initiative for chronic Obstructive Lung Disease (GOLD). Global strategy for the diagnosis, management, and prevention of COPD. Available from http://www.goldcopd.org/.
33. Murray LA, Grainge C, Wark PA, Knight DA. Use of biologics to treat exacerbations and manage disease in asthma, COPD, and IPF. *Pharmacol Ther.* 2017;169:1–12.
34. Abdo WF, Heunks LMA. Oxygen-induced hypercapnia in COPD: myths and facts. *Crit Care.* 2012;16:323–328.
35. Celli BR, MacNee W. Standards for the diagnosis and treatment of patients with COPD: a summary of the ATS/ESR position paper. *Eur Resp J.* 2004;23:932–946.
36. Lightowler JV, Wedzicha JA, Elliot MW, Ram FSF. Non-invasive positive pressure ventilation to treat respiratory failure resulting from exacerbations of chronic obstructive pulmonary disease. *BMJ.* 2003;326:185.
37. Cowl CT, Prakash UB, Kruger BR. The role of anticholinergics in bronchoscopy. A randomised clinical trial. *Chest.* 2000;118:188–192.
38. Bucknall C, Miller G, Lloyd S, et al. Glasgow supported self-management trial (GSuST) for patients with moderate to severe COPD: randomized, controlled trial. *BMJ.* 2012;344:e1060.
39. Sarkiss M. Anesthesia for bronchoscopy and interventional pulmonology: from moderate sedation to jet ventilation. *Curr Opin Pulm Med.* 2011;17:274–278.
40. Gramatica L, Brasesco OE, Mercado Luna A, et al. Laparoscopic cholecystectomy performed under regional anesthesia in patients with chronic obstructive pulmonary disease. *Surg Endosc.* 2002;16:472–475.
41. Sarkiss M. Anesthesia for bronchoscopy and interventional pulmonology: from moderate sedation to jet ventilation. *Curr Opin Pulm Med.* 2011;17:274–278.
42. Van Lier F, van der Geest PJ, Hoeks SE, et al. Epidural analgesia is associated with improved health outcomes of surgical patients with chronic obstructive pulmonary disease. *Anesthesiology.* 2011; 115:315–321.
43. Matyal R, Montealegre-Gallegos M, Shnider M, et al. Pre-emptive ultrasound-guided paravertebral block and immediate postoperative lung function. *Gen Thorac Cardiovasc Surg.* 2015; 63:43–48.
44. Majid A, Gaurav K, Sanchez JM, et al. Evaluation of tracheobronchomalacia by dynamic flexible bronchoscopy. A pilot study. *Ann Am Thorac Soc.* 2014;11:951–955.
45. Casal RF, Ost DE, Eapen GA. Flexible bronchoscopy. *Clin Chest Med.* 2013;34:341–352.
46. Cujino IF, Velásquez M, Ariza F, Loaiza JH. Awake epidural anesthesia for thoracoscopic pleurodesis: a prospective cohort study. *Rev Columb Anes.* 2013;41:10–15.
47. Ali AH, Toba H, Sakiyama S, Kondo K. Holter ECG monitoring of sympathovagal fluctuation during bronchoscopy. *Clin Respir J.* 2016;10:204–210.
48. Gaisl T, Bratton DJ, Heuss LT, et al. Sedation during bronchoscopy: data from a nationwide sedation and monitoring survey. *BMC Pulm Med.* 2016;16:113–120.
49. Arias S, Lee HJ. The future of interventional pulmonology. *Semin Respir Crit Care Med.* 2014;35:763–768.
50. Beaudoin EL, Chee A, Stather DR. Interventional pulmonology: an update for internal medicine physicians. *Minerva Med.* 2014;105:197–209.
51. Jose RJ, Shaefi S, Navani N. Sedation for flexible bronchoscopy: current and emerging evidence. *Eur Respir Rev Off J Respir Soc.* 2013;22:106–116.
52. Jose RJ, Shaefi S, Navani N. Anesthesia for bronchoscopy. *Curr Opin Anaesthesiol.* 2014;27:453–457.
53. Grendelmeier P, Tamm M, Pflimlin E, Stolz D. Propofol sedation for flexible bronchoscopy: a randomised, noninferiority trial. *Eur Respir J.* 2014;43:591–601.
54. Pawlowski J. Anesthetic considerations for interventional pulmonary procedures. *Curr Opin Anesthesiol.* 2013;26:6–12.
55. Liao R, Li JY, Liu GY. Comparison of sevoflurane volatile induction/maintenance anaesthesia and propofol-remifentanil total intravenous anesthesia for rigid bronchoscopy under spontaneous breathing for tracheal/bronchial foreign body removal in children. *Eur J Anaesthesiol.* 2010;27:930–934.
56. Goudra BG, Singh PM, Borle A, Farid N, Harris K. Anesthesia for advanced bronchoscopic procedures: state-of-the-art review. *Lung.* 2015;193:453–465.
57. Reddy C, Majid A, Michaud G, Feller-Kopman D, Eberhardt R, Herth F, Ernst A. Gas embolism following bronchoscopic argon beam coagulation: a case series. *Chest.* 2008;134:1066–1069.
58. Smith LP, Roy S. Operating room fires in otolaryngology: risk factors and prevention. *Am J Otolaryngol.* 2011;32:109–114.
59. Alraiyes AH, Machusak MS. Rigid bronchoscopy. *Semin Respir Crit Care Med.* 2014;35:671–680.
60. Goyal R, Nayar S, Gogia P, Garg M. Extraction of tracheo-bronchial foreign bodies in children and adults with rigid and flexible bronchoscopy. *J Bronchol Interv Pulmonol.* 2012;19:35–43.
61. Shen X, Hu CB, Ye M, Chen YZ. Propofol-remifentanil intravenous anesthesia and spontaneous ventilation for airway foreign body removal in children with preoperative respiratory impairment. *Paediatr Anaesth.* 2012;22:1166–1170.
62. Pathak V, Welsby I, Mahmood K, Wahadi M, MacIntyre N, Shofer S. Ventilation and anesthetic approaches for rigid bronchoscopy. *Ann Am Thor Soc.* 2014;11:628–634.

63. Slutsky AS, Drazen JM. Ventilation with small tidal volumes. *N Engl J Med.* 2002;347:630–631.
64. Putz L, Mayne A, Dincq AS. Jet ventilation during rigid bronchoscopy in adults: a focused review. *BioMed Res Int.* 2016;4234861:6.
65. Numata T, Nakayama K, Fujii S, et al. Risk factors of postoperative pulmonary complications in patients with asthma and COPD. *BMC Pulm Med.* 2018;18:4–12.
66. Jin F, Mu D, Chu D, Fu E, Xie Y, Liu T. Severe complications of bronchoscopy. *Respir Int Rev Thorac Dis.* 2008;76:429–433.
67. Sastre JA, Cordovilla R, Jimenez MF, Lopez T. Management of transbronchial cryobiopsy using the i-gel airway and the Arndt endobronchial blocker. *Can J Anesth.* 2014;61:886–888.
68. Cordasco EM, Mehta AC, Ahmad M. Bronchoscopically induced bleeding. A summary of nine year's Cleveland Clinic experience and review of the literature. *Chest.* 1991;100:1141–1147.
69. Zhou GW, Zhang W, Dong YC, et al. bronchoscopy-induced massive bleeding: a 12-year multicentre retrospective cohort study. *Respirol Carlton Vic.* 2016;21:927–931.
70. Ernst A, Simoff M, Ost D, Goldman Y, Herth FJ. Prospective risk-adjusted morbidity and mortality outcome analysis after therapeutic bronchoscopic procedures: results of a multi-institutional outcomes database. *Chest.* 2008;134:514–519.
71. Ost DE, Ernst A, Grosu HB, et al. Complications following therapeutic bronchoscopy for malignant central airway obstruction: results of the AQuIRE Registry. *Chest.* 2015148:450–471.
72. Brodsky JB. Anesthetic considerations for bronchoscopic procedures in patients with central-airway obstruction. *J Bronchol Interv Pulmonol.* 2001;8:36–43.
73. Slebos D-J, Shah PL, Herth FJF, Valipour A. Endobronchial valves for endoscopic lung volume reduction: best practice recommendations from expert panel on endoscopic lung volume reduction. *Respir Int Rev Thorac Dis.* 2017;93:138–150.
74. De Lima A, Kheir F, Majid A, Pawlowski J. Anesthesia for interventional pulmonary procedures: a review of advanced diagnostic and therapeutic bronchoscopy. *Can J Anesth.* 201865:822–836.
75. Selzer AR, Murrell M, Shostak E. New trends in interventional pulmonology. *Curr Opin Anaesthesiol.* 2017;30:17–22.

33 Thoracic Trauma

ALF KOZIAN, MORITZ A. KRETZSCHMAR

Introduction

Thoracic trauma is the cause of 25% to 50% of all fatal injuries, making it the leading cause of death in the first 3 decades of life.[1,2] In addition, injuries to the thorax are accountable for more than 50% of deaths in children. Thoracic trauma is the third leading cause of death after neoplasms and atherosclerosis for all age groups.[3]

The mortality from thoracic injuries is about 10%.[2] Blunt thoracic trauma accounts for 96.3%, whereas penetrating injuries account for only 3.7% of cases. The most common causes are motor vehicle accidents (70%), suicides (10%), falls (8%), homicides (7%), and other (5%).

The peri- and intraoperative management of patients with thoracic injuries is a difficult task for any anaesthetist.[4] The causes of perioperative morbidity and mortality include respiratory obstructions, respiratory arrest, and often difficult-to-control bleeding. In most cases, those affected present with an unstable cardiopulmonary situation and have complex, life-threatening injuries. Therefore evaluation, intervention, and possibly resuscitation take place under considerable time pressure. In close cooperation between the specialist areas, abdominal or neurologic injuries must also be treated with the same urgency and with a high priority.

The thorax protects vital organs, including the heart, lungs, large vessels close to the heart, and airways. To damage these structures, considerable force is usually required. Thoracic injuries can lead to fatal bleeding, and air or blood in the pleural space or pericardium can rapidly lead to cardiovascular collapse.

The perforation of the chest is often an isolated injury, but significant blunt trauma may be associated with multiple injuries. However, blunt and perforating mechanisms lead to a common pathway of inadequate supply of oxygen to peripheral tissues and consecutive metabolic failure.

Massive pulmonary or cardiac injuries are rare, but are usually lethal if present. Less severe injuries often result in the impairment of vital organ function, but because of the functional reserve of the organs there is often time for diagnosis and therapy.

Injuries, such as pneumothorax or cardiac tamponade, combine the effects of direct heart or lung injury, which further compromises organ functions. Hemorrhages, swelling of damaged tissues because of fluid retention, or neurogenic shock from spinal cord injuries can also contribute impaired oxygen delivery to tissues.

For example, tension pneumothorax not only affects gas exchange, but also can affect the venous return to the heart. In addition to impaired cardiac function, a cardiac tamponade also reduces venous return. The direct injury to the chest or diaphragm, usually associated with severe pain, may impair both the respiratory mechanics and gas exchange.

Perioperative management therefore requires anticipation, early detection, temporary support, and conservative or surgical care for thoracic injuries.[4]

Categories of (Blunt) Thoracic Trauma

Thoracic trauma can be divided into different categories based on the injured structures. Each category can occur on its own or in combination with other injuries, each of which has different anesthesiologic implications.

- Tracheobronchial injury/laryngeal injury
- Rib fractures, flail chest
- Lung contusion, pneumothorax, hemothorax
- Mediastinal widening
- Aortic rupture
- Cardiac contusion/myocardial trauma/pericardial tamponade
- Diaphragmatic rupture
- Esophageal perforation/rupture

Tracheobronchial Injury

In patients with blunt thoracic trauma, one must consider additional injuries to the head, face, cervical spine, and upper and lower respiratory tract injuries. Tracheobronchial injuries are rare with a frequency of 0.8%.[5] Unfortunately, most patients with this pattern of injuries die at the scene of the accident. In the patients who arrive at the trauma center, failure to diagnose early can lead to disastrous acute or delayed complications (Figs. 33.1 and 33.2).[6] Cardinal symptoms are hemoptysis and/or subcutaneous emphysema. Pneumothorax and pneumomediastinum are radiologic correlates of intrathoracic tracheobronchial injuries.[7] Impaired consciousness (Glasgow Coma Scale [GCS] <9),

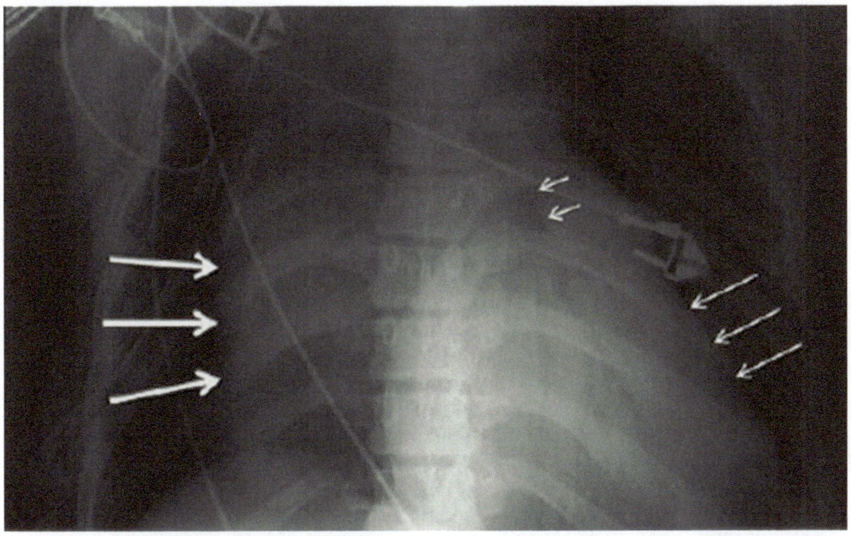

• **Fig. 33.1** Tracheobronchial injuries: chest radiography shows a collapsed right lung (*thick arrows*), left deviated trachea (*short arrows*), and shifted heart (*narrow long arrows*). (From Altinok T, Can A. Management of tracheobronchial injuries. *Eurasian J Med.* 2014;46(3):209–215.)

respiratory obstruction, or insufficient or impossible mask ventilation require immediate endotracheal intubation or the immediate establishment of surgical airways.

A tracheobronchial injury must be considered when a pneumothorax with massive air leakage cannot be drained or reduced in size with the insertion of a chest tube. The extent of the injury is confirmed by fiberoptic bronchoscopy. Control and splinting of the respiratory tract, injuries of the main bronchi, large air leaks, and/or hemoptysis is frequently established with insertion of a double-lumen tube (DLT). Regardless of the type of endotracheal tube used, placement should be carried out under direct fiberoptic visualization. The injury can be accurately diagnosed and documented by bronchoscopy to avoid further aggravation of the lesion.[8]

The need for cervical immobilization, the uncertain nil per os (NPO) status, and the trauma related disturbed gastric emptying usually necessitate a "rapid sequence induction" or, more safely, an awake intubation (direct laryngoscopy, or with fiberoptic bronchoscopy).

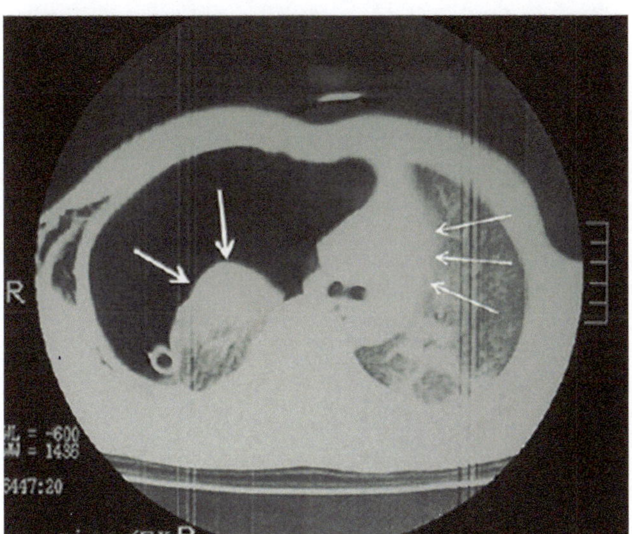

• **Fig. 33.2** Tracheobronchial injuries: computed tomography of the chest illustrating the collapsed right lung (*thick arrows*) and shifted heart (*narrow long arrows*). (From Altinok T, Can A. Management of tracheobronchial injuries. *Eurasian J Med.* 2014;46(3):209–215.)

Injuries to the Larynx

Blunt injuries to the larynx are rare[2,9] at about 0.3%,[2,10] its estimated incidence varying between 1:5000 and 1:137,000 trauma patients.[1–5,7,11] However, recent data suggest that its incidence may be higher than previously reported and fractures of the laryngeal skeleton may be diagnosed in almost 1% of all neck-trauma patients imaged with multidetector computed tomography (CT) in the emergency setting.[8] Prompt management is paramount to avoid patient death or long-term impairment of breathing, swallowing, and speaking. Classic signs of laryngeal injury are:

- hoarseness
- subcutaneous neck emphysema
- hemoptysis

Injuries to the respiratory system must be excluded at the initial presentation of the patient (e.g., trauma bay). Even in the absence of airway and breathing problems and lack of further obvious respiratory injuries. The inspection and examination of the upper respiratory tract by endoscopy and/or CT is necessary to determine the degree of occult injury and to make a prognosis as to whether airway obstruction in the further course can be anticipated.[9]

Patients with laryngeal injuries may seemingly present with normal respiratory findings, but and can develop life-threatening obstruction of the upper respiratory tract within a very short period of time. Early tracheal intubation should be considered dependent on the laryngoscopic finding. In addition, early tracheostomy should be considered in all patients with respiratory injury.[12,13]

Rib Fracture

The most common blunt thoracic injury in both adults and children with 67.3% incidence are rib fractures.[2,11,14] Often rib fractures are associated with other injuries, such as

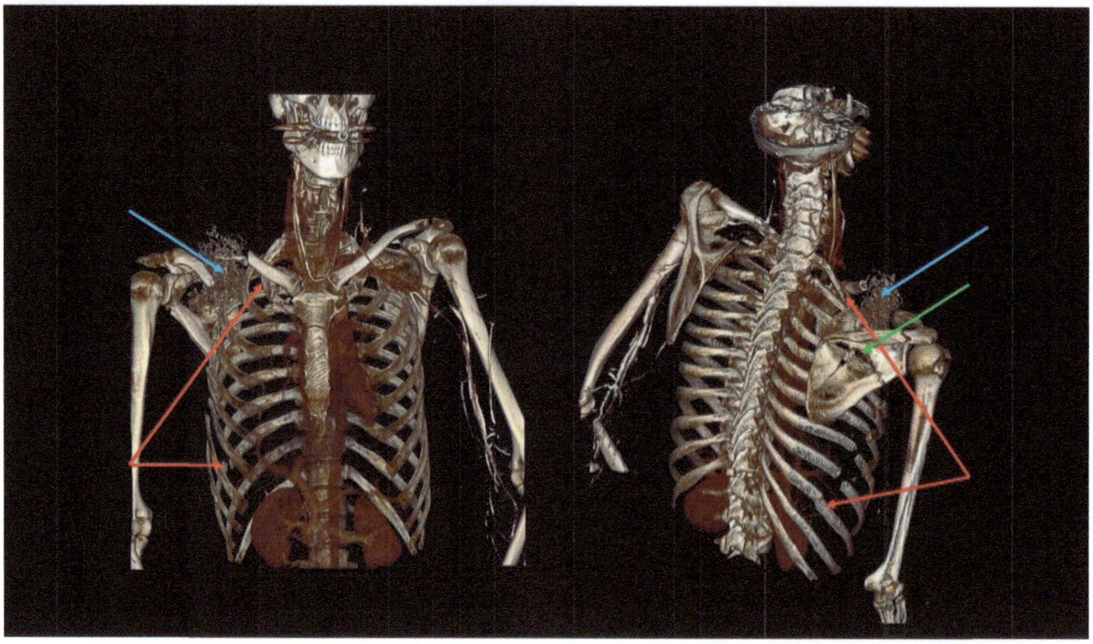

• **Fig. 33.3** Rib fracture: 36-year-old male patient polytraumatized after motorcycle accident. III° open fracture of the right clavicle and tear of the right brachial plexus and the right subclavian artery (*blue arrows*). Fractures of the first to 10th rib (*red arrows*) and right scapula (*green arrow*) with hematopneumothorax, lung contusion, and tissue emphysema. Pictures show cropped three-dimensional reconstruction of the initial trauma scan.

thoracic instability (flail chest), lung contusion, and pneumothorax. Pronounced pain can lead to shallow breathing and thus results in secondary atelectasis formation and secretion retention.[15] Perioperative pain management is therefore of eminent importance.[16]

In awake patients, a rib fracture can be easily detected clinically. However, preoperative thoracic x-ray imaging is not only used to detect the fracture, but also to detect associated injuries, such as pneumothorax, hemothorax, or lung contusion, as these need preferential treatment.

The greatest perioperative risk (besides the risk of bleeding) is the injury of the pleura by bone fragments, which may lead to the formation of a tension pneumothorax during the transition from spontaneous breathing to mechanical positive pressure ventilation. The placement of a chest tube before the induction of general anesthesia seems warranted (Fig. 33.3).

Thoracic Instability

Thoracic instability occurs when several adjacent ribs (rib series fracture) are affected, creating a mobile segment of the thoracic wall. During spontaneous inspiration, the segment moves paradoxically in the opposite direction of the uninjured thoracic wall (Figs. 33.4 and 33.5). An unstable thorax is therefore a purely clinical diagnosis that can only be made during spontaneous breathing and affects 23.1% of patients with blunt thoracic trauma in the operating room.[2] Because of the high elasticity of the ribs in childhood, the incidence in pediatric patients is extremely low[14] and is an indicator of excessive force.

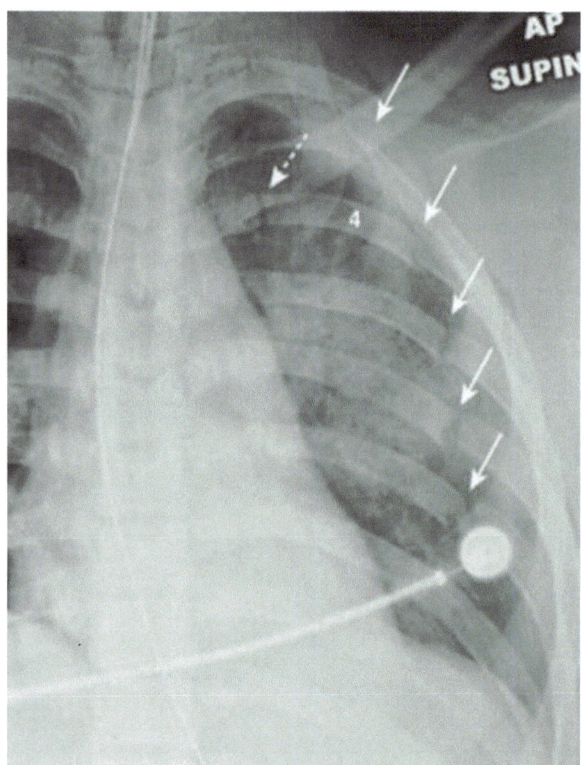

• **Fig. 33.4** Flailed chest: section of chest x-ray showing double fractures of the right ribs 3 to 6, leading to a flailed chest. (From Radiology Key: Fastest Radiology Insight Engine.)

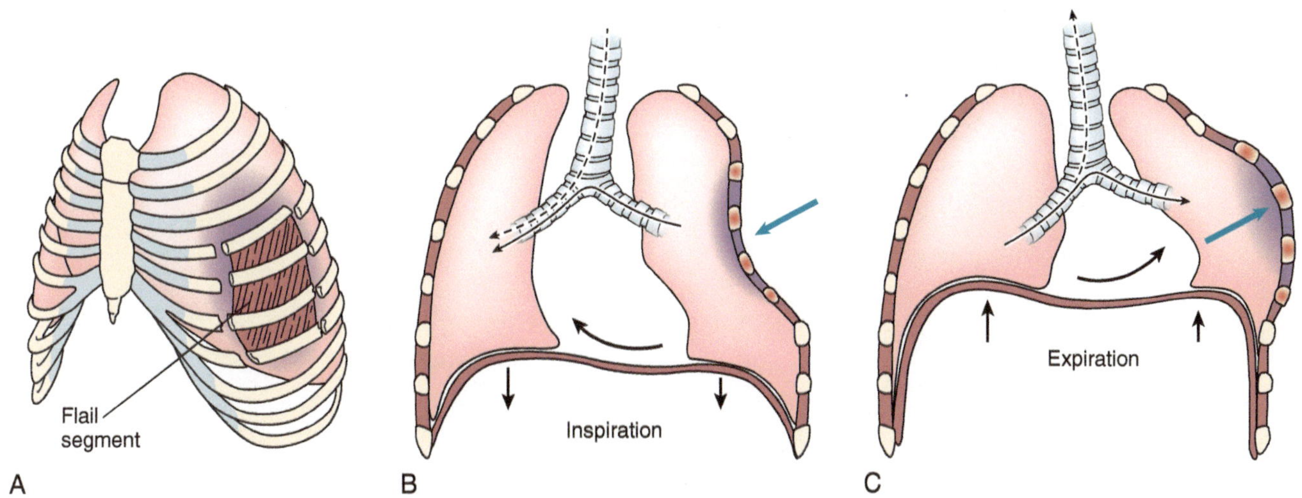

• **Fig. 33.5** Flailed chest: schematic visualization (**A**) of flailed chest effects on respiratory function illustrating paradoxical chest movement (**B** and **C**). (From 2021 UpToDate, Inc. and/or its affiliates. All Rights Reserved. (https://www.uptodate.com/contents/initial-evaluation-and-management-of-chest-wall-trauma-in-adults#H15009025).)

Thoracic instability is usually associated with a contusion of adjacent lung structures. Shallow breathing and accompanying pulmonary contusion lead to increased work of breathing, an increase in intrapulmonary shunt volume, and hypoxemia. Anesthetic management primarily includes pain control and intermittent overpressure ventilation.[17] The criteria for endotracheal intubation and mechanical ventilation are:[18]

- arterial partial pressure of oxygen (PaO2) under 70 mm Hg under supplemental oxygen (reservoir)
- PaCO2 over 50 mm Hg
- Respiratory rate over 35 breaths per minute
- Vital capacity under 15 mL/kg
- Negative inspiratory strength less than 20 cm H_2O

Pulmonary Contusion

A contusion of the lungs often becomes apparent as hypoxemia. The frequency in adult patients in emergency surgery is 65%.[2] The therapy consists of supplemental oxygen and the application of positive airway pressure, either with the help of a continuous positive airway pressure (CPAP) mask or by intubation and mechanical ventilation with positive end-expiratory pressure (PEEP).

Lung contusion causes a significant disturbance of vascular integrity through intraparenchymal and alveolar hemorrhage, which results in reduced pulmonary compliance and increased shunt fraction.[19] Intraalveolar hemorrhage can result in severe acute respiratory distress syndrome (ARDS) by inducing profound inflammation and causing severe bronchiolitis. Because of inconclusive clinical signs, the diagnosis is usually made radiologically, presenting as diffuse, nonsegmental lung consolidation on the anteroposterior thoracic x-ray image.

Hemorrhage in the tracheobronchial tree can be observed in about 10% of patients. An important measure in the therapy of bleeding is frequent endotracheal suction via the endotracheal tube. In about 33% of patients with respiratory hemorrhage, lung isolation with DLT to prevent blood spillage is required.[2] Alternative treatment methods, such as diuretics and corticosteroid application, have not shown benefits.[18] PEEP ventilation improves hypoxemia, but not the underlying contusion.[19]

The treatment of rib fractures requires a sufficient treatment of pain (parenteral analgesics, interpleural anesthetics, or epidural/regional anesthesia). The affected lung is susceptible to the formation of a capillary leak; therefore careful fluid management is indicated.[20] Intraalveolar hemorrhage resulting from severe pulmonary parenchymal trauma caused aspiration pneumonitis intraoperatively that resulted in severe ARDS following surgical stabilization of rib fractures (SSRF). Risk factors for this include lateral decubitus position, early SSRF (within 5 days of injury), and the use of a single lumen tube during the procedure. Care should be taken in performing SSRF in patients with significant traumatic lung parenchymal injury, and intraoperative lung isolation should be exercised in these patients (Fig. 33.6).[21]

Pneumothorax

Blunt thoracic trauma should always lead to suspicion of a pneumothorax. In adults, the incidence of a pneumothorax in emergency interventions is 30%.[2]

Possible causes include alveolar rupture with perivascular spread of air to the hilus and the connection of the distal airways to the pleural space.[22] Under general anesthesia, with positive pressure ventilation, a viable risk that a simple pneumothorax will result in a life-threatening tension pneumothorax exists (Fig. 33.7). The increase in pressure in the pleural space on the one hand leads to hypoventilation and hypoxemia, and on the other hand, the venous return is reduced by kinking of the pulmonary veins and the vena cava and results in a pronounced hypotension. If untreated promptly, this may lead to cardiac arrest.

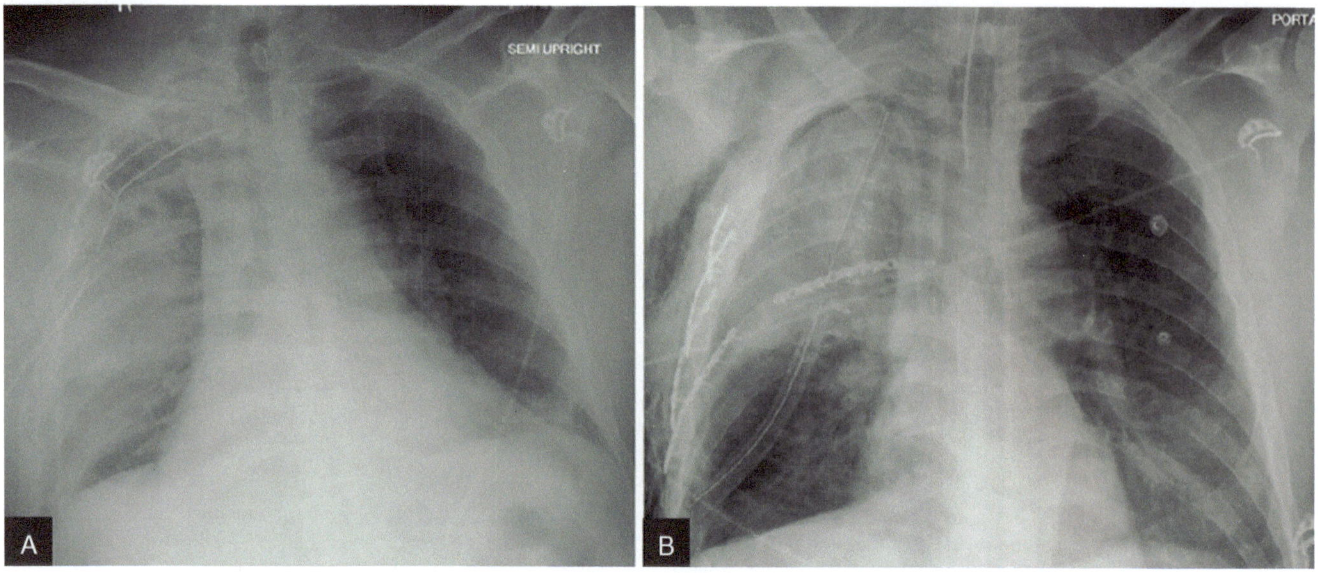

• **Fig. 33.6** Pulmonary contusion: preoperative anteroposterior view plain chest radiograph showing severe right-sided opacification from pulmonary contusion (**A**). The same patient immediately following surgical stabilization of rib fractures showing marked opacification of the contralateral lung fields (**B**). (From Tumminello M, Smith A, McGrew P, et al. Complications from pulmonary contusions after rib plating: a case series and lessons learned. *J Cardiothorac Trauma.* 2019;4(1):35–40.)

Diagnosis of pneumothorax under general anesthesia is difficult. Controlled mechanical ventilation and ambient noise make it difficult to diagnose by auscultation.[22] Frequently, pneumothorax is only suspected when symptoms, such as hypotension, tachycardia, increased airway pressure, increased jugular venous pressure, and trachea deviation, occur.

The suspicion alone calls for the placement of a thoracic drain to prevent a lethal complication. Patients with multiple rib fractures may have a subclinical pneumothorax, and therefore prophylactic thoracic drainage should be performed.[23]

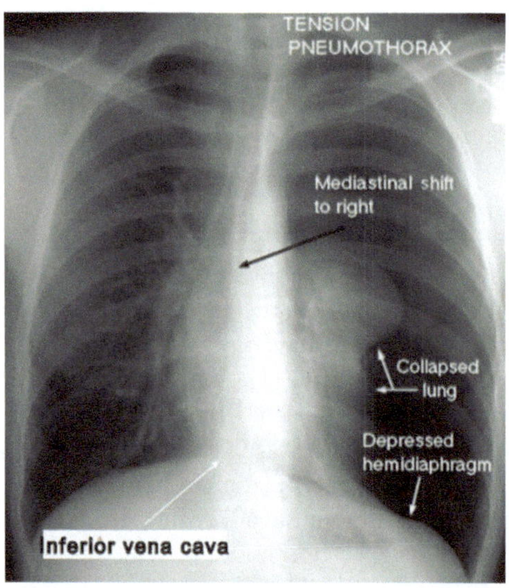

• **Fig. 33.7** Tension pneumothorax: anteroposterior view plain chest radiograph showing left-sided tension pneumothorax with collapsed lung and depressed hemidiaphragm (*white arrows*) resulting in mediastinal shift to the right side (*black arrow*). (From ALFA (Assisted Learning for All Med Surg II).)

With lung ultrasound, it is possible to accurately rule in or rule out pneumothorax at the bedside in almost all clinical scenarios.[24,25] Alternatively, if the patient is clinically stable, a thoracic x-ray can secure the diagnosis preoperatively.

Hemothorax

The frequency of hemothorax in adult patients following thoracic trauma is 26%.[10] Bleeding can be minimal or massive, as a hemithorax can hold up to 30% to 40% of the total blood volume. This massive bleeding (Fig. 33.8) is usually caused by a laceration of the heart or of the large vessels in proximity to the heart.[23] A massive hemothorax is defined as a collection of more than 1500 mL of free blood in the pleural space, which inevitably results in hypovolemic shock. The mediastinal shift leads to further cardiovascular depression and ultimately to cardiovascular collapse. Clinical diagnosis in the operating room is difficult, yet symptoms, such as missing or attenuated breath sound, as well as contralateral tracheal displacement should always raise suspicion of the presence of hemothorax. The diagnosis is confirmed by ultrasound at the bedside or by an x-ray with shading of the entire hemithorax. Placement of a large diameter thoracic drainage is the therapy of choice.[26] This makes it possible to improve ventilation and control thoracic blood loss. Intraoperatively, the patient is best managed with a DLT and one-lung ventilation if necessary.[27]

Mediastinal Widening

The widening of the mediastinum in an x-ray image after blunt thoracic trauma is often associated with thoracic aortic injury. However, because of the vulnerability of thoracic

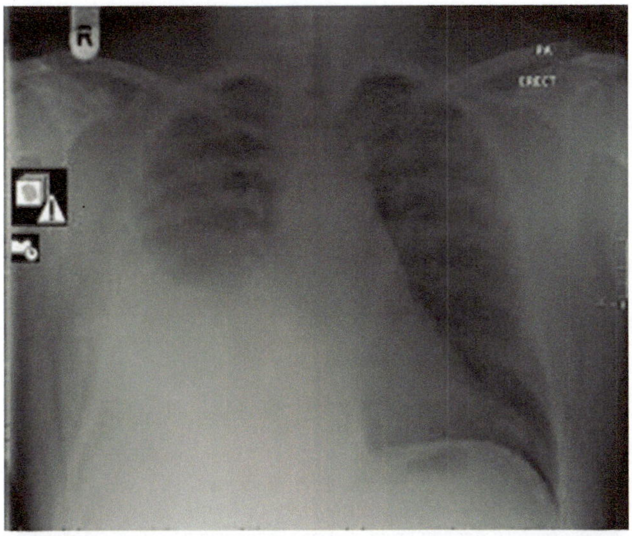

• **Fig. 33.8** Hemothorax: anteroposterior supine view plain chest radiograph showing right-sided opacification from massive (>500 mL) collection of fluid (blood) caused by gunshot wound (bullet projects on to ninth rib). (From Yap D, Ng M, Chaudhury M, Mbakada N. Longest delayed hemothorax reported after blunt chest injury. *Am J Emerg Med.* 2018;36(1):171.e1–171.e3. doi: 10.1016/j.ajem.2017.10.025. Epub 2017 Oct 16. PMID: 29079373.)

x-ray diagnostics to artifacts, the diagnosis should be secured by a CT examination. The loss of aortic contour, the displacement of the esophagus to the right, and a mediastinal widening are corresponding radiologic signs.[28,29]

Thoracic Aortal Injury

The incidence of traumatic aortic rupture is 4.8%.[10] About 90% of these patients die at the scene of the accident. About 10% may have minimal symptoms and reach the hospital alive, as the tunica adventitia of the aorta remains intact.[28]

An initial suspicion must therefore always be excluded or confirmed by CT-angiography. Morbidity and mortality of the injury are directly associated with prompt diagnosis.

The rupture usually takes place at the aortic isthmus, distal of the exit of the left subclavian artery. If hemodynamic stabilization is not established, emergency interventions have a high mortality. Although the traditional therapy for blunt traumatic rupture of the thoracic aorta (TRA) is immediate operative repair, there may be a selective role for delayed repair, particularly in patients with head trauma, respiratory failure, or cardiac dysfunction. Maggisano et al.[24] evaluated 59 consecutive three groups of patients with aortic isthmus TRA at a regional trauma unit: group I (n = 12) included patients who either arrived in extremis or rapidly became unstable during triage; group II (n = 3) included patients who had no contraindications to early repair and underwent repair at the time of diagnosis; and group III (n = 44) consisted of patients who, because of concomitant injuries or sepsis, required initial admission and management in the intensive care unit until their clinical status had improved sufficiently to allow for deliberate delayed operative repair of the TRA. Overall survival rates in groups I, II, and III were 17%, 100%, and 82%, respectively. The authors concluded that TRA may not require immediate operative repair in all cases, but may instead be managed selectively depending on the patient's clinical status.

Intraoperatively, advanced hemodynamic monitoring and equipment is recommended which includes:

- invasive blood pressure measurement in the right radial or brachial artery
- additional invasive blood pressure measurement in a femoral artery
- large bore central venous access
- consider pulmonary artery catheter
- transesophageal echocardiography
- multiple large bore peripheral venous access
- "rapid-infusion" system
- in-line fluid warmer

If an aortic injury is suspected, blood pressure must be continuously monitored. Hypertensive episodes must be avoided; mean arterial pressure should be maintained between 70 and 80 mm Hg using beta blockers and vasodilators.[28]

For the purpose of lung isolation, primary intubation with a DLT is advisable not only for surgical exposure but also to enhance clearance of bloody secretion. Hypertensive phases can be controlled with vasodilators and/or beta blockers during (partial) clamping of the aorta. Hypotonic phases after release of the clamping are treated with fluids and reduction of vasodilators.

Strategies for interdisciplinary renal/spinal stabilization[28,30,31] are, for example:

- short aortic clamping time
- femoral arteriovenous bypass
- intravenous application of Mannitol
- thoracic epidural anesthesia

Blunt Cardiac Trauma

Real structural injuries to the heart resulting from blunt trauma are rare.[23] The incidence of myocardial contusion in patients with thoracic trauma is 2.6%, based on radionuclide examinations, angiographic, or autopsy diagnoses.[32] The incidence of this injury in patients with blunt thoracic trauma who underwent emergency surgery was 5.7%. In combination with additional injuries, the mortality rate is significantly increased. The incidence of hypotension or dysrhythmia is similar with or without myocardial contusion. The leading intraoperative cause of death in adults with cardiac contusion is hypovolemia, not heart injury. Devitt et al.[20] examined the frequency and importance of intraoperative mortality, arrhythmias, and hypotension in the presence of thoracic trauma to determine the effect of myocardial contusion on these perioperative complications. Patients were also studied for the presence of myocardial injury with radionuclide angiography, at autopsy or at thoracotomy. A total of 201 patients were studied. The intraoperative and overall mortality was 7.9% and 22.9%, respectively. Of the operating room survivors, the incidence of intraoperative arrhythmias and hypotension was 3.8% and 26.5%, respectively. Only 5.9% of patients had a suspected or confirmed myocardial contusion. All patients with blunt thoracic injury may develop intraoperative arrhythmias or hypotension. Children seem to tolerate cardiac contusion without major complications.[33]

Blunt heart trauma includes a broad clinical spectrum of disorders, such as the disturbance of electrical formation or conduction in the heart to cardiac rupture and death. The right atrium and the right ventricle are the most frequently injured chambers because of their anterior position in the thorax, followed by the left atrium and the left ventricle. A rupture of a chamber is survived by about 40% of patients. Mortality increases rapidly when multiple chambers are affected. The diagnosis is made by echocardiography.[34]

Cardiac Contusion

Patients with suspected myocardial contusion do not need to be routinely monitored in an intensive care unit. If electro- and echocardiogram are normal and there are no further injuries, the patient can be discharged from hospital after 12 hours. Young patients show hardly any cardiac complications after cardiac contusion. The importance of diagnostic procedures remains controversial. The electrocardiogram is unreliable unless an ST elevation is visible. The appearance of creatine kinase (CK)-MB isoenzymes cannot be used diagnostically because it tends to cause more confusion than clarification in trauma situations.[35] Cardiac troponin I (specific for myocardial damage) has not been adequately investigated. Echocardiography is valuable in the detection of wall motion disorders and pericardial effusions and can indicate complications in combination with changes in CK-MB isoenzymes. Radionuclide angiography can also be predictive for further complications. Thallium scintigraphy can detect areas with reduced perfusion, but cannot distinguish an acute from an existing lesion.[36,37]

Pericardial Tamponade

The pericardial space enclosed between the two serosal layers normally contains up to 50 mL of plasma ultrafiltrate. The pericardium may be affected by all categories of diseases, including infectious, autoimmune, neoplastic, iatrogenic, traumatic, and metabolic.[1] Pericardial effusions may develop acutely, such as in thoracic trauma, or more gradually. A pericardial tamponade must be suspected if an existing hypotension cannot be plausibly explained by other findings (pneumothorax, hemothorax, abdominal, or other bleeding).

The causes may be cardiac or aortic rupture, as well as myocardial contusion without rupture.[20,23,34] If fluid accumulation is gradual, pericardial pressure remains low because the pericardium can increase its compliance by undergoing stretch, which is accomplished by an increase in surface area and mass. Rapid accumulation of blood from thoracic trauma usually results in impaired cardiac filling and cardiac tamponade (Fig. 33.9). Cardiac tamponade patients presents with shortness of breath, tachycardia,

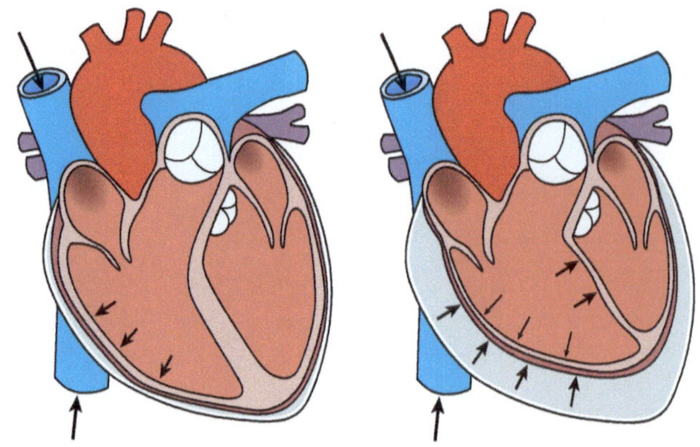

• **Fig. 33.9** Pericardial tamponade: figure schematically displays accumulation of fluid in the pericardial space (tamponade) with impaired filling of the right ventricle resulting in insufficient cardiac output in comparison to a healthy heart. (From Diseasedic.com (last accessed 02.12.2021) https://diseasesdic.com/cardiac-tamponade-overview-causes-and-diagnosis/)

hypotension with a narrow pulse pressure, and pulsus paradoxus (an inspiratory fall of systolic blood pressure of more than 10 mm Hg during normal spontaneous breathing), which is an important diagnostic finding in CT. Jugular venous distention, marked hypotension, and muffled heart sounds (Beck's triad) are the three classic signs of cardiac tamponade. **Hemodynamic** instability is usually present because of heart compression caused by the accumulation of fluid and blood, in the pericardial space. Electrocardiography may show signs of large pericardial effusion, with especially low QRS voltage and electrical alternans (an alternating amplitude or axis of the QRS complexes in any or all leads). Echocardiography is the main diagnostic method for detection of pericardial effusion and tamponade. The main echocardiographic sign of cardiac tamponade is the presence of pericardial effusion, with collapse of the low-pressure cardiac chambers with the thin walls (namely the right atria at end-diastole and the right ventricle outflow tract) at early diastole. The primary therapy consists of immediate surgical drainage via a window in the pericardium (pericardiocentesis), which should be performed under fluoroscopic or echocardiographic guidance. Alternatively, a pericardial drain can be inserted under ultrasound guidance in local anesthesia. Hemodynamic changes are best tolerated by spontaneously breathing patients.

Diaphragmatic Rupture

In blunt thoracic trauma, the incidence of a diaphragm rupture in the operating room is 9.1%.[10] Symptoms are similar to pneumothorax with lung compression and hypoxemia.

The diaphragmatic rupture is probably a direct result of a sudden massive increase in intraabdominal pressure. If the tear in the diaphragm is large enough, the negative pleural pressure during spontaneous breathing promotes the herniation of the abdominal organs into the thoracic cavity with

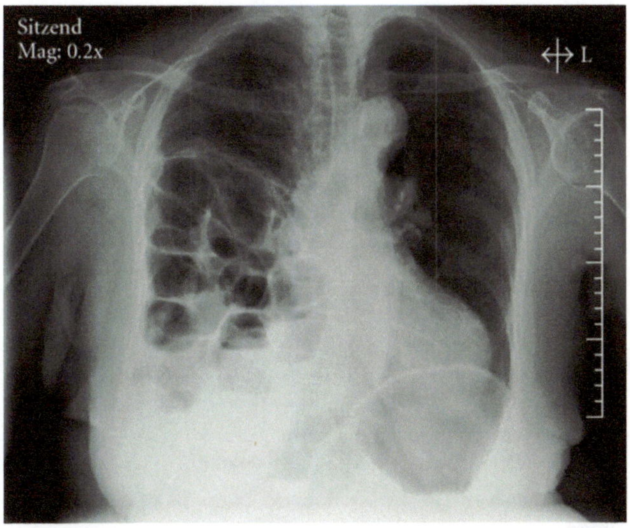

• **Fig. 33.10** Diaphragmatic rupture with herniation of bowel into the right hemithorax after blunt trauma: chest radiograph shows a herniation of bowel into the right hemithorax with consecutive ileus signs 4 days after blunt thoracic trauma with diaphragmatic rupture.

subsequent compression of the adjacent pulmonary areas leading to shortness of breath (Fig. 33.10).[38]

Diaphragm injuries are more common on the left side because the liver provides some protection to the right hemidiaphragm. Physical examination is not very helpful with the diagnosis. The thoracic x-ray shows an elevation of the left diaphragmatic dome and an arc-shaped shadow indicating an unusually high diaphragm on the left side. The shift of the heart and mediastinal structures to the opposite side of the defect also indicate a diaphragm injury. The diagnosis is confirmed when the tip of a gastric probe can be detected in the intrathoracic stomach.[29]

With intrathoracic herniation of abdominal structures, the risk of aspiration is high. Sufficient oxygenation requires intubation and mechanical positive pressure ventilation, also to protect the airways. If a concomitant hemothorax is present, a rupture of the spleen has to be suspected.[23,29]

Penetrating Thoracic Trauma

Blunt trauma is the dominating mechanism for injuries to the thorax, although penetrating thoracic trauma is not rare. U.S. Centers for Disease Control and Prevention records for 2016 show that deaths from gunshot wounds in the United States were comparable to the number of deaths from motor vehicle accidents. Tissue damage resulting from penetrating injuries may be complex and is dependent on characteristics of the penetrating object.[39]

Categorization of penetrating thoracic trauma is slightly different from blunt trauma. All entities are described in detail in the blunt trauma section. Basically, all combinations of injured structures may occur. Based on the injured structures it can be divided in:

- tracheobronchial injury/esophageal injury
- gunshot wounds/stab wounds
- pericardial tamponade
- hemothorax/pneumothorax
- diaphragmatic injury

In general, one can divide penetrating trauma into low, medium, or high velocity injuries, where low velocity (nonballistic) injury is caused by sharp, impaling objects (stabbing), and medium/high velocity (ballistic) injuries result from projectiles (arrows, shrapnel, bullets). Nonballistic injury is characterized by lacerations along the trajectory of the penetrating object, whereas ballistic injuries can cause tissue disruptions greatly exceeding the original path. Any single injury or combinations thereof can lead to decompensation and follow common pathophysiologic pathways (Fig. 33.11).[40]

Most penetrating injuries to the chest in civilian patients can be treated initially with the insertion of a chest tube, yet although stable, these patients should be thoroughly evaluated for the presence of occult life-threatening conditions because there is the potential for rapid decompensation and demise resulting from initially unrecognized intrathoracic injuries.

The standard Advanced Trauma Life Support protocol should be followed expeditiously. Intubation and intravenous access should be quickly and efficiently performed.

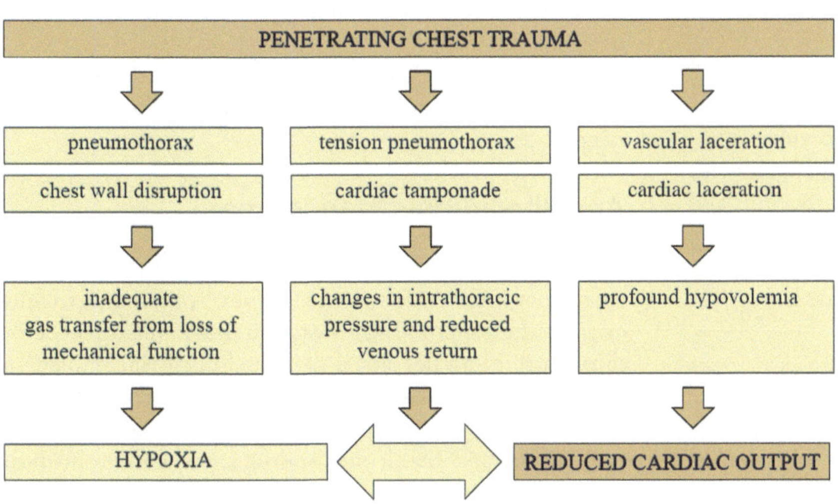

• **Fig. 33.11** Pathophysiologic consequences of penetrating chest trauma: initial injury to the thorax leads via different pathophysiologic pathways to common clinical consequences. (From Hunt PA, Greaves I, Owens WA. Emergency thoracotomy in thoracic trauma—a review. *Injury.* 2006;37(1):1–19.)

Patients with life-threatening cardiac injuries can present as relatively stable, only to decompensate quickly. All injuries inside the "cardiac box" (defined as inferior to the clavicles, superior to the costal margin, and medial to the midclavicular line) are highly suspicious of cardiac association and should be assessed at least with a point-of-care ultrasound examination. Wounds outside the cardiac box do not rule out cardiac involvement, and cardiac injuries should be initially suspected and ruled out in all unstable patients.[41]

Preoperative Evaluation

A & B: Airway and Breathing

The careful clinical evaluation of the ventilation of the traumatized patient must include inspection of the upper airway, respiratory rate, paradox movements of the chest wall, and obvious thoracic wounds. Palpation of the thorax should provide evidence of pain, crepitation, and subcutaneous emphysema as indication of the underlying pathology. The auscultation of the lungs should identify a pneumothorax or hemothorax before a radiologic diagnosis can be carried out and additionally assess the sufficiency of ventilation. Percussion, although theoretically useful, can help in the discrimination between pneumo- and hemothorax, but is practically difficult to perform in the typical shock room atmosphere. Point-of-care sonography, however, should be performed as early as possible. Best-known applications include focused abdominal sonography for trauma and focused echocardiographic evaluation in life support. The technology is almost ubiquitously available and can be performed during resuscitation.[42]

Circulation

In thoracic trauma, hypotension is usually associated with hypovolemia and should initially be treated aggressively with volume substitution (crystalloids), whereas other possible causes (e.g., pneumothorax, cardiac tamponade, and cardiac contusion) must be diagnosed or excluded. The presence of arrhythmia increases the suspicion of blunt cardiac trauma (contusion).[37,43] Arterial hypertension can dramatically worsen from bleeding in the thorax and should therefore be treated immediately.

Laboratory Diagnostics

Preoperative (e.g., in the emergency room) laboratory examinations should include at least a complete blood count with coagulation, electrolyte status, glucose, urea, creatinine, and if necessary, urinalysis. The immediate determination of the blood group and the provision of erythrocyte concentrates and clotting preparations is highly recommended.

Radiologic Diagnostics

Radiologic diagnostics should be commenced immediately after controlling and securing of vital functions. The method of choice is, almost ubiquitously available, a spiral CT, possibly using contrast agents in case of suspicion of vascular involvement. All injuries to the bony thorax, usually the surrounding soft tissues, as well as the thoracic organs can be detected.

The CT of the thorax can also indicate aortic injuries and confirm pneumothorax that are not visible in the simple x-ray imaging. Angiography is used to precisely locate the source of bleeding from vascular injuries.[28,29]

Ultrasound Diagnostics

Ultrasound is a standard procedure in the diagnosis of thoracic organs. The assessment of the heart (kinetics, injury, pericardial tamponade) is certainly possible early on. Echocardiography, either transthoracic or transesophageal, is useful in assessing the pericardium (effusions), the valve, and wall movements of the heart, as well as the presence and extent of a possible aortic injury (see Chapter 54).

Chest Radiography

The thoracic X-ray image in two planes is still of great importance in the care of thoracic trauma if no CT or ultrasound examination is possible. Only life-threatening situations should delay it.[29] Because of the speed of modern CT scanners and increasing availability of scans in the trauma bay, conventional x-ray studies are losing their standard place in the assessment of trauma patients. Nevertheless, a short overview of the possible findings follows because sometimes CT scans are unavailable.

The systematic examination of x-rays can detect both suspected and unexpected pathologic changes. The bony thorax, including the ribs, collarbones, shoulder blades, and spine, should be examined for fractures. Soft tissues should be evaluated in relation to emphysema or shading. The pulmonary fields can indicate pneumothorax, hemothorax, and a consolidation that indicate lung contusion. X-ray anomalies of the mediastinum, in particular pneumomediastinum, widening, or displacement, indicate a respiratory rupture, aortic injury, and a tension pneumothorax.

Radiologic evidence of an injury to the thoracic aorta may include an extension of the upper mediastinum, the loss of the aortic button, and right or left apical deviation of a gastric tube.

Finally, assessing the heart silhouette can help diagnose a blunt myocardial injury, including the detection of a pericardial tamponade.

Anesthesiologic Management

Surgery in patients with blunt thoracic trauma is usually an emergency intervention. There is generally little time to fully evaluate the patient. The history can often only be collected through third parties and is therefore usually incomplete or totally unknown. Useful information from an anesthesiologic perspective includes the mechanism of injury, a recent food intake, possible alcohol or drug abuse, current medication, and all known concomitant diseases (heart, circulation, lungs, metabolic disorders, etc.). SAMPLER mnemonic comprises: (S, Signs/Symptoms; A, Allergies; M, Medications; P, Past pertinent medical history; L, Last oral intake; E, Events leading up to present injury; R, risk factors).

Preoperative evaluation should include a short neurologic evaluation (pupil reaction, neurologic reflex status, and motor reactions), careful assessment of the respiratory tract, and an examination of the thorax. Evidence of injuries, such as hemothorax, pneumothorax, tension pneumothorax, rib fractures, and thoracic stability, must be investigated.

Preoperative diagnostics should include thoracic radiography (CT is preferred), blood count, coagulation status, electrolyte status, and arterial blood gas analysis.[2]

Basic monitoring has to meet the minimum required American Society of Anesthesiologists standard such as among others pulse oximetry, electrocardiogram, noninvasive blood pressure, temperature, airway pressure, and end-tidal CO2. Advanced hemodynamic monitoring with arterial blood pressure, central venous catheter, and bladder catheterization is crucial for critically ill patients. In addition to continuous blood pressure monitoring, a permanent artery catheter enables intermittent blood gas analysis, as well as the monitoring of other hematologic and laboratory chemical parameters. In addition, it allows the hands of the anesthetist to be free for possible resuscitation measures. Other procedures, such as echocardiography or the insertion of a pulmonary artery catheter, must not cause any delay in any vital measures and are components of the further management.

Additional complications, such as a pneumothorax, can develop intraoperatively; therefore the prophylactic thoracic drain on the affected side (e.g., in the case of rib fractures) must initially be taken into account. This also allows the anesthesiologist to sufficiently monitor any blood loss from the affected hemithorax.[10]

Initial airway management remains controversial. In emergency surgery, up to 30% of patients with blunt thoracic trauma have respiratory compromise resulting from lower jaw and/or upper jaw fractures, cervical spine and/or thoracic and lumbar spine injuries. Because of the urgency and extent of the injuries, the cervical spine often cannot be fully examined before surgery.

The frequency of cervical spine injuries in surgical patients is about 12%.[10] A cervical spine injury must be suspected in all patients with blunt trauma until proven otherwise.

To protect the cervical spine, either if injury is confirmed or at least suspected, intubation should be performed with limited to no motion in the cervical spine. When immobilized in a rigid collar, one can assume difficulties in laryngeal visualization. Different airway management techniques have to be available, their advantages and disadvantages known.

For instance, (awake) fiberoptic intubation greatly limits spine movement, yet needs operator proficiency, patient cooperation, takes time, and is hindered by blood and secretions in the upper airway. Also the placement of DLT via fiberoptic intubation is a great challenge. An excellent alternative is video laryngoscopy with different bladed because the indirect view allows for less mouth opening and limit the neck extension, although blood/secretions can also limit the view and training is required. Even with these limitations, some studies suggest better first-attempt success rates with video laryngoscopy versus direct laryngoscopy.[44]

When the option of video assistance is not available, conventional direct laryngoscopy has been proven safe and remarkably effective. A review of over 32,000 emergent intubations by experienced anesthesiologists, where over 6000 were within the first hour of admission, found only one suspected case of compromised neurologic outcome because of intubation.[45]

Concomitant injuries in thoracic trauma are often found in the abdomen and the head/face.

Intraoperative ventilation problems initially impress as an increase in airway pressure and decrease in oxygen saturation. The causes are usually bleeding in the airways, pulmonary edema after aggressive resuscitation, and occurrence of intraoperative pneumothorax.

Blood accumulation in the airways can lead to a compromisation of the healthy lungs and thus to severe hypoxia. The isolation of the hemorrhagic lung is paramount.[10]

Victims of blunt force to the thorax regularly have hypovolemia (hypovolemic shock) when they arrive at the operating room. Adequate volume substitution is therefore required before induction of general anesthesia. Negative inotropic drugs or peripheral vasodilating pharmaceuticals should be used with caution, in reduced dosage, or be avoided all together.

Using specific anesthetics for induction and maintenance of anesthesia is far less important than knowledge of the corresponding physiologic and pharmacologic principles in polytraumatized patients under shock.

Exsanguination remains the main cause of intraoperative death in patients with blunt thoracic trauma.[10,23] Several large-bore peripheral lines should be placed initially because the massive transfusion of blood and clotting preparations is often necessary.

Coagulation management focuses primarily on the treatment of an underlying or acute coagulopathy, of hypothermia and hypocalcemia. Coagulopathies after massive transfusions are common, and their clinical diagnosis and therapy are confirmed and guided by laboratory chemical tests, ideally including bedside thromboelastography. This is caused by dilution as a result of volume substitution, as well as the increased consumption of platelets and coagulation factors.

Disseminated intravascular coagulation (DIC) can occur as a result of shock and coagulopathy should the state of hemorrhagic shock persist. After exchanging the entire blood volume, the platelet count may be low enough to maintain coagulopathy alone. When the double blood volume is substituted, coagulation factors are diluted to the extent that coagulopathy inevitably results. With prolongation of prothrombin and partial thromboplastin time and absence of DIC, hypofibrinogenemia is likely. The management of dilution coagulopathy requires the substitution of platelet concentrates and individual factors. However, causal therapy consists in (surgical) stopping of the underlying bleeding; the substitution of factors is only supportive.[46]

Permissive hypotension can be considered in individual cases to reduce blood loss if surgical control of the hemorrhage is difficult and prolonged,[47,48] although large randomized trials to support it's use is still lacking.

Hypothermia in trauma patients is frequent because of external environmental influences at the time of injury, rapid infusion of cold fluids and blood, altered homeostasis because of anesthesia, and intraoperative exposure of the abdominal and thoracic organs. The body temperature is determined by the balance of heat loss and heat gain. The anesthesiologist and surgeon can aggravate the heat loss by inhibiting the heat-producing mechanisms. The following mechanisms contribute to heat loss to varying extent:

- Radiation (energy loss because of thermal radiation, 40%–50%)
- Convection (energy loss via body surface through air movement, 25%–35%)
- Evaporation (heat loss via water vapor, 10%–20%)
- Conduction (direct contact with cold surfaces, 5%–15%)

The body's acute responses to a cold stimulus are limited. These include behavioral change for heat preservation, superficial vasoconstriction, trembling, and nontrembling thermogenesis. The application of anesthetics accelerates heat loss by preventing physiologic vasoconstriction, trembling, and the reduction of thermogenesis by suppressing appropriate behavioral reactions. The main factor, however, is radiation and convective heat loss; therefore controlling the room and ambient temperature is the most efficient way of maintaining and controlling the patient's temperature.

Respiratory gas conditioning also reduces heat loss by about 10% to 15%. The heating of blood and intravenous fluids is also essential during high volume turnover. Forced air warming and heat pads are less efficient, but in the context of thermal management they are an important factor.[49]

The occurrence of hypocalcemia is rare, but can be associated with massive transfusion (an erythrocyte concentrates every 5 minutes), persistent hypovolemic shock with insufficient perfusion of the liver, hypothermia, and clamping of the portal vein to control the liver hemorrhage. If laboratory values are not available, an unclear arterial hypotension with extended QT interval in the electrocardiogram is suspicious of hypocalcemia.[2]

One-Lung Ventilation

The following situations may necessitate the isolation of a lung, a lobe, or segment:[50]

- Avoiding contamination of the contralateral lung with blood or secretion
- Large bronchopleural or bronchoalveolar fistula
- Surgical factors (diagnostic or surgical treatment of lung injuries)
- Surgery of the thoracic aorta or esophagus

Several alternative methods are available for this purpose:

- Advancing a single lumen tube into a main bronchus
- DLT
- Different types of bronchial blockers

The DLT is regarded as the gold standard in clinical practice. A left-sided DLT is much easier to place and has a lower dislocation rate than a right-sided DLT. The correct position must be controlled fiberoptically because only 20% to 48% of the DLT are in the correct position after "blind" insertion.

With fiberoptic bronchoscopy, the correct position of the tube can be verified when looking at the main carina in the tracheal lumen. The bronchial cuff is blocked from a bronchoscopic point of view, thus preventing herniation and obstruction of the contralateral bronchus. Via the bronchial lumen, it is necessary to confirm that lobar bronchi are not obstructed. The functional isolation of the lungs is carried out by selective clamping and venting of an arm of the DLT. Bronchoscopy, inspection, and auscultation confirm the success of lung separation.

Rare, albeit serious, complications during insertion of a DLT include traumatic damage to the tracheobronchial tree and larynx. Malpositioning can lead to insufficient pulmonary separation or herniation of the bronchial cuff with obstruction of the contralateral main bronchus at the carinal level. The most serious complication is the rupture of the trachea. The following reasons for malpositioning have been identified[51]:

- Membranous portion of the trachea (98%)
- Female (86%)
- Involvement of the carina (79%)
- Age over 50 years (66%)

Other methods of lung separation are the use of endobronchial blockers (Univent Blocker, Arndt Blocker, Cohen Blocker, etc.) or embolectomy catheters in children. The EZ blocker (Teleflex Medical) is a Y-shaped catheter with 2 distal extension which overcome the need to steer the blocker into the selected bronchus. It can be positioned without FB which is useful in cases of hemoptysis (Chapters 16,17).

Here, it is possible to vent the collapsed lung via the inner lumen of the blocker or to apply a CPAP. After insertion and after each change of patient position, immediate bronchoscopy to confirm the blocker position is mandatory.

As a last resort, a bronchus can be surgically clamped to prevent ventilation, or the ventilation can be intermittently halted. A tracheal rupture may require high frequency jet ventilation via the operating field.

Postoperative Care

In general, postoperative care requires an intensive care unit. Patients with emergency surgery for blunt thoracic trauma frequently need to be ventilated postoperatively. The indication for continued ventilation is supported by a combination of severe thoracic and/or head injuries. In addition, coexisting injuries of the abdominal organs and the spinal cord must be taken into account.[10]

Postoperative Pain Therapy

Systemic opioid application, transcutaneous electrical nerve stimulation, nonsteroidal antiinflammatory medication, or regional analgesia procedures (intercostal nerve blockage, epidural analgesia, intrathecal opioid administration,

TABLE 33.1 Benefits of Thoracic Epidural Analgesia Compared With Patient Controlled Analgesia Using Opioids

	Pro	Con
Thoracic epidural analgesia	• analgesia ↑ • respiratory function ↑ • length of hospital stay ↓ • opioid side effects ↓ • myocardial infarction ↓ • pneumonia ↓ • respiratory depression ↓ • thrombotic risk ↓	• invasive • complications during placement • hypotension • epidural hematoma • infection • skill set required • masking of other injuries
Patient controlled analgesia	• easy implementation • accepted method • patient satisfaction • analgesia ↑ • safe	• ability to use system (consciousness, motor skills) • sedative • nausea, vomiting • obstipation • side effects ↑ with age • drug interaction

intrapleural analgesia, and thoracic paravertebral blockage) are available as procedures for postoperative pain therapy. Although invasive, regional analgesia techniques, in particular thoracic epidural anesthesia/analgesia (Table 33.1), have been shown to be the most effective methods with low systemic side effects.[52,53]

Conclusion

Blunt thoracic trauma counts to the serious injuries. The anesthesiologic management of emergency interventions is complex and requires a high level of (patho-) physiologic understanding, equipment, manual skills, and quick, correct decisions. The main causes of intraoperative death are persistent blood loss and asphyxia.

References

1. O'Connor JV, Adamski J. The diagnosis and treatment of non-cardiac thoracic trauma. *JRAMC.* 2010;156:5–14.
2. Moloney JT, Fowler SJ, Chang W. Anesthetic management of thoracic trauma. *Curr Opin Anaesthesiol.* 2008;21:41–46.
3. Sheffy N, Chemsian RV, Grabinsky A. Anaesthesia considerations in penetrating trauma. *Br J Anaesth.* 2014;113:276–285.
4. Kozian A, Bergmann A, Hachenberg T, Schilling T. Der Patient mit Thoraxtrauma: anästhesiologisches Management. Anasthesiologie, Intensivmedizin, Notfallmedizin, Schmerztherapie. *AINS.* 2017;52:422–435.
5. Mahmodlou R, Sepehrvand N. Tracheobronchial injury due to blunt chest trauma. *Int J Crit Ill injury Sci.* 2015;5:116–118.
6. Altinok T, Can A. Management of tracheobronchial injuries. *Euras J Med.* 2014;46:209–215.
7. Mehdiratta N, Archer M, Stewart M, Dennis B, Grogan E. Novel airway and ventilator management of tracheobronchial disruption after blunt trauma. *Ann Thorac Surg.* 2017;104:e359–e361.
8. Jalisi S, Zoccoli M. Management of laryngeal fractures—a 10-year experience. *J Voice.* 2011;25:473–479.
9. Schaefer SD. The treatment of acute external laryngeal injuries. 'State of the art'. *Arch Otolaryngol Head Neck Surg.* 1991;117:35–39.
10. Devitt JH, McLean RF, Koch JP. Anaesthetic management of acute blunt thoracic trauma. *Can J Anaesth.* 1991;38:506–510.
11. Shorr RM, Crittenden M, Indeck M, Hartunian SL, Rodriguez A. Blunt thoracic trauma. Analysis of 515 patients. *Ann Surg.* 1987;206:200–205.
12. Schaefer SD. The acute management of external laryngeal trauma. A 27-year experience. *Arch Otolaryngol Head Neck Surg.* 1992;118: 598–604.
13. Schaefer SD. Management of acute blunt and penetrating external laryngeal trauma. *Laryngoscope.* 2014;124:233–244.
14. Pearson EG, Fitzgerald CA, Santore MT. Pediatric thoracic trauma: current trends. *Semin Pediatr Surg.* 2017;26:36–42.
15. Caragounis EC, Fagevik Olsen M, Pazooki D, Granhed H. Surgical treatment of multiple rib fractures and flail chest in trauma: a one-year follow-up study. *World J Emerg Surg.* 2016;11:27.
16. Galvagno SM, Smith CE, Varon AJ, et al. Pain management for blunt thoracic trauma: a joint practice management guideline from the Eastern Association for the Surgery of Trauma and Trauma Anesthesiology Society. *J Trauma Acute Care Surg.* 2016;81: 936–951.
17. Bastos R, Baisden CE, Harker L, Calhoon JH. Penetrating thoracic trauma. *Semin Thorac Cardiovasc Surg.* 2008;20:19–25.
18. Clark GC, Schecter WP, Trunkey DD. Variables affecting outcome in blunt chest trauma: flail chest vs. pulmonary contusion. *J Trauma.* 1988;28:298–304.
19. Požgain Z, Kristek D, Lovrić I, et al. Pulmonary contusions after blunt chest trauma: clinical significance and evaluation of patient management. *Eur J Trauma Emerg Surg.* 2018;44:773–777.
20. Calhoon JH, Grover FL, Trinkle JK. Chest trauma. Approach and management. *Clin Chest Med.* 1992;13:55–67.
21. Tumminello M, Smith A, McGrew P, et al. Complications from pulmonary contusions after rib plating: a case series and lessons learned. *J Cardiothorac Trauma.* 2019;4:35.

22. McGillicuddy D, Rosen P. Diagnostic dilemmas and current controversies in blunt chest trauma. *Emerg Med Clin North Am.* 2007;25:695–711, viii–ix.
23. Devitt JH, McLean RF, McLellan BA. Perioperative cardiovascular complications associated with blunt thoracic trauma. *Can J Anaesth.* 1993;40:197–200.
24. Volpicelli G. Sonographic diagnosis of pneumothorax. *Intensive Care Med.* 2011;37:224–232.
25. Volpicelli G, Elbarbary M, Blaivas M, et al. International evidence-based recommendations for point-of-care lung ultrasound. *Intensive Care Med.* 2012;38:577–591.
26. Jones KW. Thoracic trauma. *Surg Clin North Am.* 1980;60:957–981.
27. Devitt JH, Boulanger BR. Lower airway injuries and anaesthesia. *Can J Anaesth.* 1996;43:148–159.
28. Maggisano R, Nathens A, Alexandrova NA, et al. Rupture of the thoracic aorta: should one always operate immediately? *Ann Vasc Surg.* 1995;9:44–52.
29. Eghbalzadeh K, Sabashnikov A, Zeriouh M, et al. Blunt chest trauma: a clinical chameleon. *Heart* (British Cardiac Society). 2018; 104:719–724.
30. O'Connor CJ, Rothenberg DM. Anesthetic considerations for descending thoracic aortic surgery: part 1. *J Cardiothorac Vasc Anesth.* 1995;9:581–588.
31. O'Connor CJ, Rothenberg DM. Anesthetic considerations for descending thoracic aortic surgery: part II. *J Cardiothorac Vasc Anesth.* 1995;9:734–747.
32. Holanda MS, Domínguez MJ, López-Espadas F, López M, Díaz-Regañón J, Rodríguez-Borregán JC. Cardiac contusion following blunt chest trauma. *Eur J Emerg Med.* 2006;13:373–376.
33. Ildstad ST, Tollerud DJ, Weiss RG, Cox JA, Martin LW. Cardiac contusion in pediatric patients with blunt thoracic trauma. *J Pediatr Surg.* 1990;25:287–289.
34. Perchinsky MJ, Long WB, Hill JG. Blunt cardiac rupture. The Emanuel Trauma Center experience. *Arch Surg.* 1995;130:852–856; discussion 856–857.
35. Ruppert M, van Hee R. Creatinine-kinase-MB determination in non-cardiac trauma: its difference with cardiac infarction and its restricted use in trauma situations. *Eur J Emerg Med.* 2001;8: 177–179.
36. Cachecho R, Grindlinger GA, Lee VW. The clinical significance of myocardial contusion. *J Trauma.* 1992;33:68–71; discussion 71–73.
37. Marcolini EG, Keegan J. Blunt cardiac injury. *Emerg Med Clin North Am.* 2015;33:519–527.
38. Hoffmann H, Oertli D, Heizmann O. Laparoscopic treatment of a rare right diaphragmatic rupture with small bowel herniation after blunt thoracic trauma. *Minimally Invasive Surg.* 2010;2010: 109062.
39. Durso AM, Caban K, Munera F. Penetrating thoracic injury. *Radiol Clin North Am.* 2015;53:675–693; vii–viii.
40. Hunt PA, Greaves I, Owens WA. Emergency thoracotomy in thoracic trauma—a review. *Injury.* 2006;37:1–19.
41. Casós SR, Richardson JD. Role of thoracoscopy in acute management of chest injury. *Curr Opin Crit Care.* 2006;12:584–589.
42. Stengel D, Leisterer J, Ferrada P, Ekkernkamp A, Mutze S, Hoenning A. Point-of-care ultrasonography for diagnosing thoracoabdominal injuries in patients with blunt trauma. *Cochrane Database Syst Rev.* 2018;12:CD012669.
43. Rosenthal MA, Ellis JI. Cardiac and mediastinal trauma. *Emerg Med Clin North Am.* 1995;13:887–902.
44. Mosier JM, Stolz U, Chiu S, Sakles JC. Difficult airway management in the emergency department: GlideScope videolaryngoscopy compared to direct laryngoscopy. *J Emerg Med.* 2012;42: 629–634.
45. Stephens CT, Kahntroff S, Dutton RP. The success of emergency endotracheal intubation in trauma patients: a 10-year experience at a major adult trauma referral center. *Anesth Analg.* 2009;109:866–872.
46. Holcomb JB, Jenkins D, Rhee P, et al. Damage control resuscitation: directly addressing the early coagulopathy of trauma. *J Trauma.* 2007;62:307–310.
47. Carrick MM, Leonard J, Slone DS, Mains CW, Bar-Or D. Hypotensive resuscitation among trauma patients. *BioMed Res Int.* 2016;2016:8901938.
48. Tran A, Yates J, Lau A, Lampron J, Matar M. Permissive hypotension versus conventional resuscitation strategies in adult trauma patients with hemorrhagic shock: a systematic review and meta-analysis of randomized controlled trials. *J Trauma Acute Care Surg.* 2018;84:802–808.
49. Reynolds L, Beckmann J, Kurz A. Perioperative complications of hypothermia. Best practice and research. *Clin Anaesthesiol.* 2008; 22:645–657.
50. Fouche Y, Tarantino DP. Anesthetic considerations in chest trauma. *Chest Surg Clin N Am.* 1997;7:227–238.
51. Chen EH, Logman ZM, Glass PS, Bilfinger TV. A case of tracheal injury after emergent endotracheal intubation: a review of the literature and causalities. *Anesth Analg.* 2001;93:1270–1271.
52. Ho AM, Karmakar MK, Critchley LA. Acute pain management of patients with multiple fractured ribs: a focus on regional techniques. *Curr Opin Crit Care.* 2011;17:323–327.
53. Karmakar MK, Ho AM. Acute pain management of patients with multiple fractured ribs. *J Trauma.* 2003;54:615–625.

34

Mediastinal Mass and Superior Vena Cava Syndrome

DANIEL KALOWITZ, MENACHEM M. WEINER

Introduction

An anterior mediastinal mass is one of the most challenging pathologies an anesthesiologist may face during his or her career. To safely care for these patients, it is imperative to know the relevant anatomy of the mediastinum, understand how mediastinal pathology can compromise a patient's respiratory and cardiovascular systems, and recognize how to prepare for and quickly intervene to treat these potentially life-threatening complications. In this chapter, we will present a case of an anterior mediastinal mass with superior vena cava syndrome (SVCS). We will discuss the important preoperative testing, preanesthetic considerations, risk stratification, and intraoperative anesthetic management. We will also present a flowchart with potential management strategies to assist in safely caring for the majority of these patients.

Case Presentation

A 30-year-old female with no significant past medical history presents to the emergency department with dyspnea, inability to lie flat, cough, and chest discomfort that has progressively worsened over the past few weeks. Clinical examination findings are notable for engorged neck veins with head and upper extremity swelling. Following admission to the hospital, a subsequent workup reveals a very large anterior mediastinal mass associated with both tracheal and great vessel compression. A malignancy is suspected, and the plan is to obtain a tissue sample for histologic diagnosis followed by surgical resection by a multidisciplinary team.

Review of the Literature

Anatomy and Pathophysiology

The mediastinum is the area within the chest bounded anteriorly by the sternum, posteriorly by the vertebral column, laterally by the two parietal pleura, inferiorly by the diaphragm, and superiorly by the thoracic inlet.[1] Some authors divide it into four compartments: the superior, anterior, middle, and posterior compartments. The superior compartment is bound superiorly by the thoracic inlet and inferiorly by the plane extending from the sternal angle anteriorly to the lower border of the fourth thoracic vertebrae posteriorly.[2] The anterior, middle, and posterior compartments are bound superiorly by this plane, inferiorly by the diaphragm, and are divided in the anterior to posterior direction based on the pericardium[2,3] (Fig. 34.1). Others argue that because there is no true anatomic boundary separating the superior and anterior compartments, it is considered one compartment, the anterosuperior compartment, and that the mediastinum is made up of three distinct compartments: the anterosuperior, middle, and posterior compartments[1,3] (Fig. 34.2).

Regardless of whether there are three or four mediastinal compartments, it is important to realize that these compartments cannot be treated as separate entities. Masses in one compartment often extend and affect structures in other compartments. Anterior masses often invade the middle compartment, and masses in the anterior and middle compartments may have similar effects.[4] Furthermore, many of the lesions in the superior compartment originate from or extend into the anterior compartment.[1] In addition, although the majority of complications are described for anterior mediastinal masses, masses in the middle and posterior mediastinum have also been associated with hemodynamic and respiratory collapse with induction of general anesthesia.

There are many vital structures within the mediastinum that can be affected by the presence of masses[3] (Fig. 34.3). The anterosuperior compartment contains the lower trachea, the aortic arch and its branches, the super vena cava, and the azygous vein. The middle compartment contains the heart, the carina and mainstem bronchi, the pulmonary hila, and the terminal portion of the superior vena cava. The posterior compartment contains various nerves and nerve roots, the sympathetic chain, the descending aorta, the esophagus, and the azygous vein.[1]

Mediastinal masses can be primary or metastatic tumors[5,6] (Fig. 34.4; Table 34.1). Metastatic tumors are relatively common, whereas primary tumors are quite rare and

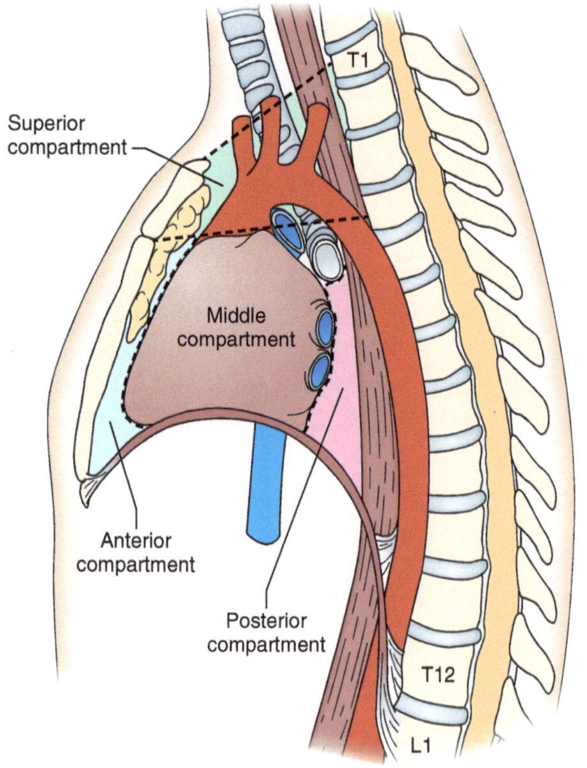

• **Fig. 34.1** Four-compartment model of the mediastinum. (From Liu W, Deslauriers J. Mediastinal divisions and compartments. *Thorac Surg Clin*. 2011;21(2):183–190.)

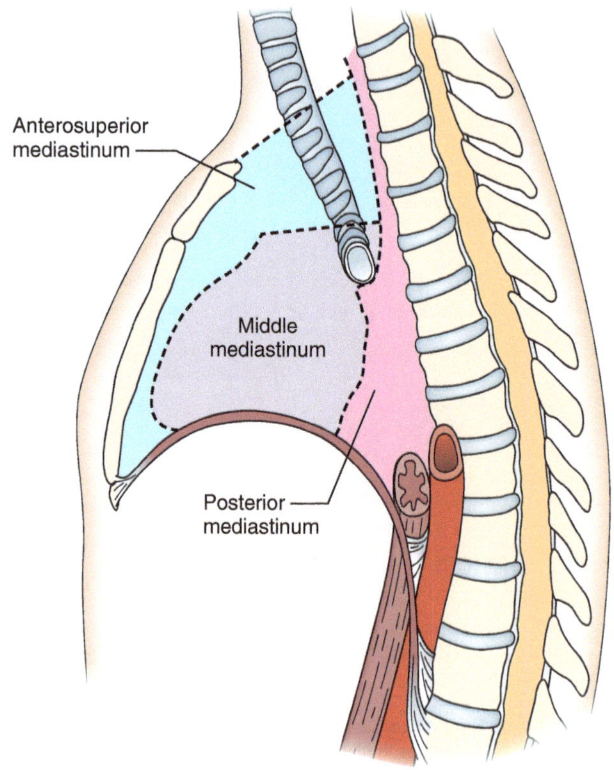

• **Fig. 34.2** Three-compartment model of the mediastinum. (From Liu W, Deslauriers J. Mediastinal divisions and compartments. *Thorac Surg Clin*. 2011;21(2):183–190.)

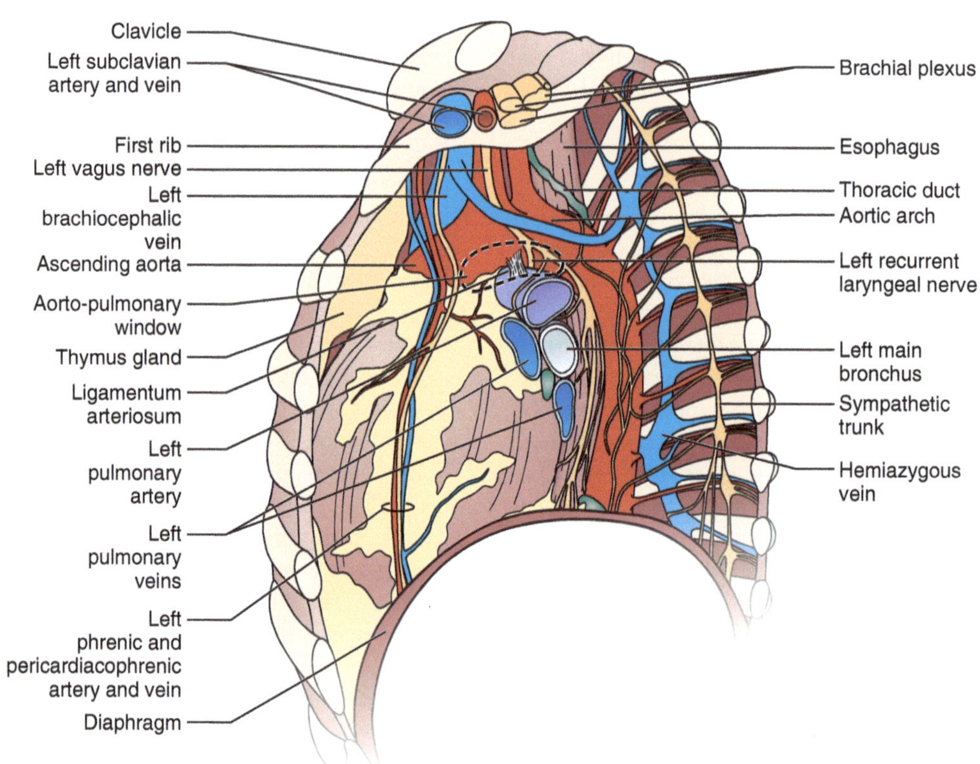

• **Fig. 34.3** Structures in the mediastinum. (From Liu W, Deslauriers J. Mediastinal divisions and compartments. *Thorac Surg Clin*. 2011;21(2):183–190.)

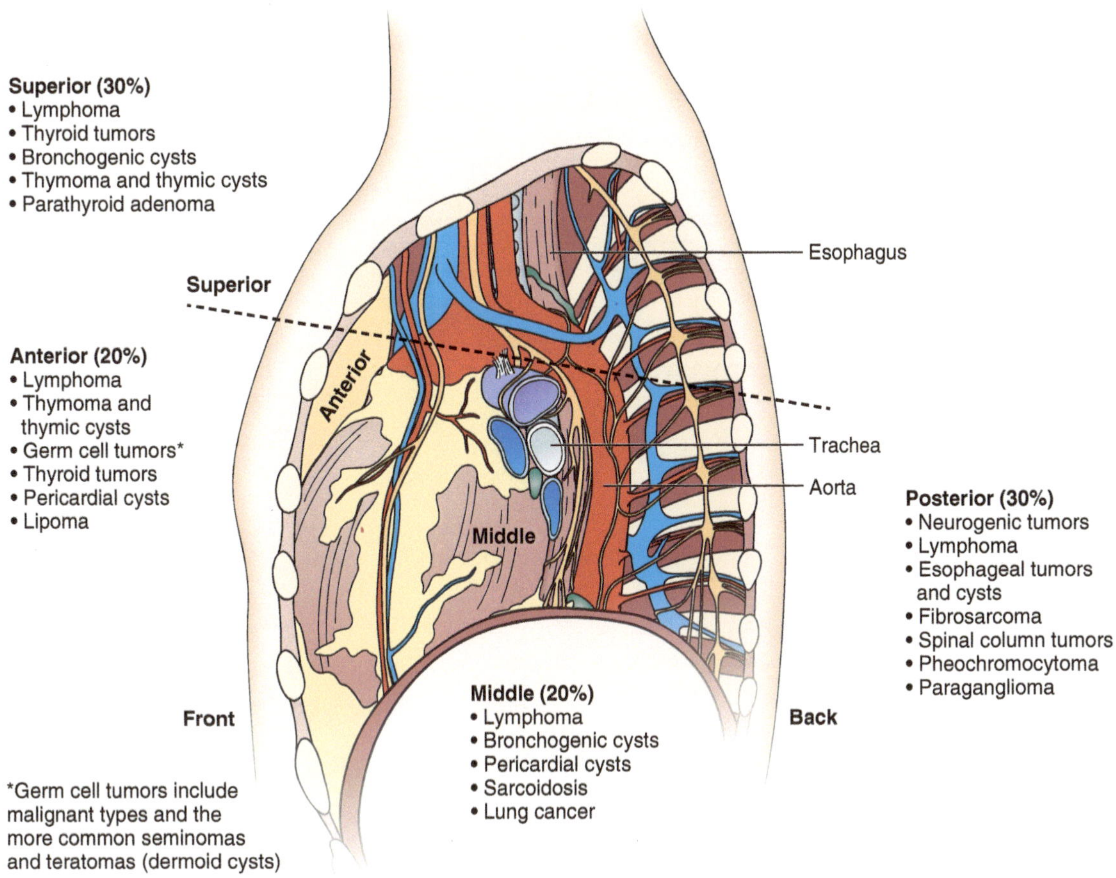

• **Fig. 34.4** Types and locations of mediastinal tumors. (From Salgia R, Blanco R, Skarin AT. Lung cancer and tumors of the heart and mediastinum. In: Skarin AT, ed. *Atlas of Diagnostic Oncology*. 4th ed. Philadelphia: Elsevier; 2010:98–159.)

are often benign.[5] The most common anatomic location and histologic type of mediastinal tumor differs by age.[4] In children, there is an increased incidence of neurogenic tumors, particularly neuroblastomas, and masses are predominantly found in the posterior mediastinum.[1,4] In adolescents, lymphomas in the anterior mediastinum are the most common.[1] In adults, masses are seen most frequently in the anterosuperior compartment,[1] and are most often thymomas and lymphomas.[7]

A growing mass in the mediastinum has the potential to interfere with many of the important structures contained within it and cause a variety of symptoms. When adding the physiologic changes seen under general anesthesia, even an asymptomatic patient can develop severe, and potentially fatal, complications.

Preanesthetic Assessment

Presenting Symptoms and Clinical Findings

Perioperative complications are associated with cardiorespiratory signs and symptoms at initial presentation.[8] An anesthesiologist caring for these patients must be able to identify the variety of clinical signs and symptoms of a mediastinal mass (Table 34.2).[1,2] The patient can also present with no symptoms at all. In children with mediastinal tumors, the incidence of symptoms at presentation is about 70%.[9] Their relatively soft airways make them more susceptible to compression by a mass, and there might be a history of cough, dyspnea, and frequent respiratory infections.[10] Roughly 40% of all tumors involving the mediastinum are asymptomatic at presentation. Consequently, these masses regularly grow to such a size that determination of the site of origin is challenging. Regardless of the definitive diagnosis, the exact size, or location, all large mediastinal and intrathoracic masses may cause mechanical compression of vital mediastinal structures, purely because of the sheer weight and volume of the tumor. Acute or chronic respiratory insufficiency may occur with compression of the airways. Hemodynamic decompensation can be caused by compression of the heart or major vessels in the mediastinum. As mentioned before, these effects can be greatly aggravated by induction of anesthesia or positional changes during surgery and can lead to life-threatening situations.[9] Those patients who are symptomatic often have vague and nonspecific complaints that can often be referred to the respiratory and/or cardiovascular systems.[2] The most common complaints in adults are cough, chest pain, dyspnea, and dysphagia.[1,10]

TABLE 34.1 Malignant and Benign Mediastinal Tumors by Location

Compartment	Malignant Tumors	Benign Tumors
Anterior	Lymphoma Mixed germ cell Seminoma Thymic carcinoma Thymic carcinoid Thyroid carcinoma	Cystic hygroma Foramen of Morgagni hernia Parathyroid adenoma Thymic cyst Thymic hyperplasia Thymolipoma Thymoma Thyroid
Middle	Esophageal cancer Lymphoma Metastases Thyroid carcinoma	Benign adenopathy Cardiac and vascular structures Cardiophrenic fat pad Cysts Ectopic thyroid Esophageal mass Foramen of Morgagni hernia Hiatal hernia Lipomatosis
Posterior	Neuroblastoma	Neurofibroma Schwannoma Chemodectoma Foramen of Bochdalek hernia Meningocele

Modified from Yoneda KY, Louie S, Shelton DK. Mediastinal tumors. *Curr Opin Pulm Med*. 2001;7(4):226–233.

SVCS is a group of symptoms caused by an obstruction of the SVC. It is seen in 28% of patients with a mediastinal mass.[7] Historically, 40% of the cases with SVCS were caused by obstruction, resulting from syphilitic aneurysms and tuberculosis mediastinitis.[11] Presently, SVCS is almost always secondary to an obstruction caused by a mediastinal tumor.[11] It is more frequently seen in patients with diffuse histiocytic lymphoma, in those with lesions on the right side of the body, and those with an obstruction below the azygous vein drainage into the SVC.[12] The most common symptom for SVCS is dyspnea, with facial and periorbital edema being an early sign of this disease process.[2] Other signs and symptoms of SVCS depend on the speed at which the obstruction progresses and can include upper extremity swelling, plethora, head and neck vein dilation, headaches, mental status changes, and visual disturbances.

TABLE 34.2 Symptoms and Clinical Findings in Patients With Mediastinal Masses and Superior Vena Cava Syndrome

Symptoms	Clinical Findings
Cough	Cyanosis
Dyspnea	Wheezing
Orthopnea	Decreased breath sounds
Hoarseness	Pleural effusions
Nasal stuffiness	Stridor
Fatigue	Vocal cord paralysis
Chest pain	Syncope
Faintness	Pulsus paradoxus
Headache	Altered mentation
Altered mentation	Horner syndrome
Distorted vision	Upper extremity swelling
Dysphagia	Head and neck vein dilation
	Papilledema

Modified from Narang S, Harte BH, Body SC. Anesthesia for patients with a mediastinal mass. *Anesthesiol Clin North Am*. 2001;19(3):559–579; and Pullerits J, Holzman R. Anaesthesia for patients with mediastinal masses. *Can J Anaesth*. 1989;36(6):681–688.

Diagnostic Testing

Early reports in the 1970s and 1980s found increased risks of respiratory complications in patients with mediastinal tumors undergoing general anesthesia.[13,14] Since then, many additional reports have been published that highlight the increased risk of cardiovascular complications as well.[15,16] Whereas many of these reports have occurred in children with mediastinal masses undergoing anesthesia, adults with mediastinal tumors are at the same risk. The correlation of perioperative complications to mediastinal mass size and location, as well as cardiorespiratory signs and symptoms at presentation, highlight the critical importance of a thorough preanesthetic clinical workup.[8,17]

Diagnostic imaging is the mainstay of the preoperative evaluation of these patients. With the exception of a true surgical emergency, all patients with suspected or known mediastinal masses should have a radiologic evaluation of the mass. Because mediastinal masses may grow quickly within 2 to 3 weeks, it is important to perform these imaging tests as close to the proposed anesthetic as possible.[1,2] The decision to use magnetic resonance (MR), computed tomography (CT),

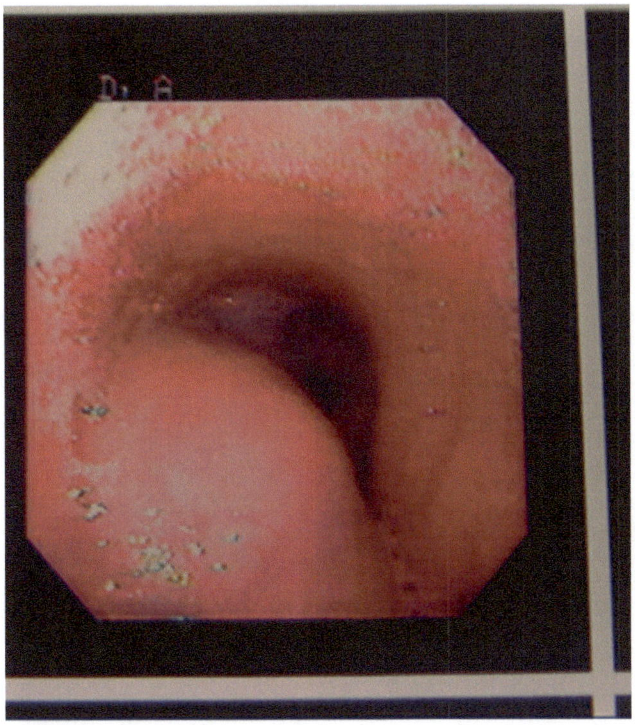

• **Fig. 34.5** Bronchoscopic image showing external tracheal compression.

x-ray, and/or angiography depends on the location and type of lesion. CT and MR imaging are especially useful for the preanesthesia evaluation, as they are performed in the supine position and may detect positional compression of the airway, heart, or great vessels by the mass that may be further accentuated under anesthesia.[1] If the compression of the trachea at any point is greater than 50% of the tracheal diameter (Fig. 34.5), it should immediately raise a red flag that will require meticulous preparation before induction of anesthesia.

Chest x-ray is often the first imaging modality to be performed and can provide valuable information. Because of the two-dimensional nature of the image, it is important to obtain both anterior-posterior and lateral images (Fig. 34.6).[18] CT is perhaps the most commonly used imaging modality, and it has been accepted that all patients with a mediastinal mass should have CT imaging.[1] CT has superior spatial resolution[9] and can determine the morphology of the tumor, its exact anatomic location, and define its relation to the surrounding mediastinal structures.[4] Intravenous contrast may be used with CT imaging to delineate the vascularity of the tumor and its surroundings[9,19] (Fig. 34.7). MR imaging is superior in identifying vascular compression and tissue invasion,[1] and distinguishing soft tissues from vascular structures.[9] In 25% of patients, MR may show more extensive disease than CT. It is the imaging modality recommended for neurogenic lesions, vascular abnormalities, and those disease processes involving the aortic arch and branches[1,4,20] (Fig. 34.8). Other uncommon modalities that may be seen are scintigraphy and positron emission tomography (PET), which is not used for primary imaging but can be used to follow up germ-cell tumors after initial treatment. Kitami et al.[21] performed a retrospective analysis of 109 patients to evaluate the usefulness of PET/CT findings in the classification and management of anterior mediastinal tumors. They found that the sensitivity, specificity, and accuracy of ^{18}F-fluorodeoxyglucose (FDG) in the detection of low-grade thymomas and thymomas with a maximum diameter of 50 mm or less and a standardized uptake value maximum of 3.4 or less (>2 is suggestive of malignancy SUV's=Standardized Uptake Values) were 85%, 48%, and 60%, respectively. The authors concluded that FDG-PET/CT is an objective and useful modality in the differential diagnosis and management of anterior mediastinal tumors.

Regardless of the imaging technique used, the anesthesiologist must personally review the images. A radiologist's report may not provide enough detail regarding the level of airway obstruction, tumor position, and cardiac compression that is crucial for the anesthesiologist for the safe care of these patients.[1]

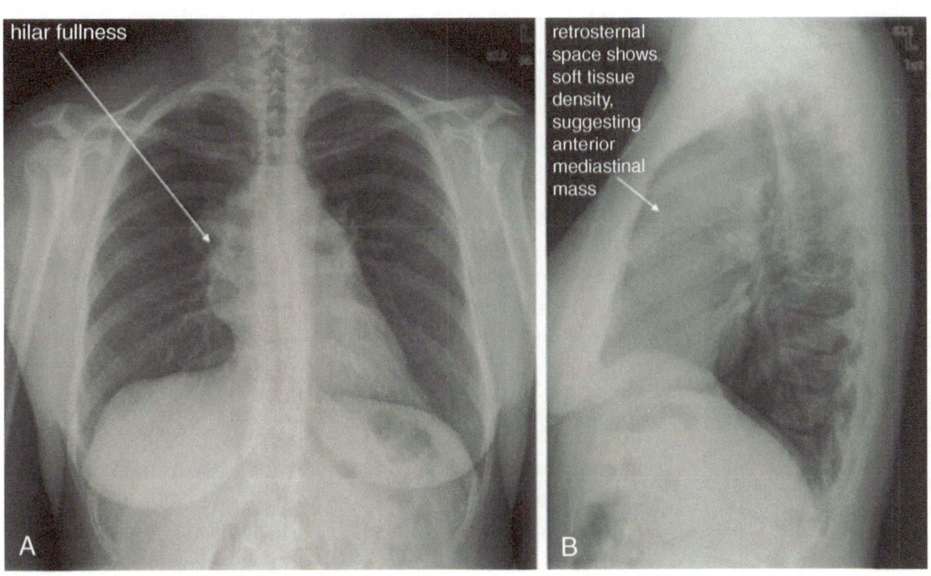

• **Fig. 34.6** Posterior-anterior (**A**) and lateral (**B**) chest x-rays in a patient with an anterior mediastinal mass and superior vena cava syndrome. (From Broder J. *Diagnostic Imaging for the Emergency Physician*. Philadelphia: Elsevier; 2011.)

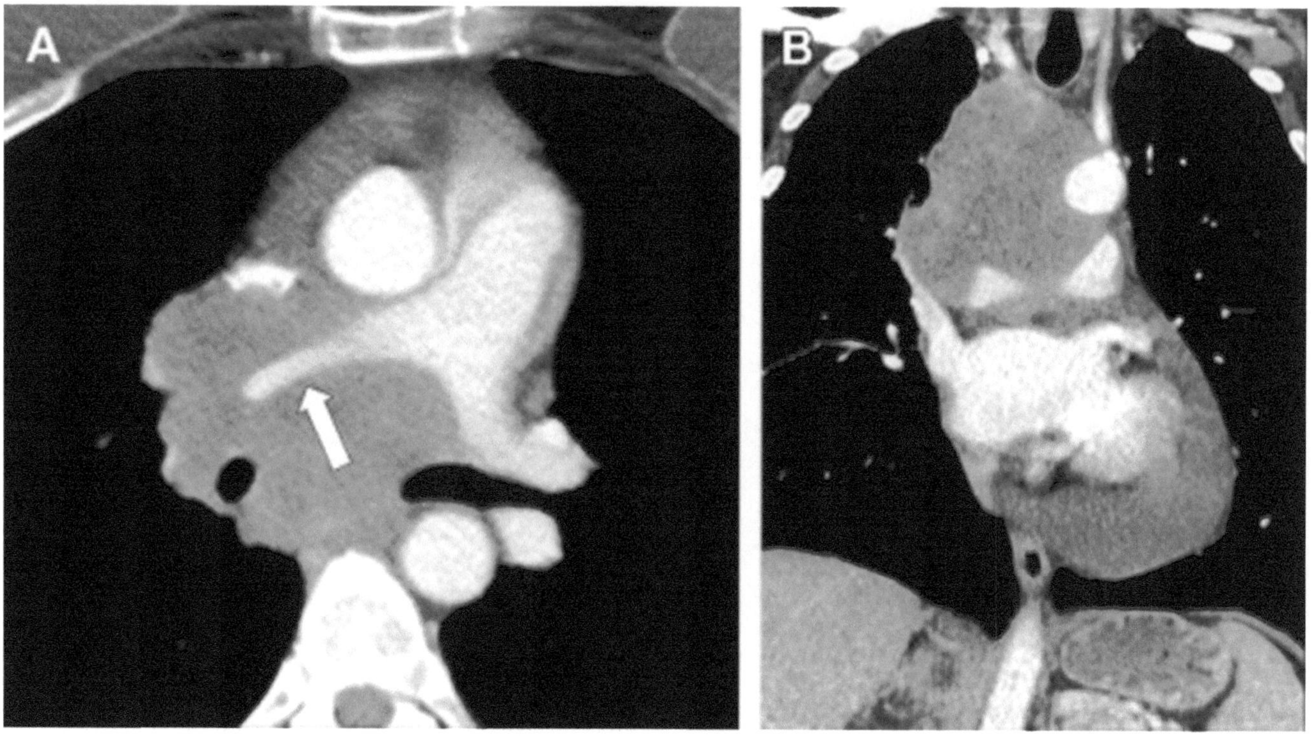

• **Fig. 34.7** Contrast enhanced computed tomography chest (**A**, axial) (**B**, coronal) showing a mediastinal mass with narrowing of the right pulmonary artery (*arrow*). (From Hayes SA, Plodkowski AJ, Ginsberg MS. Imaging of thoracic cavity tumors. *Surg Oncol Clin N Am*. 2014;23(4):709–733.)

Preoperative echocardiography is another diagnostic test that may be recommended for some patients. Echocardiography to assess a patient's cardiac structure and function can provide valuable information for the risk stratification of these patients.[9] Transthoracic echocardiography may be performed in both the supine and lateral positions to help detect positional changes on compression of the heart and the great vessels. Transesophageal echocardiography (TEE) has been shown to help detect the invasion of cardiac cavities and the vena cava. It can provide valuable information to help determine whether cardiac surgery standby is required.[22] Anderson et al.[23] reported a case of a patient with a posterior mediastinal mass requiring urgent cardiopulmonary bypass which was delineated by the perioperative TEE. Brooker et al.[24] reported a case where, after a pericardial window and chest tube placement for a pericardial effusion, TEE newly identified a mediastinal mass that encased the ascending aorta and pulmonary artery that was previously missed on preoperative chest x-ray and surface echocardiography (Fig. 34.9).[24] In addition, TEE can be a useful tool for improved staging of thymoma patients before surgery, which is the treatment of choice whenever a complete resection may be accomplished. After surgery, all thymomas, except completely encapsulated stage I tumors, should be treated with postoperative adjuvant radiation.

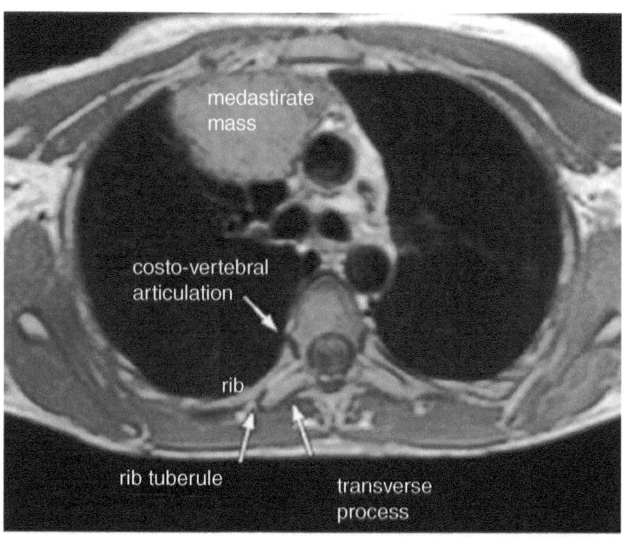

• **Fig. 34.8** Magnetic resonance imaging of the chest in a patient with a mediastinal mass. (From Carrier G, Fréchette E, Ugalde P, Deslauriers J. Correlative anatomy for the sternum and ribs, costovertebral angle, chest wall muscles and intercostal spaces, thoracic outlet. *Thorac Surg Clin*. 2007;17(4):521–528.)

The usefulness of preoperative pulmonary function tests (PFTs) appears to be the most controversial aspect of the preoperative assessment. Patients with mediastinal masses have flow volume loops that correlate with a fixed lesion because of a reduction in peak inspiratory and expiratory flows, which is usually the first value to be distorted[25,26] (Fig. 34.10). In 1984, Neuman et al.[27] stated that every patient should obtain upright and supine flow volume loops, as it is the most sensitive noninvasive way to diagnose airway obstruction. However, more recent opinions appear to disagree with this. Many have found that although PFTs can confirm the presence of obstructive or restrictive defects, they do not correlate with

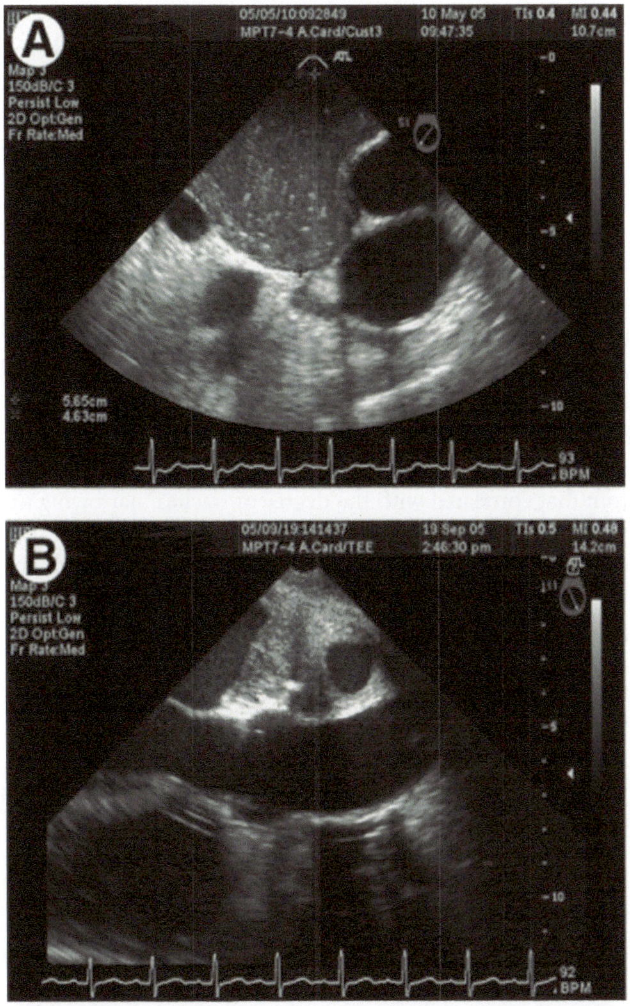

• **Fig. 34.9 Midesophageal transesophageal echocardiography imaging** (**A**, Midesophageal ascending aorta short axis view) (**B**, Midesophageal ascending aorta long-axis view) showing a mediastinal mass posterior to the ascending aorta. (From Brooker RF, Zvara DA, Roitstein A. Mediastinal mass diagnosed with intraoperative transesophageal echocardiography. *J Cardiothorac Vasc Anesth*. 2007;21(2):257–258.)

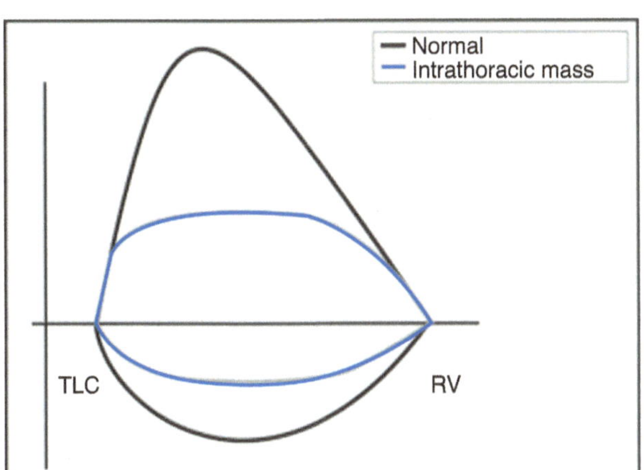

• **Fig. 34.10** Pulmonary function tests seen in patients with an intrathoracic mass. *RV,* Right ventricular; *TLC,* Total lung capacity. (From: Gerlac RM, Klafta JM. Mediastinal masses, complications in anesthesia. In: Fleisher LA, Rosenbaum SH (eds). 3rd ed. Philadelphia: Elsevier; 2018:262–265.)

perioperative outcomes or anatomic abnormalities, and provide no additional useful information compared with chest imaging,[1,4,28–31] A study by Hnatiuk et al.[32] looked at 37 patients with anterior mediastinal masses at the Walter Reed Army Medical Center over a 6-year period. Spirometry in the upright and supine positions was suggestive of possible upper airway obstruction in four patients. However, general anesthesia was used in all four patients without complications. The authors concluded that the recommendation to perform PFTs was anecdotal and PFTs were not better than imaging and symptoms at predicting perioperative complications.

It is important to note that if thymus or thyroid pathology is suspected, an anesthesiologist must recognize the endocrinologic risks associated with these abnormally functioning glands. The possibility of thyroid storm, myxedema coma, and myasthenia gravis, among other disease processes, must be considered. The management of these disorders, however, is beyond the scope of this chapter.

Risk Stratification

The increased anesthetic risk in patients with mediastinal masses is caused by the possibility of worsening compression of the pulmonary tree and/or cardiovascular structures and the subsequent effect on those systems. Compression of any part of the pulmonary tree can lead to a loss of the airway and difficulty with oxygenation and ventilation. It can lead to hypoxia, hypercarbia, ventilation-perfusion mismatch, and potential respiratory collapse. Compression of the heart or of any major vessels can lead to hypotension, decreased cardiac preload, increased afterload, and the potential for cardiovascular collapse. It is important to recognize that any or all of these complications can occur abruptly during any point during the perioperative period, although they appear to be most commonly seen on induction of anesthesia. Being able to recognize the symptoms and clinical findings that indicate a higher likelihood of perioperative complications is a tool every anesthesiologist must have in their armamentarium.

Some practitioners believe that in the absence of preoperative airway obstruction and severe clinical symptoms, general anesthesia may be safely induced in patients with anterior mediastinal masses. Ferrari et al.[33] conducted a chart review of 44 pediatric patients admitted to Memorial Sloan-Kettering Cancer Center with a diagnosis of anterior mediastinal mass that required surgery. No patient died or sustained permanent injury as a result of their anesthetic or operative experience. Of the nine patients with preoperative respiratory symptoms, two patients experienced difficulty on induction of anesthesia and required tracheal intubation with a rigid bronchoscope. Two others developed airway obstruction during anesthetic maintenance that was corrected with changes in patient position. The authors concluded that in the absence of life-threatening preoperative airway obstruction and severe clinical symptoms, general anesthesia may be safely induced before radiation therapy. Despite the authors conclusion, in that study, 4 out of 44 patients required unconventional measures to maintain

• BOX 34.1 Symptoms and Clinical Findings Associated With Increased Perioperative Risk

- Stridor
- Orthopnea
- Increased cough when supine
- Jugular venous distension
- Superior vena cava syndrome
- Syncope
- Pulmonary function tests (PFTs) with restrictive and obstructive pattern
- PFTs with peak expiratory flow <40% or <50% of predicted pericardial effusion
- Computed tomography scan with tracheal cross-sectional area <50%
- Large mediastinal masses with mediastinal mass ratio >45%
- Large mediastinal masses with standardized tumor volume >2.5

oxygenation during induction of anesthesia, using a rigid bronchoscopy or turning the patient in the lateral position to alleviate the tracheal compression. It is up to the anesthesiologist to consider the pros and cons of induction versus awake fiberoptic intubation.

However, perioperative complications can be seen in patients without preoperative symptoms or clinical findings,[34–36] and certain symptoms and clinical findings have been found to be associated with increased anesthetic risk (Box 34.1). One additional symptom to take seriously is syncope during a forced Valsalva maneuver, such as during a bowel movement, as this maneuver can further diminish venous return, and this may suggest significant cardiac or pulmonary artery compression.[2]

Bechard et al.[8] were the first to find a correlation between perioperative complications and cardiorespiratory signs and symptoms at initial presentation. They defined severe symptoms as the presence of stridor, orthopnea, cyanosis, jugular vein distension, or SVCS, which had high perioperative complication rates. Although the severity of symptoms did not remain a predictor after multivariate logistic regression analysis, they believed this was caused by a lack of statistical power. They concluded that it seems prudent to avoid general anesthesia, when possible, when severe cardiorespiratory signs and symptoms are observed. There are multiple reports of patients with SVCS who received general anesthesia and subsequently experienced perioperative events and/or death.[12,37,38]

Neuman et al.[27] state that general anesthesia should be avoided when a patient's PFTs are severely abnormal. Bechard et al.[8] found more than 10-fold increases in perioperative complications in patients with a peak expiratory flow of 40% or less. They also found increased risk in patients with combined obstructive and restrictive patterns on PFTs. As mentioned previously, others disagree and state that PFTs do not play a role in evaluating a patient's risk. Gothard[4] stated that lung function tests, including an arterial blood gas analysis, are usually performed to obtain a baseline, however, in the author and colleagues' experience, they do not play a large role in evaluating the risk of surgery. The author did note that it is important to realize that symptoms can be worse in the postoperative period, particularly following a biopsy procedure under general anesthesia, as the patient is exposed to the deleterious effects of anesthesia, including diminished lung volumes, or from positive pressure ventilation in the presence of SVCS without the benefits of tumor excision.

In regard to imaging, Azizkhan et al.[39] found that children are at risk for total airway obstruction during general anesthesia when the mediastinal masses are associated with severe tracheobronchial compression, defined in their study as greater than one-third decrease in luminal area.

Shamberger et al.[40] found in a retrospective study of 42 children that the presence of orthopnea was the only symptom that correlated with the degree of tracheal narrowing on CT scanning. Furthermore, their findings confirmed that general endotracheal anesthesia was safe in patients with anterior mediastinal masses and a tracheal cross-sectional area greater than 50%. It is important to note, however, that in this study, the majority of patients with a tracheal cross-sectional area of less than 50% received either local anesthesia, preoperative radiation to shrink the tumor size, or were kept spontaneously breathing. The same authors, in a prospective study, found no respiratory collapse when using only local anesthesia for patients with a tracheal cross-sectional area less than 50% or a peak expiratory flow less than 50%. They concluded that while the criteria may be too restrictive, it is not too permissive.[25]

King et al.,[28] in a retrospective study of 51 children, confirmed Shamberger's findings that patients with evidence of tracheal narrowing of greater than 50% of CT scanning are at the greatest perioperative risk. Furthermore, they found tumor size to be the most important factor for the incidence of complications. A mediastinal mass ratio (MMR), defined as the maximum width of the mediastinal mass divided by the maximum intrathoracic width as seen on anterior-posterior chest films, was calculated for all patients. None of the patients with a small mass, defined as an MMR of less than or equal to 30%, experienced airway collapse. Large masses were defined as greater than or equal to an MMR of 45%, and the average MMR of those experiencing airway obstruction was 56%. They also found respiratory symptoms to be a reasonable indicator of airway compression and risks with general anesthesia.

Bechard et al.[8] found pericardial effusions to be associated with intraoperative complications and confirmed that, in their patients, tracheal compression greater than 50% on preoperative CT was associated with postoperative respiratory complications.

Kawaguchi et al.[41] retrospectively evaluated 31 pediatric patients and compared those who experienced respiratory collapse to those who did not. Their analysis revealed that all eight patients with tracheal collapse had large tumors in the anterior mediastinum. Size was calculated using a standardized tumor volume (STV), a formula adapted from the formula for the volume of an ellipsoid. Using an STV cutoff value of 2.5, the sensitivity and specificity were 0.86 for predicting airway collapse under general anesthesia.

A large clinical experience in the literature discusses perioperative management and complications in children or those with anterior mediastinal masses, as these are the most common cases. Identifying the risk factors that may indicate potentially increased perioperative complication rates is key to the safe anesthetic management of a patient with a mediastinal mass. Risk stratifying these patients, and determining an appropriate anesthetic plan, is a complex process. Every patient needs his or her own "individually tailored" perioperative plan. A preoperative interdisciplinary discussion between the anesthesiologist, the surgeon, and frequently the radiologist, should be a requirement for all patients.[35,42] The varying degrees of clinical presentation, ranging from patients who are completely asymptomatic to those who present with complete cardiovascular or cardiopulmonary collapse, is of particular concern. As mentioned previously, a lack of symptoms during clinical examination does not guarantee an uneventful anesthetic course once general anesthesia is initiated.

Those patients with any of the findings listed in Box 34.1 should be treated with caution. Although general anesthesia may be administered safely in those without any of the findings listed in Box 34.1, extreme caution and constant vigilance is essential.[43] Complications may even occur despite the most conservative perioperative management and in those considered low risk and without symptoms.[35,43–46] There is numerous evidence from previous reports that complications can occur at any moment, both intraoperatively and postoperatively, regardless of the size and location of the mediastinal mass.[2,30,42,44,47] These patients can also present for emergency surgery unrelated to their mediastinal mass.[48]

Szokol et al.[36] presented a case of a 29-year-old patient in her 32nd week of twin gestation with anemia secondary to a gastrointestinal bleed (GIB). Because she had several episodes of bloody emesis, an emergency cesarean delivery was performed under general anesthesia followed by twin delivery. During an upper endoscopy to identify the source of the GIB, it became difficult to ventilate the patient once the endoscope was advanced into the esophagus. When the endoscope was pulled back, ventilation improved. At this point, there was concern of a possible chest mass with tracheal compression exacerbated by the endoscope. The patient was taken for chest CT which demonstrated a 6.4 × 6.9-cm mediastinal mass with significant compression of the right pulmonary artery, SVC, trachea, right mainstem bronchus, and right upper lobe bronchus, all of which were unrecognized before the induction of anesthesia.

Anesthetic Management

Preoperative Treatment Considerations

Once a patient's preoperative workup has been completed and the risks have been established, an anesthetic plan can be devised. As mentioned previously, a preoperative interdisciplinary team should be established as soon as possible to discuss the patient's management.[35,42] This team should include a member from anesthesiology, surgery, radiology, pathology, and oncology. The involvement of additional team members should be patient-specific. This team can help determine whether the goal is to obtain a small tissue sample for histologic diagnosis to establish a radiation or chemotherapy treatment plan to shrink the mass before complete excision. The next step is to consider is whether general anesthesia is necessary. If only a tissue biopsy of the mass is necessary, it is reasonable to obtain a sample using only local anesthesia in the operating room or in an international radiology suite.[28,39,49] Samples for histologic diagnosis may also be obtained by other methods, such as via pleural fluid, bone marrow aspiration, lymph node biopsy, and peripheral blood sample.[49,50] If this is not possible, or if the plan is for mass excision, general anesthesia may be necessary.

In those patients needing general anesthesia, or in those high-risk patients receiving local anesthesia or minimal sedation, preoperative treatment with chemotherapy, radiation, and/or steroids should be considered.[2,39] Depending on the histologic diagnosis, neoadjuvant therapy can be helpful in reducing tumor burden, potentially leading to resectability in initially inoperable cases, or greatly facilitating surgical resection. On one hand, those in favor of preoperative treatment argue that many tumors, especially lymphomas, are very sensitive to radiotherapy and will shrink after minimal treatment, thereby reducing the incidence of perioperative complications and improving overall anesthetic risk.[2,17,33] On the other hand, those against pretreatment argue that a good sample is needed for accurate diagnosis and optimal treatment, and pretreatment risks interfering with obtaining an adequate sample, distorting cellular morphology, and impairing accurate histologic diagnosis.[2,33,40] When lymphoma is suspected, the use of steroids can interfere with proper diagnosis.[2] Some authors have concluded that when pretreatment is necessary, treatment with radiation is favored over steroids.[2,40] A reasonable approach in these situations may be to exclude some tissue from the radiation field so that an accurate sample and diagnosis can be made at a later stage.[2,40,51]

Tracheal stenting may be another consideration to decrease the chances of compression of the tracheobronchial tree, which may be aggravated in the supine position and with use of muscle relaxants. Flexible metal tracheal stents have been placed through a laryngeal mask airway with a patient under propofol and sevoflurane general anesthesia.[52] An awake intubation using dexmedetomidine sedation, followed by general anesthesia using higher doses of dexmedetomidine, has also successfully been used to place a silicone Y stent through a rigid bronchoscope.[53] In patients with SVCS, the preoperative placement of an SVC stent using fluoroscopy, to relieve the obstruction and improve symptomatology, should be considered as well (Fig. 34.11).

Monitors, Access, and Positioning Considerations

Before anesthesia induction, all patients with mediastinal masses should receive an arterial line for continuous blood pressure monitoring. Large bore intravenous access should be placed as well to administer medications and fluids. Placement of central venous access is another consideration,

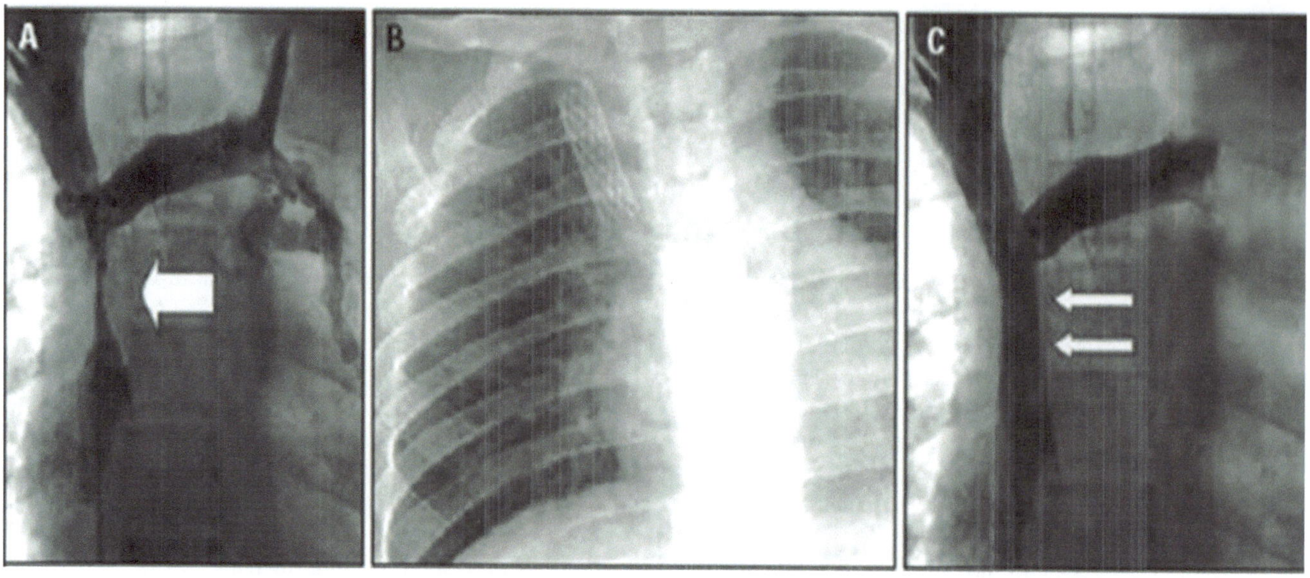

• **Fig. 34.11** Preoperative placement of a superior vena cava stent using fluoroscopy, to relieve obstruction. (**A**) Superior Vena Cavogram demonstrating obstruction (*arrow*). (**B**) Fluouroscopic image of a stent placed to relieve the obstrction. (**C**) Superior Vena Cavogram with the obstruction relieved (*arrows*).

especially in patients believed to be at risk of complications.[35] All other standard monitors, including continuous electrocardiography, pulse oximetry, and end-tidal carbon dioxide monitoring, should be used.

In cases when SVC involvement is suspected preoperatively, or where an SVC cross-clamp or innominate vein to right atrium bypass may be used, additional monitoring modalities to assess adequacy of cerebral perfusion, preferably cerebral oximetry with near-infrared spectroscopy or transcranial Doppler in combination with simultaneous monitoring of jugular vein pressure, should be strongly considered.[9] Depending on the extent of SVC involvement, partial resection or complete resection followed by reconstruction with prosthetic grafts or vein grafts, can be performed. Spaggiari et al.[54] advocated partial resection if less than 50% of the circumference of the SVC is affected, with a pericardial patch repair when needed. Although partial resection can be performed with partial clamping alone when SVC involvement is minimal, cross-clamping of the SVC with systematic heparinization is the most used technique for reconstruction. The authors reported a series of 70 consecutive patients[52] with lung cancer and 18 with mediastinal tumors who underwent SVC resection secondary to SVC involvement. There were 25 replacements (36%) of the SVC by prosthesis, whereas the remaining underwent partial resection. Major postoperative morbidity and mortality rates in lung cancer patients were 23% and 7.7%, respectively, and 50% and 5.6% in patients with mediastinal tumors.

Planning the ideal location for these lines and monitors is important. In patients with SVCS, all intravenous access should be placed in the lower extremity. This will ensure adequate and timely delivery of medication and fluid or blood to the patient.[11,34,35,37] Placing the pulse oximeter and the arterial line on opposite arms may be prudent. This may help to quickly diagnose an area or vessel being compressed. Using a noninvasive blood pressure cuff for this purpose is less desirable because the data are not continuous. The compression might go unrecognized, and the diagnosis may be delayed.

Patient positioning during transportation and on arrival to the operating room is also important. With SVCS, having the patient sitting upright will help reduce the facial, airway, and upper extremity swelling.[34,35,37] This may be particularly helpful when airway manipulation is attempted. Every patient should be asked for his/her position of greatest comfort, such as lying prone or lying on the right or left side.[35,55] Knowing this will provide a clue of the dynamic nature of the patient's intrathoracic mass. If complications are seen, tilting the operating room table, or moving the patient into the position of greatest comfort, may relieve the obstruction, while other, more permanent, measures are sought.[45,56,57]

Equipment Considerations

It is necessary to ensure that all possible necessary medications and equipment are present and easily accessible. This includes both anesthetic equipment, as well as surgical equipment. When complications from a mediastinal mass occur, the effects are quick and potentially life-threatening. Having to wait even moments for rescue medications or equipment can be life-threatening.

All possible medications that may be needed, including inotropes and vasopressors, should be drawn up and readily available. Multiple laryngoscopes and endotracheal tubes (ETTs) should be present in the operating room. This includes ETTs of different sizes, different lengths, such as microlaryngeal tubes, and different types, such as reinforced and double lumen tubes (DLTs). There are numerous reports of respiratory complications being relieved by laryngoscopy,[58] advancing an ETT, passing a smaller diameter ETT, or passing a longer ETT beyond the area of compression.[10,37,56,59] If necessary, using a

DLT may provide a more stable patent airway than a standard polyvinyl chloride ETT because it is more rigid.[45]

Having a rigid bronchoscope in the room, with an experienced provider ready to use it, is another important piece of equipment that must be present and can be a life-saving device. A rigid bronchoscope, which is more solid and sturdy than an ETT, has a higher likelihood of being able to displace a mass that is causing airway compression. The rigid bronchoscope will also enable the surgeon to stent open the airway, thereby enabling patient oxygenation and ventilation through the rigid bronchoscope.[56,59] The mode of ventilation to be used with the rigid bronchoscope, such as high-frequency jet ventilation, should be planned in advance, and the ventilator should be readily available and tested before the induction of anesthesia.

Cardiopulmonary bypass (CPB), as well as staff capable of initiating and maintaining CPB, must be considered for high-risk patients. This involves having a cardiac surgeon and perfusionist present. The use of CPB can maintain patient oxygenation, ventilation, and perfusion if any or all of these functions become compromised. If a mediastinal mass were to compress the airway, the CPB can be initiated to replace the role of the lungs.[60] If the mass were to obstruct the inflow or outflow of the heart, CPB can maintain adequate perfusion.

The approaches that have been used with CPB range from having everything "standby" in the room to cannulating the patient and initiating CPB before induction of anesthesia. Although there are reports of unexpected cardiopulmonary collapse and the use of CPB as a rescue maneuver, cannulation and initiation of CPB using a femorofemoral approach takes approximately 20 minutes, even with the most experienced providers.[29,42,55] Most reports seem to agree that CPB standby is not an acceptable rescue measure for symptomatic or high-risk patients, as the time it takes to initiate CPB increases the risk of neurologic injury and death.[30,42,61,62] Some argue that placing wires into the femoral vessels is adequate, as this can save time and provide quicker cannulation.[29] However, these wires may be lost, kinked, or dislocated during attempted emergency cannulation.[42] Therefore when the need for cardiopulmonary collapse is likely, patients should have their femoral vessels cannulated awake, under local anesthesia, before induction of anesthesia. In severe cases, CPB may be initiated while the patient is awake and maintained until CPB is no longer needed.[44,63–66] Alternative locations for the CPB cannulas can also be used depending on the nature of the situation. For example, a jugulosaphenous venovenous shunt can be used in cases of SVCS to relieve and avoid an increase in venous pressure and prevent complications because of respiratory compression.[67]

Having TEE present, with a provider who is able to obtain appropriate images and interpret them quickly, should be considered. TEE has been used in patients with mediastinal masses during moments of hemodynamic instability to help guide intraoperative management.[29,42,68–70] TEE is a valuable tool to help monitor real-time cardiac function and as mentioned previously, can provide valuable information on the extent of the mass and possible cardiac or great vessels invasion.

Last, Linnaus et al.[71] report using a sternal hook connected to a sternal elevator to lift the chest and temporarily reverse the respiratory complications seen with an anterior mediastinal mass.

Considerations for General Anesthesia Induction

Induction of general anesthesia causes a reduction in lung volumes, particularly functional residual capacity, especially in the supine position.[25,27,61,72] Relaxation of bronchial smooth muscle and the loss of chest wall muscle tone cause greater compressibility.[2] Muscle paralysis and the loss of spontaneous diaphragmatic movement lead to increased ventilation-perfusion mismatch[72] and reduces the normal transpleural pressure gradient that normally helps stent the airways open.[51,61] These changes are more pronounced in patients with mediastinal masses with extrinsic compression of the pulmonary or cardiovascular system by the mediastinal mass and limited reserve.[2] These effects increase the risks of respiratory complications in patients who are already at risk.

As mentioned earlier, patient positioning is key in preparation for anesthesia induction. A priori knowledge of a position that the patient finds most comfortable may be helpful.[35] During general anesthesia, the loss of muscle tone from muscle relaxant makes the airways susceptible to collapse because of external compression by mediastinal masses. Furthermore, the supine position leads to cephalic displacement of the diaphragm and reduces thoracic anteroposterior diameter. Therefore patient repositioning can ameliorate airway obstruction by an anterior mediastinal tumor during general anesthesia. If ventilatory compromise occurs following anesthesia induction, changing the patient's position to the lateral decubitus position is immediately feasible until other interventions to resolve the tumor-related cardiorespiratory complications can be initiated. During the preoperative evaluation of images, the location of the mediastinal mass should be clearly established. Should complications occur, the patient should be turned so that the dependent hemithorax is the one most occupied by the mass. This would theoretically displace the mass away from the trachea and alleviate the tracheal compressing because of gravity.[73]

Furthermore, increases in intrathoracic pressure, such as during a Valsalva maneuver or with patient bucking, must be avoided in the presence of SVCS. Patients with SVCS should also remain in the upright position to help with venous drainage. Preoperative sedatives that may cause respiratory depression or muscle relaxation should be avoided.

A number of concerns must be addressed before anesthesia induction and airway management in patients with mediastinal masses. The first is whether paralysis will be used or if the patient should remain spontaneously breathing throughout the case. Although low-risk patients will often tolerate standard intravenous induction (with or without muscle relaxation), patients at intermediate or high risk of airway compression should be kept spontaneously breathing at least until one is certain that paralysis and controlled ventilation are safe. This can be accomplished with either an inhalational induction or small intravenous boluses of induction agents. However, airway collapse has been reported even in cases of maintaining spontaneous ventilation, thus the highest risk patients should not be induced without consideration for the use of CPB.

In contrast to the classical teaching that these patients should be kept spontaneously breathing, Hartigan et al.[74] showed, via a video bronchoscopy of the carina in patients with anterior mediastinal masses, an increase in airway area following paralysis and positive pressure ventilation. Despite this finding, it is recommended to maintain spontaneous respiration in all patients with mediastinal masses until one is absolutely certain that paralysis and positive pressure ventilation can be safely administered without any respiratory or cardiovascular complications.

The relationship of laminar and turbulent airway flow in these patients must also be considered. As the size of the airway narrows, velocity increases to maintain the same flow rate. Once a threshold velocity is reached, flow changes from laminar to turbulent flow. Once past the obstruction or narrowing, flow must resume laminar flow to reach the distal airways. However, if the pressures and turbulent flows are too high and unable to resume laminar flow, ventilation of the distal airways may not be achievable. An anesthesiologist's first reaction is to hand ventilate with higher pressures when issues with oxygenation or ventilation are seen. This reaction may not be helpful, and may be harmful, for these patients.[51]

Another consideration with anesthesia induction is whether the patient needs an awake fiberoptic intubation or if a standard asleep induction can be used. The decision should be made based on the patient's preoperative airway assessment and whether additional information would be gained from observing the status and the diameter of the patient's airway. Some encourage continuous bronchoscopic airway monitoring to provide an early warning of airway collapse.[75]

Anesthesia can be safely induced and maintained with any combination of the commonly used anesthetic medications today. These may include the inhaled anesthetics, opioids, ketamine, dexmedetomidine, and propofol.[51,53,57,76] The patient must be closely monitored, and the drugs administered must be carefully titrated to maintain the desired depth of anesthesia. This is particularly crucial when the maintenance of spontaneous respiration is desired to prevent apnea and respiratory collapse. Vasoactive drugs should be immediately available to treat any cardiovascular instability.

Much of this discussion is summarized in our process flow diagram (Fig. 34.12) that displays one approach to these complex patients.

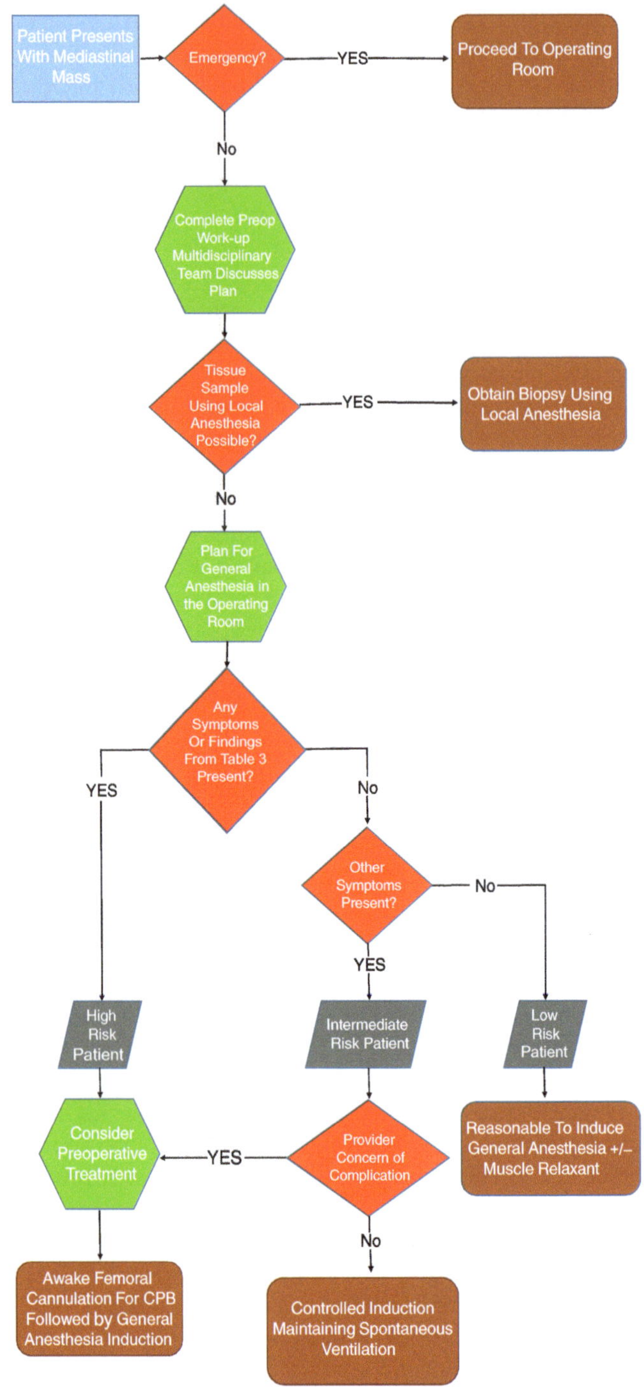

• **Fig. 34.12** Management flowchart for anesthetic care of patients with mediastinal masses.

Potential Complications

In patients with mediastinal masses, the most feared complications are related to compression of pulmonary and/or cardiovascular structures. Regardless of the reason behind the new onset or acute change in compression, hemodynamic and respiratory collapse can ensue, possibly followed shortly thereafter with patient death. Even with the most conservative approach, complications can occur.[44] One must always be prepared. **Most importantly, never burn your bridges!** Always define a backup plan that is familiar to the entire team should the initial plan fail.

A wheeze should not automatically be interpreted as peripheral bronchospasm, as it may reflect tracheal or bronchial compression.[38] With large mediastinal masses, difficult intubation is a possibility because of the anatomic changes from tracheal compression. Airway swelling when the mediastinal mass is associated with SVCS may make intubation challenging. This airway edema may still be present after surgery, which can complicate extubation as well. When preparing for extubation in patients with SVCS, patients should be spontaneously breathing, to avoid the increases in intrathoracic pressure seen with positive pressure ventilation, and positioned in the sitting position to assist with venous drainage and decrease upper body swelling.

The recurrent laryngeal nerve may be damaged during surgery in the chest, thereby complicating patient extubation from vocal cord involvement. Furthermore, tracheomalacia can occur from prolonged compression of the airway, which may present as a tracheal collapse during expiration. As such, it is prudent to extubate over an intubating stylet with racemic epinephrine in certain situations.[35] Observation in an intensive care unit postoperatively is prudent.

Other complications that can occur are major hemorrhage, especially in the presence of increased venous pressures seen with SVCS or during the use of CPB because of the systemic heparinization required.[9,77] As with any chest surgery, pleural effusion, hemothorax, chylothorax, and/or pneumothorax can be seen.

Managing Our Case

The case presented involves a 30-year-old female with an anterior mediastinal mass. Her physical examination indicated orthopnea and SVCS, and her preoperative imaging included a CT scan showing a tracheal cross-sectional area less than 50%, all of which are severe features consistent with increased perioperative morbidity and mortality. A multidisciplinary team was formed to discuss her case. The team included an oncologist, thoracic surgeon, anesthesiologist, radiologist, and pathologist. Because the patient was cooperative and the location of the mass was amenable to CT-guided biopsy, it was determined that a CT-guided biopsy was the safest approach. The concern was the patient's ability to be positioned properly and lie flat enough to enter the CT scanner.

When the patient was brought to the CT suite, she was positioned comfortably in a semi-recumbent position using pillows. She was able to lie flat enough to fit into the CT scanner without causing her symptoms to worsen. She tolerated the procedure well without complication. An adequate tissue sample was obtained and a diagnosis of lymphoma was made by the pathologist. The oncologists soon started her on a chemotherapy and radiation treatment regimen.

Her symptoms significantly improved. She was able to lie nearly fully supine and her cough was no longer present. However, although her facial and upper extremity swelling improved, SVCS was still present. Follow-up imaging showed a reduction in the size of her mass, but still with some compression of the trachea and great vessels remained. The multidisciplinary team determined that the mass should be resected.

The patient was brought to the operating room. No sedation was administered. An arterial line and large bore lower extremity intravenous access were placed. Because of the fact that severe symptoms and clinical findings remained, her femoral artery and vein were cannulated with the patient awake using local anesthesia for potential need of femorofemoral bypass. A careful combination of dexmedetomidine and propofol infusions, titrated slowly, were then used to induce general anesthesia while keeping the patient spontaneously breathing. Once under general anesthesia, the patient was intubated with a reinforced ETT using a fiberoptic scope to evaluate her trachea. She tolerated anesthesia induction without any complications. A TEE probe was then placed as well to monitor her cardiac function and any effects by the mass. The operation proceeded via a median sternotomy without any evidence of cardiopulmonary compromise. CPB was not used and no blood products were administered. Upon completion of the procedure and decannulation of her femoral vessels, she was brought intubated to the intensive care unit where she was extubated later that evening.

Conclusion

Mediastinal masses can present in a number of ways. Recognizing them and ensuring proper evaluation of a patient with a mediastinal mass is important to safely manage these patients. Improved knowledge and understanding of the pathophysiology have reduced the perioperative morbidity and mortality in this patient population. According to the American Society of Anesthesiologists Closed Claims project database, there were only five pediatric claims in patients with anterior mediastinal masses, all of which were in the 1980s.[78] Over the past few decades, fewer reports of intraoperative fatalities and decreased morbidity indicate that perioperative management of these patients has improved. Airway complications are now more likely to occur postoperatively.[30]

Thorough preoperative assessment and knowledge of the location and the size of the mass and its relationship to adjacent structures are critical for anesthesia planning. One should always err on the side of caution, as these masses can be unpredictable with severe complications. Some may find it difficult to perform these procedures awake or to cannulate the femoral vessels for CPB when it may not end up being necessary. It is always better to have it and not need it rather than need it and not have it. Finally, close communication with the surgical team, thorough risk assessment, and formulating a plan in advance for intraoperative respiratory or cardiovascular complications all contribute to the successful management of these complex cases.

References

1. Narang S, Harte BH, Body SC. Anesthesia for patients with a mediastinal mass. *Anesthesiol Clin North Am*. 2001;19(3):559–579.
2. Pullerits J, Holzman R. Anaesthesia for patients with mediastinal masses. *Can J Anaesth*. 1989;36(6):681–688.
3. Liu W, Deslauriers J. Mediastinal divisions and compartments. *Thorac Surg Clin*. 2011;21(2):183–190.
4. Gothard JW. Anesthetic considerations for patients with anterior mediastinal masses. *Anesthesiol Clin*. 2008;26(2):305–314, vi.
5. Salgia R, Blanco R, Skarin AT. Lung cancer and tumors of the heart and mediastinum. In: Skarin AT, ed. *Atlas of Diagnostic Oncology*. 4th ed. Philadelphia: Elsevier; 2010:98–159.
6. Yoneda KY, Louie S, Shelton DK. Mediastinal tumors. *Curr Opin Pulm Med*. 2001;7(4):226–233.
7. Dubashi B, Cyriac S, Tenali SG. Clinicopathological analysis and outcome of primary mediastinal malignancies—a report of 91 cases from a single institute. *Ann Thorac Med*. 2009;4(3):140–142.
8. Béchard P, Létourneau L, Lacasse Y, Côté D, Bussières JS. Perioperative cardiorespiratory complications in adults with mediastinal mass: incidence and risk factors. *Anesthesiology*. 2004;100(4): 826–834.
9. Li WW, Van boven WJ, Annema JT, Eberl S, Klomp HM, De mol BA. Management of large mediastinal masses: surgical and anesthesiological considerations. *J Thorac Dis*. 2016;8(3):E175–E184.
10. Thakur P, Bhatia P, Sitalakshmi N, Virmani P. Anaesthesia for mediastinal mass. *Indian J Anaesth*. 2014;58(2):215–217.
11. Lokich J, Goodman R. Superior vena cava syndrome. *JAMA*. 1975;231(1):58–61.
12. Northrip DR, Bohman BK, Tsueda K. Total airway occlusion and superior vena cava syndrome in a child with an anterior mediastinal tumor. *Anesth Analg*. 1986;65(10):1079–1082.
13. Amaha K, Okutsu Y, Nakamura Y. Major airway obstruction by mediastinal tumour. A case report. *Br J Anaesth*. 1973;45(10): 1082–1084.
14. Bittar D. Respiratory obstruction associated with induction of general anesthesia in a patient with mediastinal Hodgkin's disease. *Anesth Analg*. 1975;54(3):399–403.
15. Keon TP. Death on induction of anesthesia for cervical node biopsy. *Anesthesiology*. 1981;55(4):471–472.
16. Levin H, Bursztein S, Heifetz M. Cardiac arrest in a child with an anterior mediastinal mass. *Anesth Analg*. 1985;64(11):1129–1130.
17. Piro AJ, Weiss DR, Hellman S. Mediastinal Hodgkin's disease: a possible danger for intubation anesthesia. Intubation danger in Hodgkin's disease. *Int J Radiat Oncol Biol Phys*. 1976;1(5–6): 415–419.
18. Broder J. *Diagnostic Imaging for the Emergency Physician*. Philadelphia: Elsevier; 2011.
19. Hayes SA, Plodkowski AJ, Ginsberg MS. Imaging of thoracic cavity tumors. *Surg Oncol Clin N Am*. 2014;23(4):709–733.
20. Carrier G, Fréchette E, Ugalde P, Deslauriers J. Correlative anatomy for the sternum and ribs, costovertebral angle, chest wall muscles and intercostal spaces, thoracic outlet. *Thorac Surg Clin*. 2007; 17(4):521–528.
21. Kitami A, Sano F, Ohashi S, et al. The usefulness of positron-emission tomography findings in the management of anterior mediastinal tumors. *Ann Thorac Cardiovasc Surg*. 2017;23(1):26–30.
22. Oneglia C, Di fabio D, Bonora-ottoni D, Rusconi C. Is transesophageal echocardiography useful in planning surgery of mediastinal thymomas? Transesophageal investigation of a mediastinal thymoma. *Int J Cardiol*. 2007;121(3):312–314.
23. Anderson DM, Dimitrova GT, Awad H. Patient with posterior mediastinal mass requiring urgent cardiopulmonary bypass. *Anesthesiology*. 2011;114(6):1488–1493.
24. Brooker RF, Zvara DA, Roitstein A. Mediastinal mass diagnosed with intraoperative transesophageal echocardiography. *J Cardiothorac Vasc Anesth*. 2007;21(2):257–258.
25. Shamberger RC, Holzman RS, Griscom NT, Tarbell NJ, Weinstein HJ, Wohl ME. Prospective evaluation by computed tomography and pulmonary function tests of children with mediastinal masses. *Surgery*. 1995;118(3):468–471.
26. Gerlac RM, Klafta JM. Mediastinal masses, complications in anesthesia. In: Fleisher LA, Rosenbaum SH, eds. *Complications in Anesthesia*. 3rd ed. Philadelphia: Elsevier; 2018:262–265.
27. Neuman GG, Weingarten AE, Abramowitz RM, Kushins LG, Abramson AL, Ladner W. The anesthetic management of the patient with an anterior mediastinal mass. *Anesthesiology*. 1984;60(2):144–147.
28. King DR, Patrick LE, Ginn-Pease ME, Mccoy KS, Klopfenstein K. Pulmonary function is compromised in children with mediastinal lymphoma. *J Pediatr Surg*. 1997;32(2):294–299.
29. Rath L, Gullahorn G, Connolly N, Pratt T, Boswell G, Cornelissen C. Anterior mediastinal mass biopsy and resection: anesthetic techniques and perioperative concerns. *Semin Cardiothorac Vasc Anesth*. 2012;16(4):235–242.
30. Slinger P, Karsli C. Management of the patient with a large anterior mediastinal mass: recurring myths. *Curr Opin Anaesthesiol*. 2007;20(1):1–3.
31. Vander Els NJ, Sorhage F, Bach AM, Straus DJ, White DA. Abnormal flow volume loops in patients with intrathoracic Hodgkin's disease. *Chest*. 2000;117(5):1256–1261.
32. Hnatiuk OW, Corcoran PC, Sierra A. Spirometry in surgery for anterior mediastinal masses. *Chest*. 2001;120(4):1152–1156.
33. Ferrari LR, Bedford RF. General anesthesia prior to treatment of anterior mediastinal masses in pediatric cancer patients. *Anesthesiology*. 1990;72(6):991–995.
34. Dubey PK, Tripathi N. Anesthetic considerations in a patient with large anterior mediastinal mass. *J Cardiothorac Vasc Anesth*. 2019;33(4):1073–1075.
35. Erdös G, Tzanova I. Perioperative anaesthetic management of mediastinal mass in adults. *Eur J Anaesthesiol*. 2009;26(8):627–632.
36. Szokol JW, Alspach D, Mehta MK, Parilla BV, Liptay MJ. Intermittent airway obstruction and superior vena cava syndrome in a patient with an undiagnosed mediastinal mass after cesarean delivery. *Anesth Analg*. 2003;97(3):883–884.
37. Chaudhary K, Gupta A, Wadhawan S, Jain D, Bhadoria P. Anesthetic management of superior vena cava syndrome due to anterior mediastinal mass. *J Anaesthesiol Clin Pharmacol*. 2012;28(2): 242–246.
38. Mackie AM, Watson CB. Anaesthesia and mediastinal masses. A case report and review of the literature. *Anaesthesia*. 1984;39(9): 899–903.
39. Azizkhan RG, Dudgeon DL, Buck JR, et al. Life-threatening airway obstruction as a complication to the management of mediastinal masses in children. *J Pediatr Surg*. 1985;20(6):816–822.
40. Shamberger RC, Holzman RS, Griscom NT, Tarbell NJ, Weinstein HJ. CT quantitation of tracheal cross-sectional area as a guide to the surgical and anesthetic management of children with anterior mediastinal masses. *J Pediatr Surg*. 1991;26(2):138–142.
41. Kawaguchi Y, Saito T, Mitsunaga T, et al. Prediction of respiratory collapse among pediatric patients with mediastinal tumors during induction of general anesthesia. *J Pediatr Surg*. 2018;53(7): 1365–1368.

42. Anderson DM, Dimitrova GT, Awad H. Patient with posterior mediastinal mass requiring urgent cardiopulmonary bypass. *Anesthesiology*. 2011;114(6):1488–1493.
43. Takeda S, Miyoshi S, Omori K, Okumura M, Matsuda H. Surgical rescue for life-threatening hypoxemia caused by a mediastinal tumor. *Ann Thorac Surg*. 1999;68(6):2324–2326.
44. Gardner JC, Royster RL. Airway collapse with an anterior mediastinal mass despite spontaneous ventilation in an adult. *Anesth Analg*. 2011;113(2):239–242.
45. Lee J, Rim YC, In J. An anterior mediastinal mass: delayed airway compression and using a double lumen tube for airway patency. *J Thorac Dis*. 2014;6(6):E99–E103.
46. Stricker PA, Gurnaney HG, Litman RS. Anesthetic management of children with an anterior mediastinal mass. *J Clin Anesth*. 2010; 22(3):159–163.
47. Shapiro BP, Sprung J, Scott K, Arendt K, Krowka MJ, Afessa B. Cardiovascular collapse induced by position-dependent pulmonary vein occlusion in a patient with fibrosing mediastinitis. *Anesthesiology*. 2005;103(3):661–663.
48. Shi D, Webb CA, Wagner M, Dizdarevic A. Anesthetic evaluation and perioperative management in a patient with new onset mediastinal mass syndrome presenting for emergency surgery. *Case Rep Anesthesiol*. 2011;2011:782391.
49. Acker SN, Linton J, Tan GM, et al. A multidisciplinary approach to the management of anterior mediastinal masses in children. *J Pediatr Surg*. 2015;50(5):875–878.
50. Malik R, Mullassery D, Kleine-Brueggeney M, et al. Anterior mediastinal masses - A multidisciplinary pathway for safe diagnostic procedures. *J Pediatr Surg*. 2019;54(2):251–254.
51. Sibert KS, Biondi JW, Hirsch NP. Spontaneous respiration during thoracotomy in a patient with a mediastinal mass. *Anesth Analg*. 1987;66(9):904–907.
52. Rajagopalan S, Harbott M, Ortiz J, Bandi V. Anesthetic management of a large mediastinal mass for tracheal stent placement. *Braz J Anesthesiol*. 2016;66(2):215–218.
53. Abdelmalak B, Marcanthony N, Abdelmalak J, Machuzak MS, Gildea TR, Doyle DJ. Dexmedetomidine for anesthetic management of anterior mediastinal mass. *J Anesth*. 2010;24(4):607–610.
54. Spaggiari L, Leo F, Veronesi G, et al. Superior vena cava resection for lung and mediastinal malignancies: a single-center experience with 70 cases. *Ann Thorac Surg*. 2007;83(1):223–229.
55. Asai T. Emergency cardiopulmonary bypass in a patient with a mediastinal mass. *Anaesthesia*. 2007;62(8):859–860.
56. Bray RJ, Fernandes FJ. Mediastinal tumour causing airway obstruction in anaesthetised children. *Anaesthesia*. 1982;37:571–575.
57. Sharifian Attar A, Jalaeian Taghaddomi R, Bagheri R. Anesthetic management of patients with anterior mediastinal masses undergoing chamberlain procedure (anterior mediastinostomy). *Iran Red Crescent Med J*. 2013;15(4):373–374.
58. Desoto H. Direct laryngoscopy as an aid to relieve airway obstruction in a patient with a mediastinal mass. *Anesthesiology*. 1987; 67(1):116–117.
59. John RE, Narang VP. A boy with an anterior mediastinal mass. *Anaesthesia*. 1988;43(10):864–866.
60. Hong Y, Jo KW, Lyu J, et al. Use of venovenous extracorporeal membrane oxygenation in central airway obstruction to facilitate interventions leading to definitive airway security. *J Crit Care*. 2013;28(5):669–674.
61. Goh MH, Liu XY, Goh YS. Anterior mediastinal masses: an anaesthetic challenge. *Anaesthesia*. 1999;54(7):670–674.
62. Tempe DK, Arya R, Dubey S, et al. Mediastinal mass resection: femorofemoral cardiopulmonary bypass before induction of anesthesia in the management of airway obstruction. *J Cardiothorac Vasc Anesth*. 2001;15(2):233–236.
63. Herring K, Sreelatha P, et al. Perioperative airway management of a mediastinal mass through early intervention with extracorporeal membrane oxygenation (ECMO). *Int J Clin Anesth*. 2014;2(1): 1022–1024.
64. Said SM, Telesz BJ, Makdisi G, et al. Awake cardiopulmonary bypass to prevent hemodynamic collapse and loss of airway in a severely symptomatic patient with a mediastinal mass. *Ann Thorac Surg*. 2014;98(4):e87–e90.
65. Sendasgupta C, Sengupta G, Ghosh K, Munshi A, Goswami A. Femoro-femoral cardiopulmonary bypass for the resection of an anterior mediastinal mass. *Indian J Anaesth*. 2010;54(6):565–568.
66. Wang G, Lin S, Yang L, Wang Z, Sun Z. Surgical management of tracheal compression caused by mediastinal goiter: is extracorporeal circulation requisite? *J Thorac Dis*. 2009;1(1):48–50.
67. Radauceanu DS, Dunn JO, Lagattolla N, Farquhar-Thomson D. Temporary extracorporeal jugulosaphenous bypass for the peri-operative management of patients with superior vena caval obstruction: a report of three cases. *Anaesthesia*. 2009;64(11): 1246–1249.
68. Lin CM, Hsu JC. Anterior mediastinal tumour identified by intraoperative transesophageal echocardiography. *Can J Anaesth*. 2001;48(1):78–80.
69. Redford DT, Kim AS, Barber BJ, Copeland JG. Transesophageal echocardiography for the intraoperative evaluation of a large anterior mediastinal mass. *Anesth Analg*. 2006;103(3):578–579.
70. Yang YL, Lu HI, Huang HW, Tseng CC. Mediastinal tumor resection under the guidance of transoesophageal echocardiography. *Anaesth Intensive Care*. 2007;35(2):312.
71. Linnaus ME, Morray J, Bae J, Fraser JD. Use of a sternal elevator to reverse complete airway obstruction secondary to anterior mediastinal mass in an anesthetized child. *J Pediatr Surg Case Rep*. 2016;8:42–45.
72. Froese AB, Bryan AC. Effects of anesthesia and paralysis on diaphragmatic mechanics in man. *Anesthesiology*. 1974;41(3):242–255.
73. Choi WJ, Kim YH, Mok JM, Choi SI, Kim HS. Patient repositioning and the amelioration of airway obstruction by an anterior mediastinal tumor during general anesthesia - A case report. *Korean J Anesthesiol*. 2010;59(3):206–209.
74. Hartigan PM, Ng JM, Gill RR. Anesthesia in a patient with a large mediastinal mass. *N Engl J Med*. 2018;379(6):587–588.
75. Hartigan PM, Ng JM, Gill RR. More on anesthesia with a large mediastinal mass. *N Engl J Med*. 2018;379(22):2183–2184.
76. Elmatite W, Upadhyay S, Alfahel W, Mireles R, Ramsdell R, et al. Anesthetic management for anterior mediastinal mass with strong family history of malignant hyperthermia. *Am J Anesth Clin Res*. 2018;4(1):015–018.
77. Park BJ, Flores R, Downey RJ, Bains MS, Rusch VW. Management of major hemorrhage during mediastinoscopy. *J Thorac Cardiovasc Surg*. 2003;126(3):726–731.
78. Maranets I, Wang SM. Anterior mediastinal masses and anesthesia in children: how far have we come along? *J Clin Anesth*. 2010;22(3):157–158.

35

Mediastinoscopy

ELIZABETH MAY VUE, NICOLE MORIKAWA, JONATHAN LEFF

Introduction

Cancer is the second leading cause of death in the United States; of these, lung cancer is the most common cause in both males and females.[1] Although the lung cancer death rate has declined over the years primarily because of a reduction in smoking, the 5-year relative survival rate remains comparatively low at 19%. Early detection and treatment improves survival rates and can possibly offer a cure depending on the type and extent of lung cancer. Unfortunately, because of the lack of symptoms during the early stage, most lung cancers are diagnosed at advanced stages. Accurate cancer staging plays a crucial role in the prognosis and selection of appropriate treatment modality.[2,3]

Mediastinoscopy is an invasive diagnostic procedure for mediastinal lesions and is effective in clinically staging lung carcinoma. There are minimal to noninvasive modalities useful in clinical staging,[4–8] and these have precluded the need for routine tissue confirmation via mediastinoscopy. Nevertheless, the sensitivity and specificity for these procedures are subpar compared with mediastinoscopy,[6,9] which remains the gold standard[4,6] because of its reliability. Cervical mediastinoscopy (CM) is the conventional approach; alternatives include a left anterior mediastinoscopy and variations of the CM procedure, such as an extended cervical mediastinoscopy (ECM) and video-assisted mediastinoscopy (VAM).

Patients undergoing mediastinoscopy can pose an unusual and potentially dangerous challenge to anesthesiologists. Anterior mediastinal masses could cause significant cardiopulmonary obstruction, resulting in hemodynamic changes that may become exacerbated during induction and maintenance of general anesthesia. The anesthetic management of anterior mediastinal masses is discussed in Chapter 34. Surgical instrument manipulation can potentially result in ischemia, strokes, arrhythmia, and massive hemorrhage. Therefore it is important to understand the surgical procedure and its implications on the anesthetic management.

Case Presentation

A 69-year-old male with a medical history significant for hypertension, type 2 diabetes mellitus on insulin, and 15 pack-years of active cigarette smoking presented with shortness of breath. He had a normal chest x-ray (CXR). Further workup revealed a right upper lobe pulmonary nodule with spiculate margins on chest computed tomography (CT). Positron-emission tomography (PET) showed avid uptake in the right upper lobe nodule in addition to mediastinal and hilar lymph nodes suspicious for metastatic malignancy. An endobronchial ultrasonographic fine-needle aspiration (EBUS-FNA) procedure was negative for malignancy at the hilar and subcarinal stations (average of 3.5 passes). Because of the high suspicion for malignancy, the patient then presented for a standard CM.

Additional preoperative evaluation revealed mild obstructive lung disease on the pulmonary function test and normal cardiac function on the echocardiogram. Preoperative labs were within normal ranges, including a complete blood count, chemistry, and coagulation.

Case Management

The patient was preoperatively evaluated, confirming the nil per os (NPO) status and a reassuring airway with no signs of airway obstruction. Availability of blood products and appropriate vasoactive medications and setup were confirmed before induction. A five-lead electrocardiogram (ECG) was placed to monitor for arrhythmia and cardiac ischemia. The pulse oximeter was placed on the right hand and the noninvasive blood pressure cuff on the contralateral arm. After obtaining peripheral access and preoxygenation, intravenous induction was commenced, followed by a single lumen endotracheal tube (ETT) intubation. The ETT was securely taped and positioned away from the direction of the anticipated mediastinoscope. Additional vascular access was established with a large bore peripheral intravenous (PIV) line. Anesthesia was maintained with an inhalational volatile agent and paralysis via an intermittent neuromuscular blockade agent titrated by twitch monitor.

During the diagnostic mediastinocopy procedure, desaturation was noted with flattening of the continuous pulse oximeter waveform. Ventilator parameters and hemodynamics remained unchanged and stable. The surgeon was immediately notified, and the mediastinoscope position was readjusted. The pulse oximeter waveform returned to baseline. The patient maintained normal saturations and hemodynamics throughout the procedure. Lymph node biopsies were successfully obtained with minimal bleeding. Seven paratracheal and five subcarinal lymph nodes were obtained and sent for pathology. The right upper lobe nodule was left untouched. Hemostasis was ensured with assistance of cautery as the mediastinoscope was slowly withdrawn. The incision was subsequently sutured closed. A sterile bandage was applied. The head of the bed was then rotated back to the anesthesiologist for emergence.

After meeting extubation criteria, the patient was successfully extubated and transported to the recovery room for continuous perioperative monitoring, specifically assessing for any hoarseness, stridor, shortness of breath, neurologic changes, and bleeding. He remained neurologically intact postoperatively and reported minimal pain at the incision site. In addition, there was no pneumothorax on his postoperative CXR. After an uneventful postoperative recovery, the patient was discharged to the inpatient floor.

Review of Literature

Indications

According to the guidelines from the European Society of Thoracic Surgeons and American College of Chest Physicians, tissue confirmation to assess nodal involvement should be considered for nonsmall cell lung cancer (NSCLC) except in patients with peripheral carcinomas of 3 cm or smaller and no evidence of nodal involvement on diagnostic imaging. Imaging modalities, such as CT and PET, can provide information on the clinical staging of mediastinal masses and help avoid unnecessary procedures and noncurative resections.[3] Minimally invasive diagnostic procedures are often recommended as the first surgical diagnostic tool, if available[3,6]; even considering the limitations. Most importantly, the sensitivity of EBUS-FNA and endoscopic ultrasound FNA (EUS-FNA) are 89% and 89%, respectively. Combined, the sensitivity increases to 93%.[5,6]

Mediastinal lymph nodes can be accessed from the airway or esophagus under real-time ultrasound guidance.[5,6,10] EBUS permits access to the paratracheal, subcarinal, and hilar nodes. Paraesophageal nodes can be accessed through the EUS approach. In contrast, CM is limited to the paratracheal and subcarinal nodes for sampling,[8] and extends to paraaortic nodes in ECM.[11] In addition, minor complication rates occur in less than 1% (vs. 6% in mediastinoscopy).[5,6] Uncommon major complications include pneumothorax, empyema, and hemopneumomediastinum. Given that endosonography has a similar sensitivity but lower complication risk to that of mediastinoscopy, EBUS-FNA or EUS-FNA is recommended as the first diagnostic and staging approach. The procedure is usually performed under local anesthesia and moderate sedation at an outpatient center. A flexible ultrasonic bronchoscope is inserted through the mouth and into the trachea (EBUS) or the esophagus (EUS) to locations of known nodal stations (Fig. 35.1). Once lymph nodes are detected, transbronchial or transesophageal needle aspiration is performed. Sampling errors may occur if there is a small amount of tumor present in the node, resulting in a false negative.[10] Thus it is common to perform multiple passes through different parts of the node (average of three passes). The negative predictive value (NPV) remains lower than desired in endosonography at 60%.[5] Negative findings should be surgically validated if clinical suspicion remains high. Mediastinoscopy following a negative EBUS/EUS improves overall sensitivity from 85% to 94%, and NPV 93%. The staging algorithm for NSCLC and diagnostic indications is out of the scope of this chapter and is discussed in Chapter 4.

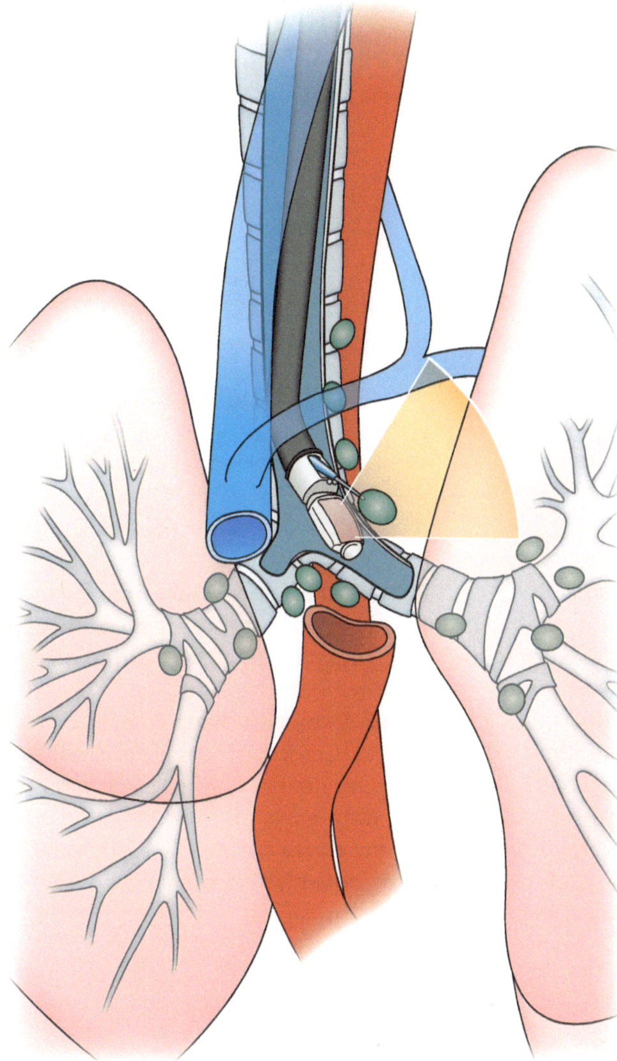

• **Fig. 35.1** Endobronchial ultrasound illustrating mediastinal lymph node imaging and transbronchial biopsy. Note that the flexible bronchoscope is in the airway. In contrast, the endoscope is in the esophagus for endoscopy ultrasound.

Clinical staging of NSCLC is the most common indication for mediastinoscopy.[3,6,8] This includes obtaining tissue to diagnose the pathology and assess the level of nodal involvement. Mediastinoscopy is recommended if minimally invasive methods, as discussed previously, are negative. It may be the preferred diagnostic tool for central tumors or

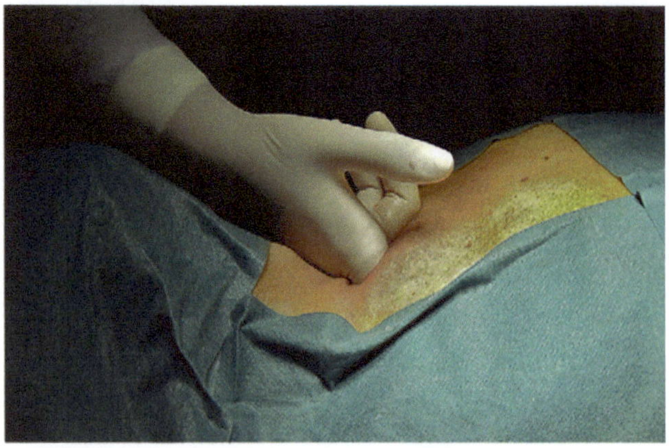

• **Fig. 35.2** This image illustrates the incisional location for cervical mediastinoscopy. A passage has been created along the cervical and pretracheal fascia as seen by the insertion of the finger.

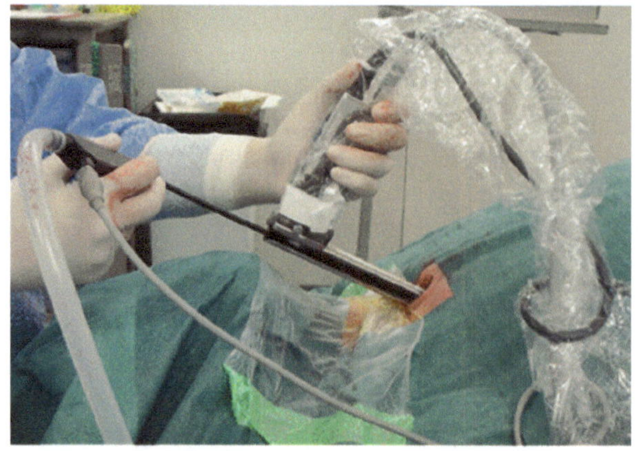

• **Fig. 35.3** This image depicts the insertion of the scope in a cervical mediastinoscopy procedure.

tumors over 3 cm.[8] It can also be used in the clinical staging of small cell lung carcinoma[12] and other mediastinal malignancies, including mesothelioma. Mediastinoscopy may be combined with other thoracic procedures in the resection of lung carcinoma and radical lymphadenectomy. Contraindications to mediastinoscopy include inaccessible lymph nodes, cervical spine disease (limited neck extension), thoracic aortic aneurysm, prior chest radiation or mediastinoscopy, and superior vena cava (SVC) syndrome, which carries the risk of potential bleeding from an increase in venous pressure.

Mediastinoscopy Procedure

A CM is approached via a 3-cm midline transverse incision in the suprasternal notch, as depicted in Fig. 35.2. Continuous dissection along the cervical and pretracheal fascia to the anterior trachea creates a passage for the advancement of the rigid mediastinoscope into the superior mediastinum, anterior to trachea and posterior to the great vessels[13] (Fig. 35.3). The pretracheal, paratracheal, and anterior subcarinal lymph nodes are predominantly accessible for tissue sampling.[11] The anatomic position of the rigid scope between the trachea and right innominate artery places the artery and trachea at risk for compression (Figs. 35.4 and 35.5).

ECM is a variation of the CM. ECM uses the same cervical incision as CM and continues with blunt dissection down the left carotid and innominate arteries to the aortic arch and left innominate vein.[8,11,14] A mediastinoscope can be inserted obliquely over the aortic arch to allow access to the paraaortic and subaortic nodal stations. VAM is also a variation of CM. Through the same cervical incision as CM, a mediastinoscope incorporated with optic fibers can be used for its improved bimanual surgical mobility and optimum visualization for dissection and sampling of lymph nodes.

The left anterior mediastinotomy, also known as transthoracic or Chamberlain's procedure, is performed through a vertical parasternal incision of the second or third intercostal space with removal of the intercostal cartilage.[14,15] Alternatively, a mediastinoscope may be used to visualize and obtain paraaortic lymph nodes through the incision. This method avoids the need for intercostal cartilage removal. Care is taken to avoid injuring the left internal

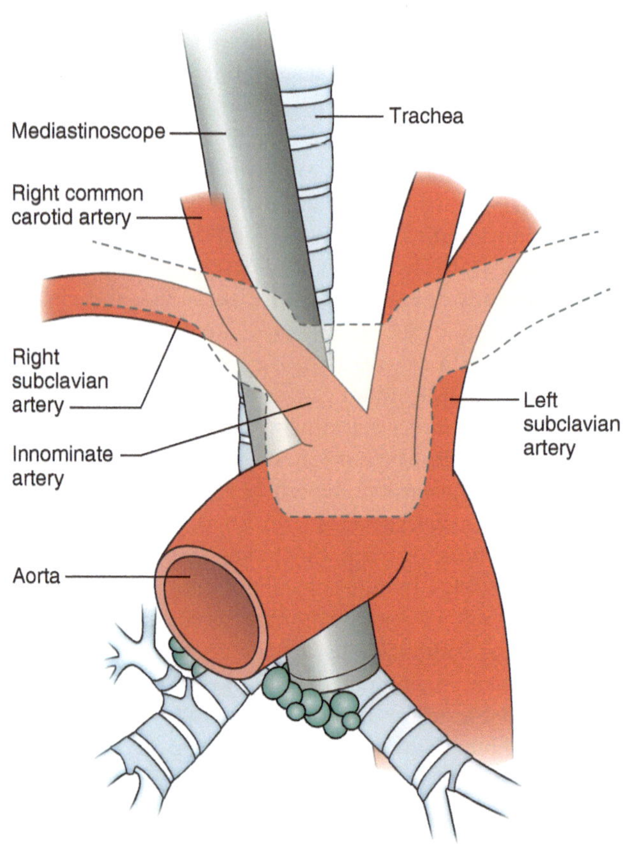

• **Fig. 35.4** The anatomic relation of the mediastinoscope to vital structures. Note the close position of the scope behind the right innominate artery and anterior to the trachea. (From Eisenkraft JB, Neustein E, Cohen E. Anesthesia for thoracic surgery. In: Barash PG, Cullen BF and Stoelting RK eds. *Clinical Anesthesia*, 7th ed. Philadelphia, PA: Lippincott Company; 2016).

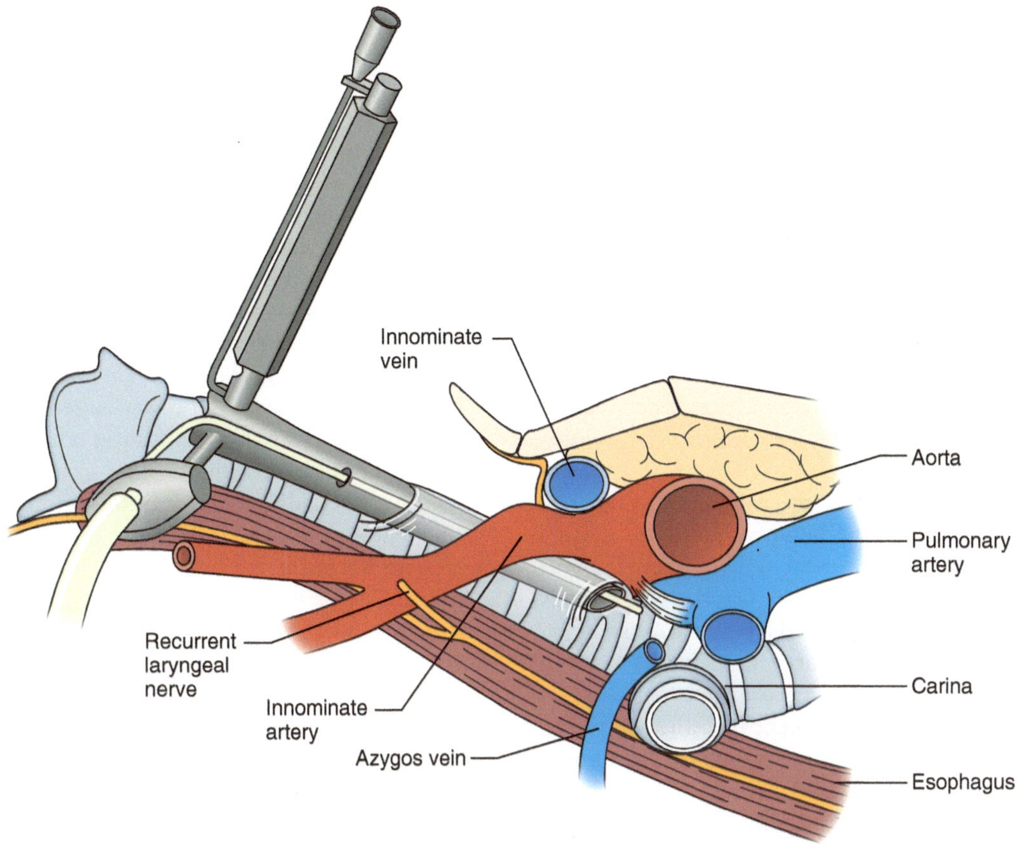

• **Fig. 35.5** A sagittal view of the placement of the mediastinoscope relative to right innominate artery and aortic arch.

mammary artery during dissection. This procedure is helpful in a patient with limited neck extension, in which the conventional mediastinoscopy is sometime impossible.

Preoperative Considerations

Medical History

A thorough history is essential to understanding the clinical picture. Knowledge of the location and sizes of the mediastinal masses in relation to important structures will help guide the preoperative assessment and anesthetic plan. Patients with masses concerning for tracheobronchial compression and SVC syndrome should be clinically assessed for severity of symptoms. Mediastinal masses may cause fixed compression of adjacent vital structures independent of positioning. Patients may be asymptomatic, but cardiopulmonary collapse may occur on induction or paralysis.[16,17] A review of CT images and pulmonary function tests (PFTs) can help identify these patients who are at high risk. The anterior mediastinal masses present a high risk for airway obstruction from tracheal compression. Patients with bronchial or tracheal obstruction may present with cough, dyspnea, wheezing, history of frequent respiratory infections, and changes in symptoms with positioning (from supine to sitting upright). A physical examination in the supine and sitting position to assess symptoms may be warranted to help guide the induction and airway plan. Awake fiberoptic intubation may be needed if potential airway obstruction is present. Patients who have facial flushing or distended jugular veins should be evaluated for SVC syndrome. Enlarged lymph nodes or mediastinal masses may be obstructing the SVC, causing edema of the tongue and larynx and making laryngoscopy and intubation difficult.

Smoking is the most common cause of lung cancer.[1] A smoking history and comorbidities associated with smoking including coronary artery disease, hypertension, cerebral vascular disease, peripheral vascular disease, and chronic obstructive lung disease, should be assessed. Peripheral vascular access may be difficult, necessitating the need for ultrasound guidance. Last, systemic effects from mediastinal carcinomas should also be investigated. Mediastinal tumors may be associated with paraneoplastic syndromes because of the secretion of endocrine hormones or substances that may impact the anesthetic management, such as antibodies to presynaptic voltage-gated calcium channels at the neuromuscular junction in Lambert-Eaton myasthenic syndrome.[18]

Investigations

A routine workup should include hematology, chemistry, type and screen, and an electrocardiogram. Chest x-ray and CT imaging are important in evaluating the size and relationship of the mass to structures, and to assess for any other abnormalities such as tracheal compression. PFTs and flow-volume loops are useful to evaluate pulmonary physiology and potential mass effects. An echocardiogram or stress test may be indicated to evaluate cardiac function and wall motion under stress. Imaging assessment for atherosclerosis and patency of the carotid arteries, in particular the left carotid, should be considered because of the elevated risk for an intraoperative stroke from right innominate compression and an occluded left carotid artery.[14]

Monitoring

A five-lead ECG should be used to monitor for arrhythmia and ischemia. Consideration should be taken when placing a continuous plethysmograph on the right upper extremity, such as a pulse oximeter and/or arterial line, to monitor for innominate compression by the rigid mediastinoscope during the procedure.[14,19] The noninvasive blood pressure cuff should be on the contralateral arm to reflect the true blood pressure. It is not the author's practice to routinely place arterial lines, unless indicated by medical history or clinical status. An arterial line placement is reasonable if there is concern for hemodynamic changes, high risk for hemorrhage, or the need for frequent blood gas monitoring. A preinduction arterial line insertion in the right upper extremity is encouraged if there is concern for significant hemodynamic instability on induction. Cerebral oximetry with near-infrared spectroscopy (NIRS) may also be considered to monitor for cerebral ischemia.[20] There is a paucity of data looking at the use of NIRS in mediastinoscopy, and it is not the author's routine practice. In patients undergoing general anesthesia, neuromuscular monitoring is vital to ensure patient safety in the critical moments, and is mandatory in patients with neuromuscular diseases like Lambert-Eaton syndrome. Airway pressures should be monitored in the event of tracheal or bronchial compression by the mediastinoscope.

Anesthetic Management

Surgical Plan

Communication and coordination with the surgical team is important because anesthetic plans can range from local anesthesia to general anesthesia with extracorporeal support. Understanding the indication and surgical plan is important in guiding the anesthetic plan. As previously discussed, mediastinoscopy may be combined with other thoracic procedures, such as a video-assisted thoracoscopic lung carcinoma resection, where one-lung ventilation is necessary. In patients at elevated risk for cardiopulmonary collapse, preinduction extracorporeal access or support[17] may be indicated. The overall anesthetic plan should take into consideration all surgical components.

General Anesthesia

CM is usually performed under general anesthesia with paralysis. Cross-matched blood should be ready in the event of hemorrhage, and a sternotomy setup should be available. Asymptomatic patients may be preoxygenated and intravenously induced. After intubation, the ETT should be taped securely and away from the position of the mediastinoscope to avoid kinks and compression during the procedure. A single-lumen ETT, preferably reinforced, is adequate for the procedure. Typically, the head of the bed is rotated 90-degrees away from the anesthesiologist with the surgeon at the head. Access to the airway is limited. There should be adequate breathing circuit length to accommodate the positioning.

Adequate large bore PIVs should be placed in preparation for possible resuscitation. The arms may be available at the side or tucked in. A lower extremity PIV should be considered for resuscitative measures. The lower body drains into the heart via the inferior vena cava. In the event of an SVC injury, fluids and medications administered through the upper extremity access will not be reliable.

General anesthesia can be maintained intravenously, inhalationally, or with a combination. Paralysis is necessary until the end of the procedure. Coughing or moving will increase risk of damage to nearby vital structures. Patients who do not tolerate positive pressure ventilation may need spontaneous breathing, and paralysis should be avoided in these patients. However, a deeper level of anesthetic is needed to minimize the risk of sudden movement. In turn, fluids and vasoactive drugs may be indicated to compensate for the anesthetic-induced hypotension. Other hemodynamic changes may occur because of compression of the trachea, causing bradycardia or hypertension and tachycardia from sympathetic chain stimulation or pain.[14] Perioperative pain can be managed by short-acting opioids, local anesthetic, and nonopioid analgesics.

Patients should meet extubation criteria before removing the ETT. Full recovery of reflexes and strength should be established. Signs of stridor, hypoventilation, and hypoxia should be monitored during transport to the recovery room. A postoperative CXR should be performed to assess for pneumothorax. Depending on the clinical status, patients may be admitted and discharged home on the same day.

Alternative Methods

Local anesthesia may be the preferred anesthetic technique in certain cases. For patients where the risks of general anesthesia outweigh the benefits, such as tracheal compression, local or regional anesthesia may be the safer alternative.[16] This requires effectively managing the patient's expectations to prepare for a safe procedure. The decision to supplement with additional sedation should be patient-dependent.

Risks and Benefits

Mediastinoscopy requires minimal to no movement during the surgical dissection and biopsy. Inopportune patient movements may cause injury to nearby vital structures in the mediastinum. General anesthesia allows for the securement of the airway at the beginning of the case and the administration of muscle relaxants to inhibit movement. In the event of vascular injury and hemorrhage, efforts could be comfortably focused on resuscitation. However, general anesthesia and/or paralysis may cause pulmonary and hemodynamic instability in select patients. Symptomatic patients with mechanical compression of the airway or vital structures are at elevated risk for adverse events.

Local or regional anesthesia may be considered in select patients and procedures, although it is not the preferred anesthetic technique. It has been described in the Chamberlain's procedure[15] but less commonly in CM. Local anesthesia can provide intraoperative and postoperative analgesia without a sedative effect. Surgeons are able to perform the procedure with minimal discomfort, while the patient maintains spontaneous respiration. Mental status can be evaluated throughout the case if there is concern for cerebral ischemia. Patient selection is important if performing local anesthesia. Typically, patients are placed in the supine position with neck extension and the head turned slightly to the side, which can present discomfort for the patient. Immobility is critical to ensure patient safety, therefore patients may need to be constantly reminded to remain still. Moreover, given the patients are sterilely draped from head to toe, patients with claustrophobia are usually intolerant to having their faces covered.

Complications and Management

Complications from CM include bleeding, vascular compression, airway obstruction, cerebral ischemia, hoarseness, stridor, arrhythmia, pneumothorax, and postoperative infection. Close proximity of the bronchoscope to the SVC, innominate artery, and aorta increases the potential for vascular compression, resulting in SVC obstruction, cerebral ischemia, and hypotension. Hemodynamics and airway parameters should be closely monitored, and the surgeon promptly notified to relieve the mechanical compression. During dissection, vascular injury to these major vessels may also occur. The anesthesiologists should be prepared to resuscitate if major hemorrhage occurs. Sternotomy may be necessary to obtain hemostasis. Of the many of the presumed biopsies of the targeted lymph node, sometime a vessel can be reflected through the mediastinoscopy as a lymph node and mistakably biopsied. In addition, laceration of a large vein by the biopsy forceps can be more difficult to control than an arterial laceration, where the source of bleeding can be easily identified by the blood stream from the lacerated artery. The venous laceration is more diffuse, and it is difficult to identify the source of the bleeding.

Dissection between the trachea and large vessels to access the mediastinal lymph nodes could potentially result in airway compromise. This includes tracheal compression from mechanical compression and pneumothorax from invasion into the pleural space. An intraoperative pneumothorax should be suspected if the patients become hypotensive with unexplained tachycardia, an increase in peak airway pressure, and sudden change in end-tidal CO2. Chest auscultation will confirm the reduced breath sound at the side of the pneumothorax. If chest sonography is available, the presence of pneumothorax can be confirmed intraoperatively. A postoperative CXR should follow to evaluate for pneumothorax and to determine the need for a chest tube insertion. Hoarseness is common after extubation, however, new-onset hoarseness and dysphonia may indicate vocal cord dysfunction owing to recurrent laryngeal nerve (RLN) injury during dissection.[21,22] Vocal cord dysfunction is the most common adverse event in CM at an incidence of 0.6% because of its location along the tracheoesophageal groove. Incidence of hoarseness was higher in VAM than in CM. According to one case report, bilateral vocal cord paralysis may also occur because of the spread of local anesthetic injected by the surgeon at the incision site.[22] Horner syndrome is a potential complication, which most likely resolves in 2 to 3 days postoperatively. Anterior neck hematoma formation compressing the airway, RLN, and nearby structures should also be considered. Management will depend on the clinical status and should aim at maintaining a patent airway.

Conclusion

Lung cancer deaths have declined over the years primarily from smoking cessation. If diagnosed early, survival rates are high. Unfortunately, most lung cancers not caught until the advanced stages. Accurate diagnosis and clinical staging are needed to help guide the optimal treatment course of the patients. Diagnostic tissue samples by minimally invasive procedures are typically the first option; however, surgical mediastinoscopy is recommended if there is high suspicion for malignancy. Sedation for select patients can be considered, but should be approached with caution; general anesthesia is often the preferred technique in most cases. Appropriate placement of monitors can detect early signs of mechanical compressions and help minimize risk for adverse events. The potential perioperative complications may be detrimental. Communication between the surgical and anesthesiology teams is key for the safe management of these patients.

References

1. Howlader N, Noone AM, Krapcho M, et al. SEER Cancer Statistics Review, 1975–2016. Bethesda, MD; National Cancer Institute; 2016.
2. Cho JH, Kim J, Kim K, Choi YS, Kim HK, Shim YM. A comparative analysis of video-assisted mediastinoscopy and conventional mediastinoscopy. *Ann Thorac Surg*. 2011;92:1007–1011.
3. Detterbeck FC, Postmus PE, Tanoue LT. The stage classification of lung cancer: diagnosis and management of lung cancer, 3rd ed: American College of Chest Physicians evidence-based clinical practice guidelines. *Chest*. 2013;143:e191S–e210S.
4. Silvestri GA, Gonzalez AV, Jantz MA, et al. Methods for staging non-small cell lung cancer: diagnosis and management of lung cancer, 3rd ed: American College of Chest Physicians evidence-based clinical practice guidelines. *Chest*. 2013;143:e211S–e250S.

5. Annema JT, van Meerbeeck JP, Rintoul RC, et al. Mediastinoscopy vs endosonography for mediastinal nodal staging of lung cancer: a randomized trial. *JAMA*. 2010;304:2245–2252.
6. De Leyn P, Dooms C, Kuzdzal J, et al. Revised ESTS guidelines for preoperative mediastinal lymph node staging for non-small-cell lung cancer. *Eur J Cardiothorac Surg*. 2014;45:787–798.
7. Anraku M, Miyata R, Compeau C, Shargall Y. Video-assisted mediastinoscopy compared with conventional mediastinoscopy: are we doing better? *Ann Thorac Surg*. 2010;89:1577–1581.
8. Call S, Obiols C, Rami-Porta R. Present indications of surgical exploration of the mediastinum. *J Thorac Dis*. 2018;10:S2601–S2610.
9. Kimura H, Iwai N, Ando S, Kakizawa K, Yamamoto N, Hoshino H, Anayama T. A prospective study of indications for mediastinoscopy in lung cancer with CT findings, tumor size, and tumor markers. *Ann Thorac Surg*. 2003;75:1734–1739.
10. Rintoul RC, Tournoy KG, El Daly H, et al. EBUS-TBNA for the clarification of PET positive intra-thoracic lymph nodes-an international multi-centre experience. *J Thorac Oncol*. 2009;4:44–48.
11. Metin M, Citak N, Sayar A, et al. The role of extended cervical mediastinoscopy in staging of non-small cell lung cancer of the left lung and a comparison with integrated positron emission tomography and computed tomography: does integrated positron emission tomography and computed tomography reduce the need for invasive procedures? *J Thorac Oncol*. 2011;6:1713–1719.
12. Inoue M, Nakagawa K, Fujiwara K, Fukuhara K, Yasumitsu T. Results of preoperative mediastinoscopy for small cell lung cancer. *Ann Thorac Surg*. 2000;70:1620–1623.
13. Foster ED, Munro DD, Dobell AR. Mediastinoscopy. A review of anatomical relationships and complications. *Ann Thorac Surg*. 1972;13:273–286.
14. Cata JP, Lasala J, Mena GE, Mehran JR. Anesthetic considerations for mediastinal staging procedures for lung cancer. *J Cardiothorac Vasc Anesth*. 2018;32:893–900.
15. Apostolakis E, Papakonstantinou NA, Chlapoutakis S, Prokakis C. Save or sacrifice the internal mammary pedicle during anterior mediastinotomy? *Ann Thorac Med*. 2014;9:138–143.
16. Bechard P, Letourneau L, Lacasse Y, Cote D, Bussieres JS. Perioperative cardiorespiratory complications in adults with mediastinal mass: incidence and risk factors. *Anesthesiology*. 2004;100:826–834; discussion 5A.
17. Said SM, Telesz BJ, Makdisi G, et al. Awake cardiopulmonary bypass to prevent hemodynamic collapse and loss of airway in a severely symptomatic patient with a mediastinal mass. *Ann Thorac Surg*. 2014;98:e87–e90.
18. Bukhari S, Soomro R, Fawwad S, Alvarez C, Wallach S. Adenocarcinoma of lung presenting as Lambert-Eaton myasthenic syndrome. *J Invest Med High Impact Case Rep*. 2017;5:2324709617721251.
19. Petty C. Right radial artery pressure during mediastinoscopy. *Anesth Analg*. 1979;58:428–430.
20. Li WW, van Boven WJ, Annema JT, Eberl S, Klomp HM, de Mol BA. Management of large mediastinal masses: surgical and anesthesiological considerations. *J Thorac Dis*. 2016;8:E175–E184.
21. Lemaire A, Nikolic I, Petersen T, et al. Nine-year single center experience with cervical mediastinoscopy: complications and false negative rate. *Ann Thorac Surg*. 2006;82:1185–1189; discussion 1189–1190.
22. Velez-Cubian FO, Toosi K, Glover J, Pancholy B, Hong E. Transient aphonia after mediastinoscopy. *Ann Thorac Surg*. 2017;103:e549–e550.

36

Lung Resection and Pulmonary Hypertension

LEILA HOSSEINIAN, BENJAMIN S. SALTER

Introduction

Pulmonary hypertension (PH) has become an increasingly common diagnosis among patients presenting for surgery. With advances pertaining to the diagnosis and treatment of PH, these patients are now living longer with an improved quality of life. Although surgery still poses a significant risk, patients with PH can safely undergo noncardiac surgery. Patients with precapillary PH undergoing noncardiac surgery have a mortality rate ranging from 1% to 9.7% and a high perioperative morbidity rate range from 24% to 42% despite improvements in the quality of treatment and optimization.[1–5] Common complications include respiratory failure (7%–28%), congestive heart failure and/or volume overload (10%–13.5%), arrhythmia (12%), hemodynamic instability (8%), acute kidney injury (7%–10%), and myocardial ischemia (4%).[1,4,5] Emergency procedures, particularly those with the potential for rapid blood loss, thoracic surgery, and laparoscopic surgery are all associated with highest risk.[1] Changes in intrathoracic pressure, oxygenation, airway pressure, and the need for one-lung ventilation (OLV), all can acutely increase pulmonary vascular resistance (PVR) and suppress right ventricular (RV) function, which poses an increased risk to patients with PH patients undergoing thoracic surgery. However, with diligent preoperative optimization and careful intraoperative management, lung resections on patients with PH have been performed with no increase in morbidity or mortality.[6] Successful intraoperative management of thoracic surgical patients with PH requires a thorough understanding of the disease process, assessment of the severity of the disease and comorbidities. Proper optimization, understanding the nature of the procedure being performed and a team approach to unified anesthetic plan considering the increased risk of cardiac and pulmonary complications is essential.

Definition

PH is defined as a persistent elevation of mean pulmonary artery pressure (MPAP) 25 mm Hg or more at rest measured by right heart catheterization. This definition was established at the World Symposium on PH organized by the World Health Organization. During the sixth World Symposium on PH in 2018, experts reconsidered MPAP of 20 mm Hg as the new cut off.[7] PH is divided into five different groups (Table 36.1) and can further be divided into three different categories based on the hemodynamic implications of the disease process (Table 36.2). Anesthesiologists need to be aware of these classifications as they impact the available treatment and management strategies.

Classification/Pathophysiology

Group 1 pulmonary arterial hypertension (PAH) is associated with an alteration of pulmonary vasculature, including pulmonary arterial vasoconstriction smooth muscle hypertrophy, intimal and adventitial proliferation with eventual fibrosis, complex plexiform lesions, and thrombotic lesions.[8–10] Endothelial dysfunction disrupts the balance between the production of vasodilators and vasoconstrictors. There are various sources stimulating endothelial dysfunction and include free radicals, hypoxia, inflammatory mediators, acidosis, stress from left-to-right intracardiac shunts, and fibrin from thromboembolism.[8] Eventually this results in an overexpression of vasoconstrictor and proliferative substances, such as thromboxane A2 and endothelin-1 (ET-1). ET-1 is both a potent vasoconstrictor but also stimulates smooth muscle proliferation, resulting in smooth muscle hypertrophy of the pulmonary vasculature. On the other hand, there is a downregulation of vasodilator and antiproliferative substances, such as nitric oxide (NO) and prostacyclin. Platelets also take part in the pathogenesis of PAH by occluding vessels through the production of thrombotic lesions and vasoconstrictive mediators.[8–10] These changes result in an elevation of MPAP and PVR with a normal pulmonary capillary wedge pressure (PCWP) and is known as precapillary PH (Fig. 36.1).

Group 2 comprises PH caused by left heart disease. Hemodynamically, this group has elevated MPAP and PCWP with a normal PVR and is known as postcapillary PH. The elevation of MPAP is caused by passive back pressure from an elevation in left atrial pressure. Initially, the transpulmonary

TABLE 36.1 Classification of Pulmonary Hypertension

Pulmonary Hypertension				
World Health Organization (WHO) Group 1 Pulmonary Arterial Hypertension	WHO Group 2 Pulmonary Hypertension Caused by Left-Sided Heart Disease	WHO Group 3 Pulmonary Hypertension Caused by Lung Disease or Hypoxia	WHO Group 4 Chronic Thromboembolic Pulmonary Hypertension and Other Pulmonary Artery Obstructions	WHO Group 5 Pulmonary Hypertension With Multifactorial Mechanisms
• Idiopathic • Heritable • Drug and toxin induced Associated with: • Connective tissue disease • HIV infection • Portal hypertension • Congenital heart disease • Schistosomiasis • WHO Group I (pulmonary veno-occlusive disease and pulmonary capillary hemangiomatous) • WHO Group I (persistent pulmonary hypertension of the newborn)	• Left ventricular systolic dysfunction • Left ventricular diastolic dysfunction • Valvular heart disease • Specific congenital abnormalities	• Chronic obstructive pulmonary disease • Interstitial lung diseases • Other mixed restrictive or obstructive lung disease • Sleep-disordered breathing • Alveolar hypoventilation disorders • Chronic exposure to high altitude • Developmental lung diseases	• Chronic thromboembolic pulmonary hypertension • Other pulmonary artery obstructions (e.g., angiosarcoma, other intravascular tumors, arteritis, congenital stenoses, and parasites)	• Hematologic disorders (e.g., sickle cell disease) • Systemic disorders (e.g., sarcoidosis, Langerhans cell granulomatosis) • Metabolic disorders (e.g., Gaucher disease) • Others (e.g., renal disease)

From Hoeper MM, Humbert M, Souza R, Idrees M, Kawut SM, Sliwa-Hahnle K, et al. A global view of pulmonary hypertension. *Lancet Respir Med.* 2016;4:306–322. With permission.

gradient is low but eventually with longstanding disease, the increase in MPAP is caused by the increase in left atrial pressure which results in vascular remodeling and pulmonary arterial vasoconstriction and consequently an increase in the transpulmonary pressure gradient.[11] Careful consideration needs to be taken with the use of pulmonary vasodilators in this group of patients who are at risk of associated pulmonary edema from elevated pulmonary venous pressure.

Groups 3, 4, and 5 also fall under the category of precapillary PH. **Group 3** represents PH secondary to lung disease. Hypoxia is the main driving factor causing pulmonary vasoconstriction. Hypoxia induces endothelial cell damage

TABLE 36.2 Hemodynamic Definitions of Pulmonary Hypertension

Definition	Characteristics	Clinical Group
Precapillary PH	MPAP >20 mm Hg PCWP ≤15 mm Hg PVR ≥3WU	1, 3, 4, and 5
Isolated postcapillary PH	MPAP >20 mm Hg PCWP >15 mm Hg PVR <3WU	2 and 5
Combined pre- and postcapillary PH	MPAP >20 mm Hg PCWP >15 mm Hg PVR ≥3WU	2 and 5

MPAP, Mean pulmonary artery pressure; *PCWP*, pulmonary capillary wedge pressure; *PH*, pulmonary hypertension; *PVR*, pulmonary vascular resistance; *WU*, wood units.

Modified from Simonneau G, Montani D, Celermajer DS, et al. Haemodynamic definitions and updated clinical classification of pulmonary hypertension. *Eur Respir J*. 2019;53.

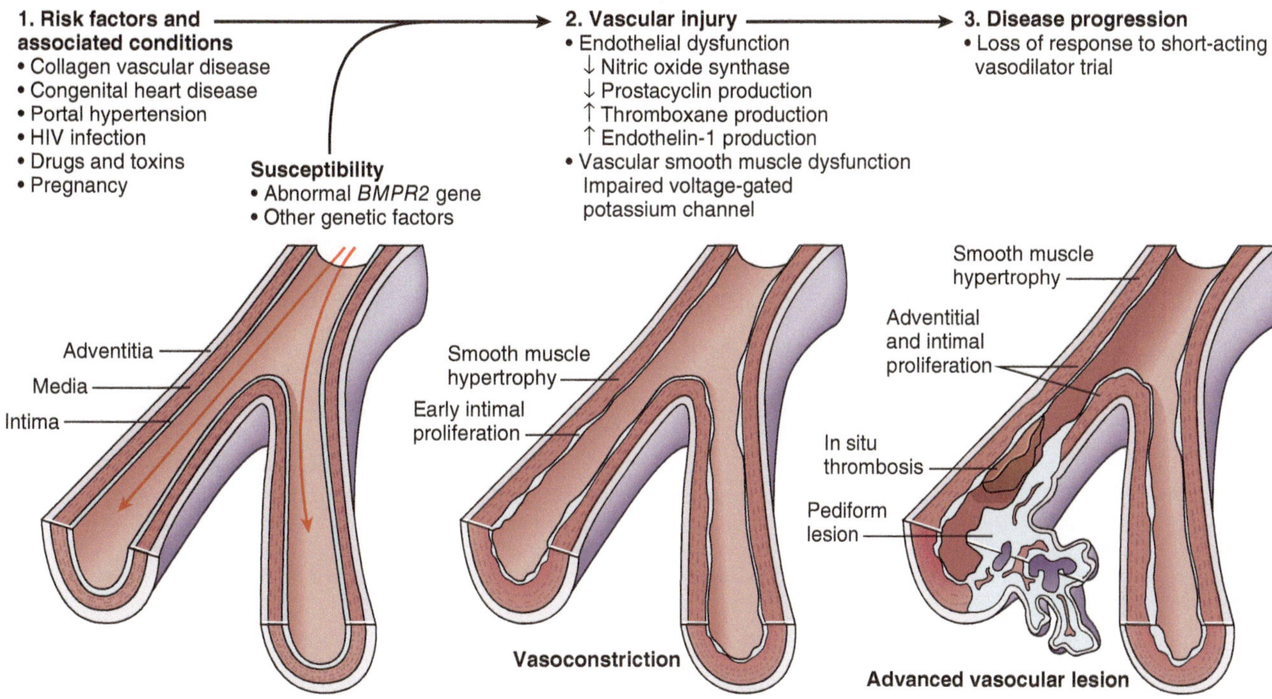

• **Fig. 36.1** Pathogenesis of pulmonary arterial hypertension. (From Rubenfire M, Bayram M, Hector-Word Z. Pulmonary hypertension in the critical care setting: classification, pathophysiology, diagnosis, and management. *Crit Care Clin*. 2007;23:801–834.)

causing release of vasoconstrictors, such as ET-1, that lead to smooth muscle vasospasm and proliferation. Also there is eventually intimal thickening, medial, hypertrophy, and adventitial collagen deposition.[10] Interestingly, although sleep disordered breathing is part of this group, relatively only a minority (17%) of patients with obstructive sleep apnea go on to develop PH. The likelihood however increases when the patient has associated underlying lung disease.[12] **Group 4** includes patients with thromboembolic obstruction of the pulmonary arteries. They may develop partial or complete occlusion of the pulmonary arteries through the formation of mural thrombi. These patients have an abnormal mechanism of fibrinolysis or have underlying hematologic or autoimmune disorders resulting in a hypercoagulable state.[8,10] Interestingly, vascular remodeling also occurs in vessel regions not affected by thrombi which may be related to sheer stress.[11] Only a fraction of patients with acute pulmonary emboli develop chronic thromboembolic PH (CTEPH). Surgical intervention with pulmonary thromboendarterectomy is potentially curative.[10] Anticoagulation is the main medical therapy for these patients. Finally, **Group 5** is PH resulting from idiopathic or multifactorial mechanisms which include, sarcoidosis, splenectomy, and myeloproliferative disorders.

Preoperative Evaluation

Patients with PH presenting for thoracic surgery require an extensive preoperative workup. A team approach composed of multiple specialists including internists, pulmonologists, and cardiologists commonly care for these patients and a team discussion is imperative to ensure medical optimization before surgery. Considering the increased risk of thoracic surgery, a discussion with the thoracic surgeon preoperatively will help to design an anesthetic technique that best mitigates risk.

The goal of a thorough preoperative evaluation for patients undergoing thoracic surgery is to identify and optimize any current medical conditions and implement additional treatment strategies to decrease the patient's perioperative risk. Intraoperative complications include, but are not limited to, those involving cardiac, neurologic, metabolic, and respiratory insults. A more thorough discussion of the preoperative assessment of patients undergoing thoracic surgery is covered in Chapter 8; however, a brief summary with attention to the supplemental testing required for patients with PH will be presented here.

No single test has the ability to precisely predict outcomes in thoracic surgery, so clinicians use the results from several different predictive tests to define the thresholds necessary for minimizing risk. These tests, creatively referred to as the "three-legged stool" of respiratory assessment, encompass lung mechanical function, pulmonary parenchymal function, and cardiopulmonary reserve.[13] **Functional tests** of lung mechanics include forced expiratory volume in 1 second (FEV_1), forced vital capacity (FVC), maximal voluntary ventilation (MVV), and residual volume/total lung capacity (RV/TLC) ratio; of these, the predicted postoperative FEV_1 (ppoFEV_1%) is the most validated for predicting complications. **Pulmonary tissue function** is commonly assessed using the results of arterial blood gases, spirometry, and plethysmography; however, the diffusion capacity of carbon monoxide (DLCO) remains the most useful measurement. Finally, a patient's **cardiopulmonary reserve** is assessed

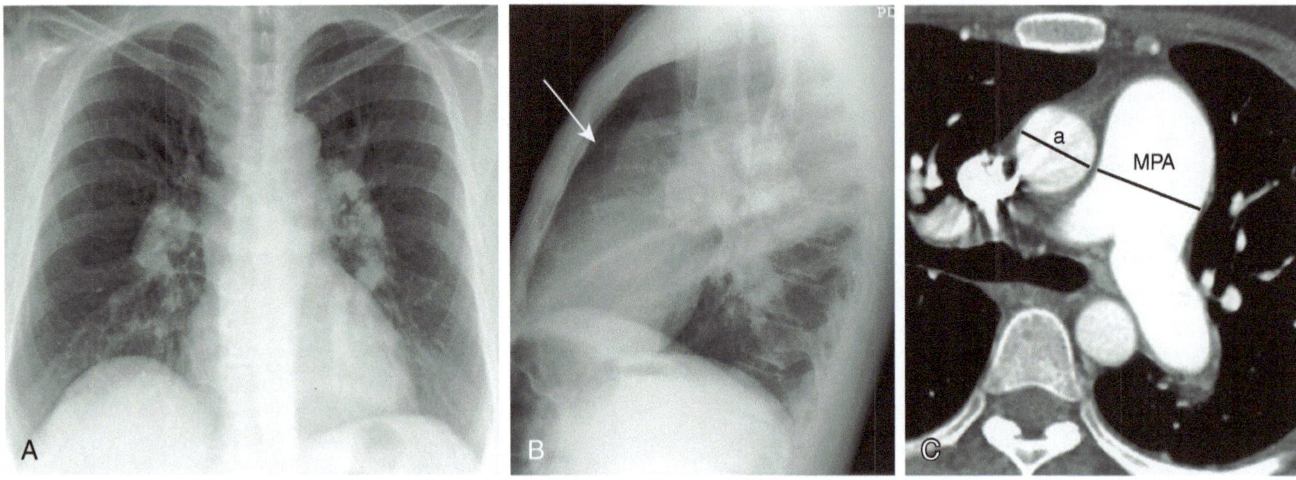

• **Fig. 36.2** Frontal (**A**) and lateral (**B**) chest radiographs showing bilateral, symmetrical central pulmonary arterial enlargement. (B) reveals filling of the substernal regions representing enlargement of the right ventricular outflow graft (*arrow*). **C.** Axial enhanced chest CT shows enlargement of the main pulmonary artery, (MPA) consistent with elevated pulmonary arterial pressure. *a,* Aorta. (Modified from *Murray and Nadel's Textbook of Respiratory Medicine* (978-1455733835). With permission.)

using either a bicycle or treadmill to generate a maximal oxygen consumption (VO2 max) or the more simple, self-paced 6-minute walking test (6MWT).[13–15]

The preoperative assessment in addition to the aforementioned "three-legged stool" of respiratory assessment, should also include an evaluation of the multisystemic sequelae of PH. Signs and symptoms are dynamic and fluctuate throughout the course of the disease, thus qualification of the severity of PH is necessary to optimize the patient and assess surgical risk. Additional tests can include a preoperative chest x-ray (CXR), electrocardiogram (ECG), echocardiogram, and often a right heart catheterization. The CXR can reveal the stigmata of PH, including enlargement of the pulmonary arteries and a boot-shaped or globular heart representing an elevated cardiac apex because of RV hypertrophy or pulmonary edema resulting from worsening heart failure[16] (Fig. 36.2). The ECG can show evidence of RV hypertrophy, right-heart failure, including right axis deviation, a large R wave in V1, an increase in the P wave amplitude in lead II, a right bundle branch block, and possible diffuse repolarization abnormalities[11,17] (Fig. 36.3). The echocardiogram offers clinicians a noninvasive method for diagnosing PH. Patients with chronic PH may have evidence of a pericardial effusion and signs of RV pressure overload, including hypertrophy, dilation, impaired function, tricuspid valve regurgitation, and flattening of the interventricular septum with possible left ventricular dysfunction (Fig. 36.4). In addition, estimates of pulmonary artery pressures can be made based on the presence and severity of tricuspid and pulmonic valve regurgitation. These echocardiographic findings, along with decreased tricuspid annular plane systolic excursion (TAPSE), Tei index (a myocardial performance index to express global diastolic and systolic function), peak systolic tricuspid lateral annular velocity, isovolumic contraction velocity and abnormal RV free wall strain are all predictors of a poor prognosis in patients with PH.[18,19]

The gold standard test for assessment of PH is a right heart catheterization. PAP, PCWP, right atrial and ventricular pressures, cardiac output (CO), mixed venous oxygen saturation, and PVR are all critically important values to understand the severity of the patient's PH. In addition, during the right heart catheterization, vasoreactivity testing (which is a decrease of at least 10 mm Hg in MPAP with a short-acting agent, such as inhaled NO or iloprost) is performed which will help the anesthesiologist to predict the perioperative effectiveness of intraoperative vasodilators.[18,20,21]

Finally, routine hematologic, biochemical, and thyroid function tests are required in all patients. Acutely worsening measures of end organ function, such as liver function tests or creatinine, can be a sign of worsening heart failure and should be addressed before proceeding with surgery. In addition, plasma brain natriuretic peptide (BNP) and N-terminal pro-BNP are useful markers of RV strain and can be used to guide clinical decision making and response to treatment. They have also been studied as independent predictors of mortality.[18,22]

With regard to preoperative medications, all PH therapies should be continued in the operating room with the exception of anticoagulation which in certain circumstances may need to be converted to short-acting intravenous (IV) therapy.[23] The most common therapies include prostaglandin analogs (epoprostenol, iloprost), endothelin receptor antagonists (bosentan), and phosphodiesterase inhibitors (sildenafil). The abrupt discontinuation of pulmonary vasodilators could lead to an acute PH crisis.

Intraoperative Management

Monitoring

Although there are no guidelines for monitoring patients with PH undergoing thoracic surgery, serious consideration should be made for the use of invasive monitoring. Invasive blood pressure monitoring is a must and will enable the

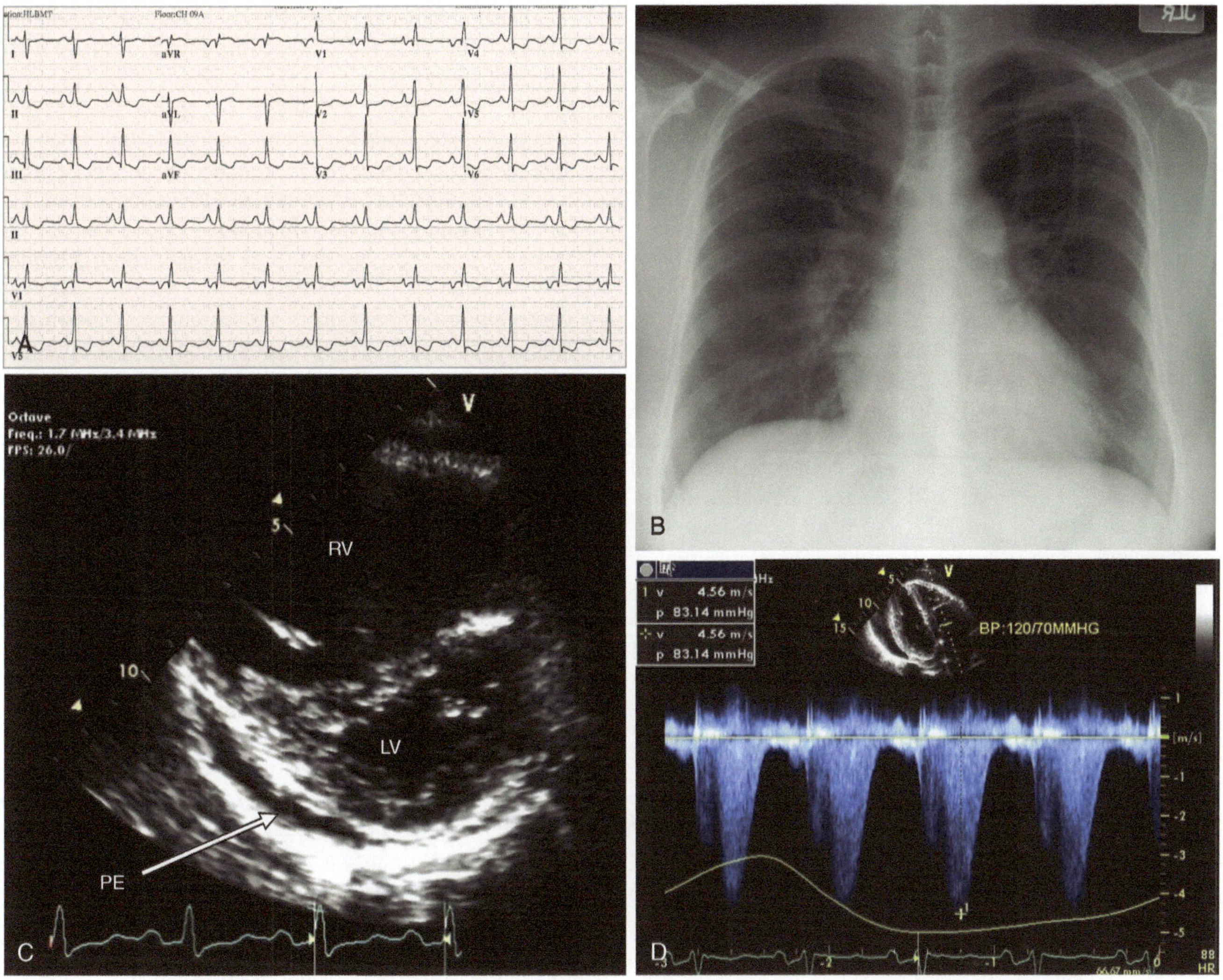

• **Fig. 36.3** **A**: Electrocardiogram in a patient with pulmonary arterial hypertension. Typical findings include right axis deviation, right atrial enlargement, and right ventricular hypertrophy. **B**; CXR with Pericardial effusion (PE). C:D: Echo image of pericardial effusion (From Dubrock, Hilary et al. *Heart Failure: A Companion to Braunwald's Heart Disease* (978-1455733835). With permission.)

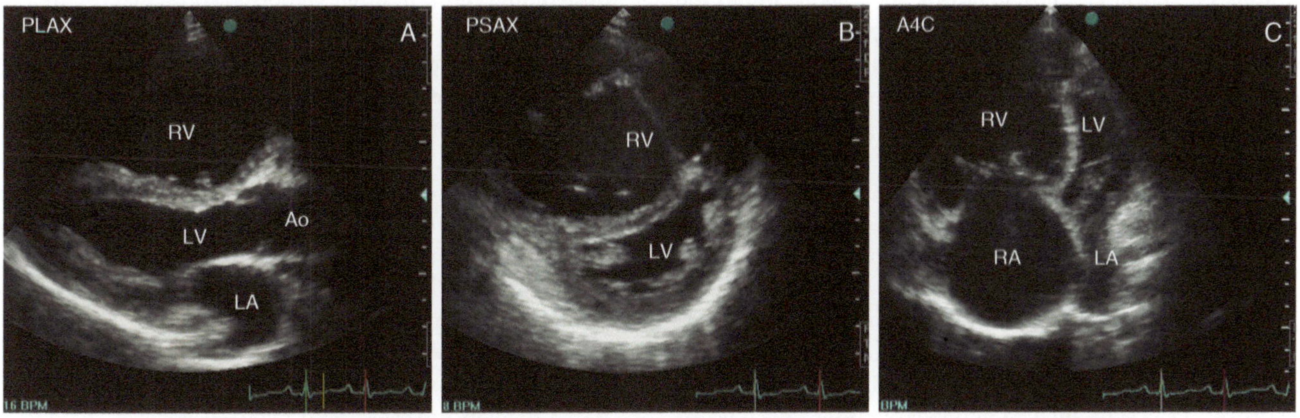

• **Fig. 36.4** Echocardiographic signs of pulmonary hypertension include severe right ventricular (*RV*) dilation with the ventricular septum compressed toward the left ventricle in systole, limiting left ventricular (*LV*) size. (**A**) Parasternal long axis; (**B**) short-axis; and (**C**) the apical 4-chamber. *Ao:* Aorta *RA:* Right Atrium *LA:* Left Atrium. (From Celemajer DS, Playford D. Pulmonary hypertension: role of echocardiography in diagnosis and patient management. *Pract Clin Echocardiogr*. 2017:633–650. With permission.)

anesthesiologist not only to rapidly recognize hemodynamic deterioration, but also to facilitate monitoring and maintenance of adequate oxygenation and normocarbia. Pulse pressure variation on an arterial line can help to distinguish hypovolemia or tamponade (respiratory fluctuation) from a low stroke volume caused by cardiogenic shock (diminished pulse pressure). A central venous catheter can be helpful, not only for monitoring of right heart filling pressures, which can help to guide volume management, but also for the delivery of vasopressors and inotropes. In addition, central venous oxygenation values help measure the level of end organ perfusion. For select patients with severe PH undergoing more extensive thoracic surgical procedures, a pulmonary arterial catheter (PAC) provides additional information regarding the patient's CO/index, PAP and mixed venous oxygen saturation. Although its utility has been questioned by the results of numerous trials and there is no data exploring its benefit in PH patients, following the changes in pulmonary pressures during the surgical procedure is extremely important.[24] There is a greater risk of PA rupture when floating a PA catheter in a patient with PH.[25] However, the ability to monitor PAP and CO and assess the outcome of therapeutic interventions can be beneficial in this patient population. Finally, the use of transesophageal echocardiography (TEE) monitoring allows for real-time monitoring of cardiac contractility, estimation of systolic PAPs and volume status (see Chapter 55).[26] The TEE allows for quick assessment of both left- and right-sided cardiac function, as well as helping to assess for other causes of hypotension. No guidelines exist for the role of intraoperative TEE monitoring in PH patients undergoing noncardiac surgery.

Anesthetic Technique

There are no specific anesthetic techniques proven to be safest in patients with PH. Instead, the anesthetic plan should focus on preserving the patient's hemodynamics, oxygenation, and ventilation. Furthermore, the principles management that apply to all patients undergoing thoracic surgery also apply to those with PH with the goal to provide adequate anesthesia and analgesia without further increasing their perioperative risk.

Choosing an anesthetic technique is dependent on the planned procedure and severity of PH symptoms. For example, although regional anesthesia can allow maintenance of spontaneous breathing, patients with RV heart failure or significant lung disease may not tolerate the supine/decubitus position necessary for surgery.[27] Thus general anesthesia (GA) performed alongside a regional or neuraxial technique may be better suited for these patients.

GA is usually the anesthetic of choice in this patient population as it provides adequate oxygenation, controlled ventilation, the ability to perform intraoperative TEE, and a delivery vehicle for inhaled pulmonary vasodilators if necessary. There are however several disadvantages to GA, most notably the blood pressure variability associated with anesthetic induction and the critical hemodynamic and respiratory consequences of emergence. Moreover, mechanical ventilation, specifically positive pressure delivery, and anesthetic-induced hypotension can significantly compromise coronary perfusion and contractility.[11]

Standard intravenous anesthetic agents like propofol and etomidate, along with nonhistamine releasing narcotics (i.e., sufentanil, fentanyl) are theoretically all safe to use for a slow, controlled induction in this patient population. PVR can significantly decrease when using etomidate and propofol for induction but return to normal within 5 minutes postintubation.[28] That being said, any agent in excess can compromise hemodynamics and coronary perfusion pressure especially. Furthermore, nonhistamine releasing paralytics, such as rocuronium and cisatracurium, can be used safely as well. The use of ketamine in patients with PH is debatable as it has been reported to increase PVR; however, several authors and case reports cite its value as part of a balanced anesthetic in these patients.[29–31]

Although nearly all of the inhaled anesthetics induce vascular relaxation and blunting of hypoxic pulmonary vasoconstriction (HPV), data does suggest volatile anesthetics (up to 1 MAC) can be administered without any significant adverse effects on pulmonary resistance and pressure.[11,32,33] Nitrous oxide, on the other hand should be avoided as it is well known to increase PVR, especially in patients with existing PH.[33]

Regional anesthesia can be an excellent complement to GA for thoracic surgery. Neuraxial techniques provide excellent analgesia and limit the systemic effect of IV medications; however, PH patients are commonly on anticoagulation therapy and current guidelines must be considered.[34] Furthermore, adequate postoperative pain control allows for improved respiratory mechanics and can mitigate the risk of respiratory acidosis and hypoxemia from splinting or the use of narcotics. More recently, fascial plane blocks, such as the erector spinae block and serratus anterior block, have come into vogue as safe and effective alternatives to neuraxial analgesia. Early studies are promising; however, large, quality trials are necessary to provide formal recommendations.[35,36]

OLV certainly complicates the management of patients undergoing thoracic surgery and the consequences are even more severe in patients with PH. For most patients, OLV is tolerated because of HPV as it reduces pulmonary shunting and improves oxygenation. However, in patients with PH, OLV can cause a significant increase in PVR and PAP.[37] Clamping of PA branches will increase the PAP, PVR, and myocardial oxygen consumption by acutely decreasing the pulmonary vascular bed area.[38] It is important to recognize that PVR is lowest at functional residual capacity, so tidal volumes should be adjusted accordingly. Both hyperinflation and atelectasis should be avoided as they lead to compression of alveolar vessels causing increased PVR.[37] Positive end-expiratory pressure (PEEP) should be individually titrated to avoid atelectasis and hypoxia; however, high levels of PEEP will compress the capillaries in the well-ventilated areas of the lung and divert flow to less well-ventilated areas (V/Q mismatch) which can result in decreased arterial oxygen partial pressure (PaO2) and increase in PVR.[8]

Recently, optimization of driving pressure (DP) has been considered as a tool to optimize mechanical ventilation during surgery and to improve outcome. DP is defined as the difference between plateau pressure and PEEP (Plat – PEEP), and can also be expressed as the ratio of tidal volume to respiratory system compliance. DP is derived from the interaction between the ventilatory parameters set by the physician and the patient's total thoracic compliance. The level of PEEP can be titrated to achieve the lowest DP which will avoid atelectasis or overdistension.[39,40]

Finally, the lateral decubitus position which is commonly used in thoracic surgery can also have an impact on oxygenation intraoperatively. Patients with unilateral lung disease should be positioned with the diseased side up; however, some patients may not tolerate both OLV and the lateral decubitus position because of significant increase in PAP.[41] Fundamentally, avoidance of hypoxia and hypercarbia is paramount to tolerating OLV. If PAP pressures significantly increase with OLV, the anesthesiologist must consider the use of pulmonary vasodilators and discuss with the surgeon regarding limiting the time using OLV.

Hemodynamic Management

Patients with PH have marginal cardiac reserve so tight control of hemodynamic parameters is critical to ensuring their safety. The goal of an anesthesiologist is to maintain systemic and coronary perfusion pressure by promptly recognizing and treating intra-operative hypotension. Blaise et al. also recommend that the intra-operative mean pulmonary artery pressure should not fluctuate beyond 15% above or below the initial preoperative value.[42] There are five factors that are generally responsible for hypotension in these patients: afterload, preload, contractility, rhythm and rate[26] (Fig. 36.5).

Increased RV afterload is the primary culprit for hypotension in these patients. Hypoxia, hypercarbia, acidosis, hyperinflation of the lungs, atelectasis, hypothermia, and pain can all cause an increase in PVR. If RV afterload is not decreased with improvement of the earlier factors, initiation of vasodilators can be helpful. Vasodilators can improve forward flow in the RV by decreasing afterload. IV vasodilators are first line for afterload reduction in patients with an adequate systemic vascular resistance (SVR). However, a drop in mean systemic blood pressure to the degree that it impairs RV perfusion can cause ischemia especially among patients with RV hypertrophy and must be avoided. Another concern regarding IV vasodilators is that they can exacerbate V/Q mismatch by inhibiting HPV. In those instances, inhaled pulmonary vasodilators are preferred as they primarily dilate the pulmonary vasculature without causing significant systemic vasodilation. Another benefit of inhaled pulmonary vasodilators is that selectively dilate the pulmonary vessels in well-ventilated regions, thereby improving V/Q matching and oxygenation. The use of pulmonary vasodilators should be carried out with caution in patients with group 2 PH because it can lead to pulmonary edema and left heart failure.[27] Table 36.3 lists the most commonly used IV and inhaled vasodilators.

A hypertrophied RV is preload dependent, so a sudden drop in preload is not well tolerated. On the other hand,

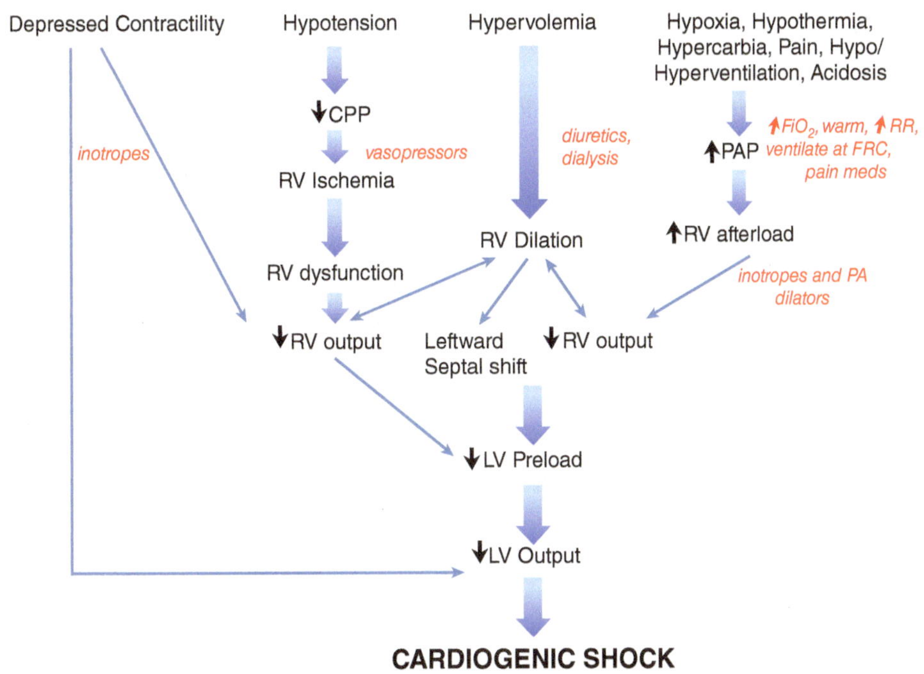

• **Fig. 36.5** The anesthetic management of pulmonary hypertension (PH) requires maintenance of RV contractility, avoidance of hypotension and hypervolemia, and elevations of PAP. *CPP*, Coronary perfusion pressure; *FRC*, functional residual capacity; *LV*, left ventricle; *PA*, pulmonary artery; *PAP*, pulmonary artery pressure; *RR*, respiratory rate; *RV*, right ventricle. (Modified from Hosseinian L. Pulmonary hypertension and noncardiac surgery: Implications for the anesthesiologist. *J Cardiothorac Vasc Anesth.* 2014;28:1064–1074. With permission.)

TABLE 36.3 Inhaled and Intravenous Vasodilators

Name	Administration	Comments
Nitroglycerin	IV infusion	2–10 mcg/kg/min
Nitroprusside	IV infusion	0.2–0.3 mcg/kg/min
Sildenafil (PDE-5 inhibitor)	IV bolus	Bolus 3 times a day up to 1.6 mg/kg/day
Milrinone (PDE-3 inhibitor)	Nebulized IV infusion	2–5 mg for 10–15 minutes 25–50 mcg/kg bolus followed by 0.25–0.75 mcg/kg/min infusion
Epoprostenol	Inhaled IV infusion	Continuous 10–50 ng/kg/min 2–10 ng/kg/min
Iloprost	Nebulized IV infusion	5–10 mg, administered every 2–4 hours 1–3 ng/kg/min
Nitric oxide	Inhaled	Continuous 5–40 ppm

IV, Intravenous; *kg*, kilograms; *mcg*, micrograms; *mg*, milligrams; *ng*, nanograms; *PDE*, phosphodiesterase; *ppm*, parts per million.
(Modified from Sarkar MS, Desai PM. Pulmonary hypertension and cardiac anesthesia: Anesthesiologist's perspective. *Ann Card Anaesth*. 2018;21:116–122.)

over aggressive volume resuscitation must also be avoided as it can worsen RV failure, increasing the shifting of the intraventricular septum toward the left, further compromising left ventricular filling and thus decreasing CO. Diuresis, conservative volume management, and eventually the use of inotropes will be necessary to improve RV function. Although there is no perfect monitor to determine euvolemia, the use of central venous pressure, PA catheter, and TEE can be useful to guide determination of fluid status.

Many anesthetic agents have negative inotropic effects, which can further exacerbate RV dysfunction in PH. Intraoperative increases in PVR or changes in volume status can also worsen **RV contractility**. Inotropes should be considered if there is evidence of inadequate oxygen delivery because of myocardial depression. Dobutamine, epinephrine, and milrinone have all been used to increase contractility. Milrinone and dobutamine have the added benefit of reducing PVR which can help to offload the RV. They also however drop SVR, but this can be offset by the use of vasopressors. Vasopressin is a vasoconstrictor that can restore systemic perfusion pressure and coronary artery perfusion pressure without marked increases in PVR. In experimental models, vasopressin has been shown to bind to peripheral V_1 receptors and cause systemic vasoconstriction while also stimulating nitric oxide release and vasodilatation to the pulmonary circulation. However, for patients with RV dysfunction as well as hypotension, a vasopressor with inotropic properties such as norepinephrine and epinephrine, may be a better option.[43,44]

Each one of these drugs has the potential to cause tachyarrhythmias, which can be hemodynamically detrimental. These patients, particularly ones with precapillary PH are prone to developing atrial flutter.[43] **Maintaining sinus rhythm** is ideal to optimize RV preload and CO. Chemical or electrical cardioversion may be necessary to restore sinus rhythm and improve patient's hemodynamics.[43] A heart rate between 60 and 90 beats per minute is also recommended to maintain optimal RV performance and CO. Significant tachycardia must be avoided because it reduces time in diastole, resulting in inadequate ventricular filling and stroke volume.

Close post-operative monitoring is critical because these patients are at risk for cardiac and respiratory complications. Serious consideration should be made to transferring PH patients post thoracic surgery to an intensive care unit. Postoperative management should include the prevention of factors which exacerbate PVR, such as hypoxia, hypercapnia, acidosis, hypothermia, and pain. Vasodilator therapy started in the operating room should be continued and eventually transitioned to the patient's home regimen. Inotropes and vasopressors should be gradually weaned and conservative fluid management continued in the perioperative period to avoid a drop in CO. Finally, a plan for postoperative pain control should be established. High-dose opiates should be avoided as they can cause respiratory depression, hypoxia, and hypercarbia. Use of nonopiate medications, as well as nerve blocks with continuous catheters or epidurals should be continued postoperatively.

Conclusion

Patients with PH undergoing thoracic surgery have a higher morbidity and mortality compared with other procedures. However, when a specialized and focused multidisciplinary care team performs their assessment, optimization, intraoperative management, and postoperative monitoring, these procedures can be safely performed.

References

1. Ramakrishna G, Sprung J, Ravi BS, Chandrasekaran K, McGoon MD. Impact of pulmonary hypertension on the outcomes of noncardiac surgery: predictors of perioperative morbidity and mortality. *J Am Coll Cardiol.* 2005;45:1691–1699.
2. Meyer S, McLaughlin VV, Seyfarth H-J, et al. Outcomes of noncardiac, nonobstetric surgery in patients with PAH: an international prospective survey. *Eur Respir J.* 2013;41:1302–1307.
3. Price LC, Montani D, Jaïs X, et al. Noncardiothoracic nonobstetric surgery in mild-to-moderate pulmonary hypertension. *Eur Respir J.* 2010;35:1294–1302.
4. Kaw R, Pasupuleti V, Deshpande A, Hamieh T, Walker E, Minai OA. Pulmonary hypertension: an important predictor of outcomes in patients undergoing non-cardiac surgery. *Respir Med.* 2011;105:619–624.
5. Lai H-C, Lai H-C, Wang K-Y, Lee W-L, Ting C-T, Liu T-J. Severe pulmonary hypertension complicates postoperative outcome of non-cardiac surgery. *Br J Anaesth.* 2007;99:184–190.
6. Wei B, D'amico T, Samad Z, Hasan R, Berry MF. The impact of pulmonary hypertension on morbidity and mortality following major lung resection. *Eur J Cardiothorac Surg.* 2014;45:1028–1033.
7. Simonneau G, Montani D, Celermajer DS, et al. Haemodynamic definitions and updated clinical classification of pulmonary hypertension. *Eur Respir J.* 2019:53.
8. Fischer LG, Van Aken H, Bürkle H. Management of pulmonary hypertension: physiological and pharmacological considerations for anesthesiologists. *Anesth Analg.* 2003;96:1603–1616.
9. Galiè N, Humbert M, Vachiery J-L, et al. 2015 ESC/ERS Guidelines for the diagnosis and treatment of pulmonary hypertension: The Joint Task Force for the Diagnosis and Treatment of Pulmonary Hypertension of the European Society of Cardiology (ESC) and the European Respiratory Society (ERS)Endorsed by: Association for European Paediatric and Congenital Cardiology (AEPC), International Society for Heart and Lung Transplantation (ISHLT). *Eur Respir J.* 2015;46:903–975.
10. Sysol JR, Machado RF. Classification and pathophysiology of pulmonary hypertension. *Continu Cardiol Educ.* 2018;4(1).
11. Gille J, Seyfarth H-J, Gerlach S, Malcharek M, Czeslick E, Sablotzki A. Perioperative anesthesiological management of patients with pulmonary hypertension. *Anesth Res Pract.* 2012; 2012:356982.
12. Friedman SE, Andrus BW. Obesity and pulmonary hypertension: a review of pathophysiologic mechanisms. *J Obes.* 2012 2012.
13. Slinger P, Darling G. *Preanesthetic Assessment for Thoracic Surgery, Principles and Practice of Anesthesia for Thoracic Surgery.* New York, NY: Springer; 2011:11–34.
14. Brunelli A, Kim AW, Berger KI, DJ Addrizzo-Harris. Physiologic evaluation of the patient with lung cancer being considered for resectional surgery: diagnosis and management of lung cancer, 3rd ed. American College of Chest Physicians Evidence-Based Clinical Practice Guidelines. *Chest.* 2013;143:e166S–e190S.
15. ATS Committee on Proficiency Standards for Clinical Pulmonary Function Laboratories: ATS statement: guidelines for the six-minute walk test. *Am J Respir Crit Care Med.* 2002;166:111–117.
16. Altschul E, Remy-Jardin M, Machnicki S, et al. Imaging of pulmonary hypertension: pictorial essay. *Chest.* 2019; 156:211–227.
17. Henkens IR, Scherptong RWC, van Kralingen KW, Said SAM, Vliegen HW. Pulmonary hypertension: the role of the electrocardiogram. *Neth Heart J.* 2008;16:250–254.
18. Thenappan T, Ormiston ML, Ryan JJ, Archer SL. Pulmonary arterial hypertension: pathogenesis and clinical management. *BMJ.* 2018:360.
19. Cordina RL, Playford D, Lang I, Celermajer DS. State-of-the-art review: echocardiography in pulmonary hypertension. *Heart Lung Circ.* 2019;28:1351–1364.
20. Ginoux M, Cottin V, Glérant J-C, et al. Safety of right heart catheterization for pulmonary hypertension in very elderly patients. *Pulm Circ.* 2018;8.
21. Grignola JC. Hemodynamic assessment of pulmonary hypertension. *World J Cardiol.* 2011;3:10–17.
22. Sahay S. Evaluation and classification of pulmonary arterial hypertension. *J Thorac Dis.* 2019;11:S1789–S1799.
23. Pilkington SA, Taboada D, Martinez G. Pulmonary hypertension and its management in patients undergoing non-cardiac surgery. *Anaesthesia.* 2015;70:56–70.
24. Sandham JD, Hull RD, Brant RF, et al. Canadian Critical Care Clinical Trials Group. A randomized, controlled trial of the use of pulmonary-artery catheters in high-risk surgical patients. *N Engl J Med.* 2003;348:5–14.
25. Bussières JS. Iatrogenic pulmonary artery rupture. *Curr Opin Anaesthesiol.* 2007;20:48–52.
26. Hosseinian L. Pulmonary hypertension and noncardiac surgery: implications for the anesthesiologist. *J Cardiothorac Vasc Anesth.* 2014;28:1064–1074.
27. Sarkar MS, Desai PM. Pulmonary hypertension and cardiac anesthesia: anesthesiologist's perspective. *Ann Card Anaesth.* 2018;21:116–122.
28. Kaushal RP, Vatal A, Pathak R. Effect of etomidate and propofol induction on hemodynamic and endocrine response in patients undergoing coronary artery bypass grafting/mitral valve and aortic valve replacement surgery on cardiopulmonary bypass. *Ann Card Anaesth.* 2015;18:172–178.
29. Strumpher J, Jacobsohn E. Response to Drs Maxwell and Jackson. *J Cardiothorac Vasc Anesth.* 2012;26:e25–e26.
30. Ogawa K, Tanaka S, Murray PA. Inhibitory effects of etomidate and ketamine on endothelium-dependent relaxation in canine pulmonary artery. *Anesthesiology.* 2001;94:668–677.
31. Williams GD, Philip BM, Chu LF, et al. Ketamine does not increase pulmonary vascular resistance in children with pulmonary hypertension undergoing sevoflurane anesthesia and spontaneous ventilation. *Anesth Analg.* 2007;105:1578–1584.
32. Pritts CD, Pearl RG. Anesthesia for patients with pulmonary hypertension. *Curr Opin Anesthesiol.* 2010;23:411–416.
33. Saraswat V. Effects of anaesthesia techniques and drugs on pulmonary function. *Indian J Anaesth.* 2015;59:557–564.
34. Horlocker TT, Vandermeulen E, Kopp SL, Gogarten W, Leffert LR, Benzon HT. Regional anesthesia in the patient receiving antithrombotic or thrombolytic therapy. *Reg Anesth Pain Med.* 2018;43:263–309.
35. Saad FS, Baradie SYE, Aliem MAWA, Ali MM, Kotb TAM. Ultrasound-guided serratus anterior plane block versus thoracic paravertebral block for perioperative analgesia in thoracotomy. *Saudi J Anaesth.* 2018;12:565–570.
36. Marciniak D, Kelava M, Hargrave J. Fascial plane blocks in thoracic surgery. *Curr Opin Anaesthesiol.* 2020;33:1–9.
37. Ross AF, Ueda K. Pulmonary hypertension in thoracic surgical patients. *Curr Opin Anaesthesiol.* 2010;23:25–33.
38. Nonaka DF, Grichnik KP, Whitener GB. Pulmonary hypertension and thoracic surgery: diagnostics and advances in therapy and intraoperative management. *Curr Anesthesiol Rep.* 2014;4:135–141.

39. Bugedo G, Retamal J, Bruhn A. Driving pressure: a marker of severity, a safety limit, or a goal for mechanical ventilation? *Crit Care.* 2017;21.
40. Park M, Ahn HJ, Kim JA, et al. Driving pressure during thoracic surgery: a randomized clinical trial. *Anesthesiology.* 2019;130:385–393.
41. Ichinokawa M, Hida Y, Kaga K, Kawada M, Niizeki H, Kondo S. A case of primary pulmonary hypertension with pulmonary tumor. *Ann Thorac Cardiovasc Surg.* 2010;16:3.
42. Blaise G, Langleben D, Hubert B. Pulmonary arterial hypertension: Pathophysiology and anesthetic approach. *Anesthesiology.* 2003;99(6):1415–1432.
43. Condliffe R, Kiely DG. Critical care management of pulmonary hypertension. *BJA Education.* 2017;17(7):228–234.
44. McGlothlin D, Ivascu N, Heerdt PM. Anesthesia and pulmonary hypertension. *Prog Cardiovasc Dis.* 2012;55:199–217.

37

Tubeless Thoracic Procedures

JIAXI HE,# DIEGO GONZALEZ-RIVAS,# HUI LIU, QINGLONG DONG, LIXIA LIANG, JIANXING HE, SHUBEN LI, EDMOND COHEN

Tubeless thoracic procedures are performed without an endotracheal tube while the patient is spontaneously breathing. Initially it was defined as an "awake" thoracic procedure, but the term was updated to "tubeless" because these procedures are performed with sedation and/or regional block of variable extent while maintaining spontaneous ventilation.

For decades, the use of a double-lumen tube (DLT) and the insertion of chest tube drainage were considered mandatory for thoracoscopic pulmonary resection. Recently, an alternative minimally invasive tubeless approach to thoracic procedures is gaining popularity. The initial concern was that the iatrogenic surgical pneumothorax can be detrimental and not tolerated by a spontaneously breathing patient. In 2004 Pompeo et al.[1] reported the resection of pulmonary nodules by conventional video-assisted thoracic surgery (VATS) under intravenous anesthesia without endotracheal intubation. In addition, under direct thoracoscopic vision, vagus nerve block and lidocaine sprayed on the surface of the lung are used to effectively abolish the cough reflex. Avoiding the positive pressure ventilation fulfills the goal of performing a less traumatic, safe operation with decreased postoperative pain and expeditious postoperative recovery.

Airway management of thoracic surgery is crucial, and the challenge increases if the patients receive tubeless anesthesia. Previous studies show that airway-related emergencies occurred frequently during thoracic and tracheal surgeries.[2,3] Therefore a thorough and meticulous airway management is indispensable, including preoperative evaluation, preparation, intraoperative monitoring, manipulation, and postoperative precaution.

Preoperative Evaluation

A detailed preoperative airway evaluation is crucial for tubeless anesthetic thoracic surgery. The anesthesiologist should review the patient medical history and symptoms and carefully evaluate any underlying respiratory diseases, which may put the patient at risk or jeopardize the procedure.[4] In addition to the preoperative evaluation, pulmonary and cardiac function tests are indispensable in patients with hypersensitivity syndrome, asthma, chronic obstructive pulmonary disease (COPD) or a long-term smoking history. A bronchodilator challenge is recommended, depending on the patient medical history and his current medication. Furthermore, these underlying diseases should be evaluated preoperatively as a team approach in collaboration with the surgeon and the pulmonologists. The patients with poorly controlled respiratory diseases or pulmonary infection, including AECOPD (acute exacerbated COPD), should have a preoperative adequate antibiotics regime and surgery should be postponed until the therapy is completed. When tracheal or laryngeal surgeries are planned, characteristic signs and symptoms including stridor, hoarseness, and shortness of breath should raise a red flag as they usually indicate the presence of upper respiratory tract obstruction.[5–8] A preoperative communication between anesthesiologists and surgeons is necessary for a smooth and safe procedure.

Patients with a high body mass index (BMI) are not candidates for tubeless anesthesia because these patients have high oxygen consumption and carbon dioxide production owing to the high metabolic activity of body, tissue, and an increase in respiration work.[9–11] An increased intraabdominal pressure decreases the compliance of the thoracic cavity and restricts lung expansion. Moreover, excessive adipose tissue in the pharyngolaryngeal area would cause upper airway obstruction and hypoventilation usually associated with sleep apnea. Most importantly, if indicated, they may be difficult to intubate in an emergency during the procedure. Therefore patients with a higher BMI should have an extensive evaluation and if the procedure is not urgent, they should be encouraged to lose weight.[12–14] The criteria for patient selection for tubeless procedures are depicted in Box 37.1. Most importantly the patient should not have a difficult airway if the tubeless procedure needs to be converted to general anesthesia with an endotracheal tube.

In case of emergency during the surgical procedure, a difficult airway cart should be immediately available. The cart should contain topical anesthetic medications, video laryngoscopy (Fig. 37.1A) and angulated video-bronchoscopy with all sizes of endotracheal tubes, including nasal Ring-Adair-Elwyn (RAE), oral RAE, microlaryngeal tube, flexometallic tubes and DLTs.[7,14]

• BOX 37.1 Patient Selection

- ASA class II–III
- No difficult airways
- BMI <30 kg/m^2
- No significant cardiac disease (e.g., ischemia, arrhythmia, or EF <40%)
- No hemodynamic instability
- No coagulopathy
- No asthma or significant hypoxemia (pulmonary fibrosis)
- No sleep apnea, where dedicated control of the airway is often preferable when performing a surgical procedure

ASA, American Society of Anesthesiologists; *BMI*, body mass index; *EF*, ejection fraction.

Intraoperative Management

Except for a patients with a difficult airway, laryngeal masks (see Fig. 37.1B) are used in most cases of tubeless procedures to secure the airway. After thoracotomy, topical anesthesia by spraying lidocaine on the surface of lung and hilum (see Fig. 37.2A), intercostal nerve block (see Fig. 37.2B), and vagal nerve block (see Fig. 37.2C) are highly recommended to decrease the irritation threshold to cough and tracheobronchial spasm.[15] During the tubeless procedure, spontaneous respiration is maintained and therefore phrenic nerve block should be avoided.[16,17]

During the procedure the anesthesiologist should periodically use suction to remove mucus and sputum in the trachea and bronchus. In a patient where tracheostomy or bronchial resection is performed with a sleeve or reconstruction surgeries, close communication with

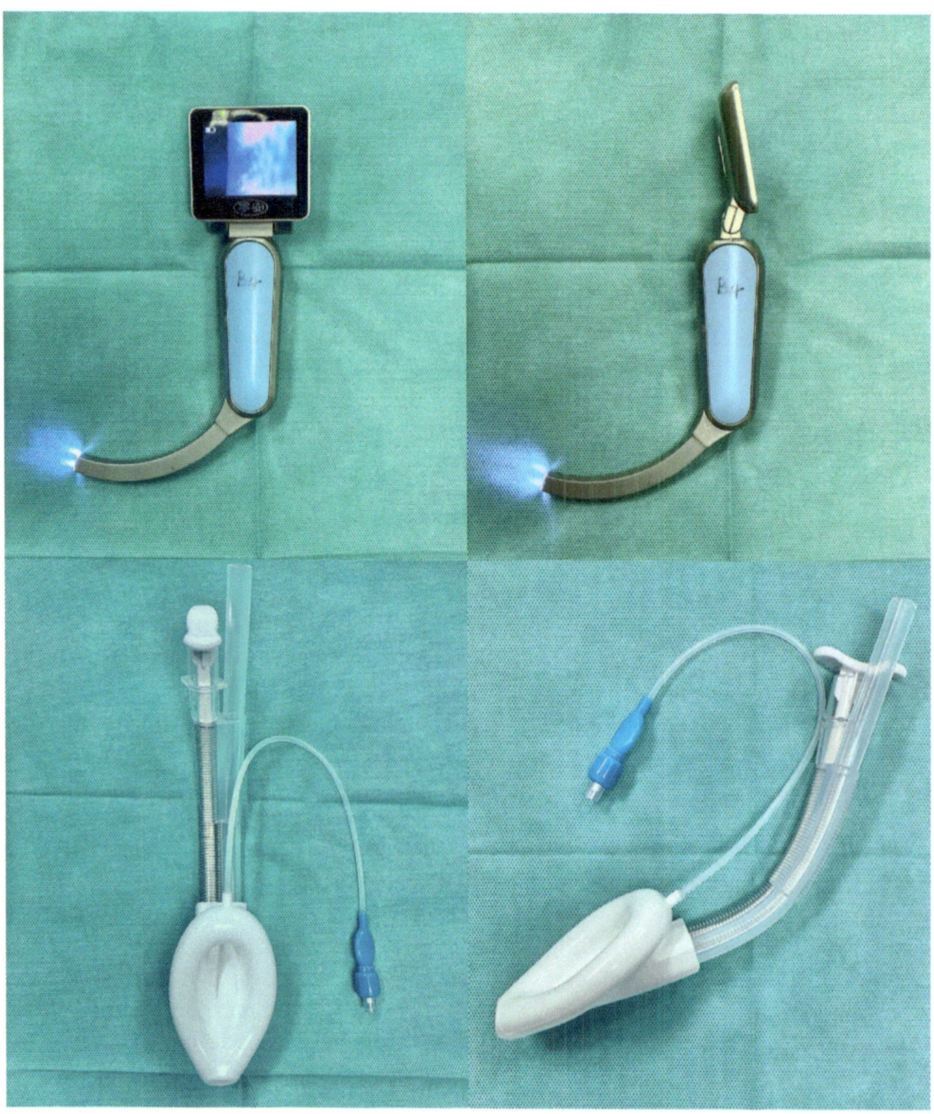

A

B

• Fig. 37.1 Tools for tubeless anesthesia. (**A**) Visualized laryngoscopy. (**B**) Double-lumen laryngeal mask.

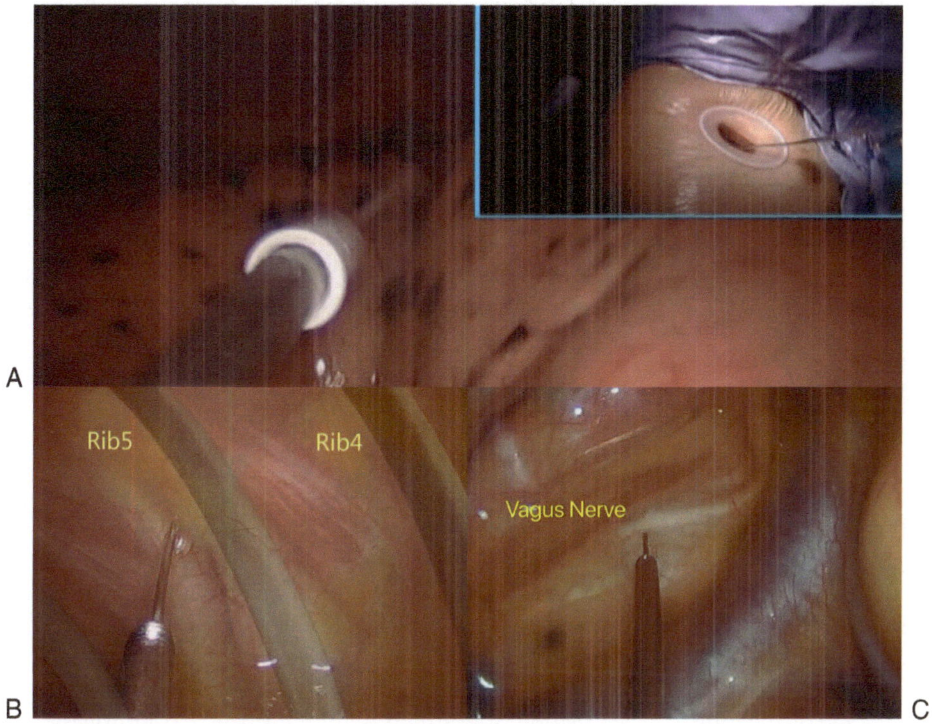

• **Fig. 37.2** Anesthetic maneuver. (**A**) Pulmonary surface spray anesthesia. (**B**) Intercostal nerve block. (**C**) Vagal nerve block.

the surgeon is crucial. When the tracheobronchial lumen is open, the oxygen concentration inside the trachea or bronchus is decreased and the blood or drainage may flow into the lumen to potentially cause an airway obstruction.[18–21] Therefore increasing the oxygen supply and meticulous suctioning before opening the bronchial lumen are helpful to minimize these risks of hypoxemia and hypercarbia.

Two phenomena occur when the patient is spontaneously breathing with an open chest that would need immediate treatment. Hypotension from mediastinal shift from vertical downward movement of the mediastinum and paradoxical breathing that causes movement of air from the nondependent lung into the dependent lung in inspiration and the opposite occurs during exhalation. This wasted ventilation results in hypoxemia and hypercarbia and can be treated by applying slight positive pressure with the face mask; this will usually immediately stabilize the patient.

An overview of the intraoperative management, including the type of regional blocks, such as epidural, paravertebral, or intercostal block and vagal nerve block, the sedation and the airway management with laryngeal mask airway (LMA), high-flow nasal cannula, or nasal continuous positive airway pressure (CPAP), is depicted in Table 37.1.

TABLE 37.1 Tubeless Thoracic Procedures

Regional Blockade	Sedation	Airway Management
• Thoracic epidural • Intercostal block • Serratus anterior plane block • Transverse thoracic plane block • Thoracic paravertebral block • Procedures perform by the surgeon • Local anesthetic infiltration • Vagal nerve blockade • Local anesthetic spray of the pleura	• Propofol infusion • Fentanyl • Remifentanil • Dexmedetomidine • Ketamine • Oxygen saturation >90% • Maintaining BIS 40–60 • Respiratory rate of 12–20 breaths per minute	• LMA • Nonrebreather oxygen mask • High-flow nasal cannula • Positive pressure nasal oxygen mask • Manual ventilation

BIS, Bispectral index; *LMA*, laryngeal mask airway.
Courtesy of Edmond Cohen, MD.

At the conclusion of the procedure, the laryngeal mask should be removed as soon as the patients regain their consciousness and the cough reflation gradually replaced by a facial mask or nasal tube instead. Saliva and secretions should be removed by gentle suction to clear the trachea and bronchus.[22] Encouraging coughs and deep breaths are also important for rapid recovery.[23] Coughs should not be encouraged after tracheal or laryngeal surgeries because of the risk of anastomotic dehiscence.

Advantages of Tubeless Thoracic Procedures (Box 37.2)

The most important advantage of tubeless thoracic procedures is the avoidance of mechanical ventilation. There is no benefit to the lung when ventilated with positive pressure. Mechanical ventilation has a number of potential side effects, such as pressure-induced injury, lung overdistension from volutrauma, the release of a variety of proinflammatory mediators, atelectasis, and potential laryngeal or tracheal injuries. Avoidance of muscle relaxants will reduce the degree of atelectasis in the dependent zone of the lung from diaphragmatic dysfunction, will keep the ventilation/perfusion (V/Q) matching, eliminating the potential for residual neuromuscular blockade. That is particularly important in the thoracic patient who may have compromised lung mechanics, COPD, compromised chest wall mechanics from hyperinflation, or a patient with myasthenia gravis. In addition, airway irritation or sore throat from intubation and chest tube or urinary catheter insertion can be avoided, and may result in shorter hospital stay and improved patient satisfaction. Another major advantage of nonintubated VATS is to offer the potential for surgery to patients who may be considered too high risk for endotracheal general anesthesia.

• BOX 37.2 Tubeless Thoracic Procedures

- Avoid intubation-related airway trauma from mechanical ventilation-induced lung injury
- OLV under spontaneous breathing preserves a better match of ventilation and perfusion
- Respiratory efficiency is increased by conserving diaphragmatic function
- No residual muscular blockade, offer surgical opportunities for patients who are too risky for intubated general anesthesia
- The quality of the pulmonary collapse obtained by iatrogenic pneumothorax via tubeless VATS is at least as good as in mechanical ventilation using a DLT or bronchial blocker
- Offer surgical opportunities for patients who are too risky for intubated general anesthesia
- The quality of the pulmonary collapse obtained by iatrogenic pneumothorax via tubeless VATS is at least as good as in mechanical ventilation using a DLT or bronchial blocker
- A faster and improved postoperative recovery and outcome
- Less postoperative nausea and vomiting

DLT, Double-lumen tube; *OLV*, one-lung ventilation; *VATS*, video-assisted thoracic surgery.
(Courtesy of Edmond Cohen, MD).

Ventilation/Perfusion With the Patient Breathing Spontaneously With an Open Chest

During the surgical procedure, patients are in the lateral decubitus position. The lung of operative hemithorax would collapse after thoracotomy. Although spontaneous respiration is maintained during tubeless procedures, the nerve block and topical anesthesia may decrease the respiration movement to some extent. This leads to decreased ventilation of well-perfused lung tissue, V/Q mismatch to results in hypoxemia, and hypercapnia.[24,25] In the lateral decubitus position, the thoracic cavity on the nonoperative side is compressed by the patient's mediastinal shift, which leads to restricted lung expansion that results in relative V/Q mismatch and hypoxemia. The transient hypoxemia or hypercapnia stimulates peripheral chemoreceptors and leads to increase respiratory rate and tidal volume. The increase in ventilation and perfusion to the nonoperative lung because of gravity and hypoxic pulmonary vasoconstriction (HPV) will improve the V/Q mismatch. To satisfy the oxygen consumption and improve the hypoxemia, incrementing oxygen supply is indicated. Because carbon dioxide has higher diffusion efficiency than oxygen, hypercapnia is uncommon during uncomplicated cases without airway obstruction or impaired diffusion.[65–68]

Risk of Carbon Dioxide Insufflation

Often, to enhance the quality of the lung collapse, the surgeon would insufflate carbon dioxide (CO2) into the operative open chest, which may induce hypotension and hypercarbia. Close communication with the surgeon to adjust the insufflation pressure is essential. The longer the operation time, the higher the risk from CO2 insufflation would be, especially in complicated open airway cases including sleeve resection, tracheal, or carinal resection and reconstruction. In spontaneously breathing patient, once the tidal volume and respiratory rate increase, which are induced by hypoxemia, CO2 rebreathing would occur. However, hypercapnia is seldomly seen in these cases because of an increased tidal volume.[29,30] Furthermore, connecting the laryngeal mask to the ventilator or increasing the oxygen supply would decrease the negative side effects from CO2 insufflation.

Monitoring

Compared with the general anesthesia, tubeless anesthesia procedure requires intense and careful monitoring. Standard monitors, which include electrocardiogram, noninvasive arterial blood pressure, respiratory rate, pulse oximetry and end-tidal carbon dioxide (EtCO2), are measured through the laryngeal mask or nasal cannula. A bispectral index (BIS) is also required to monitor the depth of sedation. Two peripheral intravenous lines should be placed during tubeless thoracic surgery.[31–33]

Because it is tubeless anesthesia, a urinary catheter, and in selected cases invasive blood pressure measurement are not placed routinely unless there are strong indications for their placement. Therefore anesthesiologists should carefully record the volume of fluid infusion and monitor the noninvasive blood pressure and heart rate to maintain a stable hemodynamic status. The anesthesiologists should be aware of the vital signs, including anesthesia induction, pharyngeal mask placement, skin incision, and thoracotomy.[34] This recommendation is derived from one of the largest series of tubeless patients from the Tor Vergata Hospital in Rome, Italy, that has formed the "Awake Thoracic Surgery Research Group" dedicated to performing thoracic operations in awake nonintubated patients. It reported that more than 1000 various tubeless thoracic procedures have been performed successfully, with a low conversion rate. Some of the procedures were performed Uniportal-tubeless.[35]

Anesthesia Sedation

The target of tubeless anesthesia is always "less is more." It means the surgeons, and anesthesiologists, goal is to achieve more with less procedure or drugs. The idea of the tubeless technique is that less procedure brings less invasiveness and less pain. Limiting drug usage leads to faster recovery. However, three major parts of anesthetic medications are necessary in any thoracic operation.

Sedation and Amnesia

Surgery may be an unpleasant experience with mental stress to the patients, with detrimental effects on their pathophysiology which may lead to alterations in vital signs.[36] Intraoperative awareness is a significant problem, may induce panic attack, have postoperative consequences, and jeopardize the safety of surgery. Therefore sedation and amnesia are most important during the thoracic surgeries, especially prolonged operations, including lobectomy, sleeve lobectomy, or tracheal surgeries. Adequate sedation would offer a stable condition for surgeons to complete the surgeries in a stress-free environment for patients.

During sedation, BIS monitoring is recommended and should be maintained between 40 and 60, for balanced respiration and hemodynamic stability. Before induction of anesthesia, midazolam and atropine are administered.[37] Subsequently, target-controlled infusion (TCI) of propofol is given aiming to maintain BIS around 60.[38,39] Inhaled anesthetics are not recommended during tubeless procedures, because it would be difficult to precisely control the depth of anesthesia under spontaneous respiration. The rate of the propofol infusion should be titrated to the patient BIS and vital signs.[33]

Analgesia

The unpleasant sensation of pain should be alleviated by analgesics administration throughout the surgical procedure. Making surgical incisions (VATS ports) from the skin to parietal pleura generates moderate to severe pain. Any manipulation of structures in the thoracic cavity cause irritation to the visceral pleura. These pain stimuli and irritations could significantly influence the stability of respiration, hemodynamic, and postoperative recovery. Therefore analgesia is crucial in every surgical procedure, especially in tubeless thoracic surgery.

Regional anesthesia is effective during thoracic surgical procedures. It can alleviate the pain of chest skin and parietal pleura, and is widely used during thoracentesis. Regional anesthesia is seldom used as the sole analgesia during tubeless thoracic surgery, and is used in combination with other anesthetic modalities to achieve better effects. Lidocaine is mostly administered for regional anesthesia from the skin to parietal pleura before incision. A total of 2% lidocaine is recommended for regional anesthesia after the skin incision is closed.[40–42]

Epidural anesthesia and paravertebral nerve block (Fig. 37.3) have been proved to have better intraoperative and postoperative pain control following traditional thoracotomy. Despite the shift from traumatic thoracotomy procedures to minimally invasive procedures, epidural anesthesia is still clinically used worldwide.[43] However, Yie et al. reported that it has no superiority over narcotic-based intravenous patient-controlled analgesia in pain control.[44] Moreover, both local (epidural hematoma, dural puncture,

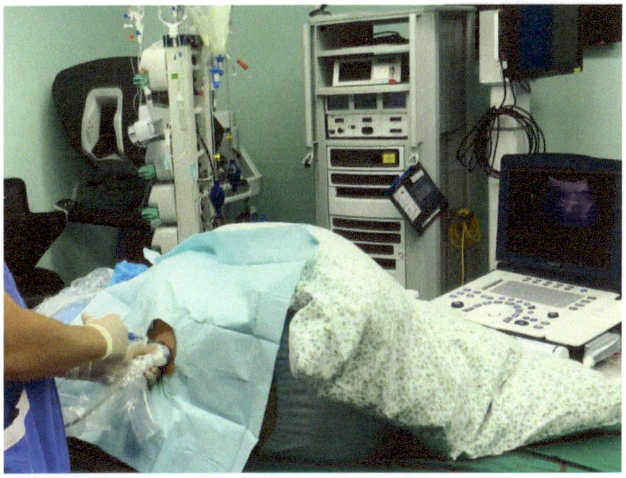

• **Fig. 37.3** Ultrasound-guided paravertebral nerve block anesthesia.

catheter malposition or displacement, infection, radiculitis, spinal trauma, medullar ischemia) and systemic (hypotension, head lightness, dizziness, headache, respiratory depression, shivering, urinary retention) complications have been previously reported in epidural anesthesia cases.

Bupivacaine, fentanyl, and its derivatives are routinely used during thoracic surgeries.[45,46] A 0.25% concentration of bupivacaine is given as a loading dose of 8 to 10 mL followed by continuously infusion (0.1 mL/kg/h). Some authors reported that 0.125% concentration is as effective with 10 mL and followed by infusion at 8 mL/h.[47,48] Levobupivacaine is an alternative for similar sensitive block, analgesia, and hemodynamic response.[49,50] Ropivacaine infusion, 0.75% or 0.25% concentration in 5 mL, was effective for postthoracotomy pain control.[51] A T4 level epidural catheter insertion is recommended. During the procedure, sensory level should frequently evaluate. Some centers have reported that the 7th or 8th thoracic intervertebral space could be also the effective puncture site. The epidural catheter should be inserted and advanced 3 cm into the epidural space followed by the administration of 2 mL of 2% lidocaine to test the sensory level.[52]

Paravertebral nerve block consists of the infiltration of local anesthetic in the cuneiform area along the vertebral column and affects the spinal nerves after egress from the intervertebral foramina[53] (see Fig. 37.2A). It is considered as unilateral epidural anesthesia because of its selectivity. Although the somatic and sympathetic nerves could be involved in this maneuver, the hemodynamic effects are less significant. It provides similar quality of analgesia, with fewer complications and better outcomes.[43,53,54] In some cases, the surgeons could perform it intraoperatively under direct vision. However, ultrasound guidance is the method of choice.[55–58] Catheter placement for continuous infusion or single dosage infiltration with long-acting anesthetic are both reported to be effective. Bupivacaine, levobupivacaine, and ropivacaine have been reported to have similar effects. Ropivacaine is administered at 0.75% while bupivacaine and levobupivacaine are used at 0.25% to 0.5%. A volume of 5 mL local anesthetics for each paravertebral space is injected. Continuous infusion is administered at the same concentration for bupivacaine and levobupivacaine (0.1 mL/kg/h or 2.5–10 mL/h).[43,54,55]

Intercostal nerve block (see Fig. 37.2B) can be performed percutaneously by the anesthesiologists blindly or echo-guided, or it can be done by surgeons "from the inside" via thoracoscopy. It is effective in reducing painful sensation after surgery. A mixture of lidocaine 1% to 2% and levobupivacaine 0.2% is used to block the level of the incision and always recommended to be extended two or three intercostal spaces above and below.[59,60] A volume of 1.5 to 2 mL is injected depending on the number of intercostal spaces which need to be covered. Adding low-dose epinephrine inhibits systemic absorption and prolongs the effect. Compared with the epidural anesthesia or paravertebral nerve block, the intercostal nerve block seems to be less effective for pain control. However, it has a lower incidence of adverse events and is easier to perform, which would shorten the anesthesia and surgery duration.

Intravenous analgesia is the prevailing approach in tubeless anesthesia because it has fast onset time and is easy to control. Consistent intravenous analgesia provides a stable condition for surgeons to perform the surgeries. During the surgical procedure, continuous infusion of remifentanil (0.03–0.05 mcg/kg/min) can be administered with dexmedetomidine (0.5–1.0 mcg/kg/h) and propofol TCI mode (1.0–3.0 mcg/mL) to maintain a stable analgesic condition and respiration. Fentanyl (50–100 mcg) or sufentanil (10 mcg) have been used during anesthesia induction.[21,61] However, no superiority has been observed in the previous studies. Preference is individual (Table 37.2).

Antireflection

Cough reflection in tubeless thoracic surgery, which is a protective mechanism, is an inevitable problem. Temporary suppression is required to prevent inference with the

TABLE 37.2 The Recommendations of Analgesics for Different Anesthesia Methods

Anesthetic Methods	Analgesics	Concentration	Dosage
Epidural Anesthesia	Ropivacaine	0.375%	10–15 mL
Incision Regional Anesthesia	Lidocaine	2%	5–10 mL
Topical Anesthesia	Lidocaine	2%	10 mL
Intercostal Nerve Block	Ropivacaine+Lidocaine (1:1)	0.375% Ropivacaine, 1% Lidocaine	1.5–2 mL each intercostal space
Vagal Nerve Block	Ropivacaine+Lidocaine (1:1)	0.375% Ropivacaine, 1% Lidocaine	5 mL
Intravenous Anesthesia	Induction: Fentanyl, Sufentanil Duration: Remifentanil	Remifentanil: 0.03–0.05 mcg/kg/min	Fentanyl: 50–100 mcg Sufentanil: 10 mcg

surgical procedure. On the other hand, it should not be oversuppressed because it is beneficial for the respiratory tract excretion and rapid recovery. Stretching the trachea, bronchus, lung, or hilum could induce cough during the operation. Vagal nerve block is usually used (2 mL levobupivacaine 0.25%). According to the anatomic difference between left and right sides, the paratracheal space on the right and the level of aortopulmonary window are chosen as the vagal block sites[62–65] (see Fig. 37.2C).

Potential Complications

Inappropriate Sedation and Pain Control

An inappropriate sedation and inadequate pain control could generate risks in the tubeless surgical procedure and ultimately lead to conversion to general anesthesia with endotracheal intubation. During the procedure, the conscious level of patients should be monitored carefully using BIS and should be maintained between 40 and 60. Besides, vital signs of patients, including body temperature, heart rate, respiratory, blood pressure, and blood gas are also crucial in monitoring the level of sedation and pain control. Close monitoring of these values and adjusting the dosage of analgesia and anesthesia are necessary to maintain stable and steady operation conditions.

Excessive Movement or Coughing

Excessive movement, including the patient's diaphragm and mediastinum, is one of the most common during tubeless anesthesia thoracic surgeries. It is closely dependent upon the team experience, and could interfere with the surgical procedure, prolong the duration of the operation, and further significantly deteriorate hemodynamic stability and respiration. Incomplete pain control and sedation account for the majority of the causes. Cough reflection can be present in cases with insufficient vagal nerve block. When the excessive movement is observed, it is best to briefly stop the procedure and possibly repeat the vagal nerve block or spray local anesthetics on the surface of the visceral pleura. The anesthesiologists could increase the analgesia and anesthesia administration according to the vital signs and BIS value.

Hemodynamic Instability

Hemodynamic instability has higher incidence in cardiothoracic surgeries than in other surgical procedures. During tubeless thoracic surgeries with the absence of central venous pressure, invasive artery pressure monitoring, or even urinary catheter, hemodynamic condition should be carefully monitored and maintained properly to prevent undesired consequences. In addition to medication and monitoring of ventilation, fluid therapy is crucial to stabilize hemodynamic conditions and optimize postoperative outcomes.[66,67] Intravascular volume directly affects cardiac output and consequently oxygen delivery. Hypervolemia can increase pulmonary complications, heart failure risk, and delay recovery. On the contrary, hypovolemia can compromise the perfusion of important organs, especially the kidney. It was reported that the incidence of acute kidney injury following thoracic surgery is between 5.9% and 6.8%.[68,69]

Hypoxia

Although muscle relaxants are avoided during tubeless thoracic surgery, sedation can still increase the risk of hypoxia owing to respiratory suppression and hypoventilation. Among the causes of hypoventilation, displacement of the laryngeal mask is commonly seen, which may lead to air leak and airway obstruction.[70] In these cases of high oxygen demand, one-lung ventilation without endotracheal intubation may be insufficient to maintain saturation. Adjustment of laryngeal mask and placement of suction tube into the trachea are effective methods. During complicated cases, such as sleeve resection or tracheal reconstruction, high-jet ventilation and cross-field intubation could be used to solve hypoxia.

Hypercapnia

Hypercapnia is seen during hypoventilation, especially in patients with COPD or neuromuscular disease (myasthenia gravis). In several studies, transient hypercapnia is reported as permissive, and conversion to general anesthesia is unnecessary. Partial pressure of CO_2 usually increases after thoracotomy and remains stable (<55 mm Hg) during the surgical process. It would return to normal gradually after wound closure. Most COPD cases can successfully be treated with mild assisted ventilation.[71,72] During long-lasting surgeries, periodical gentle assisted ventilation is recommended to lower the risk of hypercapnia. The management of hypoxemia and hypercapnia is depicted in Box 37.4.

• BOX 37.3 Reasons for Conversion to General Anesthesia

- Major bleeding, severe pleural adhesions, large tumors
- Severe hypoxemia, hypercapnia, and acidosis
- Hemodynamic instability: hypotension, cardiac index decreased, intractable arrhythmias, and right ventricular failure
- Persistent cough that creates difficulty or prevents performing surgery
- Excessive movement of the diaphragm or mediastinum, causing unsafe surgery
- Inability to collapse the lung
- Intraoperative airways injury

• BOX 37.4 Hypoxemia and Hypercarbia

The incidence of hypoxemia is low

- Intraoperative hypoxemia typically occurs after the lung at the surgical side completely collapses. If SpO2 is <90%, manually assisted ventilation or synchronized intermittent mechanical ventilation (SIMV) (FiO2 =100%, VT 3–5 mL/kg, RR 12–15 times/min, and oxygen flow 4–5 L/min) can be applied
- When the operated lung completely collapses, the airway resistance of the operated side is higher than that of the contralateral side
- During the low tidal-volume ventilation, most air will enter the contralateral lung, which does not cause the inflation of the operated lung and has negligible impact on the surgical operation

Intraoperative hypercapnia is common

- If PaCO2 is ≥60 mm Hg, manually assisted ventilation or SIMV (FiO2 = 100%, VT 3–5 mL/kg, RR 12–15 times/min, and oxygen flow 4–5 L/min) can be applied, along with the adjustment of infusion rates of propofol and remifentanil

FiO2, fraction of inspired oxygen; *PaCO2*, arterial partial pressure of carbon dioxide; *RR*, respiratory rate; *SpO2*, oxygen saturation; *VT*, tidal volume.

From He J, Liu J, Zhu C, et al. Expert consensus on tubeless video-assisted thoracoscopic surgery (Guangzhou). *J Thorac Dis.* 2019;11(10):4101–4108.

Conversion to General Anesthesia (Box 37.4)

Intraoperative conversion to general anesthesia with endotracheal intubation or cross-field intubation is inevitable in the cases of significant bleeding, massive pleural adhesion, or other sudden emergencies. The anesthesiologists should be able to convert the anesthesia mode during surgery and address a variety of complications, such as hypoxemia and hypercapnia. If the patient is hemodynamically unstable have movement or cough which interfere with the surgical procedure, or the ability to collapse the lung despite CO2 insufflation, endotracheal intubation would be necessary. Intubation in the lateral decubitus position is challenging to anesthesiologists and may require tilting the operative table to reduce the lateral position to allow laryngoscopy, most appropriately video laryngoscopy. Fiberoptic bronchoscopy intubation might be an option in the conversion to endotracheal intubation.

Expert Consensus on Tubeless Video-Assisted Thoracoscopic Surgery (Guangzhou)

Recently a group of worldwide experts with wide experience in performing tubeless thoracic procedures, (which included anesthesiologists, surgeons, and critical care providers) published an expert consensus on tubeless video-assisted thoracoscopic surgery (Guangzhou) that extensively covers the various issues in tubeless thoracic procedures.[73]

Box 37.5 depicts the inclusion criteria that were delineated in the consensus. It is clear that these criteria are more restrictive in the selection of patients for tubeless procedures. They limit the patients to American Society of Anesthesiologists (ASA) I or II and the age to below 65 years old, which eliminates a fair number of patients to qualify for tubeless procedures. In addition, there is restriction on the patient baseline PaO2 and CO2. Finally, they recommend the exclusion of patients who are likely to developed postoperative complications. As depicted in Box 37.6, the group offered a recommendation regarding the intraoperative management, including the use of LMA, assisting the intraoperative ventilation, ideal tidal volume, respiratory rate, and lung reinflation.

• BOX 37.5 Inclusion Criteria

- The operation duration is no more than 2 hours
- Aged 16–60 years
- Patients who have undergone previous surgeries, such as pulmonary bullous resection, lung biopsy, pulmonary wedge resection, pleural biopsy, thoracic sympathectomy, and/or resection of the posterior mediastinal tumor
- Patients who are unlikely to develop severe complications, such as major bleeding, respiratory obstruction, and severe postoperative pain
- Patients who have been measured as having an American Society of Anesthesiologists Standard (ASA) grade of ≤II
- There are no indications of arrhythmia, such as frequent premature ventricular contractions (PVCs) or atrial fibrillation
- For patients with suspicious or positive coronary heart disease and other high-risk conditions, coronary artery CT angiography can be performed; if the coronary artery and its branches have stenosis of ≤75%, coronary angiography is recommended
- Cardiopulmonary function (EF >50% and FEV_1% >50%) and other vital organ functions are normal. Resting blood gas analysis without oxygen inhaling shows PO2 ≥75 mm Hg and PCO2 <45 mm Hg

CT, Computed tomography; *EF*, ejection fraction; *FEV1*, forced expiratory volume in 1 second; *PCO2*, partial pressure of carbon dioxide; *PO2*, partial pressure of oxygen.

From He J, Liu J, Zhu C, et al. Expert consensus on tubeless video-assisted thoracoscopic surgery (Guangzhou). *J Thorac Dis.* 2019;11(10):4101–4108.

• BOX 37.6 Intraoperative Management

- The possibility of a positional shift of the laryngeal mask with sudden experiences inspiratory dyspnea, PetCO2 waveform suddenly becomes flat or disappears, and/or VT suddenly drops. The position of the laryngeal mask needs to be properly adjusted under deeper anesthesia.
- Reinflation of the operated lung may be difficult if air leaks from the laryngeal mask.
- Intraoperative sputum suctioning if sputum suctioning is required through the laryngeal mask.
- Repeated stimulation of the glottis should be avoided, as it may cause cough and laryngospasm.
- Excessive mediastinal bulging will affect the surgical operation. This is mainly because of one-lung breathing and the effect of the anesthetic drugs (remifentanil and propofol) on breathing after the establishment of artificial pneumothorax.
- The ideal parameters of one-lung spontaneous breathing are VT 3–4 mL/kg and RR 20–25 beats per minute. Because dexmedetomidine has a small effect on respiration, the dose of dexmedetomidine remains constant during surgery.
- The VT and RR of spontaneous breathing can be changed by adjusting the infusion rates of remifentanil and propofol.
- The BIS is maintained at 45–60. After local anesthesia + nerve block is achieved, the dose of propofol could be adjusted.

BIS, bispectral index; *PetC02*, partial pressure of end-tidal carbon dioxide; *RR*, respiratory rate; *VT*, tidal volume.
From He J, Liu J, Zhu C, et al. Expert consensus on tubeless video-assisted thoracoscopic surgery (Guangzhou). *J Thorac Dis.* 2019;11(10):4101–4108.

Conclusion

The tubeless technique in thoracic surgery has been widely used. Starting from simple cases such as sympathectomy and wedge resection, it has been applied to extensive cases, including sleeve resection and tracheal resection/reconstruction. Tubeless procedures maximized avoidance of any auxiliary catheterization and tubes placement, aimed at further reducing the surgical invasiveness and eventually make ambulatory VATS a reality in the near future. However, tubeless thoracic procedures also place higher demands on the surgical teams, and several measures should be followed in response to this. These procedures also favor rapid recovery with shorter anesthesia time, less airway inflammation, lower risk of postoperative infection, and shorter postoperative hospital stay. However, limitations of such techniques have to be recognized. Indications should be well clarified and evaluated to secure safety. Not only the expertise and experience of anesthesiologist's matter, but cooperation with other members in the surgical team is of crucial importance.

References

1. Pompeo E, Mineo D, Rogliani P, Sabato AF, Mineo TC. Feasibility and results of awake thoracoscopic resection of solitary pulmonary nodules. *Ann Thorac Surg.* 2004;78:1761–1768.
2. Moorthy SS, Gupta S, Laurent B, Weisberger EC. Management of airway in patients with laryngeal tumors. *J Clin Anesth.* 2005;17(8):604–609.
3. Wilson WM, Smith AF. The emerging role of awake videolaryngoscopy in airway management. *Anaesthesia.* 2018;73(9):1058–1061.
4. Rosenstock CV, Norskov AK, Wetterslev J, Lundstrom LH. Danish Anaesthesia Database. Emergency surgical airway management in Denmark: a cohort study of 452 461 patients registered in the Danish Anaesthesia Database. *Br J Anaesth.* 2016;117(1):i75–i82 Suppl.
5. Krecmerova M, Schutzner J, Michalek P, Johnson P, Vymazal T. Laryngeal mask for airway management in open tracheal surgery-a retrospective analysis of 54 cases. *J Thorac Dis.* 2018;10(5):2567–2572.
6. Zhu ZR, Hu ZY, Jiang YL, Xu LL, McQuillan PM. The use of a double-lumen central venous catheter for airway management in pediatric patients undergoing laryngeal papillomatosis surgery. *Paediatr Anaesth.* 2014;24(2):157–163.
7. Li SQ, Chen JL, Fu HB, Xu J, Chen LH. Airway management in pediatric patients undergoing suspension laryngoscopic surgery for severe laryngeal obstruction caused by papillomatosis. *Paediatr Anaesth.* 2010;20(12):1084–1091.
8. Okami K, Hamano T, Sakai A, et al. Airway management during the laryngoscopic surgery for the benign laryngeal obstructive disease. *Tokai J Exp Clin Med.* 2004;29(3):123–126.
9. Jones RL, Nzekwu MM. The effects of body mass index on lung volumes. *Chest.* 2006;130(3):827–833.
10. Pelosi P, Croci M, Ravagnan I, et al. The effects of body mass on lung volumes, respiratory mechanics, and gas exchange during general anesthesia. *Anesth Analg.* 1998;87(3):654–660.
11. Ezri T, Medalion B, Weisenberg M, Szmuk P, Warters RD, Charuzi I. Increased body mass index per se is not a predictor of difficult laryngoscopy. *Can J Anaesth.* 2003;50(2):179–183.
12. Calle EE, Thun MJ, Petrelli JM, Rodriguez C, Heath Jr CW. Body-mass index and mortality in a prospective cohort of U.S. adults. *N Engl J Med.* 1999;341(15):1097–1105.
13. Wang HX, Wan L, Tian M, Xue FS. A safe strategy for anesthesia induction and airway management in morbidly obese patients. *Chin Med J (Engl).* 2019;132(14):1747–1748.
14. Aceto P, Perilli V, Modesti C, Ciocchetti P, Vitale F, Sollazzi L. Airway management in obese patients. *Surg Obes Relat Dis.* 2013;9(5):809–815.

15. Hung MH, Hsu HH, Chan KC, et al. Non-intubated thoracoscopic surgery using internal intercostal nerve block, vagal block and targeted sedation. *Eur J Cardiothorac Surg*. 2014;46(4):620–625.
16. Zheng H, Hu XF, Jiang GN, Ding JA, Zhu YM. Nonintubated-awake anesthesia for Uniportal video-assisted thoracic surgery procedures. *Thorac Surg Clin*. 2017;27(4):399–406.
17. Kao MC, Lan CH, Huang CJ. Anesthesia for awake video-assisted thoracic surgery. *Acta Anaesthesiol Taiwan*. 2012;50(3):126–130.
18. Macchiarini P, Rovira I, Ferrarello S. Awake upper airway surgery. *Ann Thorac Surg*. 2010;89(2):387–390, discussion 90-1.
19. Liu J, Li S, Shen J, et al. Non-intubated resection and reconstruction of trachea for the treatment of a mass in the upper trachea. *J Thorac Dis*. 2016;8(3):594–599.
20. Peng G, Cui F, Ang KL, et al. Non-intubated combined with video-assisted thoracoscopic in carinal reconstruction. *J Thorac Dis*. 2016;8(3):586–593.
21. Li S, Liu J, He J, et al. Video-assisted thoracoscopic surgery resection and reconstruction of thoracic trachea in the management of a tracheal neoplasm. *J Thorac Dis*. 2016;8(3):600–607.
22. Hausman MS Jr, Jewell ES, Engoren M. Regional versus general anesthesia in surgical patients with chronic obstructive pulmonary disease: does avoiding general anesthesia reduce the risk of postoperative complications? *Anesth Analg*. 2015;120(6):1405–1412.
23. Mineo TC, Tacconi F. Nonintubated thoracic surgery: a lead role or just a walk on part? *Chin J Cancer Res*. 2014;26(5):507–510.
24. Grichnik KP, Clark JA. Pathophysiology and management of one-lung ventilation. *Thorac Surg Clin*. 2005;15(1):85–103.
25. Suehiro K, Okutani R. Influence of tidal volume for stroke volume variation to predict fluid responsiveness in patients undergoing one-lung ventilation. *J Anesth*. 2011;25(5):777–780.
26. Lohser J, Slinger P. Lung injury after one-lung ventilation: a review of the pathophysiologic mechanisms affecting the ventilated and the collapsed lung. *Anesth Analg*. 2015;121(2):302–318.
27. Gothard J. Lung injury after thoracic surgery and one-lung ventilation. *Curr Opin Anaesthesiol*. 2006;19(1):5–10.
28. Kozian A, Schilling T, Schutze H, Senturk M, Hachenberg T, Hedenstierna G. Ventilatory protective strategies during thoracic surgery: effects of alveolar recruitment maneuver and low-tidal volume ventilation on lung density distribution. *Anesthesiology*. 2011;114(5):1025–1035.
29. Sancheti MS, Dewan BP, Pickens A, Fernandez FG, Miller DL, Force SD. Thoracoscopy without lung isolation utilizing single lumen endotracheal tube intubation and carbon dioxide insufflation. *Ann Thorac Surg*. 2013;96(2):439–444.
30. Caso R, Kelly CH, Marshall MB. Single lumen endotracheal intubation with carbon dioxide insufflation for lung isolation in thoracic surgery. *Surg Endosc*. 2019;33(10):3287–3290.
31. Sunaga H, Blasberg JD, Heerdt PM. Anesthesia for nonintubated video-assisted thoracic surgery. *Curr Opin Anaesthesiol*. 2017;30(1):1–6.
32. Kiss G, Castillo M. Nonintubated anesthesia in thoracic surgery: general issues. *Ann Transl Med*. 2015;3(8):110.
33. Yang JT, Hung MH, Chen JS, Cheng YJ. Anesthetic consideration for nonintubated VATS. *J Thorac Dis*. 2014;6(1):10–13.
34. Solli P, Brandolini J, Bertolaccini L. Tubeless thoracic surgery: ready for prime time? *J Thorac Dis*. 2019;11(3):652–656.
35. Mineo TC, Tamburrini A, Perroni G, Ambrogi V. 1000 cases of tubeless video-assisted thoracic surgery at the Rome Tor Vergata University. *Future Oncol*. 2016;12(23s):13–18.
36. Sendelbach SE, Halm MA, Doran KA, Miller EH, Gaillard P. Effects of music therapy on physiological and psychological outcomes for patients undergoing cardiac surgery. *J Cardiovasc Nurs*. 2006;21(3):194–200.
37. Okuda K, Nakanishi R. The non-intubated anesthesia for airway surgery. *J Thorac Dis*. 2016;8(11):3414–3419.
38. Na SH, Jeong KH, Eum D, Park JH, Kim MS. Patient quality of recovery on the day of surgery after propofol total intravenous anesthesia for vitrectomy: A randomized controlled trial. *Medicine (Baltimore)*. 2018;97(40):e12699.
39. Umari M, Falini S, Segat M, et al. Anesthesia and fast-track in video-assisted thoracic surgery (VATS): from evidence to practice. *J Thorac Dis*. 2018;10(suppl 4):S542–S554.
40. De Cosmo G, Aceto P, Gualtieri E, Congedo E. Analgesia in thoracic surgery: review. *Minerva Anestesiol*. 2009;75(6):393–400.
41. Wu J, Buggy D, Fleischmann E, Parra-Sanchez I, Treschan T, Kurz A, et al. Thoracic paravertebral regional anesthesia improves analgesia after breast cancer surgery: a randomized controlled multicentre clinical trial. *Can J Anaesth*. 2015;62(3):241–251.
42. Steinthorsdottir KJ, Wildgaard L, Hansen HJ, Petersen RH, Wildgaard K. Regional analgesia for video-assisted thoracic surgery: a systematic review. *Eur J Cardiothorac Surg*. 2014;45(6):959–966.
43. Baidya DK, Khanna P, Maitra S. Analgesic efficacy and safety of thoracic paravertebral and epidural analgesia for thoracic surgery: a systematic review and meta-analysis. *Interact Cardiovasc Thorac Surg*. 2014;18(5):626–635.
44. Yie JC, Yang JT, Wu CY, Sun WZ, Cheng YJ. Patient-controlled analgesia (PCA) following video-assisted thoracoscopic lobectomy: comparison of epidural PCA and intravenous PCA. *Acta Anaesthesiol Taiwan*. 2012;50(3):92–95.
45. Manion SC, Brennan TJ. Thoracic epidural analgesia and acute pain management. *Anesthesiology*. 2011;115(1):181–188.
46. Powell ES, Cook D, Pearce AC, Davies P, Bowler GM, Naidu B, et al. A prospective, multicentre, observational cohort study of analgesia and outcome after pneumonectomy. *Br J Anaesth*. 2011;106(3):364–370.
47. Perttunen K, Nilsson E, Heinonen J, Hirvisalo EL, Salo JA, Kalso E. Extradural, paravertebral and intercostal nerve blocks for post-thoracotomy pain. *Br J Anaesth*. 1995;75(5):541–547.
48. Richardson J, Sabanathan S, Jones J, Shah RD, Cheema S, Mearns AJ. A prospective, randomized comparison of preoperative and continuous balanced epidural or paravertebral bupivacaine on post-thoracotomy pain, pulmonary function and stress responses. *Br J Anaesth*. 1999;83(3):387–392.
49. Novak-Jankovic V, Milan Z, Potocnik I, et al. A prospective, randomized, double-blinded comparison between multimodal thoracic paravertebral bupivacaine and levobupivacaine analgesia in patients undergoing lung surgery. *J Cardiothorac Vasc Anesth*. 2012;26(5):863–867.
50. Cok OY, Eker HE, Turkoz A, et al. Thoracic epidural anesthesia and analgesia during the perioperative period of thoracic surgery: levobupivacaine versus bupivacaine. *J Cardiothorac Vasc Anesth*. 2011;25(3):449–454.
51. Casati A, Alessandrini P, Nuzzi M, et al. A prospective, randomized, blinded comparison between continuous thoracic paravertebral and epidural infusion of 0.2% ropivacaine after lung resection surgery. *Eur J Anaesthesiol*. 2006;23(12):999–1004.
52. Li S, Jiang L, Ang KL, et al. New tubeless video-assisted thoracoscopic surgery for small pulmonary nodules. *Eur J Cardiothorac Surg*. 2017;51(4):689–693.
53. Piraccini E, Pretto Jr EA, Corso RM, Gambale G. Analgesia for thoracic surgery: the role of paravertebral block. *HSR Proc Intensive Care Cardiovasc Anesth*. 2011;3(3):157–160.

54. Davies RG, Myles PS, Graham JM. A comparison of the analgesic efficacy and side-effects of paravertebral vs epidural blockade for thoracotomy–a systematic review and meta-analysis of randomized trials. *Br J Anaesth*. 2006;96(4):418–426.
55. Ding X, Jin S, Niu X, Ren H, Fu S, Li Q. A comparison of the analgesia efficacy and side effects of paravertebral compared with epidural blockade for thoracotomy: an updated meta-analysis. *PLoS One*. 2014;9(5):e96233.
56. Amlong C, Guy M, Schroeder KM, Donnelly MJ. Out-of-plane ultrasound-guided paravertebral blocks improve analgesic outcomes in patients undergoing video-assisted thoracoscopic surgery. *Local Reg Anesth*. 2015;8:123–128.
57. Abdallah FW, Morgan PJ, Cil T, et al. Ultrasound-guided multilevel paravertebral blocks and total intravenous anesthesia improve the quality of recovery after ambulatory breast tumor resection. *Anesthesiology*. 2014;120(3):703–713.
58. Helms O, Mariano J, Hentz JG, et al. Intra-operative paravertebral block for postoperative analgesia in thoracotomy patients: a randomized, double-blind, placebo-controlled study. *Eur J Cardiothorac Surg*. 2011;40(4):902–906.
59. Wurnig PN, Lackner H, Teiner C, et al. Is intercostal block for pain management in thoracic surgery more successful than epidural anaesthesia? *Eur J Cardiothorac Surg*. 2002;21(6):1115–1119.
60. Bolotin G, Lazarovici H, Uretzky G, Zlotnick AY, Tamir A, Saute M. The efficacy of intraoperative internal intercostal nerve block during video-assisted thoracic surgery on postoperative pain. *Ann Thorac Surg*. 2000;70(6):1872–1875.
61. Guo Z, Yin W, Wang W, et al. Spontaneous ventilation anaesthesia: total intravenous anaesthesia with local anaesthesia or thoracic epidural anaesthesia for thoracoscopic bullectomy. *Eur J Cardiothorac Surg*. 2016;50(5):927–932.
62. Hung WT, Cheng YJ, Chen JS. Video-assisted thoracoscopic surgery lobectomy for lung cancer in nonintubated anesthesia. *Thorac Surg Clin*. 2020;30(1):73–82.
63. Chen JS, Cheng YJ, Hung MH, Tseng YD, Chen KC, Lee YC. Nonintubated thoracoscopic lobectomy for lung cancer. *Ann Surg*. 2011;254(6):1038–1043.
64. Guarracino F, Gemignani R, Pratesi G, Melfi F, Ambrosino N. Awake palliative thoracic surgery in a high-risk patient: one-lung, non-invasive ventilation combined with epidural blockade. *Anaesthesia*. 2008;63(7):761–763.
65. Pompeo E, Mineo TC. Awake operative videothoracoscopic pulmonary resections. *Thorac Surg Clin*. 2008;18(3):311–320.
66. Pedziwiatr M, Pisarska M, Major P, et al. Laparoscopic colorectal cancer surgery combined with enhanced recovery after surgery protocol (ERAS) reduces the negative impact of sarcopenia on short-term outcomes. *Eur J Surg Oncol*. 2016;42(6):779–787.
67. Gustafsson UO, Hausel J, Thorell A, et al. Adherence to the enhanced recovery after surgery protocol and outcomes after colorectal cancer surgery. *Arch Surg*. 2011;146(5):571–577.
68. Ahn HJ, Kim JA, Lee AR, Yang M, Jung HJ, Heo B. The risk of acute kidney injury from fluid restriction and hydroxyethyl starch in thoracic surgery. *Anesth Analg*. 2016;122(1):186–193.
69. Ishikawa S, Griesdale DE, Lohser J. Acute kidney injury after lung resection surgery: incidence and perioperative risk factors. *Anesth Analg*. 2012;114(6):1256–1262.
70. Pompeo E, Tacconi F, Mineo TC. Comparative results of non-resectional lung volume reduction performed by awake or non-awake anesthesia. *Eur J Cardiothorac Surg*. 2011;39(4):e51–e58.
71. Pompeo E, Rogliani P, Tacconi F, et al. Randomized comparison of awake nonresectional versus nonawake resectional lung volume reduction surgery. *J Thorac Cardiovasc Surg*. 2012;143(1):47–54, e1.
72. Mineo TC, Pompeo E, Mineo D, Tacconi F, Marino M, Sabato AF. Awake nonresectional lung volume reduction surgery. *Ann Surg*. 2006;243(1):131–136.
73. He J, Lui J, Zhu C, et al. Expert consensus on tubeless video-assisted thoracoscopic surgery (Guangzhou). *J Thorac Dis*. 2019;11(10):4101–4108.

38

Thoracic Anesthesia for the Geriatric Patient

MARIA CASTILLO

Introduction

Among the geriatric population, there is great variability in physiologic condition from person to person. Because of this variability, the patient's preoperative functional status, comorbidities, and tumor stage may influence surgical outcomes more than chronologic age alone. However, even an otherwise healthy older person will exhibit limited physiologic reserve because of the normal process of aging. Optimal management of these patients in the perioperative period will necessitate an understanding of changes in physiologic reserve and consideration of comorbid conditions and overall health status. Chronic obstructive pulmonary disease (COPD) and congestive heart failure in particular have implications for postoperative morbidity and mortality. Patient quality of life, overall life expectancy, and functional status must also be considered.

Various studies involving preoperative assessment aim to elucidate risk factors and implement resources to optimize overall patient health and physiologic condition, and thus decrease morbidity and mortality. Minimally invasive surgical techniques, extent of surgical resection, and anesthetic considerations may all play roles in achieving satisfactory outcomes in this population.

Demographics

It is predicted that by the year 2030, there will be more than 70 million United States citizens over the age of 65 years.[1] Adults 85 years old or older are the fastest growing age group in the United States. By 2060, the number of people aged 85 years and older is expected to nearly triple from 6.4 million in 2016 to 19 million.[2]

Cancer is the second leading cause of death in the United States, and the probability of developing cancer increases with age. Among people age 60 to 79 years, it is the leading cause of death.[3] The incidence of cancer is 9.8 times greater among people older than 65 years than those younger than 65 years.[4] According to the National Cancer Institute Surveillance, Epidemiology, and End Results (SEER) Program, 56% of all new cancer diagnoses were among patients older than 65 years.[1] Almost two-thirds of cancer survivors are aged 65 years or older.[5] People older than 85 years make up 2% of the population, but 8% of all new cancer diagnoses.[2] It is estimated that there were 228,150 new diagnoses of cancer of the lung or bronchus, and 142,670 deaths from these cancers in 2019. Lung cancer is the most common cause of cancer death, compromising 25% of all cancer deaths. It is the second most common cancer diagnosis for both men and women.[3] The median age of lung cancer patients presenting for surgery is greater than 70 years.[6]

The expanding geriatric population, with its increased risk of cancer compared with younger patients, will lead to an increase in elderly patients presenting for thoracic surgery. Thoracic anesthesiologists must be adept at caring for patients who may have a wide range of chronic conditions, as well as suffer from expected age-related physiologic changes.

Physiology of Aging

Elderly patients may exhibit a limited ability to respond to the stress of illness or major surgery because of the natural decline of maximal physiologic reserves. Manifestations of pathology may be blunted, and a geriatric patient may have symptoms that are atypical, diminished, or misdiagnosed as simply because of "old age."[7] The incidence of comorbidities is increased in this patient population, especially cardiovascular disease and pulmonary disease. These comorbidities superimposed on normal senescence can make management of elderly patients more complex.

Cardiovascular Changes

Interrelated molecular and structural changes occur within the myocardium, aorta, and cardiac conduction system (Table 38.1). The breakdown of elastin and increased collagen deposition and cross-linking cause vascular stiffness, which increases impedance and peripheral vascular resistance. The aorta becomes more dilated, exhibiting decreased

TABLE 38.1 Age-Related Cardiovascular Changes

Cardiac	Progressive cardiomyocyte hypertrophy Gradual development of cardiac fibrosis Increased collagen deposition and altered cross-linking
	Increased fatty infiltration and extracellular matrix degradation capacity Decreased myocardial reserve capacity Decreased left ventricular (LV) function Increased LV mass secondary to increased wall thickness and volumes Prolonged systolic contraction and diastolic relaxation
	Increased risk of conduction defects Decreased heart rate variability
	Increased stroke work Increased dependence on preload and atrial kick Decreased autophagy Accumulation of misfolded proteins and dysfunctional mitochondria
Vascular	Increased afterload Increased peripheral vascular resistance
	Increased incidence of coronary artery disease, plaques, calcification, and fixed stenosis
	Impaired vasodilation Decreased arterial elasticity
	Aortic dilation and increased pulse wave velocity Aortic thickening with decreased compliance and higher wall tension
Reflex regulation	Decreased sympathetic signaling Baroreceptor impairment
	Decreased chronotropic and inotropic response to catecholamines
	Decreased maximal cardiac output and heart rate
	Diminished autonomic control of peripheral vascular resistance

Modified from Castillo MD, Port J, Heerdt PM. Thoracic surgery in the elderly. In: Slinger P, ed. *Principles and Practice of Anesthesia for Thoracic Surgery*. 2nd ed. Switzerland: Springer; 2019; Meschiari CA, Ero OK, Pan H, Finkel T, Lindsey ML. The impact of aging on cardiac extracellular matrix. *Geroscience*. 2017;39(1):7–18; Shirakabe A, Ikeda Y, Sciaretta S, Zablocki DK, Sadoshima J. Aging and autophagy in the heart. *Circ Res*. 2016;118(10):1563–1576.

compliance associated with higher wall tension, as large elastic arteries become stiffer with an increase in pulse wave velocity and pulse pressure. This in turn is associated with an increase in left ventricular (LV) afterload with LV dilatation or reduced ejection fraction. Coronary arteries may develop plaques and calcified lesions, as well as fixed stenoses.[8]

Progressive myocyte hypertrophy, myocardial fibrosis, inflammation, valvular sclerosis, and calcification lead to increased LV mass over time and decreased compliance. Subcellular changes in myocyte calcium cycling occur that allow the ventricle to maintain tension against increased afterload,[9] which can be helpful in some situations but maladaptive under other conditions, such as in the setting of tachycardia. In such a situation, delayed relaxation can impede chamber filling. Over time, there is an accumulation of misfolded proteins and dysfunctional mitochondria, as well as decreased in dysfunctional cell components removal by autophagy. Cardiac aging is characterized by the presence of hypertrophy, fibrosis, and accumulation of misfolded proteins and dysfunctional mitochondria. Autophagy may play an important role in combating the adverse effects of aging in the heart. Autophagy is a lysosome-dependent bulk degradation mechanism that is essential for intracellular protein and organelle quality control. Autophagic flux is generally decreased in aging hearts, with loss of function that develops exacerbated cardiac dysfunction that is accompanied by accumulation of misfolded proteins and dysfunctional organelles. Stimulation of autophagy generally improves cardiac function by removing accumulated misfolded proteins, dysfunctional mitochondria, and damaged deoxyribonucleic acid, thereby improving the overall cellular environment and alleviating aging-associated pathology in the heart.[10] Increases in fatty infiltration, fibrosis, and amyloid content can result from altered collagen cross-linking that can increase the risk of conduction defects. Hypertrophic myocytes demand more energy and oxygen. As a result, cardiac performance may be maintained under normal circumstances, however, the diminished cardiac reserve may become apparent when the patient's heart is subjected to increased workload or stressors.[8]

Homeostatic reflexes are dampened, which increases the impact of the age-related decline in cardiovascular reserve.[9] Typical changes include decreased baroreceptor sensitivity, myocardial response to catecholamines, and autonomic control of peripheral vascular resistance. Maximal heart rate and cardiac output decrease as well.[11]

Pulmonary Changes

Alterations in lung parenchyma, the chest wall, and central regulation of respiration that occur with aging can contribute to decreased respiratory function (Table 38.2). Fewer alveoli and lung capillaries, enlargement of alveolar air spaces, and decreased airway size and alveolar-capillary surface area become apparent with age. These changes result in decreased elastic recoil and less negative intrapleural pressure. Weakened musculature, a stiffer rib cage, kyphosis, and a greater anteroposterior diameter of the thorax lead to decreased chest wall compliance. The pulmonary physiologic changes of the aging lung may synergize with the pathologic changes of various lung diseases to affect lung structure and function. Such synergistic effects may lead to more severe manifestations of lung disease in the

TABLE 38.2 Age-Related Respiratory Changes

Structural	Alterations in collagen fiber network Decreased number of alveoli Decreased number of lung capillaries Impairment of elastic recoil Alveolar duct dilation Enlargement of alveolar air spaces Diminished alveolar-capillary surface area Decrease in alveolar surface tension Less efficient mucociliary transport Diminished protective airway reflexes
Extrapulmonary	Loss of respiratory muscle mass Decreased diaphragmatic strength Decreased chest wall compliance because of fibrosis Stiffening of the rib cage because of calcification Decreased negative intrapleural pressure
Central regulation	Blunted ventilatory response to hypoxia Blunted ventilatory response to hypercarbia Increased periodic breathing during sleep
Functional manifestations	Increased functional residual capacity (FRC) Increased air trapping Decreased forced expiratory volume exhaled in 1 sec (FEV_1) Decreased forced vital capacity (FVC) Increased residual volume (RV) Increased closing capacity Decreased maximal voluntary ventilation (MVV) Increased work of breathing Widened alveolar-arterial gradient for oxygen Increased dead space Decreased diffusion capacity of the lung for carbon monoxide (DLCO) Increased ventilation–perfusion mismatch Decreased resting arterial partial oxygen pressure (PaO_2) More susceptible to infection and environmental stresses

Modified from Castillo MD, Port J, Heerdt PM. Thoracic surgery in the elderly. In: Slinger P, ed. *Principles and Practice of Anesthesia for Thoracic Surgery*. 2nd ed. Switzerland: Springer; 2019; Skloot GS. The effects of aging on lung structure and function. *Clin Geriatr Med*. 2017;33(4):447–457; Barnes PJ. Pulmonary diseases and ageing. *Subcell Biochem*. 2019;91:45–74.

elderly. Loss of elastic recoil of the lung is a prominent feature of aging, similar to asthma and COPD. The presence of alveolar enlargement in the aged adult likely coexists with destruction of alveolar walls and the inflammatory infiltrate found in patients with emphysema. Aging leads to changes in the expression of transforming growth factor-β and extracellular matrix composition, which may lead to increased incidence of fibrotic lung disorders in the elderly. Although total lung capacity is characteristically maintained with normal aging, because the increased residual volume is counterbalanced by the decrease in vital capacity, this is not the case in the older individual with fibrotic lung disease, given the significant decrease in vital capacity (Fig. 38.1).

Aging is associated with changes in the pulmonary circulation that occur in response to increased dead space ventilation and ventilation/perfusion mismatch, as well as to general stiffening of the pulmonary vasculature, with an increase in pulmonary arterial systolic pressure particularly pertinent during exercise. The effects on the pulmonary circulation because of aging combined with severe lung disease may worsen gas exchange and increase the work of breathing[12] (Fig. 38.2).

Secretory and immune function also wane, resulting in less efficient mucociliary transport, less robust polymorphonuclear leukocyte function, blunted delayed-type hypersensitivity response to foreign antigens, and an increased response to autologous antigens.[11] Ventilatory response to hypoxia and hypercarbia is diminished, and periodic breathing during sleep may increase. Air trapping, work of breathing, closing capacity, dead space, and ventilation-perfusion mismatch increase. Forced expiratory volume exhaled in one second (FEV_1), forced vital capacity (FVC), diffusing capacity, and maximal voluntary ventilation (MVV) decrease.[12] The alveolar-arterial gradient for oxygen widens, and resting arterial oxygen partial pressure (PaO2) decreases. As a result of these changes, lung function can additionally be compromised after thoracic surgery, particularly in patients who have a history of COPD. Splinting for pain from chest incision exacerbates these effects. Conversely, opioids can further blunt the response to hypoxia and hypercarbia (Fig. 38.3).

Hepatorenal Changes

Changes in liver and kidney function as a result of the aging process can profoundly affect metabolism and clearance (Table 38.3). Liver size can decrease by 40%, as well as renal mass by the age of 80 years.[13] Hepatic blood flow can decrease by 35% to 50%.[14] Hepatic vascular resistance increases, and portal pressure increases. Hepatocyte function deteriorates, decreasing molecular biosynthesis and clearance of toxins.[13] Decreased perfusion can affect the plasma clearance of drugs metabolized by the liver, such as opiates, benzodiazepines, propofol, etomidate, barbiturates, and most nondepolarizing neuromuscular blockers, which are commonly used during anesthesia.[15] Decreased

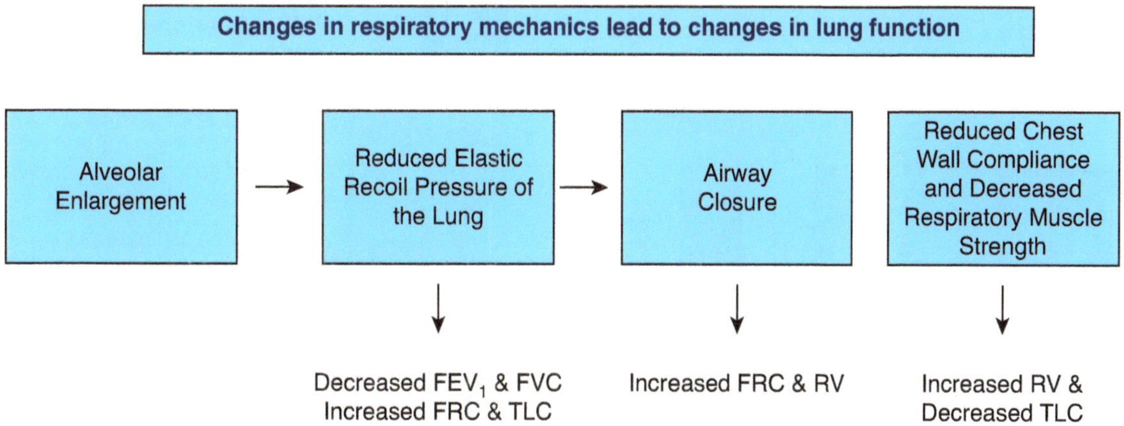

• **Fig. 38.1 Changes in respiratory mechanics lead to changes in lung function.** The reduction in elastic recoil pressure with aging causes a decrease in forced expiratory volume in 1 second (*FEV_1*) and forced vital capacity (*FVC*), and increase in functional residual capacity (*FRC*) and total lung capacity (*TLC*). The decreased elastic recoil pressure facilitates airway closure, which increases air trapping (i.e., FRC and residual volume increase). Reduced chest wall compliance and decreased respiratory muscle strength increase residual volume but tend to decrease TLC. *RV,* Residual volume. (From Skloot GS. The effects of aging on lung structure and function. *Clin Geriatr Med*. 2017;33(4):447–457.)

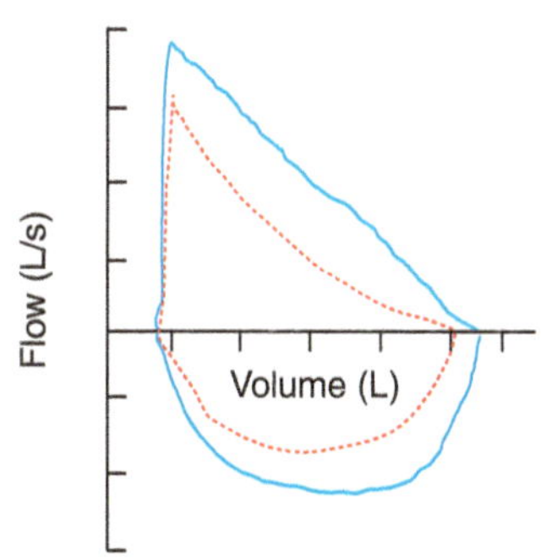

• **Fig. 38.2** The expiratory limb of the flow volume loop in an elderly subject (*dashed line*) suggests obstruction to airflow by its convex or scooped-out appearance in contrast to the flow volume loop from a younger subject (*solid line*). (From Skloot GS. The effects of aging on lung structure and function. *Clin Geriatr Med*. 2017;33(4):447–457.)

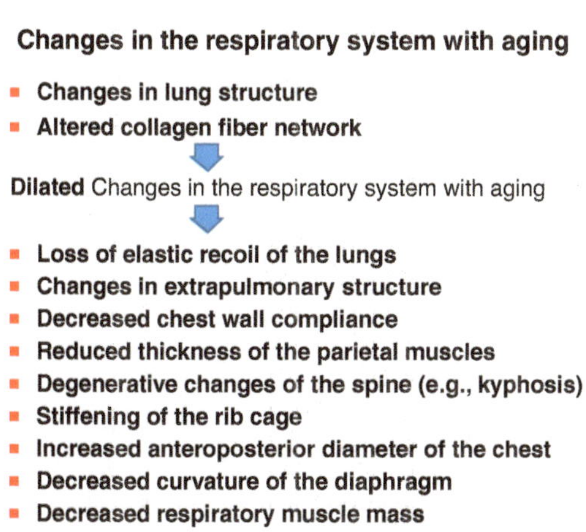

• **Fig. 38.3** Changes in the respiratory system with aging. (From Skloot GS. The effects of aging on lung structure and function. *Clin Geriatr Med*. 2017;33(4):447–457.)

cytochrome P450 activity compounds this affect. Changes in immune function can predispose elderly patients to autoimmunity, while decreasing the immune response to pathogens and malignant cells.[14]

The number of functional glomeruli decrease with aging as a result of increased nephrosclerosis, increased arterial atherosclerosis, tubular atrophy, and interstitial fibrosis. Cortical volume decreases, and there may be other structural changes, such as an increased number of cysts or focal scars. Elderly patients possess diminished renal functional reserve, putting them at higher risk for ischemia and acute kidney injury. Glomerular filtration rate (GFR) declines at a rate of 6.3 mL/min/1.73 m^2 per decade. The lowest risk of mortality is at a GFR of more than or equal to 75 mL/min/1.73 m^2 for those under 55 years but at a lower GFR of 45 to 104 mL/min/1.73 m^2 for those 65 years and over.[16] These patients experience prolonged elimination half-time of drugs, dependent on renal clearance. Reduced renal perfusion decreases GFR, creatinine clearance, and response to antidiuretic hormone aldosterone, renin, and vasopressin. Variability in individually calculated pharmacokinetic parameters increases with age, resulting in varying clearance of drugs across the geriatric population.[17] Diminished sodium reabsorption, potassium secretion, and urine concentration ability puts the geriatric patient at higher risk of volume depletion and salt retention[18] (Fig. 38.4).

Nervous System Changes

Changes in the brain that occur with age include a decrease in the number of dendrites and synapses, leading to decreased neuronal connectivity and brain volume. Older patients are at higher risk of experiencing dementia, sleep disorders, memory problems, movement disorders, and delirium.[19] Cognitive function varies greatly among the elderly in terms of reserve and baseline deficit. An association between

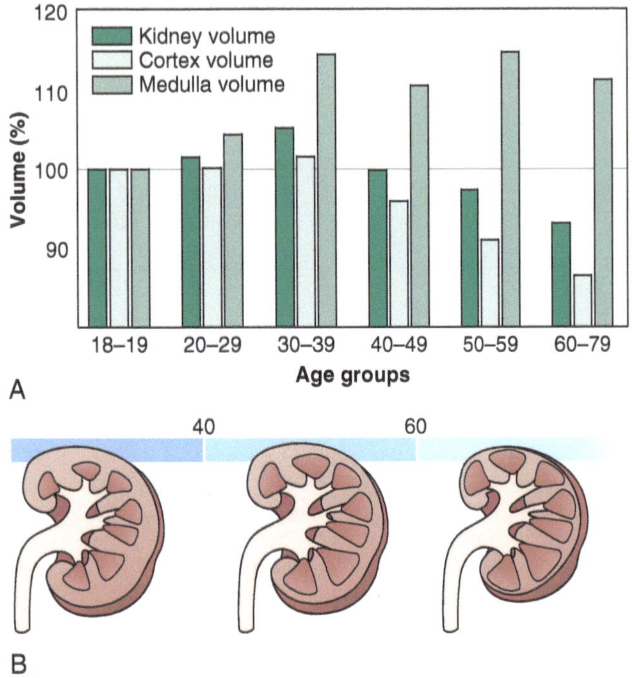

• **Fig. 38.4** Changes in the renal system with aging. **A.** Cortical volume declines, whereas medullary volume increases, making total kidney volume relatively stable until about 50 years of age. After which, medullary volume does not increase anymore and total kidney volume begins to decline. **B.** Schematic illustration of cortical and medullary volume changes with aging (From Denic A, Glassock RJ, Rule AD. Structural and functional changes with the aging kidney. *Adv Chronic Kidney Dis*. 2016;23(1):19–28.)

postoperative delirium and long-term outcome, as highlighted by recent data, suggests that short-term cognitive impairment may reflect systemic deficits. Using a series of functional and cognitive assessments, Robinson et al. found a 44% incidence of delirium in a study of 144 patients over 50 years old, of whom more than half underwent thoracic surgery.[20] Risk factors included increasing age, hypoalbuminemia, anemia, intraoperative hypotension, history of alcohol abuse, preexisting dementia, and impaired functional status. Delirium has been associated with increased length of hospital stay and a greater 6-month mortality.[21]

Medication choice and administration can have particular importance for geriatric patients. A recent study suggests that dexmedetomidine (DEX) may reduce the incidence and intensity of delirium in elderly patients after lung cancer surgery. Medical records of 346 lung cancer patients over 65 years post pulmonary resection for lung cancer were assigned to DEX or control group. Patients, care-providers, and investigators were all blinded to group assignment. DEX was administered in the preoperative and intraoperative periods. During postoperative day (POD) 1 to POD 7, delirium occurs in both groups. However, the incidence of delirium was lower in the DEX group than that in the control group, there were fewer moderate and severe delirium patients in the DEX group compared with the control group. Finally, patients in the DEX group had a shorter duration of delirium, a lower numeric pain rating scale during movement, and better sleep quality.[22] Other data support the use of total intravenous anesthesia and epidural analgesia, citing an association between these techniques and a significant decrease in the number of unplanned admissions to intensive care for patients who underwent lung resection.

TABLE 38.3 Age-Related Hepatorenal Changes

Hepatic	Decreased number of hepatocytes Deterioration in hepatocyte function Reduction of liver mass and volume Increased hepatic vascular resistance Increased portal pressure Decreased hepatic blood flow Partial loss of endothelial fenestration Increased oxidative stress Decreased cytochrome P450 activity Decreased molecular biosynthesis Decreased metabolic capacity Diminished clearance of toxins Decreased regulation of inflammation Impaired immune response to antigens and malignant cells Predisposition to autoimmunity Decreased regeneration capacity Increased susceptibility to drug-induced liver injury Increased susceptibility to ischemia
Renal	Decreased number of functional glomeruli because of nephrosclerosis Decreased cortical volume Increased kidney artery atherosclerosis, arteriosclerosis Increased tubular atrophy Increased interstitial fibrosis Decreased perfusion Increased renal vascular resistance Decreased glomerular filtration rate Decreased functional reserve Decreased autoregulation capacity Decreased creatinine clearance Decreased response to antidiuretic hormone Blunted response to aldosterone, vasopressin, and renin Decreased ability to conserve sodium or concentrate urine Increased susceptibility to renal ischemia and renal injury Increased risk of postoperative urinary retention and urinary tract infection

Modified from Tajiri K, Shimizu Y. Liver physiology and liver diseases in the elderly. *World J Gastroenterol*. 2013;19(46):8459–8467; Gekle M. Kidney and aging- a narrative review. *Exp Gerontol*. 2017;87(Pt B): 153–155; Denic A, Glassock RJ, Rule AD. Structural and functional changes with the aging kidney. *Adv Chronic Kidney Dis*. 2016;23(1):19–28; Maeso-Diaz R, Ortega-Ribera M, Fernandez-Iglesias A, et al. Effects of aging on microcirculatory function and sinusoidal phenotype. *Aging Cell*. 2018;17(6): e12829.

A total of 253 out of 11,208 patients undergoing lung resection in the study period of 2 years that had an unplanned admission to intensive care in the postoperative period, were evaluated in the United Kingdom. The incidence of intensive care unit admission was 2.3% (95% confidence interval [CI], 2.0%–2.6%). Patients who had an unplanned admission to intensive care unit had a higher mortality (29.00% vs. 0.03%, $P < .001$), and hospital length of stay was increased (26 vs. 6 days, $P < .001$). Patients receiving total intravenous anesthesia [odds ratio [OR], 0.50 (95% CI, 0.34–0.70)], and patients receiving epidural analgesia (OR 0.56 (95% CI 0.41–0.78) were less likely to have an unplanned admission to intensive care after thoracic surgery.[23]

Risk-Benefit Relationship of Surgical Intervention

Because survival rates are so low for patients with untreated lung cancer, elderly patients can benefit from surgical treatment, whether surgery alone for early stage cancer, or as part of a multimodal approach in a more advanced disease. Similarly, surgical treatment for esophageal cancer can confer benefit for elderly patients because survival with untreated esophageal cancer is extremely low. The risk-benefit relationship of surgical resection remains favorable even among octogenarians because of increasing life expectancy and advances in neoadjuvant therapy, surgical technique, and perioperative management. The prevalence of comorbidities, especially COPD and congestive heart failure, is high among patients with lung cancer, and this compounds the complexity of patient care and can have implications for perioperative management and postoperative morbidity and mortality. Among patients with lung cancer, the prevalence of comorbidities, especially COPD and congestive heart failure, was higher than patients with other types of cancer and patients in a control cohort without cancer.[24]

For patients with locally advanced stage III nonsmall cell lung cancer (NSCLC), neoadjuvant chemotherapy and radiation is increasing the pool of those who may be candidates for surgical resection. Various studies demonstrate a significant survival advantage in such patients who undergo the combination of preoperative chemotherapy and surgery compared with those undergoing surgery alone.[25–29] Another study suggested that elderly patients who received neoadjuvant therapy in conjunction with esophagectomy for esophageal cancer did not experience significantly increased mortality or major complications.[30]

Elderly patients have a higher incidence of early stage lung cancer at the initial diagnosis[31] but at the same time have a slower growing of squamous cell lung cancers. Although surgical resection is the treatment of choice for early-stage lung cancer, clinicians tend to offer less aggressive therapies to this group. However, recent advances in perioperative care and surgical technique have encouraged surgeons to offer surgical resection to more and older patients. The risk-benefit relationship of surgical intervention must be considered in terms of how the risk of surgery compares to that of other nonsurgical interventions or no intervention at all.

Birim et al. in a retrospective study concluded that for patients age 70 years or older, operative morbidity and mortality are low enough to justify surgery.[32] The Lung Cancer Study from 1983 concluded that rates of complications and mortality for patients older than 80 years were substantially higher than for those under 65 years.[33] However, more recent data indicate improved results for octogenarians undergoing lung resection.[34–36] A retrospective cohort study found that health status and tumor stage are more closely associated with better outcome and survival than chronologic age alone. The authors analyzed 174 patients aged 80 years or older with lung cancer who underwent surgical resection. Perioperative morbidity and mortality were 24.3% and 1.15%, respectively. Of 163 patients who were followed up completely, 78 (47.9%) died. The overall postoperative survival rate at 3 and 5 years was 63.6% and 48.3%, respectively. Almost half of the deaths were resulting from causes other than lung cancer recurrence, with respiratory disease accounting for the majority. Of interest, low body mass index (BMI) was a significant risk factor for death from respiratory disease after lung cancer surgery.[37] Several studies of elderly patients undergoing esophagectomy for esophageal cancer also report outcomes that were similar to that of younger patients, including mortality, postoperative complications, and long-term results.[38–42]

Goals of therapy for an older patient may differ from that of younger patients. The risks of surgical intervention increase with the severity of a person's comorbid conditions, thus shifting a patient's priorities. Quality of life, relief of symptoms, and an acceptable functional status may become more important than long-term survival. However, it is reasonable for those patients with good functional status to undergo surgical resection that is potentially curative considering that average life expectancies for 70-year-old men and women are currently an additional 14.5 and 16.7 years, respectively. Men and women who are 85 years old can expect an additional 5.9 and 7 years, respectively.[43] The life expectancy of patients with lung cancer that is not surgically resected is so dismal that resection for an 85-year-old patient can prolong life by an appreciable amount, adding years of active and independent life. A study of lung cancer patients 65 years or older using the Society of Thoracic Surgeons (STS) General Thoracic Surgery Database (GTSD) reported the median survival after lung resection was 6.7 years for pathologic stage I, 3.5 years for stage II, 2.4 years for stage III, and 2.2 years for stage IV.[44]

A study was conducted with elderly patients aged 75 years or over with stage I small cell lung cancer diagnosed histologically who were identified from the SEER database. A total of 983 patients were divided into a surgery group (received surgery, accompanied by chemotherapy, radiotherapy, or both or neither), nonsurgical group (only received radiotherapy, chemotherapy, or combination), and untreated group. Among all of the patients, 24% patients received surgery, 46.6% patients received nonsurgical treatment, and 29.4% patients received no treatment. The 5-year overall survival (OS) rates of surgery, nonsurgical, and untreated groups were 31%, 12%, and 6%, respectively ($P < .0001$). In subgroup analysis, surgery remained an independent factor for OS among patients aged 75 to 79 years and 80 to 84 years.[45] Multiple studies found lung cancer surgery outcomes acceptable even among octogenarians.[46–48] Recent data suggest that outcomes in carefully selected patients in their 80s is comparable to younger patients.[49,50]

For patients with lung cancer who are over 80 years old, more deaths will be attributed to the progression of lung cancer if left unresected rather than other causes. For patients who undergo resection, noncancer-specific mortality is a significant competing event and increases as patients age.[51]

Role of Surgical Techniques

For elderly patients, there is an association between the extent of pulmonary resection and postoperative complications, suggesting that lung-sparing techniques, such as segmentectomy and wedge resection can be considered, although it is unclear if this approach carries a higher risk of local occurrence. Mery et al. studied patients aged 75 years or older using data from the SEER database and found no difference in OS between those undergoing lobectomy versus limited resection.[31] More recent studies of elderly patients with stage I disease have echoed these findings.[52–57]

Video-assisted thoracoscopic surgery (VATS) is gaining popularity as a minimally invasive technique for lung resection and as an adjunct for esophagectomy. Compared with thoracotomy, patients who undergo VATS experience shorter hospital stays, lower narcotic requirement, and reduced shoulder dysfunction.[58] A study of 1100 VATS lobectomies reported low rates of morbidity and mortality.[59] Using the STS GTSD, Onaitis et al. found the VATS approach was associated with improved long-term survival. Analysis of 29,094 patients with a confirmed stage, 69% were stage I, 18% stage II, 11% stage III, and 2% stage IV. Median age was 73 years (interquartile range, 68–78 years). Of the procedures performed, lobectomy was performed in 69% of patients, bilobectomy in 3%, pneumonectomy in 3%, segmentectomy in 7%, sleeve lobectomy in 1%, and wedge resection in 17%. Thoracoscopic approach was performed in 47% of resections. After controlling for stage, wedge resection, segmentectomy, bilobectomy, and pneumonectomy are all associated with increased hazard of death in comparison with lobectomy. Thoracoscopic approach is associated with improved long-term survival in comparison with thoracotomy.[60] Other recent studies reported similar findings.[61,62] Emerging data comparing robotic-assisted lung resection with VATS and thoracotomy has also been encouraging.[63–67]

Recent data support the incorporation of VATS techniques, laparoscopy, and robotics when performing esophagectomies. Zhao et al. reported similar outcomes after minimally invasive esophagectomy for elderly patients was compared with those of younger patients. A total of 273 patients with esophageal squamous cell carcinoma who underwent minimally invasive esophagectomy were evaluated. Patients were divided into elderly (≥70 years) and nonelderly (<70 years) groups based on age at the time of surgery. Groups were compared with regard to general preoperative data, intraoperative data, postoperative 30-day complications and their severity, pathologic result, recurrence, OS, and disease-free survival (DFS) rates. Comparisons of other general preoperative data showed no significant differences. In addition, there were no significant differences in short-term outcomes except for postoperative 30-day complication rate, which was higher in the elderly group compared with the nonelderly group. However, the incidence of major complications such as cancer recurrence, 5-year OS, and 5-year DFS rates also were similar between both groups.[68] Esophagectomy is a stressful surgical procedure with significant associated morbidity and mortality. Various studies report that elderly patients are at higher postoperative risk than their younger counterparts, and should be carefully selected for surgery; however, advanced age alone should not be considered a limiting factor for surgery.[69–73]

Preoperative Assessment

The fundamentals of preoperative assessment apply to the geriatric patient population. However, certain aspects of perioperative planning and assessment become more important and may require different interpretations. The American College of Chest Physicians guidelines for thoracic surgery patients include a physical examination with cardiovascular evaluation and spirometry.[74] Measurement of diffusion capacity for carbon dioxide (DLCO) is particularly important for elderly patients because of age-related lung parenchymal changes and the propensity for obstructive disease. Patients with dyspnea out of proportion to the results of spirometry measurements should be carefully evaluated. Estimated postoperative FEV_1 and DLCO should be calculated for patients whose FEV_1 or DLCO are less than 80% of predicted. Estimated postoperative values of less than 40% for either measurement is a significant negative predictor of outcome in any lung resection patient, but it becomes even more important in the geriatric patient because of the reduction in intrinsic pulmonary reserve.

Cardiopulmonary exercise testing and an estimation of maximal oxygen consumption (VO2 max) is useful to assess the patient's risk. A VO2 max less than 15 mL/kg/min is a negative predictor for outcome. Substitutes for exercise testing can include stair climbing, shuttle walk, and the 6-minute walk. A patient who cannot climb one flight of stairs or perform 25 shuttles likely demonstrates a VO2 max of less than 10 mL/kg/min. Unfortunately for the geriatric patient, exercise testing may not be applicable because of comorbidities, such as arthritis or peripheral vascular disease that limit the ability to perform such tests independent of VO2 max.

Older patients are more likely to suffer from significant comorbidities, such as dementia, thromboembolic disorders, thyroid disorders, diabetes, and renal insufficiency.

Perioperative risk can be reduced by a modest exercise program and nutritional and hormonal optimization.

Risk Stratification

Older patients, particularly those with significant comorbidities, are at risk for increased postoperative complications. Predicting who is most at risk for such complications can allow for more targeted implementation of resources for prevention. Various methods of assessing patient risk have been suggested in the literature. One approach using the Comprehensive Geriatric Assessment was evaluated by a group of geriatric oncologists using a comprehensive review of the literature. They concluded that functional impairment, malnutrition, and comorbidities were independently associated with survival. However, feasibility and impact on treatment decisions remain unclear.[75] For elderly patients undergoing VATS lobectomy, Zhang et al. evaluated 441 patients who underwent thoracoscopic lobectomy for early-stage lung cancer. Clinical outcomes were compared between elderly (>70 years, $n = 176$) and younger patients ($n = 265$). They found the American Society of Anesthesiologists physical status (ASA-PS) to be a strong predictor of morbidity. In particular, the risk of pulmonary and cardiopulmonary complications for patients with an ASA-PS grade 3 was nearly 6- and 3-fold, respectively, as compared with patients with a score less than 3. In addition, they report more than an 8-fold increase in the odds of pulmonary complications in elderly men compared with elderly women.[76]

Haruki and colleagues used a Simplified Comorbidity Score (SCS) for predicting postoperative complications for patients older than 75 years undergoing VATS. It assigned various scores to the patients' comorbidities, including smoking, diabetes, renal insufficiency, respiratory disease, cardiovascular disease, neoplastic disease, and alcoholism. Using data from 216 patients, they found that patients with higher SCS scores experienced more frequent postoperative complications. Furthermore, the low SCS group experienced a 5-year OS of 79% compared with 52% for the high SCS group.[77]

Kawaguchi and colleagues devised a risk score to predict the incidence of postoperative complications among elderly lung cancer patients undergoing lobectomy. This risk score incorporated a history of coronary artery disease, a history of cerebrovascular accident, the presence of restrictive ventilator impairment, a history of interstitial pneumonia, and male sex. However, it is based on 119 patients from a single institution.[78] Further, larger scale studies would be necessary to validate these findings.

Physicians, pharmacists, nurses, and clinical psychologists at Okayama University Hospital in Japan formed a Delirium Management and Assessment Center (D-mac), which screened patients at a high-risk for delirium to offer interventions, such as pharmaceutical management and support. Murakawa et al. compared rates of postoperative delirium in patients with lung or esophageal cancer before and after the implementation of this program and found a significant decrease in the incidence of delirium with interventions in this program.[79]

Lai and colleagues conducted a prospective randomized controlled trial of 60 elderly patients undergoing lung cancer surgery. One group received exercise endurance training and inspiratory muscle training for 1 week. The mean postoperative length of stay was significantly reduced in the group that received intensive preoperative pulmonary rehabilitation training compared with the control group.[80]

Shiono et al. implemented an enhanced recovery after surgery (ERAS) program for elderly patients undergoing open thoracotomy and compared outcomes of patients who were enrolled in the ERAS program to those who were not. The program included standardized patient education, a multimodal approach to anesthesia, timing and details on postoperative oral intake, early ambulation 4 hours after surgery, and standard chest tube management. Although they did not find a significant impact on patients under 65 years of age, patients older than 65 years experienced a decreased length of stay.[81] On the other hand, data suggest that patients undergoing VATS may not necessarily derive significant benefit from an ERAS protocol.[82,83]

Frailty score is used to measure the health status of older individuals; it serves as a proxy measure of aging and vulnerability to poor outcomes. The concept of frailty as a clinical state that is characterized by an increased vulnerability to stressors could be a useful tool in the preoperative evaluation of thoracic surgery patients. A metaanalysis by Dunne and colleagues of 70 papers concluded that there was not enough evidence to support or refute frailty scoring for patients undergoing thoracic surgery, but the data suggested some correlation between higher frailty scores and increased rates of postoperative complications and mortality.[84] Hirpara et al. devised a comprehensive frailty assessment using risk stratification questionnaires and physiotherapy testing for 40 patients scheduled for lung and esophageal surgery for cancer. They found high completion rates for the questionnaires, which were easy to administer in the clinic, but lower completion rates for physiotherapy testing, which necessitated additional visits and coordination with a trained physiotherapist. Further, they found that most of the measures were not associated with the occurrence of postoperative complications.[85] Han and associates conducted a prospective cohort study of elderly patients undergoing major thoracic and abdominal surgery, assessing them for frailty. Prevalence of frailty was 26.12%. Significant differences were observed between the frail and nonfrail groups with respect to age, activities of daily living, Charlson Comorbidity Index, respiratory function, presence of malignancy, serum albumin, prealbumin, and hemoglobin levels. This group found frailty to be an effective predictor of postoperative complications and concluded that frailty assessment can improve the predictive ability of current surgical risk assessment tools.[86]

Malnutrition is more common in elderly patients and may put them at risk for increased postoperative complications and mortality. Kubo et al. found the Geriatric Nutritional Index to be associated with long-term survival after esophagectomy.[87] Takeda and colleagues reported that low BMI was an independent prognostic factor for survival after resection of stage I NSCLC.[88] Watanabe and associates describe using the prognostic nutritional index to predict outcomes of elderly patients undergoing lung cancer surgery.[89] Various studies using skeletal muscle mass measurements as an indicator of sarcopenia attempted to show an association with outcomes after resection of NSCLC, with conflicting results.[90–93] Although Siegal et al. found no association between sarcopenia and complications after esophagectomy, Nakashima and colleagues found sarcopenia to be a predictor of poor outcomes, specifically for the patients over 65 years but not for those younger than 65 years.[94,95]

Postoperative Care and Planning

Diagnostic and staging procedures, such as bronchoscopy, needle biopsy, and cervical mediastinoscopy can be performed on an outpatient basis in patients without severe preexisting illness who do not experience profound intraoperative complications. Following lobectomy and bilobectomy, even elderly patients can be admitted to a step-down care unit.[96] After more extensive procedures, such as esophagectomy, pneumonectomy, or resection of a large mediastinal mass, or thymectomy for myasthenia gravis, admission to the intensive care unit is indicted because of the increased risk of major respiratory and cardiovascular complications.

Jung and colleagues conducted a retrospective review of 1916 patients who underwent major lung resection and analyzed the data on the 63 patients who required intensive care unit admission after their initial recovery. They found that acute respiratory distress syndrome (ARDS) and delirium were independent risk factors for in-hospital mortality, and suggested that further studies could help determine if prevention of delirium and ARDS could improve outcomes.[97]

Beckert et al. conducted a prospective cohort study of 125 thoracic surgical candidates older than 60 years of age who were screened for frailty criteria, including weakness, slow gait, unintentional weight loss, self-reported exhaustion, and low self-reported physical activity. Of those, 69% were found to be frail or prefrail, which has been shown to predict surgical complications. This suggests that a large percentage of these patients could be candidates for enrollment in presurgical frailty reduction interventions.[98] Miyazaki et al. reported that among 191 patients scheduled for esophagectomy, preoperative nutritional status, particularly low BMI, was a significant risk factor for poorer prognosis.[99] Additional studies could determine if enhancing nutritional status preoperatively could improve outcomes for these patients.

Surgical treatment of cancer, as well as cancer itself, will affect a patient's quality of life. Mitigating that effect will require further research. Schwartz and colleagues reported preliminary findings on 100 patients undergoing lung resection for stage I NSCLC that indicated that lobectomy, not limited resection, had a negative impact on their quality of life and physical health, regardless of whether their surgery was performed through VATS or thoracotomy.[100] Kidane and colleagues used a Functional Assessment of Cancer Therapy-Esophagus (FACT-E) to measure health-related quality of life. FACT-E is a health-related quality of life instrument validated in patients with esophageal cancer. It is composed of a general component and an esophageal cancer subscale. The objective was to determine whether the baseline FACT-E and esophageal cancer subscale scores are associated with survival in patients with stage II and III cancer of the gastroesophageal junction or thoracic esophagus. In the 207 patients with esophageal cancer, they found that a higher baseline FACT-E was independently associated with longer survival[101] (Fig. 38.5).

A prospective population-based cohort study by Al-Ameri et al. of 249 patients having thoracic surgery found that a lower preoperative self-reported physical quality of life was associated with significantly worse survival.[102] Leach and colleagues studied 921 cancer patients matched to 4605 controls from the Medicare Health Outcomes Survey (MHOS) database and found that patients with cancer experienced greater declines in physical functioning and an increased risk of depression, with the greatest change in patients with lung cancer.[103] These studies outline the ways in which this patient population are vulnerable, and further research could guide us toward interventions that can improve patient quality of life after a cancer diagnosis.

Kent and colleagues used the SEER-MHOS linked data resource to study the patient-reported outcome (PRO) data, which included health-related quality of life, functional status, and other information from older adults with cancer. They suggest that PRO data could be useful to guide interventions. For example, older adults with cancer may be more likely to die after a fall than those without cancer, indicating that fall prevention might be a high priority with these patients. They also conclude that further research using PRO may help to elucidate the relationship between functional status and mortality in cancer survivors.[104]

A number of thoracic surgical procedures are noncurative. Freeman et al. reported that 884 of 3842 thoracic surgery procedures performed at a single institution were palliative; however, only 14% of those patients had a palliative care assessment before their thoracic surgery consultation. They suggest that thoracic surgeons should be familiar with palliative care concepts to best meet patient needs.[105]

Although not always predictable, discharge planning should be considered as early as during the initial preoperative visit. It is important to ascertain who will be providing support for the patient after discharge, as well as where the patient will be going once discharged. Patients who are self-sufficient preoperatively may be unable to care for themselves postoperatively for a certain amount of time. For these patients, early discharge planning and coordination with family members, social workers and home care services is extremely important.

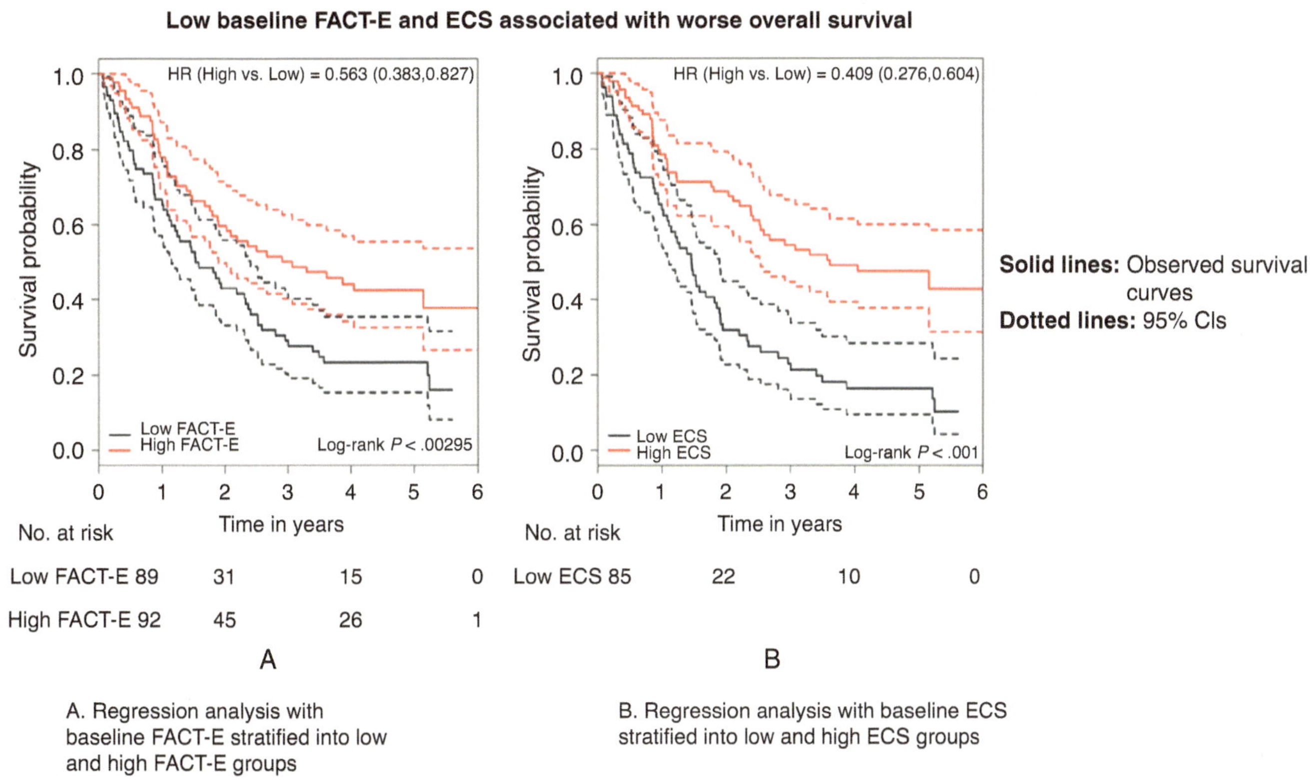

• **Fig. 38.5** Low baseline Functional Assessment of Cancer Therapy-Esophagus (*FACT-E*) and esophageal cancer surgery (*ECS*) associated with worse overall survival. **A.** Regression analysis with baseline FACT-E stratified into low and high FACT-E groups. **B.** Regression analysis with baseline ECS stratified into low and high ECS groups. (From Kidane Sulman J, Xu W, et al. Baseline measure of health-related quality of life (Functional Assessment of Cancer Therapy-Esophagus) is associated with overall survival in patients with esophageal cancer. *J Thorac Cardiovasc Surg*. 2016;151(6):1571–1580.)

Conclusion

Increasing numbers of geriatric patients will present for surgery as the population ages. The risk-benefit relationship remains favorable even among octogenarians because of recent advances in surgical techniques and neoadjuvant therapies, as well as increasing life expectancy. There are wide disparities between chronologic age and physiologic condition among the elderly, resulting in outcomes that are influenced more by tumor stage, preoperative functional status, and comorbidities than age alone. Nonetheless, the normal process of aging can limit an otherwise healthy patient's physiologic reserve. Minimally invasive surgery, lung-sparing techniques, and advances in neoadjuvant therapies are increasing the pool of surgical candidates to include older patients with more severe comorbidities. These patient population will increasingly become more common to be cared by the thoracic anesthesiologist. Further studies are needed to help target implementation of resources to optimize overall patient health and physiologic condition to decrease perioperative and postoperative morbidity and mortality, and to optimize quality of life.

References

1. Yancik R. Population aging and cancer: a cross-national concern. *Cancer J*. 2005;11(6):437–441.
2. DeSantis CE, Miller KD, Dale W, et al. Cancer statistics for adults aged 85 years and older 2019. *CA Cancer J Clin*. 2019; 69(6):452–467.
3. Siegel RL, Miller KD, Jemal A. Cancer statistics 2019. *CA Cancer J Clin*. 2019;69(1):7–34.
4. Hurria A, Kris MG. Management of lung cancer in older adults. *CA Cancer J Clin*. 2003;53(6):325–341. Review.
5. Miller KD, Nogueira L, Mariotto AB. et al. Cancer treatment and survivorship statistics, 2019. *CA Cancer J Clinic*. 2019;69(5):363–385.
6. Jemal A, Ward EM, Johnson CS, et al. Annual report to the nation on the status of cancer, 1975–2014, featuring survival. *J Natl Cancer Inst*. 2017;109(9).
7. Watters JM, McClaran JC, Man-Son-Hing M. *The Elderly Surgical Patient. ACS Surgery Principles and Practice*. New York, NY: WebMD; 2005.
8. Meschiari CA, Ero OK, Pan H, Finkel T, Lindsey ML. The impact of aging on cardiac extracellular matrix. *Geroscience*. 2017;39(1):7–18.

9. Lakatta EG, Sollott SJ. Perspectives on mammalian cardiovascular aging: humans to molecules. *Comp Biochem Physiol a Mol Integr Physiol.* 2002;132(4):699–721. Review.
10. Shirakabe A, Ikeda Y, Sciarretta S, Zablocki DK, Sadoshima J. Aging and autophagy in the heart. *Circ Res.* 2016;118(10):1563–1576.
11. Castillo MD, Port J, Heerdt PM. Thoracic surgery in the elderly editor. In: Slinger P, ed. *Principles and Practice of Anesthesia for Thoracic Surgery.* 2nd ed. Switzerland: Springer; 2019.
12. Skloot GS. The effects of aging on lung structure and function. *Clin Geriatr Med.* 2017;33(4):447–457.
13. Maeso-Diaz R, Ortega-Ribera M, Fernandez-Iglesias A, et al. Effects of aging on microcirculatory function and sinusoidal phenotype. *Aging Cell.* 2018;17(6):e12829.
14. Tajiri K, Shimizu Y. Liver physiology and liver diseases in the elderly. *World J Gastroenterol.* 2013;19(46):8459–8467.
15. Sieber FE, Pauldine R. Geriatric anesthesia. In: Miller RD, ed. *Anesthesia.* Philadelphia: Churchill Livingstone; 2009.
16. Denic A, Glassock RJ, Rule AD. Structural and functional changes with the aging kidney. *Adv Chronic Kidney Dis.* 2016; 23(1):19–28.
17. Muhlberg W, Platt D. Age-dependent changes of the kidneys: pharmacological implications. *Gerontology.* 1999;45(5):243–253.
18. Gekle M. Kidney and aging- a narrative review. *Exp Gerontol.* 2017;87(Pt B):153–155.
19. Berger M, Acker L, Deiner S. Geriatric anesthesia. In: Gropper MA, ed. *Miller's Anesthesia.* 2020.
20. Robinson TN, Raeburn CD, Tran ZV, Angles EM, Moss M. Postoperative delirium in the elderly: risk factors and outcomes. *Ann Surg.* 2009;249(1):173–178.
21. Aldecoa C, Betelli G, Bilotta F, et al. European Society of Anaesthesiology evidence-based and consensus-based guideline on postoperative delirium. *Eur J Anaesthesiol.* 2017;34(4):192–214.
22. Huyan T, Hu X, Peng H, Zhu Z, Li Q, Zhang W. Perioperative dexmedetomidine reduces delirium in elderly patients after lung cancer surgery. *Psychiatr Danub.* 2019;31(1):95–101.
23. Shelley BG, McCall PJ, Glass A, Orzechowska I, Klein AA. Association of Cardiothoracic Anaesthesia and collaborators. Association between anaesthetic technique and unplanned admission to intensive care after thoracic lung resection surgery: the second Association of Cardiothoracic Anaesthesia and Critical Care (ACTACC) National Audit. *Anaesthesia.* 2019;74(9): 1121–1129.
24. Edwards BK, Noone AM, Mariotto AB, et al. Annual report to the nation on the status of cancer, 1975-2010, featuring prevalence of comorbidity and impact on survival among persons with lung, colorectal, breast, or prostate cancer. *Cancer.* 2014;120(9): 1290–1314.
25. Roth JA, Atkinson EN, Fosella F, et al. Long-term follow-up of patients enrolled in a randomized trial comparing preoperative chemotherapy and surgery with surgery alone in resectable stage IIIA non-small-cell lung cancer. *Lung Cancer.* 1998;21(1):1–6.
26. Takeda S, Maeda H, Okada T, et al. Results of pulmonary resection following neoadjuvant therapy for locally advanced (IIIA-IIIB) lung cancer. *Eur J Cardiothorac Surg.* 2006;30(1):184–189.
27. Rosell R, Gomez-Codina J, Camps C, et al. Preresectional chemotherapy in stage IIIA non-small-cell lung cancer: a 7-year assessment of a randomized controlled trial. *Lung Cancer.* 1999; 26(1):7–14.
28. Fujita S, Katakami N, Takahashi Y, et al. Postoperative complications after induction chemoradiotherapy in patients with non-small-cell lung cancer. *Eur J Cardiothorac Surg.* 2006;29(6): 896–901.
29. Petersen RP, Pham D, Toloza EM, et al. Thoracoscopic lobectomy: a safe and effective strategy for patients receiving induction therapy for non-small cell lung cancer. *Ann Thorac Surg.* 2006; 82(1):214–218.
30. Ruol A, Portale G, Castoro C, et al. Effects of neoadjuvant therapy on perioperative morbidity in elderly patients undergoing esophagectomy for esophageal cancer. *Ann Surg Oncol.* 2007;14(11):3242–3250.
31. Mery CM, Pappas AN, Bueno R, et al. Similar long-term survival of elderly patients with non-small cell lung cancer treated with lobectomy or wedge resection within the Surveillance, Epidemiology, and End Results Database. *Chest.* 2005;128(1):237–245.
32. Birim O, Zuydendorp HM, Maaat AP, et al. Lung resection for non-small-cell lung cancer in patients older than 70: mortality, morbidity, and late survival compared with the general population. *Ann Thorac Surg.* 2003;76(6):1796–1801.
33. Ginsberg RJ, Hill LD, Eagan RT, et al. Modern thirty-day operative mortality for surgical resections in lung cancer. *J Thorac Cardiovasc Surg.* 1983;86(5):654–658.
34. Yamamoto K, Alarcon JP, Medina VC, et al. Surgical results of stage I non-small cell lung cancer: comparison between elderly and younger patients. *Eur J Cardiothorac Surg.* 2003;23(1):21–25.
35. Sullivan V, Tran T, Holmstrom A, et al. Advanced age does not exclude lobectomy for non-small cell lung carcinoma. *Chest.* 2005;128(4):2671–2676.
36. Sawada S, Komori E, Nogami N, et al. Advanced age is not correlated with either short-term or long-term postoperative results in lung cancer patients in good clinical condition. *Chest.* 2005;128:1557–1563.
37. Matsuoka K, Ueda M, Miyamoto Y. Risk factor for respiratory death after lung cancer surgery in octogenarians. *Asian Cardiovasc Thorac Ann.* 2015;23(9):1044–1049.
38. Internullo E, Moons J, Nafteux P, et al. Outcome after esophagectomy for cancer of the esophagus and GEJ in patients aged over 75 years. *Eur J Cardiothorac Surg.* 2008;33(6):1096–1104.
39. Nguyen NT, Hinojosa MW, Smith BR, Chang KJ, Gray J, Hoyt D. Minimally invasive esophagectomy: lessons learned from 104 operations. *Ann Surg.* 2008;248(6):1081–1091.
40. Ruol A, Portale G, Zaninotto G, et al. Results of esophagectomy for esophageal cancer in elderly patients: age has little influence on outcome and survival. *J Thorac Cardiovasc Surg.* 2007;133(5): 1186–1192.
41. Morita M, Egashira A, Yoshida R, et al. Esophagectomy in patients 80 years of age and older with carcinoma of the thoracic esophagus. *J Gastroenterol.* 2008;43(5):345–351.
42. Alibakhshi A, Aminian A, Misharifi R, Jahangiri Y, Dashti H, Karimian F. The effect of age on the outcome of esophageal cancer surgery. *Ann Thorac Med.* 2009;4(2):71–74.
43. Arias E, Xu J, Kochanek KD. United States life tables, 2016. *Natl Vital Stat Rep.* 2019;68(4):1–66.
44. Fernandez FG, Furnary AP, Kosinski AS, et al. Longitudinal follow-up of lung cancer resection from the Society of Thoracic Surgeons General Thoracic Surgery Database in patients 65 years or older. *Ann Thorac Surg.* 2016;101(6):2067–2076.
44. Li Y, Hu S, Xie J, Zhang X, Zong Y, Xu B, Li C. Effects of surgery on survival of elderly patients with stage I small-cell lung cancer: analysis of the SEER database. *J Cancer Res Clin Oncol.* 2019; 145(9):2397–2404.
46. Tutic-Horn M, Gambazzi F, Rocco G, et al. Curative resection for lung cancer in octogenarians is justified. *J Thorac Dis.* 2017;9(2):296–302.

47. Cohen C, Al Orainy S, Pop D, et al. Anatomical pulmonary resections for primary lung cancer in octogenarians within a dedicated protocol. *J Thorac Dis.* 2019;11(9):3732–3737.
48. Feczko A, McKeown E, Wilson JL, et al. Assessing survival and grading the severity of complications in octogenarians undergoing pulmonary lobectomy. *Can Respir J.* 2017;2017:6294895.
49. Vazirani J, Moraes J, Barnett S, et al. Outcomes following resection of non-small cell lung cancer in octogenarians. *ANZ J Surg.* 2018;88(12):1322–1327.
50. Kutluk AC, Akin H, Ceritoglu A, et al. Is the outcome of pulmonary resections due to non-small cell lung cancer in octogenarian patients worse? *Ann Thorac Cardiovasc Surg.* 2019;25(2):95–101.
51. Eguchi T, Bains S, Lee MC, Tan KS, Hristov B, Buitrago DH, et al. Impact of increasing age on cause-specific mortality and morbidity in patients with stage I non-small-cell lung cancer: a competing risks analysis. *J Clin Oncol.* 2017;35(3):281–290.
52. Razi SS, John MM, Sainathan S, Stavropoulos C. Sublobar resection is equivalent to lobectomy for T1a non-small cell lung cancer in the elderly: a Surveillance, Epidemiology, and End Results database analysis. *J Surg Res.* 2016;200(2):683–689.
53. Zhang Z, Feng H, Zhao H, et al. Sublobar resection is associated with better perioperative outcomes in elderly patients with clinical stage I non-small cell lung cancer: a multicenter retrospective cohort study. *J Thorac Dis.* 2019;11(5):1838–1848.
54. Fang Z, He J, Fang W, Ruan L, Fang F. Long-term outcomes of thoracoscopic anatomic resections and systematic lymphadenectomy for elderly high-risk patients with stage IB non-small-cell lung cancer. *Heart Lung Circ.* 2016;25(4):392–397.
55. Tsutani Y, Tsubokawa N, Ito M, et al. Postoperative complications and prognosis after lobar resection versus sublobar resection in elderly patients with clinical stage I non-small-cell lung cancer. *Eur J Cardiothorac Surg.* 2018;53(2):366–371.
56. Dong S, Roberts SA, Chen S, et al. Survival after lobectomy versus sub-lobar resection in elderly with stage I NSCLC: a meta-analysis. *BMC Surg.* 2019;19(1):38.
57. Yutaka Y, Sonobe M, Kawaguchi A, et al. Prognostic impact of preoperative comorbidities in geriatric patients with early-stage lung cancer: significance of sublobar resection as a compromise procedure. *Lung Cancer.* 2018;125:192–197.
58. Landreneau RJ, Hazelrigg SR, Mack MJ, et al. Postoperative pain-related morbidity: video-assisted thoracic surgery versus thoracotomy. *Ann Thorac Surg.* 1993;56(6):1285–1289.
59. McKenna RJ Jr, Houck W, Fuller CB. Video-assisted thoracic surgery lobectomy: experience with 1,100 cases. *Ann Thorac Surg.* 2006;81(2):421–425.
60. Onaitis MW, Furnary AP, Kosinski AS, et al. Prediction of long-term survival after lung cancer surgery for elderly patients in The Society of Thoracic Surgeons General Thoracic Surgery Database. *Ann Thorac Surg.* 2018;105(1):309–316.
61. Ezer N, Kale M, Sigel K, et al. Outcomes after video-assisted thoracoscopic lobectomy versus open lobectomy for early-stage lung cancer in older adults. *Ann Am Thorac Soc.* 2018;15(1):76–82.
62. Oda R, Okuda K, Osaga S, et al. Long-term outcomes of video-assisted thoracoscopic surgery lobectomy vs. thoracotomy lobectomy for stage IA non-small cell lung cancer. *Surg Today.* 2019;49(5):369–377.
63. Oh DS, Reddy RM, Gorrepati ML, Mehendale S, Reed MF. Robotic-assisted, video-assisted thoracoscopic and open lobectomy: propensity-matched analysis of recent premier data. *Ann Thorac Surg.* 2017;104(5):1733–1740.
64. Reddy RM, Gorrepati ML, Oh DS, Mehendale S, Reed MF. Robotic-assisted versus thoracoscopic lobectomy outcomes from high-volume thoracic surgeons. *Ann Thorac Surg.* 2018;106(3):902–908.
65. Louie BE, Wilson JL, Kim S, et al. Comparison of video-assisted thoracoscopic surgery and robotic approaches for clinical stage I and stage II non-small cell lung cancer using The Society of Thoracic Surgeons Database. *Ann Thorac Surg.* 2016;102(3):917–924.
66. Yang CJ, Kumar A, Klapper JA, et al. A national analysis of long-term survival following thoracoscopic versus open lobectomy for stage I non-small-cell lung cancer. *Ann Surg.* 2019;269(1):163–171.
67. Yang HX, Woo KM, Sima CS, et al. Long-term survival based on the surgical approach to lobectomy for clinical stage I nonsmall cell lung cancer: comparison of robotic, video-assisted thoracic surgery, and thoracotomy lobectomy. *Ann Surg.* 2017;265(2):431–437.
68. Zhao H, Liu G, Wei S, Liu H. Short- and long-term outcomes of minimally invasive esophagectomy in elderly patients with esophageal squamous cell carcinoma. *J BUON.* 2017;22(6):1540–1546.
69. Schlottman F, Strassle PD, Nayyar A, Herbella FAM, Cairns BA, Patti MG. Postoperative outcomes of esophagectomy for cancer in elderly patients. *J Surg Res.* 2018;229:9–14.
70. Motoori M, Ito Y, Miyashiro I, et al. Impact of age on long-term survival in patients with esophageal cancer who underwent transthoracic esophagectomy. *Oncology.* 2019;97(3):149–154.
71. Otero J, Arnold MR, Kao AM, et al. Short-term outcomes of esophagectomies in octogenarians- an analysis of ACS-NSQIP. *J Surg Res.* 2019;235:432–439.
72. Paulus E, Ripat C, Koshenkov V, et al. Esophagectomy for cancer in octogenarians: should we do it. *Langenbecks Arch Surg.* 2017;402(3):539–545.
73. Voncken FEM, van der Kaaii RT, Sikorska K, et al. Advanced age is not a contraindication for treatment with curative intent in esophageal cancer. *Am J Clin Oncol.* 2018;41(9):919–926.
74. Colice GJ, Shafazand S, Griffin JP, Keenan R, Bollinger CT, American College of Chest Physicians. Physiologic evaluation of the patient with lung cancer being considered for resectional surgery: ACCP evidence-based clinical practice guidelines (2nd edition), College of Chest Physicians. *Chest.* 2007;132(3 Suppl):161S-177S.
75. Caillet P, Laurent M, Bastuii-Garin S, et al. Optimal management of elderly cancer patients: usefulness of the Comprehensive Geriatric Assessment. *Clin Interv Aging.* 2014;9:1645–1660.
76. Zhang R, Kyriss T, Dippon F, Hansen M, Boedeker E, Friedel G. American Society of Anesthesiologists Physical Status facilitates risk stratification of elderly patients undergoing thoracoscopic lobectomy. *Eur J Cardiothorac Surg.* 2018;53(5):973–979.
77. Haruki T, Yurugi Y, Wakahara M, et al. Simplified comorbidity score for elderly patients undergoing thoracoscopic surgery for lung cancer. *Surg Today.* 2017;47(6):718–725.
78. Kawaguchi Y, Hanaoka J, Ohshio Y, et al. A risk score to predict postoperative complications after lobectomy. *Gen Thorac Cardiovascular Surg.* 2018;66(9):537–542.
79. Murakawa K, Kitamura Y, Watanabe S, Hongo S, Shinomiya K, Sendo T. Clinical risk factors associated with postoperative delirium and evaluation of delirium management and assessment team in lung and esophageal cancer patients. *J Pharm Health Care Sci.* 2015;1:4.

80. Lai Y, Huang J, Yang M, Su J, Liu J, Che G. Seven-day intensive preoperative rehabilitation for elderly patients with lung cancer: a randomized controlled trial. *J Surg Res.* 2017;209:30–36.
81. Shiono S, Endo M, Suzuki K, Hayasaka K. Impact of enhanced recovery after surgery on outcomes of elderly patients undergoing open thoracic surgery. *Gen Thorac Cardiovasc Surg.* 2019;67(10): 867–875.
82. Van Haren RM, Mehran RJ, Mena GE, et al. Enhanced recovery decreases pulmonary and cardiac complications after thoracotomy for lung cancer. *Ann Thorac Surg.* 2018;106(1):272–279.
83. Brunelli A, Kim AW, Berger KI, Addrizzo-Harris DJ. Physiologic evaluation of the patient with lung cancer being considered for resectional surgery: diagnosis and management of lung cancer, 3rd edition: American College of Chest Physicians evidence-based clinical practice guidelines. *Chest.* 2013;143(5 suppl):e166S–e190S.
84. Dunne MJ, Abah U, Scarci M. Frailty assessment in thoracic surgery. *Interact Cardiovasc Thorac Surg.* 2014;18(5):667–670.
85. Hirpara DH, Kidane B, Rogalla P, et al. Frailty assessment prior to thoracic surgery for lung or esophageal cancer: a feasibility study. *Support Care Cancer.* 2019;27(4):1535–1540.
86. Han B, Li Q, Chen X. Frailty and postoperative complications in older Chinese adults undergoing major thoracic and abdominal surgery. *Clin Interv Aging.* 2019;14:947–957.
87. Kubo N, Sakurai K, Tamura T, et al. The impact of geriatric nutritional risk index on surgical outcomes after esophagectomy in patients with esophageal cancer. *Esophagus.* 2019;16(2):147–154.
88. Takada K, Shimokawa M, Akamine T, et al. Association of low body mass index with poor clinical outcomes after resection of non-small cell lung cancer. *Anticancer Res.* 2019;39(4):1987–1996.
89. Watanabe I, Kanauchi N, Watanabe H. Preoperative prognostic nutritional index as a predictor of outcomes in elderly patients after surgery for lung cancer. *Jpn J Clin Oncol.* 2018;48(4):382–387.
90. Fintelmann FJ, Troschel FM, Mario J, et al. Thoracic skeletal muscle is associated with adverse outcomes after lobectomy for lung cancer. *Ann Thorac Surg.* 2018;105(5):1507–1515.
91. Nakamura R, Inage Y, Tobita R, et al. Sarcopenia in resected NCSCLC: effect on postoperative outcomes. *J Thorac Oncol.* 2018;13(7):895–903.
92. Suzuki Y, Okamoto T, Fujishita T, et al. Clinical implication of sarcopenia in patients undergoing complete resection for early non-small cell lung cancer. *Lung Cancer.* 2016;101:92–97.
93. Kim EY, Lee HY, Kim KW, et al. Preoperative computed tomograohy-determined sarcopenia and postoperative outcome after surgery for non-small cell lung cancer. *Scand J Surg.* 2018;107(3):244–251.
94. Siegal SR, Dolan JP, Dewey EN, et al. Sarcopenia is not associated with morbidity, mortality, or recurrence after esophagectomy for cancer. *Am J Surg.* 2018;215(5):813–817.
95. Nakashima Y, Saeki H, Nakanishi R, et al. Assessment of sarcopenia as a predictor of poor outcome after esophagectomy in elderly patients with esophageal cancer. *Ann Surg.* 2018;267(6):1100–1104.
96. Pedoto A, Heerdt PM. Postoperative care after pulmonary resection: postanesthesia care unit versus intensive care unit. *Curr Opin Anaesthesiol.* 2009;22(1):50–55.
97. Jung JJ, Cho JH, Hong TH, et al. Intensive care unit (ICU) readmission after major lung resection: prevalence, patterns, and mortality. Thorac Cancer. 2017;8(1):33-39.
98. Beckert AK, Huisingh-Scheetz M, Thompson K, et al. Screening for frailty in thoracic surgical patients. *Ann Thorac Surg.* 2017;103(3):956–961.
99. Miyazaki T, Sakai M, Sohda M, et al. Prognostic significance of inflammatory and nutritional parameters in patients with esophageal cancer. *Anticancer Res.* 2016;36(12):6557–6562.
100. Schwartz RM, Yip R, Flores RM, Olkin I, Taioli E, Henschke C. I-ELCAP investigators. The impact of resection method and patient factors on quality of life among stage IA non-small cell lung cancer surgical patients. *J Surg Oncol.* 2017;115(2):173–180.
101. Kidane B, Sulman J, Xu W, et al. Baseline measure of health-related quality of life (Functional Assessment of Cancer Therapy- Esophagus) is associated with overall survival in patients with esophageal cancer. *J Thorac Cardiovasc Surg.* 2016;151(6): 1571–1580.
102. Al-Ameri M, Bergman P, Franco-Cereceda A, Sartipy U. Self-reported physical quality of life before thoracic operations is associated with long-term survival. *Ann Thorac Surg.* 2017;103(2):484–490.
103. Leach CR, Bellizzi KM, Hurria A, Reeve BB. Is it my cancer or am I just getting older? impact of cancer on age-related health conditions of older cancer survivors. *Cancer.* 2016;122(12): 1946–1953.
104. Kent EE, Malinoff R, Rozjabek HM, et al. Revisiting the Surveillance Epidemiology and End Results Cancer Registry and Medicare Health Outcomes Survey (SEER-MHOS) linked data resource for patient-reported outcomes research in older adults with cancer. *J Am Geriatr Soc.* 2016;64(1):186–192.
105. Freeman RK, Arevalo G, Ascioti AJ, Dake M, Mahidhara RS. An assessment of the frequency of palliative procedures in thoracic surgery. *J Surg Educ.* 2017;74(5):878–882.

39

Thoracic Aortic Aneurysm Resection

GEORGE SILVAY, JACOB MICHAEL LURIE

Introduction

Historical Notes on Thoracic Aortic Aneurysms

The dilatation of arteries was first recognized as a disease of the cardiovascular system in Egypt in the 1550s BC, and the first to describe an abdominal aortic aneurysm was the Flemish physician Vesalius about three millennia later in 1555. Two centuries later, in 1785, the English surgeon John Hunter began to treat aneurysms of the peripheral vessels by ligation.[1] Hunter ligated the superficial femoral artery, causing a patient's popliteal aneurysm to slowly decrease in size over several weeks. Before this procedure, the options for treating such a popliteal aneurysm were to either wait for rupture or to prophylactically amputate the extremity.[2] The first attempt at percutaneous endovascular aneurysm repair was commenced by Moore and Muchison in 1864, in which a patient with a thoracic aortic aneurysm had an aneurysm cannulated and packed with a couple dozen yards of wire coils in hopes of inducing thrombosis. While the patient died, the aneurysm was noted to have partially thrombosed.[3] Accompanied by the advancement of other therapeutic modalities, in 1948, Dr. Rudolph Nissen in New York used a cellophane wrap to treat aortic aneurysms. One of the greatest scientific minds of the 20th century experienced a thoracic aortic aneurysm and was treated by Nissen: in December 1948, Albert Einstein underwent surgery for a large thoracic aortic aneurysm, and Nissen performed the procedure. He was, however, only able to wrap the anterior portion of the aneurysm with cellophane, as aortic mobilization was generally considered to be forbidden at the time. The treatment was partially effective, but despite Nissen's best efforts, Einstein died of a ruptured aneurysm 6 years later at the age of 76 years.[4]

In 1951, Dr. Charles Dubost in Paris performed the first successful resection of an abdominal aortic aneurysm, using a 15 cm long cadaver aortic homograft.[5] After this development, a new era in the surgical treatment of aortic aneurysms was launched along with the introduction and clinical application of cardiopulmonary bypass (CPB) by John Gibbon in 1953. These developments facilitated the application of various surgical techniques required for the reconstruction of the ascending aorta, including the use of aortic allografts as an aortic replacement. In the mid-1950s, other major milestones in open heart surgery were also taking place, such as the first open-heart repairs of ventricular septal defect, atrioventricular communis, and tetralogy of Fallot. Such procedures used extracorporeal cross-circulation.[6–10]

Later, a combined operation to replace the ascending thoracic aortic aneurysm, as well as the aortic valve along with the reimplantation of the coronary arteries was performed by Hugh Bentall and Antony De Bono in 1968,[11,12] and around this time, Dacron was introduced by Dr. Michael DeBakey.[13] Interestingly, DeBakey, himself a pioneering cardiac surgeon, was affected by an aortic aneurysm when he was 97 years old. He was at home while preparing a medicine lecture when he experienced symptoms that he himself recognized as those of an acute thoracic aortic aneurysm dissection. He initially refused anesthesia and surgery, but his situation deteriorated, and his wife demanded that her husband have surgery. The Ethics Committee at Methodist Hospital in Houston, Texas approved the planned surgery. His postoperative recovery was prolonged and complex. In retrospect, Dr. DeBakey publicly acknowledged that he was happy that he underwent the surgical procedure. He died of natural causes shortly before his 100th birthday in July, 2008.[14]

In the decades following DeBakey's accomplishments, developments in the realm of thoracic aortic aneurysm repair commenced. The use of one-lung ventilation (OLV) was first described by Dr. Eric Carlens, who introduced the double-lumen endobronchial tube.[15] Dr. Irving Sarot, a thoracic surgeon at the Mount Sinai Hospital, started to use the same technique in 1971.

Dr. Randall Griepp, who later became the chairman of cardiothoracic surgery at the Mount Sinai Hospital, developed the use of deep hypothermic circulatory arrest in the repair of ascending thoracic aortic aneurysms while at Stanford University Hospital. Griepp explained that "a combination of surface cooling and CPB was used to produce total body hypothermia," and subsequently "CPB was then used to warm the patient and resuscitate the heart."[16] A timeline incorporating some of the most significant events pertaining to aortic aneurysms can be seen in Fig. 39.1, including the first successful endovascular aneurysm repair, which occurred in 1990, and the first successful thoracic endovascular aortic repair, which took place in 1992.

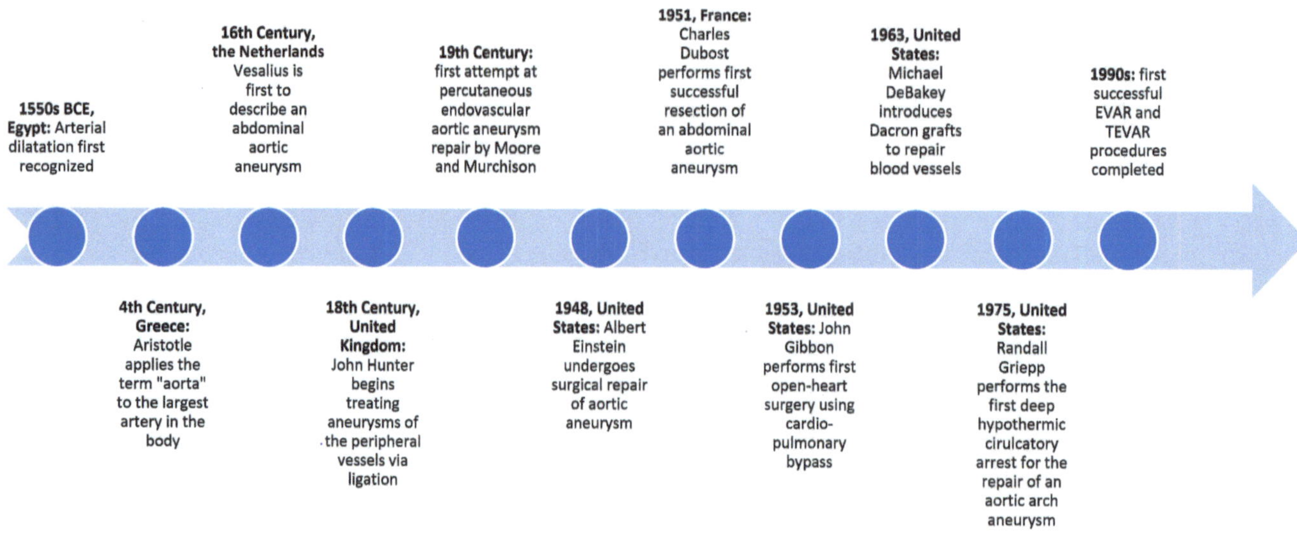

• **Fig. 39.1** Timeline of accomplishments in the treatment of aortic aneurysms. *EVAR*, Endovascular abdominal aortic aneurysm repair; *TEVAR*, thoracic endovascular aortic repair.

The repair of a thoracic aortic aneurysm is now a daily practice in cardiac surgery, and management of such cases presents challenges in the domains of anesthesia, analgesia, ventilation, perfusion, monitoring, and the surgical procedure itself.[17,18] Major milestones in the development of the contemporary clinical paradigm of the management of thoracic aortic aneurysms have included OLV, CPB, hemodilution, hypothermic circulatory arrest, cerebral perfusion, as well as advances in anesthesia, pharmacology, and monitoring, including echocardiography and cerebral oximetry.[19] These multiple advances in surgery and anesthesia facilitated the development and practice of techniques for the reconstruction of the ascending aorta and aortic arch following a dissection.[5,6,20]

Marfan Syndrome: History and Importance

Marfan syndrome is a common genetic disorder that holds implications for thoracic aortic disease.[21] The condition affects around one in 5000 people and will most likely be seen by almost all anesthesiologists during their careers. The specific mutation in Marfan syndrome is in the gene encoding the fibrillin-1 protein, a significant component of the extracellular matrix. It was previously believed that an abnormal fibrillin-1 protein decreased the strength of the extracellular matrix in tissue, such as the aortic wall, causing patients to have abnormal elasticity in the aortic wall and predisposing to dilatation.[22] Interestingly, newer evidence suggests instead that aberrant signaling pathways lead to the degeneration of the aortic wall matrix. It is thought that transforming growth factor beta (TGF-β) is particularly affected by abnormal fibrillin. In fact, the inhibition of TGF-β in these mouse models largely reverses phenotypic and pathologic disease manifestations.[23] The physical manifestations of Marfan syndrome are well-documented and include joint hypermobility, a tall, lean stature, high palate, ocular disorders, mitral valve prolapse, and aortic root dilatation. The most common cause of death in patients with Marfan syndrome is complications involving the aorta.[24] It is not uncommon for patients to be totally unaware that they have Marfan syndrome until they present with an acute aortic event.

The first description of Marfan syndrome was presented by French pediatrician Antonin-Bernard Jean Marfan at the Société Médicale des Hôpitaux de Paris on February 28, 1896 in a presentation entitled, "Un cas de deformation congénitale des quatre membres, plus prononcée aux extrémités, caractérisée par l'allongement des os avec un certain degré d'amincissement" (roughly translated as "a case of congenital deformation of the four limbs, more pronounced at the extremities, characterized by the elongation of the bones with a certain degree of thinning").[25] The presentation discussed multiple joint contractures, as well as scoliosis and abnormally long and thin limbs and fingers in a 5-year-old girl.

In 1901, Mery and Babonneix used the newly discovered tool of x-rays to further investigate this pathology. They presented newly observed skeletal features at the Société Médicale des Hôpitaux de Paris, documenting x-ray findings of the same patient described by Antonin-Bernard Jean Marfan, noting that the bones showed dévelopement hypertrophié des cartilages, or the development of hypertrophied cartilages.[26] In 1938, the patient died of tuberculosis, and no cardiac or ocular findings were mentioned. Although it is unclear whether or not this small girl actually had what would now be referred to as Marfan syndrome, she indeed had congenital contractual arachnodactyly.[27]

Descriptions further elucidating Marfan syndrome came into the literature over the next several years. A patient with hypogonadism and dolichostenomelia (i.e., lengthy limbs), in addition to mobile joints in the hands, was soon described, and his presentation was used to better characterize the condition. Also ectopia lentis (i.e., subluxation of the ocular lenses) was described in tandem with disproportionately lengthy limbs in 1914, and an association between these physical traits and hereditability was made in 1931, when Weve described *distrophia mesodermalis congenita, typus* Marfanis.[28,29] The following decade, dolichostenomelia was associated with mitral valve degeneration and aortic root dissection. The connection between aortic root dissection and skeletal abnormalities was made by Baer and colleagues in 1943,[30] and the associations between skeletal, ocular, and aortic pathologies in Marfan syndrome have since been a cornerstone in its diagnosis.[31]

It was not until 1986 that the connective tissue glycoprotein (fibrillin) was isolated from human fibroblast cell cultures. It was determined that this glycoprotein was ubiquitous throughout the human body, composing significant portions of the extracellular matrix in skin, tendons, cartilage, cardiac valves, lungs, kidneys, muscle, and corneas.[32] In 1991, the gene linked to Marfan disease, fibrillin-1(FBN1), was ultimately uncovered by researchers at the Mount Sinai Medical Center in New York City.[33] This gene structure was subsequently characterized, and these discoveries contributed to the currently available genetic testing for the diagnosis of Marfan syndrome.[34]

Thoracic Aortic Aneurysms: Prevalence, Significance, and Complications

Thoracic aortic aneurysms are oftentimes silent until catastrophe strikes, and almost 95% of patients with thoracic aortic aneurysms are undiagnosed and totally unaware of their condition.[35,36] The management of thoracic aortic aneurysms remains challenging in both the elective and emergent settings.[37] The mortality of ruptured thoracic aortic aneurysms approaches 100%,[38] and it can be a difficult decision whether or not to operate on a thoracic aortic dissection once it has been discovered. Clinician opinions differ on when to initiate aggressive surgical procedures, and these decisions hold tremendous consequences for patients. It is highly probable that reported incidences of thoracic aortic aneurysms are underestimates, as fatal thoracic aortic aneurysm ruptures can be misdiagnosed as myocardial infarctions.[39,40] No two thoracic aortic aneurysms are the same, and it is critical to understand the etiology and management of this phenomenon.[11] Historically, the only treatment option for aortic arch disease has been open arch replacement under circulatory arrest conditions with or without selective cerebral perfusion. However, this open procedure has significant morbidity and mortality, especially in elderly patients with multiple comorbidities. To potentially mitigate the risks associated with open aortic arch replacement, endovascular arch repair has gained momentum as an alternative treatment option. Currently, efforts to stent the aortic arch are being trialed in numerous international healthcare facilities around the world. Patients selected for this procedure are considered high risk for conventional open arch replacement.[41]

Thoracic aortic aneurysms affect more than 15,000 people in the United States every year, and around 60% of all thoracic aortic aneurysms are in the ascending aorta. One of the principal causes of death because of thoracic aortic aneurysms is a dissection, or a tear in the wall of the aorta, as well as total rupture. Type A aortic dissection (TAAD), for example, is specified in the Stanford classification as a dissection of the ascending aorta, regardless of the distal extent of the tear, whereas type B dissection involves the lower aorta. Overall, pooled hospital mortality from a recent systematic review and metaanalysis demonstrated that hospital mortality for all surgical repairs of TAAD was 11.9%.[42,43] Etiologies of TAAD include hypertension, atherosclerosis, connective tissue disorders, trauma, infection, and previous cardiac or vascular surgery. The inherited disorders associated with TAAD include aortopathies associated with Marfan syndrome, Ehlers-Danlos syndrome, Loeys-Dietz syndrome, and the bicuspid aortic valve.[44] Examples of other such conditions that serve as a differential diagnosis for Marfan syndrome can be seen in Box 39.1. The revised Ghent criteria for the diagnosis of Marfan syndrome in adults is found in Box 39.2. An artistic illustration of a thoracic aortic aneurysm is presented in Fig. 39.2. In addition, a computed tomography (CT) angiography of an aneurysmal thoracic aorta in Marfan syndrome is seen in Fig. 39.3.

The following Case Presentation and Case Management sections will demonstrate the preoperative, intraoperative, and postoperative care of a young man with Marfan syndrome who is found to have a thoracic aortic aneurysm. We will use this case to underscore some of the important aspects in the care of patients with thoracic aortic aneurysms and discuss some of the most up-to-date and practical literature on the topic.

• BOX 39.1 Differential Diagnosis of Marfan Syndrome

Hereditary Connective Tissue Disorders

Fibrillinopathies

- MASS (mitral valve, aorta, skeleton, skin) phenotype
- Familial mitral valve prolapse
- Familial arachnodactyly
- Familial ectopia lentis
- Shprintzen-Goldberg syndrome

Nonfibrillinopathies

- Loeys-Dietz syndrome
- Ehlers-Danlos syndrome
- Arterial tortuosity syndrome
- Aneurysm-Osteoarthritis syndrome

Nonsyndromic familial aortic aneurysms

- Bicuspid aortic valve with thoracic aortic aneurysm
- Familial aortic aneurysms and dissection
- Loeys-Dietz syndrome variants

From Cañadas V, Vilacosta I, Bruna I, Fuster V. Marfan syndrome. Part 1: pathophysiology and diagnosis. *Nat Rev Cardiol*. 2010;7(5):256; Loeys B, Matthys D, De Paepe A. Genetic fibrillinopathies: new insights in molecular diagnosis and clinical management. *Acta Clin Belg*. 2003;58(1):3–11.

• BOX 39.2 Revised Ghent Criteria Used in the Diagnosis of Marfan Syndrome

Criteria for the Diagnosis of Marfan Syndrome

In the absence of a family history of Marfan syndrome:

1. Aortic root dilatation Z score >2 and ectopia lentis
2. Aortic root dilatation Z score >2 and an *FBN1* mutation
3. Aortic root dilatation Z score >2 and a systematic score >7
4. Ectopia lentis and an *FBN1* mutation associated with aortic root dilatation

In the presence of a family history of Marfan syndrome (as defined in 1–4 earlier):

1. Ectopia lentis and a family history of Marfan syndrome (as defined earlier)
2. Systemic score > 7 and a family history of Marfan syndrome (as defined earlier)
3. Aortic root Z score >2 if above 20 years old, >3 if below 20 years old, and a family history of Marfan syndrome (as defined earlier)
4. Systemic points calculate as follows: wrist and thumb sign (3 points), wrist or thumb sign (1 point), pectus carinatum deformity (2 points), pectus excavatum or chest asymmetry (1 point), hindfoot deformity (2 points), plain flat foot (1 point), spontaneous pneumothorax (2 points), dural ectasia (2 points), protucio acetabulae (2 points), scoliosis or thoracolumbar kyphosis (1 point), reduced elbow extension (1 point), three of five facial features (1 point), skin striae (1 point), severe myopia (1 point), mitral valve prolapse (1 point).

From Von Kodolitsch Y, De Backer J, Schüler H, et al. Perspectives on the revised Ghent criteria for the diagnosis of Marfan syndrome. *Appl Clin Genet.* 2015;8:137.

Case Presentation

A 17.5-year-old male presented to the emergency department of a local hospital because of the sudden onset of sharp, substernal chest pain that he reported as 7 out of 10 in intensity. He stated that the pain did not radiate. The patient did not have any previous discomfort or history of similar symptomatology and was in his normal state of health and not active when the pain began. A basic examination revealed mild pectus excavatum and nearsightedness, which were consistent with a potential diagnosis of Marfan syndrome. The patient had a CT scan, which revealed a 7.7-cm ascending thoracic aortic aneurysm. Following this discovery, the patient was urgently transferred to the Aortic Aneurysm Surveillance Program at the Mount Sinai Medical Center in New York City.

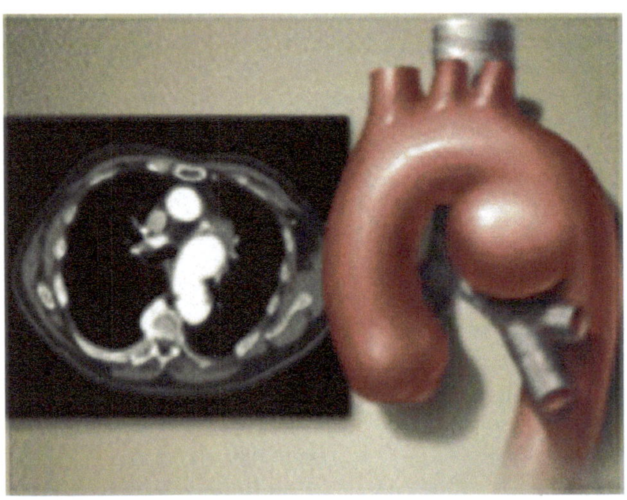

• **Fig. 39.2** An artistic rendering of a thoracic aortic aneurysm located superior to the left mainstem bronchus, as well as a computed tomography scan of the same. (From Goodwin MR, Blasius KR, Brand J, Silvay G. One-lung ventilation for surgical repair of thoracic aortic aneurysm. *Semin Cardiothorac Vasc Anesth*. 2013;17(2):146–151.)

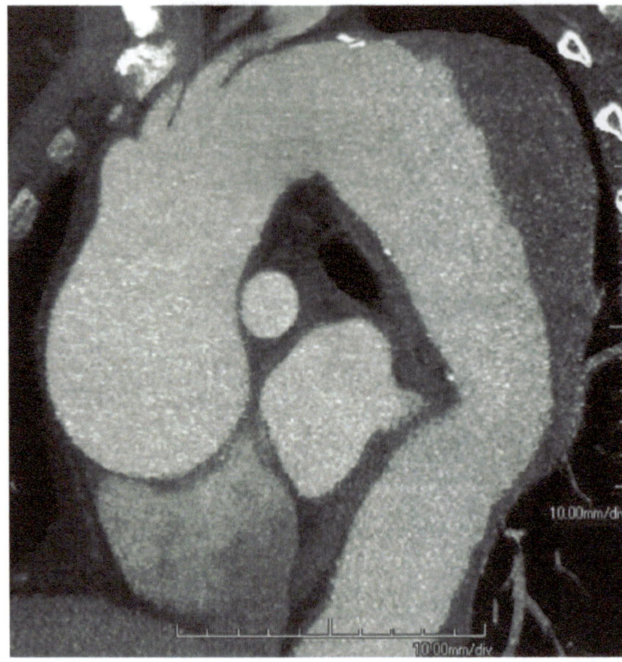

• **Fig. 39.3** A computed tomography angiography of a diffusely aneurysmal thoracic aorta in a patient with Marfan syndrome. (From Castellano JM, Silvay G, Castillo JG, editors. Marfan syndrome: clinical, surgical, and anesthetic considerations. *Semin Cardiothorac Vasc Anesth*. 2014;18(3):260–271.)

At the Aortic Aneurysm Surveillance Program, further medical history revealed that the patient did not take any medications and had no known allergies. He had no other known past medical history, and he saw a pediatrician regularly. He stated that he was a starting center on his high school's basketball team, and he had tried out for several prominent college-level basketball programs. The patient was an only child and lived with his parents. The patient's pain subsided while at the Aortic Surveillance Clinic, and he stated he felt normal.

On examination, the patient's vital signs were notable for tachycardia (115 beats per minute) and hypertension (145/85 mm Hg measured on both arms). His other vital signs were unremarkable: his respiratory rate was 14 breaths per minute, oxygen saturation (SpO2) 100%, and he was afebrile. The patient had a height of 80.5 inches and a slender build, weighing 92 kg. The patient's arms and legs were long and seemingly disproportionate to his torso. He was also noted to have a high-arched palate and slight pectus excavatum on his chest exam, which he stated had been noted by previous providers. His cardiac examination was notable for a soft, high-pitched 1-2/6 diastolic decrescendo murmur most prominent at Erb's point (the left third intercostal space), consistent with aortic regurgitation.

An electrocardiogram showed normal sinus rhythm. The patient then underwent an echocardiogram, which revealed a thoracic aortic root aneurysm with a sinus of Valsalva diameter of 7.7 cm and an aortic root of 7.6 cm. There was evidence of moderate aortic regurgitation but no evidence of aortic dissection. The left ventricle showed mild dilation with a normal ejection fraction. A trace of tricuspid regurgitation with pulmonary insufficiency was evident. Laboratory values, including a coagulation panel, were within normal limits.

The cardiology and surgical teams decided that urgent cardiac surgery was in the patient's best interest.

The patient was sent to the Preoperative Evaluation Clinic, and the operation was scheduled for the next day. Additional tests were performed to ensure the patient was in an optimized state of health before his thoracic aortic aneurysm resection. Cardiac catheterization revealed normal coronary arteries, and magnetic resonance imaging confirmed the dimensions of the aorta. The patient was informed of the risks and benefits of the operation, and informed consent was obtained. The patient and his relatives were informed about the course of the surgical treatment, including aspects of mechanical ventilation, the length of the intensive care unit stay, as well as the rehabilitation and discharge process.

On the day of surgery, a brief review of his medical status was performed, and his vital signs were checked. Vancomycin and cefazolin were administered 90 minutes before incision. Aminocaproic acid was used as the antifibrinolytic of choice. The availability of type-matched blood and fresh frozen plasma was confirmed with the blood bank. A rapid infusion system was made available in the operating room.

The patient was brought into the operating room, and anesthesia was induced with midazolam, fentanyl, etomidate, and vecuronium, with desflurane used for anesthetic maintenance. Standard anesthesia management for open heart surgery was used with OLV. Using a double lumen tube, the right lung was ventilated while the left lung was collapsed for the thoracic aortic aneurysm resection. In addition to the standard American Society of Anesthesiologists (ASA) monitors, access to the left radial artery was obtained, and near-infrared spectrometry and bispectral index leads were placed on the patient's forehead. Initial cerebral oximetry readings were 71% and 74% on the right and left hemispheres, respectively. Additional intravenous access was obtained via a 9 Fr multilumen catheter in the right internal jugular vein, as well as a pulmonary artery catheter. A coagulation monitoring system was used.

A transesophageal echocardiogram (TEE) probe was inserted. The preoperative TEE examination revealed a 2.6-cm aortic valve annulus with 1+ aortic regurgitation, with no aortic stenosis and mildly distorted aortic valve leaflets because of aortic dilation. The ascending aorta was measured as 7.6 cm in diameter, and the sinus of Valsalva was 7.7 in diameter. There was also mild mitral and tricuspid regurgitation. The left ventricular ejection fraction (LVEF) was 60%.

Surgery started with the exposure of the right axillary artery and right femoral vein. Following heparinization, a median sternotomy was performed under precautionary CPB to protect the patient from the possibility of bleeding problems because of the large thoracic aneurysm and deep pectus excavatum. The initiation of total CPB and cooling began and proceeded uneventfully. The TEE indicated sufficient blood flow into the aortic arch. The esophageal temperature was brought down to 15°C in preparation for circulatory arrest, and the jugular bulb oxygen saturation reached 97%. At this time, perfusion was stopped, and CPB was initiated. Following the induction of hypothermia and the cessation of perfusion before a short period of circulatory arrest, the valve-sparing aortic root replacement (the David procedure) was conducted uneventfully.

Rewarming was subsequently initiated, and the patient was noted to have appropriate urinary output. His hemoglobin and hematocrit levels were maintained with intraoperative cell salvage and one unit of packed red blood cells. Following careful hemostasis, the patient was gradually rewarmed, and he was weaned off CPB. Heparin was neutralized with protamine sulfate. The total bypass time was 350 minutes, and cross-clamp time was 20 minutes. The lowest temperature before deep hypothermic circulatory arrest was 15°C.

The patient was taken to the cardiothoracic intensive care unit for close monitoring. He was extubated on postoperative day one. There was increased chest tube output and a drop in hematocrit on postoperative day two, and the patient was transfused three units of packed red blood cells and one pool of platelets. The patient remained hemodynamically stable afterwards and was started on a low-dose beta blocker. The patient's neurologic and hemodynamic status was closely monitored, and he was discharged on postoperative day four.

Following discharge, the patient had additional testing to further investigate his Marfan status. He underwent genetic testing, which confirmed a diagnosis of Marfan syndrome, as well as ophthalmologic evaluation. A CT angiogram revealed a normal post-David-procedure aorta, without any evidence of dissection or thrombotic changes. The patient was asymptomatic in good health, and ultimately elected to attend his school of choice on a basketball scholarship.

Case Management

The management of patients with thoracic aortic aneurysms must involve detailed and clear communication between cardiologists, surgeons, and anesthesiologists. In concert, these physicians should develop a strategy for the preoperative, intraoperative, and postoperative complications that patients may face. In addition to every organ system being evaluated, and the administration of proper perioperative antibacterial prophylaxis, physicians should account for what may be a lengthy procedure using hypothermia and prosthetic materials to reconstruct the aorta. In nonemergent situations, preoperative evaluation before elective open thoracic aortic surgery is of paramount importance, and one must take the time to consider nearly every organ system in any assessment.[45] In both emergent and elective surgical procedures, careful anesthetic management is required for the prevention of intraoperative hypertension and aortic rupture. The anesthetic approach to the patient with a thoracic aortic aneurysm depends on the urgency of surgical intervention. One of the most difficult decisions facing patients and physicians is whether to perform surgery when a thoracic aortic aneurysm is diagnosed. There are several issues to keep in mind, as stated by Dr. John Elefteriades: "Thoracic aortic aneurysm, while lethal, is indolent. Mortality usually does not occur until after years of growth. The aneurysmal ascending thoracic aorta grows slowly: about 0.1 cm per year. Over a patient's lifetime, 'hinge points' at which the likelihood of rupture or dissection skyrockets are seen at 5.5 cm for the ascending aorta. Intervening at 5 cm diameter for the ascending thoracic aortic aneurysm prevents most adverse events. Symptomatic aneurysms require resection regardless of size. The yearly rate of rupture, dissection, or death is 14.1% for a patient with a thoracic aorta of 6 cm diameter."[46] Elective surgery for nonurgent cases may provide the best results. In cases in which surgery is not recommended, patients are followed over time and evaluated periodically until the potential benefits of surgery outweigh risks.[47,48]

Ascending Thoracic and Aortic Arch Aneurysms

Thoracic aortic aneurysms can be either acquired or inherited. Oftentimes, thoracic aneurysms of the ascending aorta are secondary to associated conditions, such as Marfan syndrome, cystic medial degeneration, the expansion of an aortic dissection, trauma, poststenotic dilatation, or dilatation following previous aortic manipulation. Such thoracic aneurysms are usually seen along with a bicuspid aortic valve, and hypertension is commonly present. Historically, advanced syphilis was associated with ascending thoracic aortic aneurysms, although this is significantly less common today.[49] Furthermore, various familial thoracic aortic aneurysm syndromes have been described.[50]

Aneurysms of the ascending thoracic aorta may extend into the aortic arch. Repair can occur via the head vessels being reinserted individually to a main graft, reimplanted as a unit, or anastomosed to a composite graft, as seen in Figure 39.4.[51,52] In these procedures, hypothermic circulatory arrest is used as the mainstay of cerebral protection.[53] Subsequently, a composite graft can be used to perform selective cerebral perfusion as the arch is reconstructed. Adjunctive therapies for cerebral protection includes the use of steroids to prevent edema, barbiturates, and retrograde cerebral perfusion, and various techniques have also been described in preparation for cerebral circulatory arrest, such as electroencephalography (EEG), jugular bulb saturation monitoring, and cerebral oximetry.[54]

Cardiovascular Considerations

Many patients undergoing thoracic aortic aneurysm resections have medical comorbidities, such as hypertension, coronary artery disease, or atherosclerosis. Others may also have congestive heart failure or ischemic heart disease. Coronary artery ischemia may result from distortions in the anatomy and physiology of the heart, resulting in decreased oxygen supply to the entire organ. Thoracic aortic aneurysms may also distort the aortic valve, leading to valve incompetence and heart failure. Before thoracic aortic aneurysm resection, several tests should be performed. For example, an electrocardiogram can demonstrate ischemia or prior myocardial events, in addition to left ventricular hypertrophy and other electrical abnormalities, suggesting some form of cardiac impairment. The thoracic aneurysm itself should be assessed via echocardiography which can accurately reveal the dimensions of the thoracic aneurysm, as well as valve function and anatomy. Angiography can be used to further visualize the thoracic aneurysm, especially in patients with coronary artery disease.[48]

Cardiovascular complications in patients with Marfan syndrome are recognized as the leading cause of morbidity and mortality. The risk of an acute aortic event in a patient with Marfan syndrome increases steadily with age, and such events result in death in up to 50% of undiagnosed patients by age 40 years.[55] Additional cardiovascular pathologies are seen in Marfan syndrome, such as mitral valve prolapse with regurgitation, pulmonary artery dilatation, and aortic valve regurgitation. About two in three patients with Marfan syndrome have an associated cardiothoracic abnormality other than aortic root dilatation, and physicians must be aware of these comorbidities.[31] In children with early-onset and severe Marfan syndrome, these pathologies are particularly alarming, and mitral valve insufficiency can lead to congestive heart failure and death.[34]

Renal Considerations

Proper perioperative fluid management is essential to the prevention of kidney injury during aortic resection surgery. Anesthesiologists should implement renal-protective strategies, such as the use of diuretics like mannitol or furosemide, as well as the possible use of low-dose dopamine to enhance renal perfusion. The use of CPB can result in some kidney dysfunction. Patients with thoracic aortic aneurysms are susceptible to kidney dysfunction. Those at highest risk for renal failure include patients with preoperative renal dysfunction, those with aneurysms extending distally to include renal artery involvement, and those with a history of congestive heart failure. In addition, transient

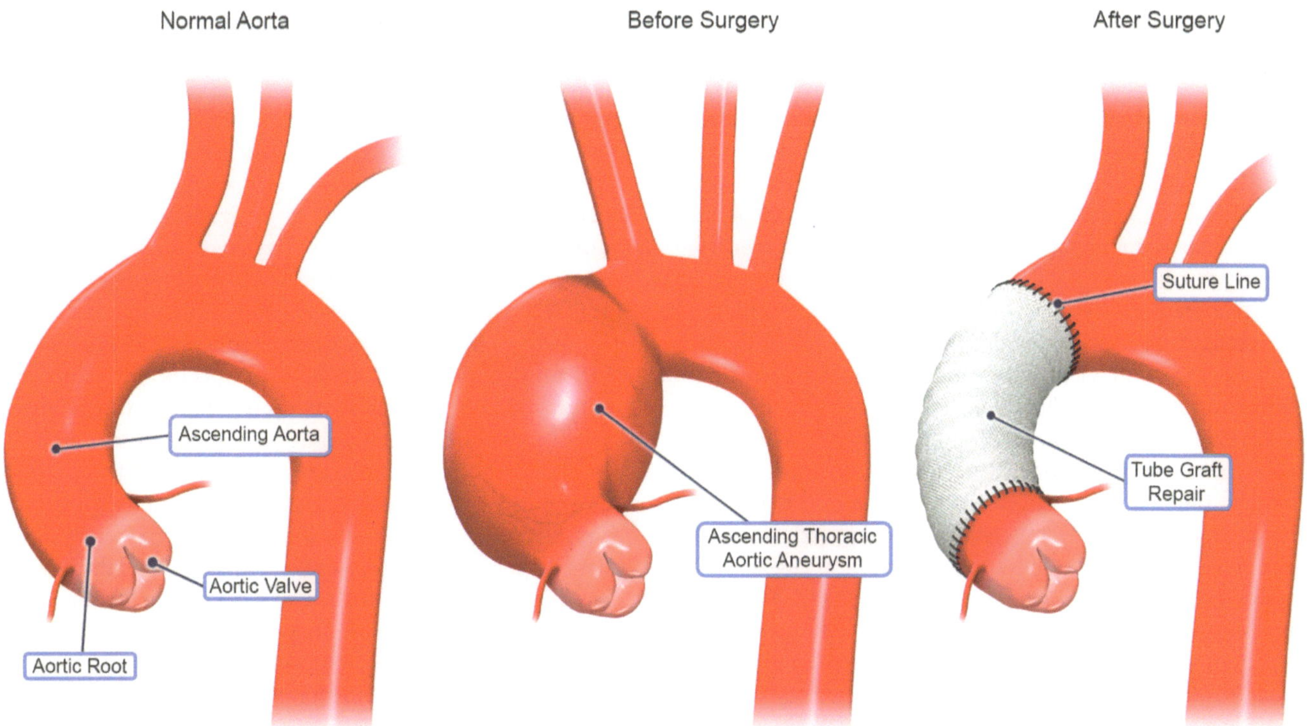

• **Fig. 39.4** An example of an ascending thoracic aortic aneurysm repair utilizing a tube graft. (From Grubb K. The patient guide to heart, lung, and esophageal surgery. *Soc Thorac Surg*. 2019.)

elevations of kidney enzymes can be seen with the administration of contrast dyes. Relevant to our patient who had an ascending thoracic aortic aneurysm, it has been demonstrated that up to 10% of ascending thoracic aortic aneurysm resections can result in kidney failure.[56] All patients should have preoperative creatinine and blood urea nitrogen measurements to attain a baseline before thoracic aortic aneurysm repair.

Pulmonary Considerations

Baseline arterial blood gas analyses and pulmonary function testing should be obtained before thoracic aortic aneurysm surgery because these data can aid in ventilator weaning following the surgical procedure. In addition, the preoperative physical examination is crucial to lung function and potential respiratory disease. For example, stridor or dyspnea may suggest compression on the trachea or bronchi, and overt hemoptysis. An x-ray depicting the compression of an airway by a large thoracic aortic aneurysm can be seen in Fig. 39.5. Hoarseness on examination may indicate a recurrent laryngeal nerve palsy in patients with ascending thoracic aortic aneurysms.[57] In addition, patients should be aware that postoperative hoarseness may occur if there is damage to the recurrent laryngeal nerve during aortic surgery. Other considerations regarding recurrent laryngeal nerve injury include predisposition to aspiration, and patients should be counseled about the seriousness of this potential but rare complication. Our patient had no hoarseness and his pulmonary examination was otherwise normal, with lungs clear to auscultation bilaterally and no wheezes or rhonchi noted.

Chronic obstructive pulmonary disease is common in patients with thoracic aortic aneurysms, as many have a lengthy

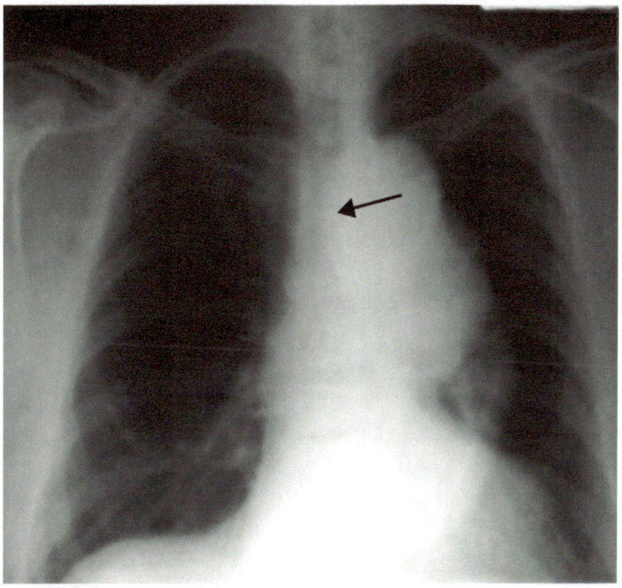

• **Fig. 39.5** A preoperative chest x-ray of a thoracic aortic aneurysm compressing the airway. (From Goodwin MR, Blasius KR, Brand J, Silvay G. One-lung ventilation for surgical repair of thoracic aortic aneurysm. *Semin Cardiothorac Vasc Anesth*. 2013;17(2):146–151.)

smoking history. A history of smoking fundamentally changes anesthetic and ventilatory parameters, and any history of smoking should be clarified with the patient. Our patient (with no smoking history) was successfully weaned without incident from the DLT. However, this process could have been far more tumultuous had the patient been a smoker, and interestingly, the most common complication of ascending and aortic arch repairs is prolonged intubation following surgery.[58]

Preoperative chest x-rays are an effective way to identify potential complications of thoracic aortic aneurysms, such as a deviated trachea or left mainstem bronchus, which are both important considerations when placing a left-sided DLT. Left-sided endotracheal tubes are overwhelmingly preferred for this procedure and not only provide a safety benefit, but also grant surgeons more space in the chest cavity to operate. The most significant complication of such endotracheal tubes is blunt trauma to the thoracic aneurysm, which could cause the aneurysm to tear. A tracheal bronchoscopy through a right-sided double-lumen tube in a patient with a thoracic aneurysm can be seen in Figs. 39.6; and 39.7A and B.

Nervous System Considerations

A thorough, detailed, and specific neurologic history should be conducted to assess for any history of cerebral vascular accidents, transient ischemic events, and seizures. Neurologic complications are not uncommon following thoracic aortic aneurysms, and a robust baseline evaluation from the patient should be obtained. Some patients may benefit from carotid angiography or duplex studies to exclude the presence of compromised carotid blood flow. Patients should be evaluated for postoperative neurologic status changes, which could indicate ischemic neurologic events or other concerning pathology. Neurologic consults can generally be considered to more thoroughly assess the patient.[59]

In 2014, the International Aortic Arch Surgery Study Group was formed to facilitate interinstitutional collaboration in exploring the impacts of surgical techniques on patient outcomes with particular attention to long-term neurologic outcomes. This organization assisted in the production of robust comparisons between institutional reports and what were otherwise piecemeal accountings and records of outcomes. Critically, this organization developed a management-orientated classification system for significant clinical end points specific for aortic arch surgery. Table 39.1 presents their grading system for the severity of clinical complications related to aortic arch surgery, and Table 39.2 presents their classification of clinical end points of the neurologic system, such as spinal cord complications, which have been underreported in the past. The International Aortic Arch Surgery Study Group has also created standardized criteria for the assessment of the cardiovascular, respiratory, renal, and gastrointestinal systems, among others, but these criteria are beyond the scope of this chapter and can be reviewed in the article by Yan et al. from 2014.[60]

Intraoperatively, monitoring cerebral oxygenation using jugular bulb oximetry can help predict when patients are at risk of developing neurologic complications. It is thought that both microembolisms and cerebral hypoperfusion contribute to neurologic complications following aortic surgery using CPB.[61,62] An imbalance between cerebral oxygen supply and cerebral metabolic demand is a likely factor contributing to neurologic complications. Jugular bulb venous oxygen saturation mirrors the overall balance between cerebral oxygen supply and demand and is normally between 55% and 75% (and sometimes up to 85%).[63,64] When this oxygen saturation falls below 50%, the oxygen supply to the cerebrum is insufficient and falls

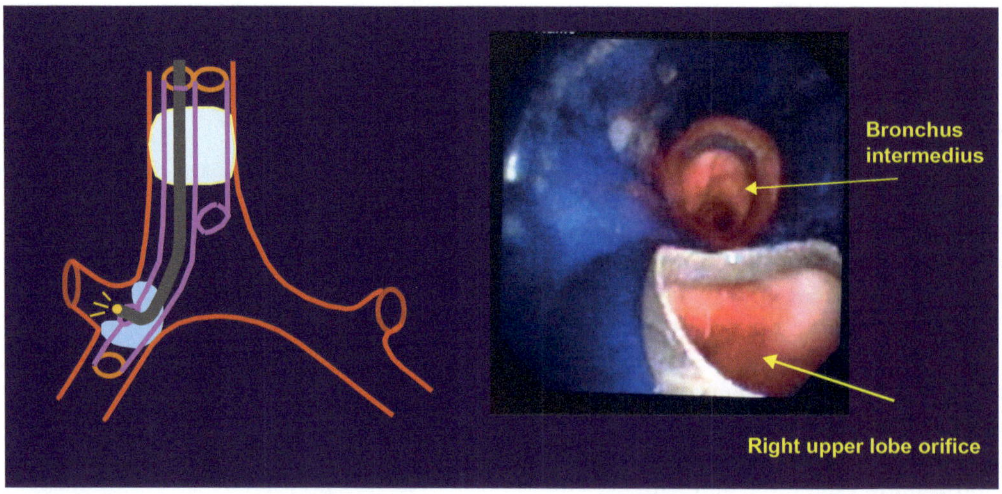

• **Fig. 39.6** A bronchoscopy through a right-sided double-lumen tube. (Courtesy of Edmond Cohen M.D.)

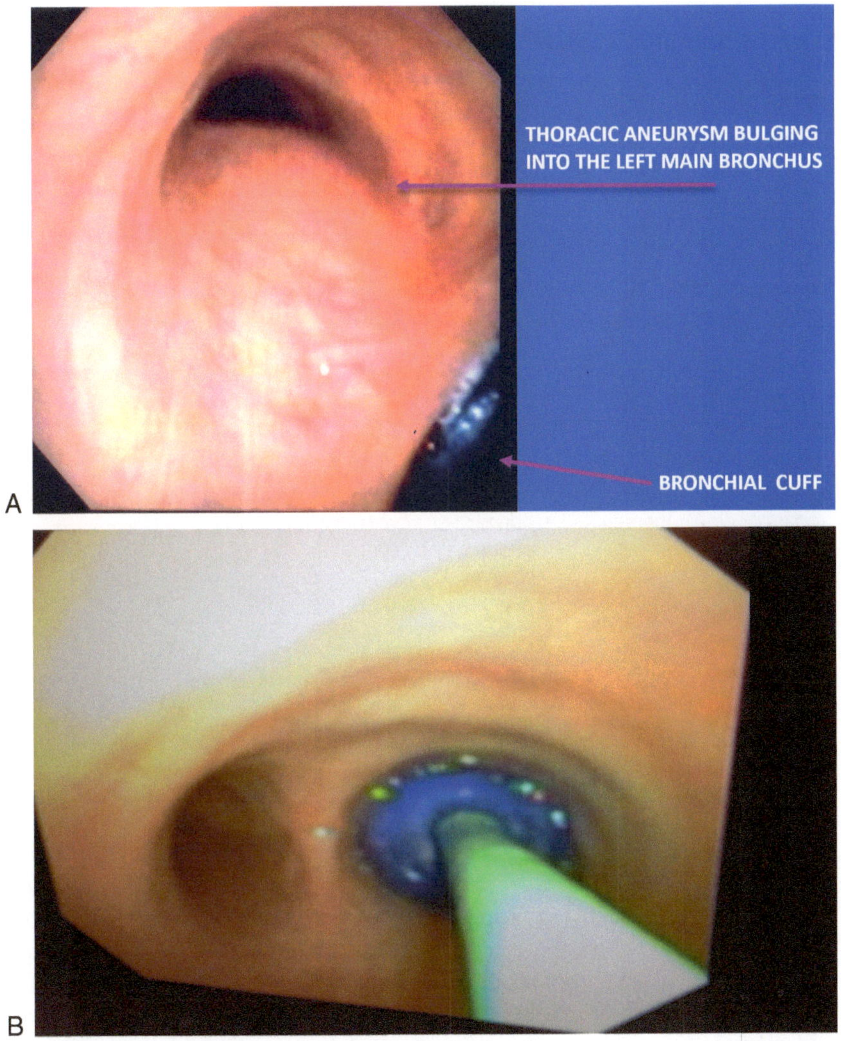

• **Fig. 39.7** **A.** A tracheal bronchoscopy through a double-lumen tube in a patient with a thoracic aortic aneurysm. **B.** An endobronchial blocker *in situ*. (Courtesy of Edmond Cohen M.D.)

below metabolic demand.[65] Such a disparity could occur because of diminished cerebral blood flow or a decrease in arterial oxygen content. Conversely, a jugular bulb oxygen saturation of greater than 75% occurs when the oxygen supply to the brain increases in relation to demand.[63] Jugular bulb venous oxygen measurements are a useful proxy for cerebral metabolic demand and provide information about responses to intraoperative interventions. Close monitoring of jugular bulb venous saturation may allow close brain monitoring during cardiac surgery.[66]

TABLE 39.1 Grading System of the Severity of Clinical Complications Related to Aortic Arch Surgery

Grade	Severity of Complications
I	Any deviation from the normal postoperative course but self-limiting or requiring simple therapeutic regimens[a]
II	Complications requiring pharmacologic treatment for resolution
III	Complications requiring surgical, endoscopic, or radiologic intervention but not requiring regional or general anesthesia or requiring interdisciplinary intervention
IV	Complications requiring surgical, endoscopic, or radiologic intervention under regional or general anesthesia, or requiring new intensive care unit admission or ongoing intensive care unit management for >7 days or hospitalization for >30 days, or causing secondary organ failure
V	Death caused by a complication

[a]Including antiemetics, antipyretics, analgesics, electrolytes, and physiotherapy

From Yan TD, Tian DH, LeMaire SA, et al. Standardizing clinical end points in aortic arch surgery: a consensus statement from the International Aortic Arch Surgery Study Group. *Circulation*. 2014;129(15):1610–1616.

TABLE 39.2 Classifications of Clinical End Points of the Neurologic System

Neurologic System	Grade I	Grade II	Grade III	Grade IV
Global neurologic deficit	Self-limiting within 24 hours	Resolving within 24–72 hours, requiring pharmacologic therapy, or requiring intubation for 24–72 hours	Requiring intubation for 3–7 days or requiring stroke rehabilitation	Requiring prolonged intubation for >7 days or tracheostomy
Focal neurologic deficit	Self-limiting within 24 hours	Resolving within 24–72 hours, requiring pharmacologic therapy, or requiring intubation for 24–72 hours	Requiring intubation for 3–7 days or requiring stroke rehabilitation	Requiring intubation for >7 days or tracheostomy or requiring radiologic or neurosurgical intervention
Spinal neurologic deficit	Self-limiting within 24 hours	Resolving within 24–72 hours, requiring pharmacologic therapy (e.g., to optimize cerebrospinal perfusion pressure)	Requiring drainage of cerebrospinal fluid to optimize cerebrospinal perfusion pressure or reversible spinal neurologic deficit requiring spinal rehabilitation	Irreversible spinal neurologic deficit

From Yan TD, Tian DH, LeMaire SA, et al. Standardizing clinical end points in aortic arch surgery: a consensus statement from the International Aortic Arch Surgery Study Group. *Circulation*. 2014;129(15):1610–1616.

Retrograde cannulation of the jugular vein is generally the method of choice to monitor jugular bulb saturation.[67,68] This technique helps to prevent contamination from extracranial sources, although contamination can also occur if jugular blood is aspirated too rapidly.[69] Thus the rate of aspiration withdrawal (i.e., slow and steady) is critical to ensuring the accuracy of a venous blood sample. One estimate suggests that oxygen saturation measurements can be up to 25% higher with faster rates of blood aspiration. The catheter tip should lie high in the jugular bulb to minimize the risk of contamination with blood from the facial veins. Radiography should be used to confirm the catheter placement, and it has been demonstrated that extracerebral contamination is lessened when the catheter tip is located less than two centimeters down from the jugular bulb.[66,70]

Limitations of jugular bulb oximetry include that precise areas of regional cerebral ischemia may not be detected, as the measurement of jugular bulb oximetry has a high specificity but a generally low sensitivity. A normal jugular bulb oximetry does not exclude the presence of regional cerebral ischemia, however, a jugular vein oxygen saturation of less than 50% is a reliable indicator that cerebral ischemia is occurring.[71] Potentially significant complications from jugular bulb oximetry include damage from placing the catheter; for example, a rupture of the carotid artery or other trauma done to nerves in the area, which can include the phrenic nerve or cervical ganglion, as well as a pneumothorax or other local tissue damage.[66,72] In addition, if a catheter is poorly maintained or left in the jugular vein, it could serve as a nidus for infection or contribute to thrombosis. Importantly, these devices are generally considered to be very safe in both children and adults.[73,74]

During hypothermic CPB, the period of most significant cerebral hypoperfusion occurs during rewarming. As the brain is rewarmed, oxygen consumption gradually increases across the cerebrum, leading to increased oxygen uptake and utilization.[75] During rewarming, oxygen saturation as measured by jugular bulb oximetry decreases to subnormal values, reflecting a state of increased metabolic demand. Thus the increase in cerebral oxygen demand temporarily outpaces oxygen availability.[76] It has been hypothesized that the oxygen imbalance may be caused by an inadequate compensatory response to the increased metabolic rate (e.g., an autoregulation problem), microemboli, cerebral vasoconstriction in response to the CPB itself, or even hemodilution secondary to the CPB, resulting in decreased cerebral oxygenation.[77] The speed of rewarming is also critical to patient outcomes. It has been demonstrated that patients who were more rapidly rewarmed had more significant reductions in jugular bulb oxygenation, revealing pace of rewarming could be a factor in the imbalance between cerebral oxygen supply and demand.[78] Rapid rewarming likely accentuates cerebral metabolic demand.[79,80] The period of rewarming must be carefully monitored and deserves critical observation. Aside from slower rewarming, mild hypercapnia has been shown to prevent jugular bulb desaturation during rewarming,[81] and there is some debate about the potential of pulsatile perfusion in preventing jugular bulb oxygenation, as well.[82,83]

More recently, because of the cost, invasiveness, and tedious application of jugular bulb oximetry, cerebral oximetry for neuroprotection in thoracic aortic aneurysm repairs has been performed via bilateral, noninvasive sensors placed on the forehead to monitor the regional oxygen saturation of the frontal cortex. This process uses noninvasive near-infrared spectroscopy (NIRS) and allows for the continuous measurement of oxygenated and deoxygenated hemoglobin. It also allows for the detection of decreases in cerebral perfusion and for the restoration of cerebral perfusion.[84] This technique is important where unilateral antegrade cerebral perfusion is the routine perfusion adjunct during aortic arch reconstruction.[85] NIRS-based cerebral oximetry allows for real-time detection of cerebral hypoxia and permits anesthesiologists to ameliorate the issue. This technique can also stratify patients preoperatively according to their risk of cerebral hypoperfusion.[86] Although not standard monitoring, the continuous measuring of cerebral oximetry in cardiovascular surgery has demonstrated that the technique has the potential to improve postoperative outcomes. Future studies should further evaluate continuous cerebral oximetry monitoring in tandem with treatments for desaturations.[87]

Hematologic Considerations

Because of the use of CPB, aortic aneurysm resections have a high incidence of coagulopathy. The use of deep hypothermia and particularly lengthy bypass times also hinder the coagulation cascade. Providers should consider the use of blood conservation strategies, such as normovolemic hemodilution, cell-saver, and preoperative autologous blood donation.[88] Postoperatively, point-of-care testing should guide the administration of blood transfusions, fresh frozen plasma, cryoprecipitate, and platelets. Many institutions use antifibrinolytics like tranexamic acid or aprotinin during thoracic aortic aneurysm resections.[48]

Gastrointestinal Considerations

Depending upon the location of a thoracic aortic aneurysm, bowel ischemia may occur because of the involvement of celiac or mesenteric arteries. In our patient, the thoracic aortic aneurysm was more proximal than these vascular structures, and this was not a large concern.

Airway Considerations

A preoperative examination of the airway is important for all patients undergoing surgery, but there are nuances for patients with Marfan syndrome, which include the potential presence of prognathism and a high palate. Both conditions can complicate intubation and should be carefully assessed in the preoperative period. During intubation, excessive pressure and traction along the temporomandibular joint should be avoided, and ideally, physicians that are experienced in airway management should perform the intubation of patients with Marfan syndrome. A fiberoptic bronchoscope should be used to inspect the airway before intubation to ensure that the thoracic aortic aneurysm will not be harmed by the endotracheal tube. The hemodynamic response associated with intubation should be blunted with the generous use of fentanyl or vasodilator drugs during induction. It is critical to reduce the stress put onto the thoracic aortic aneurysm, and this can be done by decreasing systolic blood pressure and inotropy.

Other Considerations

A thorough examination of the patient's joints is necessary, including their laxity. This can help prevent dislocations intraoperatively and other injuries because of changes in patient positioning that may not be relevant for patients that do not have Marfan syndrome.[31]

Thoracic Aortic Aneurysms and Anesthetic Management

The anesthetic management in these complex procedures is typically a regimen titrated to adequate analgesia (with a synthetic opioid), amnesia (with a volatile inhalational agent, or benzodiazepine), and neuromuscular blockade (with vecuronium or rocuronium). An appropriate titration of these anesthetics is critical in all cardiovascular procedures, but it deserves special attention in a surgery as delicate and complex as a thoracic aortic aneurysm repair. Prevention of hypertension during surgery is an important aspect of anesthetic management because hypertension can have catastrophic consequences intraoperatively as the thoracic aortic aneurysm is being resected. Standard ASA monitoring is required for this procedure, as well as both arterial and venous access, bladder catheterization, transesophageal echocardiography, multiple available locations for temperature measurements, jugular vein access, and cerebral function monitoring with oximetry.[14,36,48,89] Open surgical repair for a thoracic aortic aneurysm may require the interruption of cerebral perfusion. Deliberate hypothermia is induced with the aid of CPB to protect the viability of the brain during the period of elective circulatory arrest. Periods of deep hypothermic circulatory arrest permit surgical reconstruction of the aortic arch.[8,16,90–92] The issues of bleeding, hemostasis, and blood transfusion are important in aortic arch surgery, and a recent comprehensive update on this topic is covered in a special article by Raphael et al.[93]

Invasive Blood Pressure Monitoring

Invasive blood pressure monitoring in aortic resection procedures is critical to assessing the patient's vascular competence in real time. In general, this is accomplished with an indwelling arterial line, although the location can be variable and should be based upon the surgical plan and the condition of the patient and his or her disease. For example, in the case of an innominate artery dissection, a right-sided radial artery line should not be placed. A continuous and accurate blood pressure measurement is necessary because of the high probability of hemodynamic instability, aortic fragility, as well as the unpredictability associated with hypothermic CPB with nonpulsatile flow. Invasive monitoring also allows for frequent blood gases to be collected, which help guide anesthetic management.

Invasive Central Pressure Monitoring

Central venous cannulation indications include establishing access for volume resuscitation, the need for a reliable and timely intravenous access route for the administration of vasoactive agents, and securing access for pulmonary artery catheterization. An oximetric pulmonary arterial catheter is used to monitor central pressures, cardiac output, and systemic vascular resistance in real time in both the intraoperative and postoperative settings. Central venous pressure monitoring is also required for pressure monitoring to guide retrograde cerebral perfusion during the repair of an aortic arch. In this situation, the central venous pressure is transduced at the level of the internal jugular vein above the tip of the perfusion cannula in the superior vena cava, and the goal is to maintain a pressure in the range of 15 to 20 mm Hg to avoid cerebral edema.[58]

Temperature Monitoring

The goal of hypothermia during the repair of a thoracic aortic aneurysm is to suppress brain metabolism and therefore provide a degree of ischemic tolerance for a patient. Temperature monitoring is necessary to guide the management of hypothermic CPB for optimal neuroprotection. The nasopharyngeal temperature has been shown to closely mirror the brain temperature, and this is an ideal location from which to monitor. The distal esophagus is theoretically a more accurate location to measure temperature, but it is not generally used because of heat loss during open chest surgeries. Temperatures taken from the rectum and bladder have a significant temperature lag and are not closely reflective of a patient's brain temperature.[94] Temperatures vary from individual to individual, and therefore EEG monitoring during cooling in CPB allows for the precise determination of the effect of temperature change. However, in the emergent setting, EEG may not be readily available. In these cases, patients are generally brought to profound hypothermia or are cooled for longer than an hour.[95,96]

There are three major neuroprotective techniques in hypothermic circulatory arrest: profound hypothermia, retrograde cerebral perfusion, and antegrade cerebral perfusion.[97,98] Profound hypothermia in isolation has been shown to effectively provide neuroprotection, and in tandem with retrograde cerebral perfusion, effective neuroprotection can also be achieved, with shorter hypothermic circulatory arrest times (i.e., <30–45 minutes). Antegrade cerebral perfusion is also an effective adjunct to profound hypothermia, and this combination is particularly effective when hypothermic circulatory arrest times are prolonged (i.e., >30–45 minutes). Retrograde cerebral perfusion has additionally been used in tandem with profound hypothermia with success. Hypothermic circulatory arrest can decrease metabolic rate, and therefore it is crucial that adequate cooling be achieved.[99] Cooling should generally last for at least 30 minutes to prevent fluctuations in temperature and ensure that the cooling is maintained throughout the aortic reconstruction. Consistent intracranial temperature can be ensured by evenly packing around the patient's head with ice. Following the procedure, proper rewarming is essential and entails gradual, consistent perfusion temperatures to compensate for the patient's increasing oxygen demand. Cerebral vasoconstriction can be avoided by maintaining and meticulously monitoring hemodynamics in the postoperative period.[100]

The International Aortic Arch Surgery Study Group recommends utilizing the axillary artery as the arterial inflow route during CPB for the induction of hypothermia. This route has several advantages, including no retrograde cerebral emboli or retrograde dissections, a decreased risk of cerebral emboli, a reduced risk of malperfusion and regional hypoperfusion, and the ability to provide access for subsequent unilateral antegrade cerebral perfusion.[101,102]

Transesophageal Echocardiography

Transesophageal echocardiography is used in the perioperative evaluation of the thoracic aorta. Its advantages include high sensitivity and specificity for aortic pathologies, the ability to forgo contrast and radiation, and the ability to successfully visualize and assess the cardiac valves and ventricles. This imaging methodology assists in confirming diagnoses, reliably detecting and quantifying cardiac complications, and demonstrating new imaging findings.[103] However, it is important to note that a major limitation is the "blind spot," that is the distal ascending aorta and proximal aortic arch. These structures are obscured because of the air-filled tracheobronchial tree.[17,104] A modified TEE can help overcome this impairment via the placement of the fluid-filled balloon in the trachea. Alternatively to a modified TEE, imaging of the entire arch and blind spot can be done with epiaortic imaging in the setting of an open chest. Altogether, imaging from TEE can guide cannulation of the true lumen in the dissected ascending aorta for CPB.[17,105]

There is a major role for TEE in a thoracic aortic aneurysm repair because TEE provides a comprehensive analysis of the aortic valve to quantify the severity and mechanism of aortic regurgitation. This can help determine if the natural valve can be repaired or should be replaced. TEE can also be used during the critical phase of the operation to monitor the accuracy of cerebral perfusion (the kinetics of the intimal flap may precipitate cerebral malperfusion, which is especially important during the initiation of CPB, clamping of the ascending aorta, and during antegrade cerebral perfusion). This imaging can be achieved by withdrawing the TEE into the pharynx or by transcutaneous scanning.[85,106]

Cerebral malperfusion can then be corrected via an adjustment of the cannulation site, a surgical fenestration of the intimal flap to restore perfusion to both true and false lumen, an adjustment of arterial cannula, or the initiation of bilateral antegrade cerebral perfusion.[84,107]

Ventilation Management and Ventilatory Modalities (see Chapter 20)

OLV is the preferred modality for the open repair of a thoracic aortic aneurysm. OLV provides numerous benefits and serves as the ideal choice for the repair of a thoracic aortic aneurysm, including providing optimal space in the left chest cavity for surgical manipulation.[89,108,109] OLV can help protect the dependent lung from secretions, such as blood, pus, or lavage fluids. The use of fiberoptic bronchoscopy to confirm optimal position of the DLT is essential. Lung protective ventilation includes the use of low tidal volumes, low peak airway pressures, positive end-expiratory pressure (PEEP), and frequent recruitment maneuvers. The lowest safe fraction of inspired oxygen (FiO2) that can be used is also an important aspect of anesthetic management.[110–113]

OLV can be performed with either the intubation of the left or right mainstem bronchus.[114] In general, the use of right-sided double-lumen tubes is more complicated because of anatomic variability of the right mainstem bronchus, as well as the possibility of right upper lobe (RUL) obstruction, which can lead to poor ventilation of this lobe.[115] The right main bronchus is shorter than the left main bronchus, with a decreased margin of safety and an increased risk of upper-lobe obstruction with a right-sided double-lumen tube.[116] Thus left-sided double-lumen tubes grant anesthesiologists a wider safety range in placement. In addition, in as many as 3% of the population, the RUL originates at the carina or even the trachea, and in these cases, the use of right-sided double-lumen tubes is not recommended.[117] A right-sided DLT has the advantage of avoiding the left mainstem bronchus, although it has a lower margin of safety. It is mandatory, however, if there is a risk of rupturing a thoracic aortic aneurysm bulging into the left main bronchus. The use of double-lumen tubes is superior to the use of bronchial blockers because double-lumen tubes offer the possibility of more effective suctioning. Bronchial blockers also achieve effective lung collapse but may tend to dislodge more easily. One of the advantages of using a bronchial blocker is the elimination of the need to change the tube at the end of the procedure.[118,119]

Intraoperative Physiologic Considerations During One-Lung Ventilation

During OLV in the lateral decubitus position, a redistribution of pulmonary perfusion occurs in which the dependent lung receives significantly more perfusion. This positioning leads to shunt, which is about 20% to 25% of cardiac output.[120] Gravity and surgical manipulation contribute to decreased perfusion in the collapsed lung, and this exacerbates any pulmonary disease in the nondependent lung. In addition, during two-lung ventilation in the lateral position, over one-half of the tidal volume is delivered to the nondependent lung while an anesthetized and paralyzed patient is in the lateral decubitus position.[121] While under anesthesia, there is a reduction in the functional residual capacity of the dependent lung, as well as a decrease in its compliance.[122] Ventilation/perfusion (V/Q) mismatch occurs in this setting because the nondependent lung is better ventilated, and its functional residual capacity greater than the dependent lung. Separation of the lungs exacerbates the V/Q mismatch that is inherent to anesthesia, because of the intrapulmonary shunt through the non-dependent lung.[120,123] This scenario leads to hypoxemia, which can be further worsened by lung disease or vasculopathy.[124] The fractional blood flow to the nondependent lung decreases during OLV, whereas it increases in the dependent lung because of gravity and hypoxic pulmonary vasoconstriction.[108]

Although lower tidal volumes are linked to a decreased incidence of volume trauma, there is a concern about adequate oxygenation in this setting.[125,126] Without PEEP, OLV with low tidal volumes has been shown to increase atelectasis and provide inadequate oxygenation. During OLV, the dependent lung is at particular risk of alveolar collapse during expiration, and thus PEEP is especially recommended for OLV.[127] In addition, the initiation of high-pressure inspiration for a short period of time accompanied by PEEP has been demonstrated to prevent alveolar collapse and improve arterial oxygenation during OLV.[125] Some cases of hypoxemia can be managed with continuous positive airway pressure (CPAP) with high oxygen flow delivered to the nondependent lung, which provides apneic oxygenation, maintains the patency of alveoli, and enhances oxygenation.[128] Lower tidal volumes have been demonstrated to better maintain left ventricular and right ventricular systolic function compared with intermediate tidal volumes during mechanical ventilation, and this may help protect cardiac systolic functioning intraoperatively.[129]

Tidal volumes and ventilatory pressures can be lowered by decreasing minute ventilation, and this can prevent barotrauma in OLV.[130] In addition, a similar protective strategy using decreased minute ventilation has been found to reduce the incidence of acute lung injury.[131]

Postoperative Ventilation Considerations

A chief concern in the immediate postoperative period in patients having undergone OLV for the repair of a thoracic aortic aneurysm is adequate hemodynamic and respiratory control. The choice between a single or DLT in the immediate postoperative setting should not have a major impact on mechanical ventilation. Double-lumen tubes, used in the intraoperative setting, have been suggested to provide greater resistance to mechanical ventilation because of their two-lumen nature and therefore confer a more prolonged

$$\Delta p = \frac{8\mu LQ}{\pi R^4} = \frac{8\pi\mu LQ}{A^2}$$

• **Fig. 39.8** The Hagen-Poiseuille equation, where Δp is the pressure difference between the two ends, L is the pipe length, μ is the dynamic viscosity, Q is the volumetric flow rate, R is the pipe radius, and A is the cross section of pipe.

weaning period.[112,132] Considering a patient's overall clinical stability and respiratory parameters, the DLT can be exchanged for a single-lumen tube in the operating room before full extubation.

There are numerous advantages to the use of double-lumen tubes in thoracic aortic aneurysm procedures, although these devices pose some challenges in the postoperative ventilation period. One dilemma for physicians is whether to leave the DLT in place and when to exchange the DLT for a single-lumen tube. Nearly every patient undergoing a repair of a thoracic aortic aneurysm will require postoperative mechanical ventilation. In determining the most appropriate postoperative care, the chief concerns include a patient's airway resistance and clearance of secretion, as well as airway irritation and trauma. Airway resistance is proportional to the radius of a tube to the fourth power and is directly proportional to the length of a tube, as indicated by the Hagen-Poiseuille equation in Fig. 39.8. It has been theorized that because of the increased length of a DLT over a single-lumen tube (as well as being split into two separate lumens), it is more resistant to ventilation, potentially making it more difficult to wean from mechanical ventilation. Interestingly, however, airway resistance has been shown to differ from one type of DLT to another. For example, a 7.5-mm single-lumen tube has been shown to have a higher airway resistance than a 37 Fr Rusch or Sheridan double-lumen tube, which one would not expect simply given the Hagen-Poiseuille equation.[133] The use of a DLT postoperatively should not be expected to increase the patient's work of breathing or otherwise complicate weaning from mechanical ventilation.

Although rates of significant tracheobronchial injuries are low, a DLT may be more likely than a single-lumen tube to cause a sore throat or hoarseness postoperatively because of the increased diameter of the tube.[134] Importantly, there is no evidence that leaving a DLT in postoperatively can lead to inflammation of the airway or edema in the larynx. Proper positioning (i.e., head up) can also help prevent the accumulation of edema in and around the airway. In addition, postoperative stridor can be prevented with the use of preoperative steroids, which is generally routine practice. DLTs do cause more coughing than single-lumen tubes as they cross the carina, but this has not been well studied in a postoperative setting.[135]

Nevertheless, it is not recommended to send the patient with a DLT in place to the cardiac intensive care unit. DLTs can be exchanged for single-lumen tubes via direct laryngoscopy or video laryngoscopy. An advantage of single-lumen tubes in the postoperative setting is that intensive care unit staff (including physicians, nurses, and respiratory therapists) are accustomed to single-lumen endotracheal tubes, and they facilitate the sampling of secretions and removal of mucous plugs. Depending upon the intraoperative course, the exchanging of a DLT for a single-lumen one may be more complicated, such as when a patient has airway edema or has a limited respiratory reserve. In these situations, an airway exchange catheter can be useful. Such a device can be inserted into the bronchial lumen of the DLT and function as a guide to remove the DLT and help replace it with a single-lumen tube. A prospective study performed over a 9-year period demonstrated the safety and effectiveness of airway exchange catheters and showed a high rate of successful first attempts at reintubation. Various complications, including hypotension, low oxygen saturation, bradycardia, and esophageal intubation were far less common when reintubation was performed with an airway exchange catheter, and other studies have corroborated such outcomes.[136] By using a connector, an airway exchange catheter can also be converted to a conduit for jet ventilation and the insufflation of oxygen.[137] An example of such a connector can be seen in Fig. 39.9A and 39.9B.

Proper postoperative pain control is critical to the successful management of a patient following a thoracic aortic aneurysm procedure and can help facilitate timely extubation. Although parenteral opioids serve as the mainstay of pain management in this setting, epidural analgesia provides numerous benefits and has been shown to decrease postoperative pulmonary complications and improve lung function.[138] However, the use of epidural analgesia is limited by the risk of an epidural hematoma, which is a potentially catastrophic complication, especially in the setting of CPB with full heparinization.[139] Epidural infusions of local anesthetics can also cause sympathectomy, interfering with blood pressure goals following a thoracic aortic aneurysm repair and resulting in hypotension. An alternative is a paravertebral catheter, which has similar contraindications related to coagulopathy but results in less hypotension. Another option is an intercostal nerve block, which can provide pain control. Adjuvants include nonsteroidal antiinflammatory drugs, and although they can achieve significant pain relief, their usage is limited by the possibility of end-organ damage, as well as toxicity. Effective and safe pain control regimens should be tailored to each patient and take into account medical comorbidities, the extent of the pain, laboratory values, such as coagulation studies, hemodynamic stability, and the surgical technique itself.[113] A take-home summary for anesthesiologists to consider while performing OLV for the surgical repair of a thoracic aortic aneurysm can be found in Box 39.3.

Alternative Methods

Medical Management

Although our patient received a surgical intervention for his large ascending thoracic aortic aneurysm, medical management in a patient with less severe disease is a possibility.

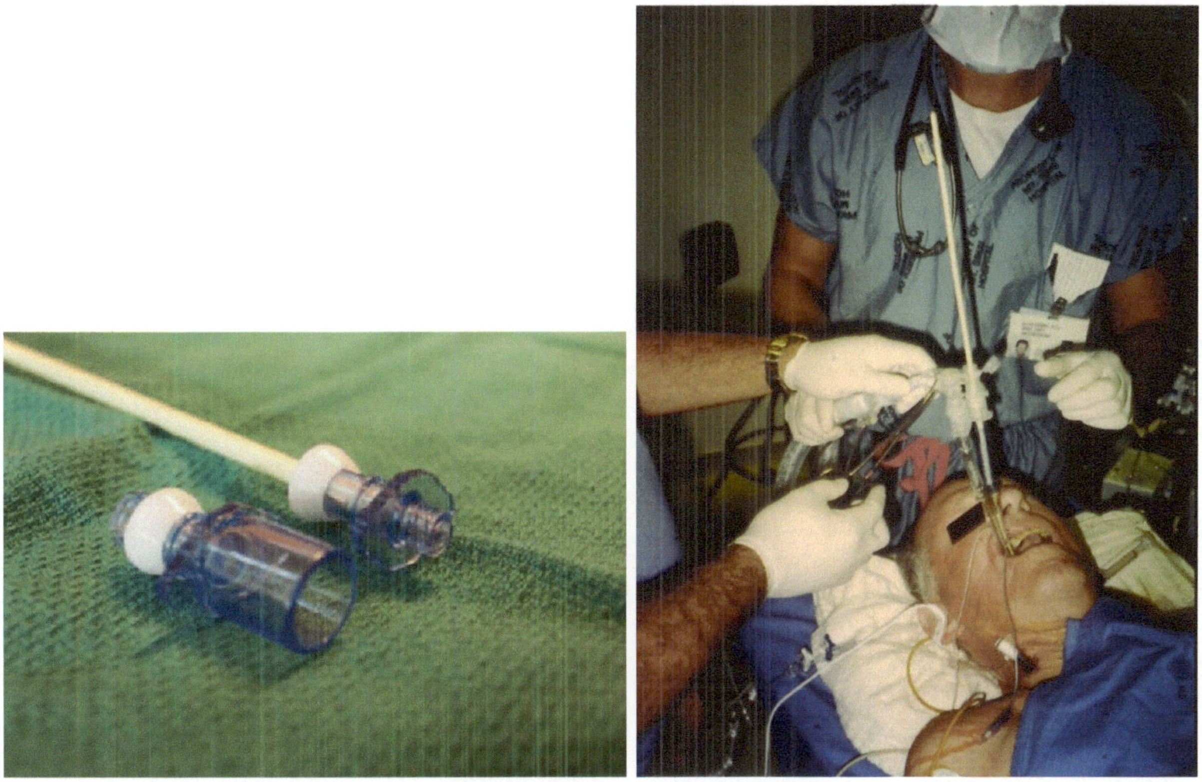

• **Fig. 39.9** (**A**) Connectors from an airway exchange catheter to a ventilator or jet ventilator. (**B**) An intubated patient connected to an airway exchange catheter. (Courtesy of Edmond Cohen M.D.)

Two mainstay medications for the medical management of a thoracic aortic aneurysm in the setting of Marfan syndrome are beta blockers and angiotensin angiotensin-converting enzyme (ACE) inhibitors.[140,141] A primary goal is to reduce the wall tension of a thoracic aortic aneurysm, which can be accomplished via beta-adrenergic blockade. Beta blockers provide a reduction in aortic wall stress because of their inotropic and negative chronotropic effects, and, although under debate, an association with reduced mortality with the use of beta blockers has been described.[142] Currently, it is recommended that all patients with Marfan syndrome be placed on beta blockers, regardless of aortic measurements. This is especially useful in pediatric populations, as the use of beta blockers may help delay surgery. As an alternative to beta blockers, ACE inhibitors and selective angiotensin II receptor blockers (ARBs) may be used to control blood pressure and help reduce the stiffness of the aortic wall.[143] Inhibition of the renin-angiotensin system prevents angiotensin II from stimulating the proliferation of smooth muscle cells, thereby reducing fibrosis. Animal models have shown that ARBs reduce TGF-β levels, interfering with elements of the pathogenesis of Marfan syndrome in the aorta.[144] Beta blockers and ARBs have been shown to be effective in pediatric populations when used in tandem, with the dilatation rate of the aortic root being significantly less in groups receiving both therapies than in those receiving beta blockers alone.[145]

• BOX 39.3 Take-Home Points for Anesthesiologists Performing One-Lung Ventilation for the Surgical Repair of a Thoracic Aortic Aneurysm

1. One-lung ventilation (OLV) provides optimal visualization and reduces reactions related to mechanical trauma that may have occurred to the left lung during surgery
2. A left-sided endobronchial tube is optimal for OLV because it is easy to position and less likely to become nonfunctional
3. A right-sided endobronchial tube for OLV may be necessary, especially if the left main bronchus is compressed by a large aneurysm, as there is a possibility for catastrophic rupture and bleeding
4. Proper tube placement during ventilation must be confirmed after positioning the patient in the left lateral decubitus position
5. OLV requires the use of the fiberoptic bronchoscope
6. Anesthesiologists must consider the status of the patient's lungs (e.g., age, disease, smoking history), monitoring, lung protective ventilation (low tidal volumes, low peak airway pressures, high positive end-expiratory pressure [PEEP], lower fraction of inspired oxygen [FiO2]), and closely follow systemic oxygenation

From Silvay G, Lurie J, Casale, M. The anaesthetic management of patients with thoracic ascending aortic aneurysms: A review. *J Perioper Pract.* 2020;1–8.

Additional Surgical Management

Marfan syndrome is associated with numerous cardiovascular complications, and two of the most common include mitral valve prolapse and aortic root aneurysm. The subvalvular apparatus enables the proper closure of the mitral valve, and four in five patients with Marfan syndrome have severe annular dilatation accompanied by degeneration of this structure. Still, however, only one in four of these patients develops mitral valve prolapse and mitral regurgitation requiring surgery.[146] Aortic root dilatation affects about one in two patients with Marfan syndrome at some point in their lives, and can result in mortality in around 50% of these patients by the age of 40 years without proper surgical intervention because of aortic dissection and frank rupture.[56]

Risks and Benefits

Prophylactic surgery to replace a thoracic aortic aneurysm in a patient with Marfan syndrome is the only way to prevent major complications, such as aortic ruptures or dissections. It is generally recommended that prophylactic surgery occur when the diameter of the ascending aorta at the level of the aortic sinus reaches 5.0 cm. Patients are also triaged into varying risk groups depending on the diameter of their aorta at this location: patients with an aortic diameter of less than 2.75 cm/m^2 are categorized as low risk of dissection, patients with an aortic diameter from 2.75 to 4.24 cm/m^2 are at moderate risk of dissection, and those with an aortic diameter greater than 4.25 cm/m^2 are at high risk of dissection.[147] Patients with risk factors may require earlier intervention, such as a known family history of aortic dissection, severe aortic regurgitation accompanied by left ventricular dilation, a rate of aortic dilation of over 2 mm per year, and the feasibility for that particular patient to undergo the surgical procedure.[148]

Thoracic aneurysms of the ascending aorta, in an acute setting, necessitate prompt surgical repair with or without optimal medical stabilization to prevent rupture with serious complications.[149] Thoracic aneurysmal dissections are a severe, life-threatening condition with a high overall mortality when untreated. The mortality rate in a TAAD has been shown to be up to 50% if surgery is delayed beyond 48 hours, with the average mortality rate at 1% to 2% per hour in this critical period.[150] The diagnosis and early treatment of a TAAD are of great importance.[36,46,151] Early diagnosis and stabilization, prompt referral to an aortic center, and early operation significantly reduce mortality, particularly with a symptomatic patient with a leaking thoracic aneurysm.[92]

Close communication between the surgeon, anesthesiologist, and perfusion team is required before and during surgery for a thoracic aortic aneurysm, integrating strategies relating to patient positioning, OLV, as well as aspects regarding cannulation, monitoring, and anticoagulation management. The anesthetic approach to the repair of a thoracic aortic aneurysm must account for the thoracic aneurysm's severity, including its size and location, etiology, as well as general condition of the patient.[92,152,153] Detailed information pertaining to the extent and location of the thoracic aneurysm, and the functional status of the heart and coronary anatomy, is critical. Most patients undergo coronary angiography before the surgery. A preoperative pulmonary workup, neurologic examination, and coagulation studies panel may also provide important information, but these may be limited in scope depending on the clinical status of the patient.[48,154] The type of repair is dictated not only by the location and extent of the disease, but also the general condition of the patient and the underlying etiology.[60]

Patients with Marfan syndrome require close monitoring and special considerations intraoperatively and postoperatively to avoid extremes in blood pressure (whether hypotension or hypertension), maintain coronary perfusion, and ensure the prevention of a thoracic aneurysmal dissection. Progressive dilation of the aortic ring can result in angina, dyspnea, and arrhythmia secondary to aortic regurgitation. Although not common, there are situations in which it may not be warranted to attempt an extubation at the end of a thoracic aortic aneurysm resection procedure, such as cases in which the airway is severely edematous. It may be undesirable to change the DLT because of the risk of lung contamination.[113]

A Review of Recent Literature

Central Nervous System Protection and Monitoring

Recent literature has addressed hypothermic circulatory arrest and its adjuncts, such as antegrade cerebral perfusion. For example, a systematic review and metaanalysis including nine comparative studies on unilateral versus bilateral antegrade cerebral perfusion in hypothermic circulatory arrest determined that no significant differences were seen in either approach with regard to mortality, permanent neurologic deficits, acute kidney injury, or reoperation for bleeding.[155] Another study determined that when comparing deep hypothermic circulatory arrest to antegrade cerebral perfusion in the surgical treatment of chronic dissection of the ascending and arch aorta, quality of life in the long-term was not dependent on the cerebral protection method used during surgery.[156] Interestingly, another group determined that antegrade selective cerebral perfusion reduced the in-hospital mortality and permanent focal neurologic deficits in patients during elective aortic arch surgery,[157] and other investigators have also determined benefits of using adjunctive cerebral perfusion.[158] However, some studies have found little difference between profound hypothermia and either antegrade or retrograde cerebral perfusion in elective aortic arch surgery.[159] In addition, a metaanalysis using 18 comparative studies focused on temperature selection in antegrade cerebral perfusion for aortic arch surgery determined that antegrade cerebral perfusion with warmer circulatory arrest temperatures could reduce the incidence of permanent neurologic deficits, among other clinical outcomes, but there were no differences in mortality or reexploration for bleeding.[160]

The safety of various degrees of hypothermia accompanied by antegrade cerebral perfusion in total aortic arch replacement is another area of recent investigation. Total aortic arch replacements typically use deep hypothermic circulatory arrest, and the impact of moderate hypothermic circulatory arrest and antegrade cerebral perfusion has been assessed. The Aortic Arch ARCH international aortic databasetic arch helped identify over 3000 patients undergoing total aortic arch replacement using antegrade cerebral perfusion, and patients were divided on lowest cooling temperature: moderate hypothermia (20°C–28°C) or deep hypothermia (12°C–20°C). There was no difference between the two cohorts in terms of neurologic outcomes or in-hospital mortality, and thus total aortic arch replacement with moderate hypothermic circulatory arrest and antegrade circulatory perfusion, the authors suggest, can be safely performed and may reduce the need for deep hypothermic circulatory arrest.[161] In addition, another study determined that higher temperatures within the range of moderate hypothermia (defined here as 20.1°C–28°C) are safe in elective proximal or total arch surgery when compared with colder temperatures,[95] whereas a study assessing moderate-to-mild hypothermia (>28°C) in surgery using antegrade cerebral perfusion for acute TAAD determined that these temperatures could safely be used and offered sufficient neurologic and other organ protection.[162]

Retrograde cerebral perfusion has also been a topic of recent research. A systematic review and metaanalysis sought to assess whether retrograde cerebral perfusion, which has become less frequently used as a method of neuroprotection during aortic surgery, was a worthwhile adjunct to hypothermic circulatory arrest. Twenty-eight comparative studies were identified. The cohort with hypothermic circulatory arrest and retrograde cerebral perfusion had a significantly reduced mortality. Stroke was also significantly more common in the hypothermic circulatory arrest cohort. These findings suggest the addition of retrograde cerebral perfusion may contribute to better outcomes, and additional data are necessary to further investigate these events.[163]

The role of EEG during moderate hypothermic circulatory arrest, accompanied by selective antegrade cerebral perfusion, has recently been investigated in a cohort undergoing hemiarch replacement, although the study only included 71 patients. About half of these patients experienced an abrupt cessation of electrocerebral activity following circulatory arrest, and although unilateral selective antegrade cerebral perfusion usually restored prearrest electrocerebral activity, intraoperative EEG has been argued to have potential value in identifying patients with persistent cerebral ischemia even after selective antegrade cerebral perfusion is initiated.[84] EEG has been used to confirm electrocerebral silence and aid in the induction of deep hypothermic circulatory arrest with retrograde or antegrade cerebral perfusion during aortic arch surgery and is thought to be a reliable monitoring tool for this procedure.[107]

Arterial Cannulation Site

There has been recent debate on the efficacy and safety of different locations for arterial cannulation in aortic arch surgery. For example, a recent propensity score analysis of right axillary and innominate artery cannulation conducted on over 900 patients undergoing elective hemiarch or total arch surgery found that the cannulation location did not independently predict operative mortality or composite adverse events (including stroke). Both cannulation sites provided similar operative death rates and composite adverse event rates, suggesting both produce similar results and can be conducted safely.[164] The safety of right axillary artery cannulation in patients with TAAD with innominate artery involvement was also assessed recently, and although there were under 200 patients in the study, results suggest that right axillary artery cannulation is as safe as nonright axillary artery cannulation in this patient population. Axillary versus femoral arterial cannulation during the repair of a TAAD have also recently been demonstrated to be comparable.[165]

Classifications of Acute Aortic Dissections

Since 2001, the Stanford classification system has been used to stratify aortic dissections into type A, which involve the ascending aorta (previously DeBakey type I and II), and type B, which do not (previously DeBakey type III).[166] Since 2009, the Penn classification system has also been used to better describe outcome risk in Stanford TAAD. According to the Penn classification system, there are four classes of type A dissections: class a, which involved the absence of ischemia, class b, which involve branch vessels with clinical regional ischemia, class c, which involve cardiovascular collapse with global ischemia, and class b + c, which involves branch vessel ischemia, as well as cardiovascular collapse, that is both regional and global ischemia.[104,167] The Penn classification has been validated in clinical trials and has shown that a higher burden of ischemia correlates with an increased risk of mortality.[168–170] Although the Penn classification system was traditionally applied to TAADs, it has now been extended to Stanford type b dissections to help elucidate outcomes in more distal thoracic aortic aneurysms. The Penn classification system has been validated in both type A and type B aortic dissections managed either surgically or medically.

Acknowledgments

Declaration of conflicting interests: The authors declared no potential conflicts of interest with respect to the research, authorship, and/or publication of this article.

Funding: The authors state no funding was received in support of this work.

References

1. Livesay JJ, Messner GN, Vaughn WK. Milestones in treatment of aortic aneurysm: Denton A. Cooley, MD, and the Texas Heart Institute. *Tex Heart I J.* 2005;32(2):130.
2. Meakins JL. A surgical history. *Can Med Assoc J.* 2005;172(13): 1713–1714.
3. Moore CH, Murchison C. On a new method of procuring the consolidation of fibrin in certain incurable aneurisms: with the report of a case in which an aneurism of the ascending aorta was treated by the insertion of wire. *Medico-Chirurgic Transact.* 1864;47:129.
4. Cervantes J. Reflections on the 50th anniversary of the first abdominal aortic aneurysm resection. *World J Surg.* 2003;27(2):246–248.
5. Dubost C, Allary M, Oeconomos N. Resection of an aneurysm of the abdominal aorta: reestablishment of the continuity by a preserved human arterial graft, with result after five months. *AMA Arch Surg.* 1952;64(3):405–408.
6. Gibbon J Jr. Application of a mechanical heart and lung apparatus to cardiac surgery, in recent advances in cardiovascular physiology and surgery. *Minnesota Med.* 1953:107–113.
7. Appoo JJ, Augoustides JG, Pochettino A, Savino JS, McGarvey ML, Cowie DC, et al. Perioperative outcome in adults undergoing elective deep hypothermic circulatory arrest with retrograde cerebral perfusion in proximal aortic arch repair: evaluation of protocol-based care. *J Cardiothorac Vasc Anesth.* 2006;20(1):3–7.
8. Augoustides J, Patel P, Ghadimi R, Choi J, Yue Y, Silvay G. Current conduct of deep hypothermic circulatory arrest in China. *HSR Proc Intensive Care Cardiovasc Anesth.* 2013;5(1):25.
9. Belway D, Tee R, Nathan H, Rubens F, Boodhwani M. Temperature management and monitoring practices during adult cardiac surgery under cardiopulmonary bypass: results of a Canadian national survey. *Perfusion.* 2011;26(5):395–400.
10. Lillehei C, Varco R, Cohen M, Warden H, Patton C, Moller JH. The first open-heart repairs of ventricular septal defect, atrioventricular communis, and tetralogy of Fallot using extracorporeal circulation by cross-circulation: a 30-year follow-up. *Ann Thorac Surg.* 1986;41(1):4–21.
11. Stehbens WE. History of aneurysms. *Med History.* 1958;2(4): 274–280.
12. Cooley DA. Aortic surgery: a historical perspective. *Semin Cardiothorac Vasc Anesth.* 2012;16(1):7–10.
13. De Bakey ME, Crawford ES, Cooley DA, Morris GC Jr, Royster TS, Abbott WP. Aneurysm of abdominal aorta analysis of results of graft replacement therapy one to eleven years after operation. *Ann Surg.* 1964;160(4):622.
14. Silvay G, Castillo J. History of anesthesia for aortic surgery in the world. In: Chiesa R, Melissano G, Setacci C, Argentieri A, eds. *History of Aortic Surgery in the World*: Edizioni Minerva Medica; 2015:58–69.
15. Carlens E. A new flexible double-lumen catheter for bronchospirometry. *J Thorac Surg.* 1949;18(5):742–746.
16. Griepp RB, Stinson EB, Hollingsworth JF, Buehler D. Prosthetic replacement of the aortic arch. *J Thorac Cardiovasc Surg.* 1975;70(6):1051–1063.
17. Tolis G, Sundt TM III. Contemporary insights into the management of type A aortic dissection. *Expert Rev Cardiovasc Ther.* 2016;14(10):1189–1196.
18. Silvay G, Khromava M, Weiner M, Augoustides JG, Castillo. Management of patients with a type A aortic dissection. *Gen Reanimatol.* 2019;15(2):36–52.
19. Gutsche J, Feinman J, Silvay G, et al. Practice variations in the conduct of hypothermic circulatory arrest for adult aortic arch repair: focus on an emerging European paradigm. *Heart Lung Vessels.* 2014;6(1):43.
20. Cooley DA, De Bakey ME. Resection of entire ascending aorta in fusiform aneurysm using cardiac bypass. *JAMA.* 1956; 162(12):1158–1159.
21. Kirpekar MK, Silvay G, Augoustides JG, et al. The adolescent minor and urgent aortic surgery: challenges and solutions with capacity and competence in informed consent. *J Cardiothorac Vasc Anesth.* 2019;33(4):1139–1145.
22. Milewicz D, Pyeritz R, Crawford ES, Byers P. Marfan syndrome: defective synthesis, secretion, and extracellular matrix formation of fibrillin by cultured dermal fibroblasts. *J Clin Invest.* 1992;89(1):79–86.
23. Lemaire R, Bayle J, Lafyatis R. Fibrillin in Marfan syndrome and tight skin mice provides new insights into transforming growth factor-β regulation and systemic sclerosis. *Curr Opin Rheumatol.* 2006;18(6):582–587.
24. Yetman AT, Bornemeier RA, McCrindle BW. Long-term outcome in patients with Marfan syndrome: is aortic dissection the only cause of sudden death? *J Am Coll Cardiol.* 2003;41(2): 329–332.
25. Marfan AB. Un cas de deformation congénitale des quatre membres, plus prononcée aux extrémités, caractérisée par l'allongement des os avec un certain degré d'amincissement. *Bull Mem Soc Med Hop Paris.* 1896;13:220.
26. Arbustini E, Disabella E. History of Marfan syndrome. In: Chiesa R MG, Setacci C, Argentieri A, eds. *History of Aortic Surgery in the World*: Edizioni Minerva Medica; 2015:88–94.
27. Léonard J, Morin C. Antonin-Bernard Jean Marfan and Gabrielle. *Arch Pediatr.* 2008;15(5):562–563.
28. Weve H. Ueber Arachnodarktylie (Dystrophia mesodermalis congenitia, typus Marfnis). *Arch Augenheilk.* 1931;104:1.
29. Arachnodactylie Achard C. *Bull Mem Soc Med Hop Paris.* 1902; 19:834.
30. Baer R, Taussig H, Oppenheimer EH. Congenital aneurysmal dilatation of the aorta associated with arachnodactyly. *Bull JHM.* 1943;72:309.
31. Castellano JM, Silvay G, Castillo JG. Marfan syndrome: clinical, surgical, and anesthetic considerations. *Semin Cardiothorac Vasc Anesth.* 2014;18(3):260–271.
32. Sakai LY, Keene DR, Engvall E. Fibrillin, a new 350-kD glycoprotein, is a component of extracellular microfibrils. *J Cell Biol.* 1986;103(6):2499–2509.
33. Lee B, Godfrey M, Vitale E, et al. Linkage of Marfan syndrome and a phenotypically related disorder to two different fibrillin genes. *Nature.* 1991;352(6333):330–334.
34. Judge DP, Dietz HC. Marfan's syndrome. The Lancet. 2005; 366(9501):1965–1976.
35. Kuzmik GA, Sang AX, Elefteriades JA. Natural history of thoracic aortic aneurysms. *J Vasc Surg.* 2012;56(2):565–571.
36. Silvay G. Thoracic aortic aneurysm: anesthesiologist's view 2009. *Rev Mex Anestesiol.* 2009;32(S1):35–36.
37. Olsson C, Thelin S, Stahle E, Ekbom A, Granath F. Thoracic aortic aneurysm and dissection. *Circulation.* 2006;114(24):2611–2618.
38. Johansson G, Markström U, Swedenborg J. Ruptured thoracic aortic aneurysms: a study of incidence and mortality rates. *J Vasc Surg.* 1995;21(6):985–988.
39. Itani Y, Watanabe S, Masuda Y, et al. Measurement of aortic diameters and detection of asymptomatic aortic aneurysms in a mass screening program using a mobile helical computed tomography unit. *Heart Vessels.* 2002;16(2):42–45.

40. Kälsch H, Lehmann N, Möhlenkamp S, et al. Body-surface adjusted aortic reference diameters for improved identification of patients with thoracic aortic aneurysms: results from the population-based Heinz Nixdorf Recall study. *Int J Cardiol.* 2013; 163(1):72–78.
41. Zoller JK, Gregory SH, Stevens TW, Sanchez LA, Hueneke R. Anesthetic considerations for aortic arch stenting. *J Cardiothorac Vasc Anesth.* 2019;33(11):3163–3175.
42. Smith HN, Boodhwani M, Ouzounian M, et al. Classification and outcomes of extended arch repair for acute type A aortic dissection: a systematic review and meta-analysis. *Interact Cardiovasc Thorac Surg.* 2017;24(3):450–459.
43. Melissano G, Chiesa R. *Aortic Complexities.* Milan, Italy: Edi Ermes; 2018.
44. Czerny M, Schmidli J, Adler S, et al. Current options and recommendations for the treatment of thoracic aortic pathologies involving the aortic arch: an expert consensus document of the European Association for Cardio-Thoracic Surgery (EACTS) and the European Society for Vascular Surgery (ESVS). *Eur J Cardiovasc Thorac Surg.* 2018;55(1):133–162.
45. Silvay G, Zafirova Z. Ten years experiences with preoperative evaluation clinic for day admission cardiac and major vascular surgical patients: model for "perioperative anesthesia and surgical home". *Semin Cardiothorac Vasc Anesth.* 2016;20(2):120–132.
46. Elefteriades JA. Thoracic aortic aneurysm: reading the enemy's playbook. *Curr Prob Cardiol.* 2008;33(5):203–277.
47. Flynn BC, de Perio M, Hughes E, Silvay G. The need for specialized preanesthesia clinics for day admission cardiac and major vascular surgery patients. *Semin Cardiothorac Vasc Anesth.* 2009; 13(4):241–248.
48. Silvay G, Stone ME. Repair of thoracic aneurysms, with special emphasis on the preoperative work-up. *Semin Cardiothorac Vasc Anesth.* 2006;10(1):11–15.
49. Nkomo VT, Enriquez-Sarano M, Ammash NM, et al. Bicuspid aortic valve associated with aortic dilatation: a community-based study. *Arterioscleros Thrombos Vasc Biol.* 2003;23(2):351–356.
50. Albornoz G, Coady MA, Roberts M, et al. Familial thoracic aortic aneurysms and dissections—incidence, modes of inheritance, and phenotypic patterns. *Ann Thorac Surg.* 2006;82(4): 1400–1405.
51. Antunes MJ, Colsen PR, Kinsley RH. Hypothermia and circulatory arrest for surgical resection of aortic arch aneurysms. *J Thorac Cardiovasc Surg.* 1983;86(4):576–581.
52. Griepp RB, Stinson EB, Hollingsworth JF, Buehler D. Prosthetic replacement of the aortic arch. *J Thorac Cardiovasc Surg.* 1975;70(6):1051–1063.
53. Kulik A, Castner CF, Kouchoukos NT. Outcomes after thoracoabdominal aortic aneurysm repair with hypothermic circulatory arrest. *J Thorac Cardiovasc Surg.* 2011;141(4):953–960.
54. Spielvogel D, Etz CD, Silovitz D, Lansman SL, Griepp RB. Aortic arch replacement with a trifurcated graft. *Ann Thorac Surg.* 2007;83(2):S791–S795.
55. Tierney ESS, Levine JC, Chen S, et al. Echocardiographic methods, quality review, and measurement accuracy in a randomized multicenter clinical trial of Marfan syndrome. *J Am Soc Echocardiogr.* 2013;26(6):657–666.
56. Moreno-Cabral CE, Miller DC, Mitchell RS, et al. Degenerative and atherosclerotic aneurysms of the thoracic aorta: determinants of early and late surgical outcome. *J Thorac Cardiovasc Surg.* 1984;88(6):1020–1032.
57. Ishii K, Adachi H, Tsubaki K, Ohta Y, Yamamoto M, Ino T. Evaluation of recurrent nerve paralysis due to thoracic aortic aneurysm and aneurysm repair. *Laryngoscope.* 2004;114(12): 2176–2181.
58. Spielvogel D, Halstead JC, Meier M, et al. Aortic arch replacement using a trifurcated graft: simple, versatile, and safe. *Ann Thorac Surg.* 2005;80(1):90–95.
59. Reich DL, Uysal S, Sliwinski M, et al. Neuropsychologic outcome after deep hypothermic circulatory arrest in adults. *J Thorac Cardiovasc Surg.* 1999;117(1):156–163.
60. Yan TD, Tian DH, LeMaire SA, et al. Standardizing clinical end points in aortic arch surgery: a consensus statement from the International Aortic Arch Surgery Study Group. *Circulation.* 2014;129(15):1610–1616.
61. Melnyk V, Fedorko L, Djaiani G. Microemboli on cardiopulmonary bypass: Should we care? *J Cardiothorac Vasc Anesth.* 2020; 34(6):1504–1505.
62. Seese L, Kilic A, Chu D. Cerebral perfusion goals during cardiopulmonary bypass—the Goldilocks effect. *JAMA Surg.* 2019; 154(9):827.
63. De Deyne C, Decruyenaere J, Colardyn F. How to interpret jugular bulb oximetry? In: Vincent J, ed. *Yearbook of Intensive Care and Emergency Medicine:* Springer, Berlin, Germany; 1996:731–741.
64. Sharma D, Lele A. Monitoring of jugular venous oxygen saturation. In: Koht A, Sloan TB, Toleikis R, eds. *Monitoring the Nervous System for Anesthesiologists and Other Health Care Professionals*: Springer, Chicago, IL; 2017:229–242.
65. Dearden NM. Jugular bulb venous oxygen saturation in the management of severe head injury. *Curr Opin Anesthesiol.* 1991; 4(2):279–286.
66. Shaaban Ali M, Harmer M, Latto I. Jugular bulb oximetry during cardiac surgery. *Anaesthesia.* 2001;56(1):24–37.
67. Andrews P, Dearden N, Miller J. Jugular bulb cannulation: description of a cannulation technique and validation of a new continuous monitor. *Br J Anesth.* 1991;67(5):553–558.
68. Abdo A, Castellanos R, Benítez Y, et al. Catheterization of jugular bulb guided by ultrasound in real time. *Rev Cuban Med Intensiva Emerg.* 2017;16(2):28–33.
69. Chaikittisilpa N, Vavilala MS, Lele AV. Jugular venous oximetry. In: Prabhakar H, ed. *Neuromonitoring Techniques*: Elsevier, London, UK; 2018:57–75.
70. Greeley WJ. Assessment of CNS function: cerebral blood flow and metabolism. *Brain Inj Pediatr Cardiac Surg.* 2019:12.
71. Matta B. Advances in monitoring cerebral oxygenation. *Curr Opin Anesthesiol.* 1996;9(5):365–370.
72. Gupta A, et al. Jugular venous oximetry. In: Gupta A, Gelb A, Duane D, Adapa R, eds. *Gupta and Gelb's Essentials of Neuroanesthesia and Neurointensive Care Cambridge: Cambridge University Press,* London, UK; 2018:328.
73. Wallin E, Larsson IM, Nordmark-Grass J, Rosenqvist I, Kristofferzon ML, Rubertsson S. Characteristics of jugular bulb oxygen saturation in patients after cardiac arrest: A prospective study. *Acta Anaesthesiol Scand.* 2018;62(9):1237–1245.
74. Goetting M, Preston G. Jugular bulb catheterization does not increase intracranial pressure. *Intensive Care Med.* 1991;17(4): 195–198.
75. Sapire KJ, Gopinath SP, Farhat G, et al. Cerebral oxygenation during warming after cardiopulmonary bypass. *Crit Care Med.* 1997;25(10):1655–1662.
76. Hu Z, Xu L, Zhu Z, Seal R, McQuillan PM. Effects of hypothermic cardiopulmonary bypass on internal jugular bulb venous oxygen saturation, cerebral oxygen saturation, and bispectral index in pediatric patients undergoing cardiac surgery: a prospective study. *Medicine (Baltimore).* 2016;95(2).

77. Hindman BJ. Jugular venous hemoglobin desaturation during rewarming on cardiopulmonary bypass what does it mean, what does it matter? *Anesthesiology.* 1998;89(1):3–5.
78. Nakajima T, Kuro M, Hayashi Y, Kitaguchi K, Uchida O, Takaki O. Clinical evaluation of cerebral oxygen balance during cardiopulmonary bypass: on-line continuous monitoring of jugular venous oxyhemoglobin saturation. *Anesth Analg.* 1992;74(5): 630–635.
79. Bibevski S, Felmly L, Kavarana MN. Cardiopulmonary bypass. In: Ungerleider R, Meliones JN, McMillan KN, Cooper DS, Jacobs JP, eds. *Critical Heart Disease in Infants and Children*: Elsevier, Philadelphia, PA; 2019:513–524.
80. Varelmann DJ. Hypothermia. In: Aglio LS, Urman RD, eds. *Anesthesiology*: Springer, Boston, MA; 2017:29–32.
81. Hanel F, von Knobelsdorff G, Werner C, am Esch JS. Hypercapnia prevents jugular bulb desaturation during rewarming from hypothermic cardiopulmonary bypass. *Anesthesiology.* 1998; 89(1):19–23.
82. Kawahara F, Kadoi Y, Saito S, Yoshikawa D, Goto F, Fujita N. Balloon pump–induced pulsatile perfusion during cardiopulmonary bypass does not improve brain oxygenation. *J Thorac Cardiovasc Surg.* 1999;118(2):361–366.
83. Mutch WAC, Lefevre GR, Warrian RK. Computer-controlled cardiopulmonary bypass increases jugular venous oxygen saturation during rewarming. *Ann Thorac Surg.* 1998;65(1):59–65.
84. Keenan JE, Wang H, Ganapathi AM, et al. Electroencephalography during hemiarch replacement with moderate hypothermic circulatory arrest. *Ann Thorac Surg.* 2016;101(2):631–637.
85. Khan NR, Smalley Z, Nesvick CL, Lee SL, Michael LM. The use of lumbar drains in preventing spinal cord injury following thoracoabdominal aortic aneurysm repair: an updated systematic review and meta-analysis. *J Neurosurg Spine.* 2016;25(3):383–393.
86. Vretzakis G, Georgopoulou S, Stamoulis K, et al. Cerebral oximetry in cardiac anesthesia. *J Thorac Dis.* 2014;6(Suppl 1):S60.
87. Green D, Kunst G. Cerebral oximetry and its role in adult cardiac, non-cardiac surgery and resuscitation from cardiac arrest. *Anaesthesia.* 2017;72:48–57.
88. Shore-Lesserson L, Reich DL, Silvay G, Griepp RB. Hemostasis in aortic and cardiothoracic surgery. *J Cardiac Surg.* 1997;12(2):232–237 Suppl.
89. Campos JH, Feider A. Hypoxia during one-lung ventilation—a review and update. *J Cardiothorac Vasc Anesth.* 2018;32(5): 2330–2338.
90. Yan TD, Bannon PG, Bavaria J, et al. Consensus on hypothermia in aortic arch surgery. *Ann Cardiothorac Surg.* 2013;2(2):163.
91. Augoustides JG, Patel PA, Savino JS, Bavaria JE. *Editorial Comment: The Heart Team Approach to Acute Type A Dissection: A New Paradigm in the Era of the Integrated Penn Classification and the Essen Concept.* Oxford University Press; 2012:404–405.
92. Guo MH, Appoo JJ, Saczkowski R, et al. Association of mortality and acute aortic events with ascending aortic aneurysm: a systematic review and meta-analysis. *JAMA.* 2018;1(4):e181281.e.
93. Raphael J, Mazer CD, Wilkey A, et al. Society of Cardiovascular Anesthesiologists (SCA) Clinical Practice Improvement (CPI) Advisory for management of perioperative bleeding and hemostasis in cardiac surgery patients. *J Cardiothorac Vasc Anesth.* 2019;33: 2887–2899.
94. Lim H, Kim B, Kim D-C, Lee S-K, Ko S. A comparison of the temperature difference according to the placement of a nasopharyngeal temperature probe. *Korean J Anesthesiol.* 2016;69(4): 357.
95. Preventza O, Coselli JS, Akvan S, et al. The impact of temperature in aortic arch surgery patients receiving antegrade cerebral perfusion for >30 minutes: How relevant is it really? *J Thorac Cardiovasc Surg.* 2017;153(4):767–776.
96. Stamou SC, Rausch LA, Kouchoukos NT, et al. Comparison between antegrade and retrograde cerebral perfusion or profound hypothermia as brain protection strategies during repair of type A aortic dissection. *Ann Cardiothorac Surg.* 2016;5(4):328.
97. Misfeld M, Leontyev S, Borger MA, et al. What is the best strategy for brain protection in patients undergoing aortic arch surgery? A single center experience of 636 patients. *Ann Thorac Surg.* 2012;93(5):1502–1508.
98. Leshnower BG, Rangaraju S, Allen JW, Stringer AY, Gleason TG, Chen EP. Deep hypothermia with retrograde cerebral perfusion versus moderate hypothermia with antegrade cerebral perfusion for arch surgery. *Ann Thorac Surg.* 2019;107(4):1104–1110.
99. Griepp RB, Di Luozzo G. Hypothermia for aortic surgery. *J Thorac Cardiovasc Surg.* 2013;145(3):S56–S58.
100. Weiss AJ, Pawale A, Griepp RB, Di Luozzo G. Deep versus mild hypothermia during thoracoabdominal aortic surgery. *Ann Cardiothorac Surg.* 2012;1(3):329.
101. Tanaka A, Safi HJ, Estrera AL. Current strategies of spinal cord protection during thoracoabdominal aortic surgery. *Gen Thorac Cardiovasc Surg.* 2018;66(6):307–314.
102. Luehr M, von Aspern K, Etz CD. Limitations of direct regional spinal cord monitoring using near-infrared spectroscopy: indirect paraspinal collateral network surveillance is the answer! *Ann Thorac Surg.* 2016;101(3):1238–1239.
103. Sandhu HK, Evans JD, Tanaka A, et al. Fluctuations in spinal cord perfusion pressure: a harbinger of delayed paraplegia after thoracoabdominal aortic repair. *Semin Thorac Cardiovasc Surg.* 2017; 29(4):451–459.
104. Kreibich M, Chen Z, Rylski B, et al. Outcome after aortic, axillary, or femoral cannulation for acute type A aortic dissection. *J Thorac Cardiovasc Surg.* 2019;158(1):27–34.
105. Serraino GF, Murphy GJ. Effects of cerebral near-infrared spectroscopy on the outcome of patients undergoing cardiac surgery: a systematic review of randomised trials. *BMJ Open.* 2017; 7(9):e016613.
106. Song S, Song S-W, Kim TH, Lee K-H, Yoo K-J. Effects of preemptive cerebrospinal fluid drainage on spinal cord protection during thoracic endovascular aortic repair. *J Thorac Dis.* 2017;9(8): 2404.
107. Murashita T, Pochettino A. Intraoperative electroencephalogram-guided deep hypothermia plus antegrade and/or retrograde cerebral perfusion during aortic arch surgery. *J Cardiac Surg.* 2016; 31(4):216–219.
108. Hickey T. One-lung ventilation. *Anesthesiology.* 2017:89–93.
109. Carlens E. A new flexible double-lumen catheter for bronchospirometry. *J Thorac Surg.* 1949;18:742–746.
110. Weigel WA, Hoaglan CD. The practical management of one-lung ventilation. *Adv Anesth.* 2013;31(1):61–85.
111. Cohen E. Management of one-lung ventilation. *Anesthesiol Clin North Am.* 2001;19(3):475–495.
112. Campos JH. Which device should be considered the best for lung isolation: double-lumen endotracheal tube versus bronchial blockers. *Curr Opin Anesthesiol.* 2007;20(1):27–31.
113. Goodwin MR, Blasius KR, Brand J, Silvay G. One-lung ventilation for surgical repair of thoracic aortic aneurysm. *Semin Cardiothorac Vasc Anesth.* 2013;17(2):146–151.
114. Slinger P. Perioperative lung injury. In: Slinger P, ed. *Principles and Practice of Anesthesia for Thoracic Surgery*: Springer, Toronto, ON; 2019:181–193.
115. Campos JH, Massa FC, Kernstine KH. The incidence of right upper-lobe collapse when comparing a right-sided double-lumen

tube versus a modified left double-lumen tube for left-sided thoracic surgery. *Anesth Analg.* 2000;90(3):535–540.

116. Yu W, Wang Z, Gao D, et al. A method for addressing right upper lobe obstruction with right-sided double-lumen endobronchial tubes during surgery: a randomized controlled trial. *BMC Anesthesiol.* 2018;18(1):130.
117. Ikeno S, Mitsuhata H, Saito K, et al. Airway management for patients with a tracheal bronchus. *Br J Anesth.* 1996;76(4):573–575.
118. Alliaume B, Coddens J, Deloof T. Reliability of auscultation in positioning of double-lumen endobronchial tubes. *Can J Anaesth.* 1992;39(7):687–690.
119. Fitzmaurice BG, Brodsky JB. Airway rupture from double-lumen tubes. *J Cardiothorac Vasc Anesth.* 1999;13(3):322–329.
120. Dunn PF. Physiology of the lateral decubitus position and one-lung ventilation. *Int Anesthesiol Clin.* 2000;38(1):25–53.
121. Lohser J, Ishikawa S. Physiology of the lateral decubitus position, open chest and one-lung ventilation. In: Slinger P, ed. *Principles and Practice of Anesthesia for Thoracic Surgery.*: Springer, Toronto, ON; 2011:71–82.
122. Carramiñana A, Ferrando C, Unzueta MC, Navarro R, Suárez-Sipmann F, Tusman G, et al. Rationale and study design for an individualized perioperative open lung ventilatory strategy in patients on one-lung ventilation (iPROVE-OLV). *J Cardiothorac Vasc Anesth.* 2019;33(9):2492–2502.
123. Grichnik KP, Clark JA. Pathophysiology and management of one-lung ventilation. *Thorac Surg Clin.* 2005;15(1):85–103.
124. Pereira SM, Tucci MR, Morais CC, et al. Individual positive end-expiratory pressure settings optimize intraoperative mechanical ventilation and reduce postoperative atelectasis. *Anesthesiology.* 2018;129(6):1070–1081.
125. Karzai W, Schwarzkopf K. Hypoxemia during one-lung Ventilation: Prediction, prevention, and treatment. *Anesthesiology.* 2009;110(6):1402–1411.
126. Lohser J, Ishikawa S. Clinical management of one-lung ventilation. In: Slinger P, ed. *Principles and Practice of Anesthesia for Thoracic Surgery.* Springer, Toronto, ON; 2011:83–101.
127. Neto AS, Schultz MJ. Optimizing the settings on the ventilator: high PEEP for all? *JAMA.* 2017;317(14):1413–1414.
128. Roze H, Lafargue M, Ouattara A. Case scenario: Management of intraoperative hypoxemia during one-lung ventilation. *Anesthesiology.* 2011;114(1):167–174.
129. Cherpanath TG, Simonis FD, Bouma BJ, et al. Myocardial function during low versus intermediate tidal volume ventilation in patients without acute respiratory distress syndrome. *Anesthesiology.* 2020;132(5):1102–1113.
130. Slinger PD. Do low tidal volumes decrease lung injury during one-lung ventilation? *J Cardiothorac Vasc Anesth.* 2017;31(5):1774–1775.
131. Lohser J, Slinger P. Lung injury after one-lung ventilation: a review of the pathophysiologic mechanisms affecting the ventilated and the collapsed lung. *Anesth Analg.* 2015;121(2):302–318.
132. Telias I, Ferguson ND. Added benefit of noninvasive ventilation to high-flow nasal oxygen to prevent reintubation in higher-risk patients. *JAMA.* 2019.
133. Slinger PD, Lesiuk L. Flow resistances of disposable double-lumen, single-lumen, and Univent tubes. *J Cardiothorac Vasc Anesth.* 1998;12(2):142–144.
134. Knoll H, Ziegeler S, Schreiber J-U, et al. Airway injuries after one-lung ventilation: a comparison between double-lumen tube and endobronchial blocker. *Anesthesiology.* 2006;105(3):471–477.
135. Sasano H, Sasano N, Hattori T, Tsubouchi H, Tsuda T, Katsuya H. Tracheal tube/laryngeal mask exchange to prevent coughing in lung volume reduction surgery. *Jap J Anesthesiol.* 2000;49(3):278–281.
136. Mort TC. Continuous airway access for the difficult extubation: the efficacy of the airway exchange catheter. *Anesth Analg.* 2007;105(5):1357–1362.
137. Popat M, Mitchell V, Dravid R, Patel A, Swampillai C, Higgs A. Difficult Airway Society Guidelines for the management of tracheal extubation. *Anaesthesia.* 2012;67(3):318–340.
138. Panaretou V, Toufektzian L, Siafaka I, et al. Postoperative pulmonary function after open abdominal aortic aneurysm repair in patients with chronic obstructive pulmonary disease: epidural versus intravenous analgesia. *Ann Vasc Surg.* 2012;26(2):149–155.
139. Svircevic V, Nierich AP, Moons KG, et al. Thoracic epidural anesthesia for cardiac surgery: a randomized trial. *Anesthesiology.* 2011;114(2):262–270.
140. Groenink M, den Hartog AW, Franken R, et al. Losartan reduces aortic dilatation rate in adults with Marfan syndrome: a randomized controlled trial. *Eur Heart J.* 2013;34(45):3491–3500.
141. Ladouceur M, Fermanian C, Lupoglazoff J-M, et al. Effect of beta-blockade on ascending aortic dilatation in children with the Marfan syndrome. *Am J Cardiol.* 2007;99(3):406–409.
142. Keane MG, Pyeritz RE. Medical management of Marfan syndrome. *Circulation.* 2008;117(21):2802–2813.
143. Cañadas V, Vilacosta I, Bruna I, Fuster V. Marfan syndrome. Part 1: pathophysiology and diagnosis. *Nat Rev Cardiol.* 2010;7(5):256.
144. Habashi JP, Judge DP, Holm TM, et al. Losartan, an AT1 antagonist, prevents aortic aneurysm in a mouse model of Marfan syndrome. *Science.* 2006;312(5770):117–121.
145. Chiu H-H, Wu M-H, Wang J-K, et al. Losartan added to β-blockade therapy for aortic root dilation in Marfan syndrome: a randomized, open-label pilot study. *Mayo Clin Proc.* 2013;88(3):271–276.
146. Lacro RV, Guey LT, Dietz HC, et al. Characteristics of children and young adults with Marfan syndrome and aortic root dilation in a randomized trial comparing atenolol and losartan therapy. *Am Heart J.* 2013;165(5):828–835.
147. Hiratzka LF, Bakris GL, Beckman JA, et al. Guidelines for the diagnosis and management of patients with thoracic aortic disease. *Anesth Analg.* 2010;111:279–315 2010.
148. Svensson LG, Adams DH, Bonow RO, et al. Aortic valve and ascending aorta guidelines for management and quality measures. *Ann Thorac Surg.* 2013;95(6):S1–S66.
149. Silvay G, Flynn BC. Innovative thinking in the care of cardiac surgical patients. *Anesthesiology.* 2009;110(2):435–436.
150. Criado FJ. Aortic dissection: a 250-year perspective. *Tex Heart I J.* 2011;38(6):694.
151. Benumof JL. Anesthesia for thoracic surgery. *Elsevier Health Sci.* 1994:1663–1755.
152. Grande B, Ganter MT. What is the best strategy for one-lung ventilation during thoracic surgery? *J Thorac Dis.* 2018;10(12):6404.
153. Chiesa R, Civilini E, Melissano G, et al. Management of thoracoabdominal aortic aneurysms. *HSR Proc Intensive Care Cardiovasc Anesth.* 2009;1(1):45–53.
154. Castillo JG, Silvay G, Fischer GW. Anesthetic management of thoraco-abdominal open procedures. In: Chiesa R, Melissano G, Zangrillo A, eds. *Thoraco-Abdominal Aorta.* Milan, Italy: Springer; 2011:253–270.

155. Tian DH, Wilson-Smith A, Koo SK, Forrest P, Kiat H, TD Yan. Unilateral versus bilateral antegrade cerebral perfusion: a meta-analysis of comparative studies. *Heart Lung Circulation.* 2019.
156. Kamenskaya OV, Klinkova AS, Chernyavsky AM, Lomivorotov VV, Meshkov IO, Karaskov AM. Deep hypothermic circulatory arrest vs. antegrade cerebral perfusion in cerebral protection during the surgical treatment of chronic dissection of the ascending and arch aorta. *J ExtraCorporeal Technol.* 2017;49(1):16.
157. Leontyev S, Davierwala PM, Semenov M, et al. Antegrade selective cerebral perfusion reduced in-hospital mortality and permanent focal neurological deficit in patients with elective aortic arch surgery. *Eur J Cardiovasc Thorac Surg.* 2019;56(5):1001–1008.
158. Englum BR, He X, Gulack BC, et al. Hypothermia and cerebral protection strategies in aortic arch surgery: a comparative effectiveness analysis from the STS Adult Cardiac Surgery Database. *Eur J Cardiovasc Thorac Surg.* 2017;52(3):492–498.
159. Poon SS, Estrera A, Oo A, Field M. Is moderate hypothermic circulatory arrest with selective antegrade cerebral perfusion superior to deep hypothermic circulatory arrest in elective aortic arch surgery? *Interact Cardiovasc Thorac Surg.* 2016;23(3):462–468.
160. Tian DH, Weller J, Hasmat S, et al. Temperature selection in antegrade cerebral perfusion for aortic arch surgery: a meta-analysis. *Ann Thorac Surg.* 2019;108(1):283–291.
161. Keeling WB, Tian DH, Leshnower BG, et al. Safety of moderate hypothermia with antegrade cerebral perfusion in total aortic arch replacement. *Ann Thorac Surg.* 2018;105(1):54–61.
162. Zierer A, El-Sayed Ahmad A, Papadopoulos N, et al. Fifteen years of surgery for acute type A aortic dissection in moderate-to-mild systemic hypothermia. *Eur J Cardiovasc Thorac Surg.* 2017;51(1):97–103.
163. Tian DH, Weller J, Hasmat S, et al. Adjunct retrograde cerebral perfusion provides superior outcomes compared with hypothermic circulatory arrest alone: a meta-analysis. *J Thorac Cardiovasc Surg.* 2018;156(4):1339–1348.
164. Preventza O, Price MD, Spiliotopoulos K, et al. In elective arch surgery with circulatory arrest, does the arterial cannulation site really matter? A propensity score analysis of right axillary and innominate artery cannulation. *J Thorac Cardiovasc Surg.* 2018;155(5):1953–1960.
165. Rylski B, Czerny M, Beyersdorf F, et al. Is right axillary artery cannulation safe in type A aortic dissection with involvement of the innominate artery? *J Thorac Cardiovasc Surg.* 2016;152(3):801–807.
166. Bavaria JE, Pochettino A, Brinster DR, et al. New paradigms and improved results for the surgical treatment of acute type A dissection. *Ann Surg.* 2001;234(3):336.
167. Augoustides JG, Geirsson A, Szeto WY, et al. Observational study of mortality risk stratification by ischemic presentation in patients with acute type A aortic dissection: the Penn classification. *Nat Clin Pract Cardiovasc Med.* 2009;6(2):140–146.
168. Pisano C, Balistreri CR, Torretta F, et al. Penn classification in acute aortic dissection patients. *Acta Cardiol.* 2016;71(2):235–240.
169. Yu P-J, Cassiere HA, Kohn N, et al. Utility of established risk models to predict surgical mortality in acute type-A aortic dissection. *J Cardiothorac Vasc Anesth.* 2016;30(1):39–43.
170. Mejàre-Berggren H, Olsson C. Validation and adjustment of the Leipzig-Halifax acute aortic dissection type A scorecard. *Ann Thorac Surg.* 2017;104(5):1577–1582.
171. Grubb K. *The patient guide to heart, lung, and esophageal surgery: Soc Thorac Surg*; 2019.
172. Loeys B, Matthys D, De Paepe A. Genetic fibrillinopathies: new insights in molecular diagnosis and clinical management. *Acta Clin Belg.* 2003;58(1):3–11.
173. Von Kodolitsch Y, De Backer J, Schüler H, et al. Perspectives on the revised Ghent criteria for the diagnosis of Marfan syndrome. *Appl Clin Genet.* 2015;8:137.
174. Silvay G, Lurie J, Casale M. The anaesthetic management of patients with thoracic ascending aortic aneurysms: A review. *J Perioper Pract.* 2020:1–8.

40

Wedge Resection, Lobectomy, Pneumonectomy

TRAVIS SCHISLER, PATRICK HECHT, JENS LOHSER

Introduction

The primary indications for resection of lung parenchyma include both malignant and benign conditions. Primary lung malignancy remains the leading cause of cancer-related deaths and lung resection surgery is the cornerstone of therapy for stage I and II (localized) primary lung nonsmall cell lung cancer malignancies, as well as for some patients presenting with stage III disease. The lung is the third most common location of metastasis from other tumor types and metastasectomy is indicated in selected cases, usually with lung sparing techniques.[1]

Benign pathology requiring lung resection may include pulmonary blebs and bullae, benign masses and nodules, bronchiectasis, infectious lung disease, including mycobacterial infection, lung reduction surgery for patients with chronic obstructive pulmonary disease (COPD) and traumatic lung injuries. Sublobar wedge resection and segmentectomy are typical options for benign disease.

The type of lung resection performed will depend on the size and location of the disease, the primary pathology and the ability to obtain a safe negative margin. Lung resection can be broadly classified into anatomic and nonanatomic approaches. Anatomic resection requires selective ligation of the feeding vessels and airway for a segment or lobe of the lung. Examples of anatomic resection include pneumonectomy, lobectomy, segmentectomy, and sleeve resection. Segmentectomy (or sublobar resection) is a lung sparing operation but does not appear to provide equivalent long-term survival outcomes when compared with lobectomy, especially for larger tumors.[2]

Nonanatomic wedge resections are accomplished without ligating individual airways and vessels. A wedge or slice of lung parenchyma containing the diseased tissue is stapled and removed using surgical linear cutting staplers.

In this chapter, the authors will provide a comprehensive overview of the perioperative care for patients undergoing lung resection surgery. We will combine relevant and recent evidence with the authors, institutional practice from a quaternary care academic center in Vancouver, Canada.

The Preoperative Evaluation of the Patient for Lung Resection Surgery (See Chapter 8)

Major respiratory and/or cardiac complications occur in up to 15% to 20% of thoracic surgery patients and are predictors of prolonged postoperative length of stay after lobectomy.[3] The broad goals of preoperative evaluation for the patient being considered for lung resection are to determine the patient's likelihood to tolerate the procedure, as well as to quantify the overall risk of morbidity and mortality.

The American College of Chest Physicians (ACCP) and the British Thoracic Society (BTS) have published guidelines for preoperative assessment.[4,5] These guidelines recommend a thorough evaluation consisting of measurements of pulmonary function, gas exchange, cardiopulmonary fitness, as well as specialized testing. Concomitant comorbidities must be evaluated in a comprehensive and multidisciplinary fashion and optimized before the surgery. All patients scheduled for major lung resection are seen in the anesthesia consult clinic for a detailed evaluation. In this setting, we review all previous pulmonary and extrapulmonary testing, and, if necessary, request additional tests or consultation with internal medicine or pneumonologist colleagues and provide education for their perioperative rehabilitation. Reviewing patients well ahead of the surgical date also provides an opportunity to discuss more challenging cases with the surgeon if the preoperative evaluation raises doubts about a patient's ability to tolerate the proposed resection, enabling additional testing or modifications to the surgical plan as required. It is at the time of the anesthetic consultation that we establish a plan for the postoperative disposition and advanced postoperative monitoring (Box 40.1).

The anesthetic preoperative evaluation includes the standard elements of preoperative evaluation including past medical history, anesthetic and surgical history, allergies, medications, social history, and review of symptoms. The goals of the history are to highlight comorbidities that require further optimization. A targeted physical examination should include an upper airway assessment to help predict ease of mask ventilation and intubation, as well as an

• BOX 40.1 Predictors of Postoperative Length of Stay After Lobectomy

Predictors of Postoperative Length of Stay After Lobectomy

- Pneumonia
- Atelectasis
- Acute respiratory distress syndrome
- Myocardial infarction
- Ileus
- Renal failure
- Pulmonary embolus
- Atrial arrhythmias
- Prolonged (>5 day) air leak

Modified from Wright CD, Gaisert HA, Grab JD, et al. Predictors of prolonged postoperative length of stay after lobectomy for lung cancer. *Ann Thorac Surg.* 2008;85:1857–1865, Table 4, page 1862, Requested.

assessment of the pulmonary and cardiac systems to evaluate for the risk of volume overload, bronchospasm, and or active pulmonary infection. Examination of the limbs for adequacy of intravenous access and the back for palpable landmarks for planning of neuraxial pain modalities are also performed.

We subscribe to the "three-legged stool" approach for the preoperative assessment of patients having pulmonary resections (Fig. 40.1). This assessment targets three areas of respiratory function: (1) respiratory mechanics, (2) pulmonary parenchymal function, and (3) cardiopulmonary reserve.[6] From a physiologic standpoint these three areas evaluate oxygen transport: (1) into the alveoli, (2) into the blood, (3) and to the tissues, respectively.

Pulmonary function testing, including the forced expiratory volume in 1 second (FEV_1) and diffusing capacity for carbon monoxide (DLCO), is routine for the vast majority of patients presenting for lung resection surgery. Minor wedge resections in otherwise healthy individuals arguably do not require formal pulmonary function testing. FEV_1 and DLCO are valiant predictors for both open and video-assisted thoracic surgery (VATS) resections.[7] The percent of predicted FEV_1 is a value that is corrected for age, sex, and height and is a strong predictor of postoperative complications and correlates with respiratory impairment in patients with COPD. The single greatest predictor of postlung resection pulmonary complications is the predicted postoperative FEV_1 ($ppoFEV_1\%$) (BTS 2001), which is calculated as follows:

$$ppoFEV_1\% = \text{preoperative } FEV_1\% \times (1 - \%\text{functional lung tissue removed} / 100)$$

There are 6, 4, and 12 subsegments in the right upper, middle and lower lobes, respectively, and 10 subsegments each in the left upper and left lower lobes (Fig. 40.2). The amount of functional lung tissue removed is calculated by the total number of subsegments associated with the lung resection and assumes that all segments contribute equally to gas exchange, which may not be the case if the segments being resected are not contributing to gas exchange. For example, a patient with a preoperative $FEV_1\%$ of 60 undergoing a left upper lobectomy will have 10 of 42 subsegments removed; his $ppoFEV_1\%$ is therefore 60 × (1 - 10/42) = 45.

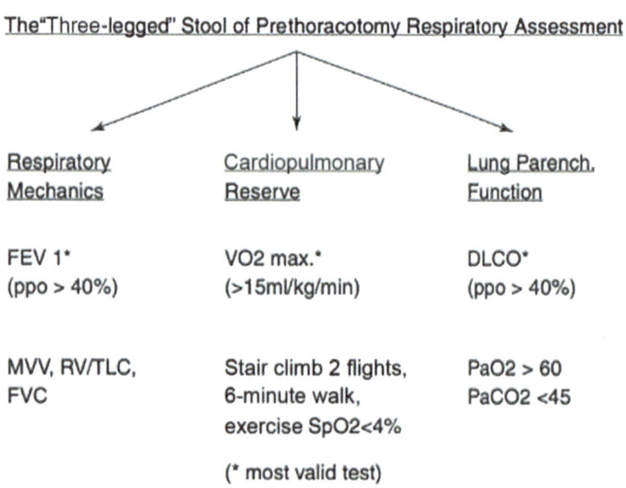

• Fig. 40.1 The three-legged stool of preoperative assessment as outlined by Peter Slinger in 2005. The three domains of respiratory assessment include respiratory mechanics, parenchymal function and cardiopulmonary reserve. *DLCO,* Diffusing capacity for carbon monoxide; *FEV 1,* forced expiratory volume in 1 second; *FVC,* forced vital capacity; *MVV,* maximal voluntary ventilation; *PaO2, PaCO2, PPO,* predictive postoperative; *RV, SpO2, TLC,* total lung capacity. (From Slinger PD and Johnston MJ. Preoperative assessment: an anesthesiologist's perspective. *Thor Surg Clin.* 2005;15(1):11–25.)

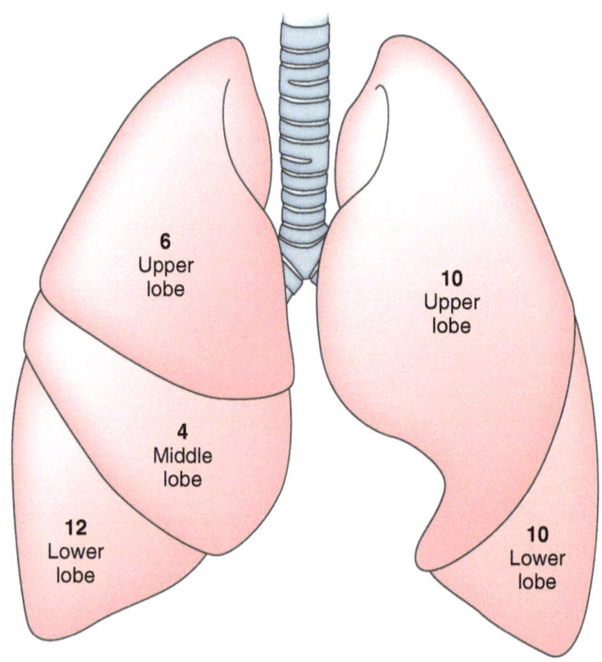

• Fig. 40.2 The number of lung subsegments present in each lobe. The number of lung subsegments removed during lung resection surgery can be used in the calculation of predicted postoperative lung function ($ppoFEV_1$ and ppoDLCO).

The same calculation can be used to determine the predicted postoperative DLCO (ppoDLCO%) to predict gas exchange abnormalities. Baseline arterial blood gas analysis is a more invasive ancillary test of gas exchange. Arterial PaO2 is not widely considered an important predictor of postoperative complications whereas baseline hypercapnia (arterial PaCO2 <45) often coexists with a low ppoFEV$_1$ or maximal oxygen consumption (VO$_2$ max) and may be a contraindication for lung resection in this population.[4]

Patients with ppoDLCO% or ppoFEV$_1$% greater than 40% have a low risk of postresection respiratory complications whereas those with values less than 30% are at high risk for postoperative morbidity.[8] Guidelines from the European Respiratory Society and the European Society of Thoracic Surgery (ERS/ESTS) use a cutoff value for ppoFEV$_1$ and ppoDLCO of 30% (rather than 40%) based on what these societies considered widespread improvements in surgical technique.[9] If either ppoFEV$_1$ or ppoDLCO are less than 30%, an exercise test is warranted to consider the decision of the suitability for resection. The lowest acceptable value of ppoFEV$_1$% to tolerate lung resection as reported by a high volume lung resection surgery center was 20%.[10] The ppoFEV$_1$% value has some limitations, including the fact that actual ppoFEV$_1$% can exceed the calculated value at 6 months following surgery because the resected segments may be diseased and/or emphysematous and therefore contribute little to preoperative lung function.

Patients at elevated risk (ppoFEV$_1$% <40) should undergo complete pulmonary function testing, ventilation/perfusion scans and a functional assessment, such as cardiopulmonary exercise testing, stair climbing or 6-minute walk test (6MWT).[11] Formal cardiopulmonary exercise testing to determine the VO$_2$ max is the most useful predictor of postresection outcome. The ACCP and the ERS/ETST both consider a VO$_2$ max less than 10 mL/kg/min to be high risk for postoperative morbidity and mortality whereas patients with a VO$_2$ max greater than 20 mL/kg/min have a low risk of postoperative respiratory complications even for pneumonectomy. VO$_2$ max values between 10 and 15 mL/kg/min indicate an increased mortality risk and suitability for surgery should therefore take into account the entirety of preoperative testing (ppoFEV$_1$, ppoDLCO) and additional patient comorbidities. Licker et al. in a retrospective observational study included 210 patients with FEV$_1$ less than 80% who were submitted to lung resection.[11a] The VO$_2$ max was a predictor of cardiopulmonary complication and death at the multivariate analysis, including preoperative clinical, surgical, and ergometric variables. Patients with a VO$_2$ max <10 mL/kg/min had a risk of total morbidity, cardiovascular morbidity, and cardiac morbidity of 65%, 39%, and 35%, respectively, in case of major resection (Fig. 40.3).

Alternatives to formal cardiorespiratory exercise testing include the 6MWT and stair climbing. The VO$_2$ max may be estimated from a 6MWT value by taking the total distance walked on flat ground in 6 minutes and dividing by 30. For example, walking 900 m total divided by 30 corresponds to a VO$_2$ max of 30 mL/kg/min. Stair climbing at

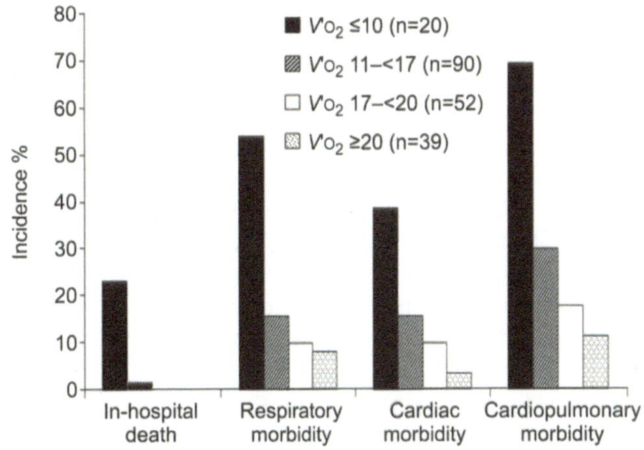

• **Fig. 40.3** Morbidity and mortality following lung resection surgery as stratified by preoperative maximal oxygen consumption ($\dot{V}O_2$ max). A VO$_2$ max less than 10 mL/kg/min significantly increases the risk for respiratory and cardiac morbidity and mortality. (From M. Licker, et al. Impact of aerobic exercise capacity and procedure-related factors in lung cancer surgery. *Eur Respir J*. 2011;37:1189–1198.)

the patient's own pace corresponds to VO$_2$ max, such that a person able to climb five flights or more has a VO$_2$ max over 20 mL/kg/min, and two flights of stairs are equivalent to 12 mL/kg/min.[12]

Regional lung function testing, such as ventilation perfusion lung scanning, is indicated in the patient undergoing major lung resection with a ppoFEV$_1$% less than 40 or when there is reason to confirm that the lung to be removed is diseased and not contributing fully to preoperative lung function. In this situation, a ppoFEV$_1$ is more accurately calculated by using the preoperative FEV$_1$% and the perfusion value of the remaining (nonresected) lung. For example, for a patient presenting for a left pneumonectomy with preoperative FEV$_1$% 74 and perfusion of the left lung 35% and right lung 65% the ppoFEV$_1$% is 74 × 0.65 = 48, which corresponds to an acceptable value (Box 40.2).

The combination of preoperative respiratory assessment tools is better than any single test and provides valuable information for the thoracic anesthesiologist to help predict postoperative outcome and to plan intra- and postoperative management. For patients with ppoFEV$_1$% greater than 40, a standard weans and extubation in the operating room would generally be considered safe. For patients with values between 30 and 40, information from functional and other ancillary tests should be factored into determining

• BOX 40.2 Predictive Postoperative Forced Expiratory Volume in 1 Second by the Perfusion Method

PPO FEV$_1$ = Preop FEV$_1$ * (1 - Fraction of total perfusion in the resected lung)

PPO FEV$_1$, Predictive postoperative forced expiratory volume in 1 second.

suitability for lung resection surgery and may require a staged wean from mechanical ventilation in the postanesthesia care unit or in the intensive care unit. As with all patients, optimal analgesia with an epidural or paravertebral catheter along with normothermia, normal metabolic parameters, and minimization of long acting sedatives will assist with extubation and early postoperative lung function. For patients with ppoFEV_1% 20 to 30, more conservative management may be warranted, including delayed extubation and planned transfer to an intensive care unit.[13]

ACCP Physiologic evaluation resection algorithm is depicted in Fig. 40.4.

Next to respiratory complications, cardiac complications are the most common source of postoperative complications in lung resection patients. The most common cardiac complications following lung resection surgery are myocardial ischemia and arrhythmias. A thorough cardiac evaluation is guided by the American College of Cardiology/American Heart Association, the European Society of Cardiology/European Society of Anaesthesiology and the Canadian Cardiovascular Society guidelines on preoperative assessment for noncardiac surgery.[14–16] These guidelines recommend a baseline electrocardiogram (ECG), assessment of functional status, determination of preoperative cardiac risk using the revised cardiac risk index (RCRI), preoperative brain natriuretic peptide (BNP) testing and selective additional cardiac risk stratification, including stress testing and echocardiography. In patients with elevated baseline risk and/or positive BNP, postoperative myocardial injury surveillance should be conducted with serial ECG and troponins on postoperative day 1 through 3. Patients should continue their cardiac medications, including beta blockers and antiarrhythmics up to the day of surgery.

In the Lee cardiac risk classification evaluated among 4513 patients, the incidence of a major cardiac complication increases with a higher cardiac risk index (1–4), which is based upon six independent predictors, including high-risk type of surgery, history of ischemic heart disease, history of heart failure, history of cerebrovascular disease, preoperative treatment with insulin, and preoperative serum creatinine over 2.0 mg/dL (177 mol/L).[17] Thoracic procedures are considered high-risk surgery, similar to major intraabdominal procedures and abdominal aortic aneurysm resections, and therefore classified at least as risk class 2.

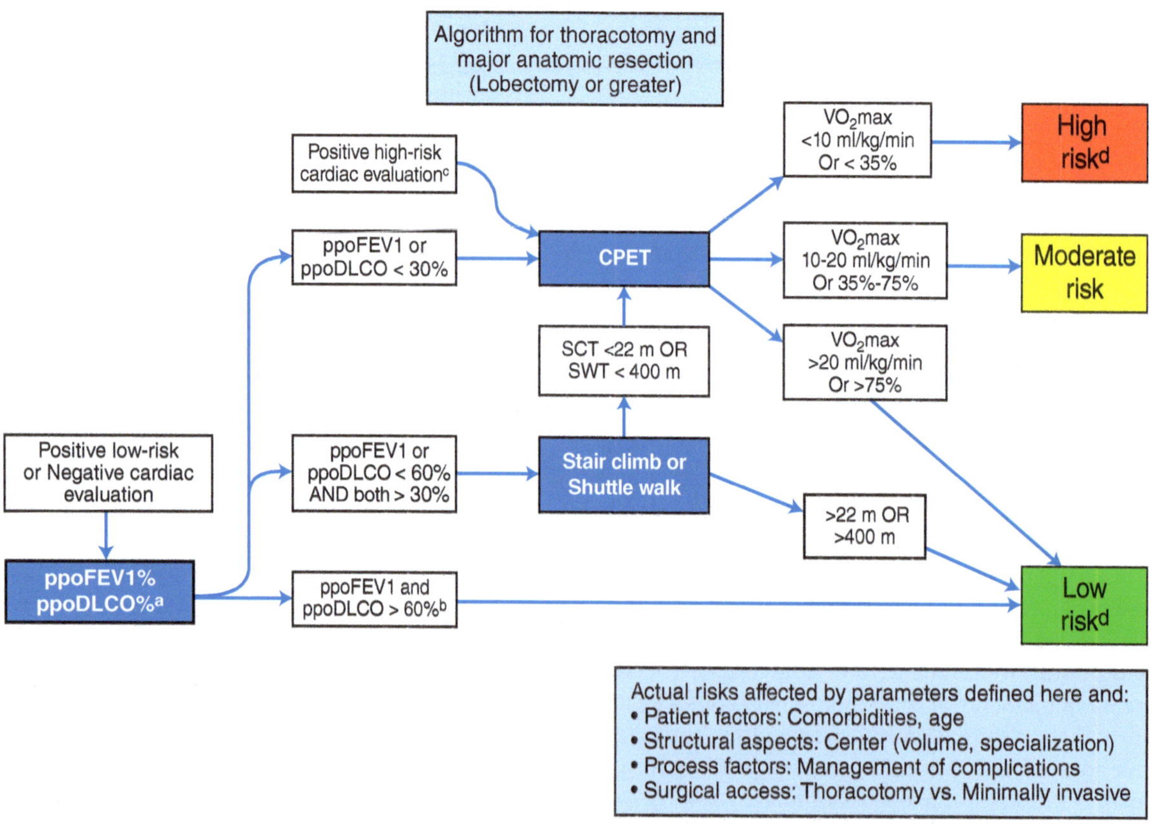

• **Fig. 40.4 The American College of Chest Physicians (ACCP) algorithm for preoperative assessment of the patient undergoing lung resection surgery.** (ppo) preoperative. Baseline spirometry values (forced expiratory volume in 1 second [FEV_1] and diffusing capacity for carbon monoxide [*DLCO*]) guide the prescription of additional functional testing to determine maximal oxygen consumption (VO_2 max) and profile the patient's perioperative risk. *CPET*, cardiopulmonary exercise testing; *ppo*, predicted postoperative; *SCT*, stair climb test; *SWT*, shuttle walk test. (From Brunelli A, Kim AW, Berger KI, Addrizzo-Harris DJ. Physiologic evaluation of the patient with lung cancer being considered for resectional surgery: diagnosis and management of lung cancer, 3rd ed: American College of Chest Physicians evidence-based clinical practice guidelines. *Chest*. 2013;143:e166S. With permission.)

Higher cardiac risk indices are indicative of a statistically significant increase in cardiac complications amongst thoracic surgery patients. COPD is a common comorbidity in patients undergoing lung resection surgery and care should be taken to thoroughly evaluate for the presence of bronchospasm, atelectasis, infection, and pulmonary edema. These comorbidities should be adequately optimized before lung resection surgery. Preoperative treatment may be required, including bronchodilators, steroids, antibiotics, and diuretics. Smoking cessation counseling is an important component of the preoperative consultation, as quitting smoking before surgery decreases wound infection postoperative pulmonary complications (PPCs) and improves pulmonary recovery.[18] Pulmonary rehabilitation before lung resection surgery, including moderate to intense exercise which improves aerobic capacity, physical fitness, and quality of life, and may reduce postoperative complications and hospital length of stay.

Pouwels et al. evaluated 11 studies with a methodologic quality ranging from poor to good. The most important finding of this systematic review was that PET based on moderate to intense exercise in patients scheduled for lung surgery has beneficial effects on aerobic capacity, physical fitness, and quality of life.[19] The patient with pulmonary malignancy may present with additional factors that may complicate care and these should be sought out and evaluated. For example, squamous cell cancers (SCC) can grow to a large size, which may produce a compression effect on adjacent airways and pulmonary vessels leading to airways obstruction, postobstructive pneumonia, superior vena cava syndrome or cavitation and hemoptysis. Hypercalcemia is sometimes seen in patients with SCC. Small cell lung cancers are associated with several paraneoplastic conditions, including hyponatremia from the syndrome of inappropriate antidiuretic hormone secretion, a Cushing syndrome from excess cortisol secretion and rarely Lambert-Eaton myasthenic syndrome. Carcinoid tumors that are found in the central airways can cause airway obstruction or hemoptysis, as well as a carcinoid syndrome from the secretion of vasoactive mediators, although rarely seen in lung cardioid, can precipitate hemodynamic collapse, coronary vasospasm, or bronchospasm.[20]

All patients with malignancy should be assessed with the 4 Ms in mind: **mass effect** of the tumor especially on airways and great vessels; the side effects of chemotherapeutic **medications**, including respiratory toxicity from bleomycin or cardiac or renal toxicity from other agents; **metabolic effects** related to paraneoplastic disorders; and other organ dysfunction related to **metastatic disease**. Finally, placement of neuraxial or regional nerve block catheters requires exclusion of pre-existing coagulopathy and discontinuation of anticoagulant medication in accordance with the American Society of Regional Anesthesia recommendations. Anticoagulant medications should therefore be reviewed and held for an appropriate preoperative interval.[21]

An important part of the preoperative evaluation is the review of the preoperative imaging, particularly the computed chest tomography (CT) scan. The preoperative CT provides valuable information that can be used to carefully plan airway management and anticipate difficulties with endobronchial tube placement, oxygenation, or ventilation during one-lung ventilation (OLV). Anesthesiologists should learn to evaluate the images themselves, as the radiologist's report may not comment on specific factors relevant to lung isolation. For example, if a left-sided resection or pneumonectomy is planned or the patient presents with a left mainstem bronchus tumor, a left-sided double lumen tube would be contraindicated. The evaluation of central airway anatomy is also important in patients presenting for a subsequent lung resection. For left-sided double lumen tube placement, the left mainstem bronchus diameter can be measured on the CT scan and be used to guide the selection of double-tumen tube size.[22] Radiologic lung pathology can be identified on chest CT and can indicate the presence of bullous lung disease or blebs, fibrotic changes, or interstitial patterns, including pulmonary edema, atelectasis, consolidation, or pleural disease including effusions. The size and precise location of any lung mass, particularly when centrally located, may yield helpful clues as to the surgical difficulty with resection and the likelihood of conversion from thoracoscopic to open approaches. Mass effect on great vessels, including the superior vena cava, brachiocephalic veins, or pulmonary arteries, can alter the plan for venous access, such as placement of additional access in the lower extremities. Extrapulmonary pathologies, including coronary artery calcification, severe cardiac chamber enlargement, pulmonary artery enlargement, or pericardial effusion, can be seen. Finally, review of the imaging will facilitate neuraxial catheter placement, both the depth of laminae for paramedian epidural placement and the absence of spinal deformities (Table 40.1).

Monitoring (See Chapters 11,12)

Basic monitoring for all patients undergoing lung resection surgery will consist of pulse oximetry, noninvasive blood pressure (NIBP) cuff and five-lead electrocardiogram and continuous end-tidal carbon dioxide ($CO2$), as well as ventilator pressure and flows after initiation of positive pressure ventilation in accordance with national society guidelines.[23–25]

Direct or invasive arterial catheter monitoring is appropriate in most patients and in particular in patients with comorbidities that require close monitoring of hemodynamics and for all patients undergoing the dissection of mediastinal vessels in more extensive procedures, such as lobectomy or pneumonectomy. Direct arterial monitoring allows for a reliable and continuous assessment of blood pressure, and intravascular volume status during lung resection surgery. Whether waveform analysis can provide information on cardiac contractility is controversial.[26,27] Arterial cannulation before the induction of anesthesia allows for baseline blood gas sampling, particularly important in patients with COPD, if not already performed, as well as periodic sampling during and after the lung resection as warranted.

Having baseline arterial blood gases (ABGs) are important to define what values are acceptable when the decision for extubation is planned. Central venous catheters are appropriate in patients for whom intra- and/or postoperative vasopressors are necessary, for more secure intravenous access or as an option for larger volume fluid administration.

Pulmonary artery catheters (PAC) and transesophageal echocardiography (TEE) are more invasive monitoring modalities that may be beneficial in certain situations. For example, a PAC in the patient with moderate to severe pulmonary hypertension and right ventricular dysfunction will better allow the anesthesiologist to titrate pulmonary vasodilator and inotropic therapies according to pulmonary artery pressure, cardiac output, and mixed venous oxygen saturation.[28] TEE is gaining more traction as a perioperative hemodynamic monitor because it is a granular technique for guiding resuscitation. It would allow continuous monitoring of both right and left ventricular systolic and diastolic function, regional wall motion, valvular heart function, intracardiac shunts, fluid responsiveness and fluid tolerance, systemic vascular resistance, mass effect during surgery, monitoring for the extent and the changes in the pericardial or pleural fluid collections, as well as diagnosing causes of hypoxemia.[29–31]

At our center we customize monitoring based on the clinical situation. In addition to the standard intraoperative monitors, all patients receive a temperature monitoring device and neuromuscular monitor. We place urinary catheters in patients undergoing major lung resections or if they receive a thoracic epidural. We place arterial catheters, usually in the dependent radial artery, for all patients undergoing lobectomy and pneumonectomy procedures and for patients with significant cardiac disease for less extensive lung resections. Central venous catheters (CVCs) are reserved for the pneumonectomy patient, the patient with a concomitant mediastinal mass, and if continuous vasopressor or inotropic therapy is thought to be necessary. The CVC is best placed on the operative (nondependent) side to avoid kinking and obstruction from the patient's head and neck. It also eliminates the potential pneumothorax in the case of dependent lung inadvertent needle puncture, although this complication is largely avoided by the use of direct continuous needle tip viewing with ultrasound. For the most part, PAC and TEE are seldom used outside of lung transplantation; however, we will consider these modalities during aggressive and extensive resections or in the patient with severe cardiac disease.

The advancements in ventilator technology have resulted in more granular monitoring of respiratory mechanics. Capnometry is mandatory and can identify inspiratory and expiratory flow patterns, airways obstruction associated with lung isolation devices, a sudden drop in cardiac output, and for the monitoring the degree of permissive hypercapnia, which is common during OLV. Spirometry allows for the continuous monitoring of flows, pressures, and volumes, which can provide valuable information on the malpositioning of airway devices, the development of autopositive end-expiratory pressure (PEEP), the severity of pulmonary air leaks following lung resection and perhaps most importantly to prevent the incidence of ventilator-associated lung injury. Respiratory compliance and driving pressure (plateau pressure—PEEP) measurements allow for the individualization of ventilatory strategy as recommended in recent guidelines. Evidence suggests that reduction of PPCs frequently associated with substantial morbidity and mortality can be reduced by using lung-protective ventilation strategies intraoperatively. Young et al. selected seven experts and produced 24 questions concerning preoperative assessment and intraoperative mechanical ventilation for patients at risk of developing PPCs. An expert consensus was reached for 22 recommendations and four statements among them: (1) a dedicated score should be used for preoperative pulmonary risk evaluation; and (2) an individualized mechanical ventilation may improve the mechanics of breathing and respiratory function, and prevent PPCs. The ventilator should initially be set to a tidal volume of 6 to 8 mL/kg predicted body weight and PEEP 5 cm H_2O. PEEP should be individualized thereafter. When recruitment maneuvers are performed, the lowest effective pressure and shortest effective time or fewest number of breaths should be used.[32] We advise individualizing both PEEP and tidal volume during OLV as guided by driving pressure and pulmonary compliance.

Methods of Lung Separation (See Chapter 16)

In brief, lung isolation is required during lung resection surgery to facilitate surgical exposure and produce a quiet surgical field. The choice of lung separation device should take into account several perioperative factors, including the nature and location of the lung resection, the upper and lower airway anatomy, the presence or risk for pulmonary infection, bleeding, or pulmonary air leak. Whether the patient is already intubated or will require postoperative ventilation, and the provider's experience and preference. Successful lung separation device placement requires a thorough understanding of tracheobronchial anatomy and expertise with fiberoptic bronchoscopy.[33] An excellent resource for anesthesiologists to improve their knowledge of airway anatomy and bronchoscopy is available online at www.thoracic-anesthesia.com.

Double-lumen tubes (DLTs) and bronchial blockers (BBs) placed through a single-lumen ETT are the two most common methods used for lung separation during lung resection surgery and each have their advantages and disadvantages (Table 40.2). Left-sided DLTs are the most commonly used device at our center for lung resection surgery because of the ease of access to either lung for bronchoscopy, suction, continuous positive airway pressure (CPAP), or ventilation. BBs can be used for anatomical or nonanatomic resections, in patients presenting to the operating room with an ETT or tracheostomy in-situ or patients with irregular tracheobronchial or difficult upper airway anatomy where DLT placement is difficult or impossible.

TABLE 40.1 **Left-Sided Double-Lumen Tube Sizing by Computed Tomography-Guided Left Bronchus Diameter**

Left Double-Lumen Tube (DLT) Size	35 Fr	37 Fr	39 Fr	41 Fr
Diameter of bronchial tube	9.5 mm	9.9 mm	10.9 mm	11.4 mm
Diameter of left bronchus on computed tomography	< 9–11 mm	11–12 mm	12–13 mm	>13 mm
Appropriate DLT size	35 Fr	37 Fr	39 Fr	41 Fr

From Hannallah M, Benumof J, Silverman P, Kelly L, Lea D. Evaluation of an approach to choosing a left double-lumen tube size based on chest computed tomographic scan measurement of left mainstem bronchial diameter. *J Cardiothorac Vasc Anesth*. 1997;11(2):168–171, Table 40.1, page 170.

Right-sided DLTs are less commonly selected because of the smaller margin of error for placement because of the shorter right mainstem bronchus and a potential tube migration resulting in inadequate ventilation or loss of isolation. In a small minority of patients, the right upper lobe bronchus may originate from the carina or within the trachea.[34] Right-sided DLTs should be placed during left pneumonectomy, distorted left mainstem bronchus anatomy (internal or external intraluminal left bronchus compression, such as in thoracic aortic aneurysm) or when the site of the surgery involves the left mainstem bronchus (sleeve resection, pneumonectomy, tracheobronchial disruption). Single-lumen tube for lung isolation may be used when immediate lung isolation is required and access to specialized lung isolation equipment is not available. Some institutions used right-sided double lumen tubes for all left-side procedures or vice versa. It is standard practice to confirm the position of the lung isolation device with a 4.0-mm fiberoptic bronchoscope; these are widely available today, also in disposable form.

Airway trauma from the placement of lung separation devices is fortunately rare but can be associated with significant morbidity and mortality.[35] Airway trauma can be reduced through a thorough assessment of tracheobronchial anatomy, by choosing an appropriately sized DLT (Table 40.3), and by using care during placement and cuff inflation. We recommend routinely reviewing the preoperative CT scan specifically for pathology and anatomic distortion of the lower airways, using bronchoscopy routinely to assist

TABLE 40.2 **Factors That Favor Choice of Lung Separation Device**

Factor	Favors Double-Lumen Tube (DLT)	Favors Bronchial Blocker
Ease of insertion	X	
Lower incidence of airway injury, sore throat		X
Need for intraoperative repositioning		X
Quality of lung deflation/reinflation	X	X
Accessibility of the nonventilated lung	X	
Ability to achieve selective lobar isolation		X
Elective lung resection	X	
Left pneumonectomy or bronchial surgery	Right-sided DLT	
Abnormal tracheobronchial anatomy		X
Need for unilateral lung protection (hemoptysis, infection, lung lavage)	X	
Endotracheal tube present		X
Tracheostomy present		X
Need for postoperative ventilation		X
Awake intubation needed		X

From Slinger P. The new bronchial blockers are not preferable to double-lumen tubes for lung isolation. *J Cardiothorac Vasc Anesth*. 2008;22(6):925–929, Table 1, page 926, Requested.

TABLE 40.3 Double-Lumen Tube Sizing by Sex and Height

Sex	Height (cm)	Double-Lumen Tube Size (Fr)
Male	>170	41
	160–170	39
	<160	37 or 39
Female	>160	37
	150–160	35
	<150	35

in placement especially when resistance is encountered and carefully inflating the cuff under direct visualization. Removing the stiff stylet after the distal tip of the DLT passes through cords and avoiding nitrous oxide are additional recommendations.

Fluid Management (See Chapter 21)

The ideal strategy for fluid administration during lung resection surgery is to balance the replacement of fluid losses to maintain cardiac output and oxygen delivery to the tissues with the avoidance of tissue hypoperfusion and potential acute kidney injury (AKI). Excessive fluid delivery is associated with expansion of the extravascular compartment and precipitates tissue edema, increases the risk of acute lung injury (ALI) and delays recovery.[36] A sensible approach to fluid management during lung resection surgery is to balance these two extremes, avoid overly restrictive or liberal fluid regimes, and maintain euvolemia.[37] This is an approach endorsed by the enhanced recovery after surgery (ERAS) and ESTS ERAS guidelines for thoracic surgery.[38]

To achieve euvolemia throughout the perioperative setting the patient should present to the operating room in a euvolemic state. This is facilitated by the consumption of an oral carbohydrate drink up to 2 hours before surgery.[39] If blood loss is minimal, we limit total intraoperative intravenous fluid to less than 6 mL/kg/h (500–1500 mL) to reduce PPC.[40] Fortunately, patients receiving less than 2 to 3 mL/kg/h of fluid intraoperatively do not experience a greater incidence of AKI, and fluid boluses to treat oliguria do not seem to affect postoperative renal function.[38] Intravenous fluids should be replaced by enteral fluids as soon as possible in the postoperative period. Balanced crystalloids are preferred to 0.9% saline solution.[41]

In the setting of hypotension related to anesthetic agents and neuraxial blockade and assuming euvolemia has been achieved, vasopressors may be used to enhance tissue perfusion although additional fluid boluses may be necessary if hypoperfusion ensues. Using cardiac output monitors including pulse contour analysis to guide fluid administration during OLV and an open chest at the present time is lacking in evidence.[42,43]

Patients scheduled for elective lobectomy at our center consume clear, carbohydrate rich fluids until their arrival to hospital and typically receive less than 1–1.5 liter of fluid in the operating room. In the setting of intraoperative hypotension or hypoperfusion, which may occur when epidural local anesthetic agents are administered, we administer boluses and/or low dose infusions of vasopressors, such as phenylephrine or norepinephrine. A maintenance intravenous fluid infusion is provided postoperatively until the patient resumes enteral nutrition. In the case of intraoperative hemorrhage or prolonged surgery, intravascular volume is replaced with a combination of balanced crystalloids, albumin and rarely packed red blood cells. Fluid administration is guided by routine monitors and clinical intuition rather than noninvasive cardiac output monitors, such as pulse contour analysis.

Intravenous Versus Inhaled Anesthesia

The ideal anesthetic for lung resection surgery is characterized by the following:

1. **Balanced anesthesia** that limits preoperative sedatives and encourages the use of multimodal and opioid-sparing analgesia.[38]
2. A **quiet surgical field** especially during the dissection and ligation of the pulmonary artery and vein, which is a delicate procedure greatly affected by sudden and unexpected breathing or coughing. Injury to these vessels can result in severe morbidity and even mortality.
3. A **rapid emergence** from anesthesia in which the patient is awake and comfortable and demonstrates favorable respiratory mechanics, oxygenation and ventilation.

The induction of anesthesia is often achieved with a combination of opioid, propofol, neuromuscular blocker, and sometimes ketamine or dexmedetomidine. Sevoflurane is the predominant agent used for the maintenance of anesthesia and is often combined with an opioid, such as fentanyl, hydromorphone, or a remifentanil infusion. Good regional anesthesia, including thoracic epidural, paravertebral, erector spinae, serratus anterior plane, or intercostal blockade, is used to spare sedatives and opioid administration and should be part of a multimodal approach to pain relief. Sevoflurane has been shown to reduce 1-year mortality, the incidence of PPCs, and lung and systemic inflammatory markers compared with propofol-based total intravenous anesthesia (TIVA) techniques. Sevoflurane is also associated with bronchodilation, more rapid elimination, and less systemic inflammation.[44,45] Beck-Schimmeret et al.[46] compared desflurane with propofol in 240 patients undergoing OLV and found no difference in complications during hospital stay and within a 6-month postoperative period. However, a recent Cochrane review by Módolo et al. concluded that the use of TIVA is a safe and acceptable alternative to volatile-based anesthesia during OLV. They included randomized controlled trials and quasi-randomized controlled trials of intravenous (e.g., propofol) versus inhalation (e.g., isoflurane, sevoflurane, desflurane) anesthesia for OLV in both surgical and intensive care participants. They included a review of 20 studies that enrolled 850 participants, all of which assessed surgical participants. No evidence indicated that the drug used to maintain anesthesia during OLV affected participant outcomes. Very little evidence suggests differences in participant outcomes with anesthesia maintained by intravenous versus inhalational anesthesia during OLV.[47]

Anesthetic adjuvants shown to decrease opioid requirements should be considered for lung resection surgery; these include acetaminophen, nonsteroidal antiinflammatory drugs, N-methyl-D-aspartate antagonists and gabapentin. Neuromuscular blocking drugs are used to optimize surgical conditions in lung resection surgery; however, because the interval between maximal surgical relaxation and emergence is short, one must ensure adequate reversal before extubation. Sugammadex has emerged as a neuromuscular blocking reversal agent that has been shown to reduce the incidence of PPCs in patients undergoing thoracoscopic lobectomy. Cho et al. obtained a medical record review of 50 patients who underwent VATS divided into two groups. The sugammadex group (group S, n = 19) was administered sugammadex 2 mg/kg, while the pyridostigmine group (group P, n = 31) received pyridostigmine 20 mg with glycopyrrolate 0.2 mg or atropine 0.5 mg. The primary endpoint measure was the overall incidence of PPCs including prolonged air leak, pneumonia, and atelectasis. The secondary endpoint measures were the length of postoperative hospital stay and duration of chest tube insertion. They concluded that the use of sugammadex, compared with pyridostigmine, showed a significantly reduced overall incidence of PPCs and decreased duration of chest tube use and postoperative hospital stay in patients undergoing VATS lobectomy, suggesting that sugammadex might be helpful in improving clinical outcomes in such patients.[48]

Methods of Ventilation (See Chapter 20)

The goals of ventilation during lung resection surgery are to facilitate a collapsed and immobile lung for optimal surgical exposure and to optimize respiratory mechanics and gas exchange of the nonsurgical lung, while at the same time minimizing the risk for ventilator-induced lung injury (VILI). Achieving complete collapse of the surgical lung in a timely fashion is possible by using the following techniques:

1. Ventilating with 100% oxygen for several minutes before initiating OLV. Replacing nitrogen with more soluble oxygen facilitates absorption atelectasis.[49]
2. Prolonged apnea (30 seconds) until the end-tidal carbon dioxide level falls to zero before initiating OLV. This ensures that the surgical lung is allowed to return to functional residual capacity and no tidal volume is trapped in the lung before commencing OLV.
3. Apnea at the time of pleural incision with the BB cuff completely deflated allowing for egress of air as the operative lung collapses.[50]
4. If a BB is used, the suction port of the BB can be capped throughout the procedure or alternatively a low level suction can be applied through the BB lumen. This technique prevents the entrainment of atmospheric gas as resorption atelectasis ensues.[51] If using a DLT, continuous suction with a suction catheter prevents passive entrainment of air. Care should be given not to advance the suction catheter beyond the tip of the DLT lumen to avoid stapling of the suction catheter.

Using the aforementioned maneuvers to optimize surgical lung collapse can have detrimental effects on the nonsurgical lung during OLV. Complete denitrogenation and prolonged apnea produces atelectasis in the nonsurgical lung, which must be reversed postprocedure to optimize gas exchange and prevent VILI. The triad of protective ventilation, using low tidal volumes, adequate PEEP to prevent the trauma associated with cyclical derecruitment of lung units (atelectrauma) and routine lung recruitment maneuvers (RM), can minimize harmful lung stress and strain.[52,53] ALI occurs in 2% of all lung resections and up to 8% after pneumonectomy with morbidity and mortality up to 40%.[54]

A lung protective ventilation strategy has been shown to lower inflammatory markers, decrease the incidence of postoperative lung dysfunction and ALI and enhance recovery.[55–57] The principles of protective ventilation during lung resection surgery and OLV are:

1. **Tidal volumes** during OLV should be reduced to 5 to 6 mL/kg ideal body weight because they are thought to be less injurious (Lohser & Slinger, 2015). Preoperative forced vital capacity (FVC) can be used to estimate safe tidal volume during OLV per the following equation: tidal volume = FVC/8.[58] Biomarkers of lung injury are reduced with lower tidal volumes although outcome data is lacking.[59] Rates of hypoxemia during OLV are low when low tidal volumes are combined with appropriate PEEP.[60]
2. An **alveolar recruitment maneuver** should be performed routinely after the initiation of OLV.[38] Blood pressure may transiently decrease with a single breath hold maneuver, and a gradual recruitment maneuver may be preferred although the decrease in blood pressure has no long-term negative consequences.[61]
3. A **PEEP** level of 5 to 10 cm H_2O is often required, but individualization of PEEP level during OLV is preferred.[62] The optimal level of PEEP during OLV is estimated when static or dynamic compliance is maximized and driving pressure (DP) is minimized.[32] Fig. 40.5 outlines an example of a PEEP decrement trial to find the optimal level of PEEP. DP is defined as the difference between plateau pressure and PEEP (Plat-PEEP). The DP depends on the tidal volume as well as on the relative balance between the amount of aerated lung at end-expiration and end-inspiration at different levels of PEEP. In randomized controlled trials of mechanical ventilation in acute respiratory distress syndrome (ARDS) patients, DP is the variable that was most strongly associated with mortality. The optimization of DP has been considered

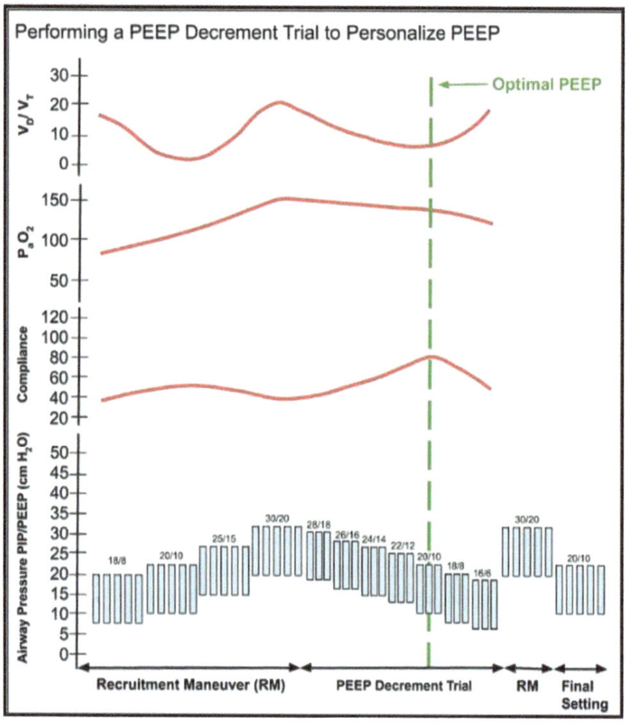

• Fig. 40.5 Performing a positive end-expiratory pressure (*PEEP*) decrement trial to individualize PEEP. A PEEP decrement trial as demonstrated in this figure results in favorable changes to lung compliance, arterial oxygenation, and physiologic dead space. This figure outlines one example of a PEEP decrement trial where inspiratory pressures are held constant and PEEP is gradually increased to produce relative lung over distension thereby optimizing the recruitment of atelectatic lung zones. This is immediately followed by a stepwise reduction in PEEP levels until the maximal lung compliance is observed.

as a tool to optimize mechanical ventilation during surgery and to improve outcome.

4. Assessing the safety of ventilation is possible with real-time compliance and **DP monitoring**.[32] DP should be limited to 15; if following an alveolar RM and PEEP titration DP exceeds 15, a reduction in tidal volume should be considered. Tidal volume and PEEP can be individualized to each patient's respiratory mechanics to lower DP. A recent study by Park et al.[63] confirmed the significance of DP during OLV. In a double-blind, randomized, controlled study of 292 patients undergoing thoracic surgery, they compared DP-guided ventilation with conventional protective ventilation. The number of patients who developed pneumonia or ARDS was smaller in the DP group than in the protective ventilation group. Therefore ventilating the lungs using the lowest DP is equivalent to ventilating according to the patient's "functional lung size."
5. **Auto-PEEP** can be detected by worsening lung compliance or if expiratory flow does not return to baseline before the next inspiratory cycle.
6. The fraction of **inspired oxygen** (F_iO2) should be set at 80% at the initiation of OLV and titrated to maintain oxygen saturation above 90% to reduce the likelihood of hyperoxia.[64] The exposure to hyperoxia can worsen absorption atelectasis, increase shunt, worsen oxygenation, and lead to oxidative stress.[32]

Hypoxemia during OLV occurs in up to 5% of cases and occurs most commonly in patients with a low arterial partial pressure of oxygen (PaO2) before OLV during left-sided OLV, normal FEV_1, and in the supine position.[65] The treatment of hypoxemia during OLV requires a thoughtful approach to diagnosing and treating the underlying cause and correcting shunt through both the surgical and nonsurgical lung.[66] The F_iO2 should be increased to 1.0 to bring the oxygen saturation above 90% and an immediate fiberoptic bronchoscopy should be used to confirm the correct position of the lung isolation device. Suctioning of secretions or blood from the major airways and optimizing cardiac output with the use of vasopressors, inotropes, or fluids may be necessary. Shunt in the ventilated lung can be treated with RM and PEEP titration.[67] Shunt through the surgical lung can be treated with the application of CPAP or passive oxygen insufflation, of which the latter may be preferred during VATS lung resection to maximize exposure of the surgical field. The beneficial effect of CPAP is through apneic oxygenation.[68,69] The surgical lung can be reinflated intermittently in the case of refractory hypoxemia or a BB can be placed selectively in the operative lobe for patients who do not tolerate OLV.[69] Rarely, reducing the shunt to the operative lung can be achieved with pulmonary artery constriction (is practical only if the surgeon has complete access to the pulmonary artery).

An example of a staged lung recruitment maneuver when it is combined with a PEEP decrement trial shows that as the recruitment and PEEP decrement trials proceed, there arc corresponding changes to lung compliance, PaO2, and V_D/V_T (dead space ventilation). The best individualized PEEP is associated with optimization of all these variables.

Open Versus Video-Assisted Surgery

The posterolateral thoracotomy at the fifth interspace is the classic surgical approach to pulmonary resection, as it provides excellent surgical exposure to both the lung and hilar structures. However, the large incision, division of the latissimus dorsi, and need for rib spreading are associated with significant postoperative pain, impairment of respiratory mechanics, and morbidity. Successful union of video technology and laparoscopy led to the first description of a minimally invasive approach to a cholecystectomy in 1987.[70] Five years later, the VATS study group was organized to explore how this technology could be applied to pathology within the chest and improve outcomes for patients.[71]

Nearly 30 years later, minimally invasive thoracic surgery (MITS) techniques have been refined, indications expanded, and now are a fundamental part of a modern thoracic surgery service. The term MITS is an umbrella term that includes VATS, approaches by 3, 2, or uniportal techniques, as well as robotic-assisted thoracic surgery. The less invasive nature of VATS manifests in improved respiratory mechanics with improved FEV_1 and FVC when compared with thoracotomy.[72] Observational studies have shown decreases in hospital stay, postoperative pain, and complications, such atrial fibrillation, air leaks, and pneumonia in patients who had a MITS procedures compared with thoracotomy.[73–75] The reduction in complications and the mortality benefit appear particularly pronounced in the elderly and more frail patients.[76,77] The extent and quality of lymph node sampling, an initial concern of MITS, has been shown to be equivalent.[78] A prospective randomized multicenter study named VIOLET is currently ongoing and hopes to firmly define the advantages for VATS lobectomy compared with an open lobectomy. This lung cancer study is a UK multicenter parallel group randomized controlled trial with blinding of outcome assessors and participants (to hospital discharge) comparing the effectiveness, cost effectiveness, and acceptability of VATS lobectomy versus open lobectomy for treatment of lung cancer.[79]

There are unique considerations to MITS compared with open surgical approaches. Although it believed to be less painful than a thoracotomy, the MITS techniques still require incisions in the intercostal spaces, significant visceral dissection and resection and need for chest tubes postoperatively. A multimodal approach to postoperative pain control including regional techniques, opiates, and nonopioid analgesics should be routine. At the author's institution and in many other practices, placement of a thoracic epidural or paravertebral catheter is used for patients presenting for VATS lobectomy. In those presenting for nonanatomic resections, such as wedge resection, a single dose of a long-acting local anesthetic in the erector spinae or serratus anterior plane may be adequate for the majority of patients.

Although the approach to lung isolation is not different, meticulous attention is needed to ensure operative lung collapse given the reduced ability to retract and manipulate the lung as with an open technique. The application of CPAP to the nondependent lung should be avoided because it will interfere with the surgeon's view of the surgical field. Occasionally, to assist with surgical visualization, the hemithorax is insufflated with CO2 under pressure and vigilance is required with adjustment of ventilation to deal with systemic absorption, as well as identifying a possible CO2 embolus. Trochar placement also requires special attention, as it can be placed inadvertently into the abdomen and can injure the liver, diaphragm, or intrathoracic structures. The port site itself can be a significant source of bleeding that may go unrecognized because it is out of the field of view for the majority of the pulmonary resection.

Possible Complications

Lung resection surgery historically was associated with extremely high morbidity and mortality. With continuous improvements in surgical and perioperative care, the incidence of complications have drastically decreased with current 30-day mortality rates for lobectomy currently reported at 1%.[80] However, adverse events related to airway, respiratory, and cardiovascular systems remain common and they significantly contribute to morbidity and increased health care costs.

Airway Injury

Lung isolation requires introduction of airway equipment into the mainstem bronchi. The most commonly used lung isolation device, the Robertshaw design disposable endobronchial DLT, is significantly larger than a single-lumen endotracheal tube and has high pressure cuffs at larger insufflation volumes. Taken together, these features increase the risk for both upper and lower airway injuries during airway manipulation. Rupture of the trachea and bronchus because of DLT is well documented. Although it remains rare with a DLT (0.05%–0.19%), it is an order of magnitude more common than with single lumen endotracheal tubes (0.005%).[81,82] In one recent prospective study of 60 patients, the rates of hoarseness and laryngeal edema with DLT and Arndt BB were 44% and 17%, respectively. However, the incidence of subclinical bronchial injury defined as redness, edema, or hematoma on bronchoscopic examination did not differ significantly between the two devices.[83] Extra care should be used when endobronchial intubation is required for patients with tracheobronchial wall pathology or leukemia, on steroid therapy, and in females over the age of 50 years.[84]

Hypoxemia/Postoperative Acute Lung Injury/Acute Respiratory Distress Syndrome/Respiratory Failure

Lung injury and hypoxemia after lung resection surgery remain one of the most common and morbid adverse events encountered postoperatively. Incidence of ALI range from 2.8% to 12% with lower rates associated with smaller nonanatomic wedge resections and higher rates with larger resections, particularly pneumonectomies.[85,86] Patients who develop ALI have dramatically increased rates of reintubation, mechanical ventilation, intensive care admission, and mortality.

Postlung resection ALI is a form of mild ARDS and its diagnostic criteria should be used to accurately identify these patients. The Berlin criteria for diagnosing ARDS include an impairment of oxygenation with a PaO2/F_iO2 less than 300 mm Hg, opacities on either chest x-ray or CT imaging and the exclusion of hydrostatic pulmonary edema caused by left-sided heart failure or congestion.[87] Factors that have been found to increase the risk of postoperative ALI include increased extent of pulmonary resection, advanced cancer stages, failure to implement lung protective ventilation,[88] severe COPD, interstitial lung disease, ischemic heart disease, greater than 4 L of fluid intake within the first 24 hours after surgery, chronic alcohol consumption, and intraoperative transfusion.[89]

Both the operative lung and ventilated lung are at risk for developing lung injury and impaired gas exchange after pulmonary resection. Abnormalities or destruction of the endothelial glycocalyx of the alveolar-capillary membrane are common to both lungs and are likely the culprit lesion to contribute to capillary leak and edema formation. The glycocalyx is a carpet of microtubules that lines the inner surface of the capillary endothelial cells, and it regulates the normal patterns of fluid fluxes across semipermeable membranes.[90] The ventilated lung is subjected to volutrauma, atelectrauma/tidal recruitment, hyperperfusion, and biotrauma.[45] The operative lung in contrast is exposed to atelectasis followed by recruitment of the lung after the resection is complete. It is also subjected to ischemia-reperfusion injury related to lung collapse and diversion of blood flow because of hypoxic vasoconstriction. Direct surgical trauma also contributes to the accumulation of interstitial edema. It has been demonstrated that increasing the surgical lung manipulation is associated with an increased potential of lung injury, which may be as damaging as the ventilation-associated injury in the nonoperative lung.[91]

The mainstay of treatment for ARDS is mainly supportive and addressing the underlying cause that precipitated the lung injury. Conservative fluid management, low tidal volume ventilation strategy between 4 and 6 mL/kg and routine use of postend expiratory pressure when mechanically ventilated have demonstrated significant mortality benefit.[92] Significant work is being done to find direct pharmocotherapies that may help with the treatment of ARDS; unfortunately none are recommended for routine administration at this time.[93]

Air Leak/Bronchopleural Fistula/ Pneumothorax (See Chapter 26)

Prolonged air leak after lung resection is defined as drainage of air via the thoracostomy tubes that persists past 5 to 7 days postoperatively.[94] This is not only associated with prolonged length of stay, but it is also one of the most common reasons for hospital readmission within 30 days of a pulmonary resection.[95] The highest risk of air leak is documented in patients after lung volume reduction surgery at a rate as high as 46%.[96] The incidence of air leak after lobectomy procedures is significantly lower, ranging from 5.6% to 26% and is lower for wedge resection at 3.5%.[97,98]

Treatment of persistent air leaks may be categorized into conservative, surgical, or nonsurgical management strategies. The ultimate goal is for full re-expansion of the lung, restoration of adequate ventilation, and oxygenation without air loss from the alveolar-pleural communication. **Conservative management** includes chest tube drainage and observation. Chest tube management is not universally agreed upon including whether the chest tube should be placed to external suction or underwater seal only. Persistent air leak that does not require suction to maintain lung expansion may be managed with a flutter valve on an outpatient basis. **Surgical approaches** typically involve the drainage of effusion or infected fluid and reinforcement of the surgical stump or leaking parenchyma.[99] Although surgery may be effective, it is associated with significant morbidity especially in elderly patients or those with significant comorbidities.[100]

Nonsurgical approaches include medical pleurodesis and bronchoscopic approaches. Although successful in the context of a spontaneous pneumothorax, attempts to use tetracycline and talc-based sclerosing agents in postoperative air leaks are much less successful because of significant recurrence rates.[101] Blood pleurodesis, where a patient's own venous blood is injected into the pleural space with the intent of coagulating and sealing over the air leak, has also been attempted. Unfortunately, studies on this technique have shown inconsistent results and are hampered by small sample volumes.[102] In patients who have failed treatment regimes or are deemed a prohibitive risk for reoperation, there are endoscopic therapies available. The initial step is the identification of the source of the air leak by bronchoscopy under general anesthesia and sequential balloon occlusion of individual lobar, segmental, and subsegmental occlusion under direct observation.[103] After identification of the most distal airway, which when occluded eliminates the leak, a one-way valve, the Spiration Valve (Olympus America), which is approved by the U.S. Food and Drug Administration for treatment of air leaks that exceed 6 days, may be placed allowing air and secretion to escape into the conducting airways but preventing air from entering into the affected bronchus. Promising results have been demonstrated in persistent air leaks of many etiologies, including postlung resection patients, but more data are required before its routine use can be recommended.[104]

Bronchopleural fistulas represent similar but distinct pathology to air leaks with a communication to the pleura from the airways that occurs more proximally, from either lobar, segmental or subsegmental bronchi. They are much less common than air leaks, occurring in 4.5% to 20% of pneumonectomies and 0.5% to 1% of lobectomies.[105] Unfortunately, spontaneous closure of these defects is unlikely to occur, requiring additional interventions. Those patients who are stable enough to return to the operating room should have surgical management that may include debridement of necrotic tissue and closure of the bronchial stump with vascularized tissue, such as omentum or muscle to cover the source of the leak.[106] Those patients who are deemed poor surgical candidates to return to the operating room may benefit from bronchoscopic therapy as described earlier. Because of the morbidity and complexity of these lesions, patients are likely to benefit from a multidisciplinary discussion between surgeon, respirologist, intensivist, and anesthesiologist.

Postpneumonectomy Syndrome

Hyperinflation of the remaining lung after pneumonectomy can result in a mediastinal shift toward the operative hemithorax with various degrees of torsion and compression of the mediastinal structures. Central airway compression may occur as the main bronchus is compressed between the vertebral column and pulmonary artery. Fig. 40.6 shows a postpneumonectomy syndrome in a 20-year-old woman who underwent right pneumonectomy for carcinoid 4 years earlier. She developed postpneumonectomy syndrome within 1 year of pneumonectomy and had mediastinal repositioning with breast implants.[107] It is not usually an

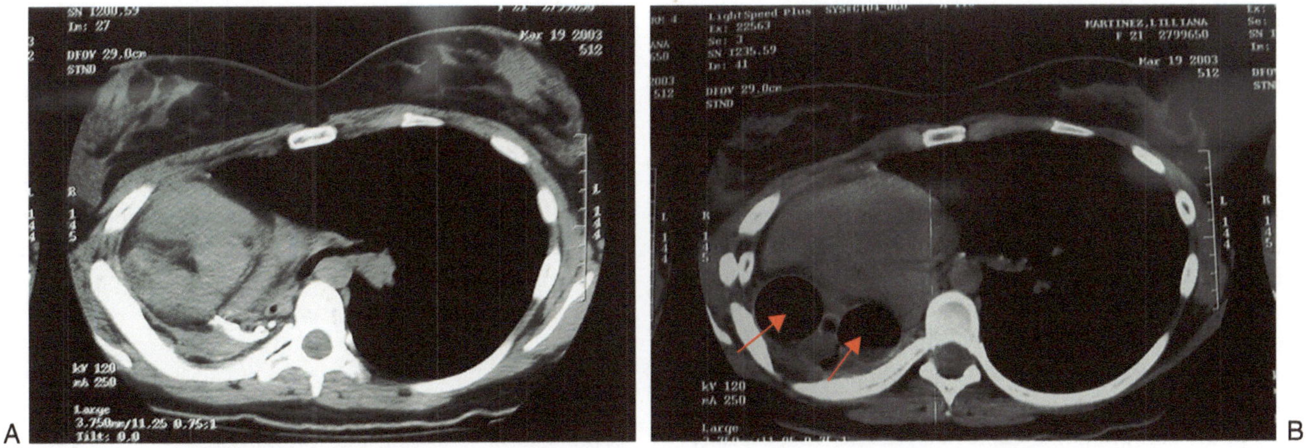

• **Fig. 40.6** (**A**) Computed tomography scan of the patient shows shift of the mediastinum to the right and posteriorly with compression of the left mainstem bronchus between the pulmonary artery and the aorta. (**B**) Despite the presence of numerous prostheses, (red arrows) the mediastinum is shifted into the pneumonectomy space. (From Shen KR, Wain JC, Wright CD, Grillo HC, Mathisen DJ. Postpneumonectomy syndrome: surgical management and long-term results. *J Thorac Cardiovasc Surg.* 2008;135(6):1210–1219.)

acute event and typically occurs after 6 months postresection. Dyspnea, cough, stridor, and recurrent pneumonia are the common symptoms that are nonspecific and require a high index of suspicion to make the diagnosis. Chest x-ray, CT imaging, or bronchoscopic examination may identify the mediastinal shift and airway compression. Esophageal and pulmonary vein compression have also been described causing dysphagia and dyspnea, respectively.[108,109] Surgical prophylaxis or treatment has been successfully achieved by repositioning of the mediastinum with placement of prostheses or by placing a saline-filled breast prosthesis in the empty hemithorax.[107]

Atrial Fibrillation (See Chapter 22)

Supraventricular arrhythmias, including atrial fibrillation and atrial flutter are a significant burden in the postoperative lung resection patient. The incidence after major lung resection (lobectomy or greater) has been reported at 10% for lobectomy and up to 43% for a right pneumonectomy.[110] It is most commonly encountered between postoperative day 2 and 4. It is typically self-limiting but may persist until 4 to 6 weeks after the resection. New onset postoperative atrial fibrillation is associated with worse outcomes secondary to increased rates of arterial thromboembolic events, pulmonary complications, or impaired tissue perfusion because of hemodynamic instability.[111] Pathophysiologic mechanisms that may contribute to the high incidence of atrial fibrillation in this surgical population include both local and systemic inflammation, increased right ventricular afterload, and increased catecholamines from both endogenous and exogenous sources.[112–114]

Risk factors for the development of atrial fibrillation include male sex, increasing age, alcohol consumption, hypertension, red cell transfusion, use of inotropes, duration, and extent of surgery and pulmonary resection via a thoracotomy incision.[110] Of note, in the retrospective review by Lee and colleagues,[110] epidural analgesia did not prevent atrial fibrillation in either the VATS or open thoracotomy population. In patients who are intermediate to high risk, the American Association for Thoracic Surgery has given a class IIa recommendation for the administration of diltiazem or amiodarone as prophylaxis against postoperative atrial fibrillation.[115] Class I recommendation is given for the continuation of beta blockade if a patient is already on it to prevent withdrawal.

Recurrent Laryngeal and Phrenic Nerve Injuries

The **phrenic nerve** descends anteriorly between the pericardium and mediastinal pleura. It may be compressed by a central malignancy or be injured during dissection near the area of an internal thoracic artery. Unilateral injury is typically identified after a procedure on chest x-ray demonstrating an elevated diaphragm on the affected side. The large majority of patients with a unilateral injury will be asymptomatic and do not require treatment. Those patients who are symptomatic or have a baseline marginal respiratory reserve may benefit from diaphragmatic plication. This surgical repair is aimed to reduce the paradoxically cephalad motion of the affected side during inspiration.[116]

The course of the **left recurrent laryngeal nerve** around the aortic arch and back up to the neck makes it particularly more vulnerable for possible invasion by pulmonary malignancy and iatrogenic injury during lung resection. One study by Filaire et al. evaluated the prevalence, the impact-related postoperative complications, and the risk factors of vocal cord dysfunction (VCD) after left lung resection for cancer in 99 consecutive patients who underwent a pneumonectomy ($n = 50$) or a lobectomy ($n = 49$). A fiberoptic laryngeal examination was performed preoperatively for all patients and within the first week postoperatively in patients with symptom(s) or sign(s) of VCD or respiratory complications:

some 31 patients (31%) had a postoperative VCD (group VCD) and 68 (68%) did not (group non-VCD). Mortality rate was 19% in group VCD and 9% in group non-VCD. The VCD patients developed more pulmonary and cardiac complications compared with group non-VCD patients. A higher rate of reintubation, pneumonia, arrhythmia, and cardiac failure was noticeable in group VCD. Preoperative radiotherapy and pneumonectomy were predictive of postoperative VCD. Hospital stay was 22 ± 16 days in group VCD and 13 ± 9 days in group non-VCD. One-third of patients who developed vocal dysfunction developed symptomatic aspiration as well.[117] This is significantly higher than in other causes for recurrent laryngeal injury and likely because of the compounding effect of a reduced vital capacity and reduced ability to generate an effective cough after lung resection.[118] A high index of suspicion for recurrent laryngeal injury is required in patients with hoarse voice after thoracic surgery as laryngeal edema secondary to airway manipulation with a double lumen endobronchial tube is common. Diagnosis can typically be made with flexible nasopharyngoscopy.

Pulmonary Torsion

Pulmonary torsion describes the rotation of a lobe around its bronchus, artery, and vein causing airway obstruction and vascular insufficiency. Although rare, prevalence is estimated at 0.1% to 0.3% with a mortality approaching 12% to 16%.[119] Diagnosis is often delayed because of nonspecific symptoms and signs, such as cough, shortness of breath, tachypnea, tachycardia, hypoxia, and fever that can be falsely attributed to multiple other more common pathologies. Unfortunately when the diagnosis is made on CT imaging or bronchoscopy, it is usually after a prolonged period of malperfusion, necessitating resection of infarcted tissue. It occurs most often in the right middle lobe after right upper lobectomy in the setting of a complete oblique fissure and long hilar pedicle. Preventative measures intra-operatively include plicating the right middle lobe to the parietal pleura or binding the right middle lobe to the right lower lobe by clips, sealants, or glue.[120]

Cardiac Herniation

Cardiac herniation is a rare and potentially life-threatening complication following intrapericardial right or left pneumonectomy. It involves herniation of the heart through the defect in the pericardium and into the empty pleural space with compression of venous and arterial vessels. Cardiac herniation is usually seen within 24 hours to 3 days of surgery. The most typical presentation is sudden onset of profound hypotension and shock, tachycardia, cyanosis, chest pain, and superior vena cava syndrome immediately after coughing, vomiting, moving, or extubation of the patient. Positive intrathoracic pressure, suction applied to the chest tubes and patient repositioning are thought to be risk factors.[121] Treatment involves lifesaving emergent thoracotomy and returning the heart to the pericardium and closure of the pericardial defect. Prevention of this complication can be accomplished by primary closure of the pericardial defect at the time of pneumonectomy, or by suturing the edges of the pericardium to the myocardium.[122]

Conclusion

Primary lung malignancy is the most frequent indication for resection of lung parenchyma. The safe and effective perioperative care of patients presenting for lung resection surgery requires careful consideration and treatment of the modifiable predictors of adverse outcomes and using various measures to support and enhance care both during and after surgery. Several preoperative assessment tools exist, which allow the anesthesiologist to better tailor care for each unique patient and surgery. The three-legged stool of preoperative pulmonary assessment is one such tool that is both simple and effective. Exciting new developments in the monitoring of mechanical ventilation have allowed providers to more safely and effectively individualize the delivery of OLV. Whereas the DLT is most frequently used to achieve lung separation during lung resection surgery, many alternative options exist and choosing the "best" device for the situation is based on both patient and surgical factors.

The goals of anesthetic care for lung resection surgery can be summarized as follows: (1) achieve effective lung isolation while protecting the nonoperative lung from VILI; (2) administer intravenous fluids sparingly and in a goal-directed fashion; (3) select anesthetic medications and practices that facilitate optimal respiratory mechanics and preservation of airway reflexes upon emergence from anesthesia; and (4) use opioid-sparing analgesia, including regional or neuraxial anesthesia. A minimally invasive approach to lung resection surgery enhances patient recovery but does carry some additional considerations for the anesthesiologist. Finally, despite dramatic improvements in 30-day mortality after lung resection surgery in the past few decades, adverse events related to the cardiorespiratory systems remain common.

References

1. Howlader N, Noone AM, Krapcho M, et al. SEER Cancer Statistics Review, 1975-2014, National Cancer Institute. Bethesda, MD, https://seer.cancer.gov/csr/1975_2014/, based on November 2016 SEER data submission, posted to the SEER web site, April 2017.
2. Roman M, Labbouz S, Valtzoglou V, et al. Lobectomy vs. segmentectomy. A propensity score matched comparison of outcomes. *Eur J Surg Oncol.* 2019;45(5):845–850.
3. Wright CD, Gaisert HA, Grab JD, O'Brien SM, Peterson ED, Allen MS. Predictors of prolonged post-operative length of stay after lobectomy for lung cancer. *Ann Thorac Surg.* 2008;85:1857–1865.

4. British Thoracic Society. Society of Cardiothoracic Surgeons of Great Britain and Ireland Working Party. Guidelines on the selection of patients with lung cancer for surgery. *Thorax.* 2001;56:89–108.
5. Brunelli A, Kim AW, Berger KI, DJ Addrizzo-Harris. Physiologic evaluation of the patient with lung cancer being considered for resectional surgery: diagnosis and management of lung cancer, 3rd ed: American College of Chest Physicians evidence-based clinical practice guidelines. *Chest.* 2013;143(5 Suppl):e166S–e190S.
6. Slinger P, Darling G. Preanesthetic assessment for thoracic surgery. In: Slinger P, ed. *Principles and Practice of Anesthesia for Thoracic Surgery.* Cham, Switzerland: Springer; 2019:13–42.
7. Zhang R, Lee SM, Wigfield C, Vigneswaran WT, Ferguson MK. Lung function predicts pulmonary complications regardless of the surgical approach. *Ann Thorac Surg.* 2015;99(5):1761–1767.
8. Nakahara K, Ohno K, Hashimoto J, et al. Prediction of postoperative respiratory failure in patients undergoing lung resection for cancer. *Ann Thorac Surg.* 1988;46:549–554.
9. Brunelli A, Charloux A, Bolliger CT, et al. ERS/ESTS clinical guidelines on fitness for radical therapy in lung cancer patients (surgery and chemo-radiotherapy). *Ann Thorac Surg.* 2009;34(1):17–41.
10. Bach PB, Cramer LD, Schrag D. The influence of hospital volume on survival after resection for lung cancer. *N Engl J Med.* 2001;345:181–188.
11. Colice GL, Shafazand S, Griffin JP, Keenan R, Bolliger CT. American College of Chest Physicians. Physiologic evaluation of the patient with lung cancer being considered for resectional surgery: ACCP evidenced-based clinical practice guidelines (2nd edition). *Chest.* 2007;132(3 Suppl):161S.
11a. Licker M, Schnyder JM, Frey JG, et al. Impact of aerobic exercise capacity and procedure-related factors in lung cancer surgery. *Eur Respir J.* 2011;37:1189–1198.
12. Olsen GN, Bolton JWR, Weiman DS, Horning CA. Stair climbing as an exercise test to predict postoperative complications of lung resection. *Chest.* 1991;99:587–590.
13. Jordan S, Evans TW. Predicting the need for intensive care following lung resection. *Thorac Surg Clin.* 2008;18:61–69.
14. Fleisher LA, Fleischmann KE, Auerbach AD, et al. 2014 ACC/AHA guideline on perioperative cardiovascular evaluation and management of patients undergoing noncardiac surgery: Executive summary: a report of the American College of Cardiology/American Heart Association Task Force on Practice Guidelines. *Circulation.* 2014;130(24):2215–2245.
15. Kristensen SD, Knuuti J, Saraste A, et al. 2014 ESC/ESA Guidelines on non-cardiac surgery: cardiovascular assessment and management: The Joint Task Force on non-cardiac surgery: cardiovascular assessment and management of the European Society of Cardiology (ESC) and the European Society of Anaesthesiology (ESA). *Eur Heart J.* 2014;35(35):2383–2431.
16. Duceppe E, Parlow J, MacDonald P, et al. Canadian Cardiovascular Society Guidelines on perioperative cardiac risk assessment and management for patients who undergo noncardiac surgery. *Can J Cardiol.* 2017;33(1):17–32.
17. Lee TH, Marcantonio ER, Mangione CM, et al. Derivation and prospective validation of a simple index for prediction of cardiac risk of major noncardiac surgery. *Circulation.* 1999;100:1043–1049.
18. Wong J, Lam DP, Abrishami A, Chan M, Chung F. Short-term preoperative smoking cessation and postoperative complications: a systematic review and meta-analysis. *Can J Anaesth.* 2012;59:268–279.
19. Pouwels S, Fiddelaers J, Teijink JA, Woorst JF, Siebenga J, Smeenk FW. Preoperative exercise therapy in lung surgery patients: a systematic review. *Respir Med.* 2015;109(12):1495–1504.
20. Vaughan DJ, Brunner MD. Anesthesia for patients with carcinoid syndrome. *Int Anesthesiol Clin.* 1997;35(4):129–142.
21. Narouze S, Benzon HT, Provenzano D, et al. Interventional spine and pain procedures in patients on antiplatelet and anticoagulant medications (Second Edition): Guidelines From the American Society of Regional Anesthesia and Pain Medicine, the European Society of Regional Anaesthesia and Pain Therapy, the American Academy of Pain Medicine, the International Neuromodulation Society, the North American Neuromodulation Society, and the World Institute of Pain. *Reg Anesth Pain Med.* 2018;43(3):225–262.
22. Hannallah M, Benumof J, Silverman P, Kelly L, Lea D. Evaluation of an approach to choosing a left double-lumen tube size based on chest computed tomographic scan measurement of left mainstem bronchial diameter. *J Cardiothorac Vasc Anesth.* 1997;11(2):168–171.
23. Checketts MR, Alladi R, Ferguson K, et al. Recommendations for standards of monitoring during anaesthesia and recovery 2015: Association of Anaesthetists of Great Britain and Ireland. *Anaesthesia.* 2016;71(1):85–93.
24. Dobson G, Chow L, Flexman A, et al. Guidelines to the practice of anesthesia—Revised Edition 2019. *Can J Anaesth.* 2019;66(1):75–108.
25. Standards for Basic Anesthetic Monitoring. Committee of Origin: Standards and Practice Parameters (Approved by the ASA House of Delegates on October 21, 1986, last amended on October 20, 2010, and last affirmed on October 28, 2016) https://www.asahq.org/~/media/Sites/ASAHQ/Files/Public/Resources/standards-guidelines/standards-for-basic-anesthetic-monitoring.pdf. Accessed on May 06, 2016.
26. Thiele RH, Durieux ME. Arterial waveform analysis for the anesthesiologist: past, present, and future concepts. *Anesth Analg.* 2011;113(4):766–776.
27. Piccioni F, Bernasconi F, Tramontano GT, Langer M. A systematic review of pulse pressure variation and stroke volume variation to predict fluid responsiveness during cardiac and thoracic surgery. *J Clin Monit Comput.* 2017;31(4):677–684.
28. Denault AY, Haddad F, Jacobsohn E, Deschamps A. Perioperative right ventricular dysfunction. *Curr Opin Anaesthesiol.* 2013;26(1):71–81.
29. Porter TR, Shillcutt SK, Adams MS, et al. Guidelines for the use of echocardiography as a monitor for therapeutic intervention in adults: a report from the American Society of Echocardiography. *J Am Soc Echocardiogr.* 2015;28(1):40–56.
30. Reeves ST, Finley AC, Skubas NJ, et al. Council on Perioperative Echocardiography of the American Society of Echocardiography and the Society of Cardiovascular Anesthesiologists. Special article: basic perioperative transesophageal echocardiography examination: a consensus statement of the American Society of Echocardiography and the Society of Cardiovascular Anesthesiologists. *Anesth Analg.* 2013;117(3):543–558.
31. Cavayas YA, Girard M, Desjardins G, Denault AY. Transesophageal lung ultrasonography: a novel technique for investigating hypoxemia. *Can J Anaesth.* 2016;63(11):1266–1276.
32. Young CC, Harris EM, Vacchiano C, et al. Lung-protective ventilation for the surgical patient: international expert panel-based consensus recommendations. *Br J Anaesth.* 2019;123(6):898–913.

33. Campos JH, Hallam EA, Van Natta T, Kernstine KH. Devices for lung isolation used by anesthesiologists with limited thoracic experience: comparison of double-lumen endotracheal tube, Univent torque control blocker, and Arndt wire-guided endobronchial blocker. *Anesthesiology*. 2006;104(2):261–266.
34. Ikeno S, Mitsuhata H, Saito K, et al. Airway management for patients with a tracheal bronchus. *Br J Anaesth*. 1996;76(4):573–575.
35. Massard G, Rougé C, Dabbagh A, et al. Tracheobronchial lacerations after intubation and tracheostomy. *Ann Thorac Surg*. 1996;61(5):1483–1487.
36. Chau EH, Slinger P. Perioperative fluid management for pulmonary resection surgery and esophagectomy. *Semin Cardiothorac Vasc Anesth*. 2014;18(1):36–44.
37. Assaad S, Kyriakides T, Tellides G, Kim AW, Perkal M, Perrino A. Extravascular lung water and tissue perfusion biomarkers after lung resection surgery under a normovolemic fluid protocol. *J Cardiothorac Vasc Anesth*. 2015;29(4):977–983.
38. Batchelor TJP, Rasburn NJ, Abdelnour-Berchtold E, et al. Guidelines for enhanced recovery after lung surgery: recommendations of the Enhanced Recovery After Surgery (ERAS®) Society and the European Society of Thoracic Surgeons (ESTS). *Eur J Cardiothorac Surg*. 2019;55(1):91–115.
39. Smith I, Kranke P, Murat I, et al. Perioperative fasting in adults and children: guidelines from the European Society of Anaesthesiology. *Eur J Anaesthesiol*. 2011;28:556–569.
40. Arslantas MK, Kara HV, Tuncer BB, et al. Effect of the amount of intraoperative fluid administration on postoperative pulmonary complications following anatomic lung resections. *J Thorac Cardiovasc Surg*. 2015;149(1):314–320.
41. Gupta R, Gan TJ. Peri-operative fluid management to enhance recovery. *Anaesthesia*. 2016;71(Suppl 1):40–45.
42. Lee JH, Jeon Y, Bahk JH, et al. Pulse pressure variation as a predictor of fluid responsiveness during one-lung ventilation for lung surgery using thoracotomy: randomised controlled study. *Eur J Anaesthesiol*. 2011;28:39–44.
43. Suehiro K, Okutani R. Stroke volume variation as a predictor of fluid responsiveness in patients undergoing one-lung ventilation. *J Cardiothorac Vasc Anesth*. 2010;24:772–775.
44. de la Gala F, Piñeiro P, Reyes A, et al. Postoperative pulmonary complications, pulmonary and systemic inflammatory responses after lung resection surgery with prolonged one-lung ventilation. Randomized controlled trial comparing intravenous and inhalational anaesthesia. *Br J Anaesth*. 2017;119:655–663.
45. Lohser J, Slinger P. Lung injury after one-lung ventilation: a review of the pathophysiologic mechanisms affecting the ventilated and the collapsed lung. *Anesth Analg*. 2015;121:302–318.
46. Beck-Schimmer B, Bonvini JM, Braun J, et al. Which anesthesia regimen is best to reduce morbidity and mortality in lung surgery? A multicenter randomized controlled trial. *Anesthesiology*. 2016;125:313–321.
47. Módolo NS, Módolo MP, Marton MA, et al. Intravenous versus inhalation anaesthesia for one-lung ventilation. *Cochrane Database Syst Rev*. 2013(7).
48. Cho HC, Lee JH, Lee SC, Park SY, Rim JC, Choi SR. Use of sugammadex in lung cancer patients undergoing video-assisted thoracoscopic lobectomy. *Korean J Anesthesiol*. 2017;70(4):420–425.
49. Grocott HP. Optimizing lung collapse with a bronchial blocker: it's not what you use, but how you use it. *J Cardiothorac Vasc Anesth*. 2017;32(4):e93–e94.
50. Bussieres JS, Somma J, Del Castillo JL, et al. Bronchial blocker versus left double-lumen endotracheal tube in video-assisted thoracoscopic surgery: a randomized-controlled trial examining time and quality of lung deflation. *Can J Anaesth*. 2016;63(7):818–827.
51. Bussières JS, Moreault O, Couture EJ, Provencher S. Optimizing lung collapse with a bronchial blocker: it's not what you use, but how you use it, Part II. *J Cardiothorac Vasc Anesth*. 2019;33(1):255.
52. Lohser J, Slinger P. Lung injury after one-lung ventilation: a review of the pathophysiologic mechanisms affecting the ventilated and the collapsed lung. *Anesth Analg*. 2015 Aug;121(2):302–318.
53. Slinger PD. Do low tidal volumes decrease lung injury during one-lung ventilation? *J Cardiothorac Vasc Anesth*. 2017;31(5):1774–1775.
54. Lohser J. Evidence-based management of one-lung ventilation. *Anesthesiol Clin*. 2008;26(2):241–272.
55. Michelet P, D'Journo XB, Roch A, et al. Protective ventilation influences systemic inflammation after esophagectomy: a randomized controlled study. *Anesthesiology*. 2006;105(5):911–919.
56. Yang M, Ahn HJ, Kim K, et al. Does a protective ventilation strategy reduce the risk of pulmonary complications after lung cancer surgery? A randomized controlled trial. *Chest*. 2011;139(3):530.
57. Licker M, Diaper J, Villiger Y, et al. Impact of intraoperative lung-protective interventions in patients undergoing lung cancer surgery. *Crit Care*. 2009;13(2):R41.
58. Hoftman N, Eikermann E, Shin J, et al. Utilizing forced vital capacity to predict low lung compliance and select intraoperative tidal volume during thoracic surgery. *Anesth Analg*. 2017;125(6):1922–1930.
59. Schilling T, Kozian A, Huth C, et al. The pulmonary immune effects of mechanical ventilation in patients undergoing thoracic surgery. *Anesth Analg*. 2005;101(4):957–965.
60. Vegh T, Juhasz M, Szatmari S, et al. Effects of different tidal volumes for one-lung ventilation on oxygenation with open chest condition and surgical manipulation: a randomised cross-over trial. *Minerva Anestesiol*. 2013;79(1):24–32.
61. Unzueta C, Tusman G, Suarez-Sipmann F, Böhm S, Moral V. Alveolar recruitment improves ventilation during thoracic surgery: a randomized controlled trial. *Br J Anaesth*. 2012;108(3):517–524.
62. Ferrando C, Mugarra A, Gutierrez A, et al. Setting individualized positive end-expiratory pressure level with a positive end-expiratory pressure decrement trial after a recruitment maneuver improves oxygenation and lung mechanics during one-lung ventilation. *Anesth Analg*. 2014;118(3):657–665.
63. Park M, Ahn HJ, Kim JA, et al. Driving pressure during thoracic surgery: a randomized clinical trial. *Anesthesiology*. 2019;130(3):385–393.
64. Suzuki S, Mihara Y, Hikasa Y, et al. Current ventilator and oxygen management during general anesthesia: a multicenter, cross-sectional observational study. *Anesthesiology*. 2018;129(1):67–76.
65. Brassard CL, Lohser J, Donati F, Bussières JS. Step-by-step clinical management of one-lung ventilation: continuing professional development. *Can J Anaesth*. 2014;61(12):1103–1121.
66. Lohser J. Managing hypoxemia during minimally invasive thoracic surgery. *Anesthesiol Clin*. 2012;30(4):683–697.
67. Ishikawa S, Lohser J. One-lung ventilation and arterial oxygenation. *Curr Opin Anaesthesiol*. 2011;24(1):24–31.

68. Lohser J. Evidence-based management of one-lung ventilation. *Anesthesiol Clin*. 2008;26(2):241–272.
69. Jung DN, Ahn HJ, Jung SH, et al. Apneic oxygen insufflation decreases the incidence of hypoxemia during one-lung ventilation in open and thoracoscopic pulmonary lobectomy: a randomized controlled trial. *J Thorac Cardiovasc Surg*. 2017;154(1): 360–366.
70. Dubois F, Icard P, Berthelot G, Levard H. Coelioscopic cholecystectomy: preliminary report of 36 cases. *Ann Surg*. 1990; 211(1):60–62.
71. Hazelrigg S, Nunchuck S, LoCicero J. Video-assisted thoracic surgery study group. *Ann Thor Surg*. 1993;56(5):1039–1044.
72. Kaseda S. Better pulmonary function and prognosis with video-assisted thoracic surgery than with thoracotomy. *Ann Thorac Surg*. 2000;70(5):1644–1646.
73. Villamizar NR, Darrabie MD, Burfeind WR, et al. Thoracoscopic lobectomy is associated with lower morbidity compared with thoracotomy. *J Thorac Cardiovasc Surg*. 2009;138(2):419–425.
74. Seder CW, Hanna K, Lucia V, et al. The safe transition from open to thoracoscopic lobectomy: a 5-year experience. *Ann Thorac Surg*. 2009;88:216–226.
75. Park BJ. Robotic lobectomy for non-small cell lung cancer (NSCLC): Multi-center registry study of long-term oncologic results. *Ann Cardiothorac Surg*. 2012;1(1):24–26.
76. Bravo Iniguez CE, Armstrong KW, Cooper Z, et al. Thirty day mortality after lobectomy in elderly patients eligible for lung cancer screening. *Ann Thorac Surg*. 2016;101(2):541–546.
77. Cattaneo SM, Park DJ, Wilton AS, et al. Use of video-assisted thoracic surgery for lobectomy in elderly results in fewer complications. *Ann Thorac Surg*. 2008;85(1):231–236.
78. Demmy TL, Yendamuri S, D'Amico TA, Burfeind WR. Oncologic equivalence of minimally invasive lobectomy: the scientific and practical arguments. *Ann Thorac Surg*. 2018;106(2):609–617.
79. Lim E, Paramasivan S, Wordsworth S, et al. Video assisted thoracoscopic lobectomy versus conventional open LobEc-Tomy for lung cancer, a multi-centre randomised controlled trial with an internal pilot. The VIOLET study. Available at https://www.journalslibrary.nihr.ac.uk/programmes/hta/130403#/. Accessed Jan 2, 2020.
80. Laursen LØ, Petersen RH, Hansen HJ, Jensen TK, Ravn J, Konge L. Video-assisted thoracoscopic surgery lobectomy for lung cancer is associated with a lower 30-day morbidity compared with lobectomy by thoracotomy. *Eur J Cardiothorac Surg*. 2016;49(3):870–875.
81. Lampl L. Tracheobronchial injuries. Conservative treatment. *Interact Cardiovasc Thorac Surg*. 2004;3(2):401–405.
82. Massard G, Rouge C, Dabbagh A, et al. Tracheobronchial lacerations after intubation and tra- cheostomy. *Ann Thorac Surg*. 1996;61(5):1483–1487.
83. Knoll H, Ziefeler S, Schreiber JU, et al. Airway injuries after one-lung ventilation: a comparison between double-lumen tube and endobronchial blocker. *Anesthesiology*. 2006;105(3):471–477.
84. Fitzmaurice B, Brodsky J. Airway rupture from double lumen tubes. *J Cardiothorac Vasc Anesth*. 1999;13(3):322–329.
85. Kim HJ, Cha SI, Kim CH, et al. Risk factors of postoperative acute lung injury following lobectomy for nonsmall cell lung cancer. *Medicine (Baltimore)*. 2019;98(13):e15078.
86. Licker MJ, Widikker I, Robert J, et al. Operative mortality and respiratory complications after lung resection for cancer: impact of chronic obstructive pulmonary disease and time trends. *Ann Thorac Surg*. 2006;81(5):1830–1837.
87. Ferguson ND, Fan E, Camporota L, et al. The Berlin definition of ARDS: an expanded rationale, justification, and supplementary material. *Intensive Care Med*. 2012;38(10):1573–1582.
88. Licker M, Diaper J, Villiger Y, et al. Impact of intraoperative lung-protective interventions in patients undergoing lung cancer surgery. *Crit Care*. 2009;13(2):R41.
89. Licker M, de Perrot M, Spiliopoulos A, et al. Risk factors for acute lung injury after thoracic surgery for lung cancer. *Anesth Analg*. 2003;97(6):1558–1565.
90. Collins SR, Blank RS, Deatherage LS, Dull RO. Special article: the endothelial glycocalyx: emerging concepts in pulmonary edema and acute lung injury. *Anesth Analg*. 2013;117(3):664–674.
91. Kozian A, Schilling T, Rocken C, Breitling C, Hachenberg T, Hedenstierna G. Increased alveolar damage after mechanical ventilation in a porcine model of thoracic surgery. *J Cardiothorac Vasc Anesth*. 2010;24(4):617–623.
92. Network Acute Respiratory Distress Syndrome, RG Brower, Matthay MA, et al. Ventilation with lower tidal volumes as compared with traditional tidal volumes for acute lung injury and the acute respiratory distress syndrome. *N Engl J Med*. 2000;342:1301–1308.
93. Duggal A, Ganapathy A, Ratnapalan M, Adhikari NK. Pharmacological treatments for acute respiratory distress syndrome: systematic review. *Minerva Anestesiol*. 2015;81(5):567–588.
94. Pompili C, Miserocchi G. Air leak after lung resection: pathophysiology and patients' implications. *J Thorac Dis*. 2016;8(suppl 1):S46–S54.
95. Salati M, Brunelli A, Xiumè F, Refai M, Pompili C, Sabbatini A. Does fast-tracking increase the readmission rate after pulmonary resection? A case-matched study. *Eur J Cardiothorac Surg*. 2012;41(5):1083–1087.
96. DeCamp MM, Blackstone EH, Naunheim KS, et al. Patient and surgical factors influencing air leak after lung volume reduction surgery: lessons learned from the National Emphysema Treatment Trial. *Ann Thorac Surg*. 2006;82(1):197–207.
97. Liberman M, Muzikansky A, Wright CD, et al. Incidence and risk factors of persistent air leak after major pulmonary resection and use of chemical pleurodesis. *Ann Thorac Surg*. 2010;89(3):891–897.
98. Abolhoda A, Liu D, Brooks A, Burt M. Prolonged air leak following radical upper lobectomy: an analysis of incidence and possible risk factors. *Chest*. 1998;113(6):1507–1510.
99. El-Sameed YA. Role of bronchoscopy in management of bronchopleural fistula. In: Mehta AC, Jain P, editors. *Interventional Bronchoscopy: A Clinical Guide*. New York: Springer Science+Business Media; 2013:211–225.
100. Lois M, Noppen M. Bronchopleural fistulas: an overview of the problem with special focus on endoscopic management. *Chest*. 2005;128(6):3955–3965.
101. Alfageme I, Moreno L, Huertas C, Vargas A, Hernandex J, Beiztegui A. Spontaneous pneumothorax. Long-term results with tetracycline pleurodesis. *Chest*. 1994;106:347–350.
102. Oliveira FH, Cataneo DC, Ruiz Jr, RL, Cataneo AJ. Persistent pleuropulmonary air leak treated with autologous blood: results from a university hospital and review of literature. *Respiration*. 2010;79(4):302–306.
103. Kovitz KL, French KD. Endobronchial valve placement and balloon occlusion for persistent air leak. *Chest*. 2013;144(2):661–665.

104. Travaline JM, McKenna RJ Jr, De Giacomo T, et al. Treatment of persistent pulmonary air leaks using endobronchial valves. *Chest.* 2009;136(2):355–360.
105. Alpert JB, Godoy MC, Degroot PM, Truong MT, Ko JP. Imaging the post-thoracotomy patient: anatomic changes and postoperative complications. *Radiol Clin North Am.* 2014;52(1):85–103.
106. Liberman M, Cassivi SD. Bronchial stump dehiscence: update on prevention and management. *Semin Thorac Cardiovasc Surg.* 2007;19:366–372.
107. Shen KR, Wain JC, Wright CD, Grillo HC, Mathisen DJ. Postpneumonectomy syndrome: surgical management and long-term results. *J Thorac Cardiovasc Surg.* 2008;135(6):1210–1219.
108. Yüksel M, Yildizeli B, Evman S, Kodalli N. Postpneumonectomy esophageal compression: an unusual complication. *Eur J Cardiothorac Surg.* 2005;28(1):180–181.
109. Partington SL, Graham A, Weeks SG. Pulmonary vein stenosis following left pneumonectomy: a variant contributor to postpneumonectomy syndrome. *Chest.* 2010;137(1):205–206.
110. Lee SH, Ahn HJ, Yeon SM, et al. Postoperative atrial fibrillation in lung resection surgery. *Anaesthesia.* 2016;71(12):1424–1430.
111. Maesen B, Nijs J, Maessen J, Allessie M, Schotten U. Post operative atrial fibrillation: a maze of mechanisms. *Europace.* 2012;14(2):159–174.
112. Hogue CW, Creswell LL, Gutterman DD, Fleisher LA. Epidemiology, mechanisms and risks: American College of Chest Physicians guidelines for the prevention and management of postoperative atrial fibrillation after cardiac surgery. *Chest.* 2005;128(2 suppl):9S–16S.
113. Boos CJ, Anderson RA, Lip GY. Is atrial fibrillation an inflammatory disorder? *Eur Heart J.* 2006;27(2):136–149.
114. Mansour Z, Kochetkova EA, Santelmo N, et al. Risk factors for early mortality and morbidity after pneumonectomy: a reappraisal. *Ann Thorac Surg.* 2009;88:1737–1743.
115. Frendl G, Sodickson AC, Chung MK, et al. 2014 AATS guidelines for the prevention and management of perioperative atrial fibrillation and flutter for thoracic surgical procedures. *J Thorac Cardiovasc Surg.* 2014;148(3):e153–e193.
116. Krasna MJ, Forti G. Nerve injury: injury to the recurrent laryngeal, phrenic, vagus, long thoracic and sympathetic nerves during thoracic surgery. *Thorac Surg Clin.* 2006;16(3):267–275.
117. Filaire M, Mom T, Laurent S, et al. Vocal cord dysfunction after left lung resection for cancer. *Eur J Cardiothorac Surg.* 2001;20(4):705–711.
118. Baldi S, Scappaticii E, Rapellino M, et al. Effect of lung resection on pulmonary function: a comparative study in different surgical procedures. *Panminerva Med.* 1989;31(1):19–21.
119. Farkas EA, Detterbeck FC. Airway complications after pulmonary resection. *Thorac Surg Clin.* 2006;16:243–251.
120. Venuta F, Anile M, de Giacomo T, Coloni GF. Prevention of middle lobe torsion after right upper lobectomy with a polymeric sealant. *J Thorac Cardiovasc Surg.* 2012;143(1):240–241.
121. Shimizu J, Ishida Y, Hirano Y, et al. Cardiac herniation following intrapericardial pneumonectomy with partial pericardiectomy for advanced lung cancer. *Ann Thorac Cardiovasc Surg.* 2003;9(1):68–72.
122. Foroulis C, Kotoulas C, Konstantinou M, Lioulias A. The use of pedicled pleural flaps for the repair of pericardial defects, resulting after intrapericardial pneumonectomy. *Eur J Cardiothorac Surg.* 2002;21(1):92–93.

41

Repair of Pectus Excavatum

JO MOURISSE, STEFAN VAN DER HEIDE

Introduction

Pectus excavatum (PE) is a congenital chest wall deformity characterized by a sternal depression, which typically begins at the manubrium and ends toward the xiphoid. Adjacent costal cartilages are displaced as well. The deformity can be symmetric or asymmetric. It is also called a funnel chest or trichterburst.

PE has an incidence of 1 to 8 per 1000 and accounts for 88% of anterior chest wall disorders. It is followed by pectus carinatum with 5%.[1] It is up to 4 times more prevalent in males.[2]

Sometimes PE is associated with connective tissue disease like Marfan syndrome, Ehlers Danlos or osteogenesis imperfecta, or with neuromuscular disease. It is also seen in some genetic disorders like Noonan syndrome and Turner syndrome.

There are a number of hypotheses for what causes PE, but the most widely adopted theory is abnormal rib or cartilage overgrowth.[3] Park et al. evaluated the costal cartilage and rib length between 18 prepubertal patients, 10 years old, with symmetric PE and 18 age-and sex-matched controls without chest wall deformity. They concluded that in patients with symmetric PE, the rib lengths in the patient group were significantly longer than in the control group for the sixth right rib and fourth, fifth, and sixth left ribs, suggesting that abnormal rib overgrowth may be a contributing factor responsible for PE rather than cartilage overgrowth.[4]

Only 22% of PE are present in the first decade of life.[2] In pubertal growth, PE deformity often worsens. A mild PE can progress in 6 to 12 months to a severe type.

At young age, the PE causes no complaints, but as they grow up and become more active, symptoms of shortness of breath on exertion, lack of endurance, and exercise tolerance appears to be problematic.

A frequent reason to seek medical attention is cosmetic concern. A severe PE may have devastating psychologic effects like depression or in rare cases even suicide. Chest pain is also often a complaint. Patients with mild PE have almost normal cardiopulmonary function and the indication is cosmetic. Severe PE produces many more symptoms as listed in Fig. 41.1.[5]

Treatment Options

Sauerbruch (1920) resected bilateral rib and cartilage with sternal osteotomy requiring external traction to prevent flail chest. This technique has since been abandoned from clinical practice.

In 1949 Ravitch described subperichondral resection of only deformed costal cartilages without entering the chest. After some modifications, the external traction was not needed, but there was a large anterior operative scar. Further modifications resulted in much smaller scars.[5]

Several modifications followed: Robicsek described the use of mesh support to stabilize the sternum. Leonard used a wire behind the sternum that is laterally externalized to be attached to a brace. Lacquet introduced a technique without prosthetic materials. All these procedures are rarely, if at all, used in clinical practice.

In 1997 Nuss introduced the insertion of a preshaped metal bar. His method is also known as the minimal invasive repair of PE (MIRPE).[5] Advantage of this method is less invasive, less blood loss, less nonunion, pseudoarthrosis, floating sternum, less acquired dystrophy, and a shorter surgical time. Some modifications followed. The first modification was the use of thoracoscopy, which allows an extensive view of the surgical field. Before that the surgeon performed a risky blind blunt dissection between the sternum and pericardial sac. Initially thoracoscopy was performed bilaterally, while current practice is limited to unilateral approach. To decrease the incidence of bar flipping. Initially, pericostal rib fixation with a suture was used, and later a stabilizer was attached to the end of the bar. Pilegaard used very short bars in an effort to decrease flipping range.[6]

Surgical alternatives for PE repair include magnet insertion upon the sternum in combination with external traction with a second magnet on a brace. For patients with low physical impact of the PE, the subcutaneous insertion of implantable custom-made prosthesis is an option. A nonsurgical alternative is external sternal suction with a vacuum bell.[7] Physical therapy aiming at improving posture and increasing chest expansion can be offered to patient with mild PE.

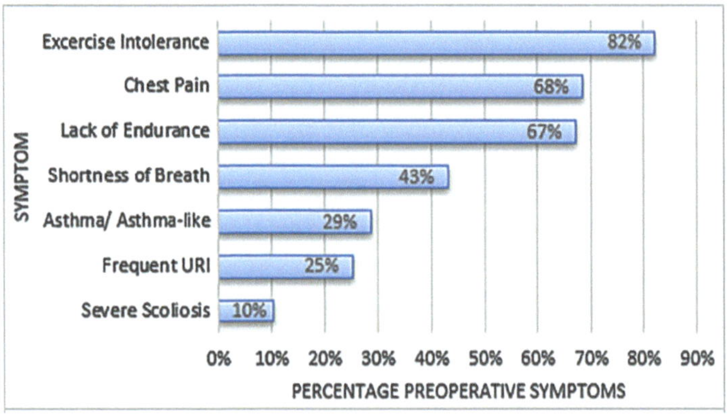

• **Fig. 41.1** Percentage preoperative symptoms in a group of 900 patients with severe pectus excavatum. *URI,* Upper respiratory infection. (From Nuss D, Kelly RE, Jr. Minimally invasive surgical correction of chest wall deformities in children (Nuss procedure). *Adv Pediatr.* 2008;55:395–410.)

Optimal Age for Treatment

At the beginning of PE repair, surgeons believed that operation was best performed early in childhood (before 20 months). Haller described in 1996 a serious complication after a Ravitch procedure: the development of a chest growth disorder or acquired asphyxiating chondrodystrophy. The restricted thoracic cage also restricts lung growth resulting in a reduction of forced vital capacity (FVC) as low as 33% to 55% of predicted.[8] Risk factors are surgery at young age and excessive resection of costal cartilage and growth centers.

Early surgery can also lead to recurrence of the abnormality. In the first publication of Nuss, the median age at surgery was 5 years. Later he recommended to operate before puberty.[5] The current practice is to correct the PE around 14 years. There are few centers that only perform the operation at 3 years; middle-aged patients are only successfully operated.[6] In adult patients aged over 30 years, the addition of open cartilage resection and open sternal osteotomy is more common.[9]

Case Presentation

At the age of 14 years, a healthy young man presented with PE, which was noticeable since a young age. At this time, he weighed 36 kg and his height is 156 cm. He had no physical complaints. Because there was only a 2-cm depression, and the growth spurt had not yet finished, the correction was postponed. At the age of 17 years, he presented again now with symptoms of shortness of breath and chest pain with deep sigh. He also felt embarrassed from his disfiguration. At this stage he was 59 kg and 184 cm. The depression had a depth of 3 cm and was slightly asymmetrically. A photograph of the chest deformity is made (Fig. 41.2). The Haller index was 4 (Fig. 41.3), FVC was 88%, and forced expiratory volume in 1 second (FEV_1) 79% of predicted.

Before the operation a thoracic epidural catheter was placed at T4–T5. The surgery, which will be detailed later in the chapter, was uneventful and a 11-inch bar with two fixation plates was placed. Following extubation, the patient went to the postanesthesia care unit and a few hours later to the ward. On chest radiograph a small bilateral apical pneumothorax (left 1 cm, right 2 cm) was observed (Fig. 41.4). Pain was managed with patient control epidural analgesia

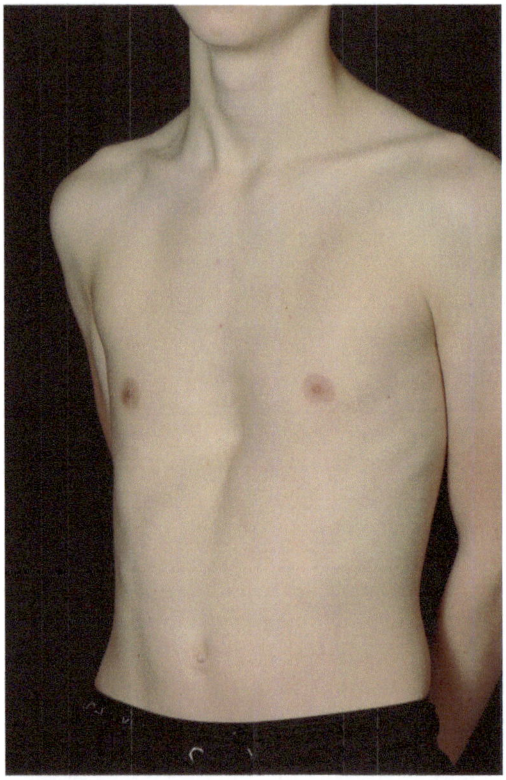

• **Fig. 41.2** Pectus excavatum deformation of a 17-year-old boy. See case presentation.

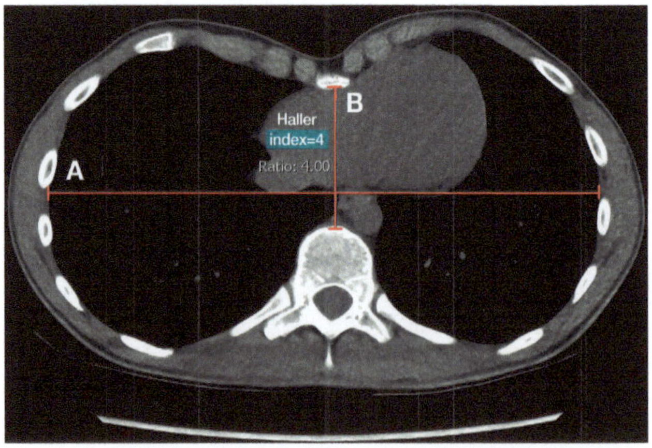

• **Fig. 41.3** Haller index or pectus severity index measurement on computed tomography-scan of the presented case: lateral diameter A divided by distance between spine and maximal depression B equals an index of 4.

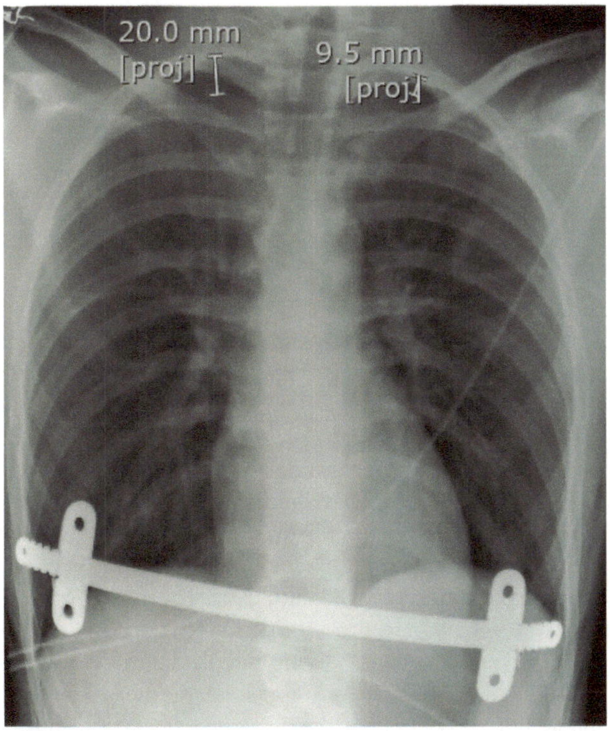

• **Fig. 41.4** Chest radiograph after Nuss bar placement in the presented case. The bar is placed somewhat oblique for optimal result. There is a small bilateral apical pneumothorax.

(PCEA) ropivacaine/sufentanil. Satisfied with the result, the patient was discharged home on the fifth postoperative day.

Case Management

Preoperative Evaluation and Indications for Surgery

The first step is to assess the severity of the deformity by inspection. The depth of the sternal depression and the asymmetry should be recorded. A depth of more than 2.5 cm is considered moderate to severe deformity. It is common practice for the chest to be imaged by photography to follow-up the progression of the PE or to illustrate the result of a treatment as the pre-surgical image is depicted in Fig. 41.2.

The practitioner must evaluate the history and progression of the PE and the presence of other symptoms, such as diminished physical activity, fatigue, shortness of breath, or pain. Psychologic and emotional complaints often play an important role to seek for medical help. In addition, associated syndromes or congenital disorders must be considered. Possible allergy to nickel and cobalt (2%) which is the composition of the metal bars must be excluded.

In mild or severe deformity or in cases of cardiorespiratory symptoms, a chest computed tomography (CT) scan is made. The pectus severity index (PSI), also known as the Haller index, is measured at the point of maximal depression and is the ratio between the lateral diameter and the distance between spine and maximal depression as illustrated in Fig. 41.3. A normal patient has a PSI of less than 2.5 and a severe PE has an PSI of equal to or more than 3.5. The mean Haller CT index, in a study of 1215 Nuss operations, was 5.15 (2.32) (mean standard deviation [SD]).[10] On a CT scan, the position of the heart, lungs, and great vessels can be easily determined. Other chest abnormalities can be observed, (often kyphotic chest) and 10% to 20% will have associated scoliosis.[5]

Cardiac function is evaluated if there is dyspnea or chest pain with exercise or when there are palpitations. Cardiac compression is found in 88% and cardiac displacement in 89% of cases whereas cardiac murmurs occur in 32%.[5] A CT scans and magnetic resonance imaging scans are normally taken in supine position, and cardiac compression is underestimated compared with the upright position particularly with exercises.[1]

Echocardiography (transthoracic or transesophageal) shows displacement of the heart to the left and this can hinders the standard views. Compression of the right ventricle outflow tract may cause a functional systolic murmur. Coln et al. evaluated retrospectively 123 patients, aged 5 to 18 years (average, 13 years) who underwent Nuss pectus repair. Symptoms related to exertion were present in 106 (86%) cases. The mean Haller chest wall index was 4.3 (2.4–10.85). Preoperative echo with exercise revealed cardiac compression in 117 (95%) cases. A mitral valve abnormality was present in 54 (44%) cases. Mitral valve prolapses occurred in 25 and mitral valve regurgitation in 29 cases. Postoperative echo was normal in 100 (93%) of those studied. Seven patients had persistent mitral valve prolapse, one had mild regurgitation. All patients were asymptomatic after surgery.[11]

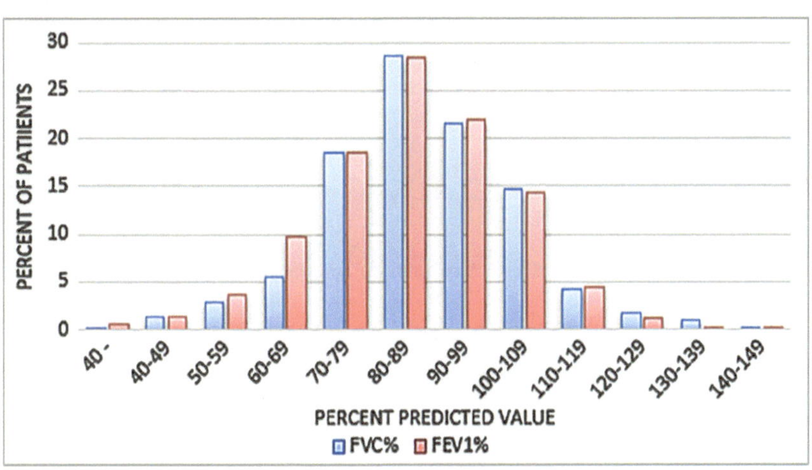

• **Fig. 41.5** Distribution forced vital capacity (*FVC*) and forced expiratory volume in 1 second (*FEV$_1$*). Static pulmonary function studies showing shift to the left in patients with severe pectus excavatum. Data collected from 750 patients. (From Nuss D, Kelly RE, Jr. Minimally invasive surgical correction of chest wall deformities in children (Nuss procedure). *Adv Pediatr.* 2008;55:395–410.)

On electrocardiogram, a right axis deviation and a ST-segment depression can be seen, which reflects the displacement and compression of the heart.

Patients with a severe deformity should undergo pulmonary function testing. Compared with the normal population, patients with PE show a shift toward smaller FVC and FEV_1 (Fig. 41.5). FVC, FEV_1, and FEF_{25-75} values were decreased by 15% below predicted value.[10] The most common finding is restrictive pulmonary function, obstructive is less common but also possible and is believed to be caused by less effective respiratory mechanics compared with normal individuals.[5] The relative fixation of the depressed sternum is compensated with increased abdominal wall movement.[1]

A large proportion of patients will not be operated on, and they are referred to a preoperative exercise program that consists of improvement of cardiopulmonary condition, improvement of posture, and increase in chest expansion. Patients have to be re-evaluated within a year following completion of the program.

Donald Nuss summarized the indications for Nuss operation[5]:

If two or more criteria apply:

- **Patient is symptomatic, has severe deformity, and has documented progression of the deformity**
- **Chest CT shows cardiac or pulmonary compression and the CT-index is 3.25 or greater**
- **Cardiology evaluation demonstrates cardiac compression or displacement with mitral valve prolapse, murmurs, or conduction abnormalities**
- **Pulmonary function studies show restrictive or obstructive lung disease**
- **Previous repair has failed**

The Surgical Procedure

Nuss

There are many modifications of the Nuss procedure. This description gives a general overview of the techniques, and details can differ in each center. The procedure starts with marking landmarks on the chest and the making of a mold of the future bar. Then there is a lateral thoracic incision to introduce the trocar (Fig. 41.6). This can be either on the right or left side depending on surgeon's preference. A subcutaneous tunnel to the top of the pectus ridge is prepared. A thoracoscope is placed in the chest cavity and some centers apply carbon dioxide (CO2) insufflation 5 to 15 mm Hg.[12] Other centers prefer to use one-lung ventilation or the combination of both. Retrosternal dissection with introducer (sword) is performed from the right side to the left side (or reversed) under thoracoscopic view. For safety, during the dissection the tip of the sword should be permanently visualized. In case of a severe PE, the sternum may be elevated with a subxiphoidal incision, sternal traction, or a sternum suction cup. Next, puncture the contralateral intercostal space from the inside and move further to the contralateral skin incision. By lifting the sword, the sternum is elevated and molded to a convex shape with manual external pressure. Umbilical tape is attached to the tip of the sword and the sword is withdrawn. The previously preshaped Nuss-bar is then introduced upside down with the tape as a guide.

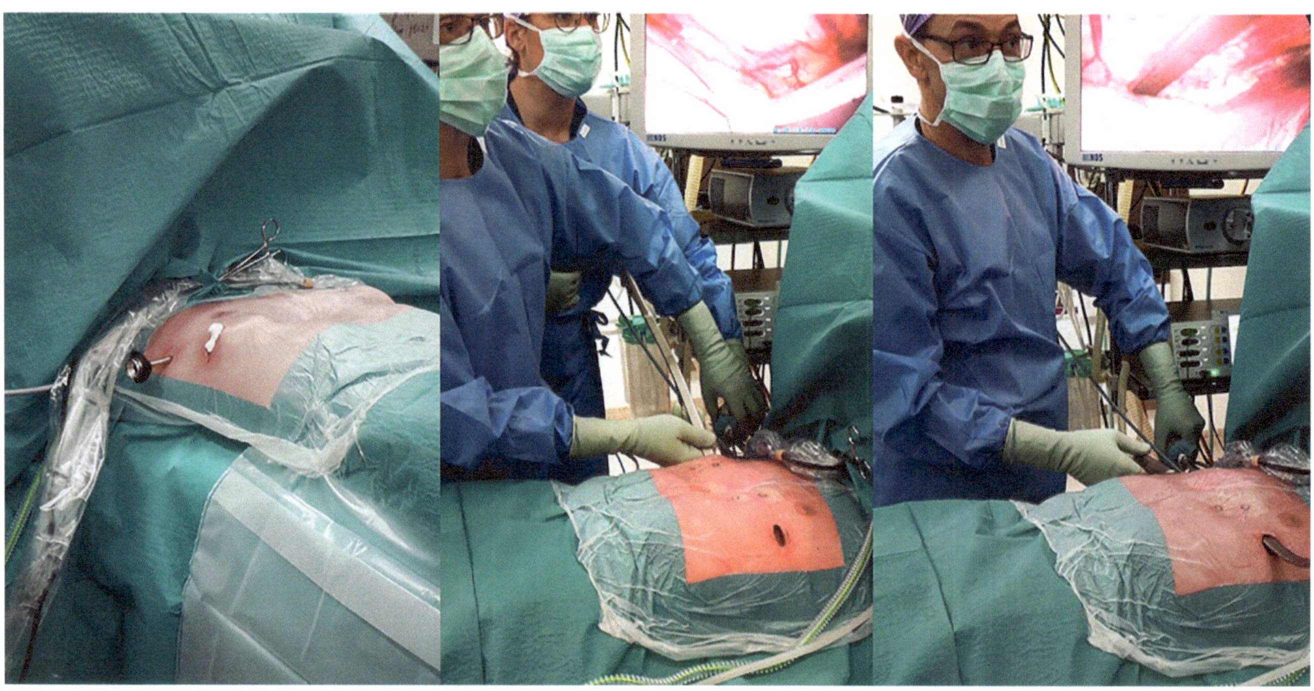

A B C

• **Fig. 41.6** Some steps of the surgery of the presented case. **A**, Two bilateral incisions and subcutaneous tunnels are already prepared and filled with gauze. More cranial, a trocar for thoracoscope is inserted. **B**, The introducer is inserted via the right sided incision under thoracoscopic view. A tunnel between sternum and pericardium is prepared. **C**, The introducer has emerged from the left sided incision. (*Continued*)

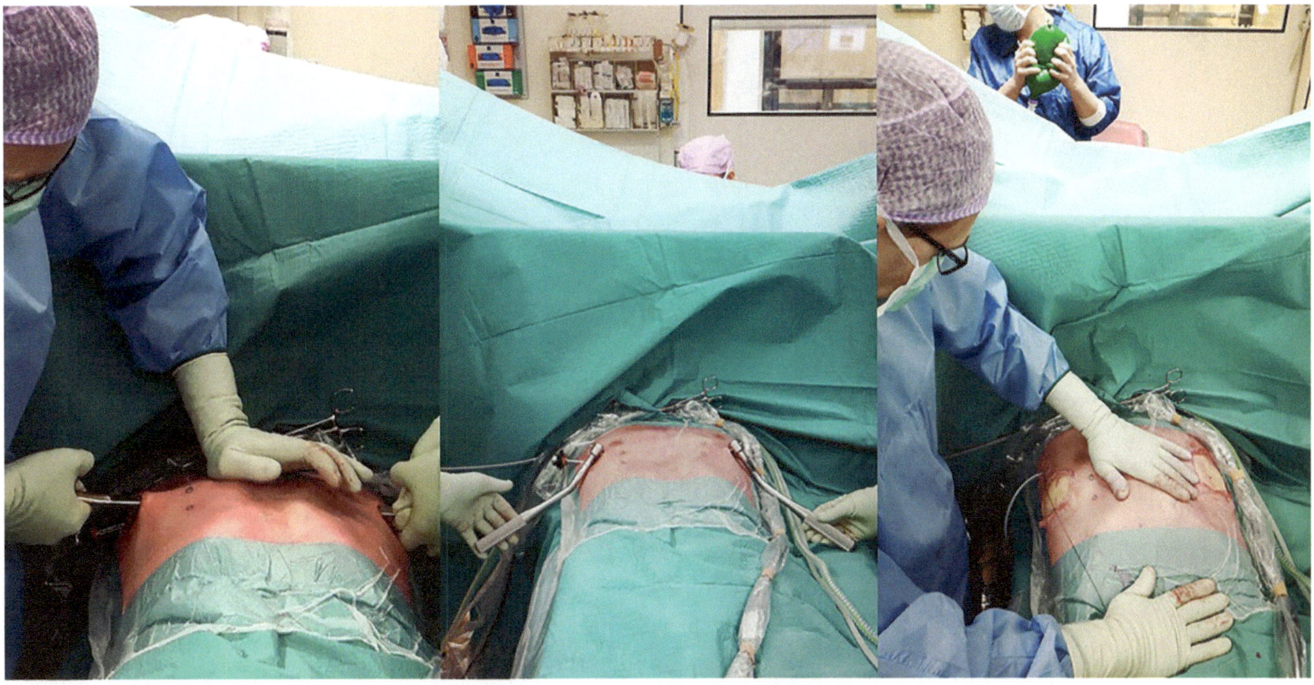

D E F

• **Fig. 41.6** *(Continued)* **D**, sternal elevation and reshaping sternum and ribs. **E**, The introducer is withdrawn after an umbilical tape was attached to it. Then the Nuss bar was inserted using that tape as a guide. Two instruments "flippers" are attached to both ends of the Nuss bar and will be rotated 180 degrees. **F**, After closure of the incisions, a small chest tube is exchanged with the trocar and the distal end is placed under water. Now continuous positive airway pressure is applied together with and chest and abdomen compression to expel residual air from the pleural cavity. Then the chest tube is quickly withdrawn.

Then the bar is flipped 180 degrees with special instruments and the chest wall convexity is obtained. The bar is stabilized with a metal plate and/or metal wire. After skin closure, the trocar for the thoracoscope is changed for a small chest tube. For evacuation of the air in the left and right thorax, positive pressure ventilation is applied, together with external thoracic and abdominal pressure by the surgeon. At the same time the proximal end of the small chest tube is held under water until no air bubbles are seen and then the chest tube is removed.

Ravitch

In our hospital, a small median incision (Fig. 41.7) is used, first detaching pectoral and rectus abdominal muscle and performing subperichondral cartilage resection. A wedge osteotomy is made at the level of angulation, leaving the posterior cortex intact. The sternum is corrected with crossed vicryl sutures in the periosteum. The perichondrium is closed and muscles refixated on the anterior chest wall. This technique avoids the use of prosthetic materials but requires intraoperative perfect muscle relaxation and the suppression of tightening the abdominal muscles in the early postoperative period.[3,13]

Results and Outcomes

Kang et al. compared Nuss and Ravitch surgery in 63 and 37 patients, respectively.[14] The Nuss procedure required a shorter operation time and shorter hospital stay than the Ravitch procedure ($P < .001$). The surveillance demonstrated that 17.6% of the Nuss group and 35.7% of the Ravitch group were not satisfied with the outcome of the surgery ($P = .072$). The most common causes of dissatisfaction were redepression in the Nuss group ($n = 5$) and incomplete correction in the Ravitch group ($n = 7$).

A meta-analysis showed that the Nuss operation duration is much shorter and had lower blood loss compared with the Ravitch procedure. Length of hospital stay was similar.[15]

After a modified Ravitch or Nuss procedure, most patients indicate an improvement in their appearance and self-image and also a subjective improvement in their exercise tolerance.[5,16–18] There is also a statistically significant improvement in exercise tolerance using validated questionnaires.[1]

The improvement in pulmonary function and cardiac output is well documented. When pulmonary function is tested while the bar is still in place, the results are initially worse. It is thought to be secondary to patient deconditioning and mostly because of the restrictive effect of the bar.[1] One year after bar removal there were modest improvements in FVC from 88% to 92% and FEV_1 from 83% to 87%.[10] Although increases are statistically significant, the clinical difference is small. After a Ravitch procedure, no improvement of lung function was observed, potentially because of disruption and calcification of the costal cartilage.[1,18–20]

Some Ravitch studies report that VO2 at submaximal exercise was increased slightly but significantly. It is unclear if this increase could be attributable to the improved physical condition 1 year after surgery.[18,21]

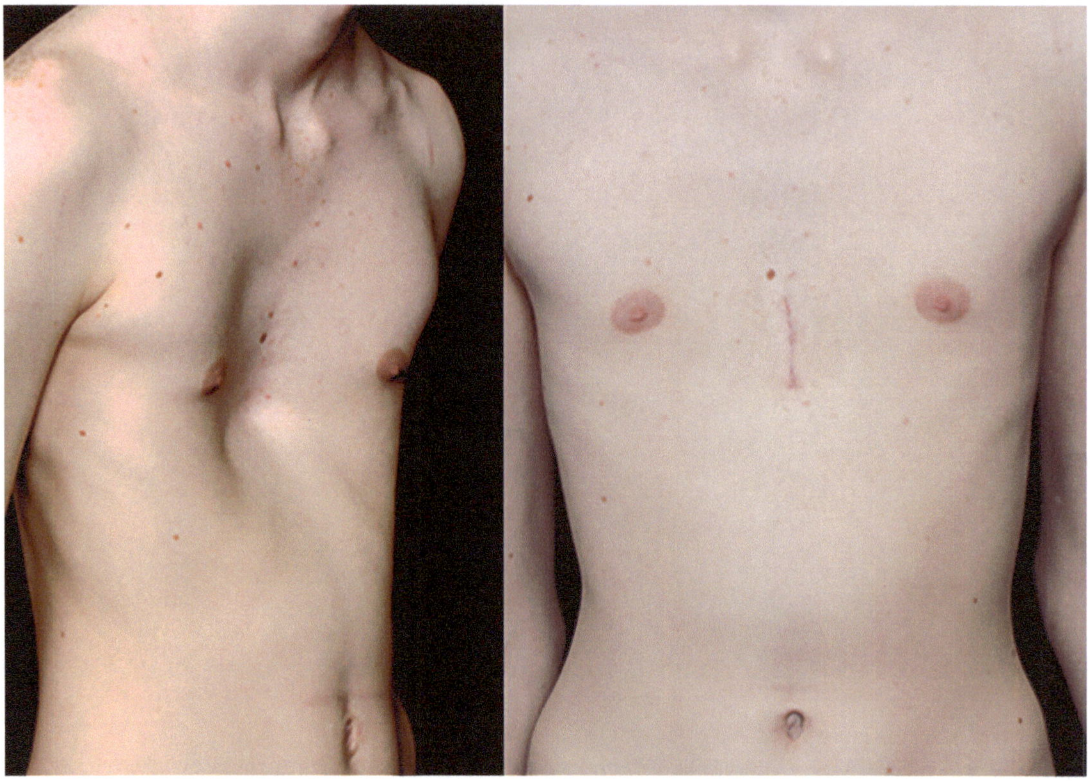

• **Fig. 41.7** An adolescent with a severe pectus excavatum, before and after the modified Ravitch operation. A small median incision is used.

The incidence of preoperative mitral valve prolapse (MVP) was 18% in a study of the Nuss operation. After the correction, almost half of the MVPs resolved.[10] Stroke volume increased after both Ravitch and Nuss procedures.[19,22] In a small study in Nuss-operated patients, stroke volume increased from 61.6 (24) to 77.5 (23) mL (SD).[22]

Surgical Complications

The overall anesthesia and surgery related complication rate is between 15% and 20%.[12,23] In Fig. 41.8, the early and late complications after the Nuss operation are shown. The true incidence of life-threatening complications and mortality

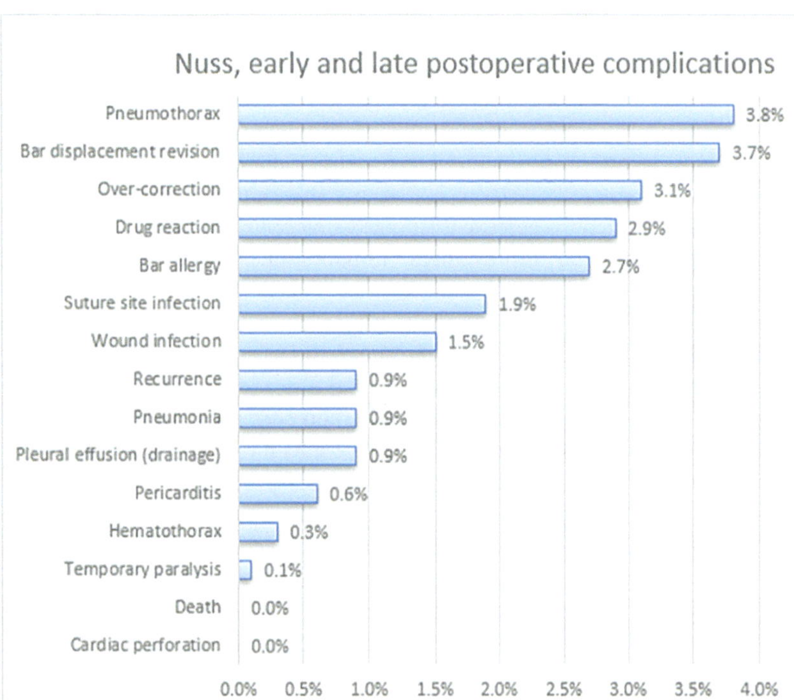

• **Fig. 41.8** Early and late postoperative complications of 1463 primary Nuss operations from 1987 until 2012 by the group of Donald Nuss. (From Nuss D, Obermeyer RJ, Kelly RE. Nuss bar procedure: past, present and future. *Ann Cardiothorac Surg.* 2016;5(5):422–433.)

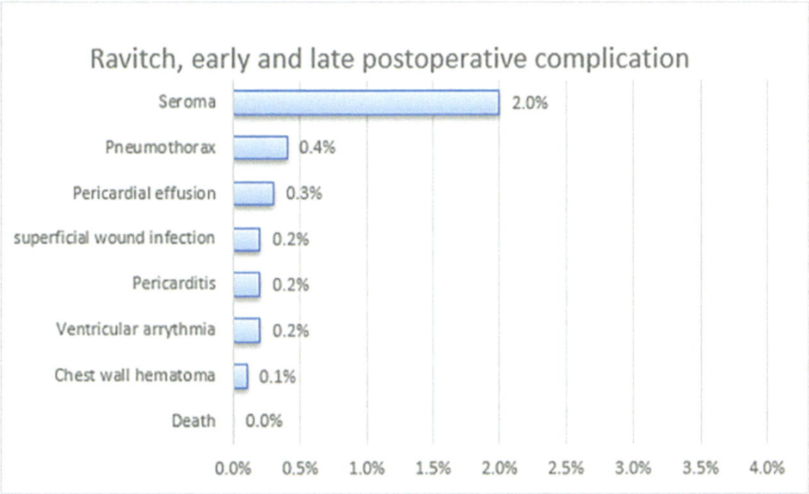

• **Fig. 41.9** Early and late postoperative complications of 912 Ravitch operations from 1969 until 2007 by the group of Fonkalsrud. (From Fonkalsrud EW. 912 open pectus excavatum repairs: changing trends, lessons learned: one surgeon's experience. *World J Surg.* 2009;33(2):180–190.)

is not known because the overall number of procedures performed worldwide is unknown. However, based on data extrapolated from survey information, the pectus bar manufacturer in the United States, literature reports, and data presented at Chest Wall International Group meetings as to the number of cases performed, it is estimated that approximately 50,000 cases have been performed and that the incidence of life-threatening complications is less than 0.1%. From 1998 to 2016, Hebra et al.[23] identified 27 published cases and 32 unreported life-threatening complications, including cardiac perforation, hemothorax, major vessel injury, lung injury, liver injury, gastrointestinal problems, and diaphragm injury. There were seven cases of major complications with bar removal. At least two cases of death during Nuss procedure are reported. With bar removal at least seven deaths are reported.[23] Practitioners should be aware about the risk of mortality and serious life-threatening complications. Risk factors are previous chest surgery, pectus severity, and inexperience of the surgeon.[23]

The most devastating complication is a **cardiac perforation.** There are several reports of cardiac perforation during retrosternal dissection during the Nuss operation.[6,24] Typically, the right atrium or the right ventricle is penetrated. In such a case, an emergence thoracotomy or sternotomy must be performed.

Hemothorax can also occur when intercostal vessels or muscles are injured.

Postoperative pericarditis or pericardial effusions, probably because of entry in the pericardial space, are reported in 0.6% to 4%.[25–27]

Arrythmia and cardiac arrest during procedures are reported. This is especially true in Nuss operations after a previous Ravitch procedure.[5]

A small **pneumothorax** is common after the Nuss operation because of thoracoscopy. It generally will be spontaneously resolved. A large pneumothorax can be caused by lung parenchymal laceration. The incidence of a severe pneumothorax requiring chest tube suction is reported to be 3%, but some series report much higher incidences.[25] Sometimes subcutaneous emphysema is observed, especially when patients are coughing rigorously.

Pleural effusion is the most common complication (63%) after the Nuss operation with an incidence of 29% of the patients in one study.[25] Most pleural effusions are caused by surgical trauma, but also later from traumatic accidents, like a fall or a punch that can cause the effusion. Symptoms are pain and dyspnea. The aspirate can be bloody or serous, although thoracocentesis or chest tube drainage is not always necessary.

Bar displacement was initially a major challenge, but now, with improvement of the technique and the increase in the surgeon's experience, it is less than 1%. Displacement can be a 90- or 180-degree posterior rotation or can be lateral.

A nickle, cobalt, or chromium containing bars may provoke an **allergic reaction.** If an allergy develops, it can be treated with low dose prednisone. Bar allergy can be prevented with the use of titanium bar.

Bar infections are rare and have been reported in less than 0.5% to 3% of cases and are treated with long-term antibiotics or bar removal.

Brachial plexus injury can be the result of suboptimal positioning during the operation.[28]

Complications of the modified Ravitch are shown in Fig. 41.9. No cases of death directly related to the Ravitch procedure are reported.[3] In a large series of 912 patients reported by Fonkalrud, no early mortality was demonstrated.[16] Overall postoperative complication rate was 8% and no serious live-threatening complication were seen.

Anesthetic Techniques

Once the indication for the procedure is established by the surgeon, the patient, frequently accompanied by parents, is invited on the preoperative screening. The goal of the evaluation is to detect any unrecognized disease and risk factors that may increase the risk of surgery and to propose strategies to reduce this risk. CT scan, echocardiography, electrocardiogram, and pulmonary function tests are performed in advance. The anesthetic procedure and postoperative care are explained. Because these patients are almost always young adolescents, special attention is given to anxiety reduction and psychologic resilience. Therefore a short acting benzodiazepine, for example, midazolam, is given 1 hour before surgery. Also, pre-emptive analgesia with paracetamol (acetaminophen) is routinely administered.

Just before surgery, the patient receives a thoracic epidural catheter at level T5–T6. Before placement, an intravenous (IV) access is created and standard monitoring attached. Extensive local infiltration with lidocaine 1% and eventual additional sedation is required to reduce discomfort. An anticholinergic agent (e.g., atropine) and a sympathomimetic agent (e.g., ephedrine) should be directly ready for injection because vasovagal collapse is not infrequent during placement of the epidural in these young patients. After correct placement, the epidural was tested with negative aspiration test and bolus injection of lidocaine 2% with epinephrine.

General anesthesia is achieved with propofol, sufentanil, rocuronium and maintained with inhaled anesthetic. Antibiotics (cefazoline) were given at induction. The probability of acute hemodynamic changes necessitates the use of an intraarterial cannula for continuous pressure monitoring and intermittent blood sampling. A bladder catheter is also inserted after induction. Antiemetics are given at the start (e.g., dexamethasone) and/or end (e.g., ondansetron) of surgery. An IV nonsteroidal antiinflammatory drug (NSAID; e.g., parecoxib) is given at the end of the operation. The epidural analgesia is topped up with sufentanil 20 mcg and ropivacaine 30 mg before incision and maintained with a continuous infusion of 4 mL ropivacaine 0.75% with 1 mcg/mL sufentanil 4 to 6 mL/hour.

We use a single-lumen endotracheal tube and spontaneous lung collapse when patient is temporarily disconnected from the ventilator. One-lung ventilation was not mandatory during this in Nuss operations. Depending on the surgeon preference, in most cases there is no need for a total collapse of the lung.[12]

However, some centers prefer to use double-lumen tubes or endobronchial blockers and apply one-lung ventilation that provide an optimal view of the surgical field.[12] Additional insufflation of CO2 to compress the ipsilateral (right) lung is also used in some centers. CO2 insufflation during the operation gives a rise in end-tidal CO2, tachycardia, and decreased mean arterial blood pressure.[12]

Original position of the Nuss procedures was with both arms abducted. This leads to brachial plexus injury in some patients.[29,30] Therefore one arm (right) is suspended in right angle at the shoulder and right angle at the elbow. The arm is attached on a pole attached to the operation table above the head (Fig. 41.10).

During insertion of the introducer and the bar, careful attention is given to arrythmia and cardiovascular instability.

Postoperative Care

Smooth and pain-free emergence from anesthesia is necessary to prevent bar dislocation. The patient must not lie on their side but stay supine. Good analgesia is necessary to prevent postoperative pulmonary complications.

Standard pain therapy in our institution is the use of the thoracic epidural infusion with ropivacaine 2% and sufentanil 1 mcg/mL 4 to 8 mL/h. In addition, a PCEA modus is used where a bolus of 2 mL each 20 minutes can be delivered. Paracetamol (1000 mg 4 dd) and NSAIDs (diclofenac 50 mg 3 dd) are given on a regularly scheme. Every day, a member of the pain team visits the patient to optimize the pain therapy. Regression of sensory and motor blockade is a well-known event during continuous epidural infusion of local anesthetics and then the infusion rate has to be increased.

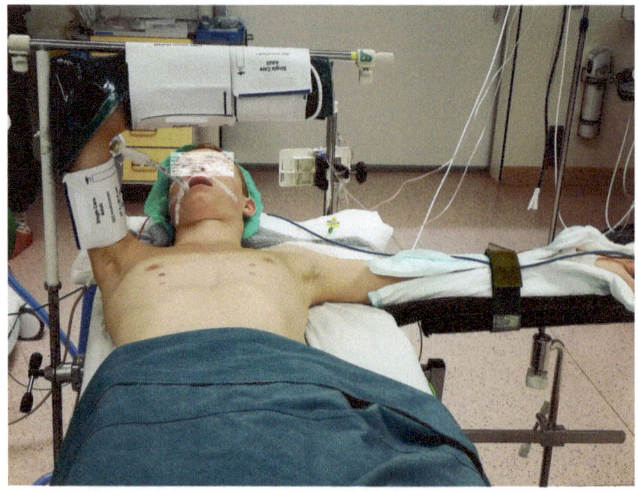

• **Fig. 41.10** Positioning for Nuss procedure for the presented case. Right arm is suspended in right angle at the shoulder and right angle at the elbow. The arm is attached above the head on a pole fixed to the operation table. Elbow and forearm are protected with gel pads. The body is positioned at the right edge of the table.

On day 2, sufentanil is removed from the epidural infusion, and oxycontin (>65 kg 10 mg 2 dd, <65 kg 5 mg 2 dd) is started. Oxynorm (5 mg 6 dd) can be given as an escape drug. Starting the scheduled oral opioid medication well in advance of stopping the epidural infusion is important for an optimal transition.

On day 3, the epidural catheter is removed, and opioid analgesics are continued as already started. If possible, these opioids are stopped on day 4 and tramadol 50 mg 3 dd is given, with an escape of an additional 50 mg. The patient leaves the hospital with paracetamol, diclofenac, and tramadol. Pantoprazol is given for prevention of peptic ulcer.

If the epidural is not effective, the patient receives morphine 2.5 mg IV and continuous infusion (maximum 0.3 mg/kg/h) or patient-controlled analgesia (PCA) with a morphine pump (2 mg/mL, lockout 5–10 minutes, bolus 1 mg). Eventually esketamine 0.1 mg/kg/h is given or clonidine 1–2 mcg/kg/h.

Intravenous antibiotics (Cefazoline) are continued for 2 days.

A physical therapist will instruct the patient how to move and get out the bed, and the patient is discharged on postoperative day 4 to 5.

To prevent bar displacement, patients must lie and sleep on their back and all sports are restricted until 6 weeks postrepair. As long as the bar is inside, contact sports are forbidden.

A bar should be left in place for at least 2 years, preferably 3 years, but not earlier than pubertal growth spurt is finished. Then it can be removed on an outpatient basis.

Review on Postoperative Pain (see Chapter 24)

Adequate pain therapy is essential to prevent discomfort and allow coughing, which is important to prevent pulmonary complications. In a practice survey published in 2014, thoracic epidural is used as a primary analgesic modality by 91% of institutions.[31]

The failure rate of epidural analgesia is up to 30% in clinical practice.[32] Factors contributing are incorrect primary placement, and also secondary migration and suboptimal dosing of local anesthetics. Failure rate is reduced if skilled anesthesiologists are responsible for placement.[33]

A thoracic epidural has some serious adverse effects and complications. The height of the block can be too large with paresis or paralysis of the upper extremities. Also, a Horner syndrome can be seen. Hypotension is possible, and in extreme situations, respiratory depression may result.

Opioids in the epidural solution can lead to drowsiness, itching, and respiratory depression. Overdose from epidural local anesthetic or intravasal injection leads to confusion, perioral tingling, hallucinations, myoclonus, loss of consciousness, and respiratory arrest. Circulatory complications are bradycardia, asystole, and other arrhythmias. The risk of overdosing is higher with impaired liver function.

Because postoperative pain has implications on length of hospital stay, activity, and quality of life, pain management is the critical component of postoperative care.

Compared with the Ravitch operation, patients undergoing the Nuss operation have slightly longer length of hospital stay.[34,35] Nuss patients also had higher average daily pain scores and received 25% more opioids, although both groups received an thoracic epidural in more than 90% of the cases.[36] It is unique that a minimally invasive technique produces more pain, which is possibly caused by crashing trauma to the intercostal nerves during the surgical manipulations. Older patients undergoing the Nuss procedure use more opioids than younger patients. This is attributed to the less compliant chest wall and therefore greater force required to elevate the sternum in older patients. There is no correlation with the Haller CT index and opioid use.[36]

Alternative Analgesic Methods

Standard care is the use of thoracic epidural analgesia (TEA). However rare potential complications that can be devastating are known to occur. In the largest retrospective review of 1215 patients undergoing the Nuss procedure, one patient developed lower extremity paralysis and loss of bowel and bladder control following thoracic epidural placement; some but not all function recovered. That group abandoned the use of thoracic epidurals and changed to PCA.[10] Paraplegia, extremely rare, following an epidural was also reported in a child undergoing a thoracotomy.[37] The predicted maximum risk of permanent neurologic damage after TEA in adults is estimated to be 0.07%.[38]

Patient-Controlled Analgesia

A prospective trial showed better pain control with TEA compared with PCA during 5 days of epidural infusion. Weber et al. evaluated 40 patients (32 male and 8 female patients) undergoing MIRPE, aged 10 to 28 years, divided in two groups. The TEA group showed lower pain scores ($P < .0001$) and required less additional pain medication in conjunction with greater wellbeing postoperatively ($P < .0001$) compared with patients receiving PCA morphine. There was no significant difference regarding the incidence of sedation ($P = .38$), nausea ($P = .10$), and pruritus ($P = .72$) in both groups.[39] A later prospective randomized trial with a shorter period of epidural infusion showed that pain control was better in the first days with TEA but better in the days thereafter with PCA.[40] The authors suggested that may be the transition from epidural to oral analgesic could be improved. Length of stay (LOS) was not different between the two groups. The greatest risk of PCA is respiratory depression.

Bilateral Intercostal Blockade

Local anesthesia may be administered via liberal infiltration around the incisions and intercostal nerve blocks. In general, this pain therapy is concomitant with PCA and multimodal analgesia. A clinical study reported much shorter LOS with oral scheduled opioids and NSAIDs in combination with intraoperative single shot intercostal block compared with a period of epidurals used.[41] Also bilateral subcutaneous catheters are used. These catheters can be used for prolonged time (e.g., maximum 7 days). Compared with TEA, daily pain scores, opioid use, and length of hospital stay were similar.[42]

Bilateral Paravertebral Block

In a retrospective analysis, continuous paravertebral block (PVB) was compared with TEA and continuous intercostal blockade. Both PVB and intercostal blockade had higher pain scores on day 1 and received more total doses of opioids. LOS was shorter because patients could go home with their continuous infusion system.[43] Compared with PCA, a single shot bilateral PVB reduced pain scores for the first 48 hours and decreased opioid use.[44]

Multimodal Analgesia

Opioids are typically used for pain therapy, but they may have many side effects like nausea, vomiting, sedation, pruritis, respiratory depression, urinary retention, and decreased bowel function. All of these complicate the postoperative care. Therefore many institutions searched for alternatives. Multimodal analgesia alleviates pain through blockade of multiple nociceptive and inflammatory pain receptors. In a retrospective comparison, multimodal analgesia (ketamine dexmedetomidine intraoperative, continuous bupivacaine wound infiltration, clonidine, and PCA postoperative) was associated with less postoperative pain, reduced opioid use, and shorter LOS compared with TEA. The addition of a single dose of methadone (0.1 mg/kg) administered at induction of anesthesia to multimodal analgesia performed even better.[33] Methadone is attractive because of its long terminal half-life of more than 24 hours (mean 35 hours [SD 22 hours]), which is 7 to 10 times longer than morphine.[45]

Costal Nerve Cryoablation

Initially, cryoablation or cryoanalgesia had been used in treating chronic pain, including neuropathic pain after thoracotomy. Otherwise, many studies targeted post-thoracotomy pain in which cryoanalgesia was applied to intercostal nerves intraoperatively by the surgeon under direct vision. The advantage of cryoanalgesia, relative to other pain-management techniques, is that the pain relief is long lasting with a single application during the operation. The anterior chest analgesia is effective for about 1 month, which is equivalent to time needed for the intercostal nerve axonal regeneration. In a review of 12 publications, the authors concluded that cryoanalgesia for postthoracotomy on its own is not effective for pain control and increases neuropathic pain postoperatively.[46] Despite the negative finding, some promising reports are published where cryoanalgesia was used during the Nuss operation. The technique of cryoanalgesia has progressed, which can explain the good results. Attention should be given on the type of cryoprobe, the duration of freezing, the time given for thawing before taking of the probe, and probably the prophylactic use of pregabalin or because analgesia after cryoablation takes several hours to be effective. All studies report lesser opioid use and shorter LOS.[47–50] Further studies, especially on long-term outcome, are necessary.

Anxiety Reduction and Mindfulness

Many patients expect that they will suffer severe pain, and therefore they are anxious. Preoperative expectations play a role in how pain is perceived and experienced postoperatively. Addressing these issues, particularly those preconditioned to expect pain intraoperatively, is important in the preoperative consultation. This includes discussing the issue of pain, its management, and the negative impact of expected pain on perceived pain. Some patients were provided training in mindfulness. It has increasingly been shown to not only provide a greater sense of wellbeing to people who practice it, but it also allows them to adapt to adverse circumstances, including how pain is perceived and experienced.

In a single center study by Schlatter et al., 173 patients following the Nuss procedure, divided in to three different analgesia approaches, had a LOS of 4.4 days (TEA), 2.2 days (PCA/intercostal nerve block), and 1.6 days (scheduled oral pain meds/intercostal nerve blocks). The current LOS for patients in this institution is 1 day. Patients successfully stop using narcotics by the end of the first week postoperatively. The authors concluded that intraoperative intercostal nerve blocks, the scheduled postoperative pain medications, and enhanced preoperative consultation aimed to educate patients about anxiety and reframe patient pain expectations, have collectively decreased LOS and reduced postoperative narcotic usage.[41] These authors believed that preoperative anxiety reduction contributes to the significantly shorter LOS. Diazepam is frequently used as needed to assist analgesia by anxiolysis and muscle relaxation.[41]

Conclusion

PE is a congenital chest wall deformity that can be repaired with either the Nuss or the Ravitch procedure. During the Nuss procedure, the surgeon and anesthesiologist should be aware of possible complications, some of which can be very serious. The Nuss procedure, although considered as minimally invasive, is known to be a painful operation. In most centers, thoracic epidural anesthesia is the preferred analgesia method, but many alternatives are possible. A hospital protocol should be established for optimal postoperative care.

References

1. Obermeyer RJ, Cohen NS, Jaroszewski DE. The physiologic impact of pectus excavatum repair. *Semin Pediatr Surg*. 2018;27(3):127–132.
2. Nuss D, Obermeyer RJ, Kelly RE, Jr. Pectus excavatum from a pediatric surgeon's perspective. *Ann Cardiothorac Surg*. 2016;5(5):493–500.
3. Morshuis WJ, Mulder H, Wapperom G, et al. Pectus excavatum—a clinical study with long-term postoperative follow-up. *Eur J Cardio-Thorac*. 1992;6(6):318–329.
4. Park CH, Kim TH, Haam SJ, Lee S. Rib overgrowth may be a contributing factor for pectus excavatum: Evaluation of prepubertal patients younger than 10 years old. *J Pediatr Surg*. 2015;50(11):1945–1948.
5. Nuss D, Kelly RE, Jr. Minimally invasive surgical correction of chest wall deformities in children (Nuss procedure). *Adv Pediatr*. 2008;55:395–410.
6. Notrica DM. Modifications to the Nuss procedure for pectus excavatum repair: a 20-year review. *Semin Pediatr Surg*. 2018;27(3):133–150.
7. Brochhausen C, Turial S, Muller FK, et al. Pectus excavatum: history, hypotheses and treatment options. *Interact Cardiovasc Thorac Surg*. 2012;14(6):801–806.
8. Haller JA, Jr., Colombani PM, Humphries CT, Azizkhan RG, Loughlin GM. Chest wall constriction after too extensive and too

early operations for pectus excavatum. *Ann Thorac Surg.* 1996; 61(6):1618–1624.

9. Jaroszewski DE, Ewais MM, Chao CJ, et al. Success of minimally invasive pectus excavatum procedures (Modified Nuss) in adult patients (>/=30 years). *Ann Thorac Surg.* 2016;102(3): 993–1003.
10. Kelly RE, Goretsky MJ, Obermeyer R, et al. Twenty-one years of experience with minimally invasive repair of pectus excavatum by the Nuss procedure in 1215 patients. *Ann Surg.* 2010;252(6): 1072–1081.
11. Coln E, Carrasco J, Coln D. Demonstrating relief of cardiac compression with the Nuss minimally invasive repair for pectus excavatum. *J Pediatr Surg.* 2006;41(4):683–686.
12. Umuroglu T, Bostanci K, Thomas DT, Yuksel M, Gogus FY. Perioperative anesthetic and surgical complications of the Nuss procedure. *J Cardiothorac Vasc Anesth.* 2013;27(3):436–440.
13. Lacquet LK. Surgical treatment of anterior chest wall deformities by sternochondroplasty and internal fixation without prosthesis. *Acta Chir Belg.* 1982;82(6):541–549.
14. Kang CH, Park S, Park IK, Kim YT, Kim JH. Long-term surveillance comparing satisfaction between the early experience of Nuss procedure vs. Ravitch procedure. *Korean J Thorac Cardiovasc Surg.* 2012;45(5):308–315.
15. Mao YZ, Tang S, Li S. Comparison of the Nuss versus Ravitch procedure for pectus excavatum repair: an updated meta-analysis. *J Pediatr Surg.* 2017;52(10):1545–1552.
16. Fonkalsrud EW. 912 open pectus excavatum repairs: changing trends, lessons learned: one surgeon's experience. *World J Surg.* 2009;33(2):180–190.
17. Gibreel W, Zendejas B, Joyce D, Moir CR, Zarroug AE. Minimally invasive repairs of pectus excavatum: surgical outcomes, quality of life, and predictors of reoperation. *J Am Coll Surg.* 2016;222(3): 245–252.
18. Morshuis W, Folgering H, Barentsz J, Vanlier H, Lacquet L. Pulmonary function before surgery for pectus excavatum and at long-term follow-up. *Chest.* 1994;105(6):1646–1652.
19. Johnson JN, Hartman TK, Pianosi PT, Driscoll DJ. Cardiorespiratory function after operation for pectus excavatum. *J Pediatr.* 2008;153(3):359–364.
20. Neviere R, Pentiah AD, Montaigne D, Wurtz A. Pectus excavatum repair improves cardiovascular function at maximal exercise by facilitating heart filling. *Eur J Cardiothorac Surg.* 2013;43(3):661.
21. Neviere R, Benhamed L, Duva Pentiah A, Wurtz A. Pectus excavatum repair improves respiratory pump efficacy and cardiovascular function at exercise. *J Thorac Cardiovasc Surg.* 2013;145(2): 605–606.
22. Sigalet DL, Montgomery M, Harder J. Cardiopulmonary effects of closed repair of pectus excavatum. *J Pediatr Surg.* 2003; 38(3):380–385.
23. Hebra A, Kelly RE, Ferro MM, Yuksel M, Campos JRM, Nuss D. Life-threatening complications and mortality of minimally invasive pectus surgery. *J Pediatr Surg.* 2018;53(4):728–732.
24. Castellani C, Schalamon J, Saxena AK, Hoellwarth ME. Early complications of the Nuss procedure for pectus excavatum: a prospective study. *Pediatr Surg Int.* 2008;24(6):659–666.
25. Castellani C, Saxena AK, Zebedin D, Hoellwarth ME. Pleural and pericardial morbidity after minimal access repair of pectus excavatum. *Langenbecks Arch Surg.* 2009;394(4):717–721.
26. Croitoru DP, Kelly RE, Jr., Goretsky MJ, Lawson ML, Swoveland B, Nuss D. Experience and modification update for the minimally invasive Nuss technique for pectus excavatum repair in 303 patients. *J Pediatr Surg.* 2002;37(3):437–445.
27. Park HJ, Lee SY, Lee CS. Complications associated with the Nuss procedure: Analysis of risk factors and suggested measures for prevention of complications. *J Pediatr Surg.* 2004;39(3): 391–394.
28. Notrica DM. The Nuss procedure for repair of pectus excavatum: 20 error traps and a culture of safety. *Semin Pediatr Surg.* 2019; 28(3):172–177.
29. de Campos JR, Fonseca MH, Werebe Ede C, Velhote MC, Jatene FB. Technical modification of the Nuss operation for the correction of pectus excavatum. *Clinics (Sao Paulo).* 2006; 61(2):185–186.
30. Fox ME, Bensard DD, Roaten JB, Hendrickson RJ. Positioning for the Nuss procedure: avoiding brachial plexus injury. *Paediatr Anaesth.* 2005;15(12):1067–1071.
31. Muhly WT, Maxwell LG, Cravero JP. Pain management following the Nuss procedure: a survey of practice and review. *Acta Anaesthesiol Scand.* 2014;58(9):1134–1139.
32. Hermanides J, Hollmann MW, Stevens MF, Lirk P. Failed epidural: causes and management. *Br J Anaesth.* 2012;109(2):144–154.
33. Singhal NR, Jones J, Semenova J, et al. Multimodal anesthesia with the addition of methadone is superior to epidural analgesia: A retrospective comparison of intraoperative anesthetic techniques and pain management for 124 pediatric patients undergoing the Nuss procedure. *J Pediatr Surg.* 2016;51(4):612–616.
34. Antonoff MB, Erickson AE, Hess DJ, Acton RD, Saltzman DA. When patients choose: comparison of Nuss, Ravitch, and Leonard procedures for primary repair of pectus excavatum. *J Pediatr Surg.* 2009;44(6):1113–1118.
35. Molik KA, Engum SA, Rescorla FJ, West KW, Scherer LR, Grosfeld JL. Pectus excavatum repair: experience with standard and minimal invasive techniques. *J Pediatr Surg.* 2001;36(2):324–328.
36. Papic JC, Finnell SM, Howenstein AM, Breckler F, Leys CM. Postoperative opioid analgesic use after Nuss versus Ravitch pectus excavatum repair. *J Pediatr Surg.* 2014;49(6):919–923.
37. Allison CE, Aronson DC, Geukers VG, van den Berg R, Schlack WS, Hollmann MW. Paraplegia after thoracotomy under combined general and epidural anesthesia in a child. *Paediatr Anaesth.* 2008;18(6):539–542.
38. Giebler RM, Scherer RU, Peters J. Incidence of neurologic complications related to thoracic epidural catheterization. *Anesthesiology.* 1997;86(1):55–63.
39. Weber T, Matzl J, Rokitansky A, et al. Superior postoperative pain relief with thoracic epidural analgesia versus intravenous patient-controlled analgesia after minimally invasive pectus excavatum repair. *J Thorac Cardiovasc Surg.* 2007;134(4):865–870.
40. St Peter SD, Weesner KA, Weissend EE, et al. Epidural vs patient-controlled analgesia for postoperative pain after pectus excavatum repair: a prospective, randomized trial. *J Pediatr Surg.* 2012;47(1):148–153.
41. Schlatter MG, Nguyen LV, Tecos M, Kalbfell EL, Gonzalez-Vega O, Vlahu T. Progressive reduction of hospital length of stay following minimally invasive repair of pectus excavatum: A retrospective comparison of three analgesia modalities, the role of addressing patient anxiety, and reframing patient expectations. *J Pediatr Surg.* 2019;54(4):663–669.
42. Jaroszewski DE, Temkit M, Ewais MM, et al. Randomized trial of epidural vs. subcutaneous catheters for managing pain after modified Nuss in adults. *J Thorac Dis.* 2016;8(8):2102–2110.
43. Loftus PD, Elder CT, Russell KW, et al. Paravertebral regional blocks decrease length of stay following surgery for pectus excavatum in children. *J Pediatr Surg.* 2016;51(1):149–153.

44. Qi J, Du B, Gurnaney H, Lu P, Zuo Y. A prospective randomized observer-blinded study to assess postoperative analgesia provided by an ultrasound-guided bilateral thoracic paravertebral block for children undergoing the Nuss procedure. *Reg Anesth Pain Med.* 2014;39(3):208–213.
45. Gourlay GK, Wilson PR, Glynn CJ. Pharmacodynamics and pharmacokinetics of methadone during the perioperative period. *Anesthesiology.* 1982;57(6):458–467.
46. Khanbhai M, Yap KH, Mohamed S, Dunning J. Is cryoanalgesia effective for post-thoracotomy pain? *Interact Cardiovasc Thorac Surg.* 2014;18(2):202–209.
47. Graves C, Idowu O, Lee S, Padilla B, Kim S. Intraoperative cryoanalgesia for managing pain after the Nuss procedure. *J Pediatr Surg.* 2017;52(6):920–924.
48. Harbaugh CM, Johnson KN, Kein CE, et al. Comparing outcomes with thoracic epidural and intercostal nerve cryoablation after Nuss procedure. *J Surg Res.* 2018;231:217–223.
49. Keller BA, Kabagambe SK, Becker JC, et al. Intercostal nerve cryoablation versus thoracic epidural catheters for postoperative analgesia following pectus excavatum repair: Preliminary outcomes in twenty-six cryoablation patients. *J Pediatr Surg.* 2016;51(12): 2033–2038.
50. Parrado R, Lee J, McMahon LE, et al. The use of cryoanalgesia in minimally invasive repair of pectus excavatum: lessons learned. *J Laparoendosc Adv Surg Tech A.* 2019;29(10):1244–1251.

42

Tracheal Resection and Reconstruction

ELIZABETH CORDES BEHRINGER, ROGER S. WILSON

Introduction

Anesthetic management of the patient who requires surgical resection of a portion of the large airways continues to challenge the skills of even the most experienced anesthesiologist. The large airways, including the trachea, carina, and major bronchi, can harbor myriad pathologic conditions that necessitate surgical resection and reconstruction.[1–3] The patient presenting for airway surgery is often complex medically. Existing disease states frequently contribute to the development of lesions of the large airways. A specific perioperative plan should be developed in concert with the surgical team, including knowledge of the extent and location of the large airway pathology, as well as the planned surgical approach. The degree of existing airway compromise must be anticipated, as coordination and sharing of the airway occurs throughout airway resection and reanastomosis. Lastly, emergence and extubation needs to be carefully timed. Perioperative care of these patients requires a multidisciplinary team approach and exemplary communication.[4]

The goals of this chapter are to review the etiology of large airway lesions; preoperative evaluation, including pulmonary function testing and radiologic evaluation; and anesthetic management techniques for tracheal resection and reconstruction. Postoperative care of this patient population is outlined.[4–7]

Historical Overview

Before 1960, management of patients with tracheal lesions was extremely conservative. Extrathoracic lesions required permanent tracheostomy, while distal lesions were managed by serial palliative dilation or, rarely, limited resection.[4] Subsequent advances in diagnosis, medical management, anesthetic and surgical techniques, and postoperative intensive care have allowed the successful primary resection and reanastomosis of a wide variety of complex large airway lesions.

Pertinent Anatomy of the Upper Airway and Trachea

The lower airway in adults includes the trachea, bronchi, and bronchi terminating in alveoli.[8] The trachea is tubular and comprised of 16 to 20 incomplete cartilages anterolaterally and a fibromuscular membrane posteriorly. As observed during bronchoscopy, the posterior fibromuscular wall of the trachea will bulge into the tracheal lumen during expiration and coughing.

The adult trachea measures 10 to 11 cm in length, and 2 cm in external diameter in males and 1.5 cm in females. It extends from the level of the sixth cervical vertebrae, which coincides with the laryngeal inlet, to the fifth thoracic vertebrae, which coincides with the carina. One-third of the length of the trachea is extrathoracic and resides above the level of the sternal notch. Flexion of the neck causes more of the trachea to reside within the mediastinum. Neck extension has the opposite effect and moves the trachea into a more cervical position. This anatomic relationship is crucial in both the surgical exposure and postoperative healing of patients undergoing tracheal resection and reconstruction.[6]

The blood supply of the trachea includes branches from the inferior thyroid, subclavian, innominate, internal thoracic, first intercostal, and bronchial arteries. These branches enter the trachea laterally. Avoiding circumferential dissection of the trachea during airway surgery maintains an adequate blood supply. Despite an extensive vascular supply and ample lymphatic drainage, the tracheal mucosa is pressure sensitive, such as those forces exerted by an endotracheal tube or its inflated cuff. Medical conditions, such as diabetes mellitus or prior radiation, may further compromise tracheal blood supply and jeopardize anastomotic healing.[6]

Lastly, the innervation of the larynx and trachea are vagally mediated via the superior and recurrent laryngeal nerves. The recurrent laryngeal nerve lies within the groove between the trachea and the esophagus. As a result, the recurrent laryngeal nerve can be injured because of tracheal pathology or surgical manipulation.[6]

Etiology of Tracheal Lesions

Tracheal lesions arise from a diverse array of pathologic causes (Box 42.1). Postintubation injuries, trauma, primary and secondary tumors, congenital anomalies, vascular lesions, infectious agents, and certain connective tissue diseases may lead to substantial tracheal pathology. Knowledge of the existing tracheal pathology is essential and invariably dictates the anesthetic regimen, as well as the surgical approach.

• Box 42.1 Etiology of Tracheal Lesions

Congenital lesions

- Tracheal agenesis/atresia
- Congenital stenosis
- Congenital chondromalacia

Neoplastic lesions

Primary neoplasms

- Squamous cell carcinoma
- Adenoid cystic carcinoma (cylindroma)
- Carcinoid adenoma
- Carcinosarcoma-chondrosarcoma

Secondary neoplasms

- Bronchogenic carcinoma
- Esophageal carcinoma
- Tracheal carcinoma
- Breast carcinoma
- Head/neck carcinoma

Postintubation injuries

- Laryngeal stenosis
- Cuff injury
- Ulceration/fistula
- Granuloma formation

Posttracheostomy injury

- Cuff lesions
- Stroma lesions

Trauma

- Penetrating
- Blunt injuries
- Cervical
- Intrathoracic

Infection

From Behringer EC, Wilson RS. Tracheal resection and reconstruction. In: Cohen EC (ed). *The Practice of Thoracic Anesthesia*. Philadelphia PA: J.B. Lippincott Co; 1995:531–561; McRae K. Tracheal resection and reconstruction. In: Slinger P. (ed). *Principles and Practice of Anesthesia for Thoracic Surgery*. Switzerland: Springer Nature; 2019:231–248.

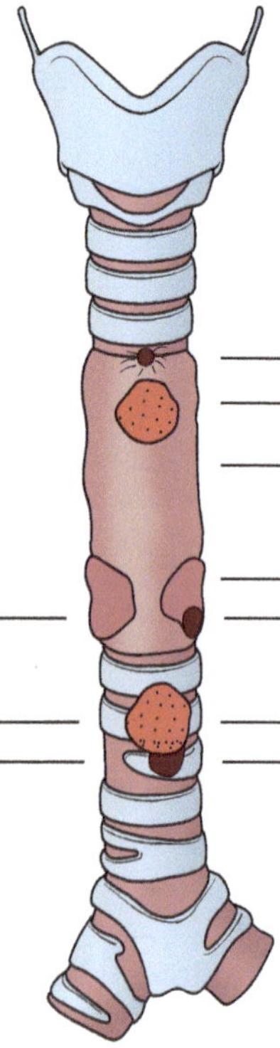

• Fig. 42.1 The most frequent types and locations of injuries in the adult trachea after intubation and tracheostomy. (From Grillo HC. The management of tracheal stenosis following assisted respiration. *J Thorac Cardiovasc Surg*. 1969;57:521. With permission.)

Postintubation injury was the leading cause of tracheal stenosis in a large series by Grillo and colleagues in a group of 503 patients. who underwent 521 tracheal resection and reconstructions for postintubation stenosis over a 27-year period.[9] There were 251 cuff-related lesions, 178 stomal lesions, 38 lesions at two levels. and 36 of undetermined origin. Postintubation tracheal lesions may occur as a result of "traumatic" intubation or secondary to prolonged pressure from an endotracheal tube cuff or tracheostomy.[9] Postintubation injuries may be apparent throughout the adult trachea, as illustrated in Fig. 42.1.[1] The locations of the postintubation injuries varied as well. Sixty-two patients with significant laryngeal injuries required complete resection of the anterior cricoid cartilage and anastomosis of the trachea to the thyroid cartilage. In 117 patients, the trachea was anastomosed to the cricoid cartilage.[9]

Factors predisposing to significant tracheal mucosal injury and the risk for the development of tracheal stenosis in an intubated patient include: (1) prolonged hypotension, (2) concurrent infection, and (3) persistent elevation of endotracheal tube or tracheostomy cuff pressures.

These factors predispose to tracheal damage by impeding mucosal blood flow, despite the widespread use of high-volume, low-pressure endotracheal tube cuffs.[7] Posterior glottic stenosis and circumferential subglottic stenosis result from direct trauma from the endotracheal tube and cuff.[7] High cuff pressures are entirely avoidable by the judicious use of the appropriate size of endotracheal or tracheostomy tube, as well as frequent monitoring of cuff pressures in all intubated patients. Cuff pressures should be maintained below 25 mm Hg whenever possible.[4] The risk of tracheal injury increases with the length of time the patient remains intubated. However, mucosal injury leading to tracheal ulceration has been noted after 2 to 3 hours in certain patients.[10]

Neoplasms are the second major indication for primary tracheal resection and reconstruction.

Over a 26-year period, 198 patients with primary tracheal tumors were evaluated. Some 147 tumors were excised (74%); 70 patients had squamous cell carcinoma (36%), 80 had adenoid cystic carcinoma (40%), and the remaining 48 (24%) had a variety of lesions.[11]

Secondary tumors of the trachea are also seen.[12] Metastatic cancers of the mediastinum comprise this group. Thyroid, esophageal, bronchogenic, and breast cancers can invade the trachea; thymomas, lymphomas, and carcinomas of the head and neck may be secondary tracheal neoplasms. Thyroid tumors occurred most frequently in this group. Such tumors cause extrinsic compression of the trachea or symptoms of upper airway obstruction by direct invasion of the trachea. Thyroid carcinomas are the most amenable to palliation and cure.

Trauma to the tracheobronchial tree may result from blunt or penetrating injuries. Failure to recognize acute airway injuries and provide an adequate airway may result in death or eventual laryngotracheal stenosis.[13] Mathisen and Grillo reported a series of 10 patients with acute laryngotracheal injuries.[13] Blunt trauma to the trachea and larynx occurred in 50% of patients with acute laryngotracheal injuries. Penetrating injuries, such as gunshot or stab wounds, affected 40% of these patients. Traumatic attempts at intubation composed the remaining 10% of acute laryngotracheal injuries. Blunt trauma to the head, neck, and chest were the most common associated injuries in patients with laryngotracheal injury. The laryngotracheal junction, the most frequent site of injury, occurred in six patients. Sudden deceleration injuries resulted in injury to the posterior membranous wall of the trachea involving the carina in two patients. All patients in this series underwent successful definitive primary repair of their airway injuries and maintained an excellent airway postoperatively. It is critical to remember that failure to identify acute laryngotracheal injury can result in progressive airway obstruction, as scarring occurs and stenosis develops.[13]

Cicala and colleagues reviewed the initial evaluation and management of upper airway injuries in a trauma population.[14] Some 46 cases of upper airway injury admitted to a large, metropolitan, university-affiliated trauma center were reviewed retrospectively over a 4-year period. A total of 26 cases of upper airway injury were the result of penetrating trauma; 17 injuries were caused by gunshot wounds and nine were resulting from knife wounds. The remaining 20 patients sustained blunt trauma to their upper airway. Motor vehicle accidents, the leading cause of this trauma, occurred in 13 patients. Diagnostic findings were varied, as illustrated in Table 42.1. The location of the injury was the larynx in 13 cases, the trachea in 24 cases, the cricoid cartilage in five cases, and multiple sites in four cases. The overall mortality rate in this series was 24%, and this rate did not vary according to patient age or mechanism of injury. Appropriate initial airway management depends on the rapid accurate diagnosis of the extent and location of the upper airway injury.[14]

Preoperative Evaluation

Thorough preoperative diagnostic evaluation of patients with obstructive lesions of the airway is mandatory. Chapter 8 describes preoperative evaluation of the thoracic surgical patient in detail. Diagnostic evaluation entails a detailed history and physical examination, pulmonary function studies, imaging studies, and bronchoscopy. The diagnostic regimen is often dictated by the severity and urgency of airway compromise. For example, in life-threatening situations in which there is a high index of suspicion as to the nature of the tracheal pathology, bronchoscopy may be the primary method of diagnosis, in addition to the detailed history and physical examination. On the contrary, the patient presenting for elective repair warrants a detailed evaluation.[7]

History and Physical Examination

A detailed history can be revealing in several areas. The physician should seek etiologies likely to produce airway compromise, such as an antecedent history of endotracheal intubation or tracheostomy. Such patients should be considered to have an organic lesion until proven otherwise.[4,6,7]

The signs and symptoms of large airway obstruction are affected by several factors. The anatomic location of the lesion, the severity of airway obstruction, and the presence of preexisting cardiopulmonary disease are important variables to consider. Clinical symptoms of airway obstruction include dyspnea, especially with effort, and

TABLE 42.1 Diagnostic Findings in Patients With Airway Injuries

	Stab Wound (*n* = 9)	Gunshot Wound (*n* = 17)	Blunt Trauma (*n* = 20)
Radiographic soft tissue air	3 (33%)	9 (53%)	10 (50%)
Subcutaneous emphysema[a]	3 (33%)	4 (24%)	8 (40%)
Airway open into wound	5 (56%)	4 (24%)	1 (11%)
Computerized tomography	0	1 (11%)	4 (24%)
Bronchoscopy	1 (11%)	1 (11%)	1 (11%)
Pneumothorax	0	2 (12%)	0
Sudden loss of airway	0	0	2 (12%)
Autopsy	0	0	1 (11%)

[a]All patients with subcutaneous emphysema also had soft tissue present on radiography.
From Cicala RS, Kudsk KA, Butts A, et al. Initial evaluation and management of upper airway injuries in trauma patients. *J Clin Anesth*. 1991;2:91–98;)

wheezing, which may present as frank stridor. Persistent cough, hoarseness, and difficulty in clearing secretions are other common symptoms. Complete airway obstruction may occur from inability to clear secretions because of an underlying organic lesion. Adult patients become symptomatic when the cross-sectional diameter of the airway is reduced to approximately 8 mm or roughly 50% of normal.[15] Extremely active adults may have symptoms with a milder degree of airway obstruction. Stridor at rest is indicative of severe airway narrowing (5–6 mm).[16,17] Patients with stridor have extremely tenuous airways. Such patients deserve close monitoring, which may warrant preoperative admission to an intensive care unit. Vocal cord or recurrent laryngeal nerve pathology is indicated by hoarseness. Direct or indirect laryngeal examination is necessary.

The symptoms described earlier are frequently misdiagnosed. Several patients, especially those with tracheal tumors, have been diagnosed as having "asthma." An alternative diagnosis is entertained only when "asthma" is unresponsive to conventional medical therapy, which often includes the use of corticosteroids.[18,19] The severity of the tracheal stenosis, graded from I to IV, is depicted in Fig. 42.2.

To review, a detailed history is essential in the patient with a known or suspected tracheal pathology. Salient points include a history of smoking, prior intubation, or tracheostomy. A precise evaluation of the patient's exercise tolerance is warranted, including any recent onset of hoarseness or stridor, inability to tolerate the supine position, persistent cough, or inability to clear secretions. The severity of preexisting cardiopulmonary disease may limit the patient's exercise tolerance. Tracheal lesions may present at an advanced stage when this occurs.

A careful physical examination entails a detailed examination of the airway. The trachea should be palpated for extrathoracic compression or deviation. Audible stridor, either at rest or with a maximal expiratory effort with an open mouth, is often elicited. Auscultation of the chest may reveal diffuse inspiratory and expiratory wheezing, which is difficult to differentiate from bronchospasm. Auscultation of the upper cervical airway may reveal high pitched inspiratory and expiratory sounds characteristic of air flow obstruction. The anesthesiologist's preoperative evaluation should include assessment for anticipated difficulty with mask ventilation, intubation, or both; the degree of airway limitation because of tracheal pathology; and any anticipated perioperative issues.[6,20]

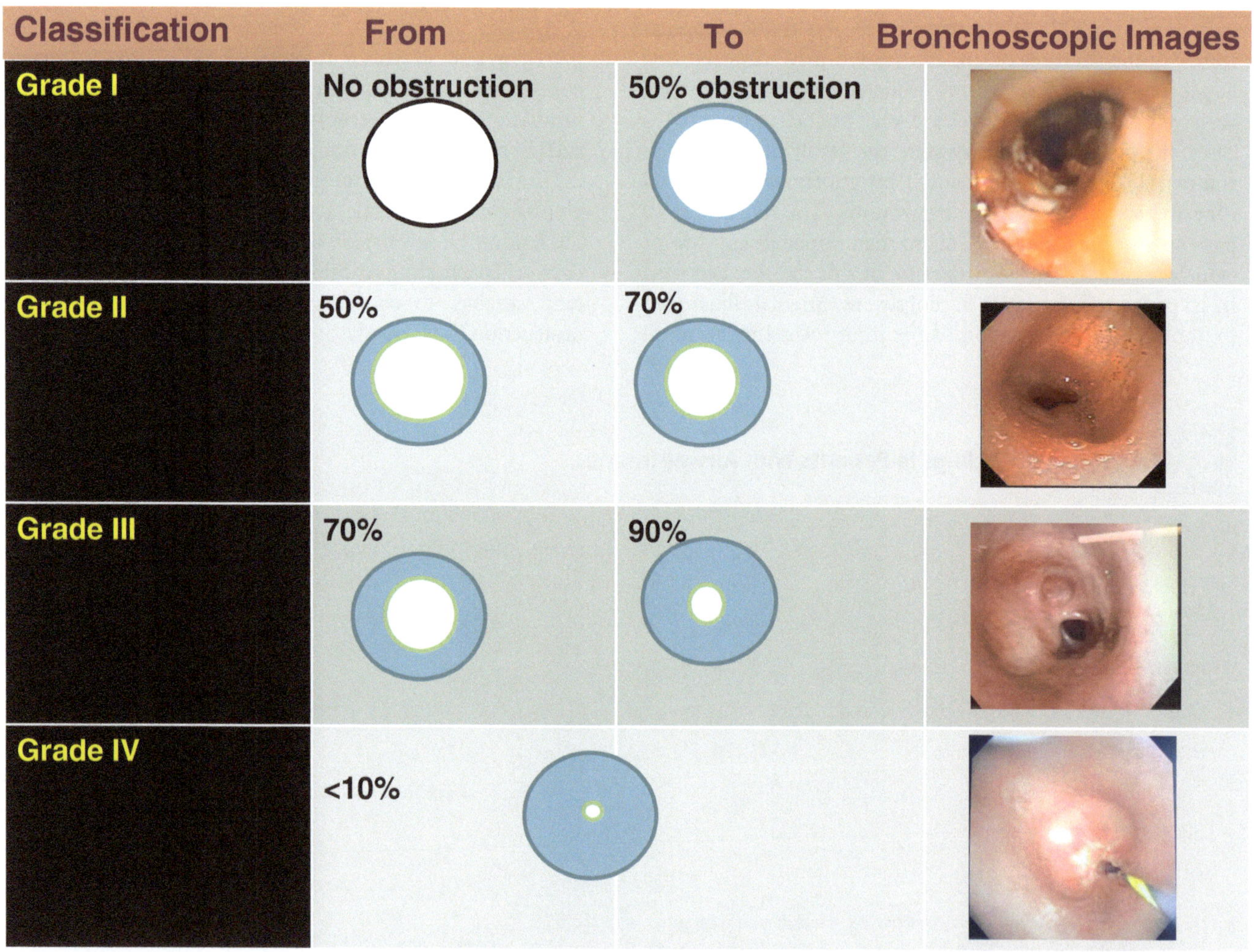

• **Fig. 42.2** The severity of tracheal stenosis, graded for I–IV. (Courtesy of Edmond Cohen, MD.)

The range of motion of the neck is an essential component of the physical examination. The patient should be able to tolerate both hyperextension and hyperflexion comfortably. Several disease states are associated with instability of the cervical spine (Box 42.2).[21,22] If the cervical spine motion limitation is in question, it should be evaluated radiographically before surgery in nonurgent cases. The type and function of the in situ tracheal appliance is important to ascertain preoperatively.[23] The patient may have a cuffed or cuffless tracheostomy tube in situ. The location of the tracheal appliance in relationship to the lesion is also important. The patient's tolerance of decannulation should be determined. The stoma should be patent and stable, and the patient should give a history of relatively stable airway if decannulated. The existing tracheal appliance may then be removed and replaced with a cuffed tube before the induction of general anesthesia. A recent tracheostomy of less than 2 weeks should only be managed by qualified team.

Diagnostic Studies

Pulmonary Function Tests

Standard spirometry may demonstrate reduction in measured air flow during inspiration and expiration, but this technique is of limited value in the diagnosis of obstructive airway lesions. The maximal expiratory and inspiratory flow is characteristically affected to a far greater degree than is the forced expiratory volume in 1 second (FEV_1). The ratio peak expiratory flow of FEV_1 is a useful index of obstruction. A ratio of 10:1 or more is suggestive of airway obstruction.

The flow-volume loop is a very reliable and specific test in diagnosis of upper airway obstruction (Fig. 42.3).[24,25] During a forced expiration from total lung capacity, the maximal flow achieved during the first 25% of the vital capacity depends on effort alone. In general, a circumferential stenosis, such as those produced by cuff lesions, is fixed in origin. Pedunculated tumors and tracheomalacia produce intermittent obstructions. In the case of fixed airway obstruction, the peak expiratory flow is markedly reduced, producing a characteristic plateau. With fixed intrathoracic and extrathoracic lesions, the inspiratory flow has the same characteristic plateau. In case of a variable obstruction, the maximal cutoff of inspiratory or expiratory flow depends on the location of the lesion. Extrathoracic or cervical lesions produce a plateau during inspiration, with minimal effect on expiratory flow. Variable intrathoracic lesions tend to demonstrate alterations in expiratory flow curve with minimal or no effect on inspiration (Fig. 42.4).

• Box 42.2 Syndromes Associated With Odontoid Hypoplasia and Conditions Associated With Atlantoaxial Subluxation

Syndromes Associated With Odontoid Hypoplasia

Morguio syndrome
Klippel-Feil syndrome
Down syndrome
Spondyloepiphyseal dysplasia
Dysproportionate dwarfism
Congenital scoliosis
Osteogenesis imperfecta
Neurofibromatosis

Conditions Associated With Atlantoaxial Subluxation

A: Congenital

Down syndrome
Odontoid anomalies
Muccopolysaccharidoses

B: Acquired

Rheumatoid arthritis
Still disease
Ankylosing spondylitis
Psoriatic arthritis
Enteropathic arthritis–Crohn disease
- Ulcerative colitis
Reiter syndrome
Trauma–odontoid fracture
- Ligamentous disruption

From Crosby E. Airway management after upper cervical spine injury: what have we learned. *Can J Anaesth*. 2002;49:733–744;

Radiologic Evaluation

Multidetector computed tomography (MDCT) is an accurate, noninvasive method for evaluating tracheal anatomy and pathology. MDCT allows for precise anatomic location of tracheal pathology, as well as information on the degree of the tracheal obstruction and on the surrounding structures. All of this information assists in surgical planning.[26] Although bronchoscopy remains an invaluable diagnostic tool, MDCT has several benefits. It is noninvasive and allows for airway evaluation distal to the area of pathology. In addition, MDCT provides detailed information of surrounding structures in the neck and chest.[26]

Other Studies

Laboratory studies obtained in the patient presenting for tracheal resection and reconstruction should consider the patient's underlying medical history. Assessment of cardiopulmonary function is particularly important. The patient may require an echocardiogram and/or myocardial perfusion imaging, in addition to an invaluable routine electrocardiogram, to evaluate a history of cardiac dysfunction, myocardial ischemic risk, and valvular and ventricular function. Room air saturation, as well as arterial blood gas, may be obtained preoperatively to serve as a guideline of baseline oxygenation and ventilation. Any documentation or anesthetic records from a recent bronchoscopy should be reviewed. It should be noted that tracheal lesions caused by either inflammation (postintubation stenosis) or tumors can quickly accelerate over a short period of time.[6]

The patient should be evaluated with the anticipation that any intraoperative difficulties associated with the

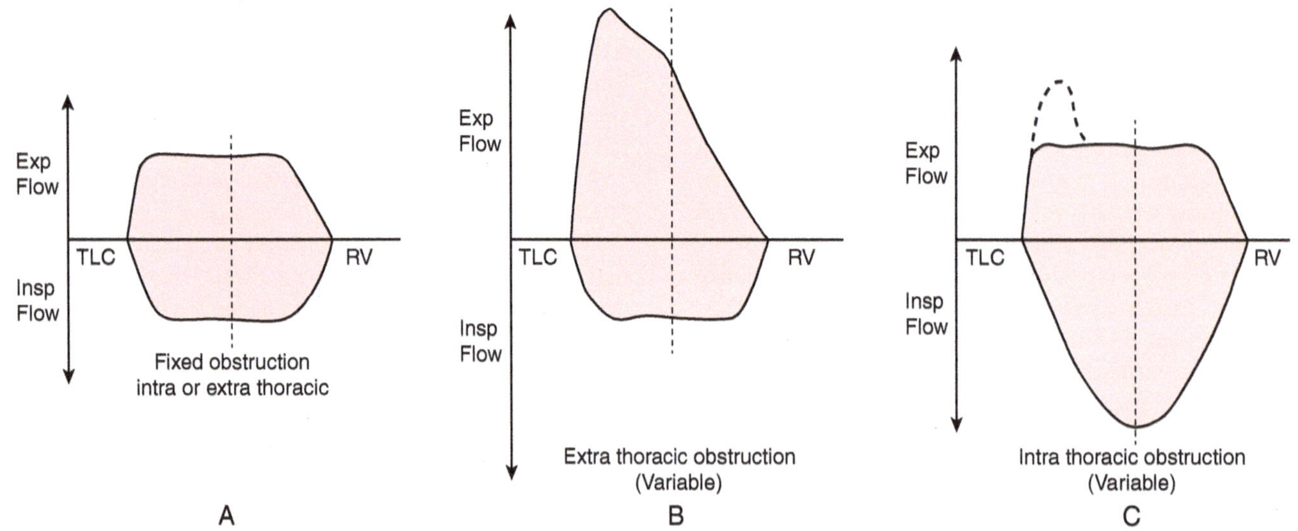

• **Fig. 42.3** Maximal inspiratory and expiratory flow-volume curves in fixed obstruction, (**A**) extrathoracic variable obstruction (**B**) and intrathoracic variable obstruction. (**C**) The *dashed line* represents a flow transient that occasionally is observed just before the plateau in intrathoracic obstruction. See text for full description. *RV*, Residual volume; *TLC*, total lung capacity.

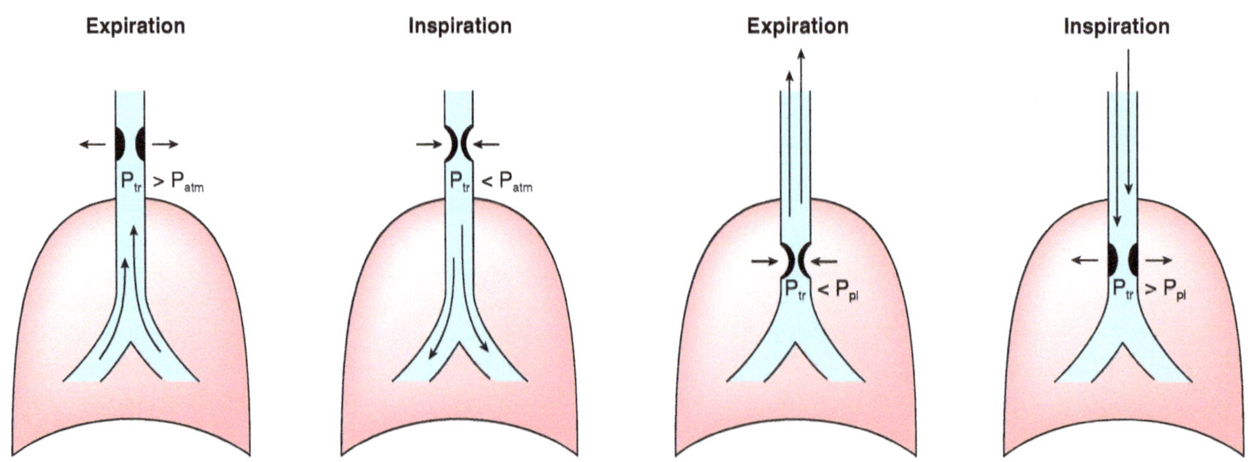

• **Fig. 42.4** Effect of the phase of respiration on an extrathoracic variable obstruction. Direction of airflow is indicated by the *long thin arrows*. During forced expiration the intratracheal, pressure (P_{tr}) is greater than the pressure around the airway (P_{atm} = atmospheric pressure), resulting in a decrease of the obstruction. During forced inspiration the pressure acting around the airway (P_{pl} = pleural pressure) may be greater than the intratracheal pressure (P_{tr}), resulting in an increase in the obstruction. During forced inspiration the intratracheal pressure is greater than the pleural pressure, thus decreasing the obstruction.

airway, as well as potential problems during induction, may expose the individual to stress from hypoxia, hypercarbia, or cardiovascular instability. Thus the anesthetic technique used and possible alternatives must be based on these factors in addition to the anticipated surgical approach.

There are a few relative contraindications to tracheal resection and reconstruction[6]:

1. Prior radiation therapy to the head and neck: as this predisposes the patient to anastomotic dehiscence
2. Steroid dependence: as this interferes with wound healing and predisposes to anastomotic dehiscence. Patients should be weaned off of steroids before surgery if feasible
3. Ventilator dependent patients: because of concerns for protracted intubation postoperatively leading to a high risk of anastomotic dehiscence

Intraoperative Management

Set-Up and Monitoring

Available equipment should include[6]:

1. A variety of endotracheal tubes (size 4.0–6.5 mm internal diameter [ID])
2. A sterile reinforced endotracheal tube for ventilation across the surgical field
3. A small size flexible scope (3.5–3.8 mm outer diameter [OD]) to confirm endotracheal tube position and so on
4. A range of rigid ventilating bronchoscopes
5. An airway exchange catheter in the event that catheter exchange of the rigid bronchoscope to an endotracheal tube is necessary[27,28]

In addition to a standard anesthetic monitoring, the following should be considered[6,7]:

1. Two functional peripheral intravenous (IV) catheters; the patient's arms will be tucked during the procedure.
2. An arterial catheter; preferably in the left radial artery. Selection of the site of arterial cannulation is governed by the availability of appropriate vessels. However, the left radial artery is preferred, as the right radial artery is often compromised owing to compression or, occasionally, deliberate sacrifice of the innominate artery.[6,7]
3. Anesthesia depth monitor because cases are often done under total intravenous anesthesia 9809.
4. Train-of-four monitoring of neuromuscular blockade.
5. A urinary catheter.
6. Central venous access is reserved for patients with a significant cardiac history or for whom use of vasoactive agents is anticipated. If a central line is warranted, the internal jugular should be avoided as its insertion site if this lies within the anticipated surgical field.[6]

There are numerous anesthetic management goals during tracheal resection and reconstruction. The primary goal is the maintenance of an adequate airway from the time of anesthetic induction through the postoperative period. An adequate airway ensures adequacy of oxygenation and ventilation, as well as secretion management. Achieving airway maintenance implies a thorough understanding of the nature and extent of the tracheal lesion, as well as detailed knowledge of the surgical approach.

It is important to recognize that the airway may become tenuous at the several stages of the operation[6,7]:

1. During the induction of general anesthesia in the patient with significant tracheal narrowing.
2. During surgical resection, when the distal airway may become obstructed with secretions and blood. Rarely, the distal trachea may be lost and withdraw into the mediastinum.
3. During the immediate postoperative period because of patient positioning or significant airway edema at the anastomotic site.

Premedication

The patient's airway anatomy and the degree of anxiety expressed during the preoperative assessment govern the approach to premedication. The preoperative visit by the anesthesiologist involved in the patient's care also serves to establish a rapport that helps diminish the need for sedative and analgesic premedication (Chs. 8,9).[29,30] A skillful, instructive, and understanding visit from the anesthesiologist to discuss the anesthetic plan and risks ensures an informed, cooperative, and calm patient.

Patients with significant tracheal narrowing, as determined by history, symptoms, pulmonary function tests, radiologic studies, or previous bronchoscopy, should receive preoperative sedation sparingly, if at all. It is crucial to avoid oversedation and central respiratory depression caused by opiates and benzodiazepines. Atropine and other agents that may produce drying of secretions should also be avoided. Inspissated mucus plugs may form and lead to near total airway obstruction. When in doubt, all premedication should be withheld in patients with critical airway narrowing until the patient arrives in the operating room (OR) under the close supervision of the anesthesiologist and surgeon. It is often prudent to have the anesthesiologist and surgeon transport the patient with a critical airway lesion from the intensive care unit to the OR.

In those patients in whom airway obstruction is minimal, or in whom airway obstruction exists but has been adequately bypassed by either an endotracheal tube or tracheostomy tube, the use of premedication is governed by the patient's needs and the conditions compatible with safe induction of anesthesia.[29,30]

Patient Positioning

Classically, the patient is placed in the supine position with both of the arms tucked and the neck extended. Use of an inflatable thyroid bag under the shoulders is often used to assist with neck extension. The occiput is positioned on a gel "doughnut." Undue neck strain should be avoided.[6,7]

Induction and Bronchoscopic Examination

In patients in whom airway obstruction is of minor significance, owing to either a good natural airway or the presence of an intratracheal appliance, anesthesia may be induced with an intravenous induction agent, such as propofol followed by a nondepolarizing neuromuscular blocking agent. Total intravenous anesthesia is a common modality.[6]

Laryngoscopy is performed, and at this time topical anesthesia, with 4% lidocaine, is applied to the oropharynx and glottis with a bronchial sprayer or its equivalent.[4] When an adequate depth of anesthesia is present, rigid bronchoscopy may be undertaken.

Rigid bronchoscopy allows for careful endoscopic examination to[6]:

1. Note the location and extent of the tracheal pathology
2. Assess the health and function of the vocal cords
3. Assess for areas of tracheal inflammation
4. Assess for areas of tracheomalacia

It is critical for the anesthesiologist to be mindful of the status of the airway with regard to the nature and the extent of the lesion. This is important in terms of appreciating the difficulty of endotracheal tube placement and selection of an appropriate-size endotracheal tube.

There are several potential problems which must be considered at this time. **Lesions involving the upper one-third of the trachea,** especially those in the subglottic region, pose special problems with endotracheal tube placement. A lesion that is located high in the airway does not allow the tube to pass because of its limited orifice, and the cuff does not pass below the cords. This results in inability to attain a complete airway seal. Selection of a tube that is small enough to pass through the lesion can pose additional problems.

The decreased ID of the tube may lead to potential airway obstruction with secretion and blood during the operative procedure.

Lesions located in the middle and lower two-thirds of the trachea have a special set of problems. The endotracheal tube may need to pass through the lesion to maintain oxygenation and ventilation until the trachea is transected. If the airway measures more than 5 mm, an endotracheal tube is generally passed to a point above the stricture in lesions of the lower two-thirds of the trachea. It may also be passed through the stricture in lesions of the upper one-third of the trachea, as previously described.

The lesion may require dilation at the time of rigid bronchoscopy to provide an adequate airway. Tracheal dilation should proceed cautiously, recognizing the risks of significant airway damage, bleeding, or perforation into adjacent structures, such as the esophagus or the great vessels. Grillo describes dilating strictures if the airway measures less than 5 mm in diameter.[31] Tracheal dilation is accomplished under direct vision with several rigid pediatric ventilating bronchoscopes. Bronchoscopes of graded size are exchanged and passed through the trachea in succession. Care should be taken, because dilators passed through a large bronchoscope may easily perforate the tracheobronchial wall, especially if the stricture is in the distal trachea.

Airway tumors must be handled with great caution because direct trauma to the tumor may occur with the passage of the endotracheal tube. The tube may dislodge a piece of the tumor, leading to near complete airway obstruction and the potential for serious hemorrhage into the airway.

Strictures of the anterior tracheal wall or stomal strictures are generally easier to manage. The mobile posterior membranous wall of the trachea usually allows passage of an endotracheal tube or sufficient gas flow beyond the lesion should the tube be positioned above it.

Once rigid bronchoscopy is completed, endotracheal intubation with the appropriate-size tube is performed. As the tube is advanced into the airway, the area of stricture can often be appreciated. A flexible pediatric fiberoptic bronchoscope may be used to confirm the adequacy and location of endotracheal tube placement. At this time, an orogastric tube should be passed to empty the stomach of gas and fluid, despite appropriate preoperative fasting. Once this maneuver is completed, the orogastric tube is removed.[4]

Management of the Critically Obstructed Airway

Serious adverse events related to airway management still occur.[32,33] In 2011 the UK Fourth National Audit Project (NAP4) found that 40% of head, neck, or tracheal cases had at least one significant airway-related adverse event.[32] Nearly 70% of adverse outcomes in the NAP4 study involved an obstructed airway. Despite excellent evidence-based guidelines for advanced airway management,[20,34] currently there is no guidance on best management strategies for the obstructed airway.[35]

Airway patency is dynamic and affected by changes to pressure within the airway. It is well known that airway obstruction can occur during normal sleep or anesthesia because of loss of pharyngeal muscle tone. If an airway lesion is present, there is loss of space within the airway lumen as well. The effects of anesthesia are therefore compounded because of increasing resistance. All anesthetic agents increase the likelihood of airway collapse to some degree.

Patients with critical airway obstruction because of a tracheal lesion may present with increased work of breathing, expiratory stridor, hypoxia, agitation and imminent respiratory failure. The management of severe airway obstruction may occur at any time of day. Management of these challenging patients may involve clinicians without significant prior experience and limited expertise in management of a critical airway. Because there is little time, to investigate these patients, it is crucial to have a preemptive management strategy in place with the entire team, including the surgical, anesthetic, respiratory therapy, and nursing staff.

Lynch and Crawley published an excellent review of the management of airway obstruction.[35]

Considerations include:

1. Identifying the urgency of the patient's status: this should be done in concert with an experienced member of the surgical team.
2. Considering symptom progression. A timeline to intervene should be in place. Respiratory distress and increasing oxygen requirement are late signs.
3. Using temporizing therapies: these may include use of high-flow nasal oxygen (HFNO), steroid therapy, nebulized epinephrine or Heliox.
4. Defining the lesion in terms of location, extent or quality (fixed or mobile), and how this may influence the approach to initial airway management.
5. Identifying where the airway can best be managed safely. Ideally, advanced airway management in the patient with a critical airway stenosis is best managed in the OR. If transport is too risky, then the airway team and the requisite equipment must be mobile.[36]

A variety of temporizing measures may be used while the entire team is mobilized. These include[35]:

1. **HFNO: High flow nasal cannula systems,** such as Optiflow (Fisher & Paykel Healthcare, Auckland, New Zealand), are widely used in critical care and anesthesia.[37] HFNO reduces patient work of breathing, provides continuous positive airway pressure (CPAP), and improves oxygenation. HFNO has numerous applications, including hypoxic respiratory insufficiency,[38,39] awake intubation,[40] prolonging safe duration of apnea without desaturation in high-risk intubation,[41] and provision of tubeless anesthesia.[42] Prolongation of apnea time using HFNO is dependent upon maintaining upper airway patency.[42] In addition, HFNO is a beneficial temporizing maneuver in the perioperative management of airway obstruction.[35]
2. **Steroid therapy:** Scientific evidence supporting the use of steroids in adults with airway obstruction is variable. Its

efficacy in pediatric croup, laryngeal edema, or postextubation stridor is published.[35,43] However, systemic steroids are used frequently as a temporalizing maneuver because of minimal risk during short-term use.[35]

3. **Nebulized epinephrine:** As a vasoconstrictor, nebulized epinephrine is often used in cases of laryngeal edema to reduce stridor.[4,35]
4. **Heliox:** Helium improves airflow as it is less dense than oxygen. Work of breathing is improved by decreasing turbulent airflow through a narrowed upper airway. The utility of Heliox is limited by the reduced availability of oxygen when admixed with helium.[44]

The literature is lacking in high quality evidence that supports any particular approach to airway management in patients with critical airway obstruction.[35] Accordingly, the airway strategy used should be individualized to the underlying pathology, as well as the expertise of the team.

A variety of techniques have been described, including[35]:

1. **Awake intubation techniques:**
   i. Awake intubation with a flexible scope requires an experienced endoscopist, adequacy of topical anesthesia, a cooperative patient, and knowledge of the intratracheal lesion through review of available information. It must be ascertained that the bronchoscope can be maneuvered around or through the lesion. Delivery of the endotracheal tube must be achieved without significant trauma. Awake flexible bronchoscopic intubation can be accomplished with the patient in the sitting position. HFNO should be administered concomitantly as the patient is breathing spontaneously.[40]

   This technique is inappropriate in patients with severe stenosis at the level of the glottis. In this case, passage of the flexible bronchoscope may cause total airway obstruction (the "cork in the bottle" phenomenon).[35]

   ii. Awake videolaryngoscopic–assisted intubation is another technique gaining acceptance.[45] As an awake technique, spontaneous respiratory effort is maintained and airway patency is not further compromised. Use of a hyperangulated blade may minimize patient discomfort.[35] As always, adequacy of topicalization of the upper airway is crucial for any "awake" technique.
2. **Awake tracheostomy:**
   i. Awake tracheostomy should be considered in patients with glottic obstruction. Although this is often considered a "gold standard" for airway management, it is not without inherent challenges.[35] There must be assurance that the level of the pathology is well above the proposed level of the tracheostomy. The patient may not be able to lie flat and the administration of sedatives risks further airway compromise. HFNO is likely beneficial as it will reduce work of breathing and patient distress.[35] Electrocautery should not be applied while HFNO is being used because of the risk of fire.[46]
3. **Inhalation induction and general anesthesia:**
   i. Inhalation induction has been the technique of choice for management of an obstructed airway in many centers.[6] There are several caveats to the use of this technique[35]:
      a. Further airway obstruction may ensue, limiting gas exchange.
      b. Inspiratory effort may induce considerable pharyngeal collapse, worsening airway obstruction. The use of pressure support or CPAP through the anesthesia circuit may assist in maintaining airway patency.
      c. Inhalation induction is a slow process to achieve sufficient anesthetic depth for instrumentation.
4. **Total intravenous anesthesia (TIVA):**
   i. Booth and colleagues published the observational STRIVE Hi study of spontaneous respiration using TIVA and HFNO during management of airway obstruction in 30 patients undergoing elective laryngotracheal surgery.[47]

The authors of this technique succeeded in preserving oxygen saturation, end-tidal carbon dioxide levels, and airway patency.[47]

Summary of the Surgical Procedure

An in-depth description of this procedure is provided elsewhere.[6,7,48] The most commonly used approach uses a small transverse cervical incision ("low collar incision"). The trachea is carefully dissected and mobilized. Care is taken to preserve the blood supply and avoid injury to the recurrent laryngeal nerve.[48]

The trachea is incised and the endotracheal tube withdrawn above the level of the tracheal pathology. A separate incision is made at the distal end of the tracheal pathology. This will tentatively form the lower portion of the anastomosis. Traction sutures around one tracheal ring assist in dissection of the posterior membranous wall of the trachea from the esophagus.

The distal trachea is intubated with a sterile reinforced endotracheal tube and cross-field ventilation occurs through connection to a sterile breathing circuit. End-tidal CO2 monitoring and visual inspection of lung inflation confirms ventilation (Fig. 42.5).

Next, the segment of trachea to be resected is dissected circumferentially and excised (Fig. 42.6). The head and neck are carefully flexed to confirm that the margins of the trachea can be anastomosed easily. The head and neck are returned to the extended position. The posterior membranous wall is sutured followed by the anterior rings. Ventilation can be sporadic at this time. Once the tracheal anastomosis is sutured but not tightly closed, the surgeon passes a sterile urethral catheter retrograde into the hypopharynx. The anesthesiologist retrieves the retrograde catheter and sutures it to the distal end of a new endotracheal tube. Reintubation occurs when the urethral catheter is gently pulled back into the surgical field, the sutures carefully removed from the new endotracheal tube.[4,6,7,48]

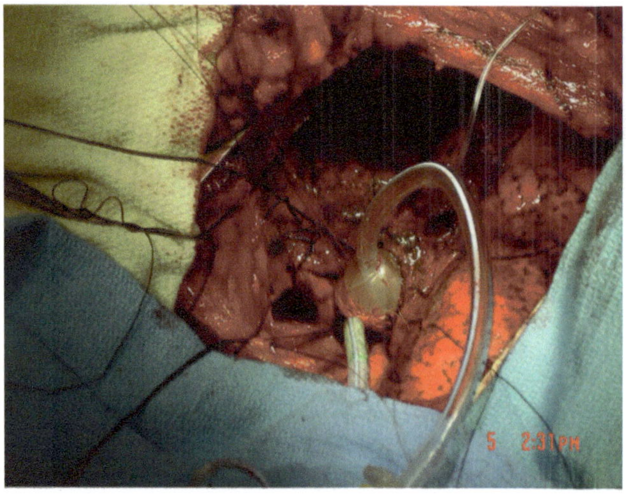

• **Fig. 42.5** Cross-field ventilation. The endotracheal tube is inserted in the distal tracheal lumen. (Courtesy of Edmond Cohen M.D,)

The head and neck are flexed by placing blankets under the patient's head. The endotracheal tube is positioned such that the cuff is distal to the anastomosis. The tracheal anastomosis is carefully closed so that the sutures do not become tangled in the endotracheal tube. This would be catastrophic as anastomotic disruption at the time of extubation would occur[7] (Fig. 42.7).

Once the tracheal anastomosis is closed, a "leak test" is performed by flooding the surgical field with sterile saline, deflating the endotracheal tube cuff and applying 30 cm H_2O pressure through the anesthetic circuit. If no bubbles are seen, the tracheal anastomosis is secure and the incision is closed. A small suction drain is placed in the pretracheal space.

A guardian suture is placed from the skin overlying the patient's manubrium to the submental space to prevent hyperextension during the initial healing phase[4,6,7,48] (Fig. 42.8).

Emergence and Extubation

The end of the procedure has several specific considerations[6]:

1. Safe extubation in the OR with full reversal of neuromuscular blockade
2. Smooth emergence, avoiding vigorous coughing and/or neck extension, which would compromise the surgical anastomosis
3. Maintaining flexion of the head and neck
4. Assessing and managing the possibility of:
   i. Tracheal bleeding
   ii. Tracheal obstruction
   iii. Laryngeal edema
   iv. Vocal cord dysfunction

Anesthetic techniques that allow for a smooth, prompt emergence with mild blunting of airway reflexes are warranted. These could include use of dexmedetomidine, sevoflurane, or low dose remifentanil.[6] Excessive narcotic administration is discouraged.

Extubation can be accomplished by one of the following methods:

1. A supraglottic airway can be placed while the patient is still anesthetized. This is used for smooth emergence,

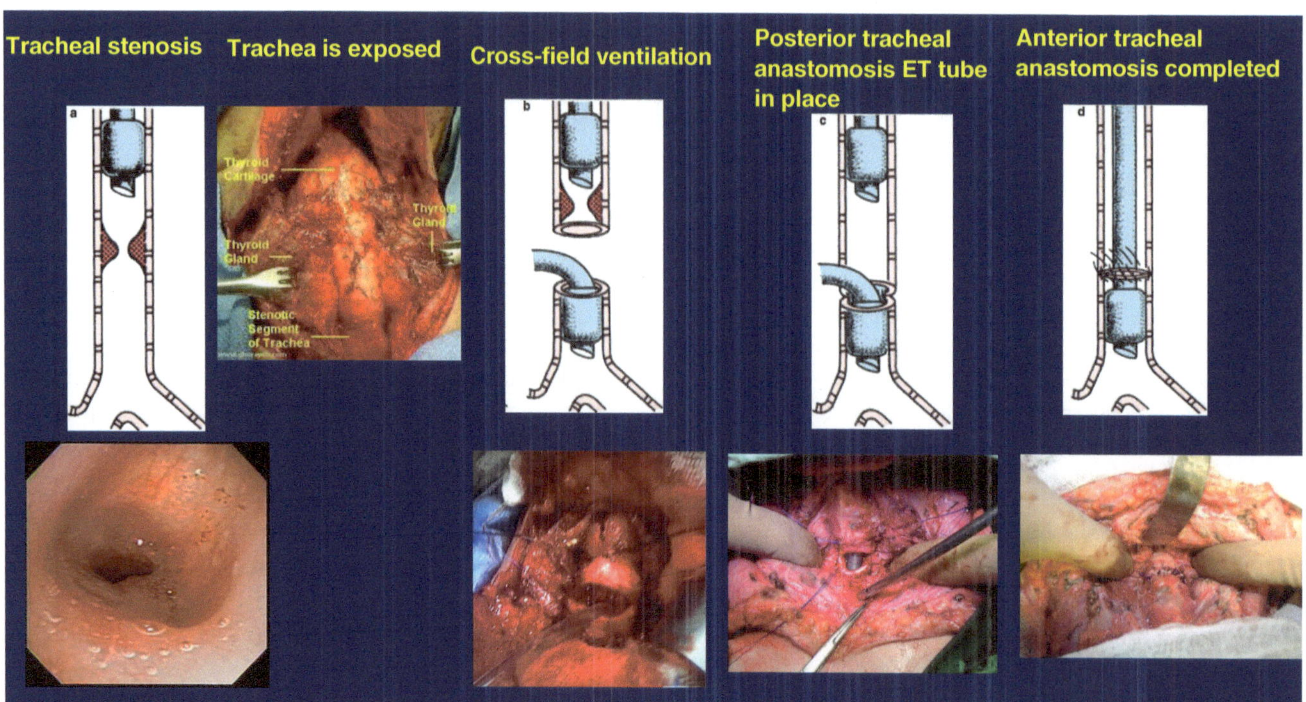

• **Fig. 42.6** Reconstruction of the upper trachea. Collar incision and extension for upper sternotomy. Dissection is carried down to isolate the damaged segment. Circumferential dissection is carried out immediately beneath the level of pathology. Traction sutures are in place and the distal airway intubated via the operating field. *ET*, Endotracheal.

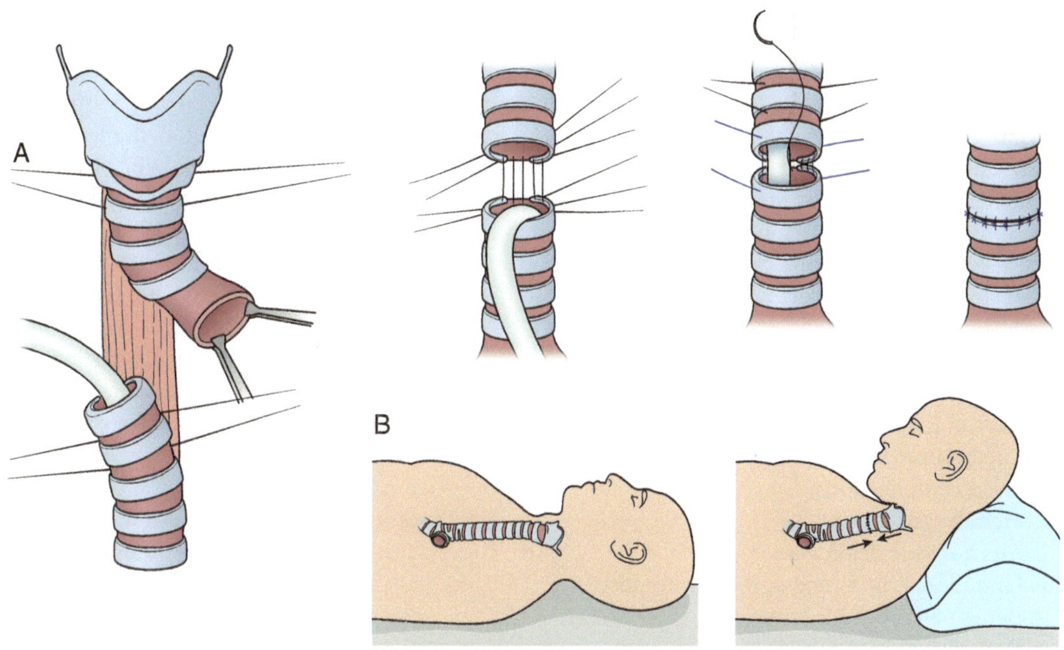

• **Fig. 42.7** Details of anastomotic technique. (**A**) Original endotracheal tube positioned in the upper trachea with the distal trachea intubated. Once all sutures are in place, the endotracheal tube is advanced and the sutures are tied in serial fashion. (**B**) With cervical flexion, the maximum amount of approximation is obtained.

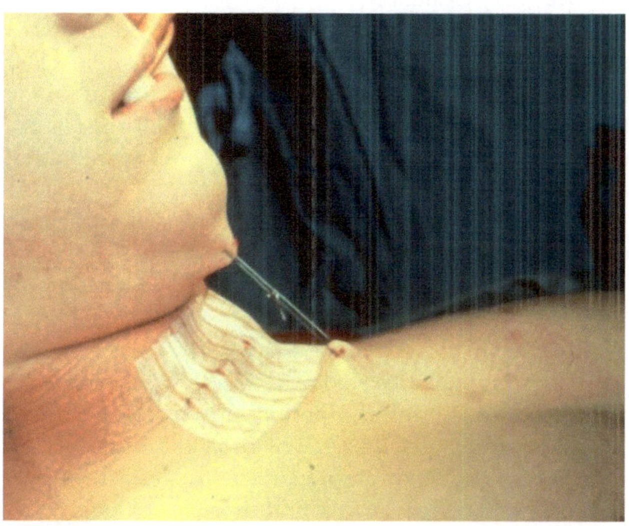

• **Fig.42.8** Guardian suture and cervical collar incision. (From Parikh D, Rajesh P (eds). *Tips and tricks in thoracic surgery*. Springer; 2018.)

fiberoptic assessment of vocal cord function, and pulmonary toilet of airway secretions.[49]

2. The endotracheal tube is simply removed once the oropharynx is suctioned, and the patient demonstrates wakefulness and adequacy of respiratory mechanics, as well as the ability to maintain an adequate airway.[6,7]

The patient is asked to vocalize following extubation to assess for any injury to the recurrent laryngeal nerve. A dedicated member of the OR team assists in gently maintaining neck flexion following extubation. The patient is positioned on the gurney in the sitting position with supplemental oxygen during transport to the intensive care unit.[48]

Schieren and colleagues recently published a systematic review and metaanalysis of approaches to airway management during tracheal resection.[50] Their review included 59 publications with 797 patients from 1965 to 2016. The most common approach was induction of general anesthesia, endotracheal tube placement, and cross-field intubation following tracheal incision (71.2% of studies). Three other approaches to airway management were identified, including regional anesthesia (25 cases), use of a supraglottic airway (4 cases) and extracorporeal support (25 cases). However, the gold standard for airway management during tracheal resection and reconstruction remains the technique described earlier.

Jet ventilation has been described as a ventilation strategy for tracheal resection and reconstruction.[6,7] Jet ventilation has been used intraoperatively to ventilate the distal tracheal across the surgical field. Advantages of this technique include better exposure of the surgical field owing to the small diameter of the jet ventilation catheter. Disadvantages include risk of barotrauma, dispersion of blood and secretions from the operative site into the OR environment and distal trachea, a less precise monitoring of end-tidal carbon dioxide. This topic is covered in Chapter 14 and in detail elsewhere.[51]

Postoperative Care and Potential Complications

Patients are admitted postoperatively to the intensive care unit. Monitoring includes electrocardiogram, pulse oximetry, and arterial pressure. A radiograph of the chest is obtained shortly after arrival to ensure that a pneumothorax is not present. Sufficient oxygen is administered with humidification via a face mask to provide adequate arterial oxygenation and thinning of secretions. The head is maintained in the flexed position with the use of several firm pillows placed behind the occiput.

Chest physical therapy and routine nursing procedures are dictated by the nature of the other underlying diseases and the ability to effectively maintain gas exchange and pulmonary toilet. Potential complications of tracheal resection and reconstruction include the following[52–54]:

1. Early complications: following extubation
   i. Respiratory failure
   ii. Vocal cord paralysis
   iii. Glottic edema
   iv. Pneumomediastinum
2. Delayed complications:
   i. Hemoptysis
   ii. Anastomotic dehiscence
   iii. Granuloma formation at the anastomosis
   iv. Benign anastomotic strictures
   v. Restenosis
   vi. Fistula formation: tracheoinnominate or tracheoesophageal
3. Rare complications:
   i. Quadriplegic because of excessive strain on the cervical spine during the operation[55]

A retrospective review studied 901 patients who underwent tracheal resection and reconstruction over a 28-year period.[54.] The authors reported a 1.2% postoperative mortality rate. The overall rate of complications was 18.2%.[54]

Postoperative respiratory failure is usually caused by one of three etiologies:

1. Oversedation with residual anesthetics/opioids
2. Insufficient reversal of neuromuscular blockade
3. Airway obstruction

Treatment for postoperative respiratory failure includes establishing a patent airway, provision of oxygen, and rapid determination of its etiology. Overnarcotized patients are treated with titrated naloxone reversal, in addition to maintaining airway patency with either a facemask or insertion of a supraglottic device.[6] Residual neuromuscular blockade is remedied with reestablishing upper airway patency with a jaw thrust or insertion of an oral or nasal airway. Insertion of a supraglottic device may be warranted in some cases whilst additional titration of reversal agent is achieved. Reintubation may be warranted if noninvasive methods of ventilation are insufficient.

Airway obstruction postoperatively falls into two categories:

1. Vocal cord edema
2. Anastomotic obstruction because of blood, secretions, or a mucosal flap.

Upper airway obstruction secondary to laryngeal edema is an infrequent complication. It has occurred most commonly when there has been a high anastomosis or previous history of laryngeal disease. Prophylactic measures should be undertaken to avoid laryngeal edema if the patient has a history of cord paralysis, if episodes of laryngeal edema occur, or if the trachea is anastomosed directly to the larynx at the level of the cricoid cartilage. Therapy includes the use of high humidity and inhalation of topical steroids and racemic epinephrine. Racemic epinephrine, 0.5 ml of 2.25% solution diluted in 3 ml NS is administered via nebulizer every 3-4 hours as needed. Dexamethasone may be inhaled or given parentally. This regimen is continued for a minimum of 24 hours, or longer if laryngeal edema, evidenced by stridor and hoarseness, persists. The patient should be maintained in a semi-sitting position to promote venous drainage.

Airway obstruction may warrant reintubation. Flexible bronchoscopy remains the gold standard for reintubation, as it maintains neck flexion, avoids undue stress on a fresh anastomosis and allows examination of the vocal cords and anastomotic site. Use of a flexible bronchoscope also allows for precise positioning of the endotracheal tube and its cuff away from the anastomotic site.

In cases in which copious secretions are a significant concern, frequent fiberoptic bronchoscopy can be a useful adjunct to pulmonary toilet. Secretions tend to pool in major bronchi without being propelled by the normal mechanisms of mucociliary clearance.

Hemoptysis in the postoperative period signifies arterial erosion into the anastomosis. Surgical reexploration and repair is warranted. Following reintubation, the cuff of the endotracheal tube is positioned at the level of the anastomosis to tamponade bleeding until surgical reexploration occurs.

Aspiration of oral contents and difficulty swallowing may occur under certain circumstances[6,7]:

1. Following tracheal resection and reconstruction of invasive tracheal tumors
2. Recurrent laryngeal nerve injury
3. Following suprathyroid laryngeal release procedures[6]

Methods to control pain postoperatively have been well described in Chapter 24, as well as in the literature.[6,7,56] Alternatives to opioids are important to consider, such as IV acetaminophen, as it is critical to avoid respiratory depression in these patients. Vigorous coughing and/or vomiting are of particular concern in the patient posttracheal resection and reconstruction, and should be treated aggressively.[57,58] Both issues can cause subcutaneous air or pneumomediastinum because of air egress through the healing tracheal anastomosis.

Patients should be kept in the intensive care unit at least overnight, until it is deemed safe to return to either the surgical ward or stepdown unit with experienced nursing care. This is dictated by the ability to discontinue cardiovascular monitoring and the need for frequent assessment of pulmonary status. Awake flexible bronchoscopy to assess the anastomosis is performed under local anesthesia before discharge.[6]

Conclusion

Patients with lesions of the large airways present for surgical repair infrequently. Such operations are performed regularly at only a few major institutions. In summary, the ability to deliver a safe anesthetic depends upon the anesthesiologist's knowledge of the anticipated surgical procedure, the etiology, and the location and extent of the lesion. The anesthesiologist must be aware of the potential complications of this surgical procedure and have a thorough understanding of the patient's other medical issues. Expert anesthesia care is an integral part of this fascinating and challenging operation.

References

1. Grillo HC. The management of tracheal stenosis following assisted respiration. *J Thorac Cardiovasc Surg*. 1969;57:521.
2. Grillo HC. Reconstruction of the trachea. Experience in 100 consecutive cases. *Thorax*. 1973;28:667.
3. Wright CD, Li S, Geller AD, et al. Postintubation tracheal stenosis: management and results 1993 to 2017. *Ann Thoracic Surg*. 2019:1471–1477.
4. Behringer EC, Wilson RS. Tracheal resection and reconstruction. In: Cohen EC, ed. *The Practice of Thoracic Anesthesia*. Philadelphia, PA: J.B. Lippincott Co; 1995:531–561.
5. Geffin B, Bland J, Grillo HC. Anesthetic management of trachea resection and reconstruction. *Anesth Analg*. 1969;48:884.
6. Hobai IA, Chhangani SV, Alfille PH. Anesthesia for tracheal resection and reconstruction. *Anesthesiology Clin*. 2012;30:709–730.
7. McRae K. Tracheal resection and reconstruction. In: Slinger P, ed. *Principles and Practice of Anesthesia for Thoracic Surgery*. Switzerland: Springer Nature; 2019:231–248.
8. Fung D, Devitt J. Anatomy, physiology, and innervation of the larynx. *Anesth Clin No Am*. 1995;13:259–276.
9. Grillo HC, Donahue DM, Mathisen DJ, et al. Postintubation tracheal stenosis: treatment and results. *J Thorac Cardiovasc Surg*. 1995;109:486–493.
10. Liu J, Zhang X, Gong W, et al. Correlations between controlled endotracheal tube cuff pressure and post procedural complications: a multicenter study. *Anesth Analg*. 2010;111:1133–1137.
11. Grillo HC, Mathisen DJ. Primary tracheal tumors: treatment and results. *Ann Thorac Surg*. 1990;49:69–77.
12. Madariaga ML, Gaissert HA. Secondary tracheal tumors: a systematic review. *Ann Cardiothorac Surg*. 2018;7:183–196.
13. Mathisen DJ, Grillo H. Laryngotracheal trauma. *Ann Thorac Surg*. 1987;43:254–262.
14. Cicala RS, Kudsk KA, Butts A, et al. Initial evaluation and management of upper airway injuries in trauma patients. *J Clin Anesth*. 1991;2:91–98.
15. Al-Bazzaz F, Grillo H, Kazemi H. Response to exercise in upper airway obstruction. *Am Rev Respir Dis*. 1975;111:631–640.
16. Geffin B, Grillo HC, Cooper JD, et al. Stenosis following tracheostomy for respiratory care. *JAMA*. 1971;216:1984–1988.
17. Lavell Jr TF, Rotman HH, Weg JG. Isoflow-volume curves in the diagnosis of upper airway obstruction. *Am Rev Respir Dis*. 1978;117:845–852.
18. Spittle N, McCluskey A. Tracheal stenosis after intubation. *BMJ*. 2000;321:1000–1002.
19. Nagappan R, Parkin G, Wright CA, et al. Adult long-segment tracheal stenosis attributable to complete tracheal rings masquerading as asthma. *Crit Care Med*. 2002;30:238–240.
20. Frerk C, Mitchell VS, McNarry AF, et al. Difficult Airway Society 2015 guidelines for management of unanticipated difficult intubation in adults. *Br J Anaesth*. 2015;115:827–848.
21. Crosby ET, Liu A. The adult cervical spine: implications for airway management. *Can J Anesth*. 1990;37:77–93.
22. Crosby E. Airway management after upper cervical spine injury: what have we learned. *Can J Anaesth*. 2002;49:733–744.
23. McGrath BA, Bates L, Atkinson D, et al. Multidisciplinary guidelines for the management of tracheostomy and laryngectomy airway emergencies. *Anaesthesia*. 2012;67:1025–1041.
24. Lunn WW, Shelter JR. Flow volume loops in the evaluation of upper airway obstruction. *Otolaryngol Clin North Am*. 1995;28:721–729.
25. Fiorelli A, Poggi C, Pia Ardo N, et al. Flow-volume curve analysis for predicting recurrence after endoscopic dilation of airway stenosis. *Ann Thorac Surg*. 2019;108:203–210.
26. Kligerman S, Sharma A. Radiologic evaluation of the trachea. *Sem Thorac Cardiovasc Surg*. 2009;21:246–254.
27. Mohyuddin N, Sulman C, Wheeler M. Management of the difficult pediatric airway: efficacy of airway exchange catheters with rigid bronchoscopy. *Ear Nose Throat J*. 2009;88:964–966.
28. Nekhendzy V, Simmonds PK. Rigid bronchoscope-assisted endotracheal intubation: yet another use of the gum elastic bougie. *Anesth Analg*. 2004;98:545–547.
29. Obianuju O, Gerlach RM, Sweitzer BJ. Preoperative evaluation for ambulatory anesthesia: what, when and how? *Anesthesiol Clin*. 2019;37:195–213.
30. Apfelbaum JL, Connis RT, et al. Practice advisory for pre-anesthesia evaluation: an updated report by the American Society of Anesthesiologists Task Force on Preanesthetic Evaluation. *Anesthesiology*. 2012;116:522–538.
31. Grillo HC. Circumferential resection and reconstruction of the mediastinal and cervical trachea. *Ann Surg*. 1965;162:374.
32. Cook TM, Nm Woodall, Frerk C. Major Complications of airway management in the UK: results of the fourth national audit project of the royal college of anaesthetists and the difficult airway society, part 1: anaesthesia. *Br J Anaesth*. 2011;106:617–631.
33. Joffe AM, Aziz MF, Posner KL, et al. Management of difficult tracheal intubation: a closed claims analysis. *Anesthesiology*. 2019;131:818–829.
34. Apfelbaum JL, Hagberg CA, Caplan RA, et al. Practice guidelines for management of the difficult airway: an updated report by the American Society of Anesthesiologists Task Force on Management of the Difficult Airway. *Anesthesiology*. 2013;118:251–270.
35. Lynch J, Crawley SM. Management of airway obstruction. *BJA Educ*. 2018;18:46–51.
36. Mark LJ, Herzer KR, Cover R, et al. Difficult Airway Response Team: a novel quality improvement program for managing hospital-wide airway emergencies. *Anesth Analg*. 2015;121:127–139.

37. Nishimura M. High-flow nasal cannula oxygen therapy devices. *Respir Care.* 2019;64:735–742.
38. Rochwerg B, Granton D, Wang DX, et al. High flow nasal cannula compared with conventional oxygen therapy for acute hypoxemic respiratory failure: a systematic review and meta-analysis. *Intensive Care Med.* 2019;45:563–572.
39. Hernandez G, Vaquero C, Colinas L, et al. Effect of postextubation high-flow nasal cannula vs noninvasive ventilation on reintubation and postextubation respiratory failure in high-risk patients: a randomized clinical trial. *JAMA.* 2016;316:1565–1574.
40. Badiger S, John M, Fernley A, et al. Optimizing oxygenation and intubation during awake fiberoptic intubation using a high flow nasal oxygen delivery system. *Br J Anaesth.* 2015:629–632.
41. Wong DT, Dallaire A, Singh KP, et al. High flow nasal oxygen improves safe apnea time in morbidly obese patients undergoing general anesthesia: a randomized controlled trial. *Anesth Analg.* 2019;129:1130–1136.
42. Patel A, Nouraei SAR. Transnasal Humidified Rapid-Insufflation Ventilatory Exchange (THRIVE): a physiological method of increasing apnoea time in patients with difficult airways. *Anaesthesia.* 2015;70:323–329.
43. Fan T, Wang G, Mao B, et al. Prophylactic administration of parental steroids for preventing airway complications after extubation in adults: meta-analysis of randomized placebo-controlled trials. *Br Med J.* 2008;337:a1841.
44. Ho AM, Dion PW, Karmakar MK, et al. Use of heliox in critical upper airway obstruction: Physical and physiologic considerations in choosing the optimal helium: oxygen mix. *Resuscitation.* 2002;52:297–300.
45. Em Fitzgerald, Hodzovic I, Smith AF. From Darkness to light: time to make awake intubation with videolaryngoscopy the primary technique for an anticipated difficult airway. *Anaesthesia.* 2015;70:387–392.
46. Adams TRP, Ricciardelli A. Airway Fire during awake tracheostomy using high-flow nasal oxygen. *Anaesth Rep.* 2020;8:25–27.
47. Booth AWG, Vidhani K, Lee PK, et al. Spontaneous respiration using intravenous anaesthesia and Hi-Flow Nasal Oxygen (STRIVE Hi) maintains oxygenation and airway patency during management of the obstructed airway: an observational study. *Br J Anaesth.* 2017;118:444–451.
48. Mathisen D. Distal tracheal resection and reconstruction: state of the art and lessons learned. *Thorac Surg Clin.* 2018;28:199–210.
49. Tan LZ, Tan DJ, Seet E. Laryngeal mask airway protector for intubation and extubation of thyroid surgeries: a case report. *Indian J Anaesth.* 2018;62:545–548.
50. Schieren M, Bohmer A, Dusse F, et al. New approaches to airway management in tracheal resections—a systematic review and meta-analysis. *J Cardiothorac Vasc Anesth.* 2017;31:1351–1358.
51. McRae K. Anesthesia for airway surgery. *Anesthesiol Clin North Am.* 2001;19:497–541.
52. Tapias LF, Mathisen DJ. Prevention and management of complications following tracheal resections-lessons learned at the Massachusetts General Hospital. *Ann Cardiothorac Surg.* 2018; 7:237–243.
53. Wright CD, Grillo HC, Wain JC, et al. Anastomotic complications after tracheal resection: prognostic factors and management. *J Thorac Cardiovasc Surg.* 2004;128:731–739.
54. Siciliani A, Rendina EA, Ibrahim M. State of the art in Tracheal Surgery: a brief literature review. *Multidiscip Respir Med.* 2018;13:34.
55. Dominguez J, Rivas JJ, Lobato RD, et al. Irreversible tetraplegia after tracheal resection. *Ann Thorac Surg.* 1996;62:278–280.
56. Uhlmann RA, Reinhart HA, Postevka E, et al. A review of postoperative pain management for thyroid and parathyroid surgery. *J Surg Res.* 2019;241:107–111.
57. Akkas M, Tiambeng C, Aksu NM, et al. Tracheal rupture as a result of coughing. *Am J Emerg Med.* 2018;36:2133.
58. Toprak V, Keles GT, Kaygisiz Z, et al. Subcutaneous emphysema following severe vomiting after emerging from general anesthesia. *Acta Anaesthesiol Scand.* 2004;48:917–918.

43 Lung Transplantation

JESSICA SPELLMAN, LAUREN SUTHERLAND

Introduction

Although many disease states result in severe lung disease, lung transplantation remains the only definitive therapy. Because of heterogeneity in underlying disease states, and significant cardiopulmonary manifestations of lung disease, lung transplantation procedures carry significant risk, and careful planning with respect to intraoperative management and postoperative care is required, with attention to hemodynamics, ventilatory parameters, immunosuppression, infection prevention, and graft dysfunction. Extracorporeal membrane oxygenation (ECMO) is increasingly being used to support patients as a bridge to lung transplantation, intraoperatively for hemodynamic and ventilatory support, and postlung transplantation in the management of graft dysfunction.

Epidemiology

Lung transplantation is the only definitive therapy for many different causes of end-stage lung disease. Between 2009 and 2016, 170 international centers performed lung transplant procedures, with 66% performed among 48 centers.[1] The number of lung transplant procedures has been steadily increasing in the United States, with 2714 lung transplants performed in 2019.[2] As with other solid organ transplants, there is inadequate organ availability, and currently more than 1300 people are awaiting lung transplantation in the United States. The median waiting time for candidates listed between 2011 and 2014 in the United States varied by blood type, but ranged from 87 days for type AB to 137 days for type O. For this time period, 58.8% of listed adults were eventually transplanted. Survival for lung transplant recipients varies based on single or double lung transplant procedure (Table 43.1).[1]

Recipient Selection

The International Society for Heart and Lung Transplantation (ISHLT) guidelines for recipient selection were updated in 2014.[3] Referral for transplant involves initial evaluation of the patient for potential as a transplant candidate; placing the patient on the active waitlist occurs when all other treatment options are exhausted, and the benefits outweigh the risks of the transplant procedure. In general, a patient should be actively listed when he or she has chronic, end-stage lung disease with greater than 50% risk of death from lung disease within 2 years, greater than 80% likelihood of 90-day survival from the transplant surgery, and greater than 80% 5-year survival from a general medical perspective.

Contraindications to lung transplantation (Table 43.2) generally include conditions that would likely lead to higher morbidity, mortality, or technical difficulty of the transplant surgery, early graft failure, or inability to manage the postoperative transplant state. Relative contraindications are less well defined, and patients who are initially deemed not to be candidates may be actively listed if medical conditions are treated or improve. For example, patients requiring invasive mechanical ventilation (IMV) or extracorporeal life

TABLE 43.1 Lung Transplant Survival 2008–2015

	1-Year Survival		5-Year Survival	
	Single	Double	Single	Double
United States	85%	87%	46%	56%
International	78%	82%	48%	59%

Reprinted with permission from Chambers DC, Yusen RD, Cherikh WS, et al, International Society for H, Lung T. The Registry of the International Society for Heart and Lung Transplantation: Thirty-Fourth Adult Lung and Heart-Lung Transplantation Report—2017; Focus Theme: Allograft ischemic time. *J Heart Lung Transplant*. 2017;36:1047–1059.

TABLE 43.2 Contraindications to Lung Transplantation

Absolute Contraindications	Relative Contraindications
Untreatable, significant dysfunction of another organ system,[a] including atherosclerotic disease, coronary disease not amenable to revascularization, and uncorrectable bleeding diathesis	Severe systemic illness
Recent history of malignancy	Age >75 years (or >65 years with low physiologic reserve)
Acute medical instability (e.g., bleeding, sepsis, myocardial infarction, or liver failure)	Medical conditions likely to result in end-stage organ damage
Chronic infection with highly virulent or resistant microbes (e.g., *Mycobacterium tuberculosis*)	Colonization or infection with highly resistant or highly virulent organisms
Severely limited functional status with poor rehabilitation potential	Severe malnutrition or osteoporosis
BMI ≥35.0 kg/m^2	BMI 30–34.9 kg/m^2
Significant chest wall or spinal deformity	Extensive prior thoracic surgery
Nonadherence to medical therapy	
Psychiatric conditions associated with the inability to cooperate with complex medical therapy	
Substance abuse or dependence	
Absence of an adequate social support system	

[a]Unless combined organ transplant can be performed. *BMI*, Body mass index.
Reprinted with permission from Weill D, Benden C, Corris PA, et al. A consensus document for the selection of lung transplant candidates: 2014–an update from the Pulmonary Transplantation Council of the International Society for Heart and Lung Transplantation. *J Heart Lung Transplant*. 2015;34:1–15.

support (ECLS) may be successfully transplanted if there is no significant evidence of another organ dysfunction. Patients with highly virulent pulmonary infections (e.g., *Burkholderia* or mycobacterium) if adequately treated and without extrapulmonary involvement may also be candidates for lung transplantation. Elderly patients who are otherwise healthy or patients with controlled medical conditions may also qualify for active listing.

Many patients listed for lung transplantation have had prior thoracic surgery, ranging from minor thoracoscopic biopsies to large thoracotomies for lung volume reduction surgery (LVRS), to cardiac surgeries with internal mammary arterial harvest. Depending on the extent of scar tissue and adhesions, surgical dissection may be significantly more challenging. Overall, this patient population has higher rates of intraoperative bleeding and phrenic nerve damage, as well as postoperative complications including renal dysfunction, primary graft dysfunction (PGD), chylothorax, and need for reexploration. Specifically, prior pleurodesis is associated with prolonged intensive care unit (ICU) length of stay and causes a significantly higher rate of bleeding. Prior LVRS is associated with more bleeding, renal dysfunction, and poorer graft function.[3] In well-selected patients with prior thoracic surgeries, there is no difference in outcome with respect to PGD and survival at 30 days, 1 year, and 5 years.[4] However, patients with multiple comorbidities and extensive prior surgeries have worse outcomes after lung transplant.[4] Lung transplant after coronary artery bypass grafting (CABG) is increasing, and prior CABG is an independent predictor of mortality at 30 days, 1 year, and 5 years in patients receiving bilateral lung transplants; however, mortality is similar to non-CABG patients for single lung transplants.[5]

Disease-Specific Selection

Chronic Obstructive Pulmonary Disease

Chronic obstructive pulmonary disease (COPD) is the most common indication for lung transplantation worldwide, accounting for 33% of all transplants. The disease is characterized by airflow limitation caused by a mixture of small airway destruction (obstructive bronchiolitis), parenchymal destruction (emphysema), and mucociliary dysfunction. Symptoms include dyspnea, chronic cough, and sputum production, and diagnosis is made through spirometry demonstrating postbronchodilator forced expiratory volume in 1 second (FEV_1)/forced vital capacity (FVC) of less than 0.70. Risk factors for COPD include smoking, environmental or occupational exposures, history of asthma or chronic respiratory disease, and the genetic disease alpha-1 antitrypsin deficiency. Chronic disease management includes smoking cessation, pharmacologic therapy with bronchodilators, beta-2 agonists, antimuscarinic drugs, inhaled corticosteroids, phosphodiesterase-4 inhibitors, and antibiotics, oxygen or noninvasive mechanical ventilation therapy, and surgical interventions (e.g., LVRS).[6]

When compared with other lung transplant indications, the clinical course of COPD often results in poor quality of life but longer pretransplant survival, as well as better survival after lung transplant.[7] Transplant evaluation should begin when the disease continues to progress despite maximal medical therapy, oxygen therapy, and pulmonary rehabilitation. In addition, hypoxia, hypercapnia, or FEV_1 less than 25% should prompt evaluation.[3] The **BODE index** is a scoring system which uses variables including **b**ody-mass index, degree of airway **o**bstruction, **d**yspnea, and **e**xercise capacity to predict survival in COPD patients. The index is calculated by tallying point values for each index variable. Higher scores indicating greater risk of death, and the hazard ratio of death per one-point increase in the BODE index is 1.34 (95% confidence interval [CI], 1.26–1.42; $P < .001$).[8]

When applied to COPD patients undergoing lung transplantation versus medical management, lung transplantation offered a better survival than predicted at 1 year (odds ratio [OR] 0.77; 95% CI, 0.65–0.89), 2 years (OR, 0.71; CI, 0.58–84), 3 years (OR, 0.67; CI, 0.54–0.8), 4 years (OR, 0.65; CI, 0.51–0.79), and 10 years (OR, 0.39; CI, 0.21–0.57)[9] with greatest benefit seen in most severe disease (BODE >7).[9,10] Patients with a BODE score of 5 to 6 are estimated a 57% 4-year survival and should undergo lung transplant evaluation. Active listing may occur when FEV_1 decreases to 15% to 20%, BODE index increases to 7 or higher, with moderate to severe pulmonary hypertension (PH), or when 3 or more major exacerbations occurred within the past year.[3]

Patients who are candidates for LVRS may be evaluated for transplantation concurrently. Those who fail to improve with LVRS may later be listed for transplantation, and at times, LVRS may improve nutritional and functional status enough to make a patient a candidate for transplant.

Interstitial Lung Disease

Interstitial lung disease (ILD) is a heterogeneous group of diseases that are characterized by the presence of cellular proliferation, infiltration, and/or fibrosis of the lung parenchyma which is not caused by infection or neoplasia.[11] ILD most often results in a restrictive pattern of pulmonary function, characterized by reduced expansion of lung parenchyma and reduced lung volumes. Causes of ILD include autoimmune and collagen vascular diseases, hypersensitivity pneumonitis because of exposures (e.g., medication, occupational, or environmental), genetic abnormalities, and idiopathic pulmonary fibrosis (IPF). ILD is the second most common indication for lung transplantation but carries the worst prognosis; IPF is the most common and life-threatening form of ILD, carrying greater mortality risk as compared with other classified ILD patients with acute respiratory failure.[12] IPF is suspected in the setting of ILD with no other identifiable cause and the following features: bilateral fibrosis on chest imaging, inspiratory crackles, age over 60 years (or, if familial fibrosis, age <60 years), history and serologic testing exclude other causes of ILD, and imaging, lavage, or biopsy exclude usual interstitial pneumonia.[13]

Patients with ILD should be referred for transplant evaluation early because of poor prognosis and the high likelihood for precipitous decline. Predictors of worse survival include older age, poor or worsening pulmonary function, PH, and concomitant emphysema. Specifically, referral should occur if FVC decreases below 80% or diffusion capacity for carbon monoxide (DLCO) below 40%, or there is development of dyspnea, functional limitation, or oxygen requirement. Active listing should occur with significant decline in FVC or DLCO, worsening 6-minute walk test (6MWT), development of PH, or clinical decompensation.[3]

Cystic Fibrosis (See Chapter 50)

Cystic fibrosis (CF) is the most common lethal genetic disease in the Caucasian population, with 30,775 patients in the United States living with the disease and 852 newly diagnosed individuals in 2018.[14] The disease is caused by a mutation in the *CFTR* gene, encoding a transmembrane chloride channel. Dysfunction or downregulation of this channel leads to dehydration of airway surfaces and accumulation of thickened secretions, inhibiting normal ciliary function and clearance of mucous. These abnormal airway secretions, as well as an abnormal host response to bacterial pathogens lead to chronic pulmonary infections, bronchiectasis, and eventual gas trapping, hypoxemia, and hypercarbia. Extrapulmonary manifestations of CF include gut malabsorption and dysmotility from impaired biliary and pancreatic secretions, diabetes from chronic pancreatic insufficiency, sinusitis, and infertility.[15]

Patients with CF have superior long-term survival after lung transplant compared with other indications.[1] Patients should be referred for transplant evaluation when frequency or severity of exacerbations increases, including need for noninvasive mechanical ventilation, diagnosis of infections with increasing antibiotic resistance, pneumothorax, life-threatening hemoptysis, or worsening nutritional status. In addition, pulmonary measures, such as an FEV_1 less than 30%, 6MWT less than 400 m, or development of PH should trigger referral. FEV_1 less than 30% is the most useful predictor of 2-year mortality. Active listing should be considered with development of chronic hypoxia or hypercapnia, PH, a need for invasive or long-term noninvasive mechanical ventilation, or overall clinical decline. Special consideration should be taken in patients with particularly virulent and resistant pulmonary infections.[1] All patients should be evaluated for nontuberculous mycobacterium, and in those with progressive pulmonary or extrapulmonary disease despite optimal therapy, lung transplantation is contraindicated. CF patients infected with *Burkholderia cenocepacia* have a more rapid progression of pulmonary decline, as well as a higher mortality posttransplant because of high risk of recurrent disease.[3]

Pulmonary Vascular Disease

Pulmonary vascular disease (PVD) refers to any process that disrupts blood flow between the heart and lungs, including pulmonary arterial hypertension (PAH), pulmonary venoocclusive disease, thromboembolic disease, pulmonary arteriovenous malformations, and pulmonary vasculitis. PVD may present acutely or chronically with signs and symptoms including dyspnea, chest pain, hypoxemia, or right heart failure (e.g., syncope, weight, edema, ascites from hepatic congestion).[16] PH is defined as mean pulmonary artery (PA) pressure of 20 mm Hg or more measured by right heart catheterization (RHC) in the supine position at rest.[17] PH can be defined by hemodynamics as pre- or postcapillary and classified further into five groups: PAH, PH caused by left heart disease, PH resulting from chronic lung disease or hypoxemia, PH caused by PA obstruction, or PH arising from multifactorial mechanisms (Box 43.1).[18]

Management of PH is targeted at the underlying pathophysiology and group classification. Patients with PAH should be assessed and risk stratified at expert PAH centers regularly.[18] The United States Registry to Evaluate Early and Long-Term PAH disease management (REVEAL) registry data created a risk score which includes the following factors: group 1 subgroup, demographics, comorbidities, functional class, vital signs, 6MWT, brain natriuretic peptide (BNP) level, echocardiogram, pulmonary function tests, and RHC findings. This scoring system was shown to effectively risk stratify and predict clinical worsening and mortality in patients who were followed 1 year or more.[19] Pharmacologic management includes prostacyclin pathway agonists (e.g., epoprostenol, trepostinil, iloprost, selexipag), endothelin receptor antagonists (e.g., ambrisentan, bosentan, macitentan), phosphosphodiesterase 5 inhibitors (e.g., sildenafil, tadalafil). A small subset of patients with group 1 PAH who respond to short-acting vasodilators with improvement in hemodynamics measured by RHC are deemed to be "vasoreactive" and should receive a trial of calcium channel blocker therapy.[18]

Patients with PVD with rapidly progressive disease, New York Heart Association (NYHA) functional class III or IV symptoms with escalating therapy, venoocclusive disease or capillary hemangiomatosis, or use of parenteral therapy (e.g., prostanoids, endothelin receptor antagonists, or phosphodiesterase inhibitors) for PAH should be evaluated for transplant. Persistent class III or IV symptoms after a 3-month trial of combination therapy, cardiac index of less than 2 L/min/m^2, or central venous pressure of greater than 15 mm Hg, worsening functional capacity, hemoptysis, pericardial effusion, or evidence of progressive right heart failure should warrant active listing.[3]

• BOX 43.1 Classification of Pulmonary Hypertension

Pulmonary Hypertension Clinical Groups

1. Pulmonary arterial hypertension
2. PH caused by left heart disease
3. PH caused by lung diseases and/or hypoxia
4. PH caused by pulmonary artery obstructions
5. PH with unclear and/or multifactorial mechanisms

PH, Pulmonary hypertension. Reprinted with permission from Galie N, Humbert M, Vachiery JL, et al, Group ESCSD. 2015 ESC/ERS Guidelines for the diagnosis and treatment of pulmonary hypertension: The Joint Task Force for the Diagnosis and Treatment of Pulmonary Hypertension of the European Society of Cardiology (ESC) and the European Respiratory Society (ERS): Endorsed by: Association for European Paediatric and Congenital Cardiology (AEPC), International Society for Heart and Lung Transplantation (ISHLT). *Eur Heart J.* 2016;37:67–119.

Special Populations

Retransplantation

Lung retransplantation makes up a small portion of lung transplants, but the proportion is increasing. Candidate selection is similar for that of initial transplant evaluation. Common indications for retransplantation include bronchiolitis obliterans syndrome (BOS), PGD, or airway complications. Survival for retransplant is inferior to original transplants, with 67% survival at 1 year and 40% at 5 years internationally,[1] and there is a higher risk of acute rejection. Renal dysfunction in this population increases mortality significantly. Consideration for removal of the prior transplant allograft should be undertaken because this can become a nidus for infection or ongoing immune stimulation. Because of this, retransplants are often done as double lung transplantations. However, removal of the prior allograft may pose greater technical difficulty surgically owing to the presence of adhesions and lead to greater operative morbidity. If a single retransplant is to be performed, generally a contralateral lung transplant is preferred.[20]

Combined Heart-Lung Transplant

In most patients with right-sided heart failure from longstanding or severe acute pulmonary disease, lung transplantation improves conditions that allow for myocardial recovery. In end-stage PH, single-center reporting of bilateral lung transplantation as compared with heart-lung transplant is associated with comparable survival.[21] However, patients with irreversible myocardial dysfunction or severe congenital defects in addition to end-stage lung disease may be candidates for combined heart-lung transplantation. Patients with intrinsic cardiac disease, such as coronary artery disease, valvular pathology, or septal defects may undergo concomitant cardiac surgery at the same time as lung transplantation rather than combined heart-lung transplant. The number of performed heart-lung transplants has generally downtrended in recent years both nationally and internationally. In the United States, 15 heart-lung transplants were performed in 2015; however, in 2019, 45 were performed, demonstrating a possible resurgence in this procedure. When indices of right ventricular (RV) function begin to decline despite maximal medical therapy, including NYHA functional class IV symptoms or cardiac index less than 2 L/min/m^2 with RA pressure over 15 mm Hg, patients should be actively listed for transplant.[3]

Pediatric Lung Transplantation

Pediatric lung transplantation is performed much less commonly than in adults. In 2019 of the 2714 total lung transplants, only 50 were in patients under 18 years of age in the

United States. Of these, most occurred in the 11 to 17 year age range.[2] CF is the most common indication for pediatric lung transplantation overall, but this varies by age. Congenital heart disease is the most common indication in infants, whereas CF and idiopathic PAH are most common between ages 1 and 10. Referral for lung transplant should occur in children with progressive lung disease on maximal medical therapy, a short-life expectancy, a poor quality of life, and when appropriate social support is in place. Nonadherence in adolescents is a common cause of graft failure, so this should be addressed at transplant assessment. Waiting times tend to be longer, especially for smaller children, so referral should occur earlier. Contraindications to transplant are similar to adult patients based on disease process. Living donor lobar transplant is an option in some pediatric cases.

Removal From the Waiting List

All patients on the waiting list should be regularly evaluated to ensure that they remain transplant candidates.[3] Patients may be temporarily or permanently delisted if their candidacy changes based on either clinical improvement or deterioration or change in social factors. Examples of causes for delisting include substantial weight loss or debilitation, renal failure, new virulent infection, and medical noncompliance. If a patient clinically improves on medical therapy, he or she may be delisted because of improved quality of life. Patients bridged with IMV or ECLS frequently have clinical changes that may result in significantly higher morbidity and mortality of the transplant procedure.

Recipient Preparation

As part of the selection process for lung transplantation, recipient candidates undergo a variety of studies to better define pulmonary disease, assess for decline in function, and exclude other systemic illness. Testing includes pulmonary function tests, chest x-ray, computed tomography (CT) scanning, nuclear medicine ventilation perfusion studies, walk or exercise testing, electrocardiogram, echocardiogram, myocardial stress testing, right and left heart catheterization, and laboratory evaluations of hematologic system, liver, and kidney function. Blood typing and comprehensive recipient human leukocyte antigen (HLA) testing is performed to allow for virtual crossmatching at the time of identification of a potential donor.[22]

Organ Allocation

Because of an organ demand that far outnumbers supply, a method of allocation was devised to distribute the available lungs in the most optimal way to both reduce waitlist mortality and improve transplant outcomes.[23] The first step in matching a donor with a recipient is based on blood type and lung size as determined by total lung capacity (TLC). Next, either national or regional location determines which recipients are eligible. In the United States, the Donation Service Area (DSA) is now a 250 nautical mile area in determining eligible recipients.[24]

• BOX 43.2 Parameters Used to Determine Lung Allocation Score

Age
Body mass index (BMI)
Pulmonary diagnosis
Functional status
Forced vital capacity (FVC)
Hemodynamic measures (e.g., pulmonary artery pressure, cardiac index)
Mechanical ventilation
Other end organ function (e.g., liver, kidney)

Reprinted with permission from UNOS. A Guide to Calculating the Lung Allocation Score.

In the United States, the Organ Procurement and Transplantation Network (OPTN) devised the lung allocation score (LAS) system in 2005 to prioritize recipients based on likelihood of transplant benefit. The LAS uses patient physiologic characteristics and statistical models to calculate a patient's waiting list urgency and expected posttransplant survival. Parameters incorporated into these calculations were updated in 2015 (Box 43.2).[25] A raw score is determined by subtracting the waiting list survival (days) from the transplant survival (days) with higher weight given to waitlist mortality, and this is converted into the LAS by normalizing between 0 and 100; a higher LAS has higher priority. Candidate information must be updated at least once every 6 months, or every 14 days for LAS scores of 50 or higher.[26] Pediatric candidates (i.e., <12 years of age) are designated priority 1 or 2 based on their medical condition and do not use the LAS system. Based on OPTN organ allocation, overall lung transplant rates increased from 87.1 per 100 waitlist years in 2009 to 172.3 in 2018.[27] Time on the waiting list was stable with 53.4% of patients transplanted after less than 90-days, and median time on the waitlist decreased from 4 to 2.5 months in 2018.[27]

Bridging to Transplantation

Patients who acutely decompensate before availability of lungs for transplantation may require bridging with either IMV or ECLS. These interventions intend to extend the interval until transplantation can occur, as well as improve clinical stability.

Invasive Mechanical Ventilation

IMV, while extending time to transplantation, may cause new clinical problems to arise, such as ventilator-associated pneumonia, immobility and deconditioning, ventilator-associated lung injury, and hemodynamic instability.[3,28] Pretransplant IMV is associated with a higher short-term mortality.[1,29] Because of high waiting list mortality and worsened mortality with pretransplant IMV, ECLS has emerged as a method of bridging to transplant to allow longer waiting list times and improved clinical stability.[3]

Extracorporeal Membrane Oxygenation (See Chapter 28)

ECMO is a form of ECLS that provides support to patients with respiratory, cardiac, or combined failure for days to weeks.[30] In 2018 in the United States, 1.6% of patients were bridged to lung transplant with IMV only, 3.3% with ECMO only, and 3.1% with both ECMO and IMV.[27] Pretransplant use of IMV and ECMO has in the past been associated with higher mortality compared with nonsupported patients,[31] but this may be attributed to higher severity of illness, as well as ventilator and ECMO-related complications and deconditioning. Studies of comparing ECMO-bridged patients to those not requiring ECLS have shown mixed results with a trend toward worse early morbidity and mortality[32–34]; however, with improvements in technology, patient selection, and management, there is evidence of high overall survival in patients bridged with ECMO,[35] especially when avoiding IMV.[36,37]

Basics

The basic ECMO circuit consists of a magnetic levitation pump, conduit tubing with drainage and return cannulas, a membrane oxygenator, and a heat exchanger.[30] Deoxygenated blood is removed via the drainage cannula, oxygenated and carbon dioxide removed by the membrane oxygenator, and returned to the body through the reinfusion cannula. ECMO may be venovenous (VV) or venoarterial (VA). **VV ECMO** both drains and returns blood to a central vein, serving a replacement for lung function in patients with inadequate oxygenation or ventilation and allowing for a reduction in ventilator settings to decrease potential for lung injury.[38] VV ECMO places the native lungs in series with the "artificial lung," so blood enters the pulmonary circulation having already been oxygenated and carbon dioxide removed. VV ECMO provides no cardiac or circulatory support (Fig. 43.1). **VA ECMO** drains blood from a central vein and returns to a central artery, supplying both cardiac and pulmonary support. The "artificial lung" runs in parallel to the native lung, with a proportion of blood pumped and oxygenated by the circuit whereas the remainder that enters the heart relies on native lung function.

VA ECMO cannulation strategies are variable, although can generally be divided into two techniques: central or peripheral (Fig. 43.2). Central VA ECMO involves direct cardiac cannulation through sternotomy or thoracotomy, similar to that of cardiopulmonary bypass (CPB), with venous cannulation of the right atrium and arterial cannulation of the ascending aorta. In peripheral VA ECMO, the drainage cannula enters either the femoral or internal jugular vein (IJV) with advancement to the junction of the inferior or superior vena cava and right atrium; arterial cannulation for reinfusion is to either the descending aorta via the femoral artery or to the subclavian artery (SCA) by way of the axillary artery. There may be combinations of central and peripheral techniques in certain clinical situations. Venoarteriovenous (VAV) ECMO involves drainage from a central vein with reinfusion flow divided between two cannulas, a central venous return and an arterial return. This configuration may be useful in a patient with both cardiac and severe pulmonary dysfunction in which additional circulatory support is required, but blood pumped through the native lungs is inadequately oxygenated and ventilated. Partial clamping of the two reinfusion cannulas allows for titration of the relative contributions of the VV and VA components.

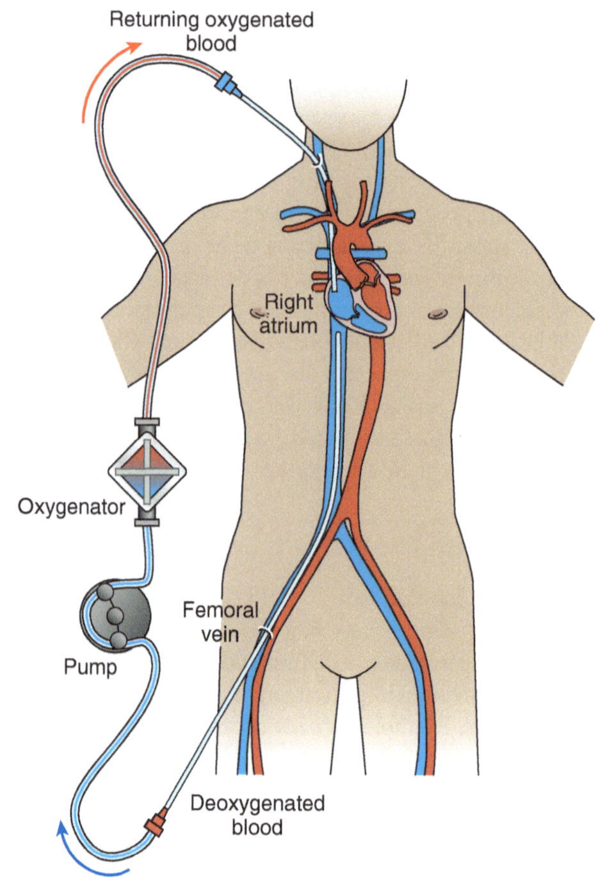

• **Fig. 43.1** In venovenous extracorporeal membrane oxygenation (*VV ECMO*), blood flows from the patient's venous system to the oxygenator and is pumped back to the patient's venous system.

Choice of cannulation strategy is based on the clinical indication, patient factors, and available vascular access. Femoral VA ECMO is more easily placed during a cardiopulmonary resuscitation situation because of access of the femoral vessels. VV ECMO cannulation on an intubated patient with acute respiratory distress syndrome (ARDS) may use femoral access; however, in a patient awaiting lung transplantation, upper body cannulation can improve mobility and even allow for ambulation. ECMO cannulation techniques as bridges to lung transplantation will be further discussed later.

Complications

Although ECMO can normalize hemodynamics, oxygenation, and acid-base status to temporize a patient while awaiting transplant, the benefits must be compared with potential harm of ECMO complications. Frequent complications of ECMO include **bleeding from cannula** or surgical sites, lower extremity ischemia distal to cannulation sites,

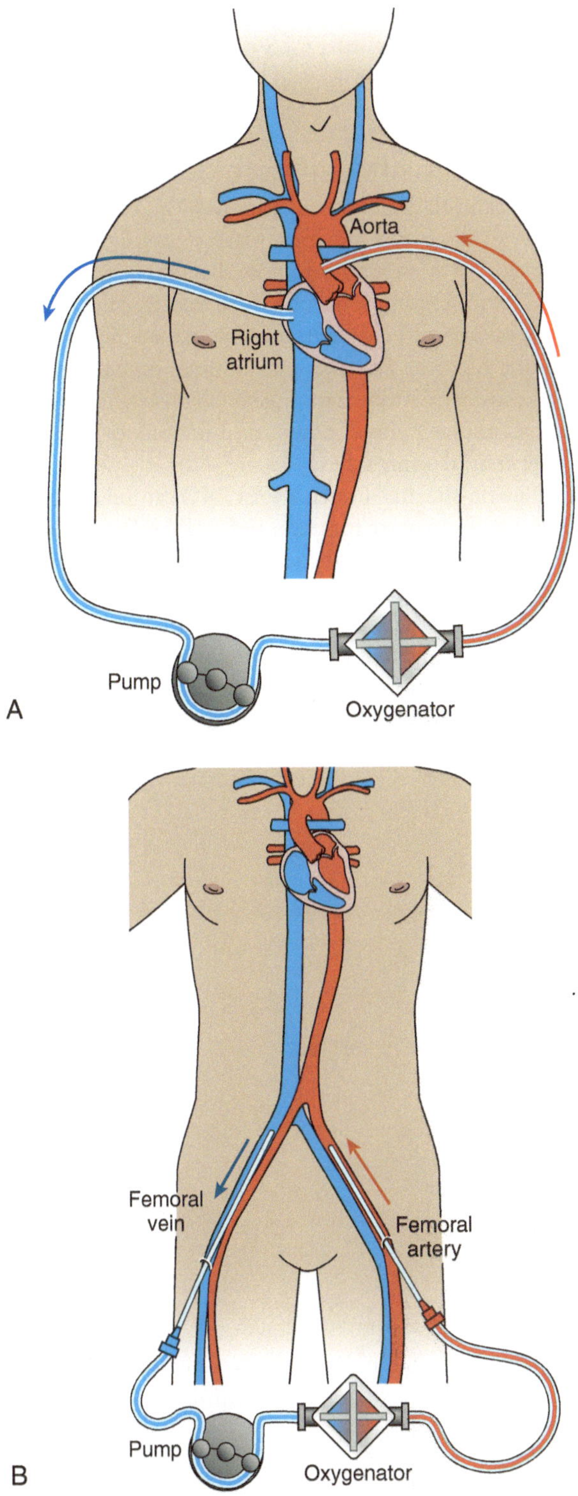

• **Fig. 43.2** In venoarterial extracorporeal membrane oxygenation (*VA ECMO*), blood flows from the patient's venous system to the oxygenator, and is pumped back to the patient's arterial system. (**A**) Central VA ECMO; (**B**) Peripheral VA ECMO.

stroke or other neurologic complications, infection, and acute kidney injury.[30] The most common sites of bleeding are cannula sites, surgical sites (e.g., mediastinal, thoracic), gastrointestinal, or central nervous system (CNS). Apparent bleeding without a clear source may also represent hemolysis. **Thromboembolic complications** include limb ischemia, intracardiac thrombus, device thrombosis including pump malfunction, oxygenator failure, or tubing obstruction, ischemic stroke, or deep vein thrombosis and pulmonary embolism. In cases of ischemia of the limb in which a cannula is placed, a distal perfusion cannula may be placed to direct a small amount of blood flow toward the limb. Vascular Doppler assessment of distal arterial vessels may be helpful, as well as vessel caliber assessment at arterial cannulation.[39]

Other complications may occur with VV and VA ECMO because of competing flow considerations with the circuit or native circulation. VV ECMO support may be ineffective if returned blood is drawn back into the drainage cannula, an issue known as **"recirculation"** which can be addressed by cannula repositioning. Peripheral VA ECMO specifically results in **high left ventricular (LV) end-diastolic pressure** because of arterial flow directed up the aorta toward the aortic valve, resulting in LV dilation, dysfunction, or failure in some patients. Failure of the LV to eject volume and resulting LV distension in these cases increase risk of stasis and thrombosis at the LV outflow tract, aortic valve, or ascending aorta. To relieve LV distention, an Impella assist-device, an intraaortic balloon pump, or transseptal left atrial drainage cannula may be placed.[38] In addition, it is important to monitor for **cerebral and coronary hypoxia** in patients with peripheral VA ECMO and lung disease. Especially in states of normal or recovering cardiac function, poorly oxygenated blood, ejected blood from the heart will preferentially supply the proximal aortic vessels (i.e., coronary and carotid arteries). In patients with peripheral VA ECMO, right radial arterial blood gases (ABGs) or saturation monitoring should be monitored as a surrogate for cerebral oxygenation.[30]

Patient Selection

In general, patients awaiting lung transplantation with severe hypercapnia, hypoxemia, or RV failure who are likely not to survive until organ availability may be bridged to lung transplant with ECMO. Those with isolated pulmonary failure benefit from VV ECMO to provide oxygenation and removal of carbon dioxide. For patients with PH or RV failure, VA ECMO provides additional cardiac output, as well as offloads preload to the right ventricle. In some cases, VV ECMO support alone can be sufficient for patients with mild PH and RV dysfunction, as the improvement in systemic oxygenation and respiratory acidosis allows for improvement in hemodynamics and RV function. In patients with PH and a large atrial septal defect (>2 cm) or atrial septostomy, VV ECMO may be effective as a bridge to transplant.[40]

Candidates with high pretransplant mortality from a pulmonary standpoint but with high likelihood of clinical improvement with cardiopulmonary support should be selected for ECMO bridging to transplantation (BTT). Those with multiorgan dysfunction or poor rehabilitation potential should not be placed on ECMO because this can present an ethical dilemma of "bridging to nowhere" if the patient does not become a transplant candidate. Except in exceptional circumstances, only patients who have been evaluated and deemed appropriate transplant candidates should be placed on ECMO as a bridge to transplant.[38]

Timing of placement on ECMO support is important and controversial. In one respect, earlier placement of ECMO may prevent development of multiorgan dysfunction and maintain candidacy for transplantation; however, complications of ECMO, such as hemorrhage, thromboembolism, infection, vascular injury, or stroke develop frequently in these patients and may preclude transplantation. Disease- and location-specific factors that result in high waitlist mortality or long waitlist times should be considered in deciding when to place a patient on ECLS while awaiting organ availability. For example, short stature has been associated with higher waitlist mortality and lower rate of transplant, so patients who fall into this category may require earlier initiation of ECMO support.[38]

Patients who are BTT with ECMO should be continuously reassessed for candidacy for transplantation, as clinical decompensation may occur rapidly, deeming these patients too unstable to undergo the procedure.[3] Patients requiring ECMO as a BTT remain good candidates if they have overall good organ function, young age, and good potential for rehabilitation; however, those with evidence of other organ system dysfunction, septic shock, advanced age, obesity, or prior prolonged ventilation are poor candidates.

Prelung Transplant Extracorporeal Membrane Oxygenation Management

In the earlier years of prelung transplant ECMO use, outcomes of lung transplant for patients BTT with ECMO were poor; however, with the improvements in technology, cannulation strategies, and management, properly selected patients benefit from ECMO support.[38] Overall goals in prelung transplant ECMO management include minimizing sedation, avoidance of endotracheal intubation, and early mobilization.[38] In many patients, ECMO support can provide sufficient oxygenation and acid-base management to allow for avoidance of or removal of IMV. Patients on ECMO who are not intubated or "awake ECMO" avoid complications related to sedation, IMV, ventilator-associated pneumonia, immobility, and artificial modes of nutrition.[38] Awake ECMO is associated with higher posttransplant survival and shorter postoperative IMV.[37] Patients with an ongoing need for IMV may undergo early tracheostomy to maximize patient comfort while minimizing sedation, allow for participation with physical therapy, and aid in clearance of respiratory secretions.[38]

Early mobilization, both in patients requiring IMV and/or ECMO, allows for improvement in physical strength and avoidance of complications related to immobility and deconditioning. This may improve physiologic reserve to tolerate the transplant procedure, as well as rehabilitation potential after surgery. Mobilization in ECMO patients as BTT has been associated with higher survival to transplant.[40] Ambulation while on ECMO is not only possible but can be done safely in properly selected patients[41,42]; a multidisciplinary team should be coordinated and guidelines or protocols developed to ensure patient safety.[43] Risk of mobilization should be weighed against potential benefit in patients with hemodynamic instability, and patients may require increased level of ECLS or medication support for ambulation.[43]

Cannulation Techniques

Although traditional VA or VV ECMO require peripheral femoral cannulation, newer cannulation strategies have evolved to allow for maximal patient mobility and early ambulation. It is important to note that emergent VV or VA ECMO cannulation should adhere to traditional approaches because of ease of placement and avoidance of the lengthy procedure required for an open, surgical approach. Configurations for early mobilization generally use single-site dual lumen cannulas, upper body cannulation, or minimally invasive central approaches.

The single-site dual lumen VV ECMO cannula (Fig. 43.3) is traditionally placed into the right IJV; bicaval drainage ports are positioned into the superior and inferior vena cava and the reinfusion port lies in the right atrium, with the jet directed toward the tricuspid valve.[38] Proper placement of this device is confirmed with fluoroscopy or transesophageal echocardiography (TEE). This device not only allows for improved mobility, but also decreased recirculation given the fixed cannula port distances.

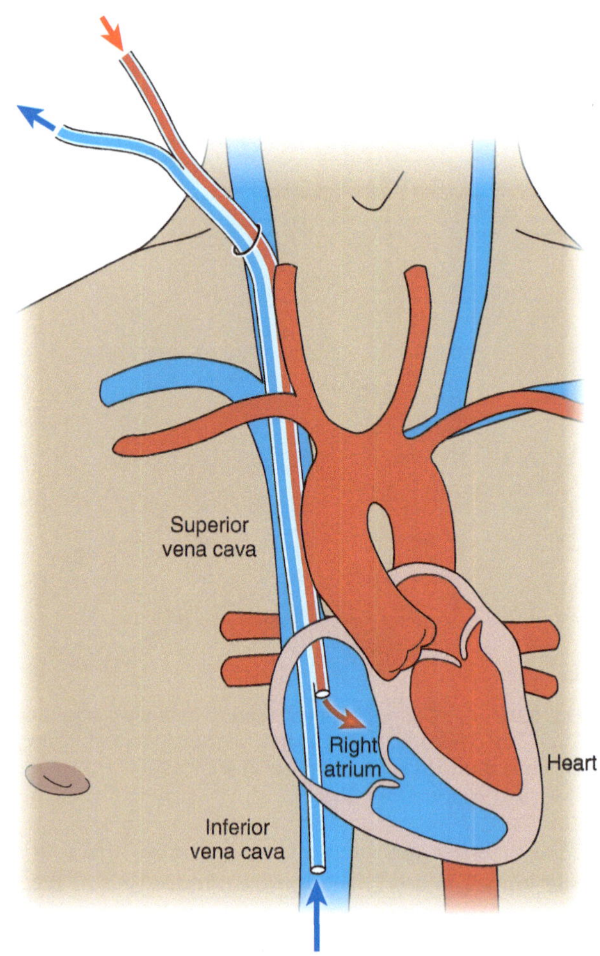

• **Fig. 43.3** Single-site dual lumen venovenous extracorporeal membrane oxygenation (*VV ECMO*).

For patients who require additional cardiac support, novel VA ECMO upper body configurations are more variable but all aim to improve upper body oxygenation in addition to maximizing patient mobility. The "sport model" approach involves IJV drainage to right SCA reinfusion[44] (Fig. 43.4). An end-to-side graft is anastomosed to the right SCA to avoid limb ischemia, and blood is reinfused down the right SCA. Unlike femoral VA ECMO where blood is directed retrograde from the femoral artery toward the aortic arch, the sport model approach ensures well-oxygenated blood flow to the carotid arteries. In patients with small or inaccessible SCAs, the innominate artery can be accessed via a miniature upper sternotomy incision for reinfusion, also known as "central sport model" ECMO.[45]

In patients with PH and a preexisting atrial septal defect or atrial septostomy, a dual-lumen VV ECMO cannula can be positioned with the reinfusion port directed over the defect, allowing oxygenated blood to shunt to the left heart and offloading the right ventricle.[38]

"Arteriovenous" ECMO using flow supported by the patient's cardiac output through a low resistance extracorporeal lung assist device (LAD) membrane ventilator circuit is also an option. This can be placed peripherally via the femoral artery to the femoral vein to support mechanical ventilation, or centrally from the PA to the left atrium.[46] Arteriovenous ECMO can also be used to gradually increase flow to the previously underfilled left heart, potentially preventing the complication of LV failure which can be seen immediately after lung transplant reperfusion in patients with severe PH.

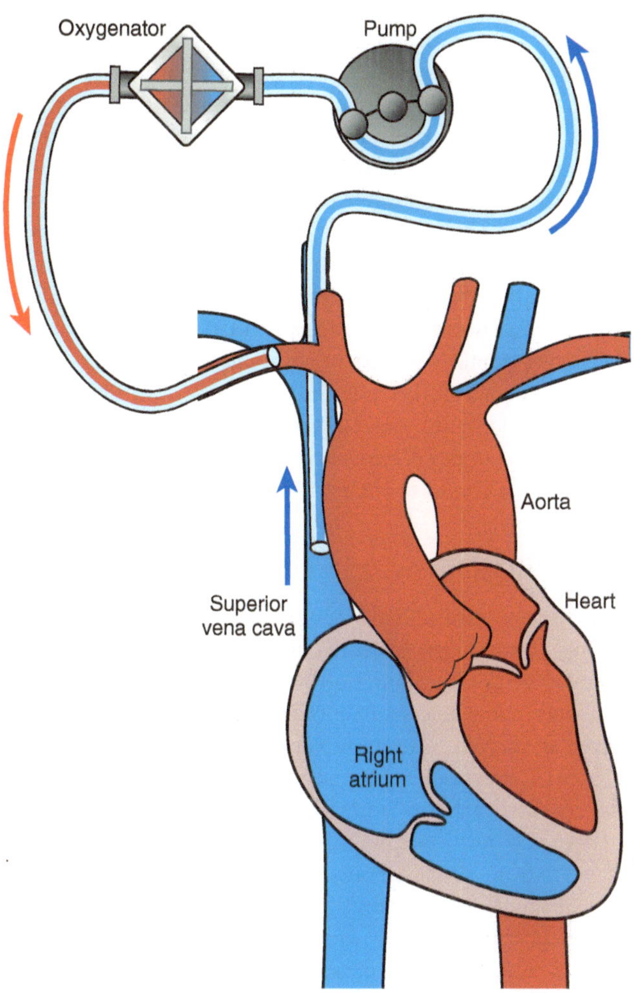

• **Fig. 43.4** Venoarterial extracorporeal membrane oxygenation (*VA ECMO*) "Sport Model".

Transfusions and Anticoagulation

Allosensitization to donor antigens from blood product transfusions can limit organ availability to patients awaiting transplant. Because of this, a more conservative transfusion strategy is preferred, targeting lower acceptable hematocrit values than in general critically ill populations.[38] In addition, although some degree of anticoagulation is required to maintain ECMO circuit patency and prevent thromboembolic complications, this must be weighed against the risk of bleeding, as well as the need for blood product transfusions. Typically, anticoagulation targets are lower in this population and short-acting, reversible anticoagulation (i.e., heparin) is preferred.

Organ Selection, Transport, and Preparation

Donor Evaluation

Lung transplant donors may be deceased or living lobar. Deceased donors include donation after brain death (DBD) and donation after circulatory determination of death (DCDD), also known as "donation after cardiac death" or "nonbeating-heart donation". Living lobar donation represents a small proportion of total lung transplantations, especially in the United States and Europe, because of high morbidity to the donors[47]; thus these procedures are most commonly performed in countries with limited deceased donor availability.

DCDD donation may be considered in patients whose life-sustaining treatment is planned for withdrawal but criteria for brain death are not met. Eligible conditions include irreversible brain injury, high spinal cord injury, and end-stage musculoskeletal disease.[48] In addition, DCDD may occur in certain unplanned situations, such as when patients unexpectedly suffer cardiac arrest from which they do not survive. For DCDD to be allowed, death must clearly precede donation, defined as cessation of all cardiopulmonary functions and irreversibility.[48] A time limit for circulatory death of up to 2 hours following withdrawal of life support is generally set to ensure viability of organs for transplantation. In selecting a patient as an appropriate donor for DCDD, clinical assessment for likelihood of circulatory death within 2 hours of withdrawal of life support should be used. Scoring systems to predict likelihood of circulatory death may be helpful.

Once the diagnosis of brain death is made or a potential DCDD donor is identified, the local procurement organization evaluates the potential donor. This organization also provides family support, obtains consent, and communicates with the United Network for Organ Sharing (UNOS) to match the donor with a recipient.

Organ Selection

Once a potential lung donor is identified, a rigorous process is undertaken to ensure graft acceptability.[49] Empiric criteria are used to identify ideal lung donors.[49] Most potential grafts are declined because of issues with donor history, chest trauma, pneumonia, aspiration, or various ICU complications.[50]

Extended donor criteria, or donor organs that do not meet this ideal donor criteria, may help increase the pool of suitable donors, while maintaining transplant outcomes in adult and pediatric lung transplantation.[51] This would include evaluation of donors of greater age range, smoking or asthma history, and certain causes of death, or other high-risk donors, if there is a continued positive trend in imaging studies and arterial partial pressure of oxygen (PaO2):fraction of inspired oxygen (F_iO2) (P/F ratio).[52] The U.S. Center for Disease Control and Prevention (CDC) labels high-risk donors as: those with exposure to human immunodeficiency virus (HIV), prison inmates, intravenous (IV) drug users, prostitution history, high-risk sexual history, and hemophiliacs. In the period of 2004 to 2010, 7% of lung transplant recipients received high-risk organs, and there was no difference in 1-year mortality as compared with nonhigh-risk organs.[53] With respect to donor age, donor graft outcome data are similar for donor ages 18 to 64 years[54]; however at the extremes of donor age, recipient pathology may play an important role in outcomes.[55]

To reduce the risk of viral transmission of SARS-CoV-2 virus (which causes COVID-19) from donor to recipient, donors are screened by polymerase chain reaction (PCR)-based testing of a nasopharyngeal or oropharyngeal swab, tracheal aspirate, or bronchoalveolar lavage (BAL), and CT scan is considered to evaluate for viral pneumonitis. It is recommended to avoid donors with positive test or CT scan results, as well as donors with exposure to confirmed or suspected SARS-CoV-2 cases in the past 14 days.[56]

Recommendations for donor and recipient size matching are based retrospective analysis and may vary based on disease state. In general, larger donor organs are preferred for recipients with hyperinflation and associated enlarged thoracic cavities and smaller organs for recipients with restrictive disease.[57] For example, it is recommended for patients with emphysema to be matched with donor lungs with 67% to 100% of the recipient actual TLC, whereas for patients with PH or CF it is recommended to match donor lungs up to 120% of the recipient predicted TLC,[58] based on height, weight, and gender. Undersized donor allografts based on of height and weight are associated with inferior posttransplant survival, with the exception of ILD in which undersized allografts experience similar survival to those that are well-matched or oversized.[59] Newer methods of three-dimensional CT lung volumetry may also provide information for size matching in lung transplantation.[60]

Donor Management

Once a potential donor is identified, a shift toward optimizing individual organ function should occur. Implementation of an intensive lung donor management protocol has been shown to increase the rate of lung procurement in DBD.[61] In addition to hemodynamic, fluid and electrolyte, and body temperature management, potential lung donors should be managed with lung-protective ventilation. Conventional ventilation strategy with high tidal volume (V_T) and low positive end-expiratory pressure (PEEP) has been associated with lower rates of eligible and harvested lungs as compared with low V_T ventilation with PEEP 8 to 10 cm H_2O.[62] Other strategies for optimizing graft function include, ventilator recruitment maneuvers with high PEEP, bronchoscopy to assess and minimize secretions, 30-degree head elevation, and adequate endotracheal cuff pressures to decrease aspiration risk.[63]

Organ Procurement

Before allograft procurement, blood sampling and bronchoscopy are performed to further assess graft function. For DCDD patients, these interventions and others including injection of heparin or phentolamine and femoral cannulation are deemed ethically appropriate as long as they do not cause harm to a prospective donor. During procurement, the lungs are excised from the PA to the pulmonary vein (PV) attachments to the left atrium, and the proximal trachea is stapled. Preservation is carried out in a fashion that will allow for allograft function along with prevention of vessel spasm and thrombosis formation. To afford this, the donor organ is preserved with a cold preservative solution, prostaglandin E1[64] (PGE1), which is administered via the PA, and the donor is anticoagulated with systemic IV heparin. The organ is transported in sterile cold preservative solution in a cooler to the recipient site.

Ischemic Time

Graft ischemic time is the time between aortic cross-clamp during donor organ procurement and lung allograft reperfusion during transplantation surgery; during bilateral lung transplant, this refers to reperfusion of the last implanted organ. In data for lung transplants performed between 2009 and 2015, median allograft ischemic time for bilateral transplants was 5.5 hours and for single lungs was 4.2 hours; median allograft ischemic times have increased over the past 25 years from about 4 hours to more than 5 hours. In addition, allografts with ischemic time >6 hours had lower Kaplan-Meyer unadjusted 30-day mortality than groups with shorter ischemic time. However, these differences were not maintained long-term, and, in multivariate analysis, allograft ischemia time is not associated with increased mortality.[1]

Ex Vivo Lung Perfusion

Ex vivo lung perfusion (EVLP) can be used to evaluate and screen compromised donor allografts that would generally be considered unsuitable or high risk for potential recovery. During EVLP, the preserved donor allograft is placed within a chamber system and perfused with a solution that is then pumped through an oxygenator, heat exchange system, and filter, simulating oxygen delivery to the body. The deoxygenated perfusate is then returned to the lungs which are ventilated with low V_T and room air oxygen. EVLP allografts can be deemed suitable for transplantation if P/F ratio is greater than 350 mm Hg and if deterioration from baseline levels of pulmonary vascular resistance, dynamic compliance, or peak inspiratory pressure is less than 15% while ventilated in the ex vivo chamber. In a study of 136 lung transplants, 23 were identified as high risk and evaluated with EVLP. After 4 hours of EVLP, 20 of the 23 EVLP allografts were deemed suitable for transplant, and outcomes as compared with the nonhigh-risk allografts had similar degrees of PGD at 72 hours (15% EVLP vs. 30% control, $P = .11$) and no differences in severe adverse events.[65] EVLP may also extend lung allograft preservation time beyond 12 hours with similar early outcome measures.[66]

Lung Transplant Procedure

Type of Surgical Procedure

Once a patient has been deemed a candidate for lung transplantation, the type of procedure may be chosen based on the disease process, as well as availability of organs. Patients may receive single or double lung transplants, a split lung bilateral lobar transplant, a living donor lobar transplant, or a combined heart and lung transplant.

Single lung transplants offer the advantage of a shorter operative and anesthetic time and allow for distribution of organs to more patients. However, single lungs provide less new, healthy lung tissue and may lead to earlier decline in function. Double lung transplants are associated with longer survival than singles.[67] Also this procedure may allow for use of less optimal grafts that would otherwise have been declined for single lung transplant. Certain disease states with high risk of infectious complications, such as CF and bronchiectasis, may only undergo double lung transplants.

Living lobar transplantation involves donation of two lower lobes from two separate donors, typically a right and a left lower lobe, to achieve a bilateral lung transplant.[47] Three operating rooms with three separate teams are typically required for simultaneous graft removal and implantation. These conditions allow for very short ischemic times; however, issues with HLA mismatching becomes more complex in situations of receiving grafts from two separate donors, and appropriate size matching must be carefully considered. Excessively small grafts can cause elevated PA pressure and pulmonary edema, whereas large grafts can lead to high airway resistance, atelectasis, and hemodynamic instability with chest closure.[68] To overcome complications of large grafts, such as when a parent donates to a small child, single lobe transplantation, graft downsizing, or delayed chest closure may be used.

Combined heart-lung transplants are reserved for patients with irreversible, end-stage heart disease in addition to lung disease. Specifically, those with left-sided heart failure may qualify for a combined procedure, as isolated right-sided heart failure often improves after lung transplantation alone. Congenital heart disease resulting in Eisenmenger syndrome (i.e., severe PH with resultant right to left shunting and cyanosis) is another common indication. For combined heart-lung transplants, the organs are transplanted en bloc. The volume of these procedures has decreased over time, with over 200 being performed internationally annually in the early 1990s to 59 procedures in 2017.[59] This low volume is likely because of increased waiting time leading to higher mortality while on the waiting list, increased risk of posttransplant morbidity (i.e., coronary artery vasculopathy and chronic lung allograft dysfunction), and the requirement for CPB for the procedure.

Surgical Procedure

For single lung transplantation, the hilum of the lung can be exposed by posterolateral thoracotomy in the lateral position or supine anterolateral thoracotomy or sternotomy; for bilateral transplantation, approaches include anterolateral thoracotomies, median sternotomy, transverse thoracosternotomy (clamshell), or modified transverse throracosternotomy.[69] The native lung is exposed and excised while supporting ventilation with either the contralateral lung or through ECMO or CPB support. Care is taken to preserve the vagus, phrenic, and recurrent laryngeal (left-sided) nerves. The donor allograft is inspected, prepared, and implanted via a posterior to anterior anastomosis technique, suturing the bronchus, the PA, and finally the PV. Before completion of the PV anastomosis, the allograft is reperfused by removing the PA clamp, and deairing is performed via the PV; after this, the anastomosis is completed. Controlled reperfusion and ventilation are generally performed over 10 minutes. For bilateral transplantation, the process is repeated for the second side. Following reperfusion, surgical hemostasis is achieved, chest tubes inserted, and the chest is closed.

Anesthetic Management

Anesthetic management, invasive monitoring preferences, and use of specific anesthetic agents vary by transplant center,[70] and a consensus on anesthetic management during lung transplantation are lacking at this time.[71] Induction of anesthesia and dosing immunosuppressive agents are deferred until final visualization and acceptance of the allograft by the donor procurement team to avoid morbidity to the recipient if the graft is deemed unacceptable. High-dose glucocorticoids are used for both reduction of reperfusion injury and initiation of immunosuppression and typically a calcineurin inhibitor (e.g., tacrolimus) and a nucleotide blocking agent (e.g., mycophenolate mofetil [MMF]) are administered immediately before or during the transplantation procedure (see immunosuppression later), as well as perioperative antibiotics.

In general, invasive arterial monitoring is required because of the high risk of hemodynamic compromise during induction of anesthesia, as well as for frequent intraoperative blood gas sampling. Central venous access is obtained for administration of vasoactive medications, and a PA catheter is placed for monitoring of PA pressures. TEE is performed to assess cardiac function and obtain baseline imaging of the native right and left PVs.

Following induction of anesthesia, the airway is secured with a single-lumen endotracheal tube, and surgical bronchoscopy is performed to review airway anatomy and clear any secretions that may impede successful one-lung ventilation. Subsequently, a double-lumen endotracheal tube is placed for allowance of lung isolation, and placement is confirmed with fiberoptic bronchoscopy. In some patients, amendobronchial blocker may be appropriate. Choice of initial ventilator settings should be disease specific, aimed at avoiding barotrauma while providing adequate gas exchange.

In the preincision time period, hemodynamic deterioration may occur as a result of anesthetic agents, positive pressure ventilation, pulmonary hypertensive crisis, RV failure, or pneumothorax if significant blebs or bullae are present. Vasoactive medications should be readily available, including vasopressors, inotropes, and pulmonary vasodilators.

Before surgical ligation of the lung, lung isolation is implemented with ventilation of the contralateral side. Time on one-lung ventilation should be minimized to avoid physiologic derangements in oxygenation and ventilation which may precipitate or worsen PH and contribute to RV failure. If significant hypoxemia occurs while utilizing one-lung ventilation, the PA of the nonventilated lung can be clamped to reduce shunt. In some situations, the ventilated lung may not be able to provide sufficient gas exchange, and intraoperative mechanical support should be considered (see "Intraoperative Mechanical Support" later).

Anesthetic Agents

There has been little formal evaluation of anesthetic agents for use during lung transplantation in humans. Evaluations in animal models suggest a lower incidence of PGD and acute rejection in donor lung allografts with volatile anesthetic gas preconditioning. In mice models of lung transplantation, sevoflurane preconditioning of the donor was associated with improved P/F ratio ($P = .03$), attenuated acute rejection scores ($P = .03$) as compared with total IV anesthesia with fentanyl and midazolam.[72] In a pig model of ischemia-reperfusion injury during lung transplantation, sevoflurane was associated with less glycocalyx destruction and lower inflammatory molecule expression as compared with propofol anesthetic,[73] suggesting preservation of lung endothelial function.

Vasoactive Medications

Vasopressor medications are titrated to support systemic circulation and coronary perfusion, and inotropes are added to assist the right ventricle if failure is noted. Short-acting agents are often preferred. In addition, pulmonary vasodilators are often used to reduce pulmonary vascular resistance and subsequent increased afterload to the right ventricle during lung transplantation. Inhaled pulmonary vasodilators include inhaled nitric oxide (iNO) and inhaled prostacyclins. iNO functions by activating intracellular guanylate cyclase to generate cyclic guanylate monophosphate, leading to vasodilation; when administered by inhaled route, it selectively vasodilates ventilated alveoli, improving V/Q matching. Use of iNO during one-lung ventilation and PA clamping is associated with reduced mean PA pressures, indexed PVR, and shunt fraction[74]; there is no evidence in lung transplantation to prove effectiveness in preventing reperfusion injury,[75] or graft dysfunction.[76]

Prostacyclins bind G-protein receptors that activate intracellular cyclic adenosine monophosphate (cAMP) and protein kinase A which causes relaxation of smooth muscles and pulmonary vasodilation. Inhaled iloprost, a prostacyclin analog, used during lung transplantation is associated with less PGD in the first 3 postoperative days ($P = .042$ on day 1, $P = .026$ on day 2, $P = .024$ on day 3).[77] Inhaled epoprostenol during lung transplantation is associated with decreased pulmonary pressures, improved P/F ratio, and decreased intrapulmonary shunting.[78] In a study comparing iNO versus inhaled prostacyclin in both heart and lung transplant patients, no significant differences hemodynamic effects were seen between the two therapies.[79] IV pulmonary vasodilators with systemic vasodilation effects are often less useful during lung transplantation because of hemodynamic instability introduced with surgical manipulation; however long-term infusions initiated before surgery are continued.

Fluid Management

In retrospective analysis of patients with PGD following lung transplantation, higher intraoperative total fluid volume ($P < .001$) and total red blood cell volume ($P = .002$) administered are associated with more severe PGD as defined by P/F ratio and radiographic diagnosis, such that each liter of volume administered increased odds for PGD grade 3 by 22%.[80] Restrictive fluid management should be balanced with risk of kidney injury or other end-organ malperfusion. Similarly, greater plasma volume received is also associated with increased patients with increased PGD (plasma volume 131 mL 95% CI, 71–191 mL, $P < .001$).[81]

Platelet transfusion, through activation and contribution to coagulation and inflammatory processes, may contribute to early inflammatory processes following allograft reperfusion,[82] and intraoperative platelet transfusion is an independent prognostic factor for in-hospital death ($P = .022$).[83] In addition, in a single-center, retrospective review of patients undergoing bilateral lung transplantation with CPB, platelet transfusion greater than the median of 1 unit was associated with increased 1-year mortality (hazard ratio 2.33; 95% CI, 1.16–4.65; $P = .017$).[84] Targeted transfusion strategies with point-of-care coagulation testing may reduce transfusion and early bleeding posttransplant, however has not been associated with reduction in in-hospital mortality ($P = .617$).[85]

TABLE 43.3 Transesophageal Echocardiography During Lung Transplantation

Structure	Transesophageal Echocardiography Assessment	Possible Findings	May Indicate
IAS	Color Doppler	Patent foramen ovale or atrial septal defect	Right to left shunt and hypoxemia
Tricuspid Valve	Color Doppler Spectral Doppler of tricuspid regurgitation jet	Tricuspid regurgitation Right ventricular systolic pressure estimate	Need for inotropic, pulmonary vasodilators, or mechanical circulatory support
Right Ventricle	Function Dilation Hypertrophy Septal position	Right ventricular failure Pulmonary hypertension	Need for inotropic, pulmonary vasodilators, or mechanical circulatory support
Pulmonary Artery	Diameter Spectral Doppler velocity	Thrombus Stenosis, kink	Embolus or anastomotic thrombus Anastomotic stricture
Pulmonary Veins	Diameter Color Doppler Spectral Doppler velocity	Thrombus Stenosis, kink	Embolus or anastomotic thrombus Anastomotic stricture
Left Ventricle	Filling	Underfilled	Hypovolemia, anastomotic stricture or thrombus, right ventricular failure

IAS, Interatrial septum.
Reprinted with permission from Tan Z, Roscoe A, Rubino A. Transesophageal echocardiography in heart and lung transplantation. *J Cardiothorac Vasc Anesth*. 2019;33:1548–1558.

Transesophageal Echocardiography

Use of TEE during lung transplantation is important for both anatomic assessment and cardiovascular monitoring. Comprehensive TEE examination should be performed utilizing a systematic approach to exclude abnormalities in the pretransplant, intraoperative and posttransplant phases that may impact care with areas of focus highlighted in Table 43.3.[86] Also incidental pretransplant TEE findings may change intraoperative surgical management, as in the case of substantial mitral regurgitation or septal defects, prompting concomitant cardiac surgery. Concomitant cardiac surgical procedures are associated with longer ventilator time and ICU length of stay[87] but do not affect allograft ischemic time, ECMO use, hospital length of stay, or 1-year mortality[88] as compared with patients undergoing lung transplantation alone.

Important points intraoperatively that warrant reassessment using TEE include induction of anesthesia, initiation of one-lung ventilation, surgical manipulation, PA clamping, reperfusion, and chest closure, as these events may result in dramatic changes to RV preload or afterload and subsequent RV failure.[86] Careful assessment after surgical anastomosis of the PA and veins or atrial cuff anastomosis is necessary to identify any flow restriction or thrombus (Figs. 43.5–43.7). In adults, a minimum PV diameter of 0.5 mm and a velocity less than 1 m/s are acceptable to ensure adequate flow,[89] although higher velocities may be seen with living-donor lobar transplants.[90] Hemodynamic context at

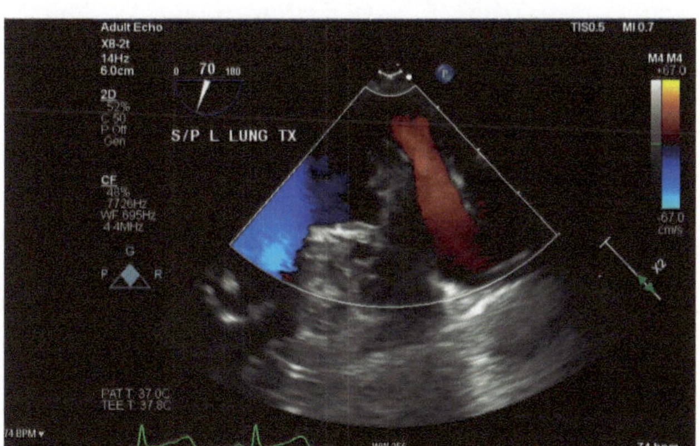

• **Fig. 43.5** Transesophageal echocardiography of left pulmonary vein color flow doppler.

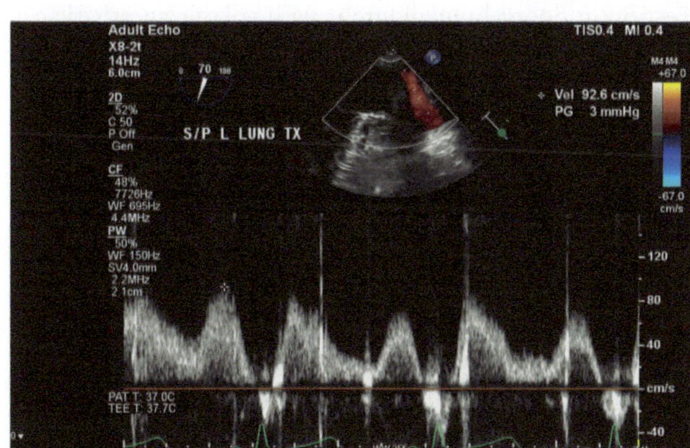

• **Fig. 43.6** Transesophageal echocardiography of left pulmonary vein spectral doppler.

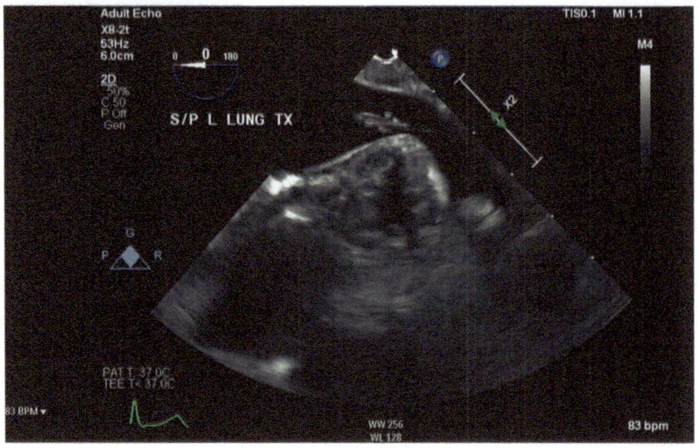

• **Fig. 43.7** Transesophageal echocardiography of left pulmonary vein thrombus.

the time of the examination should always be considered. For example, in cases of CPB or VA ECMO support, low velocities may indicate low flow state that are not caused by stenosis. Assessment of vascular anastomoses and ventricular function should be performed following discontinuation of mechanical support, and repeat assessment should occur at the time of chest closure[91] as size mismatch may compress vascular anastomosis and result in graft failure.[92]

Allograft Ventilation Management

During allograft reperfusion, F_iO2 is reduced and the graft is ventilated with room air (21% oxygen) and low airway pressures. F_iO2 greater than 40% is associated with increased risk of PGD, and PGD is increased for every 10% increase in F_iO2 during reperfusion.[93] Initial ventilator settings should be set to minimize ventilator-induced lung injury, utilizing low V_Ts and PEEP (Box 43.3).[94] Permissive hypercapnia, especially if present pretransplant, is used to ensure a normal pH. Use of inhaled or IV pulmonary vasodilators may attenuate the vasoconstriction effects of CO2 on the allograft pulmonary vasculature.

Thorough bronchoscopy should be performed after lung transplantation to assess anastomoses and clear secretions that may inhibit gas exchange. Increased airway pressures,

• BOX 43.3 Initial Ventilator Settings for Reperfused Lung Transplant Allograft

- Tidal volume 6 mL/kg donor predicted body weight, adjusted for single lung ventilation and/or lobar transplant
- PEEP of 5-cm H_2O
- Careful recruitment maneuvers, as needed
- Lowest F_iO2 possible to maintain appropriate PaO2 [>70 mm Hg] and hemoglobin oxygen saturations (SpO2) ≥92 %
- Consider keeping PaCO2 in range of pretransplant
- Bronchoscopic airway clearance

F_iO2, Fraction of inspired oxygen; *PaCO2*, arterial partial pressure of carbon dioxide; *PaO2*, arterial partial pressure of oxygen; *PEEP*, positive end-expiratory pressure; *SpO2*, oxygen saturation. Reprinted with permission from Barnes L, Reed RM, Parekh KR, Bhama JK, Pena T, Rajagopal S, et al. Mechanical ventilation for the lung transplant recipient. *Curr Pulmonol Rep*. 2015;4:88–96.

poor oxygenation, or excessively high ventilation requirements should prompt consideration for ECMO support in the early postoperative period.

Intraoperative Mechanical Support

In patients who do not tolerate one-lung ventilation because of hypercarbia, hypoxemia, PH, RV dysfunction, or hemodynamic instability with PA clamping, ECMO may be used as a supportive measure intraoperatively. A metaanalysis of use of ECMO versus CPB intraoperatively in 785 patients during lung transplantation showed that ECMO had lower rates of PGD, bleeding, renal failure requiring dialysis, tracheostomy, intraoperative transfusions, intubation time, and hospital stay.[95]

Use of CPB may be advantageous if there is a need for slow pulmonary reperfusion to both transplanted lungs simultaneously in the case of double lung transplant. Slow pulmonary reperfusion over 5 minutes with and without protective ventilation has been shown in animal models to be advantageous as compared with immediate full flow reperfusion in terms of gas exchange, airway pressures, highest oxygenation index, lung edema, and vascular leakage in the immediate posttransplant period.[96] Use of CPB may also be advantageous in small patients with suppurative disease where double-lumen tube placement is prohibitive because of need for aggressive suctioning, lavage, or clearance of secretions. In addition, if there is need for concomitant cardiac surgical procedure, such as CABG, valve replacement, heart transplant, or septal defect closure, CPB may be required. ECMO circuits can also be configured for prompt conversion from ECMO to CPB support and vice versa, as in the case of unintended surgical injury.[97]

Postoperative Care

In the early postoperative period, management goals include optimizing hemodynamics, identifying and managing bleeding, optimizing graft function including immunosuppression implementation and infection prevention, and monitoring other organ system function. Later in the postoperative course, emphasis switches to monitoring for later transplant complications, rehabilitation, and education in preparation for discharge. Frequent and early communication between ICU, surgical, and pulmonology teams is necessary for optimal management. In addition, involvement of physical therapy, occupational therapy, social work, and transplant educators may help facilitate recovery and rehabilitation in the posttransplant period.

Hemodynamic Management in The ICU

On immediate arrival to the ICU postoperatively, patients require close monitoring as hemodynamic changes may occur suddenly. Arterial blood pressure, arterial lactate, and chest tube drainage and urine output should be monitored closely to quickly identify early signs of shock because of hypovolemia, cardiogenic dysfunction, or vasoplegia. Evaluation of cardiac filling pressures through use of a PA catheter can be useful in distinguishing between these processes. In patients with sudden hemodynamic changes, early echocardiographic assessment for evidence of LV or RV dysfunction, vascular anastomotic complications, pericardial effusion, or hypovolemia (further discussed later) should occur; TEE assessment is advantageous because of superior image quality of vital cardiopulmonary structures.

For patients with vasodilatory shock, vasopressors (preferentially norepinephrine and vasopressin) should be used for blood pressure support to maintain end-organ perfusion. In cases of LV or RV dysfunction, inotropy with dobutamine, milrinone, or epinephrine should be used. Inhaled pulmonary vasodilators, such as NO or prostaglandins may be trialed for afterload reduction in cases of severe RV dysfunction.

Ventilator Management

In the early postoperative period, frequent ventilator and ABG assessment is needed to identify changes oxygenation, carbon dioxide elimination, and compliance. End tidal CO2 should be monitored and correlated with arterial PCO2 to assess dead space ventilation. Close attention should be paid to burden and consistency of respiratory secretions, and gentle suctioning should be performed as needed.

Ventilatory management mimics that of ARDS,[98] utilizing lung-protective ventilation to reduce ventilator-induced lung injury and prevent PGD.[63] Low V_T ventilation (i.e., starting with 6 mL/kg of ideal body weight) with 5 to 10 cm H_2O of PEEP is used targeting plateau pressures less than 30 cm H_2O; assist control mode in either volume control or pressure control may be used. F_iO2 should be minimized to prevent oxygen toxicity, and an appropriate respiratory rate should be set to maintain adequate minute ventilation. Especially in cases of small donor lung size, V_Ts should target the donor's rather than recipient's ideal body weight to prevent volutrauma to the graft. Of note, patients with chronic preoperative hypoventilation and resultant elevated serum bicarbonate levels may initially require relative hypoventilation to achieve a normal serum pH. Management of severe hypoxemia and hypercapnia will be discussed later in "Primary Graft Dysfunction" section.

In cases of single lung transplantation, a native lung still remains and must be considered in the ventilation strategy. For example, in cases where COPD is the indication for transplant, the native lung may become overly distended with high levels of PEEP or with inadequate expiratory time. Typically, the donor lung will have both improved ventilation and lower pulmonary vascular resistance than the diseased lung; it should therefore receive the majority of blood flow, naturally improving ventilation-perfusion matching.

In intubated patients, periodic bronchoscopic evaluation of the graft airways should occur, both for diagnosis of bronchial pathology (e.g., ischemia, rejection, or occlusion) and therapeutic removal of debris or secretions. Nebulized albuterol or ipratropium may be used in cases of bronchospasm or wheezing, and saline flushes may aid in clearing thick bronchial secretions. Typical ventilator-associated-pneumonia "bundles" including chlorhexidine mouthwash and head of bed elevation remain important in minimizing risk in this vulnerable population.

In the majority of patients, graft function will be adequate for ventilator weaning early postoperatively. Once adequate oxygenation and ventilation, hemodynamics, and hemostasis have been ensured, a spontaneous breathing trial should be attempted and, if successful, extubation performed. In general, bronchoscopy is performed before extubation to clear secretions and improve chances of a successful extubation. For those patients with graft dysfunction or severe deconditioning, early tracheostomy may be helpful in ventilator weaning and pulmonary toilet while allowing for early mobilization. For patients requiring inhaled pulmonary vasodilators or ECMO postoperatively (discussed later in "Extracorporeal Membrane Oxygenation in the Postoperative Period"), extubation is generally delayed until after weaning or decannulation.

Following extubation, pulmonary toilet remains extremely important for maintaining graft function. Chest physiotherapy should be performed to aid in secretion clearance. Patients should be encouraged to cough to bring up secretions and to use an incentive spirometer to recruit lung tissue and prevent atelectasis. Early mobilization should occur to decrease atelectasis and risk for venous thromboembolism (VTE).

Chest Tube Management

Chest tubes are placed on the operative side because of pleural space entry and high likelihood of pneumothorax, pleural effusion, or hemothorax postoperatively. Chest tubes are placed to suction initially to ensure lung expansion and drainage of accumulated blood or fluid. Output is monitored hourly for evidence of bleeding, and 100 cc/h or more is particularly concerning and may prompt blood product transfusions and chest exploration. In addition, if chest tube drainage abruptly stops, there should be suspicion for a clogged or clotted tube and inadequate drainage of the pleural space. With lack of drainage for extended times and significant postoperative bleeding, tension hemothorax may develop.

Later in the postoperative period, chest tubes serve to drain fluid or air that may accumulate in the pleural space. Pleural effusions occur universally because of increased vascular permeability and lack of lymphatic drainage. Pneumothoraces are highly common owing to air leaks from bronchial anastomotic sites or injury to lung tissue. A chylothorax, or the accumulation of chyle in the pleural space, may develop early or late following lung transplantation as a result of disruption of the thoracic duct. Chest tubes are left in place until drainage becomes minimal, pneumothoraces improve, and air leaks resolve, generally about 7 to 10 days postoperatively.

Fluid Management

Fluid management should target adequate organ perfusion while limiting excessive volume administration that may contribute to excessive graft edema; hemodynamic variables, as well as oxygenation, arterial lactate, and urine output should be considered. Typically, isotonic crystalloid is used for fluid resuscitation when necessary. For patients with evidence of active bleeding, blood product transfusion should be guided by laboratory values, as well as clinically based on hemodynamics and chest tube output, patient comorbidities, and recent operative course. A restrictive transfusion strategy may be preferable in patients without evidence of acute bleeding to avoid complications, such as transfusion reactions or transfusion-related lung injury (TRALI).

Sedation and Analgesia

On initial ICU arrival, a deep level of sedation should be targeted while evaluating for bleeding, hemodynamic changes, and initial graft function. As the clinical condition improves, sedation should be weaned for neurologic assessment and eventual spontaneous awakening trial. When safe, sedation should be kept to the minimal level required for patient comfort.

Adequate analgesia is of high importance following lung transplant surgery to allow for optimal respiratory mechanics; patients with high pain levels will typically take shallow, rapid breaths, leading to inadequate gas exchange and worsening atelectasis. Multimodal analgesia including opioids, nonopioid analgesics, and regional or neuraxial local anesthetic techniques should be considered.

Immunosuppression

Immunosuppression is important for prevention of acute and chronic graft rejection. Induction dosing begins just before or during transplant surgery, and maintenance doses are continued after ICU arrival. Risk of graft rejection is highest in the first 6 months after transplantation and gradually declines over time. Because immunosuppressive agents increase risk of infection and malignancy and often have significant toxicities, it is important not to overimmunosuppress. Ideally, immunosuppressive medications are chosen to block different aspects of the immune response pathways without significant overlap in mechanism of action or side effect profiles. Some immunosuppressive agents are tailored to a specific patient's risk for or history of rejection, whereas others are standardized for the type of organ transplant. There is no official consensus on immunosuppression immediately following lung transplantation, but a typical regimen includes an induction agent and triple therapy with a glucocorticoid, a calcineurin inhibitor, and a nucleotide blocking agent.[99] In cases of HLA-sensitization, antihumoral therapy is added.

Induction Immunosuppression Agents

Induction therapy is commonly used during lung transplant surgery to reduce the T cell response to the allograft, the primary mediator of rejection. Induction agents function to either deplete T cells or interrupt T cell activation and proliferation. Monoclonal antibody induction agents are typically interleukin (IL)-2 receptor antagonists (e.g., basilixumab, alemtuzumab), and polyclonal agents include antithymocyte or antilymphocyte globulins. Use of an induction agent during lung transplantation remains controversial as studies are small or retrospective, but trends suggest a decrease in acute rejection and improvement in long-term outcomes without a significant increase in infectious risk.[99] Induction therapy has increased significantly over the past 10 years. Basilixumab is generally dosed intraoperatively and again on the fourth postoperative day and tends to be well-tolerated. Antithymocyte globulin is dosed interprocedurally and again two to three times in the early postoperative period. It can cause a cytokine release syndrome of fever, rash, myalgias, and tachycardia and requires premedication with glucocorticoids, antihistamines, and antipyretics; other side effects include pancytopenia, glomerulonephritis, and serum sickness. Alemtuzumab can also cause a cytokine release syndrome, but it is currently not commercially available in the United States and Europe.

Glucocorticoids

Glucocorticoids inhibit both humoral and cell-mediated immunity by suppressing transcription of inflammatory-mediated genes. This leads to decreased T cell proliferation, macrophage activation, cytokine production, and altered lymphocyte migration.[99] Typically following an intraoperative dose, methylprednisolone 0.5 to 1 mg/kg daily is administered IV postoperatively; once enteral absorption is confirmed, this is converted to an equivalent dose of prednisone. Prednisone is slowly tapered over the first post-transplant year to (or if tolerated, within the first 3 months) to a minimum of 5 to 10 mg daily. If suspicion for rejection arises, high-dose glucocorticoids will be administered followed by a taper over a period of weeks. Side effects of glucocorticoids include hyperglycemia, susceptibility to infection, poor wound-healing, fluid-retention, hyperlipidemia, psychiatric disturbances, and osteoporosis.

Calcineurin Inhibitors

Calcineurin inhibitors (CNIs) target calcineurin, a protein phosphatase involved in activation of T-cells. CNIs include cyclosporine, the original in its class, and tacrolimus. Cyclosporine has many adverse effects, such as acute and chronic nephrotoxicity, hypertension, hyperlipidemia, neurotoxicity (e.g., posterior reversible encephalopathic syndrome, seizures, tremor), electrolyte abnormalities, hyperglycemia, hirsutism, gingival hyperplasia, limiting its tolerability. Tacrolimus became available later on, is more potent, and has much surpassed cyclosporine in use. It causes less nephrotoxicity, and there is some evidence of reduced rejection over cyclosporine. Both CNIs have poor oral absorption, variable bioavailability, and a narrow therapeutic window, so monitoring for a therapeutic drug level is essential. Target trough levels vary by institution, patient risk factors, and time from transplant surgery but typically are between 5 and 15 ng/mL. In most cases, tacrolimus is dosed immediately preoperatively and resumed within 1 day postoperatively, either enterally or sublingually. IV dosing has been associated with infusion reactions and increased neuro- and nephrotoxicity.

Antiproliferative Agents

This class can be divided into nucleotide blocking agents and mechanistic target of rapamycin (mTOR) inhibitors. Nucleotide blocking agents include MMF and azathioprine (AZA). MMF depletes guanosine nucleotides whereas AZA prevents de novo synthesis of purines, both inhibiting proliferation of T and B cells. Although there are limited data in the lung transplant population, MMF is preferentially used over AZA at most institutions. MMF is typically dosed immediately preoperatively and continued during the perioperative period. Doses range between 1 to 1.5 g twice daily, either orally or intravenously. Adverse effects include leukopenia, thrombocytopenia, and gastrointestinal disturbances.

mTOR inhibitors are a newer class of antiproliferative drugs including sirolimus and everolimus which interrupt deoxyribonucleic acid (DNA) and protein synthesis involved in proliferation of natural killer, T, and B cells. Although mTOR inhibitors are generally not used in a typical lung transplant immunosuppressive regimen, they are considered in special circumstances, such as patients that do not tolerate nucleotide blocking agents, those with refractory allograft rejection, or to allow for CNI dose reduction or elimination.[99] Adverse effects include poor wound healing, leukopenia, thrombocytopenia, hypertriglyceridemia, proteinuria, and pneumonitis.

Antihumoral Therapy

Most immunosuppression targets cell-mediated immune responses; however, antibody-mediated rejection can occur because of presence of donor-specific antibodies (DSA) to HLAs or other antigens. Treatment of acute and hyperacute rejection will be discussed later. Patients with antibodies to HLA antigens are "sensitized" and at higher risk of antibody-mediated rejection.[99] These patients may receive IV immunoglobulin (IVIG) intraoperatively. IVIG is a product made from pooled plasma of many donors, and it functions by blocking binding of DSA, causing B cell apoptosis, and inhibiting complement activation. IVIG is generally well-tolerated, although premedication with an antipyretic and antihistamine is frequently used to prevent an inflammatory or anaphylactoid reaction.

Infection Prevention and Management

Patients in the early posttransplant period are at high risk for bacterial, viral, and fungal infections because of the high doses of immunosuppressive drugs. In addition, patients with end-stage lung disease who undergo transplantation frequently have chronic pulmonary infections or colonization at baseline, and reactivation of latent infections may occur. Time-course following transplantation is important in predicting the type of infection that may develop.

Prophylactic antimicrobials are highly important for preventing infections in the perioperative period. Donor cultures from the time of organ harvest should be followed and microbial cultures treated in the recipient. Routine BAL cultures should be done with all surveillance bronchoscopies, and there should be a low threshold for infectious workup and initiation of broad-spectrum antimicrobials. Treatment courses for acquired infections should be tailored based on donor and recipient risk factors, culture and laboratory data, and clinical course.

For patients without known preoperative infections, prophylactic antibiotics should be continued for several days following the transplant surgery; time course depends on donor and recipient culture data and appearance on bronchoscopic evaluation. For patients with preoperative infections, especially multidrug resistant organisms, antibiotics should target previously cultured organisms and time course should be extended.

Routine antiviral prophylaxis should target cytomegalovirus (CMV), the most common opportunistic infection following solid organ transplantation.[100] CMV can either be reactivated from a previously latent infection within a host or be transmitted through the allograft. Patients at highest risk for CMV infection are those who are seronegative for CMV before transplant and receive an organ from a seropositive donor. Ganciclovir (parenteral) or valganciclovir (enteral) are typical agents used for CMV prophylaxis, with a course ranging from 3 to 12 months depending on recipient risk. Epstein-Barr virus (EBV) is another virus that can be reactivated in a host or passed through an allograft, and it is associated with development of posttransplant lymphoproliferative disorder (PTLD; described later). Ganciclovir and valganciclovir also protect against EBV reactivation, as well as herpes simplex virus. Immunization for herpes zoster and hepatitis B is recommended before transplantation. In patients with a history of hepatitis B infection (i.e., hepatitis B core antibody positive), lamivudine prophylaxis should be used.

Antifungal prophylaxis typically targets *Aspergillus* and *Candida*, the most common posttransplant opportunistic fungal species, and other agents may vary by location based on endemic species. A typical regimen includes inhaled amphotericin B lipid complex for *Aspergillus* prophylaxis for at least 2 months and nystatin oral suspension to prevent oropharyngeal candidiasis for 1 year.

Pneumocystis pneumonia (PCP), caused by the fungal organism *Pneumocystis jirovecii*, used to be a frequent postlung transplant complication.[100] With use of trimethoprim-sulfamethoxazole prophylaxis (TMP-SMX), PCP has become exceedingly rare. PCP prophylaxis is generally lifelong.

Venous Thromboembolism Prevention

Many postlung transplant patients, especially in the immediate-postoperative period, are at high risk for VTE because of immobility, advanced age, history of VTE, and use of mechanical circulatory support. This risk must be weighed against that of acute bleeding following a major surgical procedure. Typically, VTE prophylaxis with subcutaneous heparin is initiated on the first postoperative day as long as major bleeding is not apparent. In patients with a history of VTE or other condition requiring anticoagulation, therapeutic anticoagulation may be accomplished with a heparin infusion until later in the postoperative period; this allows for close monitoring and rapid reversal in case of bleeding.

Nutritional Support and Stress Ulcer Prophylaxis

Although not studied specifically in the lung transplant population, stress ulcer prophylaxis should be considered for all ventilated patients and potentially continued because of chronic steroid use. Enteral access should be obtained early in the postoperative course to allow for dosing of medications and early nutrition if extubation is delayed. Swallowing ability should be assessed following extubation to limit the likelihood of an aspiration event. For patients who are unable to swallow effectively, enteral feeding should be considering within the first few postoperative days to prevent development of malnutrition. Early bowel regimen implementation may be helpful in preventing constipation in the setting of opioid analgesia, especially in the CF population which is prone to constipation and intestinal obstruction.[15]

Early Postoperative Complications

Complications in the early postoperative period may be pulmonary or extrapulmonary. Pulmonary complications include graft dysfunction, rejection, anastomotic complications, pleural complications, phrenic nerve and diaphragmatic dysfunction, and pulmonary infection. Extrapulmonary complications include infection, VTE, hyperammonemia, myocardial infarction, arrhythmia, renal insufficiency, and delirium.

Graft Dysfunction

Early graft dysfunction manifests as hypoxemia, difficult or inadequate ventilation, or pulmonary infiltrates. Causes of graft dysfunction are broad and include volume overload, TRALI, acute antibody-mediated rejection, vascular or anastomotic complications, infection, and PGD. Often, graft infiltrates postoperatively are multifactorial rather than attributable to a single cause.

Some degree of pulmonary edema is expected in all immediately postoperative lung transplant patients because of ischemia-reperfusion injury, increased vascular permeability, and surgically interrupted lymphatic drainage. Severe pulmonary edema can result from volume overload, especially in cases of high-volume fluid administration intraoperatively or in patients with LV dysfunction. Pulmonary infiltrates caused by TRALI occur within 6 hours of blood product transfusion, specifically after high-plasma volume blood components are given; this etiology of graft dysfunction may be more common after a challenging surgical dissection with high intraoperative blood loss and transfusion requirement. Especially in patients with preexisting infections, worsening pneumonia may develop in the setting of high levels of immunosuppressive medications, and this may contribute to graft dysfunction.

Diagnostic workup and management of graft dysfunction should be tailored to the clinical scenario, considering preoperative recipient comorbidities, intraoperative complications, and common postoperative issues. An early infectious workup is prudent, and attention should be paid to ensuring proper antimicrobial coverage of any known resistant organisms that the recipient has cultured in the past. Bronchoscopy is useful to assess bronchial anastomoses for evidence of bleeding or ischemic injury, as well as to obtain culture samples and clear secretions. TEE can be useful in diagnosing vascular anastomotic complications or LV dysfunction; in cases of elevated left atrial filling pressures or diuresis should be considered to optimize volume status. In some cases, CT angiogram may be necessary to better visualize lung parenchyma, airways, and pulmonary vasculature.

Primary Graft Dysfunction

PGD is a syndrome of acute lung injury occurring within the first 72 hours of lung transplantation characterized and graded by diffuse pulmonary infiltrates and hypoxemia[101] (Fig. 43.8). PGD is thought to be caused by ischemia-reperfusion injury that alters the alveolar and vascular endothelium, leading to pulmonary edema, reduced lung compliance, and poor gas exchange.[102] PGD occurs following 30% of lung transplantation procedures and is the leading cause of early mortality after lung transplantation; it is associated with longer IMV time, ICU length of stay, and hospital length of stay. PGD is classified into different grades depending on the severity of radiographic findings and hypoxemia (Table 43.4), and grade 3 PGD is associated with the worst outcomes,[101] and can be distinguished from or accompany other causes of hypoxemia in the immediate posttransplant period (Table 43.5). Risk factors for grade 3 PGD include donor factors, such as smoking history or lung contusion, undersize of the donor relative to recipient, and heavy alcohol use. The primary diagnosis of the transplant

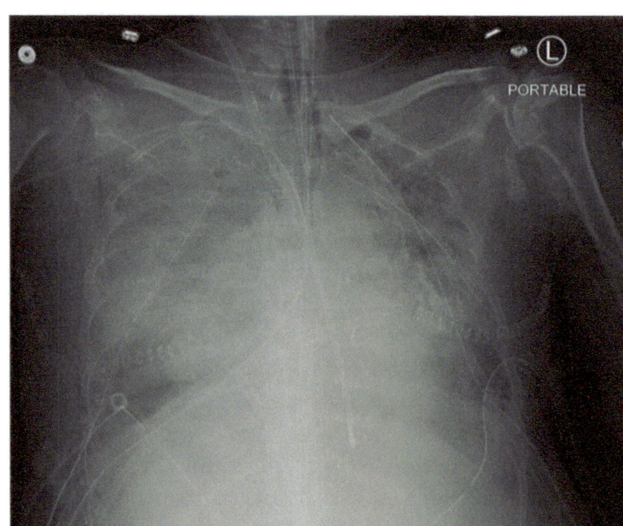

• **Fig. 43.8** Chest x-ray demonstrating severe bilateral pulmonary infiltrates in a patient with primary graft dysfunction.

TABLE 43.4 Primary Graft Dysfunction Grading System

Grade	Chest X-Ray Findings	PaO2/FiO2 Ratio
Grade 0	Normal	Any
Grade 1	Diffuse infiltrates	>300
Grade 2	Diffuse infiltrates	200–300
Grade 3	Diffuse infiltrates	<200

FiO2, Fraction of inspired oxygen; *PaO2*, arterial partial pressure of oxygen.
Modified with permission from Snell GI, Yusen RD, Weill D, et al. Report of the ISHLT Working Group on Primary Lung Graft Dysfunction, Part I: Definition and grading-A 2016 Consensus Group statement of the International Society for Heart and Lung Transplantation. *J Heart Lung Transplant*. 2017;36:1097–1103.

TABLE 43.5 Differential Diagnosis of Hypoxemia With Pulmonary Infiltrates Immediately Following Lung Transplantation

Diagnosis	Key Features	Evaluation	Treatment
Volume overload or TACO	– High fluid or blood product administration – LV dysfunction or high LA pressure – Possible pleural effusions	– Evaluation of pulmonary capillary wedge pressure – Echocardiography – BNP, troponin	– Diuresis – Inotropic support for poor LV function
TRALI	– Occurs during or within 6 hours of a transfusion – More common with high-plasma volume blood products (i.e., FFP) – May also present with fever, hypotension	– Evaluation of pulmonary capillary wedge pressure – Echocardiography – BNP, troponin	– Stop transfusion if still in progress – Report to blood bank for transfusion reaction workup
Pneumonia or aspiration	– History of recent infection (e.g., cystic fibrosis patients) – Witnessed aspiration event – Fevers, elevated white blood cell count, hypotension	– Bronchoscopy with bronchoalveolar lavage culture – Culture for bloodstream infection – Viral respiratory PCR – CMV PCR – Fungal culture/PCR	– Broad spectrum antibiotics, antiviral, or antifungal coverage targeted to prior culture data or patient/donor risk factors
Hyperacute antibody-mediated rejection	– Rapid onset, within minutes to 24 hours of allograft reperfusion	– Review pretransplant HLA antibody testing and crossmatch – New HLA antibody screen – Consider transbronchial biopsy	– Plasmapheresis – IVIG – Rituximab, bortezomib
PA flow obstruction (e.g., kinking, stenosis, thrombosis, embolism)	– Hypotension, hemodynamic instability – RV dysfunction	– CT angiography – TEE	– Surgical repair (e.g., lung repositioning, thrombectomy) – Anticoagulation
PV flow obstruction (e.g., kinking, stenosis, thrombosis, embolism)	– Often unilateral – Decreased lung compliance – LA thrombus or systemic embolism	– CT angiography – TEE	– Surgical repair (e.g., repositioning, thrombectomy) – Anticoagulation
Primary graft dysfunction	– Diffuse infiltrates – Decreased lung compliance	– Exclusion of other diagnoses	– Lung protective ventilation – Empiric antibiotics – Inhaled vasodilators – ECMO

BNP, Brain natriuretic peptide; *CMV*, cytomegalovirus; *CT*, computerized tomography; *ECMO*, extracorporeal membrane oxygenation; *FFP*, fresh frozen plasma; *HLA*, human leukocyte antigen; *IVIG*, intravenous immunoglobulin; *LA*, left atrium; *LV*, left ventricle; *PA*, pulmonary artery; *PCR*, polymerase chain reaction; *RV*, right ventricle; *TACO*, transfusion-associated circulatory overload; *TEE*, transesophageal echocardiography; *TRALI*, transfusion-related acute lung injury.

recipient is one of the greatest risk factors for the development of PGD, with an incidence of PGD of 11.8% in COPD, 12.4% in CF, 18% in IPF, 30% in idiopathic pulmonary arterial hypertension (IPAH), and 50% in sarcoidosis.[93] Overweight or obese recipients also have an elevated risk of PGD. Surgical factors, such as prolonged ischemic time, use of CPB, large volume blood product transfusion, high F_iO2 during reperfusion, and single lung transplant are also independent risk factors for highest grade PGD.[103]

Management of PGD is primarily supportive, and because of similarities between PGD and ARDS, management of PGD are typically extrapolated from that of ARDS.[63] Goals are to **limit ventilator-induced lung injury**, including volutrauma, barotrauma, and oxygen toxicity; lung-protective ventilation with PEEP is used. **Fluid restriction** and judicious diuresis should be used, if possible, while maintaining adequate perfusion. **Inhaled pulmonary vasodilators** should not be used routinely but may be trialed in situations of severe hypoxemia or elevated pulmonary vascular resistance. Both iNO and prostaglandins can improve pulmonary vasodilation in areas of lung tissue that are well-ventilated, improving ventilation-perfusion matching. In situations of severe PGD, refractory to all medical management, **postoperative ECMO** may be temporarily used (described later in "Extracorporeal Membrane Oxygenation in the Postoperative Period"). In rare situations, if severe PGD fails to improve, early retransplantation may be necessary. Because of worse overall survival in retransplantation, especially those indicated for severe PGD, and limited allograft availability, this should be reserved for situations of last resort.[63]

Acute Rejection

Between 2004 and 2016, 28% of lung transplant recipients experienced at least one episode of acute rejection in the first year.[1] Lung allografts are more prone to rejection than other solid organ transplants, possibly because of more vulnerability to ischemic injury, recurrent infections, and constant environmental exposures.[104] Although acute rejection is rarely fatal on its own, it leads to other adverse outcomes, such as increased risk of infection with its management and increased risk of chronic airflow obstruction (discussed later in "Long-term Complications of Lung Transplant").[104] Risk factors for acute rejection include HLA mismatching, certain genetic polymorphisms, and immunosuppression regimen. Signs and symptoms include cough, dyspnea, sputum production, ARDS, fever, or hypoxemia. Workup should include radiographic imaging and pulmonary function tests, as well as bronchoscopy with BAL and transbronchial biopsies. Treatment should be guided by histologic appearance of rejection in addition to severity of clinical symptoms.

Lung allograft rejection can occur by two mechanisms: cellular or humoral. Cellular rejection, the predominant type, is caused by T-cell recognition of HLA. Acute cellular rejection is diagnosed based on histopathologic changes and can be categorized as either perivascular and interstitial (A-grade) or airway (B-grade, also known as lymphocytic bronchiolitis) rejection (Table 43.6).[104,105] Acute cellular rejection is typically managed with a pulse of high-dose corticosteroids, followed by a taper over 2 to 3 weeks. Management of refractory acute cellular rejection is more varied but may include additional pulse steroids, antithymocyte globulin, or alemtuzumab, a

TABLE 43.6 Pathologic Grading of Lung Transplant Rejection

Category of Rejection	Grade	Severity	Histology
Grade A: Acute rejection	0	None	Normal lung
	1	Minimal	Small mononuclear perivascular infiltrates
	2	Mild	More frequent perivascular infiltrates, eosinophils may be present
	3	Moderate	Dense perivascular infiltrates, extending into interstitial space. Eosinophils and neutrophils
	4	Severe	Diffuse perivascular, interstitial, and air-space infiltrates with lung injury. Neutrophils may be present
Grade B: Airway inflammation	0	None	No evidence of bronchiolar inflammation
	1R	Low grade	Infrequent, scattered, or single-layer mononuclear cells in bronchiolar submucosa
	2R	High grade	Larger infiltrates of activated lymphocytes in bronchiolar submucosa; can involve eosinophils and plasmacytoid cells
Grade C: Chronic airway rejection—obliterative	0	Absent	
	1	Present	Intraluminal airway obliteration with fibrous connective tissue

Modified with permission from Martinu T, Pavlisko EN, Chen DF, Palmer SM. Acute allograft rejection: cellular and humoral processes. *Clin Chest Med.* 2011;32:295–310.

monoclonal antibody targeting the CD52 antigen present on B and T lymphocytes.

Antibody-mediated rejection occurs following lung transplant because of DSA against HLA, leading to both complement-dependent and independent pathways of immune activation.[106] Hyperacute rejection, a fulminant form occurring within the first 24 hours following reperfusion because of presence of preformed DSA, has become exceedingly rare because of preoperative HLA antibody screening and donor-specific cross-matching. Histologically, antibody-mediated rejection demonstrates neutrophil infiltration and complement component C4d deposition in alveolar capillaries.[106]

Management of acute antibody-mediated rejection includes plasmapheresis, IVIG, rituximab (a monoclonal antibody targeting B-cells), bortezomib (a proteosome inhibitor that cause apoptosis of plasma cells), as well as pulse glucocorticoids or increase in antiproliferative agents; hyperacute rejection involves use of several immunosuppressant therapies simultaneously.

Anastomotic Complications

Anastomotic complications include vascular complications, such as complications including PA or PV kinking, stenosis, thrombosis, or embolism, and airway complications, such as bronchial necrosis and dehiscence, stenosis, fistulas, or infection.

Obstruction to PA blood flow generally presents as worsening PH and RV failure with hemodynamic instability. Kinking or thrombosis of a PV anastomosis typically occurs very early in the postoperative course. It is rare but can result in significant morbidity if not identified and treated quickly. PV thrombosis results in severe unilateral pulmonary edema (unless occurring in anastomoses in both transplanted lungs), leading to hypoxemia and decreased pulmonary compliance. Patients who experience PV thromboses are at high risk for systemic embolization, leading to stroke, limb or bowel ischemia, or other embolic complications. PV thrombosis is often diagnosed through TEE following reperfusion of the allograft in the operating room, or CT angiogram if it develops later. Unstable patients may require emergent thrombectomy and surgical revision of the anastomosis, whereas more stable patients benefit from systemic anticoagulation.

Because of interruption of normal bronchial blood supply during transplantation, airway anastomoses are especially prone to ischemic injury. Airway complications occur in up to 10% to 15% of lung transplants.[107] Risk factors include surgical technique (e.g., excessive donor bronchial length), PGD, acute rejection within the first year, certain pulmonary infections, prolonged mechanical ventilation, single lung transplant, and some immunosuppressive medications.[107] Airway complications are frequently identified on surveillance bronchoscopy but may also be visible on CT scan.

Necrosis caused by ischemic injury can be a normal part of the healing process but typically resolves several weeks after transplantation; if healing fails, dehiscence occurs. This should be suspected in patients with prolonged air leaks. More severe bronchial dehiscence requires bronchoscopic or surgical repair. Bronchial stenosis is the most common airway complication and typically occurs at the suture line and extending distally. **Severe narrowing of the bronchus intermedius** can lead to vanishing bronchus intermedius syndrome which causes high morbidity and mortality. Bronchial stenosis may be asymptomatic or lead to dyspnea, cough, wheezing, frequent pneumonia, or reduction in forced expiratory flow, and treatment involves dilations, stenting, or airway ablations. **Bronchial fistulas** are rare and may develop between the airway and pleura, mediastinum, or vasculature; depending on the location, these can result in dyspnea, infection, pneumothorax, subcutaneous emphysema, or persistent air leak. These can often be fatal depending on ability to close the fistula and associated complications.

Intrathoracic Complications

Phrenic nerve injury and resulting ipsilateral diaphragmatic paralysis can occur from lung transplantation surgery and can lead to longer mechanical ventilation and hospital length of stay.[108] This diagnosis should be suspected in patients with dyspnea, hypoventilation, failure to wean from the ventilator and elevated hemidiaphragm on chest imaging. Unilateral paralysis may be more clinically significant in patients with single lung transplants. Management involves ventilator support, and in cases with persistent inability to wean from the ventilator, surgical plication or diaphragmatic pacing may be considered. **Pleural complications** including pneumothorax, chylothorax, hemothorax, and pleural effusions (see "Chest Tube Management" later) and pneumonia (see "Infection Prevention and Management") may also be present.

Extrapulmonary Complications

As in any major intrathoracic surgery, lung transplantation can result in common postsurgical complications including infection, VTE, myocardial infarction, arrhythmia, and delirium. Renal dysfunction is especially prevalent following lung transplantation with a cumulative incidence of 24.6% of patients developing severe renal dysfunction in the first 10 years.[109] Some 4.8% of patients develop severe **renal dysfunction** within the first year, although the prevalence is substantially decreased from 7.6% before 2004.[109] Cyclosporine as opposed to tacrolimus used in the first 6 months and hypertension are associated with worsening renal function. **Hypertension** may also be related to corticosteroid and calcineurin inhibitor use.[110] The high incidence of renal dysfunction following lung transplantation is likely related to ischemic injury, as well as nephrotoxins, such as CNIs used during the perioperative period.

Hyperammonemia is a rare complication following lung transplantation surgery and the mechanism is poorly understood. Possibly etiologies include liver dysfunction, urea cycle deficiencies, or systemic infection with *Mycoplasma hominis* or *Ureaplasma*. Symptoms are primarily neurologic, including somnolence, confusion, or agitation. Mortality is high, necessitating screening for early diagnosis; some lung transplant protocols now include measurement of serum ammonia even in asymptomatic patients. If hyperammonemia is diagnosed, BAL samples should be tested for presence of *Mycoplasma hominis* or *Ureaplasma* and empiric antibiotics started.[111] In addition, ammonia levels should be managed with bowel decontamination and lactulose to facilitate clearance. Hemodialysis can be considered in severe cases for ammonia clearance.

Extracorporeal Membrane Oxygenation in the Postoperative Period

ECMO may be used in the postoperative period either as a continuation of intraoperative support or as supportive therapy in cases of refractory, life-threatening PGD. In patients who require ECMO utilization during the transplant procedure, weaning may be attempted intraoperatively following reperfusion of the allografts. In cases where weaning is not tolerated because of hypoxemia, hypercarbia, or hemodynamic instability, ECMO support should be maintained during the early postoperative period. Weaning and decannulation may be attempted when respiratory mechanics, ABGs, and hemodynamics improve. ECMO may be initiated during the postoperative period to augment gas exchange or pulmonary hemodynamics, or to prevent ventilator-associated lung injury. For example, a surgically complicated procedure requiring large-volume fluid resuscitation may develop worsening pulmonary edema requiring temporary ECMO support. Typically, ECMO support is reserved for patients with severe PGD refractory to optimal ventilator and medical support, however, early initiation is associated with improved outcomes.[63]

Utilization of VV ECMO is preferable to VA ECMO because of fewer complications, such as bleeding and stroke.[5] In addition, high VA ECMO flows can result in insufficient flow through the newly transplanted lung. Peripheral VA ECMO can lead to LV distension from high afterload or poor cerebral oxygenation if carotid artery perfusion occurs with poorly-oxygenated transcardiac flow rather than well-oxygenated ECMO flow. VA ECMO may be preferentially used in severe RV dysfunction or in the subset of patients with preoperative severe PH to prevent LV volume overload.

Long-Term Complications of Lung Transplant

According to the ISHLT 2018 report, median survival in adults who underwent lung transplantation between 2009 and 2016 was 6.2 years.[109] Long-term survival after lung transplantation remains poor because of graft-related issues including chronic lung allograft dysfunction (CLAD) and graft failure. In addition, nongraft-related processes, such as infection, malignancy, renal dysfunction, diabetes, and cardiovascular disease are other major contributors to morbidity and mortality following lung transplantation.

Chronic Lung Allograft Dysfunction

CLAD is defined as a persistent decline in FEV_1 by at least 20% from the baseline postoperative value that cannot be explained by other pathologic processes (e.g., surgical, mechanical, infection, rejection, arterial strictures or emboli, tumor, drug-induced toxicity, recurrent pretransplant disease, aspiration, or normal aging).[112] Staging is defined as CLAD from 0 to 4 based on percentage of baseline FEV_1, with CLAD 4 being the most severe form. It may present with an obstructive (i.e., BOS), restrictive (i.e., restrictive allograft syndrome [RAS]), or mixed pattern. CLAD is the leading cause of mortality in lung transplant patients after the first year.[109]

BOS is the most common manifestation of CLAD, with a prevalence of 8.5% at 1-year posttransplant.[109] BOS is defined by an obstructive defect on spirometry (i.e., FEV_1/FVC < 0.7) without radiologic airspace opacities. On pathology, BOS demonstrates excess subepithelial fibrous tissue with eventual obliteration of bronchial lumens. RAS occurs in about 30% of patients with CLAD and is defined by restrictive spirometry (i.e., TLC ≤90% of baseline) with persistent airspace opacities on chest imaging. Pathologically, RAS demonstrates diffuse alveolar damage and fibroelastosis which may be pleuroparenchymal or scattered in the parenchyma.

Diagnosis of CLAD involves clinical symptoms, as well as transbronchial biopsy and BAL. There are few treatment options for CLAD, and it remains the leading cause of posttransplant mortality, accounting for 20% to 30% of deaths.[109] Patients with BOS may benefit from switching from cyclosporine to tacrolimus or from a trial of azithromycin therapy for at least 8 weeks.[109] Retransplantation may be necessary in select patients.

Malignancy

Because of chronic use of immunosuppression, lung transplant patients are at higher risk of malignancy compared with the general population. Malignancy accounts for a substantial portion of long-term mortality in lung transplant patients, with lymphoma causing 1.9% and other malignancy 15.4% of deaths in the 5- to 10-year range.[109] Common malignancies in this population include skin cancers, PTLD, and lung cancers.

The majority of skin cancers in postlung transplant patients are squamous cell carcinoma, and factors, such as male gender, advanced age, COPD, and use of a three-drug immunosuppressive regimen are associated with increased risk.[113] PTLD is a class of lymphoproliferative disease, including lymphoma, that arises from recipient lymphoid cells because of infection with oncogenic viruses, most commonly EBV. The risk of PTLD increases with cumulative level of immunosuppression, and there is potential for disease regression in some cases with tapering.[113] Lung cancer may develop in patients following lung transplantation, either in the native lung following single lung transplant or in the transplanted lung. Patients who undergo single lung transplant often have indications that place them at risk for native lung cancer, including smoking history or idiopathic fibrosis; bronchogenic carcinoma is 6-fold more common in single lung transplants than double.[113]

Infection

Infection is a leading cause of mortality in the posttransplant population, accounting for 33% in the first transplant year and 16% to 20% between 1 and 10 years.[109] Because of the immunosuppressed state, patients following lung transplantation are at high risk for bacterial, fungal, and viral pathogens, including opportunistic organisms, and prophylaxis for many of these organisms is implemented shortly after surgery (see "Infection Prevention and Management" section). Patients may be colonized with virulent organisms before transplantation or become colonized nosocomially, or reactivation of latent infections may occur. Based on the time since transplant surgery, different categories of pathogens should be considered as most-likely to cause infection. Donor or recipient infections present before transplant are most common in the first month, as well as nosocomial catheter or surgical site infections; from 1 to 6 months, opportunistic infections or latent reactivations are most likely; at 6 months following transplant, community-acquired infections are of highest concern.[100] Pneumonia and bronchitis are the overall most common infections following lung transplantation, other sites of infection should be considered.

Diagnosis of infection in lung transplant patients may be more challenging because of the immunosuppressed state masking more typical symptoms, such as fever, fatigue, night sweats, or pain or signs, such as an elevated white blood cell count; a low index of suspicion is necessary to identify infections early, before resulting in significant morbidity. Chest CT is useful in diagnosing pneumonia, and BAL and transbronchial biopsies can aid in identifying pathogens. Surveillance cultures are useful, especially during the first year following lung transplant. Aggressive antimicrobial therapy targeting known or suspected organisms is important in preventing morbidity and mortality.

Diabetes Mellitus

Diabetes mellitus is common following lung transplantation because of glucocorticoid and calcineurin inhibitor use, although prevalence of diabetes at 1-year posttransplant has decreased from 24% to 17% in the modern era.[109] Patients taking tacrolimus are at higher risk than those taking cyclosporine, although this is rarely an indication for switching medications. Risk factors for posttransplant diabetes include older age, obesity, and rejection.[114]

Monitoring and Follow-Up After Discharge

Following lung transplantation, patients require lifelong routine, close monitoring for complications that may result in morbidity or mortality. This monitoring includes clinician check-ups and contact with a nurse coordinator, lung function monitoring, and monitoring of immunosuppression regimen. Patients frequently undergo a rehabilitation program after initial discharge to allow for monitoring of lung function and other potential complications, as well as to improve physical strength. Following discharge, lung function is monitored with home, hand-held personal spirometers, as well as routine chest radiography, spirometry, and bronchoscopy; these can aid in early detection of rejection or infection. Maintenance immunosuppression requires monitoring for appropriate drug levels, potential side effects, and development infection or malignancy.

References

1. Chambers DC, Yusen RD, Cherikh WS, et al. The Registry of the International Society for Heart and Lung Transplantation: Thirty-Fourth Adult Lung and Heart-Lung Transplantation Report—/2017; Focus Theme: Allograft ischemic time. *J Heart Lung Transplant.* 2017;36:1047–1059.
2. Organ Procurement & Transplantation Network, National Data: Lung. Edited by Administration UDoHaHSHRaS.
3. Weill D, Benden C, Corris PA, et al. A consensus document for the selection of lung transplant candidates: 2014—an update from the Pulmonary Transplantation Council of the International Society for Heart and Lung Transplantation. *J Heart Lung Transplant.* 2015;34:1–15.
4. Omara M, Okamoto T, Arafat A, Thuita L, Blackstone EH, McCurry KR. Lung transplantation in patients who have undergone prior cardiothoracic procedures. *J Heart Lung Transplant.* 2016;35:1462–1470.
5. McKellar SH, Bowen ME, Baird BC, Raman S, Cahill BC, Selzman CH. Lung transplantation following coronary artery bypass surgery-improved outcomes following single-lung transplant. *J Heart Lung Transplant.* 2016;35:1289–1294.
6. Vogelmeier CF, Criner GJ, Martinez FJ, et al. Global strategy for the diagnosis, management, and prevention of chronic obstructive lung disease 2017 report: GOLD executive summary. *Eur Respir J.* 2017:49.
7. Weill D. Lung transplantation: indications and contraindications. *J Thorac Dis.* 2018;10:4574–4587.
8. Celli BR, Cote CG, Marin JM, et al. The body-mass index, airflow obstruction, dyspnea, and exercise capacity index in chronic obstructive pulmonary disease. *N Engl J Med.* 2004;350:1005–1012.
9. Lahzami S, Bridevaux PO, Soccal PM, et al. Survival impact of lung transplantation for COPD. *Eur Respir J.* 2010;36:74–80.
10. Reed RM, Cabral HJ, Dransfield MT, et al. Survival of lung transplant candidates with COPD: BODE score reconsidered. *Chest.* 2018;153:697–701.

11. Rosas IO, Dellaripa PF, Lederer DJ, Khanna D, Young LR, Martinez FJ. Interstitial lung disease: NHLBI Workshop on the Primary Prevention of Chronic Lung Diseases. *Ann Am Thorac Soc.* 2014;11(3):S169–S177.
12. Gannon WD, Lederer DJ, Biscotti M, et al. Outcomes and mortality prediction model of critically ill adults with acute respiratory failure and interstitial lung disease. *Chest.* 2018;153:1387–1395.
13. Raghu G, Remy-Jardin M, Myers JL, et al. Latin American Thoracic S. Diagnosis of idiopathic pulmonary fibrosis. An Official ATS/ERS/JRS/ALAT Clinical Practice Guideline. *Am J Respir Crit Care Med.* 2018;198:e44–e68.
14. 2018 Patient Registry Annual Data Report. Edited by Registry CFFP, 2018.
15. O'Sullivan BP, Freedman SD. Cystic fibrosis. *Lancet.* 2009;373:1891–1904.
16. Cummings KW, Bhalla S. Pulmonary vascular diseases. *Clin Chest Med.* 2015;36:235–248 viii.
17. Simonneau G, Montani D, Celermajer DS, et al. Haemodynamic definitions and updated clinical classification of pulmonary hypertension. *Eur Respir J.* 2019;53:1081913.
18. Galie N, Humbert M, Vachiery JL, et al. ESC Scientific Document Group. 2015 ESC/ERS Guidelines for the diagnosis and treatment of pulmonary hypertension: The Joint Task Force for the Diagnosis and Treatment of Pulmonary Hypertension of the European Society of Cardiology (ESC) and the European Respiratory Society (ERS): Endorsed by: Association for European Paediatric and Congenital Cardiology (AEPC), International Society for Heart and Lung Transplantation (ISHLT). *Eur Heart J.* 2016;37:67–119.
19. Benza RL, Gomberg-Maitland M, Elliott CG, et al. Predicting survival in patients with pulmonary arterial hypertension: The REVEAL Risk Score Calculator 2.0 and Comparison With ESC/ERS-Based Risk Assessment Strategies. *Chest.* 2019;156: 323–337.
20. Kon ZN, Bittle GJ, Pasrija C, Sanchez PG, Griffith BP, Pierson RN 3rd. The optimal procedure for retransplantation after single lung transplantation. *Ann Thorac Surg.* 2017;104:170–175.
21. Fadel E, Mercier O, Mussot S, et al. Long-term outcome of double-lung and heart-lung transplantation for pulmonary hypertension: a comparative retrospective study of 219 patients. *Eur J Cardiothorac Surg.* 2010;38:277–284.
22. Ju L, Suberbielle C, Li X, Mooney N, Charron D. HLA and lung transplantation. *Front Med.* 2019;13:298–313.
23. Gottlieb J. Lung allocation. *J Thorac Dis.* 2017;9:2670–2674.
24. (OPTN) OPaTN: Policy Notice: Eliminate the Use of DSAs in Thoracic Distribution, Thoracic Transplantation Committee.
25. UNOS. A Guide to Calculating the Lung Allocation Score. https://unos.org/wp-content/uploads/unos/Lung_Calculation.pdf.
26. UNOS. Questions and Answers for Transplant Professionals about Lung Allocation. https://unos.org/wp-content/uploads/unos/Lung_Professional.pdf.
27. Valapour M, Lehr CJ, Skeans MA, et al. OPTN/SRTR 2018 Annual Data Report: Lung. *Am J Transplant.* 2020;20 Suppl:427–508 s1.
28. Chiumello D, Coppola S, Froio S, Colombo A, Del Sorbo L. Extracorporeal life support as bridge to lung transplantation: a systematic review. *Crit Care.* 2015;19:19.
29. Singer JP, Blanc PD, Hoopes C, et al. The impact of pretransplant mechanical ventilation on short- and long-term survival after lung transplantation. *Am J Transplant.* 2011;11:2197–2204.
30. Squiers JJ, Lima B, DiMaio JM. Contemporary extracorporeal membrane oxygenation therapy in adults: fundamental principles and systematic review of the evidence. *J Thorac Cardiovasc Surg.* 2016;152:20–32.
31. Mason DP, Thuita L, Nowicki ER, Murthy SC, Pettersson GB, Blackstone EH. Should lung transplantation be performed for patients on mechanical respiratory support? The US experience. *J Thorac Cardiovasc Surg.* 2010;139:765–773 e1.
32. Shafii AE, Mason DP, Brown CR, et al. Growing experience with extracorporeal membrane oxygenation as a bridge to lung transplantation. *ASAIO J.* 2012;58:526–529.
33. Lang G, Taghavi S, Aigner C, et al. Primary lung transplantation after bridge with extracorporeal membrane oxygenation: a plea for a shift in our paradigms for indications. *Transplantation.* 2012;93:729–736.
34. Toyoda Y, Bhama JK, Shigemura N, et al. Efficacy of extracorporeal membrane oxygenation as a bridge to lung transplantation. *J Thorac Cardiovasc Surg.* 2013;145:1065–1071.
35. Hoopes CW, Kukreja J, Golden J, Davenport DL, Diaz-Guzman E, Zwischenberger JB. Extracorporeal membrane oxygenation as a bridge to pulmonary transplantation. *J Thorac Cardiovasc Surg.* 2013;145:862–867 discussion 867-8.
36. Crotti S, Iotti GA, Lissoni A, et al. Organ allocation waiting time during extracorporeal bridge to lung transplant affects outcomes. *Chest.* 2013;144:1018–1025.
37. Fuehner T, Kuehn C, Hadem J, et al. Extracorporeal membrane oxygenation in awake patients as bridge to lung transplantation. *Am J Respir Crit Care Med.* 2012;185:763–768.
38. Abrams D, Brodie D, Arcasoy SM. Extracorporeal life support in lung transplantation. *Clin Chest Med.* 2017;38:655–666.
39. Suresh Rao KG, Muralikrishna T, Balakrishnan KR. Demonstration of blood flow by color doppler in the femoral artery distal to arterial cannula during peripheral venoarterial-extracorporeal membrane oxygenation. *Ann Card Anaesth.* 2017;20:108–109.
40. Biscotti M, Gannon WD, Agerstrand C, et al. Awake extracorporeal membrane oxygenation as bridge to lung transplantation: a 9-year experience. *Ann Thorac Surg.* 2017;104:412–419.
41. Ko Y, Cho YH, Park YH, et al. Feasibility and safety of early physical therapy and active mobilization for patients on extracorporeal membrane oxygenation. *ASAIO J.* 2015;61:564–568.
42. Abrams D, Javidfar J, Farrand E, et al. Early mobilization of patients receiving extracorporeal membrane oxygenation: a retrospective cohort study. *Crit Care.* 2014;18:R38.
43. Abrams D, Garan AR, Brodie D. Awake and fully mobile patients on cardiac extracorporeal life support. *Ann Cardiothorac Surg.* 2019;8:44–53.
44. Biscotti M, Bacchetta M. The "sport model": extracorporeal membrane oxygenation using the subclavian artery. *Ann Thorac Surg.* 2014;98:1487–1489.
45. Chicotka S, Rosenzweig EB, Brodie D, Bacchetta M. The "Central Sport Model": extracorporeal membrane oxygenation using the innominate artery for smaller patients as bridge to lung transplantation. *ASAIO J.* 2017;63:e39–e44.
46. Strueber M, Hoeper MM, Fischer S, et al. Bridge to thoracic organ transplantation in patients with pulmonary arterial hypertension using a pumpless lung assist device. *Am J Transplant.* 2009;9:853–857.
47. Yusen RD, Hong BA, Messersmith EE, et al. Morbidity and mortality of live lung donation: results from the RELIVE study. *Am J Transplant.* 2014;14:1846–1852.

48. Bernat JL, D'Alessandro AM, Port FK, et al. Report of a National Conference on Donation after cardiac death. *Am J Transplant.* 2006;6:281–291.
49. Chaney J, Suzuki Y, Cantu E 3rd, van Berkel V. Lung donor selection criteria. *J Thorac Dis.* 2014;6:1032–1038.
50. Kotloff RM, Blosser S, Fulda GJ, et al. Society of Critical Care Medicine/American College of Chest Physicians/Association of Organ Procurement Organizations Donor Management Task Force. Management of the potential organ donor in the ICU: Society of Critical Care Medicine/American College of Chest Physicians/Association of Organ Procurement Organizations Consensus Statement. *Crit Care Med.* 2015;43:1291–1325.
51. Sommer W, Ius F, Muller C, et al. Extended criteria donor lungs do not impact recipient outcomes in pediatric transplantation. *J Heart Lung Transplant.* 2019;38:560–569.
52. Neizer H, Singh GB, Gupta S, Singh SK. Addressing donor-organ shortages using extended criteria in lung transplantation. *Ann Cardiothorac Surg.* 2020;9:49–50.
53. Arnaouatakis GJ, Sodha NR, Tedford RJ, Merlo CA, Milano CA, Shah AS. Centers for Disease Control 'high-risk' donors and thoracic organ transplantation: expanding the donor pool. *J Heart Lung Transplant.* 2013;32:316.
54. Bittle GJ, Sanchez PG, Kon ZN, et al. The use of lung donors older than 55 years: a review of the United Network of Organ Sharing database. *J Heart Lung Transplant.* 2013;32:760–768.
55. Sommer W, Ius F, Salman J, et al. Survival and spirometry outcomes after lung transplantation from donors aged 70 years and older. *J Heart Lung Transplant.* 2015;34:1325–1333.
56. ISHLT. Guidance from the International Society of Heart and Lung Transplantation regarding the SARS CoV-2 pandemic. *Web.* 2020.
57. Orens JB, Boehler A, de Perrot M, et al. Pulmonary Council, International Society for Heart and Lung Transplantation. A review of lung transplant donor acceptability criteria. *J Heart Lung Transplant.* 2003;22:1183–1200.
58. Barnard JB, Davies O, Curry P, et al. Size matching in lung transplantation: an evidence-based review. *J Heart Lung Transplant.* 2013;32:849–860.
59. Chambers DC, Cherikh WS, Harhay MO, et al. International Society for Heart and Lung Transplantation. The International Thoracic Organ Transplant Registry of the International Society for Heart and Lung Transplantation: Thirty-Sixth Adult Lung and Heart-Lung Transplantation Report—2019; Focus theme: Donor and recipient size match. *J Heart Lung Transplant.* 2019;38:1042–1055.
60. Konheim JA, Kon ZN, Pasrija C, et al. Predictive equations for lung volumes from computed tomography for size matching in pulmonary transplantation. *J Thorac Cardiovasc Surg.* 2016;151:1163–1169 e1.
61. Minambres E, Coll E, Duerto J, et al. Effect of an intensive lung donor-management protocol on lung transplantation outcomes. *J Heart Lung Transplant.* 2014;33:178–184.
62. Mascia L, Pasero D, Slutsky AS, et al. Effect of a lung protective strategy for organ donors on eligibility and availability of lungs for transplantation: a randomized controlled trial. *JAMA.* 2010;304:2620–2627.
63. Van Raemdonck D, Hartwig MG, Hertz MI, et al. Report of the ISHLT Working Group on primary lung graft dysfunction Part IV: Prevention and treatment: A 2016 Consensus Group statement of the International Society for Heart and Lung Transplantation. *J Heart Lung Transplant.* 2017;36:1121–1136.
64. Puskas JD, Cardoso PF, Mayer E, Shi S, Slutsky AS, Patterson GA. Equivalent eighteen-hour lung preservation with low-potassium dextran or Euro-Collins solution after prostaglandin E1 infusion. *J Thorac Cardiovasc Surg.* 1992;104:83–89.
65. Cypel M, Yeung JC, Liu M, et al. Normothermic ex vivo lung perfusion in clinical lung transplantation. *N Engl J Med.* 2011;364:1431–1440.
66. Yeung JC, Krueger T, Yasufuku K, et al. Outcomes after transplantation of lungs preserved for more than 12 h: a retrospective study. *Lancet Respir Med.* 2017;5:119–124.
67. Subramanian MP, Meyers BF. Bilateral versus single lung transplantation: are two lungs better than one? *J Thorac Dis.* 2018;10:4588–4601.
68. Date H. Current status and problems of lung transplantation in Japan. *J Thorac Dis.* 2016;8:S631–S636.
69. Costa J, Sonett JR, D'Ovidio F. Modified transverse thoracosternotomy and cost-effective reinforced sternal closure. *Ann Thorac Surg.* 2015;100:2376–2378.
70. Tomasi R, Betz D, Schlager S, et al. Intraoperative anesthetic management of lung transplantation: center-specific practices and geographic and centers size differences. *J Cardiothorac Vasc Anesth.* 2018;32:62–69.
71. Martin AK, Yalamuri SM, Wilkey BJ, et al. The impact of anesthetic management on perioperative outcomes in lung transplantation. *J Cardiothorac Vasc Anesth.* 2020;34:1669–1680.
72. Yamada Y, Laube I, Jang JH, et al. Sevoflurane preconditioning protects from posttransplant injury in mouse lung transplantation. *J Surg Res.* 2017;214:270–277.
73. Casanova J, Simon C, Vara E, et al. Sevoflurane anesthetic preconditioning protects the lung endothelial glycocalyx from ischemia reperfusion injury in an experimental lung autotransplant model. *J Anesth.* 2016;30:755–762.
74. Rocca GD, Coccia C, Pugliese F, et al. Intraoperative inhaled nitric oxide during anesthesia for lung transplant. *Transplant Proc.* 1997;29:3362–3366.
75. Ardehali A, Laks H, Levine M, et al. A prospective trial of inhaled nitric oxide in clinical lung transplantation. *Transplantation.* 2001;72:112–115.
76. Ramadan ME, Shabsigh M, Awad H. Con: inhaled pulmonary vasodilators are not indicated in patients undergoing lung transplantation. *J Cardiothorac Vasc Anesth.* 2017;31:1127–1131.
77. Lee SH, Lee JG, Lee CY, et al. Effects of intraoperative inhaled iloprost on primary graft dysfunction after lung transplantation: a retrospective single center study. *Medicine (Baltimore).* 2016;95:e3975.
78. Della Rocca G, Coccia C, Costa MG, et al. Inhaled areosolized prostacyclin and pulmonary hypertension during anesthesia for lung transplantation. *Transplant Proc.* 2001;33:1634–1636.
79. Khan TA, Schnickel G, Ross D, et al. A prospective, randomized, crossover pilot study of inhaled nitric oxide versus inhaled prostacyclin in heart transplant and lung transplant recipients. *J Thorac Cardiovasc Surg.* 2009;138:1417–1424.
80. Geube MA, Perez-Protto SE, McGrath TL, et al. Increased intraoperative fluid administration is associated with severe primary graft dysfunction after lung transplantation. *Anesth Analg.* 2016;122:1081–1088.
81. Liu Y, Liu Y, Su L, Jiang SJ. Recipient-related clinical risk factors for primary graft dysfunction after lung transplantation: a systematic review and meta-analysis. *PLoS One.* 2014;9:e92773.
82. Pena JJ, Bottiger BA, Miltiades AN. Perioperative management of bleeding and transfusion for lung transplantation. *Semin Cardiothorac Vasc Anesth.* 2020;24:74–83.

83. Zalunardo MP, Thalmann C, Seifert B, et al. Impact of preoperative right-ventricular function and platelet transfusion on outcome after lung transplantation. *Eur J Cardiothorac Surg.* 2011;39:538–542.
84. Ong LP, Thompson E, Sachdeva A, et al. Allogeneic blood transfusion in bilateral lung transplantation: impact on early function and mortality. *Eur J Cardiothorac Surg.* 2016;49:668–674, discussion 674.
85. Smith I, Pearse BL, Faulke DJ, et al. Targeted bleeding management reduces the requirements for blood component therapy in lung transplant recipients. *J Cardiothorac Vasc Anesth.* 2017;31:426–433.
86. Tan Z, Roscoe A, Rubino A. Transesophageal echocardiography in heart and lung transplantation. *J Cardiothorac Vasc Anesth.* 2019;33:1548–1558.
87. Parekh K, Meyers BF, Patterson GA, et al. Outcome of lung transplantation for patients requiring concomitant cardiac surgery. *J Thorac Cardiovasc Surg.* 2005;130:859–863.
88. Johnson SB, Allred AM, Cline AM, et al. Cardiac procedures in lung transplant recipients do not increase mortality in selected patients. *Ann Thorac Surg.* 2006;82:460–463, discussion 463-4.
89. Cartwright BL, Jackson A, Cooper J. Intraoperative pulmonary vein examination by transesophageal echocardiography: an anatomic update and review of utility. *J Cardiothorac Vasc Anesth.* 2013;27:111–120.
90. Miyaji K, Matsubara H, Nakamura K, et al. Equivalence of flow velocities through bilateral pulmonary vein anastomoses in bilateral living-donor lobar lung transplantation. *J Heart Lung Transplant.* 2005;24:860–864.
91. Iyer MH, Bhatt A, Kumar N, Hussain N, Essandoh MK. Transesophageal echocardiography for lung transplantation: a new standard of care? *J Cardiothorac Vasc Anesth.* 2020;34:741–743.
92. Abrams BA, Melnyk V, Allen WL, et al. TEE for lung transplantation: a case series and discussion of vascular complications. *J Cardiothorac Vasc Anesth.* 2020;34:733–740.
93. Diamond JM, Lee JC, Kawut SM, et al. Lung Transplant Outcomes Group. Clinical risk factors for primary graft dysfunction after lung transplantation. *Am J Respir Crit Care Med.* 2013;187:527–534.
94. Barnes L, Reed RM, Parekh KR, et al. Mechanical ventilation for the lung transplant recipient. *Curr Pulmonol Rep.* 2015;4:88–96.
95. Magouliotis DE, Tasiopoulou VS, Svokos AA, Svokos KA, Zacharoulis D. Extracorporeal membrane oxygenation versus cardiopulmonary bypass during lung transplantation: a meta-analysis. *Gen Thorac Cardiovasc Surg.* 2018;66:38–47.
96. Singh RR, Laubach VE, Ellman PI, et al. Attenuation of lung reperfusion injury by modified ventilation and reperfusion techniques. *J Heart Lung Transplant.* 2006;25:1467–1473.
97. Brazier A, Seville E, Hesford W, et al. The Wythenshawe Hybrid Circuit for lung transplantation: a previously undescribed circuit for lung transplant. *Perfusion.* 2019:267659119868664.
98. Acute Respiratory Distress Syndrome Network, Brower RG, Matthay MA, Morris A, Schoenfeld D, Thompson BT, Wheeler A. Ventilation with lower tidal volumes as compared with traditional tidal volumes for acute lung injury and the acute respiratory distress syndrome. *N Engl J Med.* 2000;342:1301–1308.
99. Scheffert JL, Raza K. Immunosuppression in lung transplantation. *J Thorac Dis.* 2014;6:1039–1053.
100. Nosotti M, Tarsia P, Morlacchi LC. Infections after lung transplantation. *J Thorac Dis.* 2018;10:3849–3868.
101. Snell GI, Yusen RD, Weill D, et al. Report of the ISHLT Working Group on Primary Lung Graft Dysfunction, Part I: definition and grading-A 2016 Consensus Group statement of the International Society for Heart and Lung Transplantation. *J Heart Lung Transplant.* 2017;36:1097–1103.
102. Gelman AE, Fisher AJ, Huang HJ, et al. Report of the ISHLT Working Group on Primary Lung Graft Dysfunction Part III: Mechanisms: A 2016 Consensus Group Statement of the International Society for Heart and Lung Transplantation. *J Heart Lung Transplant.* 2017;36:1114–1120.
103. Diamond JM, Arcasoy S, Kennedy CC, et al. Report of the International Society for Heart and Lung Transplantation Working Group on Primary Lung Graft Dysfunction, Part II: Epidemiology, risk factors, and outcomes-A 2016 Consensus Group statement of the International Society for Heart and Lung Transplantation. *J Heart Lung Transplant.* 2017;36:1104–1113.
104. Martinu T, Pavlisko EN, Chen DF, Palmer SM. Acute allograft rejection: cellular and humoral processes. *Clin Chest Med.* 2011;32:295–310.
105. Stewart S, Fishbein MC, Snell GI, et al. Revision of the 1996 working formulation for the standardization of nomenclature in the diagnosis of lung rejection. *J Heart Lung Transplant.* 2007;26:1229–1242.
106. Levine DJ, Glanville AR, Aboyoun C, et al. Antibody-mediated rejection of the lung: a consensus report of the International Society for Heart and Lung Transplantation. *J Heart Lung Transplant.* 2016;35:397–406.
107. Frye L, Machuzak M. Airway complications after lung transplantation. *Clin Chest Med.* 2017;38:693–706.
108. Ferdinande P, Bruyninckx F, Van Raemdonck D, Daenen W, Verleden G. Leuven Lung Transplant Group. Phrenic nerve dysfunction after heart-lung and lung transplantation. *J Heart Lung Transplant.* 2004;23:105–109.
109. Chambers DC, Cherikh WS, Goldfarb SB, et al. International Society for H, Lung T. The International Thoracic Organ Transplant Registry of the International Society for Heart and Lung Transplantation: Thirty-Fifth adult Lung and Heart-Lung Transplant Report—2018; Focus theme: Multiorgan Transplantation. *J Heart Lung Transplant.* 2018;37:1169–1183.
110. Ishani A, Erturk S, Hertz MI, Matas AJ, Savik K, Rosenberg ME. Predictors of renal function following lung or heart-lung transplantation. *Kidney Int.* 2002;61:2228–2234.
111. Bharat A, Cunningham SA, Scott Budinger GR, et al. Disseminated urea plasma infection as a cause of fatal hyperammonemia in humans. *Sci Transl Med.* 2015;7:284re3.
112. Verleden GM, Glanville AR, Lease ED, et al. Chronic lung allograft dysfunction: definition, diagnostic criteria, and approaches to treatment-A consensus report from the Pulmonary Council of the ISHLT. *J Heart Lung Transplant.* 2019;38:493–503.
113. Olland A, Falcoz PE, Massard G. Malignancies after lung transplantation. *J Thorac Dis.* 2018;10:3132–3140.
114. Ollech JE, Kramer MR, Peled N, et al. Post-transplant diabetes mellitus in lung transplant recipients: incidence and risk factors. *Eur J Cardiothorac Surg.* 2008;33:844–848.

44

Esophageal Procedures

WOLFGANG BAAR,# JOHANNES HELL,# TORSTEN LOOP

#These authors contributed equally to this work.

Introduction

Esophageal surgery in adults is associated with a high perioperative morbidity (52%) and mortality (12%). Postoperative complications are mainly pulmonary with an incidence of up to 52%, which significantly reduces the short- and long-term survival of patients. Although patient-specific risk factors (comorbidities, age, gender, nutritional status, etc.) are difficult to influence, perioperative management and medical care research is increasingly focusing on the optimization of procedural risk factors. Minimally invasive surgical techniques with consecutive reduction of both the duration of the operation and the amount of blood loss, are being investigated. Perioperative anesthesiologic management should focus on the anesthesia procedure (general anesthesia with or without neuraxial anesthesia), the intraoperative ventilation, and hemodynamic management strategy.

In addition to the anatomic and disease-specific basics, this chapter is intended to provide practical support for the surgical procedure and illustrate concrete recommendations to ensure patient safety.

Core Chapter

Anatomy (and Physiology)

The adult esophagus is a muscular tube, 25 to 28 cm long and approximately 2 cm in diameter, which serves as a duct for the passage of fluid and solid substances from the pharynx to the stomach (Fig. 44.1). Length is affected by age, sex, gender, and physiologic condition. In general, the esophagus is divided into three anatomic parts, **the cervical** (sixth cervical vertebra to first thoracic vertebra), **the thoracic** (first to 11th vertebra), and **the abdominal** esophagus (11th vertebra). The esophagus originates at the cricoid cartilage at the sixth cervical vertebra (C6) where it emerges from the pars laryngea of the pharynx. This is the location of the narrowest point of the esophagus at the upper esophageal sphincter (15–16 cm after maxillary central incisor teeth), at the point of the transition of the hypopharynx to the cervical esophagus. Descending through the superior mediastinum, the esophagus crosses behind the trachea, the aortic arch, a typical narrowing corresponding to the fourth and fifth thoracic vertebrae (23–25 cm after maxillary central incisor teeth), and the left recurrent laryngeal nerve. Subsequently, the esophagus passes the posterior mediastinum behind the tracheal bifurcation where the anatomic relation to the left mainstem bronchus results in a further narrow section (27.5 cm after maxillary central incisor teeth). Continuing caudal passing, the esophagus is located behind the left atrium. In front of the descending thoracic aorta, the esophagus joins the stomach at the level of the 11th thoracic vertebra. Here is the location of the last narrowing, the lower esophageal sphincter (LES, 40 cm after maxillary central incisor teeth), defined by functional aspects rather than an exact anatomic correlate, partly built by the esophageal hiatus in the diaphragm[1] (see Fig. 44.1).

The relation of the esophagus with the surrounding structures (Table. 44.1) and its emerging narrowing points result in important pathophysiologic and clinical consequences. Because of the partial coverage of the cervical esophagus by the trachea on the left side, this open margin provides natural surgical access for cervical esophagectomy. However, the relationship of the cervical esophagus to the left recurrent laryngeal nerve, crossing under the aortic arch at the ligamentum arteriosum and ascending in a groove at the junction of the trachea and the esophagus (tracheoesophageal sulcus), leads to the potential risk of harm during surgery. A unilateral injury of this nerve typically results in swallowing difficulties or hoarseness, in contrast a bilateral injury causes complete vocal fold paresis. Stridor, respiratory distress, and aphonia occurs because of the closure of the glottic aperture necessitating immediate intervention.

The proximity of the upper thoracic esophagus to the thoracic duct endangers this structure during surgical procedures. The proximity of the thoracic esophagus to the heart, especially to the left atrium, allows the anesthetist to examine the heart by the transesophageal echocardiography (TEE), revolutionizing cardiac anesthesia and perioperative hemodynamic management. Also the narrow points of the esophagus represent important landmarks with clinical implications. Typically, they build predilection sites for damage during

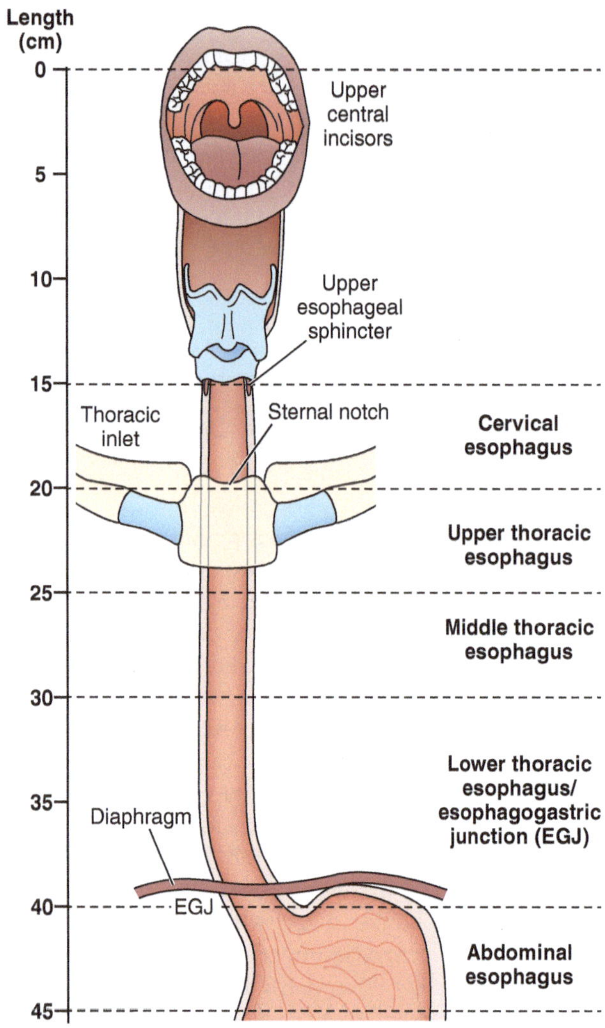

• **Fig. 44.1** Anatomy of the esophagus.

esophageal instrumentation. For example, the first narrowing in the hypopharynx is the classical zone of esophageal perforation through TEE, a rare but severe complication.[2] The vulnerable areas in the esophagus, beneath the cricoid muscle and on the left side close to the diaphragmatic hiatus, predispose for diverticula (Zenker's diverticulum or epiphrenic diverticulum) or spontaneous rupture.

The esophagus consists of four histologic layers: mucosa, submucosa, muscularis propria, and adventitia. Because no serosa is found on the esophagus, contrary to the rest of the gastrointestinal tract, infections and tumors can spread easily. The esophageal lumen is covered by nonkeratinized stratified squamous epithelium. The transition between the cells of the esophagus and the simple columnar epithelium in cardia of the stomach is called the line or squamocolumnar junction. A displacement of the squamocolumnar junction into the distal esophagus is a sign of the Barrett esophagus.

The arterial supply of the cervical esophagus is mainly achieved by branches of the inferior thyroid arteries. Blood circulation for the thoracic segments is generated by the bronchial arteries, from esophageal branches of the aorta and right intercostal arteries. The abdominal portion receives blood from the left gastric artery, short gastric arteries, and descending branch of left phrenic artery.

The venous drainage of the esophagus is more variable than the arterial supply. Cervical portions empty into inferior thyroid veins, whereas thoracic segment's venous drainage empties mainly into the azygos and right brachiocephalic vein. Venous drainage of the abdominal esophagus empties primarily into left gastric veins, additional venous drainage ensues over short gastric veins, splenic vein, and left gastroepiploic vein, all tributary of the portal vein. Therefore lower esophageal veins communicate with caval venous and portal venous systems. Impairment of portal venous blood flow, for instance because of hepatic cirrhosis, could lead to retrograde flow through this shunt system, causing venous dilatation and varices, which may result in fatal bleeding.

Esophageal peristalsis is a complex interplay of straited muscle in the upper third and smooth muscle in the remaining parts of the esophagus, behaving as a single functional unit, producing peristalsis at will (**primary peristalsis**) in contrast to the intestine. Beside primary peristalsis, local stimulation by distension at any point in the body of the esophagus will elicit peristaltic wave (**secondary peristalsis**). The neuronal control of esophageal peristalsis takes place in the central nervous system, especially in the brain stem, as well as in local nerves, modified by autonomic reflexes, and sympathetic and parasympathetic systems. In selected procedures like esophageal anastomosis, suppression of secondary peristalsis is needed. Therefore perioperative administration of hyoscine butylbromide is required.[3]

TABLE 44.1 Relation of the Esophagus to the Surrounding Structures

Relative Position to the Esophagus	Related Structures
Anterior	Trachea, aortic arch, right pulmonary artery, left main bronchus, plexus of esophagus, left atrium, anterior vagus nerve
Posterior	Vertebral column, longus coli muscle, posterior intercostal arteries, azygos vein, hemiazygos vein, anterior wall of descending aorta, posterior vagal nerve, thoracic duct, pleura
Left	Aortic arch, left subclavian artery, left inferior laryngeal nerve, left vagus nerve, thoracic ductus, and the thoracic part of aorta, carotid artery
Right	Azygos vein, pleura, right main bronchus, right vagus nerve

Esophageal sphincters: For adequate function of the esophagus, coordinated activity of the UES and LES is essential. The UES is a high-pressure zone, relaxing in precise intervals, owing to distraction and preventing the passage of air into the stomach.[4] The LES builds a pressure barrier, ranging between 15 and 35 mm Hg, at the gastroesophageal junction, to prevent gastroesophageal reflux. However, accurately timed relaxation during swallowing is crucial for ingestion. Regulation of LES tone and its relaxation is controlled by parasympathetic and sympathetic nerve fibers and modulated by a variety of neurohormonal influences. Furthermore, transient lower esophageal sphincter relaxations (TLESRs) account for physiologic gastroesophageal reflux, provoked by gastric distension.[5] Dysfunction of the LES leads to gastroesophageal reflux or esophageal achalasia, and muscarinic receptor agonists or α-adrenergic agonist could increase LES tone, β-adrenergic agonists, nitric oxide donors, or inhibitors of phosphodiesterase-5 could reduce LES contraction. Opioids and tricyclic antidepressant medications could decrease LES pressure, whereas metoclopramide or metoprolol could increase LES tone.

Esophageal Pathologies and Surgical Therapies

Benign Disease of the Esophagus

Esophageal Diverticula (Pharyngoesophageal Diverticulum, Epiphrenic Diverticulum)

Esophageal diverticula are a rare disease of the esophagus, which is divided into the rarer true diverticula, a protrusion of all layers of the esophageal wall by traction, typically in the middle third of the thoracic esophagus, and the more common false or pseudodiverticula, a bulge without muscular covering, located in muscularly weak regions, such as the hypopharynx (Zenker's diverticula) or the distal esophagus (epiphrenic diverticula), because of an emulsion caused by increased intraluminal pressure, which causes herniation. The prevalence of esophageal diverticula is between 0.015% and 3%, whereas Zenker's diverticula is the most common form of esophageal diverticula, accounting for 70%.[6] Genuine diverticula, which are usually caused by mediastinal disease, such as tuberculous lymphadenitis or sarcoidosis, are caused by motility disorders. Zenker's diverticula in particular are mainly caused by insufficient relaxation of the UES.[7] However, some studies show abnormal esophageal motility even in true esophageal diverticula, although it is unclear whether the motility abnormality is primarily or secondarily resulting from the presence of the diverticulum.[8] Achalasia is also associated with epiphrenic esophageal diverticula followed by diffuse esophageal spasms.[9]

In general, dysphagia, regurgitation of undigested food, bad breath, and a history of silent aspiration with recurrent pneumonia are typical symptoms of esophageal diverticula. However, patients with small diverticula are often asymptomatic until the pouch becomes enlarged. In rare cases, patients with long-lasting dysphagia caused by esophageal diverticula experience weight loss and malnutrition. Large Zenker's diverticula can lead to a complete obstruction of the esophagus because the retained contents press anteriorly. In addition, patients with Zenker's diverticula are often associated with hiatal hernia and gastroesophageal reflux disease (GERD; 72%).[10]

The diagnosis is confirmed by radiologic imaging, such as barium esophagography, endoscopy, and esophageal manometry. In addition, transcutaneous sonography may be an alternative method for diagnosing Zenker's diverticulum in experienced hands.

Despite an improvement in surgical therapy, mortality from esophageal diverticulum surgery is still 1% to 5%.[11] Surgical therapy is usually indicated in patients with esophageal diverticulum, but some authors recommend surgery only in symptomatic patients.[12] The Zenker's diverticulum could be resected through an open left cervical or transoral access with rigid or flexible endoscopy. Diverticulectomy or diverticulopexy could be performed, including myotomy of the cricopharyngeal muscle to treat UES dysfunction.[12] Diverticula located in the middle of the esophagus require a transthoracic approach. The operation can usually be performed by thoracoscopy or thoracotomy from the left side.[13] An additional myotomy may also be necessary. For diverticula of the lower esophagus, especially epiphrenic diverticula, transabdominal laparoscopic surgery with transhiatal access is recommended. Diverticulectomy and additional myotomy/cardiomyotomy imply the need for antireflux procedures, such as partial fundoplication. In some patients, dilatation of the inferior esophageal sphincter may be an alternative to myotomy and the required antireflux procedure, but the clinical evidence is not conclusive.[11–13]

Esophageal Fistula (Tracheo- and Bronchoesophageal Fistula) (see Chapter 45)

A fistula from the airways to the upper gastrointestinal tract bypasses the normal protection provided by intact laryngeal reflexes and could lead to significant morbidity and mortality. There are connections between the esophagus and the trachea or large bronchi, all of which are grouped together as tracheoesophageal fistula (TEF). In adults, most acquired TEFs are associated with malignant diseases, such as esophageal or lung cancer, and surgical procedures, such as esophagectomy,[14] radiotherapy, or chemotherapy.[15,16] TEFs rarely occur because of benign diseases, such as prolonged endotracheal intubation, dilatation tracheotomy, endoscopic procedures (e.g., endobronchial laser or cryotherapy, esophageal stenting), infectious diseases, or trauma. Particularly in anesthesia and intensive care units (ICUs), injury mechanisms, such as traumatic intubation, suction of the airways, and vascular compression of the tracheal wall, which is caused by prolonged overinflation of the endotracheal cuff leading to ischemia and subsequent ulceration. Most congenital TEFs are typically associated with esophageal atresia (90% with esophageal atresia have an esophageal fistula).

Symptoms when spontaneously breathing include postprandial coughing, recurrent pneumonia, hoarseness, and dysphagia. The Ohno sign, postprandial cough with fluid intake, is pathognomonic.[17] Acquired TEF should be considered in any ventilated patient with recurrent chest infections and recurrent weaning disorders and weight loss.

Radiologic imaging, such as chest x-rays enhanced by barium swallowing, thoracic computed tomography (CT) with oral contrast agent, or magnetic resonance imaging, facilitates the localization of TEFs and the identification of their likely etiology. Bronchoscopy or gastrointestinal endoscopy should be performed to confirm TEFs, whereas oral instillation of methylene blue helps to identify even small TEFs.

The therapy of TEFs depends on the etiology and localization of the fistula. Spontaneous closure of TEFs is rare, and surgical therapy is therefore necessary. In the majority of patients with acquired, nonmalignant TEFs, successful closure could be safely achieved by a single repair of the esophagus and trachea supported by tissue flaps.[18] Surgical access is via a cervical incision or thoracotomy, depending on the location of the TEF. Esophageal stenting is the dominant treatment of TEFs in malignant or critically ill patients with a high perioperative mortality rate.[19] Stenting of the esophagus, trachea, or both (double stenting) may be necessary to achieve closure of the fistula. A congenital fistula, especially in combination with esophageal atresia, usually requires neonatal surgery, which is performed as a thoracotomy or thoracoscopy with comparable complications and a total mortality rate of 3.2%.[20] The outcome in patients with benign TEF who are successfully operated on is usually good; in patients with malignant TEF, the treatment may reduce dysphagia, repeated episodes of pneumonia, and improvement of palliative care.

Esophageal Rupture and Perforation

Esophageal perforation affects a wide range of conditions characterized by the transmural disruption of the esophagus.[21] It occurs in 65% of cases as a result of iatrogenic interventions. These include endoscopy of upper gastrointestinal tract, endoscopic sclerotherapy, surgery to adjoining tissue, traumatic placement of esophageal dilators, nasogastric tubes, misplaced endotracheal tubes, or TEE. Esophageal perforation also results from external trauma or postoperatively, as well as by foreign bodies or chemically compounds—whereas alkaline compounds cause more damage than acidic compounds. Hospital mortality in patients with esophageal perforation tends to be around 17.5%, whereas 3-year survival rates are 67%.[22]

Esophageal rupture results from a sudden increase of intraabdominal pressure while the relaxation of the cricopharyngeal muscle is incomplete. Spontaneous esophageal rupture during vomiting is known as **Boerhaave syndrome** because it was first described by the Dutch physician Hermann Boerhaave in 1724. It is a very rare pathology; a study in Iceland demonstrated an incidence of 3.1/1,000,000 per year of overall esophageal rupture and of that, only 24% of cases were categorized as spontaneous ruptures.[23] Spontaneous esophageal ruptures occur more frequently in men than women and typically affect men aged 40 to 70 years who overindulge in alcohol and food.[24] Only 5% of patients with Boerhaave syndrome are considered to be healthy with no underlying etiology. The perforation is mostly located on the left posterior part of the distal esophagus, 2 to 3 cm proximally to the gastroesophageal junction.[25]

Patients with Boerhaave syndrome usually present with severe chest pain after an episode of violent vomiting. Although pain is often the primary symptom, other symptoms can include dyspnea, voice changes, dysphagia, and subcutaneous emphysema. **Mackler's triad,** often associated with spontaneous esophageal rupture, includes chest pain, vomiting, and subcutaneous emphysema. To determine the diagnosis, a chest x-ray is helpful because patients with Boerhaave syndrome will have an abnormal x-ray in 81% to 90% of cases, although within the first 6 hours of the perforation, 10% to 33% of patients may have normal chest x-ray findings.[24] To confirm the diagnosis, gastrointestinal tract contrast CT has a better sensitivity than an upper gastrointestinal tract contrast study. Esophageal endoscopy also provides up to 100% sensitivity, but insufflation can be seen as an additional risk to the tear.[26]

A spontaneous esophageal rupture is rare, but it is a serious disease with a mortality rate as high as 80%, although current improvements in detection and treatment lower the mortality rates to 2% to 20%. The mortality rate doubles if treatment is delayed after 24 hours, so timely detection is a cornerstone of the therapy.[27] Surgical treatment is still a basic modality of therapy for esophageal perforation and rupture, but conservative treatment and endoscopic therapies can also be chosen. The treatment strategy should be carefully tailored according to individual severity of the disease and the location of perforation. In this context, a severity scoring system based on 10 clinical and radiologic factors—the **Pittsburgh Classification**—has been developed to stratify treatment options; an approach to esophageal perforation based on injury severity and the degree of mediastinal and pleural contamination is of paramount importance. Although operative management remains the standard in the majority of patients with esophageal perforation, nonoperative management may be successfully implemented in selected patients with a low morbidity and mortality.[28] The score was validated in a multinational study, and it was suggested that patients with a low score (≤2) could be considered for nonsurgical management. Perforation-related morbidity, length of stay, frequency of operative treatment, and mortality increased with increasing perforation severity score (PSS) strata. Patients with high PSS were 3.37 times more likely to be treated surgically compared with low PSS.[29] New interventional endoscopic techniques, including endoscopic clips, covered metal stents, and endoluminal vacuum therapy have been developed in recent years to manage esophageal perforation reducing the associated morbidity and mortality. These interventions demonstrated the usefulness of conservative treatment of esophageal rupture.[28,30,31] Endoscopic clip placement is currently the standard method for closing small (<2 cm) luminal perforations.[32] Endoscopic

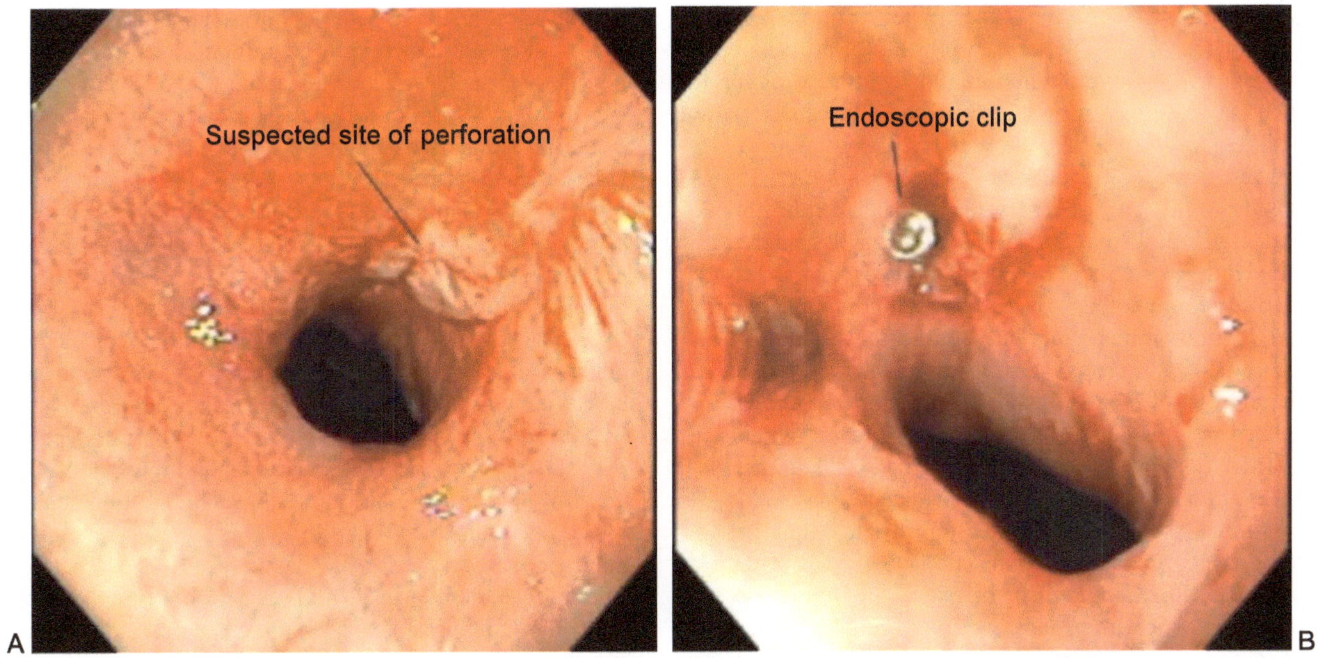

• **Fig. 44.2** Endoscopic clip application to closure of mature esophageal perforation with fistulae. (**A**) Gastro-esophageal junction with a 9-mm stricture and an area of mucosal edema suspected to be the site of perforation. (**B**) Perforation site after placement of first endoclip.

treatment is also the gold standard for closing perforations in the esophagus that occur and are detected during an endoscopic procedure[33] (Fig. 44.2).[34]

Endoscopically inserted stents (partially or fully covered self-expandable metal stents, self-expandable plastic stents) can be used to cover larger defects or to completely cover an unsatisfactory clip closure. Nonsurgical management of esophageal perforation may be considered in stable patients with early presentation, limited esophageal rupture, and minimal contamination of surrounding spaces if highly specialized monitoring is available.[33]

Esophageal emergency guidelines published in 2019 defined that patients eligible for nonsurgical management (Table 44.2) should be kept empty stomach, and administered broad spectrum antibiotics and proton pump inhibitor therapy. The early introduction of enteral nutrition or total parenteral nutrition is also essential for esophageal healing. Therefore the endoscopic placement of a nasogastric tube is recommended. Although antiinfective treatment is considered a cornerstone of esophageal perforation management, there is no consensus on the optimal antibiotic regimen and duration of treatment.

Surgery should be performed in all patients who do not meet the criteria for nonsurgical management listed in Table 44.2.[33]

If surgery is indicated for a perforation or rupture of the esophagus, patients should be taken to the operating room as soon as possible because slight delays in surgical treatment can increase morbidity and mortality. Mortality of patients

TABLE 44.2 Criteria for Nonsurgical Management of Esophageal Perforations

Delay in management	Early: <24 h
Clinical presentation	Absence of symptoms and signs of sepsis
Radiologic criteria	Cervical or thoracic location of the esophageal perforation
	Contained perforation by surrounding tissues:
	- Intramural
	- Minimal periesophageal extravasation of contrast material with intraesophageal drainage
	- Absence of massive pleural contamination
Esophageal characteristics	No preexistent esophageal disease
Other	Possibility of close surveillance by expert esophageal team
	Availability of round the clock surgical and radiologic skills

treated within 24 hours of esophageal perforation is less than 10% compared with 30% after this time.[22,26,28] Surgical repair of esophageal perforation by a minimally invasive approach, such as laparoscopy or thoracoscopy, should be considered.

The goal of surgical treatment includes a lavage drainage and suture closure of the perforation, and in some cases the formation of a gastrointestinal fistula, depending on the patient's clinical condition. Surgical therapy is generally divided into transthoracic or transhiatal procedures. To decide on a surgical method, it is extremely important to identify the location of the perforation. Thoracotomy is still mainly performed as the conventional surgical method. However, the number of reports of thoracoscopic procedures has increased recently, and are becoming more common and an effective therapy particularly for Boerhaave syndrome. Another approach to suture the tear is laparoscopic transhiatal simple closure. Laparoscopic transhiatal simple closure of all layers is considered a practical, less invasive surgical procedure for the treatment of esophageal rupture in patients who meet the following conditions: stable general condition, no intrathoracic perforation, and the perforation site is identified by preoperative examination at the lower esophagus. In summary, surgical approaches or conservative methods must be considered for thoracic or abdominal esophageal perforations. If the area of injury is diseased or direct repair of thoracic esophageal perforation is not feasible (hemodynamic instability, delayed surgical exploration, extensive esophageal damage), an emergent esophagectomy may be required, which is a safe option for the treatment of esophageal perforation with a mortality rate comparable to that of elective esophagectomy.[33,35]

Achalasia and Esophageal Stricture

Achalasia is a progressive impairment of the autonomic motor function of the esophagus, leading to failure of relaxation of the LES with hypercontractility and loss of peristalsis in the distal esophagus because of a loss of function of the myenteric plexus ganglion cells in the distal esophagus. The degeneration of the myenteric plexus ganglion cells is suspected to be caused either by an autoimmune process or as a consequence of a systemic infectious disease, such as Chagas disease.[36] In addition, achalasia is associated with other systemic secondary movement disorders, such as neuromuscular diseases, scleroderma, amyloidosis, and Parkinson disease. Achalasia is a relatively rare disease with a prevalence of 10 cases per 100,000 people and an incidence of about one case per 100,000 people.[37]

Because of the slow progression and unspecific symptoms of achalasia, patients with achalasia often seek medical advice in advanced stages of the disease. Typical esophageal symptoms are dysphagia, first with solid, later even with liquid foods, heartburn, regurgitation or vomiting, epigastric or chest pain. Other associated signs are unintentional weight loss or history of aspiration, such as chronic cough or asthma, pneumonia, or hoarseness.[36]

The gold standard for the diagnosis of achalasia is high-resolution manometry with topographic pressure imaging. A barium esophageal is only recommended if a manometry is not conclusive because of its lower sensitivity.[38] In addition, endoscopy is recommended in all patients with symptoms of achalasia to exclude other associate diseases.

There is no curative medical therapy for achalasia by various conservative symptomatic therapeutic approaches. Surgical treatment consists of cardiomyotomy and esophagomyotomy (Heller myotomy), which aims to interrupt spastic LES, followed by a partial antireflux procedure (fundoplication). Laparoscopy is the preferred surgical approach because of its lower morbidity and comparable long-term outcome compared with esophagomyotomy via left-sided thoracotomy.[39] Peroral endoscopic myotomy is a surgical procedure that is gaining popularity worldwide as a less invasive endoscopic treatment with comparable efficacy to Heller myotomy.[40] The procedure consists of creating a submucous tunnel from the middle esophagus to the proximal stomach, followed by total or partial myotomy of the muscle without an accompanying antireflux procedure (Fig. 44.3).[41] Therefore in patients

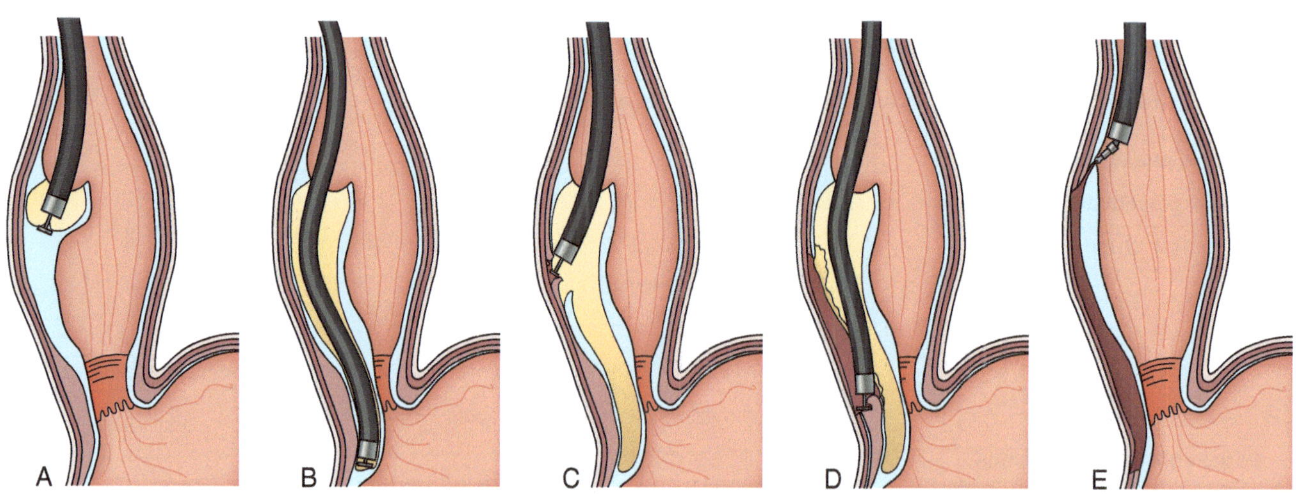

• **Fig. 44.3** Peroral endoscopic myotomy (POEM) for esophageal achalasia. Steps of POEM: (**A**) Mucosal entry; (**B**) Create submucosal tunnel; (**C** and **D**) Myotomy; (**E**) Closure mucosal entry. (©Inoue H. Showa University Northern Yokohama, 2010.)

at high risk of GERD, a Heller myotomy may be preferred after the procedure,[38] but the evidence is mixed.[42] Because of the high risk of complications, esophagectomy should only be considered in the case of end-stage achalasia if all other treatments were permanently ineffective.[43]

Gastroesophageal Reflux Disease and Hiatal Hernia

The transition between esophagus and stomach is formed by the LES, the diaphragm, the His angle, the Gubaroff valve (mucosal fold at the entrance to the stomach) and the phreno-esophageal membrane and acts as a barrier.[44] A malfunction of any of these barriers may lead to a reflux of stomach contents into the esophagus. Although some degree of gastroesophageal reflux is normal, the occurrence of frequent or severe symptoms is referred to as GERD. Lifestyle and diet, as well as increased intraabdominal pressure, such as obesity or pregnancy, sensomotoric disturbances, such as impaired esophageal peristalsis or, rarely, excessive secretion of stomach acid (Zollinger-Ellison syndrome) may all promote the symphyses of GERD. The incidence is high in developed countries and affects both the quality of life and socioeconomic aspects. Typical symptoms are heartburn, regurgitation, and dropsy.[45] Because of the disruption of various antireflux mechanisms, diaphragmatic hernia is a particular risk factor. Particularly large hiatal hernias are often associated with GERD, which is caused by an increased frequency of transient lower esophageal sphincter relaxation (TLESR), lower LES tone, and reduced esophageal motility. Hiatal hernias comprise four anatomic types. Type I, the sliding hiatal hernia, accounts for more than 90% of cases of hiatal hernia, with symmetrical ascent of the stomach through the diaphragmatic crust. They are often associated with severe degrees of esophagitis and Barrett esophagus. Types II–IV are called paraoesophageal hernias with asymmetrical ascent, and their main clinical significance depends on the anatomic deposition of the stomach, which carries the risk of ischemia, obstruction, or volvulus.[46]

The management of GERD follows a step-by-step approach. Besides lifestyle interventions, the main principle is the medical reduction of esophageal luminal acid reflux by local neutralization or by suppressing gastric acid secretion. Surgery is rarely indicated but may be considered in refractory GERD or, if associated, large hiatal hernia.[47]

There are several surgical approaches to treat GERD and associated hiatal hernia. Laparoscopic transabdominal **Nissen fundoplication (total fundoplication),** which creates a 360-degree wrap of the fundus around the lower esophagus, is the most common surgical procedure for the treatment of GERD.[48] **Partial fundoplication,** such as 180-degree fundoplication anterior or 270-degree fundoplication posterior (toupee fundoplication) has been developed to reduce postfundoplication symptoms. In patients with previous abdominal surgery, long disease duration with severe peptic strictures, or extremely large hiatal hernia, **transthoracic fundoplication** through a left lateral thoracotomy is preferred. In this case, the anesthetist must advance an esophageal dilator through the gastroesophageal junction to bring the stomach into the thorax after mobilization of the distal esophagus by the surgeon. After fundoplication, the dilator is removed and the fundoplication wrap is placed under the diaphragm.

The combination of GERD and hiatal hernia, especially paraoesophageal hernia, implies the need for surgical treatment. The repair of paraoesophageal hernia can be challenging, depending on its size and the abnormalities associated with the organ hernias. The standard procedure is currently hiatal repair and laparoscopic fundoplication.[46] The combination of this procedure with a collis gastroplasty to lengthen the esophagus contracted by the chronic inflammation to allow tension-free fundoplication may be necessary and is classically performed transthoracically.[49] In addition, the use of a net for hiatal hernia repair is favored to reduce the recurrence rate of hernia even if the evidence is weak. Robotic surgery is also developing in hiatosurgery, offering improved visualization and optimized ergonomics with low complication rates. Arcerito M et al. evaluated 75 patients (23 males and 47 females), preoperatively diagnosed with a large paraesophageal hiatal hernia, who were treated with a robotic approach. Biosynthetic tissue absorbable mesh was applied for hiatal closure reinforcement. Some 58 patients underwent total fundoplication, 11 patients had partial fundoplication, and one patient had a Collis-Nissen fundoplication for acquired short esophagus. The authors reported that all procedures were completed robotically, without laparoscopic or open conversion. Mean operative time was 223 minutes, mean length of stay was 38 hours. Moderate postoperative dysphagia was noted in eight patients, all of which resolved after 3 months without esophageal dilation. No mesh-related complications were detected. They concluded that robotic surgical treatment of GERD with large paraoesophageal hernias may afford the surgeon increased dexterity and is feasible with comparable outcomes compared with traditional laparoscopic approaches.[50]

Alternatively, endoscopic treatments for GERD have been developed in recent decades, such as transoral incisionless fundoplication or the delivery of radiofrequency energy to the LES. The Stretta procedure is a minimally invasive endoscopic procedure for the treatment of GERD that delivers radiofrequency energy in the form of electromagnetic waves through electrodes at the end of a catheter to the LES and the gastric cardia.[51] The absence of an abdominal incision and short intervention times are the advantages of these new methods, and comparable short-term results have been demonstrated.

Esophageal Tumors

Esophageal tumors can be divided into benign tumors and precursors and malignant tumors (Table 44.3).

Squamous epithelial papilloma is rare in benign tumors and precursors, and its causes include chronic mucosal irritation, human papilloma virus infection, and genetic syndromes.[52] The therapy is resection, and it does not occur afterwards. More important is **Barrett dysplasia,** which is a neoplastic epithelium restricted to the metaplastic esophageal mucosa without invasion. It can be divided

TABLE 44.3 Tumors of the Esophagus

Benign tumors and precursors	Squamous papilloma
	Barrett dysplasia
	Squamous dysplasia
Malignant tumors	Adenocarcinoma
	Adenoid cystic carcinoma
	Adenosquamous and mucoepidermoid carcinoma
	Squamous cell carcinoma
	Undifferentiated carcinoma
	Neuroendocrine neoplasms

into low-grade dysplasia and high-grade dysplasia. The observed rates of progression of low- to high-grade dysplasia or cancer range from 3% to 23%.[53,54] The symptoms of the patients are those of GERD. Risk factors are those of adenocarcinoma (see later). The current practice is to perform ablation instead of surgery in Barrett dysplasia. **Squamous cell dysplasia** is a neoplastic alteration of the squamous epithelium of the esophagus without invasion. The reported prevalence varies between 3% and 38% in different parts of the world.[55] Risk factors are those of developing squamous cell carcinoma (see later). Most patients are generally asymptomatic and the progression rates over 3.5 years from dysplasia to carcinoma vary between 5% and 65%, depending on the preexisting dysplastic status.[56]

Esophageal cancer is one of the leading causes of cancer mortality worldwide.[57,58] Despite the decline in age-standardized incidence and mortality rates, esophageal cancer remains one of the leading causes of cancer mortality and burden worldwide.[59] There are two main histologic subtypes of esophageal cancer: esophageal adenocarcinoma and esophageal squamous cell carcinoma. The diagnosis is always confirmed by endoscopic biopsy and histologic analysis. All other types of esophageal carcinoma are extremely rare and are therefore not discussed further in this book.

Almost all **adenocarcinomas** occur in the lower esophagus and the esophagogastric junction. The global incidence rate of esophageal adenocarcinoma is 0.7 cases per 100,000 people per year, with the highest incidences in North America, Northern and Western Europe, Australia, and New Zealand.[60] Risk factors for esophageal adenocarcinoma include GERD, obesity, male gender, smoking, drugs, such as nonsteroidal antiinflammatory drugs, and dietary factors. *Helicobacter pylori* infection is instead inversely associated with the risk of adenocarcinoma.[61,62] About half of patients with adenocarcinoma of the esophagus receive neoadjuvant chemoradiation therapy, and the guidelines for perioperative care in esophageal resection state that the optimal time for surgery is 6 to 10 weeks after the last day of radiotherapy.[63]

Worldwide, more than 85% of all esophageal cancer cases are esophageal **squamous cell carcinoma**, and it is the sixth most common cause of cancer-related death worldwide.[60] The highest incidence rates are found in the Asian esophageal cancer belt, which extends from East to Central Asia.[64] Squamous cell carcinoma is most commonly located in the middle third of the esophagus.[65] Risk factors include low socioeconomic status, smoking or chewing tobacco, alcohol consumption, drinking very hot beverages, dietary factors, and genetic factors. An increased body mass index is associated with a lower risk, whereas Plummer-Vinson syndrome, achalasia, radiotherapy of the chest, and injury from corrosive ingestion increase the risk of squamous cell carcinoma of the esophagus.[66] The most common symptom is dysphagia, but chest pain, odynophagia, and weight loss may also occur. Most patients with advanced esophageal squamous cell carcinoma are treated with neoadjuvant chemoradiation therapy before surgical resection, but the 5-year survival rate for this entity is less than 15%, while the 5-year survival rate for superficial disease is about 85%.[65]

Surgical Approaches (Endoscopic Resection, Open Esophagectomy, Hybrid Minimally Invasive Esophagectomy, Total Minimally Invasive Esophagectomy, Robotic Surgery)

Esophagectomy represents the current standard of care for patients with localized esophageal cancer of stage T1sm/N+ or higher.[67] Other indications include curative resection of high-grade dysplasia and severe nonmalignant diseases, such as esophageal injury, nondilatable stricture, severe recurrent GERD, and achalasia.[68,69] The standard surgical approach to esophagectomy has always been a laparotomy or a combined laparotomy and thoracotomy.[70] The three classical approaches to perform an open esophagectomy (OE) are (Table 44.4): (1) transhiatal laparotomy; (2) two-incision techniques via laparotomy and right thoracotomy (Ivor Lewis approach); and (3) three-incision techniques via laparotomy, right thoracotomy and a cervical incision for anastomosis (McKeown approach). Today, most centers perform esophagectomies using hybrid or totally minimally invasive techniques—replacing either the laparotomy with a laparoscopy or the thoracotomy with a thoracoscopy (hybrid minimally invasive esophagectomy [HMIE]). The most common surgical procedure today is the combination of laparoscopy to mobilize the stomach and the lower esophagus followed by right thoracoscopy to complete

TABLE 44.4 Approaches to Open Esophagectomy

Transhiatal Approach	Laparotomy
Two-incision approach (Ivor Lewis)	Laparotomy and right thoracotomy
Three-incision approach (McKeown)	Laparotomy, right thoracotomy, and cervical incision for anastomosis

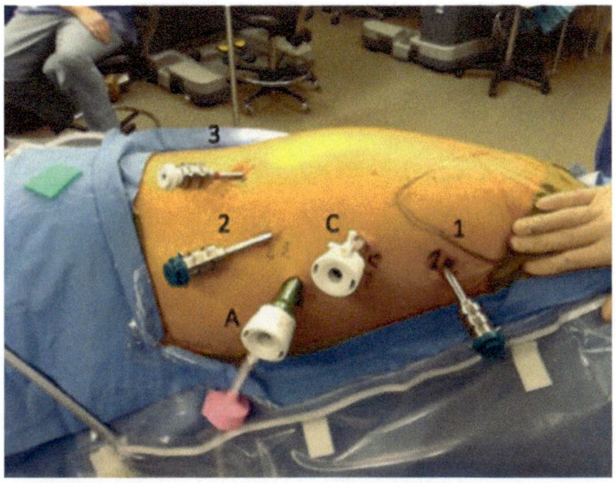

• **Fig. 44.4** Positioning and port placement for thoracic phase of robotic esophagectomy.

the resection and to carry the intrathoracic anastomosis (total minimally invasive esophagectomy [TMIE]). Robot-assisted minimally invasive thoracolaparoscopic esophagectomy (RAMIE) is also becoming increasingly common (Fig. 44.4).[71]

Both transhiatal esophagectomy (THE) and transhiatal laparoscopic esophagectomy can be performed throughout the entire esophagus, but are usually the preferred approach for tumors of the lower esophagus. Surgical extent of resection depends tumor-node-metastasis (TNM)-stadium and is illustrated in Fig. 44.5.[72,73] The purpose is to avoid thoracic access via a thoracotomy or thoracoscopy. A metaanalysis showed that THE is associated with a decrease in hospitalization, hospital mortality, surgery time, and blood loss during surgery.[74] Apart from these surgical benefits, there was no clear evidence that THE has an additional benefit in esophagogastric cancer, in fact, even fewer lymph node dissection can be obtained with this surgical option.[74] A comparison of perioperative morbidity and mortality in open THE and open Ivor Lewis esophagectomy is similar. Paymond et al. reviewed the Society of Thoracic Surgeons General Thoracic Surgery of 4321 esophagectomies that were performed by 164 participating centers. The most common procedures included Ivor Lewis (32.5%), transhiatal (21.7%), minimally invasive esophagectomy, Ivor Lewis type (21.4%), and McKeown (10.0%). The 30 days inpatient mortality was

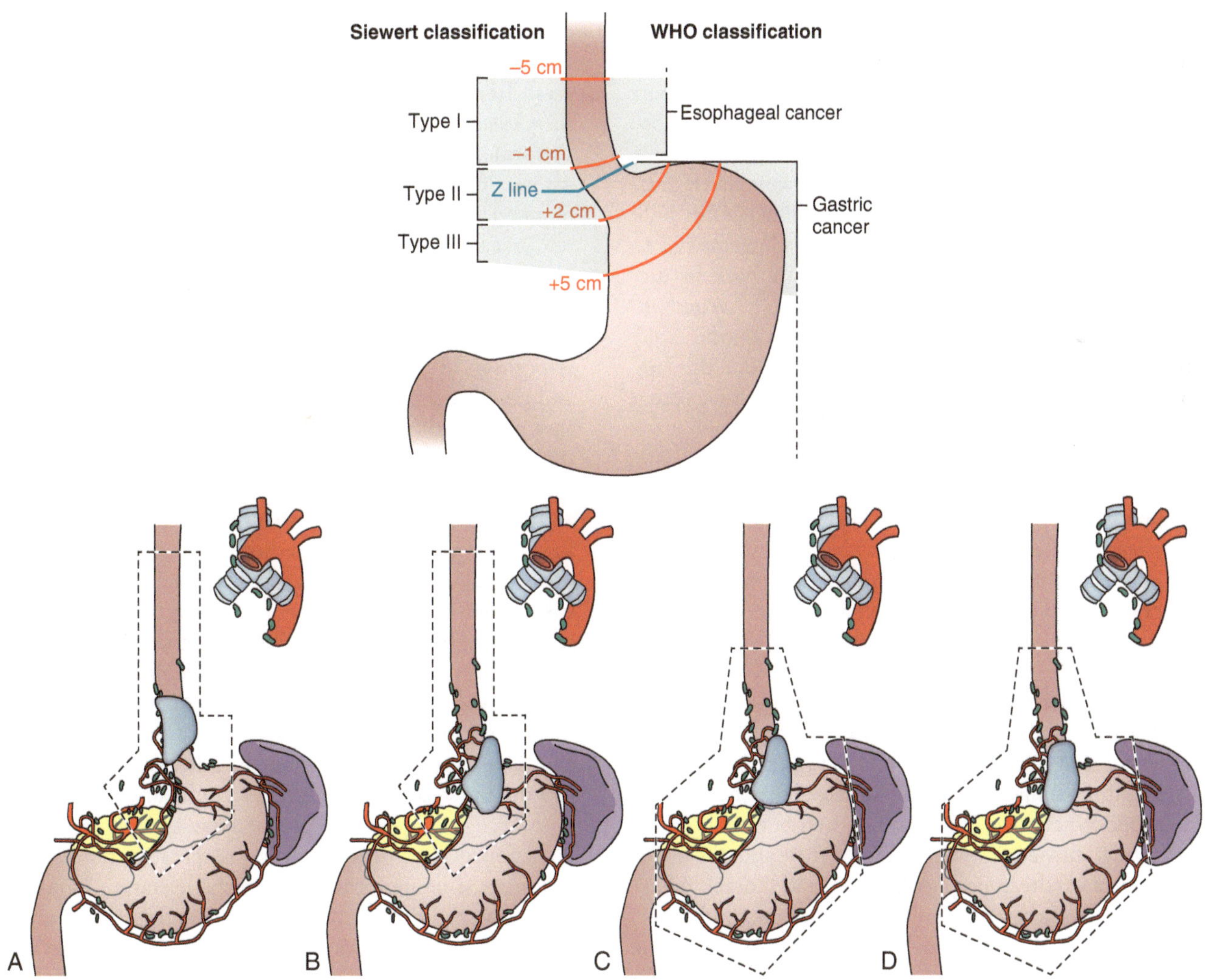

• **Fig. 44.5** Siewert classification of esophagogastric junctional cancers and recommended extent of surgical resection. **(A)** Type I (subtotal esophagectomy with polar gastrectomy), **(B)** type II (subtotal esophagectomy with polar gastrectomy or **(C)** total gastrectomy with inferior esophagectomy, and **(D)** type III (total gastrectomy).

3.4%. Major morbidity occurred in 1429 patients (33.1%), which included unexpected return to operating (15.6%), anastomotic leak (12.9%), reintubation (12.2%), initial ventilation beyond 48 hours (3.5%), pneumonia (12.2%), renal failure (2.0%), and recurrent laryngeal nerve paresis (2.0%). Predictors of combined major morbidity or mortality included age over 65 years, body mass index 35 kg/m^2 or greater, preoperative congestive heart failure, McKeown esophagectomy, current or former smoker, and squamous cell histology.[75,76] Instead, transthoracic esophagectomy was associated with longer hospitalization and higher rates of respiratory complications and wound infection, although both open approaches (McKeown and Ivor Lewis esophagectomy) were not further differentiated, but McKeown is a more risky approach than Ivor Lewis.[75,77]

Transthoracic esophagectomy is the most common approach that requires an abdominal incision to mobilize the stomach and form a gastric tube and a right thoracotomy to resect the diseased esophagus and perform the anastomosis. Subsequently, thoracoscopy and laparoscopy have been increasingly used in patients requiring esophagectomy either as TMIE or in a variety of hybrid combinations with traditional open access (e.g., HMIE).[63] Several metaanalyses showed that TMIE was associated with a statistically significant reduction in perioperative blood loss and a decrease in pulmonary infections.[78,79] Similar leakage rates, shorter hospital stays, similar mortality, similar or even higher lymph node counts and equivalent overall survival were also found. However, some studies have not found differences in pulmonary complication rates and have shown increased rates of anastomotic leakage and reintervention in patients undergoing minimally invasive esophagectomy.[78,79] Attempts have been made to explain this phenomenon by the rapid introduction and implementation of TMIE, but this approach has a significant learning curve, as a retrospective multicenter study has shown.[80,81]

The most frequently performed hybrid procedure is a modification of the classic Ivor-Lewis approach, in which the laparotomy is replaced by a laparoscopy for gastric tube preparation and celiac lymphadenectomy.[67] In addition to TMIE, a reduction in postoperative complications and perioperative blood loss, as well as a shortening of the hospital stay could be demonstrated for HMIE compared with OE.[82]

TMIE has been further developed through the use of robotic assistance (e.g., RAMIE) (see Fig. 44.4).[83] Robot-assisted surgical systems offer some surgical advantages, such as a three-dimensional magnified view of the surgical field, superior hand-eye coordination, tremor filtering, motion scaling, and ergonomic benefits. They also allow the surgeon to reach the upper mediastinum and thoracic opening more easily. Recently, the ROBOT study was published comparing RAMIE with OE: RAMIE was associated with lower intraoperative blood loss, a lower total postoperative complication rate, shorter hospital stay, better short-term quality of life and faster functional recovery, whereas lymph node yield, radicality, and survival were comparable.[84]

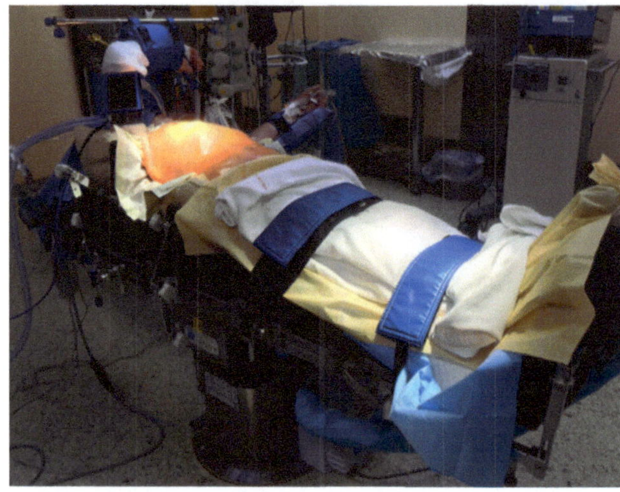

• **Fig. 44.6** Positioning for hybrid minimally invasive esophagectomy. The patient is in the supine position with the right chest elevated.

Positioning. The positioning of the patient depends on the preferred approach. With the HMIE, the patient can remain in a supine position, slightly twisted, and the right side of the chest should be elevated to allow a right thoracotomy without repositioning the patient (Fig. 44.6). For laparoscopy, the patient should be positioned in the reverse Trendelenburg position. It is also possible to change the patient's position—especially when RAMIE or TMIE is performed; laparoscopy is performed in a supine position, whereas for thoracoscopy, a left-sided decubitus position is required. Although uncommon, some centers also use the semi-recumbent or prone position for TMIE.[67]

Esophageal Reconstruction. The most commonly used replacement after esophagectomy is a gastric channel.[70] Other potential substitutes are the colon and jejunum interposition. All of these substitutes have specific advantages and disadvantages: advantages of a **gastric channel** include easy mobilization to reach the thorax or even the neck and the need for only one anastomosis, whereas disadvantages include sensitive vascularization, a tendency to chronic acid and bile reflux, and the fact that the fundus was typically in the area of preoperative radiotherapy, which could compromise the blood supply and affect healing at the anastomosis site. When comparing the whole stomach with the reconstruction of the gastric tube after an esophagectomy, patients with a gastric tube show a lower risk of delayed gastric emptying, fewer reflux symptoms, and a better quality of life.[85]

If the gastric channel is not feasible, a **colonic interposition** is usually the next option. Its advantages are the long length, the relative resistance to acids, and the excellent blood supply. Typically, a preoperative examination to rule out anomalies or tumors and a preoperative bowel preparation must be performed before the use as an esophageal replacement. Disadvantages of colon interposition are the longer operating time and the necessity of three gastrointestinal anastomoses with the possibility of compromised blood supply.

Jejunal conduits have some theoretical advantages over colon interpositions: their diameter is closer to that of the original esophagus and they are usually disease-free. Other advantages are the antegrade segmental contraction and a low leakage rate. The disadvantages are similar to those of colonic interposition: longer operating time and the need for three anastomoses. In addition, it requires technically complex, overloaded microvascular anastomoses to reach the upper thorax or neck.

Postoperative Complications (Anastomosis Insufficiency, Esophageal Conduit Necrosis, Ulcer, Stenosis)

The complication rates after esophagectomy are as high as 50%, although large-volume centers could achieve a low total mortality of 5%.[86,87] The most common intraoperative complications in esophageal surgery are hypotension and hypoxemia, usually caused by compression of the heart or large vessels by the surgeon or by retractors.[88] In esophageal surgery in particular, the maneuver of translocating the severed stomach through the hiatus into the thorax provokes temporary hypotension and cardiac arrythmias. Close communication with the surgeon is crucial. Continuous thoracic insufflation of carbon dioxide (CO_2) for minimally invasive esophageal surgery or robotic esophageal surgery could also affect hemodynamics in a pressure-dependent manner.[89] In general, a right-sided capnothorax seems to reduce venous return and cardiac output more than a left-sided thoracic CO_2 insufflation.[89] In transabdominal laparoscopic esophageal surgery, the increased pressure in the abdominal cavity caused by the pneumoperitoneum and the reverse Trendelenburg position impair hemodynamics. Particularly increased intraabdominal pressures (>15 mm Hg) hinder the venous return of the lower half of the body, which leads to hypotension. In addition, laparoscopic surgery and dissection of the gastroesophageal junction often leads to an invasion of CO_2 into the thoracic cavity, resulting in increased pleural and mediastinal pressure. Cardiac arrhythmias are frequent during esophageal surgery, widely resulting in hypotension. Typical arrhythmias are atrial fibrillation, bradycardia because of vagal stimulation by pneumoperitoneum or esophageal dissection, and premature ventricular contractions caused by intrathoracic manipulation. Fortunately, intraoperative cardiac dysrhythmias are of self-limited entity, however, almost 15% of atrial dysrhythmias require interventions.[87] As for the close relationship of the esophagus to the large vessels, acute life-threatening hemorrhage can occur at any time during the operation, leading to severe hypotension. However, the total perioperative blood loss in modern minimally invasive esophageal surgery is usually small. A number of patients who are candidates for esophagectomy with esophageal cancer have concomitant cardiovascular or preexisting coronary heart disease.[90] Therefore perioperative hypotension, tachyarrhythmias, or anemia should be avoided to reduce the incidence of serious adverse cardiovascular events.

To avoid perioperative hypotension, close communication with the surgeon and adjustment of the intraperitoneal or intrathoracic pressure of CO_2 insufflation is recommended. The anesthetist must be familiar with special surgical maneuvers, such as the translocation of the stomach into the thorax, which can lead to short episodes of hypotension.

The causes of hypoxemia during esophageal surgery also depend on the patient's comorbidities and the surgical procedure. In general, pulmonary complications are the leading cause of mortality during esophageal surgery.[91,92] In laparoscopic transabdominal accesses, increased abdominal pressure leads to cranial translocation of the diaphragm, impairs the respiratory mechanics, and provokes basal atelectasis of the lung. Therefore adjustment of peak airway pressure and positive end-expiratory pressure (PEEP) is necessary to avoid hypoxemia. In addition, surgery at the gastroesophageal junction often leads to pleural insufflation of CO_2, resulting in pneumothorax. Fortunately, a tension component is rare, and assuming a peak airway pressure to restore adequate tidal volume and adjusting the PEEP level is sufficient to avoid hypoxemia during surgery. Peritoneal absorption of insufflated CO_2 during pneumoperitoneum causes an increase in the arterial CO_2 concentration that can be offset by increasing the respiratory rate. The acceptance of permissive hypercapnia is recommended to maintain lung protective ventilation.

Venous thromboembolic events, such as deep vein thrombosis and pulmonary embolism, are common in cancer patients. In particular, patients with esophageal cancer who may have an increased risk of venous thromboembolic events before surgery or within 30 days after surgery.[93] Most pulmonary embolism events are subclinical without hemodynamic impairment, and intraoperative oxygenation is rarely affected by pulmonary embolism, but mortality in the postoperative phase is significantly increased in patients with venous thromboembolic events. Therefore prophylactic measures, such as thrombosis prophylaxis are important and in addition, intermittent mechanical compression during surgery may be helpful.[94]

Typical complications during the postoperative phase could be divided into pulmonary, cardiac, and surgical complications. **Pulmonary complications** are the most common postoperative problems with significant impact on mortality. Pneumonia occurs in one-quarter of patients after esophagectomy, followed by pleural effusion requiring drainage and pneumothorax.[87] Acute respiratory distress syndrome occurs in about 2% to 10% of patients, triggered by several factors.[87] In addition, patients have an increased risk of aspiration after esophageal surgery. To reduce postoperative respiratory complications, adequate pain therapy to facilitate effective coughing and early chest physiotherapy is therefore important. If the patient is clinically stable, early extubation of a normothermic patient following complete reversal of the neuromuscular blockade is desirable. Noninvasive positive pressure ventilation (NIV) after esophageal surgery is controversially discussed because damage to the esophageal anastomosis and gastric distension can be a major problem. However, the positive effect of NIV in reducing pulmonary complications after major surgery has been clearly demonstrated, and gentle intermittent use of NIV with a nasogastric tube to protect against overstretching is recommended.[95] Measures to reduce the risk of aspiration, such as chest elevation, use of a nasogastric tube, and early mobilization are recommended. It is important to closely monitor lung function after esophageal surgery, consisting of repeated blood gas analysis and pulmonary imaging as pulmonary ultrasound, or, if necessary, chest x-ray.

Up to 60% of patients experience postoperative surgical complications after esophageal surgery.[87] Besides postoperative bleeding, which is a life-threatening complication and requires immediate therapy, **anastomotic leakage** and anastomotic necrosis are the most serious complications after esophagectomy. An endoscopic examination of the neoesophagus is necessary if symptoms of sepsis and suspicious effusion through drains occur 5 to 10 days after surgery.[96] Signs of necrosis of the anastomosis requires immediate surgery unless an anastomotic leak is detected without necrosis; endoscopic therapy may be appropriate. Hypotension, fluid overload, or excessive use of vasopressors may promote inadequate healing or collapse of the esophageal anastomosis.[96]

Postoperative leakage of chest tubes could be a sign of small pulmonary lesions that do not require additional therapy and usually stop rapidly with spontaneous breathing. If high leakage persists, tracheobronchial lesions must be considered, and bronchoscopy is required. Endoscopic therapy or thoracotomy followed by flap closure may be required. If the pleural effusion persists above the thoracic drainage, a chylothorax must be considered. Because of the high mortality, early surgical intervention is necessary.[97]

Thermal injury, distension, vascular compromise, or excessive lymph node dissection could lead to **recurrent injury to the laryngeal nerve** after esophageal surgery (5%–14%).[87] Symptoms that begin after extubation include inspiratory stridor, hoarseness, dysphonia, and aspiration in the case of unilateral nerve injury. If a bilateral recurrent injury to the laryngeal nerve has occurred, complete airway obstruction requires immediate reintubation followed by tracheotomy. When recurrent injury to the laryngeal nerve has occurred, the incidence of postoperative pulmonary complications increases significantly.

General Anesthetic Considerations

Preoperative Evaluation (see Chapter 8)

Patients undergoing esophagectomy often show comorbidities. In general, these comorbidities can be divided into cardiopulmonary disease and symptoms and signs of the underlying esophageal disease.

Cardiopulmonary disease should be assessed according to published American College of Cardiology/American Heart Association or European Society of Cardiology/European Society of Anaesthesiology (ACC/ACA/ESC/ESA) guidelines.[98,99] The ACC/ACA/ESC/ESA guidelines discourage random routine preoperative cardiac testing because it is time consuming, costly, resource constraining, and does not improve perioperative outcome—rather it emphasizes the importance of individualized preoperative cardiac evaluation.[100] The risk of cardiovascular complications during esophagectomy can be increased by various factors resulting from surgical and anesthetic care, such as hypoxemia, bleeding, dysrhythmia, and pain.

Preoperative assessment of the cardiopulmonary system should include a 12-lead electrocardiogram (ECG), which serves as a screening test for myocardial ischemia and arrhythmias and provides a baseline for comparison. Today's standard surgical workup includes CT of the thorax and upper abdomen, which should be viewed by the anesthesiologist to identify any lung abnormalities, and have rough assessment of cardiac abnormalities and spinal condition to evaluate the optimal placement of thoracic epidural anesthesia. The main focus of the cardiopulmonary assessment should be the patient's medical history and the metabolic equivalent of the task (MET). If the MET value is less than 4, further preoperative examinations such as echocardiography, spirometry, and treadmill or dobutamine exercise testing should be considered to optimize the preoperative status. It should also be considered that many patients receive neoadjuvant oncologic therapy before surgery. It has therefore been shown that neoadjuvant chemotherapy significantly lowers the anaerobic threshold of the patient, and this reduction in fitness may further affect perioperative morbidity.[101]

The other part of the medical history should draw the anesthesiologist's attention to the symptoms and signs of esophageal obstruction, GERD, silent aspiration, and malnutrition, which may also affect the risk of perioperative complications. Obstruction symptoms, particularly dysphagia and odynophagia, can lead to reduced oral uptake and malnutrition, which in turn can lead to increased morbidity and mortality.[102] Symptoms of severe GERD with aspiration may include hypersalivation in response to reflux, supine coughing, globus sensation, laryngitis, and asthma-like symptoms. Patients with preexisting severe GERD or other reasons for aspiration risk may benefit from prophylactic medication to increase gastric pH and reduce stomach volume—even in the absence of definitive evidence of risk reduction. Possible pharmacologic prophylaxis includes proton-pump inhibitors or H_2-receptor antagonists—both reduce gastric volume and acidity.[103]

Patients preparing for esophagectomy should be encouraged to stop smoking 4 weeks before surgery because smokers have an increased risk of perioperative morbidity, particularly of wound and pulmonary complications.[104] Postoperative complications also show a 2- to 3-fold increase among alcohol addicts with an increase in hemorrhagic, wound, and cardiopulmonary morbidity.[104]

Anesthesia Management

Airway Management

In a thoracoabdominal esophageal resection with gastric uplift as the surgical procedure, a separation of the lung with a double-lumen tube (DLT) or bronchial blocker is necessary. Please see Chapter 16 for further details. Intubation with a left-sided DLT may provide a better stability of the position during intrathoracic surgical manipulation.

However, the bronchial blocker may have the advantage if postoperative ventilatory support is required. In this case, there is no need to change the DLT to a single lumen tube because most practitioners refrain from sending a patient to the ICU with a DLT in place. Exchanging the tube is not without risk if the procedure was long and the patient has some degree of airways edema Because of the potential difficulty in exchanging the tube, the use of a tube exchanger should be considered. In addition, continuous application of positive airway pressure to the collapsed lung during the intrathoracic part of the esophagectomy would be recommended because local inflammation in the collapsed lung is inhibited and further lung injury can be avoided.[105]

Perioperative Monitoring

Intraoperative monitoring for esophageal surgery should be adapted to the intraoperative anesthetic challenges and the patient's underlying disease, comorbidities and physical condition, the extent of the surgery, and the surgical approach. Fluid management, perioperative bleeding, cardiovascular complications, lung ventilation, pulmonary complications, and temperature management are tasks that must be managed during surgery.

The occurrence of concomitant coronary artery disease is increased in patients with esophageal cancer and myocardial infarction as a significant risk factor for reduced median survival.[90,106] Therefore additional ECG recordings as a five-electrode ECG with V5 with continuous ST segment analysis may be helpful to detect myocardial ischemia.[107] The incidence of perioperative arrhythmias in esophagectomy and esophagectomy is about 20% and the occurrence of atrial arrhythmias is associated with higher perioperative mortality.[108] Continuous monitoring of lead II is recommended to detect arrhythmias.

In all advanced esophageal procedures, an arterial catheter for continuous blood pressure measurement and blood gas analysis should be placed. The determination of beat-to-beat blood pressure is important for the control of vasopressor and fluid therapy. The analysis of electrolytes could improve the therapy of cardiac arrhythmias, and the evaluation of arterial concentration of oxygen and carbon dioxide facilitates the detection of deterioration of lung function. For thoracic approaches, puncture of the radial artery on the arm opposite the surgical field is recommended because of the positioning of the arm and the improved intraoperative accessibility.

Perioperative restriction of microcirculation, hypotension, and high vasopressor consumption and fluid overload may be associated with an increased incidence of anastomosis insufficiency of blood supply and increased mortality. Therefore extended monitoring of cardiac output could support fluid and vasopressor management.[109] The use of noncalibrated pulse contour analysis is feasible, but the values should be carefully interpreted taking into account the effects of intrathoracic manipulation during surgery. Fluid and vasopressor therapy with only strict adherence to the measurement of cardiac output appears to have limited or controversial effects on postoperative outcome and is not recommended.[110,111] If the patients has a significant underline cardiac disease, using a pulmonary artery catheter is possible, particularly when the use of TEE is not feasible during esophageal surgery.

In advanced esophageal surgery, the placement of a central venous catheter is indicated for vasopressor or inotropic therapy and postoperative parenteral nutrition. The central venous pressure (CVP) measurement is influenced by many different effects and is unsuitable as a control of fluid therapy. However, the assessment of CVP changes over time and the interpretation in the context of all other available hemodynamic values during surgery may be helpful to guide hemodynamic therapy.

Patients should be given a bladder catheter with the amount of urine as an additional parameter of the hemodynamic monitoring ring and to decompress the bladder during prolonged surgery. A recommendation for bladder catheters with a temperature probe helps to monitor core body temperature throughout the surgical procedure; there is an increased risk of hypothermia because of the exposed body surface during a combined thoracoabdominal procedure and early postoperative adverse events.[112] Therefore temperature measurement and maintenance of normothermia with compressed air blankets and warming mattresses is strongly recommended.[63,113] Measurement of the depth of anesthesia by means of a processed electroencephalogram and continuous measurement of muscle relaxation is helpful in achieving and maintaining an appropriate depth of anesthesia and facilitating early postoperative extubation of the patient.

Fluid Management (see Chapter 21)

Fluid management must take into account the patient's preoperative status with its preexisting deficits, maintenance requirements, and ongoing losses (i.e., urinary, gastrointestinal, and evaporation losses, bleeding and interstitial fluid displacement). In addition, it must be considered that minimally invasive surgical access tends to require less fluid than open or hybrid accesses. Excessive perioperative intravenous fluid application leads to fluid displacement into the interstitial space, tissue edema, delayed return to normal gastrointestinal function, impaired wound healing, increased risk of pulmonary edema, and heart and lung failure.[114–116] Several studies have shown that a high positive fluid balance—both intra- and postoperatively—was associated with increased pulmonary morbidity.[116–121] In patients undergoing a thoracoscopic esophagectomy in the prone position, a higher intraoperative positive fluid balance was independently associated with a higher incidence of complications such as pneumonia, arrhythmia, thrombotic events, and acute renal injury.[119]

In addition, because of excessive crystalloid infusion, edema in the conduit and at the anastomosis can lead to inflammatory infiltration and reduced oxygenation of the tissue, possibly predisposing the anastomosis to be at greater risk of failure.[96,122] Most studies agree with the idea that fluid overload is associated with undesirable outcomes. This concept is supported by an extensive metaanalysis of studies comparing liberal with restrictive fluid management in elective procedures and reporting a strong reduction in perioperative complications in the restrictive group.[123]

Therefore the recommendation for restrictive fluid management in esophagectomy was developed. Overrestrictive fluid strategy may lead to hypovolemia and complications, such as acute renal failure (acute kidney injury [AKI]), which are associated with various gastrointestinal complications (i.e., bleeding).[124] In addition, AKI itself has been shown to be a risk factor for infection.[125] Markar et al. implemented a multidisciplinary perioperative care pathway with a target value of 1.5 to 2 L of intraoperative crystalloid application. The results showed a reduction in blood loss, length of stay in the ICU and hospital, but unchanged morbidity and mortality rates.[126]

A restrictive fluid strategy can be optimized with a targeted therapy using invasive arterial monitoring (pulse pressure variation [PPV]), cardiac output monitoring (stroke volume variation [SVV]) or esophageal Doppler (aortic blood flow). The benefit of PPV and SVV in these patients with open chest in low tidal volume ventilation is unclear and not feasible using esophageal Doppler or TEE for esophagectomy.[127,128] The usefulness of SVV in assessing volume status and responsiveness in the postoperative phase after esophagectomy remains unclear.[129] Haas et al. prospectively investigated the effects of targeted intraoperative fluid management based on SVV in thoracic surgery requiring lung ventilation. These patients did not experience pulmonary fluid overload based on the perioperative extravascular lung water index.[130] The clinically relevant aspect is the prevention of fluid overload rather than fluid restriction.[131,132]

Restrictive infusion management implies the application of vasopressors to maintain perfusion pressure in the absence of hypovolemia. In patients undergoing esophagectomy, perfusion of the gastric conduit depends on the right gastroepiploic artery, and there is a possibility that vasoconstriction may negatively affect blood flow into the gastric conduit. However, studies have shown that vasopressor therapy for sympatholytic and hypotension caused by thoracic epidural anesthesia improves blood flow in the gastric conduit.[121,133,134]

A metaanalysis of 23 studies (10 studies with an enhanced recovery after surgery [ERAS] protocol) with goal directed fluid therapy [GDFT]) in major abdominal surgery showed that in addition to the decrease in total infusion volume, lower morbidity and length of stay were observed. These differences disappeared when the GDFT was used in newer studies as part of an ERAS protocol.[135] A further metaanalysis in patients with elective open abdominal surgery showed no difference between restrictive and standard or liberal fluid therapy. However, when comparing balanced fluid therapy with unbalanced therapy, there were 59% fewer complications and 3 to 4 days less time spent in the balanced fluid group.[136]

Especially for esophagectomy, it is recommended to optimize stroke volume during the abdominal phase and to monitor stroke volume during the thoracic phase and to avoid aggressive fluid application to achieve a fluid balance.[137]

Whether colloids and/or crystalloids should be used in esophageal surgery, there are studies that conclude that the application of colloids does not lead to better clinical results than the administration of crystalloids.[138] In contrast, the colloid hydroxy-ethyl starch (HES) was well tolerated and comparable with albumin in terms of its effect on renal function during thoracic esophagectomy.[139] Although intravenous application of HES reduces the total amount of fluid infused during esophagectomy, it was associated with an increased risk of postoperative mixed complications, such as AKI.[140]

The data of Klevebro et al., on the implementation of a standardized hemodynamic protocol, showed that in 501 esophagectomy patients, the average infusion volume applied intraoperatively was 2895 mL.[141] Postoperative fluid is set at 0.5 mL/kg/h up to a maximum of 100 mL/h. The mean arterial pressure (MAP) should be above 70 mm Hg in normovolemia with phenylephrine. Clinical verification is required if the MAP is below 70 mm Hg for more than 15 minutes. The authors report that because the introduction of their standardized hemodynamic protocol in 2004, the complication rate is 53.2%, the anastomosis leakage rate 5.2%, and the conduit necrosis rate 0%.[141] Compared with the Esophageal Complications Consensus Group published results where the complication rate was 59%, the anastomosis leakage rate was 11.4% and conduit necrosis was 1.3%, their standardized hemodynamic protocol shows a significant advantage.[63]

The placement and application of an epidural catheter has an impact on fluid therapy because of its sympathetic effect and hypotension. If a patient with epidural analgesia is hypotensive but normovolemic, vasopressors should be applied.[115] In practice, perioperative "optimal" fluid therapy for esophagectomy should aim for zero to no more than 2 kg/day weight gain using balanced crystalloids and catecholamines, with a MAP of at least 70 mm Hg, and fluid intake limited to less than 30 mL/kg body weight. Typically, a minimum urine flow rate of 0.5 mL/kg/h is the accepted norm.[63,137]

In summary, a standardized hemodynamic protocol is recommended because it provides specific objectives for perioperative monitoring and a structured framework for the respective measures.[141]

Pain Therapy (see Chapter 24)

Pain therapy largely depends on surgical access to the esophagus. In patients who have open or hybrid minimally invasive accesses, thoracic epidural analgesia (TEA) remains the "gold standard" of pain management in transthoracic esophagectomy.[80] TEA provides excellent analgesia,[142] reduces the inflammatory response,[143] reduces the incidence of pneumonia and other pulmonary postoperative complications after esophagectomy,[143,144] leads to lower mortality rates,[144,145] and reduces stress reactions.[142] TEA can also reduce hospitalization period and costs.[142] TEA has been shown to enable patients to mobilize more quickly and achieve satisfactory postoperative lung function more quickly.[146] Current ERAS Society guidelines emphasize the role of TEA in postesophagectomy pain.[63] Brown et al. postulated the placement of two epidural catheters for even better analgesia, which is not the standard practice.[147] The epidural catheter is placed between the T4–T5 and T7–T8 levels to provide effective analgesia, which covers both the thoracic and abdominal surgical part.[63,144,148]

Systematic reviews indicate that thoracic paravertebral blockade (TPVB) can lead to a comparably effective analgesia with fewer side effects than TEA and can therefore be a valid alternative.[149]

In summary, it can be recommended that the benefits of TEA in open and hybrid minimally invasive esophagectomies have already been demonstrated several times. For totally minimally invasive esophagectomies or situations where TEA will not be feasible, TPVB or other nonneuraxial regional anesthesia or intravenous lidocaine are alternatives.

Typical Complications

The complication rate after esophagectomy is about 50%, and large-volume centers could achieve a total mortality of 5% depending primarily on the type of surgery and the patient's comorbidities.[87] The main intraoperative complications of esophageal surgery are hypotension and hypoxemia, which are caused by several factors. Concerning the close relation of the esophagus to major vessels, acute life-threatening blood loss could occur at any time during the operation. However, overall perioperative blood loss in modern minimal invasive esophageal surgery is normally low.

To avoid perioperative hypotension, close communication with the surgeon and adjustment of intraperitoneal or intrathoracic pressure of CO2 insufflation is recommended. Hypotensive episodes should be treated with short-acting vasopressors or inotropes if required. **Anesthetists have to be familiar with special surgical maneuvers as translocation of the stomach to the thorax generating short episodes of hypotension to avoid excessive volume application.** Recommendations to reduce cardiac dysrhythmias during esophageal surgery are lacking, however, electrolyte imbalances should be treated and application of magnesium with its low side effects could be considered to reduce supraventricular arrhythmias.[63]

Pulmonary complications are the most common postoperative source of complications with significant impact on mortality. Therefore careful evaluation of the risk of aspiration and rapid sequence induction is advised. We would generally advise a gentle elevation of the chest for induction and extubation. If one-lung ventilation (OLV) is required, the anesthetist should be familiar with OLV and the procedures to manage hypoxia during OLV. We further recommend early postoperative extubation after careful evaluation of complete reversal of neuromuscular blocking agents.

Pneumonia occurs in one-quarter of patients after esophagectomy, followed by pleural effusion requiring drainage procedure and pneumothorax.[87] Furthermore, patients after esophageal surgery have an increased risk of aspiration. Therefore to reduce postoperative respiratory complications, adequate pain therapy to facilitate sufficient coughing and early chest physiotherapy is important. Also early extubation of a normothermic patient after complete reversal of neuromuscular blockade is recommended. NIV after esophageal surgery is controversial because harm of esophageal anastomosis and gastric distension is a major concern. However, the positive effect of NIV to reduce pulmonary complications after major surgery is clearly shown, therefore gentle intermittent application of NIV under protection of overdistension with a nasogastric tube can be applied.[150] Measures to reduce risk of aspiration include elevation of the chest, use of nasogastric tubes, and early mobilization. Close monitoring of pulmonary function after esophageal surgery is important, consisting of repetitive blood gas analysis and pulmonary imaging, such as lung ultrasound or chest radiography if required.

Postoperative hypotension after esophageal surgery is common because of inadequate fluid substitution, sympathectomy by thoracic epidural analgesia, hemorrhage, cardiac dysrhythmias, or congestive heart failure. Here, atrial fibrillation requiring intervention occurs in 15% of patients after esophagectomy and about 1% sustain myocardial infarction or cardiac arrest.[87] Therefore careful hemodynamic assessment is advised to stabilize patients, avoiding fluid overload or inadequate use of vasopressors or inotropes. Substitution of electrolyte imbalances could be necessary to stabilize cardiac rhythm. Prophylactic antiarrhythmic therapy with amiodarone may reduce postoperative atrial fibrillation, but evidence does not support beneficial effects on mortality.[63] Postoperative initiation of beta-blockade could be considered in patient with recurrent episodes of atrial fibrillation if not contraindicated.

Patients after esophagectomy have an increased risk for **venous thromboembolism**. Therefore pharmacologic and mechanical measures should be initiated immediately after esophagectomy.[63] Adequate interruption of antithrombotic therapy before and after insertion and removal of thoracic epidural catheter have to be considered.

Up to 60% of patients after esophageal surgery sustain minor or major **postoperative surgical complications.**[87] Postoperative bleeding, which is a life-threatening complication requiring immediate therapy, anastomotic leak, and anastomotic necrosis are the most serious complications after esophagectomy. Endoscopic evaluation of the esophagus is required if symptoms of sepsis and suspicious effusion through drainage tubes occur 5 to 10 days after surgery. Signs of necrosis of the anastomosis requires immediate surgery. If anastomotic leak without necrosis is detected, endoscopic therapy could be expedient. Hypotension, fluid overload, or excessive vasopressor use could promote inadequate healing or breakdown of esophageal anastomosis.[96]

Postoperative leakage of chest drains could be a sign of small pulmonary lesions, not requiring additional therapy and usually cease rapidly under spontaneous breathing. If high leakage persists, tracheobronchial lesions must be considered, and bronchoscopy is necessary. Endoscopic therapy or thoracotomy with subsequent coverage with a flap could be required.

If pleural effusion over chest drain persists, chylothorax has to be considered. Because of high mortality, early surgical intervention is required.

Thermal injury, stretching, vascular compromise, or excessive lymph node dissection could lead to recurrent laryngeal nerve injury after esophageal surgery (5%–14%).[87] Symptoms starting after extubation are inspiratory stridor, hoarseness, dysphonia, and aspiration in unilateral nerve injury. If bilateral recurrent laryngeal nerve injury occurrs, complete airway obstruction requires immediate reintubation followed by tracheotomy. If recurrent laryngeal nerve injury occurrs, incidence of postoperative pulmonary complications significantly increase.[151]

Risk reduction of postoperative pulmonary complications after transthoracic esophageal resection can be achieved by the following procedures:

- General anesthesia performed either as a balanced technique with sevoflurane or as total intravenous anesthesia with propofol.
- The application of thoracic epidural anesthesia as a component of general anesthesia is a key element in reducing pulmonary complications because improved pulmonary function has a causal significance in addition to more effective analgesia.
- Lung protective ventilation during OLV should be set at a PEEP greater than 5 (5–8) mbar and the tidal volume should not exceed 5 mL/kg body weight and frequent recruitment maneuvers.
- There is no clear evidence for a recommendation of an intraoperative target-oriented therapy by a general use of extended hemodynamic monitoring to reduce postoperative pulmonary complications. High-risk patients seem to benefit from an algorithm-based hemodynamic therapy with extended monitoring. The total infusion volume applied intraoperatively should be kept below 3000 mL and adjusted to the length of surgery and the amount of blood lost. The intraoperative application of HES, as well as the transfusion of erythrocyte concentrates should only be performed after strict indication.

References

1. Oezcelik A, DeMeester SR. General anatomy of the esophagus. *Thorac Surg Clin*. 2011;21(2):289–297.
2. Sainathan S, Andaz S. A systematic review of transesophageal echocardiography-induced esophageal perforation. *Echocardiography*. 2013;30(8):977–983.
3. Goyal RK, Chaudhury A. Physiology of normal esophageal motility. *J Clin Gastroenterol*. 2008;42(5):610–619.
4. Chitose SI, Shin Y, Sato K, et al. Three-dimensional imaging of upper esophageal sphincter resting pressure. *Laryngoscope Investig Otolaryngol*. 2019;4(6):645–652.
5. Straathof JW, van Veen MM, Masclee AA. Provocation of transient lower esophageal sphincter relaxations during continuous gastric distension. *Scand J Gastroenterol*. 2002;37(10):1140–1143.
6. Thomas ML, Anthony AA, Fosh BG, Finch JG, Maddern GJ. Oesophageal diverticula. *Br J Surg*. 2001;88(5):629–642.
7. Cook IJ. Cricopharyngeal function and dysfunction. *Dysphagia*. 1993;8(3):244–251.
8. do Nascimento FA, Lemme EM, Costa MM. Esophageal diverticula: pathogenesis, clinical aspects, and natural history. *Dysphagia*. 2006;21(3):198–205.
9. D'Journo XB, Ferraro P, Martin J, Chen LQ, Duranceau A. Lower oesophageal sphincter dysfunction is part of the functional abnormality in epiphrenic diverticulum. *Br J Surg*. 2009;96(8):892–900.
10. Morales-Divo C, Jecker P, Lippert B, Mann WJ. Extraesophageal reflux in patients suffering from Zenker's diverticulum. *HNO*. 2007;55(7):546–550.
11. Gutschow CA, Schmidt H. Esophageal diverticula (excluding cricopharyngeal diverticula). *Chirurg*. 2018;89(5):401–412.
12. Herbella FA, Patti MG. Modern pathophysiology and treatment of esophageal diverticula. *Langenbecks Arch Surg*. 2012;397(1):29–35.
13. Chan DSY, Foliaki A, Lewis WG, Clark GWB, Blackshaw G. Systematic review and meta-analysis of surgical treatment of non-zenker's oesophageal diverticula. *J Gastrointest Surg*. 2017;21(6):1067–1075.
14. Maruyama K, Motoyama S, Sato Y, et al. Tracheobronchial lesions following esophagectomy: erosions, ulcers, and fistulae, and the predictive value of lymph node-related factors. *World J Surg*. 2009;33(4):778–784.
15. Bartels HE, Stein HJ, Siewert JR. Tracheobronchial lesions following oesophagectomy: prevalence, predisposing factors and outcome. *Br J Surg*. 1998;85(3):403–406.
16. Reed MF, Mathisen DJ. Tracheoesophageal fistula. *Chest Surg Clin N Am*. 2003;13(2):271–289.
17. Risher WH, Arensman RM, Ochsner JL. Congenital bronchoesophageal fistula. *Ann Thorac Surg*. 1990;49(3):500–505.
18. Muniappan A, Wain JC, Wright CD, Donahue DM, Gaissert H, Lanuti M, et al. Surgical treatment of nonmalignant tracheoesophageal fistula: a thirty-five year experience. *Ann Thorac Surg*. 2013;95(4):1141–1146.
19. Ebigbo A, Karstensen JG, Aabakken L, et al. Esophageal stenting for benign and malignant disease: European Society of Gastrointestinal Endoscopy (ESGE) Cascade Guideline. *Endosc Int Open*. 2019;7(6):E833–E836.
20. Way C, Wayne C, Grandpierre V, Harrison BJ, Travis N, Nasr A. Thoracoscopy vs. thoracotomy for the repair of esophageal atresia and tracheoesophageal fistula: a systematic review and meta-analysis. *Pediatr Surg Int*. 2019;35(11):1167–1184.
21. Sdralis EIK, Petousis S, Rashid F, Lorenzi B, Charalabopoulos A. Epidemiology, diagnosis, and management of esophageal perforations: systematic review. *Dis Esophagus*. 2017;30(8):1–6.
22. Biancari F, Saarnio J, Mennander A, et al. Outcome of patients with esophageal perforations: a multicenter study. *World J Surg*. 2014;38(4):902–909.
23. Vidarsdottir H, Blondal S, Alfredsson H, Geirsson A, Gudbjartsson T. Oesophageal perforations in Iceland: a whole population study on incidence, aetiology and surgical outcome. *Thorac Cardiovasc Surg*. 2010;58(8):476–480.
24. Carrozza F, Dragean C. Spontaneous esophageal rupture or Boerhaave's syndrome. *J Belg Soc Radiol*. 2020;104(1):1.
25. Tonolini M, Bianco R. Spontaneous esophageal perforation (Boerhaave syndrome): diagnosis with CT-esophagography. *J Emerg Trauma Shock*. 2013;6(1):58–60.
26. Chirica M, Champault A, Dray X, et al. Esophageal perforations. *J Visc Surg*. 2010;147(3):e117–e128.

27. Shaker H, Elsayed H, Whittle I, Hussein S, Shackcloth M. The influence of the 'golden 24-h rule' on the prognosis of oesophageal perforation in the modern era. *Eur J Cardiothorac Surg.* 2010;38(2):216–222.
28. Abbas G, Schuchert MJ, Pettiford BL, et al. Contemporaneous management of esophageal perforation. *Surgery.* 2009; 146(4):749–755.
29. Schweigert M, Sousa HS, Solymosi N, et al. Spotlight on esophageal perforation: a multinational study using the Pittsburgh esophageal perforation severity scoring system. *J Thorac Cardiovasc Surg.* 2016;151(4):1002–1009.
30. Sudarshan M, Elharram M, Spicer J, Mulder D, Ferri LE. Management of esophageal perforation in the endoscopic era: Is operative repair still relevant? *Surgery.* 2016;160(4): 1104–1110.
31. Watkins JR, Farivar AS. Endoluminal therapies for esophageal perforations and leaks. *Thorac Surg Clin.* 2018;28(4):541–554.
32. Mangiavillano B, Viaggi P, Masci E. Endoscopic closure of acute iatrogenic perforations during diagnostic and therapeutic endoscopy in the gastrointestinal tract using metallic clips: a literature review. *J Dig Dis.* 2010;11(1):12–18.
33. Chirica M, Kelly MD, Siboni S, et al. Esophageal emergencies: WSES guidelines. *World J Emerg Surg.* 2019;14:26.
34. Raymer GS, Sadana A, Campbell DB, WA Rowe. Endoscopic clip application as an adjunct to closure of mature esophageal perforation with fistulae. *Clin Gastroenterol Hepatol.* 2003; 1(1):44–50.
35. Seo YD, Lin J, Chang AC, Orringer MB, Lynch WR, Reddy RM. Emergent esophagectomy for esophageal perforations: a safe option. *Ann Thorac Surg.* 2015;100(3):905–909.
36. Pandolfino JE, Gawron AJ. Achalasia: a systematic review. *JAMA.* 2015;313(18):1841–1852.
37. Sadowski DC, Ackah F, Jiang B, Svenson LW. Achalasia: incidence, prevalence and survival. A population-based study. *Neurogastroenterol Motil.* 2010;22(9):e256–e261.
38. Oude Nijhuis RAB, Zaninotto G, Roman S, et al. European guidelines on achalasia: United European Gastroenterology and European Society of Neurogastroenterology and Motility recommendations. *United Eur Gastroenterol J.* 2020;8(1):13–33.
39. Campos GM, Vittinghoff E, Rabl C, et al. Endoscopic and surgical treatments for achalasia: a systematic review and meta-analysis. *Ann Surg.* 2009;249(1):45–57.
40. Martins RK, Ribeiro IB, Hathorn KE, Bernardo WM. Peroral (POEM) or surgical myotomy for the treatment of achalasia: a systematic review and meta-analysis. *Arq Gastroenterol.* 2020; 57(1):79–86.
41. Phalanusitthepha C, Inoue H, Ikeda H, Sato H, Sato C, Hokierti C. Peroral endoscopic myotomy for esophageal achalasia. *Ann Transl Med.* 2014;2(3):31.
42. Cappell MS, Stavropoulos SN, Friedel D. Updated systematic review of achalasia, with a focus on POEM therapy. *Dig Dis Sci.* 2020;65(1):38–65.
43. Aiolfi A, Asti E, Bonitta G, Bonavina L. Esophagectomy for end-stage achalasia: systematic review and meta-analysis. *World J Surg.* 2018;42(5):1469–1476.
44. Herbella FA, Patti MG. Gastroesophageal reflux disease: from pathophysiology to treatment. *World J Gastroenterol.* 2010; 16(30):3745–3749.
45. Bruley des Varannes S, Cestari R, et al. Classification of adults suffering from typical gastroesophageal reflux disease symptoms: contribution of latent class analysis in a European observational study. *BMC Gastroenterol.* 2014;14:112.
46. Roman S, Kahrilas PJ. The diagnosis and management of hiatus hernia. *BMJ.* 2014;349:g6154.
47. Hunt R, Armstrong D, Katelaris P, et al. World Gastroenterology Organisation Global Guidelines: GERD global perspective on gastroesophageal reflux disease. *J Clin Gastroenterol.* 2017;51(6):467–478.
48. Marshall-Webb M, Peters MDJ, Bright T, Watson DI. Effectiveness of Nissen fundoplication versus anterior and posterior partial fundoplications for treatment of gastro-esophageal reflux disease: a systematic review protocol. *JBI Database System Rev Implement Rep.* 2018;16(5):1095–1102.
49. Patel HJ, Tan BB, Yee J, Orringer MB, Iannettoni MD. A 25-year experience with open primary transthoracic repair of paraesophageal hiatal hernia. *J Thorac Cardiovasc Surg.* 2004; 127(3):843–849.
50. Arcerito M, Perez MG, Kaur H, Annoreno KM, Moon JT. Robotic fundoplication for large paraesophageal hiatal hernias. *JSLS.* 2020;24(1).
51. Young A, Kumar MA, Thota PN. GERD: a practical approach. *Cleve Clin J Med.* 2020;87(4):223–230.
52. d'Huart MC, Chevaux JB, Bressenot AM, et al. Prevalence of esophageal squamous papilloma (ESP) and associated cancer in northeastern France. *Endosc Int Open.* 2015;3(2):E101–E106.
53. Ronkainen J, Aro P, Storskrubb T, et al. Prevalence of Barrett's esophagus in the general population: an endoscopic study. *Gastroenterology.* 2005;129(6):1825–1831.
54. Sharma P, Falk GW, Weston AP, Reker D, Johnston M, Sampliner RE. Dysplasia and cancer in a large multicenter cohort of patients with Barrett's esophagus. *Clin Gastroenterol Hepatol.* 2006;4(5):566–572.
55. Hamashige N, Doi Y, Yonezawa Y, et al. Noninvasive detection and prognosis of coronary artery disease in elderly patients; usefulness of dipyridamole-loading myocardial scintigraphy. *Nihon Naika Gakkai Zasshi.* 1987;76(8):1230–1237.
56. Dawsey SM, Lewin KJ, Wang GQ, et al. Squamous esophageal histology and subsequent risk of squamous cell carcinoma of the esophagus. A prospective follow-up study from Linxian. *China. Cancer.* 1994;74(6):1686–1692.
57. Global Burden of Disease Cancer Collaboration, Fitzmaurice C, Allen C, et al. Global, regional, and national cancer incidence, mortality, years of life lost, years lived with disability, and disability-adjusted life-years for 32 cancer groups, 1990 to 2015: a systematic analysis for the global burden of disease study. *JAMA Oncol.* 2017;3(4):524–548.
58. Bray F, Ferlay J, Soerjomataram I, Siegel RL, Torre LA, Jemal A. Global cancer statistics 2018: GLOBOCAN estimates of incidence and mortality worldwide for 36 cancers in 185 countries. *CA Cancer J Clin.* 2018;68(6):394–424.
59. Global Burden of Disease Cancer Collaboration, Fitzmaurice C, Abate D, et al. Global, regional, and national cancer incidence, mortality, years of life lost, years lived with disability, and disability-adjusted life-years for 29 cancer groups, 1990 to 2017: a systematic analysis for the global burden of disease study. *JAMA Oncol.* 2019;5(12):1749–1768.
60. Arnold M, Soerjomataram I, Ferlay J, Forman D. Global incidence of oesophageal cancer by histological subtype in 2012. *Gut.* 2015;64(3):381–387.
61. Thrift AP. Barrett's esophagus and esophageal adenocarcinoma: how common are they really? *Dig Dis Sci.* 2018;63(8):1988–1996.
62. Quante M, Graham TA, Jansen M. Insights into the pathophysiology of esophageal adenocarcinoma. *Gastroenterology.* 2018;154(2):406–420.

63. Low DE, Allum W, De Manzoni G, et al. Guidelines for perioperative care in esophagectomy: Enhanced Recovery After Surgery (ERAS(R)) Society Recommendations. *World J Surg.* 2019;43(2):299–330.
64. Ferlay J, Soerjomataram I, Dikshit R, et al. Cancer incidence and mortality worldwide: sources, methods and major patterns in GLOBOCAN 2012. *Int J Cancer.* 2015;136(5):E359–E386.
65. Tachimori Y, Ozawa S, Numasaki H, et al. Comprehensive registry of esophageal cancer in Japan, 2010. *Esophagus.* 2017;14(3):189–214.
66. Abnet CC, Arnold M, Wei WQ. Epidemiology of esophageal squamous cell carcinoma. *Gastroenterology.* 2018;154(2): 360–373.
67. Bonavina L, Asti E, Sironi A, Bernardi D, Aiolfi A. Hybrid and total minimally invasive esophagectomy: how I do it. *J Thorac Dis.* 2017;9(suppl 8):S761–S772.
68. Fernando HC, Murthy SC, Hofstetter W, et al. The Society of Thoracic Surgeons practice guideline series: guidelines for the management of Barrett's esophagus with high-grade dysplasia. *Ann Thorac Surg.* 2009;87(6):1993–2002.
69. Orringer MB, Marshall B, Stirling MC. Transhiatal esophagectomy for benign and malignant disease. *J Thorac Cardiovasc Surg.* 1993;105(2):265–276.
70. Haverkamp L, Seesing MF, Ruurda JP, Boone J, VH R. Worldwide trends in surgical techniques in the treatment of esophageal and gastroesophageal junction cancer. *Dis Esophagus.* 2017;30(1):1–7.
71. Broussard B, Evans J, Wei B, Cerfolio R. Robotic esophagectomy. *J Vis Surg.* 2016;2:139.
72. Mariette C, Piessen G, Briez N, Gronnier C, Triboulet JP. Oesophagogastric junction adenocarcinoma: which therapeutic approach? *Lancet Oncol.* 2011;12(3):296–305.
73. Kauppila JH, Lagergren J. The surgical management of esophago-gastric junctional cancer. *Surg Oncol.* 2016;25(4):394–400.
74. Yan R, Dang C. Meta-analysis of transhiatal esophagectomy in carcinoma of esophagogastric junction, does it have an advantage? *Int J Surg.* 2017;42:183–190.
75. Raymond DP, Seder CW, Wright CD, et al. Predictors of major morbidity or mortality after resection for esophageal cancer: a Society of Thoracic Surgeons General Thoracic Surgery Database Risk Adjustment Model. *Ann Thorac Surg.* 2016;102(1):207–214.
76. Papenfuss WA, Kukar M, Attwood K, et al. Transhiatal versus transthoracic esophagectomy for esophageal cancer: a 2005–2011 NSQIP comparison of modern multicenter results. *J Surg Oncol.* 2014;110(3):298–301.
77. Boshier PR, Anderson O, Hanna GB. Transthoracic versus transhiatal esophagectomy for the treatment of esophagogastric cancer: a meta-analysis. *Ann Surg.* 2011;254(6):894–906.
78. Nagpal K, Ahmed K, Vats A, et al. Is minimally invasive surgery beneficial in the management of esophageal cancer? A meta-analysis. *Surg Endosc.* 2010;24(7):1621–1629.
79. Guo W, Ma X, Yang S, et al. Combined thoracoscopic-laparoscopic esophagectomy versus open esophagectomy: a meta-analysis of outcomes. *Surg Endosc.* 2016;30(9):3873–3881.
80. Seesing MFJ, Kingma BF, Weijs TJ, Ruurda JP, van Hillegersberg R. Reducing pulmonary complications after esophagectomy for cancer. *J Thorac Dis.* 2019;11(Suppl 5):S794–S798.
81. van Workum F, Stenstra M, Berkelmans GHK, et al. Learning curve and associated morbidity of minimally invasive esophagectomy: a retrospective multicenter study. *Ann Surg.* 2019;269(1):88–94.
82. Glatz T, Marjanovic G, Kulemann B, Sick O, Hopt UT, Hoeppner J. Hybrid minimally invasive esophagectomy vs. open esophagectomy: a matched case analysis in 120 patients. *Langenbecks Arch Surg.* 2017;402(2):323–331.
83. Ruurda JP, van der Sluis PC, van der Horst S, van Hilllegersberg R. Robot-assisted minimally invasive esophagectomy for esophageal cancer: a systematic review. *J Surg Oncol.* 2015;112(3):257–265.
84. van der Sluis PC, van der Horst S, May AM, et al. Robot-assisted minimally invasive thoracolaparoscopic esophagectomy versus open transthoracic esophagectomy for resectable esophageal cancer: a randomized controlled trial. *Ann Surg.* 2019;269(4):621–630.
85. Akkerman RD, Haverkamp L, van Hillegersberg R, Ruurda JP. Surgical techniques to prevent delayed gastric emptying after esophagectomy with gastric interposition: a systematic review. *Ann Thorac Surg.* 2014;98(4):1512–1519.
86. Linden PA, Towe CW, Watson TJ, et al. Mortality after esophagectomy: analysis of individual complications and their association with mortality. *J Gastrointest Surg.* 2019;24(9):1948–1954.
87. Low DE, Kuppusamy MK, Alderson D, et al. Benchmarking complications associated with esophagectomy. *Ann Surg.* 2019;269(2):291–298.
88. Nikbakhsh N, Amri P, Shakeri A, Shakeri A. Changes in blood pressure and heart rhythm during transhiatal esophagectomy. *Caspian J Intern Med.* 2012;3(4):541–545.
89. Reinius H, Borges JB, Freden F, et al. Real-time ventilation and perfusion distributions by electrical impedance tomography during one-lung ventilation with capnothorax. *Acta Anaesthesiol Scand.* 2015;59(3):354–368.
90. Schizas D, Theochari NA, Theochari CA, et al. Perioperative management of antiplatelet therapy in patients with history of coronary artery disease undergoing surgery for esophageal cancer: a single-center experience. *In Vivo.* 2019;33(2):621–626.
91. Law S, Wong KH, Kwok KF, Chu KM, Wong J. Predictive factors for postoperative pulmonary complications and mortality after esophagectomy for cancer. *Ann Surg.* 2004;240(5):791–800.
92. Wright CD, Kucharczuk JC, O'Brien SM, Grab JD, Allen MS. Society of Thoracic Surgeons General Thoracic Surgery D. Predictors of major morbidity and mortality after esophagectomy for esophageal cancer: a Society of Thoracic Surgeons General Thoracic Surgery Database Risk Adjustment Model. *J Thorac Cardiovasc Surg.* 2009;137(3):587–595.
93. Parry K, Sadeghi AH, van der Horst S, Westerink J, Ruurda JP, van Hillegersberg R. Intermittent pneumatic compression in combination with low-molecular weight heparin in the prevention of venous thromboembolic events in esophageal cancer surgery. *J Surg Oncol.* 2017;115(2):181–185.
94. Mantziari S, Gronnier C, Pasquer A, et al. Incidence and risk factors related to symptomatic venous thromboembolic events after esophagectomy for cancer. *Ann Thorac Surg.* 2016;102(3):979–984.
95. Howells PA, Aldridge KA, Parekh D, et al. ARDS following oesophagectomy: a comparison of two trials. *BMJ Open Respir Res.* 2017;4(1):e000207.
96. Bartels K, Fiegel M, Stevens Q, Ahlgren B, Weitzel N. Approaches to perioperative care for esophagectomy. *J Cardiothorac Vasc Anesth.* 2015;29(2):472–480.
97. Vecchiato M, Martino A, Sponza M, et al. Thoracic duct identification with indocyanine green fluorescence during minimally invasive esophagectomy with patient in prone position. *Dis Esophagus.* 2020;33(12):doaa030.

98. Fleisher LA, Fleischmann KE, Auerbach AD, et al. 2014 ACC/AHA guideline on perioperative cardiovascular evaluation and management of patients undergoing noncardiac surgery: executive summary: a report of the American College of Cardiology/American Heart Association Task Force on Practice Guidelines. *Circulation.* 2014;130(24):2215–2245.
99. Kristensen SD, Knuuti J, Saraste A, et al. 2014 ESC/ESA Guidelines on non-cardiac surgery: cardiovascular assessment and management: The Joint Task Force on non-cardiac surgery: cardiovascular assessment and management of the European Society of Cardiology (ESC) and the European Society of Anaesthesiology (ESA). *Eur J Anaesthesiol.* 2014;31(10):517–573.
100. Guarracino F, Baldassarri R, Priebe HJ. Revised ESC/ESA Guidelines on non-cardiac surgery: cardiovascular assessment and management. Implications for preoperative clinical evaluation. *Minerva Anestesiol.* 2015;81(2):226–233.
101. Sinclair R, Navidi M, Griffin SM, Sumpter K. The impact of neoadjuvant chemotherapy on cardiopulmonary physical fitness in gastro-oesophageal adenocarcinoma. *Ann R Coll Surg Engl.* 2016;98(6):396–400.
102. Sungurtekin H, Sungurtekin U, Balci C, Zencir M, Erdem E. The influence of nutritional status on complications after major intraabdominal surgery. *J Am Coll Nutr.* 2004;23(3):227–232.
103. Ng A, Smith G. Gastroesophageal reflux and aspiration of gastric contents in anesthetic practice. *Anesth Analg.* 2001;93(2): 494–513.
104. Mantziari S, Hubner M, Demartines N, Schafer M. Impact of preoperative risk factors on morbidity after esophagectomy: is there room for improvement? *World J Surg.* 2014;38(11):2882–2890.
105. Verhage RJ, Boone J, Rijkers GT, et al. Reduced local immune response with continuous positive airway pressure during one-lung ventilation for oesophagectomy. *Br J Anaesth.* 2014;112(5): 920–928.
106. Backemar L, Lagergren P, Johar A, Lagergren J. Impact of co-morbidity on mortality after oesophageal cancer surgery. *Br J Surg.* 2015;102(9):1097–1105.
107. London MJ, Hollenberg M, Wong MG, et al. Intraoperative myocardial ischemia: localization by continuous 12-lead electrocardiography. *Anesthesiology.* 1988;69(2):232–241.
108. Chen LT, Jiang CY. Impact of atrial arrhythmias after esophagectomy on recovery: a meta-analysis. *Medicine (Baltimore).* 2018;97(23):e10948.
109. Veelo DP, Geerts BF. Anaesthesia during oesophagectomy. *J Thorac Dis.* 2017;9(suppl 8):S705–S712.
110. Veelo DP, van Berge Henegouwen MI, Ouwehand KS, et al. Effect of goal-directed therapy on outcome after esophageal surgery: a quality improvement study. *PLoS One.* 2017;12(3): e0172806.
111. Bahlmann H, Halldestam I, Nilsson L. Goal-directed therapy during transthoracic oesophageal resection does not improve outcome: randomised controlled trial. *Eur J Anaesthesiol.* 2019;36(2):153–161.
112. Yamasaki H, Tanaka K, Funai Y, et al. The impact of intraoperative hypothermia on early postoperative adverse events after radical esophagectomy for cancer: a retrospective cohort study. *J Cardiothorac Vasc Anesth.* 2014;28(4):943–947.
113. Zhang Z, Xu M, Wu D, Zhang X, Wu J. Postoperative myocardial injury in middle-aged and elderly patients following curative resection of esophageal cancer with aggressive or standard body temperature management: a randomized controlled trial. *Anesth Analg.* 2019;129(2):352–359.
114. Holte K, Sharrock NE, Kehlet H. Pathophysiology and clinical implications of perioperative fluid excess. *Br J Anaesth.* 2002;89(4):622–632.
115. Holte K, Foss NB, Svensen C, Lund C, Madsen JL, Kehlet H. Epidural anesthesia, hypotension, and changes in intravascular volume. *Anesthesiology.* 2004;100(2):281–286.
116. Wei S, Tian J, Song X, Chen Y. Association of perioperative fluid balance and adverse surgical outcomes in esophageal cancer and esophagogastric junction cancer. *Ann Thorac Surg.* 2008;86(1):266–272.
117. Kita T, Mammoto T, Kishi Y. Fluid management and postoperative respiratory disturbances in patients with transthoracic esophagectomy for carcinoma. *J Clin Anesth.* 2002;14(4):252–256.
118. Glatz T, Kulemann B, Marjanovic G, Bregenzer S, Makowiec F, Hoeppner J. Postoperative fluid overload is a risk factor for adverse surgical outcome in patients undergoing esophagectomy for esophageal cancer: a retrospective study in 335 patients. *BMC Surg.* 2017;17(1):6.
119. Eng OS, Arlow RL, Moore D, et al. Fluid administration and morbidity in transhiatal esophagectomy. *J Surg Res.* 2016;200(1):91–97.
120. Casado D, Lopez F, Marti R. Perioperative fluid management and major respiratory complications in patients undergoing esophagectomy. *Dis Esophagus.* 2010;23(7):523–528.
121. Ashok A, Niyogi D, Ranganathan P, et al. The enhanced recovery after surgery (ERAS) protocol to promote recovery following esophageal cancer resection. *Surg Today.* 2020;50(4):323–334.
122. Kulemann B, Timme S, Seifert G, et al. Intraoperative crystalloid overload leads to substantial inflammatory infiltration of intestinal anastomoses-a histomorphological analysis. *Surgery.* 2013;154(3):596–603.
123. Schol PB, Terink IM, Lance MD, Scheepers HC. Liberal or restrictive fluid management during elective surgery: a systematic review and meta-analysis. *J Clin Anesth.* 2016;35:26–39.
124. Fiaccadori E, Maggiore U, Clima B, Melfa L, Rotelli C, Borghetti A. Incidence, risk factors, and prognosis of gastrointestinal hemorrhage complicating acute renal failure. *Kidney Int.* 2001;59(4):1510–1519.
125. Vandijck DM, Reynvoet E, Blot SI, Vandecasteele E, Hoste EA. Severe infection, sepsis and acute kidney injury. *Acta Clin Belg.* 2007;62(Suppl 2):332–336.
126. Markar SR, Schmidt H, Kunz S, Bodnar A, Hubka M, Low DE. Evolution of standardized clinical pathways: refining multidisciplinary care and process to improve outcomes of the surgical treatment of esophageal cancer. *J Gastrointest Surg.* 2014;18(7):1238–1246.
127. Suehiro K, Okutani R. Stroke volume variation as a predictor of fluid responsiveness in patients undergoing one-lung ventilation. *J Cardiothorac Vasc Anesth.* 2010;24(5):772–775.
128. Fu Q, Duan M, Zhao F, Mi W. Evaluation of stroke volume variation and pulse pressure variation as predictors of fluid responsiveness in patients undergoing protective one-lung ventilation. *Drug Discov Ther.* 2015;9(4):296–302.
129. Kobayashi M, Koh M, Irinoda T, Meguro E, Hayakawa Y, Takagane A. Stroke volume variation as a predictor of intravascular volume depression and possible hypotension during the early postoperative period after esophagectomy. *Ann Surg Oncol.* 2009;16(5):1371–1377.
130. Haas S, Eichhorn V, Hasbach T, et al. Goal-directed fluid therapy using stroke volume variation does not result in pulmonary fluid overload in thoracic surgery requiring one-lung ventilation. *Crit Care Res Pract.* 2012;2012:687018.

131. Abbas SM, Hill AG. Systematic review of the literature for the use of oesophageal Doppler monitor for fluid replacement in major abdominal surgery. *Anaesthesia.* 2008;63(1):44–51.
132. Rahbari NN, Zimmermann JB, Schmidt T, Koch M, Weigand MA, Weitz J. Meta-analysis of standard, restrictive and supplemental fluid administration in colorectal surgery. *Br J Surg.* 2009;96(4):331–341.
133. Pathak D, Pennefather SH, Russell GN, et al. Phenylephrine infusion improves blood flow to the stomach during oesophagectomy in the presence of a thoracic epidural analgesia. *Eur J Cardiothorac Surg.* 2013;44(1):130–133.
134. Al-Rawi OY, Pennefather SH, Page RD, Dave I, Russell GN. The effect of thoracic epidural bupivacaine and an intravenous adrenaline infusion on gastric tube blood flow during esophagectomy. *Anesth Analg.* 2008;106(3):884–887.
135. Rollins KE, Lobo DN. Intraoperative goal-directed fluid therapy in elective major abdominal surgery: a meta-analysis of randomized controlled trials. *Ann Surg.* 2016;263(3):465–476.
136. Varadhan KK, Lobo DN. A meta-analysis of randomised controlled trials of intravenous fluid therapy in major elective open abdominal surgery: getting the balance right. *Proc Nutr Soc.* 2010;69(4):488–498.
137. Carney A, Dickinson M. Anesthesia for esophagectomy. *Anesthesiol Clin.* 2015;33(1):143–163.
138. Senagore AJ, Emery T, Luchtefeld M, Kim D, Dujovny N, Hoedema R. Fluid management for laparoscopic colectomy: a prospective, randomized assessment of goal-directed administration of balanced salt solution or hetastarch coupled with an enhanced recovery program. *Dis Colon Rectum.* 2009;52(12):1935–1940.
139. Fujita T, Okada N, Horikiri Y, et al. Safety and efficacy of hydroxyethyl starch 6% 130/0.4/9 solution versus 5% human serum albumin in thoracic esophagectomy with 3-field lymph nodes dissection. *Surg Today.* 2019;49(5):427–434.
140. Jo JY, Kim WJ, Choi DK, Kim HR, Lee EH, Choi IC. Effect of restrictive fluid therapy with hydroxyethyl starch during esophagectomy on postoperative outcomes: a retrospective cohort study. *BMC Surg.* 2019;19(1):15.
141. Klevebro F, Boshier PR, Low DE. Application of standardized hemodynamic protocols within enhanced recovery after surgery programs to improve outcomes associated with anastomotic leak and conduit necrosis in patients undergoing esophagectomy. *J Thorac Dis.* 2019;11(suppl 5):S692–S701.
142. Li Y, Dong H, Tan S, Qian Y, Jin W. Effects of thoracic epidural anesthesia/analgesia on the stress response, pain relief, hospital stay, and treatment costs of patients with esophageal carcinoma undergoing thoracic surgery: a single-center randomized controlled trial. *Medicine (Baltimore).* 2019;98(7):e14362.
143. Li W, Li Y, Huang Q, Ye S, Rong T. Short and long-term outcomes of epidural or intravenous analgesia after esophagectomy: a propensity-matched cohort study. *PLoS One.* 2016;11(4):e0154380.
144. Kaufmann KB, Baar W, Glatz T, et al. Epidural analgesia and avoidance of blood transfusion are associated with reduced mortality in patients with postoperative pulmonary complications following thoracotomic esophagectomy: a retrospective cohort study of 335 patients. *BMC Anesthesiol.* 2019;19(1):162.
145. Cummings Iii KC, Kou TD, Chak A, et al. Surgical approach and the impact of epidural analgesia on survival after esophagectomy for cancer: a population-based retrospective cohort study. *PLoS One.* 2019;14(1):e0211125.
146. Feltracco P, Bortolato A, Barbieri S, et al. Perioperative benefit and outcome of thoracic epidural in esophageal surgery: a clinical review. *Dis Esophagus.* 2018;31(5).
147. Brown MJ, Kor DJ, Allen MS, et al. Dual-epidural catheter technique and perioperative outcomes after Ivor-Lewis esophagectomy. *Reg Anesth Pain Med.* 2013;38(1):3–8.
148. Booka E, Nakano Y, Mihara K, et al. The impact of epidural catheter insertion level on pain control after esophagectomy for esophageal cancer. *Esophagus.* 2020;17(2):175–182.
149. Yeung JH, Gates S, Naidu BV, Wilson MJ. Gao Smith F. Paravertebral block versus thoracic epidural for patients undergoing thoracotomy. *Cochrane Database Syst Rev.* 2016;2:CD009121.
150. Howells P, Bieker M, Yeung J. Oesophageal cancer and the anaesthetist. *BJA Educ.* 2016;17(2):68–73.
151. Scholtemeijer MG, Seesing MFJ, Brenkman HJF, Janssen LM, van Hillegersberg R, Ruurda JP. Recurrent laryngeal nerve injury after esophagectomy for esophageal cancer: incidence, management, and impact on short- and long-term outcomes. *J Thorac Dis.* 2017;9(suppl 8):S868–S878.

45

Airway Fistulas in Adults

DAWN P. DESIDERIO, JACOB C. JACKSON

Introduction

Fistula formation in the airway may be broadly defined as any defect that allows pathologic communication between the respiratory tract and an adjacent structure. The type of airway fistula is determined by which section of the tracheobronchial tree and which adjacent structure is involved. For example, a tracheoesophageal fistula (TEF) is a communication between the trachea and the esophagus, whereas a bronchopleural fistula (BPF) is a communication between a lobar or segmental bronchus and the pleural space. The cause of a fistula may be iatrogenic, traumatic, or secondary to a medical disorder. The fistula size, location, and the effects on ventilation are important in determining the morbidity for the patient, the options for therapeutic intervention, and the challenges the fistula may present to anesthesiology or intensive care providers. Table 45.1 provides an overview of the major airway fistula types in adults.

A large fistula of the central airways (such as TEF of the trachea or a BPF of a mainstem bronchus) that causes significant respiratory distress can be a devastating condition and frequently requires surgical intervention to prevent the development of pulmonary sepsis, which can be catastrophic. All types of airway fistulas warrant the utmost level of preoperative planning for even the most seasoned anesthesiologist. Thorough physical examination, reviewing the computed tomography (CT) scan, and bronchoscopic evaluation to localize the defect are essential in planning the anesthetic management. Airway techniques, such as jet ventilation or placement of a left- or right-sided double-lumen tube (DLT), may be necessary to avoid further injury to a central defect, preserve oxygenation and ventilation, and isolate the defect site for surgical repair.

In its own category of airway fistula is an alveolopleural or alveolar-parenchymal-pleural fistula (APF) of the distal tracheobronchial tree (beyond a segmental bronchus), which allows air to leak into the pleural space. The etiology and treatment of an APF is distinct from a BPF or tracheal fistula. If an APF does not readily heal it may lead to a persistent air leak (PAL), a condition where air continues to enter the pleural space from the lung parenchyma for an extended period, in particular if the patient is placed on positive pressure ventilation. A postoperative PAL is typically defined as one that lasts 4 postoperative days or beyond the expected postoperative hospital stay.[1,2] Whereas a PAL may lead to a prolonged hospital stay and increased mortality, the usual course is less ominous than that of a large central airway fistula, especially if the etiology of the APF is postsurgical. Most patients with a PAL after lung resection can be safely discharged home under conservative management, and a chest tube connected to a one-way (Heimlich) valve for later removal at a follow-up clinic visit.[1,3] However, some patients with an APF may need to undergo a surgical or endoscopic procedure to seal or isolate the defect to expedite the healing process.

A bronchopleural-cutaneous fistula (BPCF) describes a special condition occurring when a communication exists between the respiratory tree, the pleural space, and the subcutaneous area of the chest wall. Respired gases enter into the pleural space and then into the subcutaneous tissue to cause diffuse subcutaneous emphysema.[4] This may occur when penetrating trauma to the chest wall injures a bronchus or other airway. For a BPCF, percutaneous chest tube placement will incompletely evacuate the pleural space to reinflate the lung because of continued filling via the airway fistula during spontaneous or mechanical ventilation.

Although the features of each fistula type are unique, an understanding of the pathophysiology of each is essential for the astute thoracic anesthesiology provider. The preoperative assessment of a challenging airway fistula includes ascertaining not only the characteristics of the airway fistula, but also other coexisting patient factors, a clear procedural plan, and the assurance of the availability of support staff and equipment. Communication with the surgeon or other proceduralist before initiation of the procedure often guides airway management planning and helps avoid pitfalls during the procedure. Patients must also be informed when significant difficulties are foreseen with oxygenation and ventilation or when there is a possible need for postoperative ventilatory support. The prudent approach is to have multiple backup modalities available, which may include extracorporeal membrane oxygenation (ECMO) for the highest risk cases.[5–7] The following case presentation highlights a management paradigm for a real patient with a central airway fistula.

TABLE 45.1 **Characteristics of Acquired Airway Fistulas in Adults**

	Tracheoesophageal Fistula (TEF)	Bronchopleural Fistula (BPF)	Alveolopleural Fistula (APF)
Description	Pathologic communication between the trachea and the esophagus	Pathologic communication between a lobar or segmental bronchus and the pleural space	Pathologic communication between the distal respiratory tree and the pleural space
Etiology	Malignancy Blunt or penetrating trauma Mediastinal infection Previous surgery Corrosive fluid ingestion Poisons and inhalation burns Iatrogenic Esophageal stent injury EGD injury TEE probe injury Tracheal tube injury	Pulmonary surgery Pneumonectomy Lobectomy Segmentectomy Chest trauma Pulmonary infection Treatment of malignancy Chemoradiation Radiofrequency ablation Microwave ablation	Pulmonary surgery Lung volume reduction Segmentectomy Wedge resection Chest trauma Pulmonary infection Spontaneous pneumothorax Mechanical ventilator trauma
Sequelae	Cough after ingestion (Ono's sign) Poor nutrition Airway soilage Pneumonia Pulmonary sepsis	Persistent air leak Atelectasis Pneumothorax Tension pneumothorax Subcutaneous emphysema Pneumonia Empyema	Persistent air leak Atelectasis Pneumothorax Tension pneumothorax Subcutaneous emphysema Pneumonia Empyema
Management	Minimize aspiration Acid suppression therapy Treat pulmonary infection Pulmonary toilet Esophageal stenting Esophageal diversion Surgical repair	Chest tube thoracostomy Nutritional support Treat pulmonary infection Pulmonary toilet Optimize ventilation Bronchoscopic intervention Surgical repair	Chest tube thoracostomy Heimlich valve Blood patch pleurodesis Chemical pleurodesis Bronchoscopic intervention Surgical repair

EGD, Esophagogastroduodenoscopy; *TEE*, transesophageal echocardiography.

Case Presentation

A 64-year-old former 20 pack-year smoker underwent a successful spinal surgery to repair a traumatic back injury sustained during a snowmobile accident, but he was experiencing anorexia, mild dysphagia, and persistent nausea during the recovery period. He was referred for an esophagogastroduodenoscopy (EGD), which demonstrated Barrett's mucosa in the lower third of the esophagus and a fungating, partially obstructive mass at the gastroesophageal junction. Biopsies of the mass and further imaging confirmed a diagnosis of esophageal adenocarcinoma stage uT3N1M0. He was treated with several weeks of radiation therapy (50 Gray), neoadjuvant chemotherapy (carboplatin and paclitaxel), and nutritional support with tumor response and symptomatic improvement. He subsequently underwent a minimally invasive Ivor Lewis esophagectomy and laparoscopic jejunostomy from which he recovered well and was discharged home on the sixth postoperative day. However, at two weeks postprocedure, the patient returned to the hospital with fever, productive cough, and dyspnea. He had bilateral diffuse rales on physical exam. A CT scan of the chest showed bilateral basal predominant groundglass opacities and patchy consolidations, as well as defects in the proximal left mainstem bronchus and the esophagus that appeared to communicate (Fig. 45.1A). The patient was scheduled for an urgent EGD and flexible bronchoscopy for further assessment and treatment.

Case Management

Preoperative Assessment and Planning

The general preoperative assessment of a patient with a known or suspected airway fistula should be thorough, but it should focus on respiratory status, hemodynamics, airway assessment, and comorbidities that are likely to be significant factors in the induction and maintenance of the general anesthetic. Relevant comorbidities include major organ system dysfunction, morbid obesity, infectious processes, metabolic or hematologic derangements from oncologic treatment or ongoing pathologic process, and the presence of injuries from a recent trauma or surgery. In this case, the patient was hemodynamically stable when assessed for

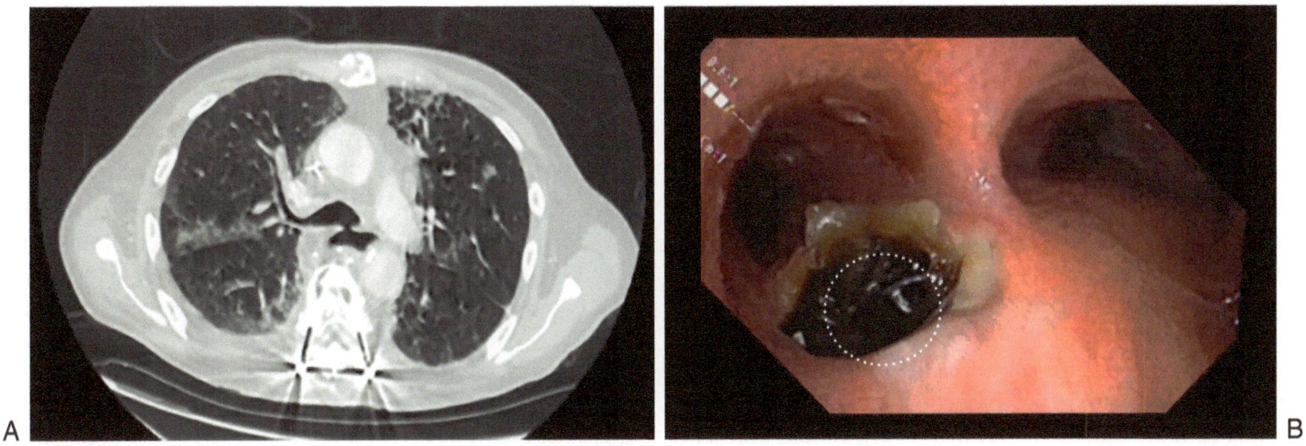

• **Fig. 45.1** (**A**) Axial computed tomography (CT) image showing a fistula in the proximal left mainstem bronchus. There are bilateral pulmonary infiltrates from soiling of the airway. (**B**) Fiberoptic bronchoscopy at the level of the carina 2 days after CT imaging. The enlarging fistula is visualized in the membranous portion of the posterior left mainstem bronchus.

surgery but had persistent fever, cough, and dyspnea suggesting the presence of pulmonary infection. The airway assessment was reassuring, he was of average body habitus, and he had no other major organ system dysfunction outside of the gastrointestinal (GI) tract before presentation. No significant metabolic or hematologic derangements were present. The CT scan suggested an anastomotic leak and soilage of the lungs bilaterally secondary to a suspected central fistula.

Impact of an airway fistula on the ability to ventilate with positive-pressure ventilation (PPV) is difficult to predict as the actual size of the fistula is only one factor to consider, along with its shape, location, and other patient-specific factors, such as lung compliance. Maintenance of spontaneous ventilation is advantageous when suitable for the patient or the planned procedure. Ventilation is especially compromised in the setting of a large fistula and noncompliant lung parenchyma, which favors respired air passing through the low-resistance fistula into dead space rather than participating in alveolar gas exchange. With a clinically significant airway fistula, the patient may experience dyspnea and a sense of air hunger in response to respiratory acidosis and ineffective respiratory mechanics because of the loss of the driving negative intrapleural pressure. If a chest drainage system is in place during preoperative assessment, it can provide additional useful information about the size of the air leak by observing the air leak chamber (Box 45.1).[8] Patients with marked respiratory distress or grade 4 air leaks are unlikely to tolerate a standard anesthetic induction or PPV via a single-lumen endotracheal tube that does not isolate the airway defect. The patient in this case was only mildly dyspneic with a small-appearing (<8 mm) fistula based on CT imaging.

When planning airway management, the anesthesia provider must appreciate that PPV in the presence of a fistula communicating with the GI tract may result in insufflation of the esophagus and stomach, possibly exacerbating reflux of gastric secretions into the lungs. PPV via a fistula communicating with the pleural space may result in a tension pneumothorax with hemodynamic collapse if a functioning chest drainage tube is not in place. A short, large-bore (≥20 Fr) chest tube should be placed for a large airway fistula communicating with the pleural space to palliate the high-volume air leak, prevent tension pneumothorax, and facilitate safer conditions for administering an anesthetic (Box 45.2).[9,10] For proximal tracheal fistulas, rapid sequence induction followed by intubation beyond the fistula site with fiberoptic bronchoscopic guidance is recommended to obviate ventilatory concerns. If possible,

• BOX 45.1 Cerfolio Classification of Air Leaks

The bubbling in the air leak chamber of a chest drainage system can provide information about the air flow through an airway fistula. Air leak only present with cough indicates a small fistula, whereas a continuous air leak indicates a large fistula.

Grade 1, FE: During forced expiration only (i.e., cough)
Grade 2, E: Expiratory only
Grade 3, I: Inspiratory only
Grade 4, C: Continuous bubbling in the air leak chamber

• BOX 45.2 The Fanning Equation

The Fanning equation describes turbulent gas flow in a tube as occurs via chest tube drainage. A shorter, larger-bore chest tube is more effective at evacuating the pleural cavity. Appropriate chest tube size selection is key to preventing tension pneumothorax development.

$$V = \frac{\pi^2 r^5 P}{fl}$$

V is the flow
P is the pressure gradient
r is the radius
f is the friction factor
l is the length

an awake fiberoptic intubation with placement of a single-lumen tube is the safest practice.

Airway Fistula Repair

In the operating room, a rapid sequence induction was performed to avoid unnecessary mask ventilation, and the patient was intubated with a single-lumen endotracheal tube. The patient was mechanically ventilated with low tidal volumes, low peak inspiratory pressures, low respiratory rate to allow for a prolong expiratory period, and no positive end-expiratory pressure (PEEP) to reduce air flow through the fistula (Box 45.3).[11,12] Bronchoscopic evaluation confirmed endotracheal tube placement above the carina and no further injury to the fistula site. The bronchial fistula measured 5 mm at this time, and the patient tolerated mechanical ventilation without difficulty. Esophagoscopy revealed partial necrosis of the gastric conduit with fistula formation at the site of anastomosis. A self-expanding metallic esophageal stent was placed to limit tracheobronchial soiling while planning for a definitive surgical repair. A chest tube thoracostomy was also performed to drain the pleural space, and the patient was placed on intravenous antibiotics.

Two days later, the patient returned to the operating room for a flexible bronchoscopy, resection of the gastric conduit via a right thoracotomy, esophageal diversion by cervical esophagostomy, and repair of the airway fistula. The patient was notably tachypneic with increased work of breathing but was hemodynamically stable. An arterial line was placed for continuous hemodynamic monitoring. Large-bore peripheral venous access and central venous access via implanted port were present. He was intubated after rapid sequence induction with a single-lumen endotracheal tube with notable air leak with PPV. A flexible bronchoscopy now showed an enlarged left mainstem bronchus fistula, likely secondary to the esophageal anastomotic leak (Fig. 45.1B). A left-sided double-lumen tube was placed gently into position in the left mainstem bronchus with fiberoptic bronchoscopic guidance to avoid further injury to the fistula site and to allow for isolation of the defect for repair via a right thoracotomy. He was extubated at the end of the procedure and underwent postanesthesia care in the intensive care unit (ICU).

• BOX 45.3 Mechanical Ventilation for Airway Fistulas

The volume of air leak through the fistula is proportional to the mean airway pressure, which is reduced with these strategies:

- Spontaneous breathing (if possible)
- Low tidal volumes
- Low peak inspiratory pressure
- Low respiratory rate
- Short inspiratory time
- Permissive hypercapnia
- Low or no positive end-expiratory pressure

Repair of a bronchial fistula has long been a major challenge for thoracic surgeons because of the limited healing potential of the poorly vascularized tracheobronchial tree.[13–18] In this case, the repair of the bronchial fistula was performed with polypropylene suture, then covered with pedicled intercostal muscle and pericardial fat pad to buttress the closure. Omentum is also sometimes used to buttress the closure and is recommended in the surgical literature.[19] Unfortunately, the closure in this case did not heal, possibly because of the patient's poorly controlled suppurative infection in the chest and compromised blood supply to the anastomosis. The patient made multiple return trips to the operating room to undergo custom silicone airway stenting, followed by a repeat attempt at surgical repair of the airway fistula when the pleural space was more thoroughly drained. However, the patient eventually succumbed to pulmonary sepsis within approximately one month of his return presentation to the hospital.

Alternative Methods

Induction of Anesthesia

The choice of a conventional or unconventional approach to the induction of anesthesia for a patient with an airway fistula is largely guided by the clinically ascertained size of the fistula (from CT imaging or bronchoscopic visualization), degree of respiratory compromise and/or the degree of air leak (if a chest tube is in place), and the predicted tolerance of PPV. When there is concern that mask ventilation or PPV via a single-lumen endotracheal tube will lead to inadequate gas exchange because of a large or unfavorably located fistula, intubation with maintenance of spontaneous ventilation represents a safer method for securing the airway. This can be achieved with local anesthetic topicalization of the airway or airway nerve blocks before direct laryngoscopy and endotracheal tube placement in an awake patient. Alternatively, intubation may be performed in a patient anesthetized in a way that preserves respiratory drive, such as by inhalational induction of general anesthesia with volatile anesthetic or intravenous sedation with dexmedetomidine or ketamine with or without judicious use of benzodiazepine. Use of opioids (e.g., a bolus or infusion of ultra-short acting remifentanil) or sub-induction doses of propofol (i.e., 0.5 mg/kg) may facilitate direct laryngoscopy and intubation but carry a higher risk of apnea. Unfortunately, many cases that warrant maintenance of spontaneous ventilation for induction of anesthesia also require placement of a DLT, which is difficult to place in a spontaneously breathing patient.

Airway and Ventilatory Management

The traditional mantra for a patient needing lung isolation with a known or suspected difficult airway is that a single-lumen tube can be placed first, followed by exchange for a DLT. Following this mantra is challenging for a large, centrally located fistula because of the potential for additional airway injury from multiple intubations and the contraindication to using an airway exchange catheter for fear of it passing into the airway fistula. Once intubated, an endobronchial blocker can be placed via a single-lumen tube under bronchoscopic guidance in select cases where the fistula site would be a safe distance from the endobronchial blocker cuff. However, an endobronchial blocker may limit the intraoperative pulmonary toilet and may be less reliable for right mainstem bronchus placement, depending on the airway anatomy. As an alternative, a single-lumen tube may be advanced into a mainstem bronchus to achieve lung isolation, although with similar drawbacks as placement of an endobronchial blocker. Mainstem placement of a single-lumen endotracheal tube is typically only used for pediatric cases, emergency situations, or in an ICU setting.

For the experienced anesthesia provider, the best plan for a large, central fistula is to use one of the aforementioned induction techniques and a combination of videolaryngoscopy and flexible bronchoscopy to guide placement of a DLT. Correct choice of right- or left-sided DLT is essential: a right-sided DLT is not suitable for a patient with a large fistula in the right mainstem bronchus because the bronchial cuff will be seated at the level of the defect, preventing a proper seal and causing further airway injury. Likewise, if the fistula is in the left mainstem bronchus, a left-sided DLT will be contraindicated. In the special case where a DLT will not suffice for ventilatory management, jet ventilation or ECMO may be considered to facilitate the planned procedure. At the conclusion of a surgical or bronchoscopic intervention, every effort should be made to extubate patients for postanesthesia care to allow more favorable respiratory mechanics and to facilitate fistula healing.

If a patient must remain intubated postoperatively, management should be undertaken in the ICU. Although conventional mechanical ventilation is preferred, lung isolation may still be required with a DLT in place. In the critical care setting, both high-frequency jet ventilation and high-frequency oscillatory ventilation have also been described, in addition to conventional mechanical ventilation and independent lung ventilation for management of patients with high-output BPF.[20–25] The review by Shekar et al. offers an overview of mechanical ventilation options for patients with clinically significant airway fistulas in the intensive care setting.[11]

Of note, placement of a chest thoracostomy tube on high suction for mechanically intubated patients with a large airway fistula may increase flow through the fistula and cause autotriggering of the ventilator when in an assist mode, thereby increasing the respiratory rate.[20,26,27] This may lead to inappropriate escalation of sedatives and/or neuromuscular blocking drugs administered to reduce perceived excessive spontaneous breathing efforts.[12,28] Thus, care should be taken to adjust the chest tubes to appropriate levels of suction.

Risks and Benefits

The risks and benefits of the anesthetic induction technique and method of airway management must be weighed on an individual patient basis, taking into consideration the nature of the planned procedure. The most serious risk is the inability to adequately ventilate by mask or invasive PPV in a patient who is no longer spontaneously breathing. The anesthesiology provider must first develop a plan to guard against this risk with backup techniques prepared and discussed with the patient or proxy and other team members in case of difficulty with the primary plan. Understanding the pathophysiology of the airway defect and optimizing preoperative conditions by treating pulmonary infection and placing a chest thoracostomy tube, if appropriate, are key steps. Each choice in care will have risks, but the goal is to chart a course with the best chance of a successful operative intervention and of a recovery that leads to fistula healing.

Review of the Literature

Incidence and Outcomes

Tracheoesophageal Fistula

Acquired TEFs in adults are most often malignant, with approximately 50% of acquired cases being the result of mediastinal malignancy.[29] Traumatic, infectious, and iatrogenic causes, such as may occur from prolonged tracheal intubation, are far less common. Among malignancy-associated TEF, 77% can be attributed to esophageal tumors.[29,30] The pathophysiology involves esophageal tumor enlargement with invasion of the adjacent trachea. Fistula formation occurs as a result of tissue necrosis and breakdown. Radiation and chemotherapy usually exacerbate the pathologic process of TEF formation. Furthermore, patients undergoing neoadjuvant chemoradiation for locally advanced esophageal carcinoma at or above the carina and who undergo subsequent transthoracic resection with extensive lymphadenectomy in the upper mediastinum have an increased risk of TEF formation. The mechanism is thought to be ischemic secondary to devascularization resulting in poor blood supply of the trachea and mainstem bronchi from the chemoradiation and from extended mediastinal lymphadenectomy.[31] Postesophagectomy patients with anastomotic leak leading to peritracheal inflammation are also predisposed to fistula formation to the trachea, typically at or close to the tracheal bifurcation. The mortality rate from each of these causes is extremely high, even with operative intervention (approaching 40%), and many patients may be too sick to tolerate a reparative procedure.[29,30] Median survival from the time of diagnosis is 1 to 6 weeks.[32] Esophageal stenting or esophageal diversion may offer palliative treatment.

Bronchoesophageal Fistula

By far, the most common etiology of BPF is a postoperative complication following lung resection, although it may also result from infectious processes, chemoradiation, and other nonmalignant etiologies.[33] BPF occurs with an incidence of up to 8.6% for right pneumonectomy, 2.3% for left pneumonectomy, 1% for lobectomy, and 0.3% for segmentectomy.[34] However, the overall incidence for postpneumonectomy BPF has been reported to range from 4.5% to as high as 20%.[34,35] Predisposing conditions to developing BPF include diabetes mellitus, hypoalbuminemia, hepatic cirrhosis, immunosuppression, residual tumor at the bronchial resection margin, and prolonged intubation.[36] Postresection BPF carries a mortality ranging from 16.4% to 71.2%.[36,37] Puskas et al. reported the factors associated with bronchopleural fistula in 42 patients, which included right pneumonectomy (n = 23), left pneumonectomy (n = 8), long bronchial stump (n = 16), pneumonia (n = 13), radiation therapy (n = 12), stapled bronchial closure (n = 8), prolonged mechanical ventilation (n = 7), recurrent carcinoma (n = 6), and tuberculosis (n = 2). The authors recommend prevention as the best measure against BPF by avoiding disruption of the bronchial blood supply, rough handling of the bronchial mucosa, and excessive suture tension, as well as to buttress closures of bronchial stumps in high-risk situations with pericardial fat pads or pedicled intercostal muscle.[19]

Alveolopleural Fistula

Primary spontaneous pneumothorax has an incidence of six per 100,000 in men and two per 100,000 in women and rarely results in PAL.[38] Secondary spontaneous pneumothorax with chronic obstructive pulmonary disease (COPD) has an incidence of 26 per 100,000 per year,[39] and PAL occurs in approximately 20% of these patients.[40,41] For postoperative air leak (APF), the incidence varies depending on the type of surgical intervention and the postoperative day. The incidence is estimated to be 25% on postoperative day 1 after lung resection and 20% on postoperative day 2.[1,42] The risk of postlung resection APF increases in patients with a low forced expiratory volume in 1 second (FEV_1), emphysema, cystic fibrosis, history of smoking, chronic steroid use, upper lobe resections, and bilobectomy compared with lobectomy.[43,44] PAL is the most common complication after pulmonary resection and has an average incidence of approximately 8% after wedge resection or segmentectomy, 10% after lobectomy, and as high as 45% after lung volume reduction surgery.[45–47] Mortality associated with PAL has been reported to be as high as 12%, potentially as a result of its correlation with other serious pulmonary complications, such as atelectasis, pneumonia, and empyema.[48,49] Although most air leaks will resolve spontaneously or with conservative management, novel endoscopic management techniques have gained in popularity for those necessitating intervention.

Endoscopic Interventions for Bronchopleural Fistula and Alveolar-Parenchymal-Pleural Fistula

There are no consensus guidelines for the treatment of BPF, leading to significant variability among clinicians in management approach. A BPF does not typically spontaneously undergo closure and requires some type of surgical or bronchoscopic intervention. Initial management focuses on recognizing and addressing life-threatening complications, such as tension pneumothorax, endobronchial contamination, and respiratory failure. Patients are managed with chest tube thoracostomy, nutritional support, pulmonary toilet, and treatment of pulmonary infection or empyema before undergoing definitive treatment. Fistula localization is done with CT imaging or fiberoptic bronchoscopy. In general, a smaller BPF (e.g., <8 mm) that is located beyond the central airways is more amenable to a bronchoscopic intervention than a large, central BPF.[11,33] Patients with large air leaks who are poor candidates for surgical repair may benefit from a bronchoscopic intervention for palliation, attempted definitive treatment, or bridge to surgery should they become a better surgical candidate in the future. Fig. 45.2 offers a suggested management paradigm for BPF.

Many bronchoscopic techniques are now available for treatment of airway fistulas, although most have a paucity of quality data on outcome. Moreover, there are no controlled studies available to show superiority of one modality over another. Choice of technique is largely dependent on institutional resources available, training of the interventionalist, and the nature of the fistula. Ablative therapy with the neodymium-doped yttrium aluminum garnet (Nd: YAG) laser has been used for small (<2 mm) proximal fistulas in the absence of tumor or infection. The laser beam is directed at the mucosa surrounding the fistula where it induces edema, denatures proteins, and causes inflammation, which facilitates closure of the fistula by fibrosis.[50,51] Endobronchial injection of sclerosing agents into the submucosa on the margins of the fistula has been performed in a few case series. Sclerosants have included ethanol, polidocanol, and tetracycline.[52–54] A nonexhaustive list of the myriad sealant materials that have been used include glutaraldehyde lead shot,[55] tissue glue methyl-2-cyanoacrylate,[56] albumin-glutaraldehyde tissue adhesive,[57,58] autologous blood patch,[59] absorbable gelatin sponge,[60] and cryoprecipitate fibrin glue.[61] These agents act first as a plug, then induce an inflammatory process with mucosal proliferation and fibrosis to create a permanent seal.

Another approach to sealing a BPF is the direct mechanical obstruction of the defect, which can be achieved with a variety of devices: angiographic coils,[62,63] airway stents,[64,65] and endobronchial valves.[66,67] Endobronchial valves were originally developed for the purpose of performing lung volume reduction in patients with lung hyperinflation from emphysema. The unidirectional valves allow for resolution of BPF or PAL by eliciting segmental or lobar atelectasis, which decreases air flow across the airway defect and allows it time to heal. The valves can be removed following resolution of the air leak. The Spiration® Intrabronchial Valve (IBV) has U.S. Food and Drug Administration (FDA) humanitarian device exemption (HDE) granted for the treatment of PAL (Fig. 45.3A). Indications for placement of the IBV include an air leak present on postoperative day seven,

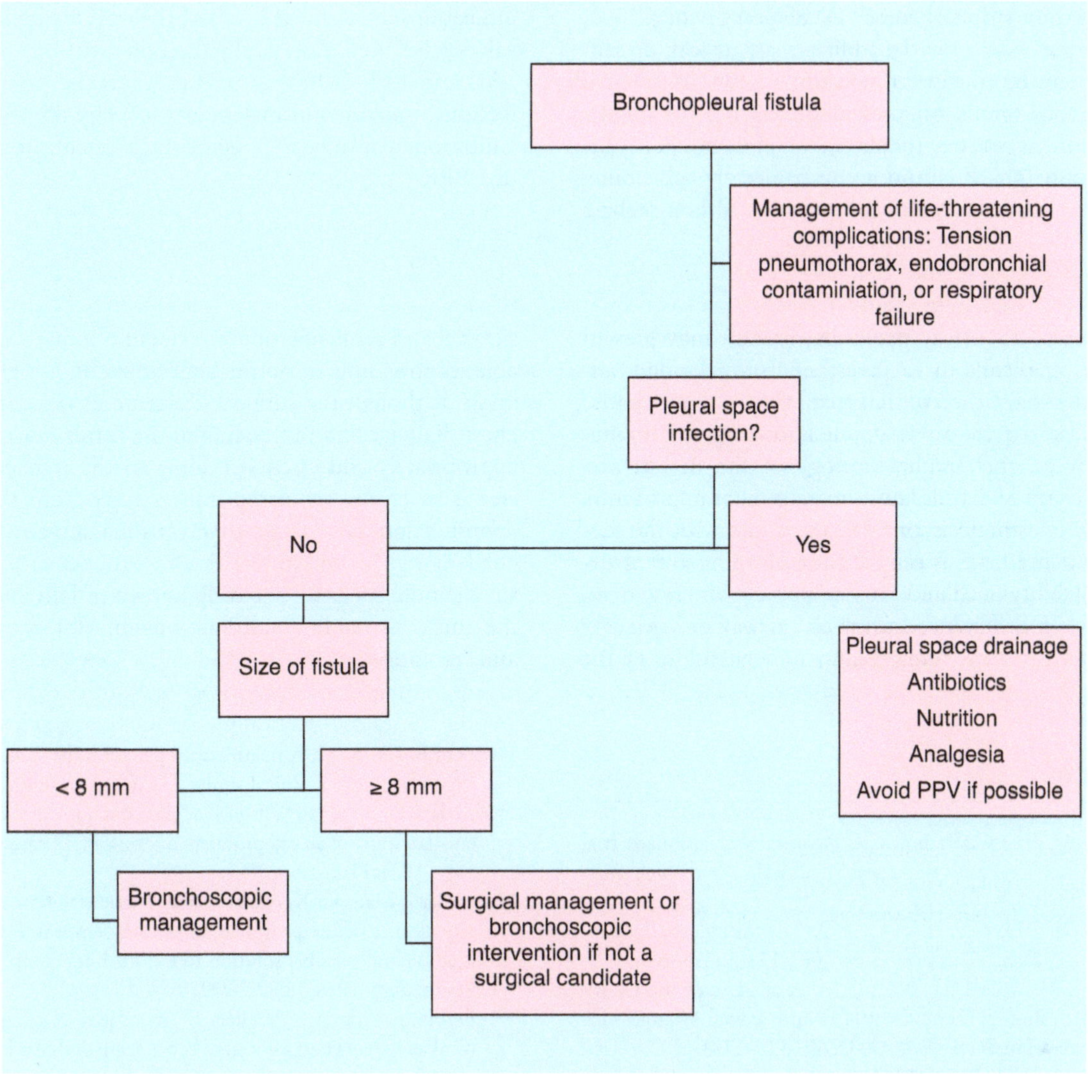

• **Fig. 45.2** Management paradigm for bronchopleural fistula (*BPF*). Recognition of life-threatening complications of BPF is the first step in management. Pleural space infections should be addressed before attempting a surgical or bronchoscopic repair to ensure successful healing of the defect. Smaller fistulas are more amenable to bronchoscopic interventions than are larger ones. *PPV*, Positive pressure ventilation.

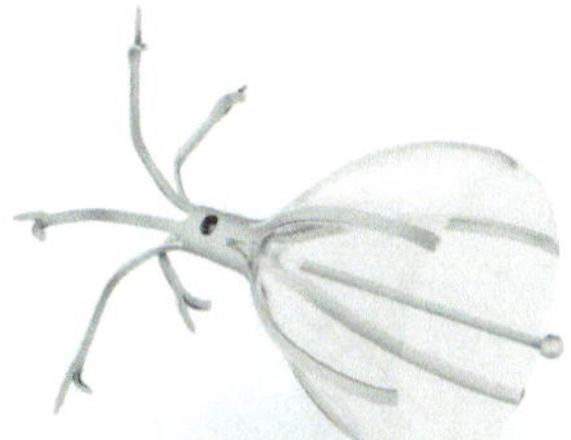

A

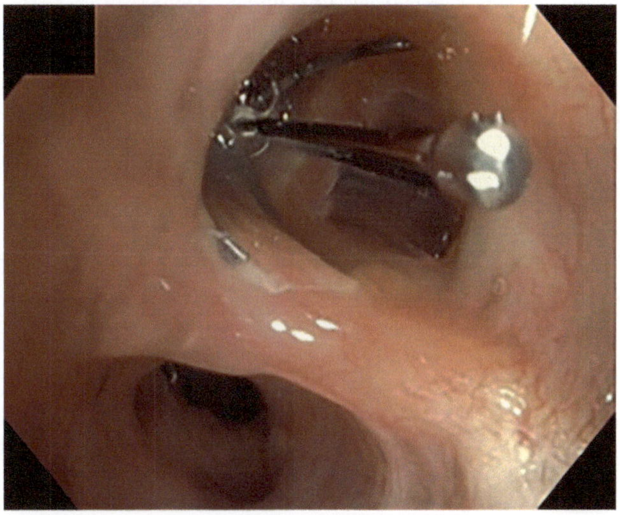

B

• **Fig. 45.3 A.** Endobronchial valves, originally designed for lung volume reduction in patients with emphysema, are now used to treat persistent air leak. The Intrabronchial Valve (IBV; pictured) reduces air flow through the leaking tissue, facilitating local tissue healing and spontaneous resolution. (*Courtesy of* Olympus America, Inc., with permission) **B.** The IBV seated in segmental bronchus. (*Courtesy of* Dr. Amit K. Mahajan with permission.)

unless present only during forced exhalation or cough (i.e., at least a grade 2 air leak). In addition, an air leak present on day five can be considered appropriate for treatment if it is continuous (grade 4), present during normal inhalation phase of inspiration (grade 3), or present upon normal exhalation (grade 2) and accompanied by subcutaneous emphysema or respiratory compromise. Although these indications are defined by the FDA's HDE, endobronchial valves have been successfully used off-label for treatment of PAL and BPF following pneumothoraces, pulmonary infections, trauma, and malignancies.[68] Fig. 45.3B shows the endobronchial valve in a segmental bronchus for treatment of a BPF.

Conclusion

The presence of an airway fistula in an adult may present a significant challenge to the anesthesia provider and surgical or pulmonary interventionalist, alike. Large, central airway fistulas require an in-depth knowledge of respiratory mechanics, the pathophysiology of the defect, and advanced airway and ventilatory management approaches. As with any anesthetic, coordination of care with the surgical and nursing team is essential for planning and assurance of availability of all necessary equipment and resources, especially when difficulty securing the airway or achieving adequate ventilation is foreseen. An understanding of the surgical and bronchoscopic treatment options is also invaluable to providing an optimal anesthetic in a high-risk situation. Although the surgical literature now recognizes that chest drainage and buttressing of the fistula closure must be appropriately addressed if healing of the tracheobronchial tree is to ensue, achieving full recovery from the dreaded complication of a large airway fistula remains extremely challenging. Postanesthesia care in patients with airway fistulas should focus on avoiding known pitfalls and ensuring the most favorable conditions possible for fistula healing and resolution.

References

1. Cerfolio RJ, Bass C, Katholi CR. Prospective randomized trial compares suction versus water seal for air leaks. *Ann Thorac Surg.* 2001;71(5):1613–1617.
2. Cerfolio RJ, Pickens A, Bass C, et al. Fast-tracking pulmonary resections. *J Thorac Cardiovasc Surg.* 2001;122(2):318–324.
3. McKenna RJ, Fischel RJ, Brenner M, et al. Use of the Heimlich valve to shorten hospital stay after lung reduction surgery for emphysema. *Ann Thorac Surg.* 2002;73:1727–1731.
4. Cahalane AM, Kelly RM, O'Neill A, et al. Bronchopleural cutaneous fistula after pulmonary radiofrequency ablation: treatment with low-adherent paraffin gauze dressing. *J Vasc Interv Radiol.* 2012;2:283–285.
5. Daoud O, Augustin P, Mordant P, et al. Extracorporeal membrane oxygenation in 5 patients with bronchial fistula with severe acute lung injury. *Ann Thorac Surg.* 2001;92:327–331.
6. Jeng EI, Piovesana G, Taylor J, et al. Extracorporeal membrane oxygenation to facilitate tracheal healing after oesophagogastric catastrophe. *Eur J Cardiothorac Surg.* 2018;52:288–289.
7. Van Drumpt AS, Kroon HM, Grüne F, et al. Surgery for a large tracheoesophageal fistula using extracorporeal membrane oxygenation. *J Thorac Dis.* 2017;9(9):E735–E738.
8. Cerfolio RJ, Bass CS, Pask AH, et al. Predictors and treatment of persistent air leaks. *Ann Thorac Surg.* 2002;73:1727–1731.
9. Swenson EW, Birath G, Ahbeck A. Resistance to air flow in bronchospirometric catheters. *J Thorac Surg.* 1957;33:275–281.
10. Baumann MH. What size chest tube? What drainage system is ideal? And other chest tube management questions. *Curr Opin Pulm Med.* 2003;9:276–281.
11. Shekar K, Foot C, Fraser J, et al. Bronchopleural fistula: an update for intensivists. *J Crit Care.* 2010;25:47–55.
12. Sarkar P, Chandak T, Shah R, et al. Diagnosis and management of bronchopleural fistula. *Indian J Chest Dis Allied Sci.* 2010;52:97–104.
13. Eggers C. The treatment of bronchial fistulae. *Ann Surg.* 1920; 72:345–347.
14. Pool E, Garlock J. A treatment of persistent bronchial fistula: an experimental and clinical study. *Ann Surg.* 1929;90:213–237.
15. Malave G, Foster E, Wilson J, et al. Bronchopleural fistula - present-day study of an old problem: a review of 52 cases. *Ann Thorac Surg.* 1971;11:1–10.
16. Miller J, Mansour K, Nahai F, et al. Single-stage complete muscle flap closure of the postpneumonectomy empyema space: a new method and possible solution to a disturbing complication. *Ann Thorac Surg.* 1984;38:227–231.
17. Eerola S, Virkula L, Varstela E. Treatment of postpneumonectomy empyema and associated bronchopleural fistula: experience of 100 consecutive post-pneumonectomy patients. *Scand J Thorac Cardiovasc Surg.* 1988;22:235–239.
18. Paiolero P, Trastek V, Allen M. Empyema and bronchopleural fistula. *Ann Thorac Surg.* 1991;51:157–158.
19. Puskas JD, Mathisen DJ, Grillo HC, et al. Treatment strategies for bronchopleural fistula. *J Thorac Cardiovasc Surg.* 1995;109:989–996.
20. Roth MD, Wright JW, Bellamy PE. Gas flows through a bronchopleural fistula. Measuring the effects of high-frequency jet ventilation and chest tube suction. *Chest.* 1988;93:210–213.
21. Campbell D, Stienmann M, Porayko L. Nitric oxide and high-frequency jet ventilation in a patient with bilateral bronchopleural fistula and ARDS. *Can J Anaesth.* 2000;47:53–57.
22. Rubio JJ, Algora-Weber A, Dominguez-de Villota E, et al. Prolonged high-frequency jet ventilation in a patient with bronchopleural fistula: an alternative mode of ventilation. *Intensive Care Med.* 1986;12:161–163.
23. Shen NH, Lu FL, Wu HD, et al. Management of tension pneumatocele with high-frequency oscillatory ventilation. *Chest.* 2002; 121:284–286.
24. Ha DV, Johnson D. High frequency oscillatory ventilation in the management of a high output bronchopleural fistula: a case report. *Can J Anaesth.* 2004;51:78–83.
25. Bishop MJ, Benson MS, Sato P, et al. Comparison of high-frequency jet ventilation with conventional mechanical ventilation for bronchopleural fistula. *Anesth Analg.* 1987;66:833–838.

26. Tilles RB, Don HF. Complications of high pleural suction in bronchopleural fistulas. *Anesthesiology*. 1975;43(4):486.
27. Zimmerman JE, Colgan DL, Mills M. Management of bronchopleural fistula complicating therapy with positive end expiratory pressure. *Chest*. 1973;64:526–529.
28. Sager JS, Eiger G, Fuchs BD. Ventilator auto-triggering in a patient with tuberculous bronchopleural fistula. *Respir Care*. 2003;48:519–521.
29. Reed MF, Mathisen DJ. Tracheoesophageal fistula. *Chest Surg Clin North Am*. 2003;13(2):271–289.
30. Couraud L, Ballester ML, Delaisment C. Acquired tracheoesophageal fistula and its management. *Semin Thorac Cardiovasc Surg*. 1998;8:392–399.
31. Bartels HE, Stein HJ, Siewert JR. Tracheobronchial lesions following oesophagectomy: prevalence, predisposing factors and outcome. *Br J Surg*. 1998;85:403–406.
32. Diddee R, Shaw IH. Acquired trachea-oesophageal fistula in adults. *Continu Educ Anaesth Crit Care Pain*. 2006;6(3):105–108.
33. Lois M, Noppen M. Bronchopleural fistulas: An overview of the problem with special focus on endoscopic management. *Chest*. 2005;128:3955–3965.
34. Cerfolio RJ. The incidence, etiology, and prevention of postresectional bronchopleural fistula. *Semin Thorac Cardiovasc Surg*. 2001;13(1):3–7.
35. Sirbu H, Busch T, Aleksic I, et al. Bronchopleural fistula in the surgery of non-small cell lung cancer: incidence, risk factors and management. *Ann Thorac Cardiovasc Surg*. 2001;7:330–336.
36. Asamura H, Naruke T, Tsuchiya R, et al. Bronchopleural fistulas associated with lung cancer operations: univariate and multivariate analysis of risk factors, management, and outcome. *J Thorac Cardiovasc Surg*. 1992;104:1456–1464.
37. Malave G, Foster E, Wilson J, et al. Bronchopleural fistula – present-day study of an old problem: a review of 52 cases. *Ann Thorac Surg*. 1971;11:1–10.
38. Dines DE, Clagett OT, Payne WS. Spontaneous pneumothorax in emphysema. *Mayo Clin Proc*. 1970;45:481–487.
39. Melton LJ, Hepper NCG, Offort KP. Incidence of spontaneous pneumothorax in Olmstead County Minnesota: 1950-1974. *Am Rev Respir Dis*. 1979;120:1379–1382.
40. George RB, Herbert SJ, Shanes JM, et al. Pneumothorax complicating pulmonary emphysema. *J Am Med Assoc*. 1975;234:389–393.
41. Videau V, Pillgram-Larsen J, Oyvind E, et al. Spontaneous pneumothorax in COPD: complications, treatment and recurrences. *Eur J Respir Dis*. 1987;71:365–371.
42. Cerfolio RJ, Tummala RP, Holman WL, et al. A prospective algorithm for the management of air leaks after pulmonary resection. *Ann Thorac Surg*. 1998;66(5):1726–1731.
43. Mueller MR, Marzluf BA. The anticipation and management of air leaks and residual spaces post lung resection. *J Thorac Dis*. 2014;6(3):271–284.
44. Dugan K, Laxmanan B, Murgu S, et al. Management of persistent air leaks. *Chest*. 2017;152(2):417–423.
45. Jones DR, Stiles BM, Denlinger CE, et al. Pulmonary segmentectomy: results and complications. *Ann Thorac Surg*. 2003;76:343–348.
46. Stolz AJ, Schützner J, Lischke R, et al. Predictors of prolonged air leak following pulmonary lobectomy. *Eur J Cardiothorac Surg*. 2005;27:334–336.
47. Ciccone A, Meyers B, Guthrie T, et al. Long-term outcome of bilateral lung volume reduction in 250 consecutive patients with emphysema. *J Thorac Cardiovasc Surg*. 2003;125:513–525.
48. Stéphan F, Boucheseiche S, Hollande J, et al. Pulmonary complications following lung resection: a comprehensive analysis of incidence and possible risk factors. *Chest*. 2000;118(5):1263–1270.
49. Brunelli A, Xiume F, Al Refai M, et al. Air leaks after lobectomy increase the risk of empyema but not of cardiopulmonary complications. *Chest*. 2006;130(4):1150–1156.
50. Wang KP, Schaeffer L, Heitmiler R, et al. Nd:YAG laser closure of a bronchopleural fistula. *Monaldi Arch Chest Dis*. 1993;48:301–303.
51. Kiriyama M, Fujii Y, Yamakawa Y, et al. Endobronchial neodymium: yttrium-aluminum garnet laser for noninvasive closure of small proximal fistula after lung resection. *Ann Thorac Surg*. 2002;73:945–948.
52. Takaoka K, Inoue S, Ohira S. Central bronchopleural fistulas closed by bronchoscopic injection of absolute ethanol. *Chest*. 2002;122:374.
53. Varoli F, Roviaro G, Grignani F, et al. Endoscopic treatment of bronchopleural fistulas. *Ann Thorac Surg*. 1998;65:807.
54. Martin WR, Siefkin AD, Allen R. Closure of bronchopleural fistula with bronchoscopic instillation of tetracycline. *Chest*. 1991;99:1040.
55. Ratliff JL, Hill JD, Tucker H, et al. Endobronchial control of bronchopleural fistulae. *Chest*. 1977;71:98–99.
56. Hartmann W, Rausch V. A new therapeutic application of the fiberoptic bronchoscope. *Chest*. 1977;71:237.
57. Potaris K, Mihos P, Gakidis I. Preliminary results with the use of an albumin-glutaraldehyde tissue adhesive. *Ann Thorac Surg*. 2004;77:325–328.
58. Lin J, Iannettoni MD. Closure of bronchopleural fistulas using albumin-glutaraldehyde tissue adhesive. *Ann Thorac Surg*. 2004;77(1):326–328.
59. Lan RS, Lee CH, Tsai YH, et al. Fiberoptic bronchial blockade in a small bronchopleural fistula. *Chest*. 1987;92(5):944–946.
60. Jones DP, David I. Gelfoam occlusion of peripheral bronchopleural fistulas. *Ann Thorac Surg*. 1986;42:334–335.
61. Glover W, Chavis TV, Daniel TM, et al. Fibrin glue application through the flexible fiberoptic bronchoscope: closure of bronchopleural fistulas. *J Thorac Cardiovasc Surg*. 1987;93(3):470–472.
62. Islam SU, Beamis JF, Choi IS. Successful closure of a bronchopleural fistula with platinum vascular occlusion coils and N-Butyl-cyanoacrylate glue. *Chest*. 2003;124:292S–293S.
63. Ponn RB, D'Agostino RS, Stern H, et al. Treatment of peripheral bronchopleural fistulas with endobronchial occlusion coils. *Ann Thorac Surg*. 1993;56:1343–1347.
64. Watanabe S, Shimokawa S, Yotsumoto G, et al. The use of a Dumon stent for the treatment of bronchopleural fistula. *Ann Thorac Surg*. 2001;72:276–278.
65. Tayama K, Eriguchi N, Futamata Y, et al. Modified Dumon stent for the treatment of bronchopleural fistula after pneumonectomy. *Ann Thorac Surg*. 2003;75:290–292.
66. Giddings O, Kuhn J, Akulian J. Endobronchial valve placement for the treatment of bronchopleural fistula: a review of the current literature. *Curr Opin Pulm Med*. 2014;20:347–351.
67. Wood DE, Cerfolio RJ, Gonzalez X, et al. Bronchoscopic management of prolonged air leak. *Clin Chest Med*. 2010;31:127–133.
68. Mahajan AK, Khandhar SJ. Bronchoscopic valves for prolonged air leak: current status and technique. *J Thorac Dis*. 2017;9(suppl 2):S110–S115.

46

Thoracic Approach to Spine Procedures

DAVID M. SHAPIRO, BARON LONNER, LILY EAKER, JONATHAN GAL

Introduction

Thoracic spine surgery can be performed from anterior, posterior, or combined approaches. Selection of the appropriate surgical approach depends on the optimal surgical procedure for the patient, the complexity of intervention to be performed, the location and extent of the pathology, and the surgeon's comfort with each technique. Thoracic spine surgery has historically been performed from a posterior approach. Recently, the anterior approach has come in and out of favor for its ability to decrease fusion levels and avoid the posterior musculature of the spine versus its higher reoperation rates and surgical complications. There has been a resurgence in the performance of anterior surgery for various pathologies, including the novel anterior vertebral body tethering (AVBT) nonfusion scoliosis correction or anterior scoliosis correction, specifically for adolescent idiopathic scoliosis (AIS). The anterior approach is predominantly used for the correction of scoliosis but is also used in the management of thoracic disc disease, vertebral fractures, malignancy (70% of spine metastases occur in the thoracic region),[1] and vertebral infections.[2]

U.S. Food and Drug Administration (FDA)-approved indications for AVBT include skeletally immature patients with a scoliosis angle between 30 and 65 degrees, although slight deviations from these indications is common. Patients diagnosed with AIS typically suffer from diminished health, poor quality of life, body image disturbance, and other psychosocial effects.[3,4] In addition, asymptomatic adolescent patients who decline early surgical intervention undergo the natural history of the disease, which may result in progressive deformity, pain, and disability. Postponing the surgical intervention in the adult often requires a greater number of levels fused and is associated with higher complication rates, longer operative times, and greater blood loss than their adolescent counterparts.[5]

To plan and perform a safe and appropriate anesthetic for anterior thoracic spine surgery, the anesthesiologist must discuss the case with the surgical and neuromonitoring teams, as well as the patient and/or guardian. The anterior approach to thoracic spine surgery has special perioperative important considerations for the anesthesiologist, including utilization of one-lung ventilation (OLV), blood conservation strategies, intraoperative neuromonitoring, and a multimodal approach to managing postoperative pain. This chapter will focus on management of scoliosis, as that is the most common indication for the anterior approach to thoracic spine surgery.

Case Presentation

The patient was a 12-year-old, 68-inch, 45-kg girl with double major idiopathic adolescent scoliosis defined as a typical double "S" shaped spinal curvature (Fig. 46.1). She did not experience pain but had progressive worsening of her spine curvatures and significant spinal deformity with expected continued worsening of the curvatures. Because of the natural history of curvatures of the size seen in this patient that will later result in back pain, as well as the potential impact on pulmonary function, surgery was recommended.

Preoperatively, the patient was seen by her pediatrician and found to be in her usual state of good health. Laboratory findings, including a basic metabolic panel, a complete blood count, and coagulation studies were all within normal limits.

The patient and her family also met with the surgeon and extensively discussed the options for treatment. Surgical options included the standard of care posterior instrumented fusion versus the more novel AVBT procedure via a thoracic approach. It was noted that the AVBT is growth and motion sparing. The surgeon had a detailed discussion with the family regarding the risks and benefits of the AVBT procedure compared with the standard of care spinal fusion. This technique places a compressive force over the convex side of the spine (slowing down growth) to permit the concave side of the spine to relatively grow more and create a straighter spine. The goals of these procedures, as opposed to spine fusion, are to correct the spinal deformity and maintain the spine motion, particularly in the low back.

The surgeon explained that because the patient had a complex double major scoliosis, she required surgical correction of the deformity through both right-sided and left-sided incisions. The planned surgical approach on the right side consisted of a 5-cm minithoracotomy between the seventh and eighth ribs at the mid-axillary line, a second mid-axillary line portal four intercostal spaces more cephalad, and an anterior axillary line portal placed in the eighth or ninth

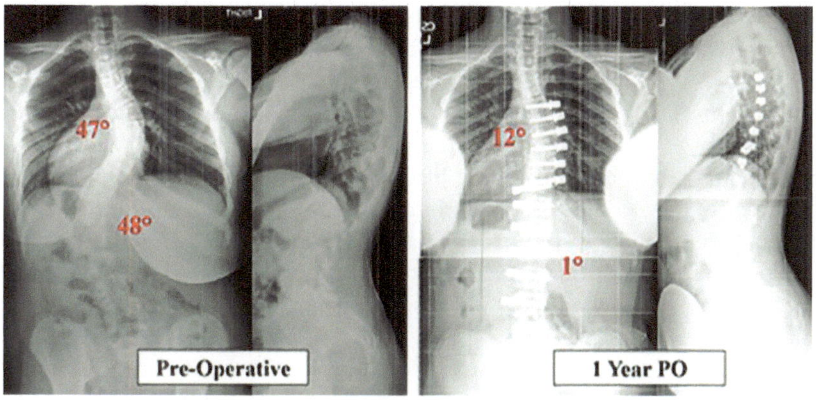

• **Fig. 46.1** Radiographs of the 12-year-old female patient with double major idiopathic scoliosis treated with a right thoracic and left thoracolumbar anterior spinal tether. The scoliosis curvatures are depicted in red.

intercostal space for introduction of the scope (Fig. 46.2). After completion of the right-sided thoracic tether from T5 through T10, the surgical team would correct the left-sided curvature. The surgical team would then perform a left-sided correction from T10 to L3 through a limited thoracotomy between the 10th and 11th ribs and a portal proximal to the thoracotomy incision in the mid-axillary line to permit access to the distal thoracic spine (Fig. 46.3).

The surgeon instructed the patient to take gabapentin 100 mg 3 times a day for 1 week before surgery.

Case Management

The patient presented for surgery in her usual state of good health. A confirmatory type and screen was drawn and 2 units of packed red blood cells were placed on hold in the blood bank. The anesthesiologist assessed the patient, discussed the anesthetic plan, including its risks, benefits, and alternatives, and answered all questions of the patient and her family. An intravenous catheter was then placed.

Before induction of anesthesia, the patient was administered three nonopioid analgesics to mitigate postoperative pain: gabapentin 300 mg by mouth (PO), acetaminophen 650 mg PO, and celecoxib 200 mg PO. She then received midazolam 4 mg for anxiolysis and anterograde amnesia and was transported to the operating room. The perioperative team assisted her into a sitting position in which a thoracic epidural was placed via a paramedian approach one to two rib spaces above the planned site of the postoperative chest tubes and above the major scoliotic curvature for ease of placement, at the T6–T7 interspace.

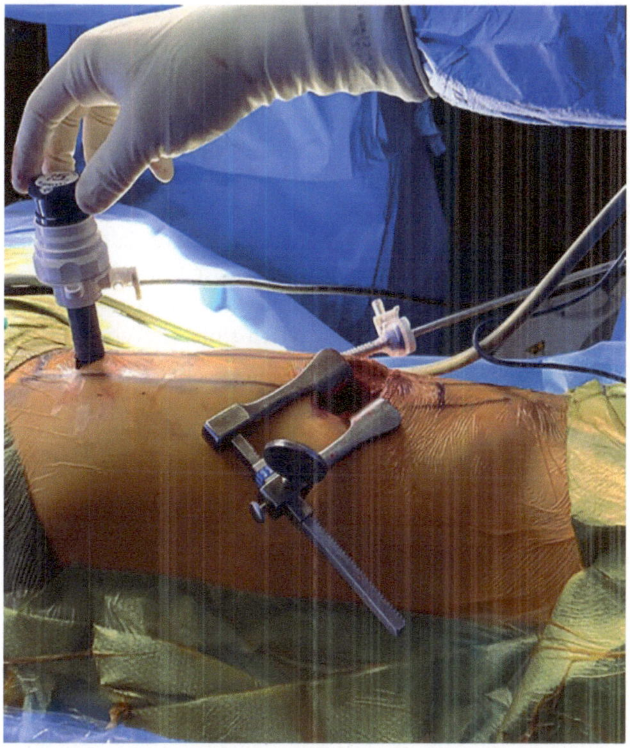

• **Fig. 46.2** Portals used for thoracic anterior vertebral body tethering with the patient in the left lateral decubitus position. Left side of image is cephalad.

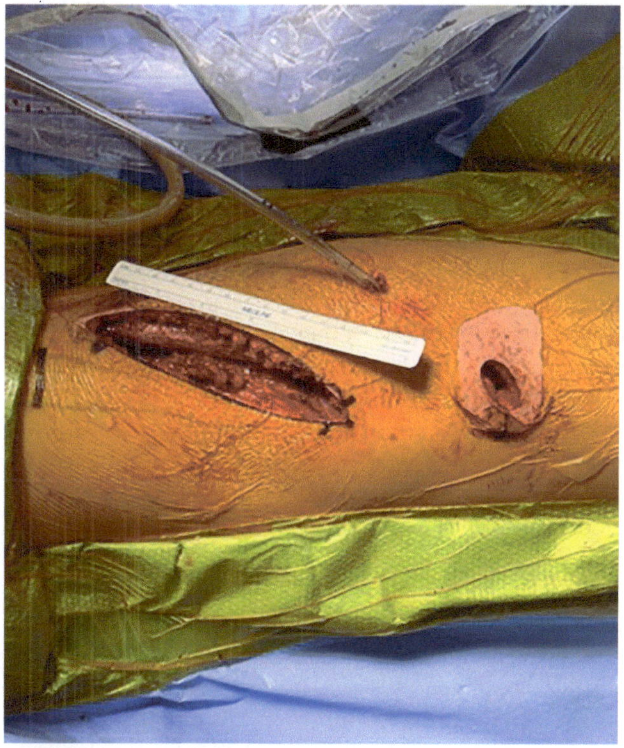

• **Fig. 46.3** Incisions for the thoracolumbar approach with the patient in the right lateral decubitus position.

The patient was then positioned supine on a Jackson table with a flat-bed insert. After placement of standard American Society of Anesthesiologists monitors and preoxygenation, general anesthesia was induced with weight-appropriate dosages of lidocaine (1.5 mg/kg), propofol (2 mg/kg), fentanyl (4 mcg/kg), ketamine (0.5 mg/kg), and succinylcholine (2 mg/kg). The patient was orally intubated with a 7.5 mm single-lumen standard cuffed endotracheal tube (ETT). After successful endotracheal intubation, the tube was secured using adhesive and umbilical tape.

Total intravenous anesthesia (TIVA) was initiated for maintenance of anesthesia. This consisted of propofol (100–150 mcg/kg/min), fentanyl (1–3 mcg/kg/h), dexmedetomidine (0.2 mcg/kg/h) and a ketamine infusion (for a total of 1.5–2.5 mg/kg during the case). A phenylephrine infusion (0.05–0.5 mcg/kg/min) was needed intermittently to maintain mean arterial pressure over 85 mm Hg at critical portions of the procedure to optimize spinal cord perfusion, particularly during placement of implants and vertebral correction. A total of 8.83 mg of phenylephrine was used during the case.

A 9-Fr bronchial blocker (BB) was placed in the lumen of the right mainstem bronchus with the aid of a 4.0 mm flexible fiberoptic bronchoscope in anticipation of the right-sided procedure. A second large-bore 18-gauge intravenous (IV) line was placed for the administration of intravenous anesthetics, fluids, and potential blood products. In addition, a radial arterial line was secured for close hemodynamic monitoring and laboratory assessment of oxygenation, hematocrit, and serum electrolytes. A neuromonitoring team placed electrodes on the patient for monitoring somatosensory evoked potentials (SSEPs), transcranial motor evoked potentials (TcMEPs), and electromyography (EMG) to continually assess spinal cord integrity for the duration of the case. A bite block was placed to protect the tongue from injury during the performance of TcMEPs.

The patient was positioned in the left lateral decubitus position and an axillary roll was placed to relieve pressure on the neurovascular plexus of the dependent arm. All pressure points on the upper and lower extremities were well-padded. Care was taken to ensure that there was no excessive pressure on the eyes and ears. A final positioning check was performed before surgical preparation and draping.

Dexamethasone 10 mg IV was administered for antiinflammatory and antiemetic effects. Cefazolin and gentamicin were dosed by weight for antimicrobial prophylaxis.

A preincisional bronchoscopy was performed to ensure proper placement of the BB in the right mainstem bronchus. Subsequently, the cuff on the BB was inflated, initiating OLV, and the lumen of the BB was placed on gentle suction to facilitate lung deflation to optimize surgical exposure. To improve oxygenation during the early stages of OLV, the patient was placed on an fraction of inspired oxygen (F_iO_2) of 100% for 15 to 30 minutes and then maintained on an F_iO_2 of 80% to 100% for the duration of the procedure with a target oxygen saturation (SpO_2) over 94%.

Vertebral body screws were placed and connected with a tethering cable to correct the scoliosis. Next, the incision was closed and a chest tube was placed in the seventh intercostal space. The BB was then deflated to reinitiate two-lung ventilation. Next, the patient was returned to the supine position and the placement of the BB in the left mainstem bronchus was facilitated by the use of fiberotic bronchoscopy. The patient was placed in the right lateral decubitus position for left-sided scoliosis correction. Once completed, a chest tube was inserted in the 10th intercostal space on the left side.

Approximately 1 hour prior to the conclusion of the procedure, the dexmedetomidine, fentanyl, and ketamine infusions were discontinued. After closure of the diaphragm and chest wall, the propofol infusion was slowly titrated down to allow for timely anesthesia emergence and extubation. At the end of the surgery, the patient was returned to the supine position and extubated. Total operative time was 300 minutes and estimated blood loss was 500 mL. In the operating room, a neurologic examination was performed by the surgical team to assess spinal cord and nerve root integrity. Subsequently, the patient was transferred to the pediatric intensive care unit (PICU) for postoperative care and observation. Note that a pediatric stepdown unit may also be appropriate depending on the institution.

Once in the PICU, the patient-controlled epidural analgesia (PCEA) infusion of hydromorphone (5 mcg/mL) at a rate of 20 mcg/h with three demand doses of 10 mcg available per hour was initiated. In addition to PCEA, the postoperative pain regimen consisted of acetaminophen (15 mg/kg IV every 6 hours; maximum 1 g/dose), ketorolac (0.5 mg/kg IV every 6 hours for 3 days) and gabapentin (100 mg PO three times daily). The acute pain service assessed the patient's pain regimen each morning and further tailored it as appropriate. Hydromorphone (0.3–0.6 mg IV q2h) for pain and diazepam (2–4 mg IV q8h) for spinal muscle spasms were administered as needed. The chest tubes were removed on postoperative day 3, after which the epidural infusion was stopped, and the catheter was removed. Once the patient's pain was well controlled on oral medications and she was able to ambulate, she was discharged home from the hospital.

The postoperative, postdischarge analgesic regimen consisted of several medications. The patient was prescribed a 10-day supply of oxycodone 5 mg PO every 4 hours (plus additional tablets for breakthrough pain as needed), diazepam 2 mg PO every 8 hours as needed for muscle spasms, ibuprofen 400 mg PO three times daily, acetaminophen 15 mg/kg PO every 6 hours, and gabapentin 100 mg PO three times daily. The patient was instructed to take polyethylene glycol 17 g PO twice a day and docusate 100 mg PO three times daily to mitigate the side effect of constipation. As an aside, note that if the patient does not tolerate oxycodone because of nausea or it does not provide adequate analgesia, the surgical team can provide an equivalent dosage of oral morphine or hydromorphone.

Risks, Benefits, and Alternatives

Preoperative Management for Postoperative Pain

Pain management for this procedure begins before the patient's arrival on the day of surgery. There is evidence that administration of preoperative oral nonopioid medications, including gabapentin,[6–10] pregabalin,[11,12] celecoxib,[7,10,11] and acetaminophen[13] improve postoperative pain scores and reduce the incidence of chronic incisional pain and postoperative opioid consumption, thereby decreasing opioid-related side effects, such as nausea, constipation, and sedation. Reducing these side effects may help improve patient satisfaction and maximize postoperative early ambulation and physical rehabilitation in patients undergoing spine surgery. Although there is a paucity of data regarding the efficacy of these agents when used specifically for anterior spine surgery, given their wide therapeutic index and minimal side effects, the benefits outweigh the risks.

Thus patients are placed on a preemptive pain regimen of gabapentin (100 mg orally, taken three times daily) 1 week before the day of surgery. On the day of surgery, the patient is given an oral multimodal nonopioid medication regimen of gabapentin 300 mg, acetaminophen 15 mg/kg, and celecoxib 200 mg. For patients over 70 kg, dosages increase to gabapentin 600 mg, acetaminophen 1000 mg, and celecoxib 400 mg.

Epidural Placement and Management

The epidural catheter is typically placed before the induction of general anesthesia. This offers the advantage of patient feedback during placement and immediate postprocedure neurologic assessment. In addition, placement is generally easier with the patient in a sitting position, whereas placement in the lateral decubitus position with the patient under general anesthesia is not recommended and is rarely performed. In cases where a young patient is unable to tolerate the awake procedure even after the administration of mild to moderate sedation, it may be reasonable to perform the procedure after the induction of general anesthesia, so long as the perceived benefits outweigh the risks. There may be an increased risk of inadvertent dural puncture or injury during placement. Proper patient positioning and epidural placement may be more challenging under general anesthesia in the lateral decubitus position, particularly in patients with a significant scoliotic curvature. Therefore in some cases it may be optimal to place the epidural catheter after the procedure and before extubation, when the spine scoliosis anatomy is corrected and straightened.

The operative side (if unilateral) and vertebral levels, targeted for correction, should dictate the approach to placement and location of the thoracic epidural for postoperative analgesia. If placing a thoracic epidural using a paramedian approach, it is prudent to perform the procedure on the ipsilateral side as the surgical exposure so as to mitigate the consequences of a pneumothorax, a rare complication of placement,[14] and to place the catheter above the site of the planned chest tubes for maximal postoperative analgesic benefit.

Postoperative epidural infusion of hydromorphone provides analgesia for the thoracotomy incisions and chest tubes that remain in place. An epidural combination of hydromorphone and a local anesthetic, such as bupivacaine, provides superior analgesia and minimizes systemic side effects of either medication by allowing for a reduced dosage of both. However, especially in spine surgery, local anesthetics may cause numbness and weakness that can confound the results of a neurologic examination and make it difficult to diagnose potential surgical complications. For this reason, an opioid-only epidural infusion is recommended.

Endotracheal Tube Choice

ETT choice and size depends on patient size, extent and laterality of surgical procedure, provider comfort and preference, as well as a careful weighing of the advantages and disadvantages of each type of tube (Table 46.1). With the exception of the youngest and smallest patients undergoing surgical correction, most patients can accommodate a 7.5-mm standard cuffed ETT, through which a 9-Fr BB may be placed on the operative side to allow for OLV.[15] Should intubation prove difficult with this size ETT, a 7.0-mm ETT, although tighter fitting with the BB and fiberoptic bronchoscope (for proper placement and visualization), is sufficient. There are rare occasions in which a double-lumen tube (DLT) is favored over a BB. These include: (1) patients who are appropriate size to accommodate a DLT (≥35 Fr), (2) those whose scoliosis curve apex is mid-thoracic (T8–T9), and (3) patients with a severe Cobb angle, the latter two making manipulation of the BB more challenging.[15] There are also 32 Fr and 28 Fr DLT that can be used for adolescents. However, they are infrequently used because they would not accommodate the standard 4.0-mm fiberoptic bronchoscope.

Before and during thoracoscopy or thoracotomy, close communication between the anesthesiologist and surgical teams is imperative. The overarching goal of using OLV is to optimize surgical exposure of the thoracic spine and facilitate performance of the procedure. This must be performed while ensuring patient safety throughout by minimizing hypoxemia, using an appropriate ventilation strategy, and managing issues in a timely manner before adverse events occur.

Hypoxemia (see Ch. 20)

Hypoxemia, typically defined as a pulse oximetry (SpO_2) reading of less than 90% (arterial partial oxygen pressure [PaO2] <60 mm Hg), is a major risk during OLV that occurs secondary to continued blood flow to the nonventilated lung. The body adapts to this condition through a process known as hypoxic pulmonary vasoconstriction (HPV), which is a defensive mechanism in which the pulmonary blood vessels supplying poorly or nonventilated areas of

TABLE 46.1 Endotracheal Tube Choice

Lung Isolation Technique	Advantages	Disadvantages
Bronchial blockers (BB)	1. Easier placement in children and known difficult airways 2. Ability to ventilate through standard ETT during placement 3. Size selection rarely an issue 4. Capability of selectively isolating lung lobes (if warranted) 5. Capacity to safely provide postoperative two lung ventilation after BB removal	1. Increased time necessary for placement and alternating side of OLV 2. Higher incidence of BB dislodgement during patient positioning and surgical manipulation 3. Requires presence of fiberoptic bronchoscope for duration of case 4. Difficulty isolating right upper lobe because of early takeoff from right mainstem bronchus 5. Inability to provide CPAP or perform bronchoscopy on isolated lung
Double-lumen tube	1. Faster initial placement 2. Reduced risk of dislodgement, repositioning less frequent 3. CPAP easily administered to isolated lung 4. Ability to perform bronchoscopy on isolated lung 5. Alternating side of lung isolation is easy	1. Not optimal for postoperative mechanical ventilation 2. Increased incidence of laryngeal and/or bronchial trauma and hoarseness[16] 3. Size selection more challenging 4. Difficult placement in patients with challenging airways

CPAP, Continuous positive airway pressure; *ETT*, endotracheal tube; *OLV*, one-lung ventilation.

lung parenchyma constrict to redirect that blood to areas of lung with higher oxygen tension. HPV can result in an up to 50% reduction in blood flow to the nonventilated lung[17] although this process can take up to 2 hours to fully stabilize. Given the slow onset of HPV, patients may experience hypoxemia (SpO_2 <90%) upon initiation of OLV, necessitating a temporary return to two lung ventilation on an F_iO_2 = 100%. Because HPV is a reflex that has a preconditioning effect, the response to subsequent hypoxic challenges after treatment upon return to OLV will be faster.

The anesthesiologist must be prepared to manage hypoxemia that may occur during OLV. Should desaturation or movement of the BB occur, most commonly because of necessary surgical manipulations, it is essential to communicate with the surgical team about the need for immediate interventions, including lung reinflation (i.e., a recruitment breath), which can disrupt the operative field. A recruitment maneuver is performed by inflating the lung to 20 to 30 cm H_2O with an F_iO_2 of 100% O_2 for 15 to 20 seconds. This may need to be repeated several times every 30 minutes.

The anesthesiologist may also need to use additional strategies to treat intraoperative hypoxemia during OLV. These include applying positive end expiratory pressure (PEEP) or administering a recruitment maneuver to the ventilated lung to open atelectatic segments of lung for subsequent participation in gas exchange. During every incidence of hypoxemia, it is prudent to reassess the positioning of the BB or DLT with the fiberoptic bronchoscope as dislodgement from its original positioning can result in occlusion of the trachea, thereby impeding adequate oxygenation and ventilation.

Right-sided blockade with the BB prevent inflation of the right upper lobe (RUL) but at the same time will slow the deflation because of the location of the BB cuff at the orifice of the RUL bronchus. This may interfere with the ability of the surgeon to adequately perform the procedure. Therefore in these circumstances, the anesthesiology and surgical teams must work in concert to pause ventilation, deflate the BB cuff, apply suction through the BB lumen or manually compress and deflate the RUL, then reinflate the BB cuff and resume OLV with the entire right lung now deflated.

There are several strategies to help promote HPV and mitigate the resultant hypoxemia. Applying continuous gentle suction to the nonventilated lung helps to promote HPV in the nonventilated lung and improve the surgical field. Care must be taken to ensure normothermia, particularly during OLV, as hypothermia can inhibit HPV. Volatile agents may potentially inhibit HPV in a dose-dependent manner. Therefore a total intravenous anesthetic technique (TIVA) is ideal for maintenance of anesthesia. Volatile agents and nitrous oxide can also impair neuromonitoring-evoked potentials and are therefore avoided during these cases. HPV response is decreased by vasodilators, such as nitroglycerin and nitroprusside. These agents are short acting and unless used for an infusion during surgery should not significantly impact HPV. Although respiratory acidosis secondary to a hypoventilation strategy does promote HPV, this strategy does not result in a net benefit to gas exchange during OLV because it results in preferential increase in pulmonary vascular tone to the ventilated lung.[18] Protective lung ventilation strategy should be applied for all the patients during the surgical procedure. The triad of low tidal volume 5 to 6 mL/kg, PEEP to the dependent lung, and frequent recruitment maneuvers are established ventilatory strategy to reduce the incidence of postoperative pulmonary complications.

Patient positioning in the lateral decubitus and using TIVA for maintenance serve to assist in mitigating the risk of hypoxemia during OLV by optimizing V/Q mismatch. Placing the patient in the lateral position is necessary for exposure of the thoracic spine via the thoracic approach, and it also improves oxygenation as more gravity dependent blood will flow to the dependent lung.

Blood Conservation Strategies

Although the anterior approach to thoracic spine surgery is associated with reduced blood loss when compared with the posterior approach, it is important to have a preoperative discussion regarding expectations of blood loss based on perceived surgical complexity and duration. This will help determine the value of using blood conservation strategies during the case. It will also aid in determining the type and size of venous access that is necessary. Allogeneic blood transfusion is associated with risks, including transfusion-related reactions, end organ damage, infection, and impaired wound healing. To actively reduce blood loss during anterior thoracic spine procedures, blood conservation strategies, including administration of antifibrinolytics, cell salvage, and deliberate hypotension, can be used.

Tranexamic acid (TXA), an antifibrinolytic, is used to minimize surgical blood loss. For surgical cases with a predicted blood loss of greater than 500 mL, 10 mg/kg TXA IV (redosed every 3 hours) can be administered to reduce blood loss and minimize the potential need for an allogenic blood transfusion. Although several recent studies noted that administration of TXA reduced estimated blood loss and allogeneic blood transfusion in patients undergoing AIS surgical correction,[19,20] the most recent Cochrane database system review from 2016 concluded that there is limited evidence of low quality to support the use of antifibrinolytics in pediatric patients undergoing scoliosis repair, based on the current data.[21] Despite limited evidence supporting the use of TXA in pediatric patients, the benefits of administration outweigh the risks given the high safety profile and limited side effects.

Cell salvage systems, also known as autologous blood recovery systems, can be used for correction cases in which the predicted blood loss is expected to be greater than 500 mL. The advantages of cell salvage include decreased need for allogeneic blood transfusions, its associated complications and costs. In fact, according to one study, one unit of cell salvaged blood costs less than half the price of a unit of allogeneic packed red blood cells.[22]

Deliberate hypotension, defined as reducing the mean arterial blood pressure of the patient of up to 30% of the patient's baseline is a technique that has been used to limit intraoperative blood loss and improve surgical field. Although deliberate hypotension may be safe to perform in select patients for short periods of time, the anesthesiologist must consider the rare but significant risks associated with its use. These include spinal cord ischemia, myocardial and kidney injury, and vision loss because of impaired perfusion. Ideally, use of deliberate hypotension should be minimized and is best reserved for posterior procedures during the spinal exposure in which blood loss can be significant.[23]

Anterior Approach to Thoracic Spine Surgery

The AVBT procedure is the first nonfusion approach for the management of scoliosis. It involves the placement of vertebral body screws attached by a tether on the convex side of the curve. When the tether is tightened, it inhibits growth on that side while still allowing growth to occur on the concave side of the curve, thereby fostering correction after the surgery during normal growth while preserving motion in the operative segments. Although still a nascent procedure, the fusionless correction lends itself to increased spinal flexibility postoperatively. To date, fewer than 30 surgeons perform the procedure nationwide. There is a paucity of data on long-term outcomes of this procedure; however, early studies evaluating safety and outcomes have been promising.[24–27] A study of 11 patients with 2-year outcomes found progressive improvement of the thoracic curvature and no major complications.[25] Comparison of AVBT and posterior surgical instrumentation and fusion (PSIF) found AVBT resulted in a large variation in the percent curve correction achieved compared with PSIF but fusion was still avoided in most patients at the 2-year follow-up.[28]

The anterior approach to the thoracic spine offers unique advantages for the patient. These include reduced blood loss and therefore transfusions (by >50%),[15,29–32] fewer fused vertebral levels (with the goal of improved postoperative mobility),[30] reduced risk of infection,[33] and improved cosmesis secondary to small, well-hidden incisions in comparison to the posterior approach.[30] In addition, patients may benefit from earlier postoperative ambulation, a reduction in postoperative pain, improved health-related quality of life, and better correction of hypokyphosis.[34,35] A retrospective matched comparison study found patients who underwent video-assisted anterior thoracoscopic spinal fusion had higher scores in the self-image, mental health, and total score domains than posterior spinal fusion patients on the SRS-22, an extensively validated questionnaire to evaluate the health-related quality of life of patients with spinal deformities. These findings are likely because of smaller surgical scars and minimal invasiveness of the anterior versus the posterior procedures.[35] Disadvantages to the anterior approach include approach related complications, such as atelectasis, pneumothorax, and chylothorax, more significant decline in pulmonary function immediately following surgery, and a greater learning curve for the surgeons that is associated with performing minimally invasive anterior correction techniques.[36–38] It is also possible that the anterior approach is associated with a higher reoperation rate when compared with PSIF.

PSIF is considered the gold standard for scoliosis treatment[39] and remains the predominant method of surgical management today in the United States. There are however several disadvantages to spinal fusion, many of which the novel AVBT was developed to address. PSIF impedes residual growth potential in the operated segments of the skeletally immature patient and eliminates spinal motion within these segments. This decrease in spinal motion is associated with the reduction in ability to play sports, particularly in patients with more distal levels of fusion.[40] In addition, noninstrumented levels adjacent to fused levels may develop disc degeneration necessitating extension of the spinal fusion in a revision surgery.[41] Regardless of whether additional operations are necessary, studies have found increased degenerative disc changes in AIS patients as compared with healthy controls and an increased incidence of disc degeneration with more distal levels of fusion.[42–45] Finally, roughly 40% of these young patients are at high risk of developing chronic postsurgical pain after this procedure.[46]

Preoperative Assessment, Testing, and Anesthetic Planning

In developing an anesthetic plan for the surgery, it is critical to review the patient's medical history and preoperative tests, and have a detailed discussion with both the surgical team and patient. In addition, it is imperative to understand the nuances of the patient's scoliosis-related pathology.

First, it is important to recognize the etiology of the scoliosis. Idiopathic scoliosis accounts for a large majority of cases (up to 85%) and is further defined by the age at which it begins to develop: infantile, juvenile, and adolescent. The latter form is the most common type seen in the United States. A minority of scoliosis cases (15%) are secondary to neuromuscular, congenital, genetic (syndromic), connective tissue, or other conditions. Patients with neuromuscular disease typically have more severe presentations of scoliosis, and surgical intervention is associated with greater perioperative complications and blood loss. In addition, there are unique anesthetic considerations for certain neuromuscular conditions.[47–49]

Age of onset of scoliosis is particularly important in determining scoliosis severity. Given that lung parenchyma continues to grow and mature until 8 years of age, the earlier the onset of scoliosis, the greater the pulmonary function impairment and reduction in lung reserve and gas exchange. This can lead to pulmonary hypertension that can encourage the development of right ventricular hypertrophy and subsequent right heart failure. If this is suspected, the patient should be evaluated with transthoracic echocardiography or right heart catheterization to further characterize the extent of pulmonary hypertension and its effects on cardiac remodeling and functioning.

Fig. 46.4 illustrates the pre- and postspine correction in an adolescent girl.

The location and severity of the pathology can have significant implications on the anesthesia plan as well. Severe scoliosis of the thoracic spine impedes the movement of ribs, reduces chest wall compliance, and increases the work of breathing in the manner of a restrictive lung disease. Although not routinely indicated for preoperative workup except in cases with severe scoliosis and/or lung pathology, pulmonary function tests will demonstrate a reduction in total lung capacity, functional residual capacity, inspiratory capacity of vital capacity on pulmonary function tests.[50,51] Patients with significant impairment in respiratory mechanics as a result of scoliosis can develop pulmonary hypertension and should be further assessed as described previously. Clinically, the patient may have a reduced exercise capacity and will desaturate faster after anesthesia induction. Involvement of the cervical vertebrae can create difficulties in airway management and may be associated with other congenital anomalies.[52] These patients are best intubated with fiberoptic bronchoscopy or with video laryngoscopy to prevent any potential cervical injury.

Neuromonitoring

There are several potential serious complications of thoracic spine surgery. These include weakness, numbness, bowel or bladder incontinence, and sexual dysfunction. According to a retrospective study examining nearly 12,000 spine surgeries, the overall incidence of major perioperative neurologic deficits after spine surgery is low 0.178%. However, it is nearly triple that rate (0.488%) after spine surgery in the thoracic region.[53] Such complications can result in physical and emotional distress, reduce quality of life, and can have profound economic implications for affected patients. Given the potential for neurologic complications, intraoperative neuromonitoring is considered necessary when performing thoracic spine surgery.

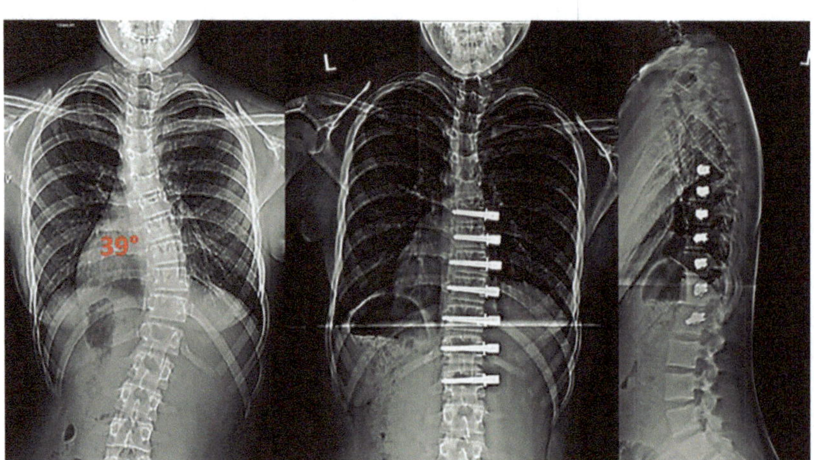

• **Fig. 46.4** A 14-year-old female, radiograph before (left image) and after surgery (middle and right image) for adolescent idiopathic scoliosis. A right-sided anterior approach was used. (From Coluna/Columna *Print version* ISSN 1808-1851 Coluna/Columna vol.13 no.1 São Paulo Jan./Mar. 2014.)

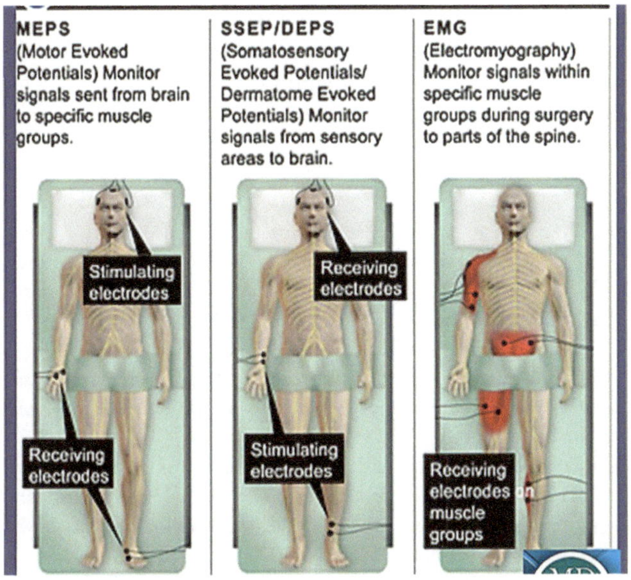

• **Fig. 46.5** Typical neuromonitoring modalities. (Reprinted with permission from MD Digitas TV.)

It is important to confirm with the surgeon and neurophysiology team how the integrity of the spinal cord will be monitored. When transcranial motor-evoked potentials are used to monitor the anterior spinal cord, a bite block should be placed between the molar teeth and secured in place to prevent injury to the tongue. In addition, long-acting neuromuscular blockade should be avoided.

Typical neuromonitoring modalities are displayed in Fig. 46.5.

There are three main neuromonitoring techniques commonly used in the United States to assess spinal cord integrity and function during spine surgery: (1) SSEPs, (2) TcMEPs, and (3) EMGs. SSEPs assess the ability of the spinal cord to conduct sensory information from peripheral nerves throughout the body to the cerebral cortex via the spinothalamic tracts within the posterior columns of the spinal cord. The **amplitude** (or strength of the conducted signal as measured within the cerebral cortex) and **latency** (the time required for the signal to travel from the peripheral nerve to the cerebral cortex) are measured and compared with the patient's baseline amplitude and latency before surgical intervention. Similarly, TcMEPs assess the ability of the spinal cord to conduct impulses from the motor cortex (using scalp electrodes), through the corticospinal tracts in the anterior (motor) columns of the spinal cord and peripheral nerves to cause muscle contractions. Again, amplitude and latency of such signals are recorded and compared with baselines. **A decrease in amplitude of 50%, increase in latency of 10%, or complete loss of the evoked potential is considered indicative of a spinal cord injury until proven otherwise**[52] and must be addressed by the perioperative care team immediately. EMG is used to monitor spinal nerve root integrity as neither SSEPs or TcMEPs are reliable techniques for doing so. EMGs are effective to prevent spinal nerve root impingement during surgical manipulation and during spine instrumentation to ensure proper placement of implants.[54]

In the event of any acute change in neuromonitoring, a team-based approach, including surgery anesthesiology, and neuromonitoring is essential in narrowing the differential diagnosis and developing a management strategy. Impaired neuromonitoring signals can be caused by direct compression or injury to neuronal structures (i.e., the spinal cord or exiting nerve roots) via surgical transection, retraction, hematoma, and/or misplaced or displaced vertebral body screws or cages. In addition, direct injury to blood vessels that supply the spinal cord can also cause similar changes in neuromonitoring. Alternatively, global signal impairment can result from hypotension or anemia-causing reduced oxygen delivery to neural structures. Physiologic derangements, including hypothermia, hypocapnia, or electrolyte imbalances (i.e., hyponatremia), can also precipitate neuronal injury or exacerbate a preexisting one. Finally, certain volatile anesthetic agents can result in reduced neuromonitoring signaling.

Whereas the surgeon assesses the operative field and appropriateness of implant placement and the neuromonitoring team evaluates lead placement and signal changes, the anesthesiologist can take several steps to aid in signal improvement and potentially mitigate ongoing neurologic injury. Such steps include augmenting the MAP to improve spinal cord and spinal nerve root perfusion by reducing the maintenance anesthetic or initiating a phenylephrine infusion, discontinuing volatile anesthetics, which can reduce amplitude and prolong latency of SSEP and TcMEP signals, ensure normothermia, and assess an arterial blood gas and correct any significant electrolyte abnormalities.[55]

Conclusion

The anterior approach to spine surgery is considered safe and has the potential for improving value in patient care. The unique advantages of the procedure, compared with PSIF, particularly when used for correction of scoliosis, include avoiding disruption of spinal musculature for surgical exposure and reducing the number of fused vertebrae (thereby preserving postoperative spinal flexibility). In addition, there is evidence to suggest that there is a reduction in the risk of infection or need for blood transfusion in the perioperative period.

Conducting a safe and appropriate anesthetic for this type of surgical approach requires careful preoperative planning with both the surgical and neurophysiology teams. Each anesthetic plan should involve appropriate patient selection in the preoperative period, an arterial line placement for hemodynamic monitoring and blood gases, as well as appropriate venous access. Intraoperative OLV to optimize the surgical field, and postoperative multimodal analgesia to help maximize early physical therapy with the goal of maintaining spine mobility. Intraoperatively, communication amongst teams and an intimate knowledge of physiology and complications of intrathoracic surgery and OLV remains essential to ensuring patient safety and a satisfactory surgical result. Although relatively few surgeons in the United States perform an anterior approach to thoracic spine surgery, it is gaining widespread favor as maintaining patient safety and outcome data continue to demonstrate that the approach offers unique advantages to the posterior approach.

References

1. Gokaslan ZL, York JE, Walsh GL, et al. Transthoracic vertebrectomy for metastatic spinal tumors. *J Neurosurg.* 1998;89:599–609.
2. Giacomo T De, Francioni F, Diso D, et al. Anterior approach to the thoracic spine. *Interact Cardiovasc Thorac Surg.* 2011;12:692–695.
3. Asher M, Lai SM, Burton D, Manna B. The influence of spine and trunk deformity on preoperative idiopathic scoliosis patients' health-related quality of life questionnaire responses. *Spine* (Phila Pa 1976). 2004;29:861–868.
4. Payne WK, Ogilvie JW, Resnick MD, Kane RL, Transfeldt EE, Blum RW. Does scoliosis have a psychological impact and does gender make a difference. *Spine* (Phila Pa 1976). 1997;22:1380–1384.
5. Lonner BS, Ren Y, Bess S, et al. Surgery for the adolescent idiopathic scoliosis patients after skeletal maturity: early versus late surgery. *Spine Deform.* 2019;7:84–92.
6. Han C, Kuang MJ, Ma JX, Ma XL. The efficacy of preoperative gabapentin in spinal surgery: a meta-analysis of randomized controlled trials. *Pain Physician.* 2017;20:649–661.
7. Haffner M, Saiz AM, Nathe R, et al. Preoperative multimodal analgesia decreases 24-hour postoperative narcotic consumption in elective spinal fusion patients. *Spine J.* 2019;19:1753–1763.
8. Trzcinski S, Rosenberg RE, Vasquez Montes D, et al. Use of gabapentin in posterior spinal fusion is associated with decreased postoperative pain and opioid use in children and adolescents. *Clin Spine Surg.* 2019;32:210–214.
9. Rusy LM, Hainsworth KR, Nelson TJ, et al. Gabapentin use in pediatric spinal fusion patients: a randomized, double-blind, controlled trial. *Anesth Analg.* 2010;110:1393–1398.
10. Vasigh A, Jaafarpour M, Khajavikhan J, Khani A. The effect of gabapentin plus celecoxib on pain and associated complications after laminectomy. *J Clin Diagn Res.* 2016;10 UC04-8.
11. Trung Kien N, Geiger P, Van Chuong H, et al. Preemptive analgesia after lumbar spine surgery by pregabalin and celecoxib: a prospective study. *Drug Des Devel Ther.* 2019;13:2145–2252.
12. Jiang H, Huang S, Song J, et al. Preoperative use of pregabalin for acute pain in spine surgery: a meta-analysis of randomized controlled trials. *Medicine* (Baltimore). 2017;96:e6129.
13. Rajpal S, Gordon DB, Pellino TA, et al. Comparison of perioperative oral multimodal analgesia versus IV PCA for spine surgery. *J Spinal Disord Tech.* 2010;23:139–145.
14. Manion SC, Brennan TJ. Thoracic epidural analgesia and acute pain management. *Anesthesiology.* 2011;115:181–188.
15. Gal JS, Curatolo CJ, Zerillo J, et al. Anesthetic considerations for a novel anterior surgical approach to pediatric scoliosis correction. *Paediatr Anaesth.* 2017;27:1028–1036.
16. Knoll H, Ziegeler S, Schreiber JU, et al. Airway injuries after one-lung ventilation: a comparison between double-lumen tube and endobronchial blocker—a randomized, prospective, controlled trial. *Anesthesiology.* 2006;105:471–477.
17. Domino K, Wetstein L, Glasser S, et al. Influence of mixed venous oxygen tension (PVO2) on blood flow to atelectatic lung. *Anesthesiology.* 1983;59:428–434.
18. Slinger P, Campos J. Anesthesia for thoracic surgery. In: Miller R, Cohen N, Eriksson L, Fleisher L, Weiner-Kronish J, Young W, eds. *Miller's Anesthesia.* 8th Ed. Philadelphia: Elsevier; 2015:1942–2006.
19. Lonner B, Ren Y, Asghar J, Shah S, Samdani A, Newton P. Antifibrinolytic therapy in surgery for adolescent idiopathic scoliosis: Does the level 1 evidence translate to practice? *Bull Hosp Joint Dis.* 2018;76:165–170.
20. Goobie SM, Zurakowski D, Glotzbecker MP, et al. Tranexamic acid is efficacious at decreasing the rate of blood loss in adolescent scoliosis surgery: A randomized placebo-controlled trial. *J Bone Jt Surg Am.* 2018;100:2024–2032.
21. Mcnicol ED, Tzortzopoulou A, Schumann R, Carr DB, Kalra A. Antifibrinolytic agents for reducing blood loss in scoliosis surgery in children. *Cochrane Database Syst Rev.* 2016;19:CD006883.
22. Waters JR, Meier HH, Waters JH. An economic analysis of costs associated with development of a cell salvage program. *Anesth Analg.* 2007;104:869–875.
23. Verma K, Lonner B, Dean L, Vecchio DLV. Reduction of mean arterial pressure at incision reduces operative blood loss in adolescent idiopathic scoliosis. *Spine Deform.* 2013;1:115–122.
24. Miyanji F, Pawelek J, Nasto LA, Parent S. A prospective, multicenter analysis of the efficacy of anterior vertebral body tethering (AVBT) in the treatment of idiopathic scoliosis. *Spine Deform.* 2018;6:820.
25. Samdani AF, Ames RJ, Kimball JS, et al. Anterior vertebral body tethering for idiopathic scoliosis. *Spine* (Phila Pa 1976). 2014;39:1688–1693.
26. Samdani AF, Ames RJ, Kimball JS, et al. Anterior vertebral body tethering for immature adolescent idiopathic scoliosis: one-year results on the first 32 patients. *Eur Spine J.* 2015;24:1533–1539.
27. Lui D, Haleem S, Lupu C, Bishop T, Bernard J. Vertebral body tethering in lumbar curves: minimum 2 year follow-up Abstract 55 Hong Kong, Hong Kong Orthopaedic Association, 2019 at hkoa.org/HKOA39/resources/Abstracts/FP08.pdf.
28. Newton P, Kluck D, Saito W, Yaszay B, Bartley C, Bastrom T. 2-Year Outcomes of Spinal Growth Tethering vs. Posterior Spinal Fusion for Scoliosis-Flexibility vs. Reliability 2017 at https://www.srs.org/whitecloud-review.
29. Lee CS, Park SJ, Chung SS, Kang KC, Jung CH, Kim YT. A comparative study between thoracoscopic surgery and posterior surgery using all-pedicle-screw constructs in the treatment of adolescent idiopathic scoliosis. *J Spinal Disord Tech.* 2013;26:325–333.
30. Lonner BS, Kondrachov D, Siddiqi F, Hayes V, Scharf C. Thoracoscopic spinal fusion compared with posterior spinal fusion for the treatment of thoracic adolescent idiopathic scoliosis. Surgical technique. *J Bone Joint Surg Am.* 2007:142–156.
31. Meert KL, Kannan S, Mooney JF. Predictors of red cell transfusion in children and adolescents undergoing spinal fusion surgery. *Spine* (Phila Pa 1976). 2002;27:2137–2142.
32. Koerner JD, Patel A, Zhao C, et al. Blood loss during posterior spinal fusion for adolescent idiopathic scoliosis. *Spine* (Phila Pa 1976). 2014;39:1479–1487.

33. Zhou J, Wang R, Huo X, Xiong W, Kang L, Xue Y. Incidence of surgical site infection after spine surgery: a systematic review and meta-analysis. *Spine* (Phila Pa 1976). 2020;45:208–216.
34. Lin Y, Chen W, Chen A, Li F, Xiong W. Anterior versus posterior selective fusion in treating adolescent idiopathic scoliosis: a systematic review and meta-analysis of radiologic parameters. *World Neurosurg*. 2018;111:e830–e844.
35. Lonner BS, Auerbach JD, Estreicher M, et al. Video-assisted anterior thoracoscopic spinal fusion versus posterior spinal fusion: a comparative study utilizing the SRS-22 outcome instrument. *Spine* (Phila Pa 1976). 2009;34:193–198.
36. Betz RR, Shufflebarger H. Controversies in spine: anterior versus posterior instrumentation for the correction of thoracic idiopathic scoliosis. *Spine* (Phila Pa 1976). 2001;26:1095–1100.
37. Lonner BS, Scharf C, Antonacci D, Goldstein Y, Panagopoulos G. The learning curve associated with thoracoscopic spinal instrumentation. *Spine* (Phila Pa 1976). 2005;30:2835–2840.
38. Sucato D, Newton P, Betz R, et al. Defining the learning curve for performing a thoracoscopic anterior spinal fusion and instrumentation for AIS: a multicenter study. *Spine J*. 2005;5:S119.
39. Ghandhari H, Ameri E, Nikouei F, Haji Agha Bozorgi M, Majdi S, Salehpour M. Long-term outcome of posterior spinal fusion for the correction of adolescent idiopathic scoliosis. *Scoliosis Spinal Disord*. 2018;13.
40. Fabricant PD, Admoni S, Green DW, Ipp LS, Widmann RF. Return to athletic activity after posterior spinal fusion for adolescent idiopathic scoliosis. *J Pediatr Orthop*. 2012;32:259–265.
41. Chang DP. *Anesthetic Implications for Pediatric Patients Undergoing Scoliosis Repair, OpenAnesthesia*. San Francisco: OpenAnesthesia; 2019 at http://www.openanesthesia.org/anesthetic-implications-for-pediatric-patients-undergoing-scoliosis-repair-with-denise-p-chang/.
42. Danielsson AJ, Nachemson AL. Back pain and function 23 years after fusion for adolescent idiopathic scoliosis: a case-control study—part II. *Spine* (Phila Pa 1976). 2003;28:E373–E383.
43. Nohara A, Kawakami N, Seki K, et al. The effects of spinal fusion on lumbar disc degeneration in patients with adolescent idiopathic scoliosis: a minimum 10-year follow-up. *Spine Deform*. 2015;3:462–468.
44. Lonner BS, Ren Y, Upasani VV, et al. Disc degeneration in unfused caudal motion segments ten years following surgery for adolescent idiopathic scoliosis. *Spine Deform*. 2018;6:684–690.
45. Danielsson AJ, Cederlund CG, Ekholm S, Nachemson AL. The prevalence of disc aging and back pain after fusion extending into the lower lumbar spine: a matched MR study twenty-five years after surgery for adolescent idiopathic scoliosis. *Acta Radiol*. 2001;42:187–197.
46. Chidambaran V, Ding L, Moore DL, et al. Predicting the pain continuum after adolescent idiopathic scoliosis surgery: a prospective cohort study. *Eur J Pain* (United Kingdom). 2017;21:1252–1265.
47. Burjek NE, Rao KE, Wieser JP, et al. Preoperative pulmonary function test results are not associated with postoperative intubation in children undergoing posterior spinal fusion for scoliosis: a retrospective observational study. *Anesth Analg*. 2019;129:184–191.
48. Cognetti D, Keeny HM, Samdani AF, et al. Neuromuscular scoliosis complication rates from 2004 to 2015: A report from the Scoliosis Research Society Morbidity and Mortality database. *Neurosurg Focus*. 2017;43:E10.
49. Flaherty DC, Lonner B, Gal JS. Successful management of a patient with x-linked myotubular myopathy for scoliosis surgery and previous cardiac arrest after prone positioning. *A Pract*. 2018;10:340–342.
50. Koumbourlis AC. Scoliosis and the respiratory system. *Paediatr Respir Rev*. 2006;7:152–160.
51. Wilton N, Anderson B. Orthopedic and spine surgery. In: Coté C, Lerman J, Anderson B, eds. *A Practice of Anesthesia for Infants and Children*. 6th ed. Philadelphia: Elsevier; 2019:727–753.
52. DelPizzo K, Zayas V. Scoliosis. In: Yao F, Malhotra V, Fong J, Skubas N, eds. *Anesthesiology Problem-Oriented Patient Management*. 8th Ed. Philadelphia: Wolters Kluwer; 2016:1072–1093.
53. Cramer DE, Maher PC, Pettigrew DB, Kuntz IV C. Major neurologic deficit immediately after adult spinal surgery: incidence and etiology over 10 years at a single training institution. *J Spinal Disord Tech*. 2009;22:565–570.
54. Brallier J, Gal J. *Neuroprotection for Spine Surgery, Neuroprotection in Critical Care and Perioperative Medicine, First*. Oxford University Press; 2017:1–26.
55. Vitale MG, Skaggs DL, Pace GI, et al. Best practices in intraoperative neuromonitoring in spine deformity surgery: development of an intraoperative checklist to optimize response. *Spine Deform*. 2014;2:333–339.

47

Myasthenia Gravis and Thymectomy

DANIEL BLECH, JAMES B. EISENKRAFT

Introduction

Myasthenia gravis (MG) is an autoimmune disorder affecting the neuromuscular junction for which patients commonly undergo surgical thymectomy as definitive treatment. It is therefore of great significance to the thoracic anesthesiologist. It is a chronic disorder characterized by fluctuating painless weakness and fatigability of voluntary muscles made worse on exertion with improvement following rest. The onset is usually slow and insidious; any skeletal muscle or muscle group may be affected. The most common onset is ocular, presenting with ptosis and diplopia. If the symptoms remain localized to the eyes for 2 years, the likelihood of progression to generalized disease is about 10%. In many cases, however, MG is generalized and may involve the bulbar musculature (muscles innervated by cranial nerves IX, X, XI, and XII), causing problems with breathing, speaking, mastication, and swallowing. Proximal muscles are more commonly involved than distal. Peripheral muscle weakness may manifest as clumsiness, difficulty holding up the head, or in ambulating. Respiratory muscle weakness may cause dyspnea, as well as a decrease in the ability to cough and clear secretions.[1]

The annual incidence of MG is estimated at 7 to 23 new cases per 1,000,000 people per year; the prevalence is 150 to 250 per one million.[1,2] It occurs more commonly in women than men. The disease affects all ages, but the age of onset has a bimodal distribution displaying an early peak in the second and third decades (female predominance) and a late peak in the sixth to eighth decades (male predominance).[3]

Etiology and Pathophysiology

In normal neuromuscular transmission, the acetylcholine (ACh) released from the motor nerve terminal stimulates postsynaptic nicotinic receptors at the motor end plate to generate an action potential leading to depolarization of the membrane and contraction of the motor unit. The normal neuromuscular junction has a very large number of postsynaptic acetylcholine receptors (AChRs) such that muscle weakness only becomes apparent when 75% or more of the receptors have been blocked. This excess of receptors has been termed the "margin of safety of neuromuscular transmission." MG patients have a significant decrease in the number of postsynaptic AChRs at the end plates of affected muscles resulting in a decreased margin of safety of neuromuscular transmission.[4]

MG is an autoimmune disorder, and about 80% of affected patients have detectable circulating antibodies to the nicotinic AChR. These anti-AChR antibodies may cause complement-mediated lysis of the postsynaptic membrane, directly block the receptors, or may modulate the receptor turnover such that the rate of degradation exceeds the rate of resynthesis. Studies of the motor end plate area show loss of synaptic folds and a widening of the synaptic cleft. Approximately 10% of MG patients who do not have anti-AChR antibodies have antibodies to muscle-specific tyrosine kinase (MuSK). The MuSK-antibody-positive MG patients often develop prominent oculobulbar muscle weakness, but the MG is not limited to the eyes. In MuSK-antibody-positive individuals cholinesterase inhibitors have no effect and may even exacerbate symptoms.[5]

The cause of MG is unknown but appears to be related in some way to the thymus gland. It has been suggested that thymic T cells are stimulated to produce antibodies following sensitization by a protein similar to the AChR. MG patients also have a higher incidence of other autoimmune diseases including autoimmune thyroid disease, rheumatoid arthritis, and systemic lupus erythematosus.[6]

Clinical Classification

The original clinical classification by Osserman and Genkins[7] outlined four classes and two subclasses according to the progressive involvement of different muscle groups and the severity of presentation. The classification now most commonly used is that of the Medical Scientific Advisory Board of the Myasthenia Gravis Foundation of America, summarized in Table 47.1.[8] Note that each class is defined by the most predominant or "severe" symptoms and may include symptoms from a "lesser" class.

Clinical and Differential Diagnosis

The diagnosis of MG is suspected from the patient's history and confirmed by clinical, electrophysiologic, pharmacologic, or immunologic testing. Typically, the patient

TABLE 47.1 **Clinical Classification of Myasthenia Gravis**

Myasthenia Gravis Class	Symptoms
I	Isolated ocular muscle weakness
IIa	Mild weakness predominantly affecting limb/axial muscles
IIb	Mild weakness predominantly affecting oropharyngeal/respiratory muscles
IIIa	Moderate weakness predominantly affecting limb/axial muscles
IIIb	Moderate weakness predominantly affecting oropharyngeal/respiratory muscles
IVa	Severe weakness predominantly affecting limb/axial muscles
IVb	Severe weakness predominantly affecting oropharyngeal/respiratory muscles
V	Requiring intubation and/or mechanical respiratory support

From Jaretzki A 3rd, Barohn RJ, Ernstoff RM, et al. Myasthenia gravis: recommendations for clinical research standards. Task Force of the Medical Scientific Advisory Board of the Myasthenia Gravis Foundation of America. *Neurology.* 2000;55(1):16–23. With permission.

cannot sustain or repeat muscular contraction. Clinical tests of fatigability include maintaining an upward gaze, holding out an affected limb, and respiratory function testing (vital capacity, maximum breathing capacity).

The electrical counterpart of fatigability is demonstrated by the repetitive nerve stimulation (RNS) test. The RNS involves the application of supramaximal stimulation to a peripheral nerve at 2 to 5 Hz. If a decrement of 10% or more is observed in the compound muscle action potential amplitude between the first and the fourth or fifth waveforms, this is considered diagnostic of MG. This is the most specific neurophysiologic test for MG, but it can be performed only on certain muscles, which may not be the ones affected in an individual patient. A more sensitive electrophysiologic test is single-fiber electromyography (EMG) which examines the variability in time interval or "jitter" between two single muscle fibers from the same motor unit.[9,10]

Historically, pharmacologic testing for MG was performed by administering the anticholinesterase edrophonium (Tensilon) and observing a rapid improvement in function; mechanical and electrical (e.g., EMG) decrements improve with 2 to 10 mg of intravenous edrophonium (Tensilon test). At time of writing, this medication is no longer available in the United States but an equivalent dose of neostigmine or pyridostigmine should produce a similar improvement.

Antibodies to the AChR are detectable in 80% of patients with MG. In equivocal cases, a positive result of a test for anti-AChR or MuSK antibodies is considered diagnostic.

A number of disorders can mimic MG and should be included in the initial differential diagnosis. Thyroiditis and resulting thyrotoxicosis can present with generalized weakness and abnormal thyroid function. Patients with neurasthenia characteristically have weakness, which disappears when individual muscle groups are tested. Progressive external ophthalmoplegia, restrictive cardiomyopathies, muscular dystrophies, brain tumors, amyotrophic lateral sclerosis, and myasthenic polymyopathy with hypersensitivity to neostigmine can all cause MG-like symptoms, as can drugs such as D-penicillamine, aminoglycosides, quinine, procainamide, and calcium channel blockers.[1,6]

Lambert-Eaton myasthenic syndrome (LEMS) is a very rare immune-mediated disorder of neuromuscular transmission, associated with antibodies to the presynaptic voltage-gated calcium channel. The prevalence is estimated to be about 3 to 4 per million. It is associated with small cell carcinoma of the lung in 50% to 60% of cases. Complaints of weakness may be mistaken for MG, but the symptoms of LEMS do not respond to administration of anticholinesterases or steroids, and activity improves strength.[11] The defect in this condition is prejunctional, is associated with diminished release of ACh from motor nerve terminals, and is improved by "facilitating" agents, such as 4-aminopyridine or 2,3-diaminopyridine that potentiate the release of ACh. Affected patients are particularly sensitive to the effects of nondepolarizing muscle relaxants, which should be used with great caution or avoided entirely.[12] The possibility of LEMS should be considered in all patients with known malignant disease and those patients undergoing diagnostic procedures for suspected carcinoma of the lung.

The major differences between MG and LEMS are specified in Table 47.2.[13]

Medical Treatment

Mary Walker was the first physician to report the similarity in presentation between MG and curare poisoning and to use an anticholinesterase to treat MG.[14] Anticholinesterases prolong the action of ACh at the postsynaptic membrane and may also exert their own agonist effect at the postsynaptic AChRs. They are the most commonly used therapy in MG. No randomized controlled trial has been conducted on the use of acetylcholinesterase inhibitors in patients with MG because the response in observational studies was such that a placebo group could not be justified. MG patients learn to regulate their acetylcholinesterase medication and titrate dose to optimum effect over time. If several muscle groups/functions are affected, the patient titrates therapy according to the most important group. Acetylcholinesterase overdose causes the muscarinic effects of ACh and may cause a cholinergic crisis. Excessive amounts of ACh at the neuromuscular junction cause persistent depolarization of the muscle membrane. In comparison, underdosing can lead to weakness or

TABLE 47.2 Comparison of Myasthenia Gravis and Lambert-Eaton Myasthenic Syndrome

	Myasthenia Gravis	Lambert-Eaton Myasthenic Syndrome
Primary weakness	Ocular, bulbar, facial muscles	Proximal limbs
Response to exercise	Increased fatigue	Improved strength
Muscle pain	Unusual	Common
Reflexes	Normal	Diminished
Gender ratio	Female predominance	Male predominance
Associated pathology	Thymoma	Small cell lung cancer
Response to neuromuscular blockade	Resistant to depolarizing NMBDs, sensitive to nondepolarizing NMBDs	Sensitive to depolarizing and nondepolarizing NMBDs

NMBDs, Neuromuscular blocking drugs.
From Dierdorf SF, Walton JS, Stasic AF. Rare coexisting diseases. In: Barash PG, Cullen BF, Stoelting RK, Calahan MK, Stock MC, Ortega R, Eds. *Clinical Anesthesia*. 7th edn. Philadelphia: Wolters Kluwer/Lippincott Williams & Wilkins; 2013:612–640. With permission.

a myasthenic crisis. Distinction between myasthenic and cholinergic crisis may be made by titrating small doses of neostigmine, or by examining pupil size, which will be large (mydriatic) in a myasthenic crisis but small (miotic) in a cholinergic crisis. Muscarinic side effects (bradycardia, bronchospasm, oral and respiratory tract secretions, and gastrointestinal cramps) are treatable with atropine; however, many MG patients treated with anticholinesterases seem to develop a resistance to the muscarinic effects.[15]

Pyridostigmine (Mestinon) is the anticholinesterase drug most commonly used to treat MG and has fewer muscarinic side effects than neostigmine (Prostigmin). Its onset of action following oral administration is 15 to 30 minutes, effect peaks at 1 to 2 hours, and duration of action is 3 to 4 hours. Daily dosage is typically 30 to 120 mg orally given in divided doses. For patients who are weak upon awakening in the morning, a long-acting formulation of 180 mg is available and can be taken at bedtime. MG patients whose disease subtypes are characterized by identifiable non-AChR antibodies generally have a limited response to anticholinesterase medications.

The immunologic basis of MG has led to the use of short- and long-term immunosuppressive drugs. Patients who do not meet treatment goals typically require immunosuppressive therapy. First-line therapy is generally a steroid combined with an immunomodulatory agent. Prolonged use of steroids may produce unwanted effects, such as peptic ulcer disease and osteoporosis. Alternate day dosing of either prednisone or prednisolone is generally prescribed to reduce side effects. Steroids often produce initial deterioration before an improvement. For long-term effect, immunomodulatory agents, such as azathioprine, cyclophosphamide, cyclosporine, methotrexate, mycophenolate mofetil, rituximab, and tacrolimus have been used. Rapid short-term immunomodulation has been achieved in acute exacerbations or to improve muscle strength before surgery. Plasma exchange or plasmapheresis may produce dramatic but transient improvements in muscle strength with decreases in anti-AChR and anti-MuSK titers, as well as other inflammatory mediators. Intravenous immunoglobulin (IVIG) and plasma exchange is usually reserved for severe MG—both have been found to be equally effective therapies.[16] Plasma exchange has been shown to improve respiratory function in both postoperative and nonoperative patients with MG. Plasmapheresis also causes a decrease in plasma cholinesterase levels, which may prolong the effect of drugs normally metabolized by this system, such as succinylcholine.

Thymectomy

Surgical thymectomy is always indicated in MG patients with thymoma and is now considered the treatment of choice in most patients with MG, excluding those with only ocular myasthenia. A recent randomized control trial has demonstrated a benefit of thymectomy in adults with AChR-antibody-positive, nonthymomatous MG with the addition of glucocorticoids, versus glucocorticoid therapy alone. Overall, these patients required less glucocorticoid over the 3-year study period, had an improvement in symptoms, and had fewer hospitalizations for management of MG symptoms. Patients who have non-AChR antibody-positive disease do not benefit from a thymectomy. Approximately 70% of MG patients demonstrate thymic hyperplasia; 10% have a thymoma.[17]

Table 47.3 delineates the current understanding of when thymectomy is indicated for MG.[18] Regardless of disease subtype, the medical treatments discussed earlier in this chapter are typically tried and evaluated for their individual effectiveness as symptoms necessitate.

Preoperative Evaluation and Management

When evaluating patients for thymectomy and concurrent anesthesia, one must consider their history of MG, any anticipated issues related to video-assisted thoracoscopic

TABLE 47.3 Indications for Thymectomy by Myasthenia Gravis Disease Subtype

Myasthenia Gravis Type	Age of Onset	Thymus Findings	Antibodies	Thymectomy?
"Early-onset"	<50 years	Hyperplasia	AChR	Yes
"Late-onset"	>50 years	Atrophy	AChR	Unclear
Thymoma	Any	Thymoma	AChR	Yes
MuSK antibody	Any	Normal	MuSK	No
LRP4 antibody	Any	Normal	LRP4	No
Seronegative	Any	Variable	None detected	No
Ocular	Any	Variable	Variable	No

AChR, Acetylcholine receptor; *LRP4*, low-density lipoprotein receptor-related protein 4; *MuSK*, muscle-specific tyrosine kinase.

From Cata JP, Lasala JD, Williams W, Mena GE. Myasthenia gravis and thymoma surgery: a clinical update for the cardiothoracic anesthesiologist. *J Cardiothorac Vasc Anesth*. 2019;33:2537–2545. With permission.

surgery with the patient in either the left or right lateral decubitus position, and anxiety/understanding related to their planned operative and postoperative course.[18]

The preoperative interview should be used to identify factors that suggest increased risk for postoperative mechanical ventilation after thymectomy. These factors are listed in Table 47.4.[19]

This information can guide the anesthesiologist in formulating the anesthetic plan, selection of preoperative medications, and arranging for postoperative care. When possible, patients with MG should be scheduled for elective surgery while in remission. Ideally, patients with MG should be scheduled to be the first case of the day in the operating room. Attempts should be made to optimize the patient's physical and emotional states before the day of surgery. Current drug therapy should be reviewed, and possible drug interactions considered. The patient should be well-informed regarding the possible need for postoperative intubation and ventilation.[1]

Laboratory studies should be individualized to the patient. In addition to routine preoperative laboratory data,

TABLE 47.4 Factors Predicting Need for Postoperative Mechanical Ventilation in Myasthenia Gravis Patients

More severe disease classification (likelihood increases with increasing degree of severity)
Presence of anti-AChR antibodies
History of prior myasthenic crisis
Decreased vital capacity on PFTs (<2.9 L)
Presence of thymoma

AChR, Acetylcholine receptor; *PFTs*, pulmonary function tests; *L*, liters.

From Chigurupati K, Gadhinglajkar S, Sreedhar R, Nair M, Unnikrishnan M, Pillai M. Criteria for postoperative mechanical ventilation after thymectomy in patients with myasthenia gravis: a retrospective analysis. *J Cardiothorac Vasc Anesth*. 2018;32:325–30. With permission.

electrolyte abnormalities, particularly hypokalemia, which can exacerbate weakenss, should be ruled out. If the patient is or has recently been receiving corticosteroids, blood glucose levels should be determined. Preoperative arterial blood gas analysis and pulmonary function testing are useful to help determine individualized extubation criteria. A respiratory therapist should educate the patient about breathing exercises and the use of an incentive spirometer.[5]

The management of anticholinesterase medication preoperatively should be individualized to the patient. Anticholinesterase therapy is generally continued throughout the perioperative period, especially if the patient is physically or psychologically dependent on it for normal functioning. A long-standing traditional practice is the withholding of pyridostigmine therapy on the morning of surgery so that the patient is weak on arrival to the operating room. This avoids interactions with other drugs used in the operating room. For example, anticholinesterase inhibits both plasma cholinesterase and acetylcholinesterase; therefore the metabolism of succinylcholine will be slowed. Others recommend continuing pyridostigmine, including an oral dose just before induction.[5] The risks and benefits can be weighed by the clinician on an individualized basis.

Preoperative plasmapheresis is considered an excessive use of scarce resources in the stable patient as many sessions are required to potentially achieve a salutary effect.[18] Anxiolysis can be satisfactorily achieved with a benzodiazepine. Opioids are usually avoided because of the potential for causing respiratory depression.

Operative Approaches

Classically, thymectomy is an open surgery performed via midline sternotomy. The transcervical thymectomy was the first attempt to reduce the morbidity and invasiveness of the surgical approach. More recently, a number of different video-assisted and robotic-assisted approaches have been used using axillary, midline, and/or suprasternal incisions. Minimally invasive surgical (MIS) techniques have been shown to be an effective option with fewer myasthenic and surgical complications, as well as decreased blood loss, postoperative pain, and hospital length-of-stay.[18] The many benefits of MIS must be weighed with the potential risk of incomplete surgical visualization (and thus incomplete thymectomy) on an individual patient basis.[20]

Approach to Induction and Maintenance of Anesthesia

If the surgical approach necessitates one-lung ventilation, general endotracheal anesthesia (GETA) is a requirement. Certain procedures may be possible with purely regional or local anesthesia, and in those cases utilization of those methods should be prioritized. For any case and especially GETA, short-acting and easily titratable medications are preferred, along with avoidance of neuromuscular blocking drugs (NMBDs) whenever possible. In anticipation of providing opioid-sparing postoperative analgesia, preoperative placement of a thoracic epidural catheter should be considered and discussed with the patient. At the discretion of the anesthesiologist, the catheter may be used to provide analgesia intraoperatively as well.[5,18]

Standard American Society of Anesthesiologists (ASA) monitors must be used. An arterial line is useful to draw arterial blood samples for gas analysis intraoperatively and postoperatively and is standard at most institutions for any invasive intrathoracic procedure. A peripheral nerve stimulator should be used in conjunction with a device that measures quantitative neuromuscular response to electrical stimulation (e.g., EMG, accelerometer, kinemyography). The chosen device should be used from the outset of the case even if NMBDs are avoided completely, as inhaled anesthetics also depress neuromuscular transmission. An inhalational anesthetic may be chosen or avoided specifically for this reason in favor of total intravenous anesthesia (TIVA), depending on individual patient and surgical considerations. If a TIVA is used, a processed electroencephalogram monitor is helpful to evaluate depth of anesthesia and prevent patient awareness.

Barring comorbid airway issues that necessitate either an awake fiberoptic intubation or the preservation of spontaneous ventilation during airway management (see Chapter 34 for a more complete discussion of this issue), most thymectomy patients may be tracheally intubated after the induction of general anesthesia. Before induction, the patient should be preoxygenated with 100% oxygen until the end-tidal oxygen concentration is greater than 90%. Induction of anesthesia may be achieved with the IV agent most familiar to the anesthesiologist—none of those commonly in use have profound neuromuscular effects. In most cases, the full range of effects required for intubation may be achieved using a potent inhaled anesthetic agent, because MG renders patients more susceptible to the neuromuscular depressant effects of these agents.[5] Anesthetic depth is increased using the potent inhaled agent and the trachea intubated under its effect. In patients with MG, isoflurane at 1.9 minimum alveolar concentration (MAC) end-tidal concentration decreased train-of-four ratio by 41%, whereas halothane at 1.8 MAC decreased train-of-four ratio by 28%. The less soluble inhaled agents, sevoflurane and desflurane, are even more rapidly taken up and withdrawn; they are now the most commonly used anesthetic drugs for patients with MG.[21] Whichever agent is used, it is discontinued at the end of the procedure and recovery of neuromuscular function begins.[22]

Another strategy to achieve adequate intubating conditions without the use of NMBDs includes the use of propofol and remifentanil (3–5 mcg/kg). "High-dose" remifentanil can provide intubating conditions similar to those of true neuromuscular blockade, although there is no guarantee of vocal fold relaxation. In addition, a remifentanil maintenance infusion (0.1–0.3 mcg/kg/min) can provide excellent surgical conditions with near-total abolition of patient movement and respiratory effort. Of note, remifentanil can cause significant blunting of sympathetic tone with hemodynamically significant bradycardia, so patients may benefit from coadministration of ephedrine or glycopyrrolate at the time of induction. The major advantage of remifentanil is its extremely reliable metabolism by plasma esterases, which results in a short and predictable context-sensitive half-time—allaying potential concerns about respiratory depression from lingering opioid effect.[23]

Once the patient is asleep, baseline (ideally quantitative) recordings of neuromuscular response to train-of-four should be obtained. In MG patients, fade in response to train-of-four and tetanic stimulation occurs in the affected muscles at baseline.[5]

Utilization and Reversal of Neuromuscular Blockade

If a patient cannot tolerate the depth of anesthesia needed to produce muscular relaxation using a potent inhaled agent or TIVA with remifentanil, NMBDs may be used, titrating dose against monitored effect. Patients with MG are sensitive (i.e., show a decrease in effective dose as defined by the $[ED]_{50}$ and $[ED]_{95}$ when compared with non-MG patients) to the nondepolarizing NMBDs because of the decreased number of postsynaptic receptors at the motor end plate. All nondepolarizing relaxants have been successfully and uneventfully used with careful monitoring in patients with MG. Because the sensitivity of any individual MG patient is unknown, these drugs should be titrated in 1/10 of the usual dose. Sensitivity to nondepolarizing NMBDs is increased during the coadministration of a potent inhaled anesthetic. Upon completion of the surgical procedure, the residual relaxation may be reversed using incremental doses of an anticholinesterase drug while neuromuscular transmission is carefully monitored to obtain maximum antagonism yet avoid a cholinergic crisis.[24]

Sugammadex is a novel γ-cyclodextrin drug that was designed to bind rocuronium with a great affinity; it also binds vecuronium. Before the introduction of sugammadex, anticholinesterase drugs were the only options for antagonism of residual nondepolarizing neuromuscular blockade, and in MG patients, anticholinesterases must be administered with caution so as to avoid myasthenic or cholinergic crises. Sugammadex has been reported to safely reverse rocuronium-induced neuromuscular blockade within 117 seconds in patients with MG at various levels of neuromuscular blockade.[25] It offers significant advantages in the management of the MG patient by allowing the practitioner to avoid the risks of anticholinesterase drugs. For reversal of neuromuscular blockade, the recommended doses of sugammadex are 2 mg/kg in patients who have two twitches present on train-of-four stimulation, 4 mg/kg in patients who have one to two post-tetanic twitches, and 16 mg/kg for immediate reversal in patients who have just received an intubating dose of 1.2 mg/kg of rocuronium.[26] If sugammadex is not available, cisatracurium may be the preferred NMBD because of its short elimination half-life, small volume of distribution, lack of cumulative effect, and high clearance.[27]

MG patients are resistant to the neuromuscular blocking effects of succinylcholine because of the decrease in number of postsynaptic receptors at the motor end plate. The ED_{95} is 2.6 times normal (0.8 mg/kg vs. 0.3 mg/kg) in these patients. Clinically, however, the use of succinylcholine has been without incident, with the usual clinical doses producing adequate relaxation for endotracheal intubation and a normal recovery time, despite the occasionally reported early onset of phase II block. Doses of 0.2 to 1.0 mg/kg have been used in a number of patients with MG, and most did not show fasciculation before becoming paralyzed. Fade in response to train-of-four stimulation was observed in some patients during recovery, but recovery was not delayed. Prior administration of an anticholinesterase may complicate the response to succinylcholine by delaying its metabolism.[28]

Although it is well established that MG patients are sensitive to nondepolarizing and resistant to depolarizing NMBDs, there is no consensus on the response to these drugs during a remission. It is therefore prudent to manage the patient as if he or she had active disease and titrate NMBDs to effect while monitoring the responses.[29,30]

Extubation

Postoperative weakness is the greatest contributing factor to perioperative respiratory failure in MG patients. As such, it is important to establish that the patient is fully awake and alert before attempting extubation and that any residual neuromuscular blockade has been completely reversed. If a quantitative neuromuscular monitoring device is used, a train-of-four ratio greater than 0.9 should be achieved before extubation. Adequate respiratory effort should be confirmed by ability to generate a negative inspiratory pressure of at least –20 cm H_2O. Although MG patients often experience improvement in respiratory function and other MG symptoms after thymectomy, it is more difficult to predict response to surgeries unrelated to MG. After extubation, it is essential to monitor the patient closely for signs of fatigue, weakness, or evidence of deteriorating respiratory status (hypercarbia, hypoxemia, tachypnea). If the patient was taking pyridostigmine preoperatively, oral dosing should be reestablished as soon as possible after extubation; if necessary, alternative anticholinesterase medications may be used as a bridging measure.[5,18] The dosage equivalents are shown in Table 47.5.

TABLE 47.5 Dosing Equivalents in Milligrams for Common Acetylcholinesterase Inhibitors Used in Treatment of Myasthenia Gravis

Drug	Oral	IV	IM	Efficacy
Pyridostigmine (Mestinon)	60	2	2–4	1
Neostigmine (Prostigmin)	1.5	0.5	0.7–1.0	1

IM, Intramuscular; *IV*, intravenous.

Care should be taken to ensure that somnolence related to opioid administration does not place the patient at increased risk of hypoventilation. In addition, vigilance is required to ensure that impending myasthenic crisis is not masked by intraoperative reversal agents that may wear off in the postanesthesia care unit.

Postoperative Analgesia

MG patients are especially sensitive to the central respiratory depressive effects of parenteral opioid administration. Consideration of this unique trait is paramount, but inadequately treated postsurgical pain can inhibit respiratory effort and thus can also worsen respiratory status. Non-opioid pain regimens should be used whenever possible. When feasible, MG patients benefit from thoracic epidural analgesia, and epidural catheter placement preoperatively is the gold standard.[5] Neuraxial anesthesia, when appropriate, greatly reduces the total dose of opioid required to achieve adequate analgesic effect. Regional anesthesia can also have a profound salutary effect. Paravertebral blocks have been demonstrated to decrease pulmonary complications, such as atelectasis and pneumonia, following thoracotomy.[31] More recently, continuous erector spinae plane blocks have been used to effectively control postoperative pain after thoracotomy.[32] Intravenous nonsteroidal anti-inflammatory drug regimens have also been effective in controlling pain in MG patients without causing respiratory depression.[33] If oral or parenteral opioids are used, the dose should be decreased for MG patients receiving anticholinesterase therapy because these medications have been reported to increase the efficacy of opioids.

Postoperative Myasthenic and Cholinergic Crises

The postsurgical state is uniquely perilous to the MG patient, and all should be observed carefully for respiratory decompensation after extubation. Cases have been reported in which previously undetected MG was diagnosed as a result of unexpected respiratory failure in the postoperative period.[34] Suggested criteria for reintubation have included tachypnea (respiratory rate greater than 40 breaths/min), respiratory acidosis not due to opioids, and vital capacity of 8 mL/kg or less.[35] For a patient in myasthenic crisis, inspiratory and expiratory forces are a better indicator of muscle strength, although the presence of a radiologic finding of atelectasis is the strongest predictor of need for reintubation.

A myasthenic crisis and a cholinergic crisis may both present with muscle weakness, salivation, and sweating, although secretory symptoms are most classically associated with parasympathetic excess. Cholinergic crisis is comparatively a very rare complication. If available, the preferred therapies for myasthenic crisis are IVIG and plasmapheresis. Anticholinesterase therapy can also be administered and titrated to effect; however, if IVIG or plasmapheresis are available, anticholinesterase medications should be decreased or discontinued to reduce pulmonary secretions.[36] The treatment for cholinergic crisis may incorporate antimuscarinic drugs (atropine, glycopyrrolate) to treat salivation and sweating but is mostly supportive and may require mechanical ventilation until the crisis is resolved.[18]

Because myasthenic and cholinergic crisis may occasionally be so difficult to distinguish that formal neurophysiologic studies are required, the true cornerstones of safe postoperative care are timely recognition of respiratory failure and excellent supportive care.

Future Directions

The increasing utilization and success of minimally invasive approaches to thymectomy, along with advances in anesthetic drug development, has empowered thoracic anesthesiologists to attempt new techniques that may decrease anesthetic morbidity in vulnerable MG patients. In addition to the use of sugammadex and remifentanil (discussed earlier), there is a small but growing body of evidence for the feasibility and advantageousness of preserving spontaneous ventilation and using a laryngeal mask airway during thoracoscopic thymectomy.[37,38]

A summary of anesthetic techniques to avoid residual opioid and NMBD effects thus far discussed is provided in Table 47.6. Each technique must be carefully considered relative to its risk/benefit profile, surgical parameters, and the individual patient. This table combines long-standing approaches to care with more novel or as-yet experimental techniques into a single framework for consideration by the thoughtful anesthesiologist attempting to optimize patient care.

TABLE 47.6 Summary of Potential Strategies to Reduce Respiratory Morbidity From the Use of Opioids and Neuromuscular Blocking Drugs in Myasthenia Gravis Patients Undergoing Surgery

Prioritization of neuraxial and/or regional analgesic techniques
Use of remifentanil in lieu of long-acting opioid or in lieu of NMBD entirely
Use of sugammadex rather than acetylcholinesterase inhibitors for NMBD reversal
Mindful utilization of the NMB effects of the potent inhaled anesthetics
Preservation of spontaneous ventilation for minimally invasive surgery; facilitates LMA use

LMA, Laryngeal mask airway; *NMB*, neuromuscular-blocking; *NMBD*, neuromuscular blocking drug.

References

1. Gilhus NE. Myasthenia gravis. *N Engl J Med.* 2016;375:2570–2581.
2. McGrogan A, Sneddon S, de Vries CS. The incidence of myasthenia gravis: a systematic literature review. *Neuroepidemiology.* 2010;34(3):171–183.
3. Carr AS, Cardwell CR, McCarron PO, McConville J. A systematic review of population based epidemiological studies in myasthenia gravis. *BMC Neurol.* 2010;10:46.
4. Paton WD, Waud DR. The margin of safety of neuromuscular transmission. *J Physiol.* 1967;191(1):59–90.
5. Blichfeldt-Lauridsen L, Hansen BD. Anesthesia and myasthenia gravis. *Acta Anaesthesiol Scand.* 2012;56(1):17–22.
6. Gilhus NE, Nacu A, Andersen JB, Owe JF. Myasthenia gravis and risks for comorbidity. *Eur J Neurol.* 2015;22(1):17–23.
7. Osserman KE, Genkins G. Studies in myasthenia gravis: review of a twenty-year experience in over 1200 patients. *Mt Sinai J Med.* 1971;38(6):497–537.
8. Jaretzki A 3rd, Barohn RJ, Ernstoff RM, et al. Myasthenia gravis: recommendations for clinical research standards. Task Force of the Medical Scientific Advisory Board of the Myasthenia Gravis Foundation of America. *Neurology.* 2000; 55(1):16–23.
9. Abraham A, Alabdali M, Alsulaiman A, et al. Repetitive nerve stimulation cutoff values for the diagnosis of myasthenia gravis. *Muscle Nerve.* 2017;55(2):166–170.
10. Stalberg E, Ekstedt J, Broman A. Neuromuscular transmission in myasthenia gravis studied with single fibre electromyography. *J Neurol Neurosur Ps.* 1974;37(5):540–547.
11. Schoser B, Eymard B, Datt J, Mantegazza R. Lambert-Eaton myasthenic syndrome (LEMS): a rare autoimmune presynaptic disorder often associated with cancer. *J Neurol.* 2017;264(9):1854–1863.

12. Weingarten TN, Araka CN, Mogensen ME, et al. Lambert-Eaton myasthenic syndrome during anesthesia: a report of 37 patients. *J Clin Anesth*. 2014;26(8):648–653.
13. Dierdorf SF, Walton JS, Stasic AF. Rare coexisting diseases. In: Barash PG, Cullen BF, Stoelting RK, Calahan MK, Stock MC, Ortega R, eds. *Clinical Anesthesia*. 7th edn. Philadelphia: Wolters Kluwer/Lippincott Williams & Wilkins; 2013:612–640.
14. Walker MB. Case showing the effect of prostigmin on myasthenia gravis. *Proc R Soc Med*. 1935;28(6):759–761.
15. Mehndiratta MM, Pandey S, Kuntzer T. Acetylcholinesterase inhibitor treatment for myasthenia gravis. *Cochrane Database Syst Rev*. 2011(2):CD006986.
16. Barth D, Nabavi Nouri M, Ng E, Nwe P, Bril V. Comparison of IVIG and PLEX in patients with myasthenia gravis. *Neurology*. 2011;76(23):2017–2023.
17. Wolfe GI, Kaminski NJ, Aban IB, et al. Randomized trial of thymectomy in myasthenia gravis. *N Engl J Med*. 2016;375(6):511–522.
18. Cata JP, Lasala JD, Williams W, Mena GE. Myasthenia gravis and thymoma surgery: a clinical update for the cardiothoracic anesthesiologist. *J Cardiothorac Vasc Anesth*. 2019;33:2537–2545.
19. Chigurupati K, Gadhinglajkar S, Sreedhar R, Nair M, Unnikrishnan M, Pillai M. Criteria for postoperative mechanical ventilation after thymectomy in patients with myasthenia gravis: a retrospective analysis. *J Cardiothorac Vasc Anesth*. 2018;32:325–330.
20. Jaretzki A. Thymectomy for myasthenia gravis: analysis of controversies—patient management. *Neurologist*. 2003;9:77–92.
21. Nilsson E, Muller K. Neuromuscular effects of isoflurane in patients with myasthenia gravis. *Acta Anaesthesiol Scand*. 1990; 34(2):126–131.
22. Nitahara K, Sugi Y, Higa K, Shono S, Hamada T. Neuromuscular effects of sevoflurane in myasthenia gravis patients. *Br J Anaesth*. 2007;98(3):337–341.
23. Imani F, Alebouyeh MR, Taghipour Anvari Z, Faiz SH. Use of remifentanil and alfentanil in endotracheal intubation: a comparative study. *Anesth Pain Med*. 2011;1(2):61–65.
24. Eisenkraft JB, Book WJ, Papatestas AE. Sensitivity to vecuronium in myasthenia gravis: a dose-response study. *Can J Anaesth*. 1990; 37(3):301–306.
25. Vymazal T, Krecmerova M, Bicek V, Lischke R. Feasibility of full and rapid neuromuscular blockade recovery with sugammadex in myasthenia gravis patients undergoing surgery - a series of 117 cases. *Ther Clin Risk Manag*. 2015;11:1593–1596.
26. Keating GM. Sugammadex: a review of neuromuscular blockade reversal. *Drugs*. 2016;76(10):1041–1052.
27. Baraka AS, Taha SK, Kawkabani NI. Neuromuscular interaction of sevoflurane–cisatracurium in a myasthenic patient. *Can J Anaesth*. 2000;47(6):562–565.
28. Eisenkraft JB, Book WJ, Mann SM, Papatestas AE, Hubbard M. Resistance to succinylcholine in myasthenia gravis: a dose-response study. *Anesthesiology*. 1988;69(5):760–763.
29. Abel M, Eisenkraft JB, Patel N. Response to suxamethonium in a myasthenic patient during remission. *Anaesthesia*. 1991;46(1): 30–32.
30. Basaranoglu G, Erden V, Delatioglu H. Anesthesia of a patient with cured myasthenia gravis. *Anesth Analg*. 2003;96(6):1842–1843.
31. Joshi GP, Bonnet F, Shah R, et al. A systematic review of randomized trials evaluating regional techniques for postthoracotomy analgesia. *Anesth Analg*. 2008;107(3):1026–1040.
32. Raft J, Chin KJ, Belanger ME, Clairoux A, Richebe P, Brulotte V. Continuous erector spinae plane block for thoracotomy analgesia after epidural failure. *J Clin Anesth*. 2018;54:132–133.
33. Su C, Su Y, Chou CW, et al. Intravenous flurbiprofen for post-thymectomy pain relief in patients with myasthenia gravis. *J Cardiothorac Surg*. 2012;7:98.
34. Cheng SP, Liu SC, Chou CL, Liu HC, Lee JJ. An uncommon cause of postthyroidectomy respiratory failure. *Thyroid*. 2009; 19(10):1129–1130.
35. Gorback MS, Moon RE, Massey JM. Extubation after transsternal thymectomy for myasthenia gravis: a prospective analysis. *South Med J*. 1991;84(6):701–706.
36. Wendell LC, Levine JM. Myasthenic crisis. *Neurohospitalist*. 2011; 1(1):16–22.
37. Jiang L, Depypere L, Rocco G, et al. Spontaneous ventilation thoracoscopic thymectomy without muscle relaxant for myasthenia gravis: comparison with "standard" thoracoscopic thymectomy. *J Thorac Cardiovasc Surg*. 2018;155:1882–1889.
38. Liu Z, Yang R, Sun Y. Nonintubated uniportal thoracoscopic thymectomy with laryngeal mask. *Thorac Cardiovasc Surg*. 2020;68(5): 449–454.

48

Hemoptysis, Empyema

MOHAMED R. EL TAHAN

Hemoptysis

Key Points

- Severe hemoptysis is a life-threatening medical emergency.
- Careful systematic workup is needed to identify the origin and reason for hemoptysis.
- The anesthesiologist should play an important role in identifying the severity and origin of hemoptysis, initiation first-aid management, and follow a systematic therapeutic plan according to the severity of hemoptysis.
- The anesthesiologist should select the best option for securing airway and sealing the source of bleeding from lung.
- There is no consensus on the best lung isolation tool in patients with hemoptysis, and it should depend upon the clinical scenario.

Introduction

Hemoptysis may present as mild or as a life-threatening condition. Massive hemoptysis, a major medical emergency associated with a high mortality,[1] has been defined in the literature by several different criteria, ranging from 100 to 600 mL of blood over wide-ranging periods of time.[2,3] These variations in definition are impacted by the difficulty in quantifying the amount of blood expectorated, which may be overestimated by patients.[3] In general, any hemoptysis that jeopardizes respiratory function should be considered a life-threatening medical emergency.[1]

Case Presentation

A 22-year-old male sustained several stab wounds to the back which penetrated into the right chest. He presented to the emergency department agitated and confused with severe hemoptysis, tachycardia, tachypnoea, and dyspnea. Physical examination revealed cyanosis, signs of respiratory distress, and absent breath sounds on the right chest. The arterial oxygen saturation was 83%, with a nonrebreather mask supplying oxygen at 15 L/min. Hemoglobin concentration was 7.5 g/dL and lactic acid was 3.7 mmol/L. Point-of-care sonography and chest radiograph showed a right hemopneumothorax. Electrocardiogram and transthoracic echocardiography showed no abnormalities.

Case Management

A chest tube was inserted to the right chest and a total of 1.2 L of blood was drained. Lactated Ringer's solution 2.0 L and 2 units of type-crossmatched packed red blood cells were administered and was followed with improved blood pressure and the level of consciousness. Chest radiography and computed tomography (CT) confirmed the presence of right hemopneumothorax. Cervical and abdominal CT scanning showed no abnormalities. The patient was brought to the operating room (OR) for emergency exploration via right posterolateral thoracotomy.

Problem A: How Can We Reduce Risk by Intraoperative Monitoring?

Routine monitors included five-lead electrocardiograph with ST segment analysis, processed electroencephalographic-based control the depth of anesthesia, and train-of-four stimulation of the ulnar nerve. Transcutaneous multifunction pads for monitoring, defibrillation, and pacing were connected to the chest wall. The radial artery was cannulated and connected to a fluid responsiveness monitoring system to guide hemodynamic parameters. An 8.0-F cordis was placed in the right internal jugular vein, and a urethral Foley's catheter was placed.

Rapid sequence induction was considered, a left-side double-lumen tube (DLT) was placed, and the proper DLT position was confirmed using a flexible 4.0-mm bronchoscope in both supine and lateral decubitus positions. Bronchoscopic examination showed significant bleeding from the right lower lobe, and the presence of major trachea-bronchial injury was ruled out. Surgery consisted of right thoracotomy and repair of the right lower lobe bronchial injury. The patient was extubated at the end of the procedure and postoperative course were uneventful.

Cause of Hemoptysis

Several causes for hemoptysis are presented in Table 48.1.

TABLE 48.1 **Common Causes of Hemoptysis**

Origin	Causes	References
Esophagus	Transesophageal echocardiography-induced injury of the bronchus	94
Pulmonary vessels	Vasculitis (e.g., long-standing vasculitis, Churg-Strauss syndrome)	95,96
	Following the Fontan procedure	97
	Pulmonary artery aneurysm	98,99
	Pulmonary vein obstruction and stenosis	100
	Arteriovenous malformation	101
	Pulmonary artery rupture by pulmonary artery catheter	2
Tracheobronchial tree	Traumatic intubation (e.g., violent intubation, deeply inserted a bougie intubating catheter in a patient with underlying endobronchial pathology	54,102
	Traumatic lower airway injuries	103,104
	Acquired trachea-bronchomalacia	105
	Tracheal bronchus	106
	Bronchopleural fistula	2
Alveolar	Tuberculosis	
	Cavitating lung abscess	107
	Neoplasm	2
	Bullae	108
	Diffuse alveolar hemorrhage secondary to negative-pressure pulmonary edema, cannabis, or sevoflurane anesthesia	109,110
	Pulmonary aspergilloma	111
	Lymphangiomyomatosis	112
	Intrapulmonary sequestration	113
Cardiac	Congenital heart disease	97
	Mitral stenosis or heart failure	2
Infradiaphragmatic	Intrathoracic rupture of hepatic hydatid cyst	114
	Thoracic endometriosis (catamenial hemoptysis)	2

Preoperative Assessment

Suspected hemoptysis must be confirmed, its severity established, the origin of bleeding located, and the cause determined.[3]

The diagnostic workup and management of severe hemoptysis is often challenging and includes chest x-ray (CXR), lung sonography, CT scanning, angiography, and importantly, bronchoscopy to identify the origin of bleeding.[2,3]

Detailed clinical history and physical examination should be emphasized on the initial causes and severity of hemoptysis to guide the diagnostic and therapeutic measures.[1,4]

Confirmation of hemoptysis is based on the direct observation of bleeding or as they are reported by the patient. Hemoptysis should be differentiated from hematemesis or bleeding from the oral cavity and nasal fossa.[5] Endoscopic examinations, such as rhinolaryngoscopy, gastroscopy, and bronchoscopy, may be needed to confirm the origin of the bleeding.

Location of origin and etiology can be identified and quantified during the initial efforts to control bleeding or when the patient condition has been stabilized.

Diagnostic tests should include[3,5–7]:

1. Clinical laboratory tests including complete blood count, coagulation parameters, and biochemistry.
2. Pulse oximetry and arterial blood gases to determine the impact of hemoptysis on oxygenation and ventilation.
3. If indicated once bleeding is controlled, spirometry can be done to determine the patient's pulmonary function. Spirometry should not be used in patients with active hemoptysis.[6]
4. Electrocardiogram to rule out pulmonary thromboembolism.

5. Transthoracic echocardiogram to detect endocarditis, mitral valve stenosis, congenital heart diseases, pulmonary hypertension, aortic aneurysm, or the presence of shunts because of arteriovenous malformations.
6. Cytologic study and sputum microbiology (e.g., Gram and Ziehl-Neelsen usual cultures and Lowëstein-Jensen).[5] Mantoux in patients with suspected tuberculosis.[5]
7. Blood cultures or serologies if infectious disease is suspected.[5]
8. Anterior-posterior and lateral CXR are the usual initial imaging tests performed in patients with hemoptysis.[3,5] CXR determines the site of bleeding in 45% to 65% of the cases and the cause in 25% to 35%.[2,7,8] However, as much as 10% of pulmonary malignancies are occult on CXR, whereas 96% of which will be detected by CT.[8]
9. Chest multidetector CT[3] must be performed in all patients with gross hemoptysis. It is useful to locate the origin of bleeding and give an idea about the proper isolation tool used (e.g., type of bronchial blocker [particularly in case of early takeoff origin of the right main bronchus] and proper size and side of double lumen tube [e.g., using the right-sided DLT in case of obstructed passage of the left main bronchus with a mass]).
10. Angiomultidetector CT is useful for identifying arteries which are the source of bleeding in hemoptysis and determining whether bronchial artery embolization is indicated or whether conservative treatment is sufficient.[3,9] Performing a CT requires the patient to be transported into a remote setting where it may be challenging to manage a massive bleed. In certain situations, it is preferable to prophylactically secure the patient's airway before transportation to the radiology suite, particularly for patients with life-threatening conditions[2] (Fig. 48.1).
11. Flexible bronchoscopy has an important role in identifying the severity (from blood-streaked sputum to gross hemoptysis), cause, and origin of hemoptysis. It can be performed rapidly at the patient's bedside in the intensive care unit (ICU) or in the OR.[1,3] It can also be used for collecting samples for cytology and microbiologic studies, bronchial aspirate, or bronchoalveolar lavage.
12. Rigid bronchoscopy obviously provides better scope for suctioning but does not generally allow visualization of upper lobes and peripheral lesions.[1,10] It allows localization of bleeding and provide a wide conduit for the instruments and catheters or materials instilled into the airways through the bronchoscope.[11,12] However, rigid bronchoscopy is performed in the OR and ventilation is best with intermittent jet ventilation.

Therapeutic Options[3]

1. **General Initial Management**
   Caution should be exercised for the classic ABCDE approach for management of patients with life-threatening hemoptysis (Box 48.1).

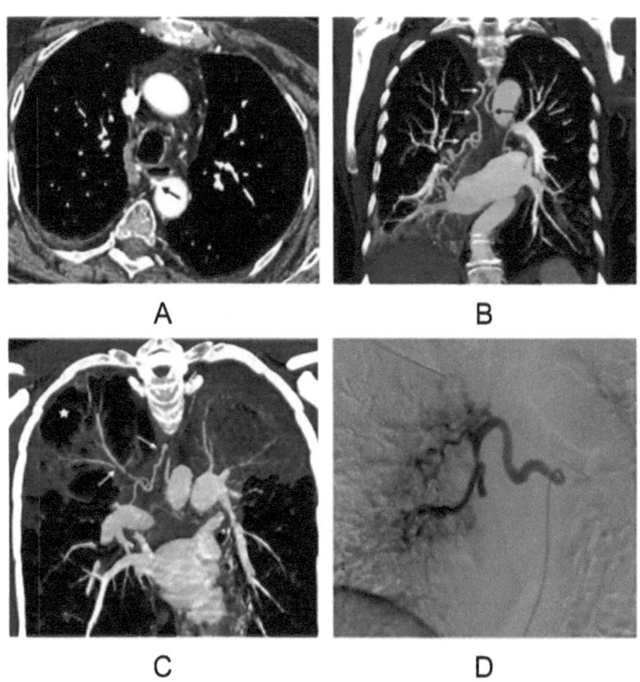

(A) Axial 1-mm-thick CT scan just below the aortic arch shows enlarged bronchial arteries (arrow) manifesting as avidly enhancing nodules in the paratracheal and retrobronchial regions of the mediastinum.

(B) Coronal thin-section MIP image demonstrates an enlarged intercostobronchial artery (arrows) coursing into the pulmonary parenchyma parallel to the bronchial airways

(C) Coronal thin-section MIP image obtained in a different patient provides a detailed analysis of the entire intrapulmonary course of an intercostobronchial artery (arrows) intracavitary mycetoma

(D) Reformatted image demonstrates how CT angiography can provide anatomic information that is useful for planning subsequent bronchial artery embolization.

MIP: maximum intensity projection

• **Fig. 48.1** Images from a thoracic computed tomography angiographic study performed with a 16–detector row scanner. (From Bruzzi JF, Rémy-Jardin M, Delhaye D, Teisseire A, Khalil C, Rémy J. Multi-detector row CT of hemoptysis. *RadioGraphics.* 2006;26:3–22.)

• BOX 48.1 General Initial Measures for Patients With Hemoptysis

ABCDE Approach

A: Secure airway with a large ETT or DLT.
B: Supplementary oxygen, if required. Monitor respiratory rate, oxygen saturation, and quantification of the hemoptysis.
C: Monitoring of vital signs (blood pressure, heart rate, capillary refilling time). Placement of large caliber venous access for fluid management, and if required, red blood cell transfusion. Type and crossmatching for RBCs or type O negative in emergency situations.
D: Lateral decubitus bed rest on the affected side. Chest physical therapy techniques must be avoided.
E: Bedside x-ray findings can be used to narrow down the site of the lesion.

Other Measures

1. Administration of antitussives to control coughing.
2. Empiric antibiotic treatment, useful in hemoptysis associated with respiratory infection and, in general, to prevent subsequent complications.
3. Antifibrinolytics (aminocaproic acid, tranexamic acid [TA])
4. Plasma-rich platelets
5. Desmopressin

DLT, Double-lumen tube; *ETT*, endotracheal tube; *RBCs*, red blood cells.

ABCDE Approach

Airway: Maintain the patency of airway. Intubation with a single-lumen tube (SLT) is recommended until the origin of bleeding is localized. In patients with lateralized or localized persistent bleeding, immediate control of the airway may be achieved by insertion of a DLT to isolate and ventilate the lungs and prevent spillage of blood to the contralateral lung, separately, or by endobronchial tamponade with a bronchial blocker.[1,13]

Breathing: Supplementary oxygen should be provided to every patient with hemoptysis. Respiratory rate and oxygen saturation should be closely monitored, and the amount of the hemoptysis should be quantified.[1,3]

Circulation: Monitoring of vital signs (blood pressure, heart rate, and capillary refill time) and placement of a large caliber venous access for rapid fluid administration and, if necessary, blood transfusion should be considered to stabilize the hemodynamic status. The use of uncrossmatched units of either type specific or group O packed red blood cells (PRBCs) can be used in emergency bleeding situations.[1,3]

Disability/Position: If the bleeding site is identified, the patient should be placed with the bleeding side down, to prevent blood contamination into the uninvolved lung. Chest physical therapy techniques must be avoided.[1,3]

Exposure: Bedside x-ray can be used to narrow down the origin of hemoptysis although it often inconclusive.

2. Other Measures to be Considered in the Management of Hemoptysis Include[3]:

A. Administration of antitussives to control coughing, however, oversedation should be avoided owing to the fear of airway obstruction.[5]

B. Empiric antibiotic treatment, useful in hemoptysis associated with respiratory infection and, in general, to prevent subsequent complications.

Antifibrinolytics (e.g., aminocaproic acid, tranexamic acid [TA]).[3] The clinical benefit of using TA has mixed results in the literature. Tscheikuna et al. enrolled 46 patients with hemoptysis completed the study. There were 21 in the TA group and 25 in the placebo group. The placebo group had a tendency not to have underlying lung disease and more patients who had a normal CXR. The benefit of TA in shortening the days of hemoptysis were not shown in this study.[14] Some investigators demonstrated that TA is effective in shortening the duration and volume of hemoptysis with low risk of thromboembolic complications. Moen et al. performed an analysis of 13 publication that represented the best evidence to answer the clinical question. Main outcomes included bleeding time, bleeding volume, and occurrence of thromboembolic complications after start of treatment. Based on results from the metaanalysis, no difference in remission of bleeding within 1 week was found between the TA and placebo groups. However, overall bleeding time was significantly shorter for the TA group. The authors concluded that limited research on the use of TA for treatment of hemoptysis exists. Because etiology of hemoptysis, as well as length of treatment, dosage, and form of TA administration varied between the studies, strong recommendations are difficult to give. Current best evidence, however, indicates that **TA may reduce both the duration and volume of bleeding, with low risk of short-term thromboembolic complications** in patients with hemoptysis.[15] Interestingly, inhaled TA (500 mg 3 times daily) can be used safely and effectively to control bleeding in patients with nonmassive hemoptysis.[16]

C. Autologous plasma rich platelets have been shown to stop bleeding immediately in 14 out of 20 patients with massive hemoptysis for 7 days.[17]

D. Desmopressin, a fast-acting blood-saving agent, can be used to control hemoptysis in various hereditary and acquired clotting disorders.[18]

3. Specific Treatment

A coordinated emergency team response is essential to guarantee the best chances of patient survival.[7] A systematic approach for definitive treatment of the patients with or without life-threatening hemoptysis has been developed from the previous reviews,[2,3,5,19,20] as shown in Fig. 48.2. The main steps are as follows:

A. Massive life-threatening hemoptysis:

i. In patients with unstable hemodynamic status, initial general treatment measures are considered to stabilize the patient's conditions. Immediate bronchoscopy should be performed in a well-equipped area (e.g., OR or ICU) to identify the cause and origin of the bleeding, secure the airway,

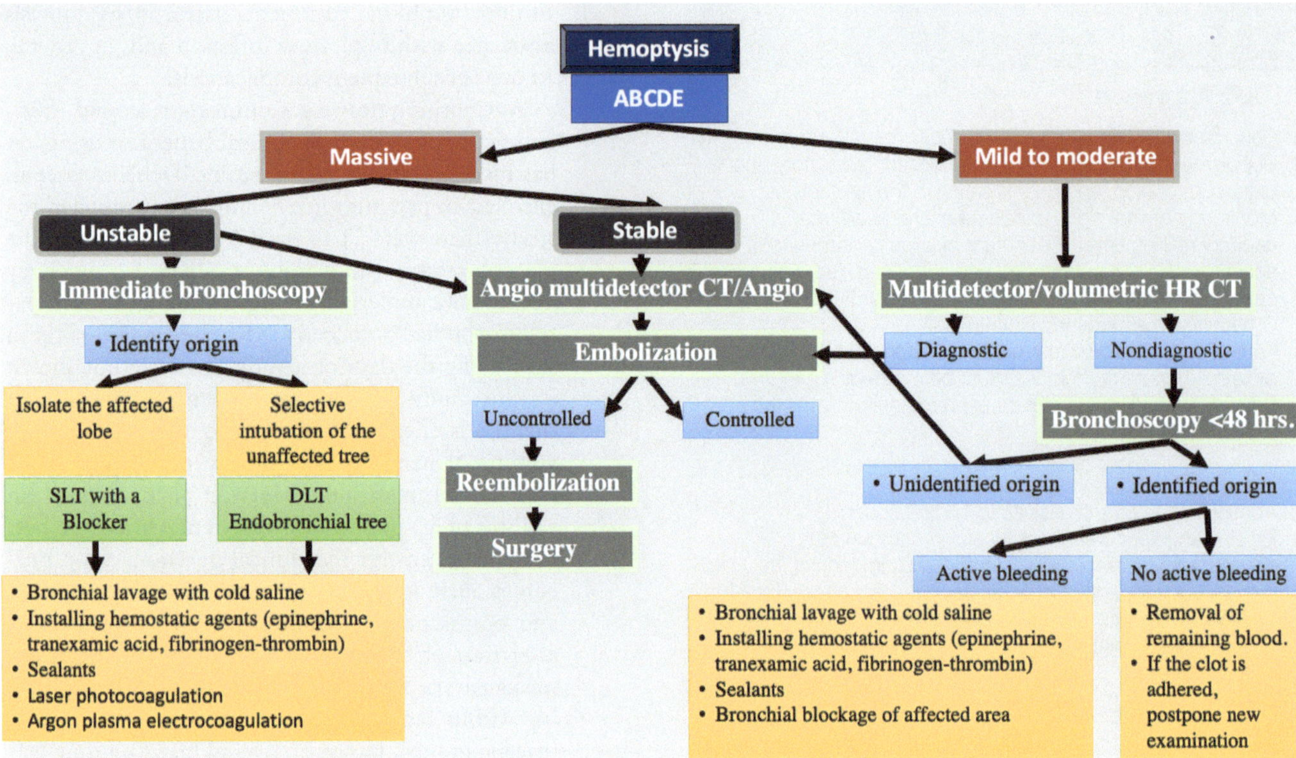

• **Fig. 48.2** A systematic definitive treatment approach for patients with or without life-threatening hemoptysis. It is produced from the previous reviews.[2,3,5,19,20] *CT*, Computed tomography; *DLT*, double-lumen endobronchial tube; *SLT*, single-lumen tube. ABCDE are the general measures as shown in Box 48.1.

administering topical measures to control bleeding (e.g., bronchial lavage, cryotherapy),[21,22] and applying topical hemostatic agents (e.g., cold saline[3] or less effective epinephrine diluted at 1:20,000[23]), sealants (e.g., Fibrinogen-thrombin [Tissucol], oxidized regenerated cellulose mesh [Surgicel] or silicone plugs [Watanabe spigot]),[3] laser photocoagulation,[24] or argon plasma electrocoagulation.[3] More definitive treatment options include angiographic embolization,[25,26] emergency surgery for lung resection,[27] or bronchial artery ligation surgery.[28] Extracorporeal membrane oxygenation (ECMO) could be considered as a rescue strategy in case of life-threatening aortobronchial fistula.[29]

ii. Patients with stable hemodynamic status should be subjected to either angiographic multidetector CT scanning or angiography to predict the value of bronchial artery embolization (Fig. 48.3). Reembolization or emergency surgery could have an

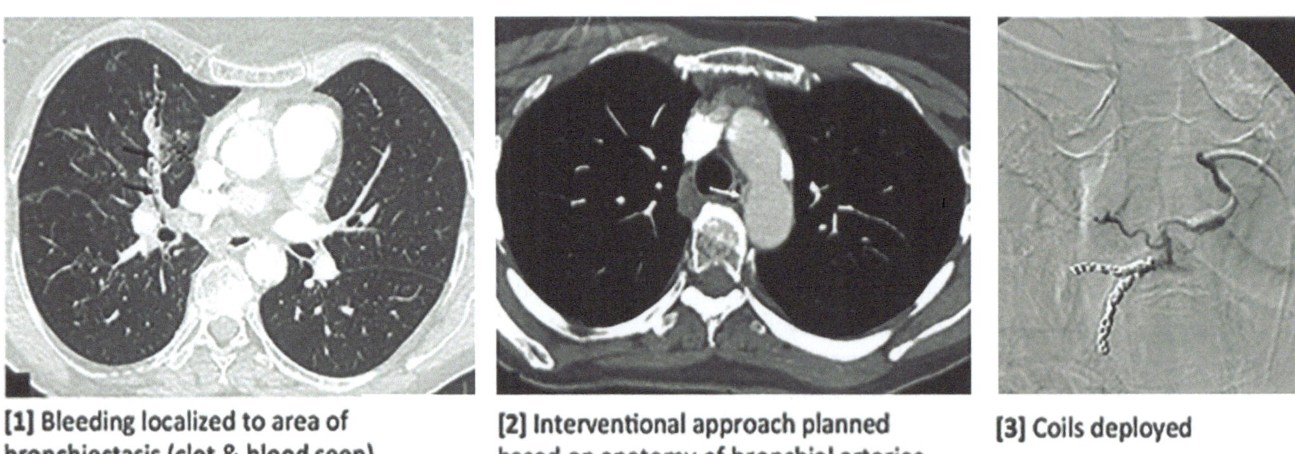

• **Fig. 48.3** Management of massive hemoptysis guided by early multidetector computed tomography scan. (From Khalil A, Fedida B, Parrot A, Haddad S, Fartoukh M, Carette M-F. Severe hemoptysis: from diagnosis to embolization. *Diag Inter Radiol*. 2015;96:775.)

important role in case of uncontrolled bleeding after embolization.

B. Mild to moderate hemoptysis:
   i. Multidetector or volumetric high-resolution CT scanning should be considered as a diagnostic tool.
   ii. Early bronchoscopy within 48 hours after presentation should be considered if the origin of bleeding could not be identified. Bronchial lavage, cryotherapy, applying topical hemostatic agents or sealants, or selective bronchial blockage of the affected area should be considered in patients with active bleeding. Caution should be exercised in patients with no active bleeding during removal of remaining blood and examination should be postponed if the clot is adhered.

Airway Protection

Objectives

Securing the airway by using the largest SLT possible (≥8.0 mm inner diameter) is the most important priority to enable passage of a flexible bronchoscope with a large working channel allowing extraction of obstructing blood clots and placement of bronchial blockers.[7,19] The main goals of anesthesia include volume resuscitation, isolating the bleeding lung or lobe to protect the normal lung, and providing sufficient oxygenation.[30]

Preparations and Monitoring

Rescue medications and equipment, including two rigid, large-bore Yankauer-type suction catheters attached to separate suction devices should be available.[31]

In addition to the standard monitors, including heart rate, noninvasive blood pressure, and pulse oximetry, invasive arterial catheterization and central venous catheterization are recommended. Large diameter intravenous catheters should be placed to allow for rapid fluid administration.[30]

The patient should be placed with the bleeding side down,[7,20,30] until lung isolation can be achieved.

Awake Endotracheal Intubation

Awake endotracheal intubation should be considered in emergency life-threatening hemoptysis with risks of airway obstruction, asphyxiation caused by flooding of the alveoli with blood, which might cause irreversible progressive hypoxia,[32] or bronchospasm during rapid sequence induction of anesthesia.[20,33,34]

Massive hemoptysis, usually accompanied with the patient's agitation, might preclude the use of awake fiberoptic intubation.[30]

The use of video laryngoscopes might offer new merits for awake endotracheal intubation in patients with massive hemoptysis.[31,35,36] Moreover, the video laryngoscopes could allow awake endobronchial intubation using the DLT although it maybe more difficult than intubation with an SLT.[37]

Rapid Sequence Induction

Rapid sequence induction of anesthesia might be considered in nonlife-threatening situations with ensuring the accessibility of rescue equipment and medications. Short active muscle relaxants should be used only if the airway is reassuring. Any concern regarding control of the airway should be managed with awake intubation. The practitioner should never burn his bridges.[33,34] Etomidate or ketamine are appropriate for induction of general anesthesia in patients with unstable hemodynamic status.[31]

Isolation of the Bleeding Lung/Lobar (see Chapter 16)

There is no consensus on the best method of lung isolation for patients with hemoptysis (Case Studies shown in Fig 48.4).

1. **Bronchial Blockers**

   Bronchial blockers can be used for isolating the main bronchus or selective lobar bronchus blockade to allow control of the bleeding lung or lobe, respectively by tamponade. The bronchial blockers are usually available in 7.0 F or 9.0 F for adult patients who require tracheal intubation with a SLT with a minimum size of 7.5 or 8.0 mm inner diameter, respectively. That allows the insertion of the flexible bronchoscopes with a size of 3.8 to 4.0 mm outer diameter.[38] The use of video laryngoscopes allows effective suctioning of blood and direct visualization of tracheal intubation with the bronchial blocker before placement of the SLT. Bronchial blockers could be placed through tracheostomy tube in patients with tracheostomies.[39]

   Bronchial blockers are more expensive than DLTs may take longer time to placement, and could be associated with more frequent dislodgement.[40,41] The use of bronchial blockers limits the effective suctioning of blood because of their narrow inner lumens. In addition, blood stagnation in the lung distal to the blocker's inflated cuff has long-term side effects.[42] However, if the patient is bleeding with the SLT in place and there is a concern regarding control of airways while converting to a DLT, it is best to use a bronchial blocker to tamponade the main bronchus of the bleeding side.

   There are several types of blockers as summarized subsequently and in Table 48.2.

   A. Fogarty Embolectomy Catheter: High-pressure low volume Fogarty embolectomy catheter (size 9.0 F in adults and 5.0 F in pediatrics) is currently used by some pulmonologists for patients with hemoptysis.[39] However, placement of the reformed rigid tip of Fogarty catheter in the right upper lobe can be challenging, particularly can not be used for suctioning without deflating the cuff. In light of availability of several types of blockers, it is almost never used and is limited for selective blockade in small children because of the risks for tracheobronchial injury owing to its low volume high pressure cuff.[43,44]
   B. The Fuji Uniblocker allows flexible high torque control and good control of the catheter tip and can be easily directed to block a selective lobar bronchus (see Table 48.2). The 1.8-mm lumen allows better suctioning of blood than other blockers but less than a DLT.

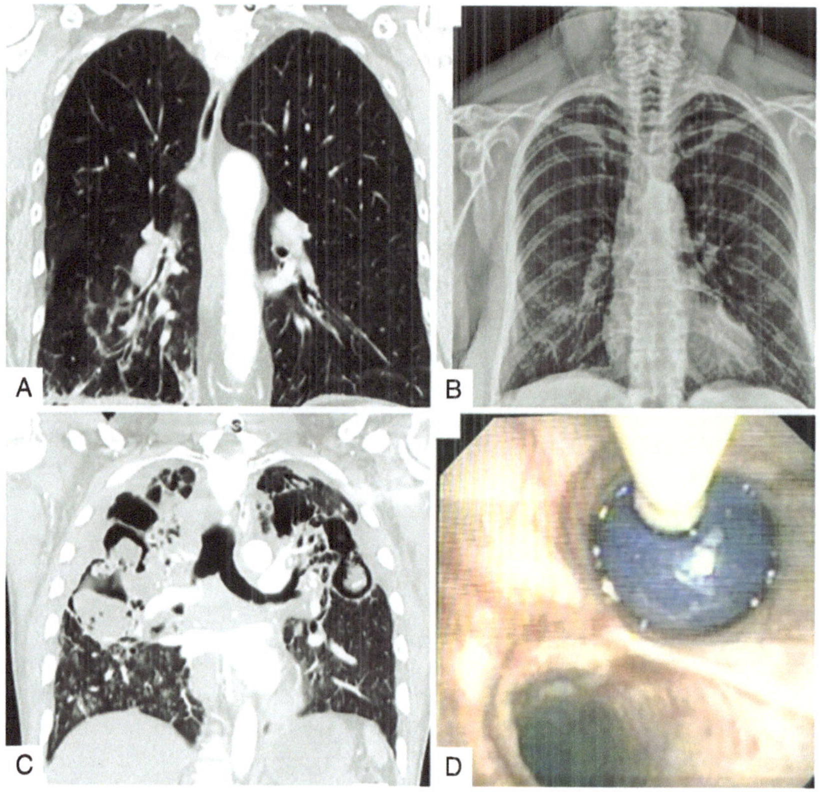

• **Fig. 48.4** Case studies—a systematic approach to the management of massive hemoptysis. **A,B,** A 59-year-old female with massive hemoptysis and bilateral bronchiectasis. Bronchoscopy revealed right lower lobe as a source of hemorrhage. **C,** A 47-year-old male with bilateral cavitation and mycetoma. Right upper lobe was identified as source of bleeding by FOB. **D,** Both subjects were stabilized by ETT intubation and right-sided bronchial blockade prior to bronchial artery embolization. (From Radchenko C, Alraiyes AH, Shojaee S. A systematic approach to the management of massive hemoptysis. *Journal of Thoracic Disease* (2017): S1069-S86. https://jtd.amegroups.com/article/view/15576.)

C. The Arndt wire-guided endobronchial blocker, available in 7.0 and 9.0 F sizes for adult patients, could be directed to any of the lobar bronchi.[45,46] It has a Tuohy-Borst–type valve that locks the blocker in place and maintains an airtight seal.

D. The Cohen flexitip endobronchial blocker, available in 9.0 F size, has a narrow central lumen of 1.6-mm in diameter. A 2-cm external plastic sleeve (gripper) improves manual control of blocker tip rotation during placement into the desired bronchus.[13,42,47] As

TABLE 48.2 Author's Recommended Choices for Selective Lung/Lobar Blockade Based on the Current Evidences Available

Lung/Lobe	Double-Lumen Tube Side	Fuji Uniblocker Torque Control	Arndt Wired Tip	Cohen Deflecting Tip	EZ Blocker	Coopdech Angled Tip
Right lung	Left or right	Green	Green	Green	Green	Green
Right upper lobe	Left	Yellow	Green	Yellow	Yellow	Yellow
Tracheal bronchus	Left	Yellow	Yellow	Yellow	Red	Yellow
Right middle lobe	Left or right	Green	Green	Green	Red	Green
Right lower lobe	Left or right	Green	Green	Green	Red	Green
Left lung	Left or right	Green	Green	Green	Green	Green
Left upper lobe	Left or right	Green	Green	Green	Red	Green
Left lower lobe	Left or right	Green	Green	Green	Red	Green
References	42	40,115	45,46	13,42	48,49	50–54

This is based on the traffic light symbols as follows; **Green**: the tool absolutely could be useful. **Yellow**: the tool would be useful. **Red**: the evidence is not important enough to support using the tool.

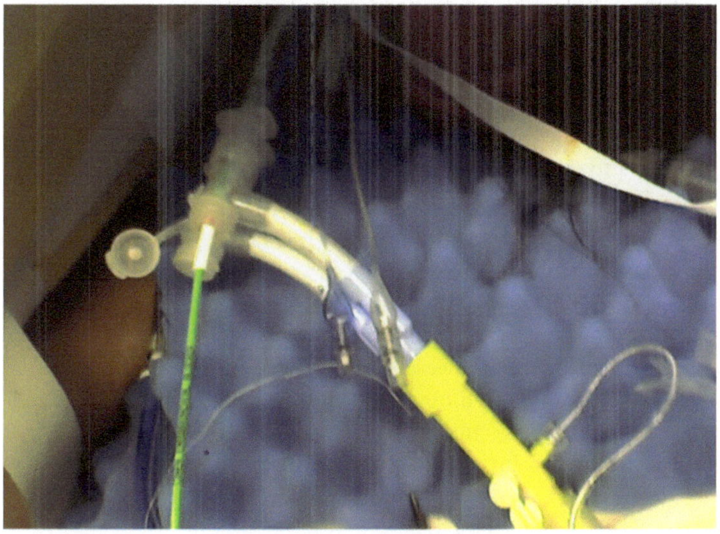

• **Fig. 48.5** The Cohen blocker is placed through the tracheal lumen of a double lumen tube to assist with control of a right lung bleeding (Courtesy of Edmond Cohen, MD).

depicted in Fig. 48.5, the Cohen blocker is placed through the tracheal lumen of a double lumen tube to assist with control of a right lung bleeding.

E. The EZ blocker has a unique Y-shaped distal end that mirrors the bifurcation of the trachea. It has been described for lung isolation in patients with tracheal bronchus.[48,49] With massive hemoptysis, the view is limited if not impossible through the bronchoscope. The EZ blocker has a distinct advantage over the other blockers because it would not necessarily require the use of a fiberoptic bronchoscope for correct positioning but instead can be placed using clinical signs.

F. The Coopdech blocker has a preformed angulated distal tip which allows selective blockade.[50–54] However, the tip can be damaged at the Murphy's eye of the endotracheal tube or at the carina.[55]

2. Double-Lumen Endobronchial Tubes

Endobronchial intubation using a DLT is a vital method in saving lives in massive hemoptysis.[56,57] In addition to allowing selective ventilation of both lungs, the DLT positioning does not require the initial identification of the side from which the bleeding originates.[2] The DLT could be used for hemoptysis originating from either lung except in patients with a tracheal takeoff of the right upper lobe, which is a rare anatomic variant, because of the associated risks for spillage of blood into the right middle and lower lobes (see Table 48.2).

The right-sided DLT requires a longer time to position and has a smaller margin of safety with regard to the right upper lobe ventilation, which may result in collapse from right upper lobe orifice obstruction.[42]

There is an increased use of the DLT outside operating theater settings particularly in the ICU. However, some ICU clinicians are reluctant to use the DLT for lung isolation in cases of hemoptysis because of being less skilled than anesthesiologists in using them or the risks for misplacement and leakage with soiling the healthy lung.[13,58] In addition, the DLT has narrow lumens that do not permit efficient evacuation of clots or use of the standard-sized 6.0-mm flexible bronchoscopes with large working channels to allow evacuating hemorrhage and blood clots from airways.[7,19]

Massive hemoptysis precludes visualization the airway when using the small-size flexible bronchoscopes for placement of the DLT.[20,30]

The skills of the clinicians in using the DLT could be built up through structured training courses. The identification of variations in bronchial anatomy before placement of DLTs and routine use of fiberoptic bronchoscope would reduce the incidence of misplacements and spillage.[59,60]

3. Selective Endobronchial Intubation

This involves advancing an endobronchial tube into the mainstem bronchus contralateral to the bleeding site under direct visualization with the bronchoscope. It has the risk of nonventilating the right upper lobe, when the shorter right mainstem bronchus is intubated.[2]

Tips for optimum sealing:

The use of a DLT to secure the airways in the presence of hemoptysis is the gold standard. The DLT clearly provides the best lung isolation with protection of the nondiseased lung from spillage of blood in case of hemoptysis, of pus in case of empyema, or of water when lung lavage is being performed. Endobronchial spillage of blood into a normal healthy lung or lobes can be prevented using the following suggestions:

A. The proper position of the tip of the DLT or bronchial blocker in the targeted main or lobar bronchus should be ensured. This requires identification of the variations in bronchial anatomy from chest radiography and bronchoscopic examination, selection of the optimum isolation tool, and the use of a flexible bronchoscope to confirm the proper tip position.[59,60]

B. Water-tight seal: Lung isolation using saline rather than air for balloon inflation of the bronchial blockers, such as Arndt Endobronchial Blocker or the Cohen Tip Deflecting Endobronchial Blocker, is a well-described technique for consistent balloon inflation for the management of massive hemoptysis.[13] Similarly, Hannallah et al.[58] demonstrated that neither an air-tight bronchial seal nor cuff pressure of 25 cm H_2O guaranteed protection against aspiration. The risk of aspiration was greatest when the DLT was positioned in the dependent lung and when the bronchial cuff volume was less than 1 mL, which most likely would not provide an appropriate seal of the bronchus lumen.

C. Lubricating the cuff with lubricant gel: A small study looked at using an artificial tracheobronchial tree that was intubated with a DLT, and showed that lubricant gel coating on the endobronchial cuff can effectively reduce the lung-to-lung aspiration.[61]

Life-Threatening Refractory Hypoxemia

Takahashi et al. demonstrated successful combined use of emergency thoracic endovascular aortic repair (TEVAR) and venovenous ECMO in a life-threatening hemoptysis in a patient with an aortobronchial fistula.[29] However, that treatment modality should be considered with extreme caution because massive hemoptysis itself is still a rare complication of ECMO that requires discontinuation of anticoagulation during increased hemoptysis.[62]

Conclusion

A systematic approach should be accomplished through a multidisciplinary team to diagnose and treat severe life-threatening hemoptysis. Attention should be paid to awake tracheal intubation in patients with massive hemoptysis airway. Lung or lobar isolation could be established using a bronchial blocker or DLT.

Empyema

Key Points

- Empyema, a common disease in developing countries, can be caused by a wide range of pathogens.
- An anesthesiologist, as a perioperative physician, should identify the risk factors for empyema, patients with sepsis or septic shock, stage of empyema, and proper timing for surgical intervention including the need for conversion to open surgery.
- Treatment modalities for empyema, including chest tube drainage, intrapleural fibrinolysis, thoracoscopic, or open surgery are chosen according to the stage of the disease.
- Lung isolation can be accomplished by using DLTs, bronchial blockers, or combination.
- Attention should be paid to expand the long-standing collapsed lung or lobe.
- Nonintubated (tubeless) thoracoscopic surgery might open new merits for unstable patients with empyema.

Introduction

Empyema is an accumulation of pus in the pleural space. Empyema cannot be coughed out and must be drained by a chest tube insertion needle or surgery. The incidence of empyema, defined as pus with a positive culture from nonpurulent pleural fluid, is increasing across all age groups.[63]

Case Presentation

A 48-year-old male presented with a left-side empyema following an explorative thoracotomy for traumatic hemothorax. He had a history of traumatic aortic injury treated with TEVAR, dorsal and lumbar spine injury, and bilateral lower limbs paresis following a road traffic accident 90 days earlier. On examination, he was mechanically ventilated at an inspired oxygen fraction of 0.35 through a placed tracheostomy tube. His Glasgow Coma Scale was 11/15, heart rate was 125 beats per minute; he had normal blood pressure and cardiac troponin levels. White blood cells were 4.7 /µmL, sodium was 138 mmol/L, albumin was 2.2 g/dL, lactic acid 1.1 mmol/L, and procalcitonin was 17.47 mcg/L. He was scheduled for a left pleural decortication and drainage.

Case Management

Initially, the risks for sepsis, stage or empyema, optimum timing and type of surgical procedure must be established.

The patient had signs of severe sepsis with normal lactate level. Hypoalbuminemia can be identified as a risk factor for empyema.

From the history, it appeared that patient had a stage 3 empyema because he underwent an explorative left thoracotomy surgery 90 days earlier, that was complicated with immediate pleural collection and fever. That indicated the need for pleural decortication through an open thoracotomy rather than thoracoscopy. Procalcitonin level was higher than 0.25 mcg/L indicating that it was not the proper timing for pleural decortication.[64]

Management

Securing the airway, lung isolation, correcting hypoxemia, and establishing venous access for the early administration of fluids and antibiotics are priorities in the management of patients with sepsis. An arterial catheter and central venous catheter were placed. Fluid resuscitation was guided with monitoring pulse contour derived cardiac index and stroke volume variation. A Fuji Uniblocker 9.0 F was placed in the left main stem bronchus through the tracheostomy tube under flexible bronchoscopic guidance. Surgery revealed a retained missed lap tape from the first surgery at another hospital. Intraoperative course was complicated with development of septic shock, which requires treatment with fluids, norepinephrine, and vasopressin, which were discontinued on the postoperative day 2.

Causes of Empyema

There are different causes of empyema as demonstrated in Table 48.3 and Fig. 48.6.

Preoperative risk identification and preparation

1. **Identifying Risk Factors for Empyema**
   Low serum albumin (<30 g/L), sodium (<130 mmol/L) levels, raised C-reactive protein (CRP) (>100 mg/L) and platelet count (>400 × 10^9 platelets/L), intravenous drug use, and chronic alcohol abuse[65] are independent

TABLE 48.3 Common Causes of Empyema

Origin	Causes	References
Gram-positive pathogens	*Staphylococcus aureus* *Streptococcus milleri* *Streptococcus anginosus*	66,116,117 118 119
Gram-negative pathogens	*Acinetobacter baumannii* *Legionella pneumophila*	116,117 120
Mycobacterium	*Mycobacterium tuberculosis*	121
Anaerobes	Peptostreptococci *Prevotella* species *Bacteroides fragilis*	119,122
Fungal	*Aspergillus fumigatus*	123
Polymicrobial empyema	S. anginosus group and anaerobes are frequent pathogens in empyema, and polymicrobial etiology	119
Posttraumatic empyema	That usually occurs in the severely injured critically ill patients with diverse pathogens and polymicrobial flora	122,124
Infradiaphragmatic	Spontaneous bacterial empyema caused by Enterobacteriaceae (e.g., *Escherichia coli* and *Klebsiella pneumoniae*) in patients with cirrhosis and hepatic hydrothorax	125,126
Others	*Salmonella houtenae*	127

1. Translocation of microorganisms from alveoli
2. Hematogenous spread (e.g., secondary to bacteremia)
3. Direct inoculation (e.g., surgical or nonsurgical trauma)
4. Diaphragmatic translocation of microorganisms from the abdomen
5. Contiguous spread from a mediastinal focus of infection
6. Reactivation of infection that is dormant adjacent to the pleural space (e.g., tuberculosis)

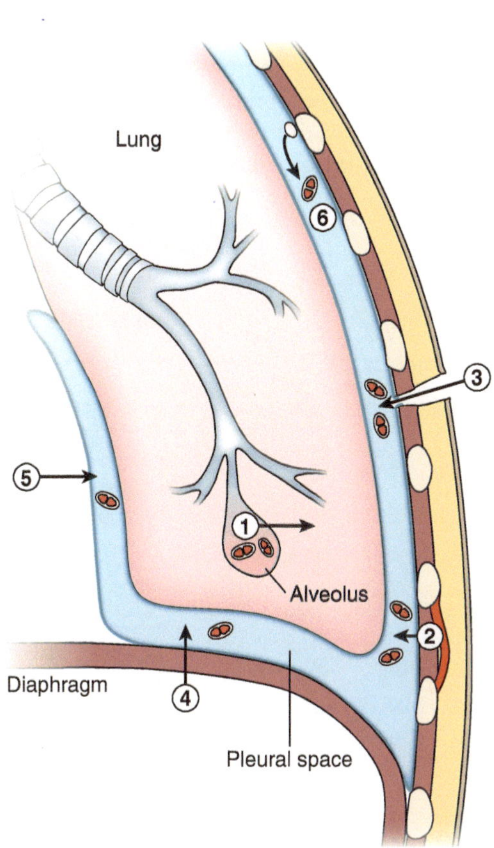

• **Fig. 48.6** Translocation of microorganisms from the alveolar space into the pleural space. (From https://www.uptodate.com/contents/image?imageKey=PULM%2F121168&topicKey=PULM%2F6702&source=see_link. © 2020 UpToDate.)

predictors of the development of pleural infection following community-acquired pneumonia.[66]

2. **Identifying Patients With Signs of Sepsis and Septic Shock**
   Patients with pleural empyema show the clinical signs of infections consisting of fever, chest pain, dyspnea, leukocytosis, and elevation of CRP. However, white blood cells and CRP are not appropriate enough to recognize bacterial infections or to distinguish between systemic and local infections.[64] Patients with sepsis and septic shock should be identified, and the sepsis "hour-1 bundle" should be initiated immediately to lessen the global burden of sepsis. The 3-hour and 6-hour bundles have been combined into a single "hour-1 bundle" with the explicit intention of beginning resuscitation and management immediately. This reflects the clinical reality at the bedside of these seriously ill patients with sepsis and septic shock—that clinicians begin treatment immediately, rather than waiting or extending resuscitation measures over a longer period. More than 1 hour may be required for resuscitation to be completed, but initiation of resuscitation and treatment such as obtaining blood for measuring lactate and blood cultures, administration of fluids and antibiotics, and in the case of life-threatening hypotension, initiation of vasopressor therapy should all be initiated immediately.[67]
3. **Identifying the Stage of Empyema**
   There are three stages/phases of empyema as presented in Table 48.4. Patients with stage 3 and pulmonary fibrosis have an increased risk of pneumothorax with markedly delayed resolution because of the high negative pleural pressures necessary for the expansion of stiff, fibrotic lungs. In these cases, prolonged chest-tube drainage in turn predisposes to the development of an organizing empyema, which frequently requires thoracotomy and definitive lung decortication, rather than a simpler thoracoscopic procedure, which is appropriate for early empyema.[68]
4. **Proper Timing of Surgery**
   The optimal time for surgical management of "parapneumonic" empyema in need of pleurectomy and decortication could be defined as the time from diagnosis of empyema and reaching procalcitonin levels under 0.25 mg/L, a preoperative blood marker for guidance of antibiotic therapy in lower respiratory tract infection with antibiotic treatment. Caviezel et al. attempted to define if the surgical outcomes will be better when procalcitonin (PCT) levels have dropped to normal ranges as evidence for resolution of the underlying pneumonia. They retrospectively analyzed outcomes of 38 patients with advanced parapneumonic empyema who underwent open decortication and pleurectomy with available preoperative PCT (pPCT) values. Patients were divided into two groups based on the pPCT cut-off of 0.25 mcg/L. Patients with a pPCT of 0.25 mcg/L or higher had a significantly longer total length of stay compared with patients with a pPCT level under 0.25 mcg/L. Eight patients in the pPCT 0.25 mcg/L or higher group had postoperative complications with two deaths, while no complications occurred in the PCT under 0.25 mcg/L group.[64] That typically should be within 4 weeks from the start of symptoms.[69]
5. **Predicting Surgical Approach**
   An anesthesiologist, as a perioperative physician, plays an important role in identifying the risk factors for predicting the need for conversion from thoracoscopic to open thoracotomy surgery. These predictive factors include a prolonged delay from diagnosis to operation, the presence of fever or frank pus during thoracentesis,[70] and of pleural thickness on CT images.[71,72] Of note, the duration of surgery and postoperative complications are significantly higher for thoracotomy patients.[71] That would help in preoperative planning for the appropriate postoperative pain control regimen.

TABLE 48.4 Stages/Phases of Empyema

	Phase/Stage 1	Phase/Stage 2	Phase/Stage 3
Name	Parapneumonic effusion	Fibrinopurulent stage	Chronic organizing stage
Pleural fluid/ space	A free-flowing exudate	Loculated fluids rich in fibrin	• Scar tissue (pleural cortex) formation • In the later stages, a solid fibrous pleural cortex begins to form, which may encase the lung, preventing reexpansion
Contents	• Low white cell count • LDH level less than half that in the serum • Normal pH • Glucose level: normal	• With or without white cells (pus) • LDH >1000 IU/L • pH <7.20 • Glucose level <2.2 mmol/L	
Microorganism	None	Bacterial invasion across the damaged lung epithelium	

LDH, Lactate dehydrogenase.

From Scarci M, Abah U, Solli P, et al. EACTS expert consensus statement for surgical management of pleural empyema. *Eur J Cardiothorac Surg.* 2015;48(5):642–653.

6. **Patients With Lung Cancer**

Special caution should be exercised in patients with empyema with associated lung cancer. Lung resection surgery, if possible, can provide full control of the infection. Preoperative pleural drainage through a chest tube might be required for 20 to 30 days, until there is no existing signs of infection.[73]

Diagnostic Tests

1. Pleural ultrasound confirms the presence and estimates the volume of pleural fluid, differentiates between pleural fluid and thickening, and assists in performing thoracentesis.[74]
2. CT is helpful in assessment of the extent of the pleura thickening and chest tube position if existing, expecting the stage of the empyema, and differentiation between lung abscesses and empyema. It is useful in choosing the appropriate type and size of DLT.[74]
3. Bronchoscopy is usually performed at the time of surgery to examine the variation in the anatomy of tracheobronchial tree and sputum or mucus plug removal before decortication will facilitate lung reexpansion in case of observed mass or lung volume loss on imaging.[74]

Treatment Modalities

1. Patients With Severe Sepsis or Septic Shock

The sepsis "hour-1 bundle"[67] should be initiated including: (1) measurement of lactate level and remeasurement if the initial lactate level is over 2 mmol/L, (2) obtain blood cultures before administration of antibiotics, (3) immediate administration of broad spectrum antibiotics less than 1 hour after sepsis diagnosis,[75] (4) fluid resuscitation (up to 30 mL/kg of crystalloids) for hypotension and a lactate level 4 mmol/L or higher, and (5) early infusions of vasopressors to maintain mean arterial blood pressure greater than 65 mm Hg to limit the need for overzealous fluid therapy.[67] The initial fluid resuscitation should be guided with monitoring of the fluid responsiveness using a transpulmonary thermodilution technique to avoid the harmful effects of fluid overload in patients with noncompliant lungs secondary to pleural empyema.[76,77]

2. Treatment options are based on the stage of pleural empyema as follows:

Stage 1: Parapneumonic effusion

Standard therapy in the treatment of early pleural space infection includes:

A. **Chest tube drainage and systemic antibiotics**

All patients with a pleural effusion identified on CXR in association with sepsis or a pneumonic illness require a prompt diagnostic pleural fluid sampling because it is impossible clinically to differentiate the presence of a complicated parapneumonic effusion requiring chest tube drainage from a simple effusion that may resolve with antibiotics alone.[74]

Patients with frankly purulent or turbid/cloudy pleural fluid on sampling should receive prompt chest tube drainage. The efficacy of drainage is assessed by a complete lung expansion and a resolution of symptoms.[65,74]

B. **Intrapleural fibrinolysis**[65,74]

The introduction of fibrinolytic agents (streptokinase, urokinase, and alteplase) into the pleural space might cleave fibrous septations and improve the drainage of fibrinopurulent empyema.[65,74] It usually will be reserved for the patients unsuitable for surgery who would not be able to tolerate one-lung ventilation. The common dosages are 250,000 IU of streptokinase or 100,000 IU of urokinase daily for 3 to 5 days.[65] The recombinant tissue plasminogen activator in combination with deoxyribonuclease could be used as an alternative therapy.[78]

Stages 2 and 3: Fibrinopurulent and Chronic organizing stages

Surgical approaches

A. Video-assisted thoracoscopic surgery (VATS) for pleural debridement and decortication, particularly for those with loculated empyema.[79] The need for intraoperative conversion from VATS to thoracotomy correlates with the stage of disease and time from symptom onset.[65,74] Therefore the optimal timing of thoracoscopic drainage and decortication for empyema is in patients with symptom durations of less than 4 weeks.[69]
B. Open thoracotomy for evacuation of all purulent material and thorough decortication of the parietal and visceral pleura together with complete separation of the diaphragm from the lung.[65,74]

Indications of surgical treatment[74]

A. VATS is indicated in patients with stages 2 and 3 and are fit enough to undergo a surgical intervention because the empyema is not going to resolve with medical treatment (class I, level B).
B. Patients with stage 2 empyema with dual agents; intrapleural fibrinolysis may be considered as an alternative to surgery (class IIa, level B).
C. Open pleural decortication, which is an extensive intervention, is indicated in patients with stage 3 empyema with a prolonged period since the start of symptoms (class IIb, level C).

Perioperative Considerations

1. **Lung Isolation Versus Separation**

Collapsing the operative lung is a commonly used technique to facilitate surgical visualization and to provide lung isolation during thoracic surgical procedures for patients with empyema.

However, the surgical technique for pleural decortication is demanding and requires intermittent inflation-deflation sequences for the surgical lung to identify the correct plane and dissection, which often is difficult to identify. Identifying the correct dissection plane is crucial for avoiding laceration of the lung parenchyma. In addition, because the lung parenchyma inevitably will lacerate during the visceral pleura decortication, there is risk of fire. The oxygen rich mixture typically used during OLV can leak into the chest cavity, which may promote fire ignition.

The presence of abscess or bronchiectasis in patients with empyema have the risk of contaminating the healthy lobes or lung with infectious secretions and require careful "isolation" of the diseased lung or lobe. The latter is challenging during the need for inflation-deflation sequences because of the risk of healthy lung soiling with pus during two-lung ventilation periods.

2. **Lung Separation/Isolation Tool**

A. DLT

The DLT is mostly used by anesthesiologists as shown in previous regional surveys. The wide lumen of the DLT facilitates suctioning of thick pus from both lungs and alternation of one- and two-lung ventilations.

Primieri et al. described a rare blocking of the bronchial lumen opening by redundant inflamed tissue on the lateral wall of the left main stem bronchus in a patient with empyema.[80]

B. Bronchial blockers

They offer good alternative to the DLT for isolating the surgical lung, particularly in pediatric and tracheostomized patients.[81,82] In addition, the bronchial blocker could be used for selective blockade of the lobar bronchus of the diseased lobe particularly in patients who undergo previous pulmonary resection.[40,41] However, the bronchial blockers have some disadvantages in patients with empyema and pulmonary infection. First, the small lumen of the bronchial blocker can be easily blocked by thick pus.[83] Second, the thick purulent secretions could be collected distal to the inflated bronchial cuff with the risk of postoperative atelectasis and arterial oxygen desaturation.[83] Third, the healthy lung might be soiled during alternation of one- and two-lung ventilations. Careful bronchoalveolar lavage using a large caliber flexible bronchoscope is required after completion of surgery, particularly in cases of using the bronchial blocker. For all these reasons, and particularly because the bronchial blocker cuff is not reliable to provide an adequate seal to prevent the spread of a pus, bronchial blockers are not recommended to be used for lung isolation for emphysema.

C. Combined use of DLT and bronchial blockers for selective lobar blockade

The combined use of a DLT and bronchial blocker has been described for efficient lobal blockade in patients with empyema.[52,84] The DLT is first placed into the main bronchus then a bronchial blocker is placed either through[52,84] or outside the lumen of the DLT under bronchoscopic guidance to selectively blocking the infected lobe.[52] That technique has the potential for providing optimum sealing performance, reducing postoperative complications, and improving arterial oxygenation.[84]

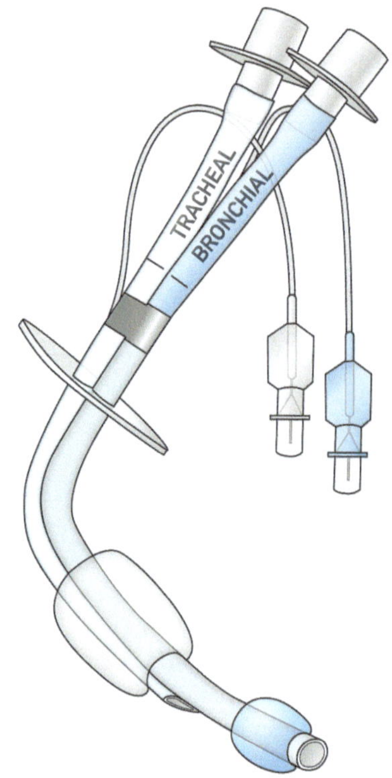

• **Fig. 48.7** Double-lumen tubes for tracheostomized patients. (Rüsch Tracheoparts, Teleflex Medical Europe Ltd.)

D. Endobronchial tube (see Fig. 48.5)

A previous study demonstrated the feasibility and safety of the combined use of an endobronchial tube and a retained airway exchange catheter (AEC) in children with empyema. The indwelling AEC allows readjustment of the tube position to provide alternation of one- and two-lung ventilations during the thoracoscopic procedure.[85]

E. Patients with tracheostomy

In patients undergoing thoracic surgery with a tracheostomy stoma in situ, the bronchial blocker can be placed through the tracheostomy tube to selectively block a lung or a lobar bronchus. There is a short version of DLT designed for the use through the tracheostomy stoma (Rüsch Tracheoparts, Teleflex Medical Europe Ltd., Athlone, Co Westmeath, Ireland). It is available in Europe but not in the United States (Fig. 48.7). In addition, oral intubation with a DLT, if oral intubation is possible, could be an alternative choice in tracheostomized patients.[86]

3. **Expanding the Collapsed Lobe or Lung**

Recruitment of the collapsed lung or lobe for a long time following pleural decortication might require using higher inflation pressures or a staircase or static recruitment strategy.[87]

Unilateral ipsilateral pulmonary edema in the remaining parenchyma after pleural decortication has been described following lung expansion.[88]

Recruiting the nonsurgical lung using apneic oxygenation or continuous positive airway pressure might be helpful to prevent or treat occasional hypoxemia during one-lung ventilation.[68]

Attention should be paid to identify significant air leak after pleural decortication.[89] Air leak (%) can be calculated as [(inspiratory tidal volume – expiratory tidal volume)/ inspiratory tidal volume × 100] and should be measured after restart of two-lung ventilation.[90] Spontaneous ventilation is best for avoiding air leak. It is there to best extubate the patient as soon as possible to avoid positive pressure ventilation.

4. Nonintubated VATS for Pleural Decortication

A regional European survey showed that 59% of respondents experienced nonintubated thoracic surgery, including pleural decortication.[91] Tubeless thoracoscopic pleural decortication could offer a feasible alternative for surgery under general anesthesia because spontaneous ventilation facilitates both identification of the correct plane and dissection, thus resulting in less surgical injury of the underlying lung. It results in satisfactory lung reexpansion in 95% of the patients.[92] Tubeless surgery under local anesthesia offers a good alternative for the debridement of a complicated parapneumonic effusion using a single-trocar thoracoscopy.[93]

Conclusion

The roles of anesthesiologists are not limited to providing optimum lung isolation and safe intraoperative anesthesia, but extends to improving postoperative patient's outcomes, helps in identification of the proper timing for surgical intervention, and considers the feasibility of VATS surgery. Recruiting the collapsed lung or lobes following pleural decortication should be accomplished with increasing airway pressures with ruling out significant air leak.

References

1. Hakanson E, Konstantinov E, Fransson SG, et al. Management of life-threatening haemoptysis. *Br J Anaesth.* 2002;88(2):291–295.
2. Gagnon S, Quigley N, Dutau H, et al. Approach to hemoptysis in the modern era. *Can Respir J.* 2017;2017:1565030.
3. Cordovilla R, de Miguel BE, Ares AN, et al. Diagnosis and treatment of hemoptysis. *Arch Bronconeumol.* 2016;52(7):368–377.
4. Estarriol MH, Sanchez MV, Goday MR, et al. [Utility of the clinical history, physical examination and radiography in the localization of bleeding in patients with hemoptysis]. *Ann Med Interna.* 2002;19(6):289–295.
5. Johnson JL. Manifestations of hemoptysis. How to manage minor, moderate, and massive bleeding. *Postgrad Med.* 2002;112(4): 101–106, 108–109, 113.
6. Jean-Baptiste E. Clinical assessment and management of massive hemoptysis. *Crit Care Med.* 2000;28(5):1642–1167.
7. Davidson K, Shojaee S. Managing massive hemoptysis. *Chest.* 2019;177(1):77–88.
8. Thirumaran M, Sundar R, Sutcliffe M, et al. Is investigation of patients with haemoptysis and normal chest radiograph justified? *Thorax.* 2009;64(10):854–856.
9. Mori H, Ohno Y, Tsuge Y, et al. Use of multidetector row CT to evaluate the need for bronchial arterial embolization in hemoptysis patients. *Respiration.* 2010;80(1):24–31.
10. Batra H, Yarmus L. Indications and complications of rigid bronchoscopy. *Expert Rev Respir Med.* 2018;12(6):509–520.
11. Dweik RA, Stoller JK. Role of bronchoscopy in massive hemoptysis. *Clin Chest Med.* 1999;20(1):89–105.
12. Alraiyes AH, Machuzak MS. Rigid bronchoscopy. *Semin Respir Crit Care Med.* 2014;35(6):671–680.
13. Gilbert CR, Mallow C, Wishire CL, et al. A prospective, ex vivo trial of endobronchial blockade management utilizing 3 commonly available bronchial blockers. *Anesth Analg.* 2019;129(6):1692–1698.
14. Tscheikuna J, Chvaychoo B, Naruman C, et al. Tranexamic acid in patients with hemoptysis. *J Med Assoc Thai.* 2002;85(4): 399–404.
15. Moen CA, Burrell A, Dunning J. Does tranexamic acid stop haemoptysis? *Interact Cardiovasc Thorac Surg.* 2013;17(6):991–994.
16. Wand O, Guber E, Guber A, et al. Inhaled tranexamic acid for hemoptysis treatment: a randomized controlled trial. *Chest.* 2018;154(6):1379–1384.
17. Sarmiento AGC, Danguilan JLJ, Mariano ZM, et al. Use of autologous platelet rich plasma (PRP) in stopping massive hemoptysis at the Lung Center of the Philippines: a pilot study. *J Vis Surg.* 2017;3:111.
18. Pea L, Roda L, Boussaud V, et al. Desmopressin therapy for massive hemoptysis associated with severe leptospirosis. *Am J Respir Crit Care Med.* 2003;167(5):726–728.
19. Yendamuri S. Massive airway hemorrhage. *Thorac Surg Clin.* 2015;25(3):255–260.
20. Cahill BC, Ingbar DH. Massive hemoptysis. Assessment and management. *Clin Chest Med.* 1994;15(1):147–167.
21. Ma Q, Shi B, Tian Y, et al. [Fibro-bronchoscopic cryosurgery for unresectable endobronchial tumors]. *Zhongguo Fei Ai Za Zhi.* 2014;17(7):545–549.
22. Rojas-Tula DG, Gomez-Fernandez M, Garcia-Lopez JJ, et al. Endobronchial cryotherapy for a mycetoma. *J Bronchol Interv Pulmonol.* 2013;20(4):330–332.
23. Schaal JV, Dubost C, De Rudnicki S, et al. Intratracheal instillation of epinephrine in life-threatening hemoptysis. *Minerva Anestesiol.* 2011;77(7):758.
24. Cheng Y, Zhang W, Zhang H, et al. [Holmium: yttrium-aluminum-garnet (Ho: YAG) laser lithotripsy in the treatment of broncholithiasis]. *Zhonghua Jie He He Hu Xi Za Zhi.* 2017;40(1):29–33.
25. Fellows KE, Stigol L, Shuster S, et al. Selective bronchial arteriography in patients with cystic fibrosis and massive hemoptysis. *Radiology.* 1975;114(3):551–556.
26. Kho SS, Chan SK, Yong MC, et al. Endobronchial embolization for life-threatening hemoptysis with Endobronchial Watanabe Spigot. *BMC Res Notes.* 2017;10(1):304.
27. Cheng BC. [Emergency lung resection in patients with massive hemoptysis]. *Zhonghua Wai Ke Za Zhi.* 1992;30(8): 490-1, 510.

28. Kaukuntla HK, Amer KM, Honeybourne D, et al. Extrapleural bronchial artery ligation for life-threatening hemoptysis in cystic fibrosis—a case report. *Angiology*. 2000;51(9):787–792.
29. Takahashi K, Kajitani M, Kamada T, et al. Endovascular repair with extracorporeal membrane oxygenation as a rescue strategy for aortobronchial fistula: a case report. *JA Clin Rep*. 2017;3(1):34.
30. Hatipoglu Z, Turktan M, Avci A. The anesthesia of trachea and bronchus surgery. *J Thorac Dis*. 2016;8(11):3442–3451.
31. Kristensen MS, McGuire B. Managing and securing the bleeding upper airway: a narrative review. *Can J Anaesth*. 2020;67(1): 128–140.
32. Maguire MF, Berry CB, Gellett L, et al. Catastrophic haemoptysis during rigid bronchoscopy: a discussion of treatment options to salvage patients during catastrophic haemoptysis at rigid bronchoscopy. *Interact Cardiovasc Thorac Surg*. 2004;3(2):222–225.
33. Carron H, Hill S. Anesthetic management of lobectomy for massive pulmonary hemorrhage. *Anesthesiology*. 1972;37(6): 658–659.
34. Peris A, Cianchi G, Bonizzoli M, et al. Anesthetic management of massive life-threatening hemoptysis. *Minerva Anestesiol*. 2010;76(9):765.
35. Brar MS. Airway management in a bleeding adult following tonsillectomy: a case report. *AANA J*. 2009;77(6):428–430.
36. Alhomary M, Ramadan E, Curran E, et al. Videolaryngoscopy vs. fibreoptic bronchoscopy for awake tracheal intubation: a systematic review and meta-analysis. *Anaesthesia*. 2018;73(9): 1151–1161.
37. Herbozo ES, Planas B, Ramasco F, et al. [Double lumen tube insertion in awake patients through the AirTraq laryngoscope in 2 cases of expected difficult airway]. *Rev Esp Anestesiol Reanim*. 2011;58(5):315–317.
38. Khidr AM, El Tahan MR, Doyle DJ, et al. Combined use of a fiberscope and fuji uniblocker for removal of retained bronchial tissue glue after repair of a disrupted left main bronchus. *Semin Cardiothorac Vasc Anesth*. 2019;23(3):333–337.
39. Spicek-Macan J, Hodoba N, Nikolic I, et al. Exsanguinating tuberculosis-related hemoptysis: bronchial blocker introduced through percutaneous tracheostomy. *Minerva Anestesiol*. 2009;75(6):405–408.
40. Campos JH. Update on selective lobar blockade during pulmonary resections. *Curr Opin Anaesthesiol*. 2009;22(1):18–22.
41. Campos JH. Which device should be considered the best for lung isolation: double-lumen endotracheal tube versus bronchial blockers. *Curr Opin Anaesthesiol*. 2007;20(1):27–31.
42. Awad H, Malik O, Hollis K, et al. Bronchial blocker versus double-lumen tube for lung isolation with massive hemoptysis during cardiac surgery. *J Cardiothorac Vasc Anesth*. 2013;27(3):e26–e28.
43. Toker A, Tanju S, Bayrak Y, et al. Life-threatening hemoptysis in a child: the only symptom. *Ann Thorac Surg*. 2004;77(1): 336–338.
44. Sharma A, Sinha S, Khanna S, et al. A novel technique to prevent endobronchial spillage during video assisted thoracoscopic lobectomy. *Ann Cardiol Anaesth*. 2014;17(2):164–166.
45. Espi C, Garcia-Guasch R, Ibanez C, et al. [Selective lobar blockade using an arndt endobronchial blocker in 2 patients with respiratory compromise who underwent lung resection]. *Arch Bronconeumol*. 2007;43(6):346–348.
46. Ng JM, Hartigan PM. Selective lobar bronchial blockade following contralateral pneumonectomy. *Anesthesiology*. 2003;98(1): 268–270.
47. Cohen E. The Cohen flexitip endobronchial blocker: an alternative to a double lumen tube. *Anesth Analg*. 2005;101(6):1877–1879.
48. Jain P, Nguyen DM, Fermin L, et al. Tracheal bronchus: anesthetic implications and importance of early recognition in the context of bronchial blocker use for lung isolation. *J Cardiothorac Vasc Anesth*. 2019;34(4):1019–1022.
49. Freitag L, Tekolf E, Stamatis G, et al. Three years experience with a new balloon catheter for the management of haemoptysis. *Eur Respir J*. 1994;7(11):2033–2037.
50. Cruz P, Orozco HD, Martinez IG, et al. [Selective lobar blockade with a Coopdech blocker combined with a double-lumen endotracheal tube for lung metastases resection by laser]. *Rev Bras Anestesiol*. 2018;68(2):200–204.
51. Ye J, Gu MN, Zhang CQ, et al. [Effects of selective left lower lobar blockade by Coopdech endobronchial blocker tube on intrapulmonary shunt and arterial oxygenation: a comparison with double-lumen endobronchial tube]. *Nan Fang Yi Ke Da Xue Xue Bao*. 2009;29(11):2244–2247.
52. Sumitani M, Matsubara Y, Mashimo T, et al. Selective lobar bronchial blockade using a double-lumen endotracheal tube and bronchial blocker. *Gen Thorac Cardiovasc Surg*. 2007;55(5):225–227.
53. Jing Y, Miaoning G, Chaoqun Z, et al. Selective left lower lobar blockade for lower oesophageal surgery. *Anaesth Intensive Care*. 2010;38(4):782–783.
54. Son M, Lee S, Lee SH, et al. Experience of hemostasis in tracheal bleeding very close to the carina by the bronchial blocker: a case report. *Korean J Anesthesiol*. 2016;69(3):270–274.
55. Venkataraju A, Rozario C, Saravanan P. Accidental fracture of the tip of the Coopdech bronchial blocker during insertion for one lung ventilation. *Can J Anaesth*. 2010;57(4):350–354.
56. Santana-Cabrera L, Arroyo MF, Rodriguez AU, et al. Double-lumen endobronchial tube in the emergency management of massive hemoptysis. *J Emerg Trauma Shock*. 2010;3(3):305.
57. Jean-Vivien S, Clement D, Jean-Pierre T, et al. Double-lumen endobronchial tube and alternatives in massive hemoptysis: How do you want to save lives? *J Emerg Trauma Shock*. 2011;4(3):438.
58. Hannallah MS, Gharagozloo F, Gomes MN, et al. A comparison of the reliability of two techniques of left double-lumen tube bronchial cuff inflation in producing water-tight seal of the left mainstem bronchus. *Anesth Analg*. 1998;87(5):1027–1031.
59. Slinger P. Lung isolation in thoracic anesthesia, state of the art. *Can J Anaesth*. 2001;48(suppl 1):R13–r15.
60. Slinger PD. Fiberoptic bronchoscopic positioning of double-lumen tubes. *J Cardiothorac Anesth*. 1989;3(4):486–496.
61. Hwang JY, Baik J, Nahm SF, et al. Prevention of lung-to-lung aspiration during emergency thoracic surgery: an experimental study. *World J Emerg Surg*. 2015;10:9.
62. Pitcher HT, Harrison MA, Shaw C, et al. Management considerations of massive hemoptysis while on extracorporeal membrane oxygenation. *Perfusion*. 2016;31(8):653–658.
63. Anthonisen NR. Empyema. *Can Respir J*. 2008;15(2):69–70.
64. Caviezel C, Schuetz P, Gerdes S, et al. Procalcitonin as preoperative marker for surgery in advanced parapneumonic empyema. *J Thorac Dis*. 2017;9(3):734–741.
65. Hofmann HS. Modern management of empyema thoracis. *Semin Thorac Cardiovasc Surg*. 2013;25(4):287–291.
66. Chalmers JD, Singanayagam A, Murray MP, et al. Risk factors for complicated parapneumonic effusion and empyema on presentation to hospital with community-acquired pneumonia. *Thorax*. 2009;64(7):592–597.

67. Levy MM, Evans LE, Rhodes A. The surviving sepsis campaign bundle: 2018 update. *Crit Care Med.* 2018;46(6): 997–1000.
68. Pfitzner J, Stevens HJ, Rao V, et al. One-lung ventilation in a patient with an organizing empyema and severe idiopathic pulmonary fibrosis. *Br J Anaesth.* 2006;97(2):266–268.
69. Chung JH, Lee SH, Kim KT, et al. Optimal timing of thoracoscopic drainage and decortication for empyema. *Ann Thorac Surg.* 2014;97(1):224–229.
70. Jagelavicius Z, Jovaisas V, Mataciunas M, et al. Preoperative predictors of conversion in thoracoscopic surgery for pleural empyema. *Eur J Cardiothorac Surg.* 2017;52(1):70–75.
71. Stefani A, Aramini B, della Casa G, et al. Preoperative predictors of successful surgical treatment in the management of parapneumonic empyema. *Ann Thorac Surg.* 2013;96(5):1812–1819.
72. Bongiolatti S, Voltolini L, Borgianni S, et al. Uniportal thoracoscopic decortication for pleural empyema and the role of ultrasonographic preoperative staging. *Interact Cardiovasc Thorac Surg.* 2017;24(4):560–566.
73. Subotic D, Petrov D, Gajic M. Lung resection for lung cancer after pleural empyema. *Thorac Cardiovasc Surg.* 2013;61(7): 612–618.
74. Scarci M, Abah U, Solli P, et al. EACTS expert consensus statement for surgical management of pleural empyema. *Eur J Cardiothorac Surg.* 2015;48(5):642–653.
75. Xantus G, Allen P, Norman S, et al. Antibiotics administered within 1 hour to adult emergency department patients screened positive for sepsis: a systematic review. *Eur J Emerg Med.* 2020;27(4):260–267.
76. Truong TN, Dunn AS, McCardle K, et al. Adherence to fluid resuscitation guidelines and outcomes in patients with septic shock: reassessing the "one-size-fits-all" approach. *J Crit Care.* 2019;51:94–98.
77. Chang P, Peng S, Zhou J, et al. [Fluid resuscitation strategy in septic shock following urinary infection with severe pulmonary capillary leakage]. *Zhonghua Wei Zhong Bing Ji Jiu Yi Xue.* 2013;25(1):14–18.
78. Ferreiro L, Porcel JM, Bielsa S, et al. Management of pleural infections. *Expert Rev Respir Med.* 2018;12(6):521–535.
79. Coote N. Surgical versus non-surgical management of pleural empyema. *Cochrane Database Syst Rev.* 2002(2):CD001956.
80. Primieri P, Ancona P, Gualtieri E. Unusual airways management during one-lung ventilation in thoracic surgery. *Saudi J Anaesth.* 2017;11(2):225–227.
81. Ho ACY, Chen C, Yang M, et al. Use of the Arndt wire-guided endobronchial blocker to facilitate one-lung ventilation for pediatric empyema during video-assisted thoracoscopy. *Chang Gung Med J.* 2005;28(2):104–110.
82. Tobias JD. Variations on one-lung ventilation. *J Clin Anesth.* 2001; 13(1):35–39.
83. Yu H, Liu B. Pulmonary soiling by pus after one-lung ventilation with a Univent tube. *Acta Anaesthesiol Scand.* 2004;48(10):1342.
84. Kim J, Lee H, Park H, et al. Combined use of a double-lumen tube and Fogarty catheter to prevent the endobronchial spread of infection: a case report. *Korean J Anesthesiol.* 2016;69(6): 619–622.
85. Ho ACY, Chung HS, Lu PP, et al. Facilitation of alternative one-lung and two-lung ventilation by use of an endotracheal tube exchanger for pediatric empyema during video-assisted thoracoscopy. *Surg Endosc.* 2004;18(12):1752–1756.
86. Campos JH, Musselman ED, Hanada S, et al. Lung isolation techniques in patients with early-stage or long-term tracheostomy: a case series report of 70 cases and recommendations. *J Cardiothorac Vasc Anesth.* 2019;33(2):433–439.
87. Hartland BL, Newell TJ, Damico N. Alveolar recruitment maneuvers under general anesthesia: a systematic review of the literature. *Respir Care.* 2015;60(4):609–620.
88. Attinger B, Buchmann P, Largiader F, et al. [Uni- and ipsilateral pulmonary edema after surgery on the lung]. *Helv Chir Acta.* 1991;58(1–2):181–185.
89. Chen B, Zhang J, Ye Z, et al. Outcomes of video-assisted thoracic surgical decortication in 274 patients with tuberculous empyema. *Ann Thorac Cardiovasc Surg.* 2015;21(3):223–228.
90. Kim WH, Lee HC, Ryu HG, et al. Intraoperative ventilatory leak predicts prolonged air leak after lung resection: a retrospective observational study. *PLoS One.* 2017;12(11):e0187598.
91. Pompeo E, Sorge R, Akopov A, et al. Non-intubated thoracic surgery—a survey from the European Society of Thoracic Surgeons. *Ann Transl Med.* 2015;3(3):37.
92. Tacconi F, Pompeo E, Fabbi E, et al. Awake video-assisted pleural decortication for empyema thoracis. *Eur J Cardiothorac Surg.* 2010;37(3):594–601.
93. Ohuchi M, Inoue S, Ozaki Y, et al. Single-trocar thoracoscopy under local anesthesia for pleural space infection. *Gen Thorac Cardiovasc Surg.* 2014;62(8):503–510.
94. Callahan SJ, Jones RM, Albon D, et al. A case of massive hemoptysis following transesophageal echocardiogram. *Respir Med Case Rep.* 2017;21:142–144.
95. Bali C, Ozmete O, Ergenoglu P, et al. A patient with Churg-Strauss syndrome complicated with pulmonary hemoptysis. *J Clin Anesth.* 2016;30:6–7.
96. Berman Dj, Knibbs N, Friedman L, et al. Postpartum hemoptysis as presenting sign of longstanding vasculitis. *Int J Obstet Anesth.* 2018;36:122–125.
97. Deisenberg M, Stayer SA. Severe hemoptysis in a child after the Fontan procedure. *Paediatr Anaesth.* 2005;15(6):515–518.
98. Heijkoop B, Gillespie H, Kiroff G. Emergency management of massive haemoptysis. *BMJ Case Rep.* 2019;12(1).
99. Haj-Yahia S, Sbaih M, Bali K, et al. Case report and management approach in idiopathic pulmonary arteries aneurysm. *J Cardiothorac Surg.* 2018;13(1):110.
100. Arora NR, Maddali MM, Al-Farqani A, et al. Hemoptysis in a patient with persistent left upper lobe consolidation. *J Cardiothorac Vasc Anesth.* 2018;32(2):1093–1095.
101. Loke GPY, Story DA, Liskaser F, et al. Pulmonary arteriovenous malformation causing massive haemoptysis and complicated by coronary air embolism. *Anaesth Intensive Care.* 2006;34(1):75–78.
102. Alter M, Peake B, Grodski S, et al. Massive haemoptysis from a bougie intubating catheter in a patient with endobronchial sarcoid. *BMJ Case Rep.* 2016:2016.
103. Devitt JH, Boulanger BH. Lower airway injuries and anaesthesia. *Can J Anaesth.* 1996;43(2):148–159.
104. Bourdereau JM, Mathe D, Voultoury JC. [Massive traumatic hemoptysis]. *Ann Fr Anesth Reanim.* 1985;4(3):308–309.
105. Jokinen K, Palva T, Sutinen S, et al. Acquired tracheobronchomalacia. *Ann Clin Res.* 1977;9(2):52–57.
106. Panigrahi MK, Pradhan G, Mohapatra PR. Tracheal bronchus presenting with recurrent haemoptysis in an adult female. *Adv Respir Med.* 2017;85(3):155–157.
107. Pfitzner J, Peacock MJ, Tsirgiotis E, et al. Lobectomy for cavitating lung abscess with haemoptysis: strategy for protecting the contralateral lung and also the non-involved lobe of the ipsilateral lung. *Br J Anaesth.* 2000;85(5):791–794.
108. Elkhayat H, Sallam M, Farouk M, et al. Uniportal VATS for treatment of bullous lung disease. *Multimed Man Cardiothorac Surg.* 2017:2017. https://pubmed.ncbi.nlm.nih.gov/28556634/.

109. Contou D, Voiriot G, Djibre M, et al. Clinical features of patients with diffuse alveolar hemorrhage due to negative-pressure pulmonary edema. *Lung.* 2017;195(4):477–487.
110. Murray AW, Smith JD, Ibinson JW. Diffuse alveolar hemorrhage, anesthesia, and cannabis. *Ann Am Thorac Soc.* 2014;11(8): 1338–1339.
111. Ngo BN, Bang GA, Jemea B, et al. Complex pulmonary aspergilloma: surgical challenges in a third world setting. *Surg Res Pract.* 2018;2018:6570741.
112. Kim D, Lee SN, Lee SK, et al. Lymphangiomyomatosis discovered by massive hemoptysis during general anesthesia—a case report. *Korean J Anesthesiol.* 2012;62(4):371–374.
113. Kas J, Feher C, Heiler Z, et al. [Treatment of adult intrapulmonary sequestration with video-assisted thoracoscopic lobectomy]. *Magy Seb.* 2018;71(3):126–133.
114. Xanthakis DS, Katsaras E, Efthimiadis M, et al. Hydatid cyst of the liver with intrathoracic rupture. *Thorax.* 1981;36(7): 497–501.
115. Orgaz OV, Navacerrada MIR, Guerrero MC, et al. Lung isolation in patients with previous lung resections: selective sequential lobar blockade using a Fuji Uniblocker(R) endobronchial blocker. *Rev Esp Anestesiol Reanim.* 2016;63(9):539–543.
116. Tantraworasin A, Thepbunchonchai A, Siwachat S, et al. Factors associated with recurrent bacterial empyema thoracis. *Asian J Surg.* 2018;41(4):313–320.
117. Pinnola A, Kuo YH, Sciarretta JD, et al. Bacteriology and comorbidities in patients requiring surgical management of empyema. *Am Surg.* 2018;84(4):599–603.
118. Maskell NA, Davies CWH, Nunn AJ, et al. U.K. Controlled trial of intrapleural streptokinase for pleural infection. *N Engl J Med.* 2005;352(9):865–874.
119. Yamazaki A, Ito A, Ishida T, et al. Polymicrobial etiology as a prognostic factor for empyema in addition to the renal, age, purulence, infection source, and dietary factors score. *Respir Investig.* 2019;57(6):574–581.
120. Maillet F, Bonnet N, Billard-Pomares T, et al. Fatal Legionella pneumophila serogroup 1 pleural empyema: a case report. *World J Crit Care Med.* 2019;8(6):99–105.
121. Goussard P, Morrison J, Appel IN, et al. Loculated empyema due to tuberculosis in a child. *BMJ Case Rep.* 2017: 2017. https://casereports.bmj.com/content/2017/bcr-2017-220315.
122. O'Connor JV, Chi A, Joshi M, et al. Post-traumatic empyema: aetiology, surgery and outcome in 125 consecutive patients. *Injury.* 2013;44(9):1153–1158.
123. Lee HW, Kim YW, Cho J, et al. Empyema necessitatis due to Aspergillus fumigatus. *BMJ Case Rep.* 2014:2014.
124. Burton PR, Lee M, Bailey M, et al. What causes post-traumatic empyema? *Emerg Med Australas.* 2009;21(2):153–159.
125. Ninan J, Fakhran S. Spontaneous bacterial empyema: its association with liver disease. *Mayo Clin Proc.* 2016;91(4): 537–538.
126. Tu CY, Chen CH. Spontaneous bacterial empyema. *Curr Opin Pulm Med.* 2012;18(4):355–358.
127. Mukai Y, Agatsuma T, Ideura G. *Salmonella houtenae*-induced empyema complicated with chronic tuberculous empyema. *Intern Med.* 2018;57(8):1141–1144.

49

Thoracic Anesthesia in the Morbidly Obese Patient: Obstructive Sleep Apnea

GEORGE W. KANELLAKOS, JAY B. BRODSKY

Introduction

Over the past 3 decades, the world has experienced an obesity epidemic. Obesity is increasing rapidly in almost every part of the world; overweight and obesity rates are higher in the United States than in any other developed country. A recent report from the National Health and Nutrition Examination Survey—which examined a nationally representative sample of the U.S. population—revealed that more than two-thirds of the adult population (>20 years) was either overweight (body mass index [BMI] >25 kg/m^2) or obese (BMI >30 kg/m^2).[1] Anesthesiologists now must manage increasing numbers of obese patients. These patients undergo a variety of procedures, both within and outside the operating suite. The presence and the degree of obesity is usually defined by BMI. BMI is calculated by dividing the patient's weight in kilograms (kg) by the square of their height in meters (m) (BMI = kg/m^2). BMI is not a measure of body fat but rather a measure of actual weight. As such, an elevated BMI can present for reasons other than increased adiposity. Extreme or morbid obesity (MO) is considered to be present when a patient has a BMI over 40 kg/m^2. Based on this definition, more than 8% of Americans are now morbidly obese. The anesthetic management of obese patients differs in many aspects from that of normal-weight patients. Obesity alters each patient's anatomy and physiology and is associated with many medical comorbidities.[2] Obstructive sleep apnea (OSA) is very common in obese patients and further complicates their care. This chapter considers the anesthetic management of the obese patient undergoing thoracic procedures with an emphasis on patients with sleep-disordered breathing.

Preoperative Considerations

During each patient's preoperative examination, the indications for the proposed surgery are reviewed and evaluated. In addition, all other associated medical conditions must be considered. For obese patients these frequently include hypertension, cardiovascular disease, type II diabetes, sleep-disordered breathing, and osteoarthritis. The preoperative diagnosis and management of each of these comorbidities often referred as "hypermetabolic syndrome," have been extensively reviewed elsewhere.[3–5]

Preoperative documentation of the patient's height and weight is extremely important because anesthetic drugs doses are based on weight scalars, either by measured actual or total body weight (TBW), or by calculating ideal body weight (IBW) and lean body weight (LBW). In normal-weight patients (defined as BMI range between 18.5 and 24.9 kg/m^2) IBW approximates TBW. This obviously is not the case for obese patients. The formula IBW = 22 × height^2 (meters) can be used to estimate IBW for both obese men and women.[6]

Both TBW and LBW increase as obesity increases. LBW equals TBW minus the weight of fat. LBW is composed of muscles, bones, tendons, ligaments, and body water. In normal-weight patients LBW can be estimated as 80% of TBW for males and 75% of TBW for females. The increase in LBW in obesity is mainly because of muscle and body water, both of which increase to a much lesser extent than does fat. Because LBW is difficult to measure clinically,[7] in a MO patient it can be roughly estimated by adding 20% or 30% to the patient's calculated IBW.

Airway Concerns

During the preanesthetic visit, predictors of potential problems with airway management are sought. The most frequently performed tests and measurements include assigning a Mallampati score, measuring sternomental and thyromental distances, measuring neck circumference, performing an upper lip bite test, noting the presence or absence of teeth and the general state of dentition, assessing cervical range of motion, noting the presence of a receding mandible and an interincisor gap, and measuring the width of mouth opening. Unfortunately, those screening tests thought to be helpful in predicting difficulty with tracheal intubation are inconsistent and have poor predictive value in obesity.[8] Roth et al. estimated the diagnostic accuracy of commonly used bedside examination tests for assessing the airway in adult patients without apparent anatomic abnormalities scheduled to undergo general anesthesia. They included 133 studies involving 844,206 participants. They evaluated the Mallampati test, modified Mallampati test, Wilson risk score, thyromental distance, sternomental distance, mouth opening test, and the upper lip bite test. They found that all index tests had relatively low sensitivities, with high variability. Although the upper lip bite test showed the most favorable diagnostic test accuracy properties, none of the common bedside screening tests is well suited for detecting unanticipated difficult airways, as many of them are missed.[9]

Conversely, the "negative" predictive values of such tests can be helpful. If a MO patient has a combination of a Mallampati score of I or II, a neck that is not thick or short, has full cervical range of motion and normal thyromental and sternomental distances, there is usually no difficulty encountered with direct laryngoscopy (DL) for tracheal intubation.[10] Adipose distribution is different between males and females, and this reassuring clinical presentation is more often present in female patients.

Preoperatively, MO men with a combination of a very large neck circumference (>65 cm) combined with a high Mallampati scores (III or IV) and a history of OSA can be expected to experience problems with some aspect of their airway management. A history of airway management difficulties during a previous anesthetic is probably the best means for anticipating a difficult DL and tracheal intubation (Fig. 49.1).

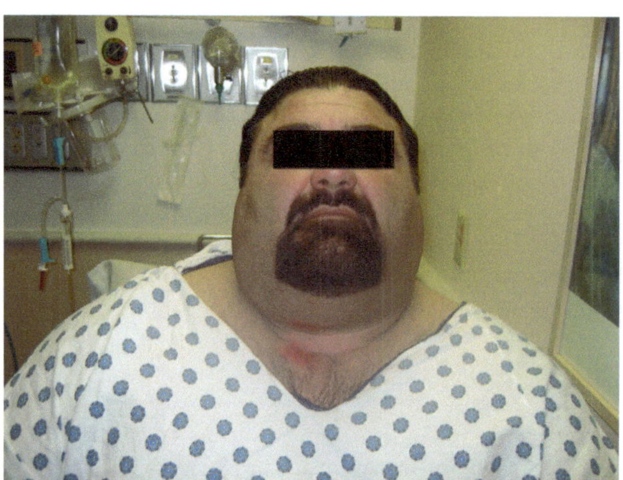

• **Fig. 49.1** Morbidly obese patients, particularly men with a very large neck circumference and a high Mallampati score (III or IV) will usually have obstructive sleep apnea. These patients can be anticipated to have difficulty with some aspect of their airway management. The presence of a beard further increases the chance of difficult mask ventilation.

Pulmonary Function

General anesthesia has a significant effect on impairing pulmonary function. These effects have also been studied in patients undergoing thoracic surgical procedures,[11] but without a focus on the obese patient. Chest wall and total pulmonary compliance decrease as patients increase in weight, leading to increased airway resistance and increased work of breathing in the spontaneously breathing MO patient. As BMI increases, pulmonary function tests reveal a restrictive ventilatory pattern with progressive decreases in functional residual capacity (FRC), which is mainly because of a decrease in expiratory reserve volume (ERV). In the supine position, these changes are associated with small airway collapse within the tidal breathing, which in turn results in air trapping, ventilation/perfusion (V/Q) mismatch, an increase in shunt fraction, and a much lower arterial partial pressure of oxygen (PaO2) than would occur in a normal weight patient.[12]

Preoperative pulmonary function testing has been used to help predict which patients can safely tolerate lung resection.[13,14] In nonobese patients, the values of 40% for both forced expiratory volume in 1 second (FEV_1) and diffusion capacity serve as acceptable guidelines for proceeding with lung resection.[15] Carbon monoxide diffusion capacity consistently appears to be the best predictor for postoperative complications.[16] These predictors are not validated in the MO patient and no predictive baseline spirometry studies in this population are currently available. For all patients, lung function decreases following surgery.[17] With increasing BMI, postoperative values for FEV_1 and FVC decrease proportionally. It is reasonable to expect even greater reductions in postoperative pulmonary function occur with the combination of thoracic operation and obesity compared with lean patients.

Sleep-Disordered Breathing

Snoring, hypopnea, OSA, OSA-hypopnea syndrome and upper airway resistance syndrome (UARS) are all disorders that fall under the umbrella of sleep-disordered breathing. OSA is characterized by repetitive collapse of the upper airway during sleep with complete cessation (apnea, lasting at least 10 seconds) or near complete cessation (hypopnea, defined as a decrease of ≥50% in airflow or ≤50% decrease for at least 10 seconds) of airflow. These events are associated with oxygen desaturation and sympathetic activation resulting in brief cortical arousals or complete awakening.[18] If there is increasing respiratory effort, apnea is described as "obstructive." In central sleep apnea there is no breathing effort.

The preoperative identification of patients who have OSA has important clinical implications. OSA is associated with day-time drowsiness, morning headaches, irritability, personality changes, depression, cognitive impairment, and visual incoordination. With severe OSA there is sleep fragmentation, transient hypoxemia and hypercapnia, large negative intrathoracic pressure swings, and marked elevations in blood pressure.[19] Recurrent hypoxic pulmonary vasoconstriction eventually results in pulmonary hypertension and right and left ventricular hypertrophy. In addition, patients with OSA may have "difficult" airways from an increased tissue mass of the oropharyngeal track. Periods of apnea or hypoventilation often result in hypercapnia and subsequent metabolic changes. This may lead to elevation in serum bicarbonate levels as a compensatory mechanism for acute respiratory acidosis.

The definitive diagnosis of OSA is made by polysomnography. Measurements during sleep include the Apnea Index (AI) (number of apneas/hour) and the Hypopnea Index (HI) (number of hypopneas/hour). The sum of the AI and HI is the Apnea-Hypopnea Index (AHI). The Arousal Index (ARI) is the number of arousals/hour that do not meet the definitions of apnea or hypopnea. The combination of ARI and AHI is the Respiratory Disturbance Index (RDI), a measure that significantly correlates with excessive daytime sleepiness. An AHI over 5 in combination with clinical symptoms is diagnostic of OSA. Bicarbonate elevation correlates with AHI, and when used in conjunction with the STOP-Bang score, the diagnosis of moderate to severe OSA significantly increases.[20]

The severity of the OSA is defined by the AHI score: moderate (AHI>5) in surgical patients, moderate to severe OSA (AHI>15) or severe (AHI >30). The prevalence of moderate to severe OSA (defined as AHI ≥15 events/hour) may be as high as 70% or even greater in MO patients, which represents a 5-fold increase compared with the general population. In the absence of a formal sleep study, the STOP and STOP-Bang Questionnaires were developed as OSA screening tools in preoperative clinics. The STOP questionnaire includes four questions related to snoring, tiredness, observed apnea, and high blood pressure. The STOP-Bang questionnaire includes the four questions used in the STOP questionnaire plus four additional demographic queries, for a total of eight questions related to features of sleep apnea (snoring, tiredness, observed apnea, high blood pressure, BMI, age, neck circumference and male gender). The total score ranges from 0 to 8 which can be used to classify OSA risk. The sensitivity of a STOP-Bang score of 3 or more to detect moderate to severe OSA (AHI >15) and severe OSA (AHI >30) is 93% and 100%, respectively.[21–23]

Moderate to severe OSA can be effectively treated with continuous positive airway pressure (CPAP). CPAP provides a pneumatic stent that opens the upper airway and maintains its patency. For patients requiring high levels of CPAP or those with chronic obstructive pulmonary disease, bilevel positive airway pressure (BiPAP) allows for independent adjustment of inspiratory and expiratory positive airway pressure.[24] CPAP treatment improves many of the associate comorbidities of OSA and should be encouraged preoperatively as early as possible. After several weeks of CPAP, benefits include the stabilization of congestive heart failure (HF), hypertension, pulmonary hypertension, and perhaps improved airway management through the reduction of tongue volume and increased pharyngeal space.

Because OSA is so common in the obese population, all MO patients should be presumed to have OSA and should be managed accordingly. The American Society of Anesthesiologists consensus guideline for the perioperative management of patients with OSA[17] and the Society of Anesthesia and Sleep Medicine Guideline on Intraoperative Management of Adult Patients With Obstructive Sleep Apnea[25] are useful resources for planning the management of any MO patient undergoing thoracic surgery.

Obesity hypoventilation syndrome (OHS) is another breathing disorder that is estimated to occur between 5% and 10% of MO patients with OSA with the highest occurrence is in superobese (BMI >50 kg/m^2) patients. OHS is defined by daytime hypercapnia ($PaCO2$ >45 mm Hg) and hypoxemia ($PaO2$ <70 mm Hg) in an obese patient (BMI >30 kg/m^2) with sleep-disordered breathing in the absence of any other cause of hypoventilation.[26] In OHS there is a diminished central ventilatory drive despite elevated PaCO2. Severe OHS has been termed "Pickwickian syndrome." OHS patients have the same symptoms as OSA patients but have greater daytime hypoxemia and is associated with more severe pulmonary hypertension.

Patients with OHS have both elevated PaCO2 and bicarbonate levels on preoperative room air arterial blood gas samples. These patients have higher risk, compared with eucapnic MO patients with OSA, of developing serious cardiovascular disease. Electrocardiographic evidence of right heart strain and hypertrophy is common. Chronic hypoxemia leads to polycythemia, further increasing an already elevated risk for postoperative pulmonary embolism.

For anesthesiologists, the management of MO patients with OHS represent one of the most challenging patient populations they will encounter. Thorough preoperative assessment with early optimization can have a significant impact in the reduction of perioperative adverse events. For OHS patients, both preoperative CPAP and noninvasive ventilation (NIV) improve clinical symptoms, gas exchange, and quality of life.[27,28] The American Thoracic Society Practice Guideline on Evaluation and Management of Obesity Hypoventilation Syndrome[29] can be a useful resource for anesthesiologists interested in optimizing the management of these challenging patients. The guideline encourages clinicians to test serum bicarbonate levels and blood gas samples to assist in the diagnosis of OHS. Stable ambulatory patients with OHS and severe OSA should receive CPAP rather than NIV as first-line treatment. Patients hospitalized with respiratory failure and suspected of having OHS should be discharged with NIV until they undergo outpatient diagnostic procedures and positive airway pressure titration in a sleep laboratory (ideally within 2–3 months). Patients with OHS are recommended to use weight-loss interventions that produce sustained weight loss of 25% to 30% of body weight. To achieve resolution of OHS by weight loss many of these patients are suggested to undergo bariatric surgery.

Cardiovascular Function

MO patients with OSA and/or OHS have an elevated risk of developing cardiac disease, that should be presumed present unless excluded by testing. MO patients frequently develop systemic hypertension because of the increase in absolute blood volume and cardiac output (hypermetabolic syndrome). The presence of OSA further increases the risks of pulmonary hypertension. Obesity is a risk factor for HF in both men and women. Severe obesity produces hemodynamic alterations that predispose to changes in cardiac morphology and ventricular function, which may lead to the development of HF. The presence of systemic hypertension, sleep apnea, and hypoventilation, comorbidities that occur commonly with severe obesity, may contribute to HF in such patients. In older MO patient's eccentric right ventricular hypertrophy, left ventricular hypertrophy, and right and left HF ("obesity cardiomyopathy") develops.[30]

A routine electrocardiogram is usually adequate for most MO patients, even those with arterial hypertension. Given that echocardiography demonstrates some degree of right ventricular dysfunction in asymptomatic patients, the presence of angina or any additional cardiac symptoms is a red flag that requires a more thorough cardiac evaluation. Moderate or severe left ventricular diastolic dysfunction was found in 50% of patients with moderate or severe OSA.[31] Long-standing or severe OSA should alert the clinician to the presence of pulmonary hypertension and potential right ventricular failure and prompt further investigations.

Intraoperative Management

Patient Position

An awake, spontaneously breathing MO patient should not be allowed to lie flat for induction of anesthesia. In the supine position, MO patients experience a further reduction in their already reduced FRC and this can result in dangerous hypoxemia, especially if they are breathing air.

The "safe apnea period" (SAP) is the duration of time between onset of apnea following preoxygenation and the administration of a neuromuscular blocking agent until pulse oximeter saturation (SpO2) falls below a safe level (usually 88%–92% in different studies). Proper patient positioning before and during the induction of general anesthesia is one of the most important means of lengthening SAP. Obese patients preoxygenated in the sitting position have significantly extended tolerance to apnea after muscle paralysis when compared with similar obese patients preoxygenated in the conventional supine position. Altermatt et al. studied 40 obese patients (BMI >35 kg/m^2) undergoing surgery with general anesthesia were randomly assigned to one of two groups: group 1 (sitting, n = 20) or group 2 (supine, n = 20). In the predetermined body position, preoxygenation was achieved with eight deep breaths within 60 s and an oxygen flow of 10 L/min. After rapid sequence induction and tracheal intubation, the patient was left apneic and disconnected from the anesthesia circuit until SpO2 decreased to 90%. Oxygen and carbon dioxide (CO2) tensions were similar between groups, both at baseline and after preoxygenation. However, the mean time to desaturation to 90% was significantly longer in the sitting group compared with the supine group (mean [standard deviation {SD}: 214 [28] vs. 162 [38] s, $P < .05$).[32]

MO patients should always be positioned in the "ramped" or **"head elevated laryngoscopy position" (HELP)** before anesthetic induction. It facilitates alignment of the pharyngeal, laryngeal, and oral axis of the airway during difficult laryngoscopy, especially in the large patient. In the MO patient, the goal is for the upper body and head to be elevated to a point that the sternum and ear are aligned in a horizontal line therefore easing the work of breathing and improving oxygen reserves.[33] In addition, if the patient is hemodynamically stable, the operating room table should be in the reverse Trendelenburg position (RTP).[34] **The semi-Fowler position** with the patient's upper body elevated 25 to 30 degrees also extends SAP but the 30 degrees RTP is better.[35,36] With the upper body elevated and the table in RTP the patient's diaphragm is "unloaded," diaphragmatic excursion is increased and the view during DL is improved. A recent study with MO volunteers confirmed that FRC is greatest in the RTP, less so in the semi-Fowler position, and least with the patient supine[37] (Fig. 49.2).

Besides maintaining the patient in a head-up, body elevated position, other strategies can be applied to the obese patient to prolong SAP. Adequate preoxygenation is most essential. Tidal volumes in a spontaneously breathing obese patient are too small to recruit lung volume. The patient must take deep vital capacity breaths. For the patient with

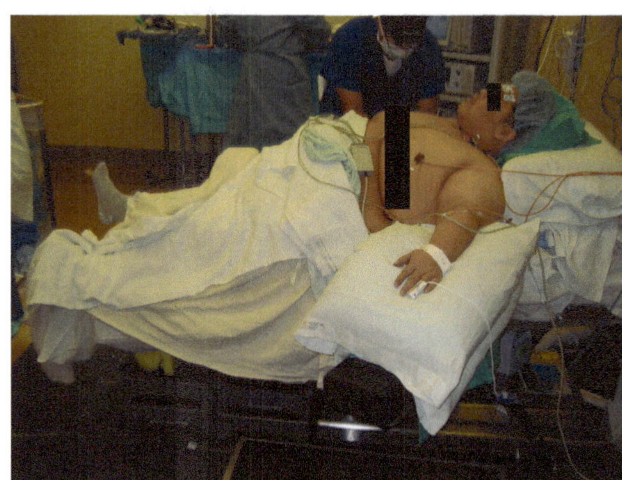

• **Fig. 49.2** Obese patients should always be positioned in the "ramped" or "head elevated laryngoscopy position" (HELP) before anesthetic induction. In this position, the upper body and head are elevated so that the sternum and ear are aligned in a horizontal line. If the patient is hemodynamically stable the operating room table should be tilted in the reverse Trendelenburg position. This arrangement will allow greater diaphragmatic excursion and improve the view during direct laryngoscopy.

an anticipated difficult airway, application of apneic or "diffusion" oxygenation should be considered.

During apnea metabolism continues and the body consumes approximately 250 mL O2/min and produces 200 mL CO2/min. Most CO2 (up to 90%) stays in the blood and will cause a respiratory acidosis. The O2 continues to be consumed from alveoli with a loss of lung volume. The resulting pressure differential allows mass movement of gas from upper airways into alveoli. Delivering a high fraction of inspired oxygen (F_iO2) at any level of the airway (pharynx, trachea, alveoli) can increase alveolar O2 and thereby increase SAP. Nasal delivery of oxygen by transnasal humidified rapid-insufflation ventilatory exchange (THRIVE),[38] through high-flow nasal cannulae,[39] and/or by the buccal route through modified endotracheal tubes (ETTs)[40] have each been used in obese patients for preoxygenation and to prevent hypoxemia during periods of apnea during upper airway procedures before the trachea being intubated. Apneic oxygenation ***cannot*** compensate for ineffective preoxygenation. The upper airway must remain patent. A nonpatent airway results in alveolar collapse with rapid desaturation. To keep the airway open the patient may require head elevation, jaw thrust, nasal prongs, or an oral airway.

Lying flat usually increases venous blood return to the heart. Cardiac output (CO), pulmonary blood flow, and an increase in arterial blood pressure can occur. The supine obese patient will experience significant increases in metabolic oxygen demand and CO2 production combined with the increases in CO and arterial and pulmonary artery pressures. For the supine MO patient with preexisting limited physiologic reserves acute and sometimes fatal cardiorespiratory decompensation, termed the **"obesity supine death syndrome,"** can result (Fig. 49.3).

Although this syndrome was first described in 1977 in two massively obese patients who were forced to lie down for medical procedures,[41] many physicians remain unaware of the great danger of placing an anesthetized or sedated obese patient in the supine position. It is postulated that the obesity supine death syndrome is the cause of unexplained deaths occurring not only in the operating room, but also at other locations, such as endoscopy, imaging, interventional radiology, or even during patient transport.[42] Unexplained deaths occur much more frequently in MO patients and in the absence of positive findings at autopsy the death is usually attributed to cardiac arrhythmia.[43] Patients at greatest risk are usually men with central obesity who have massive abdomens and who complain of shortness of breath when lying flat. When the syndrome does occur, the first response should be immediately returning the patient to a sitting or table-upright position. It is likely that in the patient with significant central obesity in the supine position the inferior vena cava can be compressed reducing venous return to the heart and causing hypotension.

Moving an anesthetized MO patient in the operating room can cause numerous injuries to the patient and is beyond the scope of this chapter. In this population, there is an additional risk to injury to the staff attempting to move

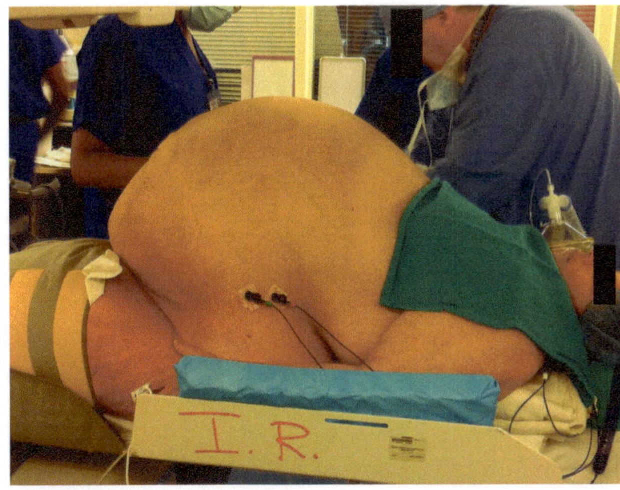

• **Fig. 49.3** When a morbidly obese patient lies flat, there is an increase in venous blood return to the heart. A further loss of functioning lung volume occurs resulting in a decrease in oxygenation, especially when breathing room air. The supine obese patient will also experience significant increases in oxygen demand and carbon dioxide production. These changes combined with increases in cardiac output and arterial and pulmonary artery pressures that occur in the supine patient can result in acute cardiorespiratory decompensation, termed the "obesity supine death syndrome." The syndrome may present not only in the operating room, but at other locations outside the operating suite, including the endoscopy unit, at imaging and interventional radiology, or even during patient transport.

the patient. The lateral position for thoracic surgery requires additional physical assistance and equipment. In that position, in addition to padding all the pressure points, special care must be taken to maintain the patient's head in a position to avoid brachial plexus stretch injuries. Because MO patients can have a short neck, supporting the head often requires extra blankets strategically placed to maintain a neutral position.

In any nonphysiologic position in an obese patient, inadequate arm support can result in brachial plexus injury. Changing to the lateral position requires larger axillary rolls and beanbags for support. The beanbag may not be large enough to adequately hold the patient. Belts or tape across the pelvis may be required to help stabilize a patient's position and special precaution should be taken when tilting the operating room table laterally (Fig. 49.4).

Airway Management

By definition, a "difficult airway" is present when a conventionally trained anesthesia provider experiences problems to get control of the patients airway which can be either bag-mask ventilation, tracheal intubation, and/or the insertion of a supraglottic airway device (SGD).[44] The association between obesity and "difficult airway" remains unresolved because the medical literature on this subject consists of heterogeneous studies with conflicting results.[45] What constitutes "problems" is not well defined and depends on what aspect of airway management is being considered and what criteria are being used to define difficulty. The

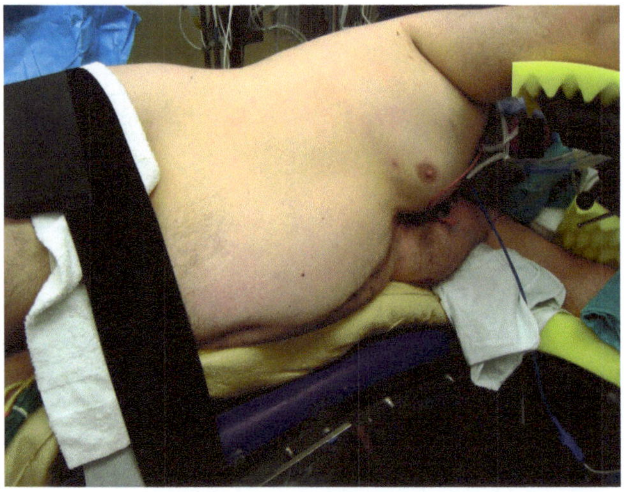

• **Fig. 49.4** The morbidly obese patient in the lateral position for thoracic surgery requires large axillary rolls and a beanbag for support. Conventional size beanbags may not be large enough to adequately hold the obese patient in place. Additional belts and tape across the pelvis are required to help stabilize the patient in the proper position.

reported incidence of "difficult" tracheal intubation in published studies widely ranges from of 1.9% to 44.4% in MO patients and from 3.2% to 20.4% in obese patients.[46]

An MO patient, especially with a history or symptoms of OSA may have a diminution of the pharyngeal space secondary to an increase in fat deposition in the pharyngeal wall, which can make airway access and bag-mask ventilation difficult. Most studies do agree that difficulty with bag-mask ventilation (DMV) is very common in obese patients. The weight of the chest wall, especially when the patient is supine, coupled with other factors, such as a poorly fitting face-mask, the presence of a beard, poor dentition, and the frequent association of OSA all complicate mask ventilation. **If any concern exists regarding the possibility of adequate mask ventilation in the patients, an awake fiberoptic intubation should be considered.**

DMV is usually defined as either mask ventilation that is inadequate to maintain oxygenation saturation SpO2 over 92%, unstable mask ventilation, or mask ventilation requiring two providers. Impossible mask ventilation is defined as the absence of end-tidal CO2 measurements and lack of perceptible chest wall movement during positive-pressure ventilation attempts despite airway adjuvants (oral or nasopharyngeal airway) and additional personnel. Obesity (BMI >30 kg/m^2) is one of many independent predictors of DMV. Other factors include age (>46 years), male gender, Mallampati score of III or IV, neck mass or radiation, limited thyromental distance, OSA, presence of teeth or beard, neck circumference >43 cm, limited cervical spine mobility and limited jaw protrusion.[47] Unlike the inconclusive data regarding obesity and difficult tracheal intubation (see later), the consistent findings from published studies is that obesity is associated with DMV.

In the past bag-mask ventilation during anesthetic induction was avoided because of concerns that insufflation of the stomach would increase the risk of aspiration. Clinically significant gastric distention does not occur during normal bag-mask ventilation, especially if peak pressures are kept low. Unless at high risk for aspiration, the anesthetic induction of the obese patient should include positive-pressure bag-mask ventilation with the application of CPAP or positive end-expiratory pressure (PEEP). Bag-mask ventilation will decrease atelectasis and increase SAP by as much as 50% in MO patients.[48]

Obesity is often listed as a factor for difficult tracheal intubation. Not a single study has ever demonstrated a direct relationship between increasing weight and/or BMI with increasing intubation difficulty.

The **Intubation Difficulty Scale (IDS)** has been used as a measure of intubation difficulty. It is based on seven variables.[49] Points are assigned as follows:

- **N1,** number of additional intubation attempts;
- **N2,** number of additional operators;
- **N3,** number of alternative intubation techniques used (e.g., SGD, change of laryngoscope blade, bougie);
- **N4,** glottic exposure as defined by Cormack and Lehane[50] (grade 1, N4 = 0; grade 2, N4 = 1; grade 3, N4 = 2; and grade 4, N4 = 3);
- **N5,** lifting force applied during laryngoscopy (N5 = 0 if "inconsiderable" and N5 = 1 if "considerable") (as assessed subjectively by the laryngoscopist);
- **N6,** need to apply external laryngeal pressure to improve glottic pressure (N6 = 0 if no external pressure or only the Sellick maneuver applied and N6 = 1 if external laryngeal pressure was used); and
- **N7,** position of the vocal cords at intubation (N7 = 0 if abducted or not visible and N7 = 1 if adducted). The IDS score is the sum of N1 through N7. An **IDS of 0** indicates intubation performed on the first attempt by the first operator using a single technique and applied minimal force to insert the ETT through a fully visualized glottis. An **IDS score from 1 to 5** indicates slight difficulty, and an IDS score over 5 indicates moderate to major difficulty.

In a study of 134 lean (BMI <30 kg/m^2) and 129 obese (BMI >35 kg/m^2) patients an IDS of 5 or more occurred in three lean (2.2%) and 20 obese (15.5%) patients during intubation by DL.[51] The conclusion was that difficult tracheal intubation is more common in obese patients based on an IDS of 5 or more. Most IDS studies consider a score of 5 to represent only "slight" difficulty. It is also important to note that the incidence of poor glottic view during laryngoscopy (Cormack-Lehane class 3 or 4) was identical between lean (10.4%) and obese (10.1%) groups, and all patients in both groups were successfully intubated by DL. A Mallampati score of III or IV was the only independent risk factor for the increased "difficulty" in the obese group and there was no relationship between increasing BMI and increasing difficulty. A similar study of 70 obese (BMI >30 kg/m^2) and 61 lean (BMI <30 kg/m^2) reported an IDS greater than 5 in 14.3% of obese and 3.0% of lean patients.[52]

These studies assessed difficult intubation by IDS criteria. By contrast, other studies using different criteria for "difficulty" have reached different conclusions. In a study of 100 consecutive MO patients (BMI >40 kg/m^2) scheduled for bariatric surgery, tracheal intubation was classified as "easy" if the product of the Cormack-Lehane graded laryngoscopy view times the number of intubation attempts was less than 3, and was classified as "problematic," that is potentially difficult, when it was 3 or more.[53] All but one patient was successfully intubated by DL without using any adjuncts. Neck circumference (>65 cm) and Mallampati score (III or IV) were the only predictors of potential difficulty with intubation. Neither absolute weight nor BMI were associated with problematic intubation.

If obesity by itself was the major factor, one would expect to see a direct relationship between increasing weight and increasing intubation difficulty and failure. None of the many studies on airway management in obesity has demonstrated such a relationship. For example, a recent study found that at a BMI greater than 30 kg/m^2, the odds of DL, simply defined as requiring more than one attempt, were greater in obese compared with lean patients. However, there was no increase in the number of intubation attempts as BMI increased. Difficult intubation was no more likely to occur in an MO patient than in a moderately obese patient. This study, like all the previous reports found that **more obesity does not convey more intubation difficulty**.[54]

There are many problems with these studies. The view obtained during DL is often used as a measure for difficult or failed intubation; however, an ETT may be easy to place despite a poor laryngoscopic view, and even with a reasonable view there can be difficulty passing an ETT. The IDS considers factors that are subjective and may lead to bias (lifting force during laryngoscopy) and factors unrelated to obesity (adduction of the vocal cords, a measure of the degree of muscle relaxation). If the laryngoscopic view and success rate with conventional laryngoscopy are used as the measure of intubation difficulty, there is little difference between lean, obese, and MO patients.

All these studies define obesity by absolute weight or BMI and fail to consider that the distribution of fat, not weight itself, can contribute to difficulty with laryngoscopy. The results can also be biased because many superobesity patients undergo elective awake fiberoptic intubation (FOI) or video-laryngoscopy (VL) and are thus excluded from the series reporting experience with DL. Finally, many of the studies are from patients undergoing bariatric surgery, which typically include a much a higher percentage of women than men.

There is a subset of obese patients that exhibit a distribution of excess adipose tissue that does directly affect airway management. This group of patients consists mostly of MO men, often with OSA, who have very thick necks and high Mallampati scores. No study has considered these patients separately in airway studies in obesity. Whereas the majority of obese and MO patients are usually not difficult to intubate, these subsets of patients can present challenging airways.

Tracheal intubation in MO patients is managed differently than in lean patients. The standard sniffing position for tracheal intubation is achieved in nonobese patients by raising their occiput 8 to 10 cm with a pillow or headrest. Obese patients, on the other hand, require much greater elevation of their head, neck, and shoulders (HELP) to produce the same alignment of axes for intubation. In studies of MO patients where the head position is suboptimal, that is not in the HELP, there are higher incidences of grade 3 and 4 Cormack–Lehane views with potentially increasing difficulty with DL.

For patients with an anticipated difficult intubation and in those in which difficult DL is encountered following induction of anesthesia, alternative methods to establish the airway should be considered. Awake FOI was once considered the "gold standard" for difficult intubation.[55] However, with the development of new airway equipment, particularly with the readily available video-laryngoscopes, FOI is now being performed less frequently.[56] FOI can be difficult in MO patients because of reduced pharyngeal space and the increase in redundant tissue which can restrict field of view, especially in the anesthetized patient when loss of pharyngeal tone further complicates the bronchoscopist's view. An "asleep FOI" compares unfavorably with other airway devices, such as video-laryngoscopes for first-intubation success. **If a difficult airway is identified in an obese patient and FOI is planned, an awake FOI should be performed.**[57] Even as a rescue strategy in the unanticipated difficult airway, FOI has now been replaced by readily available VL.

Because conventional DL is successful in the great majority of obese and MO patients, it remains unclear whether VL is superior and should be the default means for establishing an airway in obese patients.[58] A Cochrane review of 64 randomized controlled trials comparing 7044 adult patients found "moderate quality" evidence that video-scopes may reduce the number of failed intubations by improving glottic view, especially for patients with an anticipated difficult airway. Video-laryngoscopes may also reduce airway trauma and hoarseness, but there was no evidence of reduced episodes of hypoxia or mortality. Intubation success rates differed between different video-laryngoscopes. Only the C-MAC blade showed a statistically significant reduction in failed intubations, with no difference in success rates for the Glidescope, Pentax and McGrath instruments when compared with conventional DL. Although there is growing body of evidence that VL improves glottic view and reduces intubation attempts compared with Macintosh DL in obese patients, however, it is up to the practitioner to decide if to select it as a first-line use for all obese patients. Until a large, randomized trial in obese patients is performed to help determine if the routine use of VL in the obese is better than DL, factors such as provider comfort and anticipated airway difficulty should be considered when VL is used as the primary approach to intubate the trachea in obese adults. There is no strong evidence that VL reduced the number of intubation attempts, reduced the time to successful tracheal intubation, or influenced the incidence of hypoxia or respiratory complications compared with DL.[59] The success rate of VL compared with DL in obesity was not considered in this study. Another review reported weak evidence that VL may improve glottic view, reduce the number of intubation attempts, and increase the intubation success rate in obese patients. There was no evidence it reduced the time to successful intubation, a critically important concern given the short SAP in obese patients.[60]

During the past decade, there has been a steady increase in use of supraglottic devices (SGD'). The introduction of second-generation SGDs with improved oropharyngeal leak pressure and a channel for inserting a gastric tube has led to a widening of the indications for their use. The potential advantages of SGDs include ease of placement and less airway injury than an ETT. However, there is still disagreement about the role of SGDs in obese surgical patients, and their safe use in MO patients remains controversial.

The Fourth National Audit Project (NAP-4) examined the records of 2.9 million anesthetics performed in the United Kingdom. Obese and MO patients had a disproportionate incidence of airway complications.[61] Of the patients who experienced a major airway complication (death, brain damage, emergency surgical airway, or intensive care unit [ICU] admission) 42% were obese. Furthermore, patients with severe obesity were four times more likely to experience these airway problems. Regurgitation and pulmonary aspiration, which accounted for 50% of the deaths in NAP-4 occurred more frequently in MO patients. Although the use of SGDs in obesity did not differ from nonobese patients, the obese patients had an increased frequency of aspiration associated with use of an SGD. The study stated that the use of these devices in MO patients indicated "failure to respect the risks associated with airway management in obesity." Following publication of the NAP-4 report, the Society of Bariatric Anaesthetists in the United Kingdom recommended intubation with an ETT as the default airway management strategy for patients with BMI >35 kg/m^2.[62] Since NAP-4 was published, second generation SGDs have been introduced. They may have an increased role in obesity but their safe use in this population presently remains unknown.

There are indications for using an SGD in obesity. An SGD remains an important rescue tool during "cannot ventilate, cannot intubate" situations,[63] and is especially helpful in obese and MO patients as a life-saving bridge until an ETT can be placed or until a surgical airway is attempted.[64] SGDs have been used to preoxygenate obese patients to increase SAP before laryngoscopy.[65]

Anesthetic Drugs/Maintenance of Anesthesia

Sedatives and opioids decrease ventilatory response to hypoxemia and hypercarbia in every obese patient. In an MO patient with OSA these drugs will also decrease pharyngeal dilator muscle tone and activity and cause upper airway collapse. Most anesthetic agents and medications, including opioids, benzodiazepines, nitrous oxide, thiopental, propofol, and even small doses of neuromuscular blocking agents can cause pharyngeal collapse. Sedatives can have prolonged effects, and when OSA is present they increase the risk of respiratory depression even into the postoperative period. Sedative premedication should be used with caution or completely avoided.

In clinical practice, medications are dosed according to weight on a per kilogram dosing regimen. The excess weight in obesity is caused by increases in both adipose and lean tissue. Fat tissue increases to a much greater extent than lean tissue and is poorly perfused. If based on TBW, the plasma concentration of an intravenous (IV) drug administered as a bolus in an MO patient will be very high.

Propofol is now the induction agent of choice. In theory, a lipid soluble agent like propofol should be dosed according to TBW, but if followed in MO patients such large doses could result in cardiovascular collapse, particularly in the fluid restricted thoracotomy patient. **For MO patients, the induction dose of propofol should be based on LBW.** In a study of 60 MO subjects (BMI ≥40 kg/m^2) that were randomized to receive a propofol infusion (100 mg/kg/h) for induction of anesthesia based on TBW or LBW to achieve loss of conciseness (LOC). Thirty control subjects (BMI ≤25 kg/m^2) received a propofol infusion (100 mg/kg/h) based on TBW. Total propofol dose (mg/kg) required for LOC were similar between control subjects and MO subjects given propofol based on LBW. MO subjects receiving a propofol infusion based on TBW had a significantly larger propofol dose and significantly shorter time to LOC.[66]

Opioid-sparing anesthetic techniques, short-acting anesthetics, and analgesic agents and/or regional anesthesia, are better choices for the MO patient. All opioids have respiratory depressant properties and IV administration should be carefully titrated according to individual patient needs. A total intravenous anesthesia (TIVA) technique with propofol and remifentanil based on LBW in obese patients, or an inhalational technique can be used for thoracotomy. In a study of MO patients each was acceptable and neither technique was associated with intraoperative awareness.[67]

Despite claims to the contrary, there is no clear advantage between any of the common inhalational anesthetics (isoflurane, sevoflurane, desflurane) in MO patients.[68] Controversy exists as some anesthesiologists claim patients treated with desflurane take less time to emerge and to respond to commands to open their eyes and are more alert than patients treated with sevoflurane. These beliefs are supported by a meta-analysis review of 11 trials databases for randomized controlled trials that evaluated the outcome of anesthesia with desflurane, sevoflurane, isoflurane, or propofol in MO patients to assess recovery times (eye opening, hand squeezing, tracheal extubation, and stating name or birth date), time to discharge from the postanesthesia care unit (PACU), and the incidence and severity of postoperative complications. The authors found that patients given desflurane took less time to respond to commands to open their eyes, to squeeze the investigator's hand, to be prepared for tracheal extubation, and to state their name.[69] Despite these findings, there were no significant differences in PACU discharge times, nausea, or analgesic requirement and there were no differences in hemodynamics and respiratory function perioperatively using either agent.[70] The source of the controversy likely lies in how attentive clinicians are in the titration of volatile anesthetic drug doses. In procedures lasting 2 to 4 hours, emergence and recovery in MO patients receiving either desflurane or sevoflurane were similar when anesthetic concentration is carefully titrated down using bispectral index monitoring.[71] With the goal of reducing the risk of awareness, it is common practice for clinicians to deliver more volatile anesthetic than necessary[72] and the downward titration of gas is often delayed until the absolute end of a procedure. Desflurane has the lowest blood-gas partition coefficient of the agents available and its abrupt cessation, at the end of a procedure is more likely to result in earlier emergence when compared with sevoflurane. Sevoflurane is a commonly used inhalation agent in thoracic surgical procedures, including those involving obese and MO patients.

The concentration of pseudocholinesterase, the enzyme that metabolizes succinylcholine, increases with increasing weight. If succinylcholine is used for tracheal intubation in an MO patient a dose of 1 mg/kg TBW is recommended.[73]

If rocuronium is used, sugammadex should be readily available. Nondepolarizing muscle relaxants are initially dosed based on LBW, and a neuromuscular monitor is used to guide additional dosing. A reversal dose of sugammadex, 2 mg/kg TBW, is recommended by the manufacturer. Several studies have demonstrated that this amount is both unnecessary and expensive in obese patients. In one study, bariatric surgical patients received sugammadex based on either TBW or IBW. The mean dose of sugammadex in the IBW group was 4 mg/kg dosage based on IBW plus 35%, or approximately the patients' LBW. Time to complete reversal of neuromuscular blockade was not significantly different between the two groups, even though sugammadex doses were significantly lower in the IBW group.[74] Even lower doses of sugammadex have been used successfully in MO patients.[75] A single vial of sugammadex contains 200 mg of the drug, which is considered adequate for the reversal of neuromuscular blockade for most obese patients who demonstrate a "train-of four" with at least one twitch. Because MO patients are at risk for hypoventilation and upper airway obstruction following tracheal extubation, neuromuscular blockade monitoring remains essential to detect residual neuromuscular blockade or recurarization.

Lung Separation (see Ch. 16)

One of the unique skillsets of a thoracic anesthesiologist is safe isolation and selective ventilation of the lungs. Standard methods of achieving lung separation include a double-lumen tube (DLT) or a balloon-tipped bronchial blocker (BB). The choice of technique depends on the specific surgical requirements, the patient's airway, and the individual anesthesiologist's preferences and experience.[76] For successful lung separation, it is important to be familiar with airway anatomy. Bronchoscopic tracheobronchial anatomy can be reviewed online at www.thoracicanesthesia.com or www.pie.med.utoronto.ca/VB or in published reviews.[77]

The advantages and disadvantages of DLTs and BBs are covered in other chapters of this textbook. If the patient is positioned appropriately, DL and successful placement of either a DLT or ETT for bronchial blockade should be no different in an obese patient than in a lean patient.[78,79] Similar to normal-weight patients, if DL is difficult, many clinicians opt to place an ETT using another device or technique at their disposal (video-laryngoscope, an ETT through a SGD using a fiberoptic bronchoscope, or with another intubation adjunct). Once the ETT is in place, a BB can be used with the ETT, or alternatively a 100-cm long airway exchange catheter can be used to change from the ETT to a DLT. Although more challenging, a DLT can also be placed directly by fiberoptic bronchoscopy.[80] If a DLT cannot be placed, or tracheobronchial anatomy is unfavorable for a DLT, lung isolation should be possible by bronchial blockade. A BB can be advanced through an oral or in rare circumstances through a nasal ETT or through a tracheostomy tube. A blocker may be a better choice for MO patients with a high Mallampati score and thick neck who have the potential for a "difficult" intubation (Fig. 49.5).

Despite claims to the contrary, the quality of lung collapse is unaffected whether a BB or DLT is used. It may be safer to use a BB through a regular ETT if postoperative ventilation is planned, especially because exchanging a DLT for an ETT at the completion of surgery can be avoided.

Before intubation, the patient's chest radiograph or computed tomography scan should be examined to determine the tracheobronchial anatomy and airway diameters.[81] Unlike chronic obstructive lung disease, which results in a dilation of trachea and bronchi, a similar effect does not occur for the restrictive lung disease in obesity. Relatively, small tracheas are often found in very large patients.[82] Even when a smaller DLT is used, ventilating through both lumens the airway resistance should not be a concern because adult size DLTs have similar airflow resistance compared with ETTs.

One-Lung Ventilation (see Ch. 20)

During thoracic surgery requiring one-lung ventilation (OLV), the development of hypoxemia can present as a significant clinical challenge.[83] In general, OLV is not tolerated well in the supine compared with lateral position as gravity and atelectasis contribute to poor ventilation and perfusion.[84] Mechanisms for hypoxemia during OLV are accentuated in MO versus normal-weight patients. MO patients benefit from lung recruitment maneuvers following induction of anesthesia and before the institution of OLV,[85] and often require recruitment maneuvers and PEEP throughout the procedure to maintain adequate oxygenation.[86]

When patients undergo procedures in the supine, the semi-lateral decubitus, and the lateral decubitus positions, oxygenation progressively decreases with time after the start of OLV. OLV in the supine position is associated with the highest degree of hypoxemia, usually occurring approximately 10 min after initiating OLV with 100% O2.[87] Although MO patients can maintain adequate oxygenation

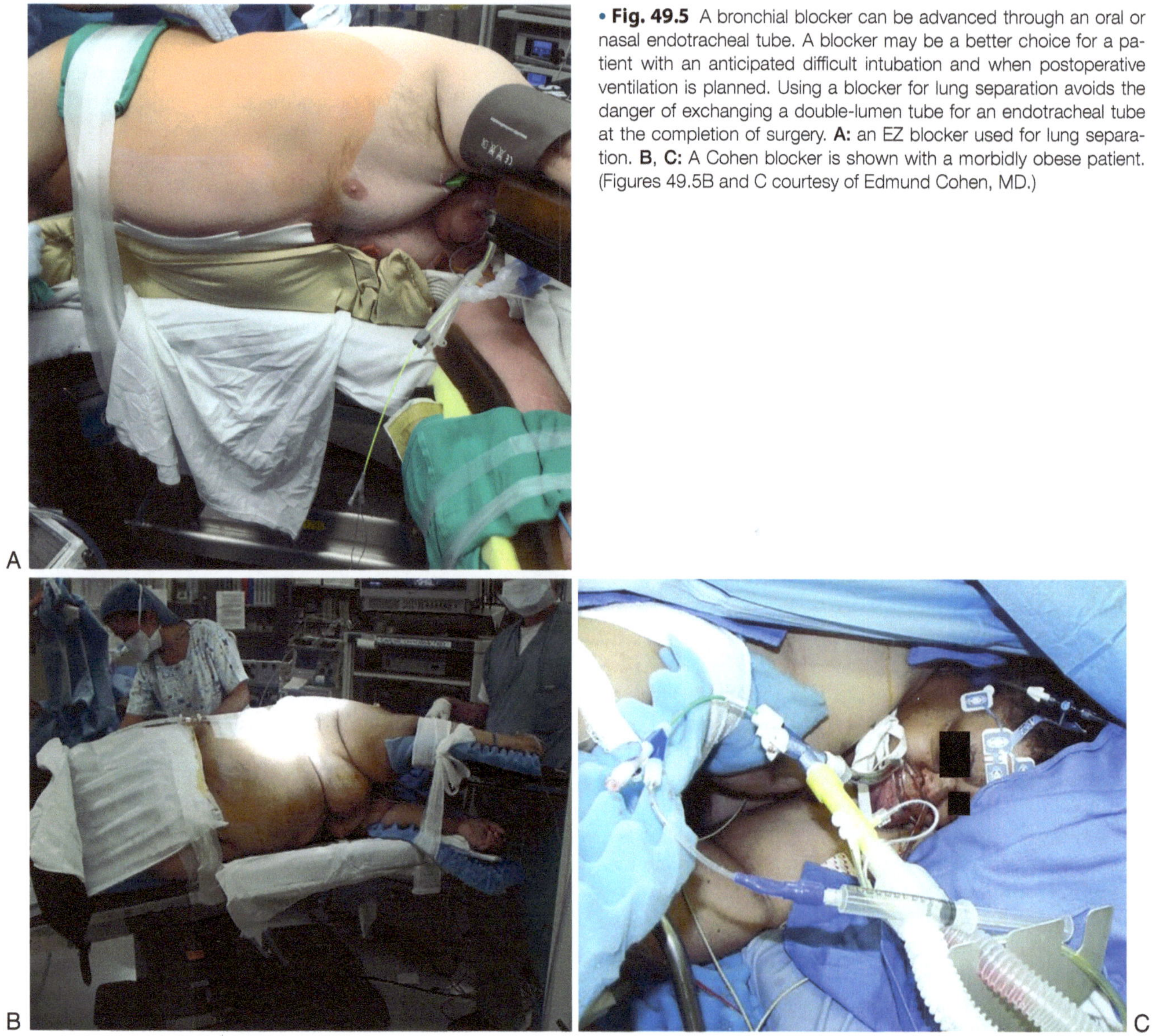

• **Fig. 49.5** A bronchial blocker can be advanced through an oral or nasal endotracheal tube. A blocker may be a better choice for a patient with an anticipated difficult intubation and when postoperative ventilation is planned. Using a blocker for lung separation avoids the danger of exchanging a double-lumen tube for an endotracheal tube at the completion of surgery. **A:** an EZ blocker used for lung separation. **B, C:** A Cohen blocker is shown with a morbidly obese patient. (Figures 49.5B and C courtesy of Edmund Cohen, MD.)

during OLV in the lateral position, arterial oxygen tension in MO patients remains significantly lower during OLV than normal-weight patients. Successful OLV in MO patients in the lateral position may be because of the panniculus being displaced laterally from the body in turn unloading the dependent diaphragm.[88]

When OLV is initiated, all patients, including the MO patients, should have lung protective ventilation strategies initiated.[89] Large tidal volumes with no recruitment maneuvers or PEEP have been associated with development of acute respiratory distress syndrome (ARDS) and other postoperative pulmonary complications, even in patients without preexisting lung disease. Ventilation with tidal volume as high as 13 mL/kg (IBW) during OLV that was used in the past does not improve oxygenation and can result in excessively high peak pressures and parenchymal damage.[90] Considering the difficulty in calculating IBW and the likelihood of clinicians roughly estimating it in the MO population, the risk of delivering an inappropriately high tidal volume is great.[91] Tidal volumes during OLV should be based on IBW (5–6 mL/kg IBW).

Another component of lung protective ventilation involves peak and plateau inspiratory pressures. Similar to lower tidal volume, lower airway pressures are protective and can reduce lung injury. Pressure control ventilation (PCV) results in lower airway pressure compared with volume control ventilation (VCV) for the same tidal volume delivered. As a result, many clinicians believe that PCV is offers greater protection and should result in less lung injury. Studies in normal-weight patients, however, fail to show differences in outcomes between the two ventilation strategies when airway pressures remain under the 25 to 30 cm H_2O range.[92]

MO patients can be more difficult to ventilate and require higher airway pressures that normal-weight patients.[93] In thoracic surgery, in an MO patient with restricted chest wall movement and impaired diaphragmatic excursion mechanical ventilation during OLV can lead to excessively high peak and plateau airway pressures. In supine abdominal laparoscopic obesity surgery, it has been demonstrated that PVC can improve oxygenation.[94] During thoracic surgery in normal-weight patients it has also been shown that PCV with PEEP during OLV may improve oxygenation and decrease peak pressures.[95] It is likely that PCV during OLV in the MO population will result in improved oxygenation and decreased airway pressures as well.

If pressure-limited OLV is used, a lower tidal volume may be delivered to MO patients who already have low lung volumes which may worsen the hypoxemia. PEEP is beneficial during two-lung ventilation in MO patients. During OLV, a mild to moderate level of PEEP to the ventilated dependent lung reduces atelectasis and improves oxygenation if it does not exceed the lower inflection point of the alveolar pressure-volume loop. Higher PEEP may result in increased pulmonary vascular resistance thereby increasing shunt to the collapsed lung and worsening hypoxemia.[96] There is no consensus regarding the optimal PEEP during OLV in the MO patients.

Recently, the driving pressure (DP) has become an important parameter in positive pressure ventilation. DP is defined as the difference between plateau pressure and PEEP (Plat-PEEP), and can also be expressed as the ratio of tidal volume to respiratory system compliance. In randomized controlled trials of mechanical ventilation in ARDS patients, DP is the variable that was most strongly associated with mortality. The optimization of DP has been considered as a tool to optimize mechanical ventilation during surgery and to improve outcome.

Park et al.[97] confirmed the significance of DP during OLV. In a double-blind, randomized, controlled study of 292 patients undergoing thoracic surgery, they compared DP-guided ventilation with conventional protective ventilation. The protective ventilation group (n = 147) received conventional protective ventilation during OLV: tidal volume 6 mL/kg, PEEP 5 cm H_2O, and recruitment maneuvers. The DP group (n = 145) received the same tidal volume and recruitment, but with titrated individualized PEEP to produce the lowest DP during OLV. The number of patients who developed pneumonia or ARDS was smaller in the DP group than in the protective ventilation group.

Presently, there are no data that has evaluated the importance of DP during thoracic procedures in MO patients.

Intravenous Fluid Management (see Ch. 21)

Historically, the routine clinical practice in thoracic surgery has been to restrict IV fluid, presumably to reduce the incidence of postoperative pulmonary edema after lung resection.[98] Therefore perioperative assessment of blood volume (BV) is particularly critical for patients undergoing thoracotomy for lung resection. The mean value for BV in lean adults is usually given as 70 mL/kg, but using this value for obese and MO patients would lead to an overestimation of BV. With progressive increases in BMI the total circulating BV also increases, but BV measured as mL/kg TBW decreases in a nonlinear manner.[99] Underestimates of BV in MO patients can lead to inadequate administration of fluids in the event of massive hemorrhage or trauma. The current recommendation for thoracic surgery is not to practice strict fluid restriction which potentially may lead to acute kidney injury, but to use "goal-directed" parameters for IV fluid administration.[100]

Emergence and Extubation

During emergence from anesthesia and following tracheal extubation, there is always a risk of acute airway obstruction. Current practice is to avoid 100% O2 and use an F_iO2 of 0.8 to 0.9 during emergence.

Emergence from anesthesia is a critical event with the potential for serious complications.[101] Tracheal extubation at the end of anesthesia is elective and should be individualized according to the unique needs of every patient.[102] During thoracic procedures normal-weight patients in the lateral position can be extubated followed by assisted mask ventilation until the patient is fully awake. Even though deep extubation is associated with more respiratory complications,[103] early extubation of the trachea at the completion of pulmonary resections lowers the risk of bronchial stump disruption and pulmonary air leaks secondary to positive pressure ventilation and airway tube trauma. In normal weight patients, complications may be transient and easily corrected.

The same practice may not be applicable to the MO patient with OSA because mask ventilation in the lateral position can be very difficult. Access to the airway if reintubation becomes necessary should be avoided in the lateral position. Similar to the preparation for induction, tracheal extubation for MO patients is best performed with the patient in HELP and the operating room table in the RTP. In preparation for extubation, a DLT completely withdrawn into the trachea is less stimulating than one in the bronchus and many anesthesiologists deflate both the tracheal and bronchial cuffs to withdraw the tube completely into the trachea. The tracheal cuff is then reinflated and the DLT used as a single-lumen tube. Even though a DLT in the bronchus is more stimulating, modern DLTs have similar flow resistances to regular ETTs and they are still well tolerated by most patients. Other anesthesiologists elect to keep a DLT in its bronchial position. If postoperative ventilation is planned, a DLT should be replaced with an ETT via an airway exchange catheter.[104] In this case, the use of a BB is advantageous because it can be pulled out from the ETT if postoperative ventilatory support is required.

A nasopharyngeal airway is less irritating and is better tolerated than a rigid oral airway. Both, however, should be inserted in the anesthetized patient with OSA before extubation, and the nasal airway should be kept in place after the oral airway is removed (Fig. 49.6).

Before tracheal extubation, airway equipment for tracheal reintubation, including a bougie and an SGD should

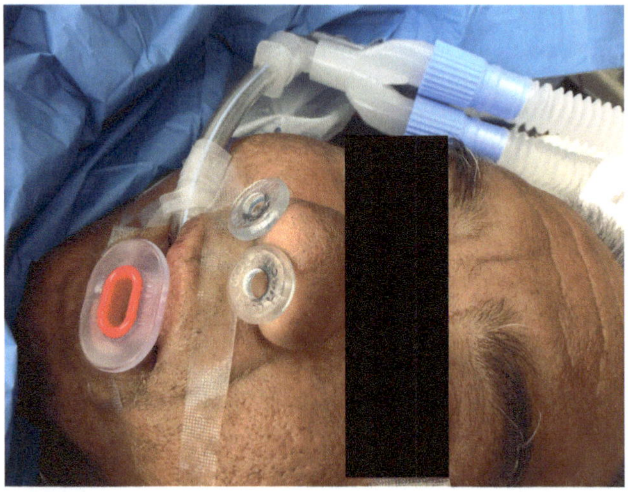

• **Fig. 49.6** Before extubating the trachea, the morbidly obese patient with obstructive sleep apnea should have both nasopharyngeal and rigid oral airways inserted to prevent airway obstruction when the endotracheal tube is removed. The patient should be completely awake and have little if any residual effects from the anesthetic gases, sedatives, and opioids before removing the breathing tube. Neuromuscular blocking agents must be completely reversed. The nasal airway is better tolerated and can be kept in place after the oral airway is removed.

always be readily available and used if needed for reintubation. For the MO patient who has been using CPAP or BiPAP preoperatively, these devices should be readily available to stent the upper airway and improve gas exchange and are supplied by respiratory therapy. Supplemental oxygen should always be administered but used with caution as oxygen therapy can increase the AHI, hypoventilation, and PaCO2 levels in a patient with OHS. Obese patients should be monitored for several hours following surgery to detect late desaturation. In most institutions, all patients with BMI above 40 kg/m^2 are transferred to a designated monitored unit (Fig. 49.7).

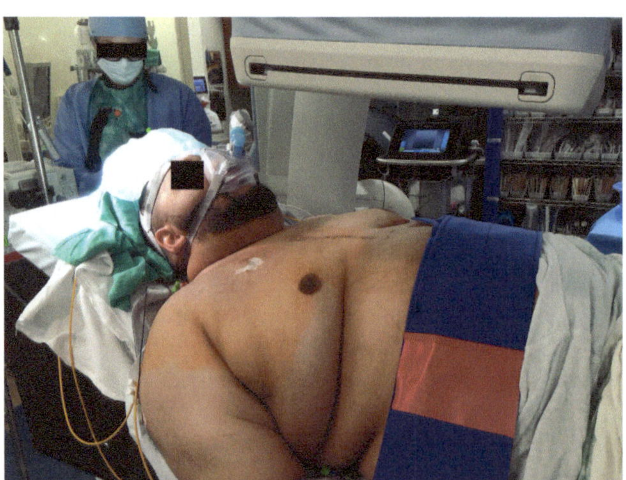

• **Fig. 49.7** Following tracheal extubation, the morbidly obese patient who has been using continuous positive airway pressure or bilevel positive airway pressure preoperatively should have the device applied to stent the upper airway and improve gas exchange.

Postoperative Management

Pain Control

Satisfactory postthoracotomy analgesia is extremely important and is covered in Chapter 25 in this book. Options include paravertebral block (PVB) and thoracic epidural analgesia (TEA), each with their own advantages and disadvantages, and to a lesser extent systemic opioids. In the MO patient, the importance of adequate pain control is further amplified because of preexisting restricted lung function.

In all patients, lung volume is significantly reduced in the postoperative period. In studies of MO patients undergoing laparotomy procedures, perioperative spirometry values decreased significantly with increasing BMI, with the greatest reduction in vital capacity immediately after tracheal extubation. It has been shown that TEA reduces this reduction in all patients, but in obese patients (BMI >30 kg/m^2) the decreases in vital capacity was significantly more pronounced than in normal patients. Similarly, recovery of spirometry values was significantly quicker in patients receiving TEA, particularly in obese patients.[17]

Epidural opioid analgesia, with or without local anesthetic, when compared with IV opioids reduces pain, improves pulmonary function and oxygenation, and reduces postthoracotomy complications.[105] Local anesthetics given epidurally also supplement general anesthesia and reduce opioid requirements during surgery.

With any analgesic technique, controlling or limiting side effects can be as important as the quality of pain control achieved. Epidural analgesia with local anesthetic is known to cause postoperative hypotension and/or motor blockade and these side effects limit the MO patient's ability to ambulate, increasing their already greater risk for pulmonary embolism.

The paravertebral space lies external to the spinal canal and a continuous infusion of local anesthetic here limits the block to the operative side and ipsilateral parasympathetic chain. A Cochrane review revealed that PVB is as effective as TEA in managing postthoracotomy incisional pain. The review evaluated 14 studies involving 698 patients which evaluated broadly if the analgesic efficacy of PVB is as effective as TEA in patients undergoing open thoracotomy. The authors found no difference between PVB and TEA in terms of death at 30 days and major complications. PVB appeared to be as effective as TEA in pain control postsurgery. TEA was associated with minor complications, such as low blood pressure, nausea and vomiting, itching, and urinary retention when compared with PVB. No difference was found in length of hospital stay between PVB and TEA.[106] Compared with an epidural, the incidence of analgesia-related complications is significantly reduced or eliminated with PVBs.[107] In some studies, the stress response to surgery is also reduced more than what is achieved by epidural analgesia.[108] These benefits, in addition to the increased challenge of successful epidural insertion in MO patients make a strong argument for PVB to be the technique of choice in the obese population. PVB may replace TEA as the preferred method of postthoracotomy pain control.[109]

Systemic opioids postthoracotomy has been shown to provide inferior pain control, regardless of the route of administration. Despite the addition of a multimodal analgesic regimen, opioid side effects, including nausea, vomiting, respiratory depression, and delirium are difficult to eliminate. In MO patients, these complications are increased because of their increased sensitivity to opioids and the previously discussed difficulty in estimating appropriate drug doses. Early institution of postoperative multimodal analgesics (including local anesthetics, interpleural local anesthetic infusions, nonsteroidal antiinflammatory agents, gabapentin, acetaminophen, ketamine, dexamethasone, and other synergistic drugs) to reduce the respiratory depressant effects of centrally acting agents is recommended for MO patients with OSA. Alpha-2 agonists (clonidine, dexmedetomidine) do not depress respiration, have analgesic properties and have been used effectively as adjuncts to epidural local anesthetics for postthoracotomy analgesia.[110]

Complications

The Society of Thoracic Surgeons General Thoracic Surgery database has been used to review surgical outcomes after thoracic operations. Following esophagectomy[111] and after elective lung resection for cancer, in a review of 41,446 patients, MO patients with a BMI greater than 40 kg/m^2 (and underweight patients with BMI <18.5 kg/m^2) had the highest incidence of complications. In contrast, being overweight or mild to moderately obese (BMI <40 kg/m^2) was associated with decreased risk of pulmonary complications and other adverse postoperative events.[112]

Patients with MO and OSA are at much higher risk for respiratory and cardiac complications in the postoperative period. As previously mentioned, opioid analgesia should be avoided if possible or used sparingly in these patients.[113] The increased incidence of postoperative desaturation and respiratory failure mandates the need for supplemental O2, and continuous O2 monitoring.[114] OSA is associated with higher odds of developing postoperative atrial fibrillation, other major adverse cardiac and cerebrovascular events, and ICU admissions than non-OSA patients.[115] In postoperative thoracic surgery patients admitted to an ICU there is a longer duration of postoperative delirium and coma in those with OSA.[116]

Rhabdomyolysis (RML) is one postoperative complication that is relatively common in MO surgical patients, but infrequent in normal-weight patients. RML results from pressure injury to skeletal muscle because of prolonged stasis in a nonphysiologic position. It has been reported in obese patients in the lateral decubitus position.[117] Long-duration surgery is the major risk factor, but other associated factors include superobesity, male gender, and a history of hypertension, diabetes and/or peripheral vascular disease. Intraoperative padding of all pressure points and close attention to patient positioning are essential to prevent RML, pressure ulcers, and neurologic damage in MO patients. Injured muscle releases myoglobin, electrolytes, and protein into the systemic circulation. Myoglobinuria can lead to acute renal failure, and electrolyte disturbances can cause dysrhythmias and even cardiac arrest.

Local signs and symptoms of RML are nonspecific and include pain, tenderness, swelling, bruising, and weakness. Complaints of numbness and muscular pain are almost always present, but epidural analgesia can mask symptoms and delay diagnosis. Myoglobinuria usually presents as "tea" or brown-colored urine. The primary diagnostic indicator of RML is elevated serum creatine phosphokinase (CPK) levels. An MO patient who complains of buttock, hip, or shoulder pain in the postoperative period and who has a serum CPK level greater than 1000 IU/L is considered to have RML. Treatment should be instituted once CPK levels increase beyond 5000 IU/L. Although intraoperative fluid replacement can reduce the risk of postoperative RML, fluid replacement is usually restricted during pulmonary resections. However, once a diagnosis of RML is made, aggressive hydration with large volumes of IV fluids and administration of diuretics are required to flush myoglobin from the kidneys.

Conclusion

An ever-increasing percentage of the thoracic surgical population is composed of obese and MO patients. With appropriate planning and management obese patients, including MO and patients with OSA, tolerate OLV during thoracic surgery. The number of published studies of MO thoracic surgical patients is slowly increasing, but the current anesthetic management for obese patients with OSA is based on experience from nonthoracic surgical procedures.

References

1. Deitel M. The International Obesity Task Force and "globesity." *Obes Surg.* 2002;12:613–614.
2. Bray GA, Kim KK, Wilding JPH. Obesity: a chronic relapsing progressive disease process. A position statement of the World Obesity Federation. *Obes Rev.* 2017;18:715–723.
3. Schumann R, Jones SB, Cooper B, et al. Update on best practice recommendations for anesthetic perioperative care and pain management in weight loss surgery, 2004–2007. *Obesity* (Silver Spring) 2009;17:889–894.
4. Ortiz VE, Kwo J. Obesity: physiologic changes and implications for preoperative management. *BMC Anesthesiol.* 2015;15:97.
5. Bohmer AB, Wappler F. Preoperative evaluation and preparation of the morbidly obese patient. *Curr Opin Anaesthesiol.* 2017;30: 126–132.
6. Lemmens HJ, Brodsky JB, Bernstein DP. Estimating ideal body weight—a new formula. *Obes Surg.* 2005;15:1082–1083.

7. Janmahasatian S, Duffull SB, Ash S, Ward LC, Byrne NM, Green B. Quantification of lean bodyweight. *Clin Pharmacokinet.* 2005;44:1051–1065.
8. Vannucci A, Cavallone LF. Bedside predictors of difficult intubation: a systematic review. *Minerva Anestesiol.* 2016;82:69–83.
9. Roth D, Pace NL, Lee A, et al. Bedside tests for predicting difficult airways: an abridged Cochrane diagnostic test accuracy systematic review. *Anaesthesia.* 2019;74:915–928.
10. Collins JS. Do all morbidly obese patients have a "difficult" airway? In: Leykin Y, Brodsky JB, eds. *Controversies in the Anesthetic Management of the Obese Surgical Patient.* Milan: Springer; 2013:145–156.
11. Seok Y, Jheon S, Cho S. Serial changes in pulmonary function after video-assisted thoracic surgery lobectomy in lung cancer patient. *Thorac Cardiovasc Surg.* 2014;62:133–139.
12. Pelosi P, Croci M, Ravagnan I, et al. The effects of body mass on lung volumes, respiratory mechanics, and gas exchange during general anesthesia. *Anesth Analg.* 1998;87:654–660.
13. Licker MJ, Widikker I, Robert J, et al. Operative mortality and respiratory complications after lung resection for cancer: impact of chronic obstructive pulmonary disease and time trends. *Ann Thorac Surg.* 2006;81:1830–1837.
14. Ferguson MK, Vigneswaran WT. Diffusing capacity predicts morbidity after lung resection in patients without obstructive lung disease. *Ann Thorac Surg.* 2008;85:1158–1164.
15. Slinger PD, Johnston MR. Preoperative assessment: an anesthesiologist's perspective. *Thorac Surg Clin.* 2005;15:11–25.
16. Kim SH, Na S, Park SY, et al. Perioperative factors for predicting the need for postoperative intensive care after major lung resection. *J Clin Med.* 2019;8(5):E744 pii.
17. von Ungern-Sternberg BS, Regli A, Reber A, Schneider MC. Effect of obesity and thoracic epidural analgesia on perioperative spirometry. *Br J Anaesth.* 2005;94:121–127.
18. Practice guidelines for the perioperative management of patients with obstructive sleep apnea: an updated report by the American Society of Anesthesiologists Task Force on Perioperative Management of patients with obstructive sleep apnea. *Anesthesiology.* 2014;120:268–286.
19. Crummy F, Piper AJ, Naughton MT. Obesity and the lung: 2. Obesity and sleep-disordered breathing. *Thorax.* 2008;63:738–746.
20. Chung F, Chau E, Yang Y, Liao P, Hall R, Mokhlesi B. Serum bicarbonate level improves specificity of STOP-Bang screening for obstructive sleep apnea. *Chest.* 2013;143:1284–1293.
21. Frey WC, Pilcher J. Obstructive sleep-related breathing disorders in patients evaluated for bariatric surgery. *Obes Surg.* 2003; 13:676–683.
22. Peppard PE, Young T, Barnet JH, Palta M, Hagen EW, Hla KM. Increased prevalence of sleep-disordered breathing in adults. *Am J Epidemiol.* 2013;177:1006–1014.
23. Chung F, Abdullah HR, Liao P. STOP-Bang Questionnaire: a practical approach to screen for obstructive sleep apnea. *Chest.* 2016;149:631–638.
24. Carlucci A, Ceriana P, Mancini M, et al. Efficacy of bilevel-auto treatment in patients with obstructive sleep apnea not responsive to or intolerant of continuous positive airway pressure ventilation. *J Clin Sleep Med.* 2015;115:981–985.
25. Memtsoudis SG, Cozowicz C, Nagappa M, et al. Society of Anesthesia and Sleep Medicine Guideline on intraoperative management of adult patients with obstructive sleep apnea. *Anesth Analg.* 2018;127:967–987.
26. Mokhlesi B. Obesity hypoventilation syndrome: a state-of-the-art review. *Respir Care.* 2010;55:1347–1362.
27. Masa JF, Pepin JL, Borel JC, Mokhlesi B, Murphy PB, Sánchez-Quiroga MÁ. Obesity hypoventilation syndrome. *Eur Respir Rev.* 2019;14:28.
28. Soghier I, Brożek JL, Afshar M, et al. Noninvasive ventilation versus CPAP as initial treatment of obesity hypoventilation syndrome. *Ann Am Thorac Soc.* 2019;16:1295 1130.
29. Mokhlesi B, Masa JF, Brozek JL, et al. Evaluation and management of obesity hypoventilation syndrome. An Official American Thoracic Society Clinical Practice Guideline. *Am J Respir Crit Care Med.* 2019;200:e6–e24.
30. Alpert MA, Lavie CJ, Agrawal H, Aggarwal KB, Kumar SA. Obesity and heart failure: epidemiology, pathophysiology, clinical manifestations, and management. *Transl Res.* 2014;164:345–356.
31. Sidana J, Aronow WS, Ravipati G, et al. Prevalence of moderate or severe left ventricular diastolic dysfunction in obese persons with obstructive sleep apnea. *Cardiology.* 2005;104:107–109.
32. Altermatt FR, Muñoz HR, Delfino AE, Cortínez LI. Preoxygenation in the obese patient: effects of position on tolerance to apnoea. *Br J Anaesth.* 2005;95:706–709.
33. Collins JS, Lemmens HJ, Brodsky JB, Brock-Utne JG, Levitan RM. Laryngoscopy and morbid obesity: a comparison of the "sniff" and "ramped" positions. *Obes Surg.* 2004;14:1171–1175.
34. Perilli V, Sollazzi L, Modesti C, et al. Determinants of improvement in oxygenation consequent to reverse Trendelenburg position in anesthetized morbidly obese patients. *Obes Surg.* 2004;14: 866–867.
35. Dixon BJ, Dixon JB, Carden JR, et al. Preoxygenation is more effective in the 25 degrees head-up position than in the supine position in severely obese patients: a randomized controlled study. *Anesthesiology.* 2005;102:1110–1115.
36. Boyce JR, Ness T, Castroman P, Gleysteen JJ. A preliminary study of the optimal anesthesia positioning for the morbidly obese patient. *Obes Surg.* 2003;13:4–9.
37. Couture EJ, Provencher S, Somma J, Lellouche F, Marceau S, Bussières JS. Effect of position and positive pressure ventilation on functional residual capacity in morbidly obese patients: a randomized trial. *Can J Anaesth.* 2018;65:522–528.
38. Patel A, Nouraei SA. Transnasal humidified rapid-insufflation ventilatory exchange (THRIVE): a physiological method of increasing apnoea time in patients with difficult airways. *Anaesthesia.* 2015;70:323–329.
39. Wong DT, Dallaire A, Singh KP, et al. High-flow nasal oxygen improves safe apnea time in morbidly obese patients undergoing general anesthesia: a randomized controlled trial. *Anesth Analg.* 2019;129:1130–1136.
40. Heard A, Toner AJ, Evans JR, Aranda Palacios AM, Lauer S. Apneic oxygenation during prolonged laryngoscopy in obese patients: a randomized controlled trial of buccal RAE tube oxygen administration. *Anesth Analg.* 2017;124:1162–1167.
41. Tsueda K, Debrand M, Zeok SS, Wright BD, Griffin WO. Obesity supine death syndrome: reports of two morbidly obese patients. *Anesth Analg.* 1979;58:345–347.
42. Lemyze M, Guerry MJ, Mallat J, Thevenin D. Obesity supine death syndrome revisited. *Eur Respir J.* 2012;40:1568–1569.
43. Lemyze M, Guiot A, Mallat J, Thevenin D. The obesity supine death syndrome (OSDS). *Obes Rev.* 2018;19:550–556.
44. Apfelbaum JL, Hagberg CA, Caplan RA, et al. American Society of Anesthesiologists Task Force on Management of the Difficult Airway. Practice guidelines for management of the difficult airway: an updated report by the American Society of Anesthesiologists Task Force on Management of the Difficult Airway. *Anesthesiology.* 2013;118:251–270.

45. Collins JS, Lemmens HJ, Brodsky JB. Obesity and difficult intubation: where is the evidence? *Anesthesiology*. 2006;104:61.
46. Dixit A, Kulshrestha M, Mathews JJ, Bhandari M. Are the obese difficult to intubate? *Br J Anaesth*. 2014;112:770–771.
47. Kheterpal S, Healy D, Aziz MF, et al. Incidence, predictors, and outcome of difficult mask ventilation combined with difficult laryngoscopy: a report from the multicenter perioperative outcomes group. *Anesthesiology*. 2013;119:1360–1369.
48. Gander S, Frascarolo P, Suter M, Spahn DR, Magnusson L. Positive end-expiratory pressure during induction of general anesthesia increases duration of nonhypoxic apnea in morbidly obese patients. *Anesth Analg*. 2005;100:580–584.
49. Adnet F, Borron SW, Racine SX, et al. The intubation difficulty scale (IDS): proposal and evaluation of a new score characterizing the complexity of endotracheal intubation. *Anesthesiology*. 1997;87: 1290–1297.
50. Cormack RS, Lehane JR, Adams AP, Carli F. Laryngoscopy grades and percentage glottic opening. *Anaesthesia*. 2000;55:184.
51. Juvin P, Lavaut E, Dupont H, et al. Difficult tracheal intubation is more common in obese than in lean patients. *Anesth Analg*. 2003;97:595–600.
52. Gonzalez H, Minville V, Delanoue K, Mazerolles M, Concina D, Fourcade O. The importance of increased neck circumference to intubation difficulties in obese patients. *Anesth Analg*. 2008;106:1132–1136.
53. Brodsky JB, Lemmens HJ, Brock-Utne JG, Vierra M, Saidman LJ. Morbid obesity and tracheal intubation. *Anesth Analg*. 2002;94:732–736.
54. Saasouh W, Laffey K, Turan A, et al. Degree of obesity is not associated with more than one intubation attempt: a large centre experience. *Br J Anaesth*. 2018;120:1110–1116.
55. Koerner IP, Brambrink AM. Fiberoptic techniques. *Best Pract Res Clin Anaesthesiol*. 2005;19:611–621.
56. Nicholson A, Smith AF, Lewis SR, Cook TM. Tracheal intubation with a flexible intubation scope versus other intubation techniques for obese patients requiring general anaesthesia. *Cochrane Database Syst Rev*. 2014(1):CD010320.
57. Wong J, Lee JSE, Wong TGL, Iqbal R, Wong P. Fibreoptic intubation in airway management: a review article. *Singapore Med J*. 2019;60:110–118.
58. King MR, Jagannathan N. Should videolaryngoscopy be the standard of care for routine tracheal intubation in obese adults? *J Clin Anesth*. 2018;45:33–34.
59. Lewis SR, Butler AR, Parker J, Cook TM, Schofield-Robinson OJ, Smith AF. Videolaryngoscopy versus direct laryngoscopy for adult patients requiring tracheal intubation: a Cochrane Systematic Review. *Br J Anaesth*. 2017;119:369–383.
60. Hoshijima H, Denawa Y, Tominage A, Nakamura C, Shiga T, Nagaska H. Videolaryngoscope versus Macintosh laryngoscope for tracheal intubation in adults with obesity: a systematic review and meta-analysis. *J Clin Anesth*. 2018;44:69–75.
61. Cook TM, Woodall N, Frerk C. Fourth National Audit Project. Major complications of airway management in the UK: results of the Fourth National Audit Project of the Royal College of Anaesthetists and the Difficult Airway Society. Part 1: anaesthesia. *Br J Anaesth*. 2011;106:617–631.
62. Nightingale CE, Cousins J, Fox WT, Kennedy N, Margarson MP, Shearer E. Comment on Fourth National Audit Project from the Society of Bariatric Anaesthetists. *Br J Anaesth*. 2021; 107:272–273.
63. Parmet JL, Colonna-Romano P, Horrow JC, Miller RF, Gonzales J. The laryngeal mask airway reliably provides rescue ventilation in cases of unanticipated difficult tracheal intubation along with difficult mask ventilation. *Anesth Analg*. 1998;87:661–665.
64. Keller C, Brimacombe J, Kleinsasser A, Brimacombe L. The Laryngeal Mask Airway Proseal™ as a temporary ventilatory device in grossly and morbidly obese patients before laryngoscope-guided tracheal intubation. *Anesth Analg*. 2002;94:737–740.
65. Sinha A, Jayaraman L, Punhani D. ProSeal™ LMA increases safe apnea period in morbidly obese patients undergoing surgery under general anesthesia. *Obes Surg*. 2013;23:580–584.
66. Ingrande J, Brodsky JB, Lemmens HJ. Lean body weight scalar for the anesthetic induction dose of propofol in morbidly obese subjects. *Anesth Analg*. 2011;113:57–62.
67. Gaszyński T, Wieczorek A. A comparison of BIS recordings during propofol-based total intravenous anaesthesia and sevoflurane-based inhalational anaesthesia in obese patients. *Anaesthesiol Intensive Ther*. 2016;48:239–247.
68. Brodsky JB, Lemmens HJ, Saidman LJ. Obesity, surgery, and inhalation anesthetics – is there a “drug of choice”? *Obes Surg*. 2006;16:734.
69. Liu FL, Cherng YG, Chen SY, et al. Postoperative recovery after anesthesia in morbidly obese patients: a systematic review and meta-analysis of randomized controlled trials. *Can J Anaesth*. 2015;62:907–917.
70. Ozdogan HK, Cetinkunar S, Karateke F, Cetinalp S, Celik M, Ozyazici S. The effects of sevoflurane and desflurane on the hemodynamics and respiratory functions in laparoscopic sleeve gastrectomy. *J Clin Anesth*. 2016;35:441–445.
71. Arain SR, Barth CD, Shankar H, Ebert TJ. Choice of volatile anesthetic for the morbidly obese patient: sevoflurane or desflurane. *J Clin Anesth*. 2005;17:413.
72. Punjasawadwong Y, Phongchiewboon A, Bunchungmongkol N. Bispectral index for improving anaesthetic delivery and postoperative recovery. *Cochrane Database Syst Rev*. 2014(6): CD003843.
73. Lemmens HJ, Brodsky JB. The dose of succinylcholine in morbid obesity. *Anesth Analg*. 2006;102:438–442.
74. Badaoui R, Cabaret A, Alami Y, et al. Reversal of neuromuscular blockade by sugammadex in laparoscopic bariatric surgery: In support of dose reduction. *Anaesth Crit Care Pain Med*. 2016;35:25–29.
75. Loupec T, Frasca D, Rousseau N, Faure JP, Mimoz O, Debaene B. Appropriate dosing of sugammadex to reverse deep rocuronium-induced neuromuscular blockade in morbidly obese patients. *Anaesthesia*. 2016;71:265–272.
76. Narayanaswamy M, McRae K, Slinger P, et al. Choosing a lung isolation device for thoracic surgery: a randomized trial of three bronchial blockers versus double-lumen tubes. *Anesth Analg*. 2009;108:1097–1101.
77. Campos JH. Update on tracheobronchial anatomy and flexible fiberoptic bronchoscopy in thoracic anesthesia. *Curr Opin Anaesthesiol*. 2009;22:4–10.
78. Campos JH. Which device should be considered the best for lung isolation: double-lumen endotracheal tube versus bronchial blockers. *Curr Opin Anaesthesiol*. 2007;20:27–31.
79. Campos JH, Hallam EA, Ueda K. Lung isolation in the morbidly obese patient: a comparison of a left-sided double-lumen tracheal tube with the Arndt® wire-guided blocker. *Br J Anaesth*. 2012;109:630–635.
80. Shulman MS, Brodsky JB, Levesque PR. Fibreoptic bronchoscopy for tracheal and endobronchial intubation with a double-lumen tube. *Can J Anaesth*. 1987;34:172–173.

81. Brodsky JB, Lemmens HJ. Tracheal width and left double-lumen tube size: a formula to estimate left-bronchial width. *J Clin Anesth*. 2005;17:267–270.
82. D'Anza B, Knight J, Greene JS. Does body mass index predict tracheal airway size? *Laryngoscope*. 2015;125:1093–1097.
83. Campos JH, Feider A. Hypoxia during one-lung ventilation-a review and update. *J Cardiothorac Vasc Anesth*. 2018;32:2330–2338.
84. Bardoczky GI, Szegedi LL, d'Hollander AA, Moures JM, de Francquen P, Yernault JC. Two-lung and one-lung ventilation in patients with chronic obstructive pulmonary disease: the effects of position and FiO2. *Anesth Analg*. 2000;90:35–41.
85. Henzler D, Rossaint R, Kuhlen R. Is there a need for a recruiting strategy in morbidly obese patients undergoing laparoscopic surgery? *Anesth Analg*. 2004;98:268.
86. Aldenkortt M, Lysakowski C, Elia N, Brochard L, Tramèr MR. Ventilation strategies in obese patients undergoing surgery: a quantitative systematic review and meta-analysis. *Br J Anaesth*. 2012;109:493–502.
87. Watanabe S, Noguchi E, Yamada S, Hamada N, Kano T. Sequential changes of arterial oxygen tension in the supine position during one-lung ventilation. *Anesth Analg*. 2000;90:28–34.
88. Brodsky JB, Wyner J, Ehrenwerth J, Merrell RC, Cohn RB. One-lung anesthesia in morbidly obese patients. *Anesthesiology*. 1982;57:132–134.
89. Lohser J. Evidence-based management of one-lung ventilation. *Anesthesiol Clin*. 2008;26:241–272.
90. Bardoczky GI, Yernault JC, Houben JJ, d'Hollander AA. Large tidal volume ventilation does not improve oxygenation in morbidly obese patients during anesthesia. *Anesth Analg*. 1995;81:385–388.
91. Jaber S, Coisel Y, Chanques G, et al. A multicentre observational study of intra-operative ventilatory management during general anaesthesia: tidal volumes and relation to body weight. *Anaesthesia*. 2012;67:999–1008.
92. Balick-Weber CC, Nicolas P, Hedreville-Montout M, Blanchet P, Stéphan F. Respiratory and haemodynamic effects of volume-controlled vs pressure-controlled ventilation during laparoscopy: a cross-over study with echocardiographic assessment. *Br J Anaesth*. 2007;99:429–435.
93. Fernandez-Bustamante A, Hashimoto S, Serpa Neto A, Moine P, Vidal Melo MF, Repine JE. Perioperative lung protective ventilation in obese patients. *BMC Anesthesiol*. 2015;6(15):56.
94. Cadi P, Guenoun T, Journois D, Chevallier JM, Diehl JL, Safran D. Pressure-controlled ventilation improves oxygenation during laparoscopic obesity surgery compared with volume-controlled ventilation. *Br J Anaesth*. 2008;100:709–716.
95. Sentürk NM, Dilek A, Camci E, et al. Effects of positive end-expiratory pressure on ventilatory and oxygenation parameters during pressure-controlled one-lung ventilation. *J Cardiothorac Vasc Anesth*. 2005;19:71–75.
96. Michelet P, Roch A, Brousse D, et al. Effects of PEEP on oxygenation and respiratory mechanics during one-lung ventilation. *Br J Anaesth*. 2005;95:267.
97. Park M, Ahn HJ, Kim JA, et al. Driving pressure during thoracic surgery: a randomized clinical trial. *Anesthesiology*. 2019;130:385–393.
98. Slinger PD. Perioperative fluid management for thoracic surgery: the puzzle of postpneumonectomy pulmonary edema. *J Cardiothorac Vasc Anesth*. 1995;9:442–541.
99. Lemmens HJ, Bernstein DP, Brodsky JB. Estimating blood volume in obese and morbidly obese patients. *Obes Surg*. 2006;16:773–776.
100. Haas S, Eichhorn V, Hasbach T, et al. Goal-directed fluid therapy using stroke volume variation does not result in pulmonary fluid overload in thoracic surgery requiring one-lung ventilation. *Crit Care Res Pract*. 2012.
101. Peterson GN, Domino KB, Caplan RA, Posner KL, Lee LA, Cheney FW. Management of the difficult airway. A closed claims analysis. *Anesthesiology*. 2005;103:33–39.
102. Difficult Airway Society Extubation Guidelines Group, Popat M, Mitchell V, Dravid R, Patel A, Swampillai C, Higgs A. Difficult Airway Society Guidelines for the management of tracheal extubation. *Anaesthesia*. 2012;67:318–340.
103. Karmarkar S, Varshney S. Tracheal extubation. *Contin Educ Anaesth Crit Care Pain*. 2008;8:214–220.
104. Brodsky JB. Lung separation and the difficult airway. *Br J Anaesth*. 2009;103(1):166–175 Supp.
105. Wu CL, Cohen SR, Richman JM, et al. Efficacy of postoperative patient-controlled and continuous infusion epidural analgesia versus intravenous patient-controlled analgesia with opioids: a meta-analysis. *Anesthesiology*. 2005;103:1079–1088.
106. Yeung JH, Gates S, Naidu BV, Wilson MJ, Gao Smith F. Paravertebral block versus thoracic epidural for patients undergoing thoracotomy. *Cochrane Database Syst Rev*. 2016;2:CD009121.
107. Davies RG, Myles PS, Graham JM. A comparison of the analgesic efficacy and side-effects of paravertebral vs epidural blockade for thoracotomy–a systematic review and meta-analysis of randomized trials. *Br J Anaesth*. 2006;96:418–426.
108. Richardson J, Sabanathan S, Jones J, Shah RD, Cheema S, Mearns AJ. A prospective, randomized comparison of preoperative and continuous balanced epidural or paravertebral bupivacaine on post-thoracotomy pain, pulmonary function and stress responses. *Br J Anaesth*. 1999;83:387–392.
109. Conlon NP, Shaw AD, Grichnik KP. Postthoracotomy paravertebral analgesia: will it replace epidural analgesia? *Anesthesiol Clin*. 2008;26:369–380.
110. Hofer RE, Sprung J, Sarr MG, Wedel DJ. Anesthesia for a patient with morbid obesity using dexmedetomidine without narcotics. *Can J Anaesth*. 2005;52:176–180.
111. Mitzman B, Schipper PH, Edwards MA, Kim S, Ferguson MK. Complications after esophagectomy are associated with extremes of body mass index. *Ann Thorac Surg*. 2018;106:973–980.
112. Williams T, Gulack BC, Kim S, Fernandez FG, Ferguson MK. Operative risk for major lung resection increases at extremes of body mass index. *Ann Thorac Surg*. 2017;103:296–302.
113. Sultana A, Torres D, Schumann R. Special indications for opioid free anaesthesia and analgesia, patient and procedure related: including obesity, sleep apnoea, chronic obstructive pulmonary disease, complex regional pain syndromes, opioid addiction and cancer surgery. *Best Pract Res Clin Anaesthesiol*. 2017;31:547–560.
114. Kaw R, Chung F, Pasupuleti V, Mehta J, Gay PC, Hernandez AV. Meta-analysis of the association between obstructive sleep apnoea and postoperative outcome. *Br J Anaesth*. 2012;109:897–906.
115. Nagappa M, Ho G, Patra J, et al. Postoperative outcomes in obstructive sleep apnea patients undergoing cardiac surgery: a systematic review and meta-analysis of comparative studies. *Anesth Analg*. 2017;125:2030–2037.
116. Wang S, Sigua NL, Manchanda S, et al. Preoperative STOP-BANG scores and postoperative delirium and coma in thoracic surgery patients. *Ann Thorac Surg*. 2018;106:966–972.
117. Kong SS, Ho ST, Huang GS, Cherng CH, Wong CS. Rhabdomyolysis after a long-term thoracic surgery in right decubitus position. *Acta Anaesthesiol Sin*. 2000;38:223–228.

50

Cystic Fibrosis

GIORGIO DELLA ROCCA, ALESSANDRA DELLA ROCCA

Clinical Case

A 17-year-old male with cystic fibrosis (CF), pancreatic insufficiency and steatorrhea and severely compromised respiratory function was evaluated for lung transplantation. An episode of bowel obstruction when he was 15 years old required a laparotomy. During the months prior to admission he suffered a gradual weight loss, severe limitation of exercise tolerance, and difficulty in performing his daily activities, with several episodes of recurrent pneumonias.

At the time of the evaluation, he was 159 cm tall and his body weight was 50 kg. Chest computed tomography (CT) scans showed bilateral bronchiectasis with peribronchial inflammation, pulmonary consolidation, and fibrosis. Areas of hyperinflation and marked parenchymal destruction were present bilaterally (Fig. 50.1). Lung scintigraphy showed a severe and bilateral deficit of perfusion with residual, irregular perfusion essentially limited to the lower lobe of the right lung.

Mild hepatosplenomegaly was diagnosed at the CT scan, but liver function tests were normal.

Respiratory function tests revealed a severe pulmonary obstructive disease: forced expiratory volume in 1 second (FEV_1) = 0.63 L/min (16% of predicted value) and forced vital capacity (FVC) = 1.69 L (39%). Arterial blood gas sample showed: pH=7.39, arterial oxygen partial pressure (PaO2) = 61 mm Hg and arterial carbon dioxide partial pressure (PaCO2) = 48.7 mm Hg with oxygen saturation (SaO2) = 90% (room air).

The electrocardiogram (ECG) was normal. The echocardiography showed increased right ventricle dimension to the upper limit of normal values and mild tricuspid regurgitation. The right heart catheterization showed a cardiac output (CO) of 4.94 L/min, mild pulmonary hypertension with a mean pulmonary arterial pressure (MPAP) of 25 mm Hg and pulmonary vascular resistance of 408 dynes/s/cm^5.

During the last year, while on the lung transplant waiting list, his lung function deteriorated because of recurrent pneumonias; he became O2-dependent, notwithstanding continuous appropriate therapy with antibiotics, bronchodilator β-adrenergic inhaled agent, pancreatic enzymes, and laxatives, together with correctly performed chest physiotherapy.

On the day of lung Tx, now 19 years old, he weighed 45 kg. He was tachypneic at rest despite oxygen therapy. Arterial gases analysis showed a PaO2/fraction of inspired oxygen (F_iO2) of 240 mm Hg and PaCO2 of 54 mm Hg with a SaO2 of 97%. Arterial invasive blood pressure (AP) was 140/80 mm Hg with a mean arterial pressure (MAP) of 100 mm Hg and heart rate (HR) of 90 beats per minute. The pulmonary catheter inserted preoperatively revealed a CO of 6 L/min with an increase in MPAP up to 33 mm Hg (PAP = 53/23 mm Hg). Only low doses of intravenous (IV) midazolam (1 mg) was administered as premedication. Before the induction of anesthesia, a thoracic peridural catheter (T4–T5 intervertebral space) was inserted for postoperative pain relief.

Induction of Anesthesia

After preoxygenation by face mask, anesthesia was induced with midazolam (0.05 mg/kg), alfentanil (0.01 mg/kg), and propofol (0.5 mg/kg), in O2 100%, and maintained with sevoflurane 1% supplemented by a continuous infusion of remifentanil (0.05–0.2 mcg/kg/min) in O2 up to 100%. Rocuronium bromide was used as neuromuscular blocking agent. The trachea was intubated with a large size single-lumen tube (outer diameter [OD] 9.5) for vigorous preoperative bronchial toilette with a flexible bronchoscope. The patient was then reintubated through an airway exchanger catheter (Cook Critical Care, Bloomington, IN, USA) with a 39 F left endobronchial tube (Bronchocath, Mallinkrodt, Covidien, Tullamore, Ireland). Ventilation was set to avoid air trapping and dynamic hyperinflation with a tidal volume (V_T) around 400 mL and a respiratory rate (RR) of 14 breaths per minute with a short inspiratory time and maximal expiratory time (I:E = 1:4), to reduce peak inflation below 30 to 40 cmH_2O and to avoid hemodynamic deterioration. Monitoring was completed with spirometry, end-tidal CO2 (EtCO2), and expiratory volatile anesthetic fraction analysis, transesophageal echocardiography (TEE), and arterial pulse contour continuous cardiac output and volumetric analysis (pulse contour cardiac output [PiCCO] System, Pulsion Medical System – Munich Germany) through the right femoral artery.

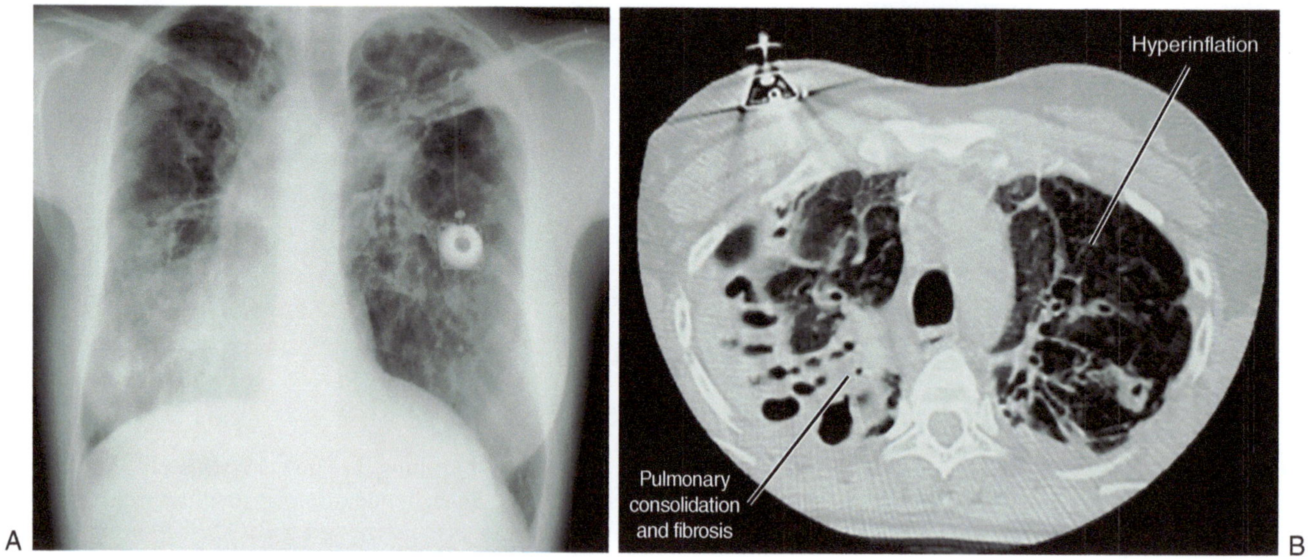

• **Fig. 50.1** Chest radiography (**A**) and chest computed tomography scan (**B**) during transplant evaluation.

Intraoperative Period

After the induction of anesthesia, in bipulmonary mechanical ventilation, hemodynamic, volumetric, and oxygenation data were: HR = 90 beats per minute, AP = 100/50 (MAP = 67) mm Hg, PAP = 48/21 (MPAP = 30) mm Hg, CO = 6.2 L/min, pH = 7.24, PaO2/F_iO2 = 350 mm Hg, PaCO2 = 74 mm Hg, intrathoracic blood volume index (ITBVI) = 850 mL/m^2 (n. v. = 800–1000), extravascular lung water index (EVLWI) = 15 mL/kg (n. v. <7). To increase right heart performance and to reduce pulmonary hypertension during surgery, dobutamine (1–10 mcg/kg/min), IV prostaglandin E1 (PGE_1) (20 ng/kg/min), inhaled nitric oxide (INO) (up to 10 ppm), inhaled aerosolized prostacyclin (IAP 10 ng/kg/min), and norepinephrine (0.05–0.3 mcg/kg/min) and ephedrine (5–10 mg/bolus) to counterbalance the systemic hypotension were administered. Frequent suctioning through the endobronchial tube was performed throughout the surgical period. Blood glucose concentration was monitored at frequent intervals. After implantation of the new lungs we observed a decrease of PAP (36/18 mm Hg), with cardiovascular stability (AP = 120/55 mm Hg, CO = 6.5 L/min, ITBVI = 750 L/min^2) and an amelioration of gas exchange (pH = 7.35, PaO2/F_iO2 = 419 mm Hg, PaCO2 = 37 mm Hg, EVLWI = 12 mL/kg).

Emergence From Anesthesia

At the end of surgery, a bolus of lidocaine 1% 8 mL was administered through the epidural catheter and a bupivacaine 0.1% (5 mL/h) continuous infusion was started. The patient was extubated in the operative room and after 30 minutes, an arterial blood gas analysis showed: pH = 7.43, PaO2/F_iO2 = 295 mm Hg, PaCO2 = 46.7 mm Hg. He was then transferred to the intensive care unit (ICU), from where he was discharged 48 hours later. The postoperative hospital length of stay was 20 days after the transplantation.

Definition

CF is the most common autosomal recessive disorder in Caucasian population, with a frequency of about one in 2500 livebirths.[1] It is caused by mutations in a 230 kb gene on chromosome 7 encoding a 1480 amino acid polypeptide, named cystic fibrosis transmembrane regulator (CFTR), which functions as a chloride channel in epithelial membranes.[2,3]

The basic defect of CF is abnormal epithelial chloride and sodium transport resulting in increased electrolyte content of secretions and in altered transluminal potential difference.[4,5] At the results of the *CFTR* gene mutation, a defect in the secretory process for sodium, chloride, and water occurs across epithelia lining of the pancreas, lungs, sweat glands, intestine, biliary system, reproductive and respiratory tracts, and salivary glands. The aberrant properties of the chloride channel disrupt osmotic gradients and transluminal potential differences, resulting in abnormally viscid secretions and obstruction of organ passages[6] (Fig. 50.2). The disease is a clinical spectrum of differing severity and patterns of organ involvement; however, increased life expectancy and the quest for a better quality of life increases the probability for anesthesiologists to encounter CF patients for complications of the disease or for unrelated surgery.[6,7,8]

CF affects multiple organs in the body (Fig. 50.3). The abnormal sweat chloride, the pulmonary disease, and the pancreatic disease constitute the classic **"diagnostic triad"** for CF, although either the pulmonary or the pancreatic disease or both may be clinically inapparent early in life.[9] The essence of CF is the chronic, suppurative, obstructive pulmonary disease that ultimately compromises the patient's life quality. Shortly after birth, many patients with CF have repeated episodes of lung infection that incites an inflammatory response that is slow to recede: the persistent lung infection and inflammation becomes self-sustaining.

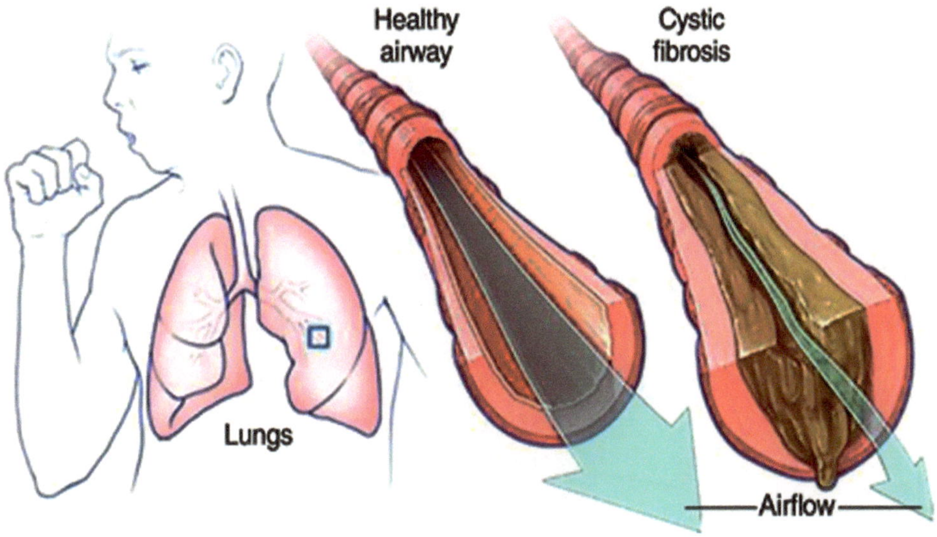

• **Fig. 50.2** Viscid secretion in CF and secretion in healthy airway.

The ongoing massive inflammatory response ultimately destroys the airways, impairs gas exchange, and may ultimately lead to death. The electrolyte transport defects of the CF airway could conspire to desiccate airway secretions that may lead to trapping of bacteria in the lung and reducing mucociliary clearance. These events results in repeated bacterial infection with recurrent episodes of pneumonia.[10]

Initially, the infant lung develops substantial small airway mucous plugging, inflammation infection, and progressive dilatation of small and large airways. As a result, children and adults develop peripherally hyperinflated lungs to compensate for the partial occlusion of the conducting airway, which fill with thick, mucopurulent exudates.[11] Bronchiectasis, a major abnormality through the course of CF, is characterized by airways with walls that are atrophic and cuffed with dense, fibroinflammatory infiltrate of lymphocytes, plasma cells, and macrophages.[12] As patients age, the airways begin to terminate in large, fibrous-walled cavities that at the visceral pleura are identified on radiographs as thin-walled cysts. These cysts are often the residual of necrotizing bronchocentric inflammation and progressive enlargement, as stenosis and mucostasis in the communicating airway function as a neck-valve to progressively trap the air in the cavity.[13] Acutely infected bronchi progress to chronic bronchiolitis, then chronic stenosing bronchiolitis and bronchiolitis obliterans.[14] Although emphysema is not a major component of early lung disease of CF, multiple areas of periseptal emphysema produce cysts or bullae, with accentuated interspersed interstitium in these areas.[15]

The earliest change in pulmonary function will result in increased air trapping, as demonstrated by decreased ratio of residual volume to total lung capacity, and changes in the maximal midexpiratory flow rates, which involve small airway disease.[9] Later, the FEV_1 is reduced out of proportion to the lung volume, indicating an obstructive ventilatory defect. The FEV_1 continues to decline throughout the life of the patient, and it is the single best predictor of mortality. Once the FEV_1 has reached 30% of predicted, the 2-year mortality is about 50%, and so this level of FEV_1 is often taken as a threshold value for referring patients for evaluation for lung Tx, which is indicated in CF when there is progressive decline in a patient's functional reserve.

Chest radiographs become abnormal early in the course of the disease. The typical stigmata of bronchiectasis (cystic changes, ring shadow, thickened airway wall) first appear in the upper lobe. Gas exchanges may be initially well-preserved into the course of the disease, whereas hypoxemia and later CO2 retention occur in a later stage. Chronic hypoxemia associated with advanced pulmonary disease may be associated with pulmonary hypertension and cor pulmonale.[16,17] This generally develops gradually, but can be precipitated acutely by infection or other physiologic stress. A progressive decrease in right ventricular ejection fraction with progressive pulmonary disease has been demonstrated in CF patients, although not universally, even in severe lung disease.[18] Although right ventricular dysfunction is characteristic, left ventricular abnormalities or a generalized cardiomyopathy have also been reported.[16]

The major morbidity and mortality associated with CF are secondary to respiratory failure and chronic pulmonary infection.[19] Airway hyperactivity is common and may be contributed to by the immune response to the prolonged and varied antigenic stimulus.[20,21] Serious respiratory complications include pneumothorax, emphysema, and hemoptysis from erosion of hypertrophic bronchial arteries, which supply the chronically infected lung. The place of pleurodesis in the management of recurrent pneumothorax has been reduced by the development of endoscopic procedures. Hemoptysis from erosion of bronchial arteries may be treated by embolization of bronchial arteries by experienced interventional radiologists.

Exocrine pancreatic insufficiency is present in about 90% of patients with CF. Pancreatic disease is thought to result from a reduced volume of pancreatic secretion with low

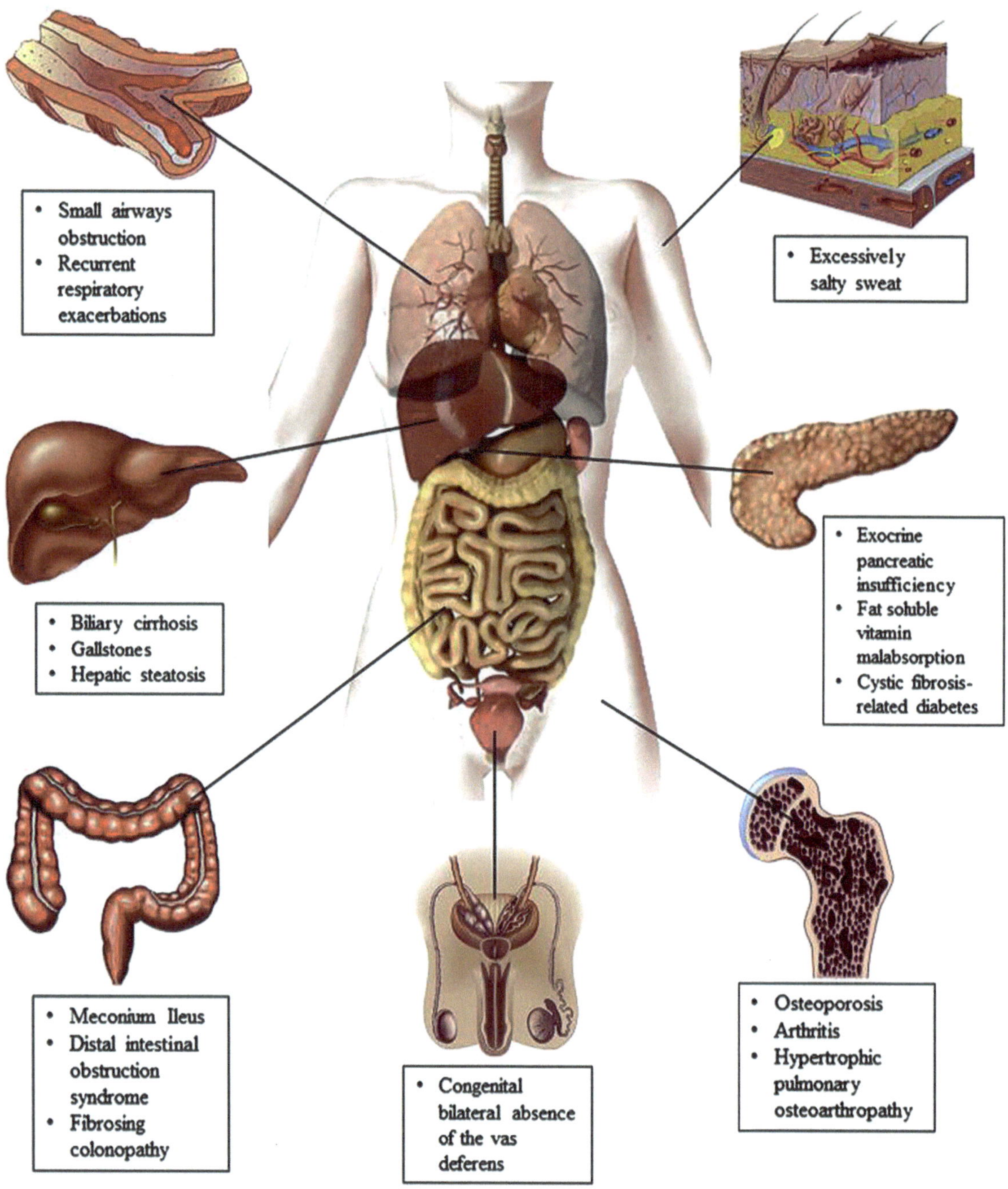

• **Fig. 50.3** Multiple organs implication in CF patients.

concentration of bicarbonate (HCO_3^-).[22] Without sufficient fluid and HCO_3^-, digestive proenzymes are retained in pancreatic ducts and prematurely activated, ultimately leading to tissue destruction and fibrosis. The pancreas secretes insufficient lipolytic and proteolytic enzymes for normal fat and protein digestion and absorption. The resulting malabsorption contributes to the failure to meet raised energy demands caused by the hypermetabolic state associated with endobronchial infection. These patients are considered "pancreatic insufficient." Commonly, patients with severe pancreatic insufficiency have more severe forms of lung disease and high sweat chloride concentrations than those with better pancreatic enzyme production.[23] Because lung infections can lead to reduced appetite and vomiting, malnutrition is further enhanced, which exacerbates lung infection, leading to a vicious cycle of malnutrition and infection. Pancreatitis or pancreatic inflammation may occur in association with pancreatic insufficiency, and diabetes develops in 1% of children and 13% of adults with CF and pancreatic insufficiency.[24,25] Diabetes in patients with CF shares features of the type 1 and 2 disorder, and a combination of reduced and delayed insulin secretion with insulin resistance is present in most patients.[26,27] It has the pattern of intermittent hyperglycemia, not associated with ketosis, which responds to insulin.[28]

CF has a profound effect on multiple segments of the gastrointestinal tract. Manifestations range from meconium ileus in the newborn infant to the distal intestinal obstruction syndrome that occurs in older children and adults. Most of the manifestations are related to insufficient secretion of pancreatic enzymes, diminished secretions from mucous glands, and the resultant viscid and adherent intestinal content.

Symptomatic liver disease is an uncommon complication of CF[29]; whereas a characteristic liver lesion of CF is focal or multilobular biliary cirrhosis, other manifestations include cholestasis secondary to common bile duct obstruction with inspissated bile, fatty infiltration of the liver, and, rarely, neonatal hepatitis.[30]

Important components in the management of CF are: (1) nutrition; (2) correction of organ dysfunction, including clearance of airway secretions, antibiotic therapy, and replacement of pancreatic enzymes; (3) genetic therapy; and (4) organ transplantation. Because the major morbidity is related to bronchial and bronchiolar disease with resultant obstructive pulmonary disease (which accounts for >90% of mortality), most therapies focus on direct antiinflammatory treatment to prevent host-mediated inflammatory obstruction, direct treatment of *Pseudomonas aeruginosa* infection, and clearance of airway secretions by overcoming the viscoelastic properties of the abnormal mucus. Respiratory therapy includes postural drainage, forced expiratory technique, bronchodilator therapy, and inhaled β-adrenergic or anticholinergic agent to improve the expiratory flow rate. Clearing the airways of tenacious, purulent secretions has been an important component of CF therapy. Postural drainage with chest percussion and vibration, applied manually or with a mechanical percussor, are the "traditional chest physiotherapy."[31] The combination of increased caloric demand at baseline, the added caloric demands of chronic lung disease, the difficulty sustaining caloric uptake because of malabsorption in patients who are pancreatic-insufficient, and anorexia. For CF patients with active lung inflammation, it may be very difficult to sustain a normal weight for height.[32]

Organ Transplantations

Until the advent of organ transplantation for patients with CF in 1984, for the majority, the inevitable outcome was death from overwhelming pulmonary sepsis. The availability of transplantation has profoundly altered the emphasis of care, and then, after transplantation, the quality of life for CF patients.[33,34]

Today, when medical treatment is failing and a patient is listed for transplantation, there is an imperative to keep the patient not only alive, but also in optimal clinical condition. The optimal perioperative management of patients with CF requires an understanding of the relevant pathophysiology and the unique challenges presented by these patients.[35] A poorly nourished, bedbound, demoralized patient is unlikely to survive the rigors to transplantation. In patients awaiting lung Tx, mechanical ventilation and extracorporeal membrane oxygenation (ECMO) are often the last ways to create a bridge to lung Tx. Both interventions are associated with a poor posttransplant outcome and survival rate. To improve the results of these patients, new "bridging-strategies" are necessary. The concept of "awake venovenous-ECMO" is feasible for the treatment of CF and can be used as a "bridging therapy" to lung Tx.[36]

It is an evident paradox that CF patients are listed for transplantation because they are unlikely to live for longer than 2 years, and yet must be presented for a lifesaving or life-threatening operation in the best possible health. The progression of pulmonary sepsis with *Pseudomonas aeruginosa* is relatively at a slow, which usually leaves sufficient time to list for transplantation the CF patient who is becoming unresponsive to treatment in a setting of multidisciplinary care. Occasionally, pulmonary sepsis will progress rapidly, and this is more commonly associated with infection with *Burkholderia cepacian*.[37]

At the end of 2018, the U.S. Food and Drug Administration approved Trikafta (elexacaftor/ivacaftor/tezacaftor), the first triple combination therapy available to treat patients with the most common CF mutation. Trikafta is approved for patients 12 years and older with CF who have at least one F508del mutation in the *CFTR* gene.[38]

Trikafta is a combination of three drugs that target the defective CFTR protein. It helps the protein made by the *CFTR* gene mutation function more effectively. Trikafta increases in the percent predicted FEV, known as $ppFEV_1$, which is an established marker of CF lung disease progression. It also results in improvements in sweat chloride, number of pulmonary exacerbations (worsening respiratory symptoms and lung function), and body mass index (weight-to-height ratio) compared with placebo.[39–43]

Currently available therapies that target the defective protein are treatment options for a limited number of patients with CF because many patients have mutations that are ineligible for treatment.

Anesthetic Considerations

Indications for surgery directly related to CF are largely age dependent and are: meconium ileus, meconium peritonitis, and intestinal atresia in neonates; nasal polypectomy, intravenous access and ear, nose, and throat surgery in children; esophageal surgery, "decortication/pleurodesis," cholecystectomy and lung Tx in adults, and more rarely liver.[44] It is unclear whether general anesthesia per se has any effect on the long-term course of the pulmonary disease. Many patients with CF have a limited respiratory reserve; therefore local and regional blocks with maintenance of spontaneous ventilation are preferred techniques if allowed by the nature of the surgical procedure.[45] Local and regional anesthesia with maintenance of spontaneous ventilation minimize the risks of aspiration, bronchospasm and barotrauma, and reduce the need for postoperative opioid analgesia, thus reducing also the related risk of postoperative constipation. The safety of continuous epidural anesthesia without endotracheal intubation cannot be determined by a single successful patient report,[46] but may be considered in patients with severe pulmonary disease. In general, children with mild to moderate CF lung disease did not experience worsening in the airway function following general anesthesia. The rate of complications was low, suggesting that the level of safety for children with CF with modern anesthesia is acceptable.[47]

Problems arise when a CF patient is scheduled for a lung Tx nearing the end of their respiratory reserve because the results are still the focus of discussion in literature. Today it is acceptable that lung Tx is still indicated in CF when there is a progressive decline in a patient's functional reserve.[48]

The official postlung Tx survival data form the International Society for Heart and Lung Transplantation Registry, not yet as promising as other solid organ transplantations, according to adult data selected for major diagnosis are reported in Fig. 50.4 and in CF adult and pediatric patients in Fig. 50.5.[49]

Preoperative Evaluation

Suggested preoperative investigations are summarized in Box 50.1. Efforts should be directed toward quantifying the level of disability and the extent of the cardiopulmonary disease preoperatively.[45]

The disease manifests as a clinical spectrum of differing severity and patterns of organ involvement. Retained secretions and recurrent respiratory infections cause the respiratory status of CF patients to change dramatically over relatively short periods of time, even in the span of a day in some cases. It is mandatory to exclude active infection at the time of elective surgery.[44] Elective operations are delayed until optimal pulmonary function can be ensured by controlling the bronchial infection and facilitating the removal of secretions from the airways. Improved pulmonary toilet lowers the airway resistance and the risk of postoperative pneumonia.

A recent preoperative chest x-ray is recommended as a baseline. It is valuable even in the absence of clinical signs because radiologic evidence of collapse or infection may be seen at imaging but not be clinically evident.[50] In addition, it could reveal asymptomatic pneumothorax, atelectasis, pulmonary bullas or blebs, beside signs of occult pneumonia. These findings would affect anesthesia management and should be reviewed by the anesthesiologists preoperatively.

Preoperative pulmonary function tests are useful to assess disease severity, but demand patients' compliance and should therefore be evaluated with caution, particularly in children. They commonly reveal an obstructive-pattern disease: increased functional residual capacity, decreased FEV_1, decreased peak expiratory flow rate and decreased vital capacity. Pulmonary fibrosis, bronchospasm, and intraluminal secretions cause low ventilation/perfusion ratios, leading to increased alveolar-arterial oxygen tension difference and lowered PaO2. Blood gases analysis is a good indicator of disease severity. PaCO2 is usually low or normal; the presence of an elevated PaCO2 often indicates advanced disease.

Sputum clearance and chest physiotherapy should continue until the patient arrives in the operating room. Some patients require a considerable period in the morning to clear secretions

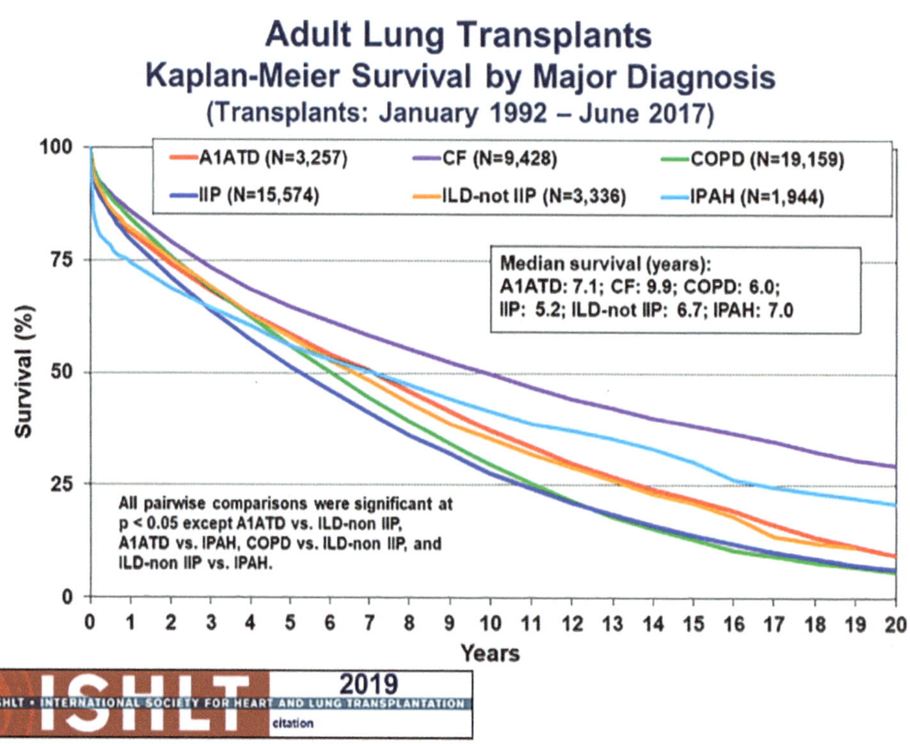

• **Fig. 50.4** Official postlung transplantation survival data from the International Society for Heart and Lung Transplantation Registry: In Adults selected for major diagnosis; *A1ATD*, Alpha-1-antitrypsin deficiency; *CF*, cystic fibrosis; *COPD*, chronic obstructive pulmonary disease; *IIP*, idiopathic interstitial pneumonia; *ILD*, Interstitial lung disease non-IIP; *IPAH*, idiopathic pulmonary arterial hypertension.

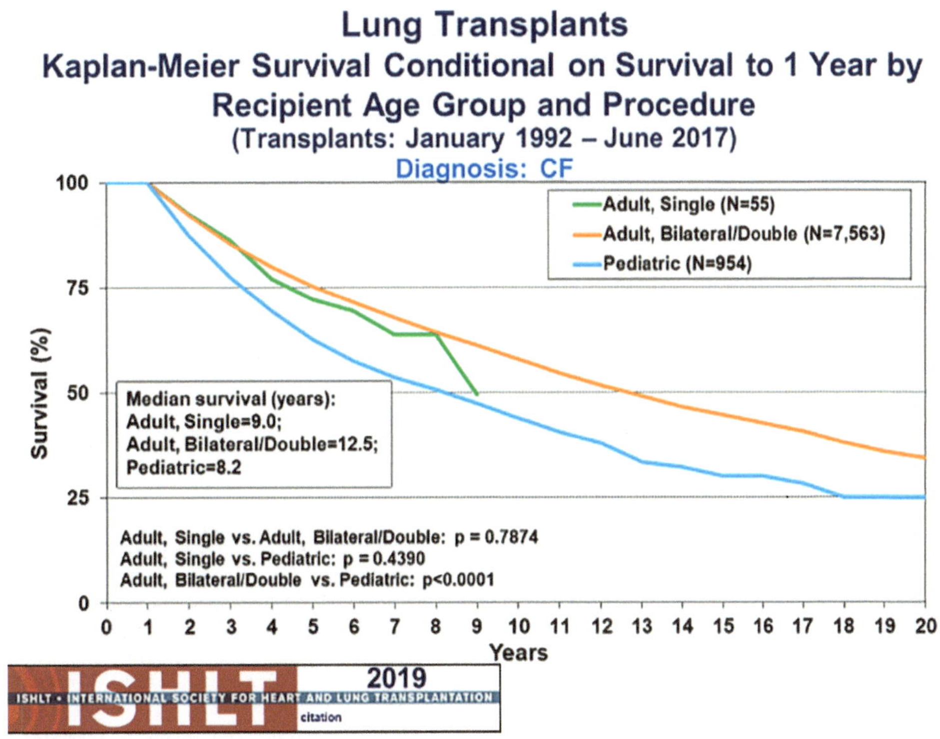

• **Fig. 50.5** Official postlung transplantation survival data from the International Society for Heart and Lung Transplantation Registry: in cystic fibrosis adult versus pediatric patients.

that accumulate during sleep. Surgical procedures are therefore best delayed until mid-morning, so that the clearance of secretions is completed before the induction of anesthesia.[45]

The ECG may show a deviation of the right axis. Clinical examination and, when appropriate, echocardiography or pulmonary artery catheterization, are more reliable methods of assessing right ventricular function and pulmonary artery hypertension.

Decreased synthesis of clotting factors by a diseased liver and impaired absorption of vitamin K from the gastrointestinal tract may include coagulopathy, prolonged prothrombin time, and partial thromboplastin time. These parameters should therefore always be evaluated.

• BOX 50.1 Investigations Necessary for Preoperative Evaluation

Preoperative Evaluation Tests

Blood count
Urea and electrolytes
Liver function tests
Chest x-ray/CT scan
Sputum culture and sensitivity
Respiratory function tests
Coagulation tests
Arterial blood gas tensions
C-reactive protein/procalcitonin
ECG
Echocardiography (with dobutamine if necessary)
Right heart catheterization (if performed)
Fasting glucose or glucose tolerance test

CT, Computed tomography; *ECG*, electrocardiogram.

Hypokalemia and hyponatremia can occur. Preoperative analgesics, sedatives, and anxiolytics are used sparingly in patients with CF, as they may lead to undesirable respiratory depression and an impaired ability to clear secretions. If premedication is tolerated, midazolam (0.04±0.07 mg/kg) can be safely used, as indicated by Kumle et al.[51]

Avoidance of postoperative constipation is a major consideration and a further reason to deflect the need for opioid analgesia. This is a serious complication because abdominal distension may severely compromise respiratory function. Prophylactic use of osmotically active laxatives will prevent constipation and obstruction in the postoperative period.

Usage of histamine-2 receptor antagonists and antiacid premedication is recommended, as the incidence of gastroesophageal reflux is high.[53]

Perioperative insulin therapy is usually not required, except when high-dose corticosteroids are used for immunosuppression of transplant recipients. Careful control of glucose administration is advised.

An appropriate decisional algorithm for the right anesthetic choice in CF patient is summarized in Fig. 50.6.

Intraoperative Period

Standard monitoring includes ECG, pulse oximetry, and capnography and noninvasive blood pressure. Advanced hemodynamic monitoring may be indicated based on the patient's individual condition and the surgical procedure (see Fig. 50.7). A central venous line (through the internal jugular vein), an arterial line and, if indicated, a pulmonary

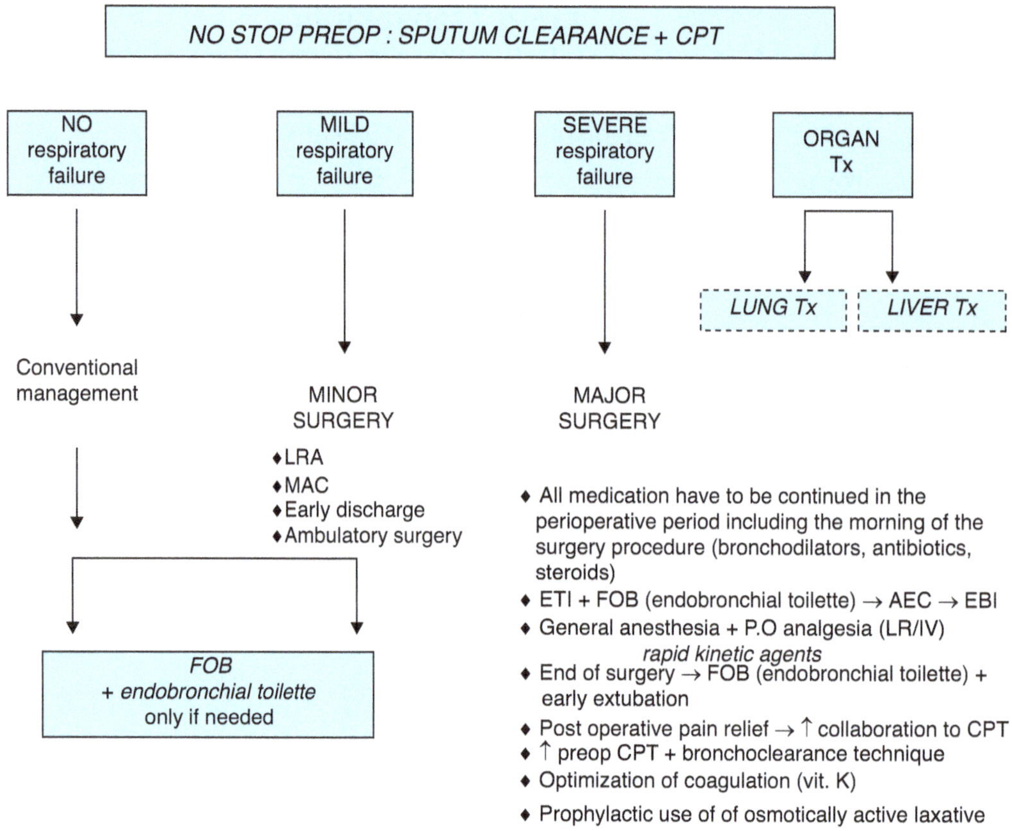

• **Fig. 50.6** Algorithm for anesthesia in cystic fibrosis patients. *AEC*, Airway exchanger catheter; *CPT*, chest physiotherapy; *EBI*, endobronchial intubation; *ETI*, endotracheal intubation; *FOB*, flexible bronchoscopy; *LR/IV*, loco regional/intravenous; *LRA*, local regional anesthesia; *MAC*, monitored anesthesia care; *PO*, postoperative.

artery catheter or a femoral artery line may be required. In selected cases, through the femoral artery, a PiCCO catheter (PiCCO System, Pulsion Medical System, Munich, Germany) computes CO continuously and is able to estimate ITBV, a preload index, and EVLW by arterial thermodilution through a single cold indicator. Arterial blood gases determinations are indicated for patients with severe disease. A TEE should be available in case of pulmonary hypertension and/or right heart dysfunction.

TEE has a central role for the patient undergoing lung Tx, and the operator needs to be aware of the key aspects to focus on pretransplant, intraprocedurally, and posttransplant.[52] Finally, during and at the end of mechanical ventilation, a lung sonography may be useful.

Induction of Anesthesia

A patient's history of clinically significant gastroesophageal reflux must be induced with a rapid sequence induction; otherwise, if no reflux is present, a standard IV or inhalational induction is acceptable.[53]

Oxygen desaturation occurs rapidly because of their reduced respiratory reserve, and preoxygenation in adults and cooperative children is particularly important whether or not a rapid sequence induction is to be used.

The rapid recovery characteristics and the absence of histamine release typical of low doses of propofol make it the most suitable choice. High functional residual capacity, small V_T (with respect to the modern protective ventilation), and ventilation-perfusion mismatch slow down induction time if inhalation drugs are chosen. Ketamine is relatively contraindicated because of its propensity to increase bronchial secretions and bronchorrhea. Agents irritating to the respiratory tract, such as isoflurane or desflurane, should be avoided during the induction of anesthesia, where sevoflurane may be indicated.[44]

The importance of adequate anesthetic depth before intubation has been stressed in view of bronchial hyperreactivity.[54,55] Local anesthesia of the vocal cords may facilitate a smoother intubation.

Induction of anesthesia should be done with caution. Malnutrition decreases the dosages of induction anesthetic drugs needed. It is preferable to administer anesthetics slowly, on demand, rather than on a body weight basis. Increased endogenous catecholamine "drive," induced by chronic hypoxia and hypercarbia, could abruptly withdraw if anesthetics are administered in large doses, resulting in circulatory collapse.[56]

Anesthetic Management

If a general anesthesia is required, maintenance of anesthesia with one of the volatile agents is advantageous, as they permit the administration of high inspired concentrations of oxygen. Bronchodilation, decreased muscle relaxant dosage, and reduced airways hyperactivity are further advantages of inhalation agents.

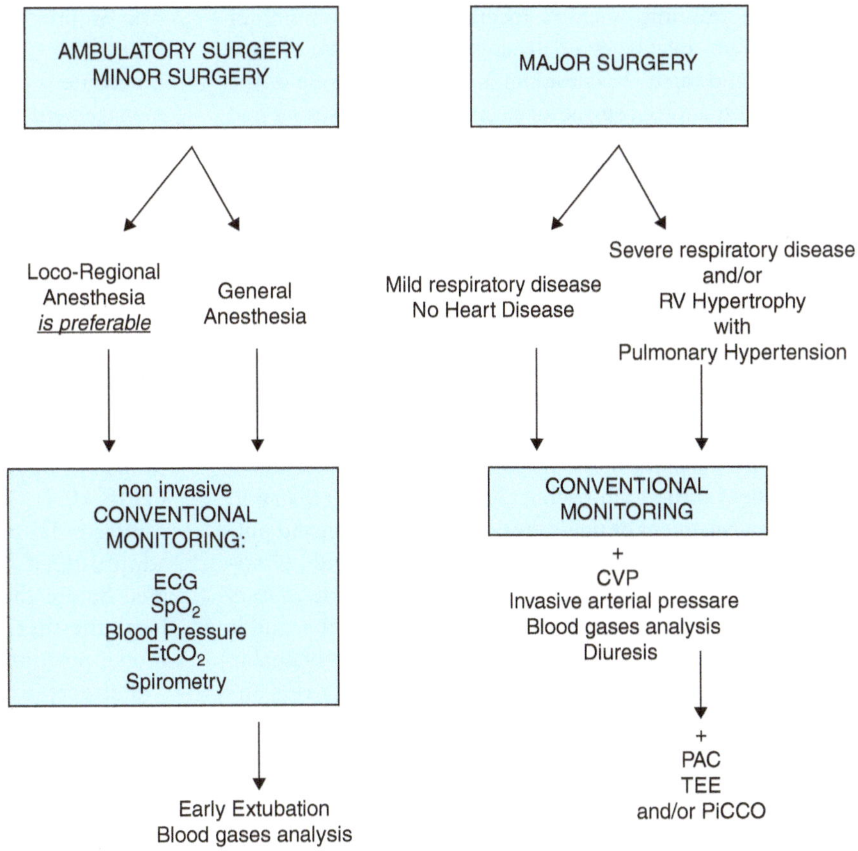

• **Fig. 50.7** Monitoring related to surgical procedure and baseline cardiovascular pathology. *CVC*, Central venous catheter; *PAC*, pulmonary artery catheter; *TEE*, transesophageal echocardiography; *PiCCO* (Pulsion, Munich Germany), pulse contour cardiac output (volumetric monitor).

The changes in ventilating pressures and breath sounds in patients with CF are dangerous due to the risk of rupture of emphysematous bullae, resulting in pneumothorax. Because the risk of pneumothorax in patients with severe disease is high, nitrous oxide should be omitted in favor of an air-oxygen mixture.

Intubation performed in a deep plane of anesthesia will avoid coughing and bronchospasm and prevent further inspissation of secretions. If nasal intubation is indicated, the turbinate should be examined preoperatively for polyps,[57] even if nasal intubation should be routinely avoided, as it may carry infections from the nasal cavity to the trachea. The largest possible single-lumen tube size should be used, which will allow this to be performed through a flexible bronchoscopy, an accurate endobronchial toilet.

Thoracic anesthesia is usually performed with a left-sided double-lumen tube that permits better suctioning of tenacious, mucopurulent secretions. Endobronchial blockers are also indicated, especially in cases of difficult airway management.

The laryngeal mask airway has been well tolerated by many patients with CF.[53] However, there is an increased risk of aspiration and airways obstruction from secretions when using this device.

Adequate and protective ventilation is necessary to avoid hypoxia, but intermittent positive pressure ventilation can lead to cardiocirculatory instability. Increased intrathoracic pressure and/or large TV reduces ventricular filling and stroke volume and increases pulmonary vascular resistance. In addition, insufficient expiration time increases air-trapping from autopositive end-expiratory pressure, and reduces heart systolic and diastolic volume; pulmonary tamponade may then occur. Pressure control ventilation and some degree of "permissive hypercarbia" in exchange for lower intrathoracic pressure are often suggested.[58] The presence of an air leak may interfere with positive pressure ventilation, but in practice, it is usually too small to make a significant difference. Thus ventilation through a tracheal tube is usually satisfactory, although it could be argued that passage of a double-lumen tube is preferable in case the air leak is of such magnitude that the ventilation has to be restricted to only one lung. One lung anesthesia, however, should be avoided if possible, in these patients, because oxygenation cannot always be ensured when one lung is ventilated, even with an oxygen concentration. In addition, delivery of the entire V_T to one lung increases the peak airway pressure, hence the risk of pneumothorax on the nondependent side (continuous positive airway pressure, high-frequency jet ventilation may be required on the nondependent lung).

Systemic hydration and humidification of inspired gases are important for maintaining secretions in a less viscous state, and frequent suctioning of the trachea throughout the surgical period is strongly indicated to minimize the accumulation of secretions.[45]

Fluid balance and plasma electrolyte concentration should be watched with care to prevent fluid overload, sodium retention, or potassium depletion.

Muscle relaxants, such as rocuronium, vecuronium, or cisatracurium, may be especially appropriate because of their clearance and safety. Rocuronium is preferred because of the introduction and the spread of sugammadex as a strong and safe antidote. Aminoglycoside antibiotics used to treat infections may prolong the neuromuscular blocking effect.[59] The high frequency of reflux mandates uses of suxamethonium or a double dose of rocuronium. Muscle pain following its administration has a high incidence in this young group and may severely compromise postoperative physiotherapy.[53] During the maintenance of anesthesia, relaxants should be administered when necessary and only in minimum doses, and a nerve stimulator should be routinely used to guide administration and assess recovery of muscle function. A qualitative neuromuscular transmission monitoring is indicated to extubate every patient with a train-of-four (TOF) ratio greater than 0.9.

The management of right ventricular dysfunction and pulmonary hypertension often require dobutamine and pulmonary vasodilators administration. Inhaled nitric oxide appears to fulfill the goal of selective pulmonary vasodilatation, and it is able to improve oxygenation in a previously unobtainable way without affecting systemic hemodynamic in patients undergoing lung Tx.[60] Its efficacy may be increased by the simultaneous additional administration of inhaled aerosolized prostacyclin.[61] Several studies have been investigated to perform a pharmacologic "modulation of pulmonary circulation" with the aim of optimizing the capability, during one-lung separation or isolation, of the dependent lung to accept blood flow through the administration of inhaled vasodilators, as well as enhancing hypoxic pulmonary vasoconstriction and diversion of blood flow from the nondependent lung through the infusion of pulmonary vasoconstrictors.[62] In case of hypotension and right ventricular failure, to avoid right ventricular ischemia and cardiac failure, norepinephrine infusion is necessary, even if it may increase pulmonary blood pressure.

Hemorrhage is occasionally a problem during pleurectomy in patients suffering from chronic, severe intrathoracic infection.

Blood glucose concentration should be monitored at frequent intervals in case of diabetes because of pancreatic insufficiency.

Postoperative Period

Extubation at the end of surgery is desirable and is usually possible in most patients, even after pulmonary resection.[63–65] Postoperative mechanical ventilation carries greater risk of infection and barotraumas. Even after lung Tx, immediate extubation can be considered when the surgical procedure is performed without major complications. Such management permits extubation of 46% of CF patients after bilateral lung Tx without an increase in postoperative risks.[66] In case of doubt, as a real point of care, a lung echography maybe useful.

At the end of surgery, all patients should be in a 30- to 40-degree sitting position, which is ideal for CF patients, as well as for all chronic obstructive pulmonary disease patients.

As active respiratory physiotherapy should be performed as soon as it is possible, anesthesia should be tailored for rapid postoperative resumption of the ability to cough and deep breathe and actively clear secretions. Postoperative residual curarization must be avoided (TOF <0.9). Provision of postoperative pain relief with nonsteroidal antiinflammatory agents and/or carefully administered opioids is mandatory and should be initiated before the skin incision, in addition to long-acting local anesthetic wound infiltration, as a standard multimodal postoperative analgesia.

Postoperative analgesia for both spontaneously breathing and mechanically ventilated patients should consist of small doses of narcotic analgesics, as nonsteroidal antiinflammatory agents may interfere with coagulation in case of decreasing of international normalized ratio value. Paracetamol (acetaminophen) is indicated in most of the cases. Local wound infiltration with longer acting local anesthetics (ropivacaine/levobupivacaine) reduces the need for opioids for postoperative analgesia. Regional analgesia and anesthesia techniques (epidural opioids and intercostal nerve blocks) are effective in preserving the pulmonary function while adequately treating postoperative pain.[57]

Throughout the immediate postoperative period, the patient with CF continues to be at risk for respiratory depression, pneumothorax, pneumonia, atelectasis, and airways obstruction[67]: therefore the patient with mild to severe respiratory failure has to be continuously monitored in a postanesthesia care unit and/or ICU.

Effective humidification is essential because viscid sputum is to be expectorated as easily as possible, and the inspired gas should be humidified during anesthesia. Humidified oxygen is used postoperatively, and additional humidification can be provided with ultrasonic nebulizers. Inhalation of nebulized iso- or hypertonic saline may help to loosen tenacious sputum.

Conclusion

Anesthesia for cystic fibrosis patient requires a skilled anesthetist, familiar with several organ dysfunctions, either during or postoperative management, of such a patient.

CF affects several organs and the balance of those disease influences the patient outcome. The thoracic anesthesia experience and familiarity in multiple organ dysfunctions play a crucial role.

A modern multispecialty approach is mandatory to manage in the right way CF patients today.

Since the preoperative evaluation, with the right intraoperative monitoring tools for the right surgical procedure, up to a protective postoperative period with a correct pain relief represent the cornerstones of a modern successful anesthesia in CF patients.

References

1. Ratjen F, Doring G. Cystic fibrosis. *Lancet.* 2003;361:681–689.
2. Rommens JM, Iannuzzi MC, Kerem BS, et al. Identification of the cystic fibrosis gene: chromosome walking and jumping. *Science.* 1989;245:1059–1065.
3. Vankeerberghen A, Cuppens H, Cassiman JJ. The cystic fibrosis transmembrane conductance regulator: an intriguing protein with pleiotropic functions. *J Cystic Fibrosis.* 2002;1:13–29.
4. Burn J, Magnay D, Claber O, et al. Population screening in cystic fibrosis. *J R Soc Med.* 1993;86(Suppl 20):2–6.
5. Knowles M, Gatzy J, Boucher R. Increased bioelectric potential difference across respiratory epithelia in cystic fibrosis. *N Engl J Med.* 1981;305:1489–1495.
6. Mc Pherson MA, Goodchild MC. The biochemical defect in cystic fibrosis. *Clin Sci.* 1988;74:337–345.
7. Helms PJ. Growing up with cystic fibrosis. *Br J Hosp Med.* 1993; 50:326–331.
8. Cystic Fibrosis Foundation: patient registry: Annual data report, Bethesda, MD: September 2000.
9. Davis PB, Drumm M, Konstan MW. Cystic fibrosis. *Am J Respir Crit Care Med.* 1996;154:1229–1256.
10. Smith JJP, Karp PH, Welsh MJ. Defective fluid transport by cystic fibrosis airway epithelia. *J Clin Invest.* 1994;93:1307–1311.
11. Wood BP. Cystic fibrosis: 1997. *Radiology.* 1997;204:1–10.
12. Tomashefski JF Jr, Konstan MW, Bruce MC, et al. The pathologic characteristics of interstitial pneumonia in cystic fibrosis: a retrospective autopsy. *Am J Clin Pathol.* 1989;91: 522–529.
13. Tomashefski JF Jr, Bruce MC, Goldberg HL, et al. Regional distribution of macroscopic lung disease in cystic fibrosis. *Am Rev Respir Dis.* 1986;133:535–540.
14. Sobonya RE, Taussing LM. Quantitative aspects of lung pathology in cystic fibrosis. *Am Rev Respir Dis.* 1986;134:290–295.
15. Konstan MW, Hilliard KA, Norvell TM, et al. Bronchiolar lavage findings in cystic fibrosis patients with stable, clinically mild lung disease suggest ongoing infection and inflammation. *Am J Respir Crit Care Med.* 1994;150:448–454.
16. Moss AJ. The cardiovascular system in cystic fibrosis. *Pediatrics.* 1982;70:728–741.
17. Slassi B, Moss AJ, Dooley R. Clinical recognition of cor pulmonale in cystic fibrosis. *J Pediatr.* 1971;78:794–805.
18. Piepsz A, Ham HR, Millet E, et al. Determinant of right ventricular ejection in children with cystic fibrosis. *Pediatr Pul.* 1987; 3:24–28.
19. Wood RE, Boat TF, Doershuk CF. Cystic fibrosis. *Am Rev Respir Dis.* 1976;113:833–878.
20. Hodson ME, Turner-Warwick M. Auto-antibodies in cystic fibrosis. *Clin Allergy.* 1981;11:565–570.
21. Collins F. Cystic fibrosis: molecular biology and therapeutic implications. *Science.* 1992;256:774–779.
22. Kopelman H, Durie P, Gaskin K, et al. Pancreatic fluid secretions and protein hyperconcentration in cystic fibrosis. *N Engl J Med.* 1985;312:329–334.
23. Fried MD, Durie PR, Tsui LC, et al. The cystic fibrosis gene and resting energy expenditure. *J Pediatr.* 1991;119:913–916.
24. Allan JL, Robbie ML, Phelan PD, et al. Familial occurrence of meconium ileus. *Eur J Paediatr.* 1981;135:291–292.
25. Lands L, Sinman R, Wise M, et al. Pancreatic function testing in meconium disease in CF: two case reports. *J Pediatr Gastroenterol Nutr.* 1988;7:276–279.
26. Lanng S, Thornsteinsson B, Lund-Anderen C, et al. Diabetes mellitus in Danish cystic fibrosis patients: prevalence and late complications. *Acta Pediatr.* 1994;83:72–77.
27. Holl RW, Wolf A, Thon A, et al. Insulin resistance with altered secretory kinetis and reduced proinsulin in cystic fibrosis patients. *J Pediatr Gastroenterol Nutr.* 1997;25:188–193.
28. Cystic Fibrosis Foundation Consensus Conference: Consensus conference on CF-related diabetes-mellitus. *Cystic Fibrosis Foundation.* 1990;1:1–8.
29. Scott-Jupp R, Lama M, Tanner MS. Prevalence of liver disease in cystic fibrosis. *Arch Dis Child.* 1991;66:698–701.
30. Furuya KN, Roberts EA, Canny GJ, et al. Neonatal hepatitis syndrome with paucity of interlobular bile ducts in cystic fibrosis. *J Pediatr Gastroenterol Nutr.* 1991;12:127–130.
31. Thomas J, Cook DJ, Brooks D. Chest physical therapy management of patient with cystic fibrosis: a meta-analysis. *Am J Respir Crit Care Med.* 1995;151:846–850.
32. MacDonald A. Nutritional management of cystic fibrosis. *Arch Dis Child.* 1996;74:81–87.
33. Yacoub MH, Banner NR, Khaghani A, et al. Heart–lung transplantation for cystic fibrosis and subsequent domino heart transplantation. *J Heart Transplant.* 1990;9:459–467.
34. Caine N, Sharples LD, Smyth, et al. Survival and quality of life of cystic fibrosis patients before and after heart-lung transplantation. *Transplant Proc.* 1991;23:1203–1204.
35. Huffmyer JL, Littlewood KE, Nemergut EC. Perioperative management of the adult with cystic fibrosis. *Anesth Analg.* 2009; 109(6):1949–1961.
36. Schmidt F1, Sasse M, Boehne M, et al. Concept of "awake venovenous extracorporeal membrane oxygenation" in pediatric patients awaiting lung transplantation. *Pediatr Transplant.* 2013; 17(3):224–230.
37. Glass S, Govan J. Pseudomonas cepacia: fatal pulmonary infection in a patient with cystic fibrosis. *J Infect.* 1986;13:157–158.
38. https://www.fda.gov/news-events/press-announcements/fda-approves-new-breakthrough-therapy-cystic-fibrosis.
39. Rowe SM, Daines C, Ringshausen FC, et al. Tezacaftor-Ivacaftor in residual-function heterozygotes with cystic fibrosis. *N Engl J Med.* 2017;377(21):2024–2035.
40. Taylor-Cousar JL, Munck A, McKone EF, et al. Tezacaftor-Ivacaftor in patients with cystic fibrosis homozygous for Phe508del. *N Engl J Med.* 2017;377(21):2013–2023.
41. Davies JC, Moskowitz SM, Brown C, et al. VX16-659-101 Study Group. VX-659-Tezacaftor-Ivacaftor in patients with cystic fibrosis and one or two Phe508del Alleles. *N Engl J Med.* 2018;379(17): 1599–1611.
42. Keating D, Marigowda G, Burr L, et al. VX16-445-001 Study Group. VX-445-Tezacaftor-Ivacaftor in patients with cystic fibrosis and one or two Phe508del Alleles. *N Engl J Med.* 2018;379(17): 1612–1620.
43. Donaldson SH, Pilewski JM, Griese M, et al. VX11-661-101 Study Group. Tezacaftor/Ivacaftor in subjects with cystic fibrosis and F508del/F508del-CFTR or F508del/G551D-CFTR. *Am J Respir Crit Care Med.* 2018;197(2):214–224.
44. Walsh TS, Young CH. Anesthesia and cystic fibrosis. *Anesthesia.* 1995;50:614–622.
45. Della Rocca G. Anesthesia in patients with cystic fibrosis. *Curr Opin Anesth.* 2002;15:95–101.
46. Edelman S. Laparoscopic cholecystectomy under continuous epidural anaesthesia in patients with cystic fibrosis. *The Pediatric Forum Jul.* 1991;145:723–724.

47. Pandit C1, Valentin R, De Lima J, et al. Effect of general anesthesia on pulmonary function and clinical status on children with cystic fibrosis. *Paediatr Anaesth.* 2014;24(2):164–169.
48. Lenihan M, Mullane D, Buggy D, Flood G, Griffin M. Anesthesia for lung transplantation in cystic fibrosis: retrospective review from the Irish National Transplantation Centre. *J Cardiothorac Vasc Anesth.* 2018;32(5):2372–2380.
49. https://ishltregistries.org/registries/slides.asp?year=2019.
50. Marom EM, McAdams HP, Palmer SM, et al. Cystic fibrosis: usefulness of thoracic CT in the examination of patients before lung transplantation. *Radiology.* 1999;213:283–288.
51. Kumle B, Breug R, Boldt J, et al. Anaesthesiologic management in the treatment of patients with cystic fibrosis. *Anaesthesiol Intensivemed Notfallmed Schmetzer Jul.* 2000;35(7):423–427.
52. Evans A1, Dwarakanath S, Hogue C, et al. Intraoperative echocardiography for patients undergoing lung transplantation. *Anesth Analg.* 2014;118(4):725–730.
53. Weeks AM, Buckland MR. Anaesthesia for adults with cystic fibrosis. *Anaesth Intensive Care.* 1995;23:332–338.
54. Doershuk CF, Reyes AL, Regan AG, et al. Anesthesia and surgery in cystic fibrosis. *Anesth Analg.* 1972;51:413–421.
55. Smith RM. Anesthetic management of patients with cystic fibrosis. *Anesth Analg.* 1965;44:143–146.
56. Truman K. Lung transplantation: historical perspective, current concepts and anesthetic considerations. *J Cardiothorac Vasc Anesth.* 1997;1(2):220–241.
57. Morray JP, Krane EJ, Geiduschek JM, et al. Anaesthesia for thoracic surgery. In: Gregory GA, ed. *Pediatric Anaesthesia.* New York, NY: Churchill Livingstone; 1994:421–464.
58. Quinlan JJ, Buffington CW. Deliberate hypoventilation in a patient with air trapping during lung transplantation. *Anesthesiology.* 1993;78:1177–1181.
59. Bauer LA, Piecoro JJ, Wilson HD, et al. Gentamicin and tobramycin pharmacokinetics in patients with cystic fibrosis. *Clin Pharm Ther.* 1983;2:262–264.
60. Della Rocca G, Passariello M, Coccia C, et al. Inhaled nitric oxide administration during one-lung ventilation in patients undergoing thoracic surgery. *J Cardiothorac Vasc Anesth.* 2001;15:218–223.
61. Della Rocca G, Coccia C, Pompei L, et al. Hemodynamic and oxygenation changes of combined therapy with inhaled nitric oxide and inhaled aerosolized prostacyclin. *J Cardiothorac Vasc Anesth.* 2001;15:224–227.
62. Cohen E. New development in thoracic anesthesia. *Review Course Lectures.* 2002.
63. Robinson DA, Brantwaite MA. Pleural surgery in patients with cystic fibrosis. *Anaesthesia.* 1984;39:655–659.
64. Marmor L, Schidlow D, Palmer J, et al. Pulmonary resection for complications of cystic fibrosis. *J Pediatr Surg.* 1983;18:811–815.
65. Della Rocca G, Coccia C, Costa MG, et al. Is very early extubation after lung transplantation feasible? *J Cardiothorac Vasc Anesth.* 2003;17:29–35.
66. Felten ML, Moyer JD, Dreyfus JF, et al. Foch Lung Transplant Group. Immediate postoperative extubation in bilateral lung transplantation: predictive factors and outcomes. *Br J Anaesth.* 2016;116(6):847–854.
67. Kheradmand F, Wiener–Kronish JP, Corry DY. Assessment of operative risk for patients with advanced lung disease. *Clin Chest Med.* 1997;18:483–494.

51

Tracheal Stents

KAREN McRAE

Introduction

An airway stent is a prosthesis inserted to maintain intraluminal integrity of a compromised conducting airway, which can consist of either relief from airway obstruction or restoration of patency of the airway, such as in the case of fistulas or airway dehiscence. Placement of central airway stents is the domain of both the thoracic surgeon and interventional pulmonologists. Both benefit from the provision of expert anesthesia care and should be experienced colleagues in management of the shared airway. Patients with a variety of challenging pathologies present for airway stenting (Table 51.1).

The ideal airway stent would be easy to place with low morbidity, while reliably reestablishing the integrity of the airway. Optimally, it would have minimal tendency to migrate, while being able to be easily removed if required. The ideal stent should have sufficient strength to support the airway, but flexible enough to allow clearance of secretions, and biologically inert to minimize the formation of granulation tissue. Long-term luminal patency should be maintained without causing ischemia, or erosion into adjacent structures would be possible. Unfortunately, to date, no currently available stent possessed all these characteristics (Table 51.2). Each patient's underlying condition and anatomy must be considered when choosing a device.[1,2]

Recently, the types and sizes of stents currently available were comprehensively reviewed.[3] There are three main varieties of stents: silicone, and self-expanding metal stents (SEMS) available in covered (typically with Silastic or polyurethane) and uncovered designs (Fig. 51.1). SEMS are generally more easily inserted; many centers routinely place them via flexible bronchoscopy. They can, however, be very difficult to remove. For malignant airway obstruction, covered models prevent tumor ingrowth. Uncovered metal stents are optimal for conditions in which the formation of granulation tissue is desirable, such as airway dehiscence. Epithelialization of the stent occurs within weeks of placement, which preserves mucociliary activity and reduces the risk of mucous plugging. An advantage of metal stents is their thin walled structure; and their internal to external diameter is larger than silicone stents. Silicone stents require placement using rigid bronchoscopy, but are far more easily removed. The rate of stent migration is higher with silicone than metal. Other characteristics of classic stent designs are outlined in Table 51.2.

Case Presentations and Management

Case 1

A 49-year-old man with esophageal carcinoma was treated with chemotherapy and radiation. He subsequently developed a tracheoesophageal fistula. An esophageal stent was placed in a community hospital; however, he developed erosion into the trachea. He was taken to the operating room for evaluation of the trachea and probable stenting.

Anesthesia was induced with 50 mg lidocaine, 20 mcg of remifentanil, 20 mg of ketamine, and 150 mg of propofol, intravenously followed by a propofol infusion of 80 mcg/kg/min. A No. 4 laryngeal mask airway (LMA Unique, Teleflex Medical) was placed, and the patient resumed spontaneous ventilation, as no muscle relaxant was administered. Upon detailed inspection, there was an obvious area in the mid to distal trachea where the stent had eroded into the membranous airway. There was also an area just proximal to the carina where a second fistula was visualized. A partially covered self-expanding Ultraflex metallic stent was placed, which was 20 mm in diameter, 45 mm in covered length, and 60 mm in total length. A guidewire was inserted into the trachea under direct vision via the bronchoscope working channel, over which the stent was threaded and deployed with the aid of fluoroscopy to confirm positioning (Fig. 51.2). The LMA was briefly removed during stent deployment, and high-flow oxygen was administered via nasal cannula until the wire was removed and the LMA replaced. After the propofol infusion was discontinued, emergence was uneventful. The procedure lasted an hour with spontaneous ventilation throughout while the fraction of inspired oxygen (FiO2) was maintained at 0.8 throughout, and there were no episodes of desaturation.

The combined esophageal and tracheal stenting was effective for some time (Fig. 51.3); however, on radiologic follow-up 3 months after tracheal stent placement, there was a suspicion of further erosion of the esophageal stent into the distal membranous portion of the trachea, extending into the left main stem bronchus (Fig. 51.4). This was

TABLE 51.1 Established Indications for Stent Placement in the Conducting Airways

Benign
Traumatic: Postintubation, blunt or penetrating trauma
Inflammatory: Amyloidosis, sarcoidosis, relapsing polychondritis, Wegener
Infectious: Tuberculosis, papillomatosis, postviral
Neoplastic: Hemangioma, hamartoma, chondroma, neurofibroma, broncholith
Anastomotic (stenosis or dehiscence): Postpulmonary transplant, sleeve resection
Vascular: Vascular rings, thoracic aneurysm
Tracheomalacia

Malignant
Endobronchial tumor: Bronchogenic, adenoid cystic, carcinoid, mucoepidermoid
Extrinsic compression by tumor or lymphadenopathy
 Primary: esophagus, thymic, thyroid, germ cell, lymphoma, sarcoma
 Metastatic: Bronchogenic, renal cell, colon, melanoma, breast
Tracheoesophageal fistula

confirmed during awake flexible bronchoscopy after upper airway topicalization. The right bronchus was normal, and on the left side, there was erosion of the esophageal stent into the membranous portion of the left main bronchus. The distal left bronchus, left upper lobe, and left lower lobe were normal. It was determined that placement of a Y-stent would be required after removal of the in situ tracheal stent. Measurement of the tracheal and bronchial lengths were made to allow acquisition of a Y stent of the appropriate dimensions.

A few days later, general anesthesia was induced with Midazolam 1 mg, Fentanyl 50 mcg, propofol 100 mg, followed by rocuronium 25 mg. A No. 4 LMA Supreme was inserted, followed by controlled positive pressure ventilation 10 cm H_2O over 4 cm H_2O of positive end-expiratory pressure (PEEP). Infusions of propofol 75 mcg/kg/min and remifentanil 0.1 mcg/kg/min were started. The airway was reexamined distal to the existing tracheal stent; the esophageal stent could be visualized in the posterior left mainstem bronchus. The LMA was removed and a size 8.5 rigid bronchoscope was inserted into the trachea. Intermitted ventilation with jets of 100% oxygen via a handheld Sanders injector device allowed ventilation via the open rigid bronchoscope with periods of apnea without desaturation. Using rigid bronchoscope forceps, the tracheal stent was grasped and removed together with the rigid bronchoscope. The LMA was reinserted. Flexible bronchoscopy revealed the membranous portion of the distal trachea extending into the left main bronchus to be absent; the esophageal stent was clearly visible. A fully covered self-expanding metallic Y-stent from Micro-Tech with the tracheal diameter of 20 mm, tracheal length of 40 mm, left main bronchus length of 30 mm, and right main bronchus length of 15 mm was placed. To accomplish this, the LMA was removed, and the trachea was again intubated with the rigid bronchoscope. Visualizing with the flexible scope through the rigid bronchoscope, a long guidewire was inserted into the left, and a shorter guidewire was then inserted into the right main bronchus. The flexible scope was removed, and the patient was preoxygenated as much as possible with jet ventilation; the rigid bronchoscope was removed, leaving the wires in place. The left and right tips of the stent were threaded over the proximal ends of the guidewires. The stent delivery system was inserted into the trachea over the guidewires. Before deployment, the flexible bronchoscope was inserted beside the apparatus to be able to visualize the tips of the stent. The stent was deployed distal ends first after ensuring that the Y portion was seated on the carina. Thereafter, the tracheal part of the stent was fully deployed. Full stent deployment took several minutes and was performed during apnea; there was a brief period of

TABLE 51.2 Types of Commonly Placed Stents

Stent Type	Advantages	Disadvantages
Silicone	Inexpensive Removable Resist external compression Least formation of granulation tissue	Require rigid bronchoscopy Higher rates of migration Thick walled so smaller inner lumen Mucus plugging Unable to conform to irregular shaped airway Flammable (risk during laser therapy)
Uncovered self-expanding metal stent (SEMS)	May be placed with flexible bronchoscopy Less migration Thinner wall, increased inner diameter Lesser impact on ciliary function	Difficult to remove Wall pressure may cause necrosis and fistula formation Tumor may regrow along length of stent May collapse with external compression
Covered SEMS	No tumor growth along length of stent May be placed with flexible bronchoscopy Less migration Thinner wall, increased inner diameter Lesser impact on ciliary function More easily removed than bare metal SEMS	Wall pressure may cause necrosis and fistula formation Formation of granulation tissue at ends may block stent Contain flammable material (risk during laser therapy) May collapse with external compression

A B C
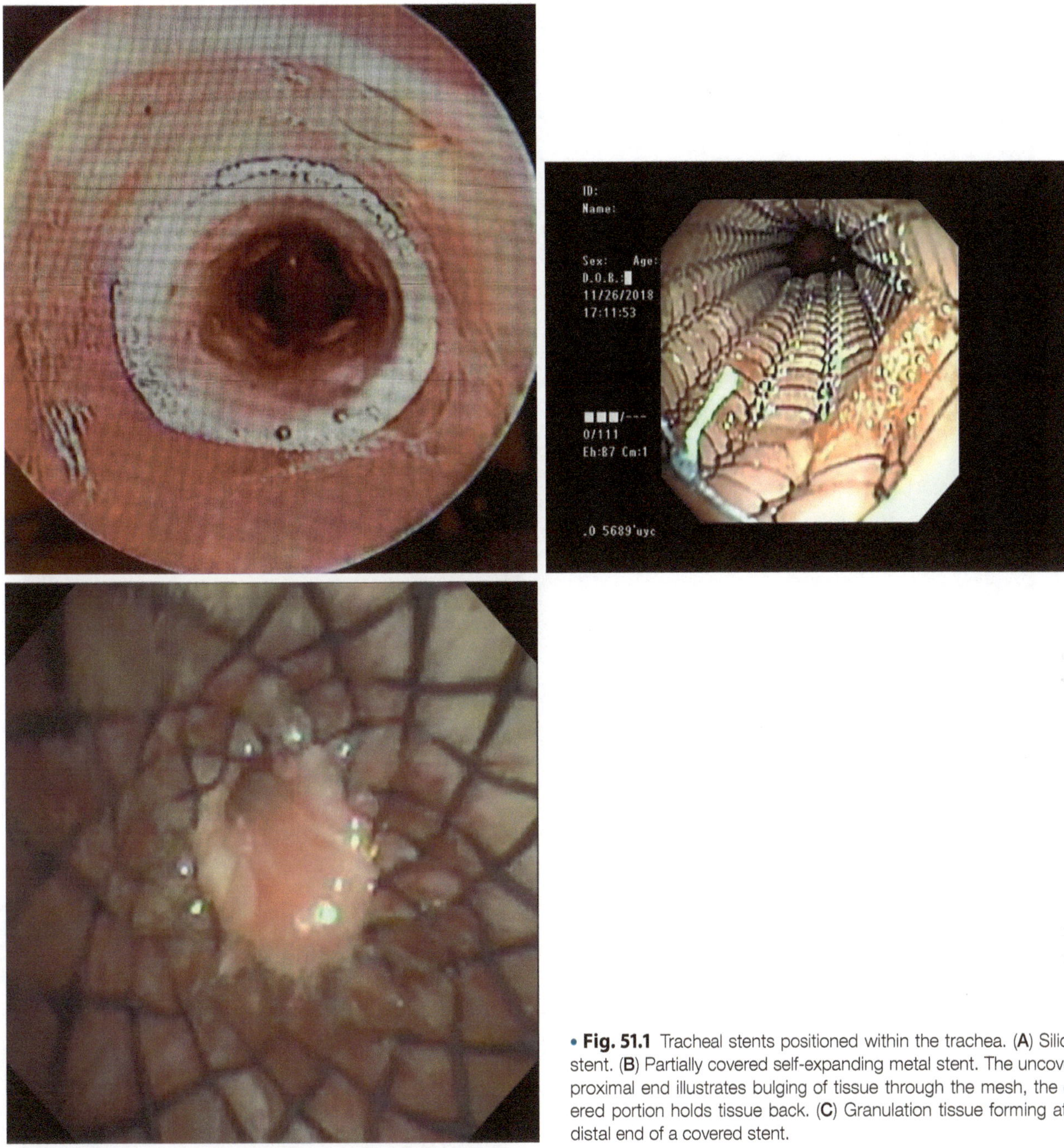

• **Fig. 51.1** Tracheal stents positioned within the trachea. (**A**) Silicone stent. (**B**) Partially covered self-expanding metal stent. The uncovered proximal end illustrates bulging of tissue through the mesh, the covered portion holds tissue back. (**C**) Granulation tissue forming at the distal end of a covered stent.

desaturation to 85%, which resolved immediately with face mask ventilation once the stent was deployed. The LMA was reinserted and flexible bronchoscopy was performed. The Y-stent had completely covered the defect in the membranous portion of the trachea, as well as extending into the left main bronchus (Fig. 51.5). Neuromuscular relaxant was reversed, and with discontinuation of propofol and remifentanil infusions, the patient emerged uneventfully from anesthesia.

This case illustrates how many patients require multiple interventions, which can include not only initial stent placement, but later stent removal, revision, and replacement. Straightforward stenting may be placed using flexible bronchoscopy, whereas more complex procedures usually require rigid bronchoscopy, facilitated by fiberoptic bronchoscopy.

Case 2

A 38-year-old patient with advanced colorectal cancer had undergone primary resection, as well as hepatic and bilateral lung metastectomies. She had developed an extensive mediastinal lymphadenopathy, presenting with significant shortness of breath and wheeze. Imaging showed near-complete occlusion of both main bronchi at the level of the carina (Fig. 51.6). She was brought to the operating room on an urgent basis because the airway narrowing appeared to be due to airway invasion, as well as from external compression. Rigid bronchoscopy for tumor debridement and stenting was planned. A lengthy and potentially difficult procedure was anticipated, and the decision was made for

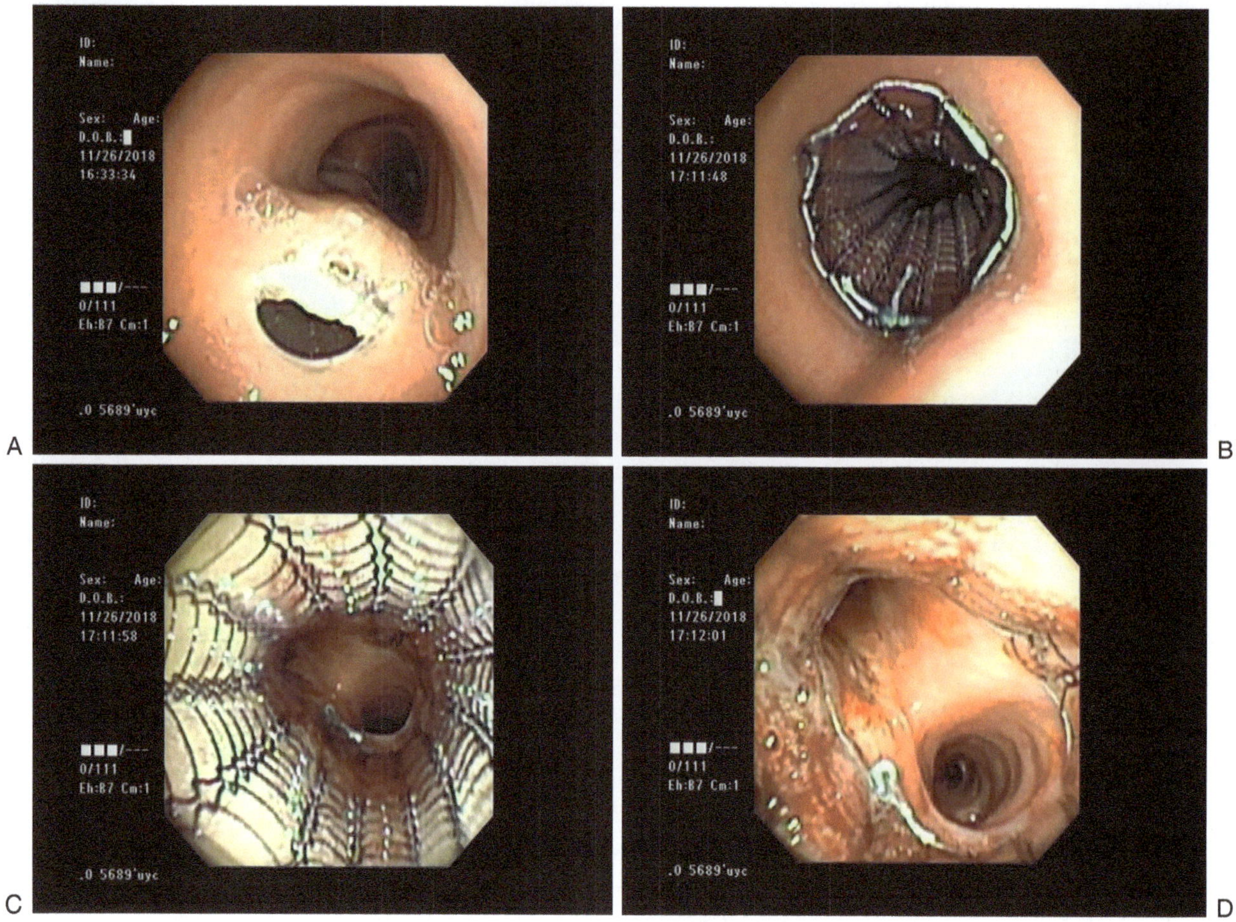

• **Fig. 51.2** A partially covered cylindrical self-expanding metallic stent is deployed in the tracheal. (**A**) The proximal fistula. (**B**) Stent just deployed. (**C**) Completely expanded. (**D**) The edge of second fistula just visible at the distal end of the stent.

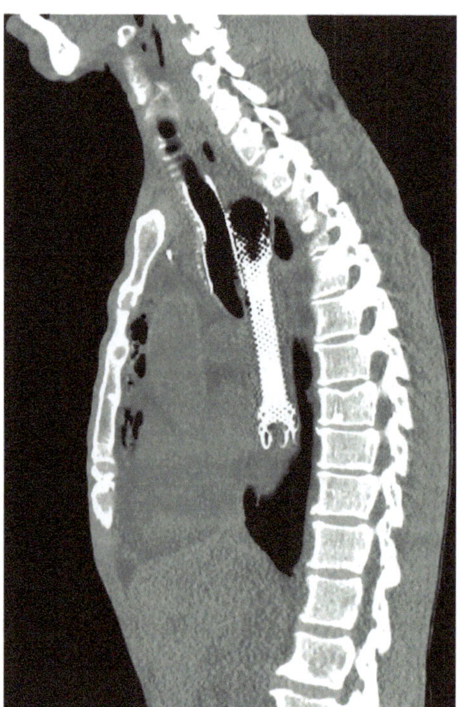

• **Fig. 51.3** Sagittal view of both stents: tracheal and esophageal.

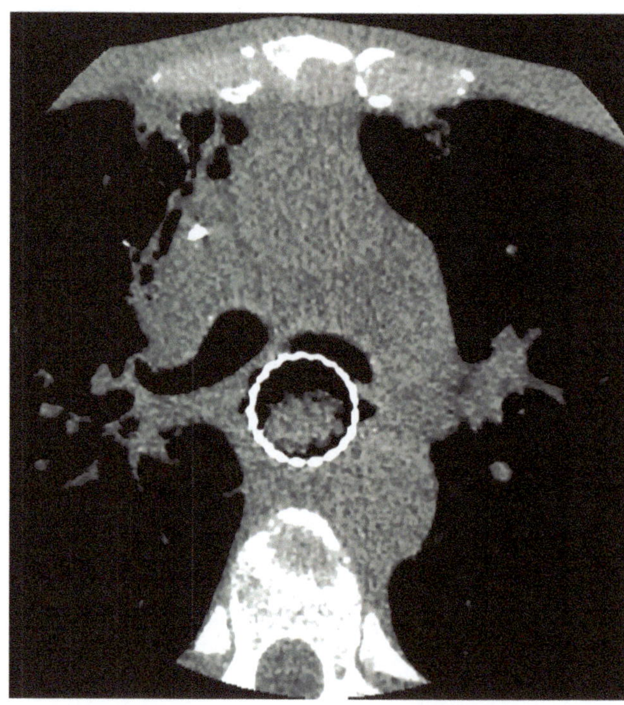

• **Fig. 51.4** Suspicion of a new fistula in the left main stem bronchus. The image shows computed tomography cut just below the carina, at the level of the takeoff of the right upper lobe bronchus.

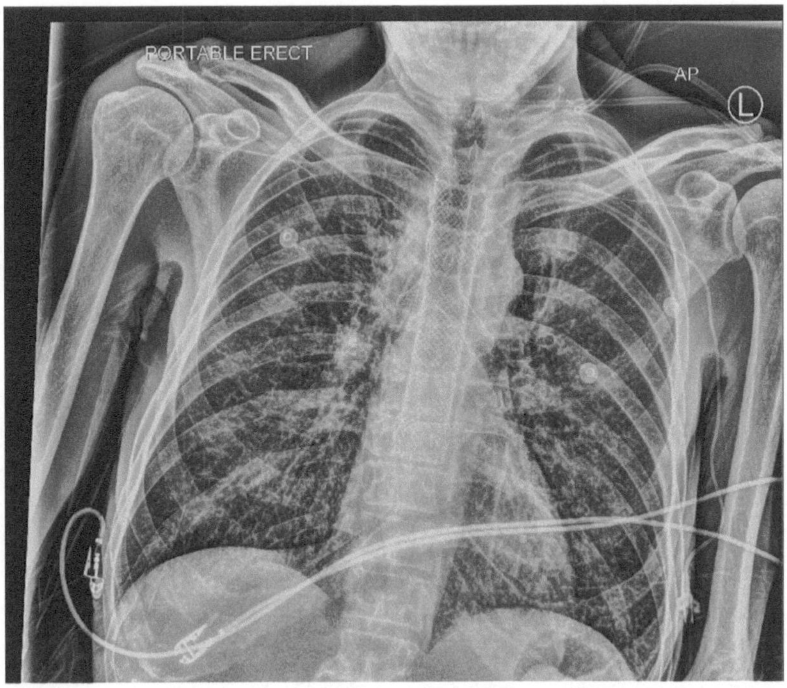

• **Fig. 51.5** After the second tracheal stenting procedure, the radiopaque esophageal stent and Y-shaped carinal stent are clearly seen.

planned use of venovenous extracorporeal membrane oxygenation (ECMO) support of gas exchange.

After a comprehensive informed consent discussion, the patient was brought to the operative room, a large bore peripheral intravenous and radial arterial catheter were placed. After preoxygenation, anesthesia was induced with lidocaine 50 mg, fentanyl 100 mcg, propofol 50 mg, ketamine 60 mg, and followed by rocuronium 60 mg. We were able to confirm immediately that she could be ventilated with positive pressure, and she was intubated with a 7.5 standard endotracheal tube (ETT). Initially, low-dose Sevoflurane was used during flexible bronchoscopy and ECMO cannulation, with conversion to total intravenous anesthesia (TIVA) with propofol infusion of 100 to 120 mcg/kg/min and remifentanil 0.05 to 0.1 mcg/kg/min titrated to effect while on ECMO.

Flexible bronchoscopy showed a very extensive tumor in the level of the carina, extending to both right- and left-main bronchi (see Fig. 51.6). A dual lumen catheter was inserted into the right jugular vein under sterile conditions with ultrasound guidance to locate the jugular vein and with verification of catheter position with fluoroscopy. A 28 Fr Crescent cannula was used and ECMO flows of 3.5 to 4 L per minute L/min were targeted (Fig. 51.7). Heparin dosing was targeted an activated clotting time (ACT) of 160 to 180; only one 4000-unit bolus was required. After initiation of apnea, blood gases were drawn and good oxygenation and ventilation were confirmed. The ETT was removed and the patient remained apneic during the stenting procedure, which lasted approximately 130 minutes (Figs. 51.8 and 51.9).

An 8.5-mm rigid bronchoscope was inserted, and extensive debridement of the tumor in the carina and both right and left bronchi was performed. Much of the endobronchial tumor was removed but there was still a significant degree of extrinsic compression, especially in the bronchus intermedius. Balloon dilatation was attempted to widen the right airways, without clear success. The decision to place a carinal Y stent was made: a Micro-tech self-expanding, fully-covered wire Y-stent was chosen. A 4 cm extension into the trachea, 2 cm into the left main bronchus, and 1.0 cm into the right main bronchus was positioned and deployed in a similar manner as described in Case 1 (Fig. 51.10). Because of the ECMO support, no interruptions for ventilation were required. The patient was hemodynamically stable throughout the procedure. The stent was placed in an optimal position without occluding the orifice of the right upper lobe bronchus. The surgeons achieved satisfactory hemostasis, especially on the right side, with a clear opening of the airway and minimal bleeding.

The patient was reintubated with a 7.5 ETT, and ventilated pressure control of 22 cm H_2O with 5 cm H_2O of PEEP; lung compliance was excellent. The ECMO gas sweep was turned off, while ventilated with FiO2 of 0.6; the patient's arterial oxygen partial pressure was 289 mm Hg. ECMO circuit was rapidly weaned and decannulated. The blood from the ECMO circuit was scavenged using a cell saver, resulting in an overall estimated blood loss of 250 mL. No protamine reversal was required. She was extubated in the operating room after reversal of neuromuscular blockade, 32 minutes after termination of ECMO, and was transferred to the postanesthesia unit breathing comfortably. Postprocedure chest x-ray (CXR) revealed reduced lower lobe aeration, potentially amenable to a future bronchial stenting of the bronchus intermedius (Fig. 51.11).

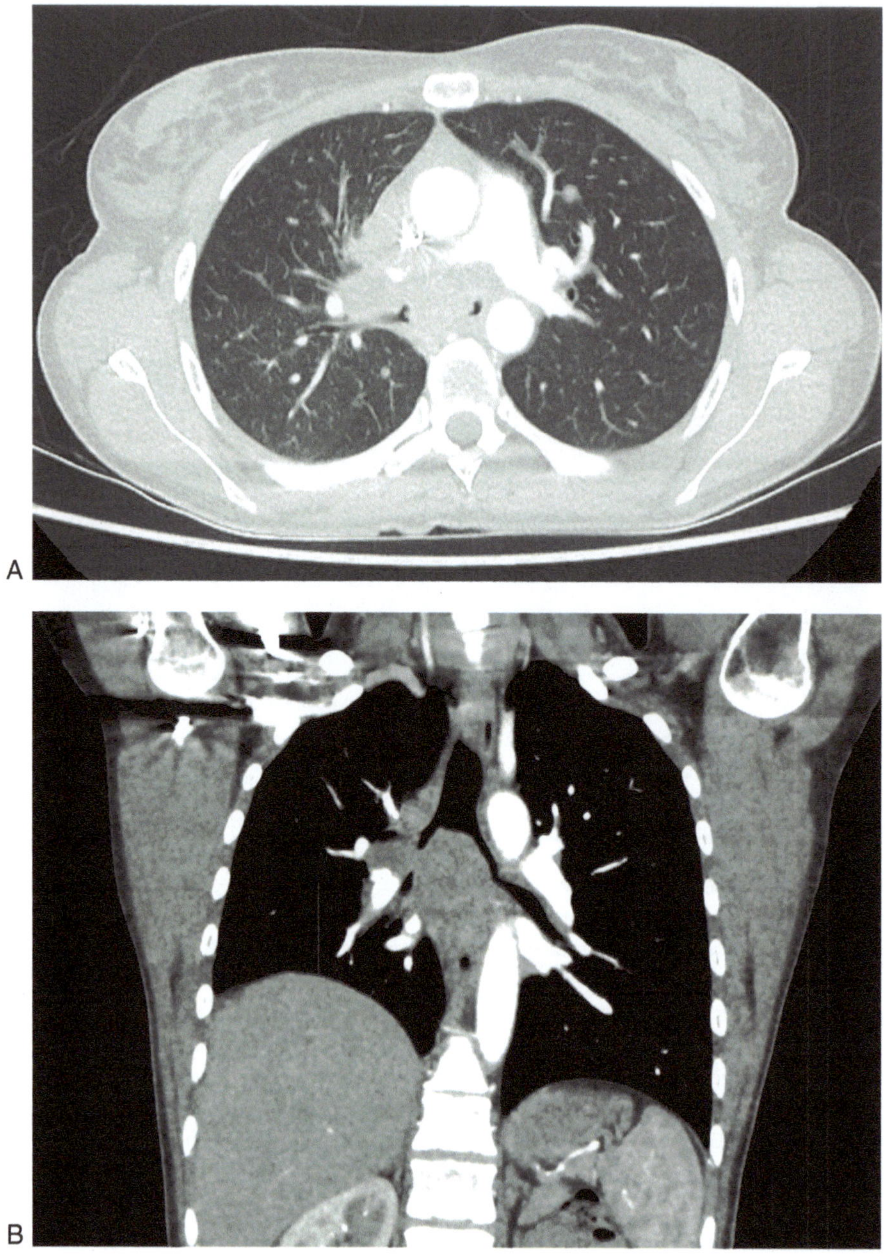

• **Fig. 51.6** A patient presenting with massive lymphadenopathy around the carina with severe distal tracheal and bilateral bronchial stenosis. (**A**) Axial view. (**B**) Coronal view on computed tomography scan.

Alternative Methods

Surgical Alternatives

Before placement of an airway stent, alternative therapy can be considered in the treatment of central airway obstruction. **Dilation** of lesions with a rigid bronchoscope can relieve acute symptoms, although recurrence is likely. When selecting the size of the scope, the largest scope that is anticipated to be able to traverse the stenosis is used, chosen after review of recent imaging, with increasing sizes used with successive dilations. In men, sizing up to an 8-mm or 9-mm scope is typical, whereas a 7-mm or 8-mm scope can be used in women. Sequential dilation with either balloons or semi-rigid dilators can be effective, and likely less traumatic to airway mucosa. **Balloon bronchoplasty** can be accomplished with flexible bronchoscopy under deep sedation. Some stenotic lesion is stiff and less amendable to dilatation. Significant debridement of the airway with forceps can only be done via a rigid bronchoscope. **Electrocautery** can be applied to pedunculated lesions via a metal snare via the bronchoscope, but must be done with appropriate electrical grounding. **Argon plasma cautery** also uses electrical current to destroy obstructive endobronchial lesions. Rather than direct tissue contact, ionized argon plasma is released at the tip of the probe by a high voltage spark from a tungsten electrode. A significant advantage is the ability to send the argon beam laterally or around corners not accessible to

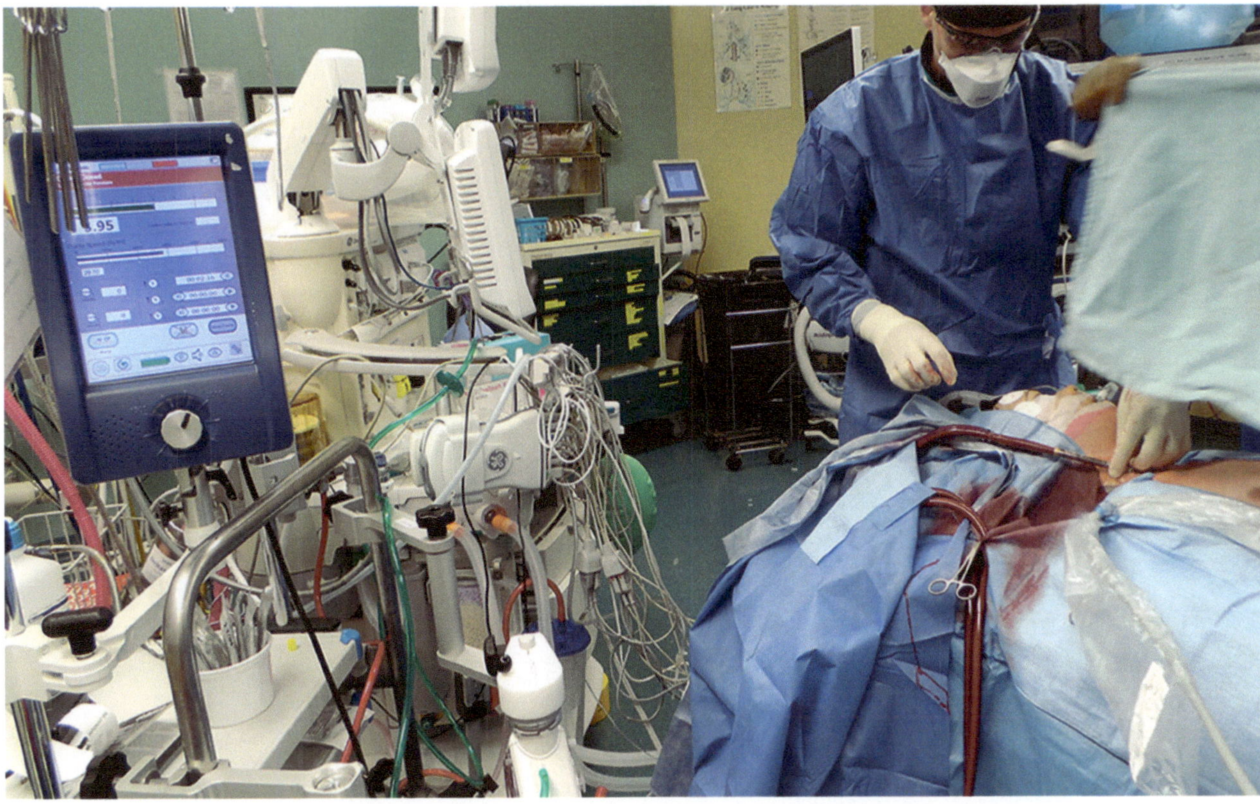

• **Fig. 51.7** Initiation of extracorporeal membrane oxygenation via a dual lumen right jugular catheter.

cautery or laser beam. **Light amplification by stimulated emission of radiation (laser)** therapy became the mainstay of endobronchial tumor treatment with the introduction of the Nd: YAG laser. The wavelength of the Nd:YAG laser (1064 nm) lies in the infrared spectrum and the filament can be advanced through the working channel of a flexible bronchoscope. Tissue penetration is up to 10 mm, so large volumes of tissue can be vaporized. Any of these alternate techniques can be used to clear the airway immediately before stent placement.[2,4]

Flexible Versus Rigid Bronchoscopy

Most experienced proceduralists will have equipment for both flexible and rigid bronchoscopy ready when placing an airway stent, a reflection of the need for the ability to fluidly transition access to the airway depending on conditions or complications. Necessarily, the ventilation strategy and anesthesia delivery may need to be modified correspondingly. Flexible bronchoscopy has the advantage of being technically straightforward and can be performed in awake or lightly

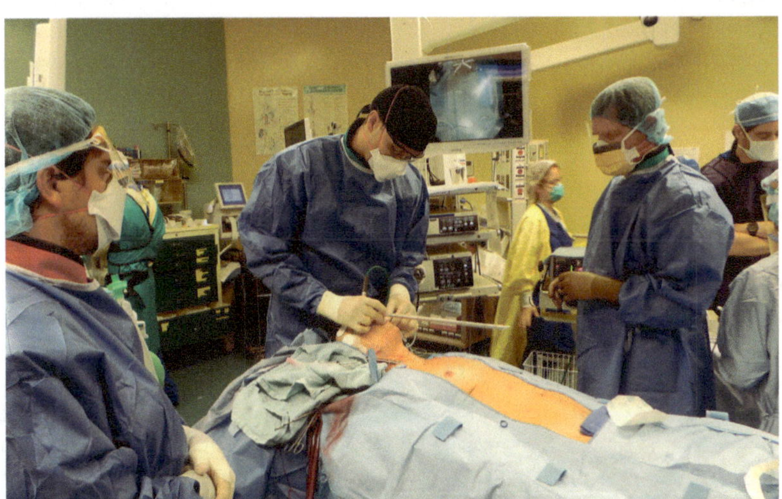

• **Fig. 51.8** Once extracorporeal membrane oxygenation is initiated, the patient is apneic and the surgeons have unobstructed access to the airway.

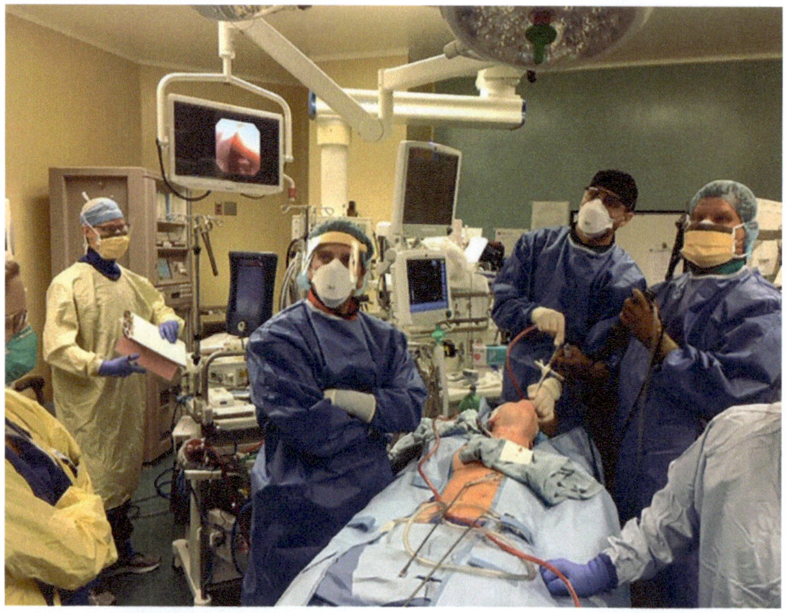

• **Fig. 51.9** There is a lot of equipment in the operating room and the configuration of the room should be planned. The extracorporeal membrane oxygenation circuit and apparatus is to the right of the patient's head, flexible and rigid bronchoscopy is on the left of the patient, the infusion pumps are at the foot of the bed during the debridement and stent placement.

sedated patients with a topicalized airway, through an LMA or ETT, or through a rigid bronchoscope. The distal airways can be accessed and there is minimal risk of trauma. Whereas the working channel of many operating bronchoscopes has a diameter of greater than 3 mm, only relatively small instruments can be inserted into the airway: snares, biopsy forceps, and laser filaments. The latest generation of SEMS include some stents that can be deployed via a flexible scope.[3]

Despite rigid bronchoscopy typically being performed by an operator with specialized training, there is a much greater risk of airway trauma than with flexible bronchoscopy. In patients with congenital or acquired diseases that cause cervical spine instability, rigid bronchoscopy is contraindicated. Down syndrome and certain forms of dwarfism can cause hypoplasia of the odontoid process of C_2 or laxity of the atlantoaxial ligament.[5] Patients with longstanding poorly controlled rheumatoid arthritis may develop atlantoaxial (C_1–C_2) subluxation from the inflammatory erosion of the ligaments which stabilize the odontoid.[6] In addition, dental injury can be caused by pressure from the rigid bronchoscope despite the placement of a protective dental guard. Rigid bronchoscopy requires general anesthesia and does not protect the airway from aspiration. The rigid scope does allow much larger instruments to be used, so is ideal for dealing with bulky tumors, larger stents, or massive hemorrhage. Once pushed past a lesion, positive pressure ventilation can be provided via the rigid scope, which is not possible with the flexible bronchoscope.

Anesthesia Alternatives

Airway topicalization and sedation may be used for lengthy flexible bronchoscopy and straightforward placement of self-expanding stents. Awake rigid bronchoscopy is almost unheard of in modern practice; however, there are occasional reports of life-saving rigid bronchoscopy and stent placement or stent revision with topicalization and minimal sedation when patients are in-extremis.[7]

When the airway circuit is closed, delivery of a potent inhaled anesthetic, usually Sevoflurane, is feasible. This option is frequently used during flexible bronchoscope via an LMA, and in some patients this is possible during rigid bronchoscopy. A ventilating rigid bronchoscope has a metal tube with a lumen equal to the bronchoscope; this is attached at a right angle as close as possible to the external end of the scope.[8,9] This side arm allows attachment of the anesthetic circuit, and a removable glass window is affixed to the external orifice of the bronchoscope to prevent leakage of inhalation agent during ventilation. The window is removed for suction or biopsy. A disadvantage of this technique is potential operating room pollution with inhaled agent and aerosol droplets, either from leaks from the glottis around the bronchoscope, or when stenting instrumentation is inserted. If jet ventilation is required, inhaled agent delivery is no longer an option.

TIVA is more commonly used. The mainstay of TIVA is currently propofol infusion, often with the addition of the ultra-short acting opioid remifentanil; however, propofol, remifentanil, lidocaine, ketamine, and dexmedetomidine may be used in combinations to accomplish effective TIVA. It can be a challenge to fully anesthetize patients with propofol and remifentanil while maintaining spontaneous ventilation. Dexmedetomidine, an α-2 adrenergic agonist, has several desirable properties for sedation while securing a critically compromised airway, including anxiolysis, analgesia, and amnesia with minimal respiratory depression.[10] It is likely the

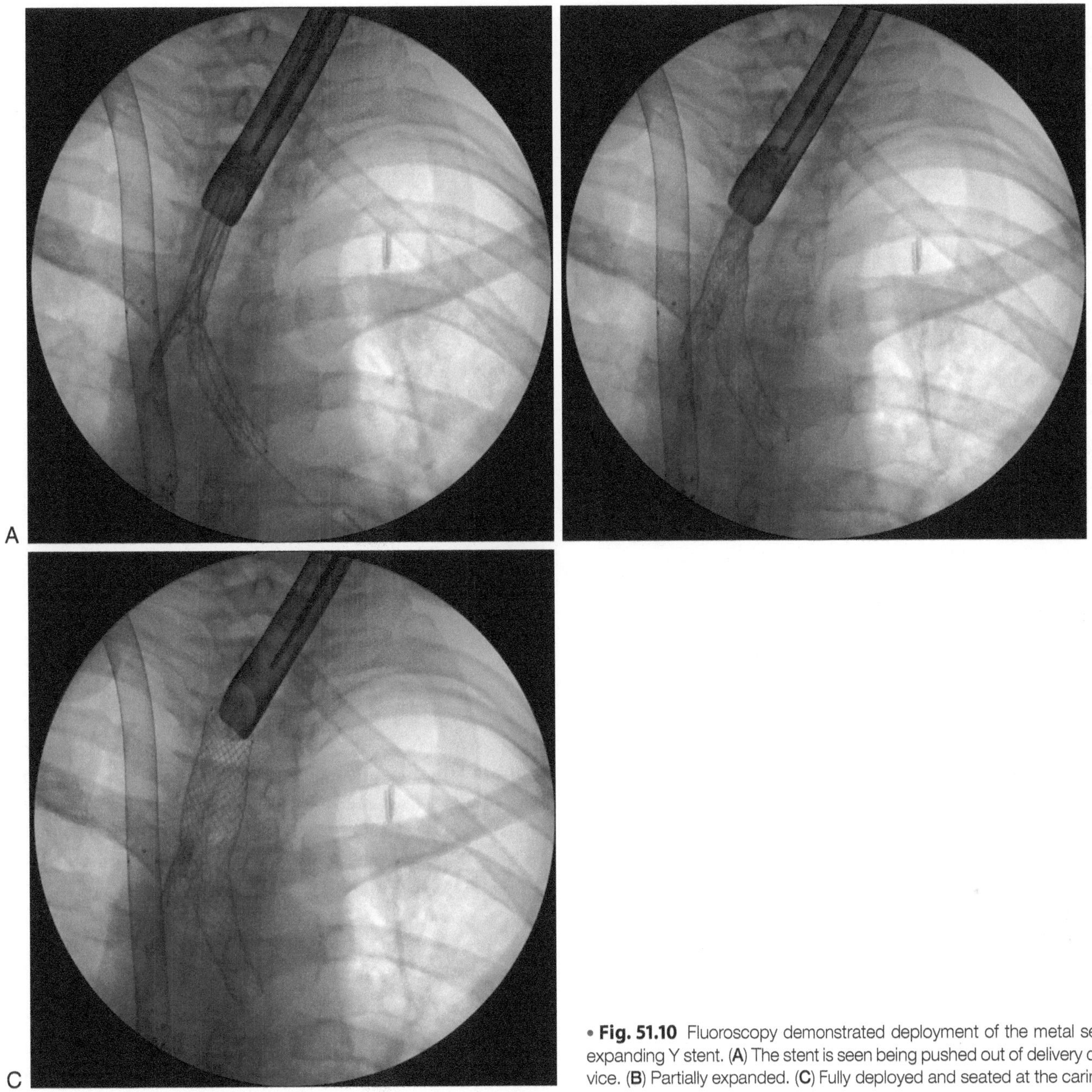

• **Fig. 51.10** Fluoroscopy demonstrated deployment of the metal self-expanding Y stent. (**A**) The stent is seen being pushed out of delivery device. (**B**) Partially expanded. (**C**) Fully deployed and seated at the carina.

sole intravenous agent that can replace inhalational induction when a spontaneous breathing technique is chosen for airway manipulation.[11] Dexmedetomidine may facilitate controlled emergence.

The use of muscle relaxant, although not always required, does facilitate the insertion of a rigid bronchoscope, improves chest wall compliance for ventilation, reduces coughing, and decreases the doses of TIVA required. Regardless of the anesthetic regimen, the choice of drugs should have rapid onset; short duration permits a deep plane of general anesthesia with prompt recovery and resumption of spontaneous ventilation, an alert state with the ability to maintain upper airway patency and to mobilize secretions. Return of full muscle strength is particularly important in patients with compromised pulmonary function or residual airway obstruction. Low to moderate doses of rocuronium are frequently chosen, neuromuscular blockade is fully and promptly reversed with the option of reversal with sugammadex. Succinylcholine is used by some practitioners to facilitate the placement of the rigid bronchoscope within the trachea, then rely on TIVA to suppress coughing. In complex procedures, the bronchoscope is repeatedly removed and reinserted, making a longer acting relaxant agent more practical. At the time of emergence, most patients breathe more comfortably in a semi-sitting position, removing the weight of abdominal contents from the diaphragm, and increasing the patient's functional lung capacity.

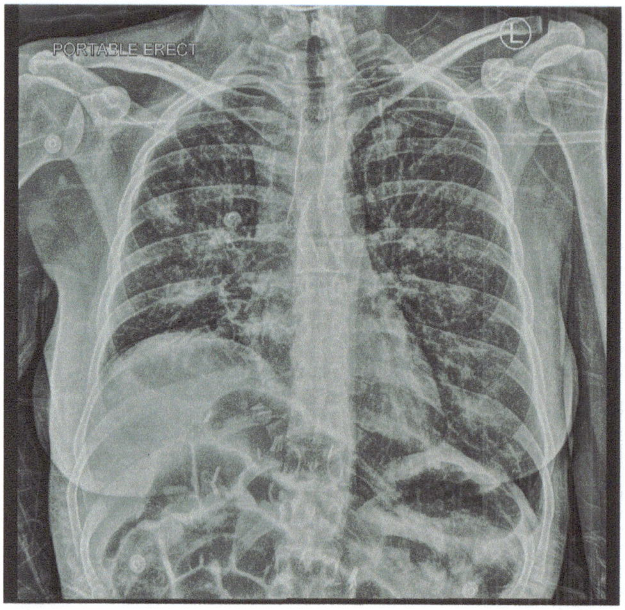

• **Fig. 51.11** Chest x-ray of postoperative position. The patient's symptoms were much improved.

Ventilation Alternatives

As part of the preprocedure checklist, a detailed plan for ventilation throughout induction, and during the period of airway examination, stent placement, and emergence must be clear to the anesthesia and surgical teams. As a general rule when dealing with airway pathologies, the anesthesiologist should never burn his/her bridges and always have a backup plan. Appropriate airway equipment should be assembled and tested to ensure that it is in good working order, including rigid bronchoscopes of a variety of diameters and a way of ventilation through the bronchoscope. A variety of ETTs of different sizes should be available. A supraglottic airway device, usually an LMA should be available. If necessary, ETTs may be placed orotracheally at the end of the procedure for emergence if the stent is not too proximal in the trachea, which would increase the risk of dislodgement. A critical decision is if and when it is safe to transition from spontaneous to controlled ventilation when the central airway is severely compromised. The decision will depend on the status of the patient, experience of the team caring for the patient, and the availability of assistance. Some teams may choose to attempt to maintain spontaneous ventilation throughout the procedure. Depending on the experience of the team, they may induce a deep plane of anesthesia, and the use of muscle relaxation to facilitate placement of the rigid bronchoscope through which conventional ventilation can be delivered via the side arm. Alternatively, a jet ventilation can be applied down the axis of the bronchoscope after the surgeon has verified the position within the airway tree. Both low-frequency jet ventilation (LFJV) via a Sanders injector, and high-frequency jet ventilation (HFJV) using a specialized ventilator, have been shown to adequately ventilate patients with severe tracheal stenosis, and have been described in detail in Chapter 14.[12,13] Both techniques, which allow the ventilation of an open airway system, require high gas flows and are intended not to generate high airway pressures. Nonetheless barotrauma can still occur. Respiratory monitoring during both LFJV and HFJV are imprecise, room air gas entrainment dilutes the delivered oxygen fraction to a variable degree, and sampling end-tidal CO2 is impractical (Table 51.3). An arterial line is indicated for any lengthy or difficult procedure, particularly in patients with severe pulmonary compromise, to monitor serial blood gases. In select tertiary care centers, ECMO is available for critical airway obstruction or anticipated technically difficult stent placement, as in Case 2.[14] ECMO has been used electively, or initiated under emergency circumstance as life-saving therapy.[15,16] This form of ventilatory assist is amenable to peripheral cannulation via jugular or femoral vessels and reduced levels of anticoagulation in the case of hemorrhage. The technical challenge of placing cannula awake in a decompensated patient should not be underestimated, particularly if the patient is unable to lie flat.

It should be emphasized that awake fiberoptic intubation is not a technique of choice for planned stenting of severe central airway obstruction. Even if a small ETT can be inserted by bronchoscopy, it will need to be immediately removed to allow dilation, debridement, or stent insertion. In the specific case of large tracheoesophageal fistulas stented under general anesthesia with conventional positive pressure, ventilation may be ineffective because of gas inflation of the gastrointestinal tract. Spontaneous ventilation using an inhaled induction may be useful until insertion of the bronchoscope. Jet ventilation directed axially past the defect in the tracheal should allow the muscle relaxants as needed.

Risk/Benefit

Risk of Rigid Bronchoscopy

Rigid bronchoscopy is an important tool for tracheal stenting; however, even in experienced hands, mechanical complications can occur. These include trauma to teeth, oropharynx, vocal cords, and other glottic structures, and to the major conducting airways. Systemic complications include vasovagal response, hypotension, hypertension, and disruption to ventilation causing hypercarbia or hypoxia. Postprocedure sore throat, laryngospasm, and bronchospasm can occur. Unanticipated postoperative respiratory difficulties should prompt a CXR to rule out pneumothorax.[17] Airway edema may occur from repeated instrumentation, further compromising airway caliber. Perioperative steroid use is empirical; controlled studies are entirely lacking. Dexamethasone (4–10 mg) is a frequent choice and is routinely used for its antiemetic properties. In selected patients with clinically significant edema, nebulized epinephrine has mucosal vasoconstrictive properties and can be helpful. The racemic form is increasingly unavailable; the more common 1% levoepinephrine is proposed to be equally effective.[18]

TABLE 51.3 Characteristics of Modes of Ventilation During Airway Procedures

	Able to Ventilate Open Airway	Immobility of Operative Field	Specialized Equipment Required	Airway Pressure Monitoring	Potential for Barotrauma	Gas Entrainment	Airway Gas Composition
IPPV	No	No	No	Pressure dependent on ventilator settings, reliable monitoring	Minor	No	Stable, accurate monitoring
LFJV	Yes	No	No	Intermittently can be high, difficult to monitor	High	Yes	Variable, difficult to monitor
HFJV	Yes	Yes	Yes	Can be high, gas trapping common, difficult to monitor delivered pressure	Yes	Yes	Variable, difficult to monitor

HFJV, High-frequency jet ventilation; *IPPV*, intermittent positive pressure ventilation; *LFJV*, low-frequency jet ventilation.

Risk of Stent Placement

Placement of airway stents does result in a high rate of complications (Table 51.4). Immediate problems with stenting include the failure to place the device in the desired location, particularly in case of complex anatomy. Initial malpositioning and/or later migration can precipitate central airway obstruction, requiring an emergent response. Airway injury or perforation can occur not only from the stent itself, but also from the tracheal pathology. The incidence of late complications, including stent migration, mucus plugging, and obstruction from granulation tissue, is in the range of 20% to 50% of patients. Fortunately, mortality from stent placement remains low.[19] For patients with advanced malignancies and with specific goals for palliative benefit, discussion of potential complications associated with airway stenting with patients and their families is warranted, as is documentation of their wishes for end-of-life care.[20]

Risks of Thermal Therapies

Thermal therapies, including electrocautery, argon beam, and laser therapy, allow debulking of intraluminal lesions before stent placement. A limitation to their use is the required drop in inspired oxygen fraction (<30%) to prevent airway fires, which may not be tolerated by some patients. Eye protection should be worn by patients and healthcare workers to avoid inadvertent retinal injury from the laser beam.[4]

Infectious Risk

The ongoing COVID-19 pandemic has increased focus on the risk to healthcare workers participating in aerosol generating procedures, such as bronchoscopy, airway suctioning, and stent placement. Particular risk is attributed to open tube rigid bronchoscopy, jet ventilation, and interruption of an otherwise closed ventilation circuit with repeated removal and reintroduction of a bronchoscope. These maneuvers generate high gas flow and high shear conditions, which generate aerosol droplets. Known or suspected COVID-19 is considered to be a relative contraindication to bronchoscopy, and that only essential emergent procedures be performed, given the clear risks to participating healthcare workers. Indications for emergent bronchoscopy include stenting of severe or symptomatic tracheal stenosis

TABLE 51.4 Complications of Airway Stent Placement

Early
Stent malposition
Hemorrhage
Airway rupture during placement

Late
Stent migration
Mucoid impaction
Infection
Formation of granulation tissue
Stent fracture
Airway erosion

and central airway obstruction from migrated stent.[21] Protective measures against infectious aerosols include use of respirator-level respiratory protection, negative pressure rooms where feasible, controlled handling of specimens, and minimization of involved personnel. Other serious aerosol transmitted infections include severe acute respiratory syndrome (SARS), Middle East respiratory syndrome (MERS) and influenza; similar precautions are warranted. When tracheal stenting is combined with laser debridement, the plume generated by the laser has been shown to be able to harbor the human papilloma virus (HPV), with documented cases of transmission to healthcare workers; however, the risk appears to be low.[22] Nonetheless evacuation of plume from the surgical field is recommended, as is the use of protective respirator masks when the patient has known HPV.

Review of the Literature

The modern history of airway stents began with the first report in 1960 by Montgomery of a T-tube for support of the subglottic airway.[23] Early reports of first-generation expandable metallic stents appeared in the 1980s with subsequent development of SEMS, both bare metal and partially covered, considered the second generation. Silicone stents were described in the 1990s by Dumon.[24] The relative advantages of the stents in the classic categories were previously presented, as are their drawbacks (see Table 51.2). Stents are manufactured in a large variety of lengths and diameters, and in cylindrical shapes and Y-shaped configurations for carinal lesions. The prospect of minimizing long-term complication rates from airway stents is driving development of novel designs using newer medical-grade materials. Hybrid fully covered SEMS, usually made from nitinol with a polymer covering, such as silicone or polyurethane, are considered third generation, and are increasingly used. Metallic stents for benign disease are still under a U.S. Food and Drug Administration (FDA) warning because of multiple reports of complications. "Our concern about complications from using metallic tracheal stents in patients with benign airway disorders stems from a review of recently published literature, medical device reports that we have received, and information from physicians. These complications include obstructive granulation tissue, stenosis at the ends of the stent, migration of the stent, mucous plugging, infection, and stent fracture."[25] It should be noted that at the time of FDA recommendation (2005), the available metallic stents were mostly uncovered and with limited biomechanical properties. With advancements in manufacturing, third-generation metallic stents have since been used to treat benign airway stenosis with a satisfactory safety profile.

Current research aims to combine the advantages of various stent designs. A newly available line of stents uses a polyester mesh embedded in silicone to achieve the luminal patency of metal stents with the option of easy removal of silicone stents. In the last decade, several groups have created temporary bioabsorbable stents; however, these must be regarded as investigational.[26] By inhibiting fibroblast growth, drug-eluting stents target the formation of granulation tissue and are currently in human trials.[3] Complex cases present airways that are deformed with areas that are narrowed, and twisted and present irregular profiles. Commercially available stents will not conform to the airway, and may create excessive radial forces on the airway mucosa, provoking granulation tissue. The feasibility of three-dimensional (3D)-printed bespoke airway stents is being explored[27,28] (Fig. 51.12). Planning patient management will in the future be influenced by 3D printing technology; models of subglottic stenosis have been found to improve clinicians' accuracy in grading the degree of stenosis and making better choices of treatment strategy[29] (Fig. 51.13).

Many innovations in anesthesia care for bronchoscopy and stent placement in adults are described in the form of case reports or small case series. There is a dearth of high-quality studies comparing choices of anesthetic, use of relaxants and ventilation technique. There is more evidence in pediatrics populations; it is usually children undergoing rigid bronchoscopy for foreign body removal, a fairly homogeneous clinical group. A recent randomized study concludes that intravenous dexmedetomidine, with lidocaine topicalization and spontaneous ventilation, provided better procedural conditions than propofol, fentanyl, and succinylcholine with manual LFJV; however, the dexmedetomidine regimen required significantly longer duration of induction and prolonged recovery time.[30] Another study concluded that higher dose remifentanil infusion (0.2 vs. 0.1 mcg/kg/min) reduced the required infusion dose of propofol, with improved hemodynamic stability and reduced recovery times.[31] It is unclear if these conclusions can be applied to adult populations undergoing airway stenting, who present a more diverse spectrum of clinical conditions. A randomized study of adults undergoing a variety of tracheobronchial interventions via rigid bronchoscopy concluded that the use of low-dose rocuronium (0.25 mg/kg) with sugammadex reversal provided better patient satisfaction than low-dose succinylcholine (0.5 mg/kg) as result of less postoperative myalgia. However, intubating conditions were superior with succinylcholine.[32]

The extent and location of the central airway obstruction will influence the clinical presentation. Milder symptoms include cough, wheezing, and shortness of breath on exertion. Expiratory wheezing is generally a sign of intrathoracic airway obstruction, whereas stridor is more likely related to extrathoracic obstruction. When evaluating patients with central airway obstruction, it should be noted that the trachea is typically significantly narrowed to less than 8 mm, before exertional dyspnea occurs. Once the lumen is less than 5 mm, symptoms present at rest. Because of the significant loss of airway cross-section before the development of symptoms, approximately half of patients with tracheal stenosis have respiratory distress at the time of first presentation.[2] Flow-volume loops, although potentially helpful for the referring physician

A

B

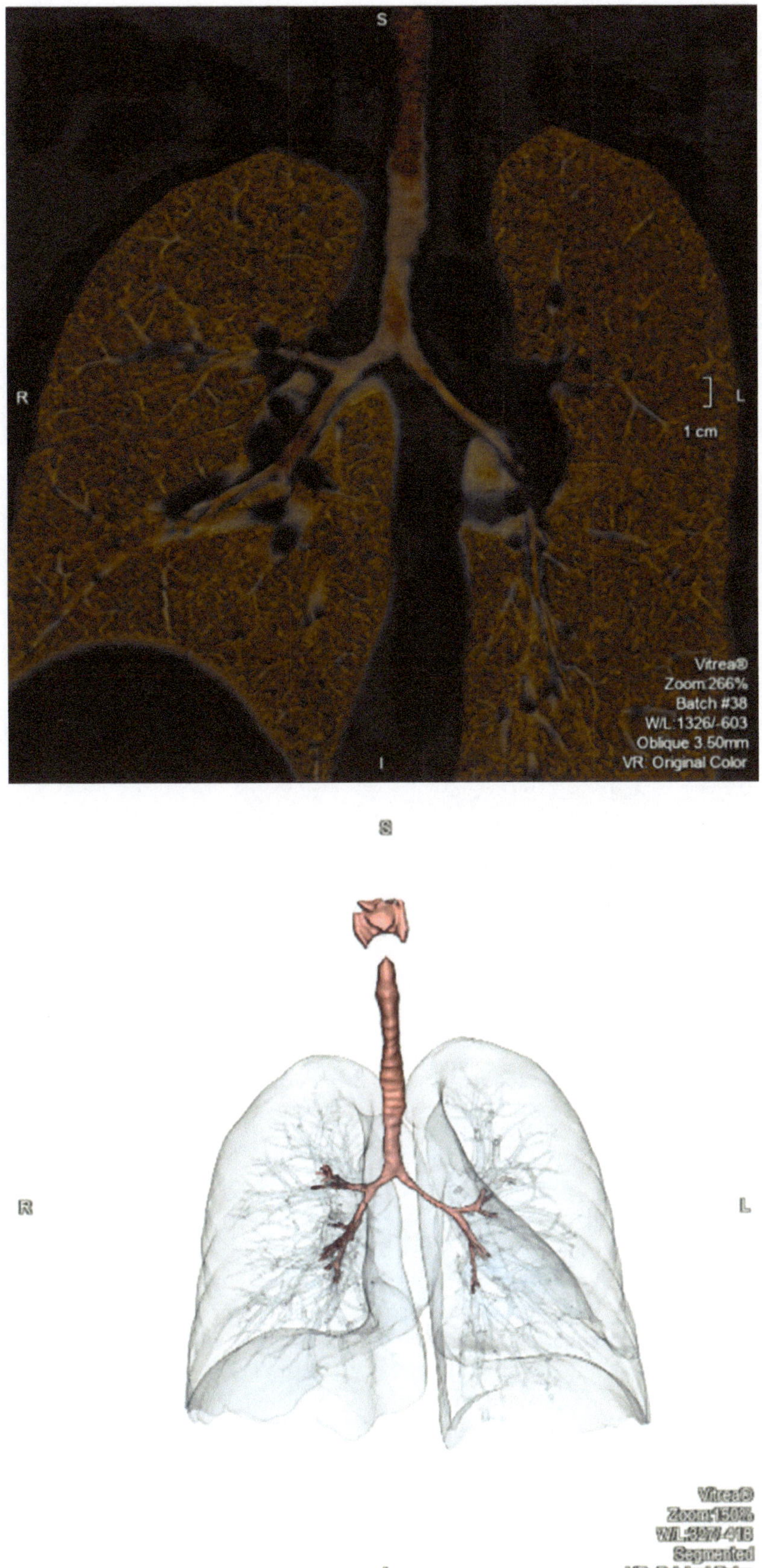

• **Fig. 51.12** Diffuse airway involvement with relapsing polychondritis. (**A**) Computed tomography image processing allows a precise description of airway anatomy. (**B**) Programmed for three-dimensional (3D) printing of airway model. Applications include surgical planning and 3D-printing of personalized airway stents.

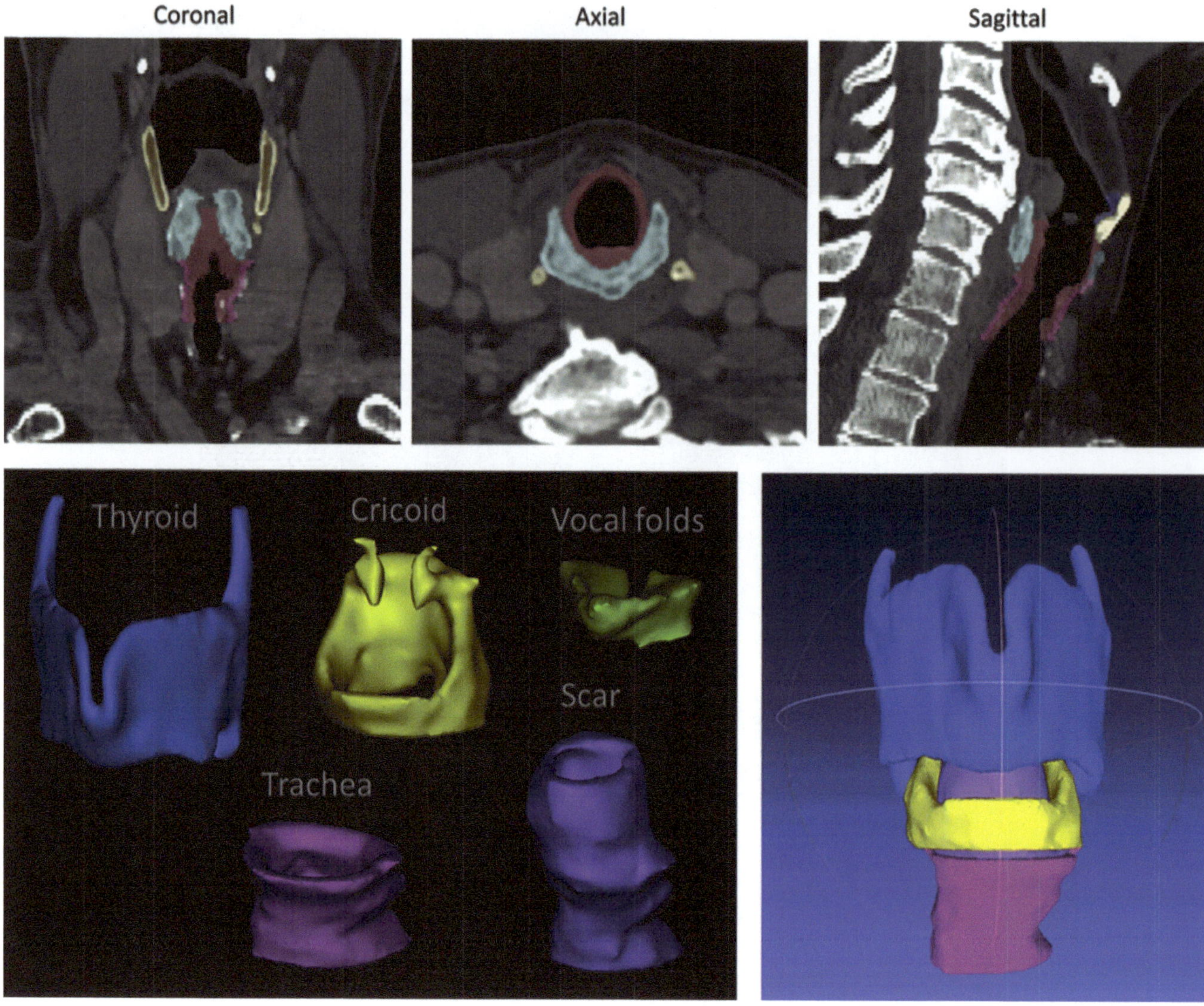

• **Fig. 51.13** Production steps of three-dimensional (3D) model of subglottic stenosis. Anatomic structures are highlighted on a computed tomography scan and rendered in a multicolor 3D model. The endoluminal stenosis is clearly represented. (From Hoetzenecker K, Chan H, Frommlet F, et al. 3D models in the diagnosis of subglottic airway stenosis. *Ann Thorac Surg.* 2019;107:1060–1865. With permission.)

to assess pulmonary function before and after stenting, does not contribute to planning intraoperative management, which relies heavily on high quality imaging of the airway tree, usually computed tomography. Extensive preoperative workup is often not possible in patients with respiratory distress and should not be attempted.

Instrumentation of the upper respiratory tract causes a significant sympathoadrenal stress response.[33] Increases in heart rate, and both systemic and pulmonary artery pressures, have been documented and may be prolonged. Myocardial oxygen consumption rises, and dysrhythmias may occur. Of patients presenting for stent placement for malignancy, many are elderly smokers with attendant risk of peripheral and coronary artery disease. The incidence of myocardial ischemia during and after rigid bronchoscopy was historically described as being as high as 10% to 15%.[34] Modern balanced anesthesia regimens allow better heart rate control as a result of routine use of remifentanil infusions during TIVA, and the availability of short acting beta blockers, such as esmolol, has reduced the incidence of ischemia, although definitive evidence is lacking.

Patients with tracheal stents in situ may present for unrelated procedures. Whenever possible, tracheal intubation should be avoided, as life-threatening complications have been reported from stent dislodgement and central airway obstruction. Regional anesthetic techniques should be used when possible. When general anesthesia is required, preference should be given to supraglottic airway support, such as an LMA. When intubation is unavoidable, placement of the ETT under fiberoptic guidance is the safest option.[35]

The care of patients with an in-situ Montgomery T-tube warrants special mention. A Montgomery T-tube stent may

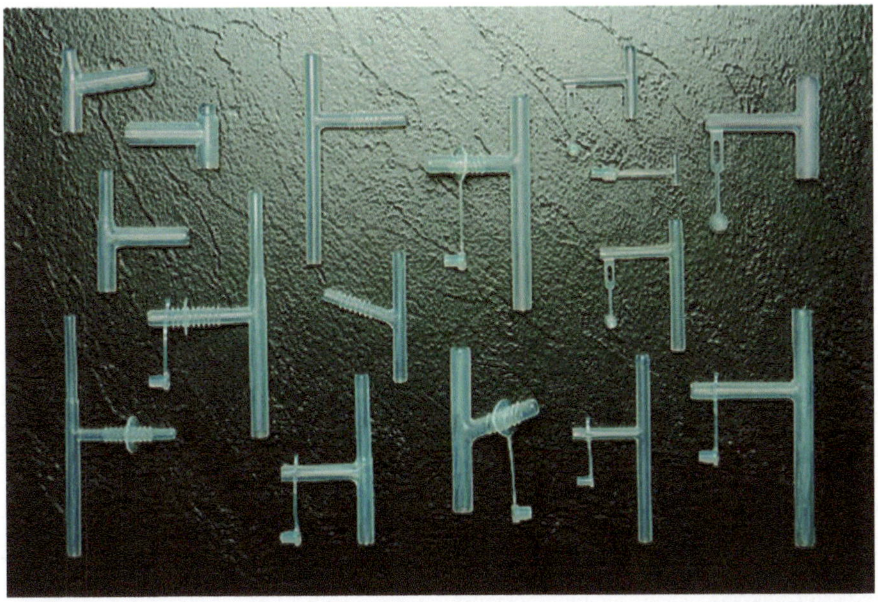

• **Fig. 51.14** Montgomery T-tubes of various sizes and configurations. T-tubes are made of silicone and can be trimmed by the surgeon before insertion to further customize them to the patient's anatomy.

be placed for a finite period of time to allow an upper airway prone to malacia or scarring to heal and stabilize, often during airway resection for subglottic stenosis (Fig. 51.14). In some patients, the T-tube becomes essentially a permanent airway support. Patients with T-tubes may require airway examination or replacement or adjustment of their T-tube, generally using rigid bronchoscopy under general anesthesia. When surgery unrelated to their airway is proposed, the T-tube presents a significant challenge to the anesthesiologist, as the presence of the upper limb of the stent just beyond the vocal chords precludes routine tracheal intubation (Fig. 51.15). The upper airway can be supported with an LMA with either spontaneous or controlled ventilation, in which the tracheostomy limb is capped. Alternatively, the use of a well seated laryngeal mask that was then capped to block the escape of gas from the proximal tracheal limb while ventilating the patient via the tracheostomy limb has been described.[36] The tracheotomy limb may be connected to a breathing circuit using the connector of a small ETT, usually size 5.5 or 6. Another reported technique is the placement of an inflated Fogarty catheter through the tracheotomy limb into the proximal limb to block egress of gas into the upper airway, with simultaneous ventilation through the tracheotomy limb. Most methods of ventilation through the T-tube offer only partial airway protection from aspiration. Awake fiberoptic telescoping of a small ETT into the proximal tracheal limb of the T-tube has been described, but aspiration around the T-tube is still possible. In a full stomach situation, there is a report of awake fiberoptic placement of a 5-mm microlaryngoscopy tube completely through the trachea proximal and distal limbs of the T-tube, with inflating of the cuff in the trachea for protection against aspiration.[37] Adult T-tube sizes vary from 8 to 16 mm external diameter. This approach may only be possible with the larger sizes. Finally, the T-tube can be removed by the patient's surgeon, and replaced by a tracheotomy tube. If the tracheotomy is left in place for any length of time, the patient could suffer a recurrence of their upper airway stenosis. T-tube replacement usually requires general anesthesia.

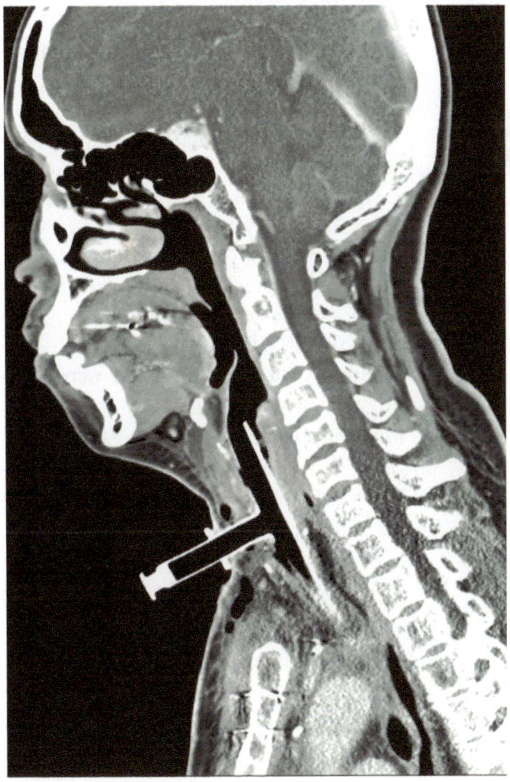

• **Fig. 51.15** A patient with Montgomery T-tube, in profile. Note in this case the slight protrusion of the proximal limb through the patient's vocal cords.

References

1. Chin C, Litle V, Yun J, Weiser T, Swanson S. Airway stents. *Ann Thorac Surg.* 2008;85:S792–S796.
2. Ernst A, Feller-Kopman D, Becker H, Mehta A. Central airway obstruction. *Am J Resp Crit Care Med.* 2004;169:1278–1297.
3. Liu L, Kong J, George C. Recent advances in airway stenting. *Shanghai Chest.* 2020;4:6.
4. Vourc'h G, Tannieres Ml, Toty L, et al. Anaesthetic management of tracheal surgery using the neodynium-yttrium-aluminium-garnet laser. *Br J Anaesth.* 1980;52:993–997.
5. Auden SM. Cervical spine instability and dwarfism: fiberoptic intubations for all. *Anesthesiology.* 1999;91:580.
6. MacArthur A, Kleinman S. Rheumatoid cervical joint disease – a challenge to the anaesthetist. *Can J Anaesth.* 1993;40:154–159.
7. Conacher I, Curran E. Local anesthesia and sedation for rigid bronchoscopy for emergency relief of central airway obstruction. *Anaesthesia.* 2004:290–292.
8. Safar P. Ventilating bronchoscope. *Anesthesiology.* 1958;19:406.
9. Sanders RD. Two ventilating attachments for bronchoscopes. *Delaware Med J.* 1967;39:170.
10. Dey S, Bhattacharyya P, Medhi J, Nellappa A. Successful tracheal stent placement for central airway obstruction using dexmedetomidine and regional airway anesthesia. *J Anaesthesiol Clin Pharmacol.* 2014;30:438–439.
11. Voscopoulos C, Kirk F, Lovrincevic M, Lema M. The use of "high-dose" dexmedetomidine in a patient with critical tracheal stenosis and anterior mediastinal mass. *Open Anesthesiology J.* 2011;5:42–49.
12. McRae K. Anesthesia for airway surgery. *Anesthesiol Clin North Am.* 2001;19:497–541.
13. Vourc'h G, Fischler M, Michon F, et al. High frequency jet ventilation v. manual jet ventilation during bronchoscopy in patients with tracheo-bronchial stenosis. *Br J Anaesth.* 1955;55:969–972.
14. McRae K, De Perrot M. Principles and indications of extracorporeal life support in general thoracic surgery. *J Thorac Dis.* 2018;10: S931–S946.
15. Park J-H, Shin J, Kim K, et al. Respiratory support with venovenous extracorporeal membrane oxygenation during stent placement for the palliation of critical airway obstruction: case series analysis. *J Thorac Dis.* 2017;9:2599–2607.
16. Ko M, dos Santos P, Machca T, Marseu Waddell T, Keshavjee S, Cypel M. Use of single-cannula veno-venous extracorporeal life support in the management of life-threatening airway obstruction. *Ann Thorac Surg.* 2015;99:e63–e65.
17. Tandon A. Rigid bronchoscopy: a general overview. *Shanghai Chest.* 2020;4:15.
18. Nutman J, Brooks LJ, Deakins KM, et al. Racemic versus l-epinephrine aerosol in the treatment of postextubation laryngeal edema: results from a prospective, randomized, double-blind study. *Crit Care Med.* 1994;22:1591–1594.
19. Pasricha V, DiBardino D, Ma K. Management of malignant central airway obstruction. *Shanghai Chest.* 2020;4:26.
20. Vonk-Noordegraaf A, Postmus PE, Sutedja TG. Tracheobronchial stenting in the terminal care of cancer patients with central airways obstruction. *Chest.* 2001;120:1811–1814.
21. Wahidi M, Shojaee S, Lamb C, et al. The use of bronchoscopy during the coronavirus disease 2019 pandemic. *Chest.* 2020;S0012–3692(20)30850–3.
22. Manson L, Damrose E. Does exposure to laser plume place the surgeon at high risk for acquiring clinical human papilloma virus infection? *Laryngoscope.* 2013:123.
23. Montgomery WW. T-tube tracheal stent. *Arch Otolaryngol.* 1965; 82:320–321.
24. Dumon JF. A dedicated tracheobronchial stent. *Chest.* 1990;97: 328–332.
25. Schultz D. FDA public health notification: Complications from metallic tracheal stents in patients with benign airway disorders. Rockville (MD): Food and Drug Administration; 2005.
26. Dutau H, Musani A, Laroumagne S, Darwiche K, Freitag L, Astoul P. Biodegradable airway stents—bench to bedside: A comprehensive review. *Respiration.* 2015;90:512–521.
27. Folch E, Stents Keyes CAirway. *Ann Cardiothorac Surg.* 2018;7: 273–283.
28. Cheng G, Folch E, Brik R, et al. Three-dimensional modeled T-tube design and insertion in a patient with tracheal dehiscence. *Chest.* 2015;148:e106–e108.
29. Hoetzenecker K, Chan H, Frommlet F, et al. 3D models in the diagnosis of subglottic airway stenosis. *Ann Thorac Surg.* 2019;107: 1060–1865.
30. Cai Y, Li W, Chen K. Efficacy and safety of spontaneous ventilation technique using dexmedetomidine for rigid bronchoscopic airway foreign body removal in children. *Pediatr Anaesth.* 2013; 23:1048–1053.
31. Teksan L, Baris S, Karakaya D, Dilek A. A dose study of remifentanil in combination with propofol during tracheobronchial foreign body removal in children. *J Clin Anesth.* 2013;25:198–201.
32. Ghezel-Ahmadi V, Ghezel-Ahmadi D, Mangen J, et al. Comparing patient satisfaction and intubating conditions using succinylcholine or low-dose rocuronium for rigid bronchoscopy: a randomized study. *Thorac Cardiovasc Surg.* 2015;63:526–532.
33. Tomori Z, Widdicombe JG. Muscular, bronchomotor and cardiovascular reflexes elicited by mechanical stimulation of the respiratory tract. *J Physiol.* 1969;200:25.
34. Hill AJ, Feneck RO, Underwood SM, et al. The haemodynamic effects of bronchoscopy, comparison of propofol and thiopentone with and without alfentanil pretreatment. *Anaesthesia.* 1991:266.
35. Davis N, Madden BP, Sheth A, et al. Airway management in patients with tracheobronchial stents. *Br J Anaesth.* 2006;96:132–135.
36. Agrawal S, Payal YS, Sharma JP, et al. Montgomery T-tube: anesthetic management. *J Clin Anesth.* 2007;19:135–137.
37. Wouters KMA, Byreddy Gleeson M, et al. New approach to anesthetizing a patient at risk of pulmonary aspiration with a Montgomery T-tube in situ. *Br J Anaesth.* 2008;101:354–357.

52 Robotic Thoracic Surgery

LASZLO L. SZEGEDI

Introduction

Robots have become increasingly present in contemporary reality. One can find them working in places where humans cannot reach because of biologic limitations, and helping people in different fields, as in the area of health care. In this regard, there is emphasis on the advances in the use of these devices in different surgical procedures, among them thoracic surgery, with good results for a variety of thoracic procedures.[1]

From the time of ancient civilizations, there have been many accounts of automated devices or automats representing humans in appearance. Through the industrial age, there appeared more practical applications, by replacing humans in performing repetitive or dangerous tasks, which humans prefer not to or are unable to do because of size limitations, or which take place in dangerous environments.

The term robot, which means forced labor in Czech language, was first used in the beginning of the last century by Karel Capek in his play entitled Rossum's Universal Robots and presented in 1921, introducing the term robot into English and other languages.

Actually, a robot means a machine capable of carrying out a complex series of actions automatically. Robots have either their control embedded within, or are guided by external, human control. Robots have become incorporated into daily life over the last half-century: what was once only science fiction has now become a reality. Robots are used widely in all kinds and types of activities and domains: from house holding, to grass movers, to leisure, to industry, and most recently medicine, enhancing the development of certain types of surgical interventions. Today, everyone living in the developed countries benefits from the advances in robotics in the daily life. Although robots were commonly used in the healthcare laboratory setting, they have been increasingly integrated into clinical medicine. Over the last 2 decades, research in surgical robotics has been continually increasing as evident from the rise in the number of manuscripts published each year. Surgical robotics is an evolving field aiming to take advantage of the features of robotics which made them so valuable in other industries.

In 1985 the first surgical application of robotic technology in medicine was described when an industrial robotic arm was modified to perform a stereotactic brain biopsy with 0.05 mm accuracy. This served as the prototype device for Neuromate (Integrated Surgical Systems, Sacramento, CA, USA), which received U.S. Food and Drug Administration (FDA) approval in 1999.[2] In 1992 the Robodoc (Integrated Surgical Systems, Sacramento, CA, USA) was introduced for use in hip replacement surgery. Whereas the Robodoc has been used in thousands of patients in Europe, it has not yet received FDA approval in the United States because of concerns regarding complication rates.[3–5] Similar devices have been designed for use in knee replacement and temporal bone surgery, but neither of these devices has yet completed clinical testing or received FDA approval.[6,7]

The potential for widespread clinical application of the newly developed telerobotic devices was commercially recognized in 1997, Intuitive Surgical's daVinci® surgical system was used to perform a laparoscopic cholecystectomy in Belgium.[8] In 1999 Computer Motion Inc. introduced the Zeus surgical system (after its predecessor AESOP, introduced in 1994), which differed from daVinci® primarily in the configuration of the surgeon's workstation. It was cleared by the FDA, but after several lawsuits against a rival medical robotics company, in 2003, Computer Motion and Intuitive Surgical merged into a single company.

The da Vinci Surgical System® is a robotic surgical system made by the American company Intuitive Surgical and approved by the FDA in 2000. It is controlled by a surgeon seated at a console which gives him a three-dimensional (3D)-image of the surgical field. The second part of the robot is the actual robot—the patient-side cart—consisting of three or four robotic arms and housing different instruments and the endoscope with incorporated camera. The third component of the system is a video monitor, including optical devices for the robot.

A full range of Endo Wrists (Surgical Intuitive) instruments are at the disposal of the surgeon for the surgical procedure. These instruments provide seven degrees of motion, which exceeds the capacity of a normal hand during open surgery and two degrees of axial wrist-like rotations.[9] The instruments are introduced via special ports and the surgeon's movements at the console are transmitted in a highly sensitive manner to the instruments attached to the arms of the robot.

Usually, a first surgeon operates the console, while the second surgeon, at the operating table, introduces and changes the trocars and the different instruments necessary for the operation.

Robotic-assisted thoracic surgery (RATS) started in a few centers in the mid-late 1990s. The first report was made at the beginning of the year 2000.[10]

Despite the fact that thoracic surgery is one of the fastest growing techniques, the results of RATS are not widely reported. Yet, we may not recognize any major advantage in the outcome when compared with video-assisted thoracic surgery (VATS), but certainly, the superior capabilities of robotic surgery could be beneficial. Gaining more experience in RATS may provide superior results in oncologic, physiologic, and life quality measurements.[11]

Advantages, Disadvantages, Learning Curves

In the beginning, RATS was mainly compared with VATS. The VATS technique gained recognition in thoracic surgery from the 1990s and some articles even reported significant improvements in comparison with open surgery. Advantages of VATS were less trauma,[12] shorter chest drainage duration, decreased hospital stay,[13–15] preservation of short-term pulmonary function,[16] reduced pain and fewer complications. Robotic surgery is of course also a minimally invasive technique, and therefore it will be difficult to show differences in performance with VATS.

Similar to the introduction of VATS several years ago, RATS is a surgical technique that is getting more and more integrated in the spectrum of thoracic surgery. The spread of initial minimally invasive techniques was slow considering limitations (limited maneuverability and unstable camera platform)[10] and poor ergonomics. Often, one specific technique, either VATS or RATS, is chosen by one particular surgeon. A minority of thoracic surgeons are trained in both minimally invasive techniques, and therefore it will be difficult to obtain large comparative studies with those equipoise experts. Also worldwide, the experience is widely differing; in some countries robotics platforms have integrated well, whereas in others, RATS programs are at the start-up point.

Of course, the costs for the use of a robotic system is an important factor. Because VATS has a less expensive price tag, its penetration became widespread faster. Unfortunately, there is no standardization of VATS, which seems to be the case with RATS. Furthermore, the learning curve for RATS is greater than for VATS (50 cases vs. 25 cases to be performed by the surgeon to be certified).[17,18] Obviously, the traditional way of surgical training must be taken into account. Previously everyone was trained for open surgery through the thoracotomy or sternotomy; later on, VATS was started up. In the group of people who have not switched to VATS, there are a number of surgeons who immediately switched to RATS, bypassing VATS. Most surgeons who switched from VATS to RATS already had a minimal invasive thoracic surgery experience.

Advantages of RATS are of course the 3D vision, the use of the robot-controlled and hinged instruments, and the ergonomic aspect for the surgeon. Movements are more precise, filtered, and scaled. Therefore improved surgical precision and accuracy are possible.

The robotic system is not perfect; disadvantages are loss of tactile feedback, increased operation time, distance between the surgeon and the patient. The significant disadvantage remains the high cost of the system and the parts that are needed for an operation. Instruments can only be used for a limited time (10–20 uses), which leads to considerable costs. Some data suggest that shorter hospital stays will offset some of the higher cost.

Another aspect is the specific training that is required. If this can be done on a dual console system, there is of course a better close guidance of the start up. The "student"-surgeon and the experienced surgeon (proctor) have the same picture and switching the instruments between the two consoles is easy. In addition, the da Vinci® robot surgical system has introduced the da Vinci skills simulator, where surgeon and surgical team can participate in the development of specific skills in a simulator center.

In case of bleeding, there is often a better control possibly because the robot's arms remain firm in the same position and are not dependent on a human factor, such as movements or distraction. An emergency thoracotomy can always be performed while the bleeding remains stable and control can be achieved better than with a VATS procedure.

The major advantage is actually for the surgeon. Ergonomics for the surgeon on the robotic console cannot be compared with the situation during a video-assisted thoracic operation. Even physically, sitting down on a comfortable chair at the console is completely different from standing with two surgeons sideways from a patient and looking at a screen.

In the meantime, the technique has been considered safe and reproducible, and there is an association with a reduced duration of stay, as well as low morbidity and mortality.[14] A recent publication confirmed that RATS achieves equally good oncologic results. Larger series show that the visualization and dissection of lymph nodes in the mediastinum can be performed more smoothly so that more nodal levels can be reached during dissection. This provides better staging of the disease and consequently a more adapted therapy.[13] The robot was primarily intended to be used during cardiac surgery, but the current clinical use of the robot covers a wide range of surgical specialties.

The Robot-Assisted Lobectomy

The lobectomy is the most commonly performed oncologic procedure, in which a precise anatomic dissection of the lung is performed. Each center has now developed a technique, usually in function of the type of the robotic system. Modern robot machines have increased from three-armed systems to four arms, which allowed better access to the patient by the caregivers. This led to more standardization (3- or 4-arm) of the technique, and it can also be used for safe resection of all lobes. The older system is more dependent on correct positioning above the patient because of less mobility of the central attachment of the robotic arms. This created situations where accessibility for the anesthesiologist to the patient was impaired, and that may be crucial in critical situations.

The mortality is comparable to the other techniques, open and video-assisted surgery. Long-term oncologic results are consistent with other large series using VATS or thoracotomy.[18] The morbidity is the same and there are no specific complications contributed to the robotic system described in the literature (in case of thoracic surgery). A retrospective study by Bao et al. compared 184 patients undergoing RATS versus VATS lung resection and found no improvement in clinical outcomes, whereas RATS procedures took longer and cost significantly more.[19]

Blood loss is not significantly different in comparative ranges between VATS and RATS.[20]

The Robot-Assisted Segmentectomy

The number and proportion of early-stage lung cancers is likely to increase because of the growth and aging of the population and the low-dose chest computed tomography screening programs of high-risk populations.

Because of the wider range of well controlled movement of the robotic arms and improved operative visualization techniques of vascular structures with indocyanine green and creation of anatomic 3D-models for preoperative planning, segmentectomy can be performed by more surgeons using this mini-invasive approach. The meticulous dissection of hilar, bronchial, and vascular lymph nodes, which is important for the correct staging of early lung cancer, was made more accessible by RATS operations.

Metastases in the lungs can thus be removed and wider resection margins can be obtained. Resections of small early lung cancers in high-risk individuals are also possible with the aid of the robot system. To determine the oncologic validation for sublobar anatomic resections in small early stage lung cancer, two studies are currently in progress, namely, CATGB 140503 (United States) and JCOG 0802 (Japan). Future results will determine whether this approach can be applied to all patients with clinical stage 1A disease without oncologic compromises. Segmentectomy has been proven safer than lobectomies,[21,22] and it carries less complications when performed thoracoscopically compared with open surgery. For that reason, some surgeons advocate that a sublobar anatomic resection has to be done thoracoscopically, and the robotic platform is useful for this operation.

The surgical technique used in our institution is a 4-arm set-up. The anesthetized, ventilated patient is positioned on a vacuum mattress in lateral decubitus. The chest is elevated with an inflatable balloon placed under the patient so that the thorax is the highest point. The robot is positioned in the back of the patient. Four ports are used and one assistant's port.

The camera is located on the intersection of the eighth or ninth intercostal space and posterior axillary line. From here, the second port is placed 8 cm to the anterior side, the third port 8 cm to the posterior side, the fourth 8 cm in 45 degrees up and posteriorly, respecting 6 cm from the midline of the spine. A 12-mm laparoscopic port is placed supradiaphragmatically, under visualization with a 30-degree camera, and after insufflation of carbon dioxide ($CO2$) at a pressure of 5–10 mm Hg. This port is used for suctioning, stapling, and retraction that will be enlarged to approximately 4 cm at the end of the operation for retraction of the specimen. Instruments that are used are the spatula in the right hand, the bipolar forceps in the right, and the tip-up forceps also in the right hand. The spatula is changed with the Cadière-forceps for passing behind structures. The assistant port is used for the stapling devices (Fig. 52.1).

After the removal of the specimen, one drain is placed in the anterior robotic port. The patients are awakened and extubated in the operating room.

The Robot-Assisted Thymectomy

Minimally invasive thymectomy is indicated for a majority of patients with myasthenia gravis and early-stage thymoma.[23] The robotic approach offers a better mediastinal dissection, may improve cosmetic results, and reduces postoperative pain, which results in accelerated recovery.[23] Size is generally accepted as a factor for the choice of operative approach, although there are no guidelines. Masses smaller than 4 cm on imaging techniques resected by RATS give better results for quality of life postoperatively. Balduyck et al. evaluated the quality of life (QoL) after robotic-assisted thoracoscopic or open anterior mediastinal tumor resection. A total of 14 patients underwent thoracoscopic resection using the da Vinci robotic system, and 22 patients, open resection through sternotomy. Questionnaires were administered before surgery and 1, 3, 6, and 12 months postoperatively: open resection by sternotomy was characterized by a significant decrease in general functioning 1 month after surgery (physical functioning $P = .001$, role functioning $P = .001$, and social functioning $P = .044$). Patients also complained of increased thoracic pain in the first 3 months after surgery. After a da Vinci robotic resection QoL scores approximated baseline preoperative values 1 month after surgery, with the exception of increase in thoracic and shoulder pain the first 3 months after surgery.[24]

The 3-arm technique is used mostly, but if the size of the patient's thorax allows it, a 4-arm technique is preferred. The patient is in dorsal decubitus on a vacuum mattress, slightly tilted (30–45 degrees) to the opposite site of the access site. The camera port is placed at the intersection of the fourth intercostal space and mid-axillary line. The second port is almost in the axilla, under the anterior axillary fold; the third is 8 cm distally of the camera port. The assistant's

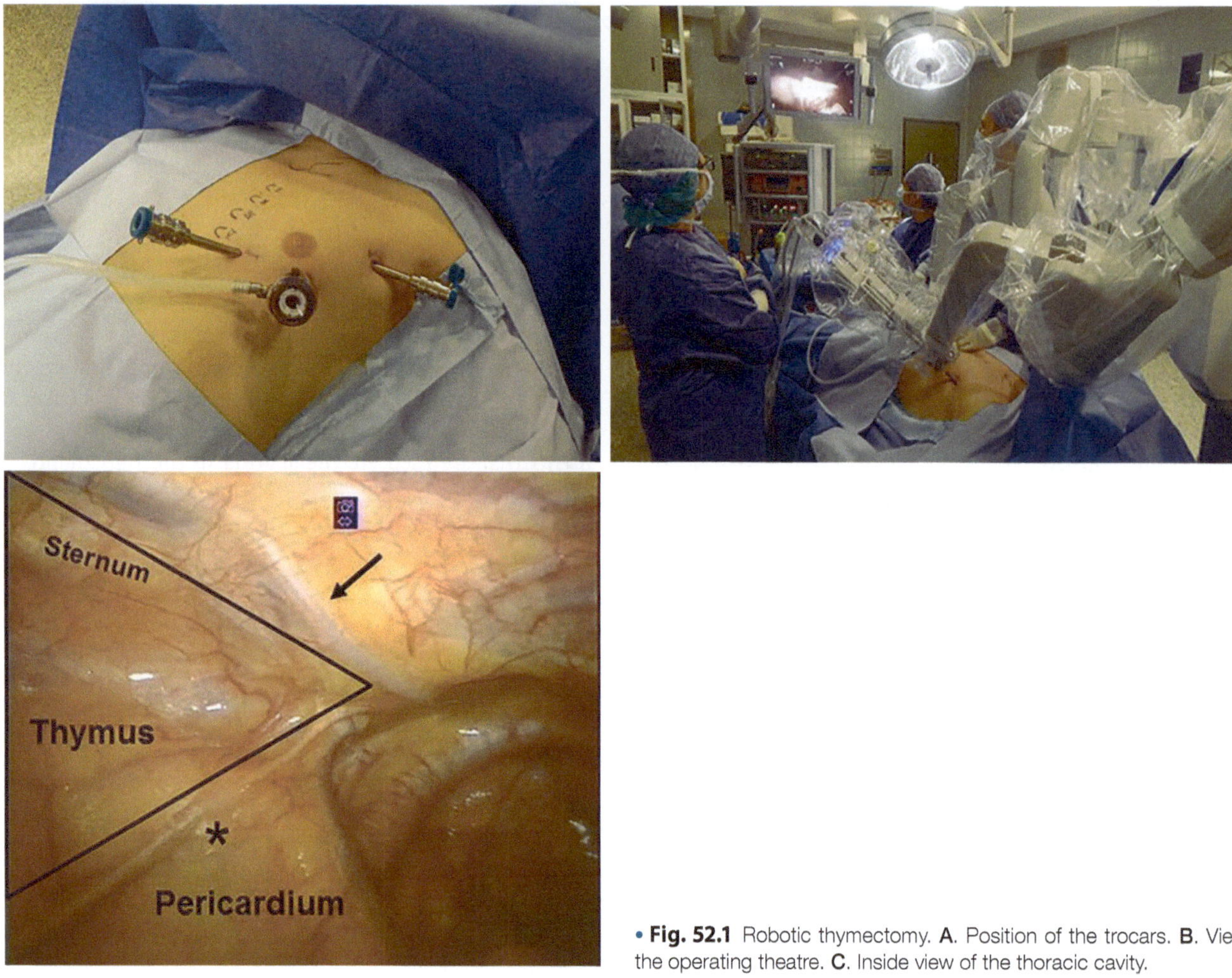

• **Fig. 52.1** Robotic thymectomy. **A**. Position of the trocars. **B**. View of the operating theatre. **C**. Inside view of the thoracic cavity.

port is placed supradiaphragmatic in the eighth or ninth intercostal space, posterior axillary line (Fig. 52.2). Insufflation of CO_2 at a pressure of 5–10 mm Hg permits a good visualization of the mediastinum. Dissection is started caudally, until the upper pols of the thymus are released. The specimen is always removed in a bag and one chest drain is placed.

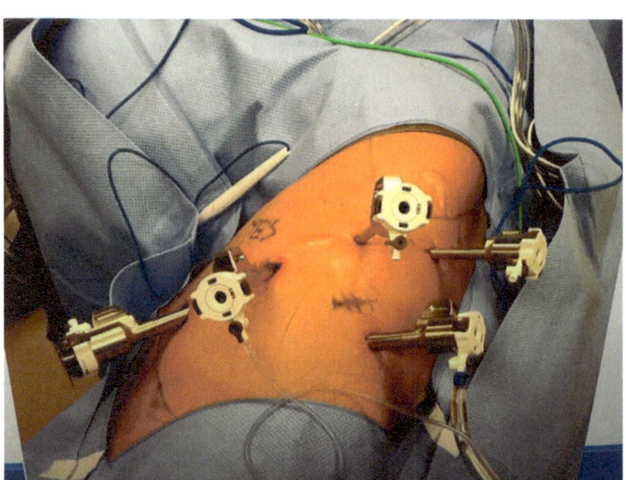

• **Fig. 52.2** The 3-arm technique.

Robotic-Assisted Esophagectomy (see Ch. 44)

Esophageal surgery is described in a dedicated chapter in this book, so here we present very briefly some specific concerns for robotic surgery.

Robotic-assisted esophagectomies are performed similarly to minimally invasive esophagectomies, by using a transhiatal route or combined transthoracic and transabdominal approach.[9,25] The experiences with robotic esophagectomies are very limited; therefore only case reports or case series were reported. No data demonstrate improved outcomes in terms of operative morbidity, pain, length of stay, operative time, or total costs, as compared with minimal invasive techniques.[9] Reported complications[26,27] after esophageal cancer surgery were conversion to open procedure because of adhesions or hemorrhage, anastomotic leakage, dysrhythmia, acute lung injury, vocal cord paralysis—this latest seems to be less frequent than in case of classical surgery.[28] Another report of a series of robotic-assisted trans-hiatal esophagectomies states that this is a safe and feasible technique. Kernstine et al.[27] and Nifong and Chitwood[29] in an editorial view have reported the necessity of a team approach in case of robotic esophagectomy, with trained nurses, surgeons, and anesthesiologists in robotic surgical procedures.

A study compared pressure versus volume controlled one-lung ventilation (OLV) during esophagectomy in prone position, without significant differences between the two ventilatory modes.[30]

Special Issues Concerning the Anesthetic Management

Given the relatively recent introduction of the RATS technique for thoracic surgery, there are few studies describing the anesthetic and analgesic technique to be used during RATS. Nevertheless, there is evidence for some differences when compared with classical VATS: some specific points, while others are common for all types of robotic surgery that should be taken into consideration.

Understanding the Surgical Technique, Equipment, and Patient Selection

First, there is the bulkiness and particularity of the robot operating technology, which can be a disturbing factor in an operating room (Figs. 52.3 and 52.4). Moreover, an increased number of operating room personnel is needed, compared with open surgeries. The thoracic robot is different from other robot-assisted surgeries because of the routine use of CO2 insufflation, artificial pneumothorax, prolonged OLV and other factors that may influence significantly the respiratory and circulatory functions. Therefore anesthesia for thoracic robotic surgery is more demanding compared with anesthesia for general robotic surgical procedures.

A full understanding of not only the surgical technique, but of the related equipment, their impact on the patient, and the corresponding pathophysiologic changes, is necessary to ensure both success of the surgery and the safety of the patient.

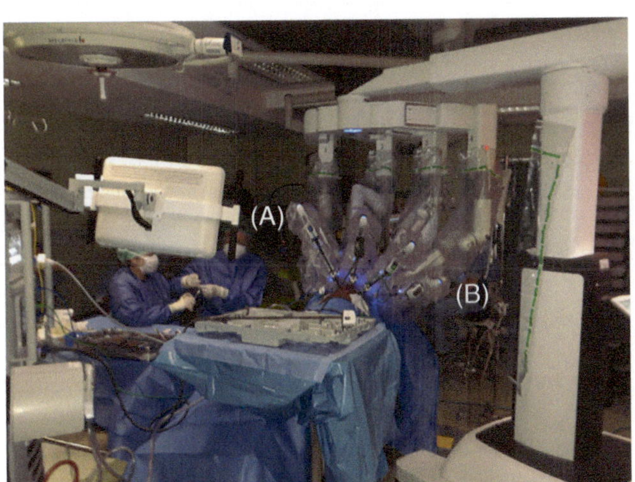

• **Fig. 52.3** An actual operation with the da Vinci® surgical robot system. Please note the space occupied by the robot, with the surgeon at the console (**A**) and anesthesiologist and anesthesia machine (**B**) barely visible.

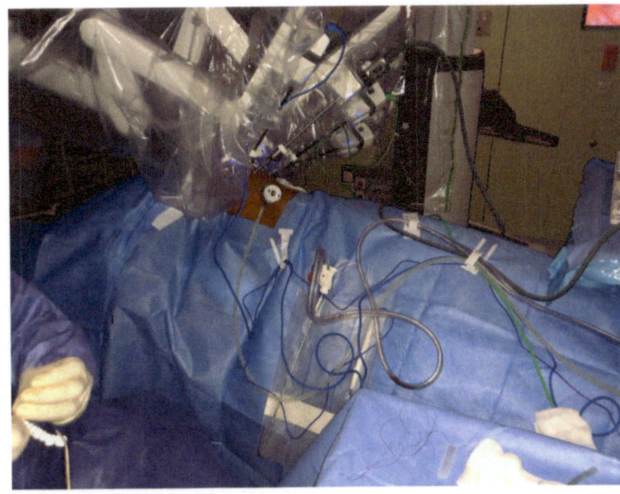

• **Fig. 52.4** The arms of the da Vinci® surgical robot system.

The patient's condition, including a height above 130 cm and a weight more than 30 kg is necessary for RATS procedures which include lobectomy, lymph node dissection, esophageal surgery, or resection of mediastinal neoplasm less than 5 cm. All patients scheduled for RATS should meet the requirements for conventional thoracotomy or thoracoscopic surgery. Lung function, arterial blood gases, chest x-ray and airway viability for endotracheal intubation, and tolerating long OLV periods are necessary. Patients with acute coronary syndrome, heart failure, serious arrhythmia, or valvular disease are best excluded from being operated on by RATS. Laboratory tests should be negative for coagulation, kidney, and liver disorders.

The duration of surgery is longer than classical VATS which consequently prolongs the period of OLV, and thus may have a negative effect on outcome. There are no clear numbers of necessary cases for surgeons to be able to reduce the duration; nevertheless, as stated before, with learning curves, the duration exceeds minimally that of a VATS procedure and 50 previous RATS operations are necessary to qualify the surgeon to perform the procedure.

Access to the Patient

Access to the patient is another major problem in addition to an extended OLV time; also, there maybe limited access the head of the patient for control of the position of the lung separating device by fiberoptic bronchoscopy.

Positioning of the Patient (see Ch. 10)

Given the long duration of surgery and the lateral position of the patient, care should be taken for the correct positioning. With the taping of the head, instead of using protecting foam devices, cases of ear injury or facial numbness were already described.

Protecting the eyes with constructed, improvised devices as "classically" done, from two eye pads and tape, is not efficient for protecting against pressure. Several companies are commercializing disposable eye protectors made from foam and having a transparent shell to protect and watch the eyes, which are available in different sizes.

With the positioning of the patient, care should be taken with the bending of the arms—in the standard lateral decubitus position, arms are restricted to a < 90 degrees angle. There should be enough room to allow the arms of the robot without touching the patient.

There are reports of robot-assisted esophagectomies performed with the patient in the prone position, but no major anesthetic complications were reported in these cases; despite a rise in central venous pressure and mean pulmonary artery pressure, no hemodynamic instabilities were mentioned.[31]

Intraoperative Monitoring, Carbon Dioxide Insufflation, Fluids

As compared with standard surgical techniques, no extra intraoperative monitoring is needed. However, it should be mentioned that given the difficulty of access to the patient and the difficulty of visualization of the "real" surgical field, intraoperative diagnosis could be altered.

An acute decrease in the arterial blood pressure can be caused by trocar insertion. However, there are other possible causes of intraoperative hypotension, for example, the position of the patient with the dependent leg bended and hanging should be evaluated also.

Insufflation of CO2 increases intrathoracic pressure, and secondary decreases preload, or even may cause pneumothorax and subcutaneous emphysema. Peak airway pressure increases and dynamic compliance of the lung decreases, without differences in tidal volume or minute ventilation during volume-controlled ventilation.[32] The anesthesiologist must be vigilant to the possibility of double-lumen endotracheal tubes (DLT) or the bronchial blocker (BB) may be dislocated from the movement of the tracheobronchial tree and frequent variation in the delivered tidal volume. Mean central venous pressure, pulmonary artery pressure, and pulmonary capillary pressures are increased, and this increase is higher when the insufflation occurs on the right side.[32,33] The insufflation pressure of CO2 should be started at not more than 5 cm H_2O and limited to a maximum of 10 cm H_2O or even less if possible in compromised patients, under low flow (<2 L/min), which is relatively safe.[34] Patients should be ventilated with high respiratory rate to offset the hypercarbia resulting from the CO2 insufflation. The potential remedies for enhanced preload should be considered, such as diminishing the insufflation pressure, inotropes and volume load, and/or repositioning the patient. One study demonstrated the positive effects of pressure-controlled ventilation as compared with volume-controlled ventilation during CO2 insufflation.

Concerning the fluids administration, although they are not the trigger of postpneumonectomy pulmonary edema, they do contribute to its worsening. A restrictive versus a goal-oriented fluid approach is still subject to debate. Thorough monitoring of fluid losses is difficult during RATS given the "closed," hidden character of the operating field, and sometimes it is difficult to evaluate the blood losses. With the long duration of surgery, the urinary output and temperature should be monitored mandatorily.

Unfortunately, in the case of RATS, and given the fact that the access to the head of the patient is limited, it is difficult to monitor transesophageal echocardiography during the surgery. Otherwise, very invasive monitoring devices of pulmonary pressures and cardiac output have been replaced by modern monitoring devices (Nicco, Picco, FloTrac, Hemosphere, etc.).

During the procedure, as compared with open or even VATS procedures, rapid diagnosis of occurring intraoperative surgical problems and complications such as bleeding or pushing with the retractor on the left atrium are difficult, despite the on-screen visualization of one or two of the operating robotic arms, but not the other arms.

Communication

The space occupied by the robot, its arms, the console of the surgeon, and the different screens not only limits the access of the anesthesiologist to the patient and surgical field (despite its visualization on screens), but makes visual and verbal communication with the surgeon difficult. Having the surgeon sitting at his console and speaking through a microphone while the others have to shout back makes verbal communication difficult, and sometimes reaction times to misunderstandings are prolonged. Although it sounds easy to just communicate, the logistics are not always adapted enough to this.

The control console can be in the direct opposite corner of the room with numerous obstacles to cross (hanging cables, portable monitors, scrub tables, etc.) (see Fig. 52.3). An arrangement of the operating room with the surgeon sitting at his console next to the anesthesiologist could be helpful for this[35] (Fig. 52.5). Clear commands, synergistic actions, and good team working are necessary for the positive outcome of the operation.

Lung Separation Techniques (see Chapter 16)

Lung separation and isolation is described in another chapter. However, as mentioned above the difficult access to the head of the patient, installed in a lateral decubitus position under the drapes, while the robot's arms are working above the patient, the possibility of displacement of the lung separation device is a present risk. The best lung separation method is the method that the anesthesiologist is most familiar and comfortable with. DLT may be used, either left- or right-sided, keeping in mind that in case of a right-sided double-lumen tube, the margin of safety for positioning is less than that of a left-sided one. An alternative for DLT, which can diminish the incidence of sore throat after anesthesia, is the use of single-lumen tubes with independent BBs. It is always best for every anesthesiologist to have an alternative for DLT in his or her "tool

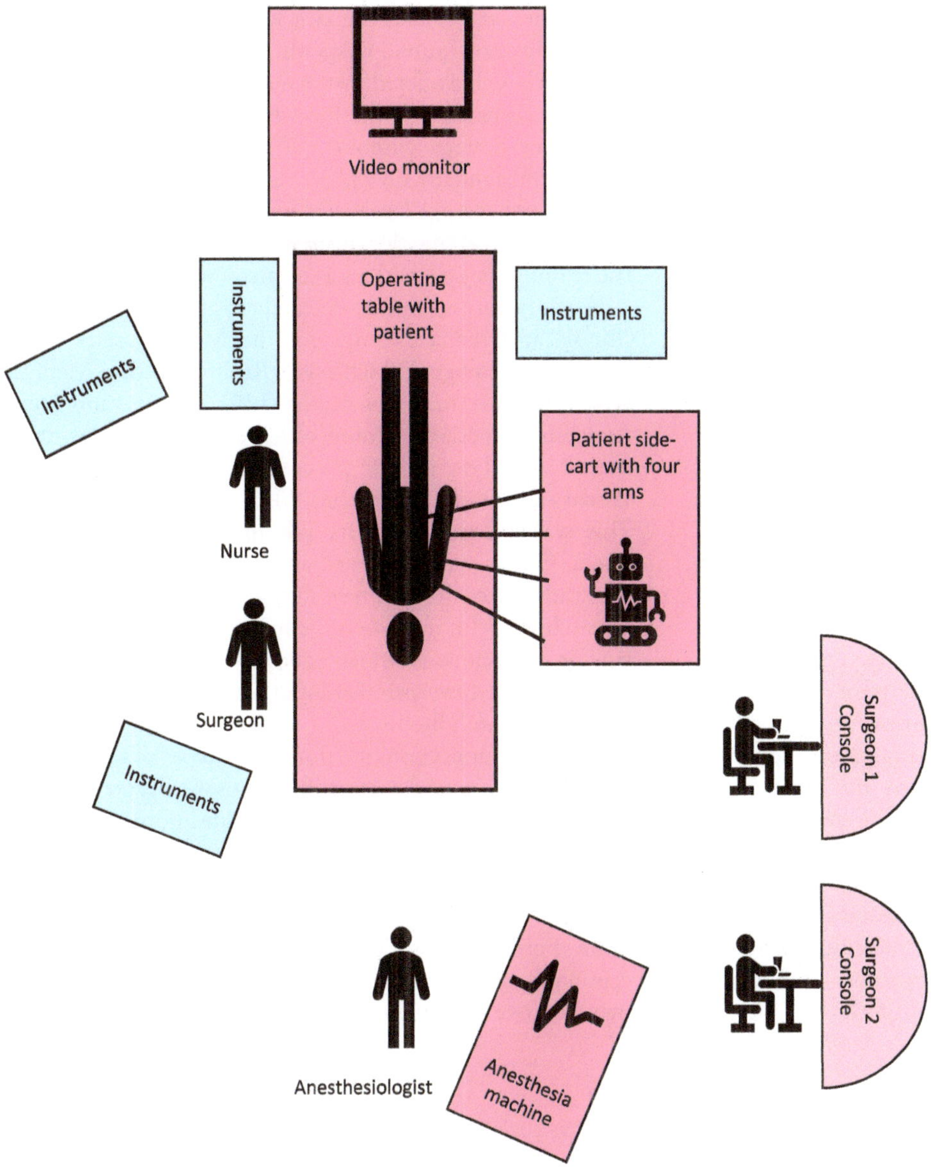

• **Fig. 52.5** The arrangement of the operating theatre used for robotic thoracic surgery. The different fiberoptic and electrical cables between consoles, robot, screens, and patient are not represented, neither the ventilator's tubing, patient's monitoring cables, fiberoptic bronchoscope, or echocardiographic device.

box".[36] A helpful method for continuous monitoring of lung separation device position might be either the recently introduced left-sided double-lumen tube with embedded camera in the tracheal limb (Viva-Sight DL, Ambu) connected to a screen, which permits continuous visualization of the position of the DLT, or a single-lumen tube with embedded (VivaSight SL, Ambu) camera and using a BB, which is described in detail in the chapter on lung separation in this book.[37,38] Moreover, a new study has found that single-use flexible bronchoscopes are more cost effective and associated with lower risk of infection than reusable flexible bronchoscopes.[39]

Pain Management

Studies on postoperative pain after RATS are lacking; nevertheless, despite the increase in number of surgical ports for the robot arms, it seems that RATS is associated with less postoperative pain most likely because the trocars used during RVAT have a smaller diameter. Indeed, patients notice less painful regions, such as pain from bladder catheters, sore throat, pain from chest tubes, and of course pain because of positioning, sometimes from cervico-facial numbness to shoulder pain. To reduce these painful regions, a BB with a single-lumen tube instead of a double-lumen tube could be used; the need for very restrictive positioning and postoperative bladder catheter should be evaluated, and infiltration of chest tube insertion places with local anesthetics should be done. Pain management after thoracic surgery is discussed in Chapter 24, but in most cases of RATS, thoracic epidural analgesia is the gold standard, whereas a paravertebral block or intercostal infiltration is a valid alternative.

Responsibility and Ethical Considerations

Although described by Capek, the one who is credited with the popularization of robotics in a collection of short stories published between 1938 and 1942 is the Russian writer

Isaac Asimov. Asimov is best known for his three laws governing robot behavior. Asimov conceived his laws of robotics to impose order on the free will of his fictional robots (Astounding Science-Fiction, March 1942, ed. John W Campbell jr, Street & Smith Publications Inc., 1942.03.00). Whether they are embedded with a control or controlled from outside, there are some robotic laws that should be respected: they should not injure a human being, they must obey orders given by a human being, and they must protect their own existence as far as it does not conflict with the first law. The laws of robotics presume that the terms "human beings" and "robots" are understood and well defined.

The human factors play an essential role in the safe delivery of patient care. They are the major contributors to adverse outcomes. The robots used in medicine and surgery, as well as for thoracic surgery, are tele-operated robots, which raises the question of responsibility in case of injury from their use.

There are no cases yet described in RATS for robot disfunction; nevertheless, there are several in other types of robot surgery.

Robotic thoracic surgery may open new perspectives in the practice of thoracic surgery. Special training and experience along with high quality assessment are required to provide state-of-the-art treatment. Although the legal basis for professional liability remains exactly the same, litigation with the use of robotic surgery may be more complex. In case of an undesirable outcome, in addition to physician and hospital, the manufacturer of the robotic system may be sued as well. In respect to ethical issues in robotic surgery, equipment safety and reliability, provision of adequate information to the patients and maintenance of confidentiality are of paramount importance. The cost of robotic surgery and the lack financial support for such systems in most public hospitals may restrict the majority from the benefits offered by the new technology. Some even raised the question of whether RATS was not just a simple marketing strategy without any beneficial effect as compared with standard VATS.

Although surgical robotics will have a significant impact on surgical practice, it presents challenges as much in the realm of law and ethics as of medicine and health care.

A study carried out by researchers at the University of Illinois at Urbana-Champaign, the Massachusetts Institute of Technology and Chicago's Rush University Medical Center[40] shows that 144 deaths, 1391 injuries, and 8061 device malfunctions were recorded out of a total of more than 1.7 million robotic procedures carried out between January 2000 and December 2013 in the United States. This was based on reports submitted by hospitals, patients, device manufacturers, and others to the FDA, and the study notes that the true number could be higher. The researchers did not, however, compare accident rates with similar operations in which robots were not used and the study has not been peer reviewed, so these data should be considered carefully.

All the complications are from other types of robotic surgery, and no serious device malfunctions were yet reported in RATS. More studies are needed to provide information about the safety and effectiveness of RATS compared with standard techniques, and to delineate the nuances of RATS relative to VATS. In spite all the issues with robotic surgery the number of these procedures is increasing, possibly because of the perception that robotic surgery is a cutting-edge technology that may improve the reputation of an institution.

Conclusion

The management of the robotic thoracic surgical patient requires the knowledge of minimally invasive surgery techniques involving the chest.

Over the past decade, robotic-assisted thoracic surgery has grown and, in the future, it will take an important place in the treatment of complex thoracic pathologies. The enhanced dexterity and 3D-visualization make it possible to do this in the small space of the thoracic cavity. Familiarity with the robotic surgical system by the anesthesiologists is mandatory.

Management of a long period of OLV with a left-sided DLT or an independent BB is required, along with flexible fiberoptic bronchoscopy techniques (best continuous monitoring).

Correct patient positioning and prevention of complications, such as eye or nerve or crashing injuries while the robotic system is used is mandatory.

Recognition of the hemodynamic effects of CO_2 during insufflation in the chest is required.

Cost is higher and outcome is not yet demonstrated to be better as compared with VATS. The possibility for conversion to open thoracotomy should be also kept in mind.

Teamwork is mandatory, as well as good communication between all the actors of the operating theatre.

We do not know what the future experiences will demonstrate for us; however, one should keep in mind the first law of robotics: "A robot may not injure a human being or, through omission, allow a human being to come to harm."

References

1. Siqueira-Batista R, Souza CR, Maia PM, Siqueira SL. Robotic surgery: bioethical aspects. *Arq Bras Cir Dig*. 2016;29(4):287–290.
2. Varma TR, Eldridge P. Use of the NeuroMate stereotactic robot in a frameless mode for functional neurosurgery. *Int J Med Robot*. 2006;2(2):107–113.
3. Nishihara S, Sugano N, Nishii T, et al. Clinical accuracy evaluation of femoral canal preparation using the ROBODOC system. *J Orthop Sci*. 2004;9(5):452–461.

4. Honl M, Dierk O, Gauck C, et al. Comparison of robotic-assisted and manual implantation of a primary total hip replacement. A prospective study. *J Bone Joint Surg Am.* 2003;85(8):1470–1478.
5. Zipper SG, Puschmann H. [Nerve injuries after computer-assisted hip replacement: case series with 29 patients]. *Z Orthop Ihre Grenzgeb.* 2005;143(4):399–402.
6. Cobb J, Henckel J, Gomes P, et al. Hands-on robotic unicompartmental knee replacement: a prospective, randomised controlled study of the acrobot system. *J Bone Joint Surg Br.* 2006;88(2): 188–197.
7. Federspil PA, Geisthoff UW, Henrich D, Plinkert PK. Development of the first force-controlled robot for otoneurosurgery. *Laryngoscope.* 2003;113(3):465–471.
8. Ballantyne GH. Robotic surgery, telerobotic surgery, telepresence, and telementoring. Review of early clinical results. *Surg Endosc.* 2002;16(10):1389–1402.
9. Watson TJ. Robotic esophagectomy: is it an advance and what is the future? *Ann Thorac Surg.* 2008;85(2):S757–S759.
10. Melfi FM, Menconi GF, Mariani AM, Angeletti CA. Early experience with robotic technology for thoracoscopic surgery. *Eur J Cardiothorac Surg.* 2002;21(5):864–868.
11. Toker A. Robotic thoracic surgery: from the perspectives of European chest surgeons. *J Thorac Dis.* 2014;6(suppl 2):S211–S216.
12. Demmy TL, Curtis JJ. Minimally invasive lobectomy directed toward frail and high-risk patients: a case-control study. *Ann Thorac Surg.* 1999;68(1):194–200.
13. Daniels LJ, Balderson SS, Onaitis MW, D'Amico TA. Thoracoscopic lobectomy: a safe and effective strategy for patients with stage I lung cancer. *Ann Thorac Surg.* 2002;74(3):860–864.
14. McKenna RJ Jr, Houck W, Fuller CB. Video-assisted thoracic surgery lobectomy: experience with 1,100 cases. *Ann Thorac Surg.* 2006;81(2):421–425; discussion 5-6.
15. Dylewski MR, Ohaeto AC, Pereira JF. Pulmonary resection using a total endoscopic robotic video-assisted approach. *Semin Thorac Cardiovasc Surg.* 2011;23(1):36–42.
16. Nagahiro I, Andou A, Aoe M, Sano Y, Date H, Shimizu N. Pulmonary function, postoperative pain, and serum cytokine level after lobectomy: a comparison of VATS and conventional procedure. *Ann Thorac Surg.* 2001;72(2):362–365.
17. Veronesi G. Robotic lobectomy and segmentectomy for lung cancer: results and operating technique. *J Thorac Dis.* 2015;7(Suppl 2): S122–S130.
18. Veronesi G. Robotic thoracic surgery: technical considerations and learning curve for pulmonary resection. *Thorac Surg Clin.* 2014; 24(2):135–141, v.
19. Bao F, Zhang C, Yang Y, He Z, Wang L, Hu J. Comparison of robotic and video-assisted thoracic surgery for lung cancer: a propensity-matched analysis. *J Thorac Dis.* 2016;8(7):1798–1803.
20. Park BJ, Melfi F, Mussi A, et al. Robotic lobectomy for non-small cell lung cancer (NSCLC): long-term oncologic results. *J Thorac Cardiovasc Surg.* 2012;143(2):383–389.
21. Pardolesi A, Park B, Petrella F, Borri A, Gasparri R, Veronesi G. Robotic anatomic segmentectomy of the lung: technical aspects and initial results. *Ann Thorac Surg.* 2012;94(3):929–934.
22. Ghaly G, Kamel M, Nasar A, et al. Video-assisted thoracoscopic surgery is a safe and effective alternative to thoracotomy for anatomical segmentectomy in patients with clinical stage I non-small cell lung cancer. *Ann Thorac Surg.* 2016;101(2):465–472; discussion 72.
23. Schwartz GS, Yang SC. Robotic thymectomy for thymic neoplasms. *Thorac Surg Clin.* 2014;24(2):197–201, vii.
24. Balduyck B, Hendriks JM, Lauwers P, Mercelis R, Ten Broecke P, Van Schil P. Quality of life after anterior mediastinal mass resection: a prospective study comparing open with robotic-assisted thoracoscopic resection. *Eur J Cardiothorac Surg.* 2011;39(4): 543–548.
25. Luketich JD, Alvelo-Rivera M, Buenaventura PO, Christie NA, McCaughan JS, Litle VR, et al. Minimally invasive esophagectomy: outcomes in 222 patients. *Ann Surg.* 2003;238(4):486–494; discussion 94–5.
26. Kernstine KH, DeArmond DT, Karimi M, et al. The robotic, 2-stage, 3-field esophagolymphadenectomy. *J Thorac Cardiovasc Surg.* 2004;127(6):1847–1849.
27. Kernstine KH, DeArmond DT, Shamoun DM, Campos JH. The first series of completely robotic esophagectomies with three-field lymphadenectomy: initial experience. *Surg Endosc.* 2007;21(12): 2285–2292.
28. Suda K, Ishida Y, Kawamura Y, et al. Robot-assisted thoracoscopic lymphadenectomy along the left recurrent laryngeal nerve for esophageal squamous cell carcinoma in the prone position: technical report and short-term outcomes. *World J Surg.* 2012;36(7): 1608–1616.
29. Nifong LW, Chitwood WR, Jr. Challenges for the anesthesiologist: robotics? *Anesth Analg.* 2003;96(1):1–2.
30. Choi YS, Shim JK, Na S, Hong SB, Hong YW, Oh YJ. Pressure-controlled versus volume-controlled ventilation during one-lung ventilation in the prone position for robot-assisted esophagectomy. *Surg Endosc.* 2009;23(10):2286–2291.
31. Kim DJ, Hyung WJ, Lee CY, et al. Thoracoscopic esophagectomy for esophageal cancer: feasibility and safety of robotic assistance in the prone position. *J Thorac Cardiovasc Surg.* 2010;139(1):53–59. e1.
32. El-Dawlatly AA, Al-Dohayan A, Samarkandi A, Algahdam F, Atef A. Right vs left side thoracoscopic sympathectomy: effects of CO2 insufflation on haemodynamics. *Ann Chir Gynaecol.* 2001;90(3):206–208.
33. Ohtsuka T, Nakajima J, Kotsuka Y, Takamoto S. Hemodynamic responses to intrapleural insufflation with hemipulmonary collapse. *Surg Endosc.* 2001;15(11):1327–1330.
34. Wolfer RS, Krasna MJ, Hasnain JU, McLaughlin JS. Hemodynamic effects of carbon dioxide insufflation during thoracoscopy. *Ann Thorac Surg.* 1994;58(2):404–407; discussion 7–8.
35. Campos JH. An update on robotic thoracic surgery and anesthesia. *Curr Opin Anaesthesiol.* 2010;23(1):1–6.
36. Campos J, Ueda K. Update on anesthetic complications of robotic thoracic surgery. *Minerva Anestesiol.* 2014;80(1):83–88.
37. Koopman EM, Barak M, Weber E, et al. Evaluation of a new double-lumen endobronchial tube with an integrated camera (VivaSight-DL): a prospective multicentre observational study. *Anaesthesia.* 2015;70(8):962–968.
38. Szarpak L, Kurowski A, Zasko P, et al. Double-lumen tube tracheal intubation in a manikin model using the VivaSight Double Lumen: a randomized controlled comparison with the Macintosh laryngoscope. *Am J Emerg Med.* 2016;34(1):103–104.
39. Mouritsen JM, Ehlers L, Kovaleva J, Ahmad I, El-Boghdadly K. A systematic review and cost effectiveness analysis of reusable vs. single-use flexible bronchoscopes. *Anaesthesia.* 2020;75(4):529–540.
40. Alemzadeh H, Raman J, Leveson N, Kalbarczyk Z, Iyer RK. Adverse events in robotic surgery: a retrospective study of 14 years of FDA data. *PLoS One.* 2016;11(4):e0151470.

53

Enhanced Recovery After Thoracic Surgery

EMILY G. TEETER, ANOUSHKA M. AFONSO, WANDA M. POPESCU

Introduction

Enhanced recovery after surgery (ERAS) refers to a comprehensive, evidence-based approach to patient-centered care in the perioperative period. The primary goals of enhanced recovery are an efficient return to baseline functional status and an avoidance of complications. Enhanced recovery has demonstrated success in multiple surgical specialties, particularly colorectal surgery. Although ERAS for thoracic surgery (ERATS) still occupies a small portion of the enhanced recovery literature, it is quickly gaining momentum. This uptick in interest has been aided by the recent release of two separate sets of enhanced recovery guidelines: one for lung resection surgery and one for esophagectomy. In this chapter, we will review the core tenets and specific components of the recent guidelines for ERATS in lung resection surgery, although the general principles for both are similar.

Background

Despite experiencing recent popularity and growth, ERAS (also referred to as enhanced recovery programs [ERPs]) is not a novel concept. Originally described in the 1990s by Kehlet et al.[1] enhanced recovery is a multidisciplinary approach to perioperative care of the surgical patient. The goal of ERPs is a smooth, efficient return to baseline functional status. A natural byproduct, therefore is an increase in the value of health care, both by improving the quality of care and at the same time decreasing its cost. An uncomplicated recovery bodes well for the patient experience, healthcare system, and outcomes. In addition, enhanced recovery in the setting of cancer also promotes an earlier return to neoadjuvant treatment.

Despite an initial shortage of evidence-based literature and lack of formal guidelines, ERATS has recently emerged as an expanding field within ERAS. In addition to several metaanalyses and descriptions of institutional experiences, 2018 saw the release of two individual sets of enhanced recovery thoracic guidelines.[2–4] The combined ERAS/European Society of Thoracic Surgeons (ESTS) guidelines were the first of their kind, and represent a review of the available literature by a multinational, multidisciplinary group of authors, including surgeons and anesthesiologists and consensus-based recommendations. In this chapter, we will focus on the ERATS guidelines for lung resection surgery, which are summarized in Table 53.1.

Fast-Track Versus Enhanced Recovery After Surgery

Often, the terms "fast-track" and enhanced recovery are used interchangeably, but an important distinction lies in the principal endpoint. Fast-track extubation and recovery, which was popularized during the 1990s, primarily focused on time to extubation and time to hospital discharge for cardiac surgery and, to a lesser degree, thoracic procedures.[5–7] However, unlike ERPs, these protocols tended to be surgeon-driven, and less focused on the collective contributions of the multidisciplinary team. In addition, although certain aspects of fast-track protocols were tailored to allow for early extubation, including minimization of opioid medications, they did not typically include sophisticated approaches to multimodal analgesia, as will be discussed in this chapter. As a final distinction, unlike enhanced recovery, the tenets of fast-track protocols did not typically span the entire perioperative period, instead largely focusing on the intraoperative and postoperative components.

Enhanced Recovery After Surgery General Overview

Several common themes and objectives persist in ERPs regardless of surgical specialty. These core components have been specifically outlined by the governing bodies for ERAS: The Enhanced Recovery after Surgery (ERAS) Society and

TABLE 53.1 Summary of Enhanced Recovery After Thoracic Surgery Components With Accompanying Levels of Evidence and Recommendation

Component	Level of Evidence	Level of Recommendation
Clear liquids up to 2 h before surgery	High	Strong
Avoidance of sedatives	Moderate	Strong
Mechanical and pharmacologic VTE prophylaxis	Moderate	Strong
Extended VTE prophylaxis in high-risk patients	Low	Weak
Perioperative antibiotic prophylaxis	High	Strong
Use of active warning	High	Strong
Continuous monitoring of core temperature	High	Strong
Lung-protective ventilation during one lung ventilation	Moderate	Strong
Combined regional and general anesthesia	Low	Strong
Short-acting anesthetic agents	Low	Strong
Nonpharmacologic PONV prophylaxis	High	Strong
Multimodal pharmacologic PONV approach	Moderate	Strong
Multimodal analgesia: Combination of acetaminophen and NSAIDs	High	Strong
Multimodal analgesia: Use of ketamine	Moderate	Strong
Multimodal analgesia: Use of dexamethasone	Low	Strong
Euvolemic fluid management	Moderate	Strong
Balanced crystalloid solutions	High	Strong
Early enteral route	Moderate	Strong

NSAIDs, Nonsteroidal antiinflammatory drugs; *PONV*, postoperative nausea and vomiting; *VTE*, venous thromboembolism.
From Teeter EG, Kolarczyk LM, Popescu WM. Examination of the enhanced recovery guidelines in thoracic surgery. *Curr Opin Anesthesiol*. 2019. With permission.

American Society of Enhanced Recovery (ASER). Outlined in Table 53.2, these components span the entire perioperative timeframe, from the patient's initial consultation to hospital discharge and potentially beyond. The **preoperative** components include: patient education and empowerment, intake of carbohydrate beverage up to 2 hours before surgery, optimization of comorbid conditions, and preemptive multimodal analgesia. **Intraoperatively**, ERAS goals include: continuation of multimodal analgesia, lung-protective ventilation, and avoidance of salt/crystalloid excess.[2,8–10] In the **postoperative** period, regardless of discipline, early enteral nutrition, mobilization, and removal of tubes and drains are essential. For comparison, Fig. 53.1 outlines components of an enhanced recovery protocol after lung resection surgery.

TABLE 53.2 Core Components of an Enhanced Recovery After Surgery Pathway

Preoperative	Intraoperative	Postoperative
Patient education and active involvement	Fluid therapy to avoid salt and crystalloid excess	Early removal of tubes and drains
Decrease in NPO interval	Minimally invasive surgical approach	Early ambulation
Carbohydrate beverage >2 hours before induction	Antibiotic and venous thromboembolism prophylaxis	Early enteral feeding
Multimodal analgesia	Multimodal analgesia	Multimodal analgesia
	Active warming	
	Defined blood pressure goals	

Enhanced Recovery After Surgery Thoracic Surgery: Justification and Applicability

Patients undergoing thoracic surgery tend to carry a substantial burden of comorbidity, in particular pulmonary and cardiovascular disease. In addition, thoracic surgery is associated with a high risk of morbidity and mortality compared with other surgeries.[11] Therefore at an individual patient

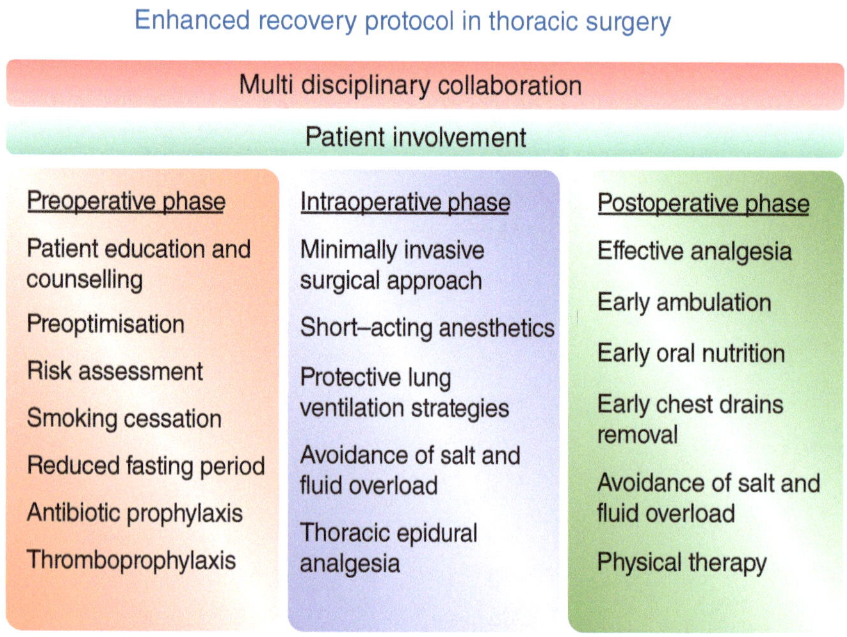

• **Fig. 53.1** Enhanced recovery protocol in lung resection surgery.

level, the potential impact of an ERP is significant. From an institutional and even larger healthcare standpoint, improving the quality and efficiency of care allows more patients to traverse through the system in a given time which also has financial implications.

Initially, the data supporting ERATS for lung resection surgery were sparse and stemmed from single institutions. Over the past decade, the literature supporting specific ERP components and overall pathways has become more rigorous, moving from retrospective reviews to meta-analyses and randomized controlled trials for certain components. Whereas colorectal surgery and other subspecialties have clearly and repeatedly demonstrated success with ERAS, it has only been in recent years that enhanced recovery for thoracic surgery has shown promise in decreasing cost, complications, and hospital length of stay.[12]

The ERAS/ESTS guidelines synthesize the available evidence for particular recommendations in ERATS. For each component, the guidelines use the GRADE system (www.gradeworkinggroup.org) to: (1) describe the strength of the literature and (2) assign a level of recommendation based upon expert consensus. Although some commonly accepted and often performed portions of ERATS do not have solid objective evidence, they may still be strongly recommended based upon the pooled opinion of the expert group who authored the guidelines.

Enhanced Recovery After Surgery Thoracic Surgery: Preoperative Components

Optimization of Comorbid Conditions

Perioperative care of the patient undergoing thoracic surgery aims to evaluate patient risk factors, stratify patients based on those risk factors, and ameliorate any conditions before surgical intervention. Through a patient-centered approach, many ERPs focus on a multidisciplinary approach, particularly in the preoperative optimization of the thoracic surgical patient.

Patient counseling, targeted education, and individualized care plans play a key role to reduce stress, fear, or anxiety and improve the morbidity of patients, allowing faster functional and psychologic recovery after thoracic surgery. Refai et al.[13] describe a patient education and care plan in thoracic surgery, noting the importance of detailed explanations. Preoperative patient counselling, performed using verbal, written, or multimedia materials, is crucial to achieve the goal of the ERAS project: making the patient a potentially active participant and the main character of his recovery, able to positively impact himself throughout the surgical and healing process.

Because thoracic surgical patients have multiple comorbidities, they are at increasing risk for developing complications after thoracic surgery. Stokes et al. systematically reviewed modifiable risk factors before elective thoracic surgery and identified pain control, nutrition, exercise/physical fitness, and smoking cessation as risk factors that can have a substantial impact on the thoracic surgical patients' perioperative course.[14] Standardized preprocedure guidance to promote patient and staff adherence with elements of an ERP will improve compliance. In thoracic surgery, a multidisciplinary team should evaluate the patient's cardiopulmonary status with stratified risk assessments of cardiac and lung function preoperatively. Models of risk assessment facilitate calculation and assessment of individual outcomes that may be discussed with the patient to make an informed decision. With the right optimization, preoperative management can shift, an otherwise unlikely surgical candidate, into one who may qualify for surgical treatment.

Tobacco and Alcohol Cessation

Smoking is the strongest risk factor for postoperative pulmonary complications (PPCs) following thoracic surgery. Development of PPCs is a leading cause of in-hospital mortality and increased hospital length of stay and cost in thoracic surgical patients.[15] Lugg et al.[16] investigated over 450 patients following resection for nonsmall cell lung cancer (NSCLC) to observe the impact of preoperative smoking cessation on long-term survival. They evaluated 462 patients which included 111 (24%) current smokers, 55 (12%) ex-smokers less than 6 weeks, 245 (53%) ex-smokers 6 weeks or longer, and 51 (11%) never smokers. PPCs occurred in 60 (13%) patients in total. Compared with never smokers, current smokers had a higher frequency of PPC (22% vs. 2%,), higher frequency of intensive care unit (ICU) admission (14% vs. 0%) and a longer hospital length of stay (LOS) (6 [5] vs. 5 [2]). In the ex-smokers there was a trend for a lower frequency of PPC (<6 weeks, 10.9% vs. ≥6 weeks, 11.8%) and ICU admission (<6 weeks, 5.5% vs. ≥6 weeks, 4.5, but there was no difference between the under 6 weeks or 6 weeks or more ex-smoking groups before surgery. There was no significant difference in long-term survival found between the groups of differing smoking status in follow-up at 29.8 months. They concluded that current smokers have a higher risk of postoperative morbidity than former smokers after lung surgery for NSCLC. Although previous studies demonstrated a further benefit past the 6-week cessation mark, this study did not observe such a difference. In a systematic review evaluating the influence of smoking cessation on prognosis of early stage lung cancer, Parsons et al. estimated that 5-year survival reaches 33% for non-quitters versus 70% for those patients who quit. Using life table modeling, the authors concluded that the mortality gain observed was most likely linked to the effects of quitting smoking on cancer progression.[17]

Another retrospective study by Fukui et al. conducted on patients undergoing resection for stage I to III primary lung cancer showed a longer period of smoking cessation may be more effective for reducing the risk of pulmonary complications, although cessation at any time is beneficial for lung cancer surgery.[18] In contrast, Matsuoka et al. showed no relationship between the length of preoperative smoking cessation period and the frequency of postoperative complications in 1248 patients who underwent lobectomy.[19] **However, recommendations from the ERAS Society suggest that smoking cessation should be at least 4 weeks before surgery.**[4]

ERPs should integrate a robust preoperative workup with dedicated counseling for patient optimization. Not only do these programs reduce mortality, but they can be cost-effective and improve quality of life in lung cancer surgery.[20]

Significant alcohol use is a modifiable perioperative risk factor in lung resections. Graf et al. reported in the Veterans Health Administration that 13% of patients undergoing lung resection reported drinking more than two drinks per day in the preoperative period, and have associated increased risk of postoperative complications.[21] In addition, patients drinking at least five drinks per day experienced an increased 30-day mortality after resection for NSCLC.[22] From an oncologic standpoint, alcohol abuse has been shown an independent predictor for decreased disease-specific and progression-free survival among patients with lung cancer.[23] Although optimal timing of alcohol cessation is unknown, the **ERATS guidelines' recommendation is to avoid alcohol for at least 4 weeks before surgery.**[4]

Prehabilitation (see Ch. 9)

The role of preoperative rehabilitation for thoracic surgery has evolved over the years. Most exercise programs focus on either supervised or unsupervised sessions of a combination of aerobic training, respiratory muscle training, and/or resistance training.[24] A recent systematic review involving 806 participants showed moderate-quality evidence that preoperative exercise significantly reduced complication rates and length of stay in patients undergoing lung resection.[25] A recently published systematic review and meta-analysis by Rosero et al. including 676 patients from 10 randomized controlled trials identified that an exercise strategy which combines aerobic, resistance and inspiratory muscle training performed at moderate levels one to three times a week for 1 to 4 weeks before thoracic surgery can improve walking endurance, decreases dyspnea, risk of hospitalization, and the incidence of PPCs.[26] Preoperative pulmonary rehabilitation programs in patients undergoing video-assisted thoracoscopic surgery (VATS) have been associated with an increase in baseline exercise tolerance and differences in exercise capacity 3 months postoperatively.[27] A small randomized clinical trial on 68 patients showed that those in the prehabilitation group had improved functional capacity both before and after esophageal surgery.[28]

Some of the high-intensity preoperative interventions can be a challenge for healthcare systems, both financially and from a systems perspective. Nonetheless, these interventions can lead to reductions in hospital length of stay and morbidity, especially in the high-risk thoracic patient population they should be considered.

Nutrition

Nutritional status plays an important role in postoperative outcomes, especially in thoracic surgery. Prevalence of malnutrition in this population is varied, with biomarkers indicating that malnutrition is present in up to 40% of pneumonectomy patients.[29] Preoperatively, there are multiple nutritional screening tools to identify malnourished patients and stratify those amenable to interventions.[30] One such tool is the Nutritional Risk Index, which uses a combination of weight, serum albumin, prealbumin for risk score calculation.[31] In major lung resection, body mass index over 30 kg/m^2 was associated with an improved overall survival.[32] Obesity may exert some protective effects in this population, either independently, or as it relates to a lower burden of smoking and tumor cachexia.[33]

Perioperative nutritional supplementation can lead to reduced risk of complications, such as infection and decreased length of stay.[31] Immunonutrition (IMN) is postulated to counteract the postoperative immune depression and improve clinical outcomes in thoracic patients. A prospective, randomized study enrolling 40 patients to evaluate the effect of perioperative immunonutritional support (7 days before and 7 days after surgery) on postoperative course and long-term survival. Although there were no differences in postoperative ICU or postoperative LOS between groups, the incidence of postoperative infectious complications were significantly lower in the immunomodulating enteral nutrition group.[34] However, the beneficial evidence for IMN overall is not well established. Although nutritional screening and oral supplementation (when warranted) are strongly recommended in thoracic surgery patients, there is no unified standard of care with an optimal nutritional approach.[4]

Enhanced Recovery After Surgery Thoracic Surgery: Intraoperative Components

Multimodal Analgesia (see Ch. 24)

Patients undergoing thoracic surgery, even VATS, are at high risk for acute and chronic pain, which is multifactorial.[35] Such pain may impact a patient's recovery, predisposing them to pulmonary and cardiovascular complications.[36] Multimodal analgesia refers to the use of multiple classes of nonopioid pain medications with synergistic mechanisms of action to decrease postoperative pain, as well as the reliance upon opioid medications. Such a pathway may decrease the adverse effects of opioid medications and also shifts the reliance from opioid medications, which is especially pertinent in the setting of the current "opioid epidemic." Multimodal analgesia should be initiated in the preoperative period and continued through hospital discharge. An excellent example of a successful implementation of a multimodal, opioid-sparing pain management pathway is described in the study by Martin et al.[9] Using this pain management strategy, which expanded over the entire perioperative period, the authors looked at video-assisted thoracic surgery (ERAS-VATS) and thoracotomy (ERAS-T). Each incorporated preoperative patient education, carbohydrate loading, opioid-sparing analgesia, conservative fluid management, and early ambulation. Patient outcomes, length of stay, pain scores, opioid use, fluid administration, and cost. Historic VATS (n = 162) were compared with 81 ERAS-VATS patients. Median postoperative morphine equivalents (86 vs. 22 mg), total fluid balance (1279 vs. 227 mL), and mean inflation adjusted hospital costs ($20,169 vs. $14,870) all decreased significantly. Historic thoracotomy patients (n = 62) were compared with 58 ERAS-T patients. Median postoperative morphine equivalents (130 vs. 54 mg), total fluid balance (788 vs. 489 mL), length of stay (6.0 vs. 4.0 days), and mean inflation adjusted hospital costs ($41,950 vs. $26,089) all decreased significantly. The authors concluded that implementation of thoracic ERAS is a dynamic process with potential to improve outcomes in thoracic surgical procedures. In the first year, the study proved a shortened length of stay, decreased opioid usage, minimized fluid overload, and decreased hospital costs.

Although multiple different classes of medication exist, the cornerstone of any multimodal pathway should be a locoregional technique, and this recommendation is reflected in the ERAS/ESTS guidelines.[4] Historically, the thoracic epidural was considered the "gold standard" of pain control for thoracic surgery, and particularly for open thoracotomy, but more recently alternative blocks have emerged. Many of these nonepidural techniques carry the advantage of a lower risk and adverse effect profile, and some may be performed despite anticoagulation status. Most notably, the paravertebral block, which may be performed by the surgeon or anesthesiologist, has proven to provide equivalent analgesia with fewer side effects than the thoracic epidural.[37] Other commonly used regional approaches include intercostal, pectoralis I and II, serratus anterior, and erector spinae blocks, and these are increasing in popularity.

Pharmacologic options for multimodal analgesia most commonly include acetaminophen, gabapentinoids, nonsteroidal antiinflammatory drugs (NSAIDs), N-methyl-D aspartate (NMDA) receptor antagonists, steroids, and alpha receptor agonists. Of these, the first three can be initiated in the preoperative period in what is referred to as "preemptive analgesia." The ERATS guidelines, as well as the American Pain Society guidelines for postoperative pain both support the use of acetaminophen and NSAIDs in lung resection surgery unless contraindicated, and suggest a potential synergistic effect between the two.[4,38] Gabapentinoids have variable support in the literature, with a recent retrospective review suggesting an opioid-sparing effect.[39] Centrally-acting alpha-2 agonists, such as dexmedetomidine, have also demonstrated a reduction in opioid requirement, as well as a potential for improved lung function for patients undergoing thoracic surgery.[40,41] NMDA receptor antagonists, such as ketamine ought to be considered, particularly for patients with a history of chronic pain.[4]

Maintenance of Anesthesia

Although multiple studies have attempted to elucidate whether any particular type of maintenance anesthetic is superior to another with regard to outcomes, no clear advantage has been found. Antiinflammatory effects of both volatile anesthetics and propofol have been described on a molecular level, and theoretically this effect would confer benefit in the prevention of reperfusion injury with one-lung ventilation. However, neither technique has demonstrated any significant difference in clinical outcomes over another, and further research is necessary.[42,43] Regardless, the ERATS guidelines do strongly recommend the avoidance of antianxiolytics whenever possible and the use of short-acting anesthetic agents to facilitate early emergence from anesthesia.[4]

Mechanical Ventilation Strategy (see Ch. 20)

Pulmonary complications are frequent in thoracic surgery patients, with an estimated incidence of 15% to 32%.[44] Thoracic patients are predisposed to such complications, both because of the underlying burden of pulmonary disease, as well as the physiology of one-lung ventilation. Intraoperative ventilatory strategy may play a role in mitigating the risk of acute respiratory distress syndrome, and the strategies to optimize mechanical ventilation for thoracic surgery patients as part of an enhanced recovery pathway are discussed.

Currently, the application of protective lung ventilation which include low tidal volume, positive end-expiratory pressure (PEEP) and frequent recruitment maneuvers is recommended. The benefit of moderate (4–8 mL/kg) tidal volumes based upon predicted body weight has been well described in the general surgery and thoracic surgery literature, and this is an important component of lung-protective ventilation.[11,45–47] More recently, attention has turned to additional components of such a strategy, such as the provision and optimization of PEEP.[44] A recent prospective study demonstrated a below-expected incidence of pulmonary complications when individually tailored PEEP was applied in conjunction with an open lung ventilation strategy for patients requiring one-lung ventilation. Driving pressure (DP) is defined as the difference between plateau pressure and PEEP (Plat-PEEP), and can also be expressed as the ratio of tidal volume to respiratory system compliance. DP is the variable that was most strongly associated with mortality. The optimization of DP has been considered as a tool to optimize mechanical ventilation during surgery and to improve outcome.[48] **The ERAS/ESTS guidelines strongly recommend the use of lung-protective ventilation, to include modest tidal volumes, adequate PEEP, and attention to limiting peak airway pressure.**[4]

Fluid Management (see Ch. 21)

Fluid management has been a subject of significant debate within thoracic surgery. Excessive fluid administration may lead to pulmonary complications, particularly in the setting of one-lung ventilation, and is directly related to the extent of the parenchymal resection. Restrictive fluid strategies have been historically linked to acute kidney injury and organ ischemia. While other ERAS pathways rely upon a goal-directed fluid therapy (GDFT) strategy, these algorithms are more difficult to apply to thoracic surgery. Dynamic monitors typically used to guide GDFT may not be valid in the setting of one-lung ventilation, low tidal volumes, open chest physiology, and lateral positioning, all of which are frequently encountered in the thoracic operating room.

As opposed to the historical tendency to keep thoracic surgery patients "dry," by using a fluid-restrictive strategy in the operating room, the ERATS guidelines recommend a zero-balance or euvolemic approach to fluid therapy, which represents a departure from the traditional approach. Such a strategy begins in the preoperative arena, with provision of clear fluids up to 2 hours before induction of anesthesia. Allowance of a carbohydrate beverage and liberalization of the fasting guidelines have associated with better patient satisfaction, decreased nausea, improved glucose tolerance, and do not portend a higher risk of aspiration.[4,9,49,50] Intraoperatively, a normovolemic pathway has been shown (in a small study) not to increase extravascular lung water, but more studies are needed to inform the conduct of fluid administration in the operating room.[51]

Other Components

While ERAS incorporates evidence-based recommendations that may upend traditional surgical dogma, the more routine parts of an anesthetic should not be overlooked. Although the thoracic-specific literature is not robust, the ERATS guidelines support the perioperative administration of venous **thromboembolism prophylaxis**, both mechanical and chemical, for thoracic surgery patients.[4,52] In addition, antibiotic prophylaxis should be provided per Surgical Care Improvement Project guidelines to decrease the incidence of surgical site infections.[9,49,53] **Active warming** and core temperature monitoring should be undertaken given the large area of exposure in lung resection surgery. In addition, hypothermia has been associated with wound infection, arrythmia, coagulopathy, and increased oxygen consumption, which could be particularly problematic in thoracic surgery patients given the preponderance of lung disease.[4,54] Lastly, **postoperative nausea and vomiting prophylaxis** should be incorporated as appropriate to facilitate smooth recovery. However, antiemetic drugs with sedating effects (droperidol, dimenhydrinate) should be avoided if possible.

Postoperative Components

Postoperatively, multimodal analgesia should be continued and even considered after hospital discharge.[55] Early mobilization, enteral feeding and removal of tubes and drains encourage an efficient return to physiologic baseline and ought to be strongly and regularly promoted by the postoperative staff. The historical model of postoperative convalescence should be traded for an active, patient-centered recovery.

Of note, heterogeneity in practice patterns exists with regard to threshold for removal of chest drains, and often persistent air leak or chest tube output limits the ability to discharge patients. Studies examining a more liberal threshold for removal of chest drains (≥200 mL/day) have shown promise, and the use of surgical sealants may be helpful as well.[56,57] Literature for lung resection surgery promotes the practice of a single chest tube rather than multiple when feasible.[58,59] Some less invasive procedure approaches, such as Uniportal thoracoscopic surgery were performed without chest tube placement, without an increase in complications.

Barriers and Strategies With Implementation

Implementing and sustaining ERPs requires knowledge of change management strategies and can be derailed if the appropriate collaborative process is not followed. Although many individual elements of enhanced recovery pathways are each simple to implement, ERPs as a whole can be challenging to adopt. Programs have a higher chance of success if there is a clear, comprehensive, and established implementation plan and guidelines.[60] Attempts to change the behavior of health professionals may be impeded by a variety of different barriers, obstacles, or determinants of practice and most importantly the traditional practice of the practitioners. Change may be more likely if implementation strategies are specifically chosen to address these determinants.

According to Pearsall and colleagues,[61] key points for success in ERPs rely on the following factors (Fig. 53.2):

1. Assessment of local barriers and enablers before implementation
2. Engagement of all of the multidisciplinary team
3. Data strategy with consistent audit and feedback mechanism to monitor real-time change

Many implementation models exist to assist ERP teams for planning change strategies.[62] Kotter's 8-step model is commonly used for implementing sustainable change, and is based on creating a sense of urgency as the first step.[63] The 8 steps include the following: (1) creating a sense of urgency, (2) forming a powerful guiding coalition, (3) create a vision, (4) communicating the vision, (5) empowering others to act on the vision, (6) planning for and creating short-term wins, (7) consolidating improvements and producing more change, (8) institutionalizing new approaches. Change management models are used to assist healthcare teams through the implementation process in a more organized manner. However, more studies are needed on change modeling and processes for sustainment and success.

An important element of ERPs is compliance and auditing. In fact, an international, multicenter ERAS registry database of 2352 colonic and rectal resections demonstrated that increasing ERP compliance was correlated with fewer complications and shorter primary hospital admission.[64] This same trend exists for thoracic surgical patients. Rogers et al.[49] examined a cohort of 422 patients who underwent lung resection. All patients followed a standardized, 15-element ERAS protocol. Key data fields included protocol compliance with individual elements, pathophysiology, and operative factors: age, lack of preoperative carbohydrate drinks, planned high dependency unit/intensive therapy unit admission, delayed mobilization, and open approach were independent predictors of delayed discharge (length of stay >5 days). There was a significant inverse relationship between protocol compliance and morbidity after surgery, with delayed mobilization as one of the independent predictors. Maintaining high compliance with elements of an enhanced recovery pathway should be one of the main goals of an ERP team.

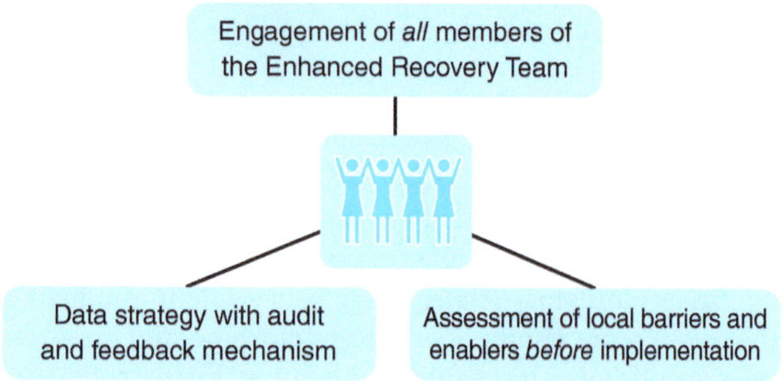

• **Fig. 53.2** Strategies for implementation success in enhanced recovery programs.

Future Direction of Enhanced Recovery After Thoracic Surgery

ERATS has experienced substantial growth in recent years, particularly with the release of the first standardized ERATS guidelines. Still, further research is needed, both for the individual components that lack strong evidentiary support and also from a bigger picture to understand how all these components interact. Ultimately, by strengthening our understanding of these pathways and their components, we can provide the most evidence-based care possible and thereby facilitate a smooth and efficient recovery for our thoracic patients.

References

1. Kehlet H. Multimodal approach to control postoperative pathophysiology and rehabilitation. *Br J Anaesth.* 1997;78:606–617.
2. Semenkovich TR, Hudson JL, Subramanian M, Kozower BD. Enhanced recovery after surgery (ERAS) in thoracic surgery. *Semin Thorac Cardiovasc Surg.* 2018;30(3):342–349.
3. Findlay JM, Gillies RS, Millo J, Sgromo B, Marshall RE, Maynard ND. Enhanced recovery for esophagectomy: a systematic review and evidence-based guidelines. *Ann Surg.* 2014;259:413–431.
4. Batchelor TJP, Rasburn NJ, Abdelnour-Berchtold E, et al. Guidelines for enhanced recovery after lung surgery: recommendations of the Enhanced Recovery After Surgery (ERAS(R)) Society and the European Society of Thoracic Surgeons (ESTS). *Eur J Cardiothorac Surg.* 2019;55:91–115.
5. Svircevic V, Nierich AP, Moons KG, et al. Fast-track anesthesia and cardiac surgery: a retrospective cohort study of 7989 patients. *Anesth Analg.* 2009;108:727–733.
6. Borracci RA, Dayan R, Rubio M, Axelrud G, Ochoa G, Rodriguez LD. [Operating room extubation (ultra fast-track anesthesia) in patients undergoing on-pump and off-pump cardiac surgery]. *Arch Cardiol Mex.* 2006;76:383–389.

7. Muehling BM, Halter GL, Schelzig H, et al. Reduction of postoperative pulmonary complications after lung surgery using a fast track clinical pathway. *Eur J Cardiothorac Surg*. 2008;34:174–180.
8. Umari M, Falini S, Segat M, et al. Anesthesia and fast-track in video-assisted thoracic surgery (VATS): from evidence to practice. *J Thorac Dis*. 2018;10:S542–S554.
9. Martin LW, Sarosiek BM, Harrison MA, et al. Implementing a thoracic enhanced recovery program: lessons learned in the first year. *Ann Thorac Surg*. 2018;105:1597–1604.
10. Ljungqvist O, Scott M, Fearon KC. Enhanced recovery after surgery: a review. *JAMA Surg*. 2017;152:292–298.
11. Ferrando C, Soro M, Unzueta C, et al. Individualized PeRIoperative Open-lung VEntilation Network. Individualised perioperative open-lung approach versus standard protective ventilation in abdominal surgery (iPROVE): a randomised controlled trial. *Lancet Respir Med*. 2018;6:193–203.
12. Li S, Zhou K, Che G, Yang M, Su J, Shen C, Yu P. Enhanced recovery programs in lung cancer surgery: systematic review and meta-analysis of randomized controlled trials. *Cancer Manag Res*. 2017;9:657–670.
13. Refai M, Andolfi M, Gentili P, Pelusi G, Manzotti F, Sabbatini A. Enhanced recovery after thoracic surgery: patient information and care-plans. *J Thorac Dis*. 2018;10:S512–S516.
14. Stokes SM, Wakeam E, Antonoff MB, et al. Optimizing health before elective thoracic surgery: systematic review of modifiable risk factors and opportunities for health services research. *J Thorac Dis*. 2019;11:S537–S554.
15. Agostini P, Cieslik H, Rathinam S, et al. Postoperative pulmonary complications following thoracic surgery: are there any modifiable risk factors? *Thorax*. 2010;65:815–818.
16. Lugg ST, Tikka T, Agostini PJ, et al. Smoking and timing of cessation on postoperative pulmonary complications after curative-intent lung cancer surgery. *J Cardiothorac Surg*. 2017;12:52.
17. Parsons A, Daley A, Begh R, Aveyard P. Influence of smoking cessation after diagnosis of early stage lung cancer on prognosis: systematic review of observational studies with meta-analysis. *BMJ*. 2010;340:b5569.
18. Fukui M, Suzuki K, Matsunaga T, Oh S, Takamochi K. Importance of smoking cessation on surgical outcome in primary lung cancer. *Ann Thorac Surg*. 2019;107:1005–1009.
19. Matsuoka K, Yamada T, Matsuoka T, Nagai S, Ueda M, Miyamoto Y. Preoperative smoking cessation period is not related to postoperative respiratory complications in patients undergoing lung cancer surgery. *Ann Thorac Cardiovasc Surg*. 2019;25:304–310.
20. Balduyck B, Sardari Nia P, Cogen A, et al. The effect of smoking cessation on quality of life after lung cancer surgery. *Eur J Cardiothorac Surg*. 2011;40:1432–1437 discussion 1437-8.
21. Graf SA, Zeliadt SB, Rise PJ, Backhus LM, Zhou XH, Williams EC. Unhealthy alcohol use is associated with postoperative complications in veterans undergoing lung resection. *J Thorac Dis*. 2018; 10:1648–1656.
22. Neuenschwander AU, Pedersen JH, Krasnik M, Tonnesen H. Impaired postoperative outcome in chronic alcohol abusers after curative resection for lung cancer. *Eur J Cardiothorac Surg*. 2002;22: 287–291.
23. Paull DE, Updyke GM, Baumann MA, Chin HW, Little AG, Adebonojo SA. Alcohol abuse predicts progression of disease and death in patients with lung cancer. *Ann Thorac Surg*. 2005;80: 1033–1039.
24. Cavalheri V, Granger C. Preoperative exercise training for patients with non-small cell lung cancer. *Cochrane Database Syst Rev*. 2017;6:CD012020.
25. Steffens D, Beckenkamp PR, Hancock M, Solomon M, Young J. Preoperative exercise halves the postoperative complication rate in patients with lung cancer: a systematic review of the effect of exercise on complications, length of stay and quality of life in patients with cancer. *Br J Sports Med*. 2018;52:344.
26. Rosero ID, Ramirez-Velez R, Lucia A, et al. Systematic review and meta-analysis of randomized, controlled trials on preoperative physical exercise interventions in patients with non-small-cell lung cancer. *Cancers* (Basel). 2019:11.
27. Sebio Garcia R, Yanez-Brage MI, Gimenez Moolhuyzen E, Salorio Riobo M, Lista Paz A, Borro Mate JM. Preoperative exercise training prevents functional decline after lung resection surgery: a randomized, single-blind controlled trial. *Clin Rehabil*. 2017;31: 1057–1067.
28. Minnella EM, Awasthi R, Loiselle SE, Agnihotram RV, Ferri LE, Carli F. Effect of exercise and nutrition prehabilitation on functional capacity in esophagogastric cancer surgery: a randomized clinical trial. *JAMA Surg*. 2018;153:1081–1089.
29. Trufa DI, Arhire LI, Nita O, Gherasim A, Nita G, Graur M. The evaluation of preoperative nutritional status in patients undergoing thoracic surgery. *Rev Med Chir Soc Med Nat Iasi*. 2014;118: 514–519.
30. van Bokhorst-de van der Schueren MA, Guaitoli PR, Jansma EP, de Vet HC. Nutrition screening tools: does one size fit all? A systematic review of screening tools for the hospital setting. *Clin Nutr*. 2014;33:39–58.
31. Veterans Affairs Total Parenteral Nutrition Cooperative Study Group Perioperative total parenteral nutrition in surgical patients. *N Engl J Med*. 1991;325:525–532.
32. Bertolaccini L, Calabrese F, Brandolini J, et al. Fat but fit for the improved survival in lung cancer surgery. *J Thorac Dis*. 2018;10: S2067–S2069.
33. Lam VK, Bentzen SM, Mohindra P, et al. Obesity is associated with long-term improved survival in definitively treated locally advanced non-small cell lung cancer (NSCLC). *Lung Cancer*. 2017;104:52–57.
34. Kanekiyo S, Takeda S, Iida M, et al. Efficacy of perioperative immunonutrition in esophageal cancer patients undergoing esophagectomy. *Nutrition*. 2019;59:96–102.
35. Mehran RJ, Martin LW, Baker CM, Mena GE, Rice DC. Pain management in an enhanced recovery pathway after thoracic surgical procedures. *Ann Thorac Surg*. 2016;102:e595–e596.
36. De Cosmo G, Aceto P, Gualtieri E, Congedo E. Analgesia in thoracic surgery: review. *Minerva Anestesiol*. 2009;75:393–400.
37. Yeung JH, Gates S, Naidu BV, Wilson MJ. Gao Smith F. Paravertebral block versus thoracic epidural for patients undergoing thoracotomy. *Cochrane Database Syst Rev*. 2016;2:CD009121.
38. Chou R, Gordon DB, de Leon-Casasola OA, et al. Management of postoperative pain: a clinical practice guideline from the American Pain Society, the American Society of Regional Anesthesia and Pain Medicine, and the American Society of Anesthesiologists' Committee on Regional Anesthesia, Executive Committee, and Administrative Council. *J Pain*. 2016;17:131–157.
39. Qiu R, Perrino AC, Jr., Zurich H, Sukumar N, Dai F, Popescu W. Effect of preoperative gabapentin and acetaminophen on opioid consumption in video-assisted thoracoscopic surgery: a retrospective study. *Rom J Anaesth Intensive Care*. 2018;25:43–48.
40. Wahlander S, Frumento RJ, Wagener G, et al. A prospective, double-blind, randomized, placebo-controlled study of dexmedetomidine as an adjunct to epidural analgesia after thoracic surgery. *J Cardiothorac Vasc Anesth*. 2005;19:630–635.
41. Lee SH, Lee CY, Lee JG, Kim N, Lee HM, Oh YJ. Intraoperative dexmedetomidine improves the quality of recovery and postop-

erative pulmonary function in patients undergoing video-assisted thoracoscopic surgery: A CONSORT-Prospective, randomized, controlled trial. *Medicine* (Baltimore). 2016;95:e2854.

42. Sugasawa Y, Yamaguchi K, Kumakura S, et al. Effects of sevoflurane and propofol on pulmonary inflammatory responses during lung resection. *J Anesth*. 2012;26:62–69.
43. Schilling T, Kozian A, Kretzschmar M, et al. Effects of propofol and desflurane anaesthesia on the alveolar inflammatory response to one-lung ventilation. *Br J Anaesth*. 2007;99:368–375.
44. Slinger PD. Optimizing one-lung ventilation: moving beyond tidal volume. *J Cardiothorac Vasc Anesth*. 2018;32(6): 2673–2675.
45. Marret E, Cinotti R, Berard L, et al., and the PPV Study Group. Protective ventilation during anaesthesia reduces major postoperative complications after lung cancer surgery: a double-blind randomised controlled trial. *Eur J Anaesthesiol*. 2018;35(10):727–735.
46. Gimenez-Mila M, Klein AA, Martinez G. Design and implementation of an enhanced recovery program in thoracic surgery. *J Thorac Dis*. 2016;8:S37–S45.
47. Brassard CL, Lohser J, Donati F, Bussieres JS. Step-by-step clinical management of one-lung ventilation: continuing professional development. *Can J Anaesth*. 2014;61:1103–1121.
48. iPROVE Network Investigators, Belda J, Ferrando C, Garutti I. The effects of an open-lung approach during one-lung ventilation on postoperative pulmonary complications and driving pressure: a descriptive, multicenter national study. *J Cardiothorac Vasc Anesth*. 2018;32:2665–2672.
49. Rogers LJ, Bleetman D, Messenger DE, et al. The impact of enhanced recovery after surgery (ERAS) protocol compliance on morbidity from resection for primary lung cancer. *J Thorac Cardiovasc Surg*. 2018;155:1843–1852.
50. Mercieri M, D'Andrilli A, Arcioni R. Improving postoperative pain management after video-assisted thoracic surgery lung resection contributes to enhanced recovery, but guidelines are still lacking. *J Thorac Dis*. 2018;10:S983–S987.
51. Assaad S, Kyriakides T, Tellides G, Kim AW, Perkal M, Perrino A. Extravascular lung water and tissue perfusion biomarkers after lung resection surgery under a normovolemic fluid protocol. *J Cardiothorac Vasc Anesth*. 2015;29:977–983.
52. Shargall Y, Brunelli A, Murthy S, et al. Venous thromboembolism prophylaxis in thoracic surgery patients: an international survey. *Eur J Cardiothorac Surg*. 2019;57(2):331–337.
53. Hawn MT, Richman JS, Vick CC, et al. Timing of surgical antibiotic prophylaxis and the risk of surgical site infection. *JAMA Surg*. 2013;148:649–657.
54. Emmert A, Franke R, Brandes IF, et al. Comparison of conductive and convective warming in patients undergoing video-assisted thoracic surgery: a prospective randomized clinical trial. *Thorac Cardiovasc Surg*. 2017;65:362–366.
55. Solak O, Metin M, Esme H, et al. Effectiveness of gabapentin in the treatment of chronic post-thoracotomy pain. *Eur J Cardiothorac Surg*. 2007;32:9–12.
56. Hessami MA, Najafi F, Hatami S. Volume threshold for chest tube removal: a randomized controlled trial. *J Inj Violence Res*. 2009;1:33–36.
57. Younes RN, Gross JL, Aguiar S, Haddad FJ, Deheinzelin D. When to remove a chest tube? A randomized study with subsequent prospective consecutive validation. *J Am Coll Surg*. 2002;195: 658–662.
58. Dawson AG, Hosmane S. Should you place one or two chest drains in patients undergoing lobectomy? *Interact Cardiovasc Thorac Surg*. 2010;11:178–181.
59. Pawelczyk K, Marciniak M, Kacprzak G, Kolodziej J. One or two drains after lobectomy? A comparison of both methods in the immediate postoperative period. *Thorac Cardiovasc Surg*. 2007;55:313–316.
60. Grol R, Grimshaw J. From best evidence to best practice: effective implementation of change in patients' care. *Lancet*. 2003; 362:1225–1230.
61. Pearsall EA, McLeod RS. Enhanced recovery after surgery: implementation strategies, barriers and facilitators. *Surg Clin North Am*. 2018;98:1201–1210.
62. Gramlich LM, Sheppard CE, Wasylak T, et al. Implementation of Enhanced Recovery After Surgery: a strategy to transform surgical care across a health system. *Implement Sci*. 2017;12:67.
63. Kotter JP. *Leading Change*. Boston, Massachusetts: Harvard Business School Press; 1996.
64. Group EC. The impact of enhanced recovery protocol compliance on elective colorectal cancer resection: results from an International Registry. *Ann Surg*. 2015;261:1153–1159.

54 Ultrasound of the Lung: Clinical Applications

MASSIMILIANO MEINERI

Introduction

Lung ultrasound (LUS)[1] has become standard of care in many clinical settings and has proven feasible at the bedside for detecting life-threatening conditions, such as pneumothorax, with a sensibility and specificity often superior to standard chest radiography.[2] For some time, the use of ultrasound (US) to assess the lung has been questioned because of the inherent physics of US and the structure of the chest and respiratory system. A normally aerated lung is constituted by more than 80% air and is surrounded by the ribcage. US waves are almost entirely reflected by the interface between soft tissue, air, or bone therefore making these two tissues impenetrable to US, and making imaging their structure not feasible.

In fact, chest US, displays images of the soft tissues between the probe and the parietal pleura and only artifacts there beyond (Fig. 54.1). The lung becomes visible only when the air is replaced by fluids (edema), tissue (infection), or the alveoli are emptied from the air (atelectasis).

For these reasons, LUS is based on the interpretation of patterns of artifacts.

Probe Selection and Scanning Protocols

LUS can be performed using any type of the US probe. The most commonly available include linear (typically used for vascular access), curved (typically used for abdominal scanning), and phased array (cardiac) probes. The microconvex array probe is a curved probe with a smaller footprint and, although not commonly available, it has been suggested to offer the best compromise for LUS.[3] The main difference among probes is the US frequency, being the highest for the linear probe and the lowest for the phased array. Probe frequency is directly related to the image resolution but inversely related to the penetration into soft tissue. For this reason, the linear probe can only be used to assess superficial structures (Fig. 54.2).

LUS is performed by placing the probe perpendicular to the ribs and pointing the probe marker toward the patient's head. LUS images can be displayed using the cardiology (image marker on the right upper corner) or the radiology (image marker on the left upper corner) convention (Fig. 54.3). This means that the marker indicates the cranial orientation.

Several protocols have been described for a complete LUS examination,[4] which include a variable number of views. Each side of the chest has been conveniently divided by the anterior and posterior axillary lines into anterior, lateral, and posterior. The anterior and posterior quadrants are further divided in half into superior and inferior, making a total of five quadrants (Fig. 54.4). Current guidelines[5] recommend a complete examination to obtain at least one US view of all quadrants on each side. Although air tends to move up and fluid follows gravity, in an emergency scenario the highest portion of the chest would be scanned to rule out pneumothorax and the lowest to rule out an effusion.

Anatomic Correlation and Normal Physiologic Findings

LUS comprises two standard views: the pleural view (Fig. 54.5) (obtained from all scanning points above the diaphragm) and the diaphragm view (Fig. 54.6) (at the level of the diaphragmatic dome). The **pleural view** is used to assess pleural sliding and underlying pleura and lung parenchyma. The **diaphragm view** is used to assess diaphragmatic movement and rule out pleural effusion.

To obtain the pleural view, the probe is positioned perpendicular to the ribs. It is first rotated to bring the ribs close together and then tilted until the pleura is best displayed. Using the linear probe, the ribs will appear on US as two black round structures, casting a shadow underneath (see Fig. 54.5). The pleural line can be identified with certainty as the first bright white line below the ribs upper contour. The space between the probe and the pleural line is filled by the intercostal muscles. This US image may be compared with an ostrich head close up where the ribs are the eyes and the pleural line the beak. This view has also been associated with the shape of a bat

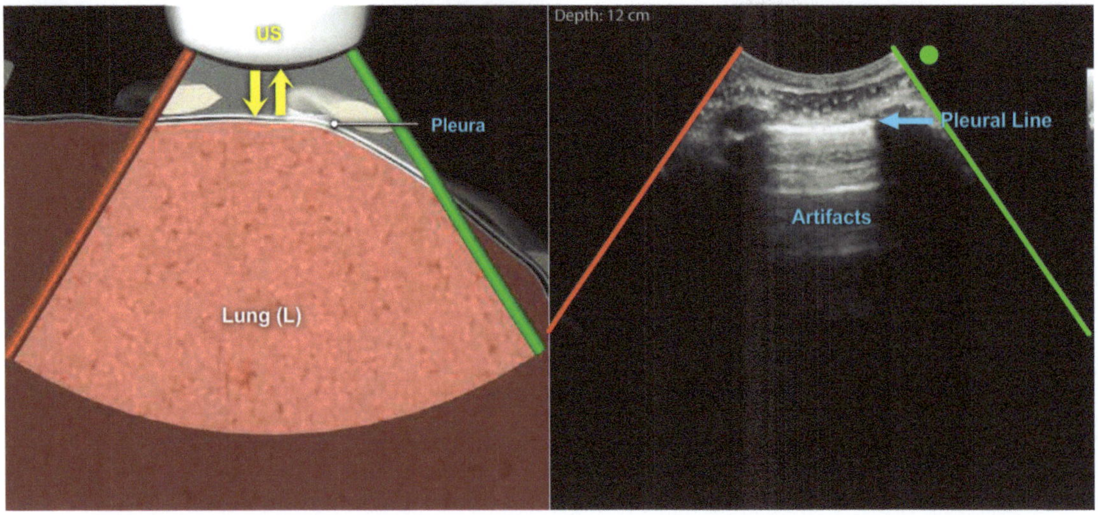

• **Fig. 54.1** Lung ultrasound image of the pleura using a curved array probe, showing the subcutaneous tissue and artifacts beyond the pleural line. (Modified from http://pie.med.utoronto.ca/POCUS/POCUS_content/lungUS.html.)

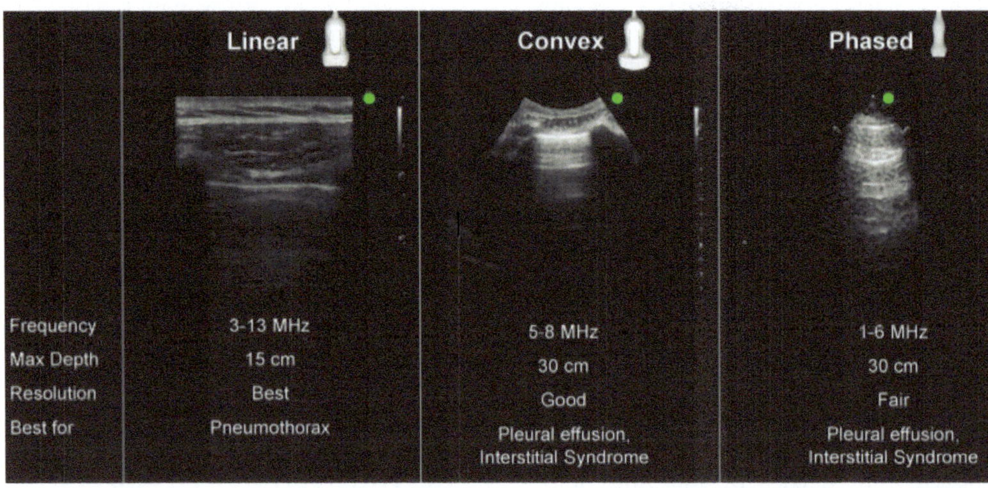

• **Fig. 54.2** Commonly available ultrasound probes and their characteristics. (Modified from http://pie.med.utoronto.ca/POCUS/POCUS_content/lungUS.html.)

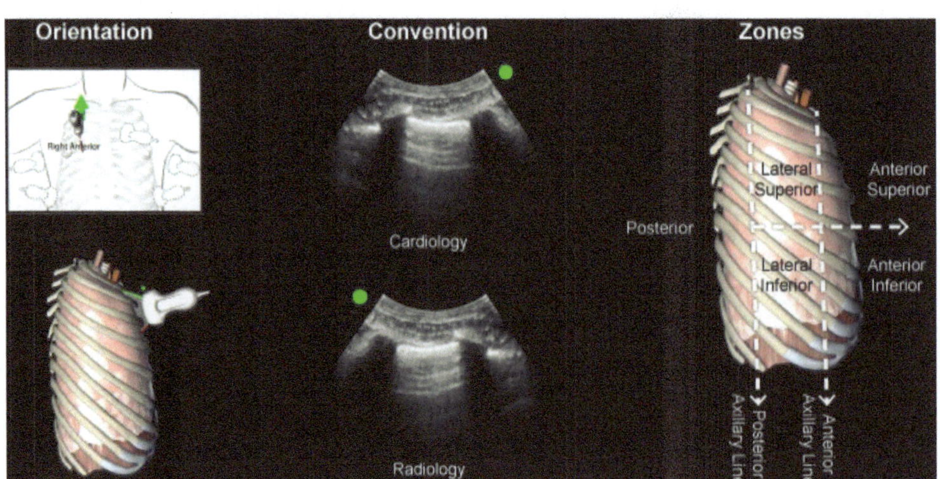

• **Fig. 54.3** Probe orientation, convention, and scanning zones. (Modified from http://pie.med.utoronto.ca/POCUS/POCUS_content/lungUS.html.)

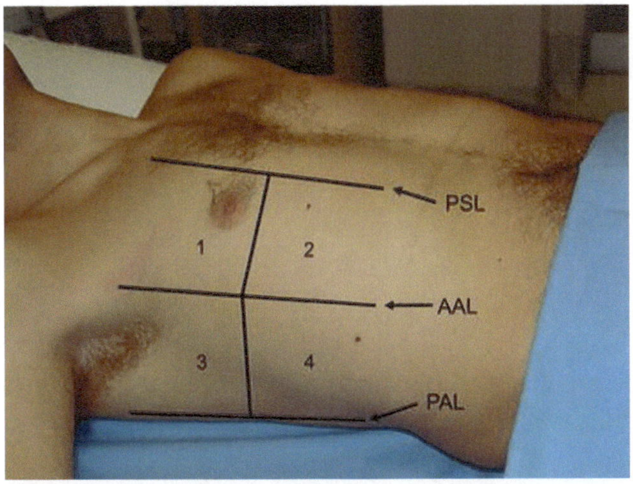

• **Fig. 54.4 Lung ultrasound scanning zones.** The four chest areas per side considered for complete eight-zone lung ultrasound examination. These areas are used to evaluate for the presence of interstitial syndrome. Areas *1* and *2* denote the upper anterior and lower anterior chest areas, respectively. Areas *3* and *4* denote the upper lateral and basal lateral chest areas, respectively. *AAL*, Anterior axillary line; *PAL*, posterior axillary line; *PSL*, parasternal line. (Modified from Volpicelli G, Elbarbary M, Blaivas M, et al. International evidence-based recommendations for point-of-care lung ultrasound. *Intensive Care Med*. 2012;38(4):577–591.)

whose wings would correspond to the upper edge of the ribs and the chest to the pleural line. A similar view can be obtained with all probes (see Fig. 54.2), however, with an increased sector depth (more than a few centimeters), a series of horizontal lines, parallel to the pleural line can be appreciated underneath. These are called **A lines**; they are considered a normal finding and are the result of a reverberation artifact. Given that the pleura is a strong reflector, the same US waves come back to the probe still very strong, bounce back off the probe toward the pleura, and travel back and forth several times. Given the duration of travel from the probe to the pleura, and back is constant, A lines are equidistant from each other at the same exact distance between the probe and the pleural line (Fig. 54.7).

The thickening of the interstitial space, as well as the presence of water in the alveoli, is responsible for the generation of reverberation of US between the most superficial alveoli and the parietal pleura resulting in vertical laser-like line originating from the pleural line, moving with the pleural sliding, and travelling to a depth of 15 cm.[5] These are called **B lines** (Fig. 54.8) and can only be displayed using a curved or a phased array probe. B lines are nonspecific signs and do not correspond to a single pathology. A single B line in one US view has no pathologic meaning and may be because of interstitial irregularities or localized atelectasis.

The **pleural line** corresponds to the parietal pleura. In a normal lung, the visceral pleura lies against the parietal pleura and slides against it with respiration. **Pleural sliding** is shown in US as a shimmering (movement of sparkles) of the pleural line. This sign has also been described as "marching ants" if we imagine the pleural line as small white and black dots moving side to side. Lung sliding identifies lung ventilation and rules out a pneumothorax.

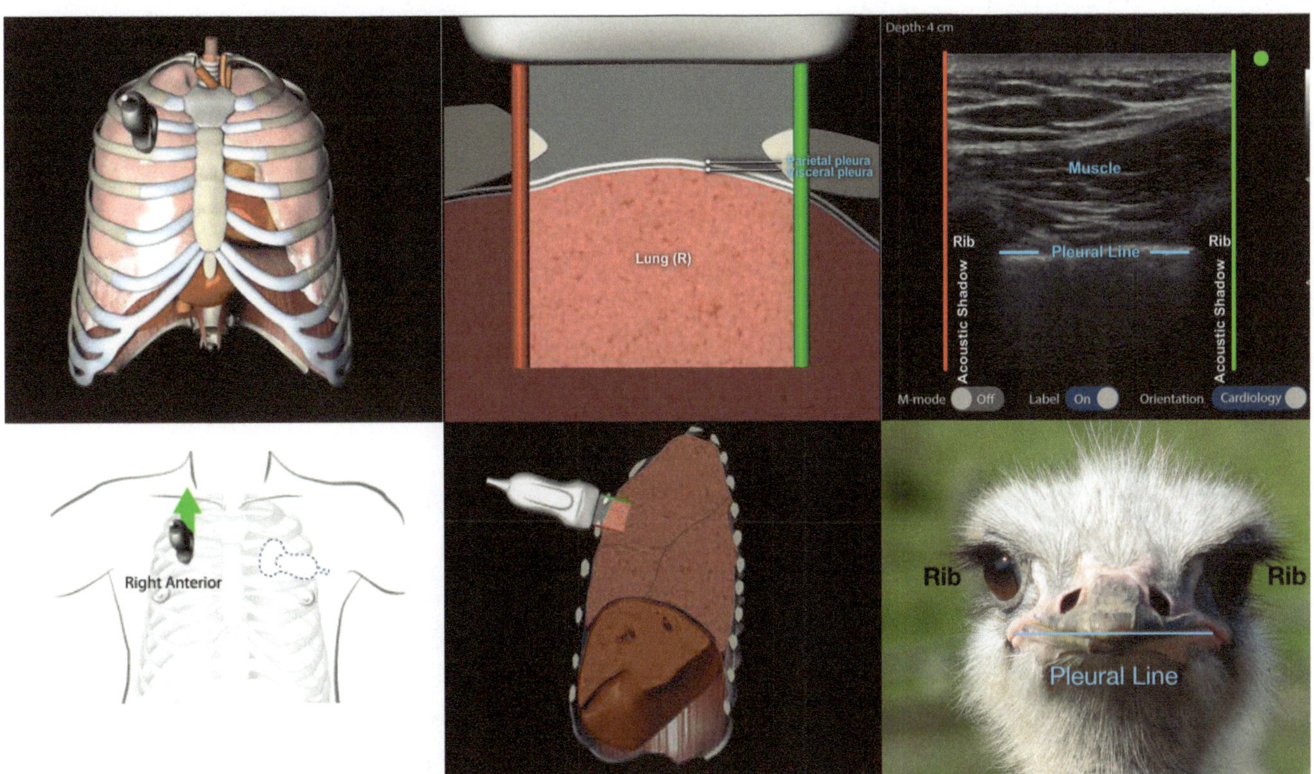

• **Fig. 54.5 Pleural view**. Probe orientation, ultrasonographic-anatomic correlation, and "ostrich" sign. (Modified from http://pie.med.utoronto.ca/POCUS/POCUS_content/lungUS.html.)

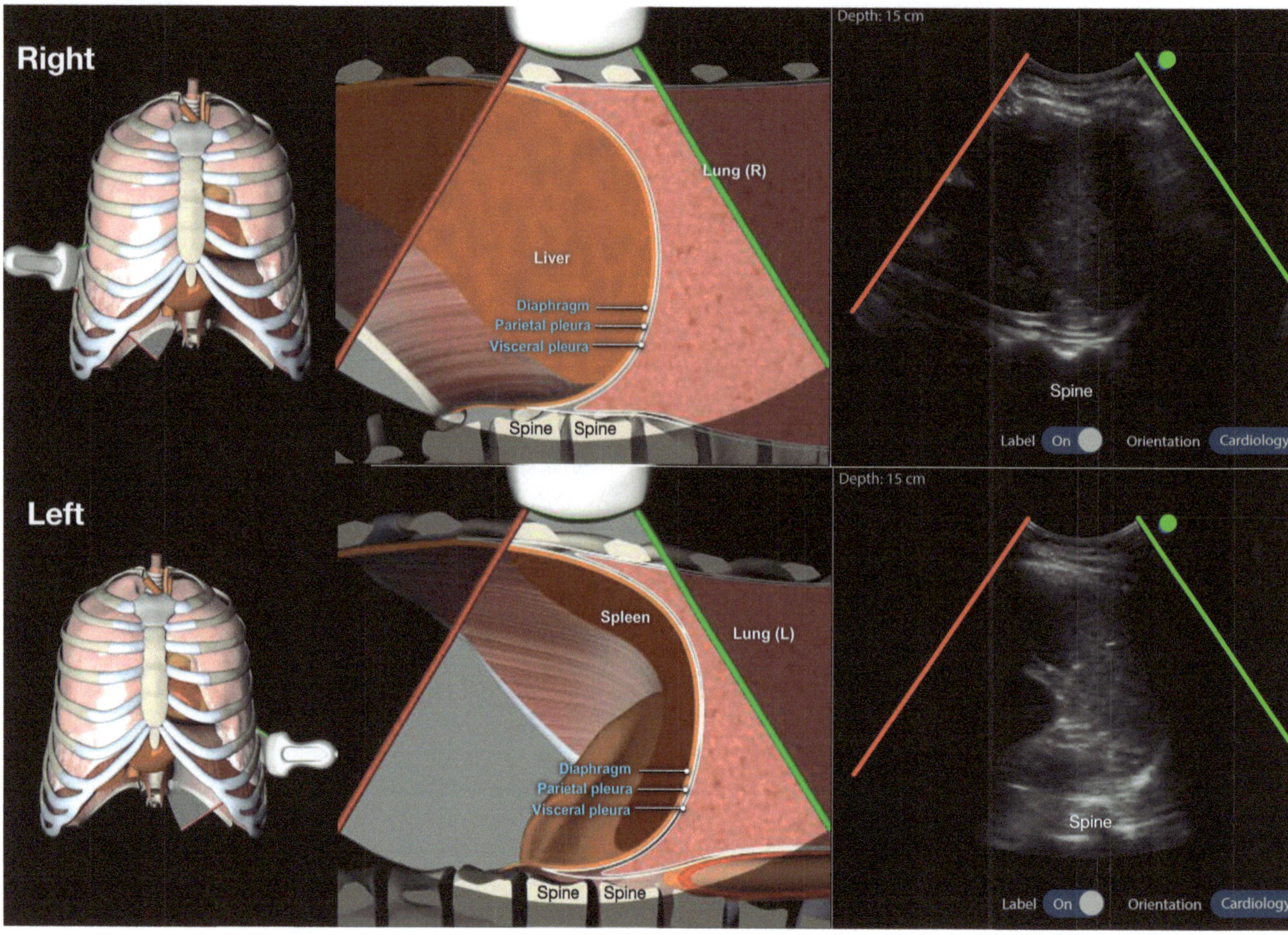

• **Fig. 54.6** Right and left pleural views and negative spine sign. The vertebral bodies can only be seen on lung ultrasound below the diaphragm. (Modified from http://pie.med.utoronto.ca/POCUS/POCUS_content/lungUS.html.)

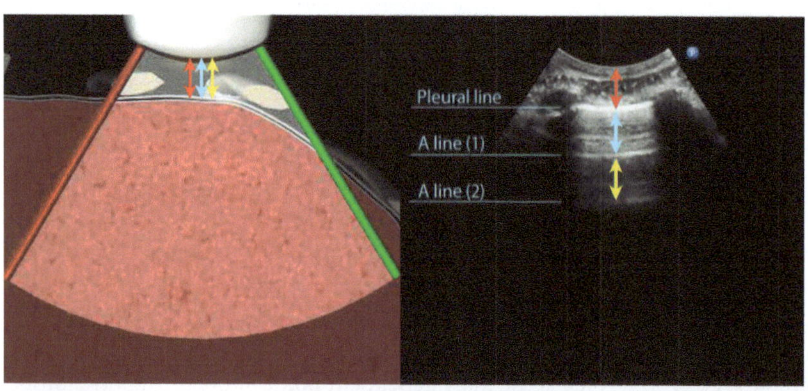

• **Fig. 54.7** A lines are caused by reverberation. The pleural line is a strong reflector and the same ultrasound waves travel multiple times (*red, blue, yellow*) back to the probe and are reflected by the probe head and return to the pleura. (Modified from http://pie.med.utoronto.ca/POCUS/POCUS_content/lungUS.html.)

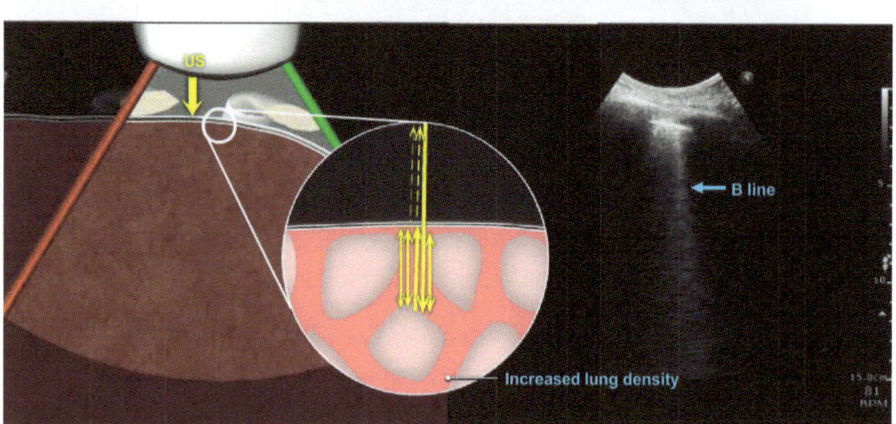

• **Fig. 54.8** **B lines** are laser-like vertical lines originating from the pleural line and are the result of increased lung density that caused reverberation of ultrasound between the interstitial space and the parietal pleura. (Modified from http://pie.med.utoronto.ca/POCUS/POCUS_content/lungUS.html.)

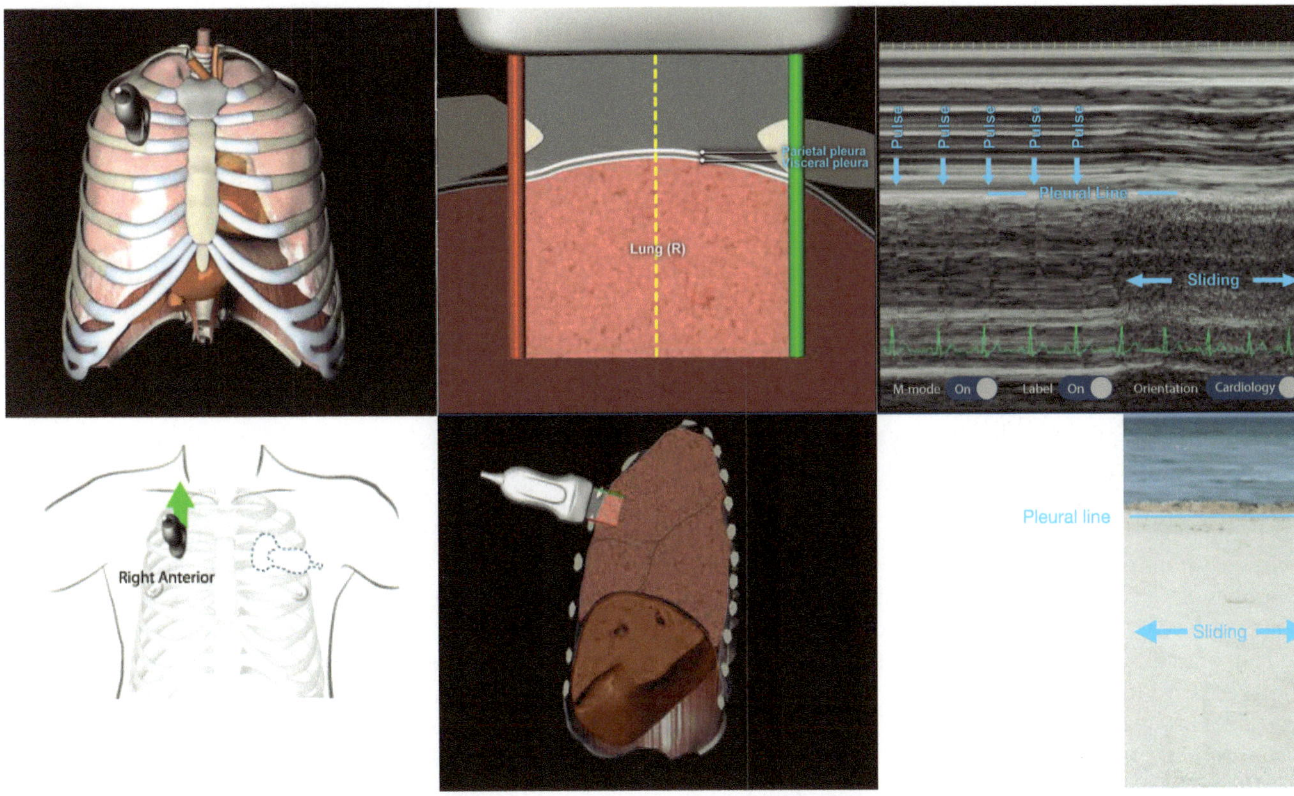

• **Fig. 54.9** M-mode demonstration of lung sliding with **"seashore" sign** and **lung pulse**. *M-mode*, Motion mode. (Modified from http://pie.med.utoronto.ca/POCUS/POCUS_content/lungUS.html.)

When a curved or a phased array probe is used, decreasing the image depth would facilitate assessment of the pleural sliding. Lung sliding rules out a pneumothorax but also confirms ipsilateral lung ventilation. LUS has been successfully used to confirm endotracheal intubation[6] and effective lung isolation.[7]

During apnea, the heartbeat is transmitted through the lung parenchyma that makes the visceral pleura slide very briefly against the parietal pleura. This brief lung sliding accompanies every heartbeat and is known as **"lung pulse"** and it is more evident on the left chest, given the proximity to the heart chambers. It results in a very brief and subtle lung sliding that can often be missed, and it is best appreciated when the pulse is palpated while observing the pleural line.

Lung sliding and lung pulse can be confirmed and better appreciated using the motion mode (M-mode) technique (see Fig. 54.8). This technique casts a vertical line in the middle of the US image. All the points along the line are dragged rightwards over time. If a dot is not moving, draw a straight line, if moving toward and then away from the probe to draw a sinusoid. In a normal lung, during respiration, the activation of M-mode with any of the probes, displays a unique view with two very different patterns above (parallel lines) and below (granules) the pleural line. The linear lines correspond to the immobile interfaces between intercostal muscle layers, and the granular pattern is generated by the lung sliding. This combination resembles a seashore (sand, ocean waves, and sky). This **seashore sign** represents normal lung ventilation. During apnea, the lung pulse is displayed on M-mode as artifacts originating from the pleural line and developing distally. When an electrocardiogram signal is available, these artifacts follow the QRS complex and are synchronous with the heartbeat (Fig. 54.9). Heart contraction: the unaverred probe movement would also result into vertical artifacts on M-mode, but they would be across the entire image (above and below the plural line) and unrelated to the heartbeat.

The diaphragm view (see Fig. 54.6) is aimed at a scan deep into the pleural cavity to visualize the posterior costophrenic angle, the most dependent point in the chest. This requires a higher scanning depth (15–20 cm) and therefore is not obtainable using the linear array probe. This view takes advantage of two parenchymal US conducting organs (the liver on the right and the spleen on the left) to visualize the spine and the adjacent posterior costophrenic angle, which is the most dependent point in the pleura. The probe is positioned on the anterior axillary line on the right and between the anterior and posterior axillary lines on the left, with the marker pointing at the patient's head. It is tilted to aim at the spine.

In absence of a pleural effusion, the US reaches the spine through the liver and the spleen but is reflected by the lung above the diaphragm. For this reason, the vertebral bodies are visible below but not above the diaphragm (negative spine sign), which rules out a pleural effusion in absence of pleural adhesions.

With the diaphragmatic movement, the lung wedges between the probe and the liver casting a shadow. This phenomenon presents as a hypoechoic artifact that wipes in from the marker side and has been described as the **"curtain" sign**. It indicates normal diaphragmatic movement and confirms ipsilateral lung ventilation.

Detection of Pneumothorax

LUS have been reported to be more sensitive and specific than standard chest x-ray in detecting pneumothorax.[2] As mentioned earlier, in a normal aerated lung, the amount of air inside the alveoli prevents the parenchyma to significantly contribute to image generation.

In other words, in a normal lung all that can be imaged is air. This means that when a layer of air separates the visceral from the parietal pleura, such as in the case of a pneumothorax, the image remains the same as in a healthy aerated lung; what change are the dynamic signs.

In presence of a pneumothorax, the visceral pleura is separated from the parietal pleura by a layer of air, therefore during lung inflation the two cannot slide while they do not touch each other, and lung sliding is no longer present also as a result of transmission of vibrations from cardiac contraction (lung pulse). On M-mode display the typical seashore sign is replaced by a series of horizontal parallel lines described as **"stratosphere" or "bar-code" sign** (Fig. 54.10).

The lack of contact between the parietal and visceral pleura does not allow formation of B lines. For this reason, a single B line excludes a pneumothorax in the field examined. International consensus on LUS[5] defines a simple diagnostic tree based on these signs (Fig. 54.11).

Although air tends to accumulate in the less dependent part of the chest wall, when ruling out a pneumothorax the patient's decubitus is of outmost importance. Most of the study demonstrated a higher sensitivity and specificity of LUS in detecting pneumothorax when performed in patients who were in supine position. That is when the least dependent point in the pleural cavity corresponds to the third-fourth intercostal space on the mid-clavicular line.[2] When the torso is elevated than 45 degrees, presence of lung sliding may not exclude a small pneumothorax at the lung apex, therefore repositioning the patient to a flat position would increase the sensitivity of the examination.

The lack of lung sliding, lung pulse, and B lines identifies the presence of a pneumothorax in the point scanned. To quantify the size of the pneumothorax, the entire hemithorax should be scanned with multiple points starting from the third to fourth intercostal space on the mid-clavicular line and moving to the next point, one intercostal space caudal and one inch lateral every time until reaching the diaphragm. In case of a full pneumothorax with retraction of the lung to the hilum, the same finding would be identified in all scanning points. In case of a partial pneumothorax, the edge of the pleural detachment can be identified by LUS with the transition between

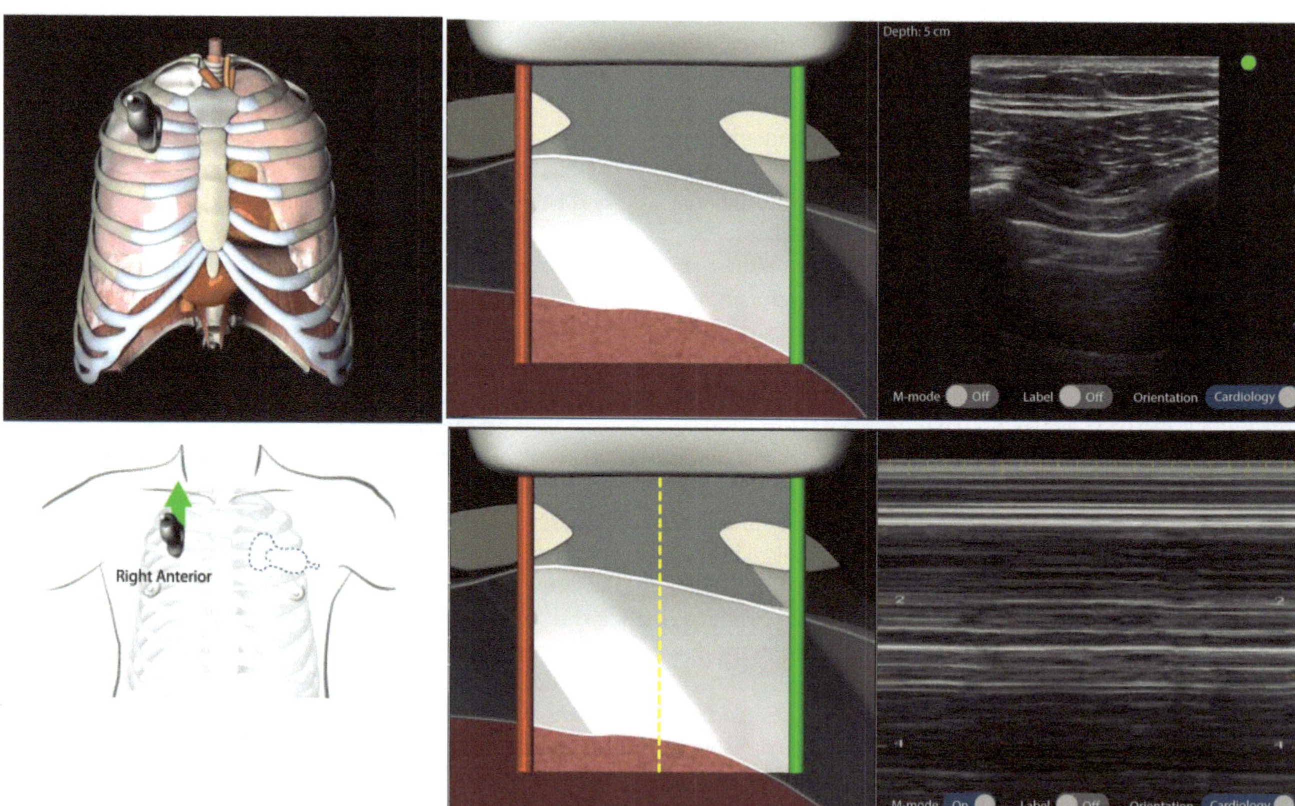

• **Fig.54.10 Demonstration of a right pneumothorax**. The lack of dynamic lung sliding results on motion mode (M-mode) in the "barcode" sign. (Modified from http://pie.med.utoronto.ca/POCUS/POCUS_content/lungUS.html.)

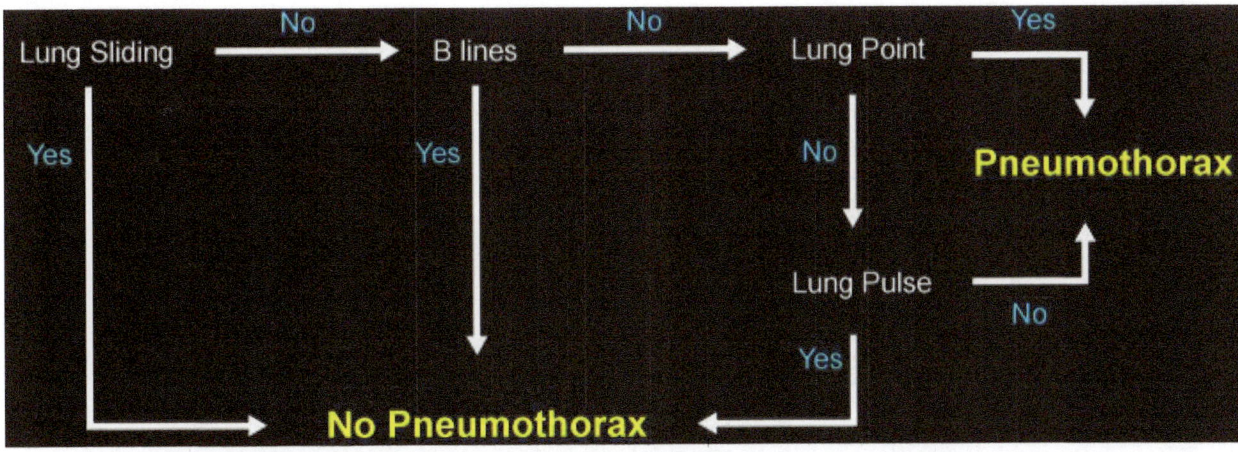

• **Fig. 54.11** Diagnostic algorithm for pneumothorax. (Modified from http://pie.med.utoronto.ca/POCUS/POCUS_content/lungUS.html.)

the presence of lung sliding and lack of sliding (Fig. 54.12). This typical US feature is called *lung point*. It is pathognomonic for a pneumothorax, and when drainage was clinically indicated should be inserted cranially to this point.

Detection of Pleural Effusion

LUS has a higher sensitivity and specificity in detecting pleural effusion than chest x-ray.[8]

On the contrary to air, fluid tends to accumulate in most dependent point in the pleura. In the absence of adhesions, this corresponds to the posterior costophrenic angle adjacent to the spine, in a semi-sitting patient. This point can be visualized in the diaphragm view using a phased or a curved array probe as described earlier (see Fig. 54.5).

This view has been integrated in the extended fast abdominal scan in trauma to rule out a hemothorax.[9] When fluid fills the costophrenic angle and the lung get displaced caudally, the US would be able to travel through the fluid and reach the spine. In this case, the spine could be seen on US below and above the diaphragm on either side of the chest. This finding is pathognomonic for pleural effusion (Fig. 54.13). The degree of cranial displacement of the lung is directly related to the amount of fluid in the pleural cavity. To estimate the volume of pleural effusion in milliliters, a simple formula suggests multiplying the maximal distance between the lung and the diaphragm in centimeters by 200 (e.g., 2 cm lung-diaphragm separation = 400 mL pleural effusion). LUS is not able to differentiate between different types of fluid as they all appear equally hypoechoic (fresh blood, exudate, transudate appear all black); however clots are more echodense and fibrin strands can be easily appreciated within the pleural fluid. Exudate can be possibly differentiated from transudate by the presence of small floating echogenic structures that gave this feature the name of **"plankton" sign**. Numerous septations and fibrin strands within pleural fluid are typically seen in cases of empyema and have been described as **"honeycomb" appearance** (Fig. 54.14). Septations are finally indicative of a complex pleural effusion that might need targeted guided drainage. LUS has also been used successfully to guide drainage of pleural effusion.

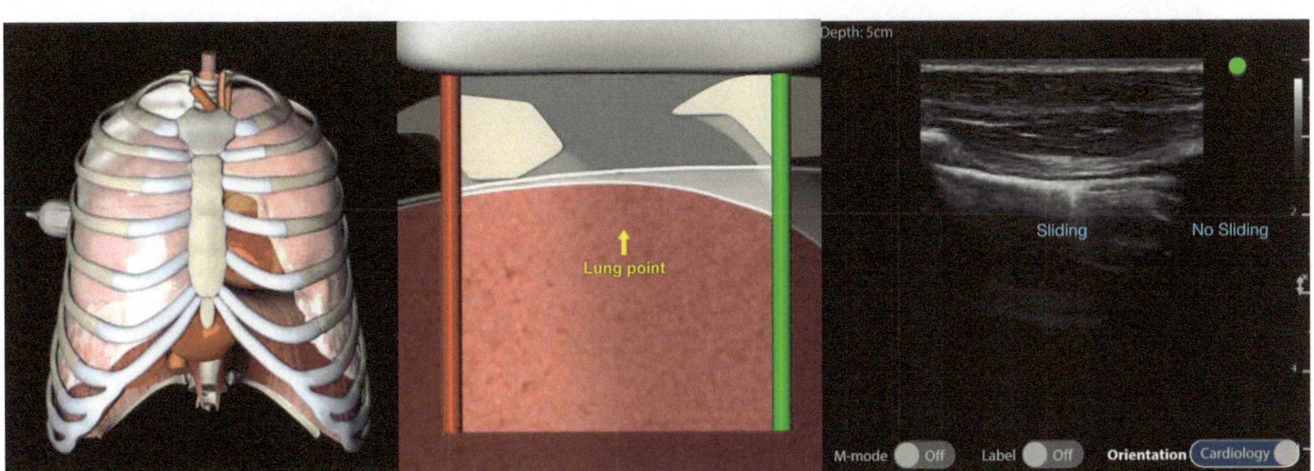

• **Fig. 54.12** Demonstration of lung point at the edge of a pneumothorax. (Modified from http://pie.med.utoronto.ca/POCUS/POCUS_content/lungUS.html.)

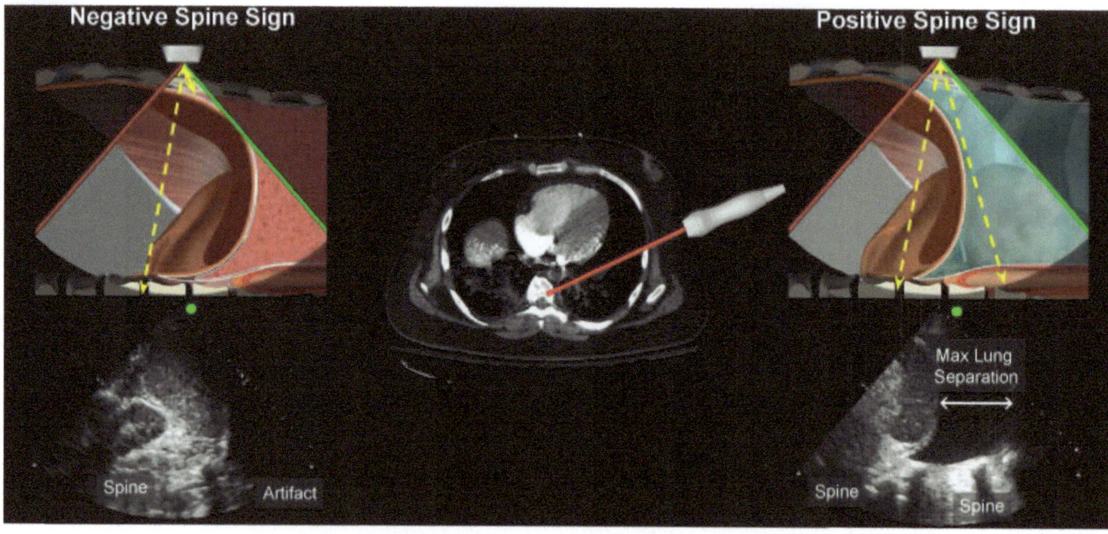

• **Fig. 54.13** Posterior costophrenic angle view and demonstration of **pleural effusion** resulting into a positive spine sign. The maximal lung separation (in cm) multiplied by 200 provides an estimate of the pleural effusion volume. (Modified from http://pie.med.utoronto.ca/POCUS/POCUS_content/lungUS.html.)

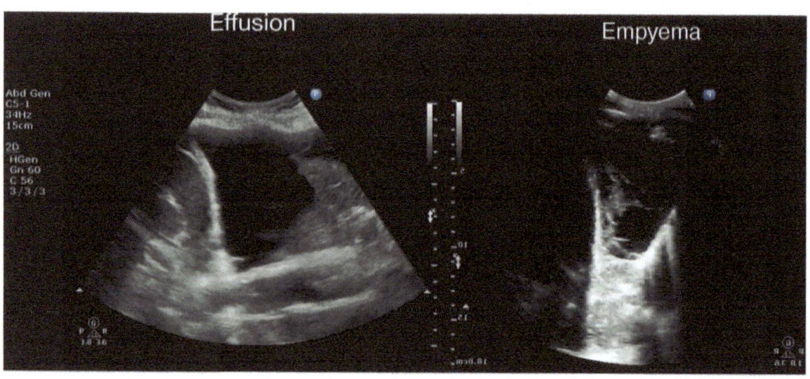

• **Fig. 54.14** A large left pleural effusion and a left pleural empyema with typical honeycomb appearance.

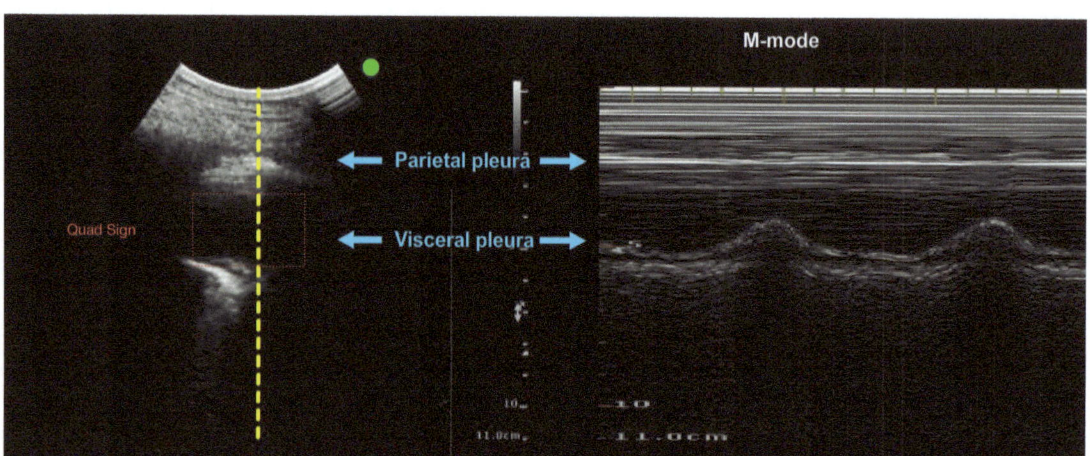

• **Fig. 54.15** The presence of pleural fluid between the visceral and parietal pleura, delimited cranially and caudally by rib shadows defines a square (quad sign); the movement of the visceral pleura toward the parietal pleural with ventilation is depicted as a sinusoid on M-mode. *M-mode*, Motion mode. (Modified from http://pie.med.utoronto.ca/POCUS/POCUS_content/lungUS.html.)

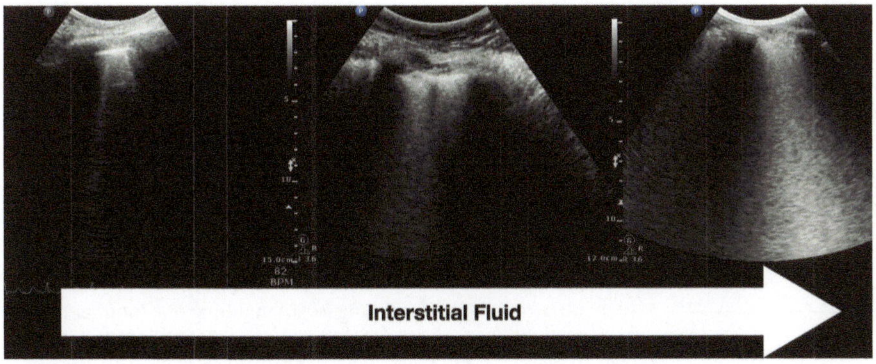

• **Fig. 54.16** Progressive increase of B lines with interstitial edema.

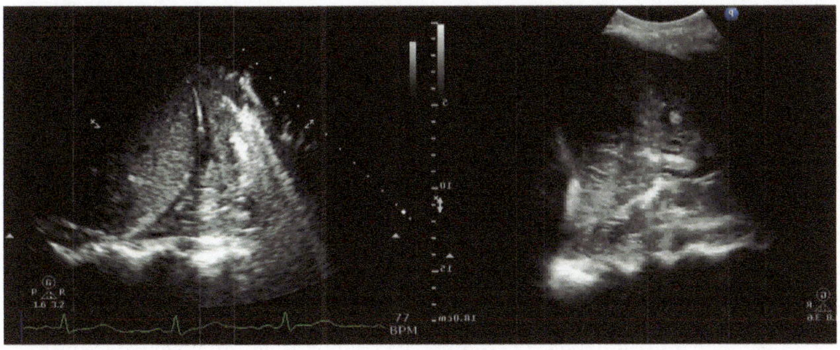

• **Fig. 54.17** One example of right lower lobe and one of left lower lobe consolidation.

A Seldinger technique would be ideal and US would safely guide needle insertion, positioning of the wire, dilatation, and advancement of the drainage.[10]

The presence of fluid between the visceral and the parietal pleura in a thoracic view create an echo-free (black) space limited laterally by the rib shadows. This is been described as a **"quad" sign**. The lung inflation results in a displacement of the visceral pleura toward the chest wall that would be depicted by M-mode as a typical sinusoid (Fig. 54.15).

Interstitial Syndrome and Lung Consolidation

As previously described, the thickening of subpleural interlobular septa results in the formation of B lines (see Fig. 54.8). These are caused by the increase in lung density, either for an increased lung weight (accumulation of fibrin, water, exudate) or decrease in air content (atelectasis).[1] B Lines are therefore nonspecific and the result of various pathologic processes that are combined under the term "interstitial syndrome".[1] The presence of three or more B lines in a single LUS view identifies a region of increased lung density. The pattern at which B lines are distributed on the chest (bilateral vs. unilateral; anterior vs. posterior) may aid differential diagnosis in cases of respiratory failure. The bedside LUS in emergency protocol combines the LUS findings in a six quadrant (anterior, lateral, and posterior) examination to nine possible phenotypes and demonstrates 95% accuracy in identifying the etiology of respiratory failure in the emergency setting.[3]

In a normal lung, the administration of crystalloids alone would result in the appearance of B lines when the patient started to be overfilled.[4] The appearance of B lines as an "ON-OFF" phenomenon has been used in the intensive care setting to guide volume administration (fluid administration limited by lung ultrasound [FALLS]).

The number of B lines is inversely related to lung aeration and has been used to quantify lung edema (Fig. 54.16).[11] It presents typically as three or more lines in a single intercostal space and progresses with a complete fusion of lines that are merged into a single broad hyperechoic artifact underlying the pleural line. LUS has been proven to detect a change in interstitial lung water as a decrease in the number of B lines as for example, after hemofiltration.[12]

When in an area of the lung the alveolar air is eliminated, the lung would appear as an echogenic consolidate parenchymal organ (like the liver). This is defined as **alveolar syndrome** and can be observed on LUS in cases of atelectasis, infective consolidations, tumors, pulmonary infarcts, and contusion. Only conditions that reach the pleura can be seen on LUS. The shape, the distribution pattern, and air-fluid bronchograms have been shown useful in determining the etiology.

In cases of infective consolidations, the presence of residual alveolar air and its movement during ventilation generates typical dynamic air bronchograms (Fig. 54.17). In the detection of lung consolidation, LUS has demonstrated a greater sensitivity and a similar sensibility to chest x-ray.[13]

Conclusion

LUS is a very powerful tool in the hands of the anesthesiologist and allows critical point of care diagnoses (such as pneumothorax) with a higher sensitivity and specificity than conventional chest x-ray. It can be performed with the available US systems and several probes. It remains operator-dependent and requires specific training. Its use must be integrated in the framework of clinical decision making to narrow diagnostic uncertainty.

References

1. Lichtenstein D, Meziere G, Biderman P, Gepner A, Barre O. The comet-tail artifact. An ultrasound sign of alveolar-interstitial syndrome. *Am J Respir Crit Care Med.* 1997;156(5):1640–1646.
2. Alrajab S, Youssef AM, Akkus NI, Caldito G. Pleural ultrasonography versus chest radiography for the diagnosis of pneumothorax: review of the literature and meta-analysis. *Crit Care.* 2013;17(5): R208.
3. Lichtenstein DA, Meziere GA. Relevance of lung ultrasound in the diagnosis of acute respiratory failure: the BLUE protocol. *Chest.* 2008;134(1):117–125.
4. Miglioranza MH, Gargani L, Sant'Anna RT, et al. Lung ultrasound for the evaluation of pulmonary congestion in outpatients: a comparison with clinical assessment, natriuretic peptides, and echocardiography. *JACC Cardiovasc Imaging.* 2013;6(11):1141–1151.
5. Volpicelli G, Elbarbary M, Blaivas M, et al. International evidence-based recommendations for point-of-care lung ultrasound. *Intensive Care Med.* 2012;38(4):577–591.
6. Sim SS, Lien WC, Chou HC, et al. Ultrasonographic lung sliding sign in confirming proper endotracheal intubation during emergency intubation. *Resuscitation.* 2012;83(3):307–312.
7. Yamaguchi Y, Moharir A, Burrier C, Tobias JD. Point-of-care lung ultrasound to evaluate lung isolation during one-lung ventilation in children: A case report. *Saudi J Anaesth.* 2019;13(3):243–245.
8. Yousefifard M, Baikpour M, Ghelichkhani P, et al. Screening performance characteristic of ultrasonography and radiography in detection of pleural effusion; a meta-analysis. *Emerg* (Tehran). 2016;4(1):1–10.
9. Zhang M, Liu ZH, Yang JX, et al. Rapid detection of pneumothorax by ultrasonography in patients with multiple trauma. *Crit Care.* 2006;10(4):R112.
10. Lichtenstein D, Hulot JS, Rabiller A, Tostivint I, Meziere G. Feasibility and safety of ultrasound-aided thoracentesis in mechanically ventilated patients. *Intensive Care Med.* 1999;25(9):955–958.
11. Via G, Lichtenstein D, Mojoli F, et al. Whole lung lavage: a unique model for ultrasound assessment of lung aeration changes. *Intensive Care Med.* 2010;36(6):999–1007.
12. Noble VE, Murray AF, Capp R, et al. Ultrasound assessment for extravascular lung water in patients undergoing hemodialysis. Time course for resolution. *Chest.* 2009;135(6):1433–1439.
13. Nazerian P, Volpicelli G, Vanni S, et al. Accuracy of lung ultrasound for the diagnosis of consolidations when compared to chest computed tomography. *Am J Emerg Med.* 2015;33(5): 620–625.

55

Transesophageal Echocardiography in Noncardiac Thoracic Surgery

BREANDAN SULLIVAN, ERIC LEIENDECKER

Introduction

The use of transesophageal echocardiography (TEE), performed by the anesthesiologist, has become commonplace in cardiac surgery operating rooms in recent years. This has been especially prominent as the use of Swan-Ganz catheters has diminished at the same time. Outside of the cardiac surgery operating room the use of TEE has, thus far, largely been reserved for cases of unexplained hypotension/hypoxia/instability or so-called "rescue TEE." However, this is changing, and more providers are electing to use TEE for hemodynamic monitoring in general surgery cases. The use of TEE in the thoracic surgery room is a natural evolution of its use in the cardiac surgery operating room because of TEE trained cardiac anesthesiologists often times providing the anesthetic for thoracic surgery patients, and the obvious interplay between the pulmonary and cardiovascular systems. In addition, as the surgical cases grow more complex and challenging, or rely on advanced therapies, such as extracorporeal membrane oxygenation (ECMO), there is an avenue to expand the use of TEE in this arena.

Thus far there is no consensus on indications for the use of TEE in thoracic surgery, save for the "rescue TEE," like there is for its use in cardiac surgery. However, practice patterns are evolving in a way that make TEE a powerful tool for guiding management of this challenging patient population.

Indications for Transesophageal Echocardiography Use

The accepted guidelines by the Society of Cardiovascular Anesthesiologists published jointly with the American Society of Echocardiographers (ASE) state that the use of TEE in noncardiac surgery is indicated for patients who have known or suspected cardiovascular pathology that may impact the outcome of the surgery. The American Society of Anesthesiologists (ASA) expands on this to state that TEE may be indicated when the patient's cardiovascular pathology may result in severe hemodynamic, pulmonary, or neurologic compromise.[1] In addition, the ASA indicates that the use of TEE is warranted in cases of unexplained life-threatening hemodynamic compromise refractory to corrective measures.[2] In cardiac surgery, the indications for TEE remain broad to include all patients undergoing open heart and in particular valvular surgeries and thoracic aortic procedures, while being indicated for select coronary artery bypass grafting (CABG) procedures. With the advent of transcatheter-based intracardiac procedures, the role of TEE has expanded to include procedural guidance during these procedures.

Beyond these, more indications for perioperative TEE are being pursued. There is growing use of TEE in the field of liver transplantation and the American Association for the Study of Liver Disease has issued a recommendation that TEE be used during orthotopic liver transplantation (OLT) to assess for the following: intracardiac chamber sizes, ventricular hypertrophy, systolic function, diastolic function, valvular function, and left ventricle (LV) outflow tract obstruction.[3] Wax et al. conducted a survey of anesthesiologists at centers performing more than 40 OLTs per year and found TEE use at least occasionally in 86% of cases and 13% of respondents use TEE for every case.[4] Furthermore, TEE findings during various phases of transplantation have been shown to be predictive of major adverse cardiac events (MACE) following surgery. For instance, the finding of intraoperative biventricular dysfunction was shown to be three times more likely than controls to suffer MACE and those with intracardiac thromboemboli were nearly five times more likely to suffer a cardiac event.[5] Most institutions that perform liver transplantation require the providers to be certified in basic TEE certification.

TEE is also used for monitoring purposes in some urologic surgeries. Recently, a published randomized controlled trial (RCT) compared TEE use during radical cystectomy to current standard of care. In that study, the authors randomized 80 patients and found that the cohort who had TEE-based monitoring received fewer central lines, had shorter durations of mechanical ventilation with fewer pulmonary complications, and showed a lower rate of cardiac arrhythmias.[6] Of course, as is the pattern nationally, one limitation of this study is that only cardiac anesthesiologists with training in advanced perioperative TEE, rather than basic, were included as the primary anesthesiologists and these results may be because of anesthesiologists selection as opposed to TEE use per se. Regardless, this highlights the search for novel uses and recognition of the value of TEE as a monitoring tool. In other urologic surgeries, such as resection of renal cell carcinoma with tumor thrombus of the inferior vena cava, TEE is used to evaluate for tumor location and extension, need for cardiopulmonary bypass, and also as a monitor for tumor embolization during the procedure.[7]

In the emergency setting, point-of-care cardiac ultrasound (US) has been widely adopted in the setting of peri- and intracardiac arrest. Systematic reviews and meta-analysis have shown US to have a high level of accuracy for identifying reversible causes and an upwards of 95% accuracy for predicting short-term survival.[8] Alternatively, the absence of cardiac activity on US is also highly predictive of the failure to achieve return of spontaneous circulation.[9] In the operating room, the so-called "rescue TEE" has been a well-established tool to evaluate refractory hemodynamic instability. This is likely caused by the high accuracy of the images obtained despite ongoing resuscitation. Diagnoses such as pericardial tamponade, pulmonary embolism (PE), aortic dissection, biventricular dysfunction, and volume status are all accurately assessed using TEE.[10] It is no surprise then that TEE during intraoperative cardiac arrests carries with it a similar benefit. This is largely because of the benefits stated previously regarding accuracy of imaging despite ongoing resuscitation.[11] Of specific benefit to TEE over transthoracic echocardiography (TTE) is that accurate image acquisition is not impeded by ongoing cardiopulmonary resuscitation and requires no interruption of chest compressions.

Despite these multiple indications, some backed up with clear evidence, there exist no randomized trials of TEE as a monitor for noncardiac thoracic surgery. Regardless, it appears that TEE can be a powerful tool in aiding both the anesthesiologist and the surgeon in managing complex patients.

Transesophageal Echocardiography as a Monitor

The ASA first directly addressed the topic of "vigilance" in a 1992 panel at the annual meeting, and this concept has evolved to make up a large portion of how the specialty is viewed.[12] This idea of vigilance in monitoring our patients in the operating room has driven countless technologic advancements seeking to allow physicians to better monitor, interpret, and respond to physiologic changes encountered (and ideally predicted) in the course of surgery. Classically, the pulmonary artery catheter (PAC) has represented the monitor of choice, though there has been growing interest in noninvasive cardiac output monitors, arterial waveform analysis, and TEE. At this time, however, the PAC remains the hemodynamic monitor most commonly used beyond the standard ASA required monitors. This use seems to persist despite lack of evidence for benefit of their use, and in at least one study potential for harm.

The goal of hemodynamic monitoring is to integrate information provided about patient variables into a plan of action that improves the outcome of the patient. In the case of PACs there has yet to be compelling evidence that supports their use in regards to improved outcomes. The Evaluation of Heart Failure and Pulmonary Artery Catheterization Effectiveness Trial (ESCAPE), published in 2005 randomized patients with heart failure to either receive a PAC to guide management or management based on clinical assessment. This study showed that patients receiving PACs were no more likely to be alive at 6 months, or did they have shorter hospitalizations.[13] This finding is congruent with multiple reports from the critical care literature showing no apparent benefit to using PACs in patient management. These studies are in agreement with the 2003 publication evaluating the use of PACs in high-risk elderly patients undergoing noncardiac surgery which showed no improvement in 6-month mortality, and showed an increased rate of PE in the treatment group. Subgroup analysis of the sampled group even showed a possible increase in mortality in the group undergoing thoracic surgery, which should lend even more scrutiny to the use of PACs in thoracic surgery.[14]

In light of this evidence showing that pulmonary artery (PA) catheters are not beneficial in managing heart failure and high-risk patients, then a natural question is "Of what benefit would echocardiography be?" This is an especially pointed question considering the large variability seen in the literature comparing PACs and TEE in one simple monitoring modality: measuring cardiac output. Su et al.[15] in 2002 did a direct comparison of esophageal Doppler and PACs in patients undergoing CABG surgery and found an excellent linear correlation between cardiac output values obtained with a PAC and that with TEE. There are retrospective studies comparing the two which showed lower levels of correlation though these have their limitations sufficient to say that with qualified users TEE can get similar values as that of PACs. More recently, there has been an emphasis on noninvasive cardiac output monitors, which appear promising. At least one group compared one device (LIDCO) to TEE and PAC during the prebypass phase of surgical aortic valve replacement for aortic stenosis and found a high degree of reliability in the device for trending cardiac output.[16] There are many more groups currently evaluating these devices and how they respond under various physiologic conditions during different phases of cardiac surgery.

Despite the results however, there is information that TEE provides the physician that a PAC or noninvasive cardiac output monitors would not provide. TEE is the only monitor that can provide instantaneous feedback about valve pathology or ventricular function. While the other monitors can provide the cardiac output, TEE has the ability to show the physician how that cardiac output is generated and if there are wall motion abnormalities or diastolic dysfunction. TEE is crucial in evaluating for pericardial disease and effusion, which goes undetected on PACs and other monitors. In addition, in the case of lung transplant TEE can provide information on the pulmonary venous anastomosis, and also indicate the function of the right ventricle (RV). In thoracic aortic surgery, TEE will evaluate for dissection and aneurysm which will of course go unnoticed on other monitors.

Clearly, there are other monitors that may provide useful information. However, the effect of these monitors (PACs) are dubious at best while some provide only very limited information (noninvasive cardiac output monitors). TEE, however, despite no RCT to validate its effect on patient outcomes, provides robust information that can help guide not only patient management by the anesthesiologist, but also surgical planning and execution with a low level of risk.

Risks of Transesophageal Echocardiography

Certainly the use of TEE carries great potential benefit, although we would be remiss if we did not speak about the potential harm of TEE use. The vast majority of the inherent risk of TEE use is related to the insertion of the echocardiogram probe into the oropharynx, around the base of the tongue, and subsequently into the esophagus. The complication that is most worrisome is direct damage to the esophagus. There are multiple reports of esophageal perforation associated with the insertion of the TEE probe. Reportedly, these most feared complications happen in 0.03% to 0.09% in large case series. The majority of these injuries (54.3%) occur in the thoracic esophagus with smaller proportions occurring in the pharyngeal or cervical regions (11.8% and 20.6%, respectively). The majority of these patients in one case series underwent repair of the perforation, though with a significant mortality of (28%) as the direct result of their injuries.[17]

Although damage to the esophagus is very worrisome, this remains a safe procedure, especially so when the patient is anesthetized in the intraoperative setting. One large case series of intraoperative TEE was done in 2001 and included over 7000 patients. These authors showed an incidence of esophageal injury of 0.01% and of upper gastrointestinal bleeding of 0.03%. In addition, they showed a low mortality rate associated with TEE of 0%. From this case series, we also see that the more common complications that arise tend to be relatively minor with odynophagia occurring in 0.1% of cases and dental injuries occurring in 0.03%.[18] More recently in 2007, Piercy et al. evaluated roughly 10,000 cardiac surgical patients and found similar rates of major complications with an incidence of about 1/1000.[19]

In light of these potential complications, which are nonzero risks, it is important to discuss safety surrounding the use of TEE and ways to avoid these potentially devastating complications. First, as with any procedure in medicine, safety begins with the physician performing a detailed history and physical exam. Largely, this interview and exam will focus on elucidating potential gastrointestinal pathology that would prevent a barrier to passing the TEE probe. A history of esophageal or stomach surgery, or a history of difficulty swallowing should raise the physician's suspicion of possible complications. If an interview elicits evidence of significant, noninvestigated, dysphagia then a barium swallow test remains the gold standard method of investigation to confirm or refute the presence of esophageal strictures or diverticula which otherwise might result in complications.[20] In addition, some attention must be given to questioning the benefit of placing the TEE probe. As discussed earlier, this can be a powerful tool that can lead in certain conditions to a change in surgical planning. However, the possibility of this must be weighed against the potential chance of causing a complication.

Safe handling of the TEE probe is a must. Once the proper screening is done, safe handling by the physician is the last line of defense in preventing a complication. Once the patient is adequately anesthetized, important as the passage of the TEE can be a strong stimulus, intubation of the esophagus can occur under direct visualization or blindly. Under direct visualization, the jaw may be thrust and tongue pulled out to expose the oropharynx through which the probe may be guided, or if done blindly one hand may insert the probe while the other guides it along the back of the tongue and into the esophagus. Occasionally, there is difficulty in passing the TEE probe necessitating direct laryngoscopy to expose the esophagus through which the probe may be inserted. In small patients or those with dysphagia, one consideration would be the use of a pediatric TEE probe, as this has a smaller bore and theoretically is less likely to cause trauma. The probe should be lubricated to reduce friction and an inserted probe should always be unlocked and in a neutral position when inserted or removed (Fig. 55.1).

Intraoperative Hemodynamic Exam

TEE is the only monitor that can provide real-time, immediate assessment of biventricular function, valve function, volume status, wall motion, or presence of effusion. To obtain all requisite information, the standard 28 views should be the minimum exam performed.[1] Although these guidelines recommend views obtained, they do not indicate timing of the examination or how often it should be repeated. In addition, there is no current recommendation for how TEE should be used for ongoing monitoring following the completion of the initial exam. It seems reasonable to continue to monitor ventricular function looking for alterations in wall motion, global function, and filling (Table 55.1).

Following the exam, the probe may be left in the mid-esophageal four-chamber (ME-4C) position as a monitor. This will provide real-time evaluation of biventricular function, which may change dramatically during periods of thoracic surgery. One-lung ventilation or selective clamping of the pulmonary artery (PA) may severely increase the

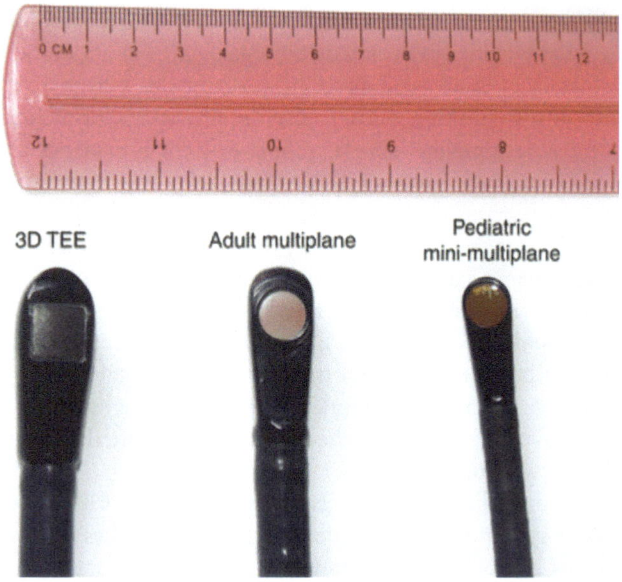

• **Fig. 55.1** Comparison of adult and pediatric transesophageal echocardiography probes with ruler for reference. *3D*, Three-dimensional; *TEE*, transesophageal echocardiography. (From Hui L, Sahn DJ. Instrumentation for transesophageal echocardiography. In: Wong P, Miller-Hance W (eds). *Transesophageal Echocardiography for Congenital Heart Disease*. Springer: London; 2014:Fig. 2.11.)

afterload on the RV, causing dysfunction. Clamping of the atrial cuff to perform anastomoses may result in coronary occlusion and regional wall motion abnormalities. All of these complications can be readily observed on TEE of basic examination images (Fig. 55.2).

Transesophageal Echocardiography Assessment of the Right Ventricle

In his 1821 work "A Treatise on Diseases of the Chest" RT Laennec pontificates that "All diseases which give rise to severe and long-continued dyspnœa produced, almost necessarily, hypertrophia or dilatation of the heart, through the constant efforts the organ is called on to perform, to propel the blood into the lungs against the resistance opposed to it by the cause of the dyspnœa."[21] Suffice to say that this physiology certainly has not changed in the nearly 200 years following his publication. Luckily, we have learned more about this physiology and the effect it has on the patient and their life. It is relatively common knowledge that pulmonary hypertension (PH) can accompany and mirror the development of severe pulmonary disease. In one series of patients undergoing workup for lung transplantation, 49% were found on right heart catheterization to have mean pulmonary artery pressure (MPAP) of at least 25 mm Hg, after eliminating those with postcapillary PH, the authors concluded that 36% of their cohort had precapillary PH. In addition, these same patients tended to have lower fraction of expiratory volume in 1 second values and higher rates of hypoxemia with lower 6-minute walk test performances. In other words, in more progressive disease, there is elevation of PAPs.[22] The reason for this rise in PAP is likely multifactorial, resulting from a combination of hypoxia, hypercapnea, and parenchymal damage leading to loss of pulmonary vessels.[23] Patients with interstitial lung disease (ILD) display a similar relationship between PH and severity of pulmonary disease, albeit with greater variability. Similar to chronic obstructive pulmonary disease (COPD), PH resulting from ILD carries a significant reduction in life expectancy urging some authors to conclude that these patients should be promptly listed for transplantation.[24]

Regardless of the etiology, this increase in RV afterload can result in varying degrees of dysfunction of the RV. Predominantly, this effect takes the form of hypertrophy of the RV with preserved systolic function, largely attributable to the slow rise in PA pressures allowing the RV to remodel. In fact, up to two-thirds of patients with COPD have evidence of this RV remodeling on autopsy.[25] Hilde and partners in 2013 showed compelling evidence that even minimal elevations of pulmonary vascular resistance and MPAP resulted in RV remodeling, dilation, and subsequently reduced RV systolic function. In addition, these investigators showed a distinct relationship between MPAP and worsening RV performance indices.[26]

Anatomically, the RV differs from the LV in its shape and structure. Instead of a thick-walled, round structure, the RV is a thin-walled conical structure that wraps around the LV septum. This structure can functionally be divided into three parts. **The inlet** is bordered by the tricuspid annulus, the chordae and the associated papillary muscles, **the apex** is made of heavily trabeculated muscle and **the outlet** which

TABLE 55.1 Intraoperative Hemodynamic Assessment can Place Patients Into Specific Profiles, the Management of Which Will Differ

Hemodynamic Assessment	Left Ventricular Contractility	Filling (Left Ventricular End-Diastolic Volume)	Diastolic Function	Right Ventricular Contractility
Normal	Normal	Normal	Normal	Normal
Left ventricular failure	Decreased	Increased	Normal or decreased	Normal
Vasoplegia	Increased or normal	Normal or decreased	Normal	Normal
Hypovolemia	Normal or increased	Decreased	Normal	Normal
Right ventricular failure	Normal	Decreased	Normal	Decreased

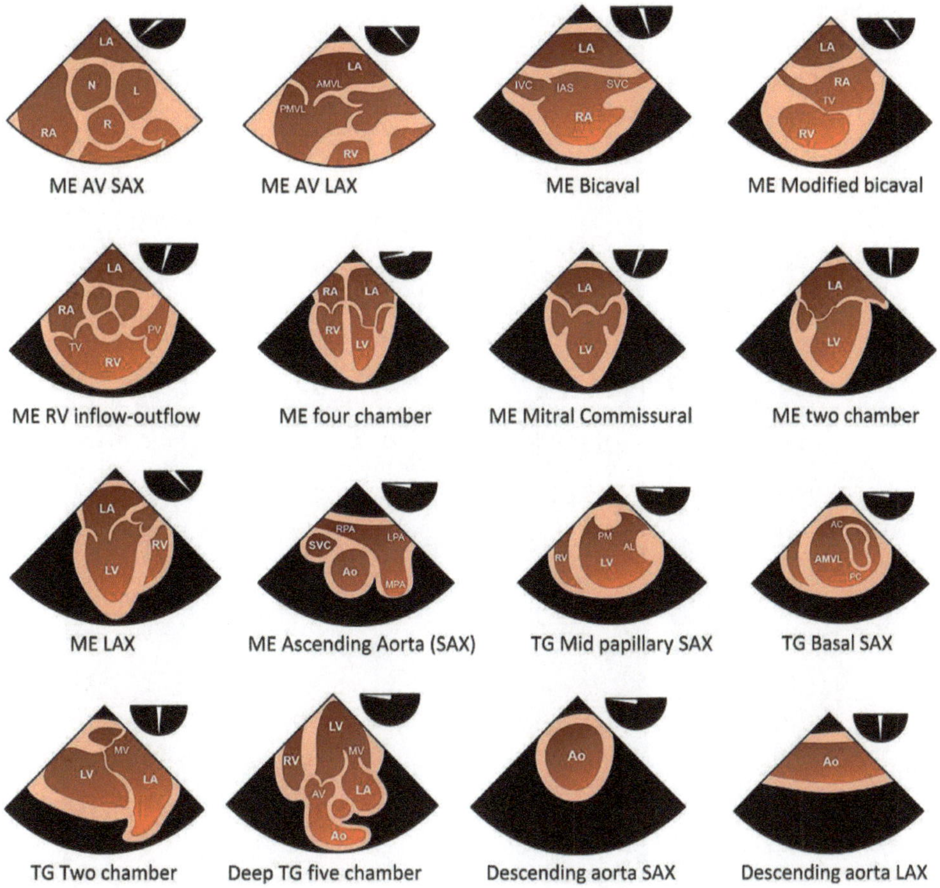

• **Fig. 55.2** Cross-sectional images of the suggested 16 views (approximate angle is indicated top right) of the transesophageal echocardiography. *AMVL,* anterior mitral valve leaflet; *Ao,* aorta; *AV,* aortic valve; *IAS,* intra-atrial septum; *IVC,* inferior vena cava; *L,* left coronary cusp; *LA,* left atrium; *LAX,* long axis; *LPA,* left pulmonary artery; *LV,* left ventricle; *ME,* mid-esophageal; *MPA,* main pulmonary artery; *MV,* mitral valve; *N,* non-coronary cusp; *PM & AL,* posteromedial and anterolateral papillary muscles; *PMVL,* posterior mitral valve leaflet; *R,* right coronary cusp; *RA,* right atrium; *RPA,* right pulmonary artery; *RV,* right ventricle; *SAX,* short axis; *SVC,* superior vena cava; *TG,* transgastric; *TV,* tricuspid valve. (From Fayad A, et al: Perioperative transesophageal echocardiography for non-cardiac surgery. Can J Anaesth. 2018 April; 65(4): 381–398.)

is essentially the smooth muscle RV outflow tract (RVOT). The function of the RV is largely dependent on systemic venous return providing preload and resistance of the balance between the pulmonary vessels providing RV afterload. These forces combine with the intrinsic contractility of the RV free wall and interventricular septum to generate RV output. RV stroke work requires much less work compared with the LV, as is evident from the pressure volume loops of the RV. These loops display a lack of isovolumetric contraction and show lower peak systolic pressures as well as simply existing at higher baseline volume levels.[27] This makes the RV relatively sensitive to physiologic perturbations.

To adequately evaluate the RV, the physician must obtain multiple views of this chamber to perform Doppler measurements, as well as anatomic measurements. These views are best obtained in the ME-4C, mid-esophageal RV inflow-outflow (MERV in-out), transgastric short axis (TG-SAX), and the transgastric RV inflow-outflow (TGRV in-out) (Fig. 55.3).

From the ME-4C view a good assessment of RV function and size can be made. In this view the RV and LV are clearly observed and the relationship of one chamber to the other can be seen. In the ME-4C view, it is easy to obtain quantification of the end-diastolic area (EDA), as well as the end-systolic area (ESA). The fractional area of change (FAC) is then defined as: (RVEDA-RVESA/RVEDA)×100. These areas are obtained by pausing the frame at the requisite point in the cardiac cycle, taking care to ensure the RV is not foreshortened and includes the apex. It is then possible to trace to RV chamber, including the trabeculae.[28] The normal value for an RV FAC is at least 35% with values under this being indicative of varying degrees of right ventricular systolic dysfunction. One limitation of this method is the likely exclusion of the RVOT which contributes at least something to the RV systolic function. The benefit, however, is that this method takes into account both longitudinal, as well as free wall contraction, thus ensuring that FAC correlates well with ejection fraction (EF) elucidated through magnetic resonance imaging (MRI).[29,30]

Also from the ME-4C view it is possible to assess RV size and shape, and relationship to the LV. The RV should appear more wedge-like as opposed to the rounded LV, with its size being roughly two-thirds that of the LV. The dilated RV will make up progressively more of the apex of the heart, as well as approach the same size as the LV. At end diastole, the areas of the two chambers are easily measured and any RV:LV ratio over 1 indicates severe dilation. As the RV dilates and becomes overloaded with pressure and/or volume, the interventricular septum shifts leftward and in the TG-SAX view will appear flattened with the LV appearing D-shaped. This shift results in two detrimental effects resulting in decreased cardiac output. First, the shift of the septum into the LV decreases this chamber size, reducing the LV end diastolic volume (LVEDV) and thus stroke volume. Second, the shift of the intraventricular septum reduces the contractility of the septum, a force that the RV depends on for its systolic performance.[30]

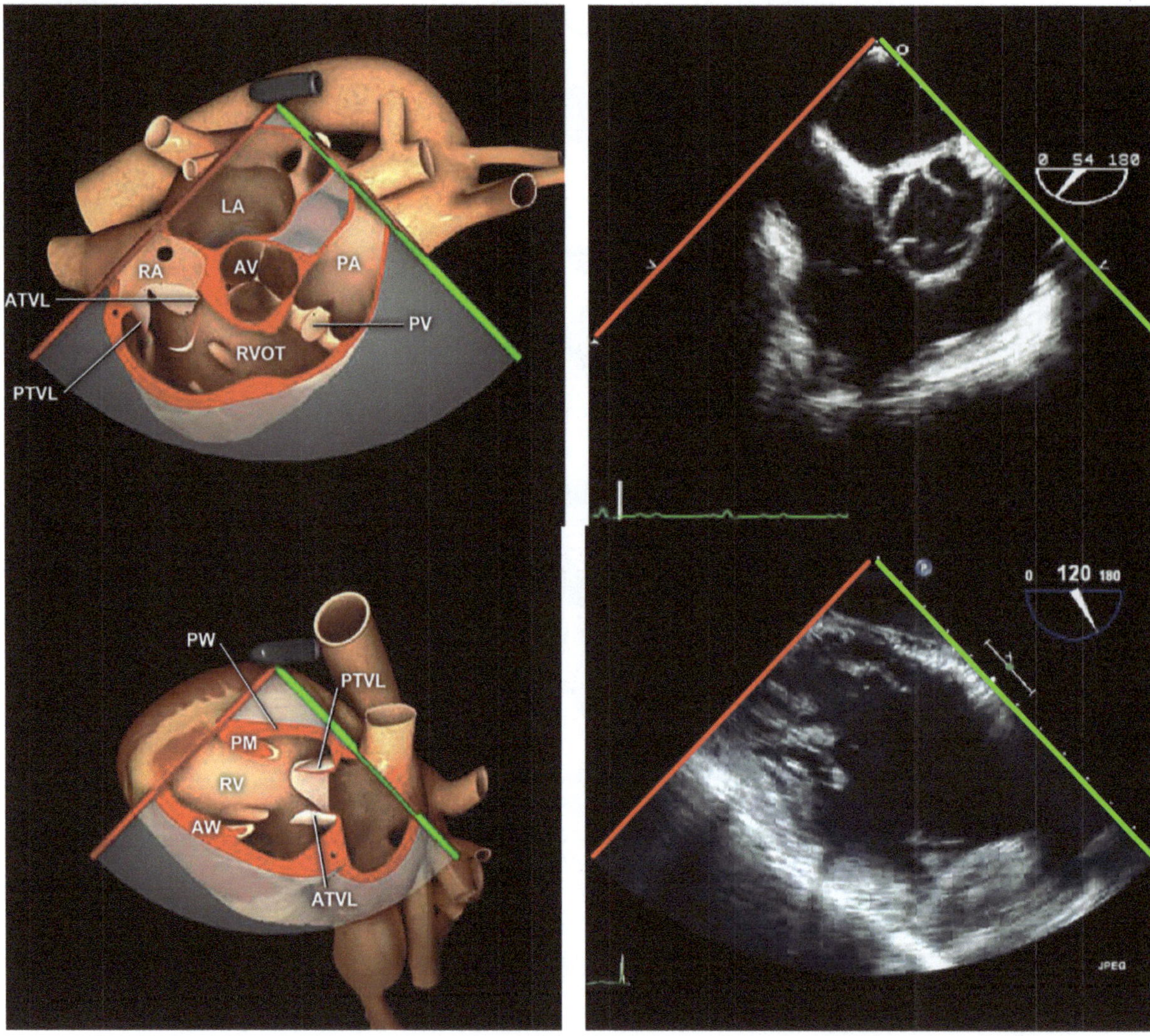

• **Fig. 55.3** The midesophageal right ventricular (*RV*) inflow-outflow and the transgastric RV inflow view that will be used in the tricuspid annular plane systolic excursion and RVs measurements. *ATML*, anterior valve leaflet; *AV*, aortic valve; *AW*, anterior wall; *LA*, left atrium; *PA*, pulmonary artery; *PTVL*, posterior valve leaflet; *PW*, pericardial wall; *RA*, right atrium; *RV*, right ventricle; *RVOT*, right ventricular outflow tract. (Reproduced with permission from http://pie.med.utoronto.ca/tee.)

Also in the ME-4C view, many physicians will attempt to measure the systolic excursion of the tricuspid valve (TV), otherwise referred to as tricuspid annular plane systolic excursion (TAPSE). This has a been a long validated method for assessing RV function in the TTE, though it has been thought to be somewhat limited in the TEE because of its dependence on obtaining a view in which the motion mode (MMode) Doppler beam could be in good alignment with the TV motion. However, there are some ways to overcome this perceived limitation and obtain a reliable TAPSE measurement.[31] Some physicians choose to make up for the poor alignment in postprocessing of the images and conducting nonlabeled measurements of the distance the tricuspid annulus moves in the cardiac cycle. Although onerous, this is one method to compensate for poor Doppler alignment. On modern machines, there is an adaptation of the traditional MMode called "anatomic MMode" corrects transducer position relative to the plane being measured. Korshin and colleagues in 2018 found that when in the TGRV in-out, anatomic MMode gave high precision and reproducibility with strong correlation to the TAPSE measured on TTE. The same method certainly can be used in the ME-4C view though with lower agreement with that of TTE.[32] Although the TAPSE is widely accepted as a marker of RV performance, it is important to note how specific disease states, that are especially relevant in thoracic surgery, can influence the prognostic and clinical effect of the TAPSE measurement. Multiple investigators have shown that TAPSE correlates with survival in patients with congestive heart failure (CHF), with one series of over 1500 patients showing a cutoff of 15.9 mm, which means that in patients with CHF who have a TAPSE of less than 15.9 mm, there is poorer prognosis than those with a higher TAPSE value. Follow-up work has demonstrated that lower TAPSE values correlate with an increase in hospitalization rates and morbidity as well. In patients with COPD, the

TABLE 55.2 These Methods of Right Ventricular Evaluation can Give Information Regarding the Performance of the Right Ventricle

Measure	Measurement	Normal Value
Tricuspid annular plane systolic excursion 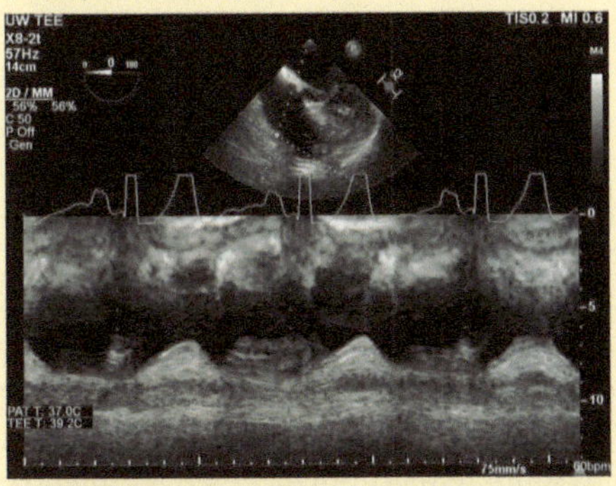	Measured in motion mode as distance between nadir and peak travel of lateral annulus of tidal volume	>1.6 cm
Fractional area of change 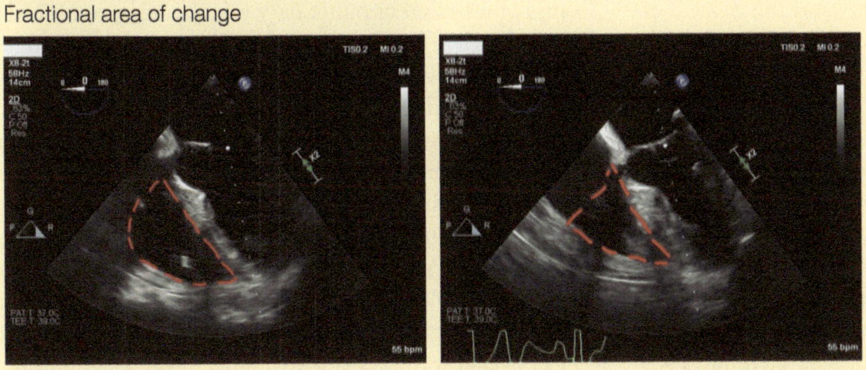 A B	((EDA – ESA)/ EDA) × 100	>35%
Longitudinal strain 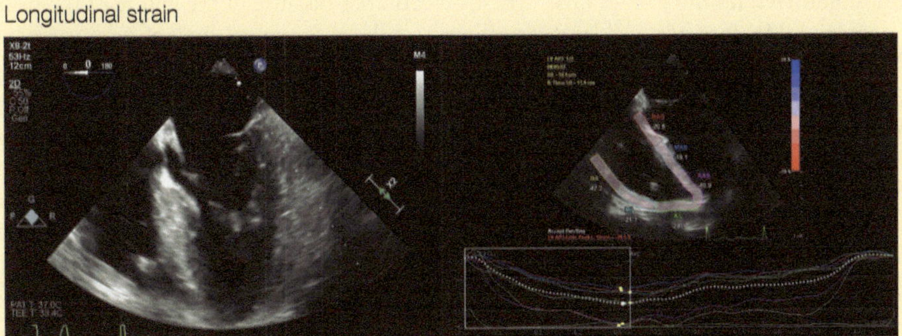	(Length in Systole – Length in Diastole)/ Length in Diastole)	More negative than –20

EDA, End-diastolic area; *ESA*, end-systolic area.

TAPSE has also been shown to correlate with poorer prognosis and higher morbidity as well (Table 55.2).[33]

While in the ME-4C view, the physician can focus on the RV by moving it to the center of the field and ensuring to limit foreshortening as much as possible. Most new TEE machines are capable of directly measuring the contraction of myocardial muscle fibers by measuring the displacement of these muscle speckles through the cardiac cycle. By doing so, it is possible to accurately quantify the longitudinal contraction as it happens from the TV annulus to the infundibulum (or RVOT). Although an in-depth discussion of this technology is well beyond the capacity of this chapter, we will briefly review it. What are termed "speckles" are actually specific patterns of interference within the myocardium, these "speckles" are then able to be tracked over time to create a measurement of strain (strain = [length in systole − length in diastole]/length in diastole). Thus as the RV free wall contracts longitudinally from the TV annulus to infundibulum. Given this, the strain measurement will be reported as a negative value with a cutoff of −20 or more negative being normal. Values less negative than −20 are considered abnormal. Two measurements of the RV can be obtained using this technique: global longitudinal strain (GLS) and free wall strain (FWS). Although both measures give a measure of longitudinal contraction, the GLS is the average value of all RV segments (3 free wall + the septum), whereas the FWS ignores the septal contribution. This technique is not angle dependent as in TAPSE; however, there is limitation when out of plane contraction is happening. This can be ameliorated by using new three-dimensional (3D) software that will measure "strain area" as opposed to longitudinal strain.[34]

The application of 3D technology to imaging the RV is relatively new, at least in the intraoperative setting. As with many RV measurements, there was concern about reproducibility and accuracy compared with TTE or MRI when extrapolating to the TEE and intraoperative setting. However, this has proven to be a valuable tool for evaluating the RV for both size and function. Fusini et al. reported a case series of 150 patients undergoing valve procedures in which the authors acquired 3D volumetric sets, which were then analyzed for RV end-systolic volume (ESV), RV end-diastolic volume (EDV), and RVEF, as well as two-dimensional (2D) measurements of FAC and TAPSE. Adequate data were acquired in 92.7% of patients and the 3D EF of these patients displayed high levels of correlation with both 2D FAC, as well as TAPSE, both of which have previously been validated compared to MRI.[35] Subsequent work has confirmed not only the feasibility of acquiring 3D data of the RV, but also the reproducibility between observers. In addition, these data sets were again found to correlate well with 2D, TTE, and MRI measurements of RV function.[36]

As the RV dilates, there is outward force applied to the TV annulus. This force changes the ellipsoid TV into a more round shape, which results in the leaflets being pulled apart leading to poor coaptation and tricuspid regurgitation (TR). It is not uncommon to see this sequence evolve acutely from pressure overload, as happens in PE, resulting in even minimal elevations of MPAP. Importantly, the degree of TR does not necessarily correlate with the degree of RV dysfunction. As the RV dilates and the function decreases the force generated will be lessened leading to a reduction in TR velocity and jet size, making this a relatively poor marker of RV performance.[37,38]

Patent Foramen Ovale

Although generally benign, patent foramen ovale (PFO) has been implicated in stroke and hypoxemia. Under normal loading conditions, the LA pressure exceeds that of the RA, creating a left to right shunt. With the rare exception, this is generally very well tolerated and inconsequential. With elevated right atrial (RA) pressure, there exists the possibility to reverse this intracardiac shunt from the RA through the PFO into the left atrium (LA). In **the case of stroke**, there are several mechanisms by which PFO is thought to be implicated. First, the PFO may serve as the path of least resistance with right to left shunting and this flow may carry with it embolic material, such as microemboli, air, or thrombus. Second, in a certain portion of patients, the PFO is associated with atrial septum aneurysm which may serve as the nidus for thrombus formation. These septal aneurysms are rare in the general population; however, they are reported on autopsy in a disproportionately high portion of patients who suffered stroke. Although somewhat peripherally related, PFO may predispose patients to atrial arrhythmias which in of themselves raise the risk of stroke.[39] Regardless of the mechanism, stroke can be a potentially devastating complication of noncardiac surgery. Unfortunately, this complication is much more prevalent in patients with preexisting atrial septal defect (ASD) or PFO. In one case series of over 600,000 noncardiac surgeries in patients who had preoperative echocardiograms, roughly 9000 patients were found to have a PFO or ASD. Over 40,000 strokes occurred perioperatively; however, 35% of those with a preexisting PFO/ASD suffered stroke compared with 6% of those with intact atrial septums.[40]

Another possible outcome of a PFO and the creation of a right to left shunt is **hypoxia.** Through this shunt, venous blood can mix with arterial blood, leading to a hypoxemic mixture. This is in turn can result in PH.[41] This mechanism has been implicated in some postthoracic surgery patients who develop hypoxia. Likely, this shunt results from increased RV afterload because of resection of pulmonary vascular beds, combined with some degree of fluid overload during surgery which can reduce RV function. These factors increase right-sided filling pressures creating the left to right shunt that contributes to hypoxia.[42] In addition, intraoperatively, the RA pressure may acutely increase as a result of one-lung ventilation induced hypercarbia raising PAP, or following clamping of the PAs.

As stated previously, a PFO is a generally irrelevant condition that is present in varying rates depending on age. In their work from 1984, Hagen and colleagues examined the hearts of 965 patients on autopsy. They found that the incidence of PFO overall was 27.3% with a range from 34.3% in the first 3 decades of life to 20.2% in the ninth and 13th decade of life.[43] These defects arise because of the failure of the primum and secundum to adhere, leaving a small passageway between the two chambers. Immediately after birth, the orifice in the muscular septum primum is covered by the mobile, more fibrous, septum secundum, and the sudden rise of LA pressure should force the two septal components against one another, allowing fusion over subsequent years. TEE with agitated saline performs well in detecting these lesions with sensitivity approaching 90% and specificity of roughly 91%.[44]

An examination intended to investigate for the presence of PFO will begin in the ME-4C view, however, 2D evaluation is unlikely to display a visually detectable PFO. The addition of color flow Doppler with the Nyquist limit of between 45 and 55cm/s will allow the physician to see evidence of flow across the septum, indicating shunting. To fully evaluate the septum for integrity, it must scan through the septum by increasing the omniplane from 0 to 130 degrees to ensure visualization of the entire structure. Ultimately, the highest sensitivity is obtained by the addition of contrast; in this setting this would be the addition of agitated saline to perform a "bubble study." Under normal loading conditions, LA pressure is greater than RA pressure, which would prevent transit through an atrial septal defect if one existed. To overcome this, a Valsalva maneuver should be applied during injection of the agitated saline, the sudden release of the Valsalva will acutely raise the preload on the RA thus increasing the RA pressure. If a PFO exists, bubbles will be seen traversing the septum and appearing in the LA.

The decision on whether or not to close an intraoperatively identified PFO is somewhat unclear at this point. Largely, there is a paucity of data examining whether to close these defects when incidentally found during surgery, and even less data indicating the preferred method of closure. The clinical significance of these PFOs is unclear and the decision of whether or not to close them appears to be dependent on surgeon preference, probability of hypoxia, and whether or not there will be a deviation in the surgical plan to accomplish this closure.[45] Those patients whose atria were already opened, mitral valve (MV) or TV repairs, and those who were younger or with prior history of stroke/transient ischemic attack were most likely to have their PFO repaired. However, there is some evidence that stroke rates increased following the repair of incidentally found PFOs.[46] This is in contrast to closure of PFOs found in patients having cryptogenic strokes. In this patient population, percutaneous closure of the septal defect has led to a lower rate of recurrent strokes when compared to those who only received medical therapy.[47]

In summary, PFO are common defects that may increase the risk of stroke in the population, though closing incidentally found PFOs appear not to reduce this risk. Intraoperatively, PFO or ASD may result in right to left shunting as the RV loading conditions change which may result in hypoxia (Fig. 55.4).

Transesophageal Echocardiography Assessment of the Left Ventricle

Intraoperative examination of LV function can provide many insights into the hemodynamic variability encountered during surgery. The basic examination should evaluate the LV for preload, global systolic function, regional systolic function, and diastolic function. To make this basic assessment, three standard views should be obtained: TG-SAX, ME-4C, and ME-2C. Getting these views will allow evaluation of all ventricle wall segments and coronary artery perfusion areas, as well as the ability to qualify diastolic function. One framework for evaluating the LV in a hemodynamic assessment would be as follows: first, evaluate preload status; second, quantify systolic function; third, estimate filling pressure; fourth, integrate these findings into a final assessment of hemodynamic status (Fig. 55.5).

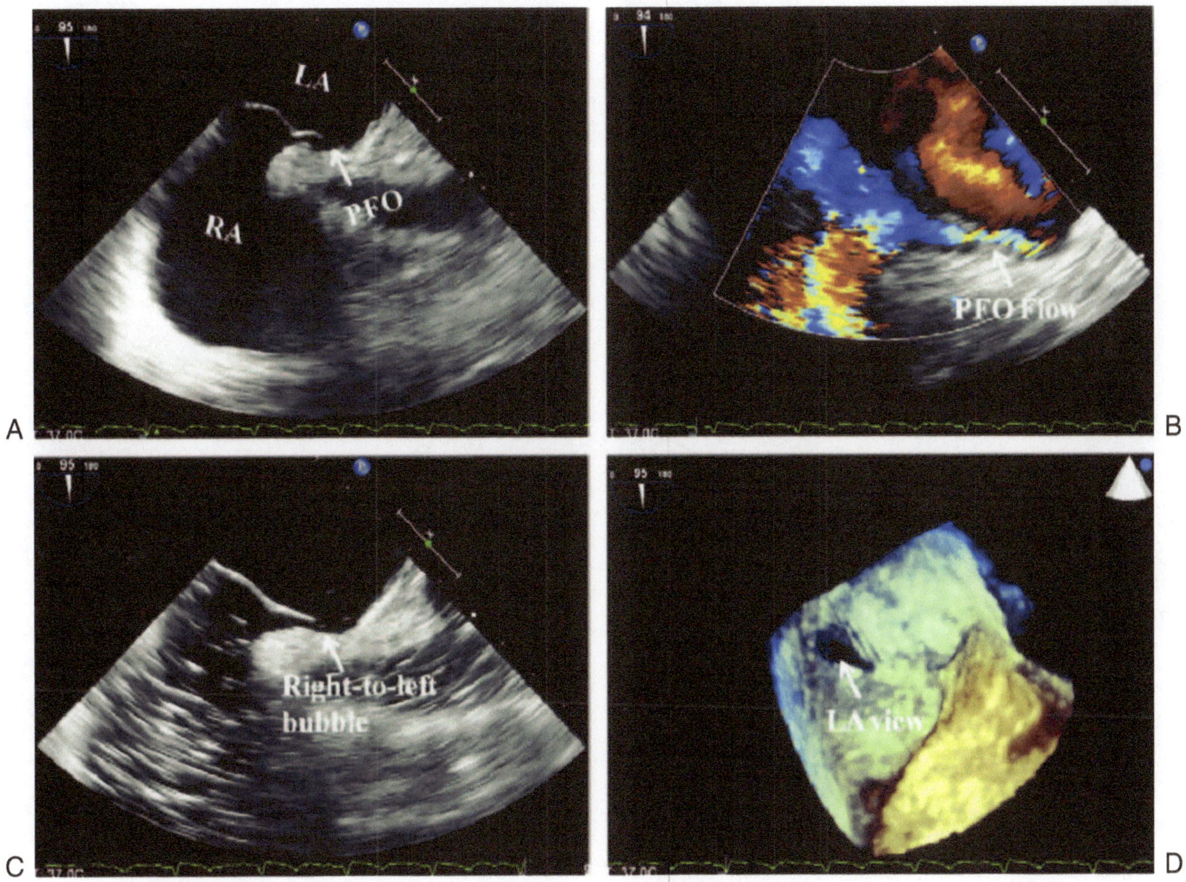

• **Fig. 55.4** **A:** Two-dimensional imaging reveals the interatrial septum (IAS) with possible defect, **B:** color flow Doppler (CFD) confirms this defect and can show directionality of the shunt. **C:** An agitated saline study can readily show right to left shunting as the bubbles traverse the IAS quick than if they had cycled through the body first. **D:** Finally, three-dimensional imaging can provide highly resolute images of the defect. *LA,* left atrium; *PFO,* patent foramen ovale; *RA,* right atrium. (From Chen Z, Li C, Li Y, Tang H, Rao Li, Wang M. Concomitant coronary and pulmonary embolism associated with patent foramen ovale: a case report. *Medicine.* 2017;96; E9480.)

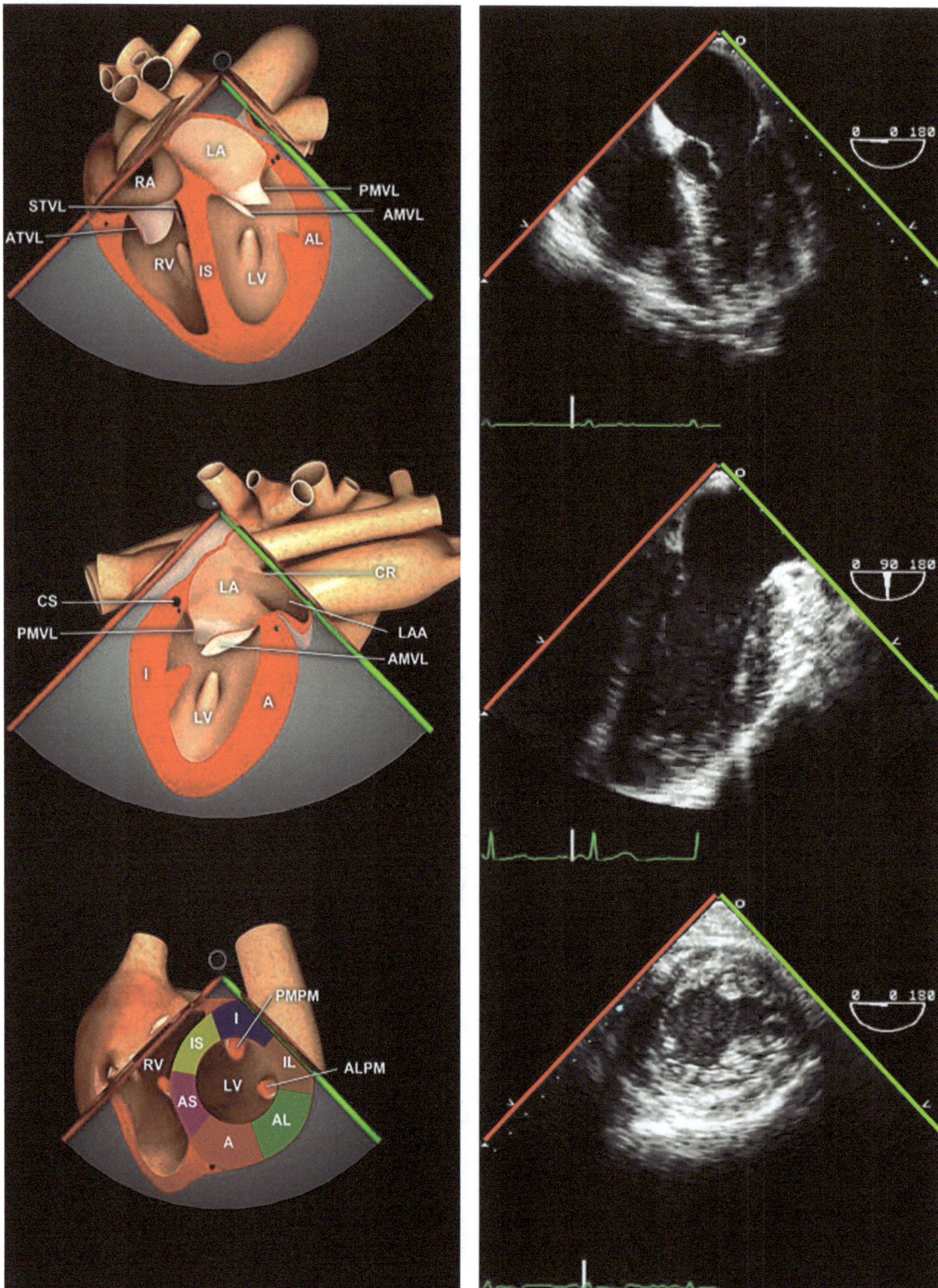

• **Fig. 55.5** Evaluation of left ventricular systolic function requires imaging of all ventricular wall segments. By obtaining mid-esophageal four chamber, mid-esophageal two chamber, and transgastric short axis this is easily accomplished. *A,* anterior; *AL,* anterolateral; *AS,* anteroseptal; *ATVL,* anterior tricuspic valve leaflet; *CR,* coonary sinus; *I,* inferior; *IL,* infrolateral; *IS,* interseptal; *LAA,* left atrial appendage; *STVL,* septal tircuspic valve leaflet. (Reproduced with permission from http://pie.med.utoronto.ca/tee.)

To **evaluate for preload of the LV**, there must be measurement of the LVEDV. Previously, LVEDV or preload would have been extrapolated from the pulmonary capillary wedge pressure (PCWP). However, it is common now to directly measure LVEDV visually on TEE and this has supplanted PCWP as the preferred, and validated, method of preload measurement.[48,49] Likely the most rudimentary method for estimating LVEDV is by using MMode. In the TG-SAX, the MMode Doppler beam can be directed through the inferior and anterior walls. Using the beginning of the QRS complex or the closure of the MV as a marker of end diastole, it is then easy to measure the LV end-diastolic dimension (LVEDD). The normal LVEDD is considered to be 3.0 to 5.6 cm with smaller than 3 cm representing an underfilled LV with a dilated LV being greater than 5.6 cm. In this same view, an LV end diastolic area (LVEDA) can also be obtained by tracing the endocardial border in end diastole. Although this is easy to perform, it must be noted that as with all echo quantification, using one single measurement is fraught with error. For example, if there is a significant wall motion abnormality, then the LVEDD may be falsely elevated, leading to the erroneous conclusion of high existing preload. Conversely, a ventricle that completely empties and continues to have a low LVEDV is likely representative of low preload.

Whereas these measure 2D areas and act as a surrogate for the LVEDV, it is possible to obtain reasonable estimates of the volume using **Simpson's method of disks**. In this method, the operator will obtain an optimal ME-4C with the LV in the center of the screen. Freezing the frame at end diastole allows the endocardial border to be highlighted. The internal chamber of the ventricle is then approximated using 20 ellipsoid stacked disks. Combining this with the same process in the ME-2C view allows for accurate quantification of ventricular volumes at both end diastole and end systole. This method has been compared with MRI imaging and found to be reliable, although with the caveat that the image must not be foreshortened and the inherent assumption of an ellipsoid LV chamber.[50]

In regards to **systolic function**, it is possible to estimate both EF, as well as strain of the LV. EF is simply the stroke volume divided by the EDV, giving a percentage of blood ejected with each contraction ([LVEDV-LVESV]/LVEDV). Of course with most TEE applications, these calculations will have to be based on 2D images. In the TG-SAX, one measure of LVEF can be obtained using FAC. This is essentially the change in chamber area expressed as a percentage. In the end diastole frame, the endocardial border is traced, yielding an area which is then used to calculate a percentage change. Normal values of the FAC are considered greater than 55%. Obviously, this is simply measuring the area of the LV chamber at a very specific location and ignoring the contribution of other areas of the ventricle, which lends itself to error (Fig. 55.6).

A more comprehensive and accurate estimation may be made using the aforementioned method of disks. In this method, the LV is imaged in both the ME-4C and ME-2C views, the volumes at diastole and systole are then estimated by tracing the endocardial border, which is then "filled" with 20 ellipsoid disks to approximate the chamber volume. Imaging in two planes, and imaging the entire ventricle helps to improve precision beyond that seen with the FAC method. However, it is important to recognize that, as with FAC, the method of disks again relies on extrapolating a 3D volume from the 2D image and is thus prone to error. Most commonly, this error is related to foreshortening and errors imaging the apex. One way to overcome these limitations is to apply 3D technology to imaging the LV which has been shown to be comparable to MRI.[51] Once an adequate 2D image of the LV is obtained in the ME-4C, a biplane view is created adding the ME-2C view, then using a multibeat image capture, an accurate 3D model is created. The benefit of this is the ability to enter into these clips and alter the orientation of the image to ensure the avoidance of foreshortening. The endocardium is then, oftentimes, detected automatically and ventricular volumes and EF are obtained with good accuracy and reproducibility (Fig. 55.7).[52]

One theoretical benefit of using PA catheters for monitoring before the advent of TEE was the ability to calculate

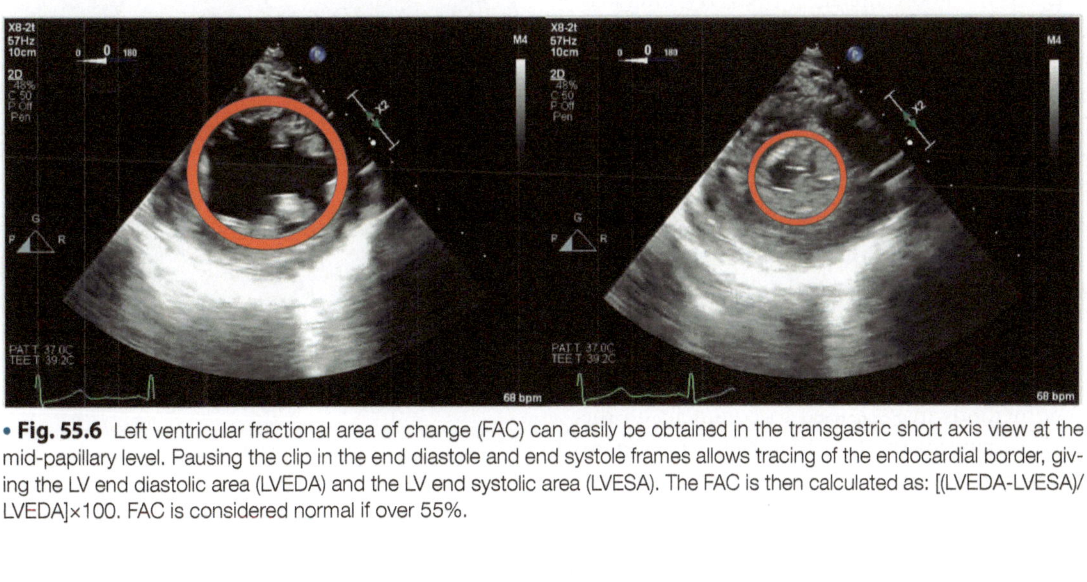

• **Fig. 55.6** Left ventricular fractional area of change (FAC) can easily be obtained in the transgastric short axis view at the mid-papillary level. Pausing the clip in the end diastole and end systole frames allows tracing of the endocardial border, giving the LV end diastolic area (LVEDA) and the LV end systolic area (LVESA). The FAC is then calculated as: [(LVEDA-LVESA)/LVEDA]×100. FAC is considered normal if over 55%.

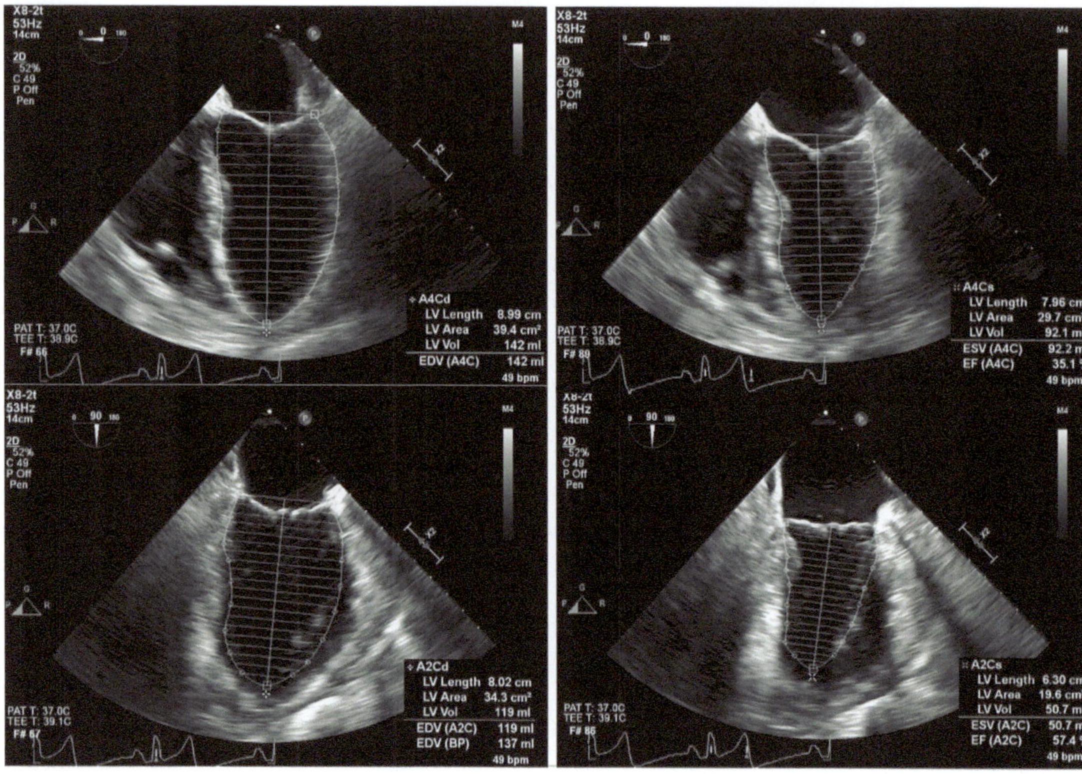

• **Fig. 55.7** Simpson's method of disks is used to obtain accurate left ventricular ejection fraction (LVEF) measurements. This method requires obtaining clips of the mid-esophageal four- and two-chamber views. The clips are then paused at end diastole and end systole, where the endocardial border is traced. The ultrasound (US) machine then places 20 "disks" in this area to calculate LV end diastolic and systolic volumes (LVEDV and LVESV). EF then is calculated by the US software. LVEF is considered normal if over 55%.

stroke volume and cardiac output intraoperatively. However, this is now information that is able to be acquired directly with TEE in a number of ways. As mentioned previously, stroke volume is able to be calculated during the calculation of the LVEF. This is possible in both the 2D, as well as the 3D modality. A somewhat less labor intensive method for estimating stroke volume involves obtaining both the LVOT area and the velocity time integral (VTI) of the LVOT and thus calculating the volume blood passing through the LVOT with each contraction. The LVOT area is obtained in the mid-esophageal (ME) AV long-axis view where the diameter may be obtained in mid-systole and then used to calculate the LVOT area. The VTI, essentially how far a column of blood moves in a unit time, is obtained in the deep TG view where pulsed wave Doppler (PWD) is placed in the LVOT. This view is optimal because of the alignment of the Doppler beam with the LVOT and path of blood flow being optimal, thus having a lower error. The stroke volume, and thus ultimately the cardiac output, may then be calculated as stroke volume = (LVOT diameter)×(LVOT VTI), with cardiac output obtained by simply multiplying the stroke volume by the heart rate (Fig. 55.8).

All of these methods may be used to comment on the global systolic function of the LV, though it is important to recognize that regional variations are necessary to investigate. Regional wall motion abnormalities can certainly impact the global function of the LV, though they also can indicate ischemic events that may be transpiring. The ASE standardizes the segments of the LV into 17 distinct segments. There are six basal segments, six mid-ventricular segments, four apical segments, and one cap on the apex.[53]

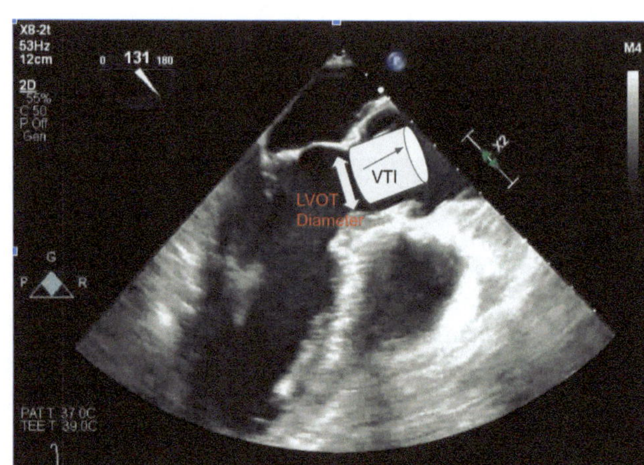

• **Fig. 55.8** Transesophageal echocardiography allows the calculation of stroke volume (SV) and subsequently cardiac output (CO). The left ventricular outflow tract (LVOT) diameter, measured in the mid-esophageal aortic valve long axis view, can be used in conjunction with the LVOT velocity time integral (VTI) from the transgastric view to obtain an SV and ultimately a CO. SV = $LVOT_{area} \times LVOT_{VTI}$. CO then is obtained by multiplying SV by heart rate.

Each of these 17 segments corresponds to the requisite coronary artery blood supply as seen later. Whereas the TG-SAX view will allow observation of all three major coronary distributions, this will only image the mid-ventricular segments. Thus ME-4C and ME-2C views must be used to thoroughly evaluate all ventricular segments (Fig. 55.9).

As mentioned earlier, 3D quantification of the LV chamber volumes and LVEF have added to the precision with which the LV may be evaluated and in investigating for dyssynchrony, this technology may also be applied. In the ME-4C view, with the LV centered and optimized for viewing, data are acquired over four or eight beats, and then 3D reconstruction of the cardiac cycle is done. With these data, each of the 16 segments (the apex is somewhat excluded) can be evaluated for dyssynchrony. The 16 segments individually are observed to achieve a maximum and minimum volume representing thickening with contraction, the timing of this cycle is compared with the other segments evaluate for dyskinetic segments. The results are reported as a "dyssynchrony index (DI)," defined as the standard deviation of the mean time of end-systolic contraction of the segment. Graphically, this can be plotted as a bullseye to identify segments that are dyssynchronous as evidenced by their elevated DI values. This technique has been well validated when compared with prior 2D techniques, such as tissue Doppler (Fig. 55.10).[54,55]

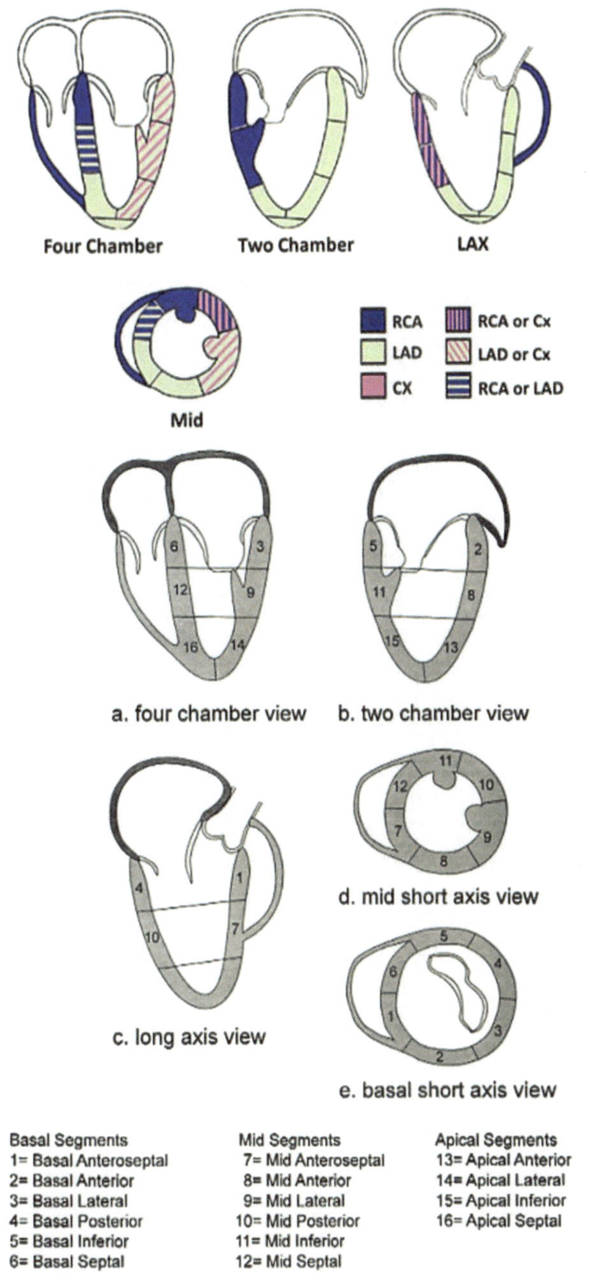

• **Fig. 55.9 American Society of Echocardiography chart showing left ventricular regional walls and coronary distributions.** (From Reeves ST, Finley AC, Skubas NJ, et al. Basic perioperative transesophageal echocardiography examination: a consensus statement of the American Society of Echocardiography and the Society of Cardiovascular Anesthesiologists. *J Am Soc Echocardiogr*. 2013;26:443–456.)

As with the RV, speckle tracking and strain measurements are valuable tools for assessing LV function. Strain has proved to be predictive of LV dysfunction post valve replacement, despite normal LVEF measurements, and may be more sensitive for detecting of subtle LV dysfunction. As with the RV, strain is measuring the longitudinal displacement of muscle fibers in the ventricle. Because strain is measuring the shortening of these muscle fibers, a negative value is reported. The more negative this value is, then the more vigorously the LV is contracting. Any value less negative than −20 represents a pathologic change in LV function.[56] In addition to providing an assessment of the global function of the LV, strain can be used to assess for regional variations that would herald the onset of ischemia or infarction. Segments with strain rates of less negative than 14 or 6 are likely to be experiencing ischemia or infarction respectively (Fig. 55.11).[57]

Finally, some attention should be paid to **evaluating LV relaxation, or diastolic function.** There is a high prevalence of diastolic dysfunction in the community with upwards of 50% of those with heart failure, actually having normal LVEF.[58] Further, the perioperative presence of diastolic dysfunction has been to be an independent predictor of MACE perioperatively.[59] In one population, vascular surgery patients, investigators found that the perioperative presence of diastolic dysfunction was independently associated with postoperative outcomes and length of stay. This was to a greater degree than was associated with even systolic function, speaking to the importance of diastology in cardiac performance.[60] Low grades (1–2) of diastolic dysfunction are unlikely to elevate LA pressure, to a significant degree, and are unlikely to be clinically relevant intraoperatively, however higher grade dysfunction may result in elevated LA pressures which should be taken into account when managing hemodynamics (Fig. 55.12).

There are four different measurements that the ASE recommends obtaining to evaluate LV diastolic function: LA size, MV inflow (E/A), MV annular e' velocities (septal and lateral), and peak TR velocity. This is an expansion of the previous practice of simply obtaining MV inflow and pulmonary vein flow Dopplers. If more

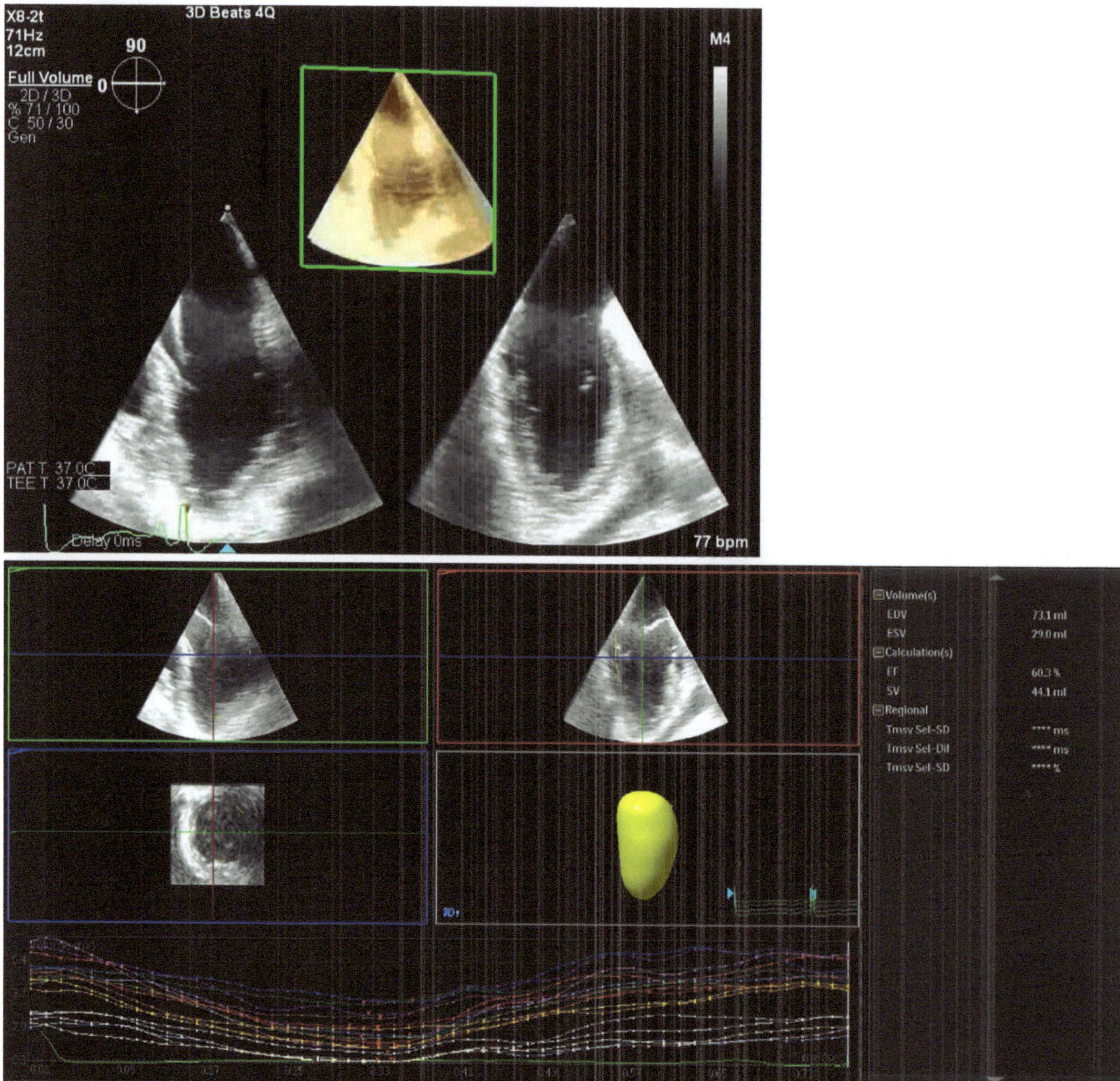

• **Fig. 55.10** Newer three-dimensional (3D) software is available on many transesophageal echocardiography machines that allows for accurate estimation of left ventricular ejection fraction (LVEF). This requires obtaining full volume 3D clips of the LV and then allowing the software to trace the endocardial border at end diastole and end systole.

than half of these variables are normal then there is no presence of diastolic dysfunction, conversely if more than half are abnormal then there is dysfunction present (Fig. 55.13).[61]

Swaminathan proposed a simplified method of monitoring for diastolic dysfunction that relies on heavily on the lateral e' value. An e' value of less than 10 cm/s was thought to represent diastolic dysfunction with the E/e' ratio delineating the degree of dysfunction.[62] This is widely accepted and has been shown to be useful in cardiac surgery, largely CABG (both on and off pump), for monitoring for onset and changes in diastolic function (Fig. 55.14).[63]

Transesophageal Echocardiography for Acute Pulmonary Hypertension

Although PH may be present in a certain population of the thoracic surgery population, the etiology can vary widely. This can be better investigated through right and left heart catheterization. However, acutely elevated PAPs during surgery are likely to be related to either PE, reduction in the vascular bed because of resection, or protamine reactions. Imaging of the PA and pulmonary valve (PV) can best be obtained in the upper esophageal aortic arch short axis (UE-Arch SAX) view (Fig. 55.15). In this view, the probe can be slightly turned

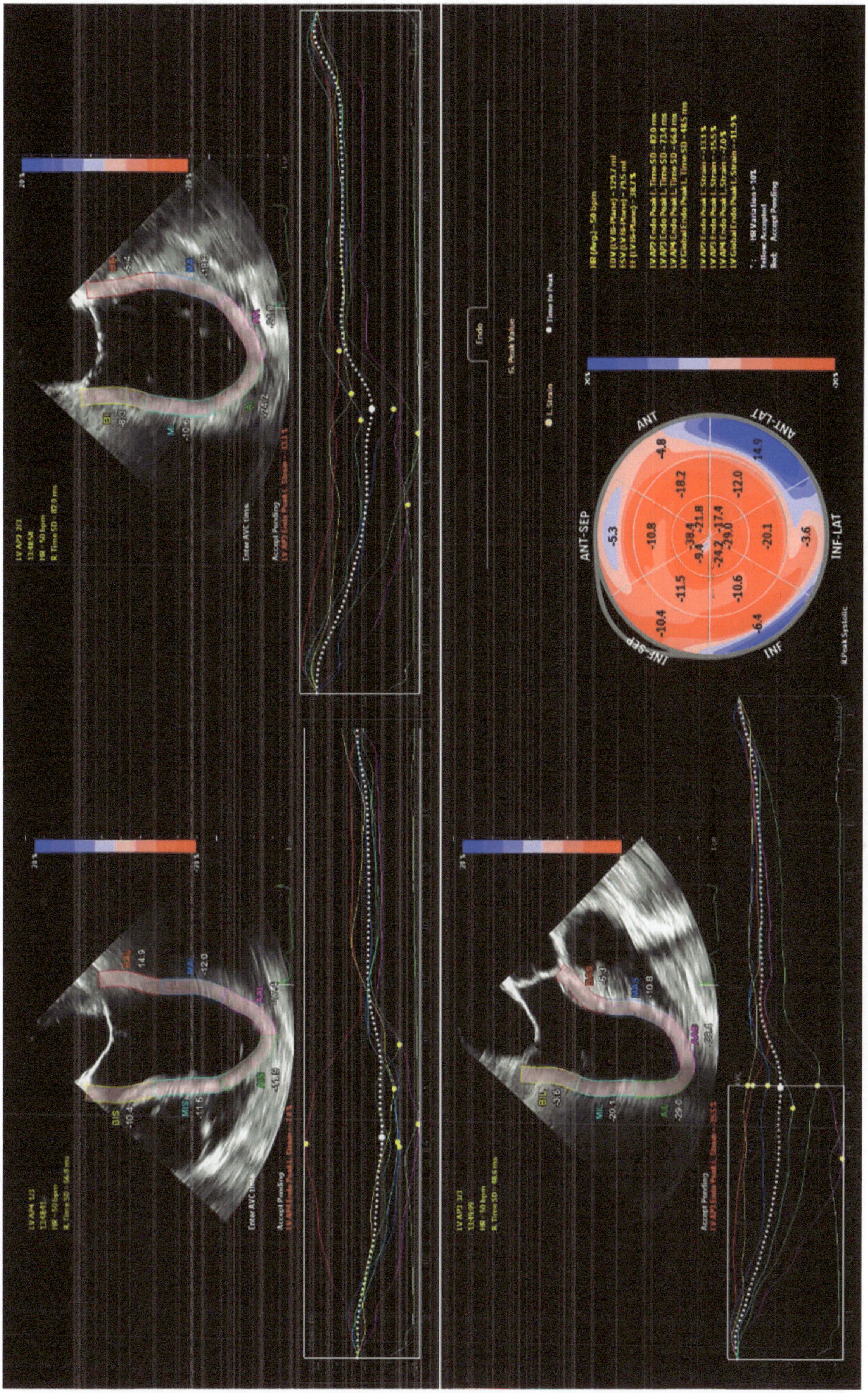

• **Fig. 55.11** Left ventricular strain measured in mid-esophageal four-chamber, mid-esophageal two-chamber, and mid-esophageal aortic valve long axis. Global longitudinal strain (GLS) of −20 or more negative are considered normal.

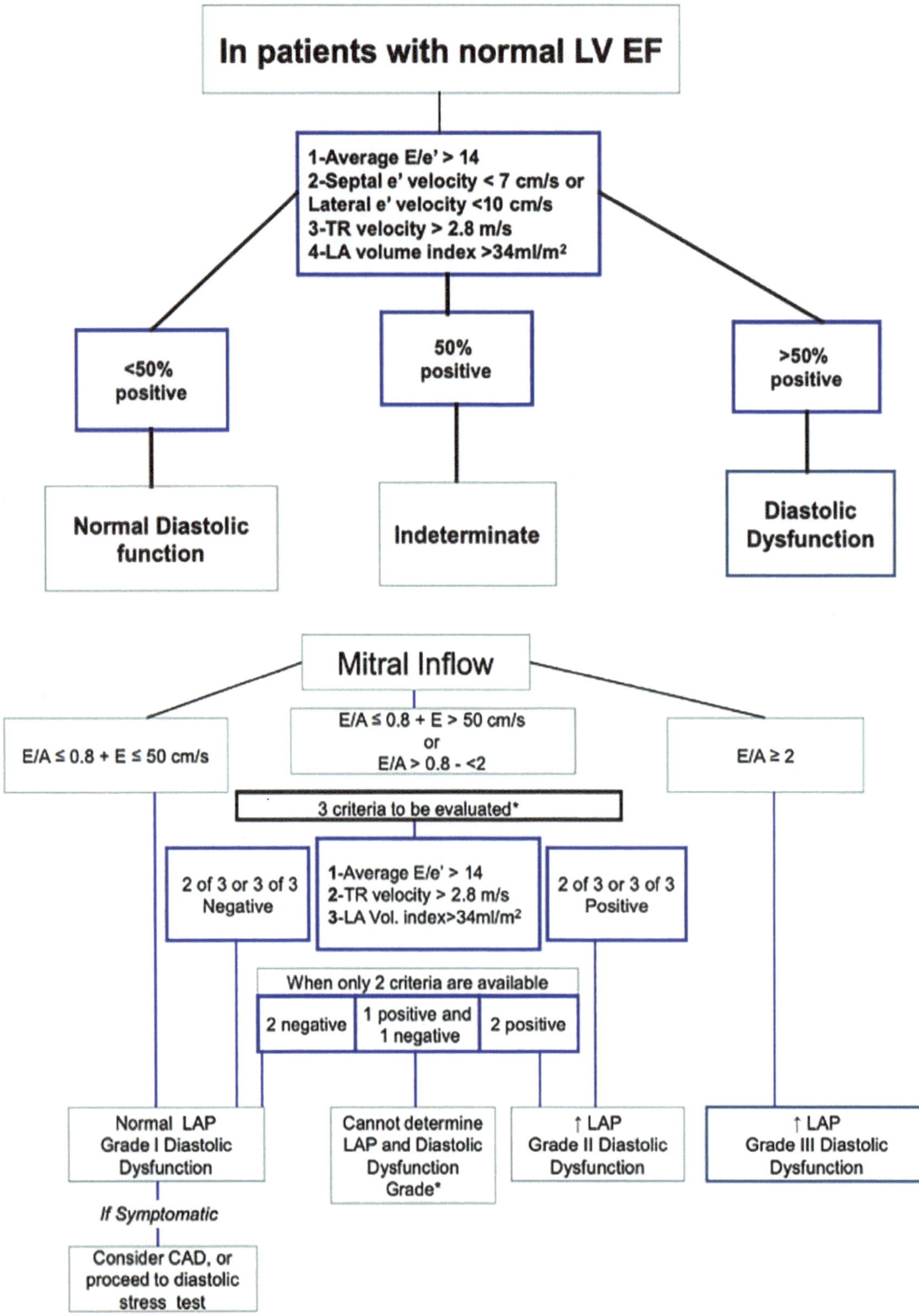

• **Fig. 55.12 Evaluation of diastolic function** as directed by the American Society of Echocardiography. (From Nagueh SF, Smiseth OA, Appleton CP, et al. Recommendations for the evaluation of left ventricular diastolic function by echocardiography: an update from the American Society of Echocardiography and the European Association of Cardiovascular Imaging. *J Am Soc Echocardiogr*. 2016;29:277–314.)

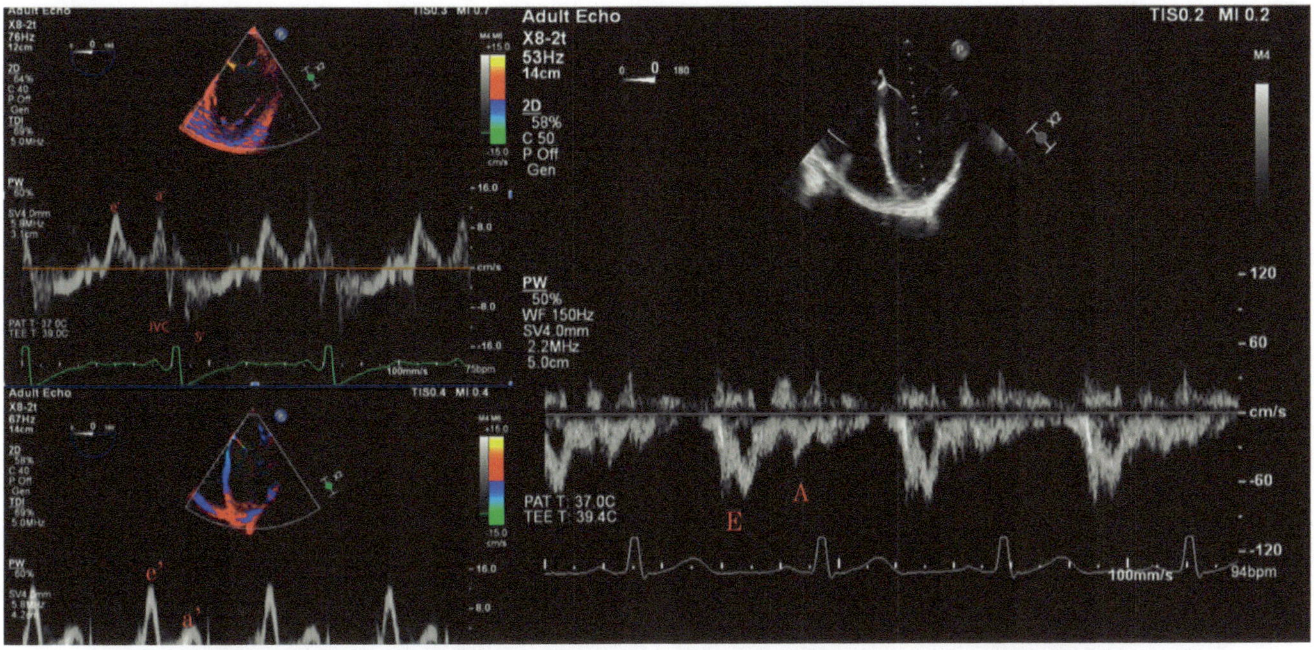

• **Fig. 55.13** The required information to make an evaluation of diastolic function consists of mitral valve (MV) E and A wave velocities, as well as septal and lateral E' velocities. MV in-flow velocities (E and A waves) with tissue Doppler of septal and lateral MV annulus (E' and e') are shown here.

to the left and retroflexed to produce optimal alignment with blood flow through the PV and into the PA. Doppler of the PA and PV can yield gradients that can be used to estimate PA pressures and RV stroke volume. A similar view is obtained in the upper esophageal ascending aorta short axis (UE-Asc SAX) view, by withdrawing the probe through the five-chamber view and anteflexing to get the aorta into short axis and the main PA with bifurcation into view. In the modified bicaval view, the TV is excellently aligned for Doppler of any TR that may be present, using Bernoulli's equation, an estimated RV systolic pressure is obtained as a surrogate for direct PAP measurement. The PA acceleration time (PAAT) can also be used to identify patients with PH.

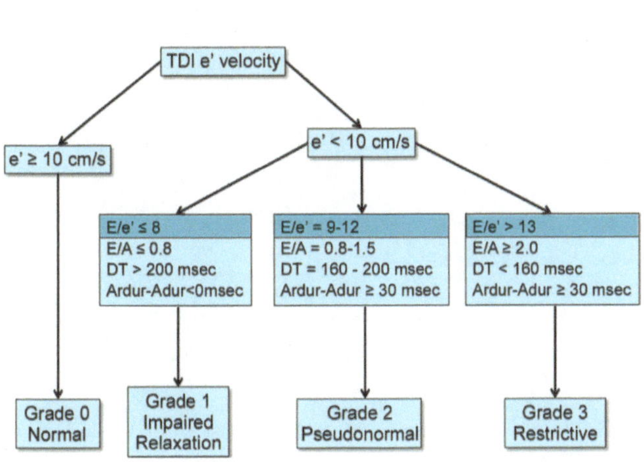

• **Fig. 55.14** Swaminathan's simplified e' based algorithm to evaluate for diastolic dysfunction in patients und. (From Swaminathan M, Nicoara A, Philips-Bute BG, et al. Utility of a simple algorithm to grade diastolic dysfunction and predict outcome after coronary artery bypass graft surgery. *Ann Thorac Surg*. 2011;91:1844–1851.)

To measure this, a PWD beam should be aligned with the blood flow through the main PA. The PAAT then is the time from beginning of ejection to peak velocity. A sharper wave, with a steeper upslope, is indicative of PH (Fig. 55.16).[64]

In the case of an acute PE resulting in elevated PAP, TEE may provide valuable information as to the etiology. Whereas outside of the operating room V/Q scan or computed tomography scanning may be the ideal modality for diagnosing an embolism, given their ability to image to the subsegmental levels, in the operating room this rarely is practical. The utility of TEE as a rescue in the acutely decompensating patient was addressed in earlier sections. Specifically, in regards to PE, there are echocardiographic signs that are especially predictive of the presence of acute embolism causing PH and/or RV decompensation. Most notably, the McConnell's sign, akinesis of the mid-free wall with normal RV apical motion, is highly specific (about 80%–90%) for PE while being poorly sensitive (~15%–30%).[65] RV/LV end-diastolic diameter ratio over 0.7 is also highly sensitive for PE, and the combination of findings adds to this power (Fig. 55.17).[66] The ability to visualize an embolism is limited by the fact that TEE can really only image the main PA into the left and right main PAs but not past this main bifurcation. There are some case reports that suggest using echo contrast can increase the yield of TEE for identifying centrally located emboli.[67] Although the topic of PFO has been addressed in an earlier section, we will mention it again in regards to PE. Paradoxical emboli certainly can raise the risk of stroke, and occasionally these can be seen in transit on TEE. Regardless, PFO should be evaluated given the association, mentioned previously, with cryptogenic stroke.

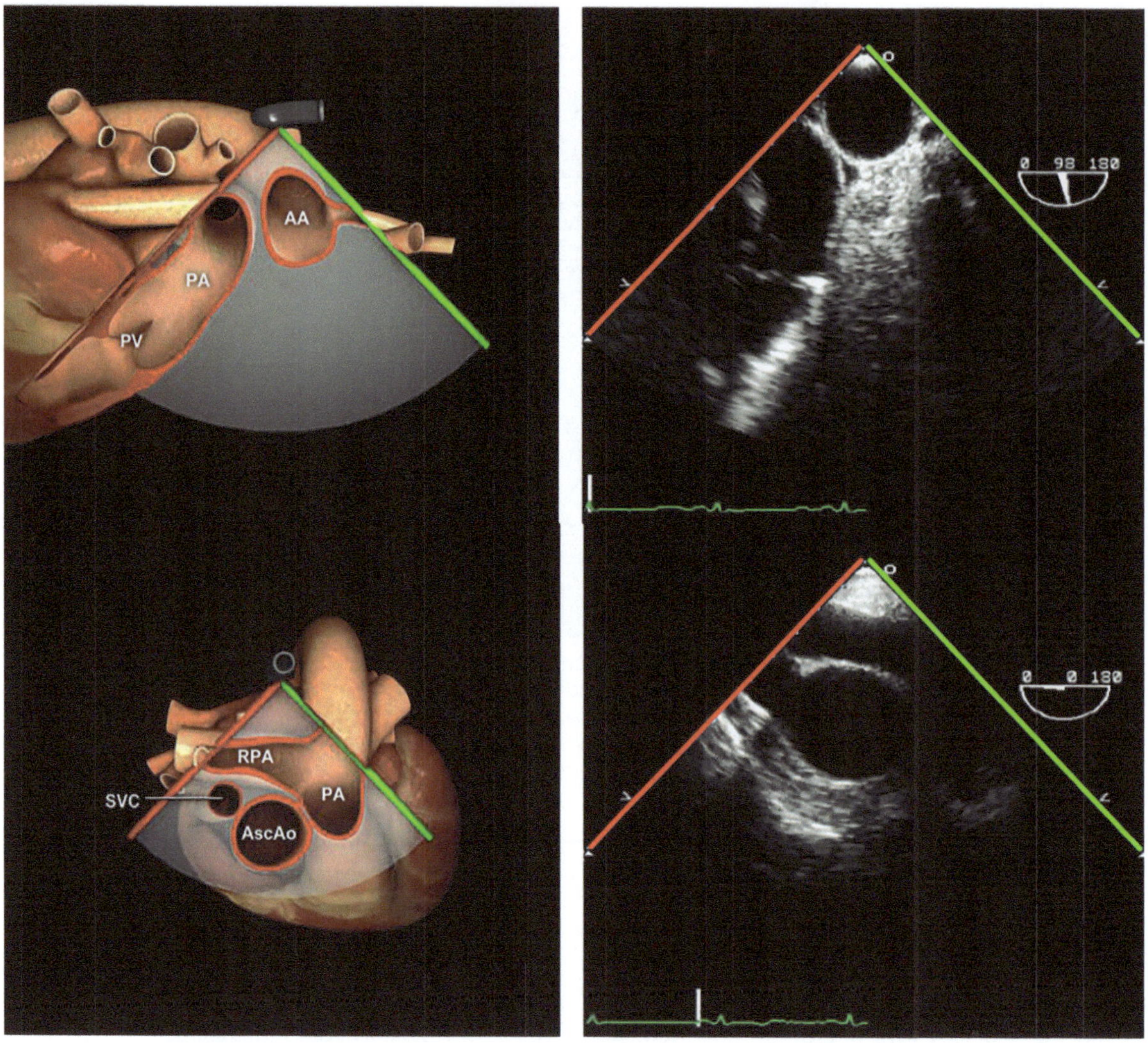

• **Fig. 55.15** The main pulmonary artery is best imaged in the upper esophageal aortic arch short axis and mid-esophageal ascending aorta short axis views. The upper esophageal window provides optimal Doppler alignment. *AscAo,* ascending aorta; *PA,* Pulmonary artery; *PV,* pulmonary vein. *RPA,* right pulmonary artery; *SVC,* Superior vena cava. (Reproduced with permission from http://pie.med.utoronto.ca/tee.)

As mentioned in earlier sections, PE can acutely raise the afterload experienced by the RV. This abrupt increase can lead to dilation of the PA, RV dilation, and TR. Chronic thromboembolic disease can result in the same physiologic changes over time. Surgical pulmonary thromboendarterectomy (PTE) remains the treatment of choice for patients who have developed PH as a result of their disease.[68] These are open procedures done on cardiopulmonary bypass with sequential periods (up to 20 minutes each) of deep hypothermic circulatory arrest (DHCA) to provide a bloodless PA. During these periods of DHCA, the PA is opened and thromboembolic disease is stripped from the artery. TEE can be used during these procedures to evaluate for changes in RV function and PAP with the expectation being improved RV function postoperatively (Fig. 55.18).

One measure of changes in the RV would be measurement of the systolic pressure. This requires evaluation of the TV and quantification of TR. In the RV in/out flow view and the modified bicaval view, Doppler can be aligned with the TR jet yielding a pressure gradient between the RA and RV. This

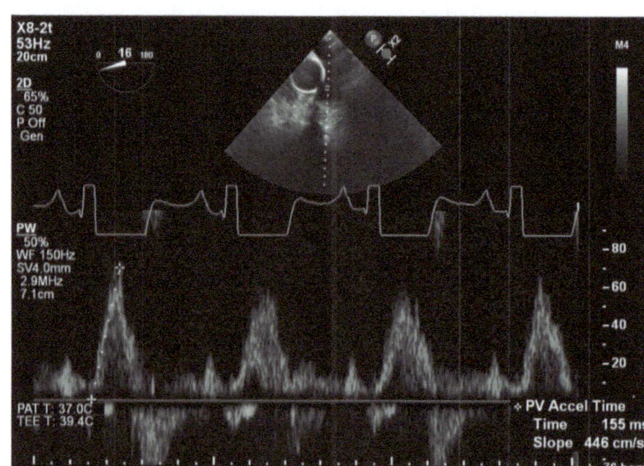

• **Fig. 55.16** By placing pulsed wave Doppler in the path of blood flow through the main pulmonary artery (MPA) a velocity time integral is captured. The pulmonary artery acceleration time (PAAT) is the time it takes for this blood flow to reach maximum velocity. In arteries with higher pressure, this will occur in a shorter period of time. This patient whose PAAT is measured at 155 ms suggesting normal PA pressures.

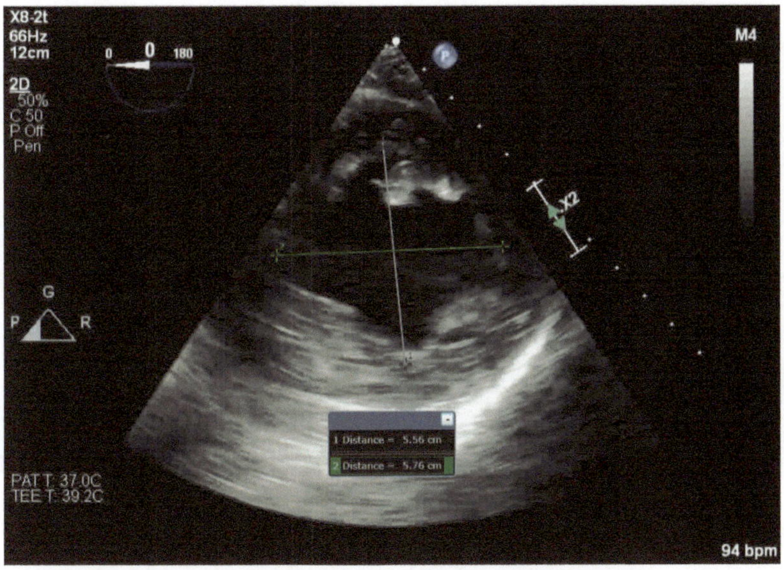

• **Fig. 55.17** Eccentricity index can provide quantification of septal flattening and is calculated as EI = D1/D2. As the septum flattens, D2 will decrease raising the EI.

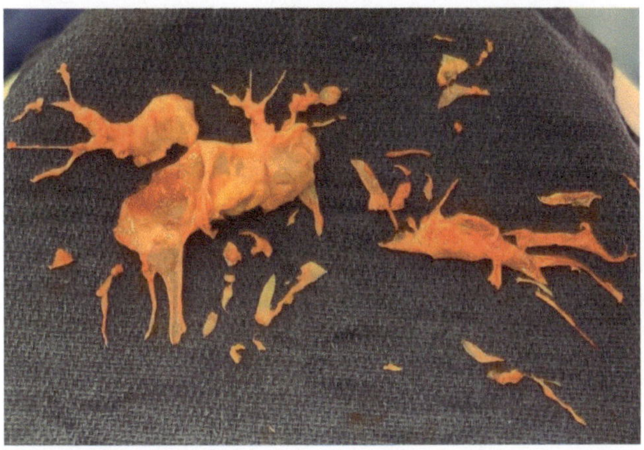

• **Fig. 55.18** Figure showing clot and casts of arterial tree removed during a pulmonary thromboendarterectomy for chronic thromboembolic pulmonary hypertension.

pressure gradient added to the RA pressure gives an estimate of the systolic pressure in the RV. At the same time, with the addition of the ME-4C view, the degree of TR should be evaluated and graded by measuring the vena contracta and jet size, and the density of the Doppler signal (Fig. 55.19).[69,70] Although the degree of TR does not necessarily correlate with the degree of RV failure, it could be expected to decrease in conjunction with the fall in RV systolic pressure as the RV afterload falls following PTE. However, note that although this is indicative of a successful surgery, the absence of these changes does not equate to a failure of the procedure. The RV may continue to remodel and adapt for the ensuing months following a successful PTE.[71]

Transesophageal Echocardiography for Lung Ultrasound (see Ch. 54)

The use of lung US for the evaluation of dyspnea or respiratory failure in the intensive care unit has been a well-established practice. Prior work has shown point-of-care lung US to perform comparably to chest radiographs in detecting common pathologies, such as pneumothorax, effusion, consolidation, or interstitial disease.[72] This transthoracic technique relies on US imaging of the lung tissue, pleura, bone, and associated artifact that are well described. The artifacts that are relevant are those arising from the pleural interface and are termed A or B lines. **A lines** are reflections of the pleura, or reverberations, that are horizontal and regularly spaced throughout the window. These are the result of the US signal being reflected back towards the probe by the acoustic impedance of the lung. This signal is then, partially, reflected back towards the pleura by the probe-patient interface, which is in turn, again, reflected by the pleura-lung interface. However, because this is a weaker signal than the initial signal leaving the probe, the time it takes to be reflected back to the probe is longer. This results in this pleural artifact being placed deeper in the image than the original pleural image. In contrast to these horizontally opposed A lines, B lines are vertical artifacts that appear comet-like extending deep from the pleura. These **B lines** are the manifestation of increased lung density that allows the US signal to penetrate the pleura and into the lung itself. The etiology of this increased denseness may be atelectasis, consolidation, or edema. Hepatization of the lung is a distinct finding of the lung parenchyma representing deaeration of the lung tissue, generally from consolidation or collapse, that is different than the artifacts listed earlier.[73]

In evaluating for the presence or absence of pneumothorax, there are four sonographic signs that should be evaluated for. The first, is the presence of lung sliding which is a bright horizontal line that will shimmer representing opposition of the visceral and parietal pleura as they move against each other. If these two pleural layers are not directly opposed, if there is air separating them, then this shimmering and subtle motion with not be seen on US examination. Second, B-lines, previously described, can be relevant in the evaluation of pneumothorax because their presence depends on the opposition of the pleural layers. Without

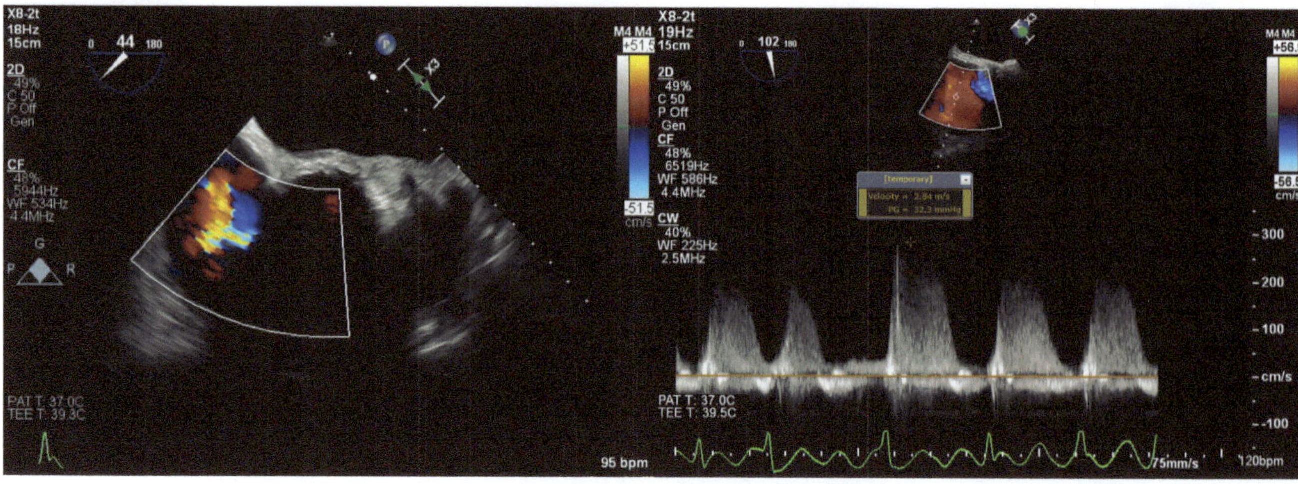

• **Fig. 55.19** Tricuspid regurgitation is seen in the right ventricular (RV) in-out flow view, increasing omniplane angle to a modified bicaval view brings this tricuspid regurgitation (TR) jet into optimal Doppler alignment. In this case, the gradient is 32.3 mm Hg which when added to the central venous pressure (15 mm Hg) gives an RV systolic pressure of 47 mm Hg which is elevated.

this contact the B lines would not be possible, and thus the presence of B lines suggests contact between the visceral and parietal lung pleura and the absence of pneumothorax with 100% certainty. Third, the lung pulse is another surrogate finding to show that contact is made between the two pleural layers. Essentially, the lung pulse is simply the heartbeat transmitted through consolidated lung tissue to the pleural interface resulting in horizontal or vertical movements on US. Because the lung pulse depends on an intact pleural interface to be seen, this finding eliminates the possibility of a pneumothorax. Finally, if there is air in the pleural space it is, at times, possible to identify a transition point where this air either appears or disappears. This transition point is referred to as the "lung point." In the supine patient, there may be suggestion of pneumothorax in the anterior field (absent B lines, absent lung sliding) and sonographic confirmation is possible by gradually evaluating laterally to a point where lung sliding and B lines again become visible. This represents the transition point from pleural separation to pleural adherence.

Most commonly, the pattern of these artifacts is used in creating a profile of the lung being viewed. The bedside lung US in emergency (BLUE) protocol is one widely used method for characterizing findings and has been shown to be highly reliable. By evaluating for the presence or absence of pneumothorax and then characterizing the lung fields by the predominant artifact seen (i.e., is there a predominance of A lines or a predominance of B lines), the physician is able, with good reliability, to deduce the underlying pathology leading to hypoxia. The BLUE protocol calls for evaluating prespecified windows on the anterior chest, with the initial emphasis being on evaluating for lung sliding. Once lung sliding is seen, attention is turned to evaluating for A lines, if there is a predominance of A lines, the veins of the groin and leg are investigated for the presence of deep vein thrombosis (DVT). This pattern of predominant A lines with a clot found in the leg veins is highly predictive of PE as the cause of hypoxia. In the absence of lower extremity DVT, attention is returned to the lung fields looking for posterolateral alveolar a pleural findings that would make pneumonia most likely, while the absence of these would elevate COPD or asthma to being highly likely. Other interstitial patterns can make acute respiratory distress syndrome very likely with a B line predominance suggesting pulmonary edema as the cause of the patient's respiratory failure (Fig. 55.20).[74]

This examination is easily performed with a standard phased array US probe and involves obtaining lung windows in three areas on either hemithorax. In each of these zones, attention is paid to whether or not lung sliding is present, whether A or B lines predominate, and whether or not there is lung consolidation or pleural effusion. Lastly, as mentioned earlier, brief scanning of the lower extremity veins can be used to evaluate for DVT. This simple exam with dichotomous questions can be organized into a decision tree, as seen later, which can be used in aiding the physician in interpretation of the profile seen. This method carries 90%+ positive and negative predictive values for the respective pathologies.[75] These data have since been expanded on and in 2012 there was publication of an international consensus that provides some guidance and standardization regarding US examination of lung pathology. **This document strongly suggests immediate use of lung US in cases where pneumothorax is on the differential, as well as evaluation in line with the BLUE protocol of patients with respiratory failure.** Interestingly, these guidelines speak to the utility of repeating the US examination to follow patient progress and evolution/resolution of their pathology.[76] This document also standardized the language used in describing the artifacts we now know as A lines and B lines, as well as what constitutes findings of pneumothorax, effusion, consolidation, and so on.

Recently, this same approach has begun being extrapolated to the use of TEE with some success. In transthoracic lung US, the interpretation of the images relies on the formation of the artifacts mentioned earlier. Because these

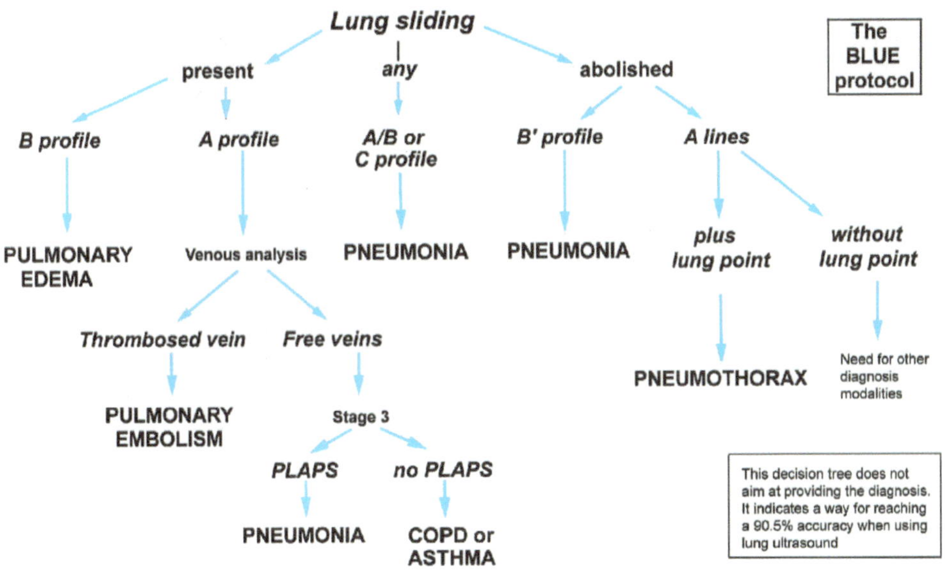

• **Fig. 55.20** The bedside lung ultrasound (US) in emergencies **(BLUE) protocol** shows that by identifying patterns of artifacts seen on bedside US examination it is possible to make an accurate assessment of the etiology of respiratory failure. (From Lichtenstein DA, Meziere GA. Relevance of lung ultrasound in the diagnosis of acute respiratory failure-The BLUE Protocol. *Chest.*2008;134:117–125.)

artifacts are created from the pleural interface, using TEE to evaluate the lungs is made more difficult. However, it is possible to still see the same artifacts used in transthoracic imaging (A lines and B lines, as well as lung sliding/pulse) in the transesophageal windows, and the relevance of these findings should be similar to that of transthoracic (Figs. 55.21 and 55.22).[77]

Transesophageal Echocardiography for Lung Transplantation (see Ch. 43)

The United Network for Organ Sharing (UNOS) tracks rates of organ transplantation. According to their data, there has been a steady increase in the number of lung transplantations occurring each year culminating with 2583 transplantations occurring in 2018. Much of this growth has been driven by the adoption of expanded donor criteria and the development of ex-vivo perfusion strategies to make donation after cardiac death a more valid option. In a series of 225 patients, there were comparable 1-year survival rates to those receiving lungs donated after brain death. The short-term morbidity and mortality were higher, however, with more frequent primary graft dysfunction (PGD) grade 3 and more ECMO use.[78] Follow-up metaanalysis corroborated these findings, with a growing experience of well over 1000 patients, showing equivalent rates of PGD and similar 1-year survival rates.[79] This adds to the growing body of evidence to advocate for expanding the criteria by which donors are evaluated. Ex-vivo lung perfusion (EVLP) has been introduced as a method to not only improve outcomes in standard criteria donations, but also expand criteria to include lungs that would have previously been rejected (Table 55.3).

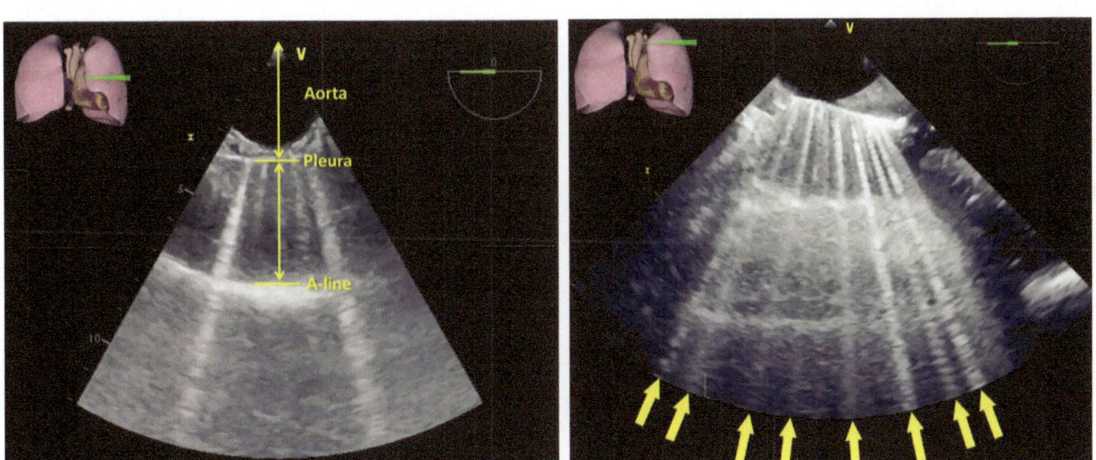

• **Fig. 55.21** **A lines** are artifacts of the pleural reflection that are horizontal in nature and occur in regular intervals. **B lines,** sometimes referred to as "comet tails" are vertical projections from the pleural interface and extending deep. (From Cavays YA, Girard M, Desjardins G, Denault AY. Transesophageal lung ultrasonography: a novel technique for investigating hypoxemia. *J Can Anesth.* 2016;63:1266–1276.)

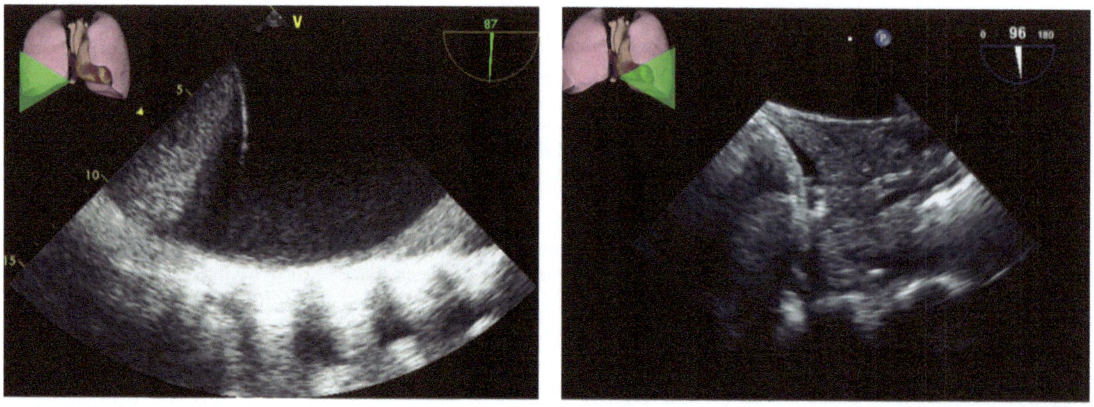

• **Fig. 55.22** Pleural effusions are easily seen, especially in the left chest, and may be associated with compressive atelectasis of the ipsilateral lung. Hepatization results in lung tissue appearing to have a liver-like quality. (From Cavays YA, Girard M, Desjardins G, Denault AY. Transesophageal lung ultrasonography: a novel technique for investigating hypoxemia. *J Can Anesth*. 2016;63:1266–1276; Figs. 3 and 7.)

Briefly, EVLP entails flushing the donated lungs with a cold preservation solution before cannulation of the left atrial cuff and PA. The lungs are then perfused with a room temperature perfusate, the temperature of which is gradually increased to 37°C. As the lungs warm to 32°C, ventilation is started at 7 breaths per minute, 7cc/kg ideal body weight, using a positive end-expiratory pressure of 5 cm H_2O and room fraction of inspired oxygen (F_iO2) of 0.21. Recruitment maneuvers are performed hourly using inspiratory holds of 20 cm H_2O and lung function is evaluated by increasing F_iO2 to 1.0 and tidal volume to 10 mL/kg at a rate of 10 breaths per minute for 10 minutes before evaluation. At the end of a predefined period of EVLP, the perfusate is cooled to 10°C, after which perfusion and ventilation are stopped, the trachea is then clamped to keep lungs inflated, and the lungs are stored at 4°C until the time of transplantation. The seminal evaluation of this technique from 2011 showed that high-risk donor lungs that underwent 4 hours of EVLP showed nearly identical outcomes compared to those conventionally selected, likely owing to the ability to optimize and reevaluate the suitability of these high-risk donors at the end of EVLP.[80] As more experience is had with expanded criteria and EVLP, it has become clear that this is a viable option, patients have nearly identical 1-, 3-, and 5-year survival compared with conventionally evaluated lungs as is their quality of life.[81]

As the donor pool has expanded, and the number of lung transplants occurring has increased, the complexity of these procedures and the comorbid conditions of the recipients has also increased. This has led to the increased use of ECMO as both a bridge to transplantation, as well as a method of support during the transplantation. Under the current lung allocation score system, those patients being supported with mechanical ventilation will receive higher scores, increasing their likelihood of receiving an organ. However, with this has come increasing issues related to patient deconditioning and posttransplantation outcomes. These issues have led to the hypothesis that in light of their worsening outcomes once needing pretransplant mechanical ventilation, then perhaps these patients are too sick to undergo transplantation and should be weaned from mechanical ventilation and rehabilitated before transplantation.[82] In some patients, the use of ECMO as support may allow for respiratory support while also allowing the patient to work with physical therapy and rehabilitation to improve their physical condition leading up to transplantation.[83] Early investigations of using ECMO as a bridge to transplant have been encouraging. A large portion of patients placed on ECMO achieve spontaneous ventilation and ambulation and in primary transplant patients shows acceptable 30-day, 1-year, and 5-year outcomes.[84]

Mechanical support, an umbrella term including ECMO, cardiopulmonary bypass, and other support devices is used at varying rates to facilitate lung transplantation. While ideally these procedures would proceed free of the need for mechanical support, this patient population can present with challenging physiology that leads to instability that necessitates using the various support options. Most commonly, this need for mechanical support is driven by refractory hypoxemia (P:F <80 mm Hg), hypercapnia (arterial carbon dioxide partial pressure [PaCO2] >80 mm Hg), PH (MPAP >30 mm Hg), or RV dysfunction. The pathology that is

TABLE 55.3 United Network for Organ Sharing Data Table for Lung Transplant Starting in 2000

	To Date	2019	2018	2017	2016	2015	2014	2013	2012	2011	2010	2009	2008	2007	2006	2005	2004	2003	2002	2001	2000
All Donor Types	40,833	2501	2530	2449	2327	2057	1925	1923	1754	1822	1769	1661	1478	1468	1405	1406	1172	1085	1042	1059	959
Deceased Donor	40,580	2501	2530	2449	2327	2057	1925	1922	1753	1821	1769	1660	1478	1465	1401	1405	1157	1070	1029	1034	941

driving the need for mechanical support will likely also dictate the choice of support used.[85] In cases of isolated hypoxia or hypercapnia without RV dysfunction, venovenous ECMO may be used safely. Conversely, in cases where PH is present or RV dysfunction is manifesting then venoarterial ECMO or full cardiopulmonary bypass should be used. Traditionally, this was thought of a dichotomous decision (i.e., on bypass or off bypass); however, the use of ECMO intraoperatively has been gaining popularity. In large part, this is caused by improved outcomes in patients whose surgery proceeds on ECMO compared with those without, a benefit thought to be related to lower anticoagulation targets while still providing adequate cardiopulmonary support. When continued for support, posttransplantation ECMO has been shown to be effective for supporting the patient through early periods of PGD and to some degree may mitigate the need for high F_iO2 and reduce otherwise elevated PAPs, which have been shown to be drivers of PGD.[86]

Regardless of how the transplantation proceeds, either with or without mechanical support, the use of TEE can provide useful information that can direct care of these complex patients. There is no trial to show the impact of TEE use in these cases, and the current ASE guidelines do not specifically mention this situation.[87] Despite the lack of clear recommendations under the category of "open-heart surgery," the use of TEE is likely beneficial given the propensity for hemodynamic changes in these cases and relatively low number of contraindications. This exam can be started immediately following intubation, allowing the bulk of the baseline exam to be completed before the use of electrocautery which can obscure the images (Table 55.4).

After confirming the findings of the preoperative transthoracic studies, attention should be paid to the RV function and the possibility of PH. Intracardiac shunts should be looked for because of the possibility of acute elevations of RV systolic pressure causing right to left shunting, which could exacerbate preexisting hypoxia. In anticipation of this shunting in response to manipulation of the heart or clamping of the PA, the decision may be made to implement cardiopulmonary bypass to correct this lesion or simply mitigate the effects of the PA clamping or manipulation. Following this baseline exam, each period of the lung transplant surgery presents specific challenges which can be evaluated for by TEE.

In general, the dissection phase will start with opening the chest via a clamshell incision to expose the heart, the native lungs with associated airways, as well as the great vessels. This phase can be fraught with hemodynamic instability that results from mechanical compression or manipulation of the heart and great vessels, and the lungs themselves. As such, the TEE examination in this phase should be directed towards biventricular function and filling which are actionable findings. In addition, the absence of other pathologies, such as regional wall motion abnormalities or new valve pathology can provide reassurance that hemodynamic perturbations are not the result of other underlying cardiac disease.

Next, the PA will be clamped to allow removal of the native lung. It is important that before the clamp actually being applied, the position of the PA catheter is evaluated to ensure its position in the main PA and out of danger of being clamped or involved in the suture line at the anastomosis. Once the left or right PA clamp is applied, there will be a sudden increase in RV afterload. This sudden increase in afterload may cause abrupt changes in RV function and filling, both of which should be evaluated for using TEE as this is a sensitive monitor of RV dysfunction.[88] In addition, as mentioned earlier, this is a point where the change in RV may incite or exacerbate right to left shunting resulting in hypoxia; this pathology should also be investigated, especially in the setting of worsening hypoxia which may necessitate the utilization of cardiopulmonary bypass.

Following the completion of the anastomoses, the graft is reperfused. Immediately following this, it is important to evaluate for causes of hemodynamic instability, which may be the result of reperfusion induced inflammatory response or entrainment of air within the vasculature of the graft. This air may return to the LV, and fill the aortic root leading to coronary air emboli and resultant wall motion abnormalities. Once stability is achieved and there is no obvious air in danger of embolizing, it becomes necessary to evaluate surgical anastomoses for patency and stenosis.

The PA anastomoses can be investigated by TEE, though the right main PA is more easily visualized, owing to the presence of the left mainstem bronchus obstructing the view of the PA. Assessment should begin with 2D imaging of the vessel with evaluation for thrombosis and simply dimension of the vessel. These anastomoses should have lumens measuring at

TABLE 55.4 Summary of the Transesophageal Echocardiography Examination During Different Points in the Process of Lung Transplantation

Induction	Dissection	Pulmonary Artery Clamping	Reperfusion	Postreperfusion
- TR - RV function - LV function - PFO/Intracardiac Shunt	- Biventricular function and filling	- RV shape - RVSP - TR - RV function	- Intracardiac air - Biventricular function	- Pulmonary veins (2D, color flow Doppler, pulsed wave Doppler) - Pulmonary Artery (2D, color flow Doppler, pulsed wave Doppler) - Biventricular function - RVSP

LV, Left ventricular; *PFO*, patent foramen ovale; *RV*, right ventricular; *RVSP*, right ventricular systolic pressure; *TR*, tricuspid regurgitation.

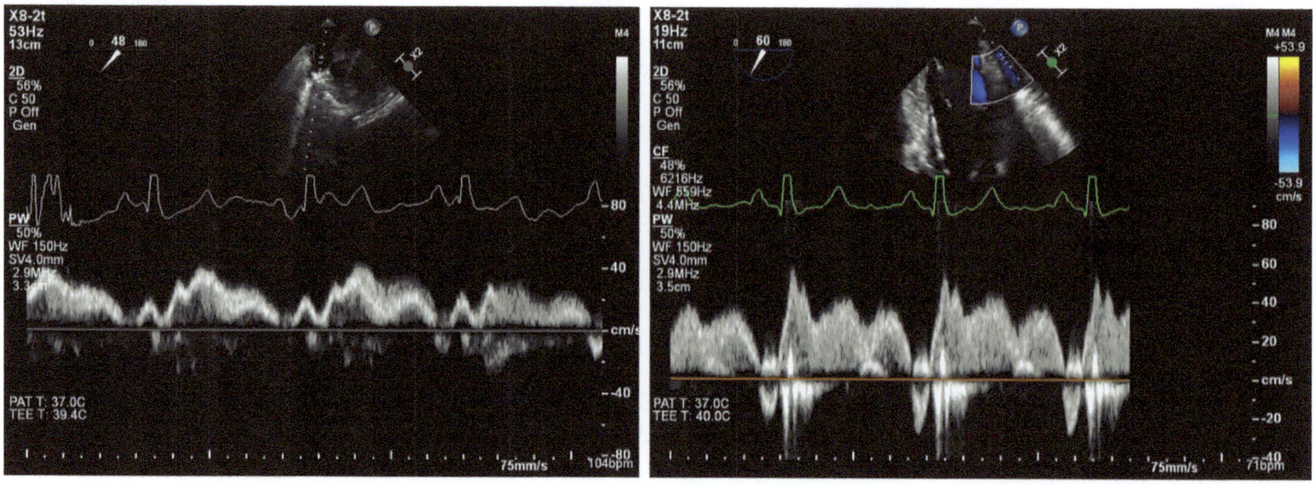

• **Fig. 55.23** Both the left and right sided pulmonary veins are imaged in two-dimensions and then color flow Doppler is applied to evaluate for turbulent flow. Doppler can then be used to deduce the velocity of blood in the respective veins. In this case both left- and right-sided veins show velocities well below the 100 cm/s cutoff that would raise concern for the status of the vein patency.

least 75% that of the diameter of the native vessel, with a lack of turbulent flow seen on color flow Doppler, to be considered normal.[89] As of now, there is no echocardiographic threshold to consider the PA anastomoses as stenotic or normal, some of which is attributed to the aforementioned difficulty with imaging right and left PAs as distally as needed to capture the anastomoses. As such, the PA catheter is likely a better indicator, outside of obvious visually appreciated narrowing or turbulent flow, for detecting trouble with the arterial anastomoses.

The main PA may be investigated starting in the RV inflow-outflow view where the RVOT, pulmonary valve, and subsequently proximal main PA can be seen. In this view, the diameter of the main PA may be measured and laminar flow confirmed using color flow Doppler. To image the distal main PA, the bifurcation, and the left and right main PAs, the ascending aorta short-axis view is obtained and the probe withdrawn slightly. A small amount of outward omniplane (5–10 degrees) may make the image more clear and bring the left main PA into view, though, as mentioned is often shadowed by the ipsilateral bronchus. Finally, the UE-Arch SAX brings the main PA into optimal alignment to allow Doppler measurements to be made.

Compared with the arterial anastomoses, the pulmonary veins are easily investigated using echocardiography. Problems in the venous anastomoses leading to poor venous drainage can result in poor graft function, pulmonary edema, hypoxia, and even death if not corrected.[90] This poor venous drainage may be the result of thrombosis in the pulmonary vein, suture in the vein, kinking of the anastomosis, or external compression. All four pulmonary veins should be evaluated, initially with 2D echo to evaluate for structure of the vessels, an effort to rule out external compression or kinking, as well as ensuring no thrombus in the lumen of the vessel. Color flow Doppler can assist in this investigation as it would be expected to show laminar flow without increased turbulence, which may indicate narrowing or a physical obstruction from a thrombus. PWD should be directed through the veins, with the expected finding being a normal S and D pattern. Velocities over 100 cm/s should raise suspicion for issues with the pulmonary vein and associated anastomosis.[91] If these veins are investigated following implantation of the first lung, it should be expected to see slightly higher velocities; this is especially true if the procedure is done free of mechanical support. This is caused by the contralateral PA remaining clamped and thus the entirety of the cardiac output is directed through the newly reperfused lung. As such, the pulmonary veins should again be evaluated following reperfusion of both lungs (Fig. 55.23).

Both stenosis and thrombosis of the pulmonary venous anastomoses have been reported and velocities under 1 m/s, a left- to right-sided venous gradient of 10 to 12 mm Hg, or a diameter of less than 5 mm are accepted cutoff values to suggest stenosis. Recent series have been published that confirm the incidence of these complications reported as 1.4% for stenosis and 2.5% for thrombosis, which although low still represents a compelling motivation to investigate these vessels intraoperatively.[92] The pulmonary veins can be imaged starting in the ME-2C view with a slight withdrawal bringing the left-upper pulmonary vein into view, lying over the left atrial appendage, and separated by the coumadin ridge. The left lower pulmonary vein can be seen by inserting the TEE probe 1 to 2 cm from the ME-2C, though this vessel often forms a common vessel with the left upper pulmonary vein. The right-sided pulmonary veins may be seen by starting in the ME-4C view, anteflexing the probe, and withdrawing slightly to create a short-axis view of the ascending aorta with the LA on the top of the screen. By turning right from here, both the right upper and right lower pulmonary veins can be seen. In all of these views, 2D images, as well as color flow Doppler and PWD measurements should be obtained.

Following reperfusion of the transplanted organ(s) TEE can be useful in managing hemodynamics as separation from mechanical support is undergone. As with any procedure involving cardiopulmonary bypass, it is essential to ensure adequate de-airing of the cardiac chambers before removal of the aortic root vent. Adequate filling and biventricular performance can be assessed as described in previous sections. Lastly, RV performance should be monitored not only for routine function assessments postcardiopulmonary bypass, but also for acute dysfunction following administration of protamine. Classically, there are three main types of protamine reactions ranging from histamine-induced hypotension to the more severe acute PH leading to RV failure.[93] If this complication is encountered, standard treatments for RV failure should be used, though ultimately it may be necessary to resume mechanical support.

Conclusion

TEE is a powerful tool that can give real-time, actionable, information to assist the physician in managing the hemodynamics of an increasingly complex patient population. The indications for TEE use and efficacy of its use are well described in cardiac surgery, and noncardiac thoracic surgery is an area where TEE use is growing though largely limited by the availability of TEE-trained physicians. Although not without risk, the most concerning of which is damage to the esophagus, TEE is the only available tool for evaluating biventricular systolic function, valve function, filling status, diastolic function, evaluation of the great vessels, and evaluation of respiratory status. Over time, TEE has replaced the PA catheter as the tool of choice for evaluating the hemodynamic status of thoracic surgery patients. The use of TEE carries specific benefits in the setting of lung transplant or chronic thromboembolic pulmonary hypertension surgery where information obtained via intraoperative TEE can influence surgical decision making and ultimately patient outcomes.

References

1. Hahn RT, Abraham T, Adams M, et al. Guidelines for performing a comprehensive transesophageal echocardiographic examination: recommendations from the American Society of Echocardiography and the Society of Cardiovascular Anesthesiologists. *J Am Soc Echocardiogr.* 2013;26:921–964.
2. Thys DM, Abel MD, Brooker RF, et al. Practice guidelines for perioperative transesophageal echocardiography. *Anesthesiology.* 2010;112:1084–1096.
3. Murray KF, Carithers RL. AASLD practice guidelines: evaluation of the patient for liver transplantation. *Hepatology.* 2005;41:1407–1432.
4. Wax DB, Torres A, Scher C, Leibowitz A. Transesophageal echocardiography utilization in high-volume liver transplantation centers in the United States. *J Cardiothorac Vasc Anesth.* 2008;22:811–813.
5. Shillcutt SK, Ringenberg KJ, Chacon MM, et al. Liver transplantation: intraoperative transesophageal echocardiography findings and relationship to major adverse cardiac events. *J Cardiothorac Vasc Anesth.* 2016;30(1):107–114.
6. Dhawan R, Shahul S, Roberts JD, Smith ND, Steinberg GD, Chaney MA. Prospective, randomized clinical trial comparing use of intraoperative transesophageal echocardiography to standard care during radical cystectomy. *Ann Card Anaesth.* 2018;21:255–261.
7. Calderone CE, Tuck BC, Gray SH, Porter KK. Rais-Bahrami S. The role of transesophageal echocardiography in the management of renal cell carcinoma with venous tumor thrombus. *Echocardiography.* 2018;35:2047–2055.
8. Tsou PY, Kurbedin J, Chen YS, et al. Accuracy of point of care focused echocardiography in predicting outcome of resuscitation in cardiac arrest patients: a systematic review and meta-analysis. *Resuscitation.* 2017;114:92–99.
9. Blyth L, Atkinson P, Gadd K, Lang E. Bedside focused echocardiography as predictor of survival in cardiac arrest patients: a systematic review. *Acad Emerg Med.* 2012;19(10):1119–1126.
10. Van Der Wouw PA, Koster RW, Delemarre BJ, De Vos R, Lampe-Schoenmaeckers AJ, Lie KI. Diagnostic accuracy of transesophageal echocardiography during cardiopulmonary resuscitation. *JACC.* 1997;30(3):780–783.
11. Memtsoudis SG, Rosenberger P, Loffler M, et al. The usefulness of transesophageal echocardiography during intraoperative cardiac arrest in non-cardiac surgery. *Anesth Analg.* 2006;102:1653–1657.
12. Edsall DW. "Vigilance" Discussed by ASA Panel. *APSF Newsletter.* 1993;8(1).
13. Binanay C, Califf RM, Hasselblad V, et al. Evaluation study of congestive heart failure and pulmonary artery catheterization effectiveness. *JAMA.* 2005;294(13):1625–1633.
14. Sandham JD, Hull RD, Brant RF, et al. A randomized, controlled trial of the use of pulmonary-artery catheters in high-risk surgical patients. *N Engl J Med.* 2003;348:5–14.
15. Su NY, Huang CJ, Tsai P, Hsu YW, Hung YC, Cheng CR. Cardiac output measurement during cardiac surgery: esophageal Doppler versus pulmonary artery catheter. *Acta Anaesthesiol Sin.* 2002;40(3):127–133.
16. Sato M, Kunisawa T. Reliability of cardiac output measurements using LiDCOrapid and calibration by transesophageal echocardiography with the continuous pulmonary artery thermodilution method in patients undergoing aortic valve replacement for aortic stenosis. *J Cardiothorac Vasc Anesth.* 2018;32(6):2495–2502.
17. Sainathan S, Andaz S. A systematic review of transesophageal echocardiography-induced esophageal perforation. *Echocardiography.* 2013;30:977–983.
18. Kallemyer I, Collard C, Fox J, Body S, Shernan S. The safety of intraoperative transesophageal echocardiography: a case series of 7200 cardiac surgical patients. *Anesth Analg.* 2001;92:1126–1130.
19. Piercy M, McNicol L, Dinh D, Story D, Smith J. Major complications related to the use of transesophageal echocardiography in cardiac surgery. *J Cardiothorac Vasc Anesth.* 2009;23(1):62–65.
20. Smith CD. Esophageal strictures and diverticula. *Surg Clin N Am.* 2015;95:669–681.
21. Lanneac RT. A treatise on the diseases of the chest, in which they are described according to their anatomical characters, and their diagnosis established on a new principle by means of acoustick instruments. London: T & G Underwood; 1821.
22. Andersen KH, Iversen M, Kjaergaard J, et al. Prevalence, predictors, and survival in pulmonary hypertension related to end-stage chronic obstructive pulmonary disease. *J Heart Lung Transplant.* 2012;31:373–380.

23. Chaouat A, Bugnet AS, Kadaoui N, et al. Severe pulmonary hypertension and chronic obstructive pulmonary disease. *Am J Respir Crit Care Med.* 2005;172:189–194.
24. Caminati A, Cassandro R, Harari S. Pulmonary hypertension in chronic interstitial lung disease. *Eur Respir Rev.* 2013;22:292–301.
25. Kolb T, Hassoun PM. Right ventricular dysfunction in chronic lung disease. *Cardiol Clin.* 2012;30:243–256.
26. Hilde JM, Skjorten I, Grotta OJ, et al. Right Ventricular Dysfunction and remodeling in chronic obstructive pulmonary disease without pulmonary hypertension. *J Am Coll Cardiol.* 2013;62: 1103–1111.
27. Konstam M, Kiernan M, Bernstein D, et al. Evaluation and management of right sided heart failure: a scientific statement from the American Heart Association. *Circulation.* 2018;137:578–622.
28. Smolarek D, Gruchala M, Sobiczewski W. Echocardiographic evaluation of right ventricular systolic function: the traditional and innovative approach. *Cardiol J.* 2017;24(5):563–572.
29. Anavekar NS, Gerson D, Skali H, Kwong RY, Yucel EK, Solomon SD. Two-dimensional assessment of right ventricular function: an echocardiographic–MRI correlative study. *Echocardiography.* 2007; 24(5):452–456.
30. Lang RM, Badano LP, Mor-Avi V, et al. Recommendations for cardiac chamber quantification by echocardiography in adults: an update from the American Society of Echocardiography and the European Association of Cardiovascular Imaging. *Eur Heart J Cardiovasc Imaging.* 2015;16:233–271.
31. Forner AF, Hasheminejad E, Sabate S, Ackermann MA, Turton EW, Ender J. Agreement of tricuspid annular systolic excursion measurement between transthoracic and transesophageal echocardiography in the perioperative setting. *Int J Cardiovasc Imaging.* 2017;33:1385–1394.
32. Korshin A, Gronlykke L, Nilsson JC, et al. The feasibility of tricuspid annular plane systolic excursion performed by transesophageal echocardiography throughout heart surgery and its interchangeability with transthoracic echocardiography. *Int J Cardiovasc Imaging.* 2018;34:1017–1028.
33. Aloia E, Cameli M, D'Ascenzi F, Sciaccaluga C, Mondillo S. TAPSE: an old but useful tool in different diseases. *Int J Cardiol.* 2016;225:177–183.
34. Silverton N, Meineri M. Speckle tracking strain of the right ventricle: an emerging tool for intraoperative echocardiography. *Anesth Analg.* 2017;125:1475–1478.
35. Fusini L, Tamborini G, Gripari P, et al. Feasibility of intraoperative three-dimensional transesophageal echocardiography in the evaluation of right ventricular volumes and function in patients undergoing cardiac surgery. *J Am Soc Echocardiogr.* 2011;24:868–877.
36. Karhausen J, Dudaryk R, Phillips-Bute B, et al. Three-dimensional transesophageal echocardiography for perioperative right ventricular assessment. *Ann Thorac Surg.* 2012;94:468–474.
37. Rodes-Cabau J, Taramasso M, O'Gara PT. Diagnosis and treatment of tricuspid valve disease: current and future perspectives. *Lancet.* 2016;388:2431–2442.
38. Mas PT, Rodriquez-Palomares JF, Antunes MJ. Secondary tricuspid valve regurgitation: a forgotten entity. *Heart.* 2015;101:1840–1848.
39. Savino K, Maiello M, Pelliccia F, Ambrosio G, Palmiero P. Patent foramen ovale and cryptogenic stroke: from studies to clinical practice. *Int J Clin Pract.* 2016;70(8):641–648.
40. Smilowitz NR, Subashchandran V, Berger JS. Atrial septal defect and the risk of ischemic stroke in the perioperative period of noncardiac surgery. *Am J Cardiol.* 2019;124:1120–1124.
41. Shanoudy H, Soliman A, Raggi P, Liu JW, Russell D, Jarmukli N. Prevalence of patent foramen ovale and its contribution to hypoxemia in patients with obstructive sleep apnea. *Chest.* 1998; 113:91–96.
42. Marini C, Miniati M, Ambrosino N, et al. Dyspnoea and hypoxaemia after lung surgery: the role of interatrial right-to-left shunt. *Eur Respir J.* 2006;28:174–181.
43. Hagen PT, Scholz DG, Edwards WD. Incidence and size of patent foramen ovale during the first 10 decades of life: an autopsy study of 965 normal hearts. *Mayo Clin Proc.* 1984;59(1):17–20.
44. Mojadidi MK, Bogush N, Caceres JD, Msaouel P, Tobis JM. Diagnostic accuracy of transesophageal echocardiogram for the detection of patent foramen ovale: a meta-analysis. *Echocardiography.* 2014;31:752–758.
45. Sukernik MR, Bennett-Guerrero E. the incidental finding of a patent foramen ovale during cardiac surgery: should it always be repaired? A core review. *Anesth Analg.* 2007;105:602–610.
46. Krasuski RK, Hart SA, Allen D, et al. Prevalence and repair of intraoperatively diagnosed patent foramen ovale and association with perioperative outcomes and long-term survival. *JAMA.* 2009;302(3):290–297.
47. Saver Jl, Carroll JD, Thaler DE, et al. Long-term outcomes of patent foramen ovale closure or medical therapy after stroke. *N Engl J Med.* 2017;377:1022–1032.
48. Rocca GD, Costa MG, Coccia C, et al. Continuous right ventricular end-diastolic volume in comparison with left ventricular end-diastolic area. *Eur J Anaesthesiol.* 2009;26:272–278.
49. Royse CF. Ultrasound-guided haemodynamic state assessment. *Best Pract Res Clin Anaesthesiol.* 2009;23:273–283.
50. Wood PW, Choy JB, Nanda NC, Becher H. Left ventricular ejection fraction and volumes: it depends on the imaging method. *Echocardiography.* 2014;31:87–100.
51. Jenkins C, Bricknell K, Hanekom L, Marwick TH. Reproducibility and accuracy of echocardiographic measurements of left ventricular parameters using real-time three-dimensional echocardiography. *J Am Coll Cardiol.* 2004;44:878–886.
52. Buccheri S, Costanzo L, Tamburino C, Monte I. Reference values for real time three-dimensional echocardiography–derived left ventricular volumes and ejection fraction: review and meta-analysis of currently available studies. *Echocardiography.* 2015;32:1841–1850.
53. Lang RM, Bierig M, Devereux RB, et al. Recommendations for chamber quantification: a report from the American Society of Echocardiography's Guidelines and Standards Committee and the Chamber Quantification Writing Group, Developed in Conjunction with the European Association of Echocardiography, a Branch of the European Society of Cardiology. *J Am Soc Echocardiogr.* 2005;18:1440–1463.
54. Liodakis E, Al Sharef O, Dawson D, Nihoyannopoulos P. The use of real-time three-dimensional echocardiography for assessing mechanical synchronicity. *Heart.* 2009;95:1865–1871.
55. Vieira ML, Cury AF, Naccarato G, et al. Analysis of left ventricular regional dyssynchrony: comparison between real time 3D echocardiography and tissue Doppler imaging. *Echocardiography.* 2009;26:675–683.
56. Tops LF, Delgado V, Marsan NA, Bax JJ. Myocardial strain to detect subtle left ventricular systolic dysfunction. *Eur J Heart Failure.* 2017;19:307–313.
57. Yang ZR, Zhou QC, Lee L, et al. Quantitative assessment of left ventricular systolic function in patients with coronary heart disease by velocity vector imaging. *Echocardiography.* 2012;29:340–345.
58. Redfield MM, Jacobsen SJ, Burnett Jr JC, Mahoney DW, Bailey KR, Rodeheffer RJ. Burden of systolic and diastolic ventricular dysfunction in the community: appreciating the scope of the heart failure epidemic. *JAMA.* 2003;289(2):194–202.

59. Fayad A, Ansari MT, Yang H, Ruddy T, Wells GA. Perioperative diastolic dysfunction in patients undergoing noncardiac surgery is an independent risk factor for cardiovascular events. *Anesthesiology*. 2016;125:72–91.
60. Matyal R, Hess PE, Subramaniam B, et al. Perioperative diastolic dysfunction during vascular surgery and its association with postoperative outcome. *J Vasc Surg*. 2009;50:70–76.
61. Nagueh SF, Smiseth OA, Appleton CP, et al. Recommendations for the evaluation of left ventricular diastolic function by echocardiography: an update from the American Society of Echocardiography and the European Association of Cardiovascular Imaging. *J Am Soc Echocardiogr*. 2016;29:277–314.
62. Swaminathan M, Nicoara A, Phillips-Bute BG, et al. Utility of a simple algorithm to grade diastolic dysfunction and predict outcome after coronary artery bypass graft surgery. *Ann Thorac Surg*. 2011;91:1844–1850.
63. Borde DP, Asegaonkar B, Apsingekar P, et al. Monitoring diastolic dysfunction using a simplified algorithm in patients undergoing off-pump coronary artery bypass grafting surgery. *Ann Card Anaesth*. 2016;19:231–239.
64. Wang YC, Huang CH, Tu YK. Pulmonary hypertension and pulmonary artery acceleration time: a systematic review and meta-analysis. *J Am Soc Echocardiogr*. 2018;31:201–210.
65. Kurzyna M, Torbicki A, Pruszczyk P, et al. Disturbed right ventricular ejection pattern as a new Doppler echocardiographic sign of acute pulmonary embolism. *Am J Cardiol*. 2002;90:507–511.
66. Lodato JA, Ward RP, Lang RM. Echocardiographic predictors of pulmonary embolism in patients referred for helical CT. *Echocardiography*. 2008;25(6):584–590.
67. Izrailtyan I, Clark J, Swaminathan M, et al. Case report: Optimizing intraoperative detection of pulmonary embolism using contrast-enhanced echocardiography. *Can J Anesth*. 2006;53:711–715.
68. Banks DA, Pretorius GV, Kerr KM, Manecke GR. Pulmonary endarterectomy: Part I. Pathophysiology, clinical manifestations, and diagnostic evaluation of chronic thromboembolic pulmonary hypertension. *Semin Cardiothorac Vasc Anesth*. 2014;18(4):319–330.
69. Zoghbi WA, Enriquez-Sarano M, Foster E, et al. Recommendations for evaluation of the severity of native valvular regurgitation with two-dimensional and Doppler echocardiography. *J Am Soc Echocardiogr*. 2003;16:777–802.
70. Luxford J, Bassin L, D'AMbra M. Echocardiography of the tricuspid valve. *Ann Cardiothorac Surg*. 2017;6(3):223–239.
71. Reesink HJ, Marcus JT, Tulevski II, Jamieson S, Kloek JJ. Reverse right ventricular remodeling after pulmonary endarterectomy in patients with chronic thromboembolic pulmonary hypertension: Utility of magnetic resonance imaging to demonstrate restoration of the right ventricle. *J Thorac Cardiovasc Surg*. 2007;133:58–64.
72. Xirouchaki N, Magkanas E, Vaporidi K, et al. Lung ultrasound in critically ill patients: comparison with bedside chest radiography. *Intensive Care Med*. 2011;37:1488–1493.
73. Lichtenstein DA, Meziere GA, Lagoueyte JF, Biderman P, Goldstein I, Gepner A. A-lines and B-lines: lung ultrasound as a bedside tool for predicting pulmonary artery occlusion pressure in the critically ill. *Chest*. 2009;136:1014–1020.
74. Lichtenstein DA. BLUE-Protocol and FALLS-Protocol two applications of lung ultrasound in the critically ill. *Chest*. 2015;147(6):1659–1670.
75. Lichtenstein DA, Meziere GA. Relevance of lung ultrasound in the diagnosis of acute respiratory failure-the BLUE protocol. *Chest*. 2008;134:117–125.
76. Volpicelli G, Elbarbary M, Blaivas M, Lichtenstein DA, Mathis G. International evidence-based recommendations for point-of-care lung ultrasound. *Intensive Care Med*. 2012;38:577–591.
77. Cavays YA, Girard M, Desjardins G, Denault AY. Transesophageal lung ultrasonography: a novel technique for investigating hypoxemia. *J Can Anesth*. 2016;63:1266–1276.
78. Sanchez PG, Rouse M, Pratt DL, et al. Lung donation after controlled circulatory determination of death: a review of current practices and outcomes. *Transplant Proc*. 2015;47:1958–1965.
79. Palleschi A, Rosso L, Musso V, Rimessi A, Bonitta G, Nosotti M. Lung transplantation from donation after controlled cardiocirculatory death. Systematic review and meta-analysis. *Transplant Rev*. 2020;30(1):100513.
80. Cypel M, Yeung JC, Liu M, et al. Normothermic ex vivo lung perfusion in clinical lung transplantation. *N Engl J Med*. 2011;364:1431–1440.
81. Tikkanen JM, Cypel M, Machuca TN, et al. Functional outcomes and quality of life after normothermic ex vivo lung perfusion lung transplantation. *J Heart Lung Transplant*. 2015;34:547–556.
82. Mason DP, Thuita L, Nowicki ER, Murthy SC, Pettersson GB, Blackstone EH. Should lung transplantation be performed for patients on mechanical respiratory support? The US experience. *J Thorac Cardiovasc Surg*. 2010;139:765–773.
83. Biscotti M, Sonett J, Bacchetta M. ECMO as bridge to lung transplant. *Thorac Surg Clin*. 2015;25:17–25.
84. Hakim AH, Ahmad U, McCurry KR, et al. Contemporary outcomes of extracorporeal membrane oxygenation used as bridge to lung transplantation. *Ann Thorac Surg*. 2018;106:192–198.
85. Garijo JM, Cypel M, McRae K, Machuca T, Cunningham V, Slinger P. The evolving role of extracorporeal membrane oxygenation in lung transplantation: implications for anesthetic management. *J Cardiothorac Vasc Anesth*. 2019;33(7):1995–2006.
86. Oto T, Rosenfeldt F, Rowland M, et al. Extracorporeal membrane oxygenation after lung transplantation: evolving technique improves outcomes. *Ann Thorac Surg*. 2004;78:1230–1235.
87. Cahalan MK, Abel M, Goldman M, et al. American Society of Echocardiography and Society of Cardiovascular Anesthesiologists task force guidelines for training in perioperative echocardiography. *Anesth Analg*. 2002;94:1384–1388.
88. Haddad F, Hunt SA, Rosenthal DN, Murphy DJ. Right ventricular function in cardiovascular disease, part I: anatomy, physiology, aging, and functional assessment of the right ventricle. *Circulation*. 2008;117:1436–1448.
89. Hausmann D, Daniel WG, Mugge A, Heublein B, Hamm M, Schafers HJ, Haverick A. Imaging of pulmonary artery and vein anastomoses by transesophageal echocardiography after lung transplantation. *Circulation*. 1992;86(suppl II);II-251–258.
90. McIlroy DR, Sesto AC, Buckland MR. Pulmonary vein thrombosis, lung transplantation, and intraoperative transesophageal echocardiography. *J Cardiothorac Vasc Anesth*. 2006;20:712–715.
91. Cartwright BL, Jackson A, Cooper J. Intraoperative pulmonary vein examination by transesophageal echocardiography: an anatomic update and review of utility. *J Cardiothorac Vasc Anesth*. 2013;27:111–120.
92. Kumar N, Essandoh M, Bhatt A, et al. Pulmonary cuff dysfunction after lung transplant surgery: a systematic review of the evidence and analysis of its clinical implications. *J Heart Lung Transplant*. 2019;38:530–544.
93. Park KW. Protamine and protamine reactions. *Int Anesthesiol Clin*. 2004;42(3):135–145.

Index

Page numbers followed by '*f*' indicate figures, '*t*' indicate tables, '*b*' indicate boxes.

A

Acetaminophen
  acute pain, postoperative management, 330
  postthoracotomy pain syndrome, 346
Achalasia, 654, 654*f*
Acute exacerbation of chronic obstructive pulmonary disease (AECOPD), 477
Acute kidney injury, 294*t*, 297
Acute kidney insufficiency, 294, 294*t*
Acute lung injury, 295*b*, 295
  fluid overload, 297. *See also* Fluid administration strategies
  hydrostatic edema, 295
  immune transfusion-related to, 298
  and multiple-hit hypothesis, 296
  postthoracotomy, risk factors, 296*b*
  revised starling and endothelial glycocalyx layer, 295
  Starling forces, 295
  transfusion-related to, 298, 299*f*
Acute pain, postoperative management
  acetaminophen, 330
  clinical advantages, 335
  complications and safety considerations, 333, 337
  controversies, 335
  erector spinae plane block, 338
  gabapentinoids, 332
  glucocorticoids, 332
  incidence, 328
  intercostal nerve block, 337, 338*f*
  intravenous lidocaine, 332
  mechanism of blockade and distribution of spread, 336
  multimodal analgesia and perioperative analgesic strategies, 329
  N-methyl-D-aspartate-receptor antagonists, 331
  nociceptive stimuli, 328
  nonsteroidal antiinflammatory drugs, 331
  opioids, 330
  regional anesthesia techniques, 332, 332*t*
  serratus anterior plane block, 339, 340*f*
  single-shot erector spinae plane *vs.* continuous erector spinae plane, 339
  sources of pain, 329*t*
  technique, 333
  thoracic epidural analgesia, 333, 334*f*
    vs. paravertebral block, 337
  thoracic paravertebral block, 335
Acute pulmonary hypertension, transesophageal echocardiography, 798, 802*f*–803*f*
Acute respiratory distress syndrome (ARDS), 279, 293, 589, 722
  Berlin definition of, 250*t*
  postthoracotomy complications, 389
Air leak, 590
  treatment, postoperative thoracic surgery, 176
Airway collapse, 508–509
Airway fistulas in adults
  alternative methods
    airway and ventilatory management, 672
    induction of anesthesia, 672
  alveolopleural/alveolar-parenchymal-pleural fistula (APF), 669
  bronchopleural-cutaneous fistula (BPCF), 669
  characteristics, 670*t*
  incidence and outcomes
    alveolopleural fistula, 674
Airway fistulas in adults (*Continued*)
    bronchoesophageal fistula, 673, 675*f*
    tracheoesophageal fistula, 673
  mechanical ventilation, 672*b*
  persistent air leak (PAL), 669
  preoperative assessment and planning, 670
  repair, 672
  risks and benefits, 673
Airway injury, 589
Airway pressures, oxygenation, 150
Airway stent, 741. *See also* Tracheal stents
  placement complications, 751*t*
Airway tumors, 62
Airway valves, 22*f*
Almitrine, 110
Almitrine besylate, 207
Alveolar component, 149
Alveolar dead space, 78
Alveolar gas spaces, 27
Alveolar-to-arterial oxygen gradient, 80
Alveolopleural fistula, 674. *See also* Airway fistulas in adults
2014 American Association of Thoracic Surgeons (AATS) guidelines, 310
American Society of Anesthesiologists (ASA), 785
American Society of Anesthesiologists Standards, 143, 144*b*
American Society of Anesthesiology Physical Classification System, 116*t*
American Society of Echocardiographers (ASE), 785
Analyzers, oxygenation, 144
Anatomic component, 149
Anemia, 128
Anesthesia effect, lung volumes, 69
Anticoagulation, 313. *See also* Postoperative atrial fibrillation (POAF)
Apnea-Hypopnea Index (AHI), 715
Apnea index (AI), 715
ARISCAT score, 288*t*, 289
  postthoracotomy complications, 378*t*
Arndt® blocker, 230
Arndt wire-guided endobronchial blocker, 702
Arousal Index (ARI), 715
Arrhythmias, 428
Arterial waveform analysis, 161
Ascending thoracic and aortic arch aneurysms, thoracic aortic aneurysms, 562
Asthma, 117
  hypoxic pulmonary vasoconstriction, 200
Atelectasis
  postoperative pulmonary complication, 260–261
  postoperative thoracic surgery, 175
  postthoracotomy complications, 387, 387*f*
Atrial fibrillation (AF), 308, 591. *See also* Postoperative atrial fibrillation (POAF)
  postthoracotomy complications
    risk, 385*t*
    and supraventricular arrhythmias, 384
    treatment, 384
Auscultation, double-lumen endotracheal tubes, 221
Awake endotracheal intubation, 701

B

Bilateral intercostal blockade, 605
Bilateral paravertebral block, 605
Bilevel positive airway pressure (BIPAP), 715

Bioimpedance, 162
Bioreactance, 162
Biotrauma, 281
Bleeding
 lung/lobar, 701
 postthoracotomy complications, 379
Blood pressure monitoring
 intraarterial catheterization, 157
 oscillometry, 154, 155*f*
 tonometry, 155
 volume clamp technique, 156
Blunt cardiac trauma, 493
BODE Index, 420
Body mass index (BMI), 533
Bradyarrhythmias, postthoracotomy complications, 386
Bronchi, 25
Bronchial blockade, 6
Bronchial blocker (BB), 584, 701–703
 lung isolation, 444
 lung separation, 227*b*, 227
 pediatric thoracic surgery, 321
 spine surgery, 680
Bronchioles, 25
Bronchoesophageal fistula, 673, 675*f*. *See also* Airway fistulas in adults
Bronchopleural-cutaneous fistula (BPCF), 669. *See also* Airway fistulas in adults
Bronchopleural fistula, 590
 treatment, postoperative thoracic surgery, 176
Bronchoscopic lung volume reduction procedures, 478–479, 479*f*
Bronchoscopy, pediatric thoracic surgery, 319
Bullae, radiology, thorax, 35, 37*f*–38*f*

C

CABG. *See* Coronary artery bypass grafting (CABG) procedures
Calcium channel blockers, 111
Capnography and capnometry, 150
Carbon dioxide
 cascade, oxygenation, 148
 insufflation, robotic thoracic surgery, 762
Carbon monoxide, diffusing capacity, 82
Cardiac arrhythmias, 308
 postthoracotomy complications, 383
  drugs used, 386*t*
Cardiac comorbidities, 129
Cardiac contusion, thoracic trauma, 494
Cardiac herniation, 592
Cardiac implantable devices and left ventricular assist devices, 430
Cardiac output (CO)
 monitoring, 159
 transesophageal echocardiography, 796*f*
Cardiopulmonary exercise testing, 83, 121
Cardiovascular considerations, thoracic aortic aneurysms, 562
Cardiovascular disease (CVD), 116
 lung resection surgery, 423
  anesthetic goals in patients with coronary artery disease, 432, 433*t*
  arrhythmias, 428
  biomarkers inclusion, 430
  cardiac implantable devices and left ventricular assist devices, 430
  congenital heart disease in adults, 428
  coronary revascularization recommendation, 430, 430*t*
  diagnostic test, 428
  DUKE activity functional status questionnaire, 429*t*
  electrocardiogram, 430
  heart failure, 426
  hypertension, 425
  hypoxemia and coronary artery disease, 431, 433*t*
  incidence, 423
  ischemic heart disease, 424
  metabolic equivalent (METS), 428, 428*t*
  nonischemic heart failure, 426*t*
  in patients with coronary artery disease, 434
  perioperative therapy recommendation, 431, 432*t*
  prosthetic valves, 427
  pulmonary hypertension, 428
  recalibrated thoracic revised cardiac index, 429*t*
Cardiovascular disease (CVD) (*Continued*)
  risk assessment, 423, 424*t*–425*t*
  risk stratification, thoracic procedures, 429, 429*t*
  valvular heart disease, 427, 427*t*
Cardiovascular drugs impact, 205
Cartilage, 24
Central nervous system protection and monitoring, 572
Central venous pressure (CVP), 157
Cerfolio classification, air leaks, 671*b*
Cervical mediastinoscopy (CM), 516, 518*f*
Chest radiographs, 33, 34*f*
Chest tube
 management, postoperative care, 354
 placement radiology, 39
Chest wall tumors, 62
Cholinergic crises, myasthenia gravis and, 694, 694*t*
Chronic lung diseases, hypoxic pulmonary vasoconstriction, 199
Chronic obstructive pulmonary disease (COPD), 117, 624, 635*t*
 anesthetic management of endoscopic treatment, 479
 consideration of anesthetic depth, 482
 endoscopic treatment, 482*t*
 incidence, 410
 monitored anesthesia care *vs.* general, 481
 preoperative treatment, 480
 regional *vs.* general, 482
 types of anesthesia, endoscopic treatment, 481
Cliny right-sided double-lumen endotracheal tubes, 225, 226*f*
Closing capacity, lung volumes, 69
Closing volume, lung volumes, 69
Cohen® Flexitip Endobronchial Blocker, 230, 702–703, 703*f*
Comprehensive geriatric assessment, frailty and, 129
Computed tomography scan, 42–43
Congenital heart disease in adults, 428
Continuous positive airway pressure (CPAP), 715
 pediatric thoracic surgery, 321
Coopdech blocker, 703
Cooximetry, 148
Cormack-Lehane graded laryngoscopy, 719
Coronary artery bypass grafting (CABG) procedures, 785
Coronary artery disease, 432, 433*t*
Coronary revascularization recommendation, 430, 430*t*
Cricoid, 24
Cricothyroid membrane, 25
Cryoablation, postthoracotomy pain syndrome, 347
Cystic fibrosis (CF), 625
 anesthesia
  emergence from, 729
  induction of, 729, 736
  intraoperative period, 735
  management, 736
  preoperative evaluation, 734, 735*b*, 737*f*
 definition, 730, 731*f*–732*f*, 736*f*
 intraoperative period, 730
 organ transplantations, 733
 postoperative period, 738

D

Dead space, 81, 149
DeBakey's accomplishments, 557, 558*f*
Dexmedetomidine, 206
Diabetes, 128
Diabetes mellitus, 645
Diaphragm, 33
Diaphragmatic rupture, 494, 495*f*
Diastolic function evaluation, 800*f*
Differential lung ventilation (DLV), 364
Differential pressure breathing, 2, 2*f*, 4*f*
Difficult airway
 double-lumen endotracheal tube, 242
 laryngeal mask airway and bronchial blocker, 242
 and lung isolation, 240
 preoperative assessment, 240
Difficulty with bag-mask ventilation (DMV), 718
Diffusion, 80
 block, 88–89

Distress syndrome, 200
Donor
  criteria, 641*t*
  evaluation, 631
  management, 632
Doppler-based techniques, 161
Double-lumen endobronchial tube, 7, 8*f*, 703
Double-lumen endotracheal tubes, 213
  auscultation, 221
  Cliny right-sided, 225, 226*f*
  complications associated with, 226
  difficult airway, 242
  flexible fiberoptic bronchoscopy, 221
  left-sided, 218
  methods of insertion, 215
  newer technology with, 223
  radiology, thorax, 41
  right-sided, 220*b*, 220
  single-lumen endotracheal tube exchange, 244
  size selection, 213
  tube exchanger technique, 242, 244*f*
  ultrasonography, 221, 223
Double-lumen tubes (DLT), 584, 585*t*–586*t*
  vs. bronchial blockers, lung isolation, 443, 444*t*
  pediatric thoracic surgery, 323
Dual lumen bicaval cannula, 398
DUKE activity functional status questionnaire, 429*t*
Dyssynchrony index (DI), 798*f*

E

Emphysema, 411
  Chartis system, 474*f*
  LIBERATE and EMPROVE, 474, 475*f*
  manifestations, 468
  pulmonx Zephyr valve, 471*f*
  radiology, thorax, 37*f*
  spiration intrabronchial valve (IBV), 472*f*
  spiration valve system (SVS), 472*f*
  surgical treatment, 469, 469*f*
  valves in treatment, 470
Empyema
  causes of, 704, 705*t*
  management, 704
  phases of, 706*t*
  stage of, 706
  timing of surgery, 706
Endobronchial intubation, 703–704
Endobronchial Valve for Emphysema Palliation Trial (VENT) study, 472, 473*f*
Endobronchial valves, 674–676
Endothelin receptor antagonists, 111
Endotracheal anesthesia, tracheal insufflation and, 3
Endotracheal intubation, and laryngoscopy, 4, 7*f*
End-stage renal disease, 294*t*
Enhanced recovery after surgery (ERAS®), 766
  barriers and strategies with implementation, 772, 772*f*
  components, 766, 767*t*
  evidence and recommendation, 767*t*
  fast-track *vs.*, 766
  postoperative components, 771
  protocol, 353
  thoracic surgery
    comorbid conditions optimization, 768
    intraoperative components, 770
    justification and applicability, 767
    nutrition, 769
    prehabilitation, 769
    preoperative components, 768
    protocol, 768*f*
    tobacco and alcohol cessation, 769
Enhanced recovery programs (ERPs), 766
Epiphrenic diverticulum, 651
ERAS. *See* Enhanced recovery after surgery (ERAS®)
ERAS for thoracic surgery (ERATS), 766
Erector spinae plane block, 338
Ergometric testing, 121
Esophageal cancer, 55
  staging TNM classification, 56*t*
Esophageal diverticula, 651
Esophageal peristalsis, 650
Esophageal reconstruction, 658
Esophageal rupture and perforation, 652, 653*f*, 653*t*
Esophageal stricture, 654
Esophageal surgery
  anesthesia management, 660
  complications, 663
  fluid management, 661
  morbidity and mortality, 649
  pain therapy, 662
  perioperative monitoring, 661
  preoperative evaluation, 660
Esophageal tumors, 655
Esophagectomy, 760
Esophagus
  anatomy, 649, 650*f*
  sphincters, 651
  surgical approaches, 656, 656*t*
  surrounding structures, 650*t*
  tumors of, 656*t*
  venous drainage of, 650
European Society of Thoracic Surgeons (ESTS) guidelines, 766
Evaluation of Heart Failure and Pulmonary Artery Catheterization Effectiveness Trial (ESCAPE)
  transesophageal echocardiography, 786
Exercise, 126
Expiratory muscles, 20*f*, 33
Expiratory reserve volume (ERV), 68, 714
Extracorporeal membrane oxygenation (ECMO) support, 669
  cannulation approaches and support modality, 395
  circuit operational parameters, 395, 396*f*
  clinical adoption, 394, 394*f*
  lung transplantation, 628, 628*f*–629*f*
    cannulation techniques, 630
    complications, 628–629
    patient selection, 629
    prelung transplant, 630
    transfusions and anticoagulation, 631
  modern, 393, 394*f*
  operational parameters, 395
  postoperative care, 371
  postoperative period, 644
  pump afterload, 397
  pump speed, 397
  during thoracic cases, positioning, 139
  tracheal stents, 745, 747*f*
Extracorporeal ventilatory therapies
  as bridge to lung transplantation, 402, 403*t*
  central venoarterial extracorporeal membrane oxygenation, 405
  clinical management, 398, 400*t*
  clinical use, 392
  experimental therapies, 407
  extracorporeal membrane oxygenation circuit
    cannulation approaches and support modality, 395
    circuit operational parameters, 395, 396*f*
    clinical adoption, 394, 394*f*
    modern, 393, 394*f*
    operational parameters, 395
    pump afterload, 397
    pump speed, 397
  failure of support and goals of care, 402
  hollow fiber membrane devices and modern oxygenators, 392
  lung disease and altered perfusion, 406
  mechanical ventilation management, 400
  peripheral venoarterial extracorporeal membrane oxygenation, 405
  persistent hypoxia, 401
  physiologic basis, 397
    as bridge to recovery in lung failure, 397
    cannulation approaches, 399*f*
    physiology of hypoxic and hypercapnic respiratory failure, 398
  pump technology, 393
  right ventricular dysfunction approach, 401

Extracorporeal ventilatory therapies (*Continued*)
  sedation management, 406
  weaning, 401
Extravascular lung water (EVLW), 164
Extubation, 693
Extubation/mechanical ventilation after surgery, 246
Ex vivo lung perfusion (EVLP), 633
EZ-blocker, 231, 703

F

Fanning equation, 671*b*
Fast-track *vs.* enhanced recovery after surgery, 766
Fell-O'Dwyer Apparatus, 5*f*
Femoral-femoral vein approach, 398
Femoral-RIJ approach, 398
Fexible fiberoptic bronchoscope (FFB), 172
  composition, 172
  contraindications, 173
  indications, 173
Fiberoptic bronchoscopy, 445
Fistula
  esophageal, 651
  formation, airway. *See* Airway fistulas in adults
  tracheal stents and, 744*f*
Flexible bronchoscopy
  airway management, 174
  anesthesia, 178
  with bronchial blockers, 175
  contraindications, 173
  presurgical diagnostics, 173
  ventilation techniques, 178
  ventilatory support during, 483
Flexible fiberoptic bronchoscopy, 221
Flexible *versus* rigid bronchoscopy, 747
Flexion, positioning, 135
Flow-time curves, 149–150
Fluid administration strategies
  choice of fluids, 302
  clinical practice, 302
  crystalloids *vs.* colloid solutions, 302
  dynamic variables, 301
  end-expiratory occlusion test, 302
  fluid challenge, 302
  fluid responsiveness, 300
  goal-directed strategies, 299, 300*f*
  hydroxyethyl starch, 302*f*
  liberal *vs.* restrictive, 299
  normovolemia as target, 299
  passive leg raising (PLR), 302
  static variables, 300
Fluid management, 586
  esophageal surgery, 661
  lung resection, 293
  postoperative care, 359*b*
Fluid responsiveness, 162
Fogarty embolectomy catheter, 701
Forced expiratory volume in one second (FEV1), 81
Forced vital capacity, 82
Fractal distribution of perfusion, 92
Frailty and comprehensive geriatric assessment, 129
Frank's Windkessel model, 161*f*
Free online bronchoscopy simulator, 236*f*
Frenckner Spiropulsator, 12*f*
Fuel cell oxygen analyzer, 144
Fuji Uniblocker®, 230, 701
Functional residual capacity (FRC), 68, 714

G

Gabapentin, 346
Gabapentinoids, 332
Gas exchange, 29, 30*f*
Gas spaces, 29
Gastroesophageal reflux disease (GERD), 655
Gastrointestinal considerations, 567
General endotracheal anesthesia (GETA), 692
Genetics, hypoxic pulmonary vasoconstriction, 199
Geriatric patient, thoracic anesthesia
  age-related respiratory changes, 546*t*
  cardiovascular changes, 544, 545*t*
  demographics, 544
  Functional Assessment of Cancer Therapy-Esophagus *(FACT-E)*, 553*f*
  hepatorenal changes, 546, 548*t*
  nervous system changes, 547
  physiology of aging, 544
  postoperative care and planning, 552
  preoperative assessment, 550
  pulmonary changes, 545
  risk stratification, 551
  surgical intervention, risk-benefit relationship, 549
  surgical techniques role, 550
Germ cell tumors, 59
Glucocorticoids, 332

H

Heart failure, 426
  postthoracotomy complications, 382
Hemodynamic monitoring, 786
Hemoptysis
  airway protection, 701
  breathing, 699
  cause of, 696, 697*t*
  circulation, 699
  disability/position, 699
  exposure, 699
  indications, 696
  initial measures for patients with, 699*b*
  management, 699, 700*f*
  postoperative thoracic surgery, 175
  preoperative assessment, 697, 698*f*
  therapeutic options, 698–701
  treatment, 699–701, 700*f*
Hemothorax, 492, 493*f*
Hiatal hernia, 655
High-flow nasal cannula oxygen therapy (HFNCOT), 365
High-frequency jet ventilation (HFJV), 182
  superimposed, 183
High-frequency oscillatory ventilation (HFOV), 183
High-frequency percussive ventilation, 184
High-frequency positive pressure ventilation, 184
High-frequency ventilation (HFV), 182, 183*t*
  airway obstructing tumor, 187
  anesthetic considerations, 189
  application, 184
  bias flow, 189
  bronchopleural fistula, 188
  cannot ventilate cannot intubate situation, 187
  contraindications, 188
  driving pressure, 189
  equipment, 185
  fraction of inspired oxygen, 189
  imaging, stereotactic procedures, and catheter ablation, 188
  indications, 186, 186*t*
  inspiratory fraction, 189
  mean airway pressure, 189
  postcardiac surgery use, 188
  postoperative care, 364
  respiratory rate, 189
  rigid bronchoscopy, 186, 187*f*
  risks and benefits, 189
  tidal volume, 189
  tracheal and carinal resection, 187
  ventilation, nondependent lung, 187
Hunsaker Mon-Jet tube, 185, 185*f*
Hypercapnia, 80
Hypertension, 425
Hypopharynx, 22
Hypopnea, 714. *See also* Sleep-disordered breathing
Hypoxemia, 80, 88, 589
  and coronary artery disease, 431, 433*t*

Hypoxemia (*Continued*)
  one-lung ventilation, 287
  pediatric thoracic surgery, 323
  thoracic spine surgery, 681
Hypoxic pulmonary vasoconstriction (HPV), 101, 193
  altitude, 199
  analgesics impact, 205
  anesthesia effects and mechanical ventilation, 200
  anesthetics impact, 205, 208
  asthma, 200
  cardiovascular drugs impact, 205
  chronic lung diseases, 199
  distress syndrome, 200
  genetics, 199
  hypoxic signal, different tissues, 193
  integrated ventilatory and perfusion changes, 202, 202*f*
  lung perfusion, 196*f*, 200
  lung volume ventilation, 201, 201*f*
  modulation, 197
  neurohumoral modulation, 197
  obstructive sleep apnea, 200
  oxygen sensing and effector mechanisms, 195
  physical factors, 198
  physiologic variations, 198
  physiology, 193
  pulmonary circulation, 198
  senescence, 198
  thoracic epidural anesthesia, 207
  time course, 195
  variations of, 199
Hypoxic signal, different tissues, 193

I

Infectious risk, tracheal stents, 751
Inhaled nitric oxide, 109
Innervation, 31
Innominate compression, 520
Inspiratory fractions of oxygen (F_iO_2), 105
Inspiratory muscles, 33
Inspiratory reserve volume, 68
Integrated ventilatory and perfusion changes, 202, 202*f*
Intercostal nerve approach, 347–348
Intercostal nerve block, 337, 338*f*
International Society for Heart and Lung Transplantation (ISHLT) guidelines, 623–624
Interstitial lung disease (ILD), 625
Interstitial syndrome, lung ultrasound, 783, 783*f*
Interventional pneumology, 177
Intraarterial catheterization, 157
Intraoperative hemodynamic exam, 787
Intraoperative monitoring, 8
Intrathoracic tumors, principles, 52
Intravenous lidocaine, 332
Intravenous *vs.* inhaled anesthesia, 586
Ischemic heart disease, 424
Ischemic time, 632

J

Jejunal conduits, 658–659

K

K-adenosine triphosphatase activity, 281
Kaplan-Meier curve, open thoracotomy, 439*f*
Ketamine, 347

L

Lambert-Eaton myasthenic syndrome, 690*t*
Laryngeal mask airway and bronchial blocker, 242
Larynx, 23, 24*f*
  injuries, 489
Lateral decubitus position, 93, 134, 134*f*
  awake, spontaneously breathing patients, 96
  chest closed, 96
Lateral decubitus position (*Continued*)
  chest open, 96
  mediastinal shift, 99
  paradoxic respiration, 100
Lateral position, 94
  anesthetized patients
    chest closed, 99
    chest open, 99
Left-sided double-lumen endotracheal tubes, 218
Left ventricle assessment
  transesophageal echocardiography, 793, 793*f*–796*f*
    dyssynchrony index (DI), 798*f*
    ME-4C and ME-2C views, 797*f*
    Swaminathan's simplified e' based algorithm, 801*f*
Left ventricular ejection fraction (LVEF) measurements, 796*f*
Life-threatening refractory hypoxemia, 704
Lobectomy
  postoperative length of stay after, 580*b*
  robotic thoracic surgery, 758
Lobe/lung segment torsions, 176
Lobe torsion, 379
Lower airway, 25
Lower extremities positioning, 134*f*, 134
Low oxygen saturation, 147
Lung atelectasis, dependent, 100
Lung cancer, 52, 53*t*, 516, 519
Lung collapse during lung isolation, 234
Lung consolidation, 783, 783*f*
Lung function, predicted postoperative, 120
Lung injury
  anesthesiologic causes, 263
  mechanical ventilation, 264
  pathogenesis of intraoperative, 263
  surgical causes, 262
Lung isolation. *See also* Video-assisted thoracic surgery (VATS)
  bronchial blockers, 444
  challenges during video-assisted thoracoscopic surgery, 443
  difficult airway and, 240
  double-Lumen tubes *vs.* bronchial blockers, 443, 444*t*
  fiberoptic bronchoscopy, 445
  history, 443
  indications, 443
  with lower airway abnormalities, 245
  total collapse of nonventilated lung, 446
  with tracheostomies, 245
  upper airway abnormalities and, 241*b*, 241
Lung mass, 34, 43
Lung perfusion, 196*f*, 200
Lung resection surgery, 523
  American College of Chest Physicians algorithm, 582*f*
  cardiovascular disease (CVD), 423
    anesthetic goals in patients with coronary artery disease, 432, 433*t*
    arrhythmias, 428
    biomarkers inclusion, 430
    cardiac implantable devices and left ventricular assist devices, 430
    congenital heart disease in adults, 428
    coronary revascularization recommendation, 430, 430*t*
    diagnostic test, 428
    DUKE activity functional status questionnaire, 429*t*
    electrocardiogram, 430
    heart failure, 426
    hypertension, 425
    hypoxemia and coronary artery disease, 431, 433*t*
    incidence, 423
    ischemic heart disease, 424
    metabolic equivalent (METS), 428, 428*t*
    nonischemic heart failure, 426*t*
    in patients with coronary artery disease, 434
    perioperative therapy recommendation, 431, 432*t*
    prosthetic valves, 427
    pulmonary hypertension, 428
    recalibrated thoracic revised cardiac index, 429*t*
    risk assessment, 423, 424*t*–425*t*
    risk stratification, thoracic procedures, 429, 429*t*
    valvular heart disease, 427, 427*t*

Lung resection surgery (*Continued*)
- central venous catheters (CVCs), 584
- lung subsegments present in each lobe, 580*f*
- monitoring, 583
- morbidity and mortality, 581*f*
- predicted postoperative DLCO (ppoDLCO%), 581
- preoperative evaluation of patient, 579
- pulmonary artery catheters (PAC), 584
- three-legged stool of preoperative assessment, 580*f*
- transesophageal echocardiography (TEE), 584

Lung separation techniques, 584, 585*t*
- Arndt® blocker, 230
- bronchial blockers, 227*b*, 227
- Cohen® Flexitip Endobronchial Blocker, 230
- complications with, 233
- double-lumen endotracheal tubes, 213
  - auscultation, 221
  - Cliny right-sided, 225, 226*f*
  - complications associated with, 226
  - flexible fiberoptic bronchoscopy, 221
  - left-sided, 218
  - methods of insertion, 215
  - newer technology with, 223
  - right-sided, 220*b*, 220
  - size selection, 213
  - ultrasonography, 221, 223
- EZ-blocker, 231
- free online bronchoscopy simulator, 236*f*
- Fuji Uniblocker®, 230
- lung collapse during lung isolation, 234
- methods of placement, 230
- robotic thoracic surgery, 762
- torque control blocker univent, 232
- trends in, 235
- VivaSight double-lumen tube, 220
- VivaSight® single-lumen tube with guided bronchial blocker, 232

Lung structure, essentials, 66

Lung transplantation
- acute rejection, 642
- allograft ventilation management, 636*f*
- anastomotic complications, 643
- anesthetic agents, 634
- anesthetic management, 633
- chronic lung allograft dysfunction, 644
- combined heart-lung transplant, 626
- contraindications, 623*t*
- cystic fibrosis, 733
- diabetes mellitus, 645
- disease-specific selection
  - chronic obstructive pulmonary disease (COPD), 624, 635*t*
  - cystic fibrosis (CF), 625
  - interstitial lung disease (ILD), 625
  - pulmonary vascular disease, 625
- donor criteria, 641*t*
- donor evaluation, 631
- donor management, 632
- epidemiology, 623
- extracorporeal membrane oxygenation, 628, 628*f*–629*f*
  - cannulation techniques, 630
  - complications, 628–629
  - patient selection, 629
  - prelung transplant, 630
  - transfusions and anticoagulation, 631
- extrapulmonary complications, 643
- ex vivo lung perfusion (EVLP), 633
- fluid management, 634
- graft dysfunction, 640
- infection, 645
- intraoperative mechanical support, 636
- intrathoracic complications, 643
- invasive mechanical ventilation, 628
- ischemic time, 632
- long-term complications, 644
- malignancy, 644
- monitoring and follow-up after discharge, 645
- organ allocation, 627*b*, 627

Lung transplantation (*Continued*)
- organ procurement, 632
- organ selection, 632
- pathologic grading, 642*t*
- pediatric, 627
- postoperative care
  - antihumoral therapy, 639
  - antiproliferative agents, 639
  - calcineurin inhibitors (CNIs), 638
  - chest tube management, 637
  - early postoperative complications, 640
  - fluid management, 637
  - glucocorticoids, 638
  - hemodynamic management, 636
  - immunosuppression, 638
  - induction immunosuppression agents, 638
  - infection prevention and management, 639
  - nutritional support and stress ulcer prophylaxis, 640
  - sedation and analgesia, 638
  - venous thromboembolism prevention, 639
  - ventilator management, 637
- primary graft dysfunction, 640, 640*f*, 641*t*
- pulmonary infiltrates, 641*t*
- recipient preparation, 627
- recipient selection, 623–624
- reperfused lung transplant allograft, 636*b*
- retransplantation, 626
- surgical procedure, 633
- survival 2008–2015, 623
- transesophageal echocardiography, 635, 635*f*, 642*t*, 805
- type of surgical procedure, 633
- vasoactive medications, 634

Lung ultrasound (LUS), 250, 775
- anatomic correlation and normal physiologic findings, 775, 777*f*
  - A lines, 778*f*
  - B lines, 778*f*
  - MMode demonstration, 779*f*
  - pleural view, 777*f*–778*f*
- atelectrauma, 255
- biotrauma, 255
- edema formation, 252
- fibroproliferative recovery phase, 253
- genotype, 251
- humoral factors, 252
- injured lung, pathophysiology of, 250, 252*f*
- interstitial syndrome and lung consolidation, 783, 783*f*
- microthrombosis, 253
- normal lung, 250
- ON-OFF phenomenon, 783
- pathologic phenotype, 251
- pleural effusion detection, 781, 781*f*–782*f*
- pneumothorax detection, 780, 780*f*–781*f*
- postoperative care, 356, 356*f*
- probes selection, 775
- protective ventilation, 256
- scanning protocols, 775, 776*f*–777*f*
- surfactant production, 252
- transesophageal echocardiography, 791*t*, 803, 805*f*–806*f*, 807*t*, 808*f*
- ventilator-induced lung injury, 253
- volutrauma, 255

Lung volume reduction surgery, 411
- anesthetic considerations
  - emergence, 418
  - intraoperative management, 416
  - maintenance and surgical procedure, 418
  - preoperative evaluation, 416
- BODE Index, 420
- early recovery, postanesthesia care unit, 419
- exclusion criteria, 415, 416*f*
- patient selection and rehabilitation, 415
- preoperative rehabilitation, 416

Lung volumes
- anesthesia effect, 69
- closing capacity, 69
- closing volume, 69
- expiratory reserve volume, 68

Lung volumes (*Continued*)
  functional residual capacity, 68
  inspiratory reserve volume, 68
  nomenclature, 67
  pulmonary function tests
    cardiopulmonary exercise testing, 83
    diffusing capacity, carbon monoxide, 82
    forced expiratory volume in one second (FEV1), 81
    forced vital capacity, 82
    recommendations, preoperative assessment, 83
  pulmonary gas exchange
    alveolar-to-arterial oxygen gradient, 80
    dead space, 81
    diffusion, 80
    hypercapnia, 80
    hypoxemia, 80
    oxygen saturation, 80
    perfusion, 77
    pulmonary blood flow (PBF), 78
    pulmonary vascular resistance, 79, 79*f*
    shunt, 80
    ventilation, 77
    ventilation-perfusion matching, 78, 80
  residual volume, 68
  respiratory mechanics, 71
    anesthesia effects, 77
    compliance, 73
    derecruitment, 76
    driving pressure, 72
    elastance, 73
    mechanical power, 76
    overdistension, 76
    resistance, 75
    strain, 75
    stress, 75
    transpulmonary pressure, 71
  tidal volume, 68
  total lung capacity, 69
Lung volume ventilation, 201, 201*f*
Lymph nodes, 516–517
  mediastinal, 517

M

Magnetic resonance imaging and pulmonary disease, 46
Major adverse cardiac events (MACE)
  postthoracotomy complications, 380
  transesophageal echocardiography, 785
Malignant pleural mesothelioma (MPM), 59
Mallampati test, 713–714
Malnutrition, 118
Marfan syndrome, 558
McKeown esophagectomy, 55
Mean airway pressure, 150
Mechanical component, 149
Mechanical ventilation, 8, 12*f*, 364*b*
Mediastinal mass
  anesthetic management
    considerations for, 511
    equipment considerations, 510
    monitors, access, and positioning considerations, 509
    preoperative treatment considerations, 509
  anterior, 505*f*
  contrast enhanced computed tomography, 506*f*
  diagnostic testing, 504
  magnetic resonance imaging, 506*f*
  malignant and benign, 504*t*
  management, 513
  potential complications, 512
  preanesthetic assessment, 503
  radiology, thorax, 35, 43
  risk stratification, 507, 508*b*
  and superior vena cava syndrome, 504*t*
  types and locations, 503*f*
Mediastinal surgery, 456
Mediastinal tumors, 58
Mediastinoscopy
  anesthetic management, 520
  cervical, 516, 518*f*
  complications and management, 521
  indications, 517, 517*f*
  nil per os (NPO) status, 516
  preoperative considerations
    investigations, 519
    medical history, 519
    monitoring, 520
  procedure, 518
  risks and benefits, 520
Mediastinum
  anatomy and pathophysiology, 501
  compartment model, 502*f*
  structures, 502*f*
Mesothelioma, 59
Metabolic equivalent (METS), 428, 428*t*
Microbolus technique, 164
Milestones, in thoracic surgery, 5
Minimal invasive repair of pectus excavatum (MIRPE), 597
Monitored anesthesia care (MAC), 143
  vs. general, 481
Monitoring blood, 145
Montgomery T-tube stent, 754–755, 755*f*
Morbid obesity (MO)
  obstructive sleep apnea, 713
  tracheal intubation in, 719
Multidetector computer tomography scan, 45
Muscle-powered air pump, 33
Muscle-specific tyrosine kinase (MuSK), 688
Myasthenia gravis (MG)
  acetylcholinesterase inhibitors, 693*t*
  and cholinergic crises, 694, 694*t*
  clinical and differential diagnosis, 688
  clinical classification, 688, 689*t*
  etiology and pathophysiology, 688
  foundation of America clinical classification, 456*t*
  incidence, 688
  vs. Lambert-Eaton myasthenic syndrome, 690*t*
  mechanical ventilation in, 691*t*
  mediastinal surgery, anesthesia in thymectomy, 456
  medical treatment, 689
  postoperative analgesia, 693
Myocardial infarction (MI), 380
Myocardial ischemia, 380

N

Nasopharynx, 22
Neck positioning, 135*f*, 135
Nervous system considerations, 564
Neurohumoral modulation, hypoxic pulmonary vasoconstriction, 197
Neuromuscular blockade, 692
N-methyl-D-aspartate-receptor antagonists, 331
Nociceptive stimuli, 328
Nondependent lung injury, 274
Noninvasive ventilation, 365, 366*t*
Nonischemic heart failure, 426*t*
Nonsmall cell lung cancer (NSCLC), 517
Nonsteroidal antiinflammatory drugs, 207
  acute pain, postoperative management, 331
  postthoracotomy pain syndrome, 347
Nonvitamin K oral anticoagulants, 315*f*
Normal tracheobronchial anatomy, 33
Nose, 20–21, 21*f*
Nuss surgical procedure, 600
Nutrition, 126

O

Obese patients, positioning, 140, 140*f*
Obesity, 118
  hypoventilation syndrome (OHS), 715
  obstructive sleep apnea, 713

Obstructive sleep apnea (OSA), 118
  hypoxic pulmonary vasoconstriction, 200
  intraoperative management
    airway management, 717, 718*f*
    anesthetic drugs/maintenance of anesthesia, 720
    emergence and extubation, 723
    intravenous fluid management, 723
    lung separation, 721
    one-lung ventilation, 721, 722*f*
    patient position, 716, 716*f*
  postoperative management
    complications, 725
    pain control, 724
  preoperative considerations, 713
    airway concerns, 713, 714*f*
    cardiovascular function, 716
    pulmonary function, 714
    sleep-disordered breathing, 714
Odontoid hypoplasia, 613*b*
Olfaction, 22
One-lung ventilation (OLV), 193, 240
  by age, 321*t*
  ARISCAT-score, 288*t*, 289
  body position, 204
  carbon dioxide during, 103
  chest opening, 204
  driving, plateau, and peak pressures, 284
  emergence of, 6
  equipment, 287*f*, 289
  during esophagectomy, 761. *See also* Robotic-assisted thoracic surgery (RATS)
  hypoxemia management during, 323
  inflammatory response, 273
  inhalational *versus* intravenous anesthetics, 453
    cancer recurrence, effects on, 454
    inflammatory response, effects on, 454
    oxygenation, effects on, 453
  inspiratory oxygen concentration, 286
  inspiratory-to-expiratory ratio, 285
  lung exclusion, 204
  lung isolation and, 320
  mechanical power, 285
  mechanical ventilation mode, 287
  nonventilated lung, 289
  obstructive sleep apnea, 721, 722*f*
  physiology of, 100
  pneumonectomy, 279
  positive end-expiratory pressure and recruitment maneuvers, 284
  protective, 281
  protective ventilation during, 267
  randomized studies, 271*t*
  rescue maneuvers, hypoxemia, 287
  respiratory rates, 283
  risks assessment, 289
  settings of protective, 282*t*
  in thoracic surgery and gas exchange, 203
  tidal recruitment, 269*f*
  tidal volume, 283
  ventilator-induced lung injury, 279, 280*f*
  during video-assisted thoracoscopic surgery. *See also* Video-assisted thoracic surgery (VATS)
    challenges, 446
    continuous positive airway pressure to the nondependent lung, 453
    fluid management and monitorization, 455
    functional hemodynamic monitors, 454
    historical and current recommendations, 447*t*
    inspiratory oxygen fraction, 453
    lung recruitment maneuvers, 448–450, 449*f*
    mechanisms of hypoxemia during, 447
    mechanisms of lung injury, 447, 448*f*
    positive end-expiratory pressure, 450, 450*t*, 451*f*–452*f*
    protective ventilation, 447
    tidal volume, 448, 449*f*
    tissue oxygenation monitoring, 455
    ventilatory modes, 453
ON-OFF phenomenon, 783
Open *vs.* video-assisted surgery, 588
Opioids, 330
  postthoracotomy pain syndrome, 347
Oral hygiene, 129
Oropharynx, 22
Orthotopic liver transplantation (OLT), 785
OSA-hypopnea syndrome, 714. *See also* Sleep-disordered breathing
Oscillometry, 154, 155*f*
Oxygenation
  analyzers, 144
  cooximetry, 148
  monitoring blood, 145
  oxygen cascade, 143
  oxygen reserve index (ORi), 148
  pulse oximetry, 145
  ventilation
    airway pressures, 150
    capnography and capnometry, 150
    carbon dioxide cascade, 148
    dead space, 149
    respiratory rate, 149
    spirometry, 149
    volume measurement, 149
Oxygen cascade, 143
Oxygen reserve index (ORi), 148
Oxygen saturation, 80
Oxygen sensing and effector mechanisms, 195
Oxygen toxicity, 275

P

Pain syndrome, postthoracotomy, 345
  clinical presentation, 345
  neuromodulation, 351
  pathophysiology, 345
  prevention, 346
  thoracic epidural analgesia, 350
  treatment
    acetaminophen, 346
    cryoablation, 347
    gabapentin, 346
    intercostal nerve approach, 347–348
    ketamine, 347
    nonsteroidal antiinflammatory drugs, 347
    opioid analgesic medications, 347
    paravertebral analgesia, 348
    pregabalin, 346
    serratus anterior plane approach, 347
    transcutaneous electrical nerve stimulation, 347
Paramagnetic oxygen analyzer, 144–145
Paravertebral analgesia, 348
Paravertebral block (PVB), 724
  thoracic epidural analgesia *vs.*, 337
Paravertebral space, 336
Partial pressure of oxygen (PaO_2), 714
Passive leg raising (PLR), 302
Patent foramen ovale (PFO), 792
Peak airway pressure, 150
Pectus excavatum (PE)
  alternative analgesic methods, 605
  anesthetic techniques, 603, 604*f*
  anxiety reduction and mindfulness, 606
  bilateral intercostal blockade, 605
  bilateral paravertebral block, 605
  costal nerve cryoablation, 606
  incidence, 597
  multimodal analgesia, 605
  optimal age for treatment, 598, 598*f*
  outcomes, 601
  patient-controlled analgesia, 605
  postoperative care, 604
  postoperative pain, 605
  preoperative evaluation and indications for surgery, 599, 600*f*–602*f*
  presentation, 598, 598*f*
  surgical complications, 602, 602*f*–603*f*

Pectus excavatum (PE) (*Continued*)
surgical procedure
Nuss, 600
Ravitch, 601
treatment options, 597
Pediatric thoracic surgery
anatomy, 318
anesthetic techniques
bronchoscopy, 319
sternotomy, 320
bronchial blocker, 321
double-lumen tube, 323
hypoxemia management during one-lung ventilation, 323
intravenous modalities, 325
monitoring, 324
one-lung ventilation by age, 321*t*
pain management, 324
physiology, 318
postoperative period, 324
preoperative evaluation, 319
regional modalities, 324
selective bronchial intubation, 321
univent tube, 323
Perfusion, 77
Pericardial effusion, 43
Pericardial tamponade, 494, 494*f*
Perioperative arrhythmias during thoracic surgery
anticoagulation, 313
management, 314*f*
monitoring, 310
nonvitamin K oral anticoagulants, 315*f*
predictive factors, 308
prevention, 310, 311*f*
rate control, 312
rhythm control, 313
treatment, 312
Perioperative lung injury
definition, 249
epidemiology, 249
imaging, 249
Perioperative nutrition screen (PONS), 126*f*
Perioperative therapy recommendation, 432*t*
Peripheral nerve injury, positioning, 138*t*
Persistent air leak (PAL), 669
Pharyngoesophageal diverticulum, 651
Phases, capnogram, 151
Phenylephrine, 207
Phosphodiesterase-5 inhibitors, 111
Plateau pressure, 150
Pleural effusion, 806*f*
detection, lung ultrasound, 781, 781*f*–782*f*
radiology, thorax, 39, 39*f*, 43
Pneumonectomy, 40
Pneumonia, postthoracotomy complications, 387
Pneumothorax, 590
detection, lung ultrasound, 780, 780*f*–781*f*
following valve insertion, 476
radiology, thorax, 38
thoracic trauma, 491
Positioning, thoracic surgery
changes in position during emergency, 139
complications to patient positioning, 137
extracorporeal mechanical oxygenation during thoracic cases, 139
flexion, 135
lateral decubitus, 134, 134*f*
lower extremities, 134, 134*f*
neck, 135*f*, 135
nerves injured, 138*t*
neutral position, 134*f*
in obese patients, 140, 140*f*
peripheral nerve injury, 138*t*
prone, 136
reverse Trendelenburg, 135, 136*f*
robotic surgery and position, 136
supine position, 133
upper extremities, 134*f*, 134–135
Positive end-expiratory pressure (PEEP), 279, 363*t*
Positive pressure ventilation, 3–5, 8
Postanesthetic care unit (PACU), 353
Postoperative acute lung injury, 589
radiology, thorax, 42
Postoperative analgesia, development of, 9
Postoperative atrial fibrillation (POAF), 117, 308
anticoagulation, 313
management, 314*f*
monitoring, 310
nonvitamin K oral anticoagulants, 315*f*
predictive factors, 308
prevention, 310, 311*f*
rate control, 312
rhythm control, 313
treatment, 312
Postoperative care
chest tubes management, 354
differential lung ventilation (DLV), 364
extracorporeal ventilatory support, 371
fluid management, 359*b*
high-flow nasal cannula oxygen therapy (HFNCOT), 365
high-frequency ventilation, 364
location and structure of, 353
lung transplantation
antihumoral therapy, 639
antiproliferative agents, 639
calcineurin inhibitors (CNIs), 638
chest tube management, 637
early postoperative complications, 640
fluid management, 637
glucocorticoids, 638
hemodynamic management, 636
immunosuppression, 638
induction immunosuppression agents, 638
infection prevention and management, 639
nutritional support and stress ulcer prophylaxis, 640
sedation and analgesia, 638
lung ultrasound as new tool, 356, 356*f*
mechanical ventilation, after thoracic surgery, 364*b*
monitoring tools, 355
noninvasive ventilation, 365, 366*t*
positive end-expiratory pressure titration, 363*t*
protective ventilation after thoracic surgery, 360
right ventricular ejection fraction (RVEF), 359
scoring systems, 354
three-bottle system, 355*f*
ventilator-associated pneumonia, 369
ventilatory support, 359
weaning, 367
Postoperative pulmonary complication
atelectasis, 260–261
characteristics, 260
definitions, 261*t*
incidence, 261
intraoperative lung injury and, 262
predisposing condition, 262
protective ventilation, 266
protective ventilation strategy and, 270
surgical causes, 262
Postoperative thoracic surgery
air leaks treatment, 176
atelectasis, 175
bronchopleural fistulas treatment, 176
hemoptysis, 175
lobe/lung segment torsions, 176
tracheal lacerations, 176
Postpneumonectomy pulmonary edema (PPPE), 293
Postpneumonectomy syndrome, 590
Postthoracotomy acute lung injury, 294
Postthoracotomy complications
acute respiratory distress syndrome, 389
ARISCAT score, 378*t*
atelectasis, 387, 387*f*

Postthoracotomy complications (*Continued*)
atrial fibrillation
risk, 385*t*
and supraventricular arrhythmias, 384
treatment, 384
bleeding, 379
bradyarrhythmias, 386
cardiac arrhythmias, 383
drugs used, 386*t*
heart failure, 382
lobe torsion, 379
major adverse cardiac events (MACE), 380
myocardial infarction (MI), 380
myocardial ischemia, 380
patient-related risk factors, 384
pneumonia, 387
postoperative pulmonary complications prediction, 376
pulmonary edema, 389
pulmonary hypertension, 389
respiratory insufficiency, 377*t*, 386
risk factors, 377, 377*f*, 379*t*, 381*t*
surgery-related risk factors, 384
valvular heart disease (VHD), 381
ventricular arrhythmia, 386
Postthoracotomy pain syndrome (PTPS), 345
clinical presentation, 345
neuromodulation, 351
pathophysiology, 345
prevention, 346
thoracic epidural analgesia, 350
treatment
acetaminophen, 346
cryoablation, 347
gabapentin, 346
intercostal nerve approach, 347–348
ketamine, 347
nonsteroidal antiinflammatory drugs, 347
opioid analgesic medications, 347
paravertebral analgesia, 348
pregabalin, 346
serratus anterior plane approach, 347
transcutaneous electrical nerve stimulation, 347
Prefusion upright position, ventilation, 89
Pregabalin, 346
Prehabilitation
anemia, 128
cardiac comorbidities, 129
diabetes, 128
exercise, 126
frailty and comprehensive geriatric assessment, 129
ideal thoracic perioperative pathway, 129
nutrition, 126
oral hygiene, 129
perioperative nutrition screen *(PONS)*, 126*f*
psychology, 127
risk prediction, 125
shared decision making *vs*. consent, 125
smoking cessation and respiratory optimization, 127
Preoperative medical assessment, 115
age, 115
Pressure control ventilation (PCV), 722
Pressure-volume loops, 150
Previous lobectomy, 39
Probes selection, 775
Prone positioning, 136
Propofol, 720
Prostacyclins, 108
Prosthetic valves, 427
Protective lung ventilation (PLV), 293
Protective ventilation after thoracic surgery, 360
Psychology, 127
Pulmonary arterial hypertension (PAH), 523, 525*f*
Pulmonary artery, 159
pressure, 159
Pulmonary artery catheter (PAC), 786
Pulmonary blood flow (PBF), 78
Pulmonary capillary wedge pressure (PCWP), 523
Pulmonary circulation
applied physiology of, 106
hypoxic pulmonary vasoconstriction, 198
intraoperative monitoring, 106
pulmonary vascular resistance, 107
regulation of, 108
ventilation-induced changes in pulmonary hemodynamics, 107
Pulmonary contusion, 490*f*, 491, 492*f*
Pulmonary disease, 34, 42
Pulmonary edema, 389
Pulmonary function tests (PFTs), 18*t*
cardiopulmonary exercise testing, 83, 121
diffusing capacity, carbon monoxide, 82
ergometric testing, 121
forced expiratory volume in one second (FEV1), 81
forced vital capacity, 82
predicted postoperative lung function, 120
preoperative, 506–507, 507*f*
recommendations, preoperative assessment, 83
spirometry and diffusing capacity, 119
tracheal resection and reconstruction, 613
Pulmonary gas exchange
alveolar-to-arterial oxygen gradient, 80
dead space, 81
diffusion, 80
hypercapnia, 80
hypoxemia, 80
oxygen saturation, 80
perfusion, 77
pulmonary blood flow (PBF), 78
pulmonary vascular resistance, 79, 79*f*
shunt, 80
ventilation, 77
ventilation-perfusion matching, 78, 80
Pulmonary hyperinflation, 410
Pulmonary hypertension (PH), 428
classification, 626*b*
classification/pathophysiology, 523, 524*t*
definition, 523
hemodynamic definitions, 524*t*, 641*t*
hemodynamic management, 529, 529*f*
inhaled and intravenous vasodilators, 530*t*
intraoperative management
anesthetic technique, 528
monitoring, 526
morbidity, 523
postthoracotomy complications, 389
preoperative evaluation, 525
Pulmonary interdependence, 27*f*
Pulmonary torsion, 592
Pulmonary vascular disease (PVD), 625
Pulmonary vascular resistance, 79, 79*f*, 107
regulation of, 108
Pulmonary vasculature, 30
Pulmonary vasodilators, 523–524, 526
administration of, 108
Pulse oximetry, 145

R

Radiology, thorax
bullae, 35, 37*f*–38*f*
chest radiographs, 33, 34*f*
chest tube placement, 39
computed tomography scan, 42–43
double-lumen endotracheal tubes, 41
emphysema, 37*f*
lung mass, 43
lung mass and, 34
magnetic resonance imaging and pulmonary disease, 46
mediastinal mass, 43
mediastinal mass and, 35
multidetector computer tomography scan, 45
normal tracheobronchial anatomy, 33

Radiology, thorax (*Continued*)
pericardial effusion, 43
pleural effusion, 39, 39*f*, 43
pneumonectomy, 40
pneumothorax, 38
postoperative acute lung injury, 42
previous lobectomy, 39
pulmonary disease, 42
and pulmonary disease, 34
single-lumen endotracheal tubes, 41
thoracic ultrasound, 47
Rapid sequence induction, 701
Ravitch surgical procedure, 601
Recurrent laryngeal and phrenic nerve injuries, 591
Regional anesthesia techniques, 332, 332*t*
Residual volume, 68
Respiratory airways, 66
Respiratory failure, 589
Respiratory insufficiency, 377*t*, 386
Respiratory mechanics, 71
anesthesia effects, 77
compliance, 73
derecruitment, 76
driving pressure, 72
elastance, 73
elastance and compliance, 73
mechanical power, 76
overdistension, 76
resistance, 75
strain, 75
stress, 75
transpulmonary pressure, 71
Respiratory optimization, 127
Respiratory rate, 149
Respiratory variation, 163
Reverse Trendelenburg positioning, 135, 136*f*
Revised cardiac risk index, 116*t*
Rhabdomyolysis (RML), 725
Rib
cage volume, 33
fracture, 489, 490*f*
motions, 19*f*
Right-sided double-lumen endotracheal tubes, 220*b*, 220
Right ventricle assessment, 788, 788*t*, 790*f*
Right ventricular ejection fraction (RVEF), 359
Rigid bronchoscopy (RB), 171
anesthesia, 178
common and specific complications of endoscopy, 484
composition, 171
indications, 171
infusion rate, 484
tracheal stents, 750
ventilation techniques, 179
ventilatory support during, 484
Risk prediction, 125
Robotic-assisted thoracic surgery (RATS)
access to patient, 761
advantages, 758
anesthetic management, 761
carbon dioxide insufflation, 762
communication, 762
disadvantages, 758
equipment, 761, 761*f*, 763*f*
esophagectomy, 760
fluids, 762
intraoperative monitoring, 762
learning curves, 758
lobectomy, 758
lung separation techniques, 762
pain management, 763
patient positioning, 761
patient selection, 761, 761*f*, 763*f*
positioning, 136
responsibility and ethical considerations, 763
segmentectomy, 759
surgical technique, 761, 761*f*, 763*f*
Robotic-assisted thoracic surgery (RATS) (*Continued*)
thymectomy, 759, 760*f*
video-assisted thoracoscopic surgery (VATS), 440

S

Safe apnea period (SAP), 716
Sanders jet ventilation, 183
Scoliosis, 678. *See also* Thoracic spine surgery
Sedation management, 406
Segmentectomy, 759, 579
Self-expanding metal stents (SEMS), 741, 744*f*, 749*f*
Senescence, hypoxic pulmonary vasoconstriction, 198
Sepsis/septic shock, 707
Serratus anterior plane
approach, postthoracotomy pain syndrome, 347
block, acute pain, postoperative management, 339, 340*f*
Shared decision making *vs.* consent, 125
Shunt, 78, 80
fraction, 89
Siewert classification, 657*f*
Silicone, tracheal stents, 741
Simpson's method, 796*f*
Single-lumen endotracheal tube
double-lumen endotracheal tube, exchange with, 244
radiology, thorax, 41
Single-shot erector spinae plane *vs.* continuous erector spinae plane, 339
Sleep-disordered breathing, 714
Smoking, 118, 519
cessation and respiratory optimization, 127
Snoring, 714. *See also* Sleep-disordered breathing
Spine surgery
anterior approach to, 683
blood conservation strategies, 683
endotracheal tube choice, 681, 682*t*
epidural placement and management, 681
hypoxemia, 681
neuromonitoring, 684
preoperative assessment, testing, and anesthetic planning, 684, 684*f*
preoperative management, postoperative pain, 681
Spirometry
and diffusing capacity, 119
oxygenation, 149
Split lung function testing
one-lung ventilation, prediction of desaturation during, 122
quantitative lung perfusion scintigraphy, 121
Squamous epithelial papilloma, 655–656
Stent placement, 751
Sternotomy, 320
Stress index, 76–77
Stroke volume (SV), 796*f*
Subxiphoid uniportal video-assisted thoracoscopic surgery (VATS), 440
Superior vena cava syndrome, 504*t*
Supine position, 133
Systemic analgesics, 331*t*
Systemic opioids postthoracotomy, 725

T

Tension pneumothorax, 492*f*
Thermal therapies, 751
Thoracic anesthesia, 1
Thoracic aortal injury, 493
Thoracic aortic aneurysms
acute aortic dissections, 573
airway considerations, 567
and anesthetic management, 567
arterial cannulation site, 573
ascending thoracic and aortic arch aneurysms, 562
cardiovascular considerations, 562
central nervous system protection and monitoring, 572
clinical end points, classifications, 566*t*
complications, 559
DeBakey's accomplishments, 557, 558*f*
differential diagnosis, 559*b*
gastrointestinal considerations, 567

Thoracic aortic aneurysms (*Continued*)
grading system, 565*t*
hematologic considerations, 567
historical notes on, 557
intraoperative physiologic considerations during one-lung ventilation, 569
invasive blood pressure monitoring, 567
invasive central pressure monitoring, 568
Marfan syndrome, 558
medical management, 570
nervous system considerations, 564
postoperative ventilation considerations, 569
prevalence, 559
pulmonary considerations, 563
renal considerations, 562
revised Ghent criteria, 560*b*
risks and benefits, 572
significance, 559
surgical management, 571
temperature monitoring, 568
transesophageal echocardiogram (TEE) probe, 561, 568
ventilation management and ventilatory modalities, 569
Thoracic epidural analgesia (TEA), 724
acute pain, postoperative management, 333, 334*f*
vs. paravertebral block, 337
Thoracic epidural anesthesia, hypoxic pulmonary vasoconstriction, 207
Thoracic instability, 490
Thoracic paravertebral block, 335
Thoracic perioperative pathway, 129
Thoracic-revised cardiac risk index, 117*t*
Thoracic spine surgery
anterior approach to, 683
blood conservation strategies, 683
endotracheal tube choice, 681, 682*t*
epidural placement and management, 681
hypoxemia, 681
neuromonitoring, 684
preoperative assessment, testing, and anesthetic planning, 684, 684*f*
preoperative management, postoperative pain, 681
Thoracic surgery
current scope of anesthesia, 10
developments in history, lung separation techniques, 13*f*
enhanced recovery after surgery
comorbid conditions optimization, 768
intraoperative components
anesthesia maintenance, 770
fluid management, 771
mechanical ventilation strategy, 771
multimodal analgesia, 770
vomiting prophylaxis, 771
justification and applicability, 767
milestones in, 5, 13*f*
nutrition, 769
prehabilitation, 769
preoperative components, 768
protocol, 768*f*
under regional anesthesia, 6
tobacco and alcohol cessation, 769
Thoracic trauma
anesthesiologic management, 496
A & B, airway and breathing, 496
blunt cardiac trauma, 493
cardiac contusion, 494
causes, 488
chest radiography, 496
circulation, 496
diaphragmatic rupture, 494, 495*f*
flailed chest, 491*f*
hemothorax, 492, 493*f*
laboratory diagnostics, 496
larynx injuries, 489
mediastinal widening, 492
mortality of, 488
one-lung ventilation, 498
patient controlled analgesia using opioids, 499*t*
penetrating, 495, 495*f*
pericardial tamponade, 494, 494*f*
Thoracic trauma (*Continued*)
pneumothorax, 491
postoperative care, 498
postoperative pain therapy, 498
preoperative evaluation, 496
pulmonary contusion, 490*f*, 491, 492*f*
radiologic diagnostics, 496
rib fracture, 489, 490*f*
tension pneumothorax, 492*f*
thoracic aortal injury, 493
thoracic instability, 490
tracheobronchial injury, 488, 489*f*
ultrasound diagnostics, 496
Thoracic ultrasound, 47
Three-bottle system, postoperative care, 355*f*
Thymectomy
approach to induction and maintenance of anesthesia, 692
general endotracheal anesthesia (GETA), 692
indications, 691*t*
mediastinal surgery, myasthenia gravis, 456
operative approaches, 691
preoperative evaluation and management, 690
robotic thoracic surgery, 759, 760*f*
Thymic tumors, 58
Thymoma
Masaoka Staging System, 59*t*
World Health Organization Classification, 59*t*
Tidal volume, 68
Tonometry, 155
Torque control blocker univent, 232
Total intravenous anesthesia (TIVA) technique, 720
propofol-based, 586–587
sevoflurane, 586–587
Total lung capacity, 69
Trachea, 25,
anatomy, 609
bifurcation, 33
Tracheal insufflation and endotracheal anesthesia, 3
Tracheal lacerations, 176
Tracheal resection and reconstruction
diagnostic findings, 611*t*
diagnostic studies, 613
emergence and extubation, 618
etiology of, 609, 610*b*
history and physical examination, 611
intraoperative management, 614
induction and bronchoscopic examination, 615
management, critically obstructed airway, 616
patient positioning, 615
setup and monitoring, 614
laboratory studies, 613
odontoid hypoplasia, 613*b*
postintubation injury, 610
postoperative care and potential complications, 619
preoperative evaluation, 611
pulmonary function tests, 613
radiologic evaluation, 613
severity of, 612*f*
surgical procedure, 617
Tracheal stenosis dilation with balloon, 172*f*
Tracheal stents
anesthesia alternatives, 748
anesthesia care for bronchoscopy, 752
central airway stents placement, 741
epithelialization, 741
extracorporeal membrane oxygenation (ECMO) support, 745, 747*f*
and fistula, 744*f*
flexible *versus* rigid bronchoscopy, 747
indications, 741, 742*t*
Montgomery T-tube stent, 754–755, 755*f*
position, 741, 743*f*, 746*f*
procedure, 745*f*
risk/benefit
airway stent placement complications, 751*t*
infectious risk, 751
rigid bronchoscopy, 750

Tracheal stents (*Continued*)
stent placement, 751
thermal therapies, 751
self-expanding metal stents (SEMS), 741, 744*f*, 749*f*
silicone, 741
surgical alternatives, 746
T-tube for support, 752
ventilation alternatives, 750, 751*t*
Tracheobronchial injury, 488, 489*f*
Tracheobronchial structure, 66
Tracheobronchial tree, 28*f*
Tracheoesophageal fistula, 673. *See also* Airway fistulas in adults
Tranexamic acid (TXA), 683
Transcutaneous electrical nerve stimulation, 347
Transesophageal echocardiography (TEE)
acute pulmonary hypertension, 798, 802*f*–803*f*
CABG, 785
cardiac output (CO), 796*f*
diastolic function evaluation, 800*f*
indications, 785
intraoperative hemodynamic exam, 787
left ventricle assessment, 793, 793*f*–796*f*
dyssynchrony index (DI), 798*f*
ME-4C and ME-2C views, 797*f*
Swaminathan's simplified e' based algorithm, 801*f*
lung transplantation, 805
lung ultrasound, 791*t*, 803, 805*f*–806*f*, 807*t*, 808*f*
mediastinal mass, 506
as monitor, 786
rescue, 785
right ventricle assessment, 788, 788*t*, 790*f*
risks, 787
stroke volume (SV), 796*f*
thoracic aortic aneurysms, 561
Transfusion-related to acute lung injury (TRALI), 295
Transhiatal esophagectomy, 55
Transpulmonary thermodilution, 159
Transthoracic echocardiography (TTE), 786
Transthoracic esophagectomy, 658
Tricuspid regurgitation, 804*f*
T-tube for support, 752
Tube exchanger technique, 242, 244*f*
Tubeless procedures, 481. *See also* Monitored anesthesia care
Tubeless thoracic procedures
advantages of, 536
airway management, 533
carbon dioxide insufflation, 536
inclusion criteria, 540
intraoperative management, 534, 541
patient selection, 534
postoperative management, 536
preoperative evaluation, 533
ventilation/perfusion with patient, 536
Two-lung ventilation
with manual retraction, 320. *See also* One-lung ventilation
vs. one-lung ventilation, 100*f*

U

Ultrasonography, double-lumen endotracheal tubes, 221, 223
Uniportal video-assisted thoracoscopic surgery (VATS), 440
United Network for Organ Sharing (UNOS), 805
Univent tube, pediatric thoracic surgery, 323
Upper airway, 20
Upper airway resistance syndrome (UARS), 714. *See also* Sleep-disordered breathing
Upper extremities positioning, 134*f*, 134–135

V

Valve treatment
persistent air leak, 477, 478*f*
practical details of, 476
Valvular heart disease (VHD), 427, 427*t*
postthoracotomy complications, 381
Vasoactive drugs, 111
Ventilation, 77
alternatives, 750, 751*t*
distribution, 89, 91
fractal distribution of perfusion, 92
lateral decubitus position, 93
lateral position, 94
supine and lateral positions, 95
improvements in, 9
lateral decubitus position, awake, spontaneously breathing patients
chest closed, 96
chest open, 96
mediastinal shift, 99
paradoxic respiration, 100
lateral position, anesthetized patients
chest closed, 99
chest open, 99
oxygenation
airway pressures, 150
capnography and capnometry, 150
carbon dioxide cascade, 148
dead space, 149
respiratory rate, 149
spirometry, 149
volume measurement, 149
prefusion upright position, 89
surgical manipulation, 101
Ventilation-induced changes in pulmonary hemodynamics, 107
Ventilation methods, 587
Ventilation-perfusion matching, 92
Ventilation/perfusion (V/Q) mismatch, 410, 714
Ventilator-associated pneumonia, 369
Ventilator-induced lung injury, 279, 280*f*, 294, 297
Ventilatory support, 359
Ventricular arrhythmia, 386
Video-assisted thoracic surgery (VATS), 707, 758. *See also* Robotic-assisted thoracic surgery (RATS)
history of, 438
with local or regional anesthesia, 457
vs. open thoracotomy, 439
postoperative analgesia after, 458
preoperative optimization and "prehabilitation," 442
preoperative risk stratification, 440, 442*f*
robotic-assisted thoracic surgery (RATS), 440
subxiphoid uniportal, 440
techniques, 438
uniportal, 440
VivaSight® double-lumen tube, 220
VivaSight® single-lumen tube, 232
Volume clamp technique, 156
Volume measurement, 149

W

Water-tight seal, 703–704
Weaning
extracorporeal ventilatory therapies, 401
postoperative care, 367
Wedge resection, 579
World Health Organization Classification, 59*t*